HANDBOOK OF PHYSIOLOGY
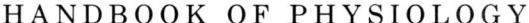

SECTION 6: The Gastrointestinal System, VOLUME I, PART 2

PUBLICATIONS COMMITTEE

PAUL C. JOHNSON, *Chairman*
FRANCOIS ABBOUD
JOHN S. COOK
MELVIN J. FREGLY
STEPHEN H. WHITE

Elizabeth M. Cowley, Ruth A. Freehling,
Melinda E. Lowy, Anna O. Trudgett,
Susie P. Mann, *Editorial Staff*

Laurie S. Chambers, *Production Manager*

Diana Witt, *Indexer*

# HANDBOOK OF PHYSIOLOGY

*A critical, comprehensive presentation of physiological knowledge and concepts*

---

## SECTION 6: The Gastrointestinal System

Formerly SECTION 6: Alimentary Canal

VOLUME I.
*Motility and Circulation, Part 2*

*Section Editor:* STANLEY G. SCHULTZ

*Volume Editor:* JACKIE D. WOOD

*Executive Editor:* BRENDA B. RAUNER

American Physiological Society, BETHESDA, MARYLAND, 1989

© Copyright 1967 (Volume I), American Physiological Society
© Copyright 1967 (Volume II), American Physiological Society
© Copyright 1968 (Volume III), American Physiological Society
© Copyright 1968 (Volume IV), American Physiological Society
© Copyright 1968 (Volume V), American Physiological Society

© Copyright 1989, American Physiological Society

Library of Congress Catalog Card Number 89-279

International Standard Book Number 0-19-520791-2

Printed in the United States of America by Waverly Press, Baltimore, Maryland 21202

Distributed by Oxford University Press, New York, New York 10016

# Preface to *The Gastrointestinal System*

The first edition of the *Handbook of Physiology*, section 6, *Alimentary Canal*, comprised five volumes published between 1967 and 1968. This completely revised, second edition of section 6, *The Gastrointestinal System*, consists of four volumes: *Motility and Circulation* (Jackie D. Wood, Volume Editor), *Neural and Endocrine Biology* (Gabriel M. Makhlouf, Volume Editor), *Salivary, Gastric, Pancreatic, and Hepatobiliary Secretion* (John G. Forte, Volume Editor), and *Intestinal Absorption and Secretion* (Michael Field and Raymond A. Frizzell, Volume Editors).

A comparison of the contents of these two editions leads to the inescapable conclusion that the past two decades represent a golden age in the long and venerable history of gastrointestinal physiology. The advent and the application of powerful technologies have led not only to an explosion of information but also to an explosion of comprehension. Many previously enigmatic phenomena are now explicable at the cellular and often at the molecular level of biological organization. No area of this diverse discipline has been left untouched by this avalanche of knowledge.

I extend my heartfelt thanks to our many authors and reviewers for their contributions to this undertaking, and my gratitude to the volume editors, without whom this project could not have been executed, can never be duly expressed. Finally, many thanks are due Laurie Chambers, Production Manager, and her staff for their expert redactory work.

STANLEY G. SCHULTZ
*Section Editor*

# Preface

This volume on *Motility and Circulation* succeeds volume IV (*Motility*) published in 1968 in section 6 (*Alimentary Canal*) of the *Handbook of Physiology* series. The 1968 volume was a critical, comprehensive presentation of the facts and concepts of motility current at that time. Still a valuable reference 20 years later, it served as a venerable foundation for the present volume on motility. This 1989 volume perpetuates the tradition by reviewing the advances in the science basic to alimentary motor function since publication of the earlier *Handbook*. Parallel progress in understanding the vascular system and lymphatics of the alimentary canal over the same two decades mandated that this subspecialty of gastrointestinal biology be included.

In the past 20 years there has been an impressive development of new information, exciting new technologies, ingenious methods, and new understanding of motility. These advances span all levels of organization from single smooth muscle cells and neurons to integrated function at the organ level, and they are expertly documented by the authors of this edition.

The first chapter on the history of gastrointestinal motility by Horace W. Davenport is a unique account by one of this century's foremost gastrointestinal physiologists. It is unlikely that anyone among the present generation of gastrointestinal scientists would be capable of telling a more comprehensive story of the historical chronology of the several facets of basic and clinical science that relates to modern concepts of gut motor function. Certainly it could not be done with the same delightful flavor of Horace Davenport.

The electrophysiology of gastrointestinal muscle was a timely topic in 1968 and a major focus in the earlier *Handbook*. Pressure electrodes, intracellular microelectrodes, and the sucrose gap were the state-of-the-art methodologies in that period. The aim was to identify the ionic currents underlying the electrical behavior of the smooth muscle. Combined sucrose-gap and voltage-clamp methods were introduced in the 1970s and rapidly became controversial. Questions on the reliability of voltage clamping long-fibered syncytia were not satisfactorily resolved prior to progress away from the method. This edition covers this period and introduces modern patch-clamp technology. The chapters by Sanders and Publicover and by Bolton include accounts of the development of techniques for enzymatic dissociation of gastrointestinal smooth muscle cells and application of patch-clamp methods. These preparations have significantly advanced understanding of the electrophysiology and pharmacology of the musculature. New insight into the operation of individual ionic channels and receptor operation of the channels has emerged from this work.

Most of our knowledge of the ultrastructure of gastrointestinal smooth muscle, the extracellular matrix, and the mechanical properties of the musculature has accrued since 1968. The chapter by Meiss presents for the first time a detailed account of the mechanics of gastrointestinal smooth muscle, and this is complimented by Gabella's expert chapter on electron microscopy and ultrastructure.

Interest in electrical slow waves dominated the reviews of the electrophysiology of intestinal muscle in the 1968 *Handbook*, and these slow waves remain an enigma in 1989. The intriguing possibility that they may not be generated by the musculature at all but by the interstitial cells of Cajal is elaborated in Thuneberg's chapter.

The neurobiology section documents exciting advances in understanding the enteric nervous system. The first microelectrode studies of the electrical and synaptic behavior of gut neurons were published in the period since 1968, and they were done both in situ and in cell culture. Burnstock and associates reviewed evidence for noncholinergic-nonadrenergic neurotransmission in the 1968 edition, which turned out to be a prelude for an explosion of information on biogenic amines, peptides, and purinergic messengers in the gut. Coverage of this new information by Daniel and associates required more pages than his classic chapter on gastrointestinal pharmacology in the original volume.

The era of immunocytochemical localization and colocalization of messenger substances and their synthetic enzymes produced a wealth of information about the gut. During this period Szurszewski and his students worked out the significance of the prevertebral sympathetic ganglia as integrative centers in control of gut function. Likewise, studies on microinjection of messengers into the brain and definition of brain-gut interactions have blossomed in the past decade.

At the organizational level of the integrated organ, the observations of the unique pattern of motility in the interdigestive state (migrating motor complex) by

Szurszewski and many subsequent investigators have dominated attention. Continued development of methodologies for manometric recording of intraluminal pressures and electrical and contractile activity of the musculature at all levels of the gastrointestinal tract is responsible for significant advances that are documented in chapters on the esophagus, the stomach, the small and large intestines, the various sphincters, and the biliary system. Included also is a current view of villous motility.

The impressive advances in the fundamentals of gastrointestinal motor function are obviously essential to understanding clinical abnormalities. Nevertheless, no major attempt is made in this edition to deal with motor disorders. On the other hand, abnormalities associated with parasitic infections, enterotoxins, emesis, and surgical perturbations provide insight into normal mechanisms and therefore receive focused attention. Chapters on parasitic infections and enterotoxins point to interactions between the intestinal immune system, musculature, and nervous system as an important determinant of altered motor function. It is becoming clear that the immune system signals the presence of antigens to the enteric nervous system, which in turn programs the effector systems for motor and secretory responses that are adaptive and beneficial in confronting foreign invasion of the gut lumen. Investigation of gastrointestinal neuroimmune relations is clearly an important area of expanding interest where major new advances can be anticipated.

Comparative physiology of gastrointestinal motility was reviewed in the 1968 edition, and an attempt to follow up is made here. Adaptations of the gastrointestinal tract to selective pressures of the environment and the ecological niche that the animal fills can provide valuable insight into the biology of the gastrointestinal tract. Nevertheless, this continues to be a neglected area, with the exception of the research on ruminants and avian species reviewed in the chapters by Ruckebusch and Duke.

The circulation section of this volume is an authoritative account of the current concepts of the specialized circulatory systems of the alimentary tract. Chapters in this section emphasize the need for recognition that these divisions of the peripheral circulation have unique aspects that are adaptive for the specialized functions of the digestive system. Multidirectional growth in knowledge of the alimentary circulation in the past two decades mandates that this be included in comprehensive coverage of gastrointestinal physiology. The circulatory system is basic to secretory and absorptive functions as well as motility, and it would have been equally appropriate to include it in the *Handbook* volume on epithelial function. Inclusion here is simply an editorial decision. The general aim is to emphasize the central role of the digestive circulation in gut function and to remove it from superficial status as a stepchild of cardiovascular physiology.

Each chapter presents major aspects of the circulatory system for which a significant body of knowledge exists. This includes introduction of basic structural and ultrastructural detail of the digestive vasculature. As is the case for motility, many of the advances in gastrointestinal circulatory function have resulted from introduction of new experimental approaches and measurement technologies that are evaluated critically by Shepherd and Kiel. Consideration of hemodynamics and regulation is subdivided into chapters on the specialized regions of the digestive circulation and the neonatal circulation. Major advances in the knowledge of neuromuscular transmission in the gut vasculature and neurohumoral control are placed in perspective in the chapters by Kreulen and Keef, Hirst, and Jodal and Lundgren. Finally, Gallavan, Parks, and Jacobson relate the basic concepts to the abnormalities of digestive circulatory function.

Overall this volume is organized to be useful for a wide spectrum of gastrointestinal interests ranging from graduate students and postdoctoral fellows to classroom instructors, active investigators, and clinicians. The book emphasizes the broad scope of research in gastrointestinal motor and circulatory function and at many junctures points to new investigative directions. I hope that the volume also conveys the excitement and significance of modern research in the many aspects of gastrointestinal physiology.

I was helped greatly with the organization of the circulatory section by consultation with D. Neil Granger, Peter R. Kvietys, and Ove Lundgren and extend my thanks to them. I am grateful to Stanley G. Schultz, the editor of this *Handbook* section on *The Gastrointestinal System*, for his support. Laurie Chambers and the book editorial staff for the American Physiological Society did a tremendous job and are likewise deserving of thanks not only from me but from all beneficiaries of the volume. I appreciate the willingness of the many who provided expert reviews of the individual chapters. Finally, I deeply thank all of the authors because the value of this book stems from their expert contributions.

JACKIE D. WOOD
*Volume Editor*

# Contents

## Part 1

**MOTILITY**

1. Gastrointestinal physiology, 1895–1975: motility
   HORACE W. DAVENPORT . . . . . . . . . . . . . . 1

*Musculature*

2. Structure of intestinal musculature
   GIORGIO GABELLA . . . . . . . . . . . . . . . . . 103
3. Distribution and exchange of electrolytes in gastrointestinal muscle cells
   R. CASTEELS
   G. DROOGMANS
   L. RAEYMAEKERS . . . . . . . . . . . . . . . . . . 141
4. Electrophysiology of dissociated gastrointestinal muscle cells
   KENTON M. SANDERS . . . . . . . . . . . . . . . 163
5. Electrophysiology of the gastric musculature
   KENTON M. SANDERS
   NELSON G. PUBLICOVER . . . . . . . . . . . . . 187
6. Electrophysiology of the intestinal musculature
   T. B. BOLTON . . . . . . . . . . . . . . . . . . . . . 217
7. Electrophysiology of colonic smooth muscle
   KENTON M. SANDERS
   TERENCE K. SMITH . . . . . . . . . . . . . . . . . 251
8. Mechanical properties of gastrointestinal smooth muscle
   RICHARD A. MEISS . . . . . . . . . . . . . . . . . 273

*Neurobiology*

9. Enteric neurons in culture
   ALAN L. WILLARD
   RAE NISHI . . . . . . . . . . . . . . . . . . . . . . 331
10. Interstitial cells of Cajal
    LARS THUNEBERG . . . . . . . . . . . . . . . . . 349
11. Identification of transmitters of functionally defined enteric neurons
    JOHN B. FURNESS
    MARCELLO COSTA . . . . . . . . . . . . . . . . . 387
12. Neurotransmitter release in the enteric nervous system
    WILLIAM M. YAU . . . . . . . . . . . . . . . . . . 403
13. Neuromuscular transmission in the gastrointestinal tract
    CHARLES H. V. HOYLE
    GEOFFREY BURNSTOCK . . . . . . . . . . . . . . 435

14. Electrical and synaptic behavior of enteric neurons
    JACKIE D. WOOD . . . . . . . . . . . . . . . . . . 465
15. Physiology of prevertebral ganglia in mammals with special reference to inferior mesenteric ganglion
    J. H. SZURSZEWSKI
    B. F. KING . . . . . . . . . . . . . . . . . . . . . . 519
16. Sensory afferents from the gastrointestinal tract
    DAVID GRUNDY
    TIM SCRATCHERD . . . . . . . . . . . . . . . . . 593
17. Control centers in the central nervous system for regulating gastrointestinal motility
    RICHARD A. GILLIS
    JOHN A. QUEST
    FRANCIS D. PAGANI
    WESLEY P. NORMAN . . . . . . . . . . . . . . . . 621
18. Central nervous system mechanisms in deglutition and emesis
    DAVID O. CARPENTER . . . . . . . . . . . . . . . 685

*Pharmacology*

19. Pharmacology of drugs acting on gastrointestinal motility
    EDWIN E. DANIEL
    STEPHEN M. COLLINS
    JO-ANN E. T. FOX
    JAN D. HUIZINGA . . . . . . . . . . . . . . . . . 715
20. Pharmacology of neuroendocrine peptides
    EDWIN E. DANIEL
    STEPHEN M. COLLINS
    JO-ANN E. T. FOX
    JAN D. HUIZINGA . . . . . . . . . . . . . . . . . 759

Index . . . . . . . . . . . . . . . . . . . . . . . . . . . . xiii

## Part 2

**MOTILITY**

*Motor Function*

21. In vivo myoelectric activity: methods, analysis, and interpretation
    SUSHIL K. SARNA . . . . . . . . . . . . . . . . . 817
22. Esophageal motility
    RAJ K. GOYAL
    WILLIAM G. PATERSON . . . . . . . . . . . . . . 865

23. Determinants of gastric emptying and transit in the small intestine
    JUAN-R. MALAGELADA
    FERNANDO AZPIROZ ............... 909
24. Colonic motility
    JAMES CHRISTENSEN ............... 939
25. Villous motility
    WILLIAM A. WOMACK
    PETER R. KVIETYS
    D. NEIL GRANGER ............... 975
26. Sphincteric function
    MARIA PAPASOVA ............... 987
27. Motor function of anorectum and pelvic floor musculature
    JACOB KRIER ............... 1025
28. Motility of the biliary system
    WYLIE J. DODDS
    WALTER J. HOGAN
    JOSEPH E. GEENEN ............... 1055
29. Pharmacology of biliary tract
    JOSE BEHAR
    PIERO BIANCANI ............... 1103

*Abnormal Motility*

30. Parasite infections and gastrointestinal motility
    GILBERT A. CASTRO ............... 1133
31. Alterations of small intestine motility by bacteria and their enterotoxins
    JOHN R. MATHIAS
    MARY H. CLENCH ............... 1153
32. Motor and myoelectric activity associated with vomiting, regurgitation, and nausea
    IVAN M. LANG
    SUSHIL K. SARNA ............... 1179
33. Adaptation to surgical perturbations
    MARIA PAPASOVA
    ELENA ATANASSOVA ............... 1199

*Comparative Physiology*

34. Gastrointestinal motor functions in ruminants
    YVES RUCKEBUSCH ............... 1225
35. Avian gastrointestinal motor function
    GARY E. DUKE ............... 1283

**CIRCULATION**

*Structure*

36. Histoanatomy and ultrastructure of vasculature of alimentary tract
    B. J. GANNON
    M. A. PERRY ............... 1301

*Hemodynamics*

37. Gastrointestinal blood flow– measuring techniques
    A. P. SHEPHERD
    J. W. KIEL ............... 1335
38. Physiology of gastric circulation
    PAUL H. GUTH
    FELIX W. LEUNG
    GORDON L. KAUFFMAN, JR. ............... 1371
39. Microcirculation of the intestinal mucosa
    D. NEIL GRANGER
    PETER R. KVIETYS
    RONALD J. KORTHUIS
    ANDRE J. PREMEN ............... 1405
40. Gastrointestinal circulation and motor function
    CHING CHUNG CHOU ............... 1475
41. Hepatic circulation
    CLIVE V. GREENWAY
    W. WAYNE LAUTT ............... 1519
42. Circulation of the pancreas and salivary glands
    PETER R. KVIETYS
    D. NEIL GRANGER
    SCOT L. HARPER ............... 1565
43. Neonatal intestinal circulation
    PHILIP T. NOWICKI ............... 1597

*Neurobiology*

44. Electrophysiological and neuromuscular relationships in extramural blood vessels
    D. L. KREULEN
    K. D. KEEF ............... 1605
45. Neuromuscular transmission in intramural blood vessels
    G. D. S. HIRST ............... 1635
46. Neurohormonal control of gastrointestinal blood flow
    MATS JODAL
    OVE LUNDGREN ............... 1667

*Abnormal Circulation*

47. Pathophysiology of gastrointestinal circulation
    ROBERT H. GALLAVAN, JR.
    DALE A. PARKS
    EUGENE D. JACOBSON ............... 1713

*Lymphatic Circulation*

48. Gastrointestinal lymphatics
    J. A. BARROWMAN
    P. TSO ............... 1733

Index ............... xiii

CHAPTER 21

# In vivo myoelectric activity: methods, analysis, and interpretation

SUSHIL K. SARNA

*Departments of Surgery and Physiology, Medical College of Wisconsin, and Department of Surgical Research, Clement J. Zablocki Veterans Administration Medical Center, Milwaukee, Wisconsin*

## CHAPTER CONTENTS

Control of Phasic Contractions
   Temporal control of phasic contractions
   Spatial control of phasic contractions
Methods of Recording
Methods of Analysis
Terminology
Spatial and Temporal Patterns of In Vivo Myoelectric Activity
   Stomach
   Small intestine
   Colon and rectum
      Electrical control activity
      Discrete electrical response activity
      Continuous electrical response activity
      Contractile electrical complex
   Esophagus
      Striated muscle esophagus
      Smooth muscle esophagus
   Sphincters and organ junctions
   Sphincters
      Upper esophageal sphincter
      Lower esophageal sphincter
      Anal sphincters
   Organ junctions
      Gastroduodenal junction (pylorus)
      Choledochoduodenal junction
      Ileocolonic junction
   Gallbladder
Special Situation Contractions
   Vomiting
   Caudad mass movement
Relaxation-Oscillator Versus Cable Model to Explain Organization of Electrical Control Activity
   Passive conduction
   Regenerative propagation
   Relaxation-oscillator propagation
Summary

---

THE MAJOR MOTOR functions of the gastrointestinal tract are *1*) physical breakdown of ingested food into smaller particles, *2*) mixing the food with secretions for chemical breakdown, *3*) agitating the intraluminal contents for uniform exposure to the mucosa, *4*) caudad propulsion of intraluminal contents at a rate consistent with the secretory and absorptive functions of the gut, *5*) prevention or regulation of reflux, *6*) expulsion of waste material at the end of digestion, *7*) rapid movement of intraluminal contents in preparation for special situations such as vomiting and defecation, and *8*) keeping the stomach and the small intestine clean of residual food, secretions, and desquamated cells in between meals.

These motor functions are accomplished by contractions of the gut wall. Basically the contractions may be of three types: *1*) phasic contractions that are present most of the time during the fasted and the fed states, *2*) tonic contractions of tissues at the junctions between different organs of the gastrointestinal tract or in special regions such as the fundus, and *3*) special situation contractions that occur infrequently during the fasted or the fed state such as those during vomiting and defecation. The phasic contractions are largely responsible for the mixing and propulsive movements of the digestive tract; the tonic contractions minimize the reflux and regulate the rate of transfer of the ingested meal between adjacent organs; and the special situation contractions are associated with rapid unidirectional movement of intraluminal contents. This chapter describes the in vivo myoelectric activity associated with contractions of the alimentary tract, methods for recording and analysis, and the interpretation of its temporal and spatial organization in individual organs.

The motor function differs in different organs of the gastrointestinal tract, and often different parts of an organ have different motor functions. For example, the major motor function of the esophagus is simply to transfer boluses of food to the stomach. The motor function of the distal esophagus is also to clear acid and other gastric contents that may reflux across the lower esophageal sphincter. These motor functions are normally achieved by single, caudad propagating contractions that are initiated by a swallow or by chemical and mechanical stimulation of esophageal receptors. The major motor functions of the gastric fundus are to act as a temporary reservoir after a meal and to transfer its contents gradually into the distal stomach. The major functions of the distal stomach are to mix the ingested food with enzymatic and acid secretions, to break it down to a fine particle size, and then to empty the chyme into the duodenum. The chyme is mixed with biliary and pancreatic secretions in the proximal small intestine and propelled distally at a rate consistent with the absorption of different food components. The propulsion rate in the proximal small intestine is faster than that in the distal small intestine and thereby spreads food over a large area rapidly to make room for further emptying from the stomach. The rate of propulsion slows down in the distal small intestine to allow more time for absorption. The motor functions of the colon are to knead its contents to uniformly expose them to the mucosal surface, propel the contents distally at a rate consistent with water and electrolyte absorption, and store them in the distal colon for voluntary defecation. The motor functions of the proximal, middle, and distal colon may indeed differ from each other, but these differences are not completely understood. Additionally the colon is required to deal with semisolid to solid contents rather than with fluid contents alone as does the small intestine. Stronger and longer duration phasic contractions may be required for this motor function of the colon (185).

The purpose of this discussion is to point out that although phasic contractions of the gut wall serve for mixing and propulsion, different temporal and spatial patterns of contractions are required for different motor functions at different levels of the gastrointestinal tract. Furthermore other characteristics of individual contractions, such as amplitude and duration, vary in response to different motor requirements. Within each organ the pattern of contraction varies in response to different compositions of the intraluminal contents because of different meals. A versatile organization of control mechanisms that can integrate sensory information from different sources and control the temporal and spatial patterns of muscle contractions is required. Such an organization of control mechanisms exists in the gut wall. Because of its complex decision-making ability, independent of the central nervous system, it is often referred to as the "gut brain" or "little brain" (192, 264, 265).

## CONTROL OF PHASIC CONTRACTIONS

Except for swallowing and defecation, the propulsive and mixing movements of the gastrointestinal tract are totally involuntary and largely under the control of phasic contractions. As pointed out previously, the extent of mixing and propulsion depends on the spatial and temporal patterns of contractions. The spatial and temporal patterns of phasic contractions are controlled by three primary control mechanisms, myogenic, neural, and chemical (Fig. 1A). The myogenic control refers to an electrical activity, called electrical control activity (ECA), generated in the smooth muscle layers of the digestive tract. The parameters of ECA that are important in the control of contractions are the resting membrane potential, frequency and amplitude of periodic oscillations of membrane potential, and the phase relationships between oscillations in adjacent cells or groups of cells. The neural control refers to the control exerted by the extrinsic and intrinsic nerves innervating the gastrointestinal tract. The chemical control refers to various peptides, neurotransmitters, and neuromediators released from nerves and the paracrine and endocrine cells and glands. The chemicals may act in the endocrine, paracrine, or the neurocrine mode to affect motor activity, as shown in Figure 1A. (97).

These three control mechanisms act in concert to control both the temporal and the spatial patterns of contractions in response to sensory information integrated from the chemical and the mechanical receptors in the gut wall (Fig. 1B). The functioning of the control mechanisms may be modulated by signals from the central nervous system and by reflex signals generated at adjacent or distant sites in the same organ or in other organs. Depending on their source, these signals may affect the smooth muscle contraction through the extrinsic nerves or intrinsic nerves or both. Endogenous chemicals may act at preganglionic sites, on the ganglia, on interneurones, at postsynaptic sites, or on smooth muscle to excite or to inhibit smooth muscle contractions.

The timing of smooth muscle contraction is controlled by ECA. In achieving the desired motor function, both temporal and spatial control of contractions is essential. The temporal control of contractions refers to the control of contractions in time in a given smooth muscle cell or a group of cells. The spatial control of contractions refers to the relationship between the onset of contractions in adjacent groups of cells.

### Temporal Control of Phasic Contractions

The two major types of electrical activities common to most of the gastrointestinal tract are ECA and electrical response activity (ERA) (184). The ECA is an omnipresent oscillation of membrane potential that controls the excitability of smooth muscle to contract (Fig. 2). The first tracing in the figure demonstrates an intracellular recording of myoelectric activity, whereas the second tracing shows its equivalent recorded with extracellular bipolar electrodes. The third tracing demonstrates contractile activity. Normally the amplitude of membrane potential oscillation is such that the plateau potential is less than the excitation threshold and the smooth muscle does not contract, as shown in the first and the third oscillations of ECA. However, when neurochemical excitation is present the plateau potential exceeds the excit-

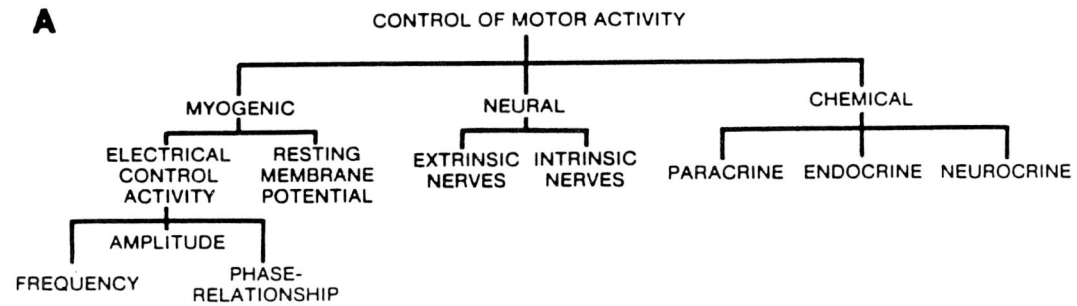

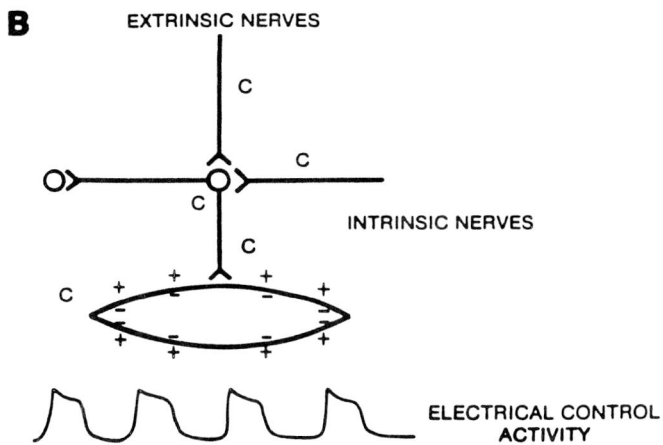

FIG. 1. *A*: hierarchy of myogenic, neural, and chemical control of gastrointestinal motor activity. *B*: interaction between myogenic neural and chemical mechanisms to control contractions of gastrointestinal smooth muscle. All extrinsic nerves are bunched together for simplicity. Evidence indicates that postganglionic sympathetic nerves may also synapse at intramural ganglia to modulate contraction of smooth muscle. *C*: sites where endogenous chemicals may act to modulate contraction of smooth muscle.

atory threshold level. When this happens, a burst of rapid oscillations of membrane potential (ERA) occurs and the smooth muscle contracts, as shown in the second, fourth, and fifth oscillations of ECA.

Two important points follow from this discussion: *1*) the gastrointestinal smooth muscle contracts only once during one cycle of ECA, and *2*) the muscle contracts only during the depolarized phase of the cycle, no matter when the neurochemical stimulus is applied. Stated differently, the maximum frequency of contractions in a given smooth muscle cell cannot exceed the frequency of its ECA. If the neurochemical stimulus is not present during every cycle of ECA, the frequency of contractions will be less than the maximal value. This process of control of contractions is referred to as temporal control of contractions because it controls contractions in the time domain at a given site.

The basic requirement for gastrointestinal smooth muscle to contract is that the membrane potential must depolarize beyond its excitation threshold level (61, 62, 235). However, it is not known whether the excitation threshold is a fixed membrane potential for a given cell or if it is a function of the resting membrane potential and the amplitude of depolarization. In several gastrointestinal tissues, such as the stomach, small intestine, and colon, in vivo depolarization of ECA above the threshold excitation level is invariably accompanied by a burst of ERA as just explained. In other tissues there may be some variations in the basic mechanism of myogenic control, for example, each and every depolarization of ECA may exceed the excitation threshold level and thereby be invariably accompanied by a contraction. Such is the case for the smooth muscle of the choledochoduodenal junction, lower esophageal sphincter, and the anal sphincter in some species. In such cases the ECA depolarization may be superimposed with ERA in some tissues, whereas in others it may not be superimposed with a burst of ERA to contract the smooth muscle. Another variation is that the frequency of phasic contractions may be such that they fuse together to result in a tonic contraction, such as in the lower esophageal and anal sphincters. These variations of the myogenic control are discussed in the individual sections on these organs.

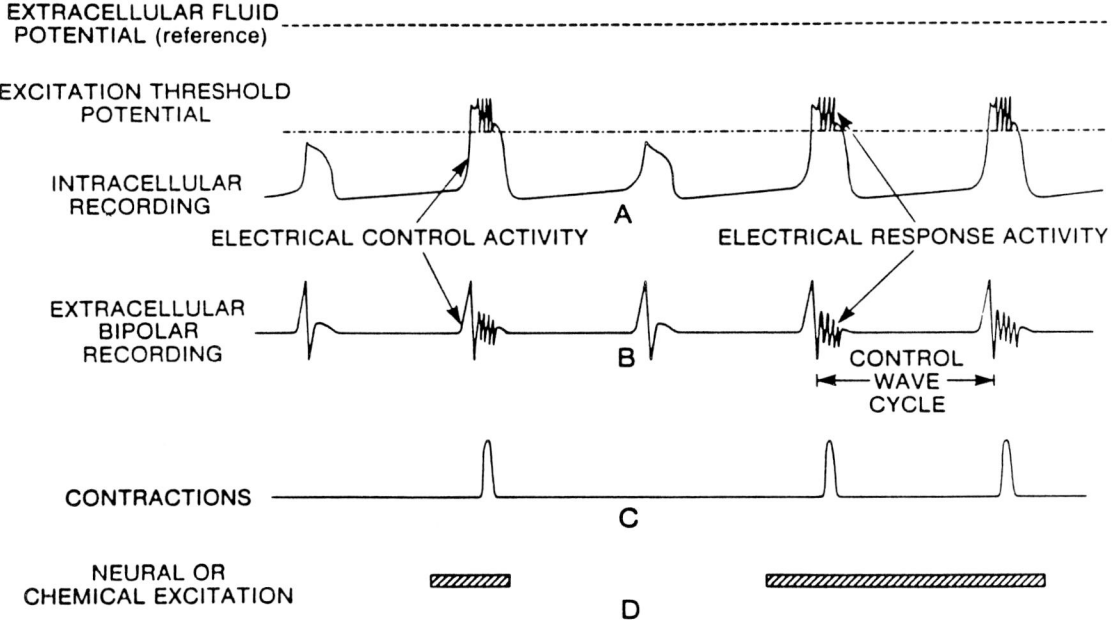

FIG. 2. Relationship between intracellular and extracellular electrical activities and contractile activity. *Resting* membrane potential in intracellular recordings is negative with respect to extracellular fluid potential (reference). Intracellularly recorded monophasic depolarizations are recorded as biphasic or triphasic depolarizations by extracellular bipolar electrodes. In intracellular recordings, electrical response activity bursts appear during depolarized phase of control potential, but in extracellular recordings they appear after initial large depolarization of control potential. However, their temporal relationship to contractile activity is the same in both types of recordings. Membrane potential depolarizations that do not exceed the excitation threshold level are not superimposed with a burst of electrical response activity and accompanied by a contraction. Neurochemical stimulation (*rectangles*) increases the amplitude of electrical control activity oscillation and results in a burst of electrical response activity and a contraction during depolarization. [Adapted from Sarna (187).]

There is a complex, incompletely understood relationship between the amplitudes and waveshapes of intracellularly and extracellularly recorded signals. The amplitude and waveshape of extracellular recordings depend on several factors, such as the size of electrodes, monopolar or bipolar recordings, spacing between the two electrodes of a bipolar electrode, propagation velocity at the site of recording, type of electrodes (wire, suction, or pressure), and whether or not the ECA being recorded is phase locked. A major component of the extracellularly recorded signal is associated with the upstroke of the membrane depolarization. The plateau portion of membrane depolarization shows very little change in extracellular recordings. Consequently, whereas the burst of ERA in intracellular recordings appears during the depolarized phase of the membrane potential, it appears after the ECA potential recorded extracellularly, as shown in Figure 2. However, the relationship between a contraction and a burst of response activity is the same in both cases. The strength and duration of contraction is related to the number and frequency of response potentials in a burst of ERA (146).

The temporal control of contractions in the gastrointestinal smooth muscle is similar in some respects to the temporal control of contractions by cardiac electrical activity in the heart muscle. Both electrical activities are omnipresent and both control contractions by periodic depolarization of muscle cells. There are two dissimilarities between them. *1*) Each depolarization of the cardiac muscle membrane potential causes a muscle contraction because every normal depolarization exceeds the excitation threshold. In several gastrointestinal organs, additional factors such as neurochemical stimulation are required for the depolarization of ECA to exceed the excitation threshold and contract the smooth muscle. *2*) The contraction of cardiac muscle is not associated with any additional type of electrical activity, but the contraction of most of the gastrointestinal smooth muscle is associated with a burst of ERA superimposed on the depolarization of ECA. The teleological reasons for the dissimilarities between the two muscles are obvious. The heart must pump blood continuously, whereas the gastrointestinal tract responds to the intermittent ingestion of meals and to special requirements between meals. The gastrointestinal smooth muscle does not need to contract continuously. The cardiovascular system has to pump more or less a consistent fluid (blood), but the gastrointestinal tract may have to respond differently to different components, different viscosities, and to different volumes of meals. Additional control mechanisms such as the enteric nervous system, the endocrine-paracrine cells, and sensory apparatus are required to handle these complexities.

*Spatial Control of Phasic Contractions*

It is apparent from the foregoing discussion that myoelectric activity in each given cell in the gastrointestinal tract controls the timing of contractions. If there is no communication between cells, each will contract independently of the others, with the result that contractions throughout the gastrointestinal tract will occur randomly. The result would be anarchy, much like fibrillation in the heart. There may be to-and-fro movement of intraluminal contents due to randomly occurring contractions, but little or no propulsion may occur. The contractions at adjacent sites must be coordinated for effective propulsion.

At this stage it is helpful to differentiate between propulsion in a closed-loop, completely filled system, such as the cardiovascular system, and in an open-loop, partially filled system, such as the gastrointestinal tract. In the cardiovascular system, most of the propulsive force for the flow of blood comes from the pressure generated by the ventricles. The cardiovascular system is equivalent to a single pump that pumps blood throughout the system. The mean pressure is greatest in the left ventricle and drops progressively in the arteries and the veins because of the resistance to flow. The gastrointestinal tract does not have a single pump; instead it is comprised of a series of peristaltic pumps. It may even be considered as a series of intelligent peristaltic pumps whose stroke length, frequency of stroking, force of propulsion, and velocity of strokes vary from one site to the next and from one stroke cycle to the next depending on the motor requirement. The net movement of contents within any segment of the gastrointestinal tract is determined mainly by the propagation of contractions rather than by pressure differentials generated in the lumen. Little or no pressure difference within an organ is recorded by various closely spaced ports of a multilumen manometric tube in the fasted or the fed state. Each perfused catheter records a pressure increase when the muscle contracts and closes the orifice. The pressure thus recorded is the resistance to outflow from the orifice, which is a function of the force of contraction. The contents are literally pushed ahead of a propagating contraction. Therefore the effectiveness of propulsion depends on the force with which a contraction occludes the lumen and on the distance that each individual contraction propagates. Thus the spatial control and coordination of contractions is an important factor in the control of gastrointestinal motility.

The spatial organization of contractions is also controlled by the three primary control mechanisms illustrated in Figure 1A. By controlling the release of endogenous substances, the neural and chemical control mechanisms determine the length of different segments in an organ that are stimulated or inhibited to contract at a given time. The spatial organization of ECA in those segments that are stimulated to contract then determines the sequence in which contractions will occur, as illustrated in Figures 3 and 4. As discussed previously, the smooth muscle contracts only during the depolarized phase of ECA. Therefore the temporal relationship between contractions in adjacent groups of cells will be the same as the temporal relationship between the depolarizations of ECA in those groups of cells. Figure 3 illustrates the spatial control of contractions by different patterns of ECA. The top half illustrates ECA recorded from four adjacent recording sites, and the bottom half illustrates contractions recorded at the corresponding sites. The site of electrode E1 is proximal and that of electrode E4 is distal. In Figure 3A, the control waves at adjacent sites are phase locked, that is, they depolarize with a more or less fixed time lag because of strong electrical coupling between adjacent cells. The ECA depolarization occurs first at electrode E1, then at electrode E2, and so on. When the neurochemical excitation is present over the entire segment covering electrodes E1 to E4, the burst of ERA and corresponding contraction occur first at the most proximal site, then at the next distal site, and so on. This is a propagated contraction. This pattern of contractions facilitates the propulsion of intraluminal contents. If the neurochemical mechanisms are activated over only a part of the segment, the contraction will propagate only over the active part of the segment, as illustrated in the fourth cycle of ECA in Figure 3A. The mean rate of propulsion of intraluminal contents over a given segment will depend on the frequency of contractions, the mean velocity of propagation of contractions and the mean distance that the contractions propagate. This pattern of ECA and contractions is present in the stomach and the proximal small intestine.

If the force of contraction is strong enough to occlude the lumen, the bolus of intraluminal contents is propelled ahead of the propagating contraction (Fig. 4A). If the force of contraction is not strong enough to occlude the lumen, some of the contents is propelled distally, whereas some escapes retrograde through the partial opening. The weaker contractions that do not occlude the lumen result in some propulsion and some mixing (Fig. 4B). One example of this type of contraction is the body of the stomach where the lumen is large and the contractions are too weak to occlude it.

The word propagation in relation to the contractions must be used with caution. In reality the contractions do not propagate because a contraction at one site does not cause a contraction at the next adjacent site. The timings of contractions at both sites are controlled by local depolarizations of ECA. If the

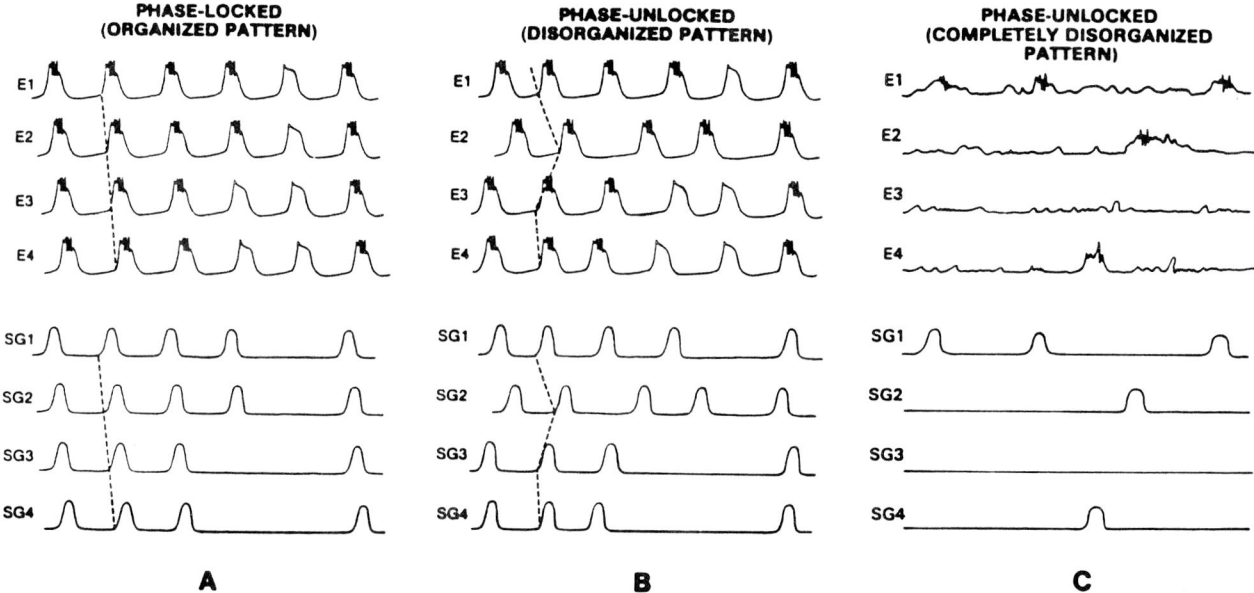

FIG. 3. Different spatial patterns of electrical control activity, electrical response activity bursts, and contractions. Electrode E1 and strain-gauge transducer SG1 represent a proximal site. Electrodes E2–E4 and strain-gauge transducers SG2–SG4 are at successively distal sites. *A*: electrical control activity is phase locked, resulting in caudad propagating contractions. *B*: electrical control activity is phase unlocked, resulting in uncoordinated contractions. *C*: electrical control activity is phase unlocked and highly variable in amplitude and waveshape, resulting in completely disorganized random contractions [Adapted from Sarna (187).]

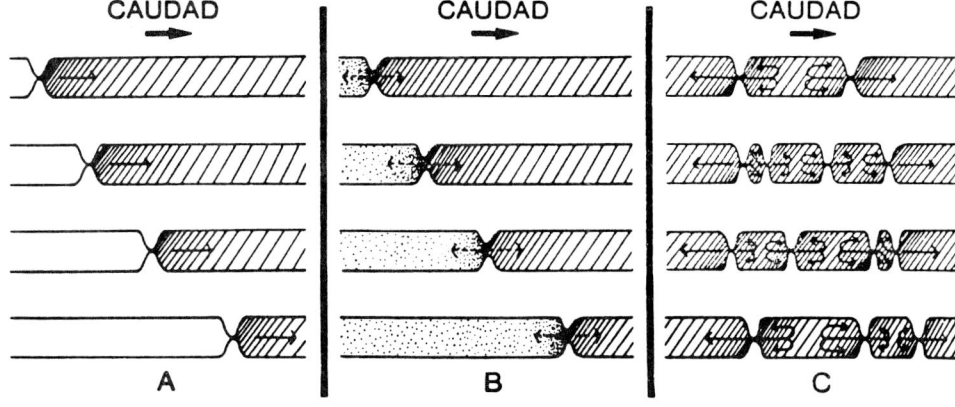

FIG. 4. Effect of different spatial patterns of contractions on mixing and propulsive movements of the gastrointestinal tract. *A*: caudad propagating lumen occluding contractions. *B*: caudad propagating nonlumen occluding contractions. *C*: disorganized lumen occluding contractions.

ECA is phase locked, then the contractions will occur sequentially and give the appearance of propagation. This appearance is much like that of light bulbs used in sign boards. The bulbs light up sequentially, giving the appearance of propagation. However, the lighting up of one bulb does not light up the next bulb; rather all bulbs are controlled by local switches.

Figure 3*B* illustrates a pattern of ECA wherein control waves at adjacent sites are not phase locked; that is, depolarizations of membrane potential at adjacent sites occur in no fixed temporal sequence, and they may occur at different frequencies. Consequently the bursts of ERA and hence contractions will also occur in an uncoordinated fashion. This pattern of contractions moves intraluminal contents back and forth resulting in mixing movements (Fig. 4*C*). Slow caudad propulsion may be associated with this pattern of contraction if the frequency of contraction at the proximal sites is greater than that at the distal sites. Additionally these contractions may propagate over short distances, resulting in a series of short propulsions that are additive. These patterns of ECA and contractions with varying degrees of discoordination are present in the middle part of the small intestine. Furthermore, if ECA becomes unstable in its amplitude and frequency, a completely disorganized pattern of contractions may occur (Fig. 3C). This pattern of contractions results largely in mixing movements. Such patterns of ECA may be present in the distal small intestine and the colon with varying degrees of instability and disorganization.

In summary, the neural and chemical control mechanisms determine whether or not contractions occur in a given segment of the gut, whereas the myogenic control mechanism determines the temporal and the spatial patterns of contractions. The remainder of this chapter deals with the in vivo myogenic control mechanism of the gastrointestinal tract. The neurochemical control mechanisms are dealt with elsewhere in this *Handbook*. In addition to the phasic contractions described previously, other types of contractions also occur in the gastrointestinal tract, for example, giant migrating contractions in the small intestine and the colon (78, 148, 170, 186), retrograde giant contractions associated with vomiting and retrograde propulsion of intestinal contents (78, 135), and long-duration phasic contractions in the colon (188, 193, 207). The myoelectric activities associated with these contractions are discussed in separate sections in this chapter.

## METHODS OF RECORDING

In vivo myoelectric activity in conscious animals is generally recorded with wire electrodes. Two types of wire electrodes have been used. One is a flexible single or multistrand wire electrode (06–.08 mm diam) usually insulated with a Teflon or Trimel coating. The electrode is inserted into the seromuscular layer along the gut circumference as shown in Figure 5A. To facilitate the placement of the flexible wire, a 23-gauge or smaller needle may be passed through the seromuscular layer and brought out at a distance of 1–1.5 cm. The flexible wire is passed through the lumen of the needle, and the needle is pulled back along with the wire. The wire is then bent back over itself and two sutures placed over it to secure it to the seromuscular layer. The excess length of the electrode is cut off. Two wires, 5–10 mm apart, are implanted in this way for bipolar recordings. The electrode wire has a bare length of 0.5–1 cm near its end. The wire is positioned so that the bare portion and a 1–2 mm length of insulated wire on each side of it is buried into the seromuscular layer. This type of electrode is particularly useful for recording from small organs such as the choledochoduodenal junction in opossums, thin-walled organs such as the gallbladder, and from the gastrointestinal tract of small animals such as the rat (108, 145, 180).

The other type of electrode consists of a pair of silver wires 0.4 mm diam embedded into a Silastic base (208, 209). The silver wire is soldered to a multistrand, 32-gauge, Teflon-coated lead wire (19 strands, 44-gauge each). The soldered joint is water-

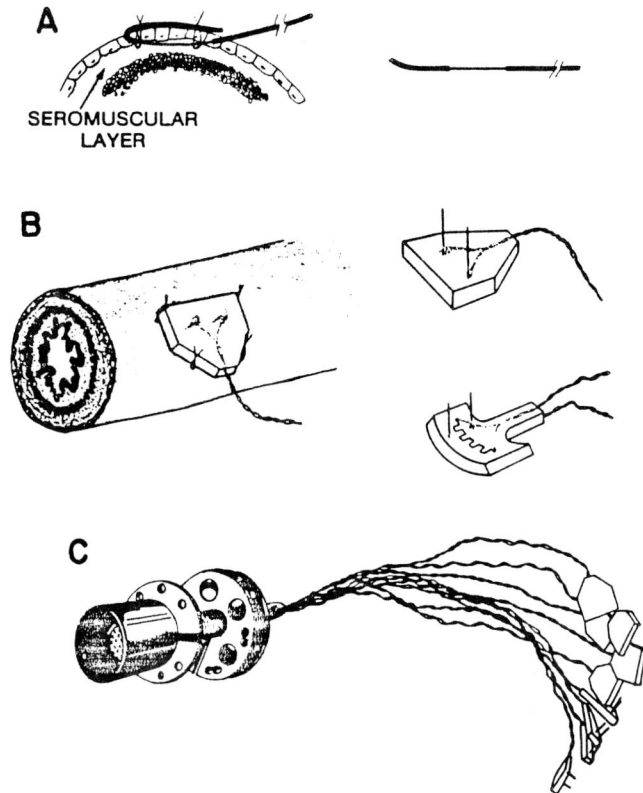

FIG. 5. *A*: preparation and implantation of flexible wire-type electrode. *B*: fabrication and implantation of Silastic base–mounted wire electrodes. *Lower inset* shows fabrication of strain gauge–electrode pair. *C*: stainless steel cannula to exteriorize lead wires. Two lower washers are sutured to inside of abdominal wall; single upper washer remains outside of abdominal wall.

proofed and encapsulated within the Silastic base. The Silastic base is positioned over the serosa, the silver wires extending 2–3 mm from the base are pressed into the intestinal wall, and the base is sutured to the seromuscular layer at each corner (Fig. 5B). The wire electrodes may also be embedded in a dental acrylic base with holes at four corners (122, 191). The Silastic is less reactive to tissue than dental acrylic. Furthermore the Silastic base can be combined with a strain-gauge transducer to record both myoelectric and contractile activities from nearly the same site as shown in Figure 5B (188). Chloriding of silver wires is usually unnecessary.

Two methods have been used to exteriorize the lead wires for either type of electrode. The wires can be tunneled subcutaneously to the subscapular region, exteriorized, and soldered to a plug (19, 146). Alternatively the lead wires are presoldered to pins in a multipin plug. The plug is embedded into a stainless steel cannula by using dental acrylic [Fig. 5C; (208, 209)]. The solder joints are protected with a coating of M-coat D followed by a coating of M-coat G, and the stem of the cannula is filled with a 50% bees wax/50% paraffin wax mixture. This combination of waxes effectively protects the plug and solder joints against corrosion by body fluids (28). The electrodes and the cannula stem are passed into the abdominal cavity through a stab wound, and the electrodes are sutured as just described. The cannula has two slip-on washers on the inside and one on the outside of the abdominal wall to prevent slippage. The inside washers are sutured to the inside of the abdominal wall through large holes. The two washers act as a lock nut, which prevents them from unscrewing after recovery of the animal. The electrode assembly with the stainless steel cannula has a longer life and is easier to maintain than the wires exteriorized at the subscapular region. The latter tends to get infected, and the wires are under a greater strain because of their longer length and frequent bending of the animal at the neck.

Myoelectric recordings can be made by monopolar or bipolar methods. Only one electrode is needed for monopolar recording from a given site, along with one common ground for all electrodes at different sites. The common ground may be an electrode implanted on the inside of the abdominal wall during surgery or a hypodermic needle inserted subcutaneously during recording. For bipolar recordings, two electrodes a few millimeters apart are used. A distance of 5–10 mm between the two wires of a bipolar electrode gives an optimal recording for both ECA and ERA. Smaller distances decrease the amplitude of ECA and distort its waveshape. The bipolar electrodes record less noise and electrocardiogram (ECG) signal than the monopolar electrodes. Figure 6 shows bipolar and monopolar recordings at different time constants from the same site in the stomach of a dog. For monopolar recordings, one wire of the bipolar electrode was grounded. The dog was also grounded by a subcutaneous electrode. The presence of ERA may sometimes be less clear in monopolar recordings than in bipolar recordings for nearly the same amplitude of contractions at that site.

In anesthetized animals, suction or pressure electrodes can be used for recording myoelectric activity as can the wire electrodes just described (7, 29, 75). Monopolar recordings are generally satisfactory when suction or pressure electrodes are used, but recordings from multiple sites with these electrodes become progressively more difficult when the number of recording sites increases.

In vivo myoelectric recordings from humans are made with intraluminal electrodes, serosal electrodes, or cutaneous electrodes (59, 86, 151, 190, 207, 218, 232, 238). Three types of intraluminal electrodes have been used: needle or wire electrodes that are held against the mucosa by suction, ring-type electrodes that simply lie in the lumen, and clip electrodes that are clipped to the mucosa. The ring-type electrodes pick up much excessive noise due to motion artifact and, in general, record reliable myoelectric activity only when the muscle is contracting strongly and the mucosa makes a satisfactory contact with the electrode wire. Therefore ERA is better recorded with ring-type electrodes than is ECA; however, if contractions due to ERA are not strong enough to occlude the lumen, these electrodes may miss some bursts of ERA. Access by clip electrodes is limited to the rectosigmoid area.

Serosal electrodes give the best recordings; however, their application in humans is limited to early postoperative recordings. Teflon-coated stainless steel

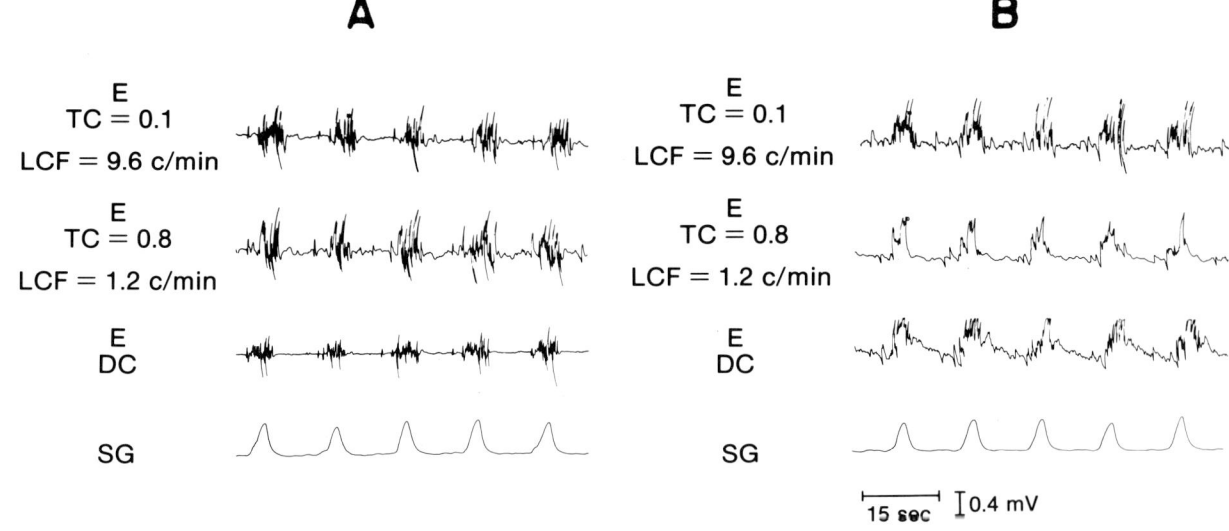

FIG. 6. Bipolar (A) and monopolar (B) recordings of gastric electrical activities from the same site at different time constants (TC). One of the wires of bipolar electrode was grounded for monopolar recordings; the dog was grounded by a subcutaneous electrode. LCF, lower cutoff frequency; E, electrical recording; SG, strain-gauge recording.

wires are used. The electrodes are held in place temporarily with absorbable sutures (190, 232). The lead wires are generally brought out through a Penrose drain or pulled out through a needle track. The electrode wires are pulled out of the subject 5–7 days after the operation.

Cutaneous electrodes are best suited for noninvasive clinical recordings; however, the signal-to-noise ratio is very low and computer analysis is essential for meaningful interpretation of the data (83, 216, 248, 249). Furthermore the only reliable information available from these electrodes is the frequency of ECA. The characteristics of propagation of ECA or of organized electrical activity such as phase III activity of migrating myoelectric complex cannot be obtained. Information about the frequency of ECA is available mostly from the antrum where the signal is the strongest.

## METHODS OF ANALYSIS

Visual analysis is often sufficient to measure ECA frequency and to detect the presence of ERA bursts in those parts of the gastrointestinal tract that have a regular and stable amplitude and frequency, such as the stomach and the proximal half of the small intestine. For other regions, such as the colon, gallbladder, or distal ileum, electronic filtering and spectral analysis with a computer are essential to precisely and objectively measure the parameters of the electric signal.

The frequency of ECA in the gastrointestinal tract of humans and most mammalian species studied thus far lies in the range of 2–40 cycles/min. The frequency of response potentials within a burst of ERA lies in the range of 0.9–10 Hz (189, 210). This separation of frequency bands allows the use of electronic filters to separate these signals. Band-pass filtering in the range of 1–10 Hz or 5–10 Hz separates out ERA from ECA (188, 208, 209). Band-pass filtering in the range of 5–10 Hz gives a clearer ERA signal without significantly attenuating its amplitude. In bipolar recordings from the stomach and the proximal small intestine, a single deflection representing the sharp rise of control potential may appear in the filtered record; however, this can be identified visually. The ECA can be separated out by using a low-pass filter with a cutoff frequency 5–10 cycles/min higher than the frequency of ECA present in the signal (188). For example, for human colonic signals in which the ECA has a frequency of 2–13 cycles/min, a low-pass filter with a cutoff frequency of 20 cycles/min gives satisfactory results (189, 207, 210).

When electrical signals are irregular in frequency and amplitude, such as those from the colon, visual analysis may be subjective and unreliable. Spectral analysis methods, such as the fast Fourier transform (FFT) and autoregressive modeling, are helpful for precise and objective analysis (23, 38, 47, 79, 93, 138, 189, 210). These methods give a power spectrum of the signal indicating the relative strengths of different frequency components. The power spectrum may be smoothed to remove spurious peaks. These methods of analysis are based on Fourier Series, which states that each complex signal can be expressed as a series of sinusoidal waves. The smallest frequency component is called the fundamental frequency of the signal. Prewritten programs for these methods are available on most computers. Computer programs and hard-wired circuits have also been used for the quantification of ERA bursts and their propagation characteristics (137, 234, 263).

The FFT and other spectral analysis methods have been used widely to analyze the frequency content of electroencephalogram (EEG), electrocardiogram (ECG), and electromyogram (EMG) signals. All of these signals have complex waveforms comprising different frequency components. The FFT method is useful not only in the frequency analysis of aperiodic signals, such as the above that deal with the power spectral density of different frequency components, but also in the analysis of transient signals that exist for only a short period, such as the seismographic signal (93). Therefore the aperiodicity of ECA in such organs as the colon and the ileum does not limit the application of this method. However, just as with any other method of analysis, care must be exercised in the interpretation of results. Spurious peaks due to respiratory artifacts, ECG, and base-line drift, if present, must be identified and discarded by visual inspection of power spectra; analysis of segments containing movement artifacts should be avoided. Finally, before assigning a physiological significance to a peak frequency, it must be confirmed that the frequency corresponds to the maximal frequency of contractions at the recording site. An understanding of the source of the signal and its method of recording also helps in meaningful interpretation of the power spectra. For example, in the stomach and small intestine where ECA is phase locked, extracellular bipolar recordings show a triphasic, pulselike waveform that corresponds to monophasic membrane potential oscillation recorded intracellularly. This triphasic waveshape may give rise to additional spurious peaks at higher frequencies that must be discarded. These spurious peaks are not due to limitation of the method but to distortion of the true signal by the recording method.

## TERMINOLOGY

Alvarez and Mahoney (4), who first reported an electrical activity in gastrointestinal smooth muscle in 1922, called it "action currents." This term was borrowed from cardiac and neurophysiology where, under physiological conditions, a depolarization of membrane potential is always accompanied by an action, that is, a contraction of cardiac muscle or striated muscle. In choosing this term, Alvarez and Mahoney intended a functional terminology because they believed at that time that the membrane depolarizations of gut smooth muscle were associated with contractions.

About a decade later, Berkson et al. (24) reported that there were fundamental differences between the electrical activity of the gut smooth muscle and that of the cardiac muscle, skeletal muscle, and nerve, which would make the use of the term action current in smooth muscle misleading. These investigators wrote, "It is conceivable that what we have observed in these experiments is not strictly comparable with the ordinary action currents."

Almost another decade later, Bozler (36) reported two types of electrical activity in gut smooth muscle and confirmed that periodic membrane depolarizations were not always accompanied by contractions. He wrote, "As pointed out by Berkson et al., these facts clearly show that the slow potential waves are not the action potentials of the rhythmic contractions of the intestine." (24). He called one type of electrical activity "slow potential waves" and the other electrical activity "action potentials." He used the terms "spike potentials" and "impulses" to describe the visual appearance of "action potentials." Bozler's terminology was based on two things, the visual appearance of the phenomenon and his feeling that the gut smooth muscle electrical activity was similar in function to cardiac and neural electrical activities. Bozler's conviction of a similarity between the electrical activity in the gut and the cardiac muscle was so strong that he even defined PQRST components of the extracellular recordings from the stomach and the small intestine. In using this terminology, Bozler confirmed the fears of Berkson et al. (24), who had written almost 14 years earlier

> From the published work in this field, one obtains the general impression that in interpreting the electrograms one may apply to smooth muscle the same principles that are involved in the electrobiology of skeletal muscle and nerve. When we first undertook this investigation, it was with the idea of employing these principles to interpret observed changes of potential in relation to mechanical movements.... We had not proceeded far, however, before it became evident that the relationship between contraction and electric change obtaining in this domain required careful scrutiny, for it presented a number of features not to be expected on the basis of the usually accepted notions regarding action currents in muscle (skeletal muscle).

The strong temptation to apply the principles of cardiac, neural, and skeletal muscle physiology to smooth muscle physiology is observed not only in terminology but also in other areas such as the controversial notion of a syncytium in gut smooth muscle and the explanation of the spread of electrical activity in smooth muscle by a cable model. In the application of such principles a tacit assumption is sometimes made that smooth muscle electrophysiology is similar to cardiac, neural, or skeletal muscle physiology. This may not be so.

The original intent of Alvarez and Mahoney (4) was to use functional terminology. Functional terminology is easy to understand and allows for fewer errors in conceptualizing and interpreting experimental findings. Code and Carlson (52) expressed similar sentiments in 1968 when they wrote, "The most satisfactory classification of contractions of the stomach would be one based on their function."

The use of a terminology based on the visual appearance of electrical activity or on the basis of the frequency of oscillation can be confusing and sometimes misleading. The term *slow* in slow wave is most often taken to mean a slow frequency. When Bozler (36) first made this observation he had only the myoelectric activity of the small intestine in mind. Since then myoelectric activities have been identified in other parts of the gastrointestinal tract, and this terminology has necessitated the use of terms such as *ultra slow wave* and *fast slow wave* (141, 252) to refer to an electrical activity that has the same function. It is now known that some smooth muscle cells in the gastrointestinal tract may have only one type of electrical activity, such as the circular muscle cells of internal anal sphincter in cats and humans (32, 153), whereas some other muscle cells like those from the colon exhibit four types of electrical activities (188, 210). The use of the term slow in such cases loses significance and meaning.

Asoh and Goyal (8) reported the presence of an electrical activity in the lower esophageal sphincter of the opossum that looked like "spikes" because of the extracellular bipolar recordings and so they called this activity spikes. However, the lower esophageal sphincter spikes differ from the spike activity elsewhere in the gastrointestinal tract. The electrical activity in the lower esophageal sphincter has a frequency of 20–30 cycles/min, which is outside the frequency range of the usual spike potentials, 0.9–10 Hz (189, 210). The spikes in the rest of the gastrointestinal tract do not occur spontaneously; however, the so-called spikes in the lower esophageal sphincter are spontaneous. Furthermore the spike activity in the lower esophageal sphincter does not occur as an intermittent burst as do the spike potentials in the rest of the gastrointestinal tract. The lower esophageal sphincter electric activity is really ECA because it is spontaneous, omnipresent, and controls individual contractions during each depolarization (107). A similar myoelectric activity in the anal sphincter has been called slow wave by other investigators (32, 153, 247). In such cases the use of a terminology based on visual appearance is deceptive.

By the late 1950s and early 1960s the function of the two types of gut electrical activities became well established. The spontaneously oscillating membrane potential controls the excitation of smooth muscle contraction. The intermittent bursts of rapid depolarizations occur in response to neurochemical stimulation and to depolarization of membrane potential.

Bass et al. (17) proposed a functional terminology for gastrointestinal electrical activity in 1961. They referred to the periodic depolarizations as "basic electric rhythm (BER)." The term *basic* referred to the persistent or fundamental property of the event (16). This term describes the omnipresence of this electrical activity yet does not describe its function, and the meaning of a fundamental property is not evident. Furthermore the basic rhythms may change with transection, electrical stimulation, or in a pathophysiological state, yet the function of the electrical activity does not change. Code and Carlson (52) proposed the term "pacesetter potential." This term implied that this activity set the pace of contractions. The term is not fully descriptive because this electrical activity determines more than the frequency of contractions; it controls their timing as well as the spatial pattern. Neither of the above two publications contained corresponding functional terms for the second type of activity, which Bozler (36) first called "action potentials," "spike potentials," or "impulses."

Sarna et al. (183, 201) proposed the terms "Electrical Control Activity (ECA)" and "Electrical Response Activity (ERA)" (183, 201). The ECA was so called because it controlled the occurrence of bursts of ERA and contractions in time and space. Each individual myoelectric signal was called a "control wave," and each individual depolarization was called a "control potential" (184). The ERA was so called because it was not spontaneous but rather occurred only in response to neurochemical stimulation and to the depolarization of the membrane potential. The individual oscillations in a burst of response activity were called response potentials.

A descriptive and precise terminology that is consistent for all of the gastrointestinal tract and relates to the function of electrical activity will help in understanding its role. This is particularly true when more than one type of electrical activity is present in an organ such as in the colon and when electrical activities with similar function are compared in different organs.

Before borrowing terms from other fields of electrophysiology, it must be confirmed that the activities not only look alike but have comparable function and identical mechanisms of initiation and propagation. Failure to do this may lead to false expectations. Berkson and colleagues (24) realized this pitfall over 50 years ago. The action potentials and spike bursts in cardiac, neural, and skeletal muscles are different from those in the gastrointestinal smooth muscle. For example, the action potentials in nerves conduct, yet the electrical activity called "action potentials" in the gastrointestinal tract does not.

## SPATIAL AND TEMPORAL PATTERNS OF IN VIVO MYOELECTRIC ACTIVITY

### Stomach

Electrophysiologically the stomach may be divided into two regions: an electrically inactive region comprising the fundus and a portion of the proximal corpus, and an electrically active region comprising the remainder of the corpus and all of the antrum (122, 201). The electrically inactive region does not have spontaneous ECA, whereas the electrically active region has omnipresent ECA. This division of stomach into regions is consistent with its motor function. The fundus acts as a temporary reservoir for the ingested meal. Regular phasic contractions that propel gastric contents distally and mix them with gastric secretions may not be required in this part of the stomach.

Spontaneous ECA is present in about the distal two-thirds of the stomach. The in vivo ECA frequency is the same at all gastric sites in all species studied (37, 59, 121, 152, 159, 201, 217); it is ~5 cycles/min in the dog stomach and ~3 cycles in the human stomach. The time lag/centimeter or phase lag/centimeter [phase lag = (time lag/cycle length) × 360°] between control waves at adjacent sites decreases distally in the stomach (Fig. 7A). This pattern of phase lag translates into a slower propagation velocity of contractions in the corpus and a higher velocity in the antrum (Fig. 7B). The higher propagation velocity of contractions in the antrum gives the appearance that the entire antrum contracts simultaneously when viewed radiographically. However, contractions recorded with strain-gauge transducers and electrical activity recorded with electrodes show a distinct time lag in the onset of contractions and ERA bursts right up to and including the pylorus (Fig. 7).

There is little or no phase lag among control waves recorded from electrodes implanted along the gastric circumference (201). Thus the smooth muscle cells along the circumference depolarize at about the same time to allow a ring of contraction to occur. The occurrence of ring contractions may be further facilitated by the segmental innervation of Latarjet's nerves that enter the stomach along the lesser curvature (64, 196). The neurochemical stimulus indicated in Figure 2 therefore may be concurrently applied to a ringlike segment.

When the electrically active region of the stomach is surgically divided into small segments by circumferential and longitudinal myotomies, each segment continues to generate ECA (201). The intrinsic frequency of the most proximal segment in the electrically active region is about the same as the frequency of the intact stomach. In the distal segments the intrinsic fre-

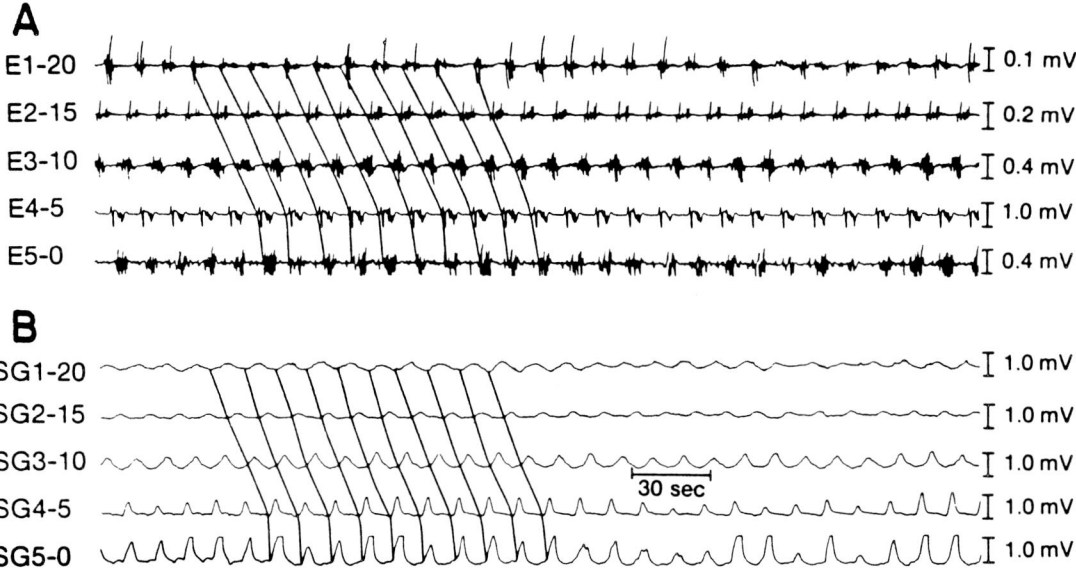

FIG. 7. Electrical and contractile activities recorded with 5 electrode–strain-gauge pairs from the stomach of an awake dog. Distances from pylorus are indicated along with electrode and strain-gauge numbers. Recording was made 60 min after a 650-kcal solid meal. Electrode E5 and strain gauge SG5 were on the pylorus. Each electrical control activity cycle was superimposed with a burst of electrical response activity and accompanied by a contraction at all recording sites. Onsets of a few caudad propagating control potentials and their corresponding contractions are joined by *solid lines*.

quency decreases progressively. For example, in the dog stomach the intrinsic frequency decreases from ~5 cycles/min in the corpus to ~1–2 cycles/min in the antrum (Fig. 8). A similar decrease of intrinsic frequency was reported in the human stomach by using in vitro techniques (82). There is a small decrease in the intrinsic frequency from the greater curvature to the lesser curvature. This finding means that the ECA in the stomach behaves like an array of relaxation oscillators (201). When the stomach is intact, the highest intrinsic frequency oscillator in the corpus near the greater curvature dominates and entrains the frequency of distal lower intrinsic frequency oscillators. The lower intrinsic frequency oscillators that are entrained by a higher intrinsic frequency oscillator always lag behind in their periodic depolarizations. Thus this gradient of intrinsic frequency ensures that smooth muscle depolarization normally occurs first in the corpus, then at a slightly distal site, and so on. This pattern of ECA then ensures that contractions in the stomach begin in the corpus and propagate distally (Fig. 7B). The negligible intrinsic frequency gradient along the gastric circumference ensures that the smooth muscle cells at the same level of the stomach depolarize with little or no phase lag and become excited to contract at about the same time.

Most of the coupling for the frequency entrainment of distal ECA oscillators in the stomach is provided by a 2–4 cm width of muscle layers along the greater curvature. The distal oscillators are uncoupled from the proximal oscillators when a circumferential myotomy is performed along this band on both sides of the stomach (202). On the other hand a circumferential myotomy beginning at the lesser curvature can be extended up to ~80% of the circumference without affecting ECA frequency at distal sites.

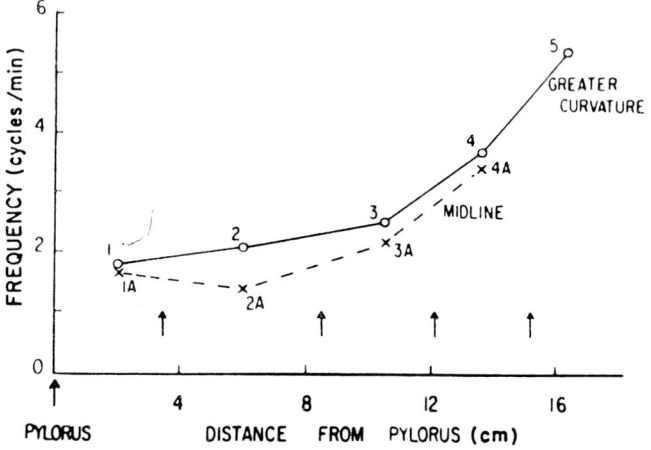

FIG. 8. Longitudinal and circumferential gradients of electrical control activity intrinsic frequency in dog stomach. *Vertical arrows*, sites of circumferential myotomies. Electrodes 1–5 were near the greater curvature and 1A to 4A on the midline. Longitudinal myotomy was made between the 2 sets of electrodes [From Sarna et al. (201).]

The ECA of the stomach can be driven by an external electrical stimulus provided that the frequency of the stimulus is slightly higher than that of

ECA (194). If this electrical stimulus is applied in the antrum, it alters the normal intrinsic frequency gradient because it artificially creates a higher intrinsic frequency oscillator in the antrum. This distal oscillator then entrains the next proximal oscillator to its own frequency, which entrains the next, and so on. Thus, the direction of phase lag among control waves is reversed. Because the propagation of contractions follows the direction of phase lag of ECA, the contractions now begin in the antrum and propagate proximally. This reversal in the direction of propagation of contractions delays gastric emptying (191).

Electrical stimulation of the proximal stomach increases the frequency of ECA in the entire stomach without a change in the direction of phase lag because the direction of the intrinsic frequency gradient is not changed. The maximum frequency to which ECA in the intact stomach can be driven is ~8 cycles/min in the dog (194). It is not known to what extent an increase in the frequency of caudad propagating gastric contractions would increase the rate of gastric emptying; the contribution of other factors that also regulate gastric emptying, such as fundic contractions, coordination of antroduodenal contractions, and enterogastric reflexes, will not be altered by electrical stimulation of ECA. Electrical stimulation in the mid stomach reverses the direction of phase lag at proximal but not at distal sites (Fig. 9). The normal organization of ECA returns a few cycles after the electrical stimulation is stopped. During this time the highest intrinsic frequency oscillator in the corpus recovers and begins to drive the next distal oscillator, which then drives the next oscillator, and so on (Fig. 9). The recovery is not instantaneous because a proximal oscillator cannot drive the distal oscillator until the distal oscillator is beyond the absolutely refractory phase of its ECA cycle (194, 201). This gradual recovery confirms that the organization of gastric ECA is due to an array of coupled relaxation oscillators rather than to conduction, as in a cable. The recovery of ECA should be instantaneous if a cable model was applicable to the stomach.

The upper limit to which the gastric ECA frequency can be driven in the intact stomach is due to the refractory properties of ECA oscillators (195, 200). The initial 30% of the ECA cycle is absolutely refractory. During this part of the ECA cycle an external stimulus does not initiate a premature control poten-

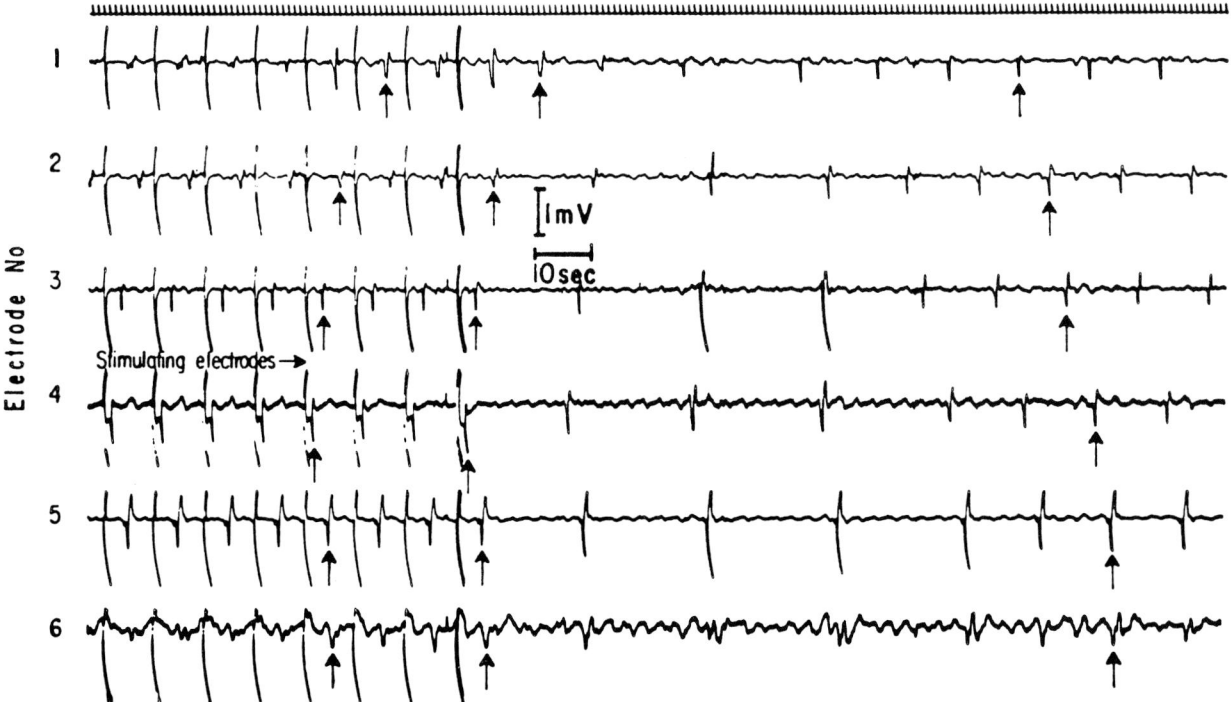

FIG. 9. Electrical stimulation of electrical control activity in the stomach. Recording electrodes 1–6 were 13.9, 10.3, 8.3, 4.6, 2.5, and 0.5 cm proximal to pylorus. Electrical stimulation at a site in between electrodes 3 and 4 entrained electrical control activity at all sites, and direction of phase lag was orad proximal to site of stimulation and caudad distal to it. *Second set of arrows* from *left* indicate last driven control potentials at each of recording sites after stimulation was stopped. Large simultaneous deflections at all recording sites indicate stimulus artifact. Normal electrical control activity frequency and caudad direction of phase lag returned a few cycles after stimulation was stopped. Electrical control activity was disorganized shortly after stimulus was stopped. [From Sarna and Daniel (194).]

tial to drive ECA (195, 200). The rest of the cycle is relatively refractory, that is, the minimum strength of stimulus required to initiate a premature control potential decreases progressively during this part of the ECA cycle.

In vitro recordings, using intracellular electrodes, show that contractions of gastric smooth muscle from the corpus and proximal antrum are related to the amplitude and duration of the plateau potential rather than to the bursts of ERA (82, 154, 235). This is not found during in vivo recordings from conscious or anesthetized dogs. As shown in Figure 7, and as reported by other investigators, contractions in vivo are always associated with bursts of ERA all the way up to the proximal corpus (119, 191). The strength of the in vivo contractions is related to the frequency and the number of response potentials in an ERA burst. The reasons for the differences between excitation-contraction couplings in vitro and in vivo are not fully understood. One of the factors that may contribute to these differences is the stretch applied to the muscle strips in vitro. Stretch is known to change membrane ionic conductance, excitation mechanisms, and resting membrane potential (39, 42, 92).

Smooth muscle cells in the fundus do not show spontaneous oscillations of ECA, but the fundus muscle does exhibit long-duration phasic contractions and a change in tone in response to a meal. The myoelectric correlates of these contractions remain to be established.

The frequency and the spatial organization of gastric ECA are disrupted in some pathological states and during recovery from abdominal surgery (27, 53, 190, 239, 266, 267). You and Chey (266) reported disorganization of ECA in patients with complaints of nausea, vomiting, and abdominal cramps. The ECA frequency in these patients was higher than normal (tachygastria), lower than normal (bradygastria), or irregular and phase unlocked (arrhythmia). Such abnormal patterns could result from ectopic, higher intrinsic frequency oscillators. However, for reasons presently unknown, when such patterns of ECA are observed, ERA bursts and contractions are usually absent. Furthermore, such abnormal patterns of ECA are normalized after ingestion of a meal, during phase III activity in the fasted state, and by cholinergic stimulation. Disorganization of ECA manifested as tachygastria, bradygastria, or arrhythmia has also been reported in subjects without the symptoms of disordered motility, nausea, or vomiting and in healthy conscious dogs (53, 98, 232). The incidence of arrhythmia increases after vagotomy (120, 158). Thus, whereas it is possible that those factors that cause nausea and vomiting may also cause ECA disorganization, it seems unlikely that disorganization of ECA causes nausea and vomiting. There is incomplete evidence for the proposal that sympathetic dominance over cholinergic activity causes ECA disorganization (65). Close intra-arterial injection of other substances such as prostaglandin $E_2$, Met-enkephalin, and glucagon also causes arrhythmias (127).

The gastric ECA is disorganized for ~12–24 h after abdominal surgery in humans (190). Contractions are generally not present during this disruption. This postoperative gastric ileus is more likely related to a neurochemical than myogenic disorder because ECA is usually quite normal intraoperative. Intraoperative recordings show that the gastric ECA frequency is not changed significantly in patients with peptic ulcer disease, gastric carcinoma, or gallbladder disease (147). Little information is available on the frequency or the organization of gastric ECA in the conscious state during fasting or after a meal in these diseases.

*Small Intestine*

The small intestine in most species studied so far (dogs, humans, cats) may be divided into two regions on an electrophysiological basis: the frequency plateau region comprising the duodenum and proximal jejunum and the variable frequency region comprising the remainder of the small intestine (Fig. 10A). (Recent evidence, however, suggests that the human small intestine may not have any well-defined frequency plateau like those in the dog and cat small intestine.) The ECA frequency is the same throughout the frequency plateau region, ~18–21 cycles/min in the dog and ~10–12 cycles/min in the human, and the control waves are phase locked (40, 51, 58, 71, 132, 199, 236). The length of the frequency plateau differs among animals of the same species (199, 236). The length of the frequency plateau decreases when the ECA frequency in the frequency plateau increases spontaneously or because of external electrical stimulation (197). In the dog the length of frequency plateau may extend to ~100 cm distal to the pylorus.

The electrical activities recorded by five extracellular bipolar electrodes, 6 cm apart, in the frequency plateau region are shown in Figure 11A. The onsets of a few successive control potentials at the five recording sites are joined by solid lines. The control waves are phase locked and stable in amplitude and waveshape; the bursts of ERA occur in a relatively fixed part of the control wave cycle. Some of the ERA bursts propagated over the entire 24-cm-long segment, whereas others started at different locations and propagated over variable lengths of the segment. This finding suggests that neurochemical excitation may be present over different lengths of intestinal segments at any given time. The distance over which ERA bursts, and hence contractions, propagate in the frequency plateau region is determined by neurochemical excitation; however, the direction of propagation, velocity of propagation, and the timing of contractions will be determined by the phase-locked ECA. The phase locking of ECA in the frequency plateau region facilitates the occurrence of propagated contractions (Fig. 3A). The ECA is phase locked in the frequency plateau

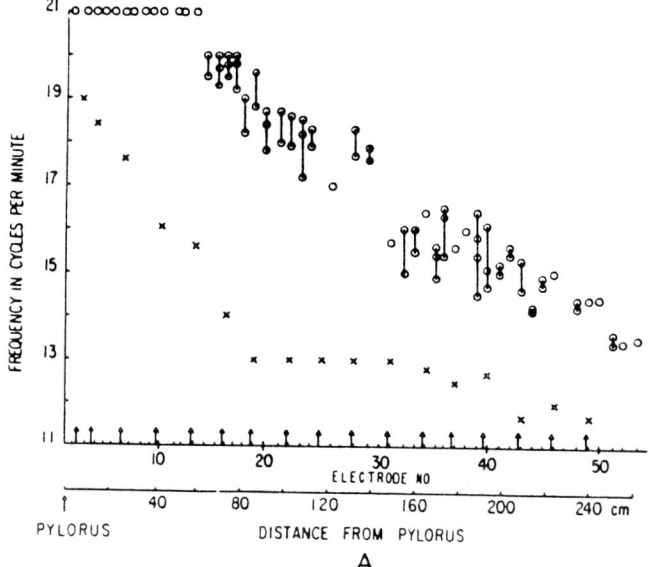

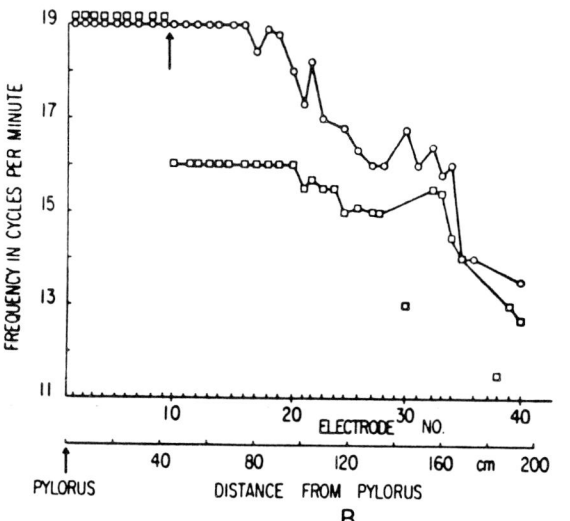

FIG. 10. *A*: intact and intrinsic frequency gradients of electrical control activity in dog small intestine. *Bars*, the range of intact frequencies. First 60 cm of small intestine was in frequency plateau region where electrical control activity frequency was the same at all sites. Remainder of small intestine was in variable frequency region. *Crosses*, mean intrinsic frequencies after complete circumferential myotomies at sites indicated by *vertical arrows*. Intrinsic frequencies decreased distally in the small intestine. *B*: effect of a single complete circumferential myotomy on frequency gradient of electrical control activity in dog small intestine. *Open circles* and *open squares*, electrical control activity frequencies before and after circumferential myotomy at site indicated by *arrow*. [From Sarna et al. (199).]

region because of the strong cell-to-cell coupling in this part (199).

The phase lag/centimeter is smaller in the proximal part of the frequency plateau than in the distal part (199). This pattern of phase lag translates into a faster propagation velocity of contractions in the duodenum than in the proximal jejunum. There is little or no phase lag among control waves recorded from different sites along the circumference in the frequency plateau region (181). This organization of ECA ensures ring-type contractions, because all smooth muscle cells along the circumference become excited at about the same time.

The ECA frequency is variable in the middle to distal jejunum and ileum. Distal to the frequency plateau region the mean frequency of ECA decreases from ~18 cycles/min to ~12–14 cycles/min in the dog and from ~10 cycles/min to ~6–7 cycles/min in humans [Fig. 10A; (58, 71, 199, 236, 253)]. There is pronounced waxing and waning of ECA amplitude at the transition from the frequency plateau region to the variable frequency region. In the variable frequency region the ECA is phase unlocked. The phase unlocking of ECA and the variability of frequency and amplitude increase distally as shown in Figure 11, *B* and *C*. The ECA recorded from the middle of the small intestine by five extracellular bipolar electrodes, 6 cm apart, is shown in Figure 11*B* and that from the terminal ileum in Figure 11*C*. The onsets of a few successive control potentials at the five recording sites are joined by solid lines in Figure 11*B*. In the middle of the small intestine, the control waves at adjacent sites slowly fall out of phase. If the whole segment was mechanically active during this time because of neurochemical excitation, some of the contractions would have propagated caudad, whereas the others would have occurred randomly or even propagated orad over short distances. In the terminal ileum the phase locking of ECA recorded from electrodes the same distance apart as in the mid small intestine is short lived or nonexistent (Fig. 11*C*).

Some investigators have reported multiple frequency plateaus in the small intestine by using only the criterion of mean frequency to define a frequency plateau (58, 71). They reported that the distal frequency plateaus continually varied in length, position, and frequency. The definition of a frequency plateau based on mean frequency alone is incomplete. The control waves must be phase locked in a frequency plateau. For example, the mean frequency of ECA at five electrodes in the middle of the small intestine in Figure 11*B* is nearly the same, yet the control waves are not phase locked. Consequently the contractions controlled by ECA at these electrodes will have very different characteristics from those in the frequency plateau region of duodenum and proximal jejunum (Fig. 11*A*).

The variable frequency and amplitude of ECA in the distal small intestine may be due to inherently unstable oscillations and to weaker cell-to-cell coupling. The irregularity of waveshape may also be due to the fact that the extracellular electrodes record from a large number of uncoordinated cells whose intrinsic frequencies may be slightly different from each other. The ECA recorded from ileal strips in vitro

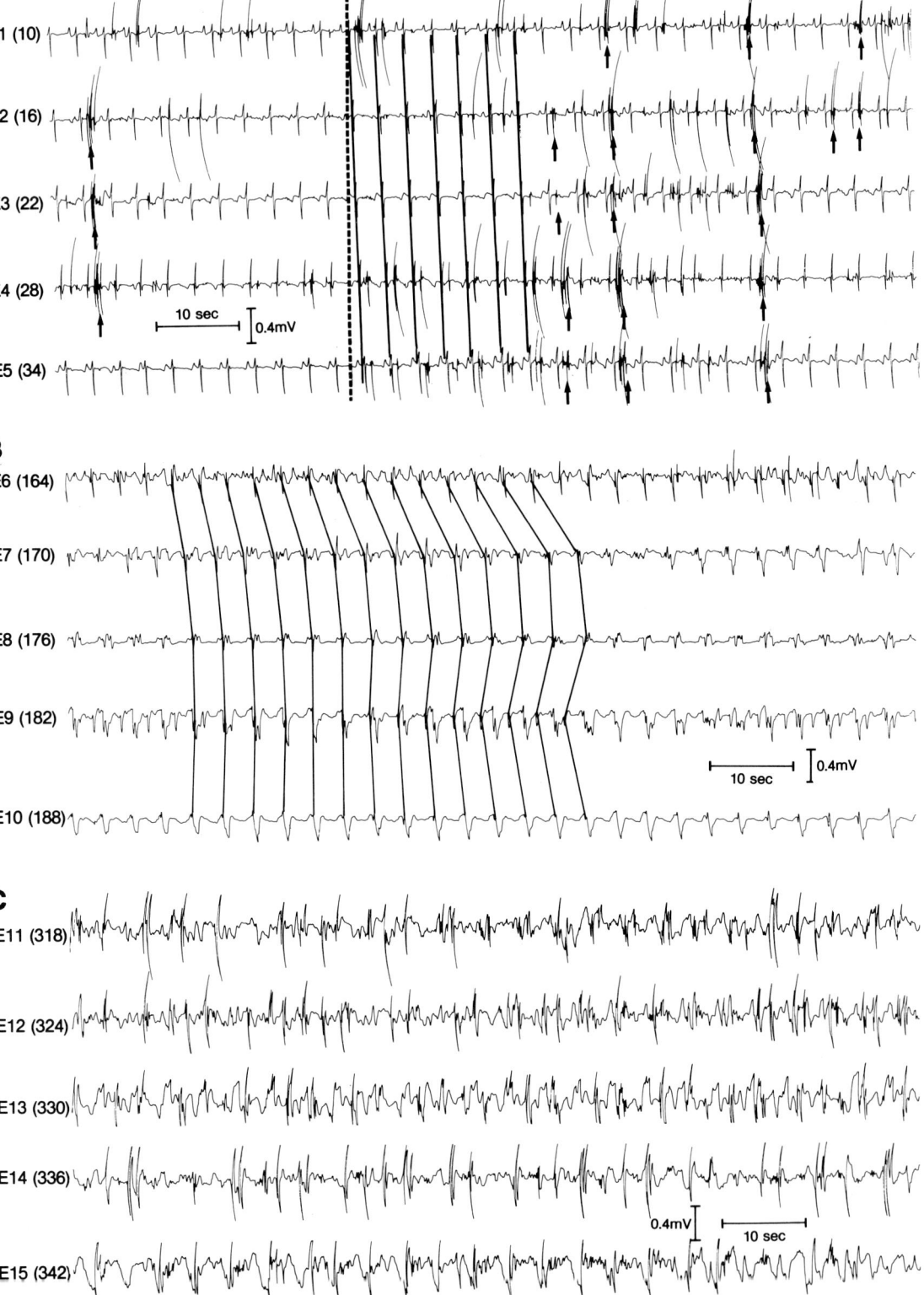

by extracellular or intracellular electrodes is generally much more regular and stable in frequency and waveshape than that recorded in vivo. It is possible that the intact nerves and circulating endogenous substances may also contribute to the instability of in vivo myoelectric activity. The irregularity of waveshape and phase unlocking of ECA results in uncoordinated contractions at adjacent sites (Fig. 3, B and C).

When the small intestine is divided into small segments by multiple complete circumferential myotomies, each segment continues to generate ECA but at a lower frequency than that in the intact state [Fig. 10A; (72, 105, 199)]. This finding means that the ECA in each small segment of the small intestine behaves as a relaxation oscillator with an intrinsic frequency of its own. When these segments are coupled to each other through cell-to-cell junctions, the highest intrinsic frequency oscillator dominates and entrains other ECA oscillators in the frequency plateau to its own frequency or a frequency slightly higher than its intrinsic frequency (199). As a result the highest intrinsic frequency oscillator depolarizes first, then the next oscillator after a short time lag, then the next, and so on. This results in a spatial pattern of ECA that facilitates propagated contractions in the proximal small intestine.

When the difference between the intrinsic frequency of the most proximal oscillator near the pylorus and the distal lower intrinsic frequency oscillators exceeds the limit that the available cell-to-cell coupling can entrain, the frequency plateau region ends. As a result, the frequency of ECA at sites distal to the frequency plateau is pulled up but not entrained. This incomplete pulling up of frequency may also contribute to the variable frequency of ECA in the distal jejunum and ileum. The distal oscillators keep falling behind a bit in each cycle and eventually lose a complete cycle. Because this phenomenon happens at different points at different times, the control waves are phase unlocked. They may temporarily be in phase over short lengths during which propagated contractions may occur. However, overall, this pattern would lead to slower transit and the bolus may be moved over shorter distances at a time. Because of a variable phase relationship among control waves, even orad propagating contractions over short distances are possible.

The foregoing explanation of the formation of frequency plateau and variable frequency regions is supported by the observation that when a single circumferential myotomy is made in the frequency plateau region, the frequency of ECA proximal to the myotomy is not affected [Fig. 10B; (199)]. Distal to the myotomy, a new frequency plateau with a lower frequency of oscillation is formed that now extends into the part of the small intestine that originally was in the variable frequency region. The reason is that after myotomy, the frequency just distal to the cut decreases to its intrinsic value. The difference between this intrinsic frequency and that of the more distal oscillators becomes less so that the available cell-to-cell coupling can entrain more distal oscillators.

The small intestinal ECA can also be driven by an externally applied electrical stimulus (2, 21, 123, 197). As in the stomach, an electrical stimulus applied at a proximal site in the doudenum increases ECA frequency without changing the direction of phase lag, but when the stimulus is applied at a distal site, the direction of phase lag is reversed at the proximal sites. At distal sites, the ECA frequency is increased without a change in the direction of phase lag. An electrical stimulus applied in the mid-frequency plateau region delays gastric emptying (21). Because of reversed phase lag of ECA, the orad propagating contractions reflux duodenal contents back into the stomach, or duodenal stasis may delay gastric emptying through enterogastric reflexes, or both.

In vitro recordings using intracellular electrodes show contractions of intestinal smooth muscle without ERA (182). These contractions are of low amplitude and occur at the frequency of ECA. Their amplitude is related to the amplitude of the plateau potential. The stronger contractions occurring spontaneously or induced by acetylcholine are, however, associated with bursts of ERA. Very-low-amplitude contractions with amplitudes of less than one-tenth the amplitude of normal phasic contractions can also be recorded in vivo using miniaturized transducers (251). It seems that the mechanisms of excitation-contraction coupling for low-amplitude contractions may be different from those for large amplitude contractions. The low-amplitude contractions may simply be due to the depolarization of membrane potential beyond a threshold level, but a burst of ERA may be essential for large amplitude contractions. It is not known if

FIG. 11. Different spatial patterns of electrical control activity and electrical response activity recorded from frequency plateau and variable frequency regions of dog small intestine. *Numbers in parentheses*, distances of electrodes from pylorus. Total length of small intestine was 372 cm. *A* ; control waves at 5 electrodes, 6 cm apart, were phase locked in the frequency plateau region. *Solid lines* connect the onset of corresponding caudad propagating control potentials. *Arrows* indicate some of the electrical control activity cycles that had electrical response activity superimposed on them. Electrical response activity bursts propagated at nearly the same velocity as control potentials. Distance of electrical response activity burst propagation ranged from <6 to 24 cm. *B*: control waves from 5 electrodes, 6 cm apart, on the middle of the small intestine (variable frequency region). *Solid lines* connecting successive electrical control activity cycles show that control waves were not phase locked. *C*: control waves from 5 electrodes, 6 cm apart, in terminal ileum (variable frequency region). Control waves were totally disorganized and unstable in frequency and amplitude.

both of these contractions are because of the same or different ionic currents. These low-amplitude contractions in vivo are hardly visible to the naked eye. Their physiological significance, if any, is not known.

Myoelectric activity of the small intestine in vivo is a fairly stable phenomenon. The frequency and organization of ECA are not affected significantly by physiological doses of most enteric peptides. Those substances that release acetylcholine may increase ECA frequency slightly by producing premature control potentials. In some cases of idiopathic intestinal pseudo-obstruction, however, the ECA has been reported to be absent most of the time or its intrinsic frequency gradient is reversed (204, 254). Each of these disorganizations may contribute to a motor disorder. The contractions will not occur if ECA is absent, and they will propagate in the orad direction if the intrinsic frequency gradient is reversed. Surgical resection of an intestinal segment decreases the ECA frequency and increases the length of frequency plateau distal to the anastomotic site. The lower ECA frequency results in a lower frequency of contractions, yet they may propagate over longer distances than before. The overall effect of these two opposite changes on intestinal propulsion is not known.

*Colon and Rectum*

Unlike the stomach and small intestine, the colon in dogs, humans, pigs, cats, and other species exhibits two types of phasic contractions: short duration and long duration (57, 80, 84, 109, 110, 116, 126, 129, 188, 207, 260, 261). In the dog colon, the long-duration phasic contractions have a mean frequency of ~1 cycle/min and a mean duration of ~50 s, whereas short-duration contractions have a mean frequency of ~4–6 cycles/min and a mean duration of ~10 s (188).

The long- and short-duration contractions in the colon are controlled by separate myoelectric mechanisms. Consequently, four types of myoelectric activities have been reported in the colon of several species studied thus far (dogs, humans, pigs, and cats). The different myoelectric activities in the colon and their counterparts, if any, in the stomach and small intestine are illustrated in Figure 12 and discussed next.

ELECTRICAL CONTROL ACTIVITY. The gradual degradation in the stability of amplitude, frequency, and waveshape of ECA that begins at the end of frequency plateau in the small intestine continues into the colon. The frequency and waveshape of in vivo ECA in the colon becomes so irregular that visual analysis of the myoelectric signals becomes difficult. Figure 13A shows the irregular ECA recorded postoperative from three electrodes implanted on the human colon (189). Spectral analysis programs like the FFT method were used to determine the frequency components of the signal (Fig. 13B). The ECA signal at electrode E2 had

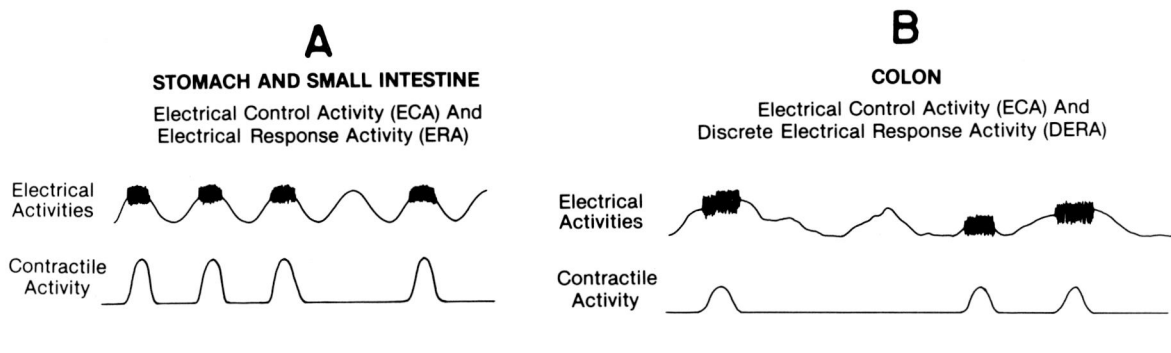

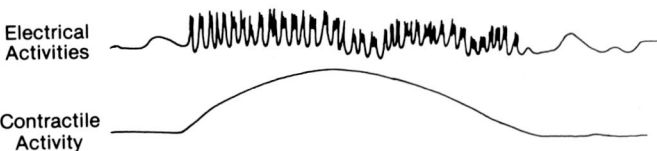

FIG. 12. Comparison of 2 types of electrical activities in the stomach and small intestine (*A*) with 4 types of electrical activities in the colon (*B*). Electrical control and response activities in the stomach and small intestine control occurrence of phasic contractions in time and space. Electrical control activity and discrete electrical response activity in the colon control short-duration contractions and contractile electrical complex and continuous electrical response activity long-duration contractions in time and space.

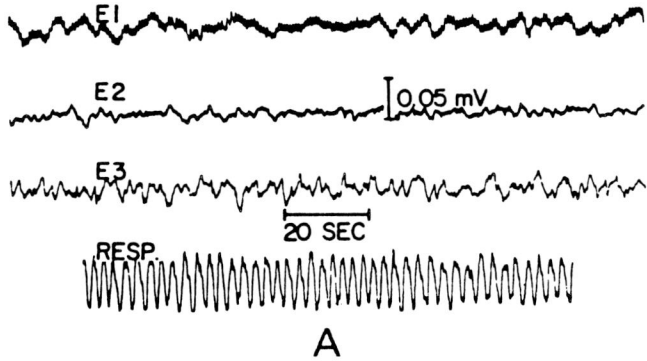

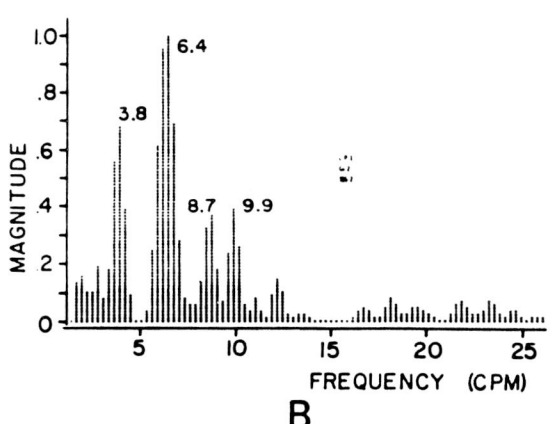

FIG. 13. *A*: postoperative electrical control activity recorded from 3 sites in human ascending colon by serosal electrodes. Distances between E1 and E2 and E2 and E3 were 5 and 3.5 cm, respectively. *B*: power spectrum of electrical control activity at electrode E2 for 1.07-min period. Power spectrum showed 4 frequency components at 3.8, 6.4, 8.7 and 9.9 cycles/min in colonic electrical control activity during this period. [From Sarna et al. (189), Copyright 1980 by The American Gastroenterological Association.]

four frequency components at 6.4, 3.8, 9.9, and 8.7 cycles/min in their decreasing order of power.

In the human colon and rectum the ECA is present in the frequency range of 2–13 cycles/min (60, 167, 189, 218, 238, 252). Within this range, frequency components in the range of 9–13 cycles/min dominate in the transverse and the descending colon, whereas in the rest of the colon components in the frequency range of 2–9 cycles/min predominate. This distribution of power of frequency components may increase the probability of contractions in the higher frequency range in the transverse and descending colon and in the lower frequency range in the rest of the colon. Other investigators have reported different ranges of ECA frequency within the above total frequency range in the human colon depending on the method of recording and the method of analysis (60, 167, 220, 238). However, the short-duration contractions controlled by ECA have been reported in the entire frequency range of ~2–13 cycles/min.

The highly variable amplitude and frequency of colonic ECA in vivo produces a variable phase relationship between control waves and the bursts of ERA; that is, bursts of ERA cannot always be identified in a fixed part of the ECA cycle as is the case in the stomach and the proximal small intestine. The waveshape and frequency of colonic ECA may vary from one cycle to the next. This variation may be due to the inherent instability of ECA in colonic smooth muscle cells and the fact that extracellular electrodes in vivo record simultaneously from a large number of uncoordinated cells. A similar but less variable relationship between ECA and ERA bursts exists in the ileum (236).

The maximum frequency of short-duration contractions and ERA bursts in the colon is the same as the corresponding ECA frequency (34, 188, 210, 218). Electronic filtering of signals in appropriate frequency ranges helps establish these relationships more clearly (Fig. 14). This figure shows that each depolarization of ECA is associated with a burst of ERA and a short-duration phasic contraction. The basic function of ECA in the colon is therefore the same as in the stomach and the small intestine, that is, to control the occurrence of bursts of ERA and hence of short-duration phasic contractions in time and space. Because there is no significant gradient of ECA frequency in the colon, and because it is highly disorganized, the resulting contractions controlled by ECA are uncoordinated and generally do not propagate.

The observed organization of colonic ECA can be explained by a chain of bidirectionally coupled relaxation oscillators (13, 139). The relaxation oscillators representing colonic ECA are inherently unstable in frequency and the coupling between them is poor.

DISCRETE ELECTRICAL RESPONSE ACTIVITY. The short- and long-duration contractions of the colon are associated with different types of ERA. The short-duration contractions are associated with bursts of discrete ERA (DERA) as shown in Figure 14. These bursts occur only during the depolarized phase of an ECA cycle and hence their mean duration is shorter than the cycle length of ECA. The discrete ERA is so called because it occurs discretely on each individual ECA cycle as opposed to continuous ERA, which occurs continuously during one or more ECA cycles. A 1:1:1 relationship between ECA depolarization, DERA bursts, and short-duration contractions has also been reported in in vitro muscle strips (80, 109, 110). Such a distinct relationship is not often visually apparent in in vivo recordings because of the variability of ECA, but the frequency of ECA and the maximum repetition rate of DERA bursts, when analyzed by computer and electronic filtering, correspond to the maximum frequency of short-duration contractions.

CONTINUOUS ELECTRICAL RESPONSE ACTIVITY. The long-duration contractions in the colon are associated with bursts of continuous ERA (CERA) as shown in Figure 15 (188). This response activity is so called because it occurs continuously through one or more cycles of ECA. The occurrence of CERA could not have been controlled by ECA because the duration of CERA is longer than the depolarized phase of ECA during which it makes the smooth muscle cells excitable to contract.

CONTRACTILE ELECTRICAL COMPLEX. The contractile electrical complex (CEC) is an intermittent burst of myoelectric oscillations in the frequency range of 25–40 cycles/min (Fig. 15). These oscillations control the occurrence of CERA and long-duration contractions. A 1:1:1 relationship between a burst of CEC, a burst of CERA, and a long-duration contraction has been reported in dog, human, and pig colon using both

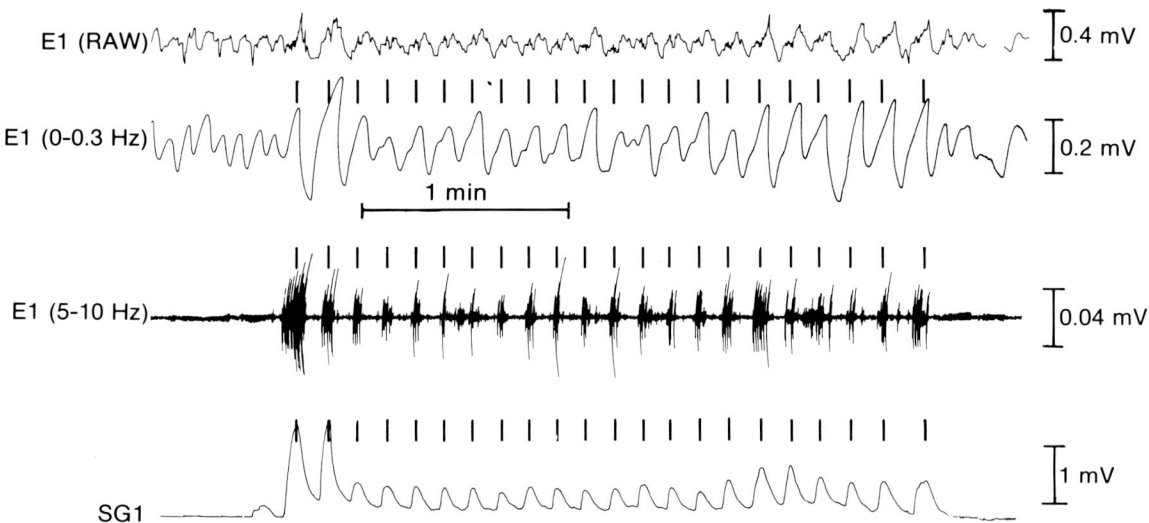

FIG. 14. Control of discrete electrical response activity and short-duration contractions by electrical control activity in dog colon. *First tracing*, raw myoelectric signal; *second tracing*, filtered electrical control activity; *third tracing*, bursts of discrete electrical response activities; and *fourth tracing*, corresponding short-duration contractions. Amplitude of contractions was related to number of response potentials in electrical response activity bursts. *Vertical lines*, correspondence between individual cycles of electrical control activity, bursts of discrete electrical response activity, and short-duration contractions. Pass bands of filters are shown in parentheses. Electrical control activity in the colon is not always regular and stable in amplitude as shown here. [From Sarna (188).]

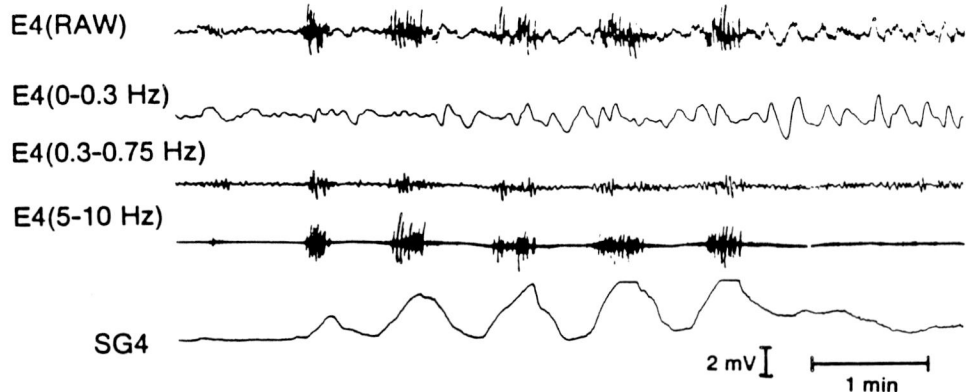

FIG. 15. Control of continuous electrical response activity and long-duration contractions by contractile electrical complex in dog colon. *First tracing*, raw myoelectric signal, *second tracing*, filtered electrical control activity; *third tracing*, bursts of contractile electrical complex; *fourth tracing*, filtered bursts of continuous electrical response activity; and *fifth tracing*, long duration contractions. Pass bands of filters are in parentheses. Each burst of contractile electrical complex was associated with a burst of continuous electrical response activity and a long-duration contraction. [From Sarna (188).]

in vivo and in vitro recording methods (80, 109, 110, 129, 188, 207). The CEC is so called because it is an electrical complex whose occurrence is invariably associated with a long-duration muscle contraction.

The mechanism of intermittent generation of bursts of CEC in vivo is not known. In vitro studies indicate that the occurrence of this complex is sensitive to tetrodotoxin and to cholinergic and adrenergic agonists and antagonists (109, 110). It is possible that nerves play a role in the intermittent generation of CEC bursts. The bursts of CEC and its associated CERA propagate in both orad and aborad directions. The long-duration contractions controlled by these myoelectric activities may play a major role in the back-and-forth movements of colonic contents and their distal propulsion.

The underlying mechanism of control of CERA and long-duration contractions by the CEC may be similar to that of control of DERA and short-duration contractions by ECA; that is, when the smooth muscle membrane potential depolarizes beyond an excitation threshold level, response activity occurs and the muscle contracts (188). Both in vivo and in vitro studies show that each oscillation of CEC may be superimposed with a burst of response potentials (188). Because of the high frequency of CEC oscillations, these bursts may fuse and give the appearance of a single continuous burst. For the same reason the muscle may not have time to relax between individual contractions associated with each oscillation of CEC, and this results in a single long-duration contraction. The characteristics of ECA and CEC are compared in Table 1.

Some investigators have used the term *slow wave* to refer to the CEC. This may not be appropriate because there are important differences between the two myoelectric control mechanisms. Electrical control activity is omnipresent, whereas the CEC occurs in intermittent bursts. Not every cycle of ECA is accompanied by response activity and short-duration contractions: a burst of CEC is invariably associated with response activity and long-duration contraction in the pig and the dog colon, but in the human colon the CEC may be directly associated with long-duration contractions (109, 188, 207). Cholinergic antagonists do not inhibit ECA but they inhibit contractile electrical complex (109, 110).

Fioramonti et al. (84) have used the terms short and long spike bursts for discrete and continuous response activities, respectively, based on an arbitrary duration of 3 s. Such an arbitrary definition can be misleading. They reported that in the ascending colon of the dog, the long spike bursts occurred at the frequency of ECA, whereas in the distal colon the long spike bursts were not related to ECA. The duration of long spike bursts on the transverse and descending colon in their study was ~14–37 s, which is much longer than the duration of an ECA cycle in the dog colon, which is ~10–15 s for a frequency range of 4–6 cycles/min. As discussed earlier, the ERA controlled by ECA can occur only during the depolarized phase of ECA and hence only on a part of the ECA cycle. The terminology of discrete and continuous response activities refers to the controlling mechanism. Both response activities occur in response to other spontaneous events such as ECA, CEC, and neurochemical excitation. The distinction between the two types of response activities based on their controlling mechanisms gives a mean duration of CERA that is about the same as the duration of long-duration contractions (188).

Visual analysis of colonic ECA in the human rectosigmoid suggested that ECA was present for only a part of the total recording period (220, 238). Computer analysis with the FFT method showed that ECA was present at all times just as in the stomach and the small intestine (136, 206). The irregularity of ECA frequency and amplitude in the colon may preclude an objective analysis by visual methods.

A similar visual analysis of colonic ECA led to the conclusion that a change in the percentage presence of frequency components at 3 cycles/min from ~10% to 50% of the recording period is the underlying cause of the colonic motility disorder in irritable bowel syndrome patients (218, 219, 237). Computer analysis indicated that there was no significant difference in the ECA frequency or its organization between normal and irritable bowel syndrome patients (136, 204, 206). Several arguments can be made against the possibility that a change in the percentage presence of the frequency component at 3 cycles/min of ECA may be the basis of motor disorder in this syndrome. *1*) There is no corresponding change in the incidence of contractions at 3 cycles/min in these patients (218, 219). Thus, if there is indeed a change in the percentage presence of 3 cycles/min, it has no effect on motor activity and hence it could not lead to a motility disorder. *2*) The percentage presence of frequency components at 3 cycles/min is not normalized during spontaneous or therapeutic remission of symptoms of irritable bowel syndrome (237). *3*) Electrical control

TABLE 1. *Characteristics and Functions of Colonic Electrical Control Activity and Contractile Electrical Complex*

|  | Electrical Control Activity | Contractile Electrical Complex |
|---|---|---|
| Presence | Omnipresent | Intermittent bursts |
| Frequency range, cycles/min* | 2–13 | 25–40 (during a burst) |
| Associated response activity | Discrete electrical response activity | Continuous electrical response activity |
| Associated contractile activity | Short-duration contractions | Long-duration contractions |

* Frequency range as measured in humans.

activity controls only one of the two types of contractions in the colon, that is, short-duration contractions that are largely disorganized. It seems unlikely that a major motility disorder such as irritable bowel syndrome could occur because one of the controlling mechanisms is present too much of the time. It is important to note that even if an ECA frequency component is present for a larger percentage of time, it does not mean that the colon will contract a larger percentage of time at that frequency. Whether the colon will contract or not is determined by neurochemical excitation. For example, after small intestinal resection, the frequency of contractions distal to the anastomosis is significantly decreased and yet no major motility disorder is present. Other factors such as the spatial organization of contractions, that is, whether contractions propagate or not, the distance that contractions propagate, the patterns of cyclic occurrence of contractions (193), and possible changes in the characteristics of long-duration contractions must be considered in establishing the basis of colonic motility disorders. *4)* Irritable bowel syndrome constitutes a heterogenous group of patients who may have constipation, diarrhea, or both alternatively. It is unlikely that a change in the percentage presence of 3 cycles/min frequency component could account for functionally opposite symptoms.

Thus, unlike the stomach and small intestine, the colon of several species studied demonstrates two different myoelectric control mechanisms for the control of phasic contractions, the ECA and CEC. The ECA may originate in the circular and the CEC in the longitudinal muscle layer (80). The ECA of the colon is omnipresent and controls the occurrence in time and space of bursts of discrete response activity and short-duration contractions. The CEC occurs intermittently and controls the occurrence in time and space of continuous response activity and long-duration contractions. The colonic ECA is highly irregular in amplitude and waveshape and results in uncoordinated or nonpropagated short-duration contractions. The irregularity in waveshape and amplitude of colonic ECA may be due to the inherent instability of colonic relaxation oscillators and to neural influences because the ECA becomes more regular in in vitro recordings.

## Esophagus

Unlike the rest of the gastrointestinal tract, the esophagus in several species, including humans, cats, baboons, monkeys, and opossums, is composed in part of striated muscle and in part of smooth muscle. The proximal one-third to two-thirds of the esophagus consists of striated muscle, whereas the remainder is composed of smooth muscle. In the transitional zone, the density of striated muscle cells decreases and that of smooth muscle cells increases distally. In some species, such as dogs and rats, the entire esophagus is composed of striated muscle.

STRIATED MUSCLE ESOPHAGUS. The striated muscle esophagus is under central control, that is, the sequence of contractions in the striated muscle esophagus is programmed in the swallowing center of the brain, and the messages are relayed for different segments to contract sequentially via the descending branches of the vagus nerve (44, 106, 175–178). Correspondingly the in vivo myoelectric activity of the striated muscle in esophagus has characteristics similar to those of other striated muscles. The peak frequency of spikes in a spike burst has been reported by two different groups of investigators to be in two ranges of 40–50 and 150–170 cycles/s (6, 102). The duration of individual spikes is ~5 ms. The frequency of spikes is low at the beginning of a burst and as more and more muscle fibers are recruited, the frequency increases, only to decrease toward the end of a burst (101, 102). The amplitude of spikes increases and decreases similarly during a spike burst. The onset of spike bursts in the striated muscle propagates caudad at a velocity of ~5 cm/s. The terminology for electrical activity used here is that used in skeletal muscle literature.

Although the initiation of swallow-induced spike bursts in the striated muscle esophagus is programmed centrally, continuous afferent input from the wall of the esophagus stimulated by the bolus is essential for the progression of bursts in the striated muscle esophagus (113, 114, 140). Deviation of the bolus in the striated muscle esophagus stops peristalsis distal to the deviation. Further evidence for central programming of the initiation and progression of spike bursts in the striated muscle esophagus is provided by the findings that transection and reanastomosis or the interposition of a jejunal segment in the striated muscle esophagus do not prevent caudad migration of these bursts (48, 113, 140, 257). Efferent signals in the vagus have been associated with spike bursts and peristaltic contractions in the striated muscle esophagus (176).

SMOOTH MUSCLE ESOPHAGUS. In vivo recordings with suction or wire electrodes show that a contraction of the circular muscle in the smooth muscle esophagus is associated with a depolarization of membrane potential, that is, ECA that has a superimposed burst of ERA (70, 95, 203, 233). Unlike the rest of the gastrointestinal tract, the ECA in the esophageal smooth muscle does not oscillate spontaneously; the depolarization of esophageal smooth muscle takes place only once in response to a single stimulus. Figure 16 shows swallow-induced esophageal electrical activities recorded with suction electrodes from an anesthetized opossum. A burst of ERA was superimposed on ECA depolarizations in both longitudinal and circular smooth muscle layers.

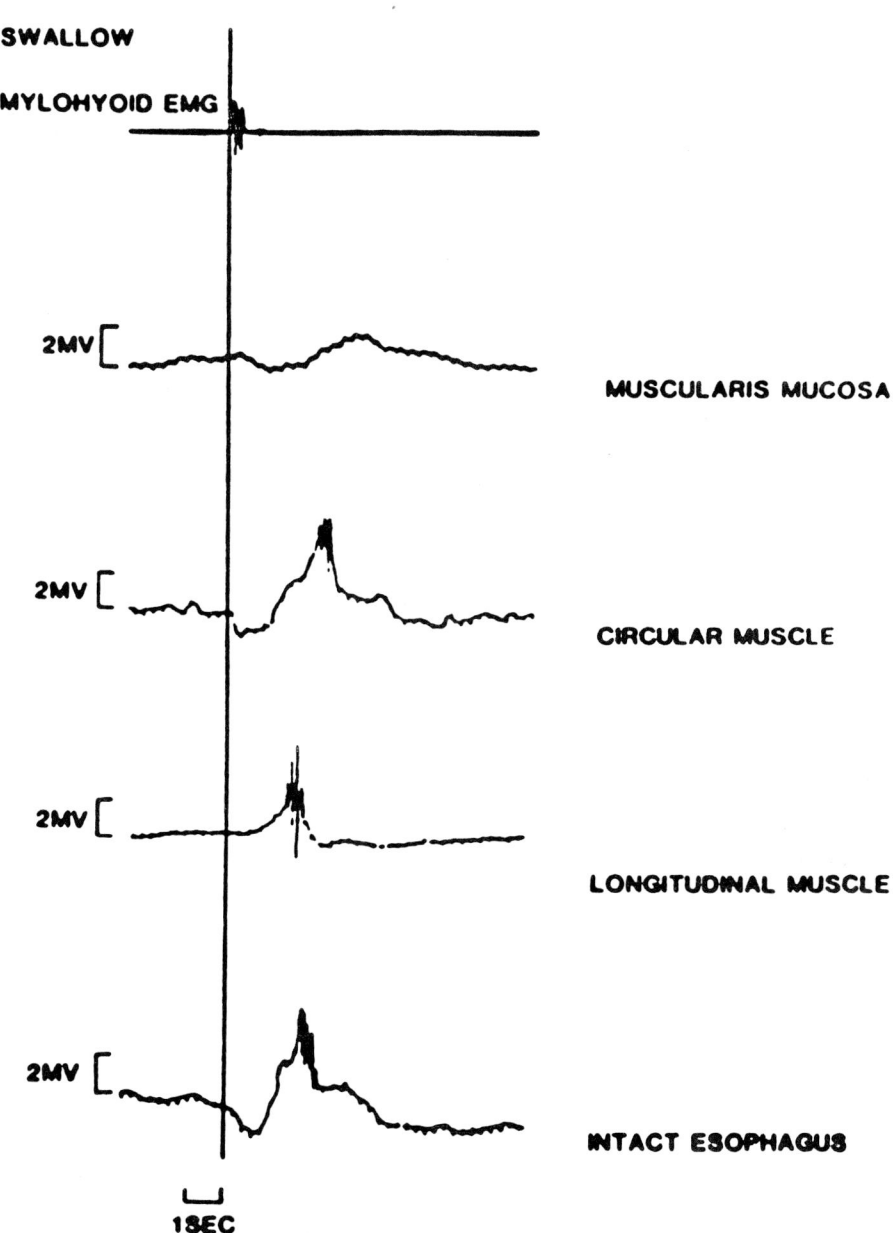

FIG. 16. Swallow-induced membrane potential changes in muscularis mucosa, circular muscle, longitudinal muscle, and intact esophagus of an anesthetized opossum. Recordings were made by a suction electrode. [From Sugarbaker et al. (233).]

It was reported that suction electrodes show a hyperpolarization of esophageal smooth muscle membrane potential that precedes depolarization and contraction (172, 233). There is no direct in vivo evidence yet that suction electrode recordings reflect membrane potential changes equivalent to those made with intracellular electrodes. Suction electrodes record the extracellular flow of currents from a group of cells as do wire electrodes. The major difference between these two types of electrodes is that the suction electrode produces injury around the recording area due to suction tip.

Esophageal electrical activity may be modeled by a chain of bidirectionally coupled one-shot oscillators (165, 166). One-shot oscillators fall under the category of forced oscillators. They oscillate only in response to an external stimulus. Normally the resting membrane potential of these oscillators is below the threshold level for oscillation. When a stimulus drives the membrane potential above this threshold level, these oscillators undergo a single all-or-none type of oscillation. This is much like the all-or-none oscillation of an action potential in a nerve. In a chain of coupled oscillators, the depolarization of one oscillator may then drive the neighboring oscillator, which then drives the next one, and so on (Fig. 17). The difference between an action potential oscillation in a nerve and a control potential oscillation in the esophagus is that

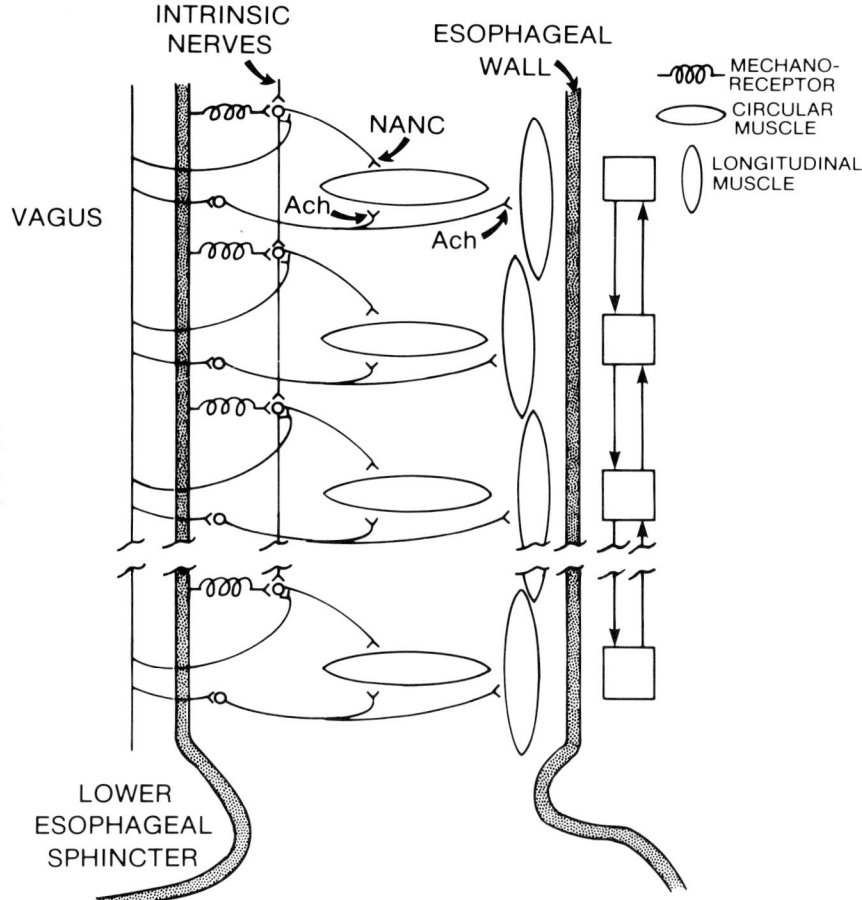

FIG. 17. Simplified model of interaction between myogenic and neural control of esophageal contractions. Smooth muscle esophagus may be considered as a chain of bidirectionally coupled, one-shot relaxation oscillators as shown at *right*. Myogenic oscillators received inputs from both intrinsic and extrinsic neurons.

the latter in turn controls the occurrence of ERA and hence smooth muscle contraction during its depolarization, whereas the former simply triggers an action potential at the adjacent site. With this model of esophageal electrical activity the most proximal oscillators in the smooth muscle esophagus may be stimulated to oscillate by the release of acetylcholine from the cholinergic neurons in response to a swallow. Thereafter each oscillator will excite the next to cause a single depolarization with superimposed ERA (Fig. 17). The evidence of such a myogenic control mechanism was provided by experiments in opossums. In the presence of tetrodotoxin, direct muscle stimulation of the opossum smooth muscle initiated contractions that propagated orad, caudad, or in both directions, depending on the site of stimulation (203).

The importance of local myogenic control of contractions in the smooth muscle esophagus is indicated by the experiments of Janssen et al. (112). Transection and reanastomosis in the smooth muscle esophagus impaired the progress of myoelectric activity and contractions across the anastomosis, partly because of the interruption of cell-to-cell connections. Unlike in the striated muscle esophagus, distal progression of myoelectric activity and contractions in the smooth muscle esophagus did not require the presence of a bolus. Furthermore, swallow-induced peristalsis persists in the smooth muscle esophagus even when the striated muscle esophagus is paralyzed by curare and after vagotomy (25, 41, 43, 73, 144, 155, 177, 241, 246). Thus the smooth muscle part of the esophagus is capable of initiating and propagating contractions independent of the central nervous system. An important difference between the one-shot oscillators in the esophagus and the spontaneous oscillators of the stomach, small intestine, and colon is that the oscillation of esophageal oscillators may be readily modulated by neural excitation, particularly the cholinergic nerves that depolarize the membrane potential and the intrinsic inhibitory nerves that hyperpolarize the smooth muscle. The depolarization of membrane potential by acetylcholine released from cholinergic nerve endings may bring the muscle closer to or above its threshold for oscillation. Hyperpolarization of membrane potential by intrinsic inhibitory nerves may hyperpolarize the smooth muscle cells and prevent their oscillation. These oscillators may undergo a rebound oscillation when the hyperpolarizing stimulus is released, much like that due to anodal excitation in axons (165, 166).

The precise interaction between myogenic and

neural control of esophageal contractions is incompletely understood. The present information in the literature may be integrated as shown by a simplified model in Figure 17. Vagal stimulation may activate both cholinergic and intrinsic inhibitory neurons (nonadrenergic noncholinergic) innervating the circular muscle. The net result would be depolarization or hyperpolarization depending on the relative degree of stimulation of these two types of neurons. Either excitation will act on the one-shot oscillators of the circular muscle to modulate their membrane potential and contraction as described previously. Once a depolarization is initiated in the proximal portion of the smooth muscle esophagus, it will propagate through coupled one-shot oscillators. The circular muscle cells may be coupled by cell-to-cell junctions between them or through the longitudinal muscle layer or both, as in the rest of the gastrointestinal tract. A richer excitatory innervation of the proximal circular muscle oscillators than that of the distal circular muscle oscillators may ensure that the oscillation begins first at the most proximal site, then at the next distal site, and so on (76, 77).

The net result of balloon distension in the esophagus may be to stimulate interneurons and postsynaptic inhibitory nerves through mechanoreceptors [Fig. 17; (49, 50)]. This stimulation hyperpolarizes circular smooth muscle cells. When the balloon distension is released, the circular smooth muscle cells undergo a rebound depolarization with increasing latency in the caudad direction because of different inherent characteristics (257, 258). Glial or Schwann-like cells have been reported to be in intimate contact with axons and varicosities of the nerve plexuses (62, 88). These cells, called hybrid cells, are positioned to conveniently transmit mechanical information from the circular muscle layer to the nerves.

The esophageal smooth muscle may contract at the onset of vagal stimulation, called an "on" contraction, or at the termination of the stimulus, called an "off" contraction. The on contractions propagate slower than off contractions (76, 77, 172). Also the velocity of propagation of on contractions increases at higher intensities of vagal stimulation. The one-shot relaxation oscillator may explain these differences in velocities of propagation. When the cervical vagus is stimulated at low intensities, acetylcholine released at all sites in the smooth muscle esophagus may depolarize smooth muscle cells. This depolarization will bring the smooth muscle cells closer to their threshold level for oscillation, and when the stimulus arrives from the proximal oscillators in the chain, the distal oscillators will reach their threshold level quicker than before, resulting in a higher propagation velocity. For higher intensities of stimulation, acetylcholine release may depolarize the oscillators at each level even closer to their excitation threshold and result in a still faster propagation velocity. Electrical stimulation of the vagus nerve also stimulates postsynaptic intrinsic inhibitory neurons, which hyperpolarize the esophageal smooth muscle cells by the release of an unidentified neurotransmitter. When the stimulus is turned off, the oscillators at all levels may show rebound depolarization simultaneously and result in a nearly simultaneous contraction of the whole smooth muscle esophagus. Whether vagal stimulation results in an on or an off contraction depends on the relative excitation of the cholinergic and the intrinsic inhibitory neurons.

The contraction of the longitudinal muscle of the esophagus in response to a swallow or vagal stimulation is associated with myoelectric activities similar to those in the circular muscle (233). The longitudinal muscle shows a depolarization with superimposed ERA. The myogenic mechanisms of control of contractions in both smooth muscle layers in the esophagus therefore may be the same as in the rest of the gastrointestinal tract, that is, when the membrane potential depolarizes beyond a threshold level a burst of ERA occurs and the muscle contracts. The difference between the esophageal smooth muscle and the smooth muscle in the rest of the gastrointestinal tract is that the esophageal smooth muscle does not exhibit spontaneous oscillations but oscillates in response to a stimulus from a neighboring oscillator, an excitatory neural stimulus, or the termination of an inhibitory neural input. The esophageal smooth muscle cells are potential oscillators. They do oscillate continuously when they are depolarized by local intra-arterial injection of carbachol (Fig. 18) or when carbachol is added to a muscle bath containing an isolated smooth muscle esophagus (81, 203). After carbachol each, depolarization is superimposed with a burst of ERA and associated with a phasic contraction.

The characteristics of ERA in the smooth muscle esophagus are different from those of spikes in the striated muscle. The frequency of oscillations within a burst of ERA is in the range of 1–10 Hz and the duration of response potential is ~16–40 ms, compared with the values of 150–170 Hz and 5 ms in striated muscle (102). In contrast to striated muscle, there is no gradual increase followed by a decrease in the frequency or amplitude of ERA, indicating that the two activities are controlled differently. The characteristics of ERA in the smooth muscle esophagus are similar to those in the rest of the gastrointestinal tract. The electrical activity in the transition zone between the striated and smooth muscle esophagus is a mixture of the smooth and striated muscle electrical activities.

The normal contractions in response to a swallow are almost always associated with bursts of ERA on a 1:1 basis (95, 172, 233). There are conflicting findings about such a relationship in diffuse esophageal spasm. Using suction electrodes, Bortolotti et al. (31) reported that a 1:1 relationship existed between multiple con-

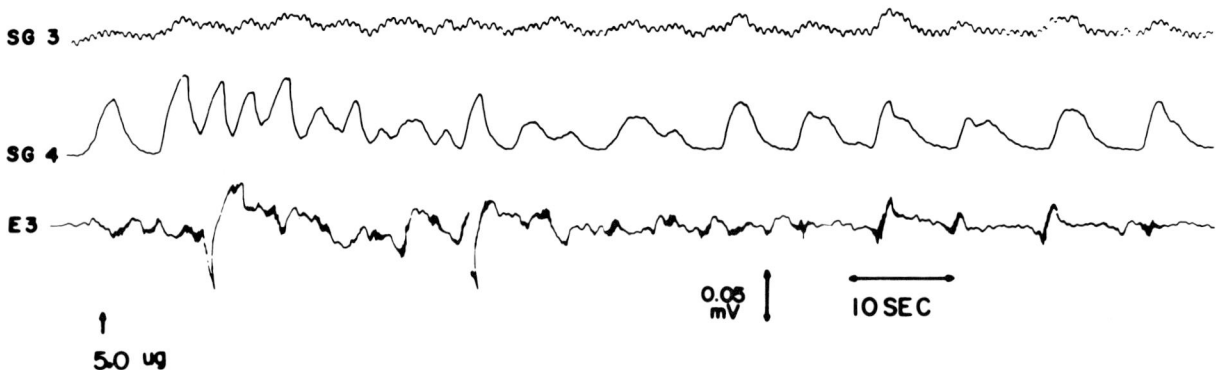

FIG. 18. Close intra-arterial injection of carbachol-induced spontaneous electrical control activity oscillations, electrical response activity bursts, and phasic contractions in an anesthetized opossum esophagus. Strain-gauge transducers SG3 and SG4 and electrode E3 were 4.3, 1.6, and 2.8 cm from the lower esophageal sphincter, respectively. [From Sarna et al. (203), Copyright 1977 by The American Gastroenterological Association.]

tractions and bursts of ERA in diffuse spasm. Using ring-type electrodes, Ouyang et al. (163) reported that 70% of contractions in diffuse esophageal spasm were not associated with ERA bursts. The difference between the two studies may be due to different recording methods. The ring-type electrodes record myoelectric activity only when the organ wall closes in tightly on them.

### Sphincters and Organ Junctions

Anatomically a sphincter is defined as a ring-like band of muscle fibers that constricts a passage or closes a natural orifice. By this definition all organ junctions and the beginning and the end of the gastrointestinal tract are sphincters. Functionally these junctional zones may be classified into two categories. The first category includes true sphincters that remain closed by active tension but open transiently by relaxation to let luminal contents pass through, such as the upper esophageal sphincter, lower esophageal sphincter, and the anal sphincters. The second category includes those junctional zones that do not remain closed most of the time but rather contract phasically to regulate the flow of contents in both directions. Such zones are located at the gastroduodenal, choledochoduodenal, and ileocolonic junctions. The junctions are not true sphincters. The two different categories of junctional zones are distinct in their myoelectric activities, as discussed next.

### Sphincters

UPPER ESOPHAGEAL SPHINCTER. The upper esophageal sphincter is a zone of high pressure at the transition from the hypopharynx to the esophagus. Its function is to prevent the reflux of esophageal contents into the pharynx and to relax during deglutition to allow the passage of food into the esophagus. This sphincter is composed of striated muscle and comprises the musculus cricopharyngeus and part of the inferior pharyngeal constrictor (7). The in vivo myoelectric activity of the upper esophageal sphincter is a continuous train of action potentials (Fig. 19; 7, 45, 250). As is typical of striated muscle, this electric activity is not myogenic in origin; its generation is dependent on continuous neural input from the pharyngeal branches of the pharyngeal plexus. These action potentials signal contractions of the sphincter muscle. The tone of the sphincteral muscle is proportional to the firing rate of action potentials. During deglutition the continuous train of action potentials is interrupted transiently and the sphincter relaxes. The amplitude and frequency of action potentials increase briefly above the resting level after deglutition and relaxation, resulting in a contraction of the upper esophageal sphincter above its basal tone, as shown in Figure 19.

LOWER ESOPHAGEAL SPHINCTER. In contrast to the upper esophageal sphincter, the lower esophageal sphincter consists of smooth muscle cells in most species studied (cats, humans, dogs, opossums). The lower esophageal sphincter in all these species exhibits two types of contractions, a tonic contraction that relaxes in response to deglutition and superimposed phasic contractions. Frequency and incidence of phasic contractions in the fasted state correspond to different phases of cyclic motor activity in the stomach (67, 107, 111).

An omnipresent membrane potential oscillation at a frequency of 20–40 cycles/min has been reported in the lower esophageal sphincter of anesthetized and awake opossums (81, 107). Each individual oscillation of this electrical activity is associated with a contraction (107). When the frequency of electrical oscillations increases because of neurochemical excitation, the individual contractions fuse to give rise to a long-

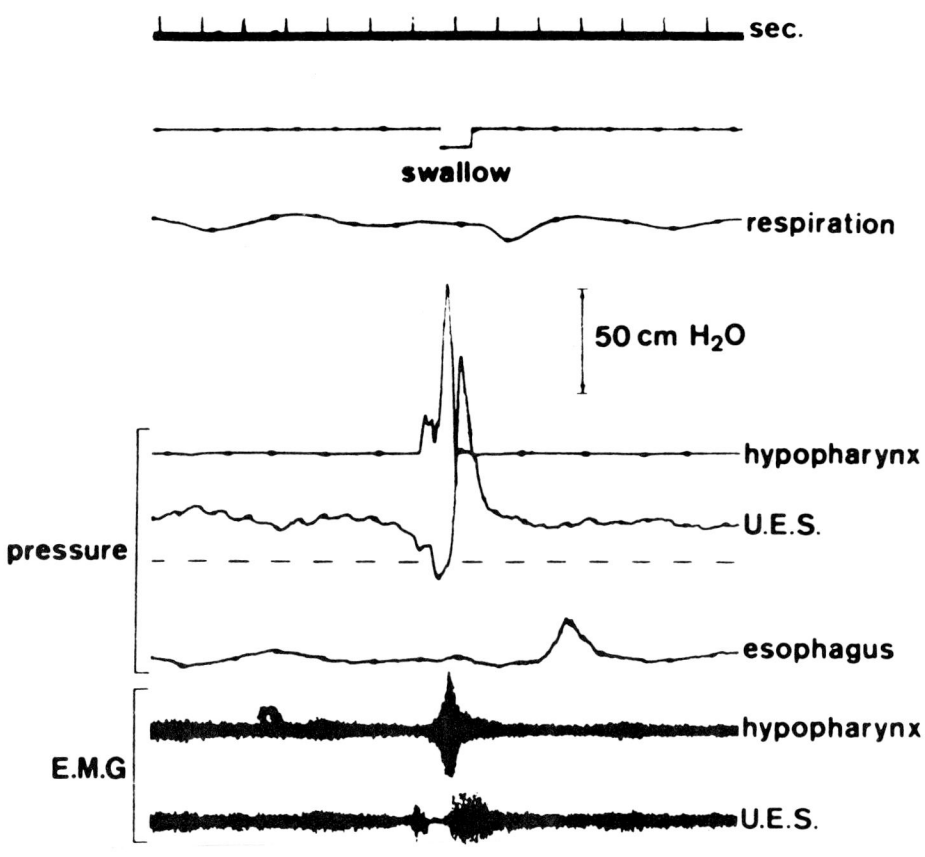

FIG. 19. Simultaneous manometric and myoelectric recording from the pharyngoesophageal segment at rest and during swallowing. Swallowing was associated with an inhibition followed by enhancement in the upper esophageal sphincter of spike activity. UES, upper esophageal sphincter; EMG, electromyogram. [From Van Overbeek et al. (250).]

duration phasic contraction, as shown in Figure 20. Some investigators have called this electrical activity "spikes," based on its visual appearance (8). However, these oscillations have no similarity to the spikes or ERA of the rest of the gastrointestinal tract. Furthermore it is uncharacteristic of smooth muscle to show spontaneous spikes without an ensuing membrane potential depolarization. These electrical oscillations are similar to the ECA of the rest of the gastrointestinal tract. The difference between them is that the ECA in the opossum lower esophageal sphincter may not be superimposed with ERA to contract smooth muscle.

A similar omnipresent ECA was reported in the cat lower esophageal sphincter (94, 174). In vivo recordings from anesthetized cats showed that vagal stimulation produced single depolarizations superimposed with bursts of ERA and associated with contraction of lower esophageal sphincter (94). The superimposition of ERA bursts on ECA depolarization in the cat, but not in the opossum, may be a species difference.

There are important differences between the interactions of the neural and myogenic control mechanisms in the lower esophageal sphincter and between those in the stomach, small intestine, and the colon. Under normal physiological conditions, the neural mechanisms in the stomach, small intestine, and colon

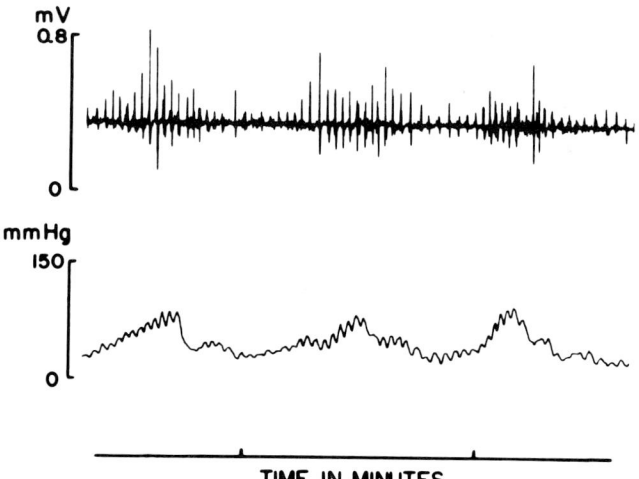

FIG. 20. Simultaneous myoelectrical and manometric recordings from the lower esophageal sphincter of an awake opossum. Each control potential was associated with a minicontraction. When frequency and amplitude of electrical control activity increased, minicontractions fused to give rise to a long-duration phasic contraction [Courtesy of W. J. Dodds.]

determine primarily whether or not ERA will occur and hence whether or not the muscle will contract. In this process the frequency of ECA does not change significantly. However, in the lower esophageal sphincter, the nerves may significantly modulate the amplitude, frequency, and even the generation of ECA to control its contraction. The ECA in the lower esophageal sphincter is obliterated during deglutition and the lower esophageal sphincter pressure collapses (8, 96, 107, 174). The response to balloon distension is similar. This obliteration of ECA is due to the activation of postsynaptic inhibitory neurons. Pharmacologically, bethanechol increases the frequency of ECA and lower esophageal sphincter pressure and isoproterenol obliterates ECA and decreases lower esophageal sphincter pressure (8, 107, 174). It is likely that the extrinsic nerves play a role in the maintenance of lower esophageal sphincter pressure in vivo through the modulation of ECA amplitude and frequency.

ANAL SPHINCTERS. The in vivo myoelectric activity of the anal sphincters has been studied largely in cats and humans. The internal anal sphincter is composed of smooth muscle cells and the external anal sphincter of striated muscle cells in both species. The in vivo myoelectric activity from the anal sphincters was recorded by wire electrodes introduced into the muscle layers by a hypodermic needle. The end of the wire was bent backward like a hook that kept the electrode in position after the needle was withdrawn (153, 247). Bouvier and Gonella (32) used pressure electrodes that were held against the circular muscle layer by spring action. The electrodes may also be held against the inner circular muscle layer by mounting them on a balloon, but balloon distension may stimulate the sphincter (247).

The smooth muscle cells of the anal sphincter in humans, cats, and other species generate spontaneous membrane potential oscillations in the frequency range of 15–35 cycles/min (mean ~20–25 cycles/min). These oscillations maintain the tonic contraction of the sphincter smooth muscle and hence constitute its ECA. In vitro recordings by the sucrose-gap technique show that each oscillation of ECA is associated with an individual phasic contraction: these contractions may fuse to produce a tonic contraction in vivo (32). The ECA of the internal anal sphincter is myogenic in nature; it is not blocked by tetrodotoxin but is blocked in the absence of $Ca^{2+}$ or when $Mn^{2+}$ is added to the muscle bath (32, 153). The ECA in the circular muscle of the internal anal sphincter is not superimposed with bursts of ERA to cause a contraction as is the case in the stomach, small intestine, and colon.

Unlike the ECA of the stomach, small intestine, and colon, the spontaneous oscillations of ECA in the internal anal sphincter are under a strong neural control. Rectal balloon distension obliterates or greatly reduces the amplitude of ECA and the internal anal sphincter relaxes (Fig. 21). A similar obliteration or reduction in amplitude of ECA is observed during spontaneous relaxation of the internal anal sphincter (153).

The ECA recorded from multiple sites in the internal anal sphincter shows a phase lag in the orad direction (32, 126). This suggests that the sphincter not only acts as a barrier to the outflow of rectal contents but also may actively propel any contents leaked into it or left during defecation back into the rectum. It is not known, however, whether the ECA in the internal anal sphincter is permanently phase locked as in the frequency plateau region of the small intestine (Fig. 11A) or whether it gradually falls out of phase as in the middle of the small intestine (Fig. 11B). The ECA amplitude of the internal anal sphincter shows significant waxing and waning.

There are some important differences between the ECA of the circular and longitudinal muscle layers of the internal anal sphincter (32, 33). Although ECA depolarization of circular muscle is not superimposed with a burst of ERA for contraction to occur, each ECA depolarization of the longitudinal muscle is superimposed with ERA and associated with a contraction. Norepinephrine enhances the frequency and amplitude of ECA of the circular muscle through its action on $\alpha$-adrenergic receptors; however, it inhibits the ECA of longitudinal muscle by its action on $\beta$-adrenergic receptors. Acetylcholine does not affect ECA of the circular muscle, whereas it enhances the frequency and amplitude of ECA of the longitudinal muscle.

Consistent with these pharmacological findings, Bouvier and Gonella (33) reported a reciprocal neural control of ECA and its associated contractions in the circular and longitudinal muscle layers of the cat internal anal sphincter. The parasympathetic nerves originating from the sacral spinal cord synapse with intramural ganglia. The postganglionic neurons innervating the circular muscle layer are nonadrenergic noncholinergic, whereas those innervating the longitudinal muscle layer are cholinergic. The electrical stimulation of pelvic nerves obliterated ECA in the circular muscle layer but increased the frequency and amplitude of ECA in the longitudinal muscle layer. The electrical stimulation of hypogastric nerves increased the amplitude and frequency of ECA in the circular muscle. This action was blocked by $\alpha$-adrenergic antagonists. On the other hand, stimulation of hypogastric nerves inhibited ECA in the longitudinal muscle through the action of norepinephrine on $\beta$-adrenergic receptors.

Although both the sympathetic and parasympathetic nerves can modulate the amplitude and frequency of ECA in the internal anal sphincter, it is not known whether a continual neural input plays a role in the maintenance of normal electrical activity and sphincter tone. The internal anal sphincter tone decreases after the hypogastric and pelvic nerves are sectioned or during spinal cord anesthesia between $T_6$ and $T_{12}$ (87). However, the sphincter tone begins to recover in ~30 min.

The interaction between the myogenic and neural

control of internal anal sphincter just described may fit well with its motor function. The myogenic ECA oscillation may generate the tonic contraction that keeps the sphincter continent. The neural input initiated by the presence of stool in the rectum via an intrinsic or an extrinsic reflex may contract the longitudinal muscle to open the sphincter and concurrently relax the circular muscle to facilitate the passage of stool. The longitudinal muscle may help in the descent of stool by shortening and widening the anal orifice and it may prevent anal prolapse by fixing the anal canal to the side wall of the pelvis (214). The exact interaction between the sympathetic and the parasympathetic nerves and the pathways for this interaction during defecation are not completely understood.

It seems that the function of nerves in the normal control of motor activity of circular muscle in the internal anal sphincter is opposite to that in the stomach, small intestine, and colon. In the circular muscle of the sphincter the amplitude of spontaneous ECA oscillations is such that each oscillation depolarizes the membrane potential above the excitation threshold, resulting in a tonic contraction. The neural excitation may reduce the amplitude of ECA or obliterate it to relax smooth muscle. In the stomach, small intestine, and colon, normal spontaneous oscillations of ECA are below the excitation threshold; neural excitation increases the amplitude of oscillation above excitation threshold to contract smooth muscle.

The external anal sphincter exhibits continuous spike activity typical of striated muscle. The spike activity is increased when the internal anal sphincter relaxes because of balloon distension of the rectum (Fig. 21). The generation of this spike activity is entirely dependent on the firing of its motoneurons (pudendal nerves) (26, 142, 213). This spike activity of the external anal sphincter and its associated tone are absent in patients with spinal cord lesions (247).

## Organ Junctions

GASTRODUODENAL JUNCTION (PYLORUS). The pylorus is a zone of thickened circular muscle and narrowed lumen at the junction between the stomach and the duodenum. Its length is estimated to be from a few millimeters to ~1 cm by using different methods in different species (22, 85, 118, 211, 212). Electrophysiologically the pylorus is indistinguishable from the terminal antrum. The frequency of ECA in the pylorus is the same as that in the rest of the stomach. The control potentials at the pylorus occur with a slight phase lag from the control potentials in the antrum (Fig. 7A).

The gastroduodenal junction is thought to play an important role in the regulation of gastric emptying and duodenogastric reflux; however, the precise mechanisms of both of these functions are largely unknown (54, 91, 115, 118). It is known that under certain circumstances antral contractions are coordinated temporarily with duodenal contractions. Two types of coordination may occur. First, the duodenal contractions may be inhibited with the occurrence of an antral contraction. This type of coordination may be present during the overlap between phase III activities of the antrum and the duodenum in the fasted state (Fig. 22A). In the second type of gastroduodenal coordination, the proximal duodenum may contract with the arrival of an antral contraction at the pylorus or shortly afterward. In between two antral contractions, the duodenum is usually quiescent. In this type of coordination the proximal duodenum contracts nearly at the frequency of the antrum. There may sometimes be two back-to-back duodenal contractions for each contraction of the antrum. This type of coordination may be present during gastric emptying after a meal (Fig. 22B). However, it is important to note that neither of these two coordinated patterns of antral and duodenal contractions is always present in the fasted or the fed state. Presumably there are other factors that may override this gastroduodenal coordination.

In most species the frequency of ECA in the duodenum is about four to five times the frequency of ECA in the stomach. This means that the maximal frequency of contractions just caudad to the pylorus may be four to five times that just orad to it. The timing of these two independently controlled contractions could be crucial in both gastric emptying and in duodenogastric reflux. If a contraction of the duodenal bulb starts when the antral contraction approaches the pylorus, this contraction may act as an obstruction to gastric emptying. If the duodenal contraction starts just after the antral contraction has emptied gastric

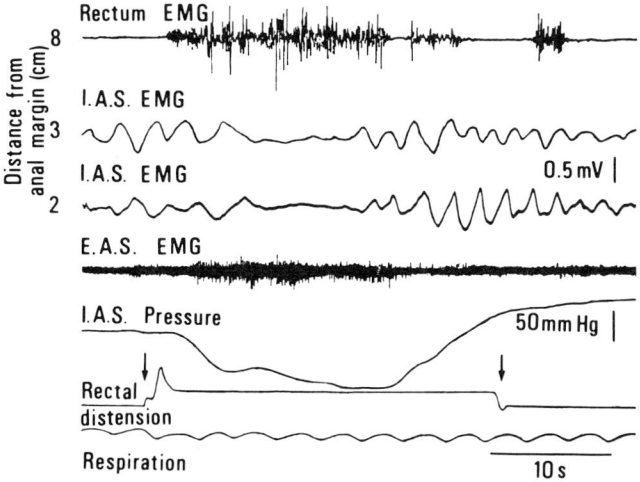

FIG. 21. Relaxation of internal anal sphincter (IAs) in humans induced by distension of a balloon in rectum and associated myoelectric activities of the IAS, external anal sphincter (EAS), and rectum. [From Monges et al. (153). In: *Gastrointestinal Motility*, edited by J. Christensen. © 1980, Raven Press, New York.]

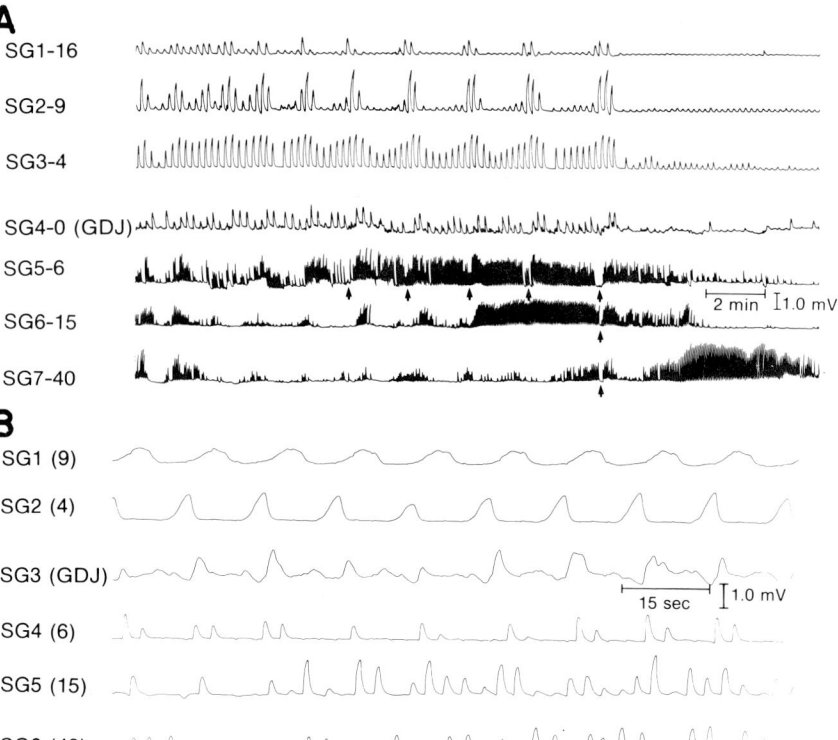

FIG. 22. *A*: Contractile activities recorded from stomach, gastroduodenal junction (GDJ), and duodenum of a dog in the fasted state. Contractions of duodenum at 19 cycles/min were inhibited when a group of contractions occurred in the stomach during phase III activity. *Arrows*, inhibition. Sometimes such inhibition extended up to 40 cm distal to GDJ. *B*: contractile activities recorded from stomach, gastroduodenal junction, and duodenum of the same dog but after a solid meal. First recording site in duodenum, 4 cm distal to GDJ, showed 1 or 2 contractions for every single contraction in stomach. Such coordinated activity was diminished or absent at distal sites.

contents into the duodenum, the duodenal contraction may aid gastric emptying by immediately removing the emptied contents from the duodenum. Likewise the timing of antral and duodenal contractions may determine whether duodenal contents reflux back into the antrum and, if refluxed, how rapidly they are returned to the duodenum.

The mechanisms of the aforementioned gastroduodenal coordination are incompletely understood, yet it seems that both myogenic and neural controls may be involved (3, 9–11, 66, 115, 160, 198, 205). Bortoff and Davis (30) reported that the amplitude of duodenal control potential that immediately follows the antral control potential has a larger amplitude than the other duodenal control potentials that occur in between two antral control potentials. The larger amplitude of duodenal control potential may increase the probability of a contraction during that ECA cycle (Fig. 2) and hence coordinate an antral contraction with a duodenal contraction (Fig. 22*B*). A computer model that coupled gastric relaxation oscillators at 5 cycles/min with duodenal relaxation oscillators at 18 cycles/min confirmed this observation (183). These findings do not support the earlier observations of Bass et al. (18) that the pylorus has no myoelectric activity and acts as an insulator between the gastric and duodenal ECA (17). Such an insulator is not necessary because relaxation oscillators with a four- to five-fold frequency difference cannot significantly alter each other's frequencies of oscillation.

Controversy exists whether the gastroduodenal junction is a true sphincter. Unlike the lower esophageal and anal sphincters, there is no myoelectric activity in the frequency range of 20–40 cycles/min that may generate a tonic contraction in the pyloric muscle. The pylorus does not normally remain shut continuously but rather contracts rhythmically. A pull through of manometric tubes shows a minimal high-pressure zone at the pylorus (85, 118). The pressure recorded during such pull throughs, however, depends on the diameter of the manometric tube, which raises the possibility that the pressure observed by this method may largely be passive because of distension of the narrow opening (118). The pyloric region is reported to have an intrinsic inhibitory innervation that is absent in adjacent strips from the antrum or the duodenum (5, 150). The presence of inhibitory nerves is not necessarily evidence of sphincter function. Such inhibitory innervation is present in other organs as well and together with the excitatory innervation and myogenic control may determine the pattern of contractions at the pylorus. Our experience is that strain-gage transducers implanted on the pylorus do not show relaxation during gastric emptying or in the fasted state, whereas similar transducers record relaxation of the lower esophageal sphincter during deglutition. The gastroduodenal junction is a dynamic structure that regulates the flow of contents through it by active contractions rather than by infrequent relaxations.

CHOLEDOCHODUODENAL JUNCTION. Anatomy and morphology of the choledochoduodenal junction vary markedly in different species. In most species (cats, dogs, humans, and guinea pigs) a major part of this junction resides within the duodenal wall (35). The opossum is an exception where most of this junction is extraduodenal. The opossum choledochoduodenal junction is also an exception in the sense that it has three smooth muscle layers: inner longitudinal, intermediate thick circular, and incomplete outer longitudinal (244). The in vivo myoelectric activity has so far been studied largely in the opossum because of easy access to its extraduodenal length. The length of this junction in the opossum is ~3–4 cm, and the terminal part has a narrow nozzle with a diameter of ~0.7 mm. The choledochoduodenal junction in the opossum does not relax as do the classic sphincters but regulates the flow of bile and pancreatic secretions by propagating contractions whose spatial and temporal patterns are controlled by ECA. The baseline pressure measured from the terminal segment by a manometric tube is highly dependent on the size of the catheter (244).

The opossum choledochoduodenal junction exhibits an omnipresent ECA with a mean frequency of ~8 cycles/min (Fig. 23). The control waves normally show a phase lag in the caudad direction and are somewhat irregular in their cycle length (20, 244). One important difference between the ECA of the choledochoduodenal junction and that of the stomach, small intestine, and colon is that in vivo, in the choledochoduodenal junction, each depolarization of ECA is superimposed with a burst of ERA (244). Presumably the absolute values of resting membrane potential and the excitation threshold levels are such that each depolarization may exceed the excitation threshold. However, neurochemical stimulation may control the frequency of ECA. Histamine and amyl nitrite abolish ECA and hence contractions, whereas bethanechol and phenylephrine increase the frequency of ECA and hence the frequency of contractions (244). The ECA of the choledochoduodenal junction is myogenic in origin; it is not abolished in the presence of tetrodotoxin (103). Distension of the choledochoduodenal junction by a balloon increases the frequency of ECA and of contractions.

The ECA of the choledochoduodenal junction also behaves like a chain of bidirectionally coupled relaxation oscillators (103). When the choledochoduodenal junction is divided into smaller segments, each segment generates independent ECAs, yet the intrinsic frequency decreases distally. This intrinsic frequency gradient ensures that a control potential occurs first at the proximal end of the choledochoduodenal junction, then at a more distal site, and so on, just as in the stomach and the frequency plateau region of the small intestine. The spatial pattern of contractions follows the spatial pattern of control potentials. Occasionally a contraction may begin at the proximal end and stop somewhere in the middle, or a contraction may begin at the distal end and propagate in the proximal direction. These findings may be explained by a marginally strong coupling between ECA oscillators at the choledochoduodenal junction, by an occasional lower than normal amplitude of depolarization of ECA at one or more sites that may not drive the next oscillator in the chain, and by an ectopic control potential at a distal site that may drive proximal oscillators.

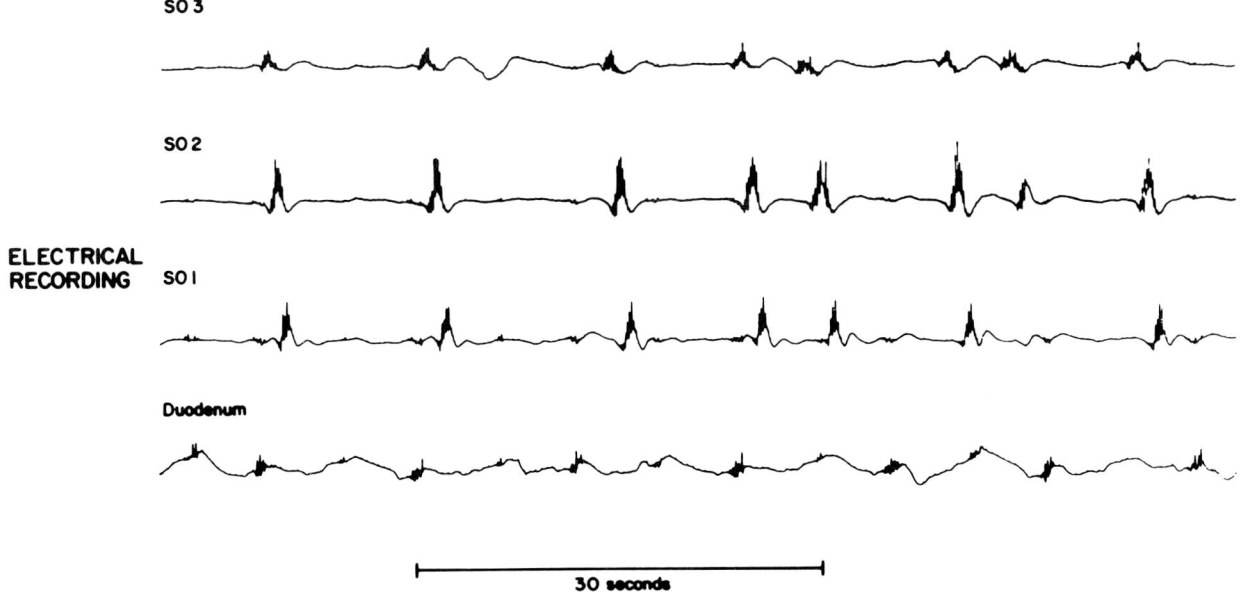

FIG. 23. Myoelectric activity recorded from choledochoduodenal junction and duodenum of an awake opossum. Electrodes SO3, SO2, and SO1 were 5 cm apart. Each electrical control activity oscillation was superimposed with a burst of electrical response activity. [From Toouli et al. (244).]

The caudad propagating contractions of the choledochoduodenal junction controlled by ECA propel its contents through the narrow opening at the distal end like a peristaltic pump and may also prevent the reflux and lodging of duodenal contents into the choledochoduodenal junction. This motor action of the choledochoduodenal junction is unlike that of classic sphincters that relax to let the contents pass through.

The in vivo myoelectric activity has not been studied in other species, but manometric recordings suggest that the in vivo myoelectric activity in humans may have an organization similar to that in the opossum (90, 245). Multilumen manometric recordings showed phasic contractions with phase lag predominantly in the caudad direction in the human choledochoduodenal junction.

ILEOCOLONIC JUNCTION. The ileocolonic junction is characterized by a narrowed lumen opening and thickened longitudinal and circular muscle at the junction between the ileum and the colon. The anatomical length of this junctional zone is ~0.5 cm, yet the physiological motor characteristics that separate this zone from the adjoining ileum and colon extend over ~2–3 cm (169).

Electrophysiologically the ileocolonic junction is indistinguishable from the terminal ileum. The frequency of ECA at the ileocolonic junction is not significantly different from that of the terminal ileum (164, 169, 171). When the individual ECA depolarizations are superimposed with ERA bursts, the ileocolonic junction shows phasic contractions (Fig. 24). When the ileocolonic junction is surgically isolated from the ileum and the colon, the frequency of ECA generation remains unchanged (164). A majority of migrating myoelectric complexes in the dog small intestine migrate right up to the end of the ileocolonic junction (171).

Balfour and Hardcastle (12) reported a myoelectrically silent zone at the ileocolonic junction. This observation seems largely a result of technical recording problems and has not been substantiated by any other group. Teleologically there is no need for a silent zone because there is an ~50% drop in ECA frequency from terminal ileum to ascending colon in most species. Such a large difference in intrinsic frequency and the generally poor coupling between oscillators in this region ensures little interaction between the ileal and colonic ECA oscillators.

Similar to the gastroduodenal junction, the ileocolonic junction has specialized innervation and receptors that are different from those in the adjacent ileal and colonic segments (46, 56, 161, 162, 179). Ileal and colonic circular muscle strips contract in response to gastrin and cholecystokinin, but the strips from the ileocolonic junction show no response. Glucagon in-

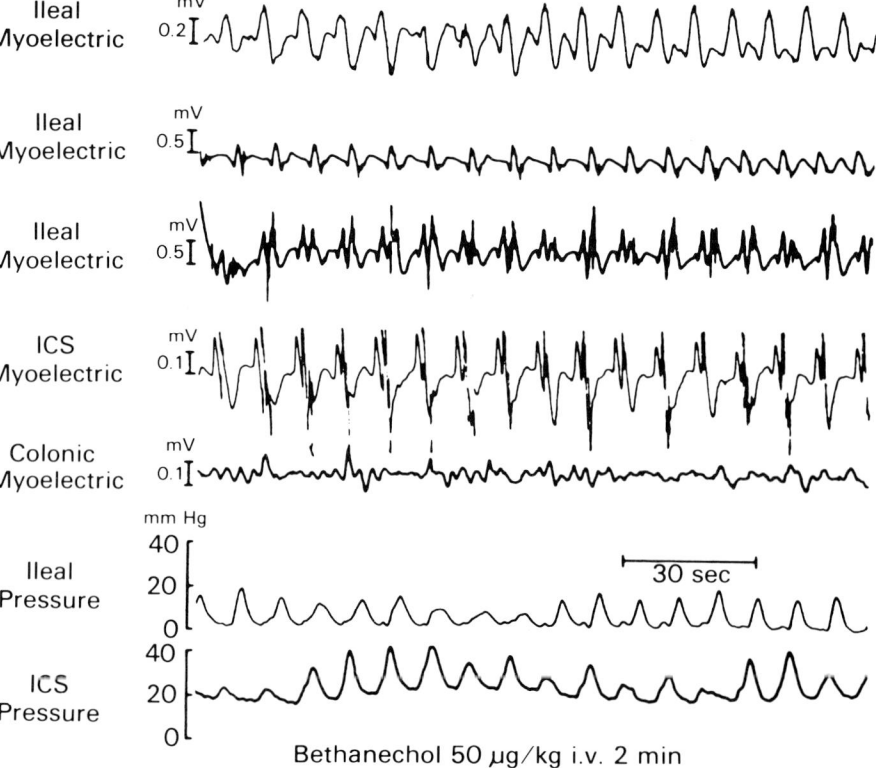

FIG. 24. Myoelectric recordings from ileum, ileocolonic junction [ileocolonic sphincter (ICS)], and colon and corresponding intraluminal pressures from ileum and ileocolonic junction after 50 µg/kg of bethanechol (iv). Myoelectric activity of ileocolonic junction is indistinguishable from that of ileum. [From Ouyang et al. (161).]

hibits ileal and colonic circular muscle contractions but has no effect on circular muscle strips from the ileocolonic junction. The ileocolonic muscle contracts in response to phenylephrine, but adjacent ileal and colonic muscle strips are inhibited. Quigley et al. (169) reported that the overall motor activity of the ileocolonic junction is significantly greater than that of the ileum and the colon. The myogenic control determines only the maximum frequency and the timing and spatial pattern of phasic contractions, whereas the neurochemical control mechanisms determine whether or not the contractions will occur (see CONTROL OF PHASIC CONTRACTIONS, p. 818). The hyperactivity of the ileocolonic junction as compared with the terminal ileum and the proximal colon may be explained on the basis of the differences in responses to neurochemical stimulation. The ileocolonic junction may regulate the flow of contents from the ileum to the colon and vice versa by active contractions rather than by simple relaxation. Wienbeck and Janssen (262) reported that some bursts of ERA are coordinated across the ileocolonic junction. However, it is not known if this coordination is because of a myogenic or neural mechanism or topical stimulation by luminal contents entering the colon.

The ileocolonic junction does not remain closed in the basal state and it does not relax when phasic contractions occur proximal to it. There are conflicting findings whether or not this junction relaxes in response to ileal balloon distension (55, 125, 169). This relaxation, if present, cannot be taken as an evidence of a true sphincter action because this myenteric reflex in response to distension is present in most of the gastrointestinal tract. The basal pressure recorded at this junction depends on the size of the manometric tube used (124). Part of the pressure thus recorded may be due to distension of the narrow lumen by the recording tube. There is some resistance to flow at the ileocolonic junction even after the death of the animal (173), which may be due to the elastic properties of the muscle at the junction.

There is evidence that the phasic contractions of the ileocolonic junction contribute to its tone (169, 171). This observation is supported by intracellular recordings that show that the circular muscle cells of the ileocolonic junction have a higher resting membrane potential than the cells of the ileum or the cecum and is closer to its threshold excitatory potential, similar to fundic smooth muscle (131, 235). These cells therefore may develop a tone when phasic contractions occur repeatedly. The mean pressure of the ileocolonic junction is lower after a meal than in the fasted state, but this may be due to a difference in the frequency and duration of phasic contractions.

*Gallbladder*

The myoelectric control of gallbladder contractions in the dog was reported recently (144). In vivo the gallbladder smooth muscle has an omnipresent ECA in the frequency range of 18–30 cycles/min. The mechanism of control of contractions seems to be by an adjustment in the amplitude of ECA oscillations. Normally the amplitude of ECA is small and the depolarizations are not accompanied by contractions. Possibly under neurochemical stimulation, when the ECA amplitude increases beyond an excitation threshold, the muscle contracts. The amplitude of ECA increases without a significant increase in ECA frequency. Electronic filtering of gallbladder electrical activity in the frequency range of 1–10 Hz did not show any ERA superimposed on ECA when the gallbladder contracted.

Figure 25 shows gallbladder ECA and its associated

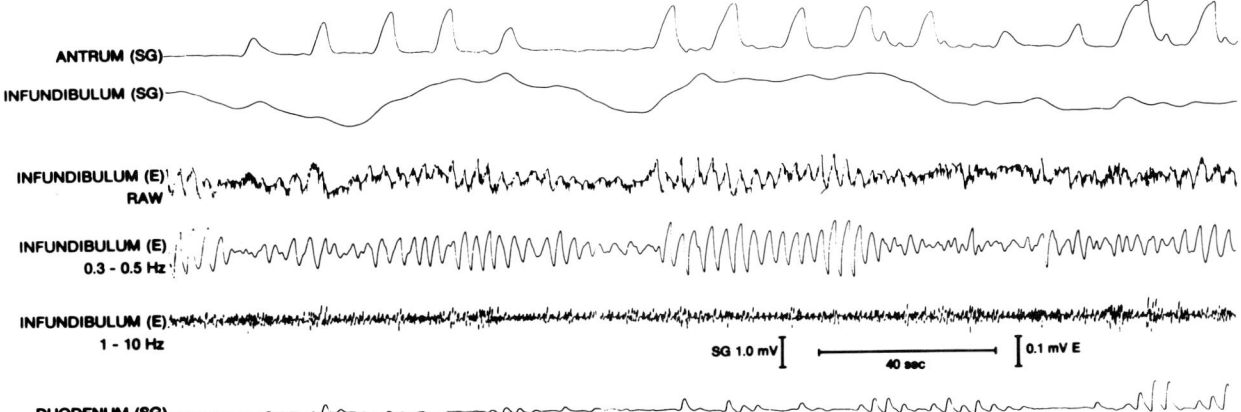

FIG. 25. *First and second tracings*, contractile activities of antrum and gallbladder infundibulum recorded with strain-gauge transducers in an awake dog; *third tracing*, raw myoelectric signal from infundibulum; *fourth tracing*, filtered electrical control activity, *fifth tracing*, no electrical response activity bursts were present in myoelectrical activity of infundibulum that could be related to its contractile activity; and *sixth tracing*, duodenal contractile activity recorded with a strain-gauge transducer. *Numbers in parentheses*, pass band of filters used.

contractions during phase III of cyclic motor activity of the gallbladder (145). Each phasic contraction is associated with an increase in the amplitude of several cycles of ECA. The amplitude of ECA was also increased after a meal or insulin administration and was associated with phasic contractions (144). The gallbladder response to insulin occurred at about the same time as the motor response in the stomach, suggesting that the response may be due to a central action of insulin mediated by the vagus nerve. The role of ECA in controlling gallbladder smooth muscle contractions was recently confirmed in in vitro strips by using intracellular electrodes and the sucrose gap technique (130).

SPECIAL SITUATION CONTRACTIONS

In general the spatial and temporal patterns of phasic contractions are such that the ingested meal moves slowly through the gastrointestinal tract. The normal mouth to anus transit time is >12 h. However, there are certain situations such as vomiting, defecation, and mass movements where the luminal contents have to be moved rapidly over long distances. This rapid shift of contents is accomplished by giant contractions, retrograde giant contractions for orad movement, and giant migrating contractions for aboral movement. The retrograde giant contraction is one of the motor correlates of vomiting (see the chapter by Lang and Sarna in this *Handbook*). This contraction is 1.3 to 1.8 times larger in amplitude and two to four times longer in duration than the phasic contractions of the migrating motor complex. This contraction begins in the middle small intestine and migrates orad at a velocity of 8–10 cm/s. This contraction rapidly retropels the contents of the proximal half of the small intestine into the stomach in preparation for vomitus expulsion.

The giant migrating contraction is associated with rapid shift of contents in the caudad direction. In the small intestine this contraction occurs infrequently and unpredictably, mostly in the distal small intestine in the healthy state. Once originated, it migrates uninterrupted to the ileocolonic junction and often into the proximal colon. The physiological role of this contraction in health is not established yet, but in the pathophysiological state the giant migrating contraction may be associated with abdominal cramping and diarrhea (186). In the colon the giant migrating contractions occur infrequently and unpredictably and are associated with mass movements and defecation (117).

*Vomiting*

The gastrointestinal motor and myoelectric correlates of vomiting have been studied largely in dogs, cats, and humans [Fig. 26; (1, 133–135, 149, 231, 240, 259)]. The gastrointestinal motor correlates of vomiting are *1*) an inhibition of spontaneous motor activity in the stomach and the small intestine; *2*) an orad-migrating giant contraction called retrograde giant contraction, which originates in the middle of the small intestine and migrates to the antrum and is followed by vomiting; *3*) a group of phasic contractions; and *4*) inhibition of motor activity in the proximal small intestine. The in vivo myoelectric correlates of these motor events have been defined in the cat and the dog (133, 135, 231, 240, 259).

Four distinct changes in myoelectric activity are associated with vomiting in dogs [Fig. 26B; (133, 134)]. *1*) The ECA frequency slows down in the small intestine and gastric antrum. The slowing of ECA frequency lasts for ~8 min in the distal small intestine and ~2 min in the gastric antrum. The duration of slowing of ECA in the small intestine decreases proximally, and the slowing of ECA may not occur in the duodenum or upper jejunum. *2*) The ECA is disrupted at the site where the retrograde giant contraction starts, and the disruption migrates orad to the antrum at a velocity of ~16 cm/s (133, 134). The disruption of ECA constitutes a marked reduction in the frequency and amplitude or total obliteration of ECA and may last ~5–20 s. The disruption begins prior to and may outlast the retrograde giant contraction. *3*) A sharp potential change associated with the onset of the retrograde giant contraction occurs first in the middle of the small intestine and migrates orad at a velocity of ~11 cm/s. Occasionally a burst of ERA lasting <1 s occurs at the peak of this potential change. Both ECA disruption and orad-migrating sharp potential change are abolished by intravenous atropine. *4*) Bursts of ERA occur on successive ECA cycles that correspond to the group of post-retrograde phasic contractions. The frequency of ECA during these bursts of ERA may be slower than normal as indicated in item one.

The myoelectric correlates of vomiting in cats are similar except that the retrograde giant contraction is associated with a sustained change in potential superimposed with a burst of ERA lasting ~4 s (231). The orad migration velocity of this myoelectric event in the cat is ~2 cm/s.

*Caudad Mass Movement*

In addition to the usual phasic contractions, the small intestine and the colon also generate large-amplitude, long-duration contractions called giant migrating contractions that have also been called prolonged propagated contractions, peristaltic rushes, and power contractions (78, 148, 170, 186). In the small intestine these contractions usually originate spontaneously in the distal portion; however, occasionally they may originate in the middle to proximal

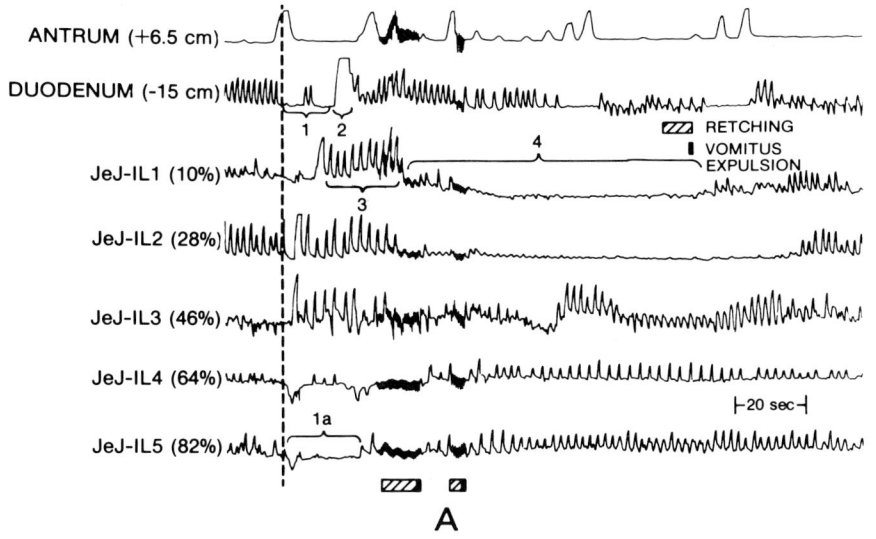

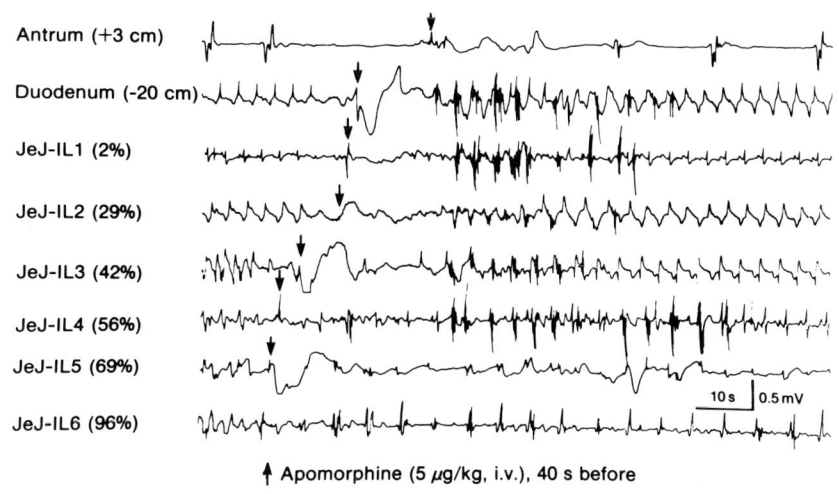

FIG. 26. *A*: motor correlates of vomiting in the dog. Percentages refer to length of small intestine between Treitz' ligament and ileocolonic junction. *1*, and *1a*, initial inhibition of motor activity; *2*, retrograde giant contraction; *3*, group of phasic contractions; and *4*, motor inhibition following group of phasic contractions. *B*: myoelectric correlates of vomiting in another dog. Arrows, the sharp deflection associated with onset of giant retrograde contractions. [Adapted from Lang et al. (135).]

jejunum and migrate caudad (186). Giant contractions can be initiated in the duodenum by different pharmacological and physiological stimuli, and then they migrate to the ileum at a velocity of ~1 cm/s (186). The mean duration of these giant migrating contractions is ~18–20 s and their amplitude is two to four times larger than that of phasic contractions during phase III of the migrating motor complex.

The initiation and migration of these giant contractions are not controlled by ECA because *1*) their duration is much longer than the cycle length of ECA (the phasic contractions controlled by ECA occur only during its depolarization and must be shorter than its cycle length), and *2*) the giant contractions migrate caudad uninterrupted at a velocity of ~1 cm/s. This uninterrupted migration is inconsistent with the fact that ECA is phase unlocked distal to the frequency plateau region.

In recordings in vivo the giant migrating contractions are usually associated with a sustained depolarization and some disruption of ECA when recorded with bipolar extracellular electrodes (Fig. 27). In most cases there is a brief burst of response activity in the electrical record at the beginning of the upstroke of a giant contraction. A single or repeated burst of response activity at ECA frequency may occur during the downstroke of the giant contraction. In between, when the peak of the contraction occurs, there is no response activity (186).

Similar giant migrating contractions have been reported in the colon (100, 117, 143). These giant migrating contractions occur spontaneously in the proximal colon but are generally present just before spontaneous or pharmacologically induced defecation. Because of their large amplitude, long duration, and rapid migration over long segments, these contrac-

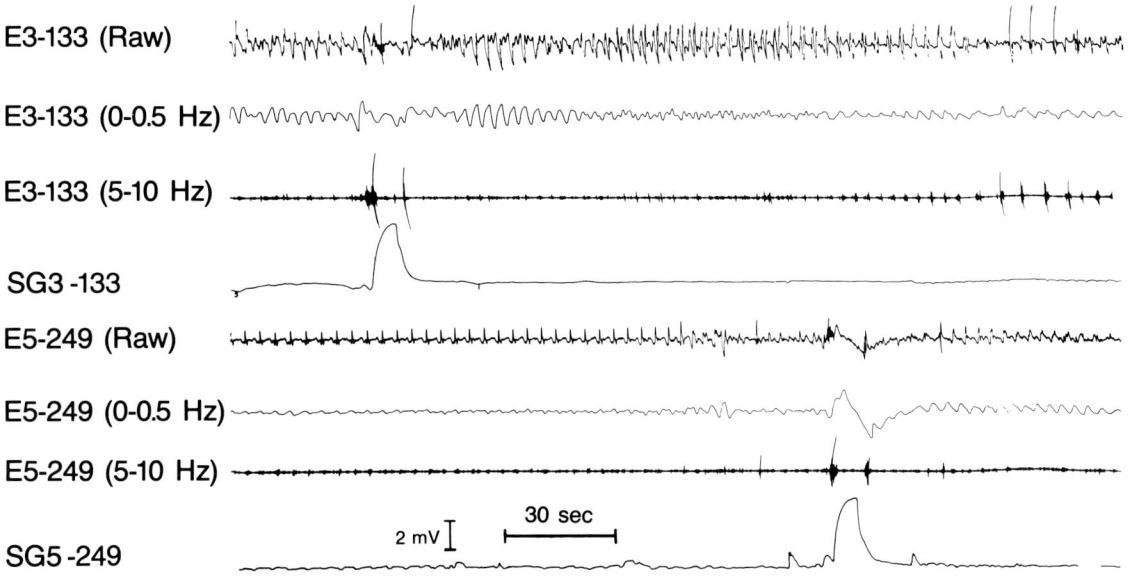

FIG. 27. Myoelectric activities associated with giant migrating contractions in small intestine. Electrode E3 and strain gauge SG3, and electrode E5 and strain gauge SG5 were pairs that recorded electrical and contractile activities from nearly the same site. Giant contraction migrated from the site of strain gauge SG3 to SG5. In each case, *top tracings*, raw signal; *middle tracings*, electrical control activity filtered in frequency range of 0–0.5 Hz; and *bottom tracings*, electrical response activity filtered in frequency range of 5–10 Hz.

tions may rapidly propel intestinal contents over long distances.

### RELAXATION-OSCILLATOR VERSUS CABLE MODEL TO EXPLAIN ORGANIZATION OF ELECTRICAL CONTROL ACTIVITY

An electric signal may be trasmitted from one point to another in one of three ways: *1*) passive conduction, *2*) regenerative propagation, and *3*) relaxation-oscillator propagation.

### Passive Conduction

In passive conduction the signal-generating source is located at one end of a passive conductor, for example, an insulated underground cable. The cable has a low impedance in the longitudinal direction, and a high impedance in the transverse direction. Most of the current flows in the direction of low impedance. The frequency of the signal at the receiving end in passive conduction is the same as that of the source at the sending end of the conductor. The salient features of this mode of transmission of an electrical signal are that the medium through which conduction takes place is totally passive and the potential at the receiving end is lower than the potential at the sending end. The differential equation that describes the signal recorded at different distances from the source is called the cable equation. This mode of conduction is commonplace in real life, such as the transmission of electricity from a power-generating plant to individual users and the transmission of audio and video signals in communication cables. In these situations the drop in the amplitude of the signal at the receiving end can be recuperated by the use of boosters or transformers. Other examples of passive conduction describable by a cable equation are conduction of heat in a rod with the heating source at one end and the diffusion of a substance in a solvent. In biological systems this type of conduction takes place in some dendrites and is called electrotonic conduction. The conducted potential is called an electrotonic potential (215).

### Regenerative Propagation

In the propagation of bioelectrical signals, such as the propagation of action potentials in nerves, it is important that the amplitude of the signal does not deteriorate during propagation, or else the signal may not perform its desired function at the receiving end. For example, a low-amplitude action potential arriving at the neuromuscular junction may not release sufficient neurotransmitter for the muscle to contract. To prevent deterioration in the amplitude of a bioelectrical signal, transmission of electrical signals in biological tissues such as a nerve or large elongated cells takes place by regenerative propagation. The anatomical structure of the tissue through which such propagation takes place resembles a cable, that is, relatively low impedance along the longitudinal axis as compared with that in the transverse axis. The inside of nerve tissue is electrochemically maintained at a potential negative to the outside. When an electrical stimulus that hyperpolarizes the membrane potential is applied at one point in the nerve, it conducts in both directions and its amplitude decreases at increasing distances from the point of stimulation. This conduction is exactly like that in a passive cable. However, this type of conduction is not the one that takes place in the normal propagation of an action potential even though the nerve has passive cablelike properties.

When a stimulus that depolarizes the nerve membrane potential beyond its excitation threshold is applied, it generates an all-or-none action potential at that site. The membrane potential change generated by the action potential conducts along the length of the nerve the same way as the hyperpolarizing stimulus; however, before conduction proceeds too far, the depolarization of membrane potential at the adjacent site initiates a new action potential of similar amplitude. The deterioration in the amplitude of the signal is prevented. The membrane potential due to the new action potential conducts again and generates another all-or-none action potential at the next adjacent site, and this process continues until the nerve ending is reached, where the last action potential acts on the neuromuscular junction. The salient feature of this mode of transmission of electrical signals is that a new but nearly identical action potential is generated at each site by local mechanisms, and therefore no deterioration takes place in the amplitude of the signal. Although a nerve has cablelike structure and properties, cablelike conduction takes place in unmyelinated nerves only over very short distances because of the regeneration of new action potentials. In myelinated nerves, true cablelike conduction during the propagation of an action potential takes place from one node of Ranvier to the next. The deterioration of amplitude from one node to the next is minimized by a 5,000-fold higher resistance and a 1,000-fold decrease in the capacitance of the myelin sheath. At each node of Ranvier, however, a new all-or-none action potential is generated. This type of saltatory conduction increases the velocity of propagation because less time is lost in regenerating new action potentials at intermediate sites. The nodes of Ranvier are about 1 mm apart.

In passive conduction the active source of signal is present only at one place. In regenerative propagation, potentially active sources of signal are present throughout the medium that generate action potentials in response to a stimulus. In other words these sources are not spontaneously active. The action potential has a physiological function only at the nerve ending; that is, to release a neurotransmitter, it performs no function at intermediate sites except to propagate itself.

Amplitude and waveshape of the signal at the receiving end in regenerative propagation do not depend on the amplitude and waveshape of the stimulus; action potentials at different sites are generated by local mechanisms. However, the frequency of the signal at the receiving end is the same as that of the stimulus at the sending end. There is a maximum frequency of stimulation up to which the above relationship is true, after which the nerve will be unable to transmit the signal faithfully because of the refractory period that follows the generation of an action potential.

*Relaxation-Oscillator Propagation*

The third mode of transmission of electrical signals is called the relaxation-oscillator mode. Here each individual cell or a group of cells is an independent spontaneous oscillator with its own intrinsic frequency. The individual oscillators are coupled to each other at the cell-to-cell junctions. These oscillators are of the relaxation type, that is, their frequency of oscillation when coupled with other oscillators may change without a significant change in other characteristics of oscillation such as amplitude and wave shape. This is an important characteristic of myoelectric oscillations in smooth muscle cells where the oscillators control a local phenomenon such as the timing of ERA bursts and phasic contractions (Fig. 2). If the contractions at a given site are to be coordinated with contractions at its adjacent sites, then only the frequency and timing of oscillations need be changed without affecting the other characteristics of oscillation that control local phenomenon. This can be achieved in a system of bidirectionally coupled relaxation oscillators.

In an array of bidirectionally coupled relaxation oscillators, the highest intrinsic frequency oscillator dominates, that is, it drives the other lower intrinsic frequency oscillators to its own frequency. This driving is a step-by-step process, unlike a cable where the potentials conduct rapidly. The oscillator with the highest intrinsic frequency drives only its adjacent oscillators to its own frequency of oscillation. The adjacent oscillators, when they have acquired a higher frequency, in turn drive their adjacent oscillators to their new frequency and the process continues until all the oscillators in the system oscillate at the frequency of the highest intrinsic frequency oscillator. This phenomenon is called frequency entrainment. Because the oscillator with the highest intrinsic frequency drives the rest of the oscillators, it has a phase lead over all other oscillators.

Figure 28 shows an array of 13 relaxation oscillators that simulate the ECA of the stomach (201). In Figure 28A, the oscillators are uncoupled from each other. This model represents the ECA of the stomach when it is divided into small segments by longitudinal and circumferential myotomies indicated by broken lines.

In this situation the highest intrinsic oscillator with a frequency of 5.5 cycles/min is located near the greater curvature in the corpus. The intrinsic frequencies of oscillation decrease distally and from the greater curvature to the lesser curvature. The intrinsic frequencies of oscillators 1 to 6 are shown in Figure 29A. When the oscillators are coupled bidirectionally as shown in Figure 28B, the model simulates the ECA of the intact stomach. Oscillator with the highest intrinsic frequency (5.5 cycles/min) entrains the frequencies of the rest of the oscillators to that of its own, and they are all phase locked as shown in Fig. 29B. The phase lag per centimeter decreases distally as shown in the inset.

The ability of a relaxation oscillator to entrain other oscillators depends on three factors: *1*) the coupling factor between oscillators, that is, how strongly one oscillator drives the next; *2*) the intrinsic frequency difference between the driver and the driven oscillators, and *3*) the refractory characteristics of the oscillators. A stronger coupling can entrain a larger intrinsic frequency difference between two relaxation oscillators (195, 201, 202). If a given coupling factor cannot entrain two relaxation oscillators, the mean frequency of the lower intrinsic frequency oscillator is pulled up, that is, it gets closer to that of the higher frequency oscillator part of the time but then it gradually decreases for a few cycles and then it increases again and the process continues. In frequency pulling, the oscillators are not phase locked. The oscillators in the variable frequency region of the small intestine are pulled up in their frequency but not entrained. Relaxation oscillator models to explain the organization of ECA in the stomach, small intestine, colon, esophagus and choledochoduodenal junction have been proposed (13, 74, 103, 139, 157, 199, 201). These models simulate all the observed characteristics of ECA in these organs.

The source of generation of ECA in the muscle layers is controversial. Different investigators have proposed the longitudinal or the circular muscle to be the source in the same species or in different species (235). The conclusions were based mainly on intracellular recordings from isolated muscle layers or muscle layers exposed by various dissection techniques. At the present time it is difficult to extrapolate these findings into a unified hypothesis of in vivo source of generation of ECA. It is possible that in vivo either one or both layers may spontaneously generate ECA, depending on the species. Whatever is the source of generation in vivo, the myoelectric activity in both muscle layers seems to be closely coupled. If both

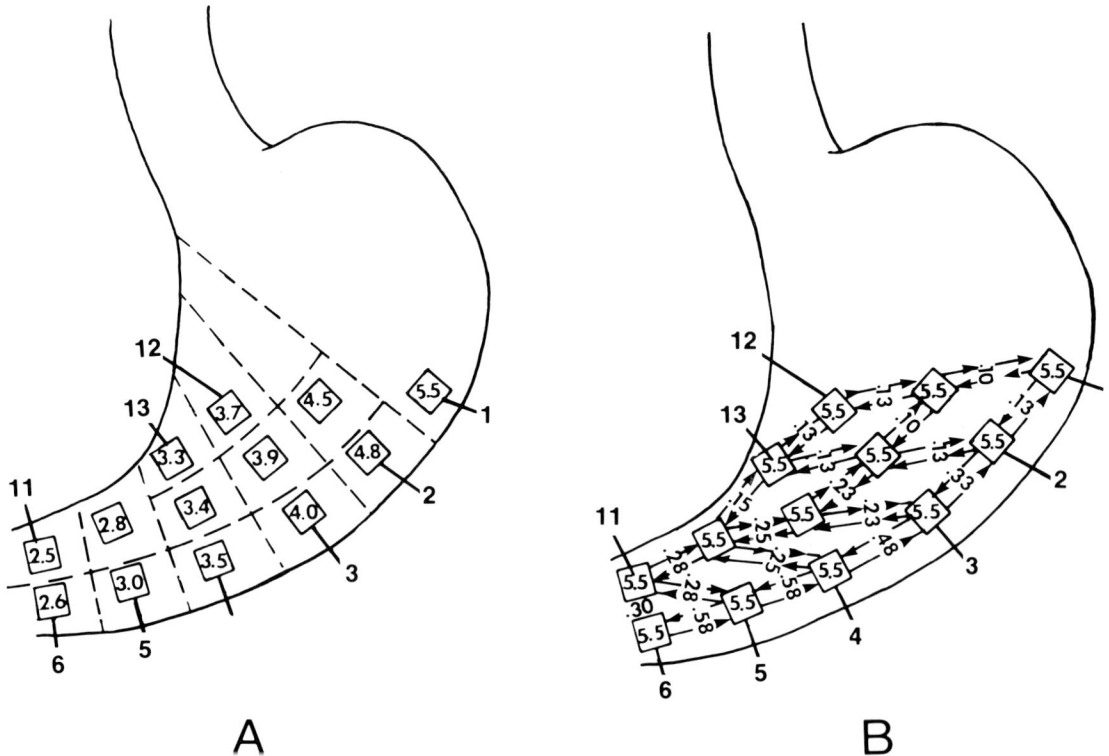

FIG. 28. *A*: relaxation oscillator model of electrical control activity in the stomach that has been divided into small segments by longitudinal and circumferential myotomies. *Broken lines*, myotomies; *numbers within boxes*, intrinsic frequencies of relaxation oscillators. *B*: bidirectionally coupled relaxation-oscillator model of intact stomach. *Numbers between boxes*, coupling factors; *numbers within boxes*, intact coupled frequencies of oscillators. [Adapted from Sarna et al. (201).]

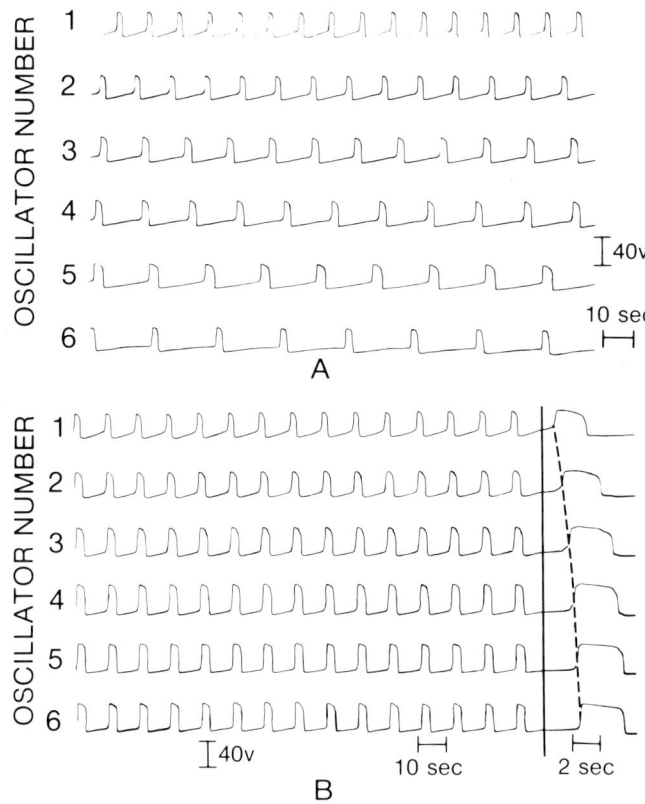

FIG. 29. *A*: intrinsic frequencies of oscillators 1–6 in model of Fig. 28 *A*. *B*: intact frequencies of oscillators 1–6 in model of Fig. 28 *B*. *Inset* shows phase lag at faster paper speed. [From Sarna et al. (201).]

layers generate spontaneous ECA, then coupling may be due to the coupling of spontaneous relaxation oscillators in both muscle layers. If only one muscle layer generates spontaneous ECA, the above coupling may be due to the coupling of spontaneous relaxation oscillators in one layer with potential relaxation oscillators in the other muscle layer. Connective tissue cells and cell-to-cell coupling has been reported between the two muscle layers, which may be the morphological basis of this coupling (89).

Following the successful application of cable equation to explain the propagation of action potential in nerves, it was proposed that the spread of myoelectric activity in the cardiac and smooth muscle cells also behaves like that in a cable. This initial hypothesis was made on the assumption that there is cytoplasmic continuity between cardiac and smooth muscle cells or that these cells are connected by low-resistance pathways (15, 68, 69).

It is now known that cardiac and smooth muscle cells are discrete, independent units (15, 89, 104). The membranes of two adjacent cells come close to each other to form a junction, but there is no membranous or cytoplasmic continuity between them. On the contrary, the fluid within the junction is continuous with the interstitial fluid. There is a gap of 10–70 nm between contiguous cells. This gap is penetrated by $L^{+3}$.

It is controversial whether these cell-to-cell junctions provide low-resistance pathways between cells. A major argument in favor of low-resistance junctions is based on the determination of long space constants of ~1–2 mm when stimulating currents are applied extracellularly to a bundle of smooth muscle cells (128, 156, 243, 256). These space constants are severalfold longer than the typical length of a cardiac or smooth muscle cell (100–200 μm). This finding suggested that smooth muscle electrical activity conducted from one cell to the next just as in an axon. The deterioration in signal amplitude from one cell to the next was small because of the long space constant. It was further assumed that extracellularly applied currents flow inside the cells and through cell junctions. However, Sperelakis (221, 223, 227) has suggested an alternate explanation of space constants determined by the extracellular application of stimulating currents. When current is applied extracellularly, it may flow largely through interstitial pathways. Sperelakis reported that a strip of closely packed cells has anisotropic properties, that is, because of physical orientation of closely packed cells in a conducting medium, the overall resistance of the bundle is lower in the axial than in the transverse direction. In other words, the flow of current in the interstitial fluid of a bundle of cells due to an extracellular stimulus will behave as that in a cable, yet this behavior may have nothing to do with the coupling between cells. Such current flow in the interstitial fluid and the anisotropic properties of closely packed cells was elegantly demonstrated in a glass rod model (221). The transverse resistance of closely packed glass rods in Tyrode's solution was several times larger than the longitudinal resistance. The ratio was higher for more closely packed rods. The glass rods are totally passive and they are not connected to each other. Thus relatively long space constants can be obtained in a bundle of fibers that are not connected by low-resistance pathways because of their anisotropic properties. Such space constants are the result of the cable properties of the muscle bundle, not of cell-to-cell connections. These findings have been confirmed by an analog computer model where it was shown that the resistance of the cell-to-cell junction had no effect on the space constant of the bundle (N. Sperelakis; personal communication). Sperelakis suggested that the cable properties of the muscle bundles must be distinguished from those of the cells.

Additional evidence against low-resistance pathways between cells and the applicability of cable models to cardiac and smooth muscle cells may be summarized as follows.

1. Interaction between two adjacent cells was studied by applying intracellular current to one cell and

recording the voltage response from the adjacent cell by another intracellular electrode (225, 230). The two intracellular electrodes were cemented together 7 μm to >100 μm apart in different experiments. When both the intracellular electrodes impaled the same cell, 100% interaction was observed. When the two intracellular electrodes impaled adjacent cells, the application of current to one cell did not affect the adjacent cell. This suggested that the smooth muscle cells do not behave as a two- or three-dimensional syncytium. Similar results were reported for cardiac muscle by other investigators (242).

The proponents of cable model argued that each cell had so many low-resistance interconnections with other cells in a three-dimensional structure that the current diffused rapidly in all directions and therefore had no measurable effect on the adjacent cells. However, this is a circuitous argument in the sense that an experiment was done to determine whether there were low-resistance connections between cells or not and then the results were dismissed by assuming that there were low-resistance connections. Furthermore, if an intracellularly applied current may diffuse to have no effect on an adjacent cell, the current generated due to changes in spontaneous membrane potential would behave similarly. If this were the case no interaction between the spontaneous oscillations of smooth muscle cells would be seen. The fact is that the electrical activities of smooth and cardiac muscle cells drive each other.

2. The input resistance between two cell interiors 0.5–1.0 mm apart is more than twice the resistance determined between one cell interior and the extracellular medium (225). If the cells were connected by low-resistance pathways, the input resistance between two cells would be much smaller than that between a single cell and the extracellular medium.

3. The specific resistances of cardiac and smooth muscle cells increase seven- to eight-fold more than that of skeletal muscle when the Tyrode solution is replaced by 10-fold dilute Tyrode made isosmotic with sucrose. This implies that the resistance to the flow of current through the intracellular pathway is higher as compared with that through the extracellular pathway. The calculated ratio of intracellular to extracellular resistance is 26.5 for intestinal smooth muscle and 2.7 for skeletal muscle (223).

4. When one of the cardiac cells in a cultured doublet was injured by impalement by a large microelectrode it depolarized and stopped oscillating, whereas the other cell maintained a substantial resting membrane potential and kept oscillating. Prior to injury, both cells were coupled and phase locked. If the two cells were connected by a low-resistance pathway, both cells would have depolarized and stopped oscillating (222).

5. In a true cable, the input resistance $R_{inp}$ is equal to $1/2\, R_{int}^{0.5} \times R_m^{0.5}$, where $R_{int}$ is the axoplasmic and junctional resistance in series and $R_m$ is the membrane resistance. If $R_{int}$ is low, $R_{inp}$ will also be low. A high $R_{inp}$ means that most of the current injected intracellularly exits close to the site of injection into the interstitial fluid. The input resistances of cat intestinal circular muscle have been reported to be ~70–100 MΩ. On the contrary, the $R_{inp}$ from the sartorius muscle fiber is ~0.5 MΩ (221). These findings suggest a high resistance at cell-to-cell junctions in smooth muscle cells.

6. When cat hearts were fixed rapidly during ventricular fibrillation, some cells were found to be contracted while the adjacent cells were relaxed (229). If there were low resistance pathways, all adjacent cells would have had nearly the same membrane potential and in nearly the same contracted state. Likewise, in the variable frequency region of small intestine and the colon, the ECA is phase unlocked at adjacent sites, which is contrary to the rapid spread of electrotonic currents through low resistance pathways.

7. In the smooth muscle, each cell is a spontaneous or a potentially spontaneous oscillator. In spontaneously active cells, one has to consider interaction between two actively depolarizing cells, not between an active region and an inactive region, as in a cable. Such interactions give rise to various possibilities such as frequency entrainment (stomach and proximal small intestine), frequency pulling (distal small intestine), or simple interaction without frequency pulling (colon). These possibilities are not adequately explained by the cable model.

8. If smooth muscle cells behaved like a cable, both ECA and ERA would conduct through them in a similar manner, yet this is not the case. It is known that ERA occurs only locally. It does not propagate as does ECA in the longitudinal or the circumferential direction. A close–intra-arterial injection of acetylcholine on the posterior side of the stomach caused a premature control potential, a burst of ERA, and a contraction on that side in the perfused segment. The premature control potential propagated to the anterior side but the ERA and its associated contraction did not (64). In the relaxation-oscillator model, the ERA from one oscillator would not spread to an adjacent oscillator because these oscillators do not respond to frequencies that are much higher than their own intrinsic frequency.

9. There is at least a partial continuity of smooth muscle at the organ junctions. If the conduction in smooth muscle occurred as in a cable or a syncytium, the ECA would conduct from one organ to the next. No such conduction has been reported. Instead the amplitude and frequency of oscillations on both sides of the junction are modulated, as would be expected in coupled relaxation oscillators.

10. The resting membrane potential of gastric smooth muscle cells varies from about −48 mV in the fundus to about −75 mV in the pyloric ring (235). Similarly, the resting membrane potential of the outer

circular muscle layer of the small intestine is ~10 mV more negative than that of the inner circular muscle layer (99). Such gradients of resting membrane potentials could not have been maintained if the cells were connected by low-resistance junctions.

In the relaxation-oscillator model, each cell or a group of cells is a spontaneous oscillator or a potential oscillator. The coupling between cells can be explained by electrical field changes in the cleft between the cells (224, 228, 226). These models do not require low-resistance pathways between cells. When one cell depolarizes, the cleft between the cells becomes electronegative with respect to the interstitual fluid surrounding the cells, and this negative cleft potential drives the next adjacent cell. The accumulation of $K^+$ at the cell junction during the depolarization may provide additional coupling to drive the adjacent cell (226). The only precondition for this type of coupling is that one cell should have a slightly higher intrinsic frequency than the other. This condition is met in both cardiac and gastrointestinal smooth muscle cells. The excitability or the coupling between cells depends on the dimensions of the cell-to-cell junctions. The basic unit of a relaxation oscillator is a single cell. Purves et al. (168) reported spontaneous oscillations from isolated single cultured smooth muscle cells of the guinea pig taenia coli. However, in vivo a large number of cells may oscillate nearly simultaneously and behave as a functional single oscillator.

## SUMMARY

There is a depolarization of ECA underlying every phasic contraction in gastrointestinal smooth muscle. The significance of ECA is to control the contractility of the smooth muscle by periodically depolarizing the membrane potential to above an excitatory threshold. The ECA controls the spatial and temporal patterns of contractions, both of which are important in the control of gastrointestinal motility. The ECA may be coupled to contractile activity in different ways in vivo. In some organs such as the stomach, small intestine, colon, gastroduodenal junction, ileocolonic junction, and the choledochoduodenal junction the depolarization of ECA is superimposed with a burst of ERA that is then associated with a contraction. In all of these organs except the choledochoduodenal junction a neurochemical stimulus may be required to increase the amplitude of depolarization to above the excitation threshold. In some other areas such as lower esophageal sphincter and the anal sphincter, each depolarization of ECA may exceed the excitation threshold level resulting in a contraction without a burst of ERA. In these sphincter zones the frequency of ECA is higher than that in adjacent organs and the characteristics of the muscle are such that the individual contractions fuse into a tonic contraction. The amplitude and generation of ECA in these sphincters is under strong neurochemical control. In the gallbladder smooth muscle the ECA is omnipresent, yet when its amplitude increases beyond an excitation threshold the smooth muscle contracts without a superimposed burst of ERA. The underlying mechanism that increases the amplitude of ECA in the gallbladder is not known yet; it is likely to be a neurochemical stimulus. In the esophagus the ECA is not spontaneous but the smooth muscle cells may undergo a single depolarization in response to a stimulus, and this depolarization is superimposed with a burst of ERA that is associated with a contraction. The colon has an additional type of intermittent oscillation called CEC, each oscillation of which may be superimposed with a burst of ERA. These colonic electrical activities are associated with long-duration phasic contractions.

In addition to the aforementioned phasic contractions and the generation of tone, the gastrointestinal tract generates giant migrating contractions that occur in special situations like vomiting, defecation, mass movement. The mechanisms of initiation and migration of these contractions and their associated myoelectric activities are incompletely understood at this time.

I acknowledge the skillful secretarial assistance of Mary Farrar in the preparation of this work and in the literature search. The skillful work done by the staff of the Medical Media Service at the Clement J. Zablocki Veterans Administration Medical Center is greatly appreciated. I gratefully acknowledge the helpful and critical comments by my colleagues in the preparation of this manuscript. Finally, I acknowledge the insatiable curiosity and unending dedication of my younger colleagues that have kept me on my toes all this time. I learn by teaching them. I am grateful that I had the opportunity of interacting with their fertile and productive minds.

This work was supported in part by Grant DK-32346 from the National Institutes of Health and Grant 7722-01P from the Veterans Administration Research Service.

## REFERENCES

1. AIZAWA, I., K. NEGISHI, T. SUZUKI, AND Z. ITOH. Gastrointestinal contractile activity associated with vomiting in the dog. In: *Gastrointestinal Motility*, edited by C. Roman. Lancaster, UK: MTP, 1984, p. 159–165.
2. AKWARI, O. E., K. A. KELLY, J. H. STEINBACH, AND C. F. CODE. Electric pacing of intact and transected canine small intestine and its computer model. *Am. J. Physiol.* 229: 1188–1197, 1975.
3. ALLEN, G. L., E. W. POOLE, AND C. F. CODE. Relationships between electrical activities of antrum and duodenum. *Am. J. Physiol.* 207: 906–910, 1964.
4. ALVAREZ, W. C., AND L. J. MAHONEY. The myogenic nature of the rhythmic contractions of the intestine. *Am. J. Physiol.* 59: 421–430, 1922.
5. ANURAS, S., A. R. COOKE, AND J. CHRISTENSEN. An inhibitory innervation at the gastroduodenal junction. *J. Clin. Invest.* 54: 529–535, 1974.
6. ARIMORI, M., C. F. CODE, J. F. SCHLEGEL, AND R. E. STRUM.

Electrical activity of the canine esophagus and gastroesophageal sphincter: its relation to intraluminal pressure and movement of material. *Am. J. Dig. Dis.* 15: 191–208, 1970.

7. ASOH, R., AND R. K. GOYAL. Manometry and electromyography of the upper esophageal sphincter in the opossum. *Gastroenterology* 74: 514–520, 1978.

8. ASOH, R., AND R. K. GOYAL. Electrical activity of the opossum lower esophageal sphincter in vivo. Its role in the basal sphincter pressure. *Gastroenterology* 74: 835–840, 1978.

9. ATANASSOVA, E. The role of the gastroduodenal junction in correlating the spike activities of the gastric and duodenal walls. *Dokl. Bolg. Akad. Nauk.* 22: 947–949, 1969.

10. ATANASSOVA, E. Bioelectrical activity of the stomach and duodenum after cutting the gastroduodenal junction. *Izv. Inst. Fiziol. Sofia* 13: 211–227, 1970.

11. ATANASSOVA, E. On the mechanism of correlation between the spike activities of the stomach and duodenum. *Izv. Inst. Fiziol. Sofia* 13: 229–242, 1970.

12. BALFOUR, T. W., AND J. D. HARDCASTLE. The identification of an electrically silent zone at the ileocaecocolic junction. In: *Gastrointestinal Motility in Health and Disease*, edited by H. L. Duthie. Lancaster: MTP, 1978, p. 407–408.

13. BARDAKJIAN, B. L., AND S. K. SARNA. A computer model of human colonic electrical control activity (ECA). *IEEE Trans. Biomed. Eng.* 27: 193–202, 1980.

14. BARR, L. Propagation in vertebrate visceral smooth muscle. *J. Theoret. Biol.* 4: 73–85, 1963.

15. BARR, L., AND M. M. DEWEY. Electrotonus and electrical transmission in smooth muscle. In: *Handbook of Physiology. Alimentary Canal Motility*, edited by Charles F. Code. Washington, DC: Am. Physiol. Soc., 1968, sect. 6, vol. 4, p. 1733–1742.

16. BASS, P. In vivo electrical activity of the small bowel. In: *Handbook of Physiology. Alimentary Canal Motility*, edited by Charles F. Code. Washington, DC: Am. Physiol. Soc., 1968, sect. 6, vol. 4, p. 2051–2074.

17. BASS, P., C. F. CODE, AND E. H. LAMBERT. Motor and electric activity of the duodenum. *Am. J. Physiol.* 201: 287–291, 1961.

18. BASS, P., C. F. CODE, AND E. H. LAMBERT. Electric activity of gastroduodenal junction. *Am. J. Physiol.* 201: 587–592, 1961.

19. BASS, P., AND J. N. WILEY. Effects of ligation and morphine on electric and motor activity of dog duodenum. *Am. J. Physiol.* 208: 908–913, 1965.

20. BECKER, J. M., F. G. MOODY, AND A. R. ZINSMEISTER. Effect of gastrointestinal hormones on the biliary sphincter of the opossum. *Gastroenterology* 82: 1300–1307, 1982.

21. BECKER, J. M., P. SAVA, K. A. KELLY, AND L. SHTURMAN. Intestinal pacing for canine postgastrectomy dumping. *Gastroenterology* 84: 383–387, 1983.

22. BEHAR, J., P. BIANCANI, AND M. P. ZABINSKI. Characterization of feline gastroduodenal junction by neural and hormonal stimulation. *Am. J. Physiol.* 236 (*Endocrinol. Metab. Gastrointest. Physiol.* 5): E45–E51, 1979.

23. BENDAT, J. S., AND A. G. PIERSOL. *Random Data: Analysis and Measurement Procedures*. New York: Wiley-Interscience, 1971.

24. BERKSON, J., E. J. BALDES, AND W. C. ALVAREZ. Electromyographic studies of the gastrointestinal tract. 1. The correlation between mechanical movement and changes in electrical potential during rhythmic contraction of the intestine. *Am. J. Physiol.* 102: 683–692, 1932.

25. BINDER, H. J., D. L. BLOOM, H. STERN, G. B. SOLITARE, W. R. THAYER, AND H. M. SPIRO. The effect of cervical vagectomy on esophageal function in the monkey. *Surgery St. Louis* 64: 1075–1083, 1968.

26. BISHOP, B., R. C. GARRY, T. D. ROBERTS, AND J. K. TODD. Control of the external sphincter of the anus in the cat. *J. Physiol. Lond.* 134: 229–240, 1956.

27. BLANK, E. L., M. KARAUS, R. GILBERT, M. GLICKLICH, S. K. SARNA, AND S. L. WERLIN. Gastrointestinal myoelectric activity in congenital idiopathic motility disorder (Abstract). *Gastroenterology* 88: 1329, 1985.

28. BORETOS, J. W. *Concise Guide to Biomedical Polymers. Their Design, Fabrication and Molding*. Springfield, IL: Thomas, 1973.

29. BORTOFF, A. Electrical activity of intestine recorded with pressure electrode. *Am. J. Physiol.* 201: 209–212, 1961.

30. BORTOFF, A., AND R. S. DAVIS. Myogenic transmission of antral slow waves across the gastroduodenal junction in situ. *Am. J. Physiol.* 215: 889–897, 1968.

31. BORTOLOTTI, M., G. LABO, R. B. BRAGAGLIA, S. MATTIOLI, AND L. POSSATI. Electromyographic study in diffuse esophageal spasm and achalasia. In: *Motility of the Digestive Tract*, edited by M. Wienbeck. New York: Raven, 1982, p. 319–326.

32. BOUVIER, M., AND J. GONELLA. Electrical activity from smooth muscle of the anal sphincteric area of the cat. *J. Physiol. Lond.* 310: 445–456, 1981.

33. BOUVIER, M., AND J. GONELLA. Nervous control of the internal anal sphincter of the cat. *J. Physiol. Lond.* 310: 457–469, 1981.

34. BOWES, K. L., N. L. SHEARIN, Y. J. KINGMA, AND Z. J. KOLES. Frequency analysis of electrical activity in dog colon. In: *Gastrointestinal Motility in Health and Disease*, edited by H. L. Duthie. Lancaster, UK: MTP, 1978, p. 251–268.

35. BOYDEN, E. A. The sphincter of Oddi in man and certain representative mammals. *Surgery St. Louis* 1: 25–37, 1937.

36. BOZLER, E. The activity of the pacemaker previous to the discharge of a muscular impulse. *Am. J. Physiol.* 136: 543–552, 1942.

37. BOZLER, E. The action potentials of the stomach. *Am. J. Physiol.* 144: 693–700, 1945.

38. BRUCE, J. D. Discrete Fourier transforms, linear filters and spectrum weighing. *IEEE Trans. Audio Electroacoust.* 16: 495–499, 1968.

39. BÜLBRING, E. Membrane potentials of smooth muscle fibres of taenia coli of guinea-pig. *J. Physiol. Lond.* 125: 302–315, 1954.

40. BUNKER, C. E., L. P. JOHNSON, AND T. S. NELSEN. Chronic in situ studies of the electrical activity of the small intestine. *Arch. Surg.* 95: 259–268, 1967.

41. BURGESS, J. N., J. F. SCHLEGEL, AND F. H. ELLIS, JR. The effect of denervation of feline esophageal function and morphology. *J. Surg. Res.* 12: 24–33, 1972.

42. BURNSTOCK, G., AND C. L. PROSSER. Responses of smooth muscles to quick stretch: relation of stretch to conduction. *Am. J. Physiol.* 198: 921–925, 1960.

43. CANNON, W. B. Esophageal peristalsis after bilateral vagotomy. *Am. J. Physiol.* 19: 436–444, 1907.

44. CAR, A., AND C. ROMAN. Etude des vitesses de conduction des fibres nerveuses motrices de l'oesophage. *C. R. Soc. Biol.* 159: 1767–1770, 1965.

45. CAR, A., AND C. ROMAN. L'activite spontanee du sphincter oesophagien superieur chez le mouton. *J. Physiol. Paris* 62: 505–511, 1970.

46. CARDWELL, B. A., M. R. RUBIN, W. J. SNAPE, JR., AND S. COHEN. Properties of the cat ileocecal sphincter muscle. *Am. J. Physiol.* 241 (*Gastrointest. Liver Physiol.* 4): G222–G226, 1981.

47. CHAMBERS, M. M., K. L. BOWES, Y. J. KINGMA, C. BANNISTER, AND K. R. COTE. In vitro electrical activity in human colon. *Gastroenterology* 81: 502–508, 1981.

48. CHRISPIN, A. R., AND G. W. FRIEDLAND. A radiological study of the neural control of oesophageal vestibular function. *Thorax* 21: 422–427, 1966.

49. CHRISTENSEN, J. Patterns and origin of some esophageal responses to stretch and electrical stimulation. *Gastroenterology* 59: 909–916, 1970.

50. CHRISTENSEN, J., AND G. F. LUND. Esophageal responses to distension and electrical stimulation. *J. Clin. Invest.* 48: 408–419, 1969.

51. CHRISTENSEN, J., H. P. SCHEDL, AND J. A. CLIFFTON. The small intestinal basic electrical rhythm (slow wave) frequency

gradient in normal men and in patients with a variety of diseases. *Gastroenterology* 50: 309–315, 1966.
52. CODE, C. F., AND H. C. CARLSON. Motor activity of the stomach. In: *Handbook of Physiology. Alimentary Canal Motility*, edited by Charles F. Code. Washington, DC: Am. Physiol. Soc., 1968, sect. 6, vol. 4, p. 1903–1916.
53. CODE, C. F., AND J. A. MARLETT. Canine tachygastria. *Mayo Clin. Proc.* 49: 325–332, 1974.
54. CODE, C. F., J. H. STEINBACH, J. F. SCHLEGEL, J. R. AMBERG, AND G. A. HALLENBECK. Pyloric and duodenal motor contributions to duodenogastric reflux. *Scand. J. Gastroenterol. Suppl.* 92: 13–16, 1984.
55. COHEN, S., L. D. HARRIS, AND R. LEVITAN. Manometric characteristics of the human ileocecal junctional zone. *Gastroenterology* 54: 72–75, 1968.
56. CONKLIN, J. L., AND J. CHRISTENSEN. Local specialization at ileocecal junction of the cat and opossum. *Am. J. Physiol.* 228: 1075–1081, 1975.
57. CONNELL, A. M. The motility of the pelvic colon. I. Motility in normals and in patients with asymptomatic duodenal ulcer. *Gut* 2: 175–186, 1961.
58. COREMANS, G., J. JANSSENS, G. VANTRAPPEN, S. CUCCHIARA, AND P. CECCATELLI. The slow wave frequency gradient of the human small intestine decreases with frequency plateaus (Abstract). *Gastroenterology* 88: 1356, 1985.
59. COUTURIER, D., C. ROZE, J. PAOLAGGI, AND C. DEBRAY. Electrical activity of the normal human stomach. A comparative study of recordings obtained from the serosal and mucosal sides. *Am. J. Dig. Dis.* 17: 969–976, 1972.
60. COUTURIER, D., C. ROZE, M. H. COUTURIER-TURPIN, AND C. DEBRAY. Electromyography of the colon in situ. An experimental study in man and in the rabbit. *Gastroenterology* 56: 317–322, 1969.
61. DANIEL, E. E. The electrical and contractile activity of the pyloric region in dogs and the effects of drugs. *Gastroenterology* 49: 403–418, 1965.
62. DANIEL, E. E. Nerves and motor activity of the gut. In: *Nerves and the Gut*, edited by F. P. Brooks and P. W. Evers. Thorofare, NJ: Slack, 1977, p. 154–196.
63. DANIEL, E. E., A. J. HONOUR, AND A. BOGOCH. Electrical activity of the longitudinal muscle of dog small intestine studied in vivo using microelectrodes. *Am. J. Physiol.* 198: 113–118, 1960.
64. DANIEL, E. E., AND S. K. SARNA. Distribution of excitatory vagal fibers in canine gastric wall to control motility. *Gastroenterology* 71: 608–613, 1976.
65. DANIEL, E. E., B. T. WACHTER, A. J. HONOUR, AND A. BOGOCH. The relationship between electrical and mechanical activity of the small intestine of dog and man. *Can. J. Biochem.* 38: 777–802, 1960.
66. DARDILLAT, C., AND Y. RUCKEBUSCH. Aspects fonctionnels de la jonction gastroduodenale chez le veau ne-ouveau-ne. *Ann. Rech. Vet.* 4: 31–56, 1973.
67. DENT, J., W. J. DODDS, T. SEKIGUCHI, W. J. HOGAN, AND R. C. ARNDORFER. Interdigestive phasic contractions of the human lower esophageal sphincter. *Gastroenterology* 84: 453–460, 1983.
68. DEWEY, M. M. The anatomical basis of propagation in smooth muscle. *Gastroenterology* 49: 395–402, 1965.
69. DEWEY, M. M., AND L. BARR. Intercellular connection between smooth muscle cells: the nexus. *Science Wash. DC.* 137: 670–672, 1962.
70. DIAMANT, N. E. Electrical activity of the cat smooth muscle esophagus: a study of hyperpolarizing responses. In: *Proc. 4th Int. Symp. Gastrointest. Motil. Alberta, Canada.* Vancouver, Canada: Mitchell, 1974, p. 593–605.
71. DIAMANT, N. E., AND A. BORTOFF. Nature of the intestinal slow-wave frequency gradient. *Am. J. Physiol.* 216: 301–307, 1969.
72. DIAMANT, N. E., AND A. BORTOFF. Effects of transection on the intestinal slow-wave frequency gradient. *Am. J. Physiol.* 216: 734–743, 1969.
73. DIAMANT, N. E., AND T. Y. EL-SHARKAWY. Neural control of esophageal peristalsis. A conceptual analysis. *Gastroenterology* 72: 546–556, 1977.
74. DIAMANT, N. E., P. K. ROSE, AND E. J. DAVISON. Computer simulation of intestinal slow-wave frequency gradient. *Am. J. Physiol.* 219: 1684–1690, 1970.
75. DIAMANT, N. E., J. WONG, AND L. CHEN. Effects of transection of small intestinal slow-wave propagation velocity. *Am. J. Physiol.* 225: 1497–1500, 1973.
76. DODDS, W. J., J. CHRISTENSEN, J. DENT, J. D. WOOD, AND R. C. ARNDORFER. Esophageal contractions induced by vagal stimulation in the opossum. *Am. J. Physiol.* 235 (*Endocrinol. Metab. Gastrointest. Physiol.* 4): E392–E401, 1978.
77. DODDS, W. J., J. J. STEF, E. T. STEWART, W. J. HOGAN, R. C. ARNDORFER, AND E. B. COHEN. Responses of feline esophagus to cervical vagal stimulation. *Am. J. Physiol.* 235 (*Endocrinol. Metab. Gastrointest. Physiol.* 4): E63–E73, 1978.
78. EHRLEIN, H. J., M. SCHEMANN, AND M. L. SIEGLE. Motor patterns of the canine small intestine (Abstract). *Dig. Dis. Sci.* 30: 767, 1985.
79. EL-CHERIF, Y. S., AND S. K. SARNA. Parametric spectral estimation of gastrointestinal signals. In: *IEEE 1981 Frontiers of Engineering in Health Care*, edited by B. A. Cohen. New York: *IEEE Trans. Biomed. Engn.* 1981, p. 132–136.
80. EL-SHARKAWY, T. Y., B. L. BARDAKJIAN, W. M. MACDONALD, AND N. E. DIAMANT. Origins of the multiple patterns of electrical control activity in the colon. In: *Motility of the Digestive Tract*, New York: Raven, 1982, p. 491–497.
81. EL-SHARKAWY, T. Y., AND N. E. DIAMANT. Contraction patterns of esophageal circular smooth muscle induced by cholinergic excitation (Abstract). *Gastroenterology* 70: 969, 1976.
82. EL-SHARKAWY, T. Y., K. G. MORGAN, AND J. H. SZURSZEWSKI. Intracellular electrical activity of canine and human gastric smooth muscle. *J. Physiol. Lond.* 279: 391–307, 1978.
83. FAMILONI, B. O., Y. J. KINGMA, I. RACHEV, AND K. L. BOWES. Noninvasive measurements of gastric electrical and contractile activity (Abstract). *Dig. Dis. Sci.* 30: 768, 1985.
84. FIORAMONTI, J., R. GARCIA-VILLAR, L. BUENO, AND Y. RUCKEBUSCH. Colonic myoelectrical activity and propulsion in the dog. *Dig. Dis. Sci.* 25: 641–646, 1980.
85. FISHER, R., AND S. COHEN. Physiological characteristics of the human pyloric sphincter. *Gastroenterology* 64: 67–75, 1973.
86. FLECKENSTEIN, P., F. KROGH, AND A. OIGAARD. The interdigestive myoelectrical complex and other migrating electrical phenomena in the human small intestine. In: *Gastrointestinal Motility in Health and Disease*, edited by H. L. Duthie. Lancaster, UK: MTP, 1978, p. 19–27.
87. FRENCKNER, B., AND T. IHRE. Influence of autonomic nerves on the internal anal sphincter in man. *Gut* 17: 306–312, 1976.
88. GABELLA, G. Special muscle cells and their innervation in the mammalian small intestine. *Cell Tissue Res.* 153: 63–77, 1974.
89. GABELLA, G. Structure of muscles and nerves in the gastrointestinal tract. In: *Physiology of the Gastrointestinal Tract*, edited by L. R. Johnson. New York: Raven, 1981, p. 197–241.
90. GEENEN, J. E., W. J. HOGAN, W. J. DODDS, E. T. STEWART, AND R. C. ARNDORFER. Intraluminal pressure recording from the human sphincter of Oddi. *Gastroenterology* 78: 317–324, 1980.
91. GILL, R. C., M.-A. PILOT, AND P. A. THOMAS. Gastroduodenal control of postprandial canine gastric motility (Abstract). *J. Physiol. Lond.* 325: 50P, 1982.
92. GILLESPIE, J. S. Spontaneous mechanical and electrical activity of stretched and unstretched intestinal smooth muscle cells and their response to sympathetic nerve stimulation. *J. Physiol. Lond.* 162: 54–75, 1962.
93. GLASER, E. M., AND D. S. RUCHKIN. *Principles of Neurobiological Signal Analysis*. New York: Academic, 1976.
94. GONELLA, J., J. P. NIEL, AND C. ROMAN. Vagal control of lower oesophageal sphincter motility in the cat. *J. Physiol. Lond.* 273: 647–664, 1977.

95. GOYAL, R. K., AND J. S. GIDDA. Relation between electrical and mechanical activity in esophageal smooth muscle. *Am. J. Physiol.* 240 (*Gastrointest. Liver Physiol.* 4): G305–G311, 1981.
96. GREENWOOD, R. K., J. F. SCHLEGEL, C. F. CODE, AND F. H. ELLIS, JR. The effect of sympathectomy, vagotomy, and oesophageal interruption on the canine gastro-oesophageal sphincter. *Thorax* 17: 310–319, 1962.
97. GROSSMAN, M. I. Neural and hormonal regulation of gastrointestinal function: an overview. *Annu. Rev. Physiol.* 41: 27–33, 1979.
98. GULLIKSON, G. W., H. OKUDA, M. SHIMIZU, AND P. BASS. Electrical arrhythmias in gastric antrum of the dog. *Am. J. Physiol.* 239 (*Gastrointest. Liver Physiol.* 2): G59–G68, 1980.
99. HARA, Y., M. KUBOTA, AND J. H. SZURSZEWSKI. Electrophysiology of smooth muscle of the small intestine of some mammals. *J. Physiol. Lond.* 372: 501–520, 1986.
100. HARDCASTLE, J. D., AND C. V. MANN. Study of large bowel peristalsis. *Gut* 9: 512–520, 1968.
101. HELLEMANS, J., AND G. VANTRAPPEN. Electromyographic studies on canine esophageal motility. *Am. J. Dig. Dis.* 12: 1240–1255, 1967.
102. HELLEMANS, J., G. VANTRAPPEN, P. VALEMBOIS, J. JANSSENS, AND J. VANDENBROUCKE. Electrical activity of straited and smooth muscle of the esophagus. *Am. J. Dig. Dis.* 13: 320–334, 1968.
103. HELM, J. F., W. J. DODDS, J. CHRISTENSEN, AND S. K. SARNA. Control mechanism of the spontaneous in vitro contractions of the opossum sphincter of Oddi. *Am. J. Physiol.* 249: (*Gastrointest. Liver Physiol.* 12): G572–G579, 1985.
104. HENDERSON, R. M., G. DUCHON, AND E. E. DANIEL. Cell contacts in duodenal smooth muscle layers. *Am. J. Physiol.* 221: 564–574, 1971.
105. HERMON-TAYLOR, J., AND C. F. CODE. Localization of the duodenal pacemaker and its role in the organization of duodenal myoelectric activity. *Gut* 12: 40–47, 1971.
106. HIGGS, B., AND F. H. ELLIS. The effect of bilateral supranodosal vagotomy on canine esophageal function. *Surgery St. Louis* 58: 828–834, 1965.
107. HOLLOWAY, R. H., E. L. BLANK, I. TAKAHASHI, W. J. DODDS, J. DENT, AND S. K. SARNA. Electrical control activity of the lower esophageal sphincter in unanesthetized opossums. *Am. J. Physiol.* 252 (*Gastrointest. Liver Physiol.* 15): G511–G521, 1987.
108. HONDA, R., J. TOOULI, W. J. DODDS, S. K. SARNA, W. J. HOGAN, AND Z. ITOH. Relationship of sphincter of Oddi spike bursts to gastrointestinal myoelectric activity in conscious opossums. *J. Clin. Invest.* 69: 770–778, 1982.
109. HUIZINGA, J. D., N. E. DIAMANT, AND T. Y. EL-SHARKAWY. Electrical basis of contractions in the muscle layers of the pig colon. *Am. J. Physiol.* 245 (*Gastrointest. Liver Physiol.* 8): G482–G491, 1983.
110. HUIZINGA, J. D., H. S. STERN, E. CHOW, N. E. DIAMANT, AND T. Y. EL-SHARKAWY. Electrophysiologic control of motility in the human colon. *Gastroenterology* 88: 500–511, 1985.
111. ITOH, Z., R. HONDA, I. AIZAWA, S. TAKEUCHI, K. HIWATASHI, AND E. F. COUCH. Interdigestive motor activity of the lower esophageal sphincter in the conscious dog. *Am. J. Dig. Dis.* 23: 239–247, 1978.
112. JANSSENS, J., I. DE WEVER, G. VANTRAPPEN, AND J. HELLEMANS. Peristalsis in smooth muscle esophagus after transection and bolus deviation. *Gastroenterology* 71: 1004–1009, 1976.
113. JANSSENS, J., P. VALEMBOLIS, J. HELLEMANS, G. VANTRAPPEN, AND W. PELEMANS. Studies on the necessity of a bolus for the progression of secondary peristalsis in the canine esophagus. *Gastroenterology* 67: 245–251, 1974.
114. JANSSENS, J., P. VALEMBOLIS, G. VANTRAPPEN, J. HELLEMANS, AND W. PELEMANS. Is the primary peristaltic contraction of the canine esophagus bolus-dependent? *Gastroenterology* 65: 750–756, 1973.
115. JOHNSON, A. G. Gastroduodenal motility and synchronization. *Postgrad. Med. J.* 49, Suppl. 4: 29–38, 1973.
116. JULÉ, Y. Etude in vitro de l'activité electromyographique du colon proximal et distal du lapin. *J. Physiol. Paris* 68: 305–329, 1974.
117. KARAUS, M., AND S. K. SARNA. Giant migrating contractions during defecation in the dog colon. *Gastroenterology* 92: 925–933, 1987.
118. KAYE, M. D., S. J. MEHTA, AND J. P. SHOWALTER. Manometric studies of the human pylorus. *Gastroenterology* 70: 477–480, 1976.
119. KELLY, K. A. Motility of the stomach and gastroduodenal junction. In: *Physiology of the Gastrointestinal Tract*, edited by L. R. Johnson. New York: Raven, 1981, p. 393–410.
120. KELLY, K. A., AND C. F. CODE. Effect of transthoracic vagotomy on canine gastric electrical activity. *Gastroenterology* 57: 51–58, 1969.
121. KELLY, K. A., C. F. CODE, AND L. R. ELVEBACK. Patterns of canine gastric electrical activity. *Am. J. Physiol.* 217: 461–470, 1969.
122. KELLY, K. A., AND C. F. CODE. Canine gastric pacemaker. *Am. J. Physiol.* 220: 112–118, 1971.
123. KELLY, K. A., AND C. F. CODE. Duodenal-gastric reflux and slowed gastric emptying by electrical pacing of the canine duodenal pacesetter potential. *Gastroenterology* 72: 429–433, 1977.
124. KELLEY, M. L., JR., E. A. GORDON, AND J. A. DEWEESE. Pressure studies of the ileocolonic junctional zone of dogs. *Am. J. Physiol.* 209: 333–339, 1965.
125. KELLEY, M. L., JR., E. A. GORDON, AND J. A. DEWEESE. Pressure responses of canine ileocolonic junctional zone to intestinal distention. *Am. J. Physiol.* 211: 614–618, 1966.
126. KERREMANS, R. Electrical activity and motility of the internal anal sphincter: an "in vivo" electrophysiological study in man. *Acta Gastro-Enterol. Belg.* 31: 465–482, 1968.
127. KIM, C. H., F. AZPIROZ, A. R. ZINSMEISTER, AND J.-R. MALAGELADA. Properties of drug-induced gastric dysrhythmia (GD) in fasting and fed states (Abstract). *Dig. Dis. Sci.* 30: 777, 1985.
128. KOBAYASHI, M., C. L. PROSSER, AND T. NAGAI. Electrical properties of intestinal muscle as measured intracellularly and extracellulary. *Am. J. Physiol.* 213: 275–286, 1967.
129. KOCYLOWSKI, M., K. L. BOWES, AND Y. J. KINGMA. Electrical and mechanical activity in the ex vivo perfused total canine colon. *Gastroenterology* 77: 1021–1026, 1979.
130. KONTUREK, J. W., AND G. W. SCOTT. Intracellular myoelectrical activity of canine gallbladder (Abstract). *Dig. Dis. Sci.* 30: 778, 1985.
131. KUBOTA, M. Electrical and mechanical properties and neuroeffector transmission in the smooth muscle layer of the guinea-pig iolececal junction. *Pfluegers Arch.* 394: 355–361, 1982.
132. LABO, G., L. BARBARA, G. A. LANFRANCHI, M. BORTOLOTTI, AND M. MIGLIOLI. Modification of the electrical activity of the human intestine after serotonin and caerulein. *Am. J. Dig. Dis.* 17: 363–372, 1972.
133. LANG, I. M., S. K. SARNA AND R. E. CONDON. The myoelectric responses of the gastrointestinal tract associated with emesis in the dog. *Soc. Neurosci. Abstr.* 10: 834, 1984.
134. LANG, I. M., J. MARVIG, S. K. SARNA, AND R. E. CONDON. Gastrointestinal myoelectric correlates of vomiting in the dog. *Am. J. Physiol.* 251 (*Gastrointest. Liver Physiol.* 14): G830–G838, 1986.
135. LANG, I. M., S. K. SARNA, AND R. E. CONDON. Gastrointestinal motor correlates of vomiting in the dog: quantification and characterization as an independent phenomenon. *Gastroenterology*, 1985; 90: 40–47.
136. LATIMER, P., S. K. SARNA, D. CAMPBELL, M. LATIMER, W. WATERFALL, AND E. E. DANIEL. Colonic motor and myoelectrical activity: a comparative study of normal subject, psychoneurotic patients, and patients with irritable bowel syndrome. *Gastroenterology* 80: 893–901, 1981.
137. LATOUR, A. Quantitative analysis and measurement of myoelectrical spike activity at the gastroduodenal junction. *Ann.*

*Biol. Anim. Biochim. Biophys.* 18: 711–716, 1978.
138. LINKENS, D. A., AND A. E. CANNELL. Interactive graphics analysis of gastrointestinal electrical signals. *IEEE Trans. Biomed. Eng.* 21: 335–339, 1974.
139. LINKENS, D. A., I. TAYLOR, AND H. L. DUTHIE. Mathematical modeling of the colorectal myoelectrical activity in humans. *IEEE Trans. Biomed. Eng.* 23: 101–110, 1976.
140. LONGHI, E. H., AND P. H. JORDAN, JR. Necessity of a bolus for propagation of primary peristalsis in the canine esophagus. *Am. J. Physiol.* 220: 609–612, 1971.
141. LORD, M. G., M. HUTTON, AND D. L. WINGATE. Fast slow waves in the canine colon (Abstract). *Gastroenterology* 76: 1188, 1979.
142. MACKEL, R. Segmental and descending control of the external urethral and anal sphincters in the cat. *J. Physiol. Lond.* 294: 105–122, 1979.
143. MANN, C. V., AND J. D. HARDCASTLE. Recent studies of colonic and rectal motor action. *Dis. Colon Rectum* 13: 225–230, 1970.
144. MATSUMOTO, T., S. K. SARNA, AND R. E. CONDON. Gallbladder electrical activity in vivo (Abstract). *Gastroenterology* 88: 1493, 1985.
145. MATSUMOTO, T., S. K. SARNA, R. E. CONDON, AND W. J. DODDS. Gallbladder cyclic motor activity (Abstract). *Gastroenterology* 88: 1493, 1985.
146. MCCOY, E. J., AND P. BASS. Chronic electrical activity of gastroduodenal area: effects of food and certain catecholomines. *Am. J. Physiol.* 205: 439–445, 1963.
147. MCINTYRE, J. A., M. DEITEL, M. BAIDA, AND S. JALIL. The human electrogastrogram at operation: a preliminary report. *Can. J. Surg.* 12: 275–284, 1969.
148. MELTZER, S. J., AND J. AUER. Peristaltic rush. *Am. J. Physiol.* 20: 259–281, 1907.
149. MIOLAN, J. P., A. M. LAJARD, P. REGA, AND C. ROMAN. Vagal control of gastrointestinal tract during vomiting. In: *Gastrointestinal Motility*, edited by C. Roman. Lancaster, UK: MTP, 1984, p. 167–176.
150. MIR, S. S., G. R. MASON, AND H. S. ORMSBEE III. An inhibitory innervation at the gastroduodenal junction in anesthetized dogs. *Gastroenterology* 73: 432–434, 1977.
151. MONGES, H., AND J. SALDUCCI. A method of recording the gastric electrical activity in man. *Am. J. Dig. Dis.* 15: 271–276, 1970.
152. MONGES, H., AND J. SALDUCCI. Electrical activity of the gastric antrum in normal human subjects. *Am. J. Dig. Dis.* 16: 623–627, 1971.
153. MONGES, H., J. SALDUCCI, B. NAUDY, F. RANIER, J. GONELLA, AND M. BOUVIER. The electrical activity of the internal anal sphincter: a comparative study in man and cats. In: *Gastrointestinal Motility*, edited by J. Christensen. New York: Raven, 1980, p. 495–501.
154. MORGAN, K. G., AND J. H. SZURSZEWSKI. Mechanisms of phasic and tonic actions of pentagastrin on canine gastric smooth muscle. *J. Physiol. Lond.* 301: 229–242, 1980.
155. MUKHOPADHYAY, A. K., AND N. W. WEISBRODT. Neural organization of esophageal peristalsis: role of the vagus nerve. *Gastroenterology* 68: 444–447, 1975.
156. NAGAI, T., AND C. L. PROSSER. Electrical parameters of smooth muscle cells. *Am. J. Physiol.* 204: 915–924, 1963.
157. NELSEN, T. S., AND J. C. BECKER. Simulation of the electrical and mechanical gradient of the small intestine. *Am. J. Physiol.* 214: 749–757, 1968.
158. NELSEN, T. S., E. H. EIGENBRODT, L. A. KEOSHIAN, C. BUNKER, AND L. JOHNSON. Alterations in muscular and electrical activity of the stomach following vagotomy. *Arch. Surg.* 94: 821–835, 1967.
159. NELSEN, T. S., AND S. KOHATSU. Clinical electrogastrography and its relationship to gastric surgery. *Am. J. Surg.* 116: 215–222, 1968.
160. ORMSBEE, H. S. III, AND P. BASS. Gastroduodenal motor gradients in the dog after pyloroplasty. *Am. J. Physiol.* 230: 389–397, 1976.
161. OUYANG, A., C. J. CLAIN, W. J. SNAPE, JR., AND S. COHEN. Characterization of opiate-mediated responses of the feline ileum and ileocecal sphincter. *J. Clin. Invest.* 69: 507–515, 1982.
162. OUYANG, A., AND S. COHEN. Multiple 5-hydroxytryptamine receptors on feline ileum and ileocecal sphincter. *Am. J. Physiol.* 244 (*Gastrointest. Liver Physiol.* 7): G426–G434, 1983.
163. OUYANG, A., J. C. REYNOLDS, AND S. COHEN. Spike-associated and spike-independent esophageal contractions in patients with symptomatic diffuse esophageal spasm. *Gastroenterology* 84: 907–913, 1983.
164. OUYANG, A., W. J. SNAPE, JR., AND S. COHEN. Myoelectric properties of the cat ileocecal sphincter. *Am. J. Physiol.* 240 (*Gastrointest. Liver Physiol.* 3): G450–G458, 1981.
165. PODGORSKI, E. A Computer Model of Esophageal Electrical Activity. McMaster University, Hamilton, Ontario, Canada. May, 1980. Master's thesis.
166. PODGORSKI, E., AND S. K. SARNA. A computer model of esophageal electrical activity (Abstract). *Gastroenterology* 76: 1218, 1979.
167. PROVENZALE, L., AND M. PISANO. Methods for recording electrical activity of the human colon in vivo. Clinical applications. *Am. J. Dig. Dis.* 16: 712–722, 1971.
168. PURVES, R. D., G. E. MARK, AND G. BURNSTOCK. The electrical activity of single isolated smooth muscle cells. *Pfluegers Arch.* 341: 325–330, 1973.
169. QUIGLEY, E. M., S. F. PHILLIPS, B. CRANLEY, B. M. TAYLOR, AND J. DENT. Tone of canine ileocolonic junction: topography and response to phasic contractions. *Am. J. Physiol.* 249 (*Gastrointest. Liver Physiol.* 12): G350–G357, 1985.
170. QUIGLEY, E. M., S. F. PHILLIPS, AND J. DENT. Distinctive patterns of interdigestive motility at the canine ileocolonic junction. *Gastroenterology* 87: 836–844, 1984.
171. QUIGLEY, E. M., S. F. PHILLIPS, J. DENT, AND B. M. TAYLOR. Myoelectric activity and intraluminal pressure of the canine ileocolonic sphincter. *Gastroenterology* 85: 1054–1062, 1983.
172. RATTAN, S., J. S. GIDDA, AND R. K. GOYAL. Membrane potential and mechanical responses of the opossum esophagus to vagal stimulation and swallowing. *Gastroenterology* 85: 922–928, 1983.
173. RENDLEMAN, D. F., J. E. ANTHONY, C. DAVIS, JR., R. E. BUENGER, A. J. BROOKS, AND E. J. BEATTIE, JR. Reflux pressure studies in the ileocecal valve of dogs and humans. *Surgery* 44: 640–643, 1958.
174. REYNOLDS, J. C., A. OUYANG, AND S. COHEN. Electrically coupled intrinsic responses of feline lower esophageal sphincter. *Am. J. Physiol.* 243 (*Gastrointest. Liver Physiol.* 6): G415–G423, 1982.
175. ROMAN, C. Côntrole nerveus de péristaltisme oesophagien. *J. Physiol. Paris* 58: 79–108, 1966.
176. ROMAN, C. La commande de la motricité oesophagienne et sa régulation. Marseille, France, Université d' Aix-Marseille, Theses Doct. Sci. Nat., 1967.
177. ROMAN, C. AND L. TIEFFENBACH. Motricité de l'oesophage à musculeuse lisse après bivagotomie: étude electromyographique (E.M.G.) *J. Physiol. Paris.* 63: 733–762, 1971.
178. ROMAN, C., AND L. TIEFFENBACH. Enregistrement de l'activité unitaire des fibres motrices vagales destinées à l'oesophage du Babouin. *J. Physiol. Paris* 64: 479–506, 1972.
179. RUBIN, M. R., J. FOURNET, W. J. SNAPE, JR., AND S. COHEN. Adrenergic regulation of ileocecal sphincter function in the cat. *Gastroenterology* 78: 15–21, 1980.
180. RUCKEBUSCH, M., AND J. FIORAMONTI. Electrical spiking activity and propulsion in small intestine in fed and fasted rats. *Gastroenterology* 68: 1500–1508, 1975.
181. SANCHOLUZ, A. R., T. E. CROLEY II, J. CHRISTENSEN, E. O. MACAGNO, AND J. R. GLOVER. Phase lock of electrical slow waves and spike bursts in cat duodenum. *Am. J. Physiol.* 229: 608–612, 1975.
182. SANDERS, K. M. Excitation-contraction coupling without $Ca^{2+}$

action potentials in small intestine. *Am. J. Physiol.* 244 (*Cell Physiol.* 13): C356–C361, 1983.
183. SARNA, S. K. Computer Models of Gastrointestinal Control Activity. Edmonton, Alberta, Canada: Univ. of Alberta, 1971. PhD thesis.
184. SARNA, S. K. Gastrointestinal electrical activity: terminology. *Gastroenterology* 68: 1631–1635, 1975.
185. SARNA, S. K. The control of colonic motility. In: *Functional Disorders of the Digestive Tract*, edited by W. Y. Chey. New York: Raven, p. 277–285.
186. SARNA, S. K. Giant migrating contractions and their myoelectric correlates in the small intestine. *Am. J. Physiol* 253 (*Gastrointest. Liver Physiol.* 16): G697–G705, 1987.
187. SARNA, S. K. Small and large bowel motility and postoperative disorders. In: *Surgical Care II*, edited by R. E. Condon and J. DeCosse. Philadelphia, PA: Lea & Febiger, 1985, p. 135–149.
188. SARNA, S. K. Myoelectric correlates of colonic motor complexes and contractile activity. *Am. J. Physiol* 250 (*Gastrointest. Liver Physiol.* 13): G213–G220, 1986.
189. SARNA, S. K., B. L. BARDAKJIAN, W. E. WATERFALL, AND J. F. LIND. Human colonic electrical control activity (ECA). *Gastroenterology* 78: 1526–1536, 1980.
190. SARNA, S. K., K. L. BOWES, AND E. E. DANIEL. Post-operative gastric electrical control activity (ECA) in man. In: *Proc. 4th Int. Symp. Gastrointest. Motil., Alberta, Canada*. Vancouver, Canada: Mitchell, 1974, p. 73–83.
191. SARNA, S. K., K. L. BOWES, AND E. E. DANIEL. Gastric pacemakers. *Gastroenterology* 70: 226–231, 1976.
192. SARNA, S., R. E. CONDON, AND V. COWLES. Enteric mechanisms of initiation of migrating myoelectric complexes in dogs. *Gastroenterology* 84: 814–822, 1983.
193. SARNA, S. K., R. CONDON, AND V. COWLES. Colonic migrating and nonmigrating motor complexes in dogs. *Am. J. Physiol.* 246 (*Gastrointest. Liver Physiol.* 9): G355–G360, 1984.
194. SARNA, S. K., AND E. E. DANIEL. Electrical stimulation of gastric electrical control activity. *Am. J. Physiol.* 225: 124–131, 1973.
195. SARNA, S. K., AND E. E. DANIEL. Threshold curves and refractoriness properties of gastric relaxation oscillators. *Am. J. Physiol.* 226: 749–755, 1974.
196. SARNA, S. K., AND E. E. DANIEL. Vagal control of gastric electrical control activity and motility. *Gastroenterology* 68: 301–308, 1975.
197. SARNA, S. K., AND E. E. DANIEL. Electrical stimulation of small intestinal electrical control activity. *Gastroenterology* 69: 660–667, 1975.
198. SARNA, S. K., AND E. E. DANIEL. Neuronal control of motility in the pyloric region in dogs (Abstract). *Gastroenterology* 70: 933, 1976.
199. SARNA, S. K., E. E. DANIEL, AND Y. J. KINGMA. Simulation of slow wave electrical activity of small intestine. *Am. J. Physiol.* 221: 166–175, 1971.
200. SARNA, S. K., E. E. DANIEL, AND Y. J. KINGMA. Premature control potentials in the dog stomach and in the gastric computer model. *Am. J. Physiol.* 222: 1518–1523, 1972.
201. SARNA, S. K., E. E. DANIEL, AND Y. J. KINGMA. Simulation of the electric-control activity of the stomach by an array of relaxation oscillators. *Am. J. Dig. Dis.* 17: 299–310, 1972.
202. SARNA, S. K., E. E. DANIEL, AND Y. J. KINGMA. Effects of partial cuts on gastric electrical control activity and its computer model. *Am. J. Physiol.* 223: 332–340, 1972.
203. SARNA, S. K., E. E. DANIEL, AND W. E. WATERFALL. Myogenic and neuronal control systems for esophageal motility. *Gastroenterology* 73: 1345–1352, 1977.
204. SARNA, S. K., E. E. DANIEL, W. E. WATERFALL, T. D. LEWIS, AND L. MARZIO. Postoperative gastrointestinal electrical and mechanical activities in a patient with idiopathic intestinal pseudoobstruction. *Gastroenterology* 74: 112–120, 1978.
205. SARNA, S. K., R. KITAI, K. MUNIAPPAN, L. MARZIO, E. E. DANIEL, AND W. E. WATERFALL. Gastroduodenal coordination: a computer analysis. In: *Gastrointestinal Motility in Health and Disease*, edited by H. L. Duthie. Lancaster, UK: MTP, 1978, p. 271–272.
206. SARNA, S., P. LATIMER, D. CAMPBELL, AND W. E. WATERFALL. Effect of stress, meal and neostigmine on rectosigmoid electrical control activity (ECA) in normals and in irritable bowel syndrome patients. *Dig. Dis. Sci.* 27: 582–591, 1982.
207. SARNA, S., P. LATIMER, D. CAMPBELL, AND W. E. WATERFALL. Electrical and contractile activities of the human rectosigmoid. *Gut* 23: 698–705, 1982.
208. SARNA, S., P. NORTHCOTT, AND L. BELBECK. Mechanisms of cycling of migrating myoelectric complexes: effect of morphine. *Am. J. Physiol.* 242 (*Gastrointest. Liver Physiol.* 5): G588–G595, 1982.
209. SARNA, S. K., C. STODDARD, L. BELBECK, AND D. MCWADE. Intrinsic nervous control of migrating myoelectric complexes. *Am. J. Physiol.* 241 (*Gastrointest. Liver Physiol.* 4): G16–G23, 1981.
210. SARNA, S. K., W. E. WATERFALL, B. L. BARDAKJIAN, AND J. F. LIND. Types of human colonic electrical activities recorded postoperatively. *Gastroenterology* 81: 61–70, 1981.
211. SCHULZE-DELRIEU, K., AND S. S. SHIRAZI. Neuromuscular differentiation of the human pylorus. *Gastroenterology* 84: 287–292, 1983.
212. SCHULZE-DELRIEU, K., AND J. P. WALL. Determinants of flow across isolated gastroduodenal junctions of cats and rabbits. *Am. J. Physiol.* 245 (*Gastrointest. Liver Physiol.* 8): G257–G264, 1983.
213. SCHUSTER, M. Motor action of rectum and anal sphincters in continence and defecation. In: *Handbook of Physiology. Alimentary Canal Motility*, edited by Charles F. Code. Washington, DC: Am. Physiol. Soc., 1968, sect. 6, vol. 4, p. 2121–2146.
214. SHAFIK, A. A new concept of the anatomy of the anal sphincter mechanism and the physiology of defecation. III. The longitudinal anal muscle: anatomy and role in anal sphincter mechanism. *Invest. Urology* 13: 271–277, 1976.
215. SHEPHERD, G. M. *The Synaptic Organization of the Brain.* New York: Oxford Univ. Press, 1974.
216. SMOUT, A. J. P. M. Myoelectric Activity of the Stomach. Gastroelectromyography and electrogastrography. Amsterdam: Delft University Press, 1980. Thesis.
217. SMOUT, A. J. P. M., E. J. VAN DER SCHEE, AND J. L. GRASHUIS. Gastric pacemaker rhythm in conscious dogs. *Am. J. Physiol.* 237 (*Endocrinol. Metab. Gastrointest. Physiol.* 6): E279–E283, 1979.
218. SNAPE, W. J., JR., G. M. CARLSON, AND S. COHEN. Colonic myoelectric activity in the irritable bowel syndrome. *Gastroenterology* 70: 326–330, 1976.
219. SNAPE. W. J., JR., G. M. CARLSON, S. A. MATARAZZO, AND S. COHEN. Evidence that abnormal myoelectrical activity produces colonic motor dysfunction in the irritable bowel syndrome. *Gastroenterology* 72: 383–387, 1977.
220. SNAPE, W. J., JR., S. A. MATARAZZO, AND S. COHEN. Effect of eating and gastrointestinal hormones on human colonic myoelectrical and motor activity. *Gastroenterology* 75: 373–378, 1978.
221. SPERELAKIS, N. Lack of electrical coupling between contiguous myocardial cells in vertebrate hearts. In: *Comparative Physiology of the Heart: Current Trends*, edited by F. V. McCann. Basel: Birkhhäuser, 1969, p. 135–165.
222. SPERELAKIS, N. Electrophysiology of cultured chick heart cells. In: *Electrophysiology and Ultrastructure of the Heart*, edited by T. Sano, V. Mizuhira, and K. Matsuda. Tokyo: Bunkodo, 1967, p. 81–108.
223. SPERELAKIS, N. The possibility of propagation between myocardial cells not connected by low-resistance pathways. In: *Myocardial Injury*, edited by J. J. Spitzer. New York: Plenum, 1983, p. 1–23.
224. SPERELAKIS, N. Propagation mechanisms in heart. *Annu. Rev. Physiol.* 41: 441–457, 1979.
225. SPERELAKIS, N., T. HOSHIKO, AND R. M. BERNE. Nonsyncytial nature of cardiac muscle: membrane resistance of single

cells. *Am. J. Physiol.* 198: 531–536, 1960.
226. SPERELAKIS, N., B. LOBRACCO, JR., J. E. MANN, AND R. MARSCHALL. Accumulation de potassium dans les jonctions intercellulaires combinee aux interactions de champ electrique pour une propagation dans le muscle cardiaque. *Innov. Tech. Biol. Med.* 6: 24–43, 1985.
227. SPERELAKIS, N., AND J. E. MANN, JR. Evaluation of electric field changes in the cleft between excitable cells. *J. Theor. Biol.* 64: 71–96, 1977.
228. SPERELAKIS, N., R. A. MARSCHALL, AND J. E. MANN. Propagation down a chain of excitable cells by electric field interactions in the junctional clefts: effect of variation in extracellular resistances, including a "sucrose gap" simulation. *IEEE Trans. Biomed. Eng.* 30: 658–664, 1983.
229. SPERELAKIS, N., R. RUBIO, AND J. REDICK. Sharp discontinuity in sarcomere lengths across intercalated disks of fibrillating cat hearts. *J. Ultrastruct. Res.* 30: 503–532, 1970.
230. SPERELAKIS, N., AND M. TARR. Weak electrotonic interaction between neighboring visceral smooth muscle cells. *Am. J. Physiol.* 208: 737–747, 1965.
231. STEWART, J. J., T. F. BURKS, AND N. W. WEISBRODT. Intestinal myoelectric activity after activation of central emetic mechanism. *Am. J. Physiol.* 233 (*Endocrinol. Metab. Gastrointest. Physiol.* 2): E131–E137, 1977.
232. STODDARD, C. J., R. H. SMALLWOOD, AND H. L. DUTHIE. Electrical arrhythmias in the human stomach. *Gut* 22: 705–712, 1981.
233. SUGARBAKER, D. J., S. RATTAN, AND R. K. GOYAL. Mechanical and electrical activity of esophageal smooth muscle during peristalsis. *Am. J. Physiol.* 246 (*Gastrointest. Liver Physiol.* 9): G145–G150, 1984.
234. SUMMERS, R. W., J. CRAMER, AND A. J. FLATT. Computerized analysis of spike burst activity in the small intestine. *IEEE Trans. Biomed. Eng.* 29: 309–314, 1982.
235. SZURSZEWSKI, J. H. Electrical basis for gastrointestinal motility. In: *Physiology of the Gastrointestinal Tract*, edited by L. R. Johnson. New York: Raven, 1981, vol. 2, p. 1435–1466.
236. SZURSZEWSKI, J. H., L. R. ELVEBACK, AND C. F. CODE. Configuration and frequency gradient of electric slow wave over canine small bowel. *Am. J. Physiol.* 218: 1468–1473, 1970.
237. TAYLOR, I., C. DARBY, AND P. HAMMOND. Comparison of rectosigmoid myoelectrical activity in the irritable colon syndrome during relapses and remissions. *Gut* 19: 923–929, 1978.
238. TAYLOR, I., H. L. DUTHIE, R. SMALLWOOD, AND D. LINKENS. Large bowel myoelectrical activity in man. *Gut* 16: 808–814, 1975.
239. TELANDER, R. L., K. G. MORGAN, D. L. KREULEN, P. F. SCHMALZ, K. A. KELLY, AND J. H. SZURSZEWSKI. Human gastric atony with tachygastria and gastric retention. *Gastroenterology* 75: 497–501, 1978.
240. THOMPSON, D. G., AND J.-R. MALAGELADA. Vomiting and the small intestine. *Dig. Dis. Sci.* 27: 1121–1125, 1982.
241. TIEFFENBACH, L., AND C. ROMAN. Rôle de l'innervation extrinsique vagale dans la motricité de l'oesophage à musculeuse lisse: étude electromyographique chez le chat et le Babouin. *J. Physiol. Paris* 64: 193–226, 1972.
242. TILLE, J. Electronic interaction between muscle fibers in the rabbit ventricle. *J. Gen. Physiol.* 50: 189–202, 1966.
243. TOMITA, T. Electrophysiology of mammalian smooth muscle. *Prog. Biophys. Mol. Biol.* 30: 185–203, 1975.
244. TOOULI, J., W. J. DODDS, R. HONDA, S. SARNA, W. J. HOGAN, R. A. KOMAROWSKI, J. H. LINEHAN, AND R. C. ARNDORFER. Motor function of the opossum sphincter of Oddi. *J. Clin. Invest.* 71: 208–220, 1983.
245. TOOULI, J., J. E. GEENEN, W. J. HOGAN, W. J. DODDS, AND R. C. ARNDORFER. Sphincter of Oddi motor activity: a comparison between patients with common bile duct stones and controls. *Gastroenterology* 82: 111–117, 1982.
246. UEDA, M., J. F. SCHLEGEL, AND C. F. CODE. Electric and motor activity of innervated and vagally denervated feline esophagus. *Am. J. Dig. Dis.* 17: 1075–1088, 1972.
247. USTACH, T. J., F. TOBON, T. HAMBRECHT, D. D. BASS, AND M. M. SCHUSTER. Electrophysiological aspects of human sphincter function. *J. Clin. Invest.* 49: 41–48, 1970.
248. VAN DER SCHEE, E. J. *Electrogastrography. Signal Analytical Aspects and Interpretation.* Rotterdam: Krips Repro Meppel, 1984.
249. VAN DER SCHEE, E. J., A. J. P. M. SMOUT, AND J. L. GRASHIUS. Application of running spectrum analysis to electrogastrographic signals recorded from dogs and man. In: *Motility of the Digestive Tract*, edited by M. Wienbeck. New York: Raven, 1982, p. 241–250.
250. VAN OVERBEEK, J. J., H. P. WIT, R. H. PAPING, H. M. SEGENHOUT. Simultaneous manometry and electromyography in the pharyngoesophageal segment. *Laryngoscope* 95: 582–584, 1985.
251. VANTRAPPEN, G., J. HOSTEIN, J. JANSSENS, M. VANDEWEERD, AND I. DE WEVER. Do slow waves induce mechanical activity? (Abstract). *Gastroenterology* 84: 1341, 1983.
252. WANKLING, W. J., B. H. BROWN, C. D. COLLINS, AND H. L. DUTHIE. Basal electrical activity in the anal canal in man. *Gut* 9: 457–460, 1968.
253. WATERFALL, W. E., B. H. BROWN, H. L. DUTHIE, AND G. E. WHITTAKER. The effects of humoral agents on the myoelectrical activity of the terminal ileum. *Gut* 13: 528–534, 1972.
254. WATERFALL, W. E., G. S. CAMERON, S. K. SARNA, T. D. LEWIS, AND E. E. DANIEL. Disorganised electrical activity in a child with idiopathic intestinal pseudo-obstruction. *Gut* 22: 77–83, 1981.
255. WATERFALL, W. E., S. K. SARNA, AND J. F. LIND. Myogenic and neuronal control mechanisms in oesophageal motility. *Ann. R. Coll. Physicians Surg. Can.* 39, 1976.
256. WIEDMANN, S. Electrical coupling between myocardial cells. *Prog. Brain Res.* 21: 275–281, 1969.
257. WEISBRODT, N. W. Neuromuscular organization of esophageal and pharyngeal motility. *Arch. Intern. Med.* 136: 524–531, 1976.
258. WEISBRODT, N. W., AND J. CHRISTENSEN. Gradients of contractions in the opossum esophagus. *Gastroenterology* 62: 1159–1166, 1972.
259. WEISBRODT, N. W., AND J. CHRISTENSEN. Electrical activity of the cat duodenum in fasting and vomiting. *Gastroenterology* 63: 1004–1010, 1972.
260. WIENBECK, M. The electrical activity of the cat colon in vivo. I. The normal electrical activity and its relationship to contractile activity. *Res. Exp. Med.* 158: 268–279, 1972.
261. WIENBECK, M., J. CHRISTENSEN, AND N. W. WEISBRODT. Electromyography of the colon in the unanesthetized cat. *Am. J. Dig. Dis.* 17: 356–362, 1972.
262. WIENBECK, M., AND H. JANSSEN. Electrical control mechanisms at the ileo-colic junction. In: *Proc. 4th Int. Symp. on Gastrointest. Motil.* Vancouver, Canada: Mitchell, 1973, p. 97–106.
263. WINGATE, D., T. BARNETT, R. GREEN, AND M. ARMSTRONG-JAMES. Automated high speed analysis of gastrointestinal myoelectric activity. *Am. J. Dig. Dis.* 22: 243–251, 1977.
264. WOOD, J. D. Intrinsic neural control of intestinal motility. *Annu. Rev. Physiol.* 43: 33–51, 1981.
265. WOOD, J. D. Physiology of the enteric nervous system. In: *Physiology of the Gastrointestinal Tract*, edited by L. R. Johnson. New York: Raven, 1981, vol. 1, p. 1–37.
266. YOU, C. H., AND W. Y. CHEY. Study of electromechanical activity of the stomach in humans and in dogs with particular attention to tachygastria. *Gastroenterology* 86: 1460–1468, 1984.
267. YOU, C. H., K. Y. LEE, W. Y. CHEY, AND R. MENGUY. Electrogastrographic study of patients with unexplained nausea, bloating and vomiting. *Gastroenterology* 79: 311–314, 1980.

# CHAPTER 22

# Esophageal motility

RAJ K. GOYAL
WILLIAM G. PATERSON

*Charles A. Dana Institute and Thorndike Laboratory, Harvard Digestive Disease Center, Division of Gastroenterology, Beth Israel Hospital and Harvard Medical School, Boston, Massachusetts*

## CHAPTER CONTENTS

Overview of Esophageal Motor Function
  General anatomy
  Innervation of esophagus and sphincters
    Efferent (motor) innervation
    Intrinsic innervation
    Interstitial cells of Cajal
    Afferent (sensory) innervation
  Deglutition reflex
    Initiation of swallowing reflex
    Central organization of swallowing reflex
  Methods of study
Upper Esophageal Sphincter
  Anatomy
  Pressure profile
    Basal pressure fluctuations
    Basal sphincter pressures
    Pressures during swallowing
    Electromyographic correlates
  Control of upper esophageal sphincter
    Maintenance of resting tone
    Reflex increases in pressure
    Reflex relaxation
Esophageal Body
  Muscular anatomy
  Pressure profile
    Basal pressures
    Swallow-induced responses
    Distension-induced responses
  Central control of esophageal peristalsis
    Striated muscle portion
    Smooth muscle portion
  Peripheral control of esophageal peristalsis
    Striated muscle portion
    Smooth muscle portion
  Peripheral control of peristalsis in esophageal smooth muscle
  Peristalsis in the junctional zone
  Role of longitudinal muscle layer and muscularis mucosa in peristalsis
Lower Esophageal Sphincter
  Muscular anatomy
  Pressure profile
    Fluctuations in basal pressure
    Basal sphincter pressure
  Genesis of basal sphincter pressure
    Mechanical factors
    Basal sphincter muscle tone
  Genesis of lower esophageal sphincter muscle tone
    Tonic excitatory nerve activity
    Local release of excitatory biological agents
    Circulating excitatory hormone activity
    Intrinsic circular muscle activity
  Modulation of resting pressure in lower esophageal sphincter
  Reflex relaxation of the lower esophageal sphincter
    Cellular basis of relaxation
    Swallow-induced relaxation
    Relaxation associated with esophageal distension
  Neurotransmitters in inhibitory pathway to lower esophageal sphincter
    Synaptic transmitters
    Inhibitory neurotransmitter
    Other neurotransmitters
  Reflex contractions of the lower esophageal sphincter

---

THE ESOPHAGUS is a hollow muscular organ closed at the rostral and caudal ends by the upper and lower esophageal sphincters, respectively. The primary function of the esophagus is to propel the food or fluid boluses from the pharynx into the stomach. This is achieved through a carefully sequenced, aborally progressing peristaltic contraction in concert with appropriately timed relaxation of the sphincters. The sphincters play an important role in preventing retrograde flow of gastric and esophageal contents. The esophagus and its sphincters also participate in several other reflex activities such as vomiting, belching, and responses to esophageal distension. The purpose of this chapter is to provide a critical review of esophageal motor function with special emphasis on the physiological mechanisms involved in peristalsis and sphincteric function. Pharyngeal motility is not discussed, therefore the reader is referred to several reviews that cover this and other topics related to swallowing (13, 39, 44, 60, 61, 70, 72, 94, 95, 98, 136, 143, 164, 197, 210, 212, 218, 225, 256, 263, 342, 359, 369, 377, 419, 423, 502, 512).

This chapter is organized into two parts. The first is an overview of esophageal motor function, including general anatomy, innervation, reflex activities in which the esophagus and its sphincters participate, and methods of study. The second is a detailed discussion of the anatomy and physiology of the three distinct functional components: the upper esophageal sphincter (UES), the esophageal body, and the lower esophageal sphincter (LES).

## OVERVIEW OF ESOPHAGEAL MOTOR FUNCTION

### General Anatomy

The esophageal wall, like other regions of the gut, consists of mucosa, submucosa, and muscularis propria; however, unlike the other regions it has no serosal covering. The outer esophageal wall is bounded by a thin, poorly defined layer of connective tissue (359).

The mucosa consists of stratified squamous epithelium in all regions except the LES, where both squamous and columnar epithelium may coexist. In the pathological condition known as Barrett's esophagus, columnar epithelium is seen to extend up into the esophageal body (22). Relatively few glands are present in the esophageal mucosa, hence its secretory function is rather limited.

The muscularis propria consists of an inner circular layer and an outer longitudinal layer; contraction of the former serves to constrict the esophageal lumen, whereas contraction of the latter shortens the esophagus along its long axis. In addition to these muscle layers there is a longitudinally oriented muscle layer called the muscularis mucosa located between the muscle layers and the mucosa.

Neurons intrinsic to the esophageal wall are organized into two main plexuses as in other regions of the gut. The submucous (Meissner's) plexus lies in the submucosa, whereas the myenteric (Auerbach's) plexus is between the circular and longitudinal muscle layers.

### Innervation of Esophagus and Sphincters

EFFERENT (MOTOR) INNERVATION. The esophagus and its sphincters are controlled by efferent nerve fibers that arise from cell bodies located in the motor vagal nuclei of the brain stem. The somatic motor fibers to the striated muscles (UES and upper portion of the esophagus) arise from neurons located in the nucleus retrofacialis and most rostral portion of the nucleus ambiguus (164, 190, 248, 306, 439, 525). The preganglionic fibers that innervate the smooth muscle portion of the esophagus and LES arise from cell bodies located in the dorsal motor nucleus of the vagus as well as from cells located in the nucleus ambiguus (21, 190, 358).

The axons of the lower motoneurons that supply the pharyngeal muscles travel through the vagus nerves into the superior pharyngeal nerves, which arise from the vagal trunks at the level of the nodose ganglion. The nerves from either side form the pharyngeal plexus, which sends branches to pharyngeal muscles, including the cricopharyngeus muscle and the upper portion of the esophagus. There is some anatomical variation among species. In the dog and cat, for example, the cricopharyngeus is innervated by a separate branch of the vagus called the pharyngoesophageal nerve (261, 296, 326, 350). Similar observations have not been made in humans (327, 328).

Motor fibers to the striated muscle portion of the esophagus also arise from the vagus. These, however, originate in the upper portion of the neck. Therefore electrical stimulation of the vagus nerve in the midportion of the neck produces no response in the striated muscle segment of the esophagus. The lower motoneurons are myelinated and make direct contact with individual striated muscle fibers via the motor end plate (486). Acetylcholine is the neurotransmitter involved at the motor end plate, exerting its effects through stimulation of nicotinic cholinergic receptors (486).

The preganglionic fibers to the smooth muscle portion of the esophagus and the LES are also carried along the vagus nerves. These fibers then branch to form the esophageal plexus and finally enter the esophagus at different levels (372, 477). It appears that these preganglionic fibers travel within the esophageal wall for several centimeters before reaching the postganglionic neurons in the intramural plexuses (277, 302).

The smooth muscle portion of the esophagus and LES also receive a sympathetic nerve supply that arises from the cell bodies in the intermediolateral cell columns of spinal segments $T_1$–$T_{10}$ (358, 526). Preganglionic fibers enter the cervical sympathetic ganglia, ganglia in the thoracic sympathetic chain, and possibly the celiac ganglia. Most fibers to the lower esophagus travel in the greater splanchnic nerves to enter the celiac ganglia where they synapse with postganglionic neurons (25, 184, 358). Postganglionic branches accompany the blood vessels, and a few fibers join the vagus to reach the esophagus. Most of the postganglionic axons terminate in the myenteric plexus (25, 266) and submucosal plexus (194). Very few terminate directly on the muscle cells. The density of the adrenergic innervation is lesser in the lower sphincter than in the more proximal esophagus (25).

INTRINSIC INNERVATION. Intramural neurons and their extensions make up the intrinsic nervous system of the esophagus. The intramural nerves are arranged in layers; the myenteric plexus is located between the circular and longitudinal muscle layer, and the submucosal plexus is located in the submucosa. The myenteric plexus has been found as high as 1 cm below the cricopharyngeal muscle in humans (442). The plexus is sparse in the striated muscle region. Some speculate that it is involved in the innervation of esophageal glands or in sensory functions. The intramural ganglia are similar in structure throughout the gastrointestinal tract, but in the esophagus the intramural neurons are fewer in number and more haphazard in arrangement than elsewhere in the gut (80, 83, 193, 450, 460).

Although the intrinsic neural elements in the LES are generally similar to those in the esophageal body, certain differences do exist. When the myenteric plexus is examined in esophageal whole mounts after dissecting the longitudinal muscle layer from the circular muscle layer (peel preparation), the density of perikarya and ganglia decline as one proceeds distally in the esophagus, being lowest in the LES (83). This apparent decrease in density, however, may merely be a function of technique. When sagittal sections of the esophageal wall are examined, many more neurons are detected in the LES than in the esophageal body. Many of these neurons are misplaced; that is, they are found in areas other than between the longitudinal and circular muscle layers (450) and thus are not identified by the peel technique. Neuronal cell bodies in the LES are smaller due to the tonically contracted state of the sphincter (450).

Intramural neurons have been classified on the basis of morphological, histochemical, functional, and electrical features (214). Their affinity for silver stains divides them into argyrophilic and argyrophobic types, with the majority being argyrophobic (460). Axons from the intramural neurons branch out as they approach the smooth muscle or other effector cells. Synaptic contact is signaled by the appearance of varicosities in the nerve fibers. These varicosities are filled with neurotransmitter vesicles of various sizes, shapes, and densities (52). More than one vesicle type frequently occurs in the same nerve varicosity (52, 448). Immunocytochemical techniques have permitted the identification of a large number of potential neurotransmitters within the neurons of the esophagus (1, 2, 25, 192, 308, 447, 492, 493).

As in the esophageal body, nerve varicosities in the LES contain a mixture of small agranular and large granular synaptic vesicles (121, 448). The large granular vescicles presumably contain the noncholinergic, nonadrenergic inhibitory neurotransmitter (see ESOPHAGEAL BODY, p. 873).

INTERSTITIAL CELLS OF CAJAL. Recently there has been renewed interest in the esophageal interstitial cells of Cajal (121, 178). These cells have been well defined by electron microscopy and are neither neuronal nor musclar in origin. In the esophagus they are found interspersed between nerve varicosities and circular smooth muscle cells, forming gap-junction contact with both cell types. This anatomical evidence is consistent with the intercalation theory of Imaizumi and Hama (262), which suggests that interstitial cells of Cajal may play a role in disseminating electrical activity from the nerve to the muscle.

In the opossum, it appears that interstitial cells of Cajal make gap-junction contact with smooth muscle more commonly in the esophageal body than in the LES (81, 121).

AFFERENT (SENSORY) INNERVATION. Little is known about the sensory innervation of the pharyngeal muscles that comprise the upper esophageal sphincter; however, a $\gamma$-efferent system is not present (164). Afferent fibers are carried via the vagus to the nucleus solitarius and from there make many complicated projections within the brain (190, 438).

Sensation from the esophageal body and lower esophageal sphincter in the cat is carried via the vagus as well as the splanchnic and thoracic sympathetic nerves and the sympathetic cardiac branch from the stellate ganglion (89). The vagal afferent fibers have their cell bodies in the nodose ganglion and project to the nucleus solitarius (190, 439). Sympathetic afferents travel via dorsal root ganglia into the spinal cord at $T_1$ to $L_2$.

Ultrastructural studies by Rodrigo et al. (413–417) reveal the presence of perivascular and free nerve endings in the esophageal submucosa of cats, as well as free intraepithelial nerve endings and peculiar tape-like nerve endings within the myenteric ganglia. The latter have been termed *intraganglionic laminar endings* (414) and are thought to be ideally located to serve as mechanoreceptors (72). The afferent nature of all these endings has been confirmed by studies that show their degeneration after extirpation of the nodose ganglion (415, 416).

There is now abundant electrophysiological evidence, obtained primarily in the cat, for the existence of different types of mechanoreceptors as well as thermoreceptors in the esophageal body and LES (91–93, 171, 337, 338, 436). Most of these sensory fibers are the unmyelinated C or myelinated $A_s$ fibers (91, 93, 171, 337). Muscular mechanoreceptors are spontaneously active and slowly adapting when stimulated by stretching or muscle contraction (91–93, 175, 176, 337). Mucosal and serosal mechanoreceptors are rapidly adapting (91–93, 337). Both morphological (414) and physiological (175) studies suggest that the afferent receptors are concentrated at the upper and the lower portions of the thoracic esophagus.

Recently calcitonin gene-related peptide (CGRP) has been found within esophageal sensory neurons (417). Others, neurons presumably, contain acetylcholine as well (175). The physiological role of putative neurotransmitters in the sensory fibers within the esophagus is unknown. They may be involved in autoregulation or in various reflex functions such as the esophageal motor response to distension.

Indirect evidence indicates that, in addition to stretch receptors, osmo- and chemoreceptors may also be present in the UES, LES, and esophageal body (107, 189, 196, 255, 271, 272, 282, 323, 505). However, the precise nature of these receptors and their connections is not known.

## Deglutition Reflex

Little thought is given to the complex act of deglutition, which is performed ~600 times per day in normal adults (309). The deglutition process can be divided into voluntary and involuntary phases. The voluntary (oral) phase consists of transport of the bolus to the oropharynx. This occurs after mastication and mixing with saliva has allowed positioning of an appropriate-sized bolus in the middle of the dorsum of the tongue. A wavelike contraction then ensues, starting from the anterior part of the tongue and working backward to squeeze the bolus against the hard palate and propel it toward the oropharynx. The posterior part of the tongue is depressed to form a grooved chute. As the bolus reaches the oropharynx, sensory receptors are activated that initiate the involuntary phase of the deglutition reflex. The motor expression of the deglutition reflex is called primary peristalsis, and its onset is marked by contraction of the mylohyoid muscle. The deglutitive activity occurring in the UES, esophageal body, and LES ensues (Fig. 1).

INITIATION OF SWALLOWING REFLEX. Receptors in the base of the tongue, tonsils, anterior and posterior pillars of the fauces, soft palate, uvula, posterior pharyngeal wall, epiglottis, and larynx are involved in the initiation of the deglutition reflex (94, 164, 376, 452). There are significant interspecies differences in the relative sensitivity of these areas in initiating deglutition. In humans, the anterior and posterior tonsillar pillars and posterior wall of the pharynx appear to be the most sensitive areas for initiating the reflex (376). The nature of the receptors is unclear. They are apparently very superficial in that when fluid of different chemical composition is applied to sensitive regions, the deglutition reflex is quickly activated (452). The afferents initiating the deglutitive reflex are carried in the maxillary branch of the trigeminal nerve, the glossopharyngeal nerve, and the superior laryngeal branch of the vagus nerve (45, 485).

Swallowing can be initiated voluntarily from the cerebral cortex (56, 275, 476) but probably requires some additional sensory input from the pharynx, because voluntary deglutition is very difficult when the pharynx is anesthetized or if there is no bolus present (434). Esophageal distension may also induce swallowing in humans (329), as does perfusion of the esophagus with a fluid of low pH (329) and reflux of gastric acid (20, 137, 149, 364). These stimuli may also evoke secondary peristalsis in other species that have smooth muscle in the esophagus; however, in animals with an entirely skeletal muscle esophageal body, such as sheep, the peristaltic wave seen with esophageal distension is not secondary but is primary, resulting from activation of the deglutition reflex (94, 259, 421).

Electrical stimulation of the superior laryngeal nerve is a popular method of inducing swallowing in experimental animals. Depending on the stimulus parameters, superior laryngeal nerve afferent stimulation can also cause gagging (163). In the opossum, contraction of the cricopharyngeus, which resembles gagging, is elicited after the onset of superior laryngeal

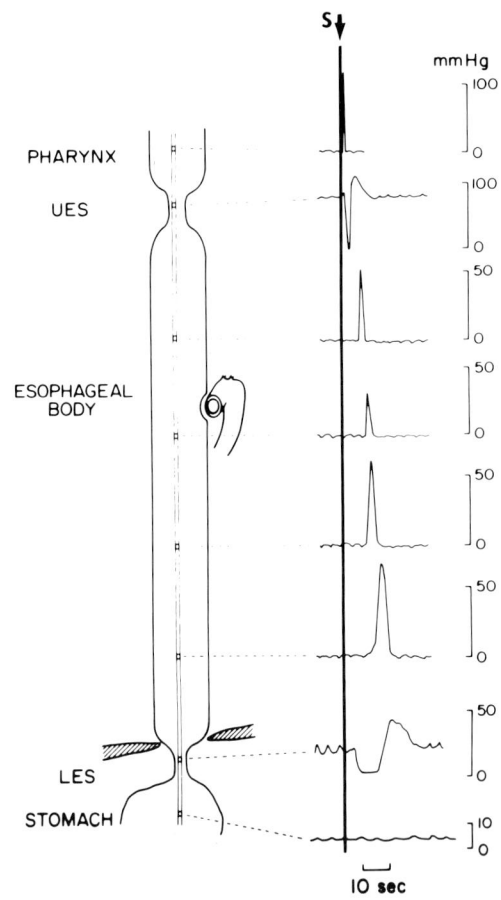

FIG. 1. Primary peristalsis as recorded by intraluminal manometry. Between swallows, pharynx reflects atmospheric, esophageal intrapleural, and stomach intra-abdominal pressures. Upper and lower esophageal sphincters (UES and LES) are identified as high-pressure zones. Swallowing causes a rapidly propagated, short-duration pharyngeal contraction coincident with abrupt relaxation of the UES, which is followed by postrelaxation UES contractions. Esophageal body shows peristaltic contraction that causes an aborally migrating pressure wave. The LES relaxes within 1–2 s of onset of swallowing and remains relaxed until esophageal pressure wave has reached distal esophagus; this usually takes 5–10 s. Lower esophageal sphincter pressure then recovers and a postrelaxation contraction occurs in upper part of sphincter in continuity with esophageal contraction. Duration of esophageal contractions increases distally. Contraction amplitude is greatest in pharynx and greater in distal smooth muscle esophagus than in proximal striated muscle esophagus. In the transition zone, where both striated and smooth muscle coexist, contraction amplitudes are the least. Propagation velocity of esophageal peristaltic wave increases in mid-esophagus and then slows to its lowest level distally. Swallowed food bolus is propelled ahead of peristaltic contraction.

stimulation. However, with continued stimulation, cricopharyngeal inhibition associated with the swallowing reflex is induced (12).

Recent studies in rats suggest that central serotonergic and muscarinic receptors are involved in the initiation of deglutition (36, 37). In humans pirenzepine, a selective $M_1$ antagonist, decreases the number of spontaneous swallows. It is not clear whether this is secondary to central blockade or inhibition of salivation (466).

CENTRAL ORGANIZATION OF SWALLOWING REFLEX. Afferent input to the swallowing center activates the swallowing reflex. The swallowing center refers to a well-organized central nervous system mechanism that executes the deglutition reflex and is located in the brain stem. It is more a functional center than a well-defined anatomical entity. Improved methods of anatomical investigation are needed to define the swallowing center (248). Once activated, the swallowing center initiates a predictable sequence of contractile events that depend on a stereotypic pattern of discharge and inhibition of various medullary motoneurons (164, 274, 276). The swallowing center interacts with other brain stem centers, most notably that which controls respiration (66, 87, 124, 164, 165, 305, 437, 475). The swallowing center can be activated to produce the deglutitive-activity reflex independent of cortical or sensory afferent input. However, it appears that the extensive afferent input that this center receives modifies the characteristics of the efferent deglutitive discharge (275, 276).

It was previously believed that the deglutition reflex was an all-or-none phenomenon; however, it now appears that the deglutition reflex can be partially activated. For example, low-intensity afferent stimulation of the deglutition center may result in LES relaxation alone or LES relaxation along with mylohyoid contraction but without pharyngeal or esophageal contraction (370).

## Methods of Study

Motility of the esophagus and its sphincters has been studied in many ways. The most readily performed technique involves the measurement of intraluminal pressure with water-filled catheters, catheter-tip miniature transducers, or small balloons. Balloons are no longer used, however, because of poor fidelity as well as other technical problems (157, 410). In the past the catheters employed were either unperfused or had high compliance. Such systems were particularly unsuitable for recording high-frequency events in the pharynx, leading to an underestimation of the amplitude of pressure transients (152, 157, 410). High-compliance perfusion-catheter systems require an excessive volume of perfusate to obtain adequate recording fidelity (55), therefore low-compliance perfusion-catheter systems (9, 224, 519) or catheter-tip transducers (254, 509) are currently the most frequently used recording methods. Dent (135) developed a perfused sleeve catheter for long-term recording of sphincter pressures. The sleeve records the highest static or oscillatory pressure acting at any point along its 6-cm length (318) and is thought to minimize the problem of axial movement of the recording site in relation to the sphincter. However, sliding of the high-pressure zone along the sleeve may introduce artifacts, and changes in pressures in the esophageal body and the stomach may modify the recorded LES pressures. For example, the duration of relaxation of the sphincter may be underestimated by this sleeve because the proximal part of the sleeve is usually located in the distal esophagus and therefore records the pressure generated by the peristaltic contraction while the sphincter itself may still be relaxed. Other catheter modifications for recording the sphincter pressure have also been described (503).

Because the esophagus is a hollow tube with potential openings at either end, the recorded pressures do not measure the true intraluminal pressures that are obtained from closed, fluid-filled cavities such as the heart or blood vessels. The pressure recorded in the esophagus is due to a direct squeeze by the esophageal muscle on the pressure-sensitive catheter tip.

Motility can also be studied by observing the passage of a swallowed barium bolus with cineradiography (14, 85, 95, 429). With film speeds in the range of 30 frames per second, the time sequence of events can be accurately determined. Simultaneously performed manometric studies show that the peristaltic contractile activity actually follows the tail of the barium bolus, and movement through the sphincters occurs while they are relaxed (95). After a barium swallow, radiographic activity may persist for 10 s, but the manometric activity lasts up to 20 s. Radioisotope techniques are now available for quantitating esophageal transit. These techniques provide a reproducible measure of bolus transport along the esophagus and may be more sensitive at detecting abnormalities of esophageal motor function than are standard manometric studies (41, 293, 297, 430, 484). In addition manometric and transit studies provide information on integrated activities of different muscle components (circular muscle, longitudinal muscle, and muscularis mucosa) in the esophageal wall. Activities of individual muscle layers can be studied in vivo in experimental animals by sewing strain gauges to the esophagus in the axis of the longitudinal or circular muscles (474).

It is also possible to record myoelectrical activity with bipolar or monopolar electrodes (8, 67, 198, 219, 235–237, 311, 421, 424). This is clearly better suited for experimental animals in whom electrodes can be sewn to the outside of the esophagus. Electrical activity has also been recorded in humans intraluminally by means of bipolar electrodes. Bipolar ring electrodes (365) are the least invasive but have the problem of loss of mucosal contact and axial movement (116). Intraluminal suction cups may reduce the problem of electrode contact with the mucosa (378), but these are difficult to use. Electrical recordings usually provide a more precise measure of the onset of muscle activity than they do of the peristaltic pressure wave itself because other pressure changes, such as those transmitted by the bolus or arising in extrinsic structures, may precede the actual peristaltic contraction. In the intact animal electrical recordings represent the sum of activities in different muscle layers.

Electrical and mechanical activity in the striated muscle segment of the esophagus are virtually simultaneous. Electrical activity is present throughout the period of contraction, and the intensity of spike activity is related to the strength of the contraction. In the smooth muscle segment, electrical and mechanical contractions are usually coupled; although electromechanical dissociation does occasionally occur (219). Electrical activity in the smooth muscle segment precedes the mechanical activity by a small latency interval (219), and the spike activity ceases at or near the peak of the muscle contraction (502). A qualitative estimation of changes in membrane potentials of cells in intact animals can be made by using suction electrodes. These studies show that swallowing is associated with immediate membrane hyperpolarization followed by depolarization and spike burst that correlates with esophageal contractions (381, 473).

Peristaltic propulsive force, that is, the force with which a solid bolus in the esophagus is moved aborally during peristalsis, has been studied with intraluminal fixed balloons attached to a device that measures the pulling force (259, 441, 521). Similarly, the strength of sphincter tone has been estimated by measuring the force required to pull a distended balloon through the tonically contracted sphincter (101).

Motor activity also can be studied in vitro by measuring the tonic and phasic contractions of muscle strips that are bathed in oxygenated physiological solutions and are connected to force transducers (64, 69, 73, 77, 78, 112, 113, 127, 325, 513). Studying the effects of pharmacological manipulation and electrical field stimulation of intramural neurons provides valuable information on the physiology and pharmacology of esophageal motor function. Longitudinal muscle, circular muscle, or muscularis mucosa can be studied separately with this technique. In addition, the electrical activity of single esophageal smooth muscle cells can be recorded with intracellular microelectrodes (114, 129, 288).

## UPPER ESOPHAGEAL SPHINCTER

### Anatomy

The upper esophageal sphincter (UES) refers to a zone of intraluminal high pressure that exists between the pharynx and the upper esophagus. Anatomically the pharynx is continuous with the esophagus, and there is no well-defined structure that can be called the UES. Thus there is controversy as to what structures constitute the UES (451).

The cricopharyngeus mucle has oblique and horizontal components (359, 366, 506). It is generally agreed that the horizontal portion of the cricopharyngeus is part of the UES. This muscle, however, is only 1 cm wide (24, 43, 94, 172) and therefore cannot itself account for the entire high-pressure zone, which measures between 2 and 4 cm (14, 94, 172, 229, 264, 366, 418, 463, 502). To account for the discrepancy between the width of the cricopharyngeus muscle and the measured length of the high-pressure zone comprising the UES, several explanations have been offered. Some investigators believe that circular muscle fibers of the proximal esophagus (172, 527) make up the remainder of the UES, whereas others believe that oblique fibers of the cricopharyngeus (also called the inferior pharyngeal constrictor muscle) contribute to the high-pressure zone (12). Still other investigators feel that both inferior pharyngeal constrictor and esophageal muscle fibers join with the cricopharyngeus in forming the UES (94, 263).

A tonically contracted striated muscle should be associated with continuous electrical spike potentials, as is evidenced in the cricopharyngeus at rest (5, 12, 57, 237, 311, 453). Studies in the opossum demonstrate that the inferior pharyngeal constrictor muscle also exhibits continuous spike activity at rest (12), whereas esophageal fibers just distal to the cricopharyngeus are quiescent at rest. Moreover the manometric high-pressure zone extended from the lower level of cricoid cartilage caudally to the lower border of the laryngeal opening orally. This area represents the anatomical extent of the cricopharyngeus and the inferior pharyngeal constrictor. These studies suggest that the UES, at least in the opossum, corresponds to the anatomic hypopharynx.

In humans, the area that extends from the laryngeal opening (bottom of the air column on a lateral X ray of pharynx) to the lower border of the cricoid cartilage is ~3.2 cm. The arytenoid and interarytenoid muscles extend vertically down 0.75 cm from the laryngeal opening (359) and the cricoid lamina extends 2.5 cm vertically below that (426). The cricopharyngeus muscle (horizontal component) extends to the lower one-third of the cartilage. It appears that if the high-pressure zone extends for ~3 cm below the air column (95), the hypopharynx along with the oblique and horizontal fibers of the cricopharyngeus muscle posterolaterally, the posterior surface of the cricoid cartilage anteriorly, and the pyriform sinuses laterally, can fully account for the UES without incriminating part of the cervical esophagus. Mucosal squeeze alone may explain the small elevation of pressure that extends further into the esophagus. Such indirect evidence indicates that the anatomic hypopharynx, in conjunction with the cricopharyngeus and inferior pharyngeal constrictor muscles, may also constitute the UES in humans.

Plain X-ray films cannot delineate the lumen of the

UES because the anterior and posterior walls of the lower hypopharynx are closely opposed (502). When barium contrast studies are performed, certain anatomic features may be observed during the swallowing phase. The uppermost portion of the cricoid cartilage may produce an indentation on the anterior wall, commencing at the $C_5$ to $C_6$ vertebral level, and the postcricoid venous plexus (375) may be seen as an impression at the lower border of the cricoid cartilage. The posterior wall of the pharynx is smooth in the upper part; however, in the lower part, the cricopharyngeus muscle may sometimes form a posterior indentation termed the *hypopharyngeal bar* at the $C_5$ to $C_7$ vertebral level (49, 446, 454, 479). Because of the upward displacement of the cricoid associated with swallowing, the cricopharyngeus is frequently seen obliquely oriented and located below the level of the lower border of the cricoid cartilage (295).

In summary, the UES mechanism is functionally comprised of the muscular cartilagenous hypopharynx along with the cricoid cartilage ventrally and the cricopharyngeus and inferior pharyngeal constrictor muscles both dorsally and laterally.

*Pressure Profile*

The closing pressure of the UES varies somewhat with the circumstances under which the measurements are made. Studies with simultaneous manometry and lateral cineradiography demonstrate that the high-pressure zone begins immediately below the pharyngeal air column and extends caudally for 2–4 cm (14, 94, 172, 195, 229, 264, 295, 366, 463, 512). If one considers even minor elevations of pressure the UES may measure close to 6 cm (418). The pressure profile along the UES shows asymmetry with a sharp ascent in its upper part and a more gradual decline in its lower part (229, 463). There is also marked radial asymmetry (12, 517, 518). The peak pressures are much higher when the recording orifice faces either anterior or posterior than when it faces laterally. With a low-compliance perfused manometric catheter with multiple radially arranged holes at the same level, Welch et al. (517) were able to construct a three-dimensional pressure profile of the UES. Not only did they record pressures to be higher in the anterior-posterior than in the lateral orientation, but they also documented a dissociation of peak pressures along the anterior and posterior aspects. The peak pressure occurs 1 cm below the upper border of the high-pressure zone anteriorly and 2 cm below the upper portion of the high-pressure zone posteriorly. The radial and axial asymmetry was not observed after laryngectomy, indicating that the rigid cartilages of the larynx forming the anterior wall of the UES are responsible for the asymmetry (517).

BASAL PRESSURE FLUCTUATIONS. When a manometric catheter is positioned at various levels in the high-pressure zone and the patient is breathing quietly, baseline pressure fluctuations are observed. Near the peak in the high-pressure zone the pressure increases with inspiration, whereas on either side of the peak, the pressure falls with inspiration (229). The average increase in peak pressure with inspiration in an unoriented catheter system is ~6.5 mmHg (229).

BASAL SPHINCTER PRESSURES. The recorded resting UES pressure may vary, depending on the radial and axial orientation of the recording device within the sphincter, the respiratory phase, the diameter of the catheter assembly, the size of the pressure-sensing hole, the fidelity of the recording system, spontaneous and reflex alterations in UES tone, and the characteristics of the normal subjects used for the studies. It is therefore difficult to provide a single value for resting UES pressure.

Reported resting UES pressures in normal subjects have ranged from 35 to 200 mmHg (152, 195, 510, 517, 518). Pressure recorded with laterally oriented manometric devices are 33% of the magnitude of pressures recorded when the device is oriented in the anterior or posterior direction. Resting UES pressures may be lower in infancy (464), in the aged (510), and during sleep (285).

PRESSURES DURING SWALLOWING. The UES opens with each swallow to permit passage of the bolus into the esophagus (see Fig. 1). Pressure recordings demonstrate a fall in UES pressure immediately after the onset of deglutition. Pressures at the nadir of relaxation may reach subatmospheric levels (14, 463) but do not reach intraesophageal levels. Occasionally, a short period (0.2 s) of slight increase in UES tone may precede the relaxation (57) and may be related to inspiratory contraction of the cricopharyngeus. This pattern is commonly recorded in laryngectomized humans (453).

The nadir in UES pressure is sometimes interrupted by a brief increase in pressure that corresponds to the backward movement of the tongue (T wave). The relaxation of the UES, recorded manometrically, lasts from 0.5 to 1.0 s (263, 418). After relaxation the UES contracts in continuity with the pharyngeal peristaltic wave, producing an elevation in pressure approximately twice that of the resting level. This aftercontraction persists for another 1 s (94) before resting UES pressure is resumed.

ELECTROMYOGRAPHIC CORRELATES. Electromyographic recordings of the cricopharyngeus muscle correlate directly with the pressure recorded intraluminally. The resting UES pressure is associated with continuous spike activity in the cricopharyngeus muscle (5, 12, 57, 311, 453, 496, 502) and in the inferior pharyngeal constrictor (12). A brief increase in spike activity lasting for ~0.2 s and corresponding to the brief inspiratory effort associated with swallowing may be observed (12, 57, 502). The intensity of spike activity is directly proportional to the intraluminal pressure. Spike activity is inhibited starting ~0.2 s after the onset of deglutition, as marked by mylohyoid activation. The inhibition persists for 0.5 s (range 0.2–0.8) and is followed by an intense spike burst that lasts for ~1 s (501, 502). Tonic basal UES spike activity returns to resting levels after this burst (Fig. 2).

*Control of Upper Esophageal Sphincter*

The UES functions to prevent the entry of air into the esophagus during inspiration, and the regurgitation of gastric and esophageal contents into the pharynx. During swallowing it must relax and open for a very short period of time to allow passage of the bolus. Proper coordination between UES relaxation and pharyngeal and esophageal contraction is imperative if the act of swallowing is to proceed smoothly. The physiological mechanisms underlying the genesis of resting UES pressure, resting-pressure modulation, and UES relaxation are controversial.

MAINTENANCE OF RESTING TONE. Several studies have demonstrated continuous electrical spike activity in the cricopharyngeus muscle (5, 12, 237, 311, 350, 453, 496). The interpretation of this activity, however, is a subject of debate. Doty concluded that resting UES closure was entirely due to passive forces caused by elasticity of the tissues, and that tonic electrical spike activity is artifactual and caused by reflex stimulation initiated by the intraluminal manometry tube (164). Asoh and Goyal (12), in contrast, performed studies in opossums indicating that continuous electrical spike activity in both the cricopharyngeus and the caudalmost fibers of the inferior pharyngeal constrictor muscle combined with passive forces are responsible for resting UES pressure. In Asoh and Goyal's study (12), when electromyographic activity in the muscle ceased, there was a significant reduction in simultaneously measured UES pressure (Fig. 2). The continuous spike activity from these muscles was present with or without an intraluminal manometry tube and therefore was not likely to be artifactual. It is noteworthy that a small amount of pressure persisted when all muscle activity had ceased, indicating that passive forces did contribute to the resting UES pressure (Fig. 3).

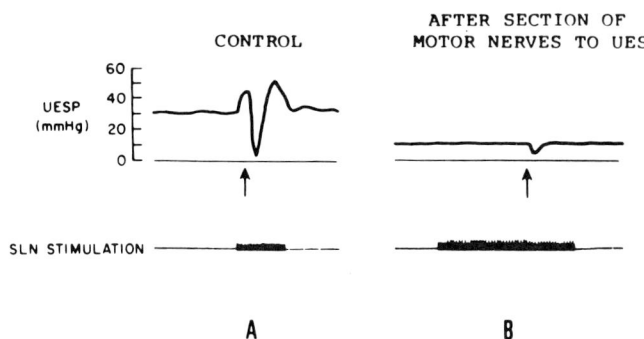

FIG. 3. Effect of transecting motor nerves to UES on resting pressures and deglutitive responses as evoked by superior laryngeal muscle (SLN) stimulation. During control period (*A*), resting UES pressure (UESP) is ~30 mmHg. Stimulation of SLN causes initial transient UES contraction, which is followed by relaxation on activation of deglutition reflex (*arrow*). After sectioning motor nerves to UES (*B*), resting UES pressure falls to ~10 mmHg and deglutition, which is induced by SLN stimulation, causes a further drop in pressure. Drop is due to opening of UES by contraction of suprahyoid muscles. [From Asoh and Goyal (12).]

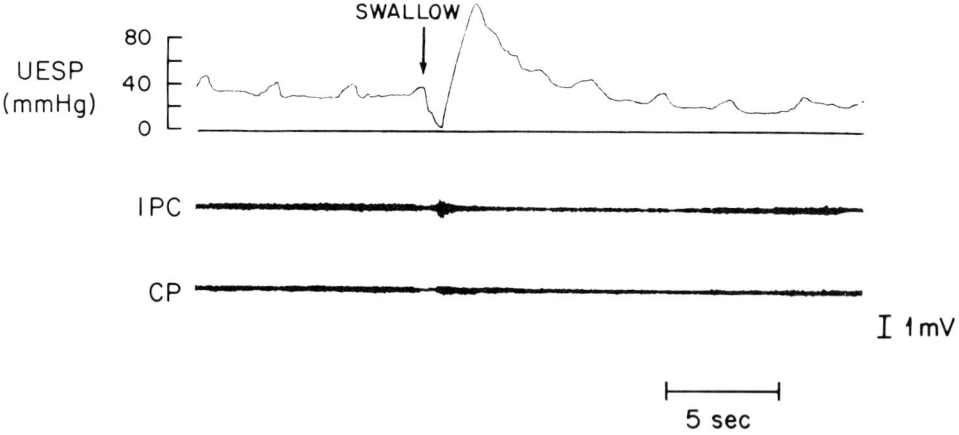

FIG. 2. Simultaneous manometric and electromyographic recordings from opossum UES. Sphincter pressure (UESP) falls abruptly on swallowing, and this is associated with cessation of tonic electrical spike activity in cricopharyngeus (CP) and inferior pharyngeal constrictor (IPC) muscles. Sphincter pressure then recovers and actually rises to well above base line (postrelaxation contraction). This corresponds to increased spike-burst activity in CP and IPC. [From Goyal and Cobb (218).]

Early investigators (296, 350) suggested that the tonic contraction of the cricopharyngeus is due to tonic sympathetic nerve activity, and that during swallowing, vagal inhibitory fibers activate relaxation of the cricopharyngeus. There is little support for this theory. In the opossum, vagal stimulation actually causes contractions of UES muscles and vagal section abolishes their activity (12). The continuous spike activity is also abolished by curare-like drugs, indicating that tonic lower motoneuron activity is responsible for the tonic cricopharyngeal activity.

The activity of the UES muscles is depressed during deep sleep and during anesthesia (12, 311, 453), and may show a phasic increase in activity with inspiration (5, 57, 290, 311).

REFLEX INCREASES IN PRESSURE. Reflex increases in UES pressure occur with esophageal distension (110, 173, 189, 230), intraesophageal acid infusion (189, 195, 196, 464), and during gastroesophageal reflux (418). The reflex increase in UES pressure induced by acid infusion or balloon distension is less marked when the more distal rather than the more proximal esophageal segments are stimulated. Bilateral cervical vagosympathetic cooling does not change the resting UES pressure but partially antagonizes the increase in pressure caused by distension and completely abolishes the increase in pressure induced by acid infusion (189). These studies suggest that the reflex increase in UES pressure caused by esophageal distension or acid infusion is largely mediated by vagal pathways. The UES pressure also increases with inspiration, glossopharyngeal breathing, gagging, and during the Valsalva maneuver when it is performed against a closed mouth and nose as opposed to a closed glottis (419). Increased resting UES pressure has also been reported in patients with the globus sensation (508); however, this has been recently refuted (322).

REFLEX RELAXATION. Relaxation of the UES occurs during deglutition, rumination, vomiting, regurgitation, and belching. During swallow-induced relaxation of the UES, the continuous spike activity of the muscles comprising the UES ceases (5, 12, 57, 453, 496). This is due to inhibition of lower motoneurons in the brain stem that innervate the upper sphincter rather than to activity of peripheral inhibitory nerves. The inhibition of tonic muscle activity is in itself not sufficient to open the UES because its closure due to passive factors persists even after cessation of all cricopharyngeal electrical activity. Elevation and anterior displacement of the larynx by the suprahyoid muscles is required to abolish this residual pressure and open the sphincter. Although in experimental settings suprahyoid muscle contraction may obliterate the UES high-pressure zone even when the cricopharyngeus continues to fire [Fig. 4; (12)], under normal circumstances the cessation of activity in the crico-

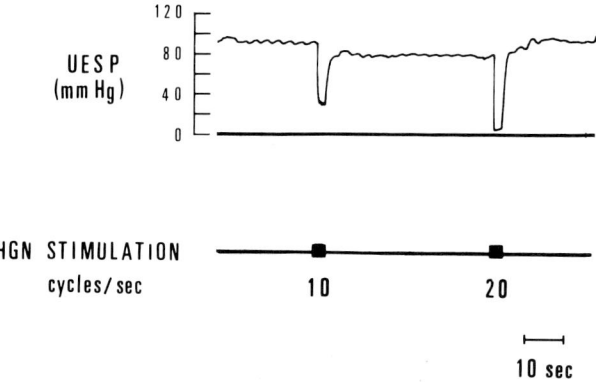

FIG. 4. Effect of geniohyoid muscle contraction on UES pressure (UESP) in opossum. Electrical stimulation of a branch of hypoglossal nerve (HGN) to geniohyoid muscle causes contraction of the muscle and precipitous fall in UES pressure. This indicates that the suprahyoid muscles function to open UES independent of relaxation of the intrinsic UES muscles. [From Asoh and Goyal (12).]

pharyngeus and contraction of the suprahyoid muscles are coordinated to ensure efficient opening of the UES. Paralysis of suprahyoid muscles significantly impairs UES opening even when the cricopharyngeus functions normally (12, 18, 257, 295). On the other hand, contraction of the suprahyoid muscles may cause considerable opening of the UES despite impaired cricopharyngeal relaxation. Because UES opening is related to two factors, it is best to distinguish between cricopharyngeal relaxation and UES opening. The relaxation component is due to the cessation of tonic activity in the cricopharyngeal and inferior pharyngeal constrictor muscles, whereas the opening is due to contraction of the suprahyoid muscles. Impaired relaxation of the cricopharyngeus muscle is responsible for the prominent cricopharyngeal bar or cricopharyngeal achalasia (49, 454, 479). In contrast, paralysis of the suprahyoid muscle and lack of opening of the upper esophageal sphincter are responsible for paralytic upper sphincter achalasia.

The unique characteristics and timing of UES function during deglutition, respiration, vomiting, and other distinct activities reveal the importance of specific nervous control mechanisms in integrating these various functions.

ESOPHAGEAL BODY

*Muscular Anatomy*

In adults the body of the esophagus, exclusive of the sphincters, is 18–22 cm long (94, 310, 502) and extends from the lower border of the UES (cricopharyngeus muscle) to the upper border of the LES. With this functional definition, the upper level of the esophageal body begins ~18 cm from the incisors and ends at 40 cm (range 36–50 cm) in males and at 37 cm (range 22–41 cm) in females (310).

Proximally, the human esophagus is composed of striated muscle in both the inner circular and outer longitudinal muscle layers. The longitudinal muscle fibers arise from the superior aspect of the median ridge on the dorsal surface of the cricoid cartilage and are joined by muscle bundles from the cricopharyngeus and posterolateral cricoid cartilage on each lateral aspect. Fibers course dorsally and caudally to join ~3 cm below the cricoid cartilage posteriorly. This arrangement leaves a triangular shaped area devoid of longitudinal muscle that is called Laimer's triangle (304). The longitudinal muscle is somewhat thicker laterally than on its anterior and posterior aspects (502). This becomes less apparent as the muscle proceeds aborally.

Smooth muscle begins to replace striated muscle ~4 cm (2–6 cm) from the proximal end of the esophageal body (7, 488, 502). Smooth and striated muscles are present in nearly equal amounts between 4 and 8 cm from the upper end. This mixture of striated and smooth muscle extends to a point 10–13 cm from the lower border of the cricopharyngeus. From that point distally is exclusively smooth muscle, so that the distal one-half to one-third of the esophagus is entirely smooth muscle in both inner circular and outer longitudinal coats (94, 310, 442). There have been rare reports of striated muscle extending the length of the entire esophagus in humans (7, 263).

Lerche (310) describes an orientation of circular fibers that varies at different levels of the esophagus. The fibers are mostly elliptical in the upper two-thirds of the esophageal body and are arranged in spirals distally. It has been suggested that both striated and smooth muscles have an orientation like an apolar screw system (194), but factual data are lacking. Also, a poorly developed oblique layer termed the *bracket fibers of Laimer* may be present on the luminal aspect of the inner circular muscle layer in the distal esophagus (310, 528). The muscle distribution in the esophageal body is similar among primates, cats, and opossum; however, in dogs, rabbits, sheep, cows, guinea pigs, rats, horses, and giraffes the esophageal body is entirely striated muscle; in amphibians, birds, and reptiles, it is exclusively smooth muscle (263). It is important to keep these anatomical differences in mind when interpreting physiological data. However, histologically comparable muscle behaves with remarkable similarity in different species.

*Pressure Profile*

BASAL PRESSURES. Basal pressures in the esophageal body fluctuate with respiration. During inspiration, pressures range from −5 to −15 mmHg and during expiration from −2 to +5 mmHg relative to atmospheric pressure (94, 256). Intraesophageal pressures have long been used by pulmonary physiologists to estimate the intrapleural pressure. However, intraesophageal pressures are usually slightly higher than intrapleural pressures recorded at the same site.

Intraluminal catheters may also record extrinsic pressures caused by the aortic and heart pulsations (489). Aortic pulsations observed in the middle and lower third of the esophagus, including the LES, are caused by the aortic arch and the descending aorta, respectively. Left atrial and ventricular pulsations may also be transmitted, as may pulsations from aberrant vessels.

SWALLOW-INDUCED RESPONSES. *Primary peristalsis.* Swallowing is associated with primary peristalsis in the esophagus, which is recognized by its association with pharyngeal peristaltic contraction and UES relaxation. A more sensitive marker of the swallowing reflex is electrical activity in the mylohyoid muscle (370).

The initial pressure change accompanying deglutition in the esophagus is a negative deflection beginning ~0.2 s after the onset of swallowing and lasting 0.3–0.5 s (500, 501). This deflection is 5–10 mmHg in magnitude and occurs simultaneously with a drop in pleural pressure. It is best recorded in the proximal esophageal body and is more frequent in elderly individuals. It is felt that a short inspiration immediately preceding swallowing accounts for this initial negative wave (164).

A small positive pressure wave often follows the initial negative deflection (53). This is also best recorded in the proximal esophagus and is attributed to transmission of pharyngeal pressures through the swallowed bolus. It occurs 0.5–1 s after the onset of swallowing. This wave may occur as a discrete peak or may plateau into a second positive wave.

The second positive wave is best demonstrated in the distal part of the esophagus and is rarely, if ever, recorded in the proximal third. Approximately one-third of swallows reveal this waveform, and its incidence can be increased by obstructing the gastroesophageal opening with a tube (500). This wave begins 1–2 s after the onset of swallowing. It is believed to be produced by compression of the lower esophageal segment between the advancing bolus and the unopened LES.

The third positive esophageal pressure wave accompanying deglutition is a large pressure transient that represents the main peristaltic wave. It is produced by a lumen-occluding contraction of the esophageal muscle. The characteristics of this wave vary with the segment of esophagus in which it is measured. The duration of the pressure wave varies from 2 to 7 s and increases in an aboral direction. The amplitude has been assigned a wide range of values by various investigators using different recording methods. Recording peak pressures with an intraesophageal transducer system reveals values of 53.4 ± 9.0 mmHg (mean ± SE) in the upper esophagus, 35.0 ± 6.4 mmHg in the midde portion, and 69.5 ± 12.1 mmHg in the lower esophagus (254). The lower pressures in the midesophagus correspond to the junction of striated and smooth muscle. The average peristaltic speed is ~4 cm/s; it is ~3 cm/s in the upper esophagus, accelerates to 5 cm/s in the midregion, and then slows again to 2.5 cm/s just above the LES [see Fig. 1; (254)].

Several factors may influence the amplitude, duration, and propagation velocity of the peristaltic wave. Within the same individual and with the same technique, peristaltic amplitude remains reasonably constant when examined serially (352). Peristaltic amplitude has been reported to be diminished in elderly people; however, this has been recently refuted (243, 510). Amplitudes of esophageal contractions are less when recorded in the upright position, with velocity increasing in the upper esophagus but decreasing in the mid- to lower esophagus in this position (292). Also, the duration and amplitude are increased and the velocity decreased when a fluid bolus is swallowed as opposed to when the bolus swallowed is dry, i.e., air (155, 191, 244, 292, 510). Increases in intra-abdominal pressure slow the speed of peristalsis (156), and bolus temperature variations may also alter peristaltic parameters (128, 171, 520) (warm boluses augment and cold boluses inhibit peristaltic contraction).

*Esophageal inhibition.* It is now increasingly apparent that primary peristalsis consists of a biphasic response consisting of inhibition followed by contraction. This inhibition preceding the contraction is called deglutitive inhibition or initial inhibition. Because there is no basal tone in the esophagus, deglutitive inhibition is not usually evident; however, it becomes evident when two swallows are taken within a few seconds of each other (495). In this situation the second swallow will inhibit the esophageal contractile activity that has been evoked by the first swallow. Repeated swallows taken at short intervals causes continuous inhibition of esophageal activity such that a peristaltic contractile sequence does not occur until after the last swallow [Fig. 5; (10, 341, 433)]. This phenomenon normally occurs during drinking, an act that consists of a train of closely spaced swallows. During normal food ingestion, when swallows are performed in rapid succession but irregularly, fewer peristaltic waves than swallows are observed. Moreover the contraction amplitudes are variable, presumably due to the phenomenon of deglutitive inhibition (340).

DISTENSION-INDUCED RESPONSES. *Secondary peristalsis.* Transient esophageal distension as occurs with rapid inflation and deflation of an intraluminal balloon is associated with peristaltic contractions in the esophagus. Esophageal distension may induce primary peristalsis. However, balloon distension in the esophagus usually produces peristalsis without

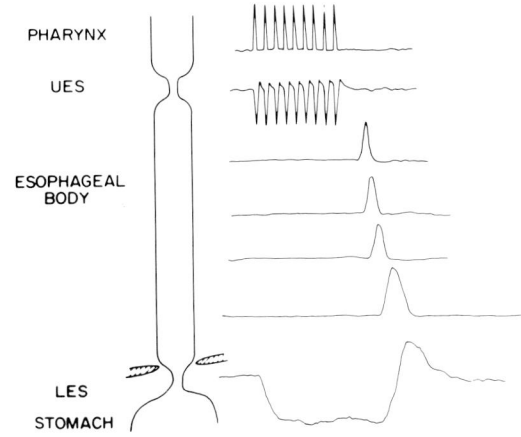

FIG. 5. Diagrammatic representation of deglutitive inhibition. Swallows taken in rapid succession are marked by repeated phasic pressure changes recorded in pharynx. The UES relaxes and recovers with each swallow on a one-to-one basis. However, peristalsis in esophageal body does not ensue until after last swallow. Also, the LES relaxes to first swallow and does not recover until after peristaltic wave initiated by last swallow has traversed the esophagus.

pharyngeal activity. The term *secondary peristalsis* is applied to esophageal distension-induced peristaltic contractions that are localized to the esophagus and not accompanied by pharyngeal peristalsis or UES relaxation. The amplitude and velocity of peristaltic contractions induced by transient esophageal distension resembles that of primary peristalsis (181).

*Esophageal propulsive force.* Peristaltic contractions of the esophageal body exert an aborally directed force on the ingested bolus, thus propelling it toward the stomach. Studies in humans have showed that the esophageal propulsive force correlates with the pressure amplitude of the peristaltic contraction (441). The esophageal propulsive force increases with increasing bolus size and is greatest in the distal esophagus (441). If a balloon is inflated in the esophageal body and prevented from moving distally, an aborally directed steady force of up to 200 g is exerted on the balloon (521). Presumably this propulsive force is produced by esophageal contraction at and just above the balloon; however, this has not been investigated in detail. During the period of fixed balloon distension, no contractions occur in the esophagus distal to the balloon; however, when restraints are removed from the balloon, the contraction producing the localized propulsive force is converted to a peristaltic sequence that progresses distally, pushing the balloon ahead of it (521).

## Central Control of Esophageal Peristalsis

Primary peristalsis is initiated by activation of the swallowing center (see OVERVIEW OF ESOPHAGEAL MOTOR FUNCTION, p. 866), which occurs either voluntarily via higher brain centers or by reflex stimulation of peripheral afferents. Stimulation of the swallowing center in turn activates neurons in several cranial nerves, including the vagi. The vagi mediate primary peristalsis in both the striated and the smooth muscle portions of the esophagus.

STRIATED MUSCLE PORTION. As with any striated muscle, the striated muscle component of the esophagus itself has no intrinsic ability to produce a contraction but is entirely dependent on excitatory nerve activity from lower motoneurons. The cell bodies of the vagal lower motoneurons that innervate the striated muscle part of the esophagus are located in the dorsal aspect of the rostral part of the nucleus ambiguus (21, 190, 248, 306, 307). Peristalsis in the striated muscle segment of the esophagus is due to sequential discharge of the motoneurons destined for progressively more distal levels (6). Bilateral cervical vagotomy above the origin of the pharyngoesophageal branches abolishes peristalsis in the striated muscle esophagus (59, 240, 260, 494, 502), although unilateral vagal nerve section has no effect, presumably because of extensive bilateral innervation (421). Experiments devised by Roman (421) in which the central portion of a sectioned vagus was used to reinnervate the sternocleidomastoid and trapezius muscles revealed that activation of deglutition induced sequential contraction of the reinnervated muscle fibers, and that this coincided with peristaltic contractions simultaneously measured by manometry.

Primary peristalsis in the striated esophageal musculature is influenced by bolus volume (155, 271, 272, 282, 323) and temperature (128, 520). In the baboon, afferent input from the esophagus affects the vagal efferent discharge as recorded in reinnervated sternocleidomastoid muscle (425). These findings indicate that esophageal sensory afferents can quantitatively affect the peristalsis in the striated muscle of the esophagus by modulating the central vagal efferent discharge.

The striated muscle portion of the esophagus usually responds on a one-to-one basis with each pharyngeal swallow; however, during rapid drinking the esophageal activity is inhibited until the last of the swallows, whereas oropharyngeal activity accompanies each swallow (10, 341). The inhibition of the striated muscle esophagus is presumably centrally mediated. A similar inhibitory effect occurs during beer guzzling, vomiting, and eructation. Reverse peristalsis is observed in ruminants and is centrally mediated in that it is abolished by vagotomy (167, 470).

Distension-induced peristalsis in the striated muscle segment of the dog (259) and sheep (421) esophagus is entirely dependent on central vagal pathways. Thus there is no difference between primary and secondary peristalsis in the striated muscle segments other than in the method of initiation and in the fact that its occurrence is independent of the oropharyngeal component. In humans esophageal balloon distension has been reported to induce UES relaxation followed by a peristaltic contraction that passes through the striated muscle segment and into the smooth muscle segment (455). Although it is unproved, it is likely that this distension-induced peristalsis involving the striated muscle portion in humans is also mediated by a central reflex.

SMOOTH MUSCLE PORTION. It is clear that swallow-induced primary peristalsis in the smooth muscle portion of the esophagus is also dependent on activation of the swallowing center and the vagal pathways to the esophagus. This is evidenced by the fact that bilateral cervical vagotomy or vagal cooling abolishes primary peristalsis in the esophagus (370, 405, 432, 482). However, unlike the striated muscle, sequential firing of vagal efferent neurons destined for progressively more caudal smooth muscle esophageal segments is not essential to activate peristalsis. This is demonstrated experimentally by simultaneously stimulating all vagal efferent fibers with an electric current and observing that peristalsis is still induced [Fig. 6; (147, 158, 198, 199, 201, 347, 422)].

Studies to define the neural mechanisms involved in peristalsis in the smooth muscle portion of the esophagus have, however, yielded conflicting data. Roman and Tieffenbach (425), for example, suggested that primary peristalsis in esophageal smooth muscle is due to sequential activation of vagal fibers. With recordings from baboon skeletal muscle that had been

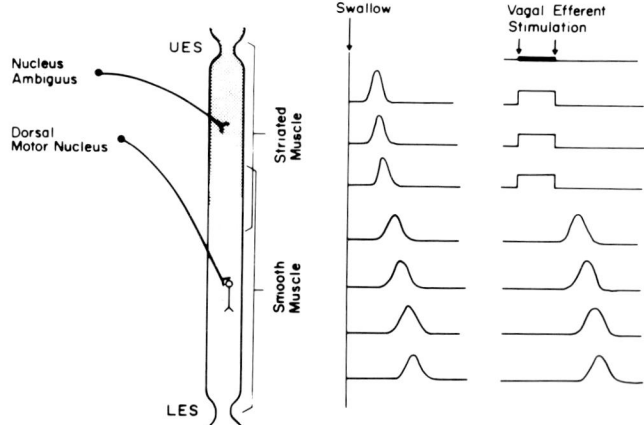

FIG. 6. Schematic representation of esophageal peristaltic contractions as evoked by swallowing and vagal efferent nerve stimulation. Swallowing evokes an aborally directed series of contractions that pass smoothly from striated to smooth muscle segment. Electrical stimulation of distal cut end of a vagus nerve, which simultaneously activates all vagal efferent fibers, evokes peristaltic contractions only in smooth muscle segment of esophagus. In striated muscle esophagus, vagal stimulation causes simultaneous contractions that occur only during period of stimulation. Striated muscle esophagus is dependent on central neuronal sequencing for its peristaltic contraction, whereas intrinsic neuronal mechanisms are capable of producing peristaltic sequence in smooth muscle segment.

reinnervated by vagal efferent fibers, they detected vagal efferent discharge that coincided with peristaltic activity in the smooth muscle esophagus. The pattern of this discharge was sequential, indicating that vagal preganglionic fibers destined to the smooth muscle esophagus are activated by a central sequencing mechanism in the same manner as is seen with the vagal lower motoneurons that supply the striated muscle esophagus. Roman and Tieffenbach (425) suggested that these preganglionic efferent fibers synapse with postganglionic cholinergic fibers in the smooth muscle esophageal wall, which, in turn, produce the peristaltic contractions.

These studies, however, do not explain the initial inhibitory discharge that occurs prior to peristaltic contraction in response to deglutition. Recent studies by Gidda and Goyal have provided new insight into these central mechanisms (200). By recording swallow-evoked potentials from single cervical vagal efferent fibers of the opossum, they were able to distinguish two types of preganglionic efferent fibers destined for the smooth muscle esophagus based on their latency distributions. Short-latency fibers began firing within 1 s of the onset of swallowing, as recorded by mylohyoid activity. Long-latency fibers had latencies to onset of discharge that ranged between 1 and 5 s (Fig. 7). The respective latency distributions indicate that short-latency discharges correlate with the initial inhibition, and the long-latency fibers correlate with the peristaltic contractions. The swallow-evoked efferent discharge in each fiber lasts ~1 s with 4–6 spikes per discharge. Moreover the spikes do not occur at a regular frequency. It is likely that in addition to ini-

tiating primary peristalsis, vagal efferent fibers also modulate speed, amplitude, and duration of the peristaltic wave. It is the intrinsic neural mechanisms, however, that are predominant in generating the peristaltic wave.

Peristalsis in the smooth muscle portion initiated by distension is independent of central pathways and is mediated by intramural neuromuscular mechanisms. This is evidenced by the fact that it is not abolished by bilateral vagotomy (302, 370, 421, 424) or vagal cooling (432), and is not accompanied by centrally controlled components of deglutition such as pharyngeal peristalsis, UES relaxation, or mylohyoid activity. Although vagal connections are not necessary, recent studies suggest that vagal pathways may exert a facilitatory influence on the intramural neuromuscular mechanisms mediating secondary peristalsis in the smooth muscle esophagus (370).

*Peripheral Control of Esophageal Peristalsis*

STRIATED MUSCLE PORTION. As stated earlier, the striated muscle portion of the esophagus has no ability to produce peristaltic contraction independent of the central nervous system. Vagal efferent stimulation of the lower motoneurons to these muscles causes contraction that occurs simultaneously in all the muscle segments. The contraction starts with the onset of the nerve stimulation, is sustained during the period of stimulation, and ceases when the nerve stimulation is stopped (see Fig. 6).

SMOOTH MUSCLE PORTION. In contrast to the striated muscle portion, the smooth muscle portion possesses an intramural neuromuscular mechanism that can produce peristalsis independent of the central nervous system.

*Peripheral Control of Peristalsis in Esophageal Smooth Muscle*

The peripheral mechanisms of peristalsis in the smooth muscle are revealed by studying the responses to *1*) distension of a balloon in the extrinsically denervated esophagus *2*) electrical vagal efferent nerve stimulation, and *3*) electrical stimulation of intramural nerves in circular muscle strips of esophageal smooth muscle.

*Localized distension of the extrinsically denervated esophagus.* Transient localized distension of the extrinsically denervated smooth muscle esophagus can produce peristaltic contractions (69, 77). A brief contraction occurs at or just proximal to the rostal margin of the balloon within 0.5 s of inflation. This contraction is resistant to tetrodotoxin, an agent that blocks action potentials in nerves and is therefore probably myogenic in origin (77). During the period of distension, the esophagus below the distending balloon re-

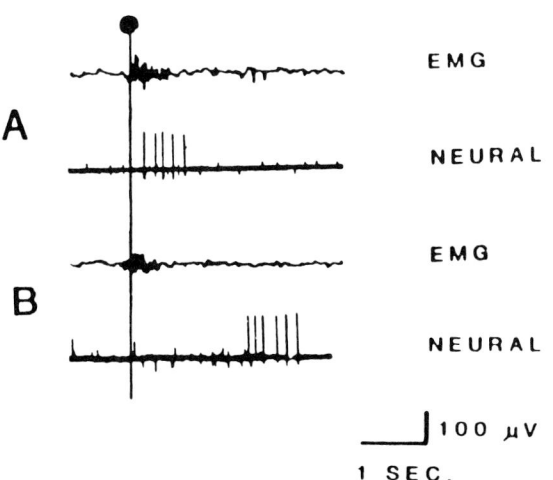

FIG. 7. Swallow-evoked discharges in 2 vagal efferent fibers, *A* and *B*. *Upper trace*, mylohyoid electromyographic (EMG) activity that marks the onset of deglutition (*vertical line*). Latency of evoked vagal efferent action potentials is short in *A* (0.21 s) as compared with *B* (1.78 s). Short-latency fibers appear to correspond to deglutitive inhibition and long-latency fibers to peristaltic contraction. [From Gidda and Goyal (200).]

mains inhibited because of smooth muscle membrane hyperpolarization (141). Contraction does not occur until after the balloon is deflated. There is a latency from the time of deflation to the onset of distal esophageal contraction, and this latency tends to increase aborally so that on deflation one sees a contraction wave that starts at the balloon and progresses toward the stomach (69, 77). This peristaltic contraction is tetrodotoxin-sensitive and is thus mediated by intramural neurons (435).

*Vagal efferent stimulation.* Electrical stimulation of vagal efferents to the smooth muscle portion of the esophagus does not produce esophageal contraction immediately after the initiation of the stimulus. The evoked esophageal contractions occur with a certain latency after the stimulus is applied. Moreover the latency of contractions is not the same throughout the length of the esophagus but progressively increases aborally (146, 147). This gradient of aborally increasing latencies of contraction manifests itself as peristalsis (see Fig. 6). The latency or latency gradient of esophageal contraction to vagal stimulation is not due to conduction delays along the nerve, as the speed of propagation of impulses along the nerve is very fast (5–6 m/s) (200) and cannot explain latencies of several seconds between the onset of vagal stimulation and the contraction of the esophagus.

Gidda and Goyal (201) showed that each esophageal contraction in response to vagal efferent stimulation is preceded by a period of active inhibition that begins promptly with the onset of vagal stimulation (initial inhibition). The duration of initial inhibition preceding the contraction increases distally along the esophagus and corresponds to the latency of esophageal contraction to vagal stimulation. It has been shown that initial inhibition is associated with hyperpolarization of the circular muscle (381).

The degree of initial inhibition is dependent on the specific parameters of vagal stimulation, with greater initial inhibition seen when larger frequencies of electrical stimulation are used (201). This corresponds to an increasing degree of hyperpolarization seen with increasing frequency of vagal stimulation (381). It has also been shown that esophageal contraction is followed by refractoriness (201, 341). Thus a short-train (e.g., 1 s) vagal efferent stimulation produces an esophageal response consisting of a sequence of three phases: initial inhibition, contraction, and refractoriness. Each one of these phases lasts ~2–5 s. Because a 1-s vagal stimulation produces an esophageal response lasting several seconds in duration, full expression of the esophageal response requires that vagal stimuli occur no more frequently than every 15 s.

If vagal stimuli occur in rapid succession, the observed esophageal responses represent a sum of simultaneously occurring inhibitory and contractile events (199). Thus, if two stimuli are applied, a contractile response to the first stimulus may be antagonized and totally blocked by the inhibition associated with the second stimulus. Similarly, if the contraction to the second stimulus falls during the refractory period of the response to the first stimulus, the contraction to the second stimulus is antagonized. Depending on the stimulus parameters and interstimulus intervals, multiple successive stimuli applied at short intervals may produce contractile responses to only the first stimulus, the last stimulus, the first and the last stimulus, or to every second or third stimulus. Moreover the contractions that do occur may show variable amplitudes. The occurrence of the contraction to the first or last stimulus in a series of successive vagal stimuli is similar to esophageal contractions seen in response to a long continuous train of electrical vagal stimulation. It is therefore reasoned that a continuous train of vagal stimulation can be conceptualized as a series of independent vagal stimuli. This explains the interesting observation of Dodds et al. (147) that, with a long-train vagal stimulation, contraction occurs only at the onset or at the end of vagal stimulation. They (147) named the contraction at the onset "A" and the one of the end "B", respectively. The A contraction may represent a response to the first stimulus and the B contraction a response to the last stimulus in the long stimulus train. Thus the A and B contractions are similar in that they both have latencies from the assumed stimulus that produced them; however, they differ from each other in that *1*) A contractions are antagonized by atropine and are therefore cholinergic, whereas B contractions are not affected by atropine; *2*) the latencies of the A contraction progressively increase aborally along the esophagus, whereas the B contractions occur almost simultaneously throughout the esophagus; and *3*) A contractions are more frequently evoked by lower stimulus frequencies, whereas B contraction occurred more frequently at higher stimulus frequencies (Fig. 8).

With a short-train (1 s) stimulus, contractions occur after the end of the stimulus and therefore appear as "off" contractions. However, these contractions may resemble either the A or B contractions. For example, short-train stimuli of low frequency cause contractions that are sensitive to atropine and have prominent distally increasing latencies of contractions, resembling A contractions, whereas short-train, high-frequency stimuli cause atropine resistant, nearly simultaneous contractions resembling B contractions (146, 147, 198). A mixture of cholinergic (A) and noncholinergic (B) responses occur at certain intermediate stimulus frequencies.

Vagal efferent nerve stimulation activates the neural mechanisms at different esophageal levels virtually simultaneously, and the local neuromuscular mechanisms are somehow responsible for the observed latencies and the latency gradient. Thus the basic mechanism of peristalsis in the smooth muscle may

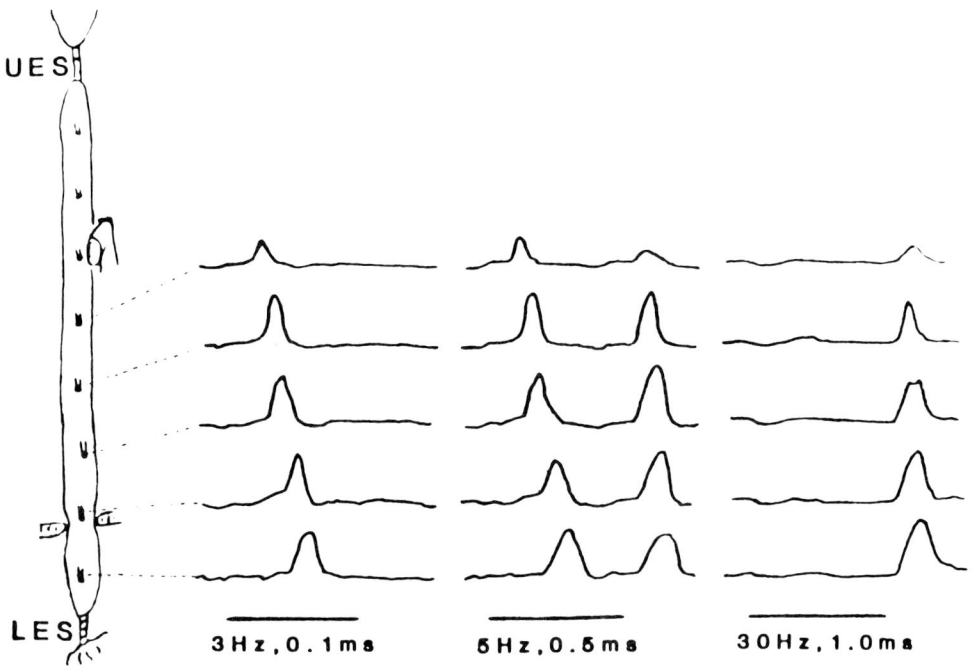

FIG. 8. Effect of long-train (8 s) vagal efferent nerve stimulation on esophageal contractions in opossum. Stimuli of low frequency and short pulse duration (*left panel*) evoke contractions during stimulus or A waves. Vagal stimulation with high frequency and longer pulse duration evoke only end-of-stimulus contractions or B waves (*right panel*). Intermediate stimulus parameters (*center panel*) evoke both A and B waves. Note that speed of propagation of A waves is significantly less than that of B waves and is closer to speed of swallow-evoked peristalsis. Pharmacologic studies indicate that the A waves are mediated by cholinergic neurons whereas neurons mediating B waves are noncholinergic and nonadrenergic. [From Dodds et al. (147).]

lie independently at each esophageal segment or it may be dependent on continuity with the adjoining esophageal segments. Studies with circular muscle strips in vitro favor the former hypothesis.

*Electrical stimulation of intramural nerves in circular smooth muscle strips.* Weisbrodt and Christensen (513) observed that transmural stimulation of intramural nerves in esophageal circular smooth muscle strips evokes contraction that starts well after the end of the stimulus. Such contractions were therefore called off contractions. A 0.5-s electrical stimulation produced an esophageal response (including latency and contraction) that occupied several seconds. They also showed that the latencies of contractions were progressively longer in the strips from more distal levels of the esophagus. This indicated that local neuromuscular mechanisms in each regional esophageal segment had built-in mechanisms that, when activated, produced peristalsislike contractions without any influence from the adjacent segments.

Christensen et al. (73, 78) observed that when long-train stimuli were applied to esophageal circular muscle strips, contraction always occurred after the end of the stimulus; that is, they were off contractions. They concluded that the off response was the main response of the esophageal circular muscle and that it was mediated by nerves that were neither cholinergic nor adrenergic.

Crist et al. (111) examined in detail the influence of long-train electrical field stimulation by using various stimulus parameters applied to circular muscle strips obtained from different sites along the opossum esophagus. Four different types of response were seen. First, a twitch response was found that is indicative of striated muscle stimulation. This was seen superimposed on other types of response in strips taken from the most proximal sites. Second, neurogenic on responses that were atropine sensitive occurred in the early period after the onset of the stimulus train and exhibited an aborally increasing latency of contraction. This latency gradient was such that at 40 Hz of electrical field stimulation the calculated speed of peristalsis was 5.2 cm/s. Third, intermediate contractions were documented. These were atropine sensitive, often multiple, and were evoked relatively infrequently. Fourth, they found off contractions that occurred at the end of the stimulus train, were tetrodotoxin sensitive but atropine resistant and did not demonstrate a large latency gradient along the esophagus. The three predominant patterns of response demonstrated in this study are depicted in Figure 9. On contractions were evoked more readily in the proximal esophagus and by higher frequency electrical stimulation, whereas off contractions predominated distally and with low-frequency stimulation. This study pointed out that the esophageal site and stimulus parameters (most notably frequency and train duration) determine whether neurogenic on or off contractions are evoked.

The on contractions in the muscle strip preparation are similar to the A waves of vagal stimulation in that both are antagonized by atropine and have prominent aborally increasing latency gradients along the esophagus. Similarly, off contractions in the circular muscle strips in vitro are much like the B contractions evoked by vagal stimulation in vivo; both are atropine resistant and the latency gradient is minimal.

*Role of on and off contractions in esophageal peristalsis.* Weisbrodt and Christensen (513) applied transmural stimulation of 0.5-s duration to circular smooth muscle strips from different levels of the esophagus. All strips contracted at the end of the stimulus, and the latency of contractions progressively increased in strips that came from the more distal regions of the esophagus. This gradient of distally increasing latencies resembled peristaltic contraction and prompted the authors to conclude that the noncholinergic off contractions were responsible for esophageal peristalsis. However, the calculated speed of peristalsis based on this off-contraction data was much faster than the speed of physiological peristalsis. Crist et al. (111) pointed out that cholinergic on and noncholinergic off contractions cannot be distinguished from each other with short-train stimuli because with short-train stimuli all responses appear as off contractions. They (111) produced on and off contractions with long-train transmural stimulation and observed that the calculated speed of propagation of an on contraction was slower than that of an off contraction and more like that seen in physiological peristalsis (Fig. 10). Dodds et al. had earlier made a similar observation in their studies with vagal efferent stimulation [see Fig. 8; (147)]. They observed that the latency gradient of A waves seen with vagal afferent stimulation increased aborally so that the speed of peristalsis was 2.66 cm/s, which is closer to the speed of physiological peristalsis seen with swallowing. On the other hand, the B wave that occurred at the end of long-train vagal stimulation had a much faster speed of peristalsis. This observation indicated that A or on contractions were involved in physiological peristalsis. However, A contractions and on contractions were sensitive to cholinergic blockade, but physiological peristalsis is only partially blocked by cholinergic antagonists (148, 182, 251, 273).

Crist et al. (112) stimulated circular muscle strips from different esophageal levels with 1-s train duration so that on and off contractions were not distinguishable because all contractions occurred after the end of the stimulus. They observed, as described by Weisbrodt and Christensen (513), that muscle strips from more distal regions of the esophagus showed progressively increasing latencies of contraction. They further examined the influence of increasing the stimulus frequency in order to recruit greater numbers of cholinergic nerves (112). This decreased the latencies in the proximal esophageal strips and increased the latencies in the distal strips (Fig. 11). This resulted in slowing of the calculated speed of peristalsis similar to that of swallow-induced peristalsis. Atropine added to the bath abolished this paradoxical response so that increasing stimulus frequencies no longer caused shortening of latencies in the proximal segments. Atropine also caused a reduction in amplitude and duration of contractions in the proximal but not in the distal esophageal strips. The authors proposed a model of the intrinsic neural mechanisms involved in peristalsis based on these results. This model suggests that there is a gradient of cholinergic and noncholinergic neurons involved in peristalsis along the

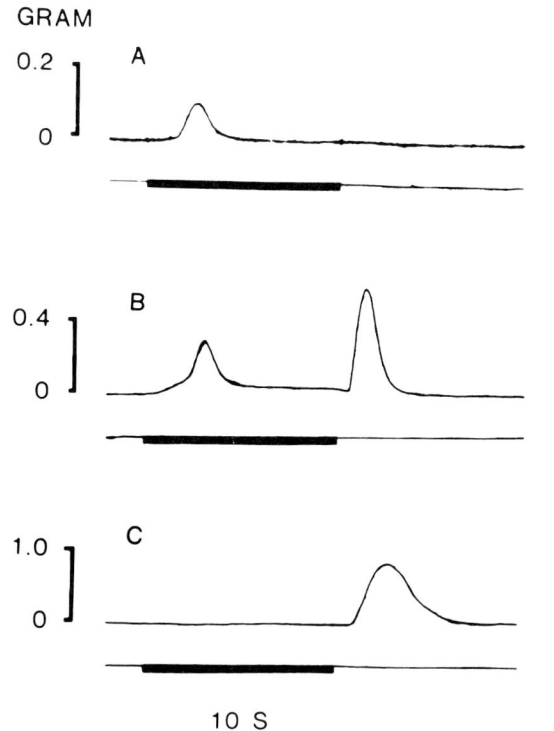

FIG. 9. Main patterns of contraction seen with transmural electrical stimulation of opossum esophageal circular smooth muscle strips. Stimulus train duration and pulse width were constant at 10 s and 1 ms, respectively. In A, stimulus of 60 V and 40 Hz resulted in only an on contraction, occurring shortly after onset of stimulus. In C, 80 V and 10 Hz evoked only an off contraction occurring after termination of stimulus. In B, 80 V and 20 Hz produced both on and off contractions. On contractions were sensitive to cholinergic blockade with atropine, whereas off contractions were not sensitive to cholinergic or adrenergic blockade. [Adapted from Crist et al. (111).]

esophagus. Cholinergic nerves dominate proximally, whereas noncholinergic nerves dominate distally (Fig. 12). Thus physiological peristalsis involves both cholinergic and noncholinergic contractions, and the predominance of cholinergic influence proximally results in earlier contraction after the initial inhibition. These two components can be experimentally separated or "electrophoresed" with long-train stimulation into on (A) and off (B) contractions.

The model explains several previously unexplained observations regarding peristalsis in animals and humans. When 1-s trains of electrical stimuli are applied to the opossum cervical vagus, atropine is seen to increase the latency of evoked contraction in the proximal smooth muscle segment of the esophagus but not in the distal esophagus. Furthermore atropine significantly delays the appearance of a primary peristaltic wave and diminishes the amplitude and duration of this wave in the proximal smooth muscle segment of the esophagus in this animal (146). In the human esophagus, cholinergic blockade also increases the latencies of contraction, particularly in the proximal smooth muscle part of the esophagus; this results in an increase in the speed of peristalsis (148). Furthermore the decreased amplitude and duration of peristaltic contraction caused by atropine are much more significant in the proximal than in the distal part of the human smooth muscle esophagus (148, 182, 251, 253, 273, 374).

These cholinergic influences on peristalsis appear to be mediated primarily by the $M_2$ muscarinic recep-

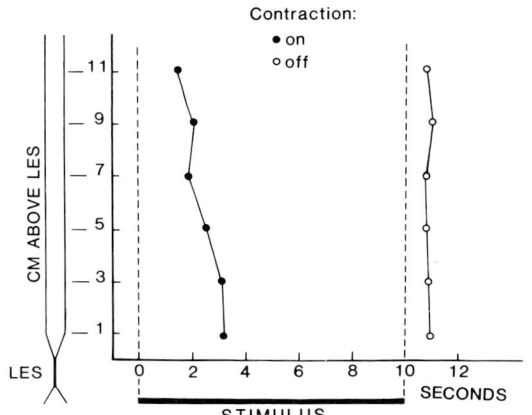

FIG. 10. Latencies of on (●) and off (○) contractions of circular smooth muscle strips from different esophageal sites. Latencies of on contractions gradually increase along esophagus in an aboral direction, whereas latencies of off contractions showed no significant change along esophagus. *Points*, represent mean of 6 on and 8 off contractions. Electrical field stimulation parameters consisted of 80 V, 40 Hz, 1-ms pulse duration and 10-s train duration. [From Crist et al. (111).]

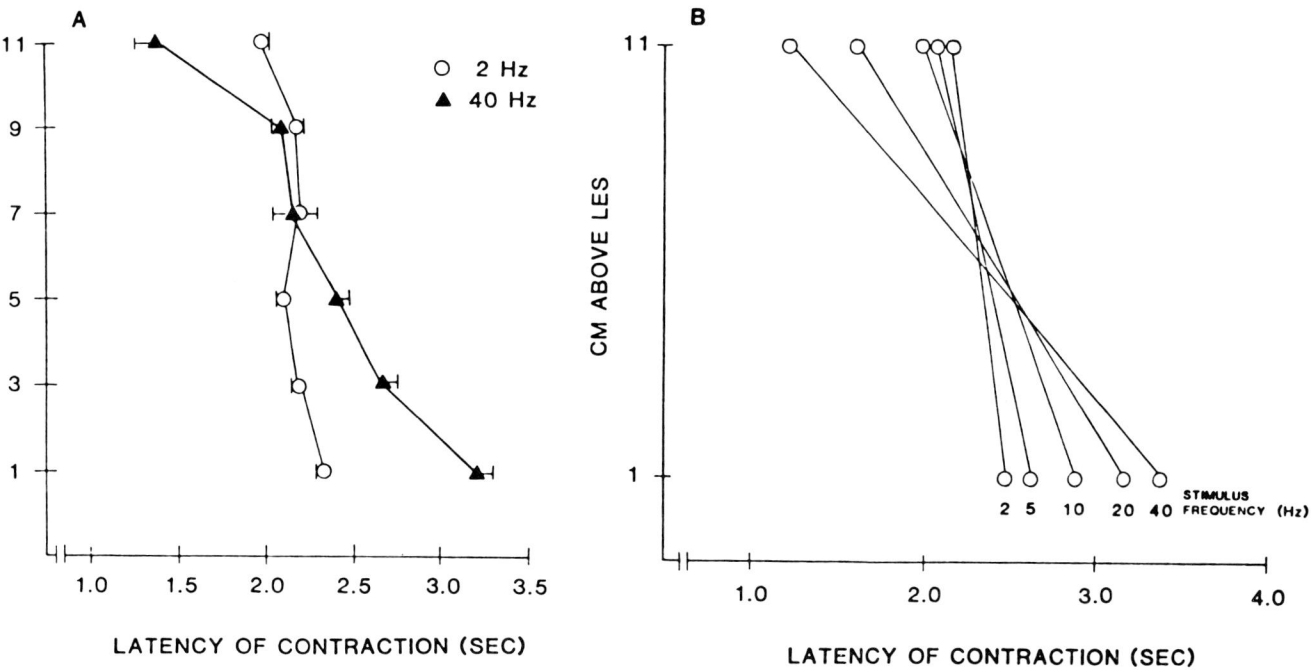

FIG. 11. *A*: effect of various stimulus frequencies on latencies of contraction of circular smooth muscle strips at different sites along opossum esophagus. Increasing stimulus frequency from 2 Hz (○) to 40 Hz (▲) resulted in decrease in latencies of contraction at more proximal sites (11, 9, and 7 cm above LES) and increase in latencies of contraction at more distal sites (5, 3, and 1 cm above LES). *B*: effect of increase in stimulus frequency (2, 5, 10, 20, and 40 Hz) on latencies of contraction of circular smooth muscle strips from sites 11 and 1 cm above LES. At 1-cm site, there is a progressive increase in latency of contraction with increases in stimulus frequency. At the 11-cm site, increasing stimulus frequency resulted in a decrease in latencies of contraction. This is due to stimulation of cholinergic neurons in the proximal esophagus. [From Crist et al. (112).]

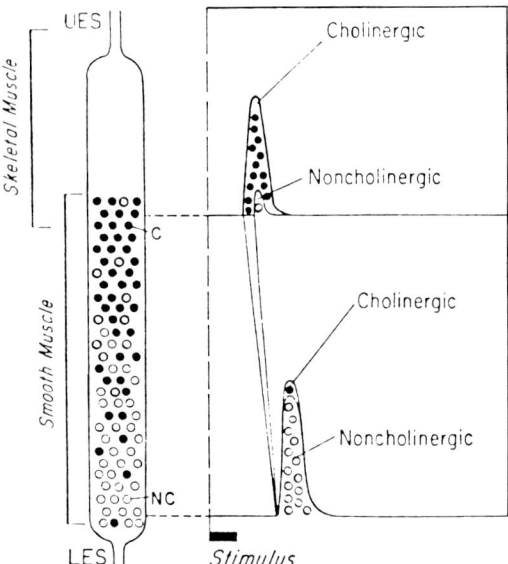

FIG. 12. Schematic drawing illustrating gradients of cholinergic (C) and noncholinergic (NC) nerve influence along smooth muscle portion of esophagus. Cholinergic influence is most prominent proximally and progressively decreases distally, whereas noncholinergic influence is most prominent distally and progressively decreases proximally. [From Crist et al. (112).]

tor in that the selective $M_1$ antagonist pirenzepine is without major effect on peristaltic amplitude and duration (40, 132, 174, 273, 466). Pirenzepine increases the latency interval of peristalsis at each site along the opossum esophagus without affecting the gradient, whereas atropine and the selective $M_2$ blocker, 4-dAMP, preferentially increase the latency interval proximally so that the latency gradient is diminished (203).

*Electrical correlates of esophageal contraction and inhibition.* The myoelectrical responses that occur during esophageal body contraction have been studied in vivo with bipolar or monopolar extracellular pressure electrodes (219, 236) or suction electrodes (114, 129, 142, 287) and in vitro with intracellular electrodes (114, 129, 288) or the sucrose-gap technique (119).

With bipolar pressure electrodes, it has been shown that electrical spike bursts coincide with phasic esophageal contractions (219, 482). Thus there is a latency gradient of these spike bursts just as there is a latency gradient of esophageal contraction. Also, the temporal relationship between the spike bursts and esophageal contraction, which is called the electromechanical delay, increases in more distal esophageal sites. This electromechanical delay can also be affected by the frequency of vagal efferent stimulation (219). Unlike skeletal muscle, dissociation between contraction and electrical spike bursts has been noted in smooth muscle (219). When contraction of the smooth muscle esophagus is evoked by high-frequency vagal efferent stimulation, contraction occasionally occurs without associated spike bursts. Conversely, spike bursts without coincident contraction have been observed at low-frequency vagal efferent stimulation [Fig. 13; (219)].

The pressure electrode is applied to the outer wall of the esophageal body and records electrical activity from all the muscle layers. However, this composite of electrical events is very similar to that recorded from the circular muscle layer alone, probably because of its larger mass (382, 473). These extracellular records are excellent for recording spike activity, but they do not provide any information on changes in membrane potential. Suction electrodes, on the other hand, can provide an estimation of membrane potential changes. Rattan et al. (382) developed a technique of recording membrane potential with suction electrodes in vivo. They found that during swallowing there is first hyperpolarization followed by depolarization and spike bursts, with the latter initiating the contraction (Fig. 14). This also occurs with vagal efferent stimulation; however, the temporal relationship of spike bursts and hyperpolarization can be altered, depending on the stimulus parameters. The amplitude of hyperpolarization increases and the rate of recovery from depolarization decreases with increased frequencies of vagal efferent stimulation, thereby prolonging the duration of hyperpolarization. The latency of onset of spike bursts decreases with increasing frequency of vagal efferent stimulation, and the corresponding contraction is of larger amplitude.

Intracellular recording from circular esophageal smooth muscle (114, 129, 288) and sucrose-gap studies (119) have revealed similar findings. Electrical field stimulation in this setting results in prompt membrane hyperpolarization, the magnitude of which depends on the intensity of the stimulus. The hyperpolarization is then followed by rebound depolarization. The spike burst is not well recorded, since, when spikes occur, the intracellular electrode often becomes dislodged secondary to the muscle contraction.

*Nature of latency and latency gradient.* From the preceding discussion it is apparent that the latency of contraction and the latency gradient along the esophagus is fundamentally important for the generation of a peristaltic sequence of contraction. At present, the mechanisms underlying the esophageal latency gradient are unclear. It is possible that the smooth muscle cell itself is different at different sites along the esophagus. In support of this, Decktor and Ryan (129) found that resting membrane potential decreases along the smooth muscle portion of the opossum smooth muscle esophagus so that the resting membrane potential is less negative distally. Furthermore a gradient in $K^+$ content along the opossum smooth muscle esophagus has also been demonstrated (444). However it is not clear how decreasing $K^+$ concentration or resting membrane potential would result in the differences in latencies. Recent studies (114) show no differences in the resting membrane potential at sites 3 and 8 cm

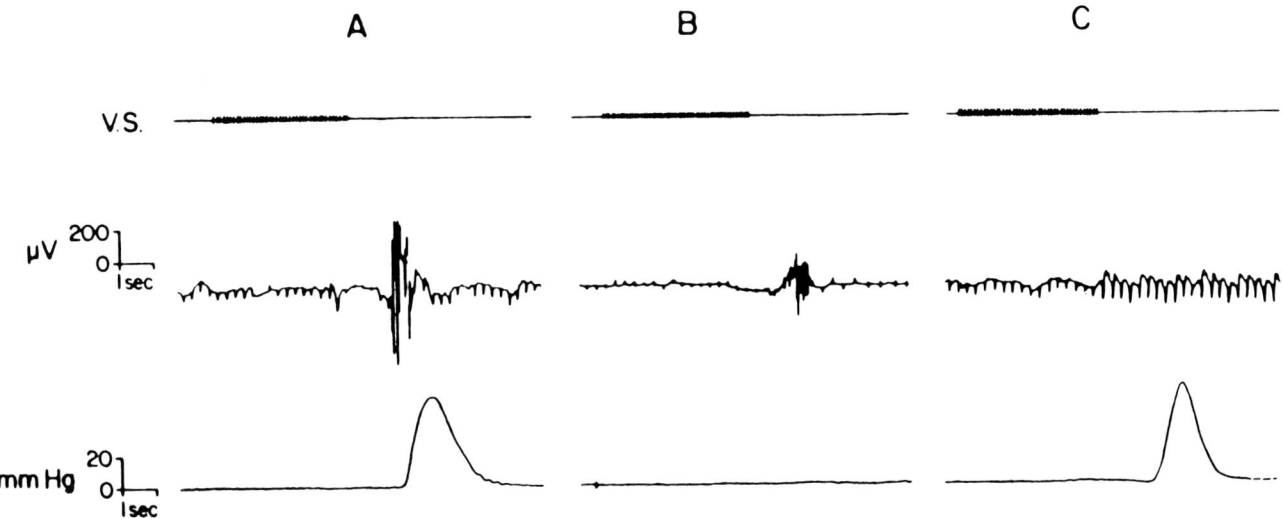

FIG. 13. Examples of electromechanically coupled (A) and uncoupled (B and C) responses to vagal efferent nerve stimulation (VS) as recorded by bipolar pressure electrodes in opossum distal esophageal body. A: electrical spike bursts precede pressure wave caused by esophageal contraction. B: spike burst occurs without esophageal contraction. However, spike burst is of low amplitude and has fewer spikes than the coupled responses A. C: vagal stimulation evokes contraction without electrical spike burst. [From Goyal and Gidda (219).]

above the LES. Moreover the length and time constants, which are measures of the passive electrical properties of the circular smooth muscle membrane, are no different at proximal and distal sites (114). Although differences may exist in the smooth muscle at different sites, this has not been confirmed and is unlikely to be of significance for the latency gradient of peristaltic contraction. Alternatively this latency gradient may be due to regional differences in intramural innervation that results in the initial inhibition being of progressively longer duration at more distal esophageal sites. The model described in Figure 12 shows how regional differences in cholinergic and noncholinergic innervation may be responsible for the latency gradient.

*Neurotransmitter(s) involved in esophageal peristalsis.* As discussed previously, there is substantial evidence that intramural cholinergic neurons are involved in the esophageal peristaltic contractions. In addition, there is a noncholinergic, nonadrenergic inhibitory neurotransmitter that is responsible for the membrane hyperpolarization or inhibitory junction potential (IJP) that plays a fundamental role in the production of initial inhibition and the latency of contractions. This hyperpolarization is followed by depolarization that is also resistant to cholinergic and adrenergic blockade. It is not clear whether this hyperpolarization-depolarization sequence, which causes inhibition followed by excitation, is produced by a single inhibitory neurotransmitter (which causes hyperpolarization and subsequent depolarization being a rebound after hyperpolarization) or separate inhibitory or excitatory nonadrenergic, noncholinergic neu-

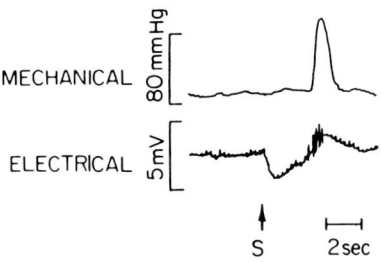

FIG. 14. Example of simultaneous recording of electrical and mechanical (intraluminal pressure) events in smooth muscle opossum esophagus in response to swallowing (S). Swallowing results in prompt fall in membrane potential (hyperpolarization) that is followed by overshoot depolarization and superimposed electrical spike bursts. Esophageal contraction occurs after onset of spike burst. This provides direct evidence that deglutition results in initial inhibition of esophagus prior to peristaltic contractions. [From Rattan et al. (381).]

rotransmitters. In any event, the identity of this (these) important neurotransmitter(s) is unknown. In the LES, the evidence supports vasoactive intestinal polypeptide (VIP) as the inhibitory transmitter (33, 228, 399). However, in the esophageal body, VIP causes contractions of the esophagus after a certain latency, and it was thus suggested that VIP may mediate esophageal peristaltic contractions (397). This view is supported by an abundance of VIP in the neurons of the esophageal body (84, 492).

With the sucrose-gap technique, Daniel et al. (119) demonstrated that neither purines nor VIP reproduced the esophageal-body smooth muscle membrane hyperpolarization-depolarization cycle seen with electrical field stimulation by using stimulus parameters that release neurotransmitters from the intramural nerves. The VIP induced repetitive contractions and membrane oscillations, as well as augmented the off response after an electrically evoked IJP. These observations do not necessarily rule out VIP as the inhibitory-excitatory neurotransmitter in the esophageal body, as the phasic oscillations of membrane potential may have actually been hyperpolarization-depolarization sequences initiated by small amounts of VIP reaching the smooth muscle cell receptor.

With circular smooth muscle strips from the cat, Behar et al. (28) found that VIP mimicked the inhibitory effect of electrical field stimulation. The VIP relaxed strips that had been contracted by bethanechol both in the presence and absence of tetrodotoxin. In vivo, VIP causes repetitive tetrodotoxin-resistant esophageal contractions when given intra-aortically to opossums (397).

It is possible that VIP applied exogenously will not mimic the smooth muscle membrane electrical changes seen when it is released from the intramural nerves. It has been speculated that an endogenously released inhibitory neurotransmitter may first act on the interstitial cells of Cajal, which in turn transmit the inhibitory electrical signals to the smooth muscle cells, whereas exogenous neurotransmitter may act directly on the circular muscle (121).

The hyperpolarization caused by release of the inhibitory neurotransmitters appears to be caused by increased $K^+$ conductance of the membrane; however, this $K^+$ channel appears unique because known $K^+$-channel antagonists such as apamin, tetraethylammonium chloride, 4-aminopyridine, and quinine do not block it (283). In sucrose-gap studies the rebound depolarization after the IJP is chloride dependent, as is the action of VIP to enhance this rebound depolarization (119). This is consistent with the view that VIP may mediate the depolarization and contraction that follow hyperpolarization. Further studies are needed to establish the role of VIP as the inhibitory-excitatory neurotransmitter that mediates peristaltic contractions in the esophageal body.

Several other neurotransmitters are present in the nerves of the esophagus (192). Many of these have clear-cut effects on esophageal contractions when used in a pharmacological setting (75); however, their physiological significance is unclear. For example, catecholamine diminishes peristaltic contraction (100), Met-enkephalin augments peristaltic contraction amplitude and duration as well as peristaltic velocity (465), and Leu-enkephalin inhibits electrical field stimulated responses in vitro (493). These enkephalins may act presynaptically to modulate the release of the neurotransmitters directly responsible for peristalsis. Substance P causes dose-dependent contraction of circular muscle strips and augments electrical field stimulation-induced contraction in vitro (308). Calcitonin and CGRP inhibit esophageal contractions (382). Certain prostaglandins (e.g., PGE) decrease peristaltic contraction amplitude and duration, an effect that is more marked in the distal esophagus (457). Interestingly galanin has been reported to cause selective inhibition of noncholinergic nerves in the esophagus (284). Further studies are required to define the physiological roles, if any, of the many neurotransmitters found in esophageal neurons.

*Peristalsis in the Junctional Zone*

Although there are fundamental differences in the mechanisms of the latency gradients in the striated versus smooth muscle segments, there is nevertheless a smooth transition as the peristaltic wave sweeps over the junctional area. For this to occur the latency gradient in the central nervous system must be precisely matched with the peripheral latency gradient in the smooth muscle. It is likely that vagal efferent fibers are involved in this transition. There is no evidence that direct coupling between striated and smooth muscle cell is involved.

Spike characteristics obtained from striated muscle are different from those obtained from smooth muscle (8, 235, 494). At 2–6 cm below the UES, spikes of the striated muscle type occur with a latency gradient and duration that coincide with the spikes of the smooth muscle type. Spikes are recorded from longitudinal striated muscle first and then from the deeper circular smooth muscle layer (236, 424).

Anticholinergic agents disrupt this normal sequence. Atropine delays the appearance of smooth muscle spikes, and a delay in the appearance of peristalsis is observed manometrically in the junctional segment (148). In monkeys, bolus distension in the transition zone is followed by spike potentials only in smooth muscle, and the striated muscle remains electrically silent (270). There is therefore no evidence that a striated muscle contribution exists in the secondary peristaltic response of the junctional zone. Clearly, further study is required to delineate the mechanisms whereby the peristaltic wave passes from the striated to the smooth muscle segment without discontinuity.

*Role of Longitudinal Muscle Layer and Muscularis Mucosa in Peristalsis*

The preceding discussion has dealt exclusively with the role of the circular muscle layer in the genesis of the peristaltic wave, because this layer is the dominant force involved in the peristaltic contraction. Nevertheless the longitudinal muscle layer and the muscularis mucosa are activated during peristalsis and may also play a role in peristalsis. Unfortunately, relatively little is known about the physiological roles of these muscle layers. The longitudinal muscle is known to contract during peristalsis and thereby shorten the esophageal body (147, 158, 474). This may serve to *1*) help slide the esophagus over the bolus and provide rigidity to the esophageal tube during peristalsis, and 2) increase the density of circular muscle fibers oral to the bolus. Recent studies in the opossum (474) have shown that longitudinal muscle, like circular muscle, contracts sequentially in an aboral direction during primary peristalsis. Unlike circular muscle, this longitudinal muscle peristalsis is mediated centrally by vagal efferents, because simultaneous contraction at all sites is seen if vagal efferents are simultaneously activated by electrical stimulation of the distal cut end of the cervical vagus. Furthermore there is a peripherally mediated, aborally increasing gradient in the duration of longitudinal muscle contraction so that contraction of the distal esophageal longitudinal muscle lasts for a much longer period than does that of the circular muscle contraction (474).

In vitro studies have shown that longitudinal muscle contracts throughout the duration of an electrical field stimulation or intramural balloon distension (77) and that this is tetrodotoxin and atropine sensitive and therefore largely due to the release of acetylcholine from intrinsic neurons. Recent studies (113) have shown that a more prolonged, more slowly developing longitudinal muscle contraction can be evoked by certain stimulus parameters and that this is mediated by release of substance P. The increased duration of longitudinal muscle contraction seen in the distal esophagus appears to be due to the substance P innervation (113).

There have been several recent studies pertaining to the pharmacology of the muscularis mucosa in various species (38, 79, 120, 286, 287, 361, 412). Electrical field stimulation induces an atropine-sensitive phasic contraction; however, as with the longitudinal layer, there is an additional tonic contraction that may also be due to the release of substance P (160). The physical role of muscularis mucosa is unknown; although in the rat it is postulated that it contributes to the genesis of intraluminal pressure (32). Whether this is the case in other species is unknown. It may function to bind down the normally loosely attached overlying mucosa and thereby prevent excessive prolapse of the mucosa during passage of the swallowed bolus.

## LOWER ESOPHAGEAL SPHINCTER

### Muscular Anatomy

The human LES is a functional structure found at the gastroesophageal junction, which can be readily identified by intraluminal manometry as a 2–4 cm zone of high pressure. The LES is composed of smooth muscle; however, the precise muscle bundles that constitute the sphincter and its anatomic landmarks are not known with certainty.

The *cardiac orifice* is the term used to describe the junction of the esophagus and stomach. Its location should mark the distal extent of the LES; however, the anatomic landmarks of the cardiac orifice are also unclear. Anatomists, radiologists, and physiologists have generated confusing verbiage to describe LES landmarks and subdivisions (188, 310, 522, 528). Figure 15 provides a simple scheme for correlating anatomic, radiographic, and manometric nomenclatures.

Anatomists have searched, largely in vain, for the area of thickened circular muscle corresponding to the lower esophageal high-pressure zone. The thickened muscle seen at autopsy in the LES is related to muscle contraction and disappears as the sphincter segment is distended to a size comparable to the esophageal body. After distension a 2–3 mm contracted band of muscle persists in some specimens (216, 220, 310) and has been termed the *inferior esophageal sphincter* (310). This area is covered by squamous epithelium and is located 2–3 cm proximal to the sling fibers that are present in the esophagogastric angle on the left side of the stomach (216). Indirect evidence from studies in human cadavers indicates that the inferior esophageal sphincter forms the uppermost portion of the LES, and its distal extent may be marked by the upper portion of the sling fibers. The inferior esophageal sphincter may correspond to a muscular ring sometimes seen on barium X rays (216, 220) and the squamocolumnar junction may be identified as a mucosal (Shatzki) ring. Frequently, however, columnar mucosa extend upward in fingerlike projections to involve distal parts of the lower esophageal sphincter. The location of the squamocolumnar junction and mucosal ring in relation to the LES has been controversial for some time (88, 213, 216, 301, 359).

Liebermann-Meffert et al. (312), in their studies with human autopsy material, found an area of muscle thickening ~3 cm wide on the greater curvature and 2.3 cm wide along the lesser curvature. Asymmetry in thickness and width was noted in this area of muscle thickening, which they termed the *gastroesophageal ring*. Subsequently this group has claimed that this anatomic area corresponds to the lower esophageal high-pressure zone as measured manometrically; however, they did not present supportive data (313). This gastroesophageal ring is similar to the "collar of Helvetius" described by earlier investigators (359). That region is covered by columnar mucosa, the squamocolumnar junction being located 2.5 cm proximally. This results in a discrepancy in that simultaneous manometric and potential difference recordings or mucosal biopsies (to identify the squamocolumnar junction) indicate that the squamocolumnar junction is located within or distal to the LES and not 2.5 cm proximal to it (170, 268, 362, 511).

The relationship between anatomic structures and their function can be more precisely studied in experimental animals. In the cat, Biancani et al. (35) have demonstrated that the manometrically defined LES is made up of a ring of thicker circular muscle. In the same species, Clerc (90) has described thickening of the muscularis mucosa and numerous annulospiral

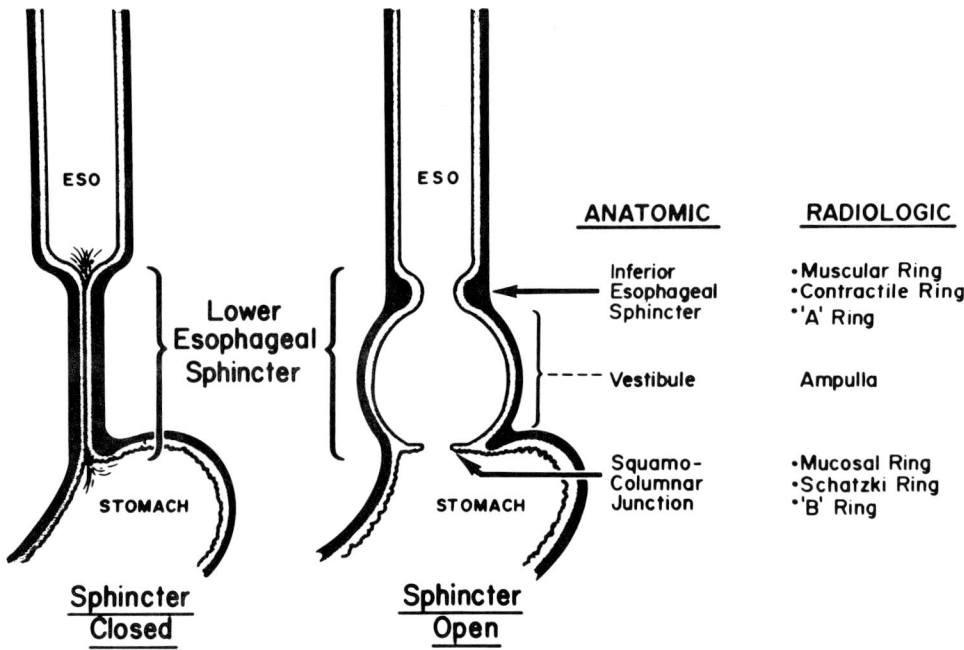

FIG. 15. Proposed scheme for anatomic radiologic landmarks of the lower esophageal sphincter. [From Goyal (212).]

elastic fibers that coil around circular muscle bundles in an area presumed to represent the LES.

The longitudinal muscle in the area of the LES shows no distinctive features. Laterally, the fibers follow the greater curvature on the left and lesser curvature on the right. Anteriorly and posteriorly, the music bundles turn upward in the direction of the fundus and interlace with fibers of the inner circular muscle layer (312, 359). Obliquely oriented bracket fibers can be found inner to the circular muscle layer in the terminal esophagus but do not extend into the stomach (216, 310).

Ultrastructural studies of the sphincter muscle in the opossum suggest that muscle cells from the LES are of larger diameter and form fewer gap junctions than do those of the esophageal body (121). These sphincter muscle cells also have irregular surfaces and evaginations that are not seen in the esophageal body. The evaginations may be related to the tonically contracted state of the sphincter muscle (448). The LES can also be distinguished from the esophageal body morphologically by the presence of more numerous intermuscular spaces containing blood vessels and connective tissue (448). It has also been reported that mitochondria and smooth endoplasmic reticulum mass is greater in the LES than in the esophageal body (82).

*Pressure Profile*

The LES is kept closed at rest and creates a zone of high pressure. A profile of LES pressure, including its length and peak amplitude, can be made by withdrawing a manometric catheter at a fixed speed across the LES. The high-pressure zone caused by the LES shows axial as well as radial asymmetry. Axially, the LES pressure has a bell-shaped configuration with a total length of between 2 and 4 cm. Pressures tend to be higher in the more distal segment of the LES.

Radial asymmetry is apparent if multiple catheters with side openings oriented in different directions are used to record LES pressure, although this asymmetry is less marked than in the UES. The LES is fairly symmetrical in its oral half, but in the aboral half, the LES shows higher pressures on the left side (515, 516). The reason for this is not fully understood. It may partly be related to mechanical factors. The terminal esophagus is not aligned in the axis of the rest of the esophagus but is angled like a hockey stick as it joins the stomach. The diaphragm makes an impression on the terminal esophagus, which is directed downward and to the right. However, some asymmetry exists even in patients with hiatal hernia or in animals with an entirely intra-abdominal LES, indicating that the diaphragm can be only partly responsible. Another possibility is that the gastric sling fibers may buttress the left side of the LES, thereby creating higher pressures in this region.

FLUCTUATIONS IN BASAL PRESSURE. The pressures recorded in the LES with a catheter positioned at a single site are not constant. Variations exist, the most common being pressure fluctuations in phase with the respiratory cycle. In humans, the pressures in the upper and lower halves of the LES are usually affected by respiration in opposite ways. In the lower part, inspiration causes a rise in LES pressure, whereas the opposite occurs in the upper part. This is thought to represent abdominal and thoracic influences at the distal and proximal locations, respectively. The point at which the respiratory pressure transition occurs is called the point of respiratory reversal or the pressure inversion point. This often occurs over a wide region that shows biphasic pressure changes with respiration. This zone is ~0.5 cm wide and is usually located in the middle of the high-pressure zone, but its precise location is variable (234).

The point of respiratory reversal may be related to the crura of the diaphragm, or the attachment of the phrenoesophageal membrane (130), which separates thoracic from abdominal cavities and provides opposing pressure environments during respiration. It may also be related to the LES itself as it separates intraesophageal from intragastric pressure.

Another source of respiratory pressure fluctuation relates to the axial movement of the esophagus relative to the recording device. The terminal esophagus moves up with expiration and down with inspiration (45, 159), and because of the bell-shaped profile of the LES high-pressure zone, the measured pressure reflects changes resulting from movement of the catheter hole in relationship to different LES sites. This phenomenon may explain in part the inspiratory increase in pressure in the lower part and inspiratory reduction in pressure in the upper part of the sphincter.

In addition, because of the position of the LES, within the diaphragmatic hiatus, the sphincter pressure may be influenced by the respiratory contractions of the crural diaphragm (46, 516). Such phasic pressure variations would be expected to have sharper peaks than the respiratory fluctuations transmitted passively to the LES. It has been shown in cats that inspiratory peaks in pressure do not occur when the crural diaphragm is inactive (46), and when this occurs, LES resting pressure equals that recorded at end expiration. In cats the crural part of the diaphragm is selectively inhibited during LES relaxation (3), a phenomenon similar to that which occurs in sheep during regurgitation (483).

The pressure inversion point is also related to the esophageal hiatus in that patients with a hiatal hernia may have a double respiratory reversal. The diaphragmatic hiatus can produce respiratory reversal when the LES is absent or displaced; however, the LES itself may produce a respiratory reversal when it is not associated with the diaphragm (234). In experimental animals, respiration-related increases in the LES pressure may occur that are related to neither axial movement nor to extrinsic pressure changes (11).

In addition to respiration-related pressure fluctuations, the LES also may show rhythmic pressure changes that occur at a rate of three to four per minute. These pressure changes have been documented during long-term recordings in the opossum (226, 245), and they also occur in humans (R. K. Goyal, unpublished observations). In addition, slow phasic contractions in phase with the gastric component of the migrating myoelectrical complex (MMC) have been described in humans and animals (140, 245, 246, 265, 462).

BASAL SPHINCTER PRESSURE. Because of the many pressure fluctuations related to respiration and other factors, it is hard to validate a single value for resting LES pressure. Furthermore the variations due to recording methods described previously for the UES also hold for the LES. As a result, several different scoring methods have been proposed to obtain a single reliable value for resting LES pressure. Some investigators use the rapid pull-through technique in which the manometric catheter is rapidly pulled through the lower esophageal high-pressure zone during suspended respiration. The major problem with this technique is that it records the LES pressure at only a single point in time. Furthermore the phase and depth of the respiratory cycle at which the rapid pull through is performed cannot be precisely controlled. Other potential sources of error with this technique include *1*) peristaltic activity going on in the esophagus at the time of the pull through may be associated with LES relaxation, and *2*) a contraction in the distal esophagus may be erroneously interpreted as representing the high-pressure zone. These problems can be partially overcome by utilizing manometry ports that detect activity simultaneously in the esophageal body (151); however, it is possible that rapid tube movement in the esophageal body stimulates minor degrees of LES relaxation without accompanying peristaltic activity (370). This may explain the lower LES pressures recorded with the rapid pull-through technique as opposed to the standard station pull-through method (515). Given these variables, it is not surprising that the rapid pull-through technique produces significant variability in the LES pressure value when repeated measurements are made in the same subject (209, 515).

The station pull-through technique is performed by withdrawing the manometry catheter in 0.5-cm stages, allowing pressure to be recorded for a period of time with the catheter set in one position. With this technique, or with the continuous slow motorized pull-through technique, sphincter pressures are recorded that demonstrate respiration-related fluctuations. It is also possible to observe the LES relaxation by having the subject swallow at each station. In such a tracing, measurement can be made at the respiratory reversal point, at the highest peak pressure, or at the highest mean pressure. The results obtained by these three methods correlate reasonably well with each other and have coefficients of variation superior to those obtained by the rapid pull through (209, 515). The scoring of the peak pressure is perhaps easiest and has the lowest interobserver variability (515). With a low-compliance perfused manometry system and the station pull-through technique, one study found resting LES pressures to range between 7 and 58 mmHg above intragastric pressure in a large group of normal volunteers (357).

The resting LES pressures are apparently not altered significantly by age (300, 464, 510), and higher LES pressures are recorded in the supine rather than in the sitting position (509). The reasons for this are unclear.

### Genesis of Basal Sphincter Pressure

Lower esophageal sphincter pressure measured in vivo is dependent on mechanical factors as well as on the basal tone in the muscle itself.

MECHANICAL FACTORS. The true resting state of the LES is undoubtedly modified when a manometric device is inserted within its lumen. Unfortunately, there is no method for measuring pressure without violating the lumen. However, this manometrically derived LES pressure seems to provide a physiologically useful measurement. LES pressures have been measured with probes of different diameters to obtain pressure-diameter curves (32, 34) that are then used to obtain tension-diameter (32) and force-of-closure–diameter (34) relationships. These studies reveal that *1*) the diameter at which active tension is developed in the LES is smaller than that in the esophageal body, *2*) tension-diameter curves of the LES are steeper than in the esophageal body, and *3*) the diameter at which maximal tension is generated occurs at a large diameter and not at the diameter of sphincter closure. These biomechanical characteristics may explain the ability of the LES to stay closed at rest with a small tension requirement and to be able to generate fairly stable pressures over a wide range of luminal diameters (32).

Normally the circular muscle of the LES is stretched slightly by folds of mucosa and underlying submucosa. These folds form a mucosal plug and probably contribute to the basal LES pressure in vivo. The precise role and importance of the mucosal plug in the competence of the LES is not known.

In vitro studies also demonstrate that length-tension curves of circular muscle from the LES are steeper than those from the esophageal body (74, 76, 319). Lower esophageal sphincter strips from the cat demonstrate higher basal and active force-generating capacity, whereas the passive-force curves are no different from those in the esophageal body (31, 35). The higher active forces appear to be due to muscle thickening, whereas higher basal forces are due partly to an increased ability of the sphincter muscle to generate stress (35). The sphincter muscle is also more sensitive than the esophageal body in its response to excitatory agents such as bethanechol and gastrin (68, 319, 440).

If the LES is in the intrahiatal position (i.e., surrounded by the crural fibers of the diaphragm), then a component of the measured resting pressure is due to phasic contraction of the crural diaphragm (46, 516). In this setting, resting pressure generated by the LES muscle itself is most closely approximated by the end-expiratory pressure (46).

These intrinsic and extrinsic mechanical factors are important, but they are clearly not responsible for generating sphincter pressure at rest. This requires the existence of active tone in the muscle itself.

BASAL SPHINCTER MUSCLE TONE. The hallmark of the sphincter muscle is its propensity to maintain tonic contraction. This property is shared with certain other tonic smooth muscles and is characterized by the muscles' ability to maintain stress for prolonged periods after the stress is developed (428). Thus it is the ability to maintain stress that distinguishes lower esophageal sphincter from esophageal body muscle. The esophageal body muscle undergoes only a transient contraction and is therefore called a phasic muscle (105). The cellular mechanisms involved in stress or tone maintenance in the LES are not fully understood. However, several distinctive properties of the sphincter muscle have been identified that may be related to tone maintenance.

Contraction in all muscles is explained on the basis of a sliding-filament model in which actin (thin filament) slides on myosin (thick filament) by an energy-requiring, myosin-$Mg^{2+}$ ATPase–mediated reaction (105). In the smooth muscle, phosphorylation of myosin on its light chain is the central determinant in the ATPase activation and hence contraction. Phosphorylation of myosin light chains is mediated by the enzyme, myosin light-chain kinase, which requires $Ca^{2+}$ and the $Ca^{2+}$-binding protein, calmodulin.

Chatterjee and Murphy (65) have reported that myosin phosphorylation increases during stress development and is correlated with the velocity of muscle shortening; however, during stress maintenance, the levels of phosphorylation decline to near-resting levels. The phenomenon of stress maintenance is called the latch phenomenon (65) and is considered to be different from the catch phenomenon as described in bivalve mollusks (428). The catch phenomenon is associated with a slowing of cross-bridge cycling between actin and myosin. This concept is supported by estimates of free intracellular $Ca^{2+}$ as determined by the $Ca^{2+}$-sensitive photoprotein aequorin. In certain tonic smooth muscles, the free intracellular $Ca^{2+}$ rises during stress development but then returns to near resting levels despite continuous force maintenance. The tone maintenance, however, is an active process and involves an as yet unknown mechanism that also requires low levels of $Ca^{2+}$.

Weisbrodt and Murphy (514) studied the phosphorylation of myosin during force development and maintenance in the opossum LES. They found that the phosphorylation rate was ~4% of maximum during the relaxed state of the sphincter, increased to 33% during tone development, and then fell to 16% during tone maintenance, supporting the role of latch phenomenon in LES tone.

Studies of free intracellular $Ca^{2+}$ concentration with the photoprotein aequorin suggest that the sphincter may have higher free intracellular $Ca^{2+}$ levels as compared with the esophageal body during the resting state (396). Several studies have examined the influence of $Ca^{2+}$-channel blockers on tone development and maintenance. It is clear that tone maintenance in the LES is dependent on intracellular as well as extracellular $Ca^{2+}$ because $Ca^{2+}$ channel–blocking drugs reduce but do not abolish the maintained tone of the sphincter (26, 42, 250, 251, 407, 408). Golenhofen (206) proposed that $Ca^{2+}$-activating systems utilized by tonic and phasic contractions were different and he called them $T$ (for tonic) and $P$ (for phasic) $Ca^{2+}$-activation systems. These two systems were distinguished on the basis of their responses to nitroprusside (which affected primarily the tonic system), and verapamil (which affected primarily the phasic system). However, maintained tone in the LES is sensitive to both nitroprusside and verapamil (127, 139, 185, 226).

Asoh and Goyal (11) showed that the opossum LES in vivo shows continuous spike activity. Moreover increases in spike activity are associated with an increase in the maintained sphincter tone and abolition of the spike activity is associated with a decrease (Fig. 16). Continuous spike activity has also been shown to be present in the cat (402, 403); however, the spike rate is lower in this species than in the opossum. The spikes in the smooth muscle are dependent on influx of extracellular $Ca^{2+}$, because agents such as verapamil abolish spike activity and reduce resting tone.

Asoh and Goyal (11) also observed that a major portion of the maintained sphincter tone in vivo persisted in the absence of any spike activity. This was called the spike-independent fraction of the sphincter tone. The basis of the spike-independent fraction of the maintained tone has been investigated by Papasova et al. (367, 368) with the sucrose-gap technique in the cat LES in vitro. These investigators found that the sphincter muscle exhibited tone in the absence of spike activity and that this spike-independent tone varied directly with the resting membrane potential. A relatively depolarized resting state of the sphincter muscle, which would result in increased tone, has been reported in studies with direct intracellular recordings. Daniel et al. (123) and Zelcer and Weisbrodt (529) reported that resting membrane potential of the sphincter smooth muscle was approximately −40 mV in contrast to the resting membrane potential of esophageal body circular muscle, which is −50 mV. It

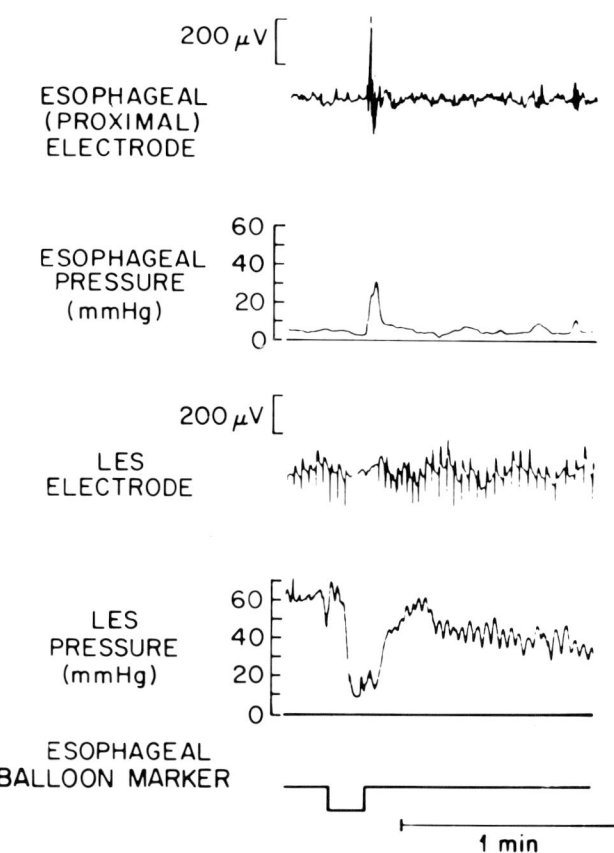

FIG. 16. Influence of inflation of an intraluminal esophageal balloon on electrical activity and pressures of distal esophageal body and LES. Balloon inflation causes a cessation of tonic LES spike activity and simultaneous fall in LES pressure. Balloon deflation causes spike activity that precedes contraction in esophageal body; in LES, tonic spike activity reappears as LES pressure returns toward base line. [From Asoh and Goyal (11).]

has been suggested that the less negative membrane potential of the sphincter muscle, in contrast to the esophageal body, is associated with a constant inward leak of $Ca^{2+}$, leading to elevated free intracellular $Ca^{2+}$ levels and thus tone maintenance. Both nitroprusside and verapamil reduced spike-independent LES tone, but the former is more effective than the latter in this regard (185, 226, 367). However, the effect of nitroprusside or verapamil on the resting membrane potential in the sphincter is not known.

Thus it is clear that tone maintenance in the sphincter is an active energy-requiring process that is associated with electrical spikes, maintained membrane depolarization without spikes, ongoing low-level phosphorylation of myosin light chains, and perhaps elevated free intracellular $Ca^{2+}$ concentration. The energy required to maintain sphincter tone is evidenced by its marked sensitivity to anoxia compared with that of esophageal body muscle (71, 445). It has been reported that the LES has lower levels of cytochrome-$c$ oxidase activity than does the esophageal body (411).

This may help explain why the LES is more dependent on exogenous $O_2$. Cytochrome-$c$ oxidase is used in oxidative metabolism, and therefore elevated levels in the esophageal body muscle would permit a greater degree of anaerobic metabolism. This does not necessarily mean that the absolute requirements for molecular $O_2$ are different in the two sites, rather the required source of $O_2$ may be different.

### Genesis of Lower Esophageal Sphincter Muscle Tone

The active tone of the LES may be due to continuous stimulation of the muscle by *1*) tonic excitatory nerve activity, *2*) locally released biologically active agents, *3*) circulating hormone(s), *4*) inherent self-stimulating properties of the smooth muscle cell, or *5*) a combination of several of these factors.

TONIC EXCITATORY NERVE ACTIVITY. Vagal or parasympathetic nerves are generally held to exert excitatory effects on smooth muscle by activating postganglionic cholinergic neurons. However, in the LES, it is clear that the major effect of vagal efferent nerves is to induce LES relaxation (86, 207, 302, 331, 383).

*Influence of nerve section or pharmacologic denervation.* Whether tonic excitatory vagal discharge plays a role in the maintenance of LES tone is controversial and depends in part on certain interspecies differences. In the opossum, bilateral cervical vagotomy causes either no change or a transient increase in resting LES pressure. Furthermore electrical stimulation of vagal efferents causes LES relaxation at all stimulus parameters. Excitatory cholinergic fibers to the LES that are carried in the vagus are not easily demonstrable experimentally (383).

In the cat the vagus may carry both inhibitory and excitatory fibers to the LES (86, 207, 404). Studies by Gonella et al. (207) suggest that vagal stimulation leads to excitatory and inhibitory LES responses, depending on the stimulus parameters. However, in this study, LES pressures were recorded with balloons, and therefore it is possible that contraction responses attributed to the LES were in fact due to contraction of the distal esophageal body. Nevertheless considerable resting LES tone remained after vagotomy, and the authors provide no evidence to support their hypothesis that the excitatory pathway to the LES is tonically active. The study by Reynolds et al. (404), in which vagal cooling was used to block the nerves in the cervical region, showed a 50% decrease in resting LES pressure; however, ventilation was apparently not controlled, and the changes seen in resting LES pressure may have been secondary to the abnormal respiration induced by vagal blockade. Other investigators have found that bilateral cervical vagotomy does not modify basal LES pressure in the cat (30, 183, 184). Furthermore, vagal stimulation causes frequency-dependent relaxation of the LES, and no parameter of vagal efferent stimulation evoked LES contraction (184). Thus, at present, there is no clear-cut evidence that tonic vagal excitatory discharge is a major determinant of basal LES tone in cats.

In the dog, cervical vagotomy abolishes basal LES pressure acutely, but it tends to recover over a period of days to weeks (277). In a study by Price et al. (379) cooling of the vagosympathetic trunks caused a drop of LES pressure in two of three dogs. Unlike the cat, stimulation of vagal efferents at certain frequencies causes contraction of the LES in the dog. Cervical vagal efferent stimulation also causes relaxation of the LES after thoracic vagotomy, indicating that vagal efferent fibers of an inhibitory nature follow an intramural path to the LES (277). In humans, the influence of cervical or high thoracic vagotomy is not known; however, high abdominal truncal vagotomy does not influence resting LES pressure (478).

There is evidence that sympathetic nerve activity plays a role in influencing resting LES pressure. In the cat, stimulation of sympathetic efferents to the LES causes contraction of the sphincter that is sensitive to atropine, hexamethonium, phentolamine, and tetrodotoxin (30, 184). Despite this, sympathetic nerve section does not modify resting LES pressure (30, 183, 184), which is evidence against tonic sympathetic nerve activity in the genesis of basal LES pressure.

It is possible that tonic intramural neuron activity could occur in the absence of tonic extrinsic nerve influence. In experiments where tetrodotoxin is used to block $Na^+$-dependent action potentials in the intramural nerves without affecting smooth muscle activity, resting LES pressure is not modified in the opossum (224). These studies suggest that tonic neural activity is not responsible for tonic LES closure in this species. However, in the cat, tetrodotoxin has been shown to cause a 25%–28% reduction in resting LES pressure (30). The effects of tetrodotoxin on LES pressure in other species has not been studied. However, spontaneous release of a neurotransmitter (i.e., not evoked by action potential) is not sensitive to tetrodotoxin, and therefore tetrodotoxin resistance does not exclude the role of spontaneous excitatory neurotransmitter release in the maintenance of tonic contraction of the LES.

*Influence of cholinergic and adrenergic antagonists.* An alternative way of examining the role of specific excitatory neurotransmitters in maintaining LES pressure is to examine the influence of selective antagonists. Despite extensive literature on the subject, there remains controversy regarding the role of cholinergic innervation in the maintenance of resting tone. In humans and animals, muscarinic agents cause contraction of the LES (420). Furthermore the LES has muscarinic cholinergic receptors demonstrable with binding studies (409), and intramural cholinergic neurons have been identified in the LES with histochemical techniques (447). It has been shown that the M$_2$ subtype of muscarinic receptor mediates LES circular smooth muscle contraction (202, 393). Atropine, however, does not antagonize resting LES pressure in opossums (148, 245, 380) and monkeys (148), although it does lower it in dogs (530). Interestingly, in dogs, cholinesterase inhibitors have been reported to produce a picture of achalasia (233). In cats and humans the effect of atropine and other anticholinergic agents on resting LES pressure is controversial (30, 148, 182, 247, 251, 280, 294, 315, 404). In humans the decline in resting LES pressure after anticholinergics is usually small and often does not reach statistical significance (182, 251, 280). In no animal species examined does atropine completely abolish the basal LES pressure.

A possible explanation for the differences in reported studies is the radial asymmetry of the LES pressure. Richardson and Welch (406) found that atropine caused a significant drop in LES pressure when the recording orifice was facing to the left but not when facing in other directions. The effect of atropine on the left side may be related to the presence of the gastric sling fibers, which bolster the left side of the LES. These fibers appear to have prominent cholinergic innervation. Another source of variability relates to the time at which LES pressure measurements are made. It has recently been shown in the opossum that atropine does not affect basal LES pressure but abolishes the MMC-related phasic pressure elevations of the LES (245).

Pharmacological studies have shown that $\alpha$-adrenergic receptor stimulation causes LES contraction. In one study adrenergic neuron destruction with 6-hydroxydopamine caused reduction in LES pressure (145). In cats $\alpha$-blockade also reduces resting LES pressure (30, 404). $\beta$-Blockade has been reported to have no affect in cats (404), but one report in humans found an increase in resting LES pressure after propranolol (481). However, these effects of antagonists on the LES are often transient, and sphincter pressure soon returns to normal levels even when adrenergic antagonism is still present. These observations do not support the view that tonic adrenergic activity is responsible for basal LES tone.

LOCAL RELEASE OF EXCITATORY BIOLOGICAL AGENTS. The tonic LES pressure may be due to release of a local hormone or biologically active agent. This may be an endogenous amine (serotonin, histamine, or dopamine), a polypeptide (substance P, enkephalin, bombesin), or a lipid (prostaglandin). Many of these have been identified in the LES.

Pharmacological studies show that dopamine decreases LES pressure (125, 348, 385), whereas histamine (23, 109, 126, 217, 303, 387), serotonin (23, 386), and opioids (392) have complex effects because of the abundance of different receptor subtypes in the nerve and muscle of the LES (225). However, the selective antagonism of these agents does not abolish basal LES pressure. For example, neither H$_1$- nor H$_2$-receptor blockade has a significant effect on resting LES pressure (19, 131, 303, 462) despite pharmacological effects of the agonist. Similarly opioid antagonist naloxone does not significantly modify LES pressure (392). These agents may play a role in modulating resting LES pressure or LES relaxation, but they clearly are not responsible for generating basal tone. It has been suggested that endogenous prostaglandins may be responsible for LES tone in vitro (117, 118); however, in vivo exogenous PGE$_1$, PGE$_2$, or arachidonic acid cause LES inhibition (144, 222, 227, 346, 458). Prostaglandin F$_{2\alpha}$ causes contraction of the LES (144, 398). Inhibition of prostaglandin synthesis by indomethacin either does not modify basal LES pressure (391) or causes a small increase in sphincter pressure (144). Thus it is unlikely that prostaglandins play a significant role in the genesis of basal LES pressure. Substance P (344), Met-enkephalin (392), galanin (394), and bombesin (345) cause LES contraction; however, it is unclear whether they have a physiological function.

CIRCULATING EXCITATORY HORMONE ACTIVITY. Several years ago there was great interest in the role of circulating gastrin in the generation of basal LES pressure (62, 96, 102, 238, 319, 320, 321). Other hormones such as secretin, cholecystokinin (CCK), and glucagon were thought to exert their effects on the LES pressure by interacting with gastrin receptors (29, 102, 179, 267). Furthermore, the modulation of LES pressure seen with feeding and antacids was thought to be secondary to changes in circulating gastrin, and various disorders of LES function were attributed to changes in levels of muscle sensitivity to circulating gastrin (104, 177).

Evidence for the physiological role of gastrin in the genesis of LES pressure was based on the observation that gastrin contracted the LES (205) and that instillation of acid into the stomach lowered the LES pressure, whereas gastric alkalinization increased LES pressure. These latter changes were thought to be due to a decrease and increase, respectively, in circulating gastrin (63). It was also reported that administration of gastrin antiserum selectively bound circulating gastrin and caused an 80% reduction in basal LES pressure (320). Subsequently, numerous studies were reported that refuted a physiological role of gastrin in the maintenance of LES tone (115, 133, 153, 187, 231, 298, 299, 332, 471, 504, 507, 524), and the studies showing a fall in basal LES pressure after administration of high-titer gastrin antiserum could not be reproduced (221). Therefore it appears unlikely that gastrin is a major determinant of basal LES pressure.

Although many other hormones may exert a modulating influence on LES pressure, they do not appear to be a major determinant of resting sphincter tone.

INTRINSIC CIRCULAR MUSCLE ACTIVITY. The fact that the LES muscle generates tone in vitro and in vivo in the presence of tetrodotoxin indicates that neural or hormonal influences are not necessary and that the muscle remains tonically contracted because of its own unique properties (i.e., mechanisms intrinsic to the muscle itself may be responsible for its sustained depolarization, spontaneous spikes, distinctive intracellular $Ca^{2+}$ mechanisms, and the latch phenomenon).

## Modulation of Resting Pressure in Lower Esophageal Sphincter

It is apparent from the foregoing discussion regarding the genesis of the LES tone that extrinsic nerves, intrinsic nerves, neuropeptides, locally released substances, and circulating hormones can modify basal LES pressure. Some of the proposed mechanisms that did not quite measure up as determinants of resting LES pressure may provide modulatory functions in regulating resting pressure. In such a system, where a multitude of excitatory and inhibitory influences are present, it is not appropriate to assign a certain proportion of the basal LES pressure to a given excitatory mechanism. For example, atropine may cause a 30% reduction in LES pressure, but this does not mean that 30% of the LES pressure at rest is due to cholinergic mechanisms. This is because, in the absence of tonic cholinergic influences, the counterbalancing inhibitory influence may cause unopposed reduction in LES pressure.

As mentioned earlier, circulating hormone and locally released agents can change the LES pressure; however, it is difficult to differentiate between physiological and pharmacological effects. The effect of various hormones and locally released agents on the LES pressure and their proposed mechanisms of action have been widely studied and are summarized in Table 1.

During pregnancy LES pressure declines (17, 48, 316, 351, 497). This appears to be due to increased circulating levels of sex hormones, most likely progesterone (180, 443, 498). Decreases in LES pressure during the luteal phase of the menstrual cycle were noted in one study (499) but not in another (356).

Many other circulating hormones and endogenous polypeptides can influence the resting LES pressure (see Table 1). Pancreatic polypeptide (330, 389), motilin (169, 232, 246, 265, 278, 339), and bombesin (106, 345) may contract the LES. In normal humans CCK relaxes the LES but causes paradoxical contraction in patients with achalasia (150). Species differences exist regarding the effect of CCK (27, 138, 395). In cats and humans the effect on the inhibitory intramural neuron predominates, causing LES relaxation, whereas in the opossum a direct effect on the circular smooth muscle predominates, causing LES contraction. A protein meal (15, 353), intraduodenal peptone (299), and gastric acidification (241, 291) have been found to cause sustained contraction of the LES. In dogs the postprandial rise in LES pressure after a protein meal seems to correlate with the release of pancreatic polypeptide (330); this effect is abolished after surgical

TABLE 1. *Effects of Some Hormones and Neuropeptides on Lower Esophageal Sphincter Pressure*

|  | Proposed Site of Action | Ref. |
|---|---|---|
| Net effect, excitatory |  |  |
|   Bombesin | Direct on CSM and indirect via release of norepinephrine from postganglionic adrenergic neuron | 106, 345 |
|   Galanin | Direct on CSM | 394 |
|   Gastrin | Direct on CSM | 205, 211, 280, 380, 431 |
|   Motilin | Preganglionic excitatory vagal efferents | 169, 232, 246, 265, 278, 339 |
|   Pancreatic polypeptide | Direct on CSM and indirect via cholinergic neurons | 330, 389 |
|   Somatostatin | Unknown | 54,† 231* |
|   Substance P | Direct on CSM and via cholinergic neurons | 108, 344 |
| Net effect, inhibitory |  |  |
|   Calcitonin gene-related peptide (CGRP) | Direct on CSM and indirect on inhibitory intramural neuron | 382 |
|   Cholecystokinin | Inhibitory intramural neuron (overrides direct excitatory effect on CSM) | 27, 138, 150,‡ 179, 395, 401, 472 |
|   Gastric inhibitory polypeptide (GIP) | Unknown | 459 |
|   Glucagon | Via release of epinephrine and norepinephrine from adrenal medulla | 29, 242, 267, 279, 456 |
|   Neurotensin | Unknown | 427, 480 |
|   Progesterone | Unknown | 180, 443 |
|   Secretin | Direct on CSM | 29, 456 |
|   Vasoactive intestinal polypeptide (VIP) | Direct on CSM | 29, 161, 399, 456 |

CSM, circular smooth muscle. * Has excitatory effect in normal humans but inhibitory effect in achalasic patients. † Has no effect on resting LESP in baboons but antagonizes increase in LESP induced by instillation of alkali or glycine into stomach. ‡ Inhibitory effect in normal humans but paradoxical excitation in achalasic patients.

exclusion of the duodenum from the chyme. Duodenal acidification in dogs causes an initial decrease in LES pressure, possibly due to secretin release, followed by a sustained increase in pressure (249). Gastric alkalinization increases LES pressure in humans, and this is apparently dependent on an intact duodenum but not on intact vagal innervation (333). Esophageal acidification has been shown to increase LES pressure in cats (403). When repeated acid infusions are used to induce experimental esophagitis in cats, the LES pressure decreases (31, 168, 215, 239). This was found to be mediated by endogenous prostaglandins in one study (168) but not in another (31). A fatty meal (354, 355) lowers LES pressure. Neurotensin infusion in doses that give blood levels comparable to those seen after a fatty meal also decreases LES pressure (427, 480). Hiatal hernia does not appear to influence LES pressure per se (314). The upright body position lowers LES pressure (16, 509) as does smoking (134, 467), chocolate (523), and coffee (99). Nicotine may mediate the inhibitory effect of smoking (384), whereas xanthine may mediate the inhibitory effect of chocolate (222, 281). Because many neurohumoral agents modify LES pressure, the final effect of these agents is likely the sum total of the different individual effects, whether they be inhibitory or excitatory (225).

*Reflex Relaxation of Lower Esophageal Sphincter*

Reflex relaxation of the LES is associated with several activities, such as swallow-related primary peristalsis and secondary peristalsis induced by esophageal distension. Relaxation of the LES also occurs during belching, retching, vomiting, and rumination (58, 94, 324, 336, 461, 469, 470, 502). During belching and vomiting, there is no esophageal contraction in association with LES relaxation. With rumination, LES relaxation is associated with reverse peristalsis. Transient lower esophageal sphincter relaxation may also occur in isolation. This is an inappropriate physiological response and is associated with gastroesophageal reflux, which may lead to reflux esophagitis (137, 149).

CELLULAR BASIS OF RELAXATION. The cellular basis of reflex LES relaxation is not fully understood. However, it is clear that it is an active process. It is associated with inhibition of continuous spike activity and hyperpolarization of the muscle cell membrane. These electrical phenomena may be related to decreases in free intracellular $Ca^{2+}$ concentration leading to cessation of myosin phosphorylation or to inhibition of the unknown proteins involved in the latch phenomenon. Agents such as isoproterenol and PGE, which increase intracellular cAMP, cause relaxation of the LES (222, 227, 391). Similarly, agents such as sodium nitroprusside that increase cGMP also cause LES relaxation (139, 226). Thus both cAMP and cGMP mediate LES relaxation (343, 489) by activating protein kinase A and G, respectively. These kinases may lower the free intracellular $Ca^{2+}$ by yet unknown mechanisms. They may also inhibit myosin phosphorylation by phosphorylating, hence inactivating, the enzyme myosin light-chain kinase.

SWALLOW-INDUCED RELAXATION. Deglutition causes relaxation of the LES, which may start with the onset of the deglutition so that both upper and lower sphincters relax almost simultaneously (see Fig. 1). Usually, LES relaxation onsets <2 s after the initiation of swallowing. At this time the swallowed bolus is in the esophagus and the peristaltic contraction is oral to the bolus in the cervical esophagus. In the upright position the swallowed bolus may reach the LES very quickly due to gravity, and when this happens, it may be transiently delayed at the sphincter before passage into the stomach. Occasionally one records a brief increase in pressure below and decrease in pressure above the respiratory reversal point just prior to relaxation of the LES. This phenomenon corresponds to that of the brief inspiration association with swallowing. The LES normally relaxes to a pressure equal to or very close to intragastric pressure (103, 289).

Relaxation of the LES may last for a total of 8–10 s (289) and is followed in the oral part of the sphincter by an aftercontraction, which is in continuity with the peristaltic contraction in the esophageal body. The aftercontraction lasts for 7–10 s. The lower part of the LES does not show aftercontractions, and the sphincter pressure simply returns to the resting level. Electrical recordings show that swallow-induced LES relaxation is associated with cessation of spike activity when present (11). Suction electrode recordings also show that swallow-induced LES relaxation is associated with membrane hyperpolarization (381).

Activation of the swallowing reflex causes LES relaxation. Relaxation of the LES is the most sensitive component of the swallowing reflex (370). Thus it is possible to have LES relaxation without any other motor evidence of the swallowing reflex. Isolated LES relaxation can be induced experimentally by applying pharyngeal tactile stimulation, which is subthreshold for producing a full swallowing response. Similarly, electrical stimulation of the superior laryngeal nerve with stimulus frequencies that fail to produce esophageal peristalsis causes isolated LES relaxation. Low-intensity stimulation of the swallowing center can also cause isolated LES relaxation (21).

Swallow-induced LES relaxation appears to be a component of deglutitive inhibition. When repeated swallows are taken in succession, as during rapid drinking, the lower esophageal sphincter remains relaxed and returns to the base-line state of tone after the last swallow (94).

The LES relaxation associated with primary peristalsis as well as isolated LES relaxation due to pharyngeal or superior laryngeal nerve stimulation is mediated by vagal efferent nerves and is abolished by bilateral cervical vagal section or cooling (370, 404, 424, 432).

RELAXATION ASSOCIATED WITH ESOPHAGEAL DISTENSION. Distension of either the striated or smooth muscle portion of the esophagus produces reflex relaxation of the LES that is associated with secondary peristalsis in the esophageal body. During prolonged localized esophageal distension, the LES may recover from relaxation despite ongoing distension (371). The sphincter relaxation due to distension in the striated muscle is centrally mediated and is abolished by vagotomy, whereas the relaxation due to distension in the smooth muscle portion is mediated by intramural nerves and remains after bilateral vagotomy. However, recent studies have shown that the vagus nerves may exert a facilitatory influence on LES relaxation, evoked by balloon distension of the smooth muscle esophagus (370, 404).

As with primary peristalsis, LES relaxation is also the most sensitive component of secondary peristalsis. Thus, isolated LES relaxation without esophageal contraction occurs with distensions that are subthreshold for activation of full secondary peristalsis (370).

The pathways involved in LES relaxation associated with vomiting, retching, or belching are not well understood. These pathways may involve the central inhibitory pathway also used in deglutition. Alternatively, they may involve intramural pathways from the stomach to the LES. It has recently been shown in vitro that electrical stimulation of intramural nerves in the stomach may cause relaxation of the LES (373). Further studies are needed to define these mechanisms.

## Neurotransmitters of Inhibitory Pathways to Lower Esophageal Sphincter

The neurotransmitters involved in the vagal inhibitory pathway to the LES have been investigated in some detail (158, 204, 223, 388). This pathway consists of a chain of at least two neurons consisting of pre- and postganglionic neurons. The preganglionic neurons are carried in the vagus and synapse on postganglionic inhibitory neurons present intramurally in the LES (Fig. 17).

SYNAPTIC TRANSMITTERS. The preganglionic neurons release predominantly acetylcholine, which activates the postganglionic inhibitory neurons by combining with both nicotininc and muscarinic receptors (223). Therefore neither hexamethonium nor atropine alone block vagally stimulated LES relaxation, but a combination of the two effectively antagonizes the response. It has been shown that the $M_1$ subtype of muscarinic receptor is involved in this transmission (202). There is also evidence that serotonin participates to a lesser degree in this synaptic transmission (388). Complete pharmacological blockade of vagally stimulated LES relaxation is produced by a combination of antagonists to nicotinic, muscarinic, and sero-

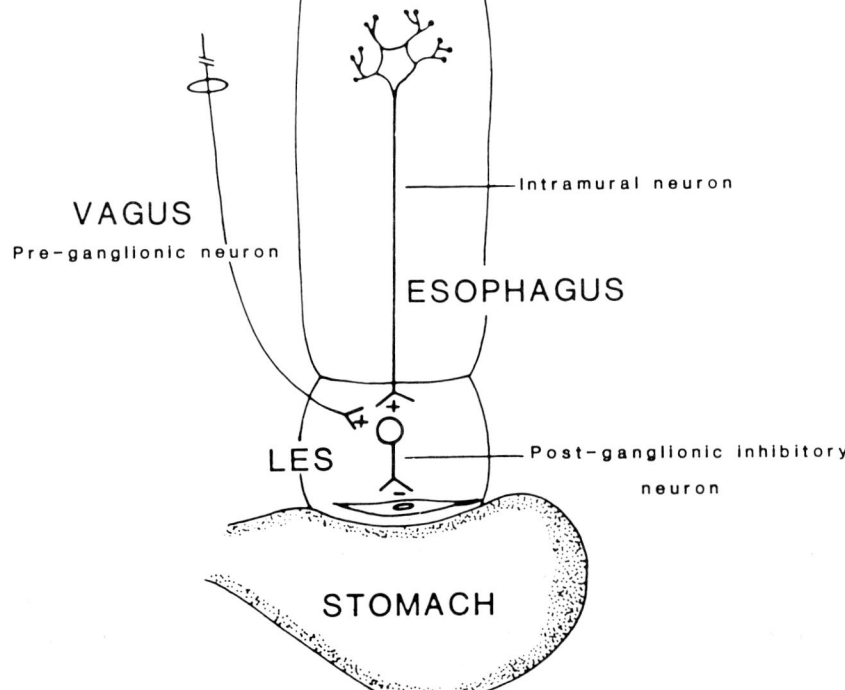

FIG. 17. Schematic representation of extrinsic (vagal) and intrinsic inhibitory pathways to LES. Vagal preganglionic efferent neurons synapse with postganglionic inhibitory neurons within LES. Synaptic neurotransmitter is mainly acetylcholine and activates inhibitory postganglionic neurons by stimulating both nicotinic and muscarinic receptors. There is also evidence that serotonin may also be involved in synaptic transmission as complete pharmacologic blockade of vagally induced LES relaxation requires a combination of muscarinic, nicotinic, and serotonin antagonists. The postganglionic inhibitory neuron can also be activated by an intramural neuron (e.g., a mechanoreceptor); however, the neurotransmitter involved at this synapse is unknown. The postganglionic inhibitory neuron in turn releases a nonadrenergic, noncholinergic neurotransmitter (?VIP) that directly relaxes the LES smooth muscle. [Adapted from Goyal (212).]

tonergic receptors. However, the combination of these antagonists does not modify LES relaxation due to electrical stimulation of intramural inhibitory nerves. These observations show that the effect of the antagonists is exerted at the synaptic site between pre- and postganglionic neurons.

The intramural neural pathway involved in distension-induced LES relaxation is not known. However, it is likely that it is a sensory neuron that makes contact with the postganglionic inhibitory neuron either directly or indirectly via an interneuron. The neurotransmitters involved in this pathway are not known.

INHIBITORY NEUROTRANSMITTER. The nature of the inhibitory neurotransmitter released by the intramural inhibitory neurons is not known with certainty. It is clearly not cholinergic or adrenergic in nature. Hence, this neurotransmitter has been called noncholinergic, nonadrenergic (223, 490). There is evidence against it being serotonin (386, 388), histamine (387), dopamine (385), or prostaglandin (391). There was initial enthusiasm for the possibility that certain purines were the transmitters involved (51, 97); however, subsequent studies have provided strong evidence against this (390).

Three pieces of evidence indicate that VIP is the neurotransmitter of the intramural inhibitory neurons in the opossum LES. First, VIP is present in large amounts in the opossum LES (400). Second, VIP causes tetrodotoxin-resistant LES relaxation and therefore has a direct inhibitory effect on the sphincter muscle itself (399). Third, a specific high-titer VIP antiserum infused in the arterial supply of the sphincter antagonizes the LES relaxation caused by electrical stimulation of vagal efferents, electrical stimulation of intramural nerves, or pharmacological stimulation of the inhibitory neuron with nicotine (228). The antagonism is not complete; however, it is not clear whether this is due to incomplete inactivation of endogenously released VIP by the antiserum or because another neurotransmitter is also involved.

Biancani et al. (33) examined the possibility that VIP is the inhibitory transmitter in the cat LES. They showed that VIP causes relaxation of the LES that is not antagonized by tetrodotoxin. Moreover LES relaxation due to transmural nerve stimulation is associated with the release of VIP into the tissue bath, and VIP antiserum antagonizes the neurally mediated relaxation of the sphincter. This evidence indicates that, in the cat LES, VIP may also be the inhibitory neurotransmitter. Furthermore, abundant VIP-containing neurons have been reported in the cat LES (492).

It has also been shown that VIP causes LES relaxation in primates (456). In humans, there is an abundance of VIP in the neurons of the LES, (2, 4), and this is markedly reduced or absent in patients with achalasia (1), a disorder in which the LES does not relax normally. These observations support the view that VIP may be the neurotransmitter of inhibitory nerves in the human LES as well.

Despite the seemingly good evidence for VIP as the inhibitory transmitter, there are several observations that would indicate otherwise. Fox et al. (186) suggested that VIP may not be the inhibitory transmitter because it did not cause relaxation of circular muscle strips in vivo and was not released into the tissue bath on nerve stimulation. This may have been due to technical factors, because VIP from a different laboratory did cause relaxation of LES muscle strips. Daniel et al. (119) also reported that VIP does not cause hyperpolarization of the esophageal body circular muscle with the sucrose-gap technique. However, they did not study the effect of VIP on membrane potential in the LES. Ormsbee et al. (343, 363) reported that VIP-induced relaxation of the cat LES is associated with an increase in intracellular cAMP levels. However, LES relaxation associated with transmural electrical stimulation was associated with an increase in cGMP levels and no change in cAMP levels (343, 489). These observations contradict VIP as the inhibitory neurotransmitter. Further studies are clearly needed to establish the role of VIP as the inhibitory neurotransmitter of the intramural inhibitory nerves in the LES. Recently CGRP has been shown to cause inhibition of the lower esophageal sphincter (382). Moreover it has been localized to intramural nerves and therefore is another candidate for an inhibitory neurotransmitter in the LES (382).

OTHER NEUROTRANSMITTERS. The intramural inhibitory neurons of the LES circular smooth muscle have an abundance of different receptors (225). Many of these probably have no functional significance; however, some may be involved in the modulation of inhibitory LES reflexes. For example, vagally induced LES relaxation is antagonized by splanchnic nerve stimulation, as well as by cholinergic, $\alpha$-adrenergic, dopaminergic, and opioid receptor stimulation (162, 166, 183, 184, 208, 252). Some of these agents may act at presynaptic receptors to modulate the release of the inhibitory neurotransmitter.

## Reflex Contractions of the Lower Esophageal Sphincter

The upper part of the LES displays reflex contraction immediately after the peristalsis-related relaxation. This contraction occurs in continuity with the peristaltic wave of the esophageal body and may represent the response of esophageal body–type circular muscle mixed with the sphincter muscle. A similar behavior is seen in muscle strips in vitro (50). This aftercontraction may somehow be related to the level of base-line tone. Human LES circular muscle strips show prominent aftercontractions when basal tone is low, but as the tone increases the aftercontraction is abolished (335).

Short-lived increases in LES pressure also occur secondary to increases in intra-abdominal pressure. Considerable controversy exists as to whether this rise in LES pressure is due to reflex contraction or merely due to passive transmission of the increased intra-abdominal pressure (47, 154, 269, 317, 349, 360, 500). The studies that show this to be a true reflex also suggest that it is vagally mediated and dependent on cholinergic neurons (269, 315, 360).

The LES also contracts transiently, in phase with stomach contractions. This is closely tied to the phasic antral contractions that occur during different stages of the MMC (140, 245, 246, 462). During the first phase of the MMC, the LES pressure is stable, whereas during late phase II and throughout phase III large-amplitude phasic contractions occur without there being a major change in the basal pressure.

These MMC-related contractions are abolished by atropine and anesthesia (245). Recent studies suggest that they are initiated by circulating motilin (246). The effect of infused motilin is abolished by hexamethonium and markedly inhibited by atropine and the selective $M_2$ antagonist 4-DAMP. This indicates that motilin may stimulate preganglionic cholinergic fibers, which in turn activate nicotinic receptors on postganglionic cholinergic excitatory fibers. These latter neurons then release acetylcholine, which causes contraction of the sphincter muscle by stimulating $M_2$ receptors (246). Infusion of acid into the esophageal lumen also causes a neurally mediated reflex contraction of the LES. This reflex contraction involves substance P–containing nerves (403).

Current address of W. G. Paterson: Queens University, Kingston, Ontario, Canada.

## REFERENCES

1. AGGESTRUP, S., R. UDDMAN, F. SUNDLER, J. FAHRENKRUG, R. HÅKANSON, H. R. SØRENSEN, AND G. HAMBRAEUS. Lack of vasoactive intestinal polypeptide nerves in esophageal achalasia. *Gastroenterology* 84: 924–927, 1983.
2. AGGESTRUP, S., R. UDDMAN, S. L. JENSEN, F. SUNDLER, O. B. SCHAFFALITZKY DE MUCKADELL, J. J. HOLST, R. HÅKANSON, R. EKMAN, AND H. R. SØRENSEN. Regulatory peptides in the lower esophageal sphincter of man. *Regul. Pept.* 10: 167–178, 1985.
3. ALTSCHULER, S. M., J. T. BOYLE, T. E. NIXON, A. I. PACK, AND S. COHEN. Simultaneous reflex inhibition of lower esophageal sphincter and crural diaphragm in cats. *Am. J. Physiol.* 249 (*Gastrointest. Liver Physiol.* 12): G586–G591, 1985.
4. ALUMETS, J., J. FAHRENKRUG, R. HÅKANSON, O. B. SCHAFFALITZKY DE MUCKADELL, F. SUNDLER, AND R. UDDMAN. A rich VIP nerve supply characteristic of sphincters. *Nature Lond.* 280: 155–156, 1979.
5. ANDREW, B. L. The respiratory displacement of the larynx: a study of the innervation of accessory respiratory muscles. *J. Physiol. Lond.* 130: 474–487, 1955.
6. ANDREW, B. L. The nervous control of the cervical oesophagus of the rat during swallowing. *J. Physiol. Lond.* 134: 729–740, 1956.
7. AREY, L. B., AND M. J. TREMAINE. The muscle content of the lower oesophagus of man. *Anat. Rec.* 56: 315–320, 1933.
8. ARIMORI, M., C. F. CODE, J. F. SCHLEGEL, AND R. E. STURM. Electrical activity of the canine esophagus and gastroesophageal sphincter. *Am. J. Dig. Dis.* 15: 191–208, 1970.
9. ARNDORFER, R. C., J. J. STEF, W. J. DODDS, J. J. LINEHON, AND W. J. HOGAN. Improved infusion system for intraluminal esophageal manometry. *Gastroenterology* 73: 23–27, 1977.
10. ASK, P., AND L. TIBBLING. Effect of time interval between swallows on esophageal peristalsis. *Am. J. Physiol.* 238 (*Gastrointest. Liver Physiol.* 1): G485–G490, 1980.
11. ASOH, R., AND R. K. GOYAL. Electrical activity of the opossum lower esophageal sphincter in vivo. Its role in the basal sphincter pressure. *Gastroenterology* 74: 835–840, 1978.
12. ASOH, R., AND R. K. GOYAL. Manometry and electromyography of the upper esophageal sphincter in the opossum. *Gastroenterology* 74: 514–520, 1978.
13. ATANASSOVA, E., AND M. PAPASOVA. Gastrointestinal motility. In: *Gastrointestinal Physiology II*, edited by R. K. Crane. Baltimore, MD: University Park, 1977, vol. 12, p. 35–69. (*Int. Rev. Physiol. Ser.*)
14. ATKINSON, M., P. KRAMER, S. M. WYMAN, AND F. G. INGELFINGER. The dynamics of swallowing. I. Normal pharyngeal mechanisms. *J. Clin. Invest.* 36: 581–588, 1957.
15. BABKA, J. C., AND D. O. CASTELL. On the genesis of heartburn—the effect of specific foods on the lower esophageal sphincter. *Am. J. Dig. Dis.* 18: 391–397, 1973.
16. BABKA, J. C., G. W. HAGER, AND D. O. CASTELL. The effect of body position on lower esophageal sphincter pressure. *Am. J. Dig. Dis.* 18: 441–442, 1973.
17. BAINBRIDGE, E. T., S. D. NICHOLAS, J. R. NEWTON, AND J. G. TEMPLE. Gastro-oesophageal reflux in pregnancy. Altered function of the barrier to reflux in asymptomatic women during early pregnancy. *Scand. Gastroenterol.* 19: 85–89, 1984.
18. BAKER, A. B., H. A. MUTZKE, AND J. R. BROWN. Poliomyelitis. III. Bulbar poliomyelitis; a study of medullary function. *Arch. Neurol. Psychiatry* 63: 257–281, 1950.
19. BALDI, F., F. FERRARINI, R. BALESTRA, D. BORIONI, G. BRUNETTI, AND L. BARBARA. Oesophageal function after oral ranitidine: an acute double blind study in normal subjects. *Hepato-Gastroenterology* 31: 38–40, 1984.
20. BALDI, F., F. FERRARINI, R. BALESTRA, D. BORIONI, A. LONGANESI, M. MIGLIOLI, AND L. BARBARA. Oesophageal motor events at the occurrence of acid reflux and during endogenous acid exposure in healthy subjects and in patients with oesophagitis. *Gut* 26: 336–341, 1985.
21. BARONE, F. C., D. M. LOMBARDI, AND H. S. ORMSBEE III. Effects of hindbrain stimulation on lower esophageal sphincter pressure in the cat. *Am. J. Physiol.* 247 (*Gastrointest. Liver Physiol.* 10): G70–G78, 1984.
22. BARRETT, N. R. The lower esophagus lined by columnar epithelium. *Surgery* 41: 881–894, 1957.
23. BARTLET, A. L. Actions of 5-hydroxytryptamine and histamine on the neural structures and muscularis mucosae of the guinea pig oesophagus. *Br. J. Pharmacol. Chemother.* 33: 184–192, 1968.
24. BATSON, O. V. The cricopharyngeus muscle. *Ann. Otol. Rhinol. Laryngol.* 64: 47–54, 1955.
25. BAUMGARTEN, M. G., AND W. LANGE. Adrenergic innervation of the oesophagus in the cat (*Felis domestica*) and rhesus monkey (*Macacus rhesus*). *Z. Zellorsch. Mikrosk. Anat.* 95: 529–545, 1969.
26. BECKER, B. S., AND R. BURAKOFF. The effect of verapamil on the lower esophageal sphincter pressure in normal subjects and in achalasia. *Am. J. Gastroenterol.* 78: 773–775, 1983.

27. BEHAR, J., AND P. BIANCANI. Effect of cholecystokinin-octapeptide on lower esophageal sphincter. *Gastroenterology* 73: 57–61, 1977.
28. BEHAR, J., AND P. BIANCANI. Effects of vasoactive intestinal polypeptide and peptide histidine isoleucine on cat esophageal smooth circular muscle in vitro (Abstract). *Gastroenterology* 88: 1320, 1985.
29. BEHAR, J., S. FIELD, AND C. MARIN. Effect of glucagon, secretin and vasoactive intestinal polypeptide on the feline lower esophageal sphincter: mechanisms of action. *Gastroenterology* 77: 1001–1007, 1979.
30. BEHAR, J., M. KERSTEIN, AND P. BIANCANI. Neural control of the lower esophageal sphincter in the cat: studies on the excitatory pathways to the lower oesophageal sphincter. *Gastroenterology* 82: 680–688, 1982.
31. BIANCANI, P., K. BARWICK, J. SELLING, AND R. MCCALLUM. Effects of acute experimental esophagitis on mechanical properties of the lower esophageal sphincter. *Gastroenterology* 87: 8–16, 1984.
32. BIANCANI, P., R. K. GOYAL, A. PHILLIPS, AND H. M. SPIRO. Mechanics of sphincter action. Studies on the lower esophageal sphincter. *J. Clin. Invest.* 52: 2973–2978, 1973.
33. BIANCANI, P., J. H. WALSH, AND J. BEHAR. Vasoactive intestinal polypeptide: a neurotransmitter for lower esophageal sphincter relaxation. *J. Clin. Invest.* 73: 963–967, 1984.
34. BIANCANI, P., M. ZABINSKI, AND J. BEHAR. Pressure, tension, and force of closure of the human lower esophageal sphincter and esophagus. *J. Clin. Invest.* 56: 476–483, 1975.
35. BIANCANI, P., M. ZABINSKI, M. KERSTEIN, AND J. BEHAR. Lower esophageal sphincter mechanics: anatomic and physiologic relationships of the esophagogastric junction of cat. *Gastroenterology* 82: 468–475, 1982.
36. BIEGER, D. Role of bulbar serotonergic neurotransmission in the initiation of swallowing in the rat. *Neuropharmacology* 20: 1073–1083, 1981.
37. BIEGER, D. Muscarinic activation of rhombencephalic neurones controlling oesophageal peristalsis in the rat. *Neuropharmacology* 23: 1451–1464, 1984.
38. BIEGER, D., AND C. TRIGGLE. Pharmacological properties of mechanical responses of the rat oesophageal muscularis mucosae to vagal and field stimulation. *Br. J. Pharmacol.* 84: 93–106, 1985.
39. BLACKWELL, J. N., AND D. O. CASTELL. Oesophageal motility: recent advances and implications. *Clin. Sci.* 67: 145–151, 1984.
40. BLACKWELL, J. N., C. B. DALTON, AND D. O. CASTELL. Oral pirenzipine does not affect esophageal pressures in man. *Dig. Dis. Sci.* 31: 230–235, 1986.
41. BLACKWELL, J. N., W. J. HANNAN, R. D. ADAM, AND R. C. HEADING. Radionuclide transit studies in the detection of oesophageal dysmotility. *Gut* 24: 421–426, 1983.
42. BLACKWELL, J. N., S. HOLT, AND R. C. HEADING. Effect of nifedipine on oesophageal motility and gastric emptying. *Digestion* 21: 50–56, 1981.
43. BOSMA, J. F. A correlated study of the anatomy and motor activity of the upper pharynx by cadaver dissection and by cinematic study of patients after maxillofacial surgery. *Ann. Otol. Rhinol. Laryngol.* 62: 51–72, 1953.
44. BOSMA, J. F. Deglutition: pharyngeal stage. *Physiol. Rev.* 37: 275–300, 1957.
45. BOTHA, G. S. M. *The Gastro-Esophageal Junction: Clinical Application to Oesophageal and Gastric Surgery.* Boston, MA: Little, Brown, 1962.
46. BOYLE, J. T., S. M. ALTSCHULER, T. E. NIXON, D. N. TUCHMAN, A. I. PACK, AND S. COHEN. Role of the diaphragm in the genesis of lower esophageal sphincter pressure in the cat. *Gastroenterology* 88: 723–730, 1985.
47. BOYLE, J. T., AND S. COHEN. Does intrinsic LES tone increase as an adaptive response to increased intraabdominal pressure? *Dig. Dis. Sci.* 29: 760–761, 1984.
48. BROCK-UTNE, J. G., T. G. B. DOW, G. E. DIMOPOULOS, S. WELMAN, J. W. DOWNING, AND M. G. MOSHAL. Gastric and lower oesophageal sphincter (LOS) pressures in early pregnancy. *Br. J. Anaesth.* 53: 381–384, 1981.
49. BRUNNER, H. Cricopharyngeal muscle under normal and pathological conditions. *Arch. Otolaryngol.* 56: 616–634, 1952.
50. BURLEIGH, D. E. The effects of drugs and electrical field stimulation on the human lower oesophageal sphincter. *Arch. Int. Pharmacodyn. Ther.* 240: 169–176, 1979.
51. BURNSTOCK, G. Past and current evidence for the purinergic nerve hypothesis. In: *Physiological and Regulatory Function of Adenosine and Adenine Nucleotides*, edited by H. P. Baer and G. I. Drummond. New York: Raven, 1979.
52. BURNSTOCK, G. Ultrastructural identification of neurotransmitters. In: *Basic Science in Gastroenterology: Structure of the Gut*, edited by J. M. Polak, S. R. Bloom, N. A. Wright, and M. J. Daly. Norwich, England: Page, 1982, p. 1–10.
53. BUTIN, J. W., A. M. OLSEN, H. J. MOERSH, AND C. F. CODE. A study of esophageal pressures in normal persons and patients with cardiospasm. *Gastroenterology* 23: 278–293, 1953.
54. BYBEE, D. E., F. C. BROWN, L. P. GEORGES, D. O. CASTELL, AND J. E. MCGUIGAN. Somatostatin effects on lower esophageal sphincter function. *Am. J. Physiol.* 237 (*Endocrinol. Metab. Gastrointest. Physiol.* 6): E77–E81, 1979.
55. BYRNE, P. J., F. B. KEAN, AND T. P. J. HENNESSY. Oesophageal manometry. A comparison of hydraulic and syringe catheter infusion systems using a simple hydrostatic bench model. *Clin. Phys. Physiol. Meas.* 5: 185–191, 1984.
56. CAR, A. La commande corticale du centre deglutition bulbaire. *J. Physiol. Paris* 62: 361–386, 1970.
57. CAR, A., AND C. ROMAN. L'activité spontanée du sphincter oesophagier chez le mouton. Ses variations au cours de la deglutition et de la rumination. *J. Physiol. Paris* 62: 505–511, 1970.
58. CARR, D. H., P. C. SCOTT, AND D. A. TITCHEN. Manometric and electromyographic observations of the oesophagus of sheep in eructation, regurgitation and swallowing. *Q. J. Exp. Physiol. Cogn. Med. Sci.* 68: 661–674, 1983.
59. CARVETH, S. W., J. F. SCHLEGEL, AND C. F. CODE. Esophageal motility after vagotomy, phrenicotomy, myotomy, and myomectomy in dogs. *Surg. Gynecol. Obstet.* 114: 31–42, 1962.
60. CASTELL, D. O. The lower esophageal sphincter: physiologic and clinical aspects. *Ann. Intern. Med.* 83: 390–401, 1975.
61. CASTELL, D. O. Sphincters of the oesophagus. *Neth. J. Med.* 27: 234–241, 1984.
62. CASTELL, D. O., AND L. D. HARRIS. Hormonal control of gastroesophageal sphincter strength. *N. Engl. J. Med.* 282: 886–889, 1970.
63. CASTELL, D. O., AND S. M. LEVINE. A new mechanism for treatment of heartburn with antacids: lower esophageal sphincter response to gastric alkalinization. *Ann. Intern. Med.* 74: 223–227, 1971.
64. CHAN, W. W.-L., AND N. E. DIAMANT. Electrical off response of cat esophageal smooth muscle: an analog simulation. *Am. J. Physiol.* 230: 233–238, 1966.
65. CHATTERJEE, M., AND R. A. MURPHY. Calcium-dependent stress maintenance without myosin phosphorylation in skinned smooth muscle. *Science Wash. DC* 221: 464–466, 1983.
66. CHERNIACK, N. S., M. A. HAXHIU, J. MITRA, K. STROHL, AND E. VAN LUNTEREN. Response of upper airway, intercostal and diaphragm muscle activity to stimulation of oesophageal afferents in dogs. *J. Physiol. Lond.* 349: 15–25, 1984.
67. CHRISTENSEN, J. Electrical activity of the esophagus. *Gastroenterology* 52: 903–904, 1967.
68. CHRISTENSEN, J. Pharmacologic identification of the lower esophageal sphincter. *J. Clin. Invest.* 49: 681–691, 1970.
69. CHRISTENSEN, J. Patterns and origin of some esophageal responses to stretch and electrical stimulation. *Gastroenterology* 59: 909–916, 1970.
70. CHRISTENSEN, J. The innervaton and motility of the esophagus. *Front. Gastrointest. Res.* 3: 18–32, 1978.

71. CHRISTENSEN, J. Oxygen dependence of contractions in esophageal and gastric pyloric and ileocecal muscle of opossums. *Proc. Soc. Exp. Biol. Med.* 170: 194–202, 1982.
72. CHRISTENSEN, J. Origin of sensation in the esophagus. *Am. J. Physiol.* 246 (*Gastrointest. Liver Physiol.* 9): G221–G225, 1984.
73. CHRISTENSEN, J., C. ARTHUR, AND J. L. CONKLIN. Some determinants of latency of off-response to electrical field stimulation in circular layer of smooth muscle of opossum esophagus. *Gastroenterology* 77: 677–681, 1979.
74. CHRISTENSEN, J., J. L. CONKLIN, AND B. W. FREEMAN. Physiologic specialization at the esophagogastric junction in three species. *Am. J. Physiol.* 225: 1265–1270, 1973.
75. CHRISTENSEN, J., AND E. E. DANIEL. Effects of some autonomic drugs on circular esophageal smooth muscle. *J. Pharmacol. Exp. Ther.* 159: 243–249, 1968.
76. CHRISTENSEN, J., B. W. FREEMAN, AND J. K. MILLER. Some physiological characteristics of the esophagogastric junction in the opossum. *Gastroenterology* 64: 1119–1125, 1973.
77. CHRISTENSEN, J., AND G. F. LUND. Esophageal responses to distention and electrical stimulation. *J. Clin. Invest.* 48: 408–419, 1969.
78. CHRISTENSEN, J., AND M. ISKANDARANI. Neuromuscular functions in esophageal smooth muscle of opossums as differently affected by veratrum alkaloids. *Gastroenterology* 81: 866–871, 1981.
79. CHRISTENSEN, J., AND W. H. PERCY. A pharmacological study of oesophageal muscularis mucosae from the cat, dog and American opossum (*Didelphis virginiana*). *Br. J. Pharmacol.* 83: 329–336, 1984.
80. CHRISTENSEN, J., G. A. RICK, B. A. ROBISON, M. J. STILES, AND M. A. WIX. Arrangement of the myenteric plexus throughout the gastrointestinal tract of the opossum. *Gastroenterology* 85: 890–899, 1983.
81. CHRISTENSEN, J., G. A. RICK, AND D. J. SOLL. Intramural nerves and interstitial cells revealed by the Champy-Maillet stain in the opossum esophagus. *J. Auton. Nerv. Syst.* 19: 137–151, 1987.
82. CHRISTENSEN, J., AND R. L. ROBERTS. Differences between esophageal body and lower esophageal sphincter in mitochondria of smooth muscle in opossum. *Gastroenterology* 85: 650–656, 1983.
83. CHRISTENSEN, J., AND B. A. ROBISON. Anatomy of the myenteric plexus of the opossum esophagus. *Gastroenterology* 83: 1033–1042, 1982.
84. CHRISTENSEN, J., T. H. WILLIAMS, J. JEW, AND T. M. O'DORISIO. Distribution of vasoactive intestinal polypeptide immunoreactive structures in the opossum esophagus. *Gastroenterology* 92: 1007–1018, 1987.
85. CHRISTRUP, J. Normal swallowing of foodstuffs of pasty consistence. A cinefluorographic investigation of a normal material. *Dan. Med. Bull.* 11: 79–91, 1964.
86. CLARK, C. G., AND J. R. VANE. The cardiac sphincter in the cat. *Gut* 2: 252–262, 1961.
87. CLARK, G. Deglutition apnea. *J. Physiol. Lond.* 54: 59, 1920.
88. CLARK, M. D., J. A. RINALDO, AND W. R. EYLER. Correlation of manometric and radiologic data from the esophagogastric area. *Radiology* 94: 261–270, 1970.
89. CLERC, N. Afferent innervation of the lower oesophageal sphincter of the cat. An HRP study. *J. Auton. Nerv. Syst.* 9: 623–636, 1983.
90. CLERC, N. Afferent innervation of the lower esophageal sphincter of the cat. Pathways and functional characteristics. *J. Auton. Nerv. Syst.* 10: 213–216, 1984.
91. CLERC, N., AND N. MEI. Mise en evidence de mecanorecepteurs muqueux au niveau du sphincter inferieur de l'oesophage. Comparaison avec les mecanorecepteurs musculaires. *C. R. Soc. Biol. Paris* 175: 352–356, 1981.
92. CLERC, N., AND M. MEI. Thoracic esophageal mechanoreceptors connected with fibers following sympathetic pathways. *Brain Res. Bull.* 10: 1–7, 1983.
93. CLERC, N., AND N. MEI. Vagal mechanoreceptors located in the lower oesophageal sphincter of the cat. *J. Physiol. Lond.* 336: 487–498, 1983.
94. CODE, C. F., AND J. F. SCHLEGEL. Motor action of the esophagus and its sphincters. In: *Handbook of Physiology. Alimentary Canal. Motility*, edited by C. F. Code. Washington, DC: Am. Physiol. Soc., 1968, sect. 6, vol. IV, p. 1821–1839.
95. COHEN, B. R., AND B. S. WOLF. Cineradiographic and intraluminal correlations in the pharynx and esophagus. In: *Handbook of Physiology. Alimentary Canal. Motility*, edited by C. F. Code. Washington, DC: Am. Physiol. Soc., 1968, sect. 6, vol. IV, p. 1841–1860.
96. COHEN, S. Hypogastrinemia and sphincter incompetence. *N. Engl. J. Med.* 289: 215–217, 1973.
97. COHEN, S. Augmentation of the neural inhibitory response of the lower esophageal sphincter. *Proc. Soc. Exp. Biol. Med.* 145: 1004–1007, 1974.
98. COHEN, S. Motor disorders of the esophagus. *N. Engl. J. Med.* 301: 184–192, 1979.
99. COHEN, S., AND G. H. BOOTH. Gastric acid secretion and lower esophageal sphincter pressure in response to coffee and caffeine. *N. Engl. J. Med.* 293: 897–899, 1975.
100. COHEN, S., AND F. GREEN. Force velocity characteristics of esophageal muscle: effect of acetylcholine and norepinephrine. *Am. J. Physiol.* 226: 1250–1256, 1974.
101. COHEN, S., AND L. D. HARRIS. Lower esophageal sphincter pressure as an index of lower esophageal spincter strength. *Gastroenterology* 58: 157–162, 1970.
102. COHEN, S., AND W. LIPSHUTZ. Hormonal regulation of human esophageal sphincter competence: interaction of gastrin and secretin. *J. Clin. Invest.* 50: 449–454, 1971.
103. COHEN, S., AND W. LIPSHUTZ. Lower esophageal sphincter dysfunction in achalasia. *Gastroenterology* 61: 814–820, 1971.
104. COHEN, S., W. LIPSHUTZ, AND W. HUGHES. Role of gastrin supersensitivity in the pathogenesis of lower esophageal sphincter hypertension in achalasia. *J. Clin. Invest.* 50: 1241–1247, 1971.
105. CONKLIN, J., AND R. K. GOYAL. Gastrointestinal smooth muscle. In: *Gastrointestinal Disease: Pathophysiology, Diagnosis and Treatment* (4th ed.), edited by M. H. Sleisenger and J. S. Fordtran. Philadelphia, PA: Saunders, in press.
106. CORAZZIARI, E., G. DELLE FAVE, C. POZZESSERE, A. KOHN, L. DE MAGISTRIS, F. ANZINI, AND A. TORSOLI. Effect of bombesin on lower esophageal sphincter pressure in humans. *Gastroenterology* 83: 10–14, 1982.
107. CORAZZIARI, E., C. POZZESSERE, S. DANI, F. ANZINI, AND A. TORSOLI. Intraluminal pH and esophageal motility. *Gastroenterology* 75: 275–277, 1978.
108. CORUZZI, G., AND G. BERTACCINI. Effect of some vasoactive peptides on the lower esophageal sphincter. *Pharmacol. Res. Commun.* 12: 965–973, 1980.
109. CORUZZI, G., AND G. BERTACCINI. Histamine and the gastrointestinal tract. Histamine receptors in the lower esophageal sphincter (LES). *Agents Actions* 12: 157–161, 1982.
110. CREAMER, B., AND J. SCHLEGEL. Motor responses of the esophagus to distention. *J. Appl. Physiol.* 10: 498–504, 1957.
111. CRIST, J., J. S. GIDDA, AND R. K. GOYAL. Characteristics of "on" and "off" contractions in esophageal circular muscle in vitro. *Am. J. Physiol.* 246 (*Gastrointest. Liver Physiol.* 9): G137–G144, 1984.
112. CRIST, J., J. S. GIDDA, AND R. K. GOYAL. Intramural mechanism of esophageal peristalsis: Roles of cholinergic and noncholinergic nerves. *Proc. Natl. Acad. Sci. USA* 81: 3595–3599, 1984.
113. CRIST, J., J. S. GIDDA, AND R. K. GOYAL. Role of substance P nerves in longitudinal smooth muscle contractions of the esophagus. *Am. J. Physiol.* 250 (*Gastrointest. Liver Physiol.* 13): G336–G343, 1986.
114. CRIST, J., A. SUPRENANT, AND R. K. GOYAL. Intracellular studies of electrical membrane properties of esophageal circular smooth muscle in peristalsis. *Gastroenterology* 92: 987–992, 1987.

115. CSENDES, A., M. OSTER, O. BRANDSBORG, J. MOLLER, M. BRANSBORG, AND E. AMDRUP. Gastroesophageal sphincter pressure and serum gastrin: reaction to food stimulation in normal subjects and in patients with gastric or duodenal ulcer. *Scand. J. Gastroenterol.* 13: 363–368, 1978.

116. DANIEL, E. E. Esophageal spikes—to be or not to be (Letter to the editor). *Gastroenterology* 84: 1639, 1983.

117. DANIEL, E. E., J. CRANKSHAW, AND S. SARNA. Prostaglandins and myogenic control of tension in lower esophageal sphincter in vitro. *Prostaglandins* 17: 629–639, 1979.

118. DANIEL, E. E., J. CRANKSHAW, AND S. SARNA. Prostaglandins and tetrodotoxin-insensitive relaxation of opossum lower esophageal sphincter. *Am. J. Physiol.* 236 (*Endocrinol. Metab. Gastrointest. Physiol.* 5): E153–E172, 1979.

119. DANIEL, E. E., A. HELMY-ELKHOLY, L. P. JAGER, AND M. S. KANNAN. Neither a purine nor VIP is the mediator of inhibitory nerves of opossum oesophageal smooth muscle. *J. Physiol. Lond.* 336: 243–260, 1983.

120. DANIEL, E. E., J. JURY, AND K. H. ROHOTHAM. Receptors for neurotransmitters in opossum esophagus muscularis mucosa. *Br. J. Pharmacol.* 88: 707–714, 1986.

121. DANIEL, E. E., AND V. POSEY-DANIEL. Neuromuscular structures in opossum esophagus: role of interstitial cells of Cajal. *Am. J. Physiol.* 246 (*Gastrointest. Liver Physiol.* 9): G305–G315, 1984.

122. DANIEL, E. E., V. POSEY-DANIEL, L. P. JAGER, J. BENEZIN, AND J. JURY. Structural effects of exposure of smooth muscle in sucrose gap apparatus. *Am. J. Physiol.* 252 (*Cell Physiol.* 21): C77–C87, 1987.

123. DANIEL, E. E., G. S. TAYLOR, AND M. E. HOLMAN. The myogenic basis of active tension in the lower esophageal sphincter (Abstract). *Gastroenterology* 70: 874, 1976.

124. DE TROYER, A., AND J. ROSSO. Reflex inhibition of the diaphragm by esophageal afferents. *Neurosci. Lett.* 30: 43–46, 1982.

125. DECARLE, D. J., AND J. CHRISTENSEN. A dopamine receptor in esophageal smooth muscle of the opossum. *Gastroenterology* 70: 216–219, 1976.

126. DECARLE, D. J., AND J. CHRISTENSEN. Histamine receptors in esophageal smooth muscle of the opossum. *Gastroenterology* 70: 1071–1075, 1976.

127. DECARLE, D. J., J. CHRISTENSEN, A. C. SZABO, D. C. TEMPLEMAN, AND D. R. MCKINLEY. Calcium dependence of neuromuscular events in esophageal smooth muscle of the opossum. *Am. J. Physiol.* 232 (*Endocrinol. Metab. Gastrointest. Physiol.* 1): E547–E552, 1977.

128. DECARLE, D. J., A. C. SZABO, AND J. CHRISTENSEN. Temperature dependence of responses of esophageal smooth muscle to electrical field stimulation. *Am. J. Physiol.* 232 (*Endocrinol. Metab. Gastrointest. Physiol.* 1): E432–E436, 1977.

129. DECKTOR, D. L., AND J. P. RYAN. Transmembrane voltage of opossum esophageal smooth muscle and its response to electrical stimulation of intrinsic nerves. *Gastroenterology* 82: 301–308, 1982.

130. DEMEESTER, T. R., E. LAFONTAINE, B. E. JOELSSON, D. B. SKINNER, J. W. RYAN, G. C. O'SULLIVAN, B. S. BRUNSDEN, AND L. F. JOHNSON. Relationship of a hiatal hernia to the function of the body of the esophagus and the gastroesophageal junction. *J. Thorac. Cardiovasc. Surg.* 82: 547–558, 1981.

131. DENIS, PH., J. P. GALMICHE, PH. DUCROTTE, R. COLIN, P. PASQUIS, AND R. LEFRANCOIS. Effect of ranitidine on resting pressure and pentagastrin response of human lower esophageal sphincter. *Dig. Dis. Sci.* 26: 999–1002, 1981.

132. DENIS, P., J-P. GALMICHE, J-F. GIBON, R. COLIN, P. PASQUIS, AND R. LEFRANCOIS. Effet du pirenzepin sur la motricité oesophagienne chez l'adulte sain. *Gastroenterol. Clin. Biol.* 6: 27–31, 1982.

133. DENNIS, M. A., J. W. MAHER, V. CRANDALL-MOOR, AND E. R. WOODWARD. Response of the canine lower esophageal sphincter to endogenous hypergastrinemia. *J. Surg. Res.* 31: 400–403, 1981.

134. DENNISH, G., AND D. O. CASTELL. Effect of smoking on lower esophageal sphincter pressure. *N. Engl. J. Med.* 284: 1136–1137, 1971.

135. DENT, J. A new technique for continuous sphincter pressure measurement. *Gastroenterology* 71: 263–267, 1976.

136. DENT, J. What's new in the esophagus. *Dig. Dis. Sci.* 26: 161–173, 1981.

137. DENT, J., W. J. DODDS, R. H. FRIEDMAN, T. SEKIGUCHI, W. J. HOGAN, R. C. ARNDORFER, AND D. J. PETRIE. Mechanism of gastroesophageal reflux in recumbent asymptomatic human subjects. *J. Clin. Invest.* 65: 256–267, 1980.

138. DENT, J., W. J. DODDS, W. J. HOGAN, R. C. ARNDORFER, AND B. C. TEETER. Effect of cholecystokinin-octapeptide on opossum lower esophageal sphincter. *Am. J. Physiol.* 239 (*Gastrointest. Liver Physiol.* 2): G230–G235, 1980.

139. DENT, J., W. J. DODDS, W. J. HOGAN, J. D. WOOD, AND R. C. ARNDORFER. Depressant effect of sodium nitroprusside on the lower esophageal sphincter of the opossum. *Gastroenterology* 76: 784–789, 1979.

140. DENT, J., W. J. DODDS, T. SEKIGUCHI, W. J. HOGAN, AND R. C. ARNDORFER. Interdigestive phasic contractions of the human lower esophageal sphincter. *Gastroenterology* 84: 453–460, 1983.

141. DIAMANT, N. E. Electrical activity of the cat smooth muscle esophagus: a study of hyperpolarizing responses. In: *Proc. Int. Symp. Gastrointest. Motil., 4th, Banff, Alberta, Canada, 1973*, edited by E. E. Daniel. Vancouver, Canada: Mitchell, 1974, p. 593–605.

142. DIAMANT, N. E., AND W. W.-L. CHAN. The electrical off response of cat circular esophageal smooth muscle: the effect of stimulus frequency on its timing. In: *Proc. Int. Symp. Gastrointest. Motil., 5th, Leuven, Belgium, September, 1975*, edited by G. Vantrappen. Herentals, Belgium: Typoff, 1975, p. 158–163.

143. DIAMANT, N. E., AND T. Y. EL-SHARKAWY. Neural control of esophageal peristalsis. *Gastroenterology* 72: 546–556, 1977.

144. DILAWARI, J. B., A. NEWMAN, J. POLEO, AND J. S. MISIEWICZ. Response of the human cardiac sphincter to circulating prostaglandins $F_2$ and $E_2$ and to antiinflammatory drugs. *Gut* 16: 137–143, 1975.

145. DIMARINO, A. J., AND S. COHEN. The adrenergic control of lower esophageal sphincter function: an experimental model of denervation supersensitivity. *J. Clin. Invest.* 52: 2264–2271, 1973.

146. DODDS, W. J., J. CHRISTENSEN, J. DENT, R. C. ARNDORFER, AND J. D. WOOD. Pharmacologic investigation of primary peristalsis in smooth muscle portion of opossum esophagus. *Am. J. Physiol.* 237 (*Endocrinol. Metab. Gastrointest. Physiol.* 6): E561–E566, 1979.

147. DODDS, W. J., J. CHRISTENSEN, J. DENT, J. D. WOOD, AND R. C. ARNDORFER. Esophageal contractions induced by vagal stimulation in the opossum. *Am. J. Physiol.* 235 (*Endocrinol. Metab. Gastrointest. Physiol.* 4): E392–E401, 1978.

148. DODDS, W. J., J. DENT, W. J. HOGAN, AND R. C. ARNDORFER. Effect of atropine on esophageal motor function in humans. *Am. J. Physiol.* 240 (*Gastrointest. Liver Physiol.* 3): G290–G296, 1981.

149. DODDS, W. J., J. DENT, W. J. HOGAN, J. F. HELM, R. HAUSER, G. K. PATEL, AND M. S. EGIDE. Mechanisms of gastroesophageal reflux in patients with reflux esophagitis. *N. Engl. J. Med.* 307: 1547–1552, 1982.

150. DODDS, W. J., J. DENT, W. J. HOGAN, G. K. PATEL, J. TOOULI, AND R. C. ARNDORFER. Paradoxical lower esophageal sphincter contraction induced by cholecystokinin-octapeptide in patients with achalasia. *Gastroenterology* 80: 327–333, 1981.

151. DODDS, W. J., AND W. J. HOGAN. Measurement of LES pressure. *Gastroenterology* 79: 588–591, 1980.

152. DODDS, W. J., W. J. HOGAN, S. B. LYDEN, E. T. STEWART, J. J. STEF, AND R. C. ARNDORFER. Quantitation of pharyngeal motor function in normal human subjects. *J. Appl. Physiol.* 39: 692–696, 1975.

153. DODDS, W. J., W. J. HOGAN, W. N. MILLER, R. F. BARRERAS, R. C. ARNDORFER, AND J. J. STEF. Relationship between serum gastrin concentration and lower esophageal sphincter pressure. *Am. J. Dig. Dis.* 20: 201–207, 1975.
154. DODDS, W. J., W. J. HOGAN, W. N. MILLER, J. J. STEF, R. C. ARNDORFER, AND S. B. LYDEN. Effect of increased intra-abdominal pressure on lower esophageal sphincter pressure. *Am. J. Dig. Dis.* 20: 298–308, 1975.
155. DODDS, W. J., W. J. HOGAN, D. P. REID, E. T. STEWART, AND R. C. ARNDORFER. A comparison between primary esophageal peristalsis following wet and dry swallows. *J. Appl. Physiol.* 35: 851–857, 1973.
156. DODDS, W. J., W. J. HOGAN, E. T. STEWART, J. J. STEF, AND R. C. ARNDORFER. Effects of increased intra-abdominal pressure on esophageal peristalsis. *J. Appl. Physiol.* 37: 378–383, 1974.
157. DODDS, W. J., J. J. STEF, AND W. J. HOGAN. Factors determining pressure measurement accuracy by intraluminal esophageal manometry. *Gastroenterology* 70: 117–123, 1976.
158. DODDS, W. J., J. J. STEF, E. T. STEWART, W. J. HOGAN, R. C. ARNDORFER, AND E. B. COHEN. Responses of feline esophagus to cervical vagal stimulation. *Am. J. Physiol.* 235 (*Endocrinol. Metab. Gastrointest. Physiol.* 4): E63–E73, 1978.
159. DODDS, W. J., E. T. STEWART, D. HODGES, AND F. F. ZBORALSKE. Movement of the feline esophagus associated with respiration and peristalsis. *J. Clin. Invest.* 52: 1–13, 1973.
160. DOMOTO, T., J. JURY, I. BEREZIN, J. E. T. FOX, AND E. E. DANIEL. Does substance P comediate with acetylcholine in nerves of opossum esophageal muscularis mucosa? *Am. J. Physiol.* 245 (*Gastrointest. Liver Physiol.* 8): G19–G28, 1983.
161. DOMSCHKE, W., G. LUX, S. DOMSCHKE, U. STRUNZ, S. R. BLOOM, AND E. WUNSCH. Effects of vasoactive intestinal peptide on resting and pentagastrin stimulated lower esophageal sphincter pressure. *Gastroenterology* 75: 9–12, 1978.
162. DOODY, P. T. Adrenergic modulation of vagal inhibitory action: evidence for dopamine receptors (Abstract). *Gastroenterology* 70: 997, 1976.
163. DOTY, R. W. Influence of stimulus pattern on reflex deglutition. *Am. J. Physiol.* 166: 142–158, 1951.
164. DOTY, R. W. Neural organization of deglutition. In: *Handbook of Physiology. Alimentary Canal. Motility*, edited by C. F. Code. Washington, DC: Am. Physiol. Soc., 1968, sect. 6, vol. IV, p. 1861–1902.
165. DOTY, R. W., AND J. F. BOSMA. An electromyographic analysis of reflex deglutition. *J. Neurophysiol.* 19: 44–60, 1956.
166. DOWLATSHAHI, K., A. EVANDER, B. WALTHER, AND D. B. SKINNER. Influence of morphine on the distal oesophagus and the lower esophageal sphincter—a manometric study. *Gut* 26: 802–806, 1985.
167. DUNCAN, D. L. The effects of vagotomy and splanchnotomy on gastric motility in the sheep. *J. Physiol. Lond.* 119: 156–169, 1953.
168. EASTWOOD, G. L., B. D. BECK, D. O. CASTELL, F. C. BROWN, AND J. R. FLETCHER. Beneficial effect of indomethacin on acid-induced esophagitis in cats. *Dig. Dis. Sci.* 26: 601–608, 1981.
169. ECKHARDT, V., AND N. D. GRACE. Lower esophageal sphincter pressure and serum motilin. *Am. J. Dig. Dis.* 21: 1008–1011, 1967.
170. ECKHARDT, V. F., B. ADAMI, H. HUCKER, AND H. LEEDER. The esophagogastric junction in patients with lower esophageal mucosal rings. *Gastroenterology* 79: 426–430, 1980.
171. EL OUAZZANI, T., AND N. MEI. Electrophysiologic properties and role of the vagal thermoreceptors of lower esophagus and stomach of cat. *Gastroenterology* 83: 995–1001, 1982.
172. ELLIS, F. H. Upper esophageal sphincter in health and disease. *Surg. Clin. N. Am.* 51: 553–565, 1971.
173. ENZMANN, E. R., G. S. HARELL, AND F. F. ZBORALSKE. Upper esophageal responses to intraluminal distention in man. *Gastroenterology* 72: 1292–1298, 1977.
174. ERCKENBRECHT, E., W. BERGES, A. SONNENBERG, J. ERCKENBRECHT, AND M. WEINBECK. The effect of pirenzepine on esophageal motility. *Scand. J. Gastroenterol. Suppl.* 72: 185–190, 1982.
175. FALEMPIN, M., AND J. P. ROUSSEAU. Reinnervation of skeletal muscles by vagal sensory fibres in the sheep, cat and rabbit. *J. Physiol. Lond.* 335: 467–479, 1983.
176. FALEMPIN, M., AND J. P. ROUSSEAU. Activity of lingual, laryngeal and oesophageal receptors in conscious sheep. *J. Physiol. Lond.* 347: 47–58, 1984.
177. FARRELL, R. L., D. O. CASTELL, AND J. E. MCGUIGAN. Measurements and comparisons of lower esophageal sphincter pressures and serum gastrin levels in patients with gastroesophageal reflux. *Gastroenterology* 67: 415–422, 1974.
178. FAUSSONE-PELLEGRINI, M. S., AND C. CORTESINI. Ultrastructural features and localization of the interstitial cells of Cajal in the smooth muscle coat of human esophagus. *J. Submicrosc. Cytol.* 17: 187–197, 1985.
179. FISHER, R. S., A. J. DIMARINO, AND S. COHEN. Mechanism of cholecystokinin inhibition of lower esophageal sphincter pressure. *Am. J. Physiol.* 228: 1469–1473, 1975.
180. FISHER, R. S., G. S. ROBERTS, C. J. GRABOWSKI, AND S. COHEN. Inhibition of lower esophageal sphincter circular muscle by female sex hormones. *Am. J. Physiol.* 234 (*Endocrinol. Metab. Gastrointest. Physiol.* 3): E243–E247, 1978.
181. FLESHLER, B., T. R. HENDRIX, P. KRAMER, AND F. J. INGELFINGER. The characteristics and similarity of primary and secondary peristalsis in the esophagus. *J. Clin. Invest.* 38: 110–116, 1959.
182. FOURNET, J., R. BOST, J. HOSTEIN, AND B. LACHET. Effets de la propantheline sur l'activité motrice de l'oesophage chez l'homme normal. *Gastroenterol. Clin. Biol.* 7: 457–464, 1983.
183. FOURNET, J., W. J. SNAPE, JR., AND S. COHEN. Modulation of lower esophageal sphincter relaxation in the opossum. *Am. J. Physiol.* 237 (*Endocrinol. Metab. Gastrointest. Physiol.* 6): E481–E485, 1979.
184. FOURNET, J., W. J. SNAPE, JR., AND S. COHEN. Sympathetic control of lower esophageal sphincter function in the cat. Action of direct cervical and splanchnic nerve stimulation. *J. Clin. Invest.* 63: 562–570, 1979.
185. FOX, J. E. T., AND E. E. DANIEL. Role of $Ca^{2+}$ in genesis of lower esophageal sphincter tone and other active contractions. *Am. J. Physiol.* 237 (*Endocrinol. Metab. Gastrointest. Physiol.* 6): E163–E171, 1979.
186. FOX, J. E. T., S. I. SAID, AND E. E. DANIEL. Is vasoactive intestinal polypeptide (VIP) an inhibitory neurotransmitter in the lower esophageal sphincter (LES) in the North American opossum (Abstract)? *Gastroenterology* 76: 1134, 1979.
187. FREELAND, G. R., R. H. HIGGS, D. O. CASTELL, AND J. E. MCGUIGAN. Lower esophageal sphincter (LES) and gastric acid (GA) responses to intravenous infusion of synthetic human gastrin heptadecapeptide I (HGH). *Gastroenterology* 71: 570–574, 1976.
188. FRIEDLAND, G. W., D. H. MELCHER, F. R. BERRIDGE, AND G. A. GRESHAM. Debatable points in the anatomy of the lower oesophagus. *Thorax* 21: 487–498, 1966.
189. FREIMAN, J. M., T. Y. EL-SHARKAWY, AND N. E. DIAMANT. Effect of bilateral vagosympathetic nerve blockade on response of the dog upper esophageal sphincter (UES) to intraesophageal distention and acid. *Gastroenterology* 81: 78–84, 1981.
190. FRYSCAK, T., W. ZENKER, AND D. KANTNER. Afferent and efferent innervation of the rat esophagus: a tracing study with horseradish peroxidase and nuclear yellow. *Anat. Embryol.* 170: 63–70, 1984.
191. FUNCH-JENSEN, P., AND E. JACOBSEN. Esophageal peristalsis before, during and after food intake in healthy people. *Scand. J. Gastroenterol.* 16: 209–212, 1981.
192. FURNESS, J. B., AND M. COSTA. *The Enteric Nervous System.* Edinburgh: Churchill Livingstone, 1987.
193. GABELLA, G. *Structure of the Autonomic Nervous System.*

London: Chapman & Hall, 1976.
194. GEBOES, K., AND V. DESMET. Histology of the esophagus. In: *Frontiers in Gastrointestinal Research. The Esophagus*, edited by L. van der Reis. Basel: Karger, 1978, vol. 3, p. 1–17.
195. GERHARDT, D., J. HEWETT, M. MOESCHBERGER, T. SCHUCK, AND D. WINSHIP. Human upper esophageal sphincter pressure profile. *Am. J. Physiol.* 239 (*Gastrointest. Liver Physiol.* 2): G49–G52, 1980.
196. GERHARDT, D. C., T. J. SHUCK, R. H. BARDEAUX, AND D. H. WINSHIP. Human upper esophageal sphincter. Responses to volume, osmotic and acid stimuli. *Gastroenterology* 75: 268–274, 1978.
197. GIDDA, J. S. Control of esophageal peristalsis. *Viewpoints Dig. Dis.* 17: 13–16, 1985.
198. GIDDA, J. S., B. W. COBB, AND R. K. GOYAL. Modulation of esophageal peristalsis by vagal efferent stimulation in opossum. *J. Clin. Invest.* 68: 1411–1419, 1981.
199. GIDDA, J. S., AND R. K. GOYAL. Influence of successive vagal stimulations on contractions in esophageal smooth muscle of opossum. *J. Clin. Invest.* 71: 1095–1103, 1983.
200. GIDDA, J. S., AND R. K. GOYAL. Swallow-evoked action potentials in vagal preganglionic efferents. *J. Neurophysiol.* 52: 1169–1180, 1984.
201. GIDDA, J. S., AND R. K. GOYAL. Regional gradient of initial inhibition and refractoriness in esophageal smooth muscle. *Gastroenterology* 89: 843–851, 1985.
202. GILBERT, R., S. RATTAN, AND R. K. GOYAL. Pharmacologic identification, activation and antagonism of two muscarine receptor subtypes in the lower esophageal sphincter. *J. Pharmacol. Exp. Ther.* 230: 284–291, 1984.
203. GILBERT, R. J., AND W. J. DODDS. Effect of selective muscarinic antagonists on peristaltic contractions in opossum smooth muscle. *Am. J. Physiol.* 250 (*Gastrointest. Liver Physiol.* 13): G50–G59, 1986.
204. GILBERT, R. J., W. J. DODDS, AND W. J. HOGAN. Subtypes of muscarinic receptors in the vagal inhibitory pathway to the lower esophageal sphincter (Abstract). *Gastroenterology* 88: 1393, 1985.
205. GILES, G. R., M. C. MASON, C. HUMPHRIES, AND C. G. CLARK. Action of gastrin on the lower oesophageal sphincter in man. *Gut* 10: 730–734, 1969.
206. GOLENHOFEN, K. Theory of P and T systems for calcium activation in smooth muscle. In: *Physiology of Smooth Muscle*, edited by E. Bulbring and M. F. Shuba. New York: Raven, 1976, p. 197–202.
207. GONELLA, J. J., P. NIEL, AND C. ROMAN. Vagal control of lower oesophageal sphincter motility in the cat. *J. Physiol. Lond.* 273: 647–664, 1977.
208. GONELLA, J., J. P. NIEL, AND C. ROMAN. Sympathetic control of lower oesophageal sphincter motility in the cat. *J. Physiol. Lond.* 287: 177–190, 1979.
209. GOODALL, R. J. R., D. J. HAY, AND J. G. TEMPLE. Assessment of the rapid pullthrough technique in oesophageal manometry. *Gut* 21: 169–173, 1980.
210. GOYAL, R. K. Disorders of the cricopharyngeus muscle. *Otolaryngol. Clin. N. Am.* 17: 115–130, 1984.
211. GOYAL, R. K. Does gastrin act via cholinergic neurons to maintain basal lower esophageal sphincter pressure? *N. Engl. J. Med.* 291: 849–850, 1974.
212. GOYAL, R. K. The lower esophageal sphincter. *Viewpoints Dig. Dis.* 8: 1–3, 1976.
213. GOYAL, R. K. Location of the squamocolumnar junction (Letter to the editor). *Gastroenterology* 73: 194–195, 1977.
214. GOYAL, R. K., AND J. CRIST. Neurology of the gut. In: *Gastrointestinal Disease: Pathophysiology, Diagnosis, and Treatment.* (4th ed.), edited by M. H. Sleisenger and J. S. Fordtran. Philadelphia, PA: Saunders, in press.
215. GOYAL, R. K. Deleterious effects of prostaglandins on esophageal mucosa. *Gastroenterology* 78: 1085–1086, 1980.
216. GOYAL, R. K., J. L. BAUER, AND H. M. SPIRO. The nature and location of the lower esophageal ring. *N. Engl. J. Med.* 284: 1175–1180, 1971.
217. GOYAL, R. K., D. O. CASTELL, J. CHRISTENSEN, S. COHEN, AND C. E. POPE, II. Round table discussion on gastroesophageal reflux disease. *Gastroenterology* 74: 449–452, 1978.
218. GOYAL, R. K., AND B. W. COBB. Motility of the pharynx, esophagus, and esophageal sphincter. In: *Physiology of the Gastrointestinal Tract* (1st ed.), edited by L. R. Johnson. New York: Raven, 1981, p. 359–391.
219. GOYAL, R. K., AND J. S. GIDDA. Relation between electrical and mechanical activity in esophageal smooth muscle. *Am. J. Physiol.* 240 (*Gastrointest. Liver Physiol.* 3): G305–G311, 1981.
220. GOYAL, R. K., J. J. GLANCY, AND H. M. SPIRO. Lower esophageal ring. *N. Engl. J. Med.* 282: 1298–1305, 1970.
221. GOYAL, R. K., AND J. E. MCGUIGAN. Is gastrin a major determinant of basal lower esophageal sphincter pressure. A double-blind controlled study using high titer gastrin antiserum. *J. Clin. Invest.* 57: 291–300, 1976.
222. GOYAL, R. K., AND S. RATTAN. Mechanism of the lower esophageal sphincter relaxation. Action of prostaglandin $E_1$ and theophylline. *J. Clin. Invest.* 52: 337–341, 1973.
223. GOYAL, R. K., AND S. RATTAN. Nature of the vagal inhibitory innervation of the lower esophageal sphincter. *J. Clin. Invest.* 55: 1119–1126, 1975.
224. GOYAL, R. K., AND S. RATTAN. Genesis of basal sphincter pressure: effect of tetrodotoxin on lower esophageal sphincter pressure in opossum in vivo. *Gastroenterology* 71: 62–67, 1976.
225. GOYAL, R. K., AND S. RATTAN. Neurohumoral, hormonal, and drug receptors for the lower esophageal sphincter. *Gastroenterology* 74: 598–619, 1978.
226. GOYAL, R. K., AND S. RATTAN. Effects of sodium nitroprusside and verapamil on lower esophageal sphincter. *Am. J. Physiol.* 238 (*Gastrointest. Liver Physiol.* 1): G40–G44, 1980.
227. GOYAL, R. K., S. RATTAN, AND T. HERSH. Comparison of the effects of prostaglandins $E_1$, $E_2$, and $A_1$, and of hypovolemic hypotension on the lower esophageal sphincter. *Gastroenterology* 65: 608–612, 1973.
228. GOYAL, R. K., S. RATTAN, AND S. SAID. VIP as a possible neurotransmitter of non-cholinergic, non-adrenergic inhibitory neurones. *Nature Lond.* 288: 378–380, 1980.
229. GOYAL, R. K., M. H. SANGREE, AND T. HERSH. Pressure inversion point at the upper high pressure zone and its genesis. *Gastroenterology* 59: 754–759, 1970.
230. GRAY, J. E., O. LOCKARD, T. J. SHUCK, AND D. H. WINSHIP. Response of the upper esophageal sphincter and upper esophagus to intraluminal esophageal balloon distention (Abstract). *Gastroenterology* 76: 1143, 1979.
231. GRECO, A. V., A. BIANCO, L. ALTOMONTE, L. D'ACQUARICA, AND G. GHIRLANDA. Effect of somatostatin on lower esophageal sphincter (LES) pressure and serum gastrin in normal and achalasic subjects. *Horm. Metab. Res.* 14: 26–28, 1982.
232. GUTIERREZ, J. G., K. D. THANIK, W. Y. CHEY, AND H. YAJIMA. The effect of motilin on the lower esophageal sphincter of the opossum. *Am. J. Dig. Dis.* 22: 402–405, 1977.
233. HARRIS, L. D., W. D. ASHWORTH, AND F. J. INGELFINGER. Esophageal aperistalsis and achalasia produced in dogs by prolonged cholinesterase inhibition. *J. Clin. Invest.* 39: 1744–1751, 1960.
234. HARRIS, L. D., AND C. E. POPE II. The pressure inversion point: its genesis and reliability. *Gastroenterology* 51: 641–648, 1966.
235. HELLEMANS, J., AND G. VANTRAPPEN. Electromyographic studies of canine esophageal motility. *Am. J. Dig. Dis.* 12: 1240–1255, 1967.
236. HELLEMANS, J., G. VANTRAPPEN, P. VALEMBOIS, J. JANSSENS, AND J. VANDENBROUCHE. Electrical activity of striated and smooth muscle of the esophagus. *Am. J. Dig. Dis.* 13: 320–339, 1968.
237. HELLEMANS, J., G. VANTRAPPEN, AND J. VANDENBROUCHE. The electrical activity of the human esophagus (Abstract). *Gastroenterology* 58: 959, 1970.
238. HENDERSON, J. M., G. LIDGARD, D. H. OSBORNE, D. C.

CARTER, AND R. C. HEADING. Lower esophageal sphincter response to gastrin—pharmacological or physiological? *Gut* 19: 99–102, 1978.
239. HIGGS, R. H., D. O. CASTELL, AND G. L. EASTWOOD. Studies on the mechanism of esophagitis-induced lower esophageal sphincter hypotension in cats. *Gastroenterology* 71: 51–56, 1976.
240. HIGGS, B., AND F. H. ELLIS, JR. The effect of bilaterial supranodosal vagotomy on canine esophageal function. *Surgery St. Louis* 58: 828–834, 1965.
241. HIGGS, B., R. D. SMYTH, AND D. O. CASTELL. Gastric alkalinization. Effect on lower esophageal sphincter pressure and serum gastrin. *N. Engl. J. Med.* 291: 486–490, 1974.
242. HOGAN, W. J., W. J. DODDS, S. E. HOKE, D. P. REID, R. K. KALKHOFF, AND R. C. ARNDORFER. Effect of glucagon on esophageal motor function. *Gastroenterology* 69: 160–165, 1975.
243. HOLLIS, J. B., AND D. O. CASTELL. Esophageal function in elderly men. *Ann. Intern. Med.* 80: 371–374, 1974.
244. HOLLIS, J. B., AND D. O. CASTELL. Effect of dry and wet swallows of different volumes on esophageal peristalsis. *J. Appl. Physiol.* 38: 1161–1164, 1975.
245. HOLLOWAY, R. H., E. BLANK, I. TAKAHASHI, W. J. DODDS, W. J. HOGAN, AND J. DENT. Variability of lower esophageal sphincter pressure in the fasted unanesthetized opossum. *Am. J. Physiol.* 248 (*Gastrointest. Liver Physiol.* 11): G398–G406, 1985.
246. HOLLOWAY, R. H., E. BLANK, I. TAKAHASHI, W. J. DODDS, AND R. D. LAYMAN. Motilin: a mechanism incorporating the opossum lower esophageal sphincter into the migrating motor complex. *Gastroenterology* 89: 507–515, 1985.
247. HOLLOWAY, R. H., W. J. DODDS, J. F. HELM, W. J. HOGAN, J. DENT, AND R. C. ARNDORFER. Integrity of cholinergic innervation to the lower esophageal sphincter in achalasia. *Gastroenterology* 90: 924–929, 1986.
248. HOLSTEGE, G., G. GRAVELAND, C. BIJKER-BIEMOND, AND I. SCHUDDEBOOM. Location of motoneurons innervating soft palate, pharynx, and upper esophagus. Anatomical evidence for a possible swallowing center in the pontine reticular formation. *Brain Behav. Evol.* 23: 47–62, 1983.
249. HONGO, M., A. ISHIMORI, A. NAGASAKI, AND T. SATO. Effect of duodenal acidification on the lower esophageal sphincter pressure in the dog with special reference to related gastrointestinal hormones. *Tohoku J. Exp. Med.* 131: 215–219, 1980.
250. HONGO, M., M. TRAUBE, R. G. MCALLISTER, JR., AND R. W. MCCALLUM. Effects of nifedipine on esophageal motor function in humans: Correlation with plasma nifedipine concentration. *Gastroenterology* 86: 8–12, 1984.
251. HONGO, M., M. TRAUBE, AND R. W. MCCALLUM. Comparison of effects of nifedipine, propantheline bromide, and the combination on esophageal motor function in normal volunteers. *Dig. Dis. Sci.* 29: 300–304, 1984.
252. HOWARD, J. M., M. R. BELSHEIM, AND S. N. SULLIVAN. Enkephalin inhibits relaxation of the lower oesophageal sphincter. *Br. Med. J.* 285: 1605–1606, 1982.
253. HUMPHRIES, T. J., AND D. O. CASTELL. Effect of oral bethanechol on parameters of esophageal peristalsis. *Dig. Dis. Sci.* 26: 129–132, 1981.
254. HUMPHRIES, T. J., AND D. O. CASTELL. Pressure profile of esophageal peristalsis in normal humans as measured by direct intraesophageal transducers. *Am. J. Dig. Dis.* 22: 641–645, 1977.
255. HUNT, P. S., A. M. CONNELL, AND T. B. SMILEY. The cricopharyngeal sphincter in gastric reflux. *Gut* 11: 303–306, 1970.
256. HURWITZ, A. L., A. DURANCEAU, AND J. K. HADDAD. *Disorders of Esophageal Motility*. Philadelphia, PA: Saunders, 1979.
257. HURWITZ, A. L., J. A. NELSON, AND J. K. HADDAD. Oropharyngeal dysphagia: manometric and cineesophagographic findings. *Am. J. Dig. Dis.* 20: 313–324, 1975.
258. HWANG, K. Nervous control of the esophagus and cardia with observations on experimental cardiospasm. Chicago, IL: Univ. of Illinois, 1953. PhD thesis.
259. HWANG, K. Mechanism of transportation of the content of the esophagus. *J. Appl. Physiol.* 6: 781–796, 1954.
260. HWANG, K., H. E. ESSEX, AND F. C. MANN. A study of certain problems resulting from vagotomy in dogs with special emphasis to emesis. *Am. J. Physiol.* 149: 429–448, 1947.
261. HWANG, K., M. I. GROSSMAN, AND A. C. IVY. Nervous control of the cervical portion of the esophagus. *Am. J. Physiol.* 154: 343–357, 1948.
262. IMAIZUMI, M., AND K. HAMA. An electron microscopic study on the interstitial cells of the gizzard of the lovebird (*Uronloncha domestica*). *Z. Zellforsch. Mikrosk. Anat.* 97: 351–357, 1969.
263. INGELFINGER, F. J. Esophageal motility. *Physiol. Rev.* 38: 533–584, 1958.
264. ISBERG, A., M. E. NILSSON, AND H. SCHIRATZKI. Movement of the upper esophageal sphincter and a manometric device during deglutition. A cineradiographic investigation. *Acta Radiol. Diagn.* 26: 381–388, 1985.
265. ITOH, I., I. AIZAWA, R. HONDA, H. HIVATASHI, AND E. F. COUCH. Control of lower esophageal sphincter contractile activity by motilin in conscious dogs. *Am. J. Dig. Dis.* 23: 341–345, 1978.
266. JACOBOWITZ, D., AND P. NEMIR. The autonomic innervation of the esophagus of the dog. *J. Thorac. Cardiovasc. Surg.* 58: 678–684, 1969.
267. JAFFER, S. S., G. M. MAKHLOUF, B. A. SCHORR, AND A. M. ZFASS. Nature and kinetics of inhibition of lower esophageal sphincter by glucagon. *Gastroenterology* 67: 42–46, 1974.
268. JANISCH, H. D., AND V. F. ECKARDT. Oesophageal transmural potential difference in normal persons. *Digestion* 25: 180–185, 1982.
269. JANISCH, H. D., T. R. WEIHRAUCH, AND K. E. HAMPEL. Is abdominal compression a useful stimulation test for analysis of lower esophageal sphincter function? *Dig. Dis. Sci.* 29: 689–695, 1984.
270. JANSSENS, J., I. DE WEVER, G. VANTRAPPEN, AND J. HELLEMANS. Peristalsis in smooth muscle esophagus after transection and bolus deviation. *Gastroenterology* 71: 1004–1009, 1976.
271. JANSSENS, J., P. VALEMBOIS, J. HELLEMANS, G. VANTRAPPEN, AND W. PELEMANS. Studies on the necessity of a bolus for the progression of secondary peristalsis in the canine esophagus. *Gastroenterology* 67: 245–251, 1974.
272. JANSSENS, J., P. VALEMBOIS, G. VANTRAPPEN, J. HELLEMANS, AND W. PELEMANS. Is the primary peristaltic contraction of the canine esophagus bolus-dependent? *Gastroenterology* 65: 750–756, 1973.
273. JAUP, B. H., H. ABRAHAMSSON, R. VIRTANEN, AND E. IISALO. Effect of pirenzepine compared with atropine and L-hyoscyamine on esophageal peristaltic activity in humans. *Scand. J. Gastroenterol.* 17: 233–239, 1982.
274. JEAN, A. Localization et activité des neurones deglutieurs bulbaires. *J. Physiol. Paris* 64: 227–268, 1972.
275. JEAN, A., AND A. CAR. Inputs to the swallowing medullary neurons from the peripheral afferent fibers and the swallowing cortical area. *Brain Res.* 178: 567–572, 1979.
276. JEAN, A. Control of the central swallowing program by inputs from the peripheral receptors. A review. *J. Auton. Nerv. Syst.* 10: 225–233, 1984.
277. JENNEWEIN, H. M., H. HUMMELT, U. MEYER, R. SIEWERT, A. KOCH, AND F. WALDECK. The effect of vagotomy on the resting pressure and reactivity of the lower esophageal sphincter (LES) in man and dog. In: *Proc. Int. Symp. Gastrointest. Motil.* 5th, edited by G. Vantrappen. Herentals, Belgium: Typoff, 1976, p. 186–189.
278. JENNEWEIN, H. M., H. HUMMELT, R. SIEWERT, AND F. WULDECK. The motor-stimulating effect of natural motilin on the lower esophageal sphincter, fundus, antrum, and duodenum in dogs. *Digestion* 13: 246–250, 1975.
279. JENNEWEIN, H. M., F. WALDECK, R. SIEWART, F. WEISER, AND R. THIMM. The interaction of glucagon and pentagastrin

on the lower esophageal sphincter in man and dogs. *Gut* 14: 861–864, 1973.
280. JENSEN, D. M., R. MCCALLUM, AND J. H. WALSH. Failure of atropine to inhibit gastrin-17 stimulation of the lower esophageal sphincter in man. *Gastroenterology* 75: 825–827, 1978.
281. JOHANNESSON, N., K. E. ANDERSSON, B. JOELSSON, AND C. G. A. PERSSON. Relaxation of lower esophageal sphincter and stimulation of gastric secretion and diuresis by antiasthmatic xanthines: role of adenosine antagonism. *Am. Rev. Respir. Dis.* 131: 26–31, 1985.
282. JORDON, P. H., JR., AND E. H. LONGHI. Relationship between size of bolus and the act of swallowing on esophageal peristalsis in dogs. *Proc. Soc. Exp. Biol. Med.* 137: 868–871, 1971.
283. JURY, J., L. P. JAGER, AND E. E. DANIEL. Unusual potassium channels mediate nonadrenergic noncholinergic nerve-mediated inhibition in opossum esophagus. *Can. J. Physiol. Pharmacol.* 63: 107–112, 1985.
284. KACZMEREK, J., S. RATTAN, AND R. K. GOYAL. Galanin selectively inhibits noncholinergic component of peristalsis in smooth muscle portion of opossum esophagus. *Gastroenterology* 92: 1802, 1987.
285. KAHRILAS, P. J., W. J. DODDS, J. DENT, B. HAEBERLE, W. J. HOGAN, AND R. C. ARNDORFER. Effect of sleep, spontaneous gastroesophageal (GE) reflux, and a meal on UES pressure (Abstract). *Gastroenterology* 91: 897–904, 1986.
286. KANIKAWA, Y., AND Y. SHIMO. Pharmacological characterization of the opioid receptor in the submucous plexus of the guinea-pig oesophagus. *Br. J. Pharmacol.* 78: 693–699, 1983.
287. KANIKAWA, Y., AND Y. SHIMO. Contractile responses to substance P and related peptides of the isolated muscularis mucosa of guinea pig esophagus. *Br. J. Pharmacol.* 81: 143–149, 1984.
288. KANNAN, M. S., L. P. JAGER, AND E. E. DANIEL. Electrical properties of smooth muscle cell membrane of opossum esophagus. *Am. J. Physiol.* 248 (*Gastrointest. Liver Physiol.* 11): G342–G346, 1985.
289. KATZ, P. O., J. E. RICHTER, R. COWAN, AND D. O. CASTELL. Apparent complete lower esophageal sphincter relaxation in achalasia. *Gastroenterology* 90: 978–983, 1986.
290. KAWASAKI, M., J. H. OGURA, AND S. TAKENOUCHI. Neurophysiologic observations of normal glutition. I. Its relationship to the respiratory cycle. II. Its relationship to allied phenomena. *Laryngoscope* 74: 1747–1780, 1964.
291. KAYE, M. D. On the relationship between gastric pH and pressure in the normal human lower esophageal sphincter. *Gut* 20: 59–63, 1979.
292. KAYE, M. D., AND R. M. WEXLER. Alteration of esophageal peristalsis by body position. *Dig. Dis. Sci.* 26: 897–901, 1981.
293. KAZEM, I. A new scintigraphic technique for the study of the esophagus. *Am. J. Roentgenol. Radium Ther. Nucl. Med.* 115: 681–688, 1972.
294. KELLY, M. L., AND H. L. FRIEDLAND. Gastroesophageal sphincteric pressure before and after oral anticholinergic drug and placebo administration. *Am. J. Dig. Dis.* 12: 823–833, 1967.
295. KILMAN, W. J., AND R. K. GOYAL. Disorders of pharyngeal and upper esophageal sphincter motor function. *Arch. Intern. Med.* 136: 592–601, 1976.
296. KIRCHNER, J. A. The motor activity of the cricopharyngeus muscle. *Laryngoscope* 68: 1119–1159, 1958.
297. KJELLEN, G., J. B. SVEDBERG, AND L. TIBBLING. Solid bolus transit by esophageal scintigraphy in patients with dysphagia and normal manometry and radiography. *Dig. Dis. Sci.* 29: 1–5, 1984.
298. KOELZ, H. R., A. P. HOLLINGER, H. SAUBERLI, F. LARGIARDER, R. SIEWERT, AND A. L. BLUM. Effect of gastric antrum on regulation of lower esophageal sphincter pressure in dog. *Am. J. Physiol.* 234 (*Endocrinol. Metab. Gastrointest. Physiol.* 3): E157–E161, 1978.
299. KOELZ, H. R., G. LEPSIEN, A. P. HOLLINGER, H. SAUBERLI, F. LARGIARDER, R. ARNOLD, A. L. BLUM, AND R. SIEWERT. Effect of intraduodenal peptone on the lower esophageal sphincter pressure in dog. *Gastroenterology* 75: 283–285, 1978.
300. KOENIG, W., B. KEHRER, AND M. BETTEX. Le sphincter inferieur de l'oesophage chez le nouveau-né. *Chir. Pediatr.* 23: 357–362, 1982.
301. KRAMER, P. Location of the squamocolumnar junction (Letter to the editor). *Gastroenterology* 73: 194, 1977.
302. KRAVITZ, J. J., W. J. SNAPE, JR., AND S. COHEN. Effect of thoracic vagotomy and vagal stimulation on esophageal function. *Am. J. Physiol.* 234 (*Endocrinol. Metab. Gastrointest. Physiol.* 3): E359–E364, 1978.
303. KRAVITZ, J. J., W. J. SNAPE, JR., AND S. COHEN. Effect of histamine and histamine antagonists on human lower esophageal sphincter function. *Gastroenterology* 74: 435–440, 1978.
304. LAIMER, E. Beitrag zur anatomic des Oesophagus. *Med. Jahrbücher Vienna* p. 333–338, 1883.
305. LARRABEE, M. G., AND R. HODES. Cyclic changes in the respiratory center revealed by the effects of afferent impulses. *Am. J. Physiol.* 155: 147–164, 1948.
306. LAWN, A. M. The localization, by means of electrical stimulation, of the origin and path in the medulla oblongata of the motor nerve fibers of the rabbit esophagus. *J. Physiol. Lond.* 174: 232–244, 1964.
307. LAWN, A. M. The localization, in the nucleus ambiguus of the rabbit, of the cells of origin of motor nerve fibers in the glossopharyngeal nerve and various branches of the vagus nerve by means of retrograde degeneration. *J. Comp. Neurol.* 127: 293–306, 1966.
308. LEANDER, S., E. BRODIN, R. HÅKANSON, F. SUNDLER, AND R. UDDMAN. Neuronal substance P in the esophagus. Distribution and effects on motor activity. *Acta Physiol. Scand.* 115: 427–435, 1982.
309. LEAR, C. S., J. B. FLANAGAN, AND C. F. MOORREES. The frequency of deglutition in man. *Arch. Oral Biol.* 10: 83–99, 1965.
310. LERCHE, W. *The Esophagus and Pharynx in Action*. Springfield, IL: Thomas, 1950.
311. LEVITT, M. N., H. H. DEDO, AND J. H. OGURA. The cricopharyngeus muscle, an electromyographic study in the dog. *Laryngoscope* 75: 122–136, 1965.
312. LIEBERMANN-MEFFERT, D., M. ALLGÖWER, P. SCHMID, AND A. L. BLUM. Muscular equivalent of the lower esophageal sphincter. *Gastroenterology* 76: 31–38, 1979.
313. LIEBERMANN-MEFFERT, D., M. HEBERER, S. MARTINOLI, AND M. ALLGOEWER. Are there muscular structures which may contribute to closure of the gastroesophageal junction? *Scand. J. Gastroenterol. Suppl.* 67: 123, 1981.
314. LIND, J. F., D. J. COTTON, R. BLANCHARD, J. J. CRISPIN, AND G. E. DIMOPOLOS. Effect of thoracic displacement and vagotomy on the canine gastroesophageal junctional zone. *Gastroenterology* 56: 1078–1085, 1969.
315. LIND, J. F., J. S. CRISPIN, AND D. K. McIVER. The effect of atropine on the gastroesophageal sphincter. *Can. J. Physiol. Pharmacol.* 46: 233–238, 1968.
316. LIND, J. F., A. M. SMITH, D. K. McIVER, A. T. COOPLAND, AND J. S. CRISPIN. Heartburn in pregnancy—a manometric study. *Can. Med. Assoc. J.* 98: 571–574, 1968.
317. LIND, J. F., W. G. WARRIAN, AND W. J. WANKLING. Responses of the gastroesophageal junction zone to increases in abdominal pressure. *Can. J. Surg.* 9: 32–38, 1966.
318. LINEHAN, J. H., J. DENT, W. J. DODDS, AND W. J. HOGAN. Sleeve device functions as a Starling resistor to record sphincter pressure. *Am. J. Physiol.* 248 (*Gastrointest. Liver Physiol.* 11): G251–G255, 1985.
319. LIPSHUTZ, W. H., AND S. COHEN. Physiological determinants of lower esophageal sphincter function. *Gastroenterology* 61: 16–24, 1971.
320. LIPSHUTZ, W. H., W. HUGHES, AND S. COHEN. The genesis of lower esophageal sphincter pressure: its identification

through the use of gastrin antiserum. *J. Clin. Invest.* 51: 522–529, 1972.
321. LIPSHUTZ, W. H., A. F. TUCH, AND S. COHEN. A comparison of the site of action of gastrin I on lower esophageal sphincter and antral circular smooth muscle. *Gastroenterology* 61: 454–460, 1971.
322. LLOYD, D. A., Y. THUM BARIMA, AND P. GULLANE. The "globus sensation" (GS) is not caused by cricopharyngeal (CP) hypertension (Abstract). *Gastroenterology* 86: 1165, 1984.
323. LONGHI, E. H., AND P. H. JORDON, JR. Necessity of a bolus for propagation of primary peristalsis in the canine esophagus. *Am. J. Physiol.* 220: 609–612, 1971.
324. LUMSDEN, K., AND W. S. HOLDEN. The act of vomiting in man. *Gut* 10: 173–179, 1969.
325. LUND, C. F., AND J. CHRISTENSEN. Electrical stimulation of esophageal smooth muscle and effects of antagonists. *Am. J. Physiol.* 217: 1369–1374, 1969.
326. LUND, W. S. The function of the cricopharyngeal sphincter during swallowing. *Acta Otolaryngol.* 59: 497–510, 1965.
327. LUND, W. S. A study of the cricopharyngeal sphincter in man and in the dog. *Ann. R. Coll. Surg. Engl.* 37: 225–246, 1965.
328. LUND, W. S., AND G. M. ARDRAN. The motor nerve supply of the cricopharyngeal sphincter. *Ann. Otol. Rhinol. Laryngol.* 73: 599–617, 1964.
329. MADSEN, T., L. WALLIN, S. BOESBY, AND V. H. LARSEN. Oesophageal peristalsis in normal subjects. *Scand. J. Gastroenterol.* 18: 513–518, 1983.
330. MAHER, J. W., A. J. OLINDE, AND J. E. MCGUIGAN. Suppression of postprandial lower esophageal sphincter pressure and pancreatic polypeptide by duodenal exclusion. *J. Surg. Res.* 37: 467–471, 1984.
331. MATARAZZO, S. A., W. S. SNAPE, JR., J. P. RYAN, AND S. COHEN. The relationship of cervical and abdominal vagal activity in lower esophageal sphincter function. *Gastroenterology* 71: 999–1003, 1976.
332. MCCALL, I. W., R. F. HARVEY, C. J. OWENS, AND B. C. CLENDINNEN. Relationship between changes in plasma gastrin and lower esophageal sphincter pressure after meals. *Br. J. Surg.* 62: 15–18, 1975.
333. MCCALLUM, R. W. Studies on the mechanism of the lower esophageal sphincter pressure response to alkali ingestion in humans. *Am. J. Gastroenterol.* 80: 513–517, 1985.
334. MCCALLUM, R. W., AND J. H. WALSH. Relationship between lower esophageal sphincter pressure and serum gastrin concentration in Zollinger-Ellison syndrome and other clinical settings. *Gastroenterology* 76: 76–81, 1979.
335. MCKIRDY, H. C., AND R. W. MARSHALL. Effect of drugs and electrical field stimulation on circular muscle strips from human lower oesophagus. *Q. J. Exp. Physiol.* 70: 591–601, 1985.
336. MCNALLY, E. F., J. E. KELLY, AND F. J. INGELFINGER. Mechanism of belching: effects of gastric distention with air. *Gastroenterology* 46: 254–259, 1964.
337. MEI, N. Mecanorecepteurs vagaux digestifs chez le chat. *Exp. Brain Res.* 11: 502–514, 1970.
338. MEI, N., M. AUBERT, J. CROUSILLAT, AND F. RANIERI. Sensory innervation of the lower esophagus of the cat. Comparison with the other parts of the digestive system. In: *Proc. Int. Symp. on Gastrointestinal Motility*, 4th, Banff, Alberta, Canada, 1973, edited by E. E. Daniel. Vancouver, Canada: Mitchell, 1974, p. 585–591.
339. MEISSNER, A. J., K. L. BOWES, R. ZWICK, AND E. E. DANIEL. Effect of motilin on the lower esophageal sphincter. *Gut* 17: 925–932, 1976.
340. MELLOW, M. H. Esophageal motility during food ingestion: a physiologic test of esophageal motor function. *Gastroenterology* 85: 570–577, 1983.
341. MEYER, G. W., D. C. GERHARD, AND D. O. CASTELL. Human esophageal response to rapid swallowing: muscle refractory period or neural inhibition? *Am. J. Physiol.* 241 (*Gastrointest. Liver Physiol.* 4): G129–G136, 1981.
342. MILLER, A. J. Deglutition. *Physiol. Rev.* 62: 129–184, 1982.
343. MILLER, C. A., M. S. BARNETTE, H. S. ORMSBEE, III, AND T. J. TORPHY. Cyclic nucleotide-dependent protein kinases in the lower esophageal sphincter. *Am. J. Physiol.* 251 (*Gastrointest. Liver Physiol.* 14): G794–G803, 1986.
344. MUKHOPADHYAY, A. K. Effect of substance P on the lower esophageal sphincter of the opossum. *Gastroenterology* 75: 278–282, 1978.
345. MUKHOPADHYAY, A. K., AND M. KUNNEMANN. Mechanism of lower esophageal sphincter stimulation by bombesin in the opossum. *Gastroenterology* 76: 1409–1414, 1979.
346. MUKHOPADHYAY, A., S. RATTAN, AND R. K. GOYAL. Effect of prostaglandin $E_2$ on esophageal motility in man. *J. Appl. Physiol.* 39: 479–481, 1975.
347. MUKHOPADHYAY, A. K., AND N. W. WEISBRODT. Neural organization of esophageal peristalsis: role of vagus nerve. *Gastroenterology* 68: 444–447, 1975.
348. MUKHOPADHYAY, A. K., AND N. W. WEISBRODT. Effect of dopamine on esophageal motor function. *Am. J. Physiol.* 232 (*Endocrinol. Metab. Gastrointest. Physiol.* 12): E19–E24, 1977.
349. MULLER-LISSNER, S. A., AND A. L. BLUM. Fundic pressure rise lowers lower esophageal sphincter pressure in man. *Hepato-Gastroenterology* 29: 151–152, 1982.
350. MURAKAMI, Y., H. FUKUDA, AND J. A. KIRCHNER. The cricopharyngeus muscle, an electrophysiological and neuropharmacological study. *Acta Oto-Laryngol. Suppl.* 311: 1–19, 1972.
351. NAGLER, R., AND H. M. SPIRO. Heartburn in late pregnancy. Manometric studies of esophageal motor function. *J. Clin. Invest.* 40: 954–970, 1961.
352. NAGLER, R., AND H. M. SPIRO. Serial esophageal motility studies in asymptomatic young subjects. *Gastroenterology* 41: 371–380, 1961.
353. NEBEL, O. T., AND D. O. CASTELL. Lower esophageal sphincter pressure changes after food ingestion. *Gastroenterology* 63: 778–783, 1972.
354. NEBEL, O. T., AND D. O. CASTELL. Inhibition of the lower esophageal sphincter by fat—a mechanism for fatty food intolerance. *Gut* 14: 270–274, 1973.
355. NEBEL, O. T., AND D. O. CASTELL. Kinetics of fat inhibition of the lower esophageal sphincter. *J. Appl. Physiol.* 35: 6–8, 1973.
356. NELSON, J. L., J. E. RICHTER, D. N. JOHNS, D. O. CASTELL, AND G. M. CENTOLA. Esophageal contraction pressures are not affected by normal menstrual cycles. *Gastroenterology* 87: 867–871, 1984.
357. NELSON, J. L., W. C. WU, J. E. RICHTER, J. N. BLACKWELL, D. N. JOHNS, AND D. O. CASTELL. What is normal esophageal manometry (Abstract)? *Gastroenterology* 84: 1258, 1983.
358. NIEL, J. P., J. GONELLA, AND C. ROMAN. Localisation par la technique de marquage à la peroxydase des corps cellulaires des neurones ortho et parasympathiques innervant le sphincter oesophagien inferieur du chat. *J. Physiol. Paris* 76: 591–599, 1980.
359. NETTER, F. H. Digestive system: upper digestive tract. In: *The Ciba Collection of Medical Illustrations*, edited by E. Oppenheimer. New York: Ciba, 1971, sect. II, vol. 3, pt. I, plate 5.
360. OGILVIE, A. L., AND M. ATKINSON. Influence of the vagus nerve upon the reflex control of the lower esophageal sphincter. *Gut* 25: 253–258, 1984.
361. OHKAWA, H. Mechanical activity of the smooth muscle of the muscularis mucosa of the guinea pig esophagus and drug actions. *Jpn. J. Physiol.* 30: 161–177, 1980.
362. ORLANDO, R. C., D. W. POWELL, J. C. BRYSON, H. B. KINARD, C. N. CARNEY, J. D. JONES, AND E. M. BOZYMSKI. Esophageal potential difference measurements in esophageal disease. *Gastroenterology* 83: 1026–1032, 1982.
363. ORMSBEE, H. S., III, T. J. TORPHY, C. F. FINE, M. BURMAN, AND M. GROUS. Increases in cGMP are associated with nerve-mediated and drug-induced LES relaxation (Abstract). *Gastroenterology* 88: 1525, 1985.
364. ORR, W. C., L. F. JOHNSON, AND M. G. ROBINSON. Effect of sleep on swallowing, esophageal peristalsis, and acid clearance.

365. OUYANG, A., J. C. REYNOLDS, AND S. COHEN. Spike-associated and spike-independent esophageal contractions in patients with symptomatic diffuse esophageal spasm. *Gastroenterology* 84: 907–913, 1983.
366. PALMER, E. D. Disorders of the circopharyngeus muscle: a review. *Gastroenterology* 71: 510–519, 1976.
367. PAPASOVA, M., K. BOEV, A. BONEV, AND E. MILOUSHEVA. Relationship between the changes in the membrane potential and the contraction of the smooth muscles of the lower oesophageal sphincter and the ileocaecal sphincter. *Agressologie* 22: 205–208, 1981.
368. PAPASOVA, M., E. MILOUSHEVA, A. BONEV, K. BOEV, AND N. KORTEZOVA. On the changes in the membrane potential and the contractile activity of the smooth muscle of the lower esophageal and ileo-caecal sphincters upon increased $K^+$ in the nutrient solution. *Acta Physiol. Pharmacol. Bulg.* 6: 41–48, 1980.
369. PATERSON, W. G., AND R. K. GOYAL. Oesophageal motility and its disorders. *Curr. Opin. Gastroenterol.* 1: 549–559, 1985.
370. PATERSON, W. G., S. RATTAN, AND R. K. GOYAL. Experimental induction of isolated lower esophageal sphincter relaxation in anesthetized opossums. *J. Clin. Invest.* 77: 1187–1193, 1986.
371. PATERSON, W. G., S. RATTAN, AND R. K. GOYAL. Lower esophageal sphincter responses to balloon inflation, deflation and obstruction of the esophageal body (Abstract). *Gastroenterology* 90: 1579, 1986.
372. PEDEN, J. K., M. D. SCHNEIDER, AND R. D. BICKEL. Anatomic relations of the vagus nerves to the esophagus. *Am. J. Surg.* 80: 32–34, 1950.
373. PERCY, W., K. SCHULZE-DELRIEU, S. SHIRAZI, AND K. VON DERAU. Spread of mechanical activity across the isolated gastroesophageal junction (JCT) of the opossum (Abstract). *Dig. Dis. Sci.* 30: 787, 1985.
374. PHAOSAWASDI, K., L. S. MALMUD, R. D. TOLIN, F. STELZER, G. APPELGATE, AND R. S. FISHER. Cholinergic effects on esophageal transit and clearance. *Gastroenterology* 81: 915–920, 1981.
375. PITMAN, R. G., AND G. M. FRASER. The post-circoid impression on the esophagus. *Clin. Radiol.* 16: 34–39, 1965.
376. POMMERENKE, W. T. A study of the sensory areas eliciting the swallowing reflex. *Am. J. Physiol.* 84: 36–41, 1928.
377. POPE, C. E., II. The esophagus: physiology. In: *Gastrointestinal Disease* (3rd ed.), edited by M. H. Sleisenger and J. S. Fordtran, Philadelphia, PA: Saunders, 1983, p. 414–424.
378. POPE, C. E., II, P. ASK, AND L. TIBBLING. Evaluation of intraluminal EMG electrodes for the oesophagus and gastrointestinal tract. *Med. Biol. Eng. Comput.* 22: 461–464, 1984.
379. PRICE, L. M., T. Y. EL-SHARKAWY, H. Y. MUI, AND N. E. DIAMANT. Effect of bilateral cervical vagotomy on balloon-induced lower esophageal sphincter relaxation in the dog. *Gastroenterology* 77: 324–329, 1979.
380. RATTAN, S., D. COLIN, AND R. K. GOYAL. The mechanisms of action of gastrin on the lower esophageal sphincter. *Gastroenterology* 70: 828–835, 1976.
381. RATTAN, S., J. S. GIDDA, AND R. K. GOYAL. Membrane potential and mechanical responses of the opossum esophagus to vagal stimulation and swallowing. *Gastroenterology* 85: 922–928, 1983.
382. RATTAN, S., P. GONELLA, AND R. K. GOYAL. Inhibitory effect of calcitonin gene-related peptide and calcitonin on opossum esophageal smooth muscle. *Gastroenterology*. 94: 284–293, 1988.
383. RATTAN, S., AND R. K. GOYAL. Neural control of the lower esophageal sphincter: influence of the vagus nerves. *J. Clin. Invest.* 54: 899–906.
384. RATTAN, S., AND R. K. GOYAL. Effect of nicotine on LES—studies on the mechanisms of action. *Gastroenterology* 69: 154–159, 1975.
385. RATTAN, S., AND R. K. GOYAL. Effect of dopamine on the esophageal smooth muscle in vivo. *Gastroenterology* 70: 377–381, 1976.
386. RATTAN, S., AND R. K. GOYAL. Effects of 5-hydroxytryptamine on the lower esophageal sphincter in vivo. *J. Clin. Invest.* 59: 125–133, 1977.
387. RATTAN, S., AND R. K. GOYAL. Effect of histamine on the lower esophageal sphincter in vivo: evidence for action at three different sites. *J. Pharmacol. Exp. Ther.* 204: 334–342, 1978.
388. RATTAN, S., AND R. K. GOYAL. Evidence of possible 5-HT participation in the vagal inhibitory pathway to the opossum LES. *Am. J. Physiol.* 234 (*Endocrinol. Metab. Gastrointest. Physiol.* 3): E273–E276, 1978.
389. RATTAN, S., AND R. K. GOYAL. Effect of bovine pancreatic polypeptide on the opossum lower esophageal sphincter. *Gastroenterology* 77: 672–676, 1979.
390. RATTAN, S., AND R. K. GOYAL. Evidence against purinergic inhibitory nerves in the vagal pathway to the opossum lower esophageal sphincter. *Gastroenterology* 78: 898–904, 1980.
391. RATTAN, S., AND R. K. GOYAL. Role of prostaglandins in the regulation of lower esophageal sphincter. In: *Gastrointestinal Motility*, edited by J. M. Christensen. New York: Raven, 1980.
392. RATTAN, S., AND R. K. GOYAL. Identification and localization of opioid receptors in the opossum lower esophageal sphincter. *J. Pharmacol. Exp. Ther.* 224: 391–397, 1983.
393. RATTAN, S., AND R. K. GOYAL. Identification of $M_1$ and $M_2$ muscarinic receptor subtypes in the control of the lower esophageal sphincter in the opossum. *Trends Pharmacol. Sci.* Suppl.: 78–81, 1984.
394. RATTAN, S., AND R. K. GOYAL. Effect of galanin on the opossum lower esophageal sphincter. *Life Sci.* 41: 2783–2790, 1987.
395. RATTAN, S., AND R. K. GOYAL. Structure-activity relationship of subtypes of cholecystokinin receptors in the cat lower esophageal sphincter. *Gastroenterology* 90: 94–102, 1986.
396. RATTAN, S., AND R. K. GOYAL. Free intracellular calcium ($[Ca^2]_i$) in unstimulated and stimulated lower esophageal sphincter (tonic) and esophageal body (phasic) smooth muscles (Abstract). *Gastroenterology* 91: 1064, 1986.
397. RATTAN, S., M. GRADY, AND R. K. GOYAL. Vasoactive intestinal peptide causes peristaltic contractions in the esophageal body. *Life Sci.* 30: 1557–1563, 1982.
398. RATTAN, S., T. HERSH, AND R. K. GOYAL. Effect of prostaglandins $F_{2\alpha}$ and gastrin pentapeptide on the lower esophageal sphincter. *Proc. Soc. Exp. Biol. Med.* 141: 573–575, 1972.
399. RATTAN, S., S. I. SAID, AND R. K. GOYAL. Effects of vasoactive intestinal polypeptide (VIP) on lower esophageal sphincter pressure (LESP). *Proc. Soc. Exp. Biol. Med.* 155: 40–43, 1977.
400. RATTAN, S., J. WALSH, AND R. K. GOYAL. Distribution of vasoactive intestinal polypeptide (VIP) in the opossum esophagus (Abstract). *Dig. Dis. Sci.* 25: 729, 1980.
401. RESIN, H., D. H. STERN, R. A. L. STURDEVANT, AND J. I. ISENBERG. Effect of the C-terminal octapeptide of cholecystokinin on lower esophageal sphincter pressure in man. *Gastroenterology* 64: 946–949, 1973.
402. REYNOLDS, J. C., A. OUYANG, AND S. COHEN. Electrically coupled intrinsic responses of feline lower esophageal sphincter. *Am. J. Physiol.* 243 (*Gastrointest. Liver Physiol.* 6): G415–G423, 1982.
403. REYNOLDS, J. C., A. OUYANG, AND S. COHEN. A lower esophageal sphincter reflex involving substance P. *Am. J. Physiol.* 246 (*Gastrointest. Liver Physiol.* 9): G346–G354, 1984.
404. REYNOLDS, R. P. E., T. Y. EL-SHARKAWY, AND N. E. DIAMANT. Lower esophageal sphincter function in the cat: role of central innervation assessed by transient vagal blockade. *Am. J. Physiol.* 246 (*Gastrointest. Liver Physiol.* 9): G666–G674, 1984.
405. REYNOLDS, R. P. E., T. Y. EL-SHARKAWY, AND N. E. DIAMANT. Oesophageal peristalsis in the cat: the role of central innervation assessed by transient vagal blockade. *Can. J. Physiol. Pharmacol.* 63: 122–130, 1984.
406. RICHARDSON, B. J., AND B. W. WELCH. Differential effect of atropine on rightward and leftward lower sphincter pressure.

*Gastroenterology* 81: 85–89, 1981.
407. RICHTER, J. E., D. R. SINAR, C. M. CORDOVA, AND D. O. CASTELL. Verapamil—a potent inhibitor of contractions in the baboon. *Gastroenterology* 82: 882–886, 1982.
408. RICHTER, J. E., C. B. DALTON, R. G. BUICE, AND D. O. CASTELL. Nifedipine: a potent inhibitor of contractions in the body of the human esophagus. *Gastroenterology* 89: 549–554, 1985.
409. RIMELE, T. J., W. A. ROGERS, AND T. S. GAGINELLA. Characterization of muscarinic cholinergic receptors in the lower esophageal sphincter of the cat: binding of [$^3$H]quinuclidinyl benzilate. *Gastroenterology* 77: 1225–1235, 1979.
410. RINALDO, J. A., AND J. F. LEVEY. Correlation of several methods for recording esophageal sphincter pressures. *Am. J. Dig. Dis.* 13: 882–890, 1968.
411. ROBISON, B. A., W. H. PERCY, AND J. CHRISTENSEN. Differences in cytochrome-c oxidase capacity in smooth muscle of opossum esophagus and lower esophageal sphincter. *Gastroenterology* 87: 1009–1013, 1984.
412. ROBOTHAM, H., J. JURY, AND E. E. DANIEL. Capsaicin effects on muscularis mucosa of opossum esophagus: substance P release from afferent nerves? *Am. J. Physiol.* 248 (*Gastrointest. Liver Physiol.* 11): G655–G662, 1985.
413. RODRIGO, J., C. J. HERNANDEZ, M. A. VIDAL, AND J. A. PEDROSE. Vegetative innervation of the esophagus. III. Intraepithelial endings. *Acta Anat.* 92: 242–258, 1975.
414. RODRIGO, J., C. J. HERNANDEZ, M. A. VIDAL, AND J. A. PEDROSE. Vegetative innervation of the esophagus. II. Intraganglionic laminar endings. *Acta Anat.* 92: 79–100, 1975.
415. RODRIGO, J., E. M. ROBLES-CHILLIDA, J. DE FELIPE, J. A. PÉREZ ANTON, J. A. PEDROSA, AND A. ARNEDO. Sensorivagal nature of oesophageal submucous layer nerve endings: determination by surgical degeneration methods. *Acta Anat. Basel* 108: 540–550, 1980.
416. RODRIGO, J., J. DE FELIPE, E. M. ROBLES-CHILLIDA, J. A. PÉREZ ANTON, I. MAYO, AND A. GOMEZ. Sensory vagal nature and anatomical access paths to esophagus laminar nerve endings in myenteric ganglia: Determination by surgical degeneration methods. *Acta Anat.* 112: 47–57, 1982.
417. RODRIGO, J., J. M. POLAK, L. FERNANDEZ, M. A. GHATEI, P. MULDERRY, AND S. R. BLOOM. Calcitonin gene-related peptide immunoreactive sensory and motor nerves of the rat, cat and monkey esophagus. *Gastroenterology* 88: 444–451, 1985.
418. ROED-PETERSEN, K. Manometric investigations of the pharyngooesophageal sphincter. *Dan. Med. Bull.* 26: 282–287, 1979.
419. ROED-PETERSEN, K. The pharyngooesophageal sphincter. *Dan. Med. Bull.* 26: 275–281, 1979.
420. ROLING, G. T., R. L. FARRELL, AND D. O. CASTELL. Cholinergic response of the lower esophageal sphincter. *Am. J. Physiol.* 222: 967–972, 1972.
421. ROMAN, C. Nervous control of peristalsis in the esophagus. *J. Physiol. Paris* 58: 79–108, 1966.
422. ROMAN, C., AND A. CAR. Esophageal contractions produced by stimulation of the vagus or medulla oblongata. *J. Physiol. Paris* 59: 377–397, 1967.
423. ROMAN, C., AND J. GONELLA. Extrinsic control of digestive tract motility. In: *Physiology of the Gastrointestinal Tract* (2nd ed.), edited by L. R. Johnson. New York: Raven, 1987, p. 289–333.
424. ROMAN, C., AND L. TIEFFENBACH. Motricité de l'oesophage musculeuse lissé après bivagotomie: étude electromyographique. *J. Physiol. Paris* 63: 733–762, 1971.
425. ROMAN, C., AND L. TIEFFENBACH. Enregistrement de l'activité unitaire des fibres motrices vagales destiné à l'oesophagus du babouin. *J. Physiol. Paris* 64: 479–506, 1972.
426. ROMANES, G. J. *Cunningham's Textbook of Anatomy*. London: Oxford Univ. Press, 1972.
427. ROSELL, S., K. THOR, A. ROKAEUS, O. NYQUIST, A. LEWENHAUPT, L. KAGER, AND K. FOLKERS. Plasma concentration on neurotensin-like immunoreactivity (NTLI) and lower esophageal sphincter (LES) pressure in man following infusion of (Gln$^4$)-neurotensin. *Acta Physiol. Scand.* 109: 369–375, 1980.
428. RUEGG, J. C. Smooth muscle tone. *Physiol. Rev.* 51: 201–248, 1971.
429. RUSHNER, R. F., AND J. A. HENDRON. The act of deglutition: a cinefluorographic study. *J. Appl. Physiol.* 3: 622–630, 1951.
430. RUSSELL, C. O. H., L. D. HILL, E. R. HOLMES, D. A. HULL, R. GANNON, AND C. E. POPE II. Radionuclide transit: a sensitive screening test for esophageal dysfunction. *Gastroenterology* 80: 887–892, 1981.
431. RYAN, J. P., AND K. R. DUFFY. LES pressure response to pentagastrin: effect of cholinergic augmentation and inhibition. *Am. J. Physiol.* 234 (*Endocrinol. Metab. Gastrointest. Physiol.* 3): E301–E305, 1978.
432. RYAN, J. P., W. J. SNAPE, JR., AND S. COHEN. Influence of vagal cooling on esophageal function. *Am. J. Physiol.* 232 (*Endocrinol. Metab. Gastrointest. Physiol.* 1): E159–E164, 1977.
433. SANCHEZ, G. C., P. KRAMER, AND F. J. INGELFINGER. Motor mechanisms of the esophagus, particularly of its distal portion. *Gastroenterology* 25: 321–332, 1953.
434. SANDBERG, N., AND I. MANSSON. Oral-pharyngeal disturbances in deglutition. *Scand. J. Gastroenterol.* 19 Suppl. 106: 112–114, 1984.
435. SARNA, S. K., E. E. DANIEL, AND W. E. WATERFALL. Myogenic and neural control systems for esophageal motility. *Gastroenterology* 73: 1345–1352, 1977.
436. SATCHELL, P. M. Canine oesophageal mechanoreceptors. *J. Physiol. Lond.* 346: 287–300, 1984.
437. SATPATHY, N. K., AND N. A. AL-SATTAR. The effects of acute oesophageal distention on arterial blood pressure, E.C.G. and respiration in dog. *Indian J. Physiol. Pharmacol.* 28: 105–114, 1984.
438. SAWCHENKO, P. E. Central connections of the sensory and motor nuclei of the vagus nerve. *J. Auton. Nerv. Syst.* 9: 13–26, 1983.
439. SCHAROUN, S. L., F. C. BARONE, M. J. WAYNER, AND S. M. JONES. Vagal and gastric connections to the central nervous system determined by the transport of horseradish peroxidase. *Brain Res. Bull.* 13: 573–584, 1984.
440. SCHENK, E. A., AND E. L. FREDERICKSON. Pharmacologic evidence for a cardiac sphincter mechanism in the cat. *Gastroenterology* 40: 75–80, 1961.
441. SCHOEN, H. J., D. W. MORRIS, AND S. COHEN. Esophageal peristaltic force in man: response to mechanical and pharmacological alterations. *Am. J. Dig. Dis.* 22: 589–597, 1977.
442. SCHOFIELD, G. C. Anatomy of muscular and neural tissues in the alimentary canal. In: *Handbook of Physiology. Alimentary Canal. Motility*, edited by C. F. Code. Washington, DC: Am. Physiol. Soc., 1968, sect. 6, vol. IV, p. 1579–1627.
443. SCHULZE, K., AND J. CHRISTENSEN. Lower sphincter of the opossum esophagus in pseudopregnancy. *Gastroenterology* 73: 1082–1085, 1977.
444. SCHULZE, K., J. L. CONKLIN, AND J. CHRISTENSEN. A potassium gradient in smooth muscle segment of the opossum esophagus. *Am. J. Physiol.* 232 (*Endocrinol. Metab. Gastrointest. Physiol.* 1): E270–E273, 1977.
445. SCHULZE-DELRIEU, K., AND S. A. CRANE. Oxygen uptake and mechanical tension in esophageal smooth muscle from opossums and cats. *Am. J. Physiol.* 242 (*Gastrointest. Liver Physiol.* 5): G258–G262, 1982.
446. SEAMAN, W. B. Cineroentogenographic observations of the cricopharyngeus. *Am. J. Roentgenol. Radium Ther. Nucl. Med.* 96: 922–931, 1966.
447. SEELIG, L. L., JR., P. DOODY, L. BRAINARD, J. S. GIDDA, AND R. K. GOYAL. Acetylcholinesterase and choline acetyltransferase staining of neurons in the opossum esophagus. *Anat. Rec.* 209: 125–130, 1984.
448. SEELIG, L. L., JR., AND R. K. GOYAL. Morphological evaluation of opossum lower esophageal sphincter. *Gastroenterology* 75: 51–58, 1978.
449. SENGUPTA, A., AND R. K. GOYAL. Localization of galanin immunoreactivity in the opossum esophagus. *J. Auton. Nerv.*

*Syst.* 22: 49–56, 1988.
450. SENGUPTA, A., W. G. PATERSON, AND R. K. GOYAL. Atypical localization of myenteric neurons in the opossum lower esophageal sphincter. *Am. J. Anat.* 180: 342–348, 1987.
451. SHAPIRO, J., AND R. K. GOYAL. Disorders of the upper esophageal sphincter. In: *The Larynx*, edited by M. Fried. Boston, MA: Little, Brown, in press.
452. SHINGAI, T., AND K. SHIMADA. Reflex swallowing elicited by water and chemical substances applied in the oral cavity, pharynx, and larynx of the rabbit. *Jpn. J. Physiol.* 26: 445–469, 1976.
453. SHIPP, T., W. W. DEATSCH, AND K. ROBERSTON. Pharyngoesophageal muscle activity during swallowing in man. *Laryngoscope* 80: 1–16, 1970.
454. SIEBERT, T. L., J. STEIN, AND M. H. POPPEL. Variations in the roentgen appearance of the "esophageal lip." *Am. J. Roentgenol. Radium Ther. Nucl. Med.* 81: 570–575, 1959.
455. SIEGEL, C. I., AND T. R. HENDRIX. Evidence for the central mediation of secondary peristalsis in the esophagus. *Bull. Johns Hopkins Hosp.* 108: 297–307, 1961.
456. SIEGEL, S. R., F. C. BROWN, D. O. CASTELL, L. R. JOHNSON, AND S. I. SAID. Effects of vasoactive intestinal polypeptide (VIP) on lower esophageal sphincter in awake baboons: comparison with glucagon and secretin. *Dig. Dis. Sci.* 24: 345–349, 1979.
457. SINAR, D. R., C. M. CORDOVA, J. R. FLETCHER, AND D. O. CASTELL. Decreased esophageal peristaltic amplitude in response to prostaglandin $E_1$ and prostacyclin in the baboon. *Dig. Dis. Sci.* 27: 1067–1072, 1983.
458. SINAR, D. R., J. R. FLETCHER, AND D. O. CASTELL. Prostaglandin $E_1$ effects on resting and cholinergically stimulated lower esophageal sphincter pressure in cats. *Prostaglandins* 21: 581–590, 1981.
459. SINAR, D. R., T. M. O'DORISIO, E. L. MAZZAFERRI, H. MEKHJIAN, H. S. J. H. CALDWELL, AND F. B. THOMAS. Effect of gastric inhibitory polypeptide on lower esophageal sphincter pressure in cats. *Gastroenterology* 75: 263–267, 1978.
460. SMITH, B. The autonomic innervation of the oesophagus. *Clin. Gastroenterol.* 5: 1–13, 1976.
461. SMITH, C. C., AND K. R. BRIZZEE. Cineradiographic analysis of vomiting in the cat. *Gastroenterology* 40: 654–664, 1960.
462. SMOUT, A. J. P. M., J. W. BOGAARD, J. VAN HATTUM, AND L. M. A. AKKERMANS. Effects of cimetidine and ranitidine on interdigestive and postprandial lower esophageal sphincter pressures and plasma gastrin levels in normal subjects. *Gastroenterology* 88: 557–563, 1985.
463. SOKOL, E. M., P. HEITMANN, B. S. WOLF, AND B. R. COHEN. Simultaneous cineradiographics and manometric study of the pharynx, hypopharynx, and cervical esophagus. *Gastroenterology* 51: 960–974, 1966.
464. SONDHEIMER, J. M. Upper esophageal sphincter and pharyngoesophageal motor function in infants with and without gastroesophageal reflux. *Gastroenterology* 85: 301–305, 1983.
465. STACHER, G., P. BAUER, H. STEINRINGER, G. SCHMIERER, B. LANGER, AND S. WINKLEHNER. Dose-related effects of the synthetic Met-enkephalin analogue FK 33-824 on esophageal motor activity in healthy humans. *Gastroenterology* 83: 1057–1061, 1982.
466. STACHER, G., P. BAUER, G. SCHMIERER, AND H. STEINRINGER. The effect of intramuscular pirenzepine on esophageal contractile activity and lower esophageal sphincter pressure under fasting conditions and after a standard meal. A double blind study. *Int. J. Clin. Pharmacol. Biopharm.* 17: 442–448, 1979.
467. STANCIU, C., AND J. R. BENNETT. Smoking and gastro-oesophageal reflux. *Br. Med. J.* 3: 793–795, 1972.
468. STANCIU, C., AND J. R. BENNETT. Upper esophageal sphincter yield pressure in normal subjects and in patients with esophageal reflux. *Thorax* 29: 459–462, 1974.
469. STEVENS, C. E., AND A. F. SELLERS. Pressure events in bovine esophagus and reticulorumen associated with eructation, deglutition and regurgitation. *Am. J. Physiol.* 199: 598–602, 1960.
470. STEVENS, C. E., AND A. F. SELLERS. Rumination. In: *Handbook of Physiology. Alimentary Canal. Bile; Digestion; Ruminal Physiology*, edited by C. F. Code. Washington, DC: American Physiological Society, 1968, sect. 6, vol. V, p. 2699–2704.
471. STURDEVANT, R. A. L. Is gastrin the major regulator of lower esophageal sphincter pressure? *Gastroenterology* 67: 551–553, 1974.
472. STURDEVANT, R. A. L., AND T. KUN. Interaction of pentagastrin and the octapeptide of cholecystokinin on the human lower esophageal sphincter. *Gut* 15: 700–702, 1974.
473. SUGARBAKER, D. J., S. RATTAN, AND R. K. GOYAL. Mechanical and electrical activity of esophageal smooth muscle during peristalsis. *Am. J. Physiol.* 246 (*Gastrointest. Liver Physiol.* 9): G145–G150, 1984.
474. SUGARBAKER, D. J., S. RATTAN, AND R. K. GOYAL. Swallowing induces sequential activation of esophageal longitudinal smooth muscle. *Am. J. Physiol.* 247 (*Gastrointest. Liver Physiol.* 10): G515–G519, 1984.
475. SUMI, T. The activity of brain stem respiratory neurons and spinal respiratory motoneuron during swallowing. *J. Neurophysiol.* 26: 466–477, 1963.
476. SUMI, T. Some properties of cortically evoked swallowing and chewing in rabbits. *Brain Res.* 15: 107–120, 1969.
477. TAILAI, Z., T. JUNSHENG, Z. ZUXUN, Z. BAOKANG, AND M. YUNPING. Vagus nerve anatomy at the lower esophagus and stomach: a study of 100 cadavers. *Chin. Med. J. Engl. Ed.* 93: 629–636, 1980.
478. TEMPLE, J. G., R. J. R. GOODALL, D. J. HAY, AND D. MILLER. Effect of highly selective vagotomy upon the lower oesophageal sphincter. *Gut* 22: 368–370, 1981.
479. TEMPLETON, F. E., AND R. H. KREDEL. The cricopharyngeal sphincter: a roentgenologic study. *Laryngoscope* 53: 1–12, 1943.
480. THOR, K., AND A. ROKAEUS. Studies on the mechanisms by which ($Gln^4$)-neurotensin reduces lower esophageal sphincter (LES) pressure in man. *Acta Physiol. Scand.* 118: 373–377, 1983.
481. THORPE, J. A. C. Effect of propranolol on the lower oesophageal sphincter in man. *Curr. Med. Res. Opin.* 7: 91–95, 1980.
482. TIEFFENBACH, L., AND C. ROMAN. The role of extrinsic vagal innervation in the motility of the smooth muscled portion of the esophagus: electromyographic study in the cat and baboon. *J. Physiol. Paris* 64: 193–226, 1972.
483. TITCHEN, D. A. Diaphragmatic and oesophageal activity in regurgitation in sheep: an electromyographic study. *J. Physiol. Lond.* 292: 381–390, 1979.
484. TOLIN, R. D., L. S. MALMUD, J. REILLEY, AND R. S. FISHER. Esophageal scintigraphy to quantitate esophageal transit. *Gastroenterology* 76: 1402–1408, 1979.
484a. TORPHY, T. J., C. F. FINE, M. BURMAN, M. S. BARNETTE, AND H. S. ORMSBEE. Lower esophageal sphincter relaxation is associated with increased cyclic nucleotide content. *Am. J. Physiol.* 251 (*Gastrointest. Liver Physiol.* 13): G786–G793, 1986.
485. TORVIK, A. Afferent connections to the sensory trigeminal nuclei, the nucleus of the solitary tract and adjacent structures—an experimental study in the rat. *J. Comp. Neurol.* 106: 51–141, 1956.
486. TOYAMA, T., I. YOKOYAMA, AND K. NISHI. Effect of hexamethonium and other ganglionic blocking agents on electrical activity of the esophagus induced by vagal stimulation in the dog. *Eur. J. Pharmacol.* 31: 63–71, 1975.
487. TRAUBE, M., AND R. W. MCCALLUM. Calcium-channel blockers and the gastrointestinal tract. *Am. J. Gastroenterol.* 79: 892–896, 1984.
488. TREACY, W. L., H. H. BAGGENSTOSS, C. H. SLOCUMB, AND C. F. CODE. Scleroderma of the esophagus. A correlation of histologic and physiologic findings. *Ann. Intern. Med.* 59: 351–356, 1963.
489. TROP, D., R. PEETERS, AND K. P. VAN DE WOESTIJNE. Localization of recording site in the esophagus by means of

cardiac artifacts. *J. Appl. Physiol.* 29: 283–287, 1970.
490. TUCH, A., AND S. COHEN. Neurogenic basis of lower esophageal sphincter relaxation. *J. Clin. Invest.* 52: 14–20, 1973.
491. TUMA, S. N., AND A. MUKHOPADHYAY. The effect of parathyroid hormone on the esophageal smooth muscle of the opossum. *Am. J. Gastroenterol.* 74: 415–418, 1980.
492. UDDMAN, R., J. ALUMETS, L. EDVINSSON, R. HAKANSON, AND F. SUNDLER. Peptidergic (VIP) innervation of the esophagus. *Gastroenterology* 75: 5–8, 1978.
493. UDDMAN, R., J. ALUMETS, R. HAKANSON, F. SUNDLER, AND B. WALLES. Peptidergic (enkephalin) innervation of the mammalian esophagus. *Gastroenterology* 78: 732–737, 1980.
494. UEDA, M., J. F. SCHLEGEL, AND C. F. CODE. Electric and motor activity of innervated and vagally denervated feline esophagus. *Am. J. Dig. Dis.* 17: 1075–1088, 1972.
495. VANEK, A. W., AND N. E. DIAMANT. Responses of human esophagus to paired swallows. *Gastroenterology* 92: 643–650, 1987.
496. VAN OVERBEEK, J. J. M., H. P. WIT, R. H. L. PAPING, AND H. M. SEGENHOUT. Simultaneous manometry and electromyography in the pharyngoesophageal segment. *Laryngoscope* 95: 582–584, 1985.
497. VAN THIEL, D. H., J. S. GAVALER, S. N. JOSHI, R. K. SARA, AND J. STREMPLE. Heartburn of pregnancy. *Gastroenterology* 72: 666–669, 1977.
498. VAN THIEL, D. H., J. S. GAVALER, AND J. STREMPLE. Lower sphincter pressure in women using sequential oral contraceptives. *Gastroenterology* 71: 232–235, 1976.
499. VAN THIEL, D. H., J. S. GALVALER, AND J. F. STREMPLE. Lower esophageal sphincter pressure during the normal menstrual cycle. *Am. J. Obstet. Gynecol.* 134: 64–67, 1979.
500. VANTRAPPEN, G., AND E. C. TEXTER, JR. Response of the physiologic gastroesophageal sphincter to increased intra-abdominal pressure. *J. Clin. Invest.* 43: 1856–1868, 1964.
501. VANTRAPPEN, G., AND J. HELLEMANS. Studies on the normal deglutition complex. *Am. J. Dig. Dis.* 12: 255–266, 1967.
502. VANTRAPPEN, G., AND J. HELLEMANS. *Diseases of the Esophagus.* New York: Springer-Verlag, 1974.
503. WALDECK, F. A new procedure for functional analysis of the lower esophageal sphincter (LES). *Pfluegers Arch.* 335: 74–84, 1972.
504. WALKER, C. O., S. A. FRANK, J. MANTON, AND J. S. FORDTRAN. Effect of continuous infusion of pentagastrin on lower esophageal sphincter pressure and gastric acid secretion in normal subjects. *J. Clin. Invest.* 56: 218–225, 1975.
505. WALLIN, L., S. BOESBY, AND T. MADSEN. The effect of HCl infusion in the lower part of the esophagus on the pharyngoesophageal sphincter pressure in normal subjects. *Scand. J. Gastroenterol.* 13: 821–826, 1978.
506. WARWICK, R., AND P. L. WILLIAMS. *Gray's Anatomy* (35th ed.). Philadelphia, PA: Saunders, 1973.
507. WATANABE, M., C. SUGAWA, T. HATAFUKU, AND S. MORI. The effect of increased gastrin release on lower esophageal sphincter pressure. *Tohoku J. Exp. Med.* 144: 377–384, 1984.
508. WATSON, W. C., AND S. N. SULLIVAN. Hypertonicity of cricopharyngeal sphincter: cause of globus sensation. *Lancet* 2: 1417–1418, 1974.
509. WEIHRAUCH, T. R., A. BRUMMER, H. BIEWENER, AND K. EWE. Assessment of various factors influencing esophageal pressure measurement. I. Significance of methodical factors in intraluminal manometry. *Klin. Wochenschr.* 58: 279–285, 1980.
510. WEIHRAUCH, T. R., P. VALLERIUS, H. ALPERS, AND K. EWE. Assessment of various factors influencing esophageal pressure measurement. II. Significance of physiological factors in intraluminal manometry. *Klin. Wochenschr.* 58: 287–292, 1980.
511. WEINSTEIN, W. M., E. R. BOGOCH, AND K. L. BOWES. The normal human esophageal mucosa: a histologic reappraisal. *Gastroenterology* 68: 40–44, 1975.
512. WEISBRODT, N. W. Neuromuscular organization of esophageal and pharyngeal motility. *Arch. Intern. Med.* 136: 524–531, 1976.
513. WEISBRODT, N. W., AND J. CHRISTENSEN. Gradient of contractions in the opossum esophagus. *Gastroenterology* 62: 1159–1166, 1972.
514. WEISBRODT, N. W., AND R. A. MURPHY. Myosin phosphorylation and contraction of feline esophageal smooth muscle. *Am. J. Physiol.* 249: (*Cell Physiol.* 18): C9–C14, 1985.
515. WELCH, R. W., AND S. T. DRAKE. Normal lower esophageal sphincter pressure: a comparison of rapid vs. slow pull through techniques. *Gastroenterology* 78: 1446–1451, 1980.
516. WELCH, R. W., AND J. E. GRAY. Influence of respiration on recordings of lower esophageal sphincter pressure in humans. *Gastroenterology* 83: 590–594, 1982.
517. WELCH, R. W., K. LUCKMANN, P. M. RICKS, S. T. DRAKE, AND G. A. GATES. Manometry of the normal upper esophageal sphincter and its alteration in laryngectomy. *J. Clin. Invest.* 63: 1036–1041, 1979.
518. WINANS, C. S. The pharyngoesophageal closure mechanism: a manometric study. *Gastroenterology* 63: 768–777, 1972.
519. WINANS, C. S., AND L. D. HARRIS. Quantitation of lower esophageal sphincter competence. *Gastroenterology* 52: 773–778, 1967.
520. WINSHIP, D. H., S. R. DEANDRADE, AND F. F. ZBORALSKE. Influence of bolus temperature on human esophageal motor function. *J. Clin. Invest.* 49: 243–250, 1970.
521. WINSHIP, D. H., AND F. F. ZBORALSKE. The esophageal propulsive force: esophageal response to acute obstruction. *J. Clin. Invest.* 46: 1391–1401, 1967.
522. WOLF, B. S. The inferior esophageal sphincter. Anatomic, roentgenologic and manometric correlation, contraction and terminology. *Am. J. Roentgenol. Radium Ther. Nucl. Med.* 110: 260–277, 1970.
523. WRIGHT, L. E., AND D. O. CASTELL. The adverse effect of chocolate on lower esophageal sphincter pressure. *Am. J. Dig. Dis.* 20: 703–707, 1975.
524. WRIGHT, L. E., R. L. SLAUGHTER, R. G. GIBSON, AND B. I. HIRSCHOWITZ. Correlation of lower sphincter pressure and serum gastrin level in man. *Am. J. Dig. Dis.* 20: 603–606, 1975.
525. YOSHIDA, Y., T. MIYAZAKI, M. HIRANO, T. SHIN, T. TOTOKI, AND T. KANASEKI. Localization of efferent neurons innervating the pharyngeal constrictor muscles and the cervical esophagus muscle in the cat by means of the horseradish peroxidase method. *Neurosci. Lett.* 22: 91–95, 1981.
526. YOUMANS, W. B. Innervation of the gastrointestinal tract. In: *Handbook of Physiology. Alimentary Canal. Motility*, edited by C. F. Code. Washington, DC: Am. Physiol. Soc., 1968, sect. 6, vol. IV, p. 1655–1663.
527. ZAINO, C., H. G. JACOBSON, H. LEPOW, AND C. H. OZTURK. *The Pharyngeal Sphincter.* Springfield, IL: Thomas, 1970.
528. ZAINO, C., M. H. POPPEL, H. G. JACOBSON, AND H. LEPOW. *Lower Esophageal Vestibular Complex.* Springfield, IL: Thomas, 1963.
529. ZELCER, E., AND N. W. WEISBRODT. Electrical and mechanical activity in the lower esophageal sphincter of the cat. *Am. J. Physiol.* 246 (*Gastrointest. Liver Physiol.* 9): G243–G247, 1984.
530. ZWICK, R., K. L. BOWES, E. E. DANIEL, AND S. K. SARNA. Mechanism of action of pentagastrin on the lower esophageal sphincter. *J. Clin. Invest.* 57: 1644–1651, 1976.

# CHAPTER 23

# Determinants of gastric emptying and transit in the small intestine

JUAN-R. MALAGELADA

FERNANDO AZPIROZ

*Division of Gastroenterology, Mayo Clinic and Mayo Foundation, Rochester, Minnesota*

## CHAPTER CONTENTS

Functional Division of Stomach
  Methodological aspects: interrelationships among parietal force and manometric and electrical measurements of gastric motility
  Motor activity of proximal stomach
  Motor activity of distal stomach
Gastrointestinal Motility During Interdigestive Period
  Interdigestive motor pattern of stomach
  Interrelationships between gastric motility, secretion, and clearance of duodenogastric reflux during interdigestive period
Gastrointestinal Response to a Meal
  Swallowing
  Early postcibal period
  Plateau phase
  Declining phase and transition to interdigestive activity
Gastric Emptying Profile
Relationships Among Gastric Emptying, Motility, and Structure: Mechanics of Gastric Emptying
  Preliminary processing: antropyloric grinder
  Emptying function
    Tonic contraction of proximal stomach
    Antropyloroduodenal resistance to flow
    Antral transport function
    Intestinal transport function
Effects of Gravity and Body Position on Gastric Emptying
Regulation of Gastric Emptying
  Physical and chemical characteristics of meals that influence their emptying from stomach
    Energy density of the meal
    Products of digestion of nutrients
    Osmolality
    Acid
    Volume of the meal
    Size and density of solid particles and viscosity
  Interactions between gastric emptying and gastric secretion
Intestinal Motility and Its Relationship to Luminal Flow and Absorption
Physiological Measurement of Transit in Small Bowel
Effects of Opiates and Sex Hormones on Intestinal Motility and Transit
Control of Gastrointestinal Motility: Physiological and Pathophysiological Implications for Gastric Motility and Intestinal Transit
  Control at level of gut smooth muscle
  Control at level of gut intrinsic and extrinsic nervous systems
  Hormonal control
  Control at cerebral level

THE MOTOR FUNCTION of the digestive system helps to achieve three main objectives: *1*) mechanical trituation and digestion of the dietary nutrients (in conjunction with the secretory function); *2*) maximal exposure of the products of digestion to the absorptive surface of the small bowel; and *3*) clearance of residue and bacteria from the gut. Thus the stomach largely liquifies the meal (digestive function) and delivers it into the intestine at a rate that matches the processing capability of the intestine (reservoir function). The motility of the small bowel spreads out chyme, rapidly expanding the absorptive area, and subjects the luminal contents to a to-and-fro movement that facilitates mixing and absorption. During the interdigestive periods, cyclic episodes of intense motor activity clear residue from the stomach and the small intestine. The physiological processes reviewed in this chapter have been largely elucidated on the basis of experimental (animal) data. Most, but not all, aspects have been confirmed in humans. Where appropriate, it is indicated whether knowledge was obtained from human studies, animal studies, or both.

## FUNCTIONAL DIVISION OF STOMACH

Although the stomach constitutes an anatomical unit in carnivores, it is functionally divided into proximal and distal parts (Fig. 1). This functional division applies similarly to the mucosal-secretory activity and the muscular-electromechanical activity. The proximal stomach is lined by an acid-peptic secretory mucosa. The mucosa of the distal stomach produces no acid but contains gastrin-releasing cells that participate in the regulation of gastric secretion. The anatomical correspondence between the secretory and motor parts is not exact. For instance, the mucosal-secretory line of division lies caudal to the electromechanical dividing line. Both areas overlap in an imprecise transitional region with intermediate prop-

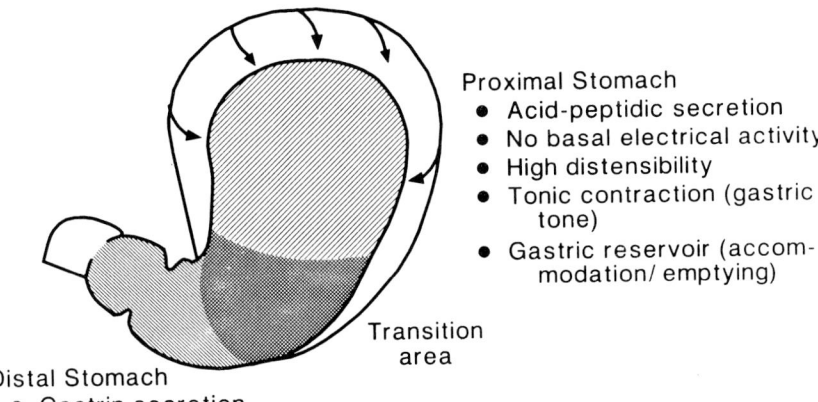

FIG. 1. Functional division of stomach as it relates to motor and secretory function.

erties, corresponding to a segment around the midstomach. Therefore the fundus and proximal gastric body form the proximal stomach, whereas the distal stomach corresponds approximately to the antrum.

On the basis of fluoroscopic studies of gastric motility, Cannon (49) was first to recognize the functional motor division between the proximal and distal stomach. The proximal stomach behaves as a reservoir and, by modulating the tonic contraction of its muscular walls, accommodates to its content. In contrast, the distal stomach (antrum) generates peristaltic phasic contractions that grind solid particles (49, 50, 91, 92). Although this concept probably represents an oversimplification of the actual physiological properties of the proximal and distal stomach (e.g., both parts may generate tonic and phasic contractions at times), it remains useful in practice.

Alvarez and Mahoney (5) and others (34, 65) demonstrated spontaneous electrical activity (slow waves or pacesetter potentials) in the canine and human stomach. Years later the absence of spontaneous electrical activity in the uppermost proximal stomach was recognized (136). Mapping the electrical activity of the canine stomach revealed an electrical dividing line between the silent proximal area and the active distal area (222). In vitro electrophysiological studies of muscle strips from different regions of the canine and human stomach subsequently established the basis for the different electrical and mechanical behavior of the two gastric parts (81, 184, 250). The membrane potential of the proximal stomach muscle is above the threshold for contraction, explaining the basal tonic contraction of muscle from this region. This tonic contraction is neurally modulated. Cholinergic stimuli induce a partial depolarization, enhancing tonic contraction, whereas nonadrenergic, noncholinergic stimuli induce repolarization and consequently decrease tonic contraction. In contrast, in the distal stomach muscle the membrane potential is far below the threshold for contraction. In response to neural cholinergic stimuli it rapidly depolarizes, causing phasic contractions. Some mechanical properties of muscle also differ between the proximal and the distal stomach. For instance, muscle strips from the proximal stomach exposed to a fixed tension undergo a larger elongation (fractional stretch) than muscle strips from the distal stomach tested under similar conditions (9). Given the greater distensibility of the proximal stomach, the gastric contents largely accommodate in this area (9, 20, 229, 234). Mechanoreceptors located in the proximal stomach signal the degree of distension, whereas antral mechanoreceptors signal information concerning the amplitude, rate, and duration of antral contractions (229). Mechanoreceptors in the transitional area exhibit properties common to both regions (229).

*Methodological Aspects: Interrelationships Among Parietal Force and Manometric and Electrical Measurements of Gastric Motility*

Physiological studies of gastric motility in humans and in experimental animals have used different measuring techniques, sometimes resulting in apparently conflicting results. Thus it seems imperative to discuss the methodologic aspects of these data and their implications vis-à-vis our understanding of gastric emptying.

MOTOR ACTIVITY OF PROXIMAL STOMACH. *Animal studies.* The study of the motor activity of the proximal stomach has been traditionally considered problematic. Although no systematic study had been performed, it was assumed, as Kelly (133) pointed out in a review in 1974, that the activity of the proximal stomach could not be recorded by conventional manometric methods. Therefore, while investigators focused on antral pressure activity, the proximal stomach was ignored for several decades. When the motor activity of the proximal stomach was eventually investigated, it was done either by isolating the proximal stomach in the form of fundic pouches (148, 198, 253) or by introducing distending bags or ballons into the cavity of the stomach (155, 158, 160). Some observations made with these methods may constitute artifacts or be of limited physiological relevance. Motor activity of the gastric body, isolated as a Heidenhain pouch, is considerably distorted compared with its motility in the original position (117). Furthermore even gastric distension of low volume (e.g., 40 ml) by an intragastric balloon substantially modified the motor activity of the proximal stomach, at least in the dog (20). Earlier studies that did not take into account such methodological pitfalls introduced a misconception still in vogue: specifically, that the proximal stomach generates slow, sustained, low-amplitude contractions (137, 180). In fact the proximal stomach generates two distinctive types of contractions: a basal tonic contraction (gastric tone) and superimposed phasic contractions. The latter can be recorded manometrically (20, 93) as strong phasic contractions that are distinct from antral contractions but that appear exclusively during fasting. Interestingly, when the motor activity of the canine gastric body was studied by implanted parietal force transducers, some of the tracings obtained corresponded to a proximal type (114, 119), whereas others corresponded to a distal type (6, 7, 212). This suggested that the transducers were implanted by different investigators on different sites of the imprecise transition zone between the proximal and distal stomach.

The study of the tonic contractile activity of the proximal stomach (gastric tone) under physiological conditions has been an elusive task. Neither intraluminal conventional manometric devices nor implanted parietal force transducers reflect tonic activity. Intraluminal pressure recordings, with or without gastric distension, do not show reproducible base-line changes, probably because variations in gastric tone produce intraluminal pressure changes too small to be discriminated from the background noise (e.g., respiratory variations and other artifacts) (20). Similarly, parietal strain gauges implanted on the proximal stomach reflect modifications of their curvature and do not differentiate between active changes (produced by muscular tonic contraction) and passive changes (produced by variations of intragastric content). We have recently taken a new approach to study the tonic activity of the proximal stomach and developed an electronic gastric barostat that maintains a low and constant gastric wall tension (by means of an air-filled intragastric bag kept at constant pressure by an electronically regulated air-injection/aspiration feedback system). With this approach, changes in intragastric volume (reduction or enlargement) quantitatively reflect motor activity (contraction or relaxation) of the proximal stomach, allowing measurement of the physiological variations in gastric tone (21).

*Human studies.* The proximal stomach of humans also exhibits distinctive tonic and phasic contractile activity, as we found by using the gastric barostat (24). However, phasic motor activity is markedly weaker than in dogs. Phasic contractions that are registered by the barostat as nearly collapsing waves are largely undetected by manometry. Therefore in humans the proximal stomach is manometrically a silent area. Phasic contractions of the canine proximal stomach are extremely propulsive and force gastric content, solid particles or injected air, into the intestine (20). It is conceivable that the weaker phasic activity of the human stomach is responsible for the gastric air bubble that is a constant feature in humans but is absent in the dog.

MOTOR ACTIVITY OF DISTAL STOMACH. During fasting the distal stomach (antrum) in the dog undergoes periods of activity characterized by forceful peristaltic contractions. These antral contractions can be visualized fluoroscopically as displacements of radiopaque markers implanted on the gastric wall, delineating both curvatures (20, 91, 92). Each contraction originates as a shallow indentation in the midstomach and propagates caudally, with progressive increase in depth, reaching the pylorus in ~20 s. These contractions can be recorded by strain-gauge force transducers implanted on the antrum (29, 78, 116, 121). In the dog, antral contractions generate a focal intraluminal pressure increase that is recorded by manometric devices [perfused catheters (16) or microtransducers (176)] in the terminal antrum. This is an intense pressure wave of ~100 mmHg or more and of ~3 s (20). In humans, optimal antral manometric recordings may be obtained in the terminal antrum, but they fade proximally. Therefore reliable recordings require the use of multiple and closely spaced manometric sites positioned across the antroduodenal area to continuously identify the antroduodenal junction and consequently the terminal antrum. Otherwise oral displacements of the manometric assembly provide a false silent (or reduced) response. Not all human manometric studies have fulfilled this technical prerequisite, and consequently the validity of some published observations is questionable.

After ingestion of solid or mixed (solid and liquid) meals, the peristaltic contractions of the distal stomach can be registered manometrically in either the dog or human (20, 208). However, after liquid meals, phasic pressure activity in the human antrum is minimal or absent (208), whereas in the dog it continues to be recorded, albeit at lower amplitude. These differences could reflect species variations in either the occlusiveness or the strength of antral peristalsis after liquid meals. Additional studies are needed to clarify this point.

## GASTROINTESTINAL MOTILITY DURING INTERDIGESTIVE PERIOD

The cyclic interdigestive activity of the gut is reviewed in the chapter by Sarna in this *Handbook*. Here the functional implications of this activity, as required for a review of the emptying process of the stomach and transit in the small bowel, is emphasized.

During fasting the gut exhibits a pattern of cyclic variations, alternating periods of quiescence with periods of activity (56, 113, 248, 278). The periods of activity appear proximally as orad as the lower esophageal sphincter (70, 97, 104, 115) and migrate caudally as far as the ileocecal junction (141, 204, 205). This interdigestive activity, or so-called fasting pattern, is constantly present during normal fasting conditions and is interrupted by ingestion of a meal and replaced by a continuous type of activity (fed pattern) (56, 99). However, factors other than a meal may interrupt the interdigestive activity during fasting, for instance, experimental manipulations (e.g., gastric distension, anesthesia, operations) (20, 73, 238). Therefore the interdigestive activity corresponds to normal basal conditions, and its absence does not necessarily imply transition to a fed pattern.

Because the interdigestive motor cycle (IMC) was first described in the small intestine, the nomenclature of its different phases still applies primarily to the small bowel. The IMC consists of a period of quiescence (phase I), followed by a period with irregularly occurring contractions (phase II), and finally a short period (5–10 min) of intense activity (phase III) with regular and forceful contractions occurring at a frequency of 10–20 contractions per minute, depending on the species and the region of intestine considered. Code and Marlett (56) consider the brief decrescendo activity with transition from phase III to phase I that may last a few minutes as phase IV. Each activity front (phase III preceded by phase II) migrates from the duodenum to the terminal ileum in about 100 min in the dog (56, 113, 233, 248), pushing forward intestinal residue (58). When the activity front reaches the terminal ileum, a new front begins in the upper gut. The duration of the motor cycle (the period between two consecutive phase IIIs) and the migration velocity of the activity front is fairly constant in the dog, whereas a high degree of variability exists in the human (210, 259, 266). The apparent origin of the activity front is also somewhat variable. In the human, the distal duodenum and proximal jejunum are the areas where activity fronts are more regularly observed (132).

### Interdigestive Motor Pattern of Stomach

The stomach exhibits alternating periods of quiescence and activity that appear to be part of the IMC. In humans the gastric activity precedes that in the midduodenum (24), whereas in dogs the period of gastric activity overlaps with the latter half of phase II and phase III in the duodenum (20, 114).

The distinction of different phases during the gastric interdigestive cycle relies on arbitrary criteria. Code and Marlett (56) initially described three phases during the canine gastric cycle (phases I, II, and III), analogous to those of the intestine. We (20, 21) and others (114, 119) observed a period of quiescence (corresponding to phase I) and a homogeneous gastric period of activity (corresponding to phases II and III) in the dog. In the human stomach, two periods—quiescence and regular intense activity—are usually recognizable in the proximal stomach, separated by a transition or intermediate period (24). In the human, distal stomach phases, I, II, and III, equivalent to those observed in the intestine, are recognizable in ~50%–80% of all duodenojejunal IMCs (210, 213).

The period of quiescence in humans and dogs is characterized by the absence of phasic contractions in the lower esophageal sphincter (70, 115), proximal stomach, antrum (20, 21), and pylorus (79) while the proximal stomach is in a state of tonic contraction (relatively high and stable level of gastric tone) (21, 23, 24).

During the period of activity, the lower esophageal sphincter exhibits phasic contractions (70, 115). The proximal stomach further increases its muscular tone (over the previous high level) and generates superimposed phasic contractions that produce high-amplitude (>50 mmHg; mean duration ~18 s in the dog) phasic pressure waves (21, 24, 93). The antrum exhibits very high amplitude (>100 mmHg) phasic peristaltic contractions that increase in frequency to a maximal rate of 5/min in dogs and 3/min in humans [Fig. 2; (113, 278)].

We studied the coordination of these different motor events in detail during the gastric period of activity by combined manometry and fluoroscopy in the dog [(Fig. 3; (18, 20)]. In the dog, phasic contractions of the lower esophageal sphincter and proximal stomach are virtually simultaneous and appear at regular intervals of 60–90 s (20, 115). The electrical correlate of these high-amplitude contractions from the proximal stomach is unknown, but a negative deflection in electrical recordings from dogs has been observed (C. H. Kim, F. Azpiroz, and J.-R. Malagelada, unpub-

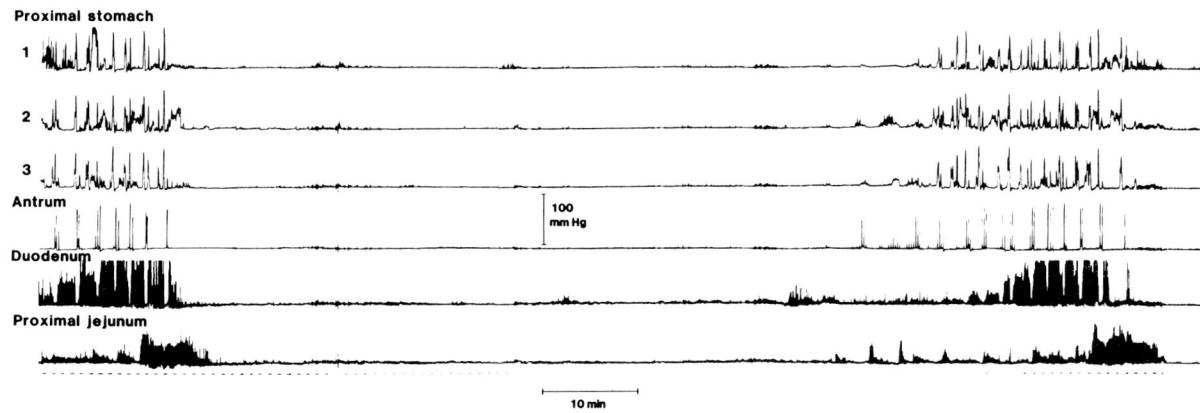

FIG. 2. Canine gastrointestinal pressure activity during fasting recorded at paper speed of 10 mm/min. Note 2 interdigestive migrating motor complexes, with participation of both proximal and distal stomach. [From Azpiroz and Malagelada (20).]

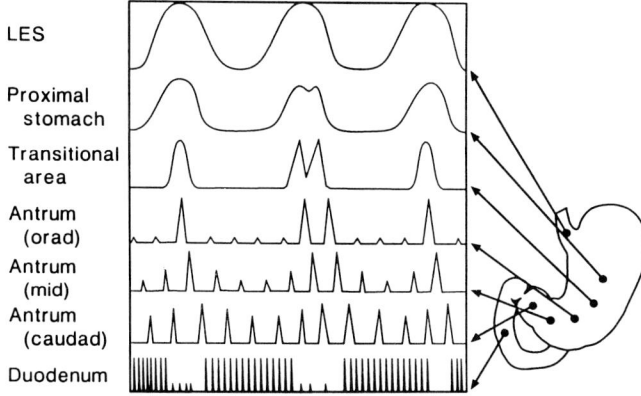

FIG. 3. Phasic pressure patterns in proximal stomach, distal stomach, and proximal duodenum during a period of motor activity. Note broad-base fundic pressure waves that propagate into distal stomach and gradually transform themselves into peaked antral waves. Antral waves that are coordinated with fundic waves are of higher amplitude than those interposed. Antral waves coordinated with fundic waves are also associated with quiescence in duodenum (noticeable during periods of duodenal regular motor activity).

lished observations). Antral contractions that coincide with such contractions of the proximal stomach have a more orad origin and are of higher amplitude than other antral waves. Therefore phasic contractile activity of the proximal and distal stomach is fused in a transitional area between both regions, where the proximal gastric phasic pressure waves appear more spike shaped and appear to propagate into the antrum (inserted in the regular antral rhythm) as high-amplitude peristaltic waves. Sometimes these high-amplitude antral waves are followed by a refractory period, with delay in the appearance of the next expected contraction. This refractory period is due to an electrical silent lapse, with delay in the appearance of the subsequent electrical slow wave (C. H. Kim, F. Azpiroz, and J.-R. Malagelada, unpublished observations). Manometric recordings in the orad antrum, where the contractions are weak and may be undetected, may only reflect the high amplitude contractions (stimulated by the proximal stomach contraction), and the antral period of activity appears then as a dozen waves or so, either single or multiple, occurring every 60–90 s. Actually this is the manometric representation of antral interdigestive activity period in humans, except for the terminal antrum, where the 3/min rhythm is often apparent during the final episode of regular intense activity (phase III).

Toward the end of the gastric period of activity, when a definite phase III develops in the duodenum, it can be observed in the dog that the regular duodenal pressure waves are interrupted by short periods of 15–20 s that coincide with the phasic gastric contractions originating in the proximal stomach [Fig. 4; (20, 28, 80)]. This phenomenon may represent an aspect of gastroduodenal motor coordination with a role in clearance of gastric residue consistent with the "housekeeper" function ascribed to the gastric component of the IMC (228).

*Interrelationships Between Gastric Motility, Secretion, and Clearance of Duodenogastric Reflux During Interdigestive Period*

Gastric, biliary, and pancreatic secretory activity increase cyclically in association with duodenal interdigestive motor activity (74, 130, 267). During duodenal phase I, secretion is low or nil, but it increases as motor activity intensifies, usually peaking during the later part of phase II or early phase III. Biliopancreatic secretion loads the duodenum and partly refluxes into the stomach. Duodenogastric reflux during fasting is probably a physiological event, at least in humans and dogs (98, 130, 168, 209). Thus, during the period of quiescence, the stomach accumulates a certain amount of swallowed saliva, gastric secretion, and refluxed biliopancreatic juice. These fasting gastric

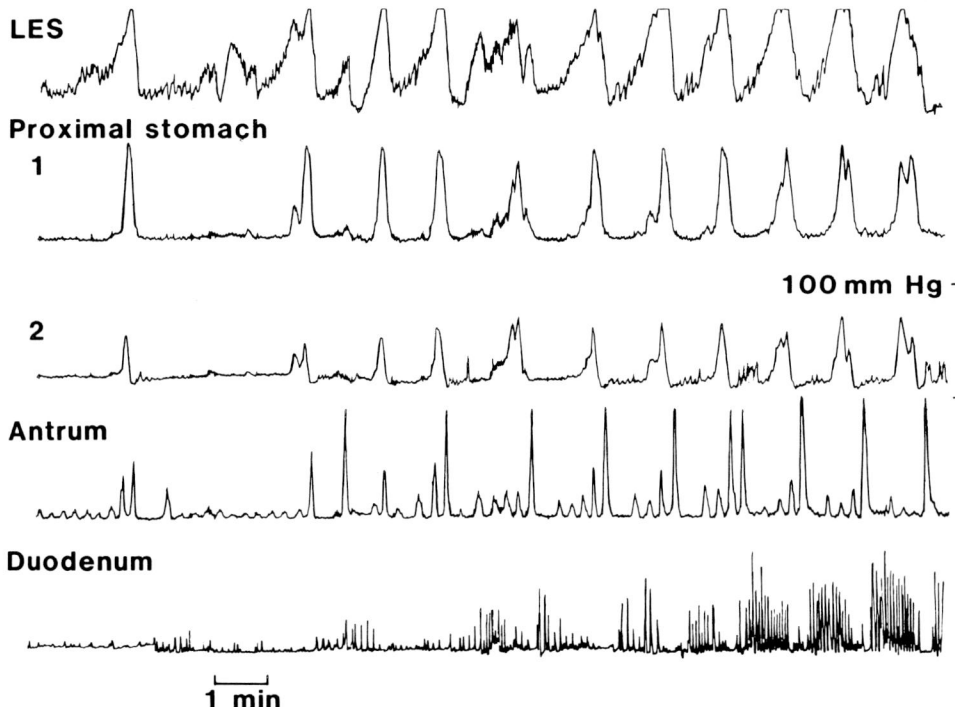

FIG. 4. Canine gastrointestinal pressure activity during fasting: lower esophageal sphincter (LES) pressure recording during period of activity in fundus at paper speed of 25 mm/min. Note relationship of fundic pressure waves with LES pressure and antral activity and with transient decrease of duodenal phase III activity. Fundic waves occur at rhythm of 25% to 20% of antral frequency. See Figure 3 for representation of this phenomenon. [From Azpiroz and Malagelada (20).]

contents are cleared during the period of activity and further swept downstream by the IMC.

GASTROINTESTINAL RESPONSE TO A MEAL

In this section the overall sequence of motor events in response to a normal meal is described. A later section describes specific responses elicited by each of the different components of a meal.

*Swallowing*

In response to deglutitions, the lower esophageal sphincter (14, 57) and the proximal stomach relax (21, 51, 148) to allow the passage and reception of the ingested material. Relaxation of the stomach during swallowing of food was first described by Cannon and Lieb (51) and termed gastric receptive relaxation. Relaxation of the fundus has also been observed in response to wet swallows (148) and esophageal distension (123).

*Early Postcibal Period*

Immediately after ingestion a profound change occurs in the whole upper digestive system. The tonic contraction of the proximal stomach is substantially reduced (decreased gastric tone) and the proximal stomach expands, with no change in gastric wall tension (intragastric pressure) (21, 122). This postcibal adaptive relaxation has been conventionally termed gastric accommodation to differentiate it from the receptive relaxation specifically elicited by swallowing (50, 133).

The lower esophageal sphincter tone tends to increase, although the net result depends on the volume and composition of gastrointestinal chyme (19). However, the phasic contractions of the lower esophageal sphincter and the proximal stomach noted during fasting disappear and do not return until interdigestive motor activity begins again at the end of the postcibal period (20, 104, 114). The distal stomach generates continuous and regular peristaltic contractions at a rate of 5/min in dogs and 3/min in humans, similar to the interdigestive activity but of lower amplitude. The small intestine develops a pattern of irregularly occurring contractions that continues throughout the postcibal period and has been termed the digestive or fed pattern (56, 114, 212). Postcibal antral and intestinal motor activity, as recorded by manometric or electromyographic techniques, resembles phase II of the interdigestive period, although its functional significance, in terms of movement of content, may be quite different (224).

Gastric, biliary, and pancreatic secretory activity begins shortly after ingestion of a normal meal (152, 153), while the liquid also begins to be rapidly emptied from the stomach. Thus during the early postcibal period the stomach is in a dynamic mode, and high rates of gastric secretion are approximately compensated by losses through the pylorus (151). As a result, intragastric volume remains relatively stable during this period, whereas nutrients remaining in the stomach are progressively diluted by an increasing proportion of secreted juice (151), providing a rich acid-peptide environment (154, 239). Thus intragastric content initially corresponds to the ingested meal, but progressively ingested liquids are replaced by secreted juice in such a way that the solid-to-liquid ratio (~1:3) stays relatively constant during the postcibal period (151).

Solids are liquified in the stomach by a grinding and mixing process that eventually delivers them as fine particles, in suspension within the liquid phase, into the intestine (101, 173, 174). However, during this early period relatively little solid material empties (solid lag phase) (48), largely because solids have not been reduced by antral phasic contractions to a particulate size small enough to allow their passage through the pylorus.

In the duodenum, chyme undergoes an elaboration process, being considerably diluted by high rates of biliopancreatic secretion. The volume of chyme entering the jejunum is thereby substantially increased and brought to neutral pH and isotonicity (~300 mosmol/kg), and the concentration of nutrients is steadied (87, 178, 179). However, these adjustments are often only partially achieved during the very early postcibal period (153).

*Plateau Phase*

Between 30 and 90 min after ingestion, some changes occur in an as yet poorly defined sequence. In dogs, gastric tone progressively increases from the previous accommodation phase and remains at a high level for most of the postcibal period [Fig. 5; (21)]. Whether similar changes in tone occur in humans is unknown. The initial peak of gastric secretion declines steadily. Although gastric outflow also decreases, the net result is a gradual decrease in intragastric volume (154). Emptying of ingested solids increases after the initial lag phase previously alluded to, and it continues thereafter at a linear rate (48). The amount of ingested solids decreases in proportion to total intragastric volume. Consequently the solid-to-liquid ratio in gas-

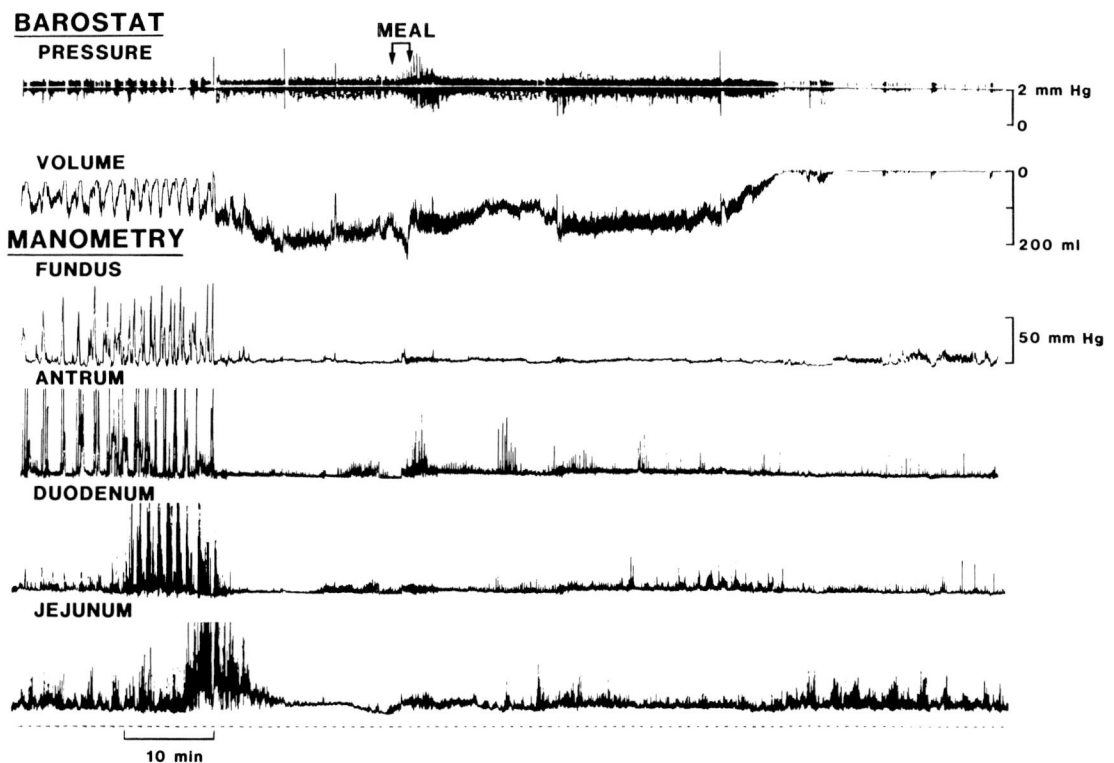

FIG. 5. Canine postcibal gastrointestinal motor activity recorded at paper speed of 10 mm/min. Barostat recorded pressure and volume of air within intragastric bag. Note postcibal volume initially remains at relatively low levels. However, later it increases gradually, reaching level higher than fasting level. [From Azpiroz and Malagelada (21).]

tric content is maintained approximately constant during the midpostcibal period (151, 152).

As the gastric outflow decreases, biliary output also decreases (as the gallbladder empties), and somewhat later pancreatic secretion also decreases (153). This results in a linear decrease of chyme flow in the duodenum (154, 178). Intestinal absorption further reduces the volume of chyme as it progresses along the small bowel. The total (cumulative) volume of gastric, biliary, and pancreatic secretion during the postcibal period is about three times the ingested volume (151, 178). About 90% of this total volume is absorbed (140, 235), and only about one-third of the original meal volume reaches the terminal ileum (87, 102). Therefore ileal flow is very much reduced compared with duodenal flow. The large volume of secreted liquids serves as a carrying medium for the suspension, digestion, and absorption of nutrients. As chyme moves toward the ileum it spreads out, increasing its exposure to the available absorptive surface. Median intestinal transit time (time for a nonabsorbable meal product to travel from the pylorus to the cecum) is ~3 h in humans (156).

*Declining Phase and Transition to Interdigestive Activity*

Toward the end of the digestive process (~3–5 h after a normal-size meal), irregular phasic contractions of the canine proximal stomach reappear, whereas antral peristalsis and intestinal motility decline (22, 114). By this time liquids ingested with the meal have been completely processed [as evidenced by the accumulation of a soluble, nonabsorbable marker ingested with dietary liquids in the distal small bowel or in the colon (156)]. Part of the ingested solids has been also processed, either absorbed in the intestine (digestible absorbable nutrients) or transported into the distal small bowel or colon (small, nonabsorbable dietary solids). After a variable period, a well-developed phase III clearly establishes the return of the interdigestive motor pattern. Nondigestible, large solid particles that have not emptied by this time are now cleared from the stomach and the small intestine by the returning IMC (188). Mojaverian et al. (182) examined in humans gastric emptying of a pH-sensitive capsule (7 by 20 mm) as a function of gastric IMC activity (not measured by itself). By inhibiting the IMC, frequent feedings (every 2–3 h) of solid meals kept the capsule in the stomach for an average of more than 14.5 h. Solid meals did so for a longer time than liquid meals.

In combined manometric and scintigraphic studies in humans, we observed that the duration of the fed motor pattern (measured from the time of ingestion of the meal to the appearance of the first well-developed phase III of the IMC) approximately correlated with gastric emptying time (meal markers remaining in the stomach). However, there was considerable intra- and interindividual variability; phase III activity reappeared sometimes even when some nutrients (usually not more than 20% of the original meal) remained in the stomach. In the context of Western dietary habits, with frequent meals distributed throughout the day, the fed pattern accounts for most of the day, and interdigestive activity develops during the night (58).

Much controversy has arisen about the nature of the stimuli, the mechanisms, and the minimal requirements of a meal to induce the gastrointestinal fed motor pattern. However, because of the imprecise and subjective definition of the fed pattern, the question remains unsolved. Stimuli such as gastric distension suppress the cyclic interdigestive pattern and elicit a fedlike activity in the gut. However, this phenomenon may well represent a distortion of the physiological activity rather than induction of a fed pattern (20). Pentagastrin (157, 254, 270, 282), cholecystokinin (CCK) (190, 282), insulin (42, 218), glucagon (280), secretin (189), neurotensin (260), or pancreatic polypeptide (96) induces a similar effect. Because blood levels of these hormones increase during the postcibal period, it has been suggested that they may constitute a mechanism inducing the fed pattern. However, it seems unlikely that the fed pattern constitutes a stereotyped response that can be elicited by a single stimulus or mechanism. Rather it is the result of multiple mechanisms triggered by ingestion of a meal.

GASTRIC EMPTYING PROFILE

Because of the highly dynamic process of gastric secretion, dilution, and emptying that occurs during digestion, a conceptual discussion of gastric emptying is warranted. Gastric emptying may indiscriminately allude to three different variables: *1*) decrease of total intragastric volume, *2*) gastric disappearance of ingested material, or *3*) gastric outflow. The total volume of ingested material in the stomach decreases during gastric emptying. However, the liquid and solid components of the meal follow a different fate. The strict physical definition of solid and liquid states does not exactly correspond with the physical phases that the stomach recognizes and discriminates as solids and liquids. Experimental observations suggest that size and consistency are the major determining factors. When a glucose solution is ingested with blenderized cooked liver, liquids and liver empty together even though the liver remains in particulate form. However, when a glucose solution is ingested with 10-mm liver cubes, liquids and liver follow a different emptying pattern (101). When water, 0.25-mm liver particles, and 10-mm liver cubes are ingested together, liver ingested as 0.25-mm particles empties twice as fast as liver ingested as 10-mm cubes but significantly slower than water (174). Therefore the gastric emptying rate of solids depends on the size of the solid particles. The critical size for solid discrimination lies between 0.03 mm and ~0.25 mm (size of particles after blenderization). The amount of liquids ingested does not appear to modify the emptying of solid particles (101, 174). Particles that are emptied into the duodenum are further digested in the intestine (277).

Gastric emptying of liquids (either dietary liquids or the mixture of meal liquids and secretions) is approximately exponential (48, 83). An exception is liquid fat, which empties more slowly than the aqueous phase and follows an approximately linear pattern resembling that for solids (63, 172). The emptying of solids presents an initial lag phase (up to 60 min from the beginning of the meal, depending on the nature of the solid) during which little emptying occurs. Subsequently emptying of solids follows a linear pattern. The time required to empty 50% of the dietary solids is about twice that required for dietary liquids. Therefore, the initial volume decrease of ingested material within the stomach corresponds to the exponential (rapid initial) liquid emptying, because solids present an initial lag time. Some investigators quantitated gastric emptying of solids, taking into account these two phases (lag time and emptying phase), whereas others measured net emptying only and included both phases in one index (for instance, time to 50% emptying). Technical issues are also important. In radioscintigraphic studies, the redistribution (posteroanterior displacement) of ingested material within the stomach needs to be taken into account; otherwise it may give a false impression of emptying (decay of activity in the gastric area) (48, 120, 175). Whether emptying is measured from the time of onset or the end of ingestion of a meal also markedly influences the duration or even the recognition of a lag time.

Gastric outflow is very high initially, even if the total intragastric volume does not change, because high rates of gastric secretion substitute for losses through the pylorus. Thus the gastric outflow rate for liquids is markedly influenced by secretory rates. In the early postcibal period, gastric outflow corresponds to ingested liquids, but as gastric dilution takes place, the proportion of secreted liquids becomes the predominant fraction. The total amount of liquids emptied from the stomach during the postcibal period (cumulative gastric outflow) is about two to three times the volume of the ingested meal [Fig. 6; (151)]. The flow through the pylorus is bidirectional, and biliopancreatic secretion partly refluxes into the stomach throughout the digestive process (139, 239). The proportion of refluxed volume diluted in gastric content progressively increases during the postcibal period (239).

RELATIONSHIPS AMONG GASTRIC EMPTYING, MOTILITY, AND STRUCTURE: MECHANICS OF GASTRIC EMPTYING

Gastric emptying is a sophisticated process determined by the coordinated motor activity of the stomach and the proximal intestine. Because the stomach delivers a liquid or semiliquid chyme into the intestine, some dietary products require a preliminary processing before being emptied. Whereas ingested liquids are readily delivered into the duodenum, ingested solids require a preliminary grinding process. Similarly, high-viscosity semisolid meals require a dilution and mixing process with gastric secretion. Once the components of the meal have been liquified, they can be emptied. Liquified means the breaking of solid foods into very small particles that are mixed and suspended in the liquid phase and follow the fate of liquids. Only a minority of solids leave the stomach with the bulk of a meal without having been subjected to this grinding process. It follows that the different emptying patterns of different solid dietary products depend partly on susceptibility to this preliminary grinding and liquefication process. The preliminary intragastric trituration and mixing processes, chiefly performed by the antropyloric grinder, and the actual emptying process are considered separately.

*Preliminary Processing: Antropyloric Grinder*

Grinding of solids is accomplished by the coordinated action of the antrum and the pylorus acting as a functional unit. The antropyloric area acts as both a discriminatory barrier (sieve) and a grinding pump, selectively retaining solid particles, based on their size, and grinding them, via a propulsion/retropulsion sequence, into fine particles. These particles, particu-

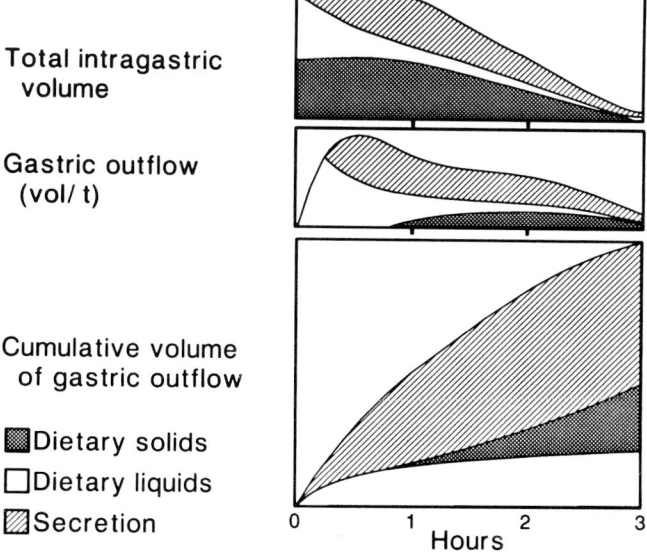

FIG. 6. Dynamics of gastric emptying. Data correspond to an idealized solid and liquid meal of ~400 ml total volume, with a liquid-to-solid ratio of 1:1 (based on data from refs. 151–154 and J.-R. Malagelada, unpublished observations).

larly those whose density is close to that of water, remain in suspension within the liquid phase by the mixing effect of gastric motility. The classic description of the antropyloric propulsion/retropulsion mechanism corresponds to Code's group (52, 54) and was lucidly described in the previous volume on motility and circulation in this *Handbook* series (55). When a peristaltic contraction originates in the midstomach as a shallow indentation (annular constriction), the pylorus is open and remains so while the antral contraction propagates caudally, with progressive acceleration and increase in depth (Fig. 7). The antral ring contraction moves smoothly along the antrum, gently pushing ahead solid particles and allowing liquids to move freely through the increasingly constricted ring. Meanwhile, the pyloric lumen, smaller than the lumen of the antral contraction, allows the passage of liquids with small solid particles in suspension into the duodenum, whereas larger particles are selectively retained in the antrum. When the antral contraction approaches the pylorus, the latter closes and the terminal antrum produces a mass contraction, called the terminal antral contraction. This mass contraction against pyloric closure forcefully retropulses antral contents (solid particles concentrated by the peristaltic wave) through the constricted antral ring. This jet ejection of antral contents into the main cavity of the stomach produces a shearing effect, with fragmentation of solid particles. It is not known whether actual pressure or hydraulic forces actually break the particles, although it is probably a combination of both. The depth of antral contractions, measured by implanted coils (37, 82), depends on the viscosity of gastric contents (202), although the matter is disputed by others (219). The size and consistency of solid particles may also have an effect on antral peristalsis by stimulating mucosal mechanoreceptors, although this finding warrants further experimental verification (31, 145, 220).

The sieving and grinding function of the antropyloric area is supported by experimental and clinical data. Large plastic spheres (7 mm in diam) are selectively retained in the canine stomach throughout the postcibal period, and they are emptied during the activity fronts after the restoration of the interdigestive pattern (188). This discriminatory function is lost after antropyloric resection and solid spheres leave the stomach prematurely (76). The canine stomach empties 70% of cooked chicken liver (ingested in 10-mm cubes) in particles smaller than 0.06 mm and 97% in particles smaller than 1 mm (174). The size of liver particles emptied significantly increases after antropyloric resection (100, 163, 174). A similar situation prevails in humans (163, 164, 173). The individual roles of the antrum and the pylorus are difficult to determine exactly, because adaptive mechanisms preserve some discriminatory function after selective antrectomy or pylorectomy (100).

After selective antral vagotomy in dogs, emptying of large plastic spheres is delayed (188), but this effect seems more likely to be the result of a disruption of the antral phase III of the IMC (which normally emptied bulky solid particles from the stomach) than of an impairment in the postcibal propulsion/retropulsion mechanism. Unfortunately, Mroz and Kelly (188) did not test emptying of digestible (fragmentable) solids in their experimental model that seems to preserve solid discrimination while selectively weakening antral motility. A clinical report of antral hypomotility associated with marked gastric retention for solids, but normal emptying of liquids, suggests that impaired antral peristalsis alters the grinding function and selectively impairs emptying of digestible solids in a normal meal (211). We subsequently identified a subgroup of patients with selective antral hypomotility, prolonged lag phase, and delayed emptying time for solids, but with normal emptying of liquids (47). These clinical studies further support the importance of the human antrum in gastric emptying of solids.

Gastric acid–peptic secretion also participates in the physical (liquefaction) digestive process, but the contribution of chemical digestion to solid trituration under normal circumstances appears to be small, at least in the dog (196).

## Emptying Function

As the dilution and liquefaction of the meal proceed, emptying takes place. Emptying involves primarily the intragastric liquid or semiliquid phase. The mechanisms involved in this emptying process are complex. Reviewed here are the contributions of the tonic contraction of the proximal stomach (gastric tone), the antropyloroduodenal resistance to flow (gastric outlet

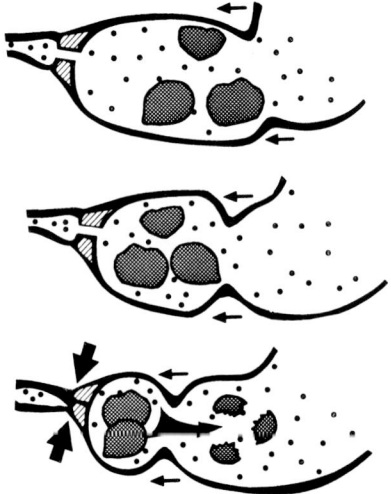

FIG. 7. Antropyloric propulsion/retropulsion mechanism. See text for full description.

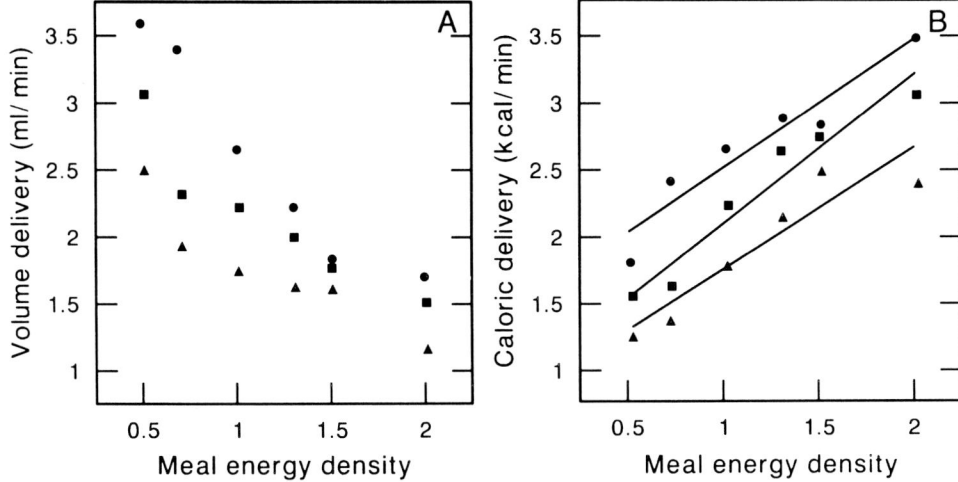

FIG. 10. Mean rates of gastric emptying (A, in ml/min; B, in kcal/min) for 18 combinations of volume and caloric density of meal fed to healthy volunteers. Rates calculated as linear slope from regression of energy delivered vs. time for all individual subjects, for each combination of meal volume and energy density. Means are plotted: ▲, 300-ml meals; ■, 400-ml meals; and ●, 600-ml meals. *Solid lines* (B), linear regressions of mean caloric rate vs. energy density for each of three volumes; slopes of these lines are not significantly different. [From Hunt et al. (110).]

the ileum (103). Among amino acids, tryptophan is particularly effective and acts on specific duodenal receptors (60). It is not clear whether specific receptors exist for other amino acids. Carbohydrate inhibition of gastric emptying is particularly potent in the ileum and is mediated by products of digestion of starch. Thus inhibition of amylase activity, which increases carbohydrate load into the distal bowel, markedly delayed gastric emptying in humans (144).

OSMOLALITY. Receptors that respond to osmotic changes in chyme are present in the duodenum (27). These receptors responded both to luminal hypertonicity and to hypotonicity (169). They may be particularly important in regulating the rapid emptying of liquids during the very early postcibal period before other regulatory mechanisms become fully operational (106).

ACID. Acid-sensitive receptors acting on neural pathways that inhibit gastric emptying are located in the first 5 cm of the duodenum (60). Acids with low-molecular-weight anions are more potent inhibitors than those with high-molecular-weight anions. The existence of acid-sensitive receptors in the jejunum is debatable.

VOLUME OF THE MEAL. It was observed that the interruption of intestinal interdigestive motility was shorter with a small meal (containing inert solid particles) than with a larger one (220). This suggests that the duration of emptying of the meal can be influenced solely by its size.

SIZE AND DENSITY OF SOLID PARTICLES AND VISCOSITY. Solid particles can be classified as digestible or nondigestible, depending on the capacity of the stomach to reduce them to a size small enough to pass through the antropyloric discriminatory mechanism previously described. In dogs and humans, radiolabeled 10-mm liver cubes (a digestible solid) empty much slower than liquids or 0.25-mm liver particles (173, 174), reflecting the time it takes for the antrum to grind the larger pieces of liver into smaller particles. As a result of the grinding and discrimination process, the majority of digestible solids (at least for liver) empty as very small particles (<2 mm in diam, and most actually are <1 mm) (31, 100, 101, 174). In contrast, indigestible plastic spheres 7 mm in diameter do not empty at all while food is in the stomach and must await the return of the interdigestive migrating motor complex in order to be evacuated.

To elucidate the emptying patterns of intermediate-size indigestible particles, Russell and Bass (220) fed 30–90 g of inert polycarbophil particles (1–3 mm in diam) to dogs. They observed that these inert solid meals elicited a fed pattern of motility and were emptied by the stomach (~50% in 4 h) before the return of the interdigestive migrating motor complex. These observations agree with human data showing that indigestible solid fiber (particles <7 mm but >1 mm), ingested either as radiolabeled bran (221) or as radiolabeled fiber strands (53), empties slowly but steadily even when food is in the stomach.

To better understand the emptying of intermediate-size inert particles ingested with food, Meyer et al. (171) fed dogs a standard meal of minced liver, steak, and water to which they added inert spheres of different sizes and densities (Fig. 11). With spheres of density 1, emptying occurred progressively faster

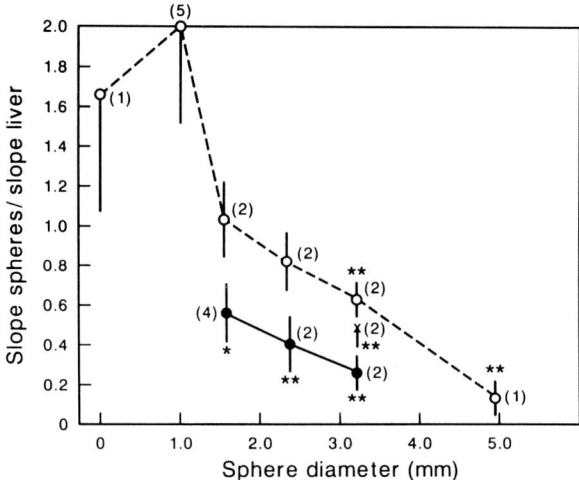

FIG. 11. Comparison of emptying of spheres with emptying of liver and of filter paper squares in dog. Slope ratios are plotted on *ordinate* as function of sphere diameter on *abscissa*. Points are means ± SE. Numbers in parentheses are numbers of repeated experiments in each group of dogs. *Open circles* and *dashed line*, spheres with density of 1; *solid circles* and *solid line*, spheres with density of 2. *Cross*, slope ratio for filter paper squares. *Asterisks*, significant differences from 1.0, i.e., from equal rates of emptying of spheres and liver. [From Meyer et al. (171).]

when their size decreased from 5 mm to 1 mm. However, spheres of 0.015 mm emptied no faster than those of 1 mml. Spheres 1.6 mm in diameter and with a density of 1 emptied at the same rate as the liver in the meal. Decreasing density below 1 or increasing density above 1 reduced emptying of the spheres. Shape and surface area of particles seemed to have little effect. Thus filter paper squares emptied at the same rate as spheres of comparable size and density (171). Increasing the viscosity of liquid meals by raising the concentration of hydrophilic fiber (psyllium or guar gum, without particulate matter) was associated with a progressive decrease in the canine gastric emptying rate (219). Holt et al. (105) have also shown in humans that psyllium and guar gum added to carbohydrate-containing meals delayed gastric emptying.

*Interactions Between Gastric Emptying and Gastric Secretion*

Physiologically it is not possible to dissociate postprandial gastric emptying from gastric secretion because gut regulatory mechanisms respond to the whole gastric contents. The gastric secretory response to a meal expands, dilutes, and acidifies gastric contents. These processes also reduce meal viscosity and relative density and bring osmolality toward isotonicity. Therefore it is apparent that changes in the gastric secretory response to a meal modify its emptying and need to be accounted for.

INTESTINAL MOTILITY AND ITS RELATIONSHIP TO LUMINAL FLOW AND ABSORPTION

The intestine behaves like a series of coupled oscillators arranged in a priority system so that a distal segment takes over when activity is absent in a more proximal one (194). By using spike-potential analysis, five main patterns of intestinal motility have been identified (162): the interdigestive migrating motor complex, the migrating spike burst, the migrating action potential complex, repetitive bursts of action potentials, and the fed pattern. Spike potentials are associated with contraction of the circular muscle. However, a contractile correlate has been demonstrated for only three of the five patterns of spike-potential activity: the migrating motor complex, the migrating spike burst, and the fed pattern. Conversely, longitudinal muscle contraction may occur in the absence of spike potentials, and it has been suggested that it could be determined by slow-wave activity (162). Contraction of the longitudinal layer of muscle may be responsible for a to-and-fro movement that is important in increasing the exposure of luminal contents to the absorptive surface of the small bowel (170).

Meals of particulate bran elicit propagated groups of contractions in the canine small bowel (41), whereas viscous meals of guar gum elicit randomly distributed contractions (219). Although the effects of these different motor patterns on transit were not studied, these studies suggested that the intestine "senses" the physical characteristics of the luminal milieu and thus participates in its self-regulation. Furthermore rabbit ileal loops exposed to bacteria or their enterotoxins developed a characteristic electrophysiological pattern: the migrating action potential complexes [see the chapter by Mathias and Clench in this *Handbook*; (161)]. This abnormal pattern can also be elicited by experimental blockade of the α-adrenergic inhibitory system (162). It is not known whether the distal intestine also reacts to colonization by normal colonic flora, but the matter deserves further study.

The relationship between normal fasting motor patterns and intestinal flow was studied by Summers et al. (247), who found the interdigestive migrating motor complex to be propulsive in dogs. Also Bueno et al. (40) observed in dogs and sheep that aboral luminal flow was associated chiefly with phase II of the interdigestive migrating motor complex and to lesser extent with phase III. In contrast, Kerlin et al. (138) reported that in humans, phase III was associated with the highest rate of flow, followed by phase II activity.

The terminal ileum appears to have distinct motor patterns and possibly different relationships between motility and flow than the more proximal small bowel. The predominant motility pattern in the terminal ileum during fasting in humans is random phasic contractions. The interdigestive migrating motor complex reaches the terminal ileum but in most instances does not propagate through the ileocecal valve (204). The migrating motor complex in the terminal ileum, as in the jejunum, is associated with increased flow (141). Two additional characteristic patterns of motility have been described in the terminal ileum: discrete clustered contractions and prolonged propagated contractions. Both types of activity are usually observed in the distal 20–30 cm of the ileum, and they have been shown in dogs and humans to be strongly propulsive (141, 204).

Retrograde pacing in dogs slowed flow and enhanced absorption in the small bowel (59). Instillation of fat into the human ileum slowed small bowel transit (103), and in a separate study it was also found to cause a reduction in jejunal contractile activity (240). Ileal fat infusion in humans was also associated with increased absorption of carbohydrate (103). However, under other circumstances slowing flow does not necessarily enhance absorption of luminal nutrients. Clearly the relationships between transit and absorption are not well understood and need further study.

## PHYSIOLOGICAL MEASUREMENT OF TRANSIT IN SMALL BOWEL

Compared with gastric emptying, relatively little is known about normal transit of chyme along the small bowel and its regulation. The reasons for the relative ignorance are largely technical and can be summarized as follows. First, input of a meal into the small bowel is variable and depends on the gastric-emptying rate. Therefore the transit time of chyme cannot be measured without simultaneously measuring gastric emptying. At the same time, intestinal transit cannot be predicted based on the rate of gastric emptying (207). Second, chyme does not progress along the small bowel as a bolus. Some parts of the meal travel to the colon faster than others. Hence the meal spreads out in the intestine as it moves aborally. Physiologically there is no single transit time but rather a spectrum of transit times that cannot be quantified by pulse techniques such as lactulose $H_2$ breath tests (102) or injections of nonabsorbable markers.

Because the stomach discriminates physiologically between liquid and solid components of a meal, meal liquids generally leave the stomach ahead of solids. Solid particles present in normal intestinal chyme are mostly small particles because large solid fragments are selectively retained in the stomach. Whether transit time from pylorus to the ileocecal valve for the liquid and solid components of intestinal chyme differs is controversial. Experimental observations in fasted dogs based on intestinal perfusion methods seem to suggest that solids move along the small bowel at a slower pace than liquids (223, 276). However, measurements performed in fed dogs did not show a difference between transit of the solid and liquid components of chyme in the small bowel (J. H. Mayer, personal communication).

Recent studies in our laboratory (156) shed some light on the normal patterns of transit of solids and liquids in the small bowel in humans. We used two radiolabeled markers, $^{99m}$Tc-labeled diethylenetriamine pentaacetic acid (DTPA)-water and $^{131}$I-labeled fiber, representing two important classes of chyme components: the luminal aqueous phase and small, particulate, nondigestible solids. The gastric-emptying rates of $^{99m}$Tc-labeled DTPA were faster than those of $^{131}$I-labeled fiber, as expected, because the fiber particles were retained longer in the stomach. However, comparison of the intestinal transit spectra of $^{131}$I-labeled fiber and $^{99m}$Tc-labeled DTPA showed that they were similar (Fig. 12). Therefore our study confirmed the conventional physiological concept that if solids and liquids are ingested together in a meal, the latter reach the colon faster. But our studies also showed that in healthy humans, the stomach, not the small bowel, is responsible for the difference.

Our studies (156) also suggested that intestinal chyme spreads over a considerable length of small bowel as it advances. This is due to the combined effects of slow emptying from the stomach and variable rates of transit between the pylorus and the ileocecal valve. It is plausible that such spreading out of chyme along the small intestine serves a useful physiological purpose, by rapidly expanding the total absorptive surface exposed to chyme. Other radioscintigraphic studies in humans further suggest that transit of radiolabeled food slows down in the ileal region where it probably interacts with receptors that slow gastric emptying and intestinal transit and suppress food intake (the "ileal brake") (136).

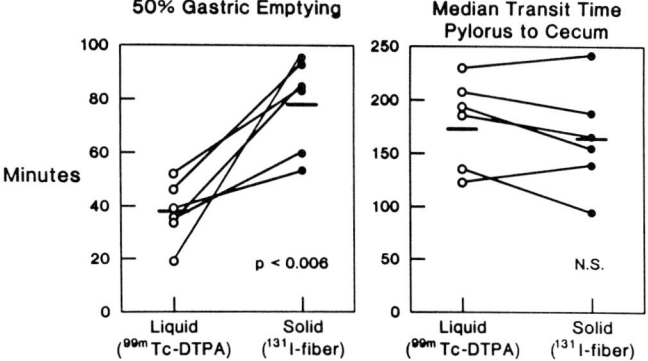

FIG. 12. Comparison of 50% gastric emptying and median small bowel transit for liquid and solid components of chyme for each of 6 healthy volunteers studied with a radioscintigraphic technique. Note that physical properties of food appear to have different influences on gastric emptying and intestinal transit: stomach selectively retains meal solids, but small bowel does not discriminate between solids and liquids. NS, not significant. DTPA, diethylenetriamine pentaacetic acid. [From Malagelada et al. (156).]

Relationships between intestinal contractile activity (the fed pattern) and transit of chyme along the human small bowel have not been well studied. However, our observations in disease indicate that when small bowel motility becomes disorganized (as in patients with the intestinal pseudo-obstruction syndrome), transit is delayed (45).

## EFFECT OF OPIATES AND SEX HORMONES ON INTESTINAL MOTILITY AND TRANSIT

In humans, both morphine and loperamide, a synthetic opiate, elicit propagated activity fronts analogous to phase III of the interdigestive migrating motor complex (32, 128, 213), thus appearing to increase cyclic interdigestive motor activity. Moreover loperamide shortened the duration of phase II–type motility preceding the activity fronts (128). Two groups of investigators (128, 227) also reported that opiates delayed transit in the jejunum, although their observations were made on the fasting not the fed state. It is not clear whether the delay in transit is because of the reduction in phase II activity reported by Kachel et al. (128), a change in the propulsive effectiveness of the motility, or the limited propagation of opiate-induced activity fronts. Furthermore apparently discrepant observations have been reported. Borody et al. (32) observed that morphine-stimulated phase III activity in the distal small bowel was associated with an early increase in flow, followed rapidly by a reduction in flow. These authors also reported that morphine had no effect on mouth-to-ileum transit of a marker mixed with a meal. It is possible that the effects of opiates on transit are different in the fasting and fed states.

During the second and third trimesters of pregnancy, mouth-to-cecum transit measured by the lactulose $H_2$-breath method is prolonged, becoming normal after delivery (143). Because gastric emptying is not affected by pregnancy (225), this prolongation is most likely attributable to delayed intestinal transit. High progesterone levels during middle and late pregnancy have been indirectly implicated, but other factors may also participate.

## CONTROL OF GASTROINTESTINAL MOTILITY: PHYSIOLOGICAL AND PATHOPHYSIOLOGICAL IMPLICATIONS FOR GASTRIC MOTILITY AND INTESTINAL TRANSIT

Control of gastrointestinal motility is exerted at various levels from the smooth muscle cell to the brain. This stratification of control includes both neural and humoral mechanisms. The effector pathways of this complex regulatory system determine changes in muscular contraction of the gut wall that, in conjunction with secretory and absorptive effects, ultimately determine movement of chyme. It is usually impossible to relate a specific control mechanism to a specific change in gastric emptying or small bowel transit because there are multiple interactions among different mechanisms. However, the probable physiological consequences of activation of certain control pathways are indicated when they are known.

### Control at Level of Gut Smooth Muscle

Control at a cellular level is determined by the electrophysiological characteristics and contractile responsiveness of smooth muscle fibers in different parts of the upper gut. In the stomach, rhythmic depolarization (slow waves) is provided by the gastric pacemaker located in the proximal body toward the greater curvature. Bauer et al. (30) recently showed that slow waves actually originate from multiple discrete foci located in the outer myenteric half of the muscle. The propagation of the slow waves toward the pylorus, which determines the peristaltic rhythm, is influenced by distension of the stomach and other maneuvers that stretch the circular muscle (136, 203). Stretch increases the propagation velocity of the slow waves. However, the actual peristaltic contraction depends on the amplitude of the plateau potential during depolarization of cells. Physiologically the action of nerves (via release of classic neurotransmitters and bioactive peptides) and hormones (reaching the smooth muscle cell from the blood) is necessary for the slow-wave depolarization to reach the threshold that converts it into an action potential and causes the muscle to contract. Paracrine substances, such as locally synthesized prostaglandins, may contribute to control of smooth muscle at the electrophysiological level. Furthermore prostaglandins, which increase spontaneous depolarization rates of stomach muscle in vitro, may be involved in the pathogenesis of gastric dysrhythmias that interfere with muscle contractile responsiveness and the coordination of peristaltic waves, thus impairing gastric emptying.

Electrophysiological activity may also control the closing of the pyloric ring that takes place synchronically with antral peristalsis, therefore affecting the antropyloric propulsion/retropulsion sequence that is key to selective retention trituration of solid particles. Szurszewski (250) pointed out that the time between the initial depolarization peak and the plateau potential (2–3 s) coincides approximately with the closure of the pylorus ahead of the approaching main peristaltic wave. Pyloric closure could then be explained on the basis of its small diameter (its edges could be brought together even by the small contraction induced by the depolarization peak) or, alternatively, because of increased contractile responsiveness of the specialized pyloric muscle.

The fundus of the stomach is myoelectrically silent.

Tone of the proximal stomach is maintained by the resting potential of muscle cells in this area, which is above the threshold for contraction. Tone inhibition, which determines relaxation, is probably mediated via neural release of vasoactive intestinal polypeptide (VIP) (95). The existence of dopaminergic inhibitory receptors is debated. Despite being electrically silent, the proximal stomach contracts phasically during fasting, and these contractions appear to be propagated into the antrum (20, 24, 93). Therefore during the interdigestive period the proximal stomach may control, to some extent, the motor activity of the distal stomach. After feeding fundic contractions disappear, whereas rhythmic antral contractions, phase locked with spike bursts, continue throughout the postprandial period in the antrum. Thus during the fed state the coordination between proximal and distal stomach is not as evident as during fasting.

The intestinal pacemaker, sited in the proximal duodenum, initiates a sequence of slow waves that migrate caudally and "capture" areas of less frequent intrinsic rhythmic activity. Contraction is determined by spike discharges superimposed on the peaks of these slow waves. The regulation of propulsive activity in the small bowel is determined by the modulation of this electrophysiological activity by the intrinsic and extrinsic nervous system. Electrophysiological control of small bowel motility and transit has not been well studied. However, diseases affecting gut smooth muscle, such as visceral myopathies (both hereditary and acquired), are associated with diminished tonic and phasic contractile activity. Consequences include delayed gastric emptying and intestinal transit of chyme.

## Control at Level of Gut Intrinsic and Extrinsic Nervous Systems

The neural control of gastric emptying and intestinal transit involves a combination of intrinsic and extrinsic reflexes. Extrinsic reflexes are probably very important in the stomach, and they have been better characterized than intrinsic reflexes.

Extrinsic innervation establishes a link between the central nervous system and the gut. It provides reflex control of the stomach and intestine in response to afferents arising in the thoracoabdominal viscera and in somatic afferents. Such reflexes relay at the level of prevertebral ganglia (251; see the chapter by Szurszewski and King in this *Handbook*), spinal cord, or medulla oblongata. The sympathetic preganglionic efferent is modulated by noradrenergic and serotoninergic inhibitory influences arising in the medulla (62). There is also evidence of descending control of parasympathetic preganglionic neurons (149).

Vagal innervation of the stomach plays a key role in the control of proximal gastric tone. Gastric tone is probably maintained under basal conditions by an excitatory cholinergic input mediated by the vagus nerve (10, 11, 23). The vagus nerve also provides an inhibitory nonadrenergic, noncholinergic input [for instance, in response to intestinal nutrients (25)], whose transmission mechanism has not been established (11, 12, 25, 125, 159, 197). Peptidergic (12, 95, 186), purinergic (13, 69), serotoninergic (90), and dopaminergic (146, 262) neurotransmitters have been suggested, although some doubts have been expressed as to the significance of dopaminergic mechanisms (12, 25). Under basal conditions, there is no adrenergic input to gastric tone; however, sympathetic stimulation, as it may occur during stress (241), induces gastric relaxation (11, 23, 94). Adrenergic gastric relaxation may involve a dual effect: inhibition of acetylcholine release from intramural cholinergic (excitatory) neurons ($\alpha$-receptors) and direct inhibition of the smooth muscle ($\beta$-receptors) (215).

Esophageal distension induces gastric relaxation. Whether this reflex is related to the phenomenon of receptive relaxation in response to swallowing remains uncertain (3, 71, 123). We recently compared the effect of esophageal distension to that of wet swallows on gastric relaxation in the dog, quantified by the gastric barostat (71). Gastric relaxation was more intense with distension. Roman and Tieffenbach (216) have shown that the presence of a solid bolus triggers more afferent activity in vagal fibers than a wet swallow. Therefore it is likely that the degree of distension of the esophagus by the bolus determines the degree of gastric relaxation. These reflexes are vagally mediated, as we showed in our vagal-cooling studies (71). However, there is a small residual nonvagal component that could be intrinsic. The physiological significance of these distension-triggered relaxatory mechanisms has not been established, but they may be physiopathologically important.

Antral distension produced a similar gastric relaxation to that observed with esophageal distension [(1, 2); F. De Ponti, F. Azpiroz, and J.-R. Malagelada unpublished observations in the dog]. Distension of the intestine (71) produced a similar effect, which was also vagally mediated. Mechanoreceptors sensitive to distension may also exist in the proximal stomach (9) and contribute to accommodation, although this has not been clearly shown. Furthermore, as noted previously, fixed-volume balloon distension of the canine stomach, although it does not cause a pressure rise, can abolish the interdigestive intestinal motor pattern (20). Whether this is part of the mechanism of conversion of fasting to fed activity after a meal or an unphysiological artifact is not known. However, it is possible that gastric accommodation coexists with reflex stimulation of pathways directed to other areas of the gastrointestinal tract.

The regulation of the antropyloric motor response to a meal depends on activation of both intramural and long reflexes. Distension of the proximal stomach (at physiological levels) stimulates antral peristalsis

(8, 13, 20, 136) by a vagovagal reflex. Indeed gastric distension produced increased discharge in vagal afferent fibers from mechanoreceptors in the proximal stomach (229) and in vagal efferent (preganglionic) fibers to the antrum (181). These discharges have also been recorded in the nucleus tractus solitarius (26) and in the dorsal vagal nucleus (84). The final path seems to be an intramural (postganglionic) excitatory cholinergic neuron (13, 249). An intramural cholinergic reflex may also participate (13). The composition of chyme delivered into the intestine plays a modulatory role. Acid, fat, and products of protein digestion decreased antral contractility stimulated by food or other stimuli (7, 36, 131, 135, 217, 226, 271). Such inhibition may constitute a feedback regulation of the liquefaction and delivery of solid nutrients into the intestine. Inhibition of antral peristalsis by intestinal nutrients appears to be vagally mediated (135, 217) by a nonadrenergic, noncholinergic mechanism; purinergic (13) and peptidergic (249) neurotransmitters have been proposed.

The rhythm of antral contractions is regulated by the intrinsic pacemaker. However, the force (amplitude) of contractions is under vagal control; this may be an excitatory cholinergic input or an inhibitory nonadrenergic, noncholinergic input (13). The sympathetic nervous system (8) may have a modulatory effect on antral peristalsis. Intraduodenal mixed amino acids or tryptophan increased pyloric contractions via opiate nerves, whereas CCK stimulated pyloric activity through a different mechanism (214).

Pathophysiologically, autonomical neuropathy is a common cause of motor dysfunction in the gut. Although it is seen most often in diabetics, it can also be observed in dysproteinemias, collagen-vascular disease, early amyloidosis, or idiopathic orthostatic hypotension. Orthostasis, urinary dysfunction, and impaired sweating are frequently associated features. Sometimes, as may be the case in advanced scleroderma and amyloidosis, muscle degeneration, infiltration of the gut wall, or both are also present, combining neuropathic and myopathic gut dysfunction. Postvagotomy gastroparesis, which probably represents an exaggeration of the usual effects of vagotomy, is another example of disturbed extrinsic neural control of gut motility. Myenteric plexus disease is emerging as a major cause of gastrointestinal motility disorders, and it represents primarily a disturbance of intrinsic nervous system control of the gut. However, given the intimate relationships between the intrinsic and extrinsic nervous systems of the gut, it is not always possible to separate conditions affecting predominantly one or the other by clinical studies. Abnormalities in gastrointestinal motility are also similar and characterized, in contrast to myopathic syndromes, by motor incoordination rather than loss of contractile force. The consequences of the motor dysfunction are impaired gastric emptying and decreased transit of chyme through the small bowel.

*Hormonal Control*

Hormones undoubtedly participate in the control of gastrointestinal motility, but their role is not well defined, in part because of the difficulty in separating pharmacological from physiological effects. It is also difficult sometimes to separate the effects of humorally released bioactive peptides from the effects, sometimes concurrent, of release of analogous peptides at a tissue level where they act as neurotransmitters or paracrine substances.

Motilin is a 23-amino acid peptide found in brain and nervous tissue of the gut; its effects on gastric and small bowel motility have been extensively studied. Peripheral blood levels of motilin increase periodically in apparent synchrony with the IMC (118). Whether this rise in motilin blood level is the cause or the consequence of the activity front remains unknown. Infusion of exogenous motilin reduces the duration of the fasting cycle (interval between sequential phase III) and induces "premature" IMCs (281), suggesting that motilin increases the responsiveness of gut smooth muscle to intrinsic neural activity. Gastrin (61, 187), CCK (185), and motilin (245) stimulate antral motility, whereas secretin and neurotensin are inhibitory (44). However, the effect of CCK may be primarily on the pylorus rather than on the antrum. Thus gut peptides seem to modulate gastric motor function, although physiologically they probably act in concert with other mechanisms, and it is difficult to ascertain which effects are physiological and which are pharmacological. However, a recent study using physiological doses of CCK administered intravenously suggested that CCK may participate in the physiological inhibitory control of gastric emptying (147). For additional information on hormonal effects on the stomach, see TONIC CONTRACTION OF PROXIMAL STOMACH, p. 919.

Hormonal regulation of intestinal motility and transit has been less well studied. Pentagastrin (270) and CCK (279) disrupt fasting motility, producing motor activity patterns resembling the fed pattern. Substance P inhibited intestinal contractility (88), whereas somatostatin induced phase III–like activity followed by motor inhibition, an effect that resembles that of opiates, and possibly is mediated via $\beta$-adrenergic receptors in the enteric nervous system. Prostaglandin $E_2$ ($PGE_2$) (30 $\mu g \cdot kg^{-1} \cdot h^{-1}$) administered intravenously to dogs delayed reappearance of the first postinfusion IMC, but it did not affect fed motility (191). Other investigators observed that either intravenous or intra-arterial $PGE_2$ and $PGI_2$ decreased intestinal motility in dogs, whereas $PGF_{2\alpha}$ increased intestinal motility, causing a fedlike pattern (261). The aforementioned effects could be pharmacological. However, intravenous indomethacin appeared to enhance intestinal motility, causing a fedlike pattern (261) and suggesting that endogenous prostaglandins might participate in the control of intestinal motility.

Substance P, somatostatins, and prostaglandins are in any case more likely to operate at a tissular than hormonal level. Furthermore both CCK and VIP have been shown to alter motility when infused into the intestinal lumen, suggesting the possible existence of enteroreceptors for these substances. For additional information on hormonal effects on the small bowel and their possible role in the conversion from a fasting into a fed motor pattern, see *Declining Phase and Transition to Interdigestive Activity*, p. 916.

*Control at Cerebral Level*

Brain centers are also involved in the regulation of gastrointestinal motility (see the chapter by Gillis et al. in this *Handbook*). They are linked with the gut via neural (parasympathetic, chiefly via the vagus nerve, and sympathetic) and humoral pathways. In the medulla oblongata, several centers concerned with the control of gut motility have been identified. There appears to be a "stomach area" within the dorsal motor nucleus of the vagus to which afferent fibers are conducted by the vagus nerve. Electrical stimulation of this area increases gastric motility (199). This area corresponds approximately with that identified in the cat by retrograde axon tracing after injection of horseradish peroxidase into the antrum (195). Not surprisingly there appears to be significant interaction between gut and other autonomic centers in the region. For instance, gastric distension, electrical stimulation, and transparietal mechanical stimulation of certain areas of the rat stomach increase blood pressure (201).

Direct injection of certain pharmacological agents into the spinal canal or into the cerebral ventriculi produces striking effects on gastrointestinal motility and transit. Galligan and Burks (89) have showed that intracerebroventricular injection of morphine in the rat delayed gastric emptying and prolonged intestinal transit. We showed that intraspinal morphine in fed dogs induced episodes of intense contractile activity that disrupted the fed pattern (255). These effects occurred at doses much smaller than those required to elicit them by the intravenous route. Neurotensin administered intracerebroventricularly to fasted dogs decreased antral motility and disrupted normal interdigestive cyclic activity in the stomach and the small bowel (39). In fed dogs, intracerebroventricular neurotensin shortened the duration of the fed pattern. These effects did not appear when neurotensin was administered intravenously, even at doses severalfold higher. Furthermore vagotomy abolished the effects of intracerebroventricular neurotensin (39). Therefore neurotensin can act centrally to control gastrointestinal motility and the effects are mediated via the vagus nerve. Bueno et al. (38) observed that the effects of intracerebroventricular neurotensin and calcitonin (which are similar to those of neurotensin) can be reproduced by $PGE_2$ and abolished by pretreatment with indomethacin. Although these results suggest that the effects of neurotensin and calcitonin are mediated via local generation of prostaglandins, the investigators also found that the somewhat similar effects of Met-enkephalin derivative were not blocked by indomethacin. Thus nonprostaglandin-mediated mechanisms are also present (38).

Central feedback mechanisms probably involve hypothalamic areas controlling feeding behavior and even the cortical level. Thus distension of the stomach by a balloon inhibits eating behavior in hungry animals exposed to food (237). In humans, inhibition of gastric emptying by perfusion of the ileum with fat increased the subjective feeling of epigastric fullness after a meal [Fig. 13; (272)].

It seems likely that medullary centers regulating gastrointestinal motility interact closely with those responsible for the emetic response (the chemoreceptor trigger zone and the vomiting center). Opiate and dopamine $D_2$ receptors are involved in the emetic center. Stimulation of these centers via an intragastric or intravenous emetic agent is normally associated with a characteristic motor sequence of events, consisting of a retrograde peristaltic contraction followed by a pause and a migrating burst of activity (142, 256). The retrograde contraction transports intestinal luminal content into the stomach (G. M. Thomforde, F. Azpiroz, and J. R. Malagelada, unpublished observations). Vomiting itself does not depend on the aforementioned motor correlates (236). The motor events of the gut can be elicited by a submaximal emetic stimulus without eliciting actual vomiting or its associated autonomic somatomotor or behavioral responses (142). Vagotomy abolishes the motor response of the gut but not vomiting itself, suggesting that the motor effects are centrally mediated (142).

The central mechanisms related to the emetic center are probably responsible for gastric stasis, nausea,

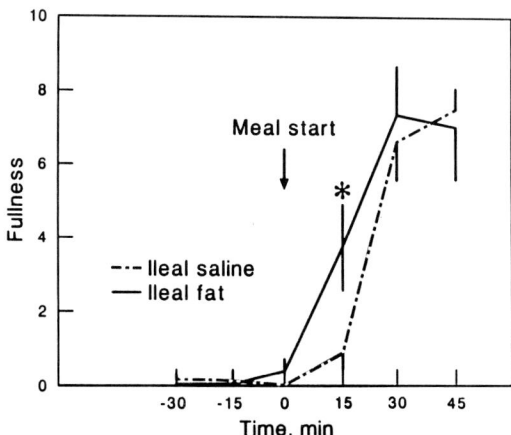

FIG. 13. Subjective scores for epigastric fullness during ingestion of meal and simultaneous infusion of either lipid emulsion (*solid line*) or saline control (*dotted line*) into ileum. Note earlier epigastric fullness with perfusion of ileal fat that delays gastric emptying (*asterisk*). Data are shown as means ± SE for 6 healthy volunteers; $P < 0.05$. [From Welch et al. (272).]

and ultimately vomiting that may be associated with metabolic disorders (e.g., electrolyte imbalances, addisonian crisis, or ketoacidosis) and certain drugs (e.g., digitalis, opiates, bromocriptine). Pharmacological studies suggest that opiate receptors and dopamine $D_2$-receptors are involved in the functioning of the emetic center, but whether they are specifically involved in the gastrointestinal response to stimulation of the center is not clear.

Behavioral studies have shown that emotions, such as anxiety or fear, may retard gastric emptying. Furthermore we recently showed that pain stress (induced by submerging one hand in cold water) has profound inhibitory effects on gastric emptying of a meal (258). Likewise direct stimulation of some brain centers, i.e., vertigo induced by labyrinthine cooling, has a similar delaying effect while at the same time inducing intestinal activity fronts similar to those previously described with selected pharmacological agents (242, 257). Whether these central effects constitute the basis for psychogenic gastroparesis and vomiting is not known. However, psychiatric disorders such as anorexia nervosa can be associated with reduced gastric emptying rates, providing an example of the blurred line of separation between psychological disturbances and objective motor abnormalities.

The present address for the authors is: Digestive System Research Unit, Vall d'Hebron Hospital, Autonomous University of Barcelona, Barcelona, Spain.

REFERENCES

1. ABRAHAMSSON, H. Vagal relaxation of the stomach induced from the gastric antrum. *Acta Physiol. Scand.* 89: 406–414, 1973.
2. ABRAHAMSSON, H., AND H. GLISE. Sympathetic nervous control of gastric motility and interaction with vagal activity. *Scand. J. Gastroenterol.* 19, Suppl. 89: 83–87, 1984.
3. ABRAHAMSSON, H., AND G. JANSSON. Elicitation of reflex vagal relaxation of the stomach from pharynx and esophagus in the cat. *Acta Physiol. Scand.* 77: 172–178, 1969.
4. AHLMAN, H., AND A. DAHLSTRÖM. Vagal mechanisms controlling serotonin release from the gastrointestinal tract and pyloric motor function. *J. Auton. Nerv. Syst.* 9: 119–140, 1983.
5. ALVAREZ, W. C., AND L. J. MAHONEY. Action currents in stomach and intestine. *Am. J. Physiol.* 58: 476–493, 1922.
6. ANDERSON, J. J., R. J. BOLT, B. M. ULLMAN, AND P. BASS. Differential response to various stimulants in the body and antrum of the canine stomach. *Am. J. Dig. Dis.* 13: 147–156, 1968.
7. ANDERSON, J. J., R. J. BOLT, B. M. ULLMAN, AND P. BASS. Effect of bile and fat on gastric motility under the influence of various stimulants. *Am. J. Dig. Dis.* 13: 157–167, 1968.
8. ANDREWS, P. L. R., D. GRUNDY, AND T. SCATCHERD. Reflex excitation of antral motility induced by gastric distension in the ferret. *J. Physiol. Lond.* 298: 79–84, 1980.
9. ANDREWS, P. L. R., D. GRUNDY, AND T. SCRATCHERD. Vagal afferent discharge from mechanoreceptors in different regions of the ferret stomach. *J. Physiol. Lond.* 298: 513–524, 1980.
10. ANDREWS, P. L. R., AND I. N. C. LAWES. The role of vagal and intramural inhibitory reflexes in the regulation of intragastric pressure in the ferret. *J. Physiol. Lond.* 326: 435–451, 1982.
11. ANDREWS, P. L. R., AND I. N. C. LAWES. Interactions between splanchnic and vagus nerves in the control of mean intragastric pressure in the ferret. *J. Physiol. Lond.* 351: 473–490, 1984.
12. ANDREWS, P. L. R., AND I. N. C. LAWES. Characteristics of the vagally driven non-adrenergic non-cholinergic inhibitory innervation of ferret gastric corpus. *J. Physiol. Lond.* 363: 1–20, 1985.
13. ANDREWS, P. L. R., AND T. SCRATCHERD. The gastric motility patterns induced by direct and reflex excitation of the vagus nerves in the anaesthetized ferret. *J. Physiol. Lond.* 302: 363–378, 1980.
14. ARIMORI, M., C. F. CODE, J. F. SCHLEGEL, AND R. E. STURM. Electrical activity of the canine esophagus and gastroesophageal sphincter: its relation to intraluminal pressure and movement of material. *Am. J. Dig. Dis.* 15: 191–208, 1970.
15. ARMITAGE, A. K., AND A. C. B. DEAN. Function of the pylorus and pyloric antrum in gastric emptying. *Gut* 4: 174–178, 1963.
16. ARNDORFER, R. C., J. J. STEF, W. J. DODDS, J. H. LINEHAN, AND W. J. HOGAN. Improved infusion system for intraluminal esophageal manometry. *Gastroenterology* 73: 23–27, 1977.
17. AUNE, S. Intragastric pressure after vagotomy in man. *Scand. J. Gastroenterol.* 4: 447–452, 1969.
18. AZPIROZ, F. Gastric Motility Physiology of Gastric Tone. Madrid: Univ. of Madrid, 1986, p. 100–108. Thesis.
19. AZPIROZ, F. Gastroesophageal reflux—the role of delayed gastric emptying and duodenogastric reflux. In: *International Trends in General Thoracic Surgery. Benign Oesophageal Disease*, edited by H. Matthews and T. R. DeMeester. Philadelphia: Saunders, vol. 3, (in press).
20. AZPIROZ, F., AND J.-R. MALAGELADA. Pressure activity patterns in the canine proximal stomach: response to distension. *Am. J. Physiol.* 247 (*Gastrointest. Liver Physiol.* 10): G265–G272, 1984.
21. AZPIROZ, F., AND J.-R. MALAGELADA. Physiological variations in canine gastric tone measured by an electronic barostat. *Am. J. Physiol.* 248 (*Gastrointest. Liver Physiol.* 11): G229–G237, 1985.
22. AZPIROZ, F., AND J.-R. MALAGELADA. Intestinal control of gastric tone. *Am. J. Physiol.* 249 (*Gastrointest. Liver Physiol.* 12): G501–G509, 1985.
23. AZPIROZ, F., AND J.-R. MALAGELADA. Importance of vagal input in maintaining gastric tone in the dog. *J. Physiol. Lond.* 384: 511–524, 1987.
24. AZPIROZ, F., AND J.-R. MALAGELADA. Gastric tone measured by an electronic barostat in health and postsurgical gastroparesis. *Gastroenterology* 92: 934–943, 1987.
25. AZPIROZ, F., AND J.-R. MALAGELADA. Vagally mediated gastric relaxation induced by intestinal nutrients in the dog. *Am. J. Physiol.* 251 (*Gastrointest. Liver Physiol.* 14): G727–G735, 1986.
26. BARBER, W. D., AND T. F. BURKS. Brain stem response to phasic gastric distension. *Am. J. Physiol.* 245 (*Gastrointest. Liver Physiol.* 8): G242–G248, 1983.
27. BARKER, G. R., G. M. COCHRANE, G. A. CORBETT, J. N. HUNT, AND S. K. ROBERTS. Actions of glucose and potassium chloride on osmoreceptors slowing gastric emptying. *J. Physiol. Lond.* 237: 183–186, 1974.
28. BASS, P. The relationship of electrical activity to contraction. In: *Gastrointestinal Motility*, edited by L. Demling and R. Ottenjann. Stuttgart, FRG: Thieme Verlag, 1971, p. 59–71. (Int. Symp. Motil. Gastrointest. Tract, Erlangen, July 15th and 16th, 1969.)
29. BASS, P., AND J. N. WILEY. Contractile force transducer for recording muscle activity in unanesthetized animals. *J. Appl. Physiol.* 32: 567–570, 1972.

30. BAUER, A. J., N. G. PUBLICOVER, AND K. M. SANDERS. Origin and spread of slow waves in canine gastric antral circular muscle. *Am. J. Physiol.* 249 (*Gastrointest. Liver Physiol.* 12): G800–G806, 1985.
31. BECKER, J. M., AND K. A. KELLY. Antral control of canine gastric emptying of solids. *Am. J. Physiol.* 245 (*Gastrointest. Liver Physiol.* 8): G334–G338, 1983.
32. BORODY, T. J., E. M. M. QUIGLEY, S. F. PHILLIPS, M. WIENBECK, R. L. TUCKER, A. HADDAD, AND A. R. ZINSMEISTER. Effects of morphine and atropine on motility and transit in the human ileum. *Gastroenterology* 89: 562–570, 1985.
33. BORTOLOTTI, M., N. PANDOLFO, C. NEBIACOLOMBO, G. LABÒ, AND F. MATTIOLI. Modifications in gastroduodenal motility induced by the extramucosal section of circular duodenal musculature in dogs. *Gastroenterology* 81: 910–914, 1981.
34. BOZLER, E. The action potentials of the stomach. *Am. J. Physiol.* 144: 693–700, 1945.
35. BRENER, W., T. R. HENDRIX, AND P. R. MCHUGH. Regulation of the gastric emptying of glucose. *Gastroenterology* 85: 76–82, 1983.
36. BRINK, B. M., J. F. SCHLEGEL, AND C. F. CODE. The pressure profile of the gastroduodenal junctional zone in dogs. *Gut* 6: 163–171, 1965.
37. BRODY, D. A., AND J. P. QUIGLEY. Application of the "inductograph" to the registration of movements, particularly of body structures such as the pyloric sphincter. *J. Lab. Clin. Med.* 29: 863–867, 1944.
38. BUENO, L., M. J. FARGEAS, J. FIORAMONTI, AND M. P. PRIMI. Central control of intestinal motility by prostaglandins: a mediator of the actions of several peptides in rats and dogs. *Gastroenterology* 88: 1888–1894, 1985.
39. BUENO, L., J. FIORAMONTI, M. J. FARGEAS, AND M. P. PRIMI. Neurotensin: a central neuromodulator of gastrointestinal motility in the dog. *Am. J. Physiol.* 248 (*Gastrointest. Liver Physiol.* 11): G15–G19, 1985.
40. BUENO, L., J. FIORAMONTI, AND Y. RUCKEBUSCH. Rate of flow of digesta and electrical activity of the small intestine in dogs and sheep. *J. Physiol. Lond.* 249: 69–85, 1975.
41. BUENO, L., F. PRADDAUDE, J. FIORAMONTI, AND Y. RUCKEBUSCH. Effect of dietary fiber on gastrointestinal motility and jejunal transit time in dogs. *Gastroenterology* 80: 701–707, 1981.
42. BUÉNO, L., AND M. RUCKEBUSCH. Insulin and jejunal electrical activity in dogs and sheep. *Am. J. Physiol.* 230: 1538–1544, 1976.
43. BURN-MURDOCH, R., M. A. FISHER, AND J. N. HUNT. Does lying on the right side increase the rate of gastric emptying? *J. Physiol. Lond.* 302: 395–398, 1980.
44. CAMERON, A. J., S. F. PHILLIPS, AND W. H. J. SUMMERSKILL. Comparison of effects of gastrin, cholecystokinin-pancreozymin, secretin, and glucagon on human stomach muscle in vitro. *Gastroenterology* 59: 539–545, 1970.
45. CAMILLERI, M., M. L. BROWN, AND J.-R. MALAGELADA. Altered gut transit in gastroparesis and pseudo-obstruction syndromes: correlation with regional motor dysfunction (Abstract). *Gastroenterology* 88: 1340, 1985.
46. CAMILLERI, M., M. L. BROWN, AND J.-R. MALAGELADA. Impaired transit of chyme in chronic intestinal pseudo-obstruction: correction by cisapride. *Gastroenterology* 91: 619–626, 1986.
47. CAMILLERI, M., M. L. BROWN, AND J.-R. MALAGELADA. Relationship between impaired gastric emptying and abnormal gastrointestinal motility. *Gastroenterology* 91: 94–99, 1986.
48. CAMILLERI, M., J.-R. MALAGELADA, M. L. BROWN, G. BECKER, AND A. R. ZINSMEISTER. Relation between antral motility and gastric emptying of solids and liquids in humans. *Am. J. Physiol.* 249 (*Gastrointest. Liver Physiol.* 12): G580–G585, 1985.
49. CANNON, W. B. The movements of the stomach studied by means of the röntgen rays. *Am. J. Physiol.* 1: 359–382, 1898.
50. CANNON, W. B. *The Mechanical Factors of Digestion.* New York: Longmans Green, 1911.
51. CANNON, W. B., AND C. W. LIEB. The receptive relaxation of the stomach. *Am. J. Physiol.* 29: 267–273, 1911.
52. CARLSON, H. C., C. F. CODE, AND R. A. NELSON. Motor action of the canine gastroduodenal junction: a cineradiographic, pressure, and electric study. *Am. J. Dig. Dis.* 11: 155–172, 1966.
53. CARRYER, P. W., M. L. BROWN, J.-R. MALAGELADA, G. L. CARLSON, AND J. T. MCCALL. Quantification of the fate of dietary fiber in humans by a newly developed radiolabeled fiber marker. *Gastroenterology* 82: 1389–1394, 1982.
54. CODE, C. F. The mystique of the gastroduodenal junction. *Rend. Romani Gastroenterol.* 2: 20–37, 1970.
55. CODE, C. F., AND H. C. CARLSON. Motor activity of the stomach: In: *Handbook of Physiology. The Alimentary Canal. Motility*, edited by C. F. Code. Washington, DC: Am. Physiol. Soc., 1967, sect. 6, vol. IV, chapt. 93, p. 1903–1916.
56. CODE, C. F., AND J. A. MARLETT. The interdigestive myoelectric complex of the stomach and small bowel of dogs. *J. Physiol. Lond.* 246: 289–309, 1975.
57. CODE, C. F., AND J. F. SCHLEGEL. Motor action of the esophagus and its sphincters. In: *Handbook of Physiology. Alimentary Canal. Motility*, edited by C. F. Code. Washington, DC: Am. Physiol. Soc., 1968, sect. 6, vol. IV, chapt. 90, p. 1821–1839.
58. CODE, C. F., AND J. F. SCHLEGEL. The gastrointestinal interdigestive housekeeper: motor correlates of the interdigestive myoelectric complex of the dog. In: *Proc. Int. Symp. Gastrointest. Motil., 4th, Banff, Alberta, Canada, 1973*, edited by E. E. Daniel. Vancouver: Mitchell, 1973, p. 631–634.
59. COLLIN, J., K. A. KELLY, AND S. F. PHILLIPS. Enhancement of absorption from the intact and transected canine small intestine by electrical pacing. *Gastroenterology* 76: 1422–1428, 1979.
60. COOKE, A. R. Localization of receptors inhibiting gastric emptying in the gut. *Gastroenterology* 72: 875–880, 1977.
61. COOKE, A. R., T. E. CHVASTA, AND N. W. WEISBRODT. Effect of pentagastrin on emptying and electrical and motor activity of the dog stomach. *Am. J. Physiol.* 223: 934–938, 1972.
62. COOTE, J. H., AND V. H. MACLEOD. The influence of bulbospinal monoaminergic pathways on sympathetic nerve activity. *J. Physiol. Lond.* 241: 453–475, 1974.
63. CORTOT, A., S. F. PHILLIPS, AND J.-R. MALAGELADA. Gastric emptying of lipids after ingestion of a solid-liquid meal in humans. *Gastroenterology* 80: 922–927, 1981.
64. CORTOT, A., S. F. PHILLIPS, AND J.-R. MALAGELADA. Parallel gastric emptying of nonhydrolzable fat and water after a solid-liquid meal in humans. *Gastroenterology* 82: 877–881, 1982.
65. COUTURIER, D., C. ROZÉ, J. PAOLAGGI, AND C. DEBRAY. Electrical activity of the normal human stomach: comparative study of recordings obtained from the serosal and mucosal sides. *Am. J. Dig. Dis.* 17: 969–976, 1972.
66. CRIDER, J. O., AND J. E. THOMAS. A study of gastric emptying with the pylorus open. *Am. J. Dig. Dis.* 4: 295–300, 1937.
67. DEBAS, H. T., O. FAROOQ, AND M. I. GROSSMAN. Inhibition of gastric emptying is a physiological action of cholecystokinin. *Gastroenterology* 68: 1211–1217, 1975.
68. DEBAS, H. T., T. YAMAGISHI, AND J. R. DRYBURGH. Motilin enhances gastric emptying of liquids in dogs. *Gastroenterology* 73: 777–780, 1977.
69. DELBRO, D., AND L. FÄNDRIKS. Inhibition of vagally induced non-adrenergic, non-cholinergic gastric relaxation by $P_2$-purinoceptor desensitization (Abstract). *Acta Physiol. Scand.* 120: 12A, 1984.
70. DENT, J., W. J. DODDS, T. SEKIGUCHI, W. J. HOGAN, AND R. C. ARNDORFER. Interdigestive phasic contractions of the human lower esophageal sphincter. *Gastroenterology* 84: 453–460, 1983.
71. DE PONTI, F., F. AZPIROZ, AND J.-R. MALAGELADA. Relaxatory responses of the canine proximal stomach to esophageal

and duodenal distention: importance of vagal pathways. *Dig. Dis. Sci.* In press.
72. DE WEVER, I., C. EECKHOUT, G. VANTRAPPEN, AND J. HELLEMANS. Disruptive effect of test meals on interdigestive motor complex in dogs. *Am. J. Physiol.* 235 (*Endocrinol. Metab.* 4): E661–E665, 1978.
73. DIAMANT, S. C., R. B. SCOTT, AND J. S. DAVISON. The effects of anaesthesia and surgery on the migrating myoelectric complex (MMC) in the ferret. *Gastroenterology* 88: 1365, 1985.
74. DIMAGNO, E. P., J. C. HENDRICKS, V. L. W. GO, AND R. R. DOZOIS. Relationships among canine fasting pancreatic and biliary secretions, pancreatic duct pressure, and duodenal phase III motor activity: Boldyreff revisited. *Dig. Dis. Sci.* 24: 689–693, 1979.
75. DOZOIS, R. R., AND K. A. KELLY. Effect of a gastrin pentapeptide on canine gastric emptying of liquids. *Am. J. Physiol.* 221: 113–117, 1971.
76. DOZOIS, R. R., K. A. KELLY, AND C. F. CODE. Effect of distal antrectomy on gastric emptying of liquids and solids. *Gastroenterology* 61: 675–681, 1971.
77. EDIN, R., J. LUNDBERG, L. TERENIUS, A. DAHLSTRÖM, T. HÖKFELT, J. KEWENTER, AND H. AHLMAN. Evidence for vagal enkephalinergic neural control of the feline pylorus and stomach. *Gastroenterology* 78: 492–497, 1980.
78. EHRLEIN, H.-J. Dehungmesstreifen zur Registrierung der Magen-Darm-Motorik bei wachen Versuchstieren. *Z. Gastroenterol.* 18: 191–197, 1980.
79. EHRLEIN, H.-J. A new technique for simultaneous radiography and recording of gastrointestinal motility in unanesthetized dogs. *Lab. Anim. Sci.* 30: 879–884, 1980.
80. EHRLEIN, H.-J., AND E. HIESINGER. Computer analysis of mechanical activity of gastroduodenal junction in unanaesthetized dogs. *Q. J. Exp. Physiol.* 67: 17–29, 1982.
81. EL-SHARKAWY, T. Y., K. G. MORGAN, AND J. H. SZURSZEWSKI. Intracellular electrical activity of canine and human gastric smooth muscle. *J. Physiol. Lond.* 279: 291–307, 1978.
82. ENGELHARDT, W., G. TOLKMITT, H.-J. EHRLEIN, AND L. H. STAHLGREN. Ein einfaches Gerät zur induktiven Messung der Darmmotilität mit implantierten Spulen. *Pfluegers Arch.* 294: 229–234, 1967.
83. ENRIQUEZ DE SALAMANCA, F., JR. Estudio de la fisiologia gastrica en él perro. *Trab. Inst. Nac. Cienc. Med. Madrid* 12: 2–64, 1949.
84. EWART, W. R., AND D. L. WINGATE. Central representation and opioid modulation of gastric mechanoreceptor activity in the rat. *Am. J. Physiol.* 244 (*Gastrointest. Liver Physiol.* 10): G27–G32, 1983.
85. FISHER, R., AND S. COHEN. Physiological characteristics of the human pyloric sphincter. *Gastroenterology* 64: 67–75, 1973.
86. FISHER, R. S., W. LIPSHUTZ, AND S. COHEN. The hormonal regulation of pyloric sphincter function. *J. Clin. Invest.* 52: 1289–1296, 1973.
87. FORDTRAN, J. S., AND T. W. LOCKLEAR. Ionic constituents and osmolality of gastric and small-intestinal fluids after eating. *Am. J. Dig. Dis.* 11: 503–521, 1966.
88. FOX, J. E. T., AND E. E. DANIEL. Substance P: a potent inhibitor of the canine small intestine in vivo. *Am. J. Physiol.* 250 (*Gastrointest. Liver Physiol.* 13): G21–G27, 1986.
89. GALLIGAN, J. J., AND T. F. BURKS. Centrally mediated inhibition of small intestinal transit and motility by morphine in the rat. *J. Pharmacol. Exp. Ther.* 226: 356–361, 1983.
90. GERSHON, M. D., AND C. F. DREYFUS. Serotoninergic neurons in the mammalian gut. In: *Nerves and the Gut*, edited by F. P. Brooks and P. L. Evers. Thorofare, NJ: Slack, 1977, p. 197–205.
91. GIANTURCO, C. Some mechanical factors of gastric physiology. Study I. The empty stomach and its various ways of filling: the pressure exerted by the gastric walls on the gastric content; the physical changes occurring to the foodstuff during digestion. *Am. J. Roentgenol.* 31: 735–744, 1934.
92. GIANTURCO, C. Some mechanical factors of gastric physiology. Study II. The pyloric mechanism: the effect of various foods on the emptying of the stomach. *Am. J. Roentgenol.* 31: 745–750, 1934.
93. GILL, R. C., M.-A. PILOT, P. A. THOMAS, AND D. L. WINGATE. Organization of fasting and postprandial myoelectric activity in stomach and duodenum of conscious dogs. *Am. J. Physiol.* 249 (*Gastrointest. Liver Physiol.* 12): G655–G661, 1985.
94. GLISE, H., AND H. ABRAHAMSSON. Reflex inhibition of gastric motility: pathophysiological aspects. *Scand. J. Gastroenterol.* 19, Suppl. 89: 77–82, 1984.
95. GRIDER, J. R., M. B. CABLE, S. I. SAID, AND G. M. MAKHLOUF. Vasoactive intestinal peptide as a neural mediator of gastric relaxation. *Am. J. Physiol.* 248 (*Gastrointest. Liver Physiol.* 11): G73–G78, 1985.
96. HALL, K. E., N. E. DIAMANT, T. Y. EL-SHARKAWY, AND G. R. GREENBERG. Effect of pancreatic polypeptide on canine migrating motor complex and plasma motilin. *Am. J. Physiol.* 245 (*Gastrointest. Liver Physiol.* 8): G178–G185, 1983.
97. HALL, K. E., T. Y. EL-SHARKAWY, AND N. E. DIAMANT. Vagal control of migrating motor complex in the dog. *Am. J. Physiol.* 243 (*Gastrointest. Liver Physiol.* 6): G276–G284, 1982.
98. HEADING, R. C. Duodenogastric reflux. *Gut* 24: 507–509, 1983.
99. HELLEMANS, J., G. VANTRAPPEN, J. JANSSENS, AND T. PEETERS. Effect of feeding and of gastrin on the interdigestive myoelectrical complex in man. In: *Gastrointestinal Motility in Health and Disease*, edited by H. L. Duthie. Baltimore, MD: University Park, 1978, p. 29–30.
100. HINDER, R. A. Individual and combined roles of the pylorus and the antrum in the canine gastric emptying of a liquid and a digestible solid. *Gastroenterology* 84: 281–286, 1983.
101. HINDER, R. A., AND K. A. KELLY. Canine gastric emptying of solids and liquids. *Am. J. Physiol.* 233: (*Endocrinol. Metab.* 2): E335–E340, 1977.
102. HOLGATE, A. M., AND N. W. READ. Relationship between small bowel transit time and absorption of a solid meal: influence of metoclopramide, magnesium sulfate, and lactulose. *Dig. Dis. Sci.* 28: 812–819, 1983.
103. HOLGATE, A. M., AND N. W. READ. Effect of ileal infusion of intralipid on gastrointestinal transit, ileal flow rate, and carbohydrate absorption in humans after ingestion of a liquid meal. *Gastroenterology* 88: 1005–1011, 1985.
104. HOLLOWAY, R. H., E. BLANK, I. TAKAHASHI, W. J. DODDS, W. J. HOGAN, AND J. DENT. Variability of lower esophageal sphincter pressure in the fasted unanesthetized opossum. *Am. J. Physiol.* 248 (*Gastrointest. Liver Physiol.* 11): G398–G406, 1985.
105. HOLT, S., R. C. HEADING, D. C. CARTER, L. F. PRESCOTT, AND P. TOTHILL. Effect of gel fibre on gastric emptying and absorption of glucose and paracetamol. *Lancet* 1: 636–639, 1979.
106. HOUPT, T. R., K. A. HOUPT, AND A. A. SWAN. Duodenal osmoconcentration and food intake in pigs after ingestion of hypertonic nutrients. *Am. J. Physiol.* 245 (*Regulatory Integrative Comp. Physiol.* 14): R181–R189, 1983.
107. HUNT, J. N. Does calcium mediate slowing of gastric emptying by fat in humans? *Am. J. Physiol.* 244 (*Gastrointest. Liver Physiol.* 7): G89–G94, 1983.
108. HUNT, J. N., AND I. MACDONALD. The influence of volume on gastric emptying. *J. Physiol. Lond.* 126: 459–474, 1954.
109. HUNT, J. N., AND N. RAMSBOTTOM. Effect of gastrin II on gastric emptying and secretion during a test meal. *Br. Med. J.* 4: 386–387, 1967.
110. HUNT, J. N., J. L. SMITH, AND C. L. JIANG. Effect of meal volume and energy density on the gastric emptying of carbohydrates. *Gastroenterology* 89: 1326–1330, 1985.
111. HUNT, J. N., AND D. F. STUBBS. The volume and energy content of meals as determinants of gastric emptying. *J. Physiol. Lond.* 245: 209–225, 1975.
112. ISENBERG, J. I., AND A. CSENDES. Effect of octapeptide of cholecystokinin on canine pyloric pressure. *Am. J. Physiol.* 222: 428–431, 1972.

113. ITOH, Z., I. AIZAWA, AND T. SEKIGUCHI. The interdigestive migrating complex and its significance in man. *Clin. Gastroenterol.* 11: 497–521, 1982.
114. ITOH, Z., I. AIZAWA, S. TAKEUCHI, AND R. TAKAYANAGI. Diurnal changes in gastric motor activity in conscious dogs. *Am. J. Dig. Dis.* 22: 117–124, 1977.
115. ITOH, Z., R. HONDA, I. AIZAWA, S. TAKEUCHI, K. HIWATASHI, AND E. F. COUCH. Interdigestive motor activity of the lower esophageal sphincter in the conscious dog. *Am. J. Dig. Dis.* 23: 239–247, 1978.
116. ITOH, Z., R. HONDA, S. TAKEUCHI, I. AIZAWA, AND R. TAKAYANAGI. An extraluminal force transducer for recording contractile activity of the gastrointestinal smooth muscle in the conscious dogs: its construction and implantation. *Gastroenterol. Jpn.* 12: 275–283, 1977.
117. ITOH, Z., R. TAKAYANAGI, S. TAKEUCHI, AND S. ISSHIKI. Interdigestive motor activity of Heidenhain pouches in relation to main stomach in conscious dogs. *Am. J. Physiol.* 234 (*Endocrinol. Metab.* 3): E333–E338, 1978.
118. ITOH, Z., S. TAKEUCHI, I. AIZAWA, K. MORI, T. TAMINATO, Y. SEINO, H. IMURA, AND N. YANAIHARA. Changes in plasma motilin concentration and gastrointestinal contractile activity in conscious dogs. *Am. J. Dig. Dis.* 23: 929–935, 1978.
119. ITOH, Z., S. TAKEUCHI, I. AIZAWA, AND R. TAKAYANAGI. Characteristic motor activity of the gastrointestinal tract in fasted conscious dogs measured by implanted force transducers. *Am. J. Dig. Dis.* 23: 229–238, 1978.
120. JACOBS, F., L. M. A. AKKERMANS, O. H. YOE, A. HOEKSTRA, AND P. WITTEBOL. A radioisotope method to quantify the function of fundus, antrum, and their contractile activity in gastric emptying of a semi-solid and solid meal. In: *Motility of the Digestive Tract*, edited by M. Wienbeck. New York: Raven, 1982, p. 233–240.
121. JACOBY, H. I., P. BASS, AND D. R. BENNETT. In vivo extraluminal contractile force transducer for gastrointestinal muscle. *J. Appl. Physiol.* 18: 658–665, 1963.
122. JAHNBERG, T., H. ABRAHAMSSON, G. JANSSON, AND J. MARTINSON. Gastric relaxatory response to feeding before and after vagotomy. *Scand. J. Gastroenterol.* 12: 225–228, 1977.
123. JAHNBERG, T., H. ABRAHAMSSON, G. JANSSON, AND J. MARTINSON. Vagal gastric relaxation in the dog. *Scand. J. Gastroenterol.* 12: 221–224, 1977.
124. JAHNBERG, T., J. MARTINSON, L. HULTÉN, AND S. FASTH. Dynamic gastric response to expansion before and after vagotomy. *Scand. J. Gastroenterol.* 10: 593–598, 1975.
125. JANSSON, G. Vago-vagal reflex relaxation of the stomach in the cat. *Acta Physiol. Scand.* 75: 245–252, 1969.
126. JIAN, R., A. PECKING, Y. NAJEAN, AND J. J. BERNIER. Étude de la progression d'un repas dans l'intestin grêle de l'homme par une méthode scintigraphique. *Gastroenterol. Clin. Biol.* 3: 755–762, 1979.
127. JIANG, C.-L., AND J. N. HUNT. The relation between freely chosen meals and body habitus. *Am. J. Clin. Nutr.* 38: 32–40, 1983.
128. KACHEL, G., H. RUPPIN, J. HAGEL, W. BARINA, M. MEINHARDT, AND W. DOMSCHKE. Human intestinal motor activity and transport: effects of a synthetic opiate. *Gastroenterology* 90: 85–93, 1986.
129. KAYE, M. D., S. J. MEHTA, AND J. P. SHOWALTER. Manometric studies of the human pylorus. *Gastroenterology* 70: 477–480, 1976.
130. KEANE, F. B., E. P. DIMAGNO, AND J.-R. MALAGELADA. Duodenogastric reflux in humans: its relationship to fasting antroduodenal motility and gastric, pancreatic, and biliary secretion. *Gastroenterology* 81: 726–731, 1981.
131. KEINKE, O., AND H.-J. EHRLEIN. Effect of oleic acid on canine gastroduodenal motility, pyloric diameter and gastric emptying. *Q. J. Exp. Physiol.* 68: 675–686, 1983.
132. KELLOW, J. E., T. J. BORODY, S. F. PHILLIPS, R. L. TUCKER, AND A. C. HADDAD. Human interdigestive motility: variations in patterns from esophagus to colon. *Gastroenterology* 91: 386–395, 1986.
133. KELLEY, K. A. Gastric motility after gastric operations. *Surg. Ann.* 6: 103–123, 1974.
134. KELLY, K. A. Gastric emptying of liquids and solids: roles of proximal and distal stomach. *Am. J. Physiol.* 239 (*Gastrointest. Liver Physiol.* 2): G71–G76, 1980.
135. KELLY, K. A., AND C. F. CODE. Effect of transthoracic vagotomy on canine gastric electrical activity. *Gastroenterology* 57: 51–58, 1969.
136. KELLY, K. A., C. F. CODE, AND L. R. ELVEBACK. Patterns of canine gastric electrical activity. *Am. J. Physiol.* 217: 461–470, 1969.
137. KELLY, K. A., J. M. ROBERTS, AND R. ROBERTS. Receptive relaxation and other motor properties of the proximal stomach. *Ital. J. Gastroenterol.* 15: 148–151, 1983.
138. KERLIN, P., A. ZINSMEISTER, AND S. PHILLIPS. Relationship of motility to flow of contents in the human small intestine. *Gastroenterology* 82: 701–706, 1982.
139. KING, P. M., R. D. ADAM, A. PRYDE, W. N. MCDICKEN, AND R. C. HEADING. Relationships of human antroduodenal motility and transpyloric fluid movement: non-invasive observations with real-time ultrasound. *Gut* 25: 1384–1391, 1984.
140. KRAMER, P., M. M. KEARNEY, AND F. J. INGELFINGER. The effect of specific foods and water loading on the ileal excreta of ileostomized human subjects. *Gastroenterology* 42: 535–545, 1962.
141. KRUIS, W., F. AZPIROZ, AND S. F. PHILLIPS. Contractile patterns and transit of fluid in canine terminal ileum. *Am. J. Physiol.* 249 (*Gastrointest. Liver Physiol.* 12): G264–G270, 1985.
142. LANG, I. M., S. K. SARNA, AND R. E. CONDON. Gastrointestinal motor correlates of vomiting in the dog: quantification and characterization as an independent phenomenon. *Gastroenterology* 90: 40–47, 1986.
143. LAWSON, M., F. KERN, JR., AND G. T. EVERSON. Gastrointestinal transit time in human pregnancy: prolongation in the second and third trimesters followed by postpartum normalization. *Gastroenterology* 89: 996–999, 1985.
144. LAYER, P., A. R. ZINSMEISTER, AND E. P. DIMAGNO. Effects of decreasing intraluminal amylase activity on starch digestion and postprandial gastrointestinal function in humans. *Gastroenterology* 91: 41–48, 1986.
145. LEEK, B. F. Abdominal and pelvic visceral receptors. *Br. Med. Bull.* 33: 163–168, 1977.
146. LEFEBVRE, R. A., J. L. WILLEMS, AND M. G. BOGAERT. Inhibitory effect of dopamine on canine gastric fundus. *Naunyn-Schmiedebergs Arch. Pharmakol.* 326: 22–28, 1984.
147. LIDDLE, R. A., E. T. MORITA, C. K. CONRAD, AND J. A. WILLIAMS. Regulation of gastric emptying in humans by cholecystokinin. *J. Clin. Invest.* 77: 992–996, 1986.
148. LIND, J. F., H. L. DUTHIE, J. F. SCHLEGEL, AND C. F. CODE. Motility of the gastric fundus. *Am. J. Physiol.* 201: 197–202, 1961.
149. LOEWY, A. D. Descending pathways to sympathetic and parasympathetic preganglionic neurons. *J. Auton. Nerv. Syst.* 3: 265–275, 1981.
150. LOUCKES, H. S., J. P. QUIGLEY, AND J. KERSEY. Inductograph method for recording muscle activity, especially pyloric sphincter physiology. *Am. J. Physiol.* 199: 301–310, 1960.
151. MALAGELADA, J.-R. Quantification of gastric solid-liquid discrimination during digestion of ordinary meals. *Gastroenterology* 72: 1264–1267, 1977.
152. MALAGELADA, J.-R. Gastric, pancreatic, and biliary responses to a meal. In: *Physiology of the Gastrointestinal Tract*, edited by L. R. Johnson, J. Christensen, M. I. Grossman, E. D. Jacobson, and S. G. Schultz. New York: Raven, 1981, p. 893–924.
153. MALAGELADA, J.-R., V. L. W. GO, AND W. H. J. SUMMERSKILL. Different gastric, pancreatic, and biliary responses to solid-liquid or homogenized meals. *Dig. Dis. Sci.* 24: 101–110, 1979.

154. MALAGELADA, J.-R., G. F. LONGSTRETH, W. H. J. SUMMERSKILL, AND V. L. W. GO. Measurement of gastric functions during digestion of ordinary solid meals in man. *Gastroenterology* 70: 203–210, 1976.
155. MALAGELADA, J.-R., W. D. W. REES, L. J. MAZZOTTA, AND V. L. W. GO. Gastric motor abnormalities in diabetic and postvagotomy gastroparesis: effect of metoclopramide and bethanechol. *Gastroenterology* 78: 286–293, 1980.
156. MALAGELADA, J.-R., J. S. ROBERTSON, M. L. BROWN, M. REMINGTON, J. A. DUENES, G. J. THOMFORDE, AND P. W. CARRYER. Intestinal transit of solid and liquid components of a meal in health. *Gastroenterology* 87: 1255–1263, 1984.
157. MARIK, F., AND C. F. CODE. Control of the interdigestive myoelectric activity in dogs by the vagus nerves and pentagastrin. *Gastroenterology* 69: 387–395, 1975.
158. MARTINSON, J. The effect of graded stimulation of efferent vagal nerve fibres on gastric motility. *Acta Physiol. Scand.* 62: 256–262, 1964.
159. MARTINSON, J. The effect of graded vagal stimulation on gastric motility, secretion and blood flow in the cat. *Acta Physiol. Scand.* 65: 300–4309, 1965.
160. MARTINSON, J., AND A. MUREN. Excitatory and inhibitory effects of vagus stimulation on gastric motility in the cat. *Acta Physiol. Scand.* 57: 309–316, 1963.
161. MATHIAS, J. R., G. M. CARLSON, A. J. DIMARINO, G. BERTIGER, H. E. MORTON, AND S. COHEN. Intestinal myoelectric activity in response to live *Vibrio cholerae* and cholera enterotoxin. *J. Clin. Invest.* 58: 91–96, 1976.
162. MATHIAS, J. R., AND C. A. SNINSKY. Motility of the small intestine: a look ahead. *Am. J. Physiol.* 248 (*Gastrointest. Liver Physiol.* 11): G495–G500, 1985.
163. MAYER, E. A., J. B. THOMSON, D. JEHN, T. REEDY, J. ELASHOFF, C. DEVENY, AND J. H. MEYER. Gastric emptying and sieving of solid food and pancreatic and biliary secretions after solid meals in patients with nonresective ulcer surgery. *Gastroenterology* 87: 1264–1271, 1984.
164. MAYER, E. A., J. B. THOMSON, D. JEHN, T. REEDY, J. ELASHOFF, AND J. H. MEYER. Gastric emptying and sieving of food and pancreatic and biliary secretion after solid meals in patients with truncal vagotomy and antrectomy. *Gastroenterology* 83: 184–192, 1982.
165. MCHUGH, P. R. Aspects of the control of feeding: application of quantitation in psychobiology. *Johns Hopkins Med. J.* 144: 147–155, 1979.
166. MEARIN, F., F. AZPIROZ, AND J.-R. MALAGELADA. Measurement of resistance to flow across the antroduodenal area during fasting. *Am. J. Physiol.* 250 (*Gastrointest. Liver Physiol.* 13): G773–G780, 1986.
167. MEARIN, F., F. AZPIROZ, AND J.-R. MALAGELADA. Pyloric contribution to antroduodenal resistance to flow in the conscious dog. *Am. J. Physiol.* 253 (*Gastrointest. Liver Physiol.* 16): G72–G78, 1987.
168. MEARIN, F., F. AZPIROZ, J.-R. MALAGELADA, AND A. R. ZINSMEISTER. Antroduodenal resistance to flow in the control of duodenogastric bile reflux during fasting. *Gastroenterology* 93: 1026–1033, 1987.
169. MEEROFF, J. C., V. L. W. GO, AND S. F. PHILLIPS. Control of gastric emptying by osmolality of duodenal contents in man. *Gastroenterology* 68: 1144–1151, 1975.
170. MELVILLE, J., E. MACAGNO, AND J. CHRISTENSEN. Longitudinal contractions in the duodenum: their fluid-mechanical function. *Am. J. Physiol.* 228: 1887–1892, 1975.
171. MEYER, J. H., J. DRESSMAN, A. FINK, AND G. AMIDON. Effect of size and density on canine gastric emptying of nondigestible solids. *Gastroenterology* 89: 805–813, 1985.
172. MEYER, J. H., E. A. MAYER, D. JEHN, Y. GU, A. S. FINK, AND M. FRIED. Gastric processing and emptying of fat. *Gastroenterology* 90: 1176–1187, 1986.
173. MEYER, J. H., H. OHASHI, D. JEHN, AND J. B. THOMSON. Size of liver particles emptied from the human stomach. *Gastroenterology* 80: 1489–1496, 1981.
174. MEYER, J. H., J. B. THOMSON, M. B. COHEN, A. SHADCHEHR, AND S. A. MANDIOLA. Sieving of solid food by the canine stomach and sieving after gastric surgery. *Gastroenterology* 76: 804–813, 1979.
175. MEYER, J. H., G. VANDEVENTER, L. S. GRAHAM, J. THOMSON, AND D. THOMASSON. Error and corrections with scintigraphic measurement of gastric emptying of solid foods. *J. Nucl. Med.* 24: 197–203, 1983.
176. MILLAR, H. D., AND L. E. BAKER. A stable ultraminiature catheter-tip pressure transducer. *Med. Biol. Eng.* 11: 86–89, 1973.
177. MILLER, J., G. KAUFFMAN, J. ELASHOFF, H. OHASHI, D. CARTER, AND J. H. MEYER. Search for resistances controlling canine gastric emptying of liquid meals. *Am. J. Physiol.* 241 (*Gastrointest. Liver Physiol.* 4): G403–G415, 1981.
178. MILLER, L. J., J.-R. MALAGELADA, AND V. L. W. GO. Postprandial duodenal function in man. *Gut* 19: 699–706, 1978.
179. MILLER, L. J., J.-R. MALAGELADA, W. F. TAYLOR, AND V. L. W. GO. Intestinal control of human postprandial gastric function: the role of components of jejunoileal chyme in regulating gastric secretion and gastric emptying. *Gastroenterology* 80: 763–769, 1981.
180. MINAMI, H., AND R. W. MCCALLUM. The physiology and pathophysiology of gastric emptying in humans. *Gastroenterology* 86: 1592–1610, 1984.
181. MIOLAN, J.-P., AND C. ROMAN. Discharge of efferent vagal fibers supplying gastric antrum: indirect study by nerve suture technique. *Am. J. Physiol.* 235 (*Endocrinol. Metab.* 4): E366–E373, 1978.
182. MOJAVERIAN, P., R. K. FERGUSON, P. H. VLASSES, M. L. ROCCI, JR., A. OREN, J. A. FIX, L. J. CALDWELL, AND C. GARDNER. Estimation of gastric residence time of the Heidelberg capsule in humans: effect of varying food composition. *Gastroenterology* 89: 392–397, 1985.
183. MOORE, J. G., P. E. CHRISTIAN, J. A. BROWN, C. BROPHY, F. DATZ, A. TAYLOR, AND N. ALAZRAKI. Influence of meal weight and caloric content on gastric emptying of meals in man. *Dig. Dis. Sci.* 29: 513–519, 1984.
184. MORGAN, K. G., T. C. MUIR, AND J. H. SZURSZEWSKI. The electrical basis for contraction and relaxation in canine fundal smooth muscle. *J. Physiol. Lond.* 311: 475–488, 1981.
185. MORGAN, K. G., P. F. SCHMALZ, V. L. W. GO, AND J. H. SZURSZEWSKI. Electrical and mechanical effects of molecular variants of CCK on antral smooth muscle. *Am. J. Physiol.* 235 (*Endocrinol. Metab.* 4): E324–E329, 1978.
186. MORGAN, K. G., P. F. SCHMALZ, AND J. H. SZURSZEWSKI. The inhibitory effects of vasoactive intestinal polypeptide on the mechanical and electrical activity of the canine antral smooth muscle. *J. Physiol. Lond.* 282: 437–450, 1978.
187. MORGAN, K. G., AND J. H. SZURSZEWSKI. Mechanisms of phasic and tonic actions of pentagastrin on canine gastric smooth muscle. *J. Physiol. Lond.* 301: 229–242, 1980.
188. MROZ, C. T., AND K. A. KELLY. The role of the extrinsic antral nerves in the regulation of gastric emptying. *Surg. Gynecol. Obstet.* 145: 369–377, 1977.
189. MUKHOPADHYAY, A. K., L. R. JOHNSON, E. M. COPELAND, AND N. W. WEISBRODT. Effect of secretin on electrical activity of small intestine. *Am. J. Physiol.* 229: 484–488, 1975.
190. MUKHOPADHYAY, A. K., P. J. THOR, E. M. COPELAND, L. R. JOHNSON, AND N. W. WEISBRODT. Effect of cholecystokinin on myoelectric activity of the small bowel of the dog. *Am. J. Physiol.* 232 (*Endocrinol. Metab.* 1): E44–E47, 1977.
191. MUKHOPADHYAY, A. K., N. W. WEISBRODT, E. D. COPELAND, AND L. R. JOHNSON. Effect of prostaglandin $E_2$ infusion on patterns of intestinal myoelectric activity (Abstract). *Gastroenterology* 66: 752, 1974.
192. MÜLLER-LISSNER, S. A., A. SONNENBERG, A. HOLLINGER, G. SCHATTENMANN, J. R. SIEWERT, AND A. L. BLUM. Gastric emptying and postprandial duodenogastric reflux in dogs with Heineke-Mikulicz pyloroplasty. *Br. J. Surg.* 69: 323–327, 1982.
193. MÜLLER-LISSNER, S. A., A. SONNENBERG, G. SCHATTEN-

MANN, A. HOLLINGER, J. R. SIEWERT, AND A. L. BLUM. Gastric emptying and postprandial duodenogastric reflux in pylorectomized dogs. *Am. J. Physiol.* 242 (*Gastrointest. Liver Physiol.* 5): G9–G14, 1982.
194. NELSEN, T. S., AND J. C. BECKER. Simulation of the electrical and mechanical gradient of the small intestine. *Am. J. Physiol.* 214: 749–757, 1968.
195. NORMAN, W. P., F. D. PAGANI, H. S. ORMSBEE, III, D. K. KASBEKAR, AND R. A. GILLIS. Use of horseradish peroxidase to identify hindbrain sites that influence gastric motility in the cat. *Gastroenterology* 88: 701–705, 1985.
196. OHASHI, H., AND J. H. MEYER. Effect of peptic digestion on emptying of cooked liver in dogs. *Gastroenterology* 79: 305–310, 1980.
197. OHGA, A., Y. NAKAZATO, AND K. SAITO. Considerations of the efferent nervous mechanism of the vago-vagal reflex relaxation of the stomach in the dog. *Jpn. J. Pharmacol.* 20: 116–130, 1970.
198. OKIKE, N., AND K. A. KELLY. Vagotomy impairs pentagastrin-induced relaxation of canine gastric fundus. *Am. J. Physiol.* 232 (*Endocrinol. Metab.* 1): E504–E509, 1977.
199. PAGANI, F. D., W. P. NORMAN, D. K. KASBEKAR, AND R. A. GILLIS. Localization of sites within dorsal motor nucleus of vagus that affect gastric motility. *Am. J. Physiol.* 249 (*Gastrointest. Liver Physiol.* 12): G73–G84, 1985.
200. PANDOLFO, N., M. BORTOLOTTI, C. NEBIACOLOMBO, G. LABÒ, AND F. MATTIOLI. Prolonged manometric study of the gastroduodenal junction in man. *Digestion* 19: 86–92, 1979.
201. POZO, F., A. FUEYO, M. M. ESTEBAN, J. M. ROJO-ORTEGA, AND B. MARÍN. Blood pressure changes after gastric mechanical and electrical stimulation in rats. *Am. J. Physiol.* 249 (*Gastrointest. Liver Physiol.* 12): G739–G744, 1985.
202. PRÖVE, J., AND H.-J. EHRLEIN. Motor function of gastric antrum and pylorus for evacuation of low and high viscosity meals in dogs. *Gut* 23: 150–156, 1982.
203. PUBLICOVER, N. G., AND K. M. SANDERS. Myogenic regulation of propagation in gastric smooth muscle. *Am. J. Physiol.* 248 (*Gastrointest. Liver Physiol.* 11): G512–G520, 1985.
204. QUIGLEY, E. M. M., T. J. BORODY, S. F. PHILLIPS, M. WIENBECK, R. L. TUCKER, AND A. HADDAD. Motility of the terminal ileum and ileocecal sphincter in healthy humans. *Gastroenterology* 87: 857–866, 1984.
205. QUIGLEY, E. M. M., S. F. PHILLIPS, AND J. DENT. Distinctive patterns of interdigestive motility at the canine ileocolonic junction. *Gastroenterology* 87: 836–844, 1984.
206. QUIGLEY, J. P., M. R. READ, K. H. RADZOW, I. MESCHAN, AND J. M. WERLE. The effect of hydrochloric acid on the pyloric sphincter, the adjacent portions of the digestive tract and on the process of gastric evacuation. *Am. J. Physiol.* 137: 153–159, 1942.
207. READ, N. W., J. CAMMACK, C. EDWARDS, A. M. HOLGATE, P. A. CANN, AND C. BROWN. Is the transit time of a meal through the small intestine related to the rate at which it leaves the stomach? *Gut* 23: 824–828, 1982.
208. REES, W. D. W., V. L. W. GO, AND J.-R. MALAGELADA. Antroduodenal motor response to solid-liquid and homogenized meals. *Gastroenterology* 76: 1438–1442, 1979.
209. REES, W. D. W., V. L. W. GO, AND J.-R. MALAGELADA. Simultaneous measurement of antroduodenal motility, gastric emptying, and duodenogastric reflux in man. *Gut* 20: 963–970, 1979.
210. REES, W. D. W., J.-R. MALAGELADA, L. J. MILLER, AND V. L. W. GO. Human interdigestive and postprandial gastrointestinal motor and gastrointestinal hormone patterns. *Dig. Dis. Sci.* 27: 321–329, 1982.
211. REES, W. D. W., L. J. MILLER, AND J.-R. MALAGELADA. Dyspepsia, antral motor dysfunction, and gastric stasis of solids. *Gastroenterology* 78: 360–365, 1980.
212. REINKE, D. A., A. H. ROSENBAUM, AND D. R. BENNETT. Patterns of dog gastrointestinal contractile activity monitored in vivo with extraluminal force transducers. *Am. J. Dig. Dis.* 12: 113–141, 1967.
213. REMINGTON, M., J.-R. MALAGELADA, A. ZINSMEISTER, AND C. R. FLEMING. Abnormalities in gastrointestinal motor activity in patients with short bowels: effect of a synthetic opiate. *Gastroenterology* 85: 629–636, 1983.
214. REYNOLDS, J. C., A. OUYANG, AND S. COHEN. Opiate nerves mediate feline pyloric response to intraduodenal amino acids. *Am. J. Physiol.* 248 (*Gastrointest. Liver Physiol.* 11): G307–G312, 1985.
215. ROMAN, C., AND J. GONELLA. Extrinsic control of digestive tract motility. In: *Physiology of the Gastrointestinal Tract*, edited by L. R. Johnson, J. Christensen, M. I. Grossman, E. D. Jacobson, and S. G. Schultz. New York: Raven, 1981, p. 289–333.
216. ROMAN, C., AND L. TIEFFENBACH. Enregistrement de l'activité unitaire des fibres motrices vagales destinées à l'oesophage du babouin. *J. Physiol. Paris* 64: 479–506, 1972.
217. ROZÉ, C., D. COUTURIER, J. CHARIOT, AND C. DEBRAY. Inhibition of gastric electrical and mechanical activity by intraduodenal agents in pigs and the effects of vagotomy. *Digestion* 15: 526–539, 1977.
218. RUCKEBUSCH, M., AND J. FIORAMONTI. Insulino-sécrétion et motricite intestinale. *C. R. Soc. Biol.* 169: 435–439, 1975.
219. RUSSELL, J., AND P. BASS. Canine gastric emptying of fiber meals: influence of meal viscosity and antroduodenal motility. *Am. J. Physiol.* 249 (*Gastrointest. Liver Physiol.* 12): G662–G667, 1985.
220. RUSSELL, J., AND P. BASS. Canine gastric emptying of polycarbophil: an indigestible, particulate substance. *Gastroenterology* 89: 307–312, 1985.
221. SAGAR, S., J. S. GRIME, W. LITTLE, M. PATTEN, P. GULLIFORD, M. CRITCHLEY, R. BENNETT, AND R. SHIELDS. Technetium-99m labelled bran: a new agent for measuring gastric emptying. *Clin. Radiol.* 34: 275–278, 1983.
222. SARNA, S. K., E. E. DANIEL, AND Y. J. KINGMA. Simulation of the electric-control activity of the stomach by an array of relaxation oscillators. *Am. J. Dig. Dis.* 17: 299–310, 1972.
223. SARR, M. G., AND K. A. KELLY. Patterns of movement of liquids and solids through canine jejunum. *Am. J. Physiol.* 239 (*Gastrointest. Liver Physiol.* 2): G497–G503, 1980.
224. SARR, M. G., K. A. KELLY, AND S. F. PHILLIPS. Canine jejunal absorption and transit during interdigestive and digestive motor states. *Am. J. Physiol.* 239 (*Gastrointest. Liver Physiol.* 2): G167–G172, 1980.
225. SCHADE, R. R., M. J. PELEKANOS, W. N. TAUXE, AND D. H. VAN THIEL. Gastric emptying during pregnancy (Abstract). *Gastroenterology* 86: 1234, 1984.
226. SCHEMANN, M., AND H.-J. EHRLEIN. The utility of cellulose meals for studies on gastrointestinal motility in dogs. *Digestion* 25: 194–196, 1982.
227. SCHILLER, L. R., G. R. DAVIS, C. A. SANTA ANA, S. G. MORAWSKI, AND J. S. FORDTRAN. Studies of the mechanism of the antidiarrheal effect of codeine. *J. Clin. Invest.* 70: 999–1008, 1982.
228. SCHLEGEL, J. F., AND C. F. CODE. The gastric peristalsis of the interdigestive housekeeper. In: *Proc. 5th Int. Symp. Gastrointest. Motil.*, edited by G. Vantrappen. Leuven, Belgium: Typoff, 1975, p. 321.
229. SCHULZE-DELRIEU, K. Volume accommodation by distension of gastric fundus (rabbit) and gastric corpus (cat). *Dig. Dis. Sci.* 28: 625–632, 1985.
230. SCHULZE-DELRIEU, K., AND C. K. BROWN. Emptying of saline meals by the cat stomach as a function of pyloric resistance. *Am. J. Physiol.* 249 (*Gastrointest. Liver Physiol.* 12): G725–G732, 1985.
231. SCHULZE-DELRIEU, K., AND S. S. SHIRAZI. Neuromuscular differentiation of the human pylorus. *Gastroenterology* 84: 287–292, 1983.
232. SCHULZE-DELRIEU, K., AND J. P. WALL. Determinants of flow across isolated gastroduodenal junctions of cats and rabbits. *Am. J. Physiol.* 245 (*Gastrointest. Liver Physiol.* 8): G257–

G264, 1983.
233. SCOTT, R. B., T. Y. EL-SHARKAWY, AND N. E. DIAMANT. Propagation of the canine migrating myoelectric complex: a mathematical model. *Am. J. Physiol.* 244 (*Gastrointest. Liver Physiol.* 7): G13–G19, 1983.
234. SEIDE, K., AND E. L. RITMAN. Three-dimensional dynamic X-ray-computed tomography imaging of stomach motility. *Am. J. Physiol.* 247 (*Gastrointest. Liver Physiol.* 10): G574–G581, 1984.
235. SMIDDY, F. G., S. D. GREGORY, I. B. SMITH, AND J. C. GOLIGHER. Faecal loss of fluid, electrolytes, and nitrogen in colitis before and after ileostomy. *Lancet* 1: 14–19, 1960.
236. SMITH, C. C., AND K. R. BRIZZEE. Cineradiographic analysis of vomiting in the cat. I. Lower esophagus, stomach, and small intestine. *Gastroenterology* 40: 654–664, 1961.
237. SMITH, G. P., AND J. GIBBS. Postprandial satiety. In: *Progress in Psychobiology and Physiological Psychology*, edited by J. M. Sprague and A. N. Epstein. New York: Academic, 1979, p. 179–242.
238. SMITH, J., K. A. KELLY, AND R. M. WEINSHILBOUM. Pathophysiology of postoperative ileus. *Arch. Surg.* 112: 203–209, 1977.
239. SONNENBERG, A., S. A. MÜLLER-LISSNER, G. SCHATTENMANN, J. R. SIEWERT, AND A. L. BLUM. Duodenogastric reflux in the dog. *Am. J. Physiol.* 242 (*Gastrointest. Liver Physiol.* 5): G603–G607, 1982.
240. SPILLER, R. C., I. F. TROTMAN, B. E. HIGGINS, M. A. GHATEI, Y. C. LEES, S. R. BLOOM, J. J. MISIEWICZ, AND D. B. A. SILK. Inhibition of jejunal motility by ileal fat infusion in man (Abstract). *Gut* 24: 472, 1983.
241. STANGHELLINI, V., J.-R. MALAGELADA, A. R. ZINSMEISTER, V. L. W. GO, AND P. C. KAO. Stress-induced gastroduodenal motor disturbances in humans: possible humoral mechanisms. *Gastroenterology* 85: 83–91, 1983.
242. STANGHELLINI, V., J.-R. MALAGELADA, A. R. ZINSMEISTER, V. L. W. GO, AND P. C. KAO. Effect of opiate and adrenergic blockers on the gut motor response to centrally acting stimuli. *Gastroenterology* 87: 1104–1113, 1984.
243. STEMPER, T. J., AND A. R. COOKE. Gastric emptying and its relationship to antral contractile activity. *Gastroenterology* 69: 649–653, 1975.
244. STEMPER, T. J., AND A. R. COOKE. Effect of a fixed pyloric opening on gastric emptying in the cat and dog. *Am. J. Physiol.* 230: 813–817, 1976.
245. STRUNZ, U., W. DOMSCHKE, P. MITZNEGG, S. DOMSCHKE, E. SCHUBERT, E. WÜNSCH, E. JAEGER, AND L. DEMLING. Analysis of the motor effects of 13-norleucine motilin on the rabbit, guinea pig, rat, and human alimentary tract in vitro. *Gastroenterology* 68: 1485–1491, 1975.
246. STRUNZ, U. T., AND M. I. GROSSMAN. Effect of intragastric pressure on gastric emptying and secretion. *Am. J. Physiol.* 235 (*Endocrinol. Metab.* 4): E552–E555, 1978.
247. SUMMERS, R. W., J. HELM, AND J. CHRISTENSEN. Intestinal propulsion in the dog: its relation to food intake and the migratory myoelectric complex. *Gastroenterology* 70: 753–758, 1976.
248. SZURSZEWSKI, J. H. A migrating electric complex of the canine small intestine. *Am. J. Physiol.* 217: 1757–1763, 1969.
249. SZURSZEWSKI, J. H. Mechanism of action of pentagastrin and acetylcholine on the longitudinal muscle of the canine antrum. *J. Physiol. Lond.* 252: 335–361, 1975.
250. SZURSZEWSKI, J. H. Electrical basis for gastrointestinal motility. In: *Physiology of the Gastrointestinal Tract*, edited by L. R. Johnson, J. Christensen, M. I. Grossman, E. D. Jacobson, and S. G. Schultz. New York: Raven, 1981, p. 1435–1466.
251. SZURSZEWSKI, J. H. Physiology of mammalian prevertebral ganglia. *Annu. Rev. Physiol.* 43: 53–68, 1981.
252. THOMAS, J. E. Mechanics and regulation of gastric emptying. *Physiol. Rev.* 37: 453–474, 1957.
253. THOMAS, P. A., AND K. A. KELLY. Hormonal control of interdigestive motor cycles of canine proximal stomach. *Am. J. Physiol.* 237 (*Endocrinol. Metab.* 6): E192–E197, 1979.
254. THOMAS, P. A., J.-C. SCHANG, K. A. KELLY, AND V. L. W. GO. Can endogenous gastrin inhibit canine interdigestive gastric motility? *Gastroenterology* 78: 716–721, 1980.
255. THOMFORDE, G. M., M. CAMILLERI, T. L. YAKSH, AND J.-R. MALAGELADA. Opioid and adrenergic effects on gastrointestinal motility: interactions within and between spinal cord and gut (Abstract). *Dig. Dis. Sci.* 30: 798, 1985.
256. THOMPSON, D. G., AND J.-R. MALAGELADA. Vomiting and the small intestine. *Dig. Dis. Sci.* 27: 1121–1125, 1982.
257. THOMPSON, D. G., E. RICHELSON, AND J.-R. MALAGELADA. Perturbation of gastric emptying and duodenal motility through the central nervous system. *Gastroenterology* 83: 1200–1206, 1982.
258. THOMPSON, D. G., E. RICHELSON, AND J.-R. MALAGELADA. Perturbation of upper gastrointestinal function by cold stress. *Gut* 24: 277–283, 1983.
259. THOMPSON, D. G., D. L. WINGATE, L. ARCHER, M. J. BENSON, W. J. GREEN, AND R. J. HARDY. Normal patterns of human upper small bowel motor activity recorded by prolonged radiotelemetry. *Gut* 21: 500–506, 1980.
260. THOR, K., S. ROSELL, Å. RÖKAEUS, AND L. KAGER. (Gln$^4$)-neurotensin changes the motility pattern of the duodenum and proximal jejunum from a fasting-type to a fed-type. *Gastroenterology* 83: 569–574, 1982.
261. THOR, P., J. W. KONTUREK, S. J. KONTUREK, AND J. H. ANDERSON. Role of prostaglandins in control of intestinal motility. *Am. J. Physiol.* 248 (*Gastrointest. Liver Physiol.* 11): G353–G359, 1985.
262. VALENZUELA, J. E. Dopamine as a possible neurotransmitter in gastric relaxation. *Gastroenterology* 71: 1019–1022, 1976.
263. VALENZUELA, J. E. Effect of intestinal hormones and peptides on intragastric pressure in dogs. *Gastroenterology* 71: 766–769, 1976.
264. VALENZUELA, J. E., C. DEFILIPPI, AND A. CSENDES. Manometric studies on the human pyloric sphincter: effect of cigarette smoking, metoclopramide, and atropine. *Gastroenterology* 70: 481–483, 1976.
265. VALENZUELA, J. E., AND M. I. GROSSMAN. Effect of pentagastrin and caerulein on intragastric pressure in the dog. *Gastroenterology* 69: 1383–1384, 1975.
266. VANTRAPPEN, G., J. JANSSENS, J. HELLEMANS, AND Y. GHOOS. The interdigestive motor complex of normal subjects and patients with bacterial overgrowth of the small intestine. *J. Clin. Invest.* 59: 1158–1166, 1977.
267. VANTRAPPEN, G. R., T. L. PEETERS, AND J. JANSSENS. The secretory component of the interdigestive migrating motor complex in man. *Scand. J. Gastroenterol.* 14: 663–667, 1979.
268. WEEMS, W. A. Intestinal wall motion, propulsion, and fluid movement: trends toward a unified theory. *Am. J. Physiol.* 243 (*Gastrointest. Liver Physiol.* 6): G177–G188, 1982.
269. WEEMS, W. A., AND G. E. SEYGAL. Fluid propulsion by cat intestinal segments under conditions requiring hydrostatic work. *Am. J. Physiol.* 240 (*Gastrointest. Liver Physiol.* 3): G147–G156, 1981.
270. WEISBRODT, N. W., E. M. COPELAND, R. W. KEARLEY, E. P. MOORE, AND L. R. JOHNSON. Effects of pentagastrin on electrical activity of small intestine of the dog. *Am. J. Physiol.* 227: 425–429, 1974.
271. WEISBRODT, N. W., J. N. WILEY, B. F. OVERHOLT, AND P. BASS. A relation between gastroduodenal muscle contractions and gastric emptying. *Gut* 10: 543–548, 1969.
272. WELCH, I., K. SAUNDERS, AND N. W. READ. Effect of ileal and intravenous infusions of fat emulsions on feeding and satiety in human volunteers. *Gastroenterology* 89: 1293–1297, 1985.
273. WILBUR, B. G., AND K. A. KELLY. Effect of proximal gastric, complete gastric, and truncal vagotomy on canine gastric electric activity, motility, and emptying. *Ann. Surg.* 178: 295–302, 1973.
274. WILBUR, B. G., AND K. A. KELLY. Gastrin pentapeptide decreases canine gastric transmural pressure. *Gastroenterology* 67: 1139–1142, 1974.

275. WILBUR, B. G., K. A. KELLY, AND C. F. CODE. Effect of gastric fundectomy on canine gastric electrical and motor activity. *Am. J. Physiol.* 226: 1445–1449, 1974.
276. WILLIAMS, N. S., D. W. JEHN, AND J. H. MEYER. Transit and digestion of liver particles in the small intestine and their relationship to fluid movement (Abstract). *Gastroenterology* 82: 1210, 1982.
277. WILLIAMS, N. S. J. H. MEYER, D. JEHN, J. MILLER, AND A. S. FINK. Canine intestinal transit and digestion of radiolabeled liver particles. *Gastroenterology* 86: 1451–1459, 1984.
278. WINGATE, D. L. Backwards and forwards with the migrating complex. *Dig. Dis. Sci.* 26: 641–665, 1981.
279. WINGATE, D. L., E. A. PEARCE, M. HUTTON, A. DAND, H. H. THOMPSON, AND E. WÜNSCH. Quantitative comparison of the effects of cholecystokinin, secretin, and pentagastrin on gastrointestinal myoelectric activity in the conscious fasted dog. *Gut* 19: 593–601, 1978.
280. WINGATE, D. L., E. A. PEARCE, P. A. THOMAS, AND B. J. BOUCHER. Glucagon stimulates intestinal myoelectric activity (Abstract). *Gastroenterology* 74: 1152, 1978.
281. WINGATE, D. L., H. RUPPIN, W. E. R. GREEN, H. H. THOMPSON, W. DOMSCHKE, E. WÜNSCH, L. DEMLING, AND H. D. RITCHIE. Motilin-induced electrical activity in the canine gastrointestinal tract. *Scand. J. Gastroenterol. Suppl.* 11: 111–118, 1976.
282. WINGATE, D. L., H. H. THOMPSON, E. A. PEARCE, AND A. DAND. The effects of exogenous cholecystokinin and pentagastrin on myoelectrical activity in the small intestine of the conscious fasted dog. In: *Gastrointestinal Motility in Health and Disease*, edited by H. L. Duthie. Baltimore, MD: University Park, 1978, p. 47–58.
283. YAMAGISHI, T., AND H. T. DEBAS. Cholecystokinin inhibits gastric emptying by acting on both proximal stomach and pylorus. *Am. J. Physiol.* 234 (*Endocrinol. Metab.* 3): E375–E378, 1978.

CHAPTER 24

# Colonic motility

JAMES CHRISTENSEN | Department of Internal Medicine, University of Iowa Hospitals and Clinics, Iowa City, Iowa

CHAPTER CONTENTS

Anatomy
    Comparative anatomy of the colon
    Development of the colon
    Gross structure of the human colon
    Muscular walls of the colon
    Nerves of the colon
Methods to Study Contractions and Flow in the Colon
Gross Patterns of Contractions and Flow in the Colon
    Rhythmic contractions
    Tonic contractions
Myogenic Factors in Colonic Contractions
    Studies in the human colon
    Relationship of slow waves, contractions, and flows
Neurogenic Factors in Colonic Contractions
    Morphological studies
    Peristaltic reflex
    Tonic neurogenic inhibition
    Intrinsic nerve stimulation
    Responses to autonomic drugs
    Extrinsic nervous control of colonic motility
Effects of Drugs on Colonic Contractions
    Adrenergic drugs
    Anticholinergic agents
    Polypeptides
    Prostaglandins
    Morphine
    γ-Aminobutyric acid
    Adenosine triphosphate
    Laxatives
    Antibiotics
    Bile acids
Anal Sphincters
    Internal anal sphincter
    External anal sphincter
Some Integrated Colonic Activities
    Response of the colon to eating
    Defecation
    Effect of emotions on the colon
Disorders of Colonic Motility
    Diverticulosis of the colon
    Aganglionosis of the colon
    Diarrhea and constipation
    Irritable colon syndrome
    Rectal incontinence
Summary

IN THE EVOLUTION OF MAMMALS, three major specializations in intestinal physiology developed in the colon. *1*) Water and electrolytes are extracted from the fluid contents of the intestinal lumen, probably to serve in the adaptation of animals to terrestrial life and, even more, to relatively dry environments. *2*) The mammalian colon contains an abundant growth of many kinds of microorganisms; the colonic flora makes an important contribution to animal biological economy and to mammalian nutrition in some species, especially in horses and probably in certain marsupials. *3*) This function is related to protection against predators: the ability of the potential quarry of a scent-oriented predator to control the placement of his fecal deposition surely has great value for the survival of that species; control of fecal deposition may also serve in identification of territories by territorial animals.

The movements of the walls of the colon exhibit special features that accomplish these three colonic functions. Wall movements are ordered in such a way as to produce very slow flow: this facilitates the extraction of water, electrolytes, and some nutrients from the fecal mass by diffusion. The slowness and the orientation of colonic wall movements allow and encourage the growth of microorganisms in the colonic lumen. The movements of the proximal colon are involuntary; the movements of the distal colon, however, are more subject to extrinsic neural control, much of which is voluntary, so that defecation is in large part under voluntary control.

The way in which colonic contractions are regulated and organized so as to accomplish the normal patterns of flow that occur in the colon is not yet completely clear. The current state of ignorance of the nature of colonic motility cannot be attributed to lack of interest, for the motions of the colon have not been wholly ignored by physiologists and physicians, nor by laymen for that matter. Rather, the ignorance of the subject is related to a variety of factors, including the intrinsic complexity of the subject, the relative inaccessibility of the colon to study, and the somewhat unattractive nature of the organ and its contents. More important, there is no ideal animal model of the human colon: the obvious and extreme differences in colonic anatomy among mammals imply that there is considerable variability in motor physiology; this makes it unwise to transpose conclusions derived from the study of one mammal to all others. A major problem is the fact that colonic motions are so very slow and recur at such very long intervals that they cannot be fully appreciated in short-term observations. The organ requires prolonged study if one is to be able to understand its full repertoire of motions.

This chapter reviews the whole topic of colonic motility, emphasizing the evidence from studies since the last such reviews (45, 120, 263).

## ANATOMY

### Comparative Anatomy of the Colon

Garry (120) was well aware of the problem in understanding colonic motor physiology raised by the extreme anatomic variability in the mammalian colon. He emphasized that carnivores have a colon in which the longitudinal muscle is of uniform thickness all about the circumference throughout the organ, so that the whole colon has the appearance of a tube of reasonably uniform caliber. He believed that the presence of taeniae and sacculation, a long cecum, and elongation of the organ were all adaptations of the colon to the herbivorous diet. This may be an oversimplification, however, because many exceptions occur (141, 162, 200, 235). For example, the colons of the horse and cow, both herbivores, are quite different from one another. That of the horse is extensively taeniated and sacculated, whereas that of the cow is less specialized. The colons of the rat and that of the opossum, both omnivores, resemble those of carnivores, whereas the colon of the pig, another omnivore, is elongated, taeniated, sacculated, and equipped with a large cecum, thus resembling the herbivore colon. Most rodents are herbivores, yet some, like mice and rats, have colons of simple structure, whereas the colon in other rodents is very complicated.

These anatomic variations probably have arisen because of variations among species in the place of the colon in the total physiological economy. Thus, for example, the enormous complexity of the colon of horses is probably related to the major contribution to the nutrition of those animals made by microbial fermentation that takes place in the cecum and ascending colon. There is a similar dependence on intraluminal microbial fermentation as a source of calories in ruminants, but this fermentation takes place in the stomach rather than in the proximal colon; in ruminants, it is the stomach that is anatomically complex.

Similarly, there seems to be a high degree of variability in the structure of the colon among birds. The familiar gallinaceous birds have two long ceca, but other birds have only one and some have none. Parrots, who are herbivorous, have no ceca and neither do woodpeckers, who are mainly insectivorous. Thus it appears that the presence of a cecum, taeniation, sacculation, and elongation of the colon are not simply results of an adaptation to the herbivorous diet.

### Development of the Colon

The various parts of the colon differ greatly in function, and there may be clues to these differences in the study of the organogenesis of the colon. The proximal colon develops from the midgut, and the distal part develops from the hindgut (184). The point at which the two join is about the point of junction of the distributions of the superior and inferior mesenteric arteries. The rectum and anal canal originate differently from the rest of the colon: those regions develop from a primitive cloaca. In development, they are separated from what is to become the urogenital tract by the urorectal septum that grows across the primitive cloaca. The cecum develops very early in life, already apparent in the 7.5-mm embryo in the form of a distinct widening in the primitive intestine (184).

The haustra and taeniae first appear quite early in the development of the human colon. Various authors report that haustra first appear as early as the 11th wk of fetal life (202), although others say they develop as late as the 3rd yr of life (11); there are other reports of intermediate ages. The evidence in favor of the earlier date is compelling, however, since both muscle layers are formed by the middle of the 3rd fetal mo and the taeniae can be seen by the 11th wk of fetal life.

### Gross Structure of the Human Colon

As measured in adult male cadavers, the human colon is ~1.5 m long, but it is likely to be somewhat shorter in life, because it probably relaxes in death. The human colon is usually designated in terms of eight segments: the appendix, the cecum, the ascending colon, the transverse colon, the descending colon, the sigmoid colon, the rectum, and the anal canal. These terms are often used for other species, where they are inappropriate, because the shape of the colon does not generally conform to the human pattern. The terms designating these segments are based on anatomy, not physiology. The cecum, from which the appendix arises, is the part of the colon that lies rostrad from the ileocolic junction; it is short in humans but very long in some other species. The ascending colon is the segment between the ileocolic junction and the hepatic flexure of the colon that lies below the liver. The transverse colon extends from the hepatic flexure to the fold at the spleen, the splenic flexure. The descending colon extends from the splenic flexure to the pelvic brim. The sigmoid colon is the segment between the pelvic brim and the point where the axis of the colon turns to lie in the rostrocaudal axis at the top of the rectum. The rectum is the region between that point and the anal canal; the anal canal is the last ~3 cm, ending at the squamocolumnar mucosal junction, called the anal verge.

*Muscular Walls of the Colon*

The human colon is a sacculated organ throughout most of its length. Sacculation is partly a result of the specialized distribution of the outer longitudinal muscle layer. The fibers of this muscle layer lie in bundles that are not uniformly distributed around the circumference of the colon, as they are in the esophagus, stomach, and small intestine. Instead, in the sacculated colon, the longitudinal muscle layer is bunched into three thick bands called the three taeniae of the colon. The longitudinal muscle layer is present between these taeniae but it is very thin in these regions. One of the taeniae lies along the line of the mesenteric insertion of the colon. The other two taeniae are placed at approximately equal distances from this mesenteric taenia. This arrangement gives the colonic lumen a triangular rather than a circular profile in the sacculated region. The saccular appearance of this part of the colon is also a consequence of the elongation of the muscle bundles of the circular muscle coat; in a cross section of the filled colon, the wall bulges in the spaces between the three taeniae. At fairly uniform intervals, narrow bands of contraction of the circular muscle layer, the plicae circulares, interrupt the bulging wall and cause this part of the colon to have the appearance of a chain of pockets, called the haustra. The bands of contracted muscle that form them are called the haustral markings. At about the point where the sigmoid colon ends, at the apex of the rectum, the three taeniae broaden and fuse, so that in the rectum the longitudinal muscle layer is uniformly thick about the circumference. The outer longitudinal muscle layer merges with the external anal sphincter at the anal canal. This sphincter is a striated muscle; the longitudinal muscle also merges into the other striated musculature of the pelvic floor. The inner circular muscle layer of the rectum ends as a thickened ring of smooth muscle, the internal anal sphincter, at the level of the external anal sphincter.

A mesentery suspends the human colon from the dorsal body wall. The width of this mesentery varies from one part of the colon to another. The cecum usually has a rather short mesentery, so that the cecum is only slightly mobile, although there is great individual variability in this. The ascending and descending parts of colon also have a comparatively narrow mesentery. Throughout the transverse colon and the sigmoid colon, the mesentery is broad so that these parts of the colon are relatively mobile. Isolated bundles of smooth muscle lie within the mesentery, joining the muscular coats of the colon to the dorsal body wall (106). Their function is not clear. The number and distribution of these bands are certainly variable and they are small, but they are especially well developed along the cecum and in the pelvis. One of these muscles, the puborectalis muscle, is particularly thick. It forms a sling about the rectum, pulling it forward to reduce the angulation between the proximal rectum and the distal rectum.

The colon, like the rest of the gut, contains a layer of muscle in the mucosa. This consists of an inner circular and an outer longitudinal layer, but the two are tightly fixed together by mixing and intertwining of fiber bundles at the interface between the two layers.

*Nerves of the Colon*

The intramural nerves in the colon are arranged into laminae that follow the general pattern of the intramural nerves. This pattern is not uniform along the colon, however, because in the cecum and in the appendix the ganglion cells of the intramural nerves are more diffusely arranged within the layers of smooth muscle (94). The functional significance of this pattern in the cecum and appendix is not clear. In the remainder of the colon, the laminae of intramural nerves, i.e., the subserous and myenteric (or intermuscular) plexuses, can be found between the circular and longitudinal muscle layers and in the submucosa.

The myenteric plexus is clearly involved in the control of colonic motility. This plexus is made up of ganglia, clusters of nerve cell bodies linked together by bundles of nerve processes. The density of distribution of nerve cell bodies in the myenteric plexus is not constant along the length of the colon. In the opossum, the nerve cell density in the cecum is about half that in the proximal colon; nerve cell distribution density declines along the distal colon to reach a value in the distal rectum that is only ~4%–5% of the ganglion cell density of the proximal colon (52). In the region of the colon where the density of nerve cells in the myenteric plexus is the greatest (ascending and proximal transverse colon), the density of nerve cells in the myenteric plexus is about the same as it is throughout the small intestine. In the rectum, the pattern of the myenteric plexus is quite different from the pattern in the rest of the colon (53). The plexus in the rectum consists of irregularly disposed coarse nerve bundles. There are relatively few ganglia, and the ganglia are small. There are knots of fine, convoluted nerve fibers among the bundles, and these knots often contain small ganglia. Some of the ganglia in the rectal myenteric plexus are located on short stalks extending from coarse nerve bundles. These have been called parafascicular ganglia because of their position relative to the nerve bundles. Similar ganglia occur in the esophagus.

The myenteric plexus of the distal colon contains other remarkable structures called the ascending nerves of the colon (247), shunt fascicles (53), or the intramural pelvic nerves (107). Although first described in 1971, they seem not to have achieved widespread recognition. These are thick nerve bundles, much thicker than those that connect the ganglia together, lying in the plane of the myenteric plexus and superimposed on the ganglia and their interconnecting fiber bundles. These ascending nerves of the colon do not pass through ganglia but give off lateral branches to adjacent ganglia that they pass by. There are several such nerves in the circumference of the colon, 6–12 in the many species that have been examined; they run straight along the long axis of the colon with little major branching to a variable distance, up to more than half the colonic length, except in rodents where they are short, thin, and few (53). These nerves are present in the human colon (247), but their extent in humans is unknown. They are clearly extensions of the extramural pelvic nerves (107), and $\leq 10\%$ of the fibers that they contain are myelinated (J. Christensen and G. A. Rick, unpublished observations). The arrangement of these intramural pelvic nerves appears to be designed to distribute preganglionic motor nerve fibers of extrinsic origin to nerve cells in the ganglia of the myenteric plexus throughout the distal half of the colon. These ascending nerves probably also receive afferent fibers from the myenteric plexus, carrying them to extrinsic centers. There is physiological evidence that the ascending nerves of the colon subserve colocolonic or colorectal reflexes that are probably independent of extrinsic nerve centers in the spinal cord or brain.

Branches from the pelvic plexus that are called the pelvic nerves constitute the major extrinsic innervation of the colon. These pass from the pelvic plexus to the level of the proximal rectum, where they ascend along the colon for a short distance and give off branches that enter into the colon wall. These branches continue as the intramural pelvic nerves or ascending nerves of the colon. The extramural pelvic nerves contain numerous ganglia: some lie on the serosal surface of the rectum and others are remote from the rectum, lying in the trunks of the pelvic nerves and in the pelvic plexus itself. The central connections of the pelvic nerves are not fully known. Onuf's nucleus in the sacral spinal cord is a center for the somatic motoneurons that supply the external anal sphincter and probably other striated muscles of the pelvic floor (180, 197). The pudendal nerves supply the external anal sphincter. They carry fibers that arise from the $L_6$ and $L_7$ spinal segments in the rhesus monkey and from the $S_1$ and $S_4$ segments in the chimpanzee (220).

The inferior mesenteric ganglion may be a major site of neural integration of movements in the distal colon, as shown by anatomical studies with horseradish peroxidase as a tracer. Such tracers are taken up by nerves and carried by axonal transport. After injection of the tracer into that ganglion, labeled cell bodies were found in the solar plexus ganglia, pelvic plexus ganglia, nodose ganglia, spinal cord, and dorsal root ganglia at the $T_{12}$–$L_4$ levels. Another tracer dye, similarly injected, stained cell bodies in myenteric and submucosal ganglia of the distal colon. Similar application of tracers to the intramural nerves in the colon labeled nerve cells in the dorsal root ganglia, in the inferior mesenteric ganglion, and in the colonic plexus ganglion (9, 70). The colonic nerves contain nerve fibers that are immunoreactive to the antibodies of the vasoactive intestinal polypeptide (VIP), to cholecystokinin (CCK), and to bombesin from the distal colon to the inferior mesenteric ganglion (71). Sympathetic nerves also project from the sacral sympathetic chain (mainly the $S_1$–$S_3$ paravertebral ganglion) through the pelvic nerves to postganglionic nerves on the surface of the colon (179). Other dry-tracer techniques have been used to trace the colonic innervation to the spinal cord (77). It has been known for a long time that vagal preganglionic fibers project to the proximal colon. This was confirmed recently in rats with studies of the fate of tracers injected into the dorsal motor nucleus (65).

## METHODS TO STUDY CONTRACTIONS AND FLOW IN THE COLON

The methods used to study colonic motility have been reviewed by Truelove (263). All of them have particular limitations and advantages.

The examination of the colon exposed at the operating table has the advantage of directness but there are several disadvantages. *1*) The technique can only rarely be used in the study of the human colon. *2*) The colon observed at operation cannot be considered to be in a normal state, for it is certainly affected by fasting, by drugs and anesthetics used in connection with operation, by reflexes excited by the opening of the peritoneum, by a subnormal body temperature, and by the effects of direct handling of the colon. *3*) No permanent record can be easily obtained, so that conclusions drawn from such methods of direct observation cannot be considered objective. Thus this method is of little use in the study of colonic motility.

Radiographic observations in animals and in humans have been made since the beginning of this century. An advantage of radiography is that variables such as the actions of drugs, the effects of reflexes, and a subnormal temperature in the organ are less problematical. The disadvantage is that in radiographic observations one is watching the flow of a luminal content that is physically and chemically very different from the normal luminal content; the radiopaque material is introduced under relatively high pressure, so that the colon is stretched, the flow is visualized rather than the wall movements themselves, and the duration of study is restricted by the limitations of radiation exposure in humans. Objectivity and quantitation are relatively hard to achieve in radiography.

Intraluminal pressures as recorded by balloon kymography have long been used to obtain an idea of the patterns of colonic movement. Balloons, introduced into the colon, are inflated and connected by a tube to a manometer or to a volume recorder; contractions of the colon against the balloon are recorded as a rise in pressure (or fall in volume) inside the balloon. Kymography offers the advantages of objectivity, quantitation, and prolonged study. Such methods, although still often used, have several disadvantages. *1)* The balloon probably evokes reflex responses or reflex modifications in contractions, so that the bowel cannot be considered to be in a completely normal state. *2)* The balloon may not yield to the contraction in the same way that normal colonic content would. *3)* The characteristics of the balloon itself may influence the signals recorded. *4)* The empty colon may not function in the same way that the full colon does.

Open-ended tubes have been used widely for manometric recording of esophageal motion in recent years and they have had some use in the study of colonic motion as well. Open-tube manometry has the advantage that the tubes can be used in animals and in humans with reasonable assurance that the motility of the colon is not being greatly influenced by the method of measurement. Objectivity, quantitation, and prolonged study are all possible with open-tube manometry. The method has the major disadvantage that the tubes record the pressure in whatever sealed cavity the open end of the tube happens to lie. It is difficult, if not impossible, to know exactly what kinds of wall movements generate the pressure changes recorded by open-ended tubes in the colon. Also, the precise location of the open end of the tube along the colon cannot be known. The tube may shift considerably during study, and this may not be apparent.

Direct recordings of contractions of the colonic wall are possible in experimental animals with chronically implanted strain gauges sewn to the colon wall. Very small strain gauges have been developed that have been used widely to study contractions of the stomach and small intestine, but these strain gauges have not been so much used to study the actions of the colon. Implanted strain gauges have the advantage that the records offer objectivity, ease of quantitation, and, probably, minimal interference with normality of function. They are not readily applied in humans.

Recordings in vitro of the contractions of colonic muscle taken from experimental animals or from humans have been made more frequently in recent years. Strips of the muscular wall of the colon are cut in either longitudinal or transverse directions and attached to a strain gauge. Their contractions are recorded isometrically or isotonically. Such methods cannot be used to depict the operation of the whole organ, but the behavior of such strips of muscle can contribute at the tissue level to the conception of how the colon works at the organ level.

The recording of the electrical signals that are generated by the colonic musculature as it contracts has been used in recent years to amplify our understanding of colonic motion. There have been few studies made with chronically implanted serosal electrodes in vivo, but mucosal electrodes, acutely implanted in the rectal mucosa in humans, have been used to record the electromyogram in various disease states. Electromyography of the human colon is still not well developed, but electromyography of the animal colon has contributed significantly to our current view of colonic motility. Electromyography has many advantages, such as ease of application, freedom from observational artifact, objectivity, quantifiability, and the opportunity for prolonged study. The disadvantage of electromyography is that the signals recorded are not yet fully interpretable in terms of actual wall movements and intralumina flows.

## GROSS PATTERNS OF CONTRACTIONS AND FLOW IN THE COLON

The gross patterns of contractions and of the flows that they produce in the colon have both been understood for a long time, because they were clearly described in two early papers on the subject. These reports seem to have been ignored for a long time but they are consistent with the results of much more recent research.

Cannon (38) in 1902 used the then new method of radiography to examine colonic motility in the cat. With bismuth subnitrate as a contrast medium, he observed the movements of the fecal mass over long periods of time. He observed patterns of movement that could be used to separate the colon into two distinctly different parts.

"The usual movement of the transverse and ascending colon is antiperistalsis," he observed. He used the term *antiperistalsis* to refer to ring contractions that move cephalad rather than caudad as they do in the small intestine. He saw that there were periods lasting 2–8 min in which cephalad-moving ring contractions occurred at a fundamental frequency of ~5.5 cycles/min in the ascending and transverse colon. Between these periods, there were periods of ~10–15 min of rest. This retrograde peristalsis drove the colonic contents backward toward or into the cecum but the contents did not pass backward through the ileocecal junction. Thus the colonic contents were churned and mixed by these wall movements within a closed compartment consisting of the cecum and the ascending colon. The entry of a new bolus of intestinal content into the colon from the ileum excited a brief period of strong contractions in the cecum and ascending colon, so that some part of the content was pushed caudad into the transverse colon, but the antiperistaltic ring contractions would soon resume. "Thus, the contents of the colon, instead of being driven immediately toward the rectum by slow peristalsis, as is the general opinion, are first repeatedly pushed toward the cecum by an antiperistaltic action," said Cannon. Cannon observed that when antiperistaltic contractions had reached a maximal intensity they started near the proximal end of the transverse colon and passed without interruption to the rostral end of the cecum.

The other part of the colon that Cannon distinguished on the basis of patterns of wall motion constitutes the areas roughly corresponding to the distal transverse and descending colon. Here "tonic contractions appear which separate the contents into a series of globular masses. These rings ... are in reality moving slowly away from the cecum, pushing the hardening contents before them," Cannon said.

The second of these important early papers is that of Elliott and Barclay-Smith (91). These investigators studied in direct observations the colons of the cat, rat, guinea pig, rabbit, dog, ferret, and hedgehog. In most cases, the animals were anesthetized, the spinal cord was destroyed, the abdomen was opened, and the colon was left in situ but made to float in a warm bath of a physiological solution. The authors excited colonic movements by putting a "thick yellow gruel—prepared by mixing pea flour with water until the whole was of precisely the same consistency as that of the food in the ileum—through an incision made in the ileum a few centimeters above the ileo-colic sphincter." Elliott and Barclay-Smith observed three main types of movement. First, in the proximal colon they observed, as had Cannon, that antiperistalsis was the dominant activity. They described this most clearly in the cat colon, where, starting from a point ~7 cm beyond the cecal apex, narrow constrictions slowly traveled retrograde toward the cecum at ~1–2 mm/s. These would repel content that had entered the colon from the ileum and would temporarily prevent the caudad flow of content. These constrictions followed one another at intervals of ~1 cm, and at frequencies of ~5–6 cycles/min. These antiperistaltic ring contractions were the main activity of the cecum and ascending colon. Such contractions were much more prominent in the rabbit (which has a big cecum) than in the dog (which has a small cecum). They were observed to churn and mix the colonic content.

In the next more distal segment of the colon, Elliott and Barclay-Smith observed the second type of movement, where coordinated peristalsis was the predominant pattern of motion, tonic contraction rings moving caudad. This pattern occurred in any part of the colon but it was the usual pattern of movement in the middle part of the colon. These slowly moving rings drove the colonic content toward the anus; the colonic content seemed to stimulate such contractions by distention of the colon.

Elliott and Barclay-Smith observed a third type of movement in the most distal colonic segment that probably corresponds to the sigmoid colon and rectum in humans. Here, the main activity that they saw was a strong contraction, a constriction moving caudad that emptied the colon. This peristaltic contraction can be directly excited by stimulation of pelvic nerves.

Thus Cannon as well as Elliott and Barclay-Smith long ago observed that greatly different patterns of contraction and of flow of luminal content can be distinguished in the three different parts of the colon. These observations are fully consistent with many other observations made subsequently in animals and in humans. For example, simple observation by radiography of the position of fecal shadows in humans suggests that there is a prolonged residence of fecal matter in the right side of the colon. Colonoscopists are well aware of the fact that the cecum and ascending colon retain colonic content with greater avidity than does the rest of the colon. Fecal shadows, seen by radiographic observation, accumulate in the right side of the abdomen, in the area of the proximal colon, and are displaced from that region by laxatives (63). From studies of transit, the cecum and sigmoid colon can be seen clearly as major points in the delay of mouth-to-anus transit. This transit may require several days (132). Presumably, the delay is caused by the dominance of antiperistalsis in that part of the colon, and this is probably a process common to many, if not all, mammalian species.

There is an extensive mixing of colonic contents during the prolonged residence of intestinal contents in the proximal colon of humans, just as it was described in the animal studies by Cannon and by Elliott and Barclay-Smith (38, 91). This has been shown by studies in which three kinds of radiopaque markers are ingested by human subjects at three separate meals, so that marker location can be subsequently monitored. Batches of radiopaque disks of three different shapes or sizes were ingested at 36, 34, and 12 h before X-ray examination of the abdomen. The three sizes of disks were observed to be thoroughly mixed throughout the colon, with some of the last that were ingested lying in advance of some of the earliest ingested ones (131). Such mixing occurred mainly in the right colon. Thus there seems to be general agreement between the laboratory studies in animals and the clinical observations made in humans that prolonged residence and mixing of intestinal content occur in the proximal colon.

In the study of Cannon (38) and that of Elliott and Barclay-Smith (91), the authors found that both the distal transverse colon and the descending colon mainly exhibit a contraction pattern in which contraction rings divide the lumen into fairly uniform segments, and that these contraction rings move slowly caudad. This pattern of motion is also supported by observations of these parts of the colon in humans. In an early radiographic study, such contractions were seen to propel the feces in both directions but over very short distances (18). Ritchie (217) used time-lapse photography with cineradiography in another, more modern study to observe the movements of segmental contractions in the human colon. Such segmental contractions were observed to form, disappear, and reform with no constant relationship to the position of fixed points on the colon wall. Ritchie observed that segmental contractions were capable of pushing contents in both antegrade and retrograde directions.

Another pattern of movement, observed neither by Cannon nor by Elliott and Barclay-Smith, has attracted a considerable degree of attention. This was called the mass movement by those who first saw it, and it is still called that. It may have been described even before the early report by Hertz (139), but the subsequent description by Holzknecht is usually cited as the classic report (147). In the course of 1,000 radiographic examinations of the colon, Holzknecht observed mass movement to occur only twice. This movement of the fecal mass was described as the sudden shift of a column of feces, a shift about one-third of the length of the colon, the fecal mass moving to the next empty segment of the colon. Segmental contractions in the region disappeared before the mass movement occurred, both in the donating segment and in the receiving segment, but the usual pattern of segmental contractions quickly returned in the receiving segment after the shift was accomplished. Such a pattern of movement was later reported by others (140), who saw mass movements more frequently than Holzknecht did; they noted that such movements were more likely to occur soon after eating. More recently, investigators have confirmed the occurrence of sudden massive shifts of colonic content. Holdstock and his colleagues (146) used various types of markers, solid radiopaque objects of various shapes, radiotelemeter capsules, capsules containing $^{51}Cr$ and free $^{51}Cr$ to observe the patterns of fecal movement in mass. They concluded that "colonic contents progress distally by a series of infrequent large movements, known as mass movements or mass peristalsis." Ritchie (218) also saw such massive periodic shifts in the fecal mass in a study that combined cinefluorography and intraluminal manometry. The colonic wall motions that induce such mass movements are very likely the same kind of contractions that Mann and Hardcastle (190) called colonic peristalsis in their manometric study of patients with colostomies. Methods to observe gross movements of the human colon are much more restrictive than are those that can be used in animals, and the exact nature of the wall contraction that produces mass movement is not clear.

The pattern of contractions of the colon critically determines the pattern of flow in the colon. In the small intestine, the patterns of flow and contraction in the fasting state are very different from the patterns that are present in the fed state. The contraction pattern seen in the small intestine in fasting is the pattern of the migrating myoelectric complex, a periodic cycling of minimal and maximal activities correlated with similar cycling in the esophagogastric sphincter, stomach, and biliary tree. Similar cycling of contractions occurs in the colon, but the cycle is not coordinated with the cycle of the small intestine. The colonic cycle lasts 32 min in the dog; it consists of the periodic recurrence of tonic contractions with superimposed phasic contractions, with intervening periods of quiescence (231).

## Rhythmic Contractions

The recording of intraluminal pressures was used widely for a long time to delineate colonic movements. The work has been reviewed before (59) and little more has been done since then. Several manometric methods have been applied in which a variety of sensing devices were used—large and small balloons, open-tip perfused catheters, and radiotelemetering capsules. Much of the writing on the subject has been devoted to a discussion of the relative merits of these methods and to details of methodology. The interpretation of records has been a matter of concern as well. The interpretation of manometric tracings requires an understanding both of the source of the signal and of the validity of the method used in detecting it. Manometric records have been subjected to interpretation as to the nature of the wall motions that they reflect, despite uncertainties in this relationship. These interpretations reflected patterns of contractions and interpretations of the quantity (both magnitude and number) of contractions.

Pattern interpretation constitutes the attempt to classify pressure peaks detected manometrically (260). Manometric tracings were made with 3-cm long balloons from the dog colon in vivo. Three waveforms were distinguished, called types 1, 2, and 3. The classification has been subsequently applied to the human colon (2, 55, 76, 212, 246) and is still alluded to. Other workers have found this classification of waves to be inadequate because of the great irregularity of the patterns seen both in tracings obtained by the use of large balloons and in those obtained with other sensing devices (42, 57, 79). The validity of the classification of pressure peaks detected manometrically may be considered to be moot, however, for no agreement has ever been reached as to what exact patterns of wall motions the pressure peaks signify.

For this reason, more recent investigators have interpreted manometric tracings in quantitative terms only, either by counting the number of peaks over time or by the integration of amplitude and time. Such methods have yielded an estimate of the "duration of activity" of the colon that is quite high and might have surprised Holzknecht (147), who thought that the colon was motionless most of the time except for the rare times when he saw mass movements occurring. The "duration of activity," i.e., the proportion of time during which pressure peaks are generated by the colon, ranges from 13% to 59% of time, as reported by Connell (59).

The manometric methods alone are unlikely to be useful in completely depicting colonic motility because of their shortcomings. Manometry might be useful in helping to describe colonic movement, however, when combined with cineradiography. These combined techniques were applied in a rigorous study by Ritchie et al. (219). The researchers examined the sigmoid colon in normal human subjects with several kinds of pressure-sensing devices, including small balloons and open-tip perfused tubes, at the same time observing movements of the wall of the sigmoid colon by cineradiography. They found that the wall movements that can produce a rise in intraluminal pressure can be exceedingly complex, and they concluded that pressure tracings alone cannot be depended on to accurately reflect wall movements either in terms of contractions or of flow. They found that colonic diameter as observed by cineradiography could undergo great changes with little change in manometrically detected pressures. They proposed a complete classification of colonic contractions, which does not, however, appear to have found general use. The considered contractions were either localized or progressive: the localized ones often recurred quite regularly with either a 5-s period or a 30-s period. Progressive contractions were seen much less commonly. These progressive (or peristaltic) contractions traveled from the descending colon to the sigmoid colon at ~2.5 cm/s in sequences of six or more, at intervals of ~20–120 s. The researchers also saw contractions that seemed to be provoked by distensions of the bowel by the displacement of intraluminal content by contractions cephalad to the point of observation. Deller and Wangel (79) also combined intraluminal manometry and cineradiography to study the colon and observed a considerable discordance between the two methods in revealing wall motions. Large movements of the colonic wall and of the colonic luminal content were observed without pressure changes detected manometrically. Deller and Wangel noted considerable temporal discordance between manometrically recorded pressure changes and wall movements observed cineradiographically. In another study combining intraluminal manometry and cineradiography to study colonic motion, only two-thirds of pressure waves recorded were associated with some form of movement of the bowel wall; when movements were seen at cineradiography, they nearly always produced a pressure peak (129). The results of these studies make it doubtful that manometry in the colon can be considered fully reliable, either as a major research technique to discover the nature of colonic motility and its controls or as a diagnostic technique for the definition of clinical disorders. Manometric methods alone have been applied recently much less than they were a few years ago.

## Tonic Contractions

The preceding discussion has dealt mainly with periodic or rhythmic contractions, which are most easily recorded manometrically. Tone, a contraction maintained at a more or less constant level over a long time, is a property that has been attributed to smooth muscle. The actual definition of tone is problematic, prolonged but limited contractions often being called "tonic." Attempts have been made, however, to measure tone in the colon in vivo by manometric methods. White et al. (273) constructed a plot of pressure against volume during the slow infusion of water into the colon. This "colonmetrogram" yielded a plot of values that was different in patients with various neurological lesions that it was in normal subjects. The limitations of such a method are severe: it is difficult to know how much of the colon is being examined, and it is difficult to control or eliminate possible retrograde flow through the ileocecal junction. Even if both these objections did not exist, the colonmetrogram would measure tone for all of the colon, and it is clear that the colon is not a single physiological entity but at least three units, as described by Elliott and Barclay-Smith (91). Lipkin et al. (185) overcame these objections by using a latex balloon to perform colonmetrography. The balloon was of such a size that at 400 cm of water pressure it held 900 ml at the dimensions of 9.7 cm in diameter and 14 cm in length. The collapsed balloon was put into the sigmoid colon and then inflated under constant pressure. The balloon was so large that a contribution of the elasticity of the balloon was not considered to be major, and so the changes in volume, within the range of the experiment, reflected chiefly the changes in the volume of the viscus. The method applied by Lipkin et al. gave reproducible results, and they were able to show consistent effects of various drugs that they used. The technique seems not to have found much further application, however, and so its value in experimental or clinical physiology remains unexplored.

Such methods seem to measure a property of the bowel wall commonly termed *tone*. This is an ancient and inexact term whose definition has been argued for a long time. Youmans defined tone in terms of the relationship between lumen volume and pressure (282). This seems to be what the colonmetrogram measures. It is not clear, however, what exact property of the muscle is reflected in measurements of tone, or indeed which muscle layer of the colon wall is responsible for tone.

## MYOGENIC FACTORS IN COLONIC CONTRACTIONS

In this section, the myogenic factors that are involved in control of contractions of the colon are discussed. It has been possible, by the use of the selective neurotoxin tetrodotoxin and of less selective agents like local anesthetics, to separate neurogenic and myogenic elements of control systems in gastrointestinal motility.

Colonic smooth muscle, like other gastrointestinal smooth muscles, generates electrical signals that are related to muscle contractions. Thus the myogenic factors that are involved in colonic motility include the following: the spontaneous electrical activities of smooth muscle cells, the electrical communications between cells, the electrical communications between muscle bundles in and between muscle layers, the sources of energy to supply various processes in smooth muscle, and the dependence of the myoelectrical events and of the contractile process on the energy metabolism of the muscle to produce colonic contractions. Not all of these factors can be discussed for the colon, because much of the necessary information is lacking.

The smooth muscle of the colonic wall, like the muscle of the walls of the stomach and small intestine, generates electrical signals that constitute the elements of the electromyogram of the colon. They may be considered to be analogous to those signals generated by cardiac muscle. The signals in the colon differ in function in one major respect from those of the heart. In the heart, the cardiac action potential has two functions: it initiates contraction in the muscle cells and it integrates contraction of the whole organ, because the cardiac action potential spreads throughout the heart according to a fixed pattern. In the heart, these two functions are assigned to a single signal but in the gut they can be assigned to two elements of the electromyographic signal. The integration of contraction is accomplished by a relatively slow electrical transient that is called the electrical slow wave. It is also called the basic electrical rhythm, the pacesetter potential, and the electrical control activity. The initiation of contraction is the function of one or more much more rapid electrical transients, the spike burst. When records are made from a single point in the gut in the regions manifesting slow waves, the electrical slow waves recur continuously at a constant frequency. The muscle at the electrode site contracts rhythmically only in relationship to these slow waves but not to all of them. Contraction occurs only with those slow waves that carry a spike burst. A spike burst occurs only at a fixed position in relation to a slow wave, i.e., slow waves restrict spike bursts to fixed points in space and time. Thus the slow wave is a mechanism restricting contractions of the muscular wall to a fixed place and time: the spike burst is an action potential, whereas the slow wave is a pacesetter.

When the electromyogram is recorded simultaneously from several points in series along the bowel, slow waves are seen to spread away from a source, as though toward a sink. Because contractions are so closely linked to slow waves, the pattern of spread of slow waves determines the pattern of spread of contractions, i.e., slow waves coordinate contractions throughout the organ. That is why they are also called the pacesetter potentials or the electrical control activity.

In stomach and small intestine, the spread of the controlling electrical event, the slow wave, generally occurs through gap junctions, or nexuses, between contiguous muscle cells, although the exact mechanism of cell-to-cell transmission is not clear. Nexuses have not been examined so thoroughly in the colon as they have been in the other viscera, but they exist. In the guinea pig colon, gap junctions are rare and small, and they are confined to the circular muscle layer (114).

In the small intestine, this relationship between the distribution of rhythmic contractions and the distribution of the electrical slow waves has been recognized for a long time. The rhythmicity of contractions in the colon was also recognized long ago, but the possibility that colonic muscle exhibits electrical slow waves like those of the small intestine and stomach seems not to have been intensely examined until after 1960. Gillespie was apparently the first to see them. He described electrical potential variations in smooth muscle from preparation taken from the rabbit colon (123, 124). His preparation was a 4-cm part of the distal colon with the mucosa intact. He made records by single-cell recording techniques from the outer longitudinal muscle layer. He described three kinds of signals: slow waves, spike bursts grouped on the slow waves, and prepotentials with each spike (123, 124). The spike bursts and accompanying contractions were phase-locked to slow waves. When the tissue was stretched, the slow waves were reduced in amplitude or disappeared, and the spiking became continuous.

This recognition of the existence of electrical slow waves in the colon that resemble those of the small intestine was advanced by a 1969 study of the cat colon (51). In that study, strips of the muscularis propria containing both muscle layers were cut from the wall of various parts of the cat colon. The mucosa was removed and the strips were arranged for simultaneous recording of contractions by an isometric strain gauge; the electromyogram was recorded by a small surface electrode from both longitudinal and circular muscle layers. The electromyogram of the inner circular muscle layer exhibited slow electrical transients very much like the slow waves found in recordings from the longitudinal muscle layer of stomach and small intestine in many species. Similar slow waves had been seen in earlier studies from France (67).

The finding that the colonic electrical slow waves originate from the circular muscle layer was a surprise, for they are associated with the longitudinal layer in other than the gastrointestinal viscera where they occur. The fact that the slow electrical transients could be better recorded from the circular muscle layer (exposed by removal of the mucosa) than from the serosal surface led to the conclusion that they originated in the circular muscle layer. Also, the slow waves were readily recorded by intracellular recording with microelectrodes in the circular muscle layer but not by similar methods from the outer longitudinal layer of smooth muscle (51). Caprilli and Onori (39) provided even stronger evidence that colonic slow waves originate in the circular muscle layer by showing that electrical slow waves were detected in isolated strips of muscle of the circular layer (separated from the longitudinal layer) but not in isolated strips of the longitudinal muscle layer. They used a variety of simple experimental techniques like those that had been used previously in the study of slow waves in the small intestine (169), and the results supported the conclusion that the electrical slow waves of the colon are generated in the inner circular muscle layer rather than in the longitudinal layer. These techniques included methods in which in strips of muscle with both layers attached the circular layer was removed from one half of each strip. Electrodes were then applied to the exposed longitudinal muscle layer at various distances from the cut edge of the circular layer. Slow-wave amplitude declined exponentially with the distance of the longitudinal muscle layer from the edge of the remaining circular muscle layer. Also, in strips containing both muscle layers, which were mounted vertically "on edge," two electrodes were applied at corresponding points on both surfaces, one on the serosal surface and one on the inner surface of the circular muscle that had been exposed by removal of the mucosa. Electrical slow waves were detected simultaneously from both surfaces. The amplitude of the simultaneously recorded slow waves was greater in the records taken from the surface of the circular muscle than it was in records from the serosal surface over the longitudinal muscle layer. Also, the slow waves recorded from the circular muscle slightly preceded those recorded at the same time from the corresponding point on the surface of the longitudinal muscle layer. Thus Caprilli and Onori (39) gave evidence to support the concept of the origin of the slow waves in the colon from the circular layer.

The patterns of propagation of the slow waves of the cat colon have also been extensively studied. Studies of the small intestine had shown that the patterns of spread of slow waves dictate the patterns of spread of contractions, so similar studies were made in the colon of the cat. Slow waves were recorded simultaneously from a series of electrodes spaced at regular intervals over the inner surface of the circular muscle layer in vitro. By the use of various configurations of distribution of such extracellular electrodes, it was found that electrical slow waves spread in both the $x$-axis and the $y$-axis of the plane of the circular muscle layer. This was seen in studies that made use of small pieces of the colon wall (48) as well as in larger segments of the colon, one-third, one-half, or more of the whole colon (50, 51). Velocity in the direction of the long axis of the circular muscle cells, along the circumference of the colon, was relatively high (1.6 cm/s), whereas velocity in the long axis of the colon across the circular muscle cells was lower (1–5 mm/s). When a segment of the proximal colon was studied with multiple closely spaced electrodes, it was seen that the slow waves of that whole segment were driven from a single pacemaker about two-thirds of the time; the rest of the time, two, three, four, or even more pacemakers were operating simultaneously. A substantial subsequent experience has suggested that a single pacemaker is the commonest situation in the proximal colon and that the emergence of multiple pacemakers may be a pathological process. When only a single pacemaker was operating in the proximal cat colon, it was usually located caudad to the study segment, so that the slow waves tended to be propagated cephalad, toward the cecum. Dominance of the proximal colon by a single pacemaker seems to be the normal state in vitro. The single pacemaker that dominates the proximal colon is usually situated near the middle of that length of the colon, but it frequently shifts in position, sometimes even to the level of the ileocecal junction. When this shift occurs, slow waves pass antegrade in the proximal colon, but the normal pattern is for slow waves to spread retrograde from this pacemaker throughout the proximal colon toward, but not into, the cecum. The cecum seems not to be invaded by slow waves, at least not in the opossum (14).

The studies discussed in the preceding paragraphs were performed in the ascending colon of the cat. Subsequently it was found that electrical slow waves occur throughout the whole of the colon in the cat (276, 277), and so it was decided that the whole colon should be studied in detail, much as the ascending colon had been; after considerable trial, a suitable preparation was devised (47). The whole abdominal colon of the cat (excluding the rectum) was everted over a tube so that the mucosa lay outermost, and a strip of the mucosa was removed to expose the circular muscle layer. Sixteen electrodes were aligned at uniform intervals along the exposed circular muscle and slow waves were recorded simultaneously from each. Slow waves were detected throughout the organ and their frequency was found to rise from 4.5 cycles/min in the most proximal 10% of the colon to 6.0 cycles/min in the most distal 10%, with intermediate values at intermediate points. The colon was cut between electrodes so that it was divided into rings ~1 cm wide, and the 16 electrodes were reapplied in their former positions. This procedure separated the segments of the muscular wall from the influences of the other segments of the colon, so that the intrinsic frequencies of the electrical slow waves of the colon could be determined. The slow-wave frequency of the most proximal 10% of the colon fell when it was separated from the rest of 44% of its value in the intact colon in vitro; frequency declined to 57% and 73% in the next two 10-percentile segments. Frequency was not changed by the division of the colon in the region of the colon that included the fifth through the ninth 10-percentile segments. It rose to 121% of control in the tenth 10-percentile segment.

Thus a gradient was found along the colon in the intrinsic frequencies of the electrical slow waves that is consistent with and accounts for the patterns of spread of slow waves found previously. This gradient is consistent with the distal-to-proximal spread of slow waves in the proximal colon from a pacemaking region in the midcolon. The gradient predicts also that, in the rest of the colon, slow-wave spread should occur only over very short distances. In this study, as in many other studies, considerable lability in the frequency of the electrical slow waves along the colon was noted. This lability of intrinsic frequencies allows slow waves occasionally to pass over rather long distances, because if one pacemaker fires first, it may capture all the others over some distance. The conclusions as to patterns of pacemaker location and patterns of slow-wave migration have not yet been confirmed in vivo.

In the earliest of these studies of the electromyogram of the cat colon (48), a short burst of rapid electrical transients often occurred on some (but not all) electrical slow waves, and it appeared that such a spike burst correlated with a rhythmic contraction of the circular muscle layer; some contractions, however, occurred without a spike burst. Thus it appeared that the electrical slow waves generally pace contractions in the circular muscle layer of the colon just as they do in that of the small intestine, but a spike burst is not a necessary electromyographic indication of contraction. In the studies of the whole colon (47), however, another kind of spike burst was seen for the first time. This spike burst was much more prolonged than the brief rhythmic spike bursts that accompanied slow waves; it spanned several slow-wave cycles and seemed to be independent of slow waves. In the studies that made use of up to 16 electrodes spaced all along the colon, this prolonged spike burst was seen to sweep along the colon, usually moving caudad but sometimes migrating cephalad as well. It was periodic, recurring every ~80 s, and it lasted at a single point along the colon ~30 s, although these values were extremely variable. The velocity of migration was ~5 mm/s. The magnitude of the spike potentials in this prolonged spike burst was low in the ascending colon, but amplitude was much greater when the signal was recorded from points caudad to the hepatic flexure. Each spike in the migrating spike burst arose from a small sinusoidal signal; at times, especially in the most proximal colon, these sinusoidal signals occurred alone without the spikes, so that the migrating spike burst was expressed as a sequence of sinusoidal oscillations alone. These migrating spike bursts were found to be associated with powerful and prolonged contractions. The migrating spike burst was proposed to be the electromyographic manifestation of the contraction that accomplishes mass movement, but that idea has not been further investigated. Subsequent studies have led to the suggestions that the migrating spike bursts and the sinusoidal signals that accompany them arise from the longitudinal muscle layer (92, 153). The phenomenon remains to be fully examined.

The cellular processes in the colonic muscle that lead to the generation of slow waves remain obscure, just as they are for the small intestine. Slow-wave frequency in the cat colon is temperature dependent: the highest frequency occurs at 37°C, and it declines both with heating and with cooling (13); frequency is also oxygen dependent. Oxygen deprivation suppresses the migrating spike bursts of the cat colon. The generation of slow waves in the cat colon is related to interactions between cAMP and calcium (12).

Although the slow waves of the colon have been most extensively studied in the cat, they have also been recorded in other species. For example, they also occur in the dog, and, as in the cat, they appear to be generated by the circular muscle layer. The maintenance of the integrity of the interface between the circular muscle layer and the submucosa seems to be critical in slow-wave generation in the dog (82). This point has not been established in the cat. The electrical activity of the longitudinal muscle layer is quite different from that of the circular muscle layer in the dog, but the two layers interact in such a way that periods of contraction in them tend to coincide (92).

The differences in the electrical activities of the longitudinal and circular muscle layers have been clearly described in both the dog (92) and the pig (152). The longitudinal muscle layer generates high-frequency (up to 30–40 cycles/min) sinusoidal oscillations: these carry spikes with small contractions that, when intense, fuse to form sustained contractions. Prolonged periodic bursts of spikes produce long contractions at intervals of minutes. These observations support the idea that the sinusoidal oscillations and the migrating spike bursts described first in the cat colon originate in the longitudinal muscle layer rather than in the circular muscle layer.

*Studies in the Human Colon*

The profound variations in the anatomy of the colon among species suggest that there may be equally great differences in function. In this connection, it is unfortunate that nearly all the work on the nature of myogenic factors in the control of colonic motility has been done in the cat and dog colon; a few studies have also been reported in other species, e.g., the opossum (14), rabbit (158, 159), and mouse (280, 281), but there is very little information about the more complex colons of other species.

Many papers describe attempts to record the electromyogram in the human colon in vivo. The most easily reached parts of the bowel—and anal canal, rectum, sigmoid or descending colon—have been the ones most commonly studied. A monopolar electrode technique has been commonly used but bipolar electrodes have been applied as well; the electrodes are usually cup electrodes attached to the mucosa by suction or clip electrodes that are pinched onto the colonic mucosa.

There are several problems in these studies of the human colonic electromyogram that dictate caution in the interpretation of the observations. *1*) Because the primate colon (including the human colon) has not been well studied in vitro (at least not to the extent that the cat colon has), the investigator does not know exactly what to expect in the human colon in vivo. *2*) It is generally assumed that an electrode on the mucosa detects electrical signals that are generated by the circular muscle layer, but it is likely that the records obtained from mucosal electrodes also contain signals generated by other tissues, such as the mucosal muscle and the longitudinal layer of the muscularis propria; also, it seems very likely that electrical records made from mucosal electrodes contain contributions from blood flow, movement artifacts, skin potentials, and transmucosal potentials (in monopolar records). *3*) It seems possible that muscle of the distal colon is quite different physiologically from the muscle of more proximal areas of the colon, and so it is not necessarily justified to blindly project "abnormalities" that are found in electromyogram of the rectum to the rest of the organ; it is quite possible that even the smooth muscle of the various parts of the distal colon alone (the sigmoid colon, rectum, and anal canal) may exhibit different physiological features from one area to another. The failure to recognize these problems may well be responsible for much of the disagreement and confusion that still attaches to studies of colonic electromyography in vivo in the human colon.

In the animal colon studied in vivo, slow waves are present constantly. In most but not all of the reported studies in the colon it has been found that slow waves are not present constantly but intermittently. In the anal canal, intermittency is not mentioned in studies of the electromyogram (265, 271), but intermittency seems to be characteristic in recordings from the rectum (67, 240). This intermittency of recording of slow waves may be real, but it is certainly possible that it is artifactual, arising from an inconstancy in electrode contact with the signal source rather than an intermittency in the generation of the signals. In the anal canal, the action of the anal sphincters is certain to hold the electrode very tightly against the mucosa, whereas such a firm contact is probably harder to achieve or maintain in the more distensible regions like the rectum and rectosigmoid. That would account for the difference in the constancy of the signal recording between the rectum and the anal canal. The reported values for duration of the slow-wave activity are very inconsistent among reported studies, which also supports the idea that the failure of slow-wave activity to appear in the records may be artifactual, due to loss of contact rather than a failure of generation of slow waves. Thus, for example, Couturier and his colleagues (67) reported that slow waves are present for only 5%–20% of the time in the rectosigmoid, whereas Snape et al. (240) reported them to be present for 46% of the time in the rectum and for 28.5% of the time in the rectosigmoid. Others found slow waves in the lower rectum 67% of the time and 25% of the time in the rectosigmoid (259). A more recent study (233) lends further support to the idea that artifactual loss of contact accounts for the inconstancy of detection of slow waves by mucosal electrodes in the colon. In this study, records were made from the proximal colon in human subjects with a mucosal suction electrode and with serosal electrodes implanted under the serosal coat of the colon at laparotomy. Slow waves were recorded from the mucosal electrodes <50% of the time, whereas they were recorded 60%–85% of the time from the implanted electrodes. This discrepancy is consistent with the idea that mucosal electrodes lose contact with the signal source more readily than do implanted electrodes. Because in colon muscle in vitro the slow-wave activity is always present both in the cat (15, 39, 47–49, 51, 276, 277) and in the dog (233), and in view of the inconsistencies cited above from the several studies in vivo in humans, it seems reasonable to conclude that the inconstancy of the slow waves seen in mucosal recordings in vivo from humans is due to intermittent loss or reduction in the contact between the mucosal electrode and the slow wave source, the circular muscle layer. The recording of slow waves could also be lost temporarily because of asynchrony of slow waves at closely adjacent points.

A second remarkable feature of the human colonic electromyogram is the variation in slow-wave frequency. This is much greater in records of slow waves recorded in situ in humans than in those recorded in vitro in colonic muscle from experimental animals. In the cat colon in situ, slow-wave frequencies have been consistently found to be in a narrow range of ~5–6 cycles/min (14, 39, 47, 48, 50, 51, 276, 277), and the frequency is very similar in the muscle of the dog colon in situ (233). In studies in vitro in the cat, the slow-wave frequency is quite labile, as compared with the frequency of slow waves in the intestine, but this lability has generally been attributed to tissue damage. However, the lability of frequency may be a characteristic of colonic muscle. Similar transient changes in frequency appear in records from colonic muscle of the dog studied in vitro. These frequency changes seen in vitro are usually brief, and, in the cat at least, they are rather uncommon. In sharp contrast, all the records obtained from the human colon in situ display a great variety of frequencies. Records from the human colon are all so badly distorted by noise that the visual recognition of the existence of a regularly recurring waveform is very difficult except for very short periods. Hence the most recent studies that attempt analysis of slow-wave frequency have made use of computers to read tape-recorded signals and to analyze the records by various automated methods of signal analysis. Wankling et al. (271) reported several frequencies in the human anal canal as detected by mucosal electrodes: "ultraslow" waves were found with frequencies of 1–2 cycles/min, whereas other slow waves had a frequency of 10–20 cycles/min (average 16.9 ± 0.9). Ustach et al. (265) in records made from the same part of the colon by a similar electrode found slow waves of 17 cycles/min with a range from ~6 to 27 cycles/min; however, they did not see the "ultraslow" waves reported by Wankling et al. In studies from more proximal levels of the colon, similar variations in frequency were found. Couturier et al. (67) reported frequencies of 8.4–10.6 cycles/min in records from the human rectosigmoid in vivo with mucosal electrodes. Snape et al. (240) reported two frequencies in records from the human rectum: slow waves were detected at 6.5 and at 3.4 cycles/min; at the rectosigmoid they were found at 7.3 and 2.9 cycles/min. Taylor et al. (259) also saw two frequencies in the human rectum, 3–4 cycles/min and 6–9 cycles/min. The presence of two different slow-wave frequencies has been repeatedly reaffirmed in reports of records from mucosal electrodes in humans by Snape et al. (241–243), and this idea has been further supported by the computer-aided analysis of real-time records (74), although it now appears that there are two very broad ranges of frequencies rather than two sharply separate discrete frequencies.

Variation in slow-wave frequency is a difficult matter to interpret. Several authors have suggested recently that abnormal colonic slow-wave frequency correlates with the existence of the functional bowel syndrome (86, 240, 242, 250). Records made by a bipolar electrode technique from the rectosigmoid area in patients with this diagnosis show an increase over normal in the fraction of time in which slow waves occur at ~3 cycles/min, as opposed to a slow-wave frequency about twice as high. The interpretation of such observations is difficult for at least two reasons. *1)* The functional bowel syndrome is so poorly defined a clinical entity that the patients who carry this diagnosis are very unlikely to constitute a homogeneous group. The different clinical features of the functional bowel syndrome—constipation, diarrhea, and postprandial abdominal pain—have been related to different patterns of colonic myoelectric activity as recorded in vivo (36). *2)* The limitations of methodology make it difficult to know the meaning of such abnormalities in frequency in terms of the basic physiological processes that give rise to slow waves in the circular muscle layer of the colon. Thus these correlations are observations that are essentially uninterpretable. Stoddard et al. (248) indicate that differences among the several computational methods used for data analysis to discover slow-wave frequency in colon electromyographic records could account for the differing incidences of different slow-wave frequencies that are reported from studies of the human colon in situ.

It is unfortunate that so much of the work on electromyogram of the human colon has been done in vivo, because the recording methods that can conveniently be used are so poor and the complex signals that they record are so noisy. It would be an advantage if one knew what to expect to find in vivo; that information could be provided by suitable recordings of colonic myoelectric activity from human colonic muscle in vitro. The methods are much easier, the signal-to-noise ratio is certainly better, and the important physiological variables can be controlled or eliminated. Such recordings from human colonic muscle in vitro has been done recently in surgically resected tissue (167). The longitudinal muscle generated high-frequency signals at 22 cycles/min with intermittent tetanic contractions. The circular muscle generated clusters of spike potentials with rhythmic contractions: slow waves were not detected at the anticipated frequency of 3–6 cycles/min. Sinusoidal oscillatory activity has been infrequent in the human colonic electromyogram, occurring only in up to about half of preparations examined (86, 178, 267). Huizinga et al. (153) found such oscillatory electrical activity at frequencies of 4.5–12 cycles/min in circular muscle from the human sigmoid colon in vitro; this activity was slowed to ~3 cycles/min by prolonged cholinergic stimulation. The frequency and amplitude of the rhythmic oscillatory activity of the electromyogram are remarkably labile spontaneously, and they are affected by stretch of the tissue and by the effects of various autonomic nerves. In this lability, colonic slow electrical signals differ greatly from those of the small intestine and stomach. The inconsistency of slow-wave frequencies and (probably) amplitude undoubtedly contributes greatly to the problem of detecting slow waves in the human colon.

*Relationship of Slow Waves, Contractions, and Flows*

A major problem in the interpretation of electromyographic records from the human colon in situ is the uncertainty that exists as to the degree of which slow waves pace the contractions of the circular muscle layer. This problem has been pointed out by Daniel (72), who emphasized that the relationships between spikes, slow waves, and contractions have not been established as clearly in the colon as they have been in the stomach and small intestine. Slow waves, spike bursts, and contractions were generally correlated in the earliest report on the study of the circular muscle coat in the cat colon (48) and in the rabbit colon (123, 124), and the relationship was thought then to be essentially the same as in the stomach and in the small bowel. In subsequent studies, including one in the dog (233), investigators have not made use of the simultaneous recording of electrical and mechanical activity, recording the electromyogram alone. In the sole study in the human colon in which manometric recordings of pressures were made at the same time as electrical records of the myoelectrical activity (243), no attempt was made to establish the correlation of myoelectric and contractile events. Thus Daniel's viewpoint expressed in his 1975 work (72) remains true. Simultaneous records must be made in situ from implanted electrodes and implanted strain gauges in the colon both in acutely anesthetized and in chronically prepared animals. Pending such studies, the degree to which slow waves are actually the major element in the control of the distribution of contractions in the colon must remain somewhat conjectural.

The idea that slow waves, contractions, and flows of colonic content are closely interrelated is implied by observations that were made some time ago in animals with diarrhea. By chance, in that study, colons were prepared for recording of the electromyogram that had been taken from cats affected by an epidemic of summer diarrhea, probably a viral enteritis. The colons were prepared for study of the electromyogram in vitro. It was found that, in such colons, a single slow-wave pacemaker did not dominate the proximal part of the colon as is the case in the normal situation (50, 51). Instead, electrodes spaced only a few millimeters apart revealed that slow waves at these points were generated independently of one another. That is, slow waves at each point had different frequencies. This could be looked on as the emergence of a great many pacemakers firing independently, or as the uncoupling of the muscle from the single pacemaker that usually dominates it. In a subsequent experiment, healthy animals were given a laxative, castor oil by mouth in a dose sufficient to induce a diarrheal state, and their colons were then removed for the recording of the electromyogram of the circular muscle layer in the ascending colon in vitro. To provide control data, other healthy cats were given equal volumes of corn oil. The control animals did not develop diarrhea, but their colons were removed at the same time interval after treatment as were those from the cats that had received the castor oil. In the cats that had received the castor oil, the same anomaly was found as had been found in the colons of the animals with viral diarrhea—the muscle of the ascending colon exhibited multiple slow-wave generators that operated independently and simultaneously, whereas a single pacemaker tended to dominate the proximal part of the colon in the animals that received the equivalent volume of corn oil. In later experiments, it was shown that a variety of laxative agents can induce such changes in the colonic electromyogram recorded in vitro. These agents include the sodium salt of the laxative principle of castor oil (sodium ricinoleate), quinine, quinidine (19), and capsaicin (15). The electromyogram in tissues exposed to such agents in vitro resembles the electrocardiogram in ventricular fibrillation. The pattern of contraction of the circular muscle is presumably altered greatly by such agents but this has not been further investigated.

## NEUROGENIC FACTORS IN COLONIC CONTRACTIONS

It is widely acknowledged that the motor innervation of colonic muscle may be of major importance in the governance of colonic motility. The nature of these nerves and the ways in which they act have only recently come under study and this remains an area of some controversy and ignorance.

### Morphological Studies

The accepted classification of the motor nerves that supply the colonic musculature is based almost entirely on the results of pharmacological studies, although there have now been limited morphological studies in some species. In general, it is accepted that there are four distinct kinds of motor nerves that can be demonstrated physiologically in colonic muscle: excitatory nerves that are cholinergic, excitatory nerves that are noncholinergic, inhibitory nerves that are adrenergic, and inhibitory nerves that are nonadrenergic (108, 110, 111).

Catecholamine-containing nerves have been described on morphological grounds by the method of catecholamine fluorescence in colonic preparations (22, 26, 40, 150). All these studies agree that most of the adrenergic innervation of the colonic wall is directed to the ganglion cells of the intramural plexuses rather than to the layers of smooth muscle. The adrenergic nerves terminate principally in a catecholamine-containing distribution around ganglion cells of the myenteric plexus, which suggests a synaptic relationship. Very few fibers seem to enter the muscle layers proper. In most species, none of the ganglion cells of the myenteric plexus exhibit catecholamine fluorescence, but there do appear to be such catecholamine-fluorescent ganglion cells in the wall of the proximal colon of the guinea pig (110). Thus species variations may exist in respect to the adrenergic innervation of the colon. The cholinergic innervation of the muscle layers of the colon originated in the ganglion cells of the myenteric plexus (150). Not all these cells exhibit the same degree of activity in the stain for cholinesterase, but the plexus certainly contains other kinds of nerve cells as well (118).

The noncholinergic excitatory nerves and the nonadrenergic inhibitory nerves that supply the colonic muscle cannot be specifically identified by any morphological method, but their existence is certainly demonstrated from both physiological and pharmacological evidence (109).

The myenteric plexus in the rabbit colon is highly organized; it contains a wide range of neuron types (morphologically) and a high ratio (approx. 2:1) of glial cells to neurons. Three types of glial cells can be identified (171). The nerve profiles in the myenteric plexus of the rabbit colon contain a wide variety of vesicle types, and the various combinations of distribution of these different types of vesicles permit the description of at least six main types of axon profiles. These different profiles cannot, however, be firmly related to the various known and postulated neurohormonal transmitters (172). It is likely that the different kinds of vesicles do not each represent a different neurotransmitter, as was once thought.

As in other parts of the gut, the nerves in the colon contain a wide variety of known and proposed neurohumoral transmitters, many of them peptides. These have been revealed both by histochemical and by immunocytochemical methods. Choline acetyltransferase has been clearly demonstrated in neurons of both the myenteric plexus and the submucous plexus in the guinea pig colon (112). Vasoactive intestinal peptide has been found in nerve cell bodies of both the myenteric plexus and the submucous plexus in the guinea pig colon, and VIP-containing fibers have been shown to project from the myenteric plexus to the taeniae of the cecum in the guinea pig (113). There is evidence that $\gamma$-aminobutyric acid (GABA) is synthesized and localized within the myenteric plexus in the cat colon (256). The release and uptake of GABA have been demonstrated in the myenteric plexus of the guinea pig colon, and GABA has been found in a subpopulation of neurons in that plexus (157, 255). Thus GABA may well be a neurotransmitter in the colonic myenteric plexus and perhaps in others parts of the gut. Other neurohormonal transmitters have been found in the transmural plexuses of the colon in humans (131, 161). These include somatostatin and serotonin. The preganglionic neurons of the sacral parasympathetic outflow to the bladder and colon contain Leu-enkephalin, and the sacral plexus nerves contain substance P, VIP, and CCK (77). Thus there are now a number of neurohormonal transmitters that may be responsible for the noncholinergic excitatory and nonadrenergic inhibitory nerve effects that can be demonstrated physiologically. Such transmitters can now be identified in nerves by various methods. These have not been applied to the colon sufficiently to allow conclusions as to their place in the control of colonic motions.

*Peristaltic Reflex*

A peristaltic reflex in the colon was first proposed in 1900 by Bayliss and Starling (23) as a result of studies that they performed on the colon of the dog and rabbit, similar to those they had done previously in the small intestine. The animals had received castor oil, "morphia and A. C. E. mixture," and had had the colon separated from the central nervous system by destruction of the spinal cord below the 10th dorsal vertebra with division of the splanchnic nerves, extirpation of the inferior mesenteric ganglia, and section of the pelvic nerves. The investigators described both the inhibition below the level of stimulation and the contraction above. A pinch of the exposed colon caused inhibition of the whole colon below the site of the pinch, but contractions above the pinch were more difficult to demonstrate. The reflex was more difficult to show in the rabbit. The authors, however, felt justified in the conclusion that the peristaltic reflex, ascending excitation, and descending inhibition in response to a pinch characterize the colon in both species. In 1934, Raiford and Mulinos (213) performed studies of the chronically exteriorized colon in unanesthetized dogs and saw no inhibitory component, only contractions resulting from mucosal stroking. Contraction of the circular muscle layer occurred above the level of the stimulus, and contraction of the longitudinal muscle layer occurred below it. These responses were blocked by the mucosal application of the local anesthetic, cocaine. The authors restated the "law of the intestine" in the colon to exclude an inhibitory response. Hukuhara and Miyaka (154) essentially confirmed the work of Bayliss and Starling in further studies in the colon in anesthetized dogs. However, there remains some uncertainty even as to the description of these reflexes, and it is unknown to what degree such reflexes are related to the governance of normal colonic motility. It is not clear that one can reasonably invoke this reflex in explaining normal colonic motions as they occur physiologically.

Distension-evoked reflexes occur in the colon. Distension of the rabbit proximal colon produces descending inhibition because of the hyperpolarizing effect of nonadrenergic, noncholinergic inhibitory nerves, and because of a serotonergic mechanism acting on the local cholinergic nerves (160). This rectorectal reflex excitatory response is partly centrally mediated and involves excitatory pelvic nerves. A lumbar inhibitory reflex that is normally overriden by the excitatory reflex is also present (253).

*Tonic Neurogenic Inhibition*

The effect of nerves on the motions of colonic muscle could also be expressed as a tonic effect, a continuously sustained and broadly applied neural influence, as opposed to a localized one that is brought about only in response to a specific stimulus such as distension. A high degree of such tonic nerve activity is suggested by experiments in which the muscle of the cat colon is exposed in vitro to the neurotoxin, tetrodotoxin, or to local anesthetics like lidocaine (46). These agents produce excitation of the muscle layers through an apparent prolongation of the electromyographic phenomenon called the migrating spike burst. Because tetrodotoxin and local anesthetics suppress nerve activity, this observation suggests that there is a tonic neurogenic inhibition of the colonic musculature; it also supports the idea that the migrating spike burst is a consequence of periodic removal of this tonic neurogenic inhibition. That is, the migrating spike burst as seen in the whole colon may in fact be a consequence of periodic neurogenic disinhibition. There may be species variation in this matter, however, since tetrodotoxin did not cause excitation of the rabbit colon in a Trendelenburg preparation (189).

*Intrinsic Nerve Stimulation*

Few studies have been made of human colonic muscle in vitro that might shed some light on the nature of the motor nerves that supply colonic muscle. Crema et al. (69) used electrical field stimulation to excite nerves in relation to both longitudinal and circular muscle layers from human colon and saw that both contractions and relaxations could occur. The effective stimuli were 1-ms pulses at 1–10 Hz. Atropine always converted the contractions into relaxations but it did not affect the relaxations themselves. The relaxations were unaffected by various adrenergic receptor antagonists and by methysergide but they were tetrodotoxin-sensitive. This inhibitory nerve response has also been seen in the guinea pig colon where it is not opposed by reserpine pretreatment, $\alpha$-methyltyrosine, perivascular denervation, or bretylium (29). The preceding reports indicate that cholinergic excitatory and nonadrenergic inhibitory nerves are present in both muscle layers of the colon wall. The transmitter of the nonadrenergic inhibitory nerves in the colon is unknown, but, as in other organs, ATP has been proposed as one candidate. In the circular muscle layer of the rabbit colon, desensitization to ATP, adenosine, and the two purines together did not affect the nonadrenergic inhibition that occurred in response to electrical field stimulation and distension of the organ, suggesting that neither of these purines is the transmitter (68).

In colonic muscle from the human colon studied in vitro, the release of acetylcholine induced by electrical field stimulation of the intrinsic innervation is inhibited by norepinephrine; this fact is consistent with the view that catecholamines that are released physiologically from adrenergic nerves may act to modify or regulate the activity of cholinergic ganglion cells. The adrenergic innervation of the colon appears mainly to be inhibitory, because ganglionic stimulants, such as nicotine and dimethylphenylpiperazine, induce relaxation, and this relaxation is sensitive both to various neurotoxins and to various adrenergic antagonists (34, 100). The existence of noncholinergic excitatory nerve fibers in the colon is suggested by the fact that some of the contractions induced in human colonic muscle in vitro by electrical field stimulation of the intrinsic nerves persist in the presence of anticholinergic agents but are tetrodotoxin sensitive.

The interrelations of these different kinds of motor innervation and their place in the integration of motor activity of the whole colon remain to be worked out. This will require the exploration of the colon by a variety of morphological methods. Few studies have been done with electrical field stimulation of nerves in colonic muscle; such possible complicating factors in the description of the motor innervation as species variation, variability between different parts of the colon, and differences between the two layers of the muscle have not been fully explored.

*Responses to Autonomic Drugs*

The use of agents that act at the selective receptors for autonomic neuroeffectors has been important in the process of understanding the way nerves are involved in the governance of contractions in the gut in general, but the colon has been neglected. Cholinergic agents usually cause colonic muscle to contract in vitro. Norepinephrine in vitro is inhibitory to colonic muscle through both $\alpha$- and $\beta$-receptor–mediated mechanisms, but there is at least one suggestion that there is an excitatory adrenergic $\alpha$-receptor mechanism (115). Serotonin is usually inhibitory in vitro to colonic muscle (28) but excitation can occur as well. Histamine is also said to cause both responses (28).

It is obvious that autonomic agents could influence motility not only by affecting the force of contractions but also through an influence on slow waves; in this way such agents could affect the duration of contractions, the integration of movements along the colon, or the direction of propagation of contractions. These relatively more subtle actions of the neuroeffectors seem not to have been looked for. Also, there is a paucity of data about the effects of such naturally occurring neuroeffector substances on colonic motility in vivo. An exception is serotonin, in the case of which results of studies in vivo generally agree with those in vitro (196).

*Extrinsic Nervous Control of Colonic Motility*

The contribution of the extrinsic nerves in the control of colonic motility seems to have been neglected until recently, probably because it is very difficult to make suitable experimental preparations. The various kinds of preparations used in the past have been unphysiological and not appropriate to studies of long duration; also, such preparations have required methods to detect contractions that yield records that are difficult or impossible to interpret in terms of the nature, magnitude, and distribution of wall movements and flows of luminal content.

Many of these methodological problems have been overcome by the use of extraluminal force strain-gauge transducers that are sewn to the serosal surface of the colon in vivo. Rostad (221–225) used such devices on the colon of the cat to examine colonic motility as it is affected by stimulation of areas of the central nervous system. The strain-gauge transducers were always sutured transversely so as to detect mainly circumferential contractions of the colon, with one transducer at the cecum, one in the midcolon, and one on the sigmoid colon. The cat colon was seldom quiet, except during deep anesthesia. Contractions of two kinds occurred: slow contractions lasting 0.5–2.0 min and rhythmic contractions at 4–7 cycles/min. Excitation from vagal stimulation and inhibition from splanchnic nerve stimulation were shown to occur throughout the cat colon, although the major effect on nerve stimulation was in the proximal part. The lumbar sympathetic nerves contained both inhibitory and excitatory fibers that were distributed to all parts of the colon. Stimulation of the hypothalamus caused either excitation or inhibition of the colon, depending on the part stimulated. In the mesencephalon, both excitation of colonic motility (mainly in the proximal colon) and inhibition of colonic motility resulted from stimulation of different regions. The combination of selective cutting of nerves and stimulation of selected areas of the brain revealed the peripheral pathways concerned in some of these effects. The excitatory effects on the colon of stimulation of the hypothalamic areas pass through both the lumbar sympathetic nerves and the parasympathetic pelvic nerves. Excitation of the colon from mesencephalic stimulation is mediated by the lumbar colonic nerves. Guanethidine blocked responses mediated through lumbar nerves, whereas atropine blocked those carried through the pelvic nerves. Some of the excitation is mediated by excitatory $\alpha$-receptors. In the telencephalon, both vagally mediated excitation and lumbar nerve–mediated inhibition were found. These observations confirm and extend the conclusions of previous studies on the subject of the central control of colonic motility; this literature was referred to by Rostad (221–225). It is thus well established that such effects of brain stimulation on colonic motility exist. It is not evident, however, how important such control mechanisms in the central nervous system are in the normal control of colonic motility. It may be that such extrinsic controls are mainly concerned in the integration of colonic activities with other functions.

Julé (159) examined the electromyographic responses of both the proximal and the distal colon of the rabbit to vagal and splanchnic nerve stimulation. In both parts of the colon, he saw evidence both for parasympathetic inhibitory nerves that were nonadrenergic and for a sympathetic inhibitory innervation that was adrenergic. Evidence for nonadrenergic as well as adrenergic inhibitory nerves has also been found in a study of the gerbil colon (126).

Stimulation of the pelvic nerves to the colon of the cat affects contractions and blood flow over a very long part of the colon (155). These effects represent the action of three distinct motor nerve systems in the colon, one excitatory cholinergic system, one excitatory enkephalinergic system, and one that mediates vasodilation through release of an unknown neurotransmitter (236). The pattern of stimulation of the pelvic nerves is important in the responses seen: continuous nerve stimulation produces colonic contractions, whereas brief periodic nerve stimulation does not (10). The vasodilation induced by pelvic nerve stimulation is probably related to the release of kinins but the contraction of the colon and the relaxation of the rectum that result from pelvic nerve stimulation are not (97). The effects of pelvic nerve stimulation may well be modified in part by events within the ganglia that lie within these nerves on the serosal surface of the distal colon (176). The vagus has long been known to reach at least the proximal colon (155) and, in the ferret, it has been shown to contain excitatory motor pathways that can be reflexly activated by a vagal afferent input: one of these contractile nerve effects is cholinergically mediated, whereas the other is not (56).

### EFFECTS OF DRUGS ON COLONIC CONTRACTIONS

Many drugs influence colonic motility. For the most part, the effects of these agents, if they have been investigated at all, are still difficult to relate directly to the control of colonic motor activity as a whole.

### Adrenergic Drugs

$\alpha$-Adrenergic excitation excites contractions in the circular muscle but it inhibits contractions in the longitudinal muscle of the cat colon. $\beta$-Agonists and dopamine are inhibitory (15). The inhibitory $\beta_1$-adrenoceptors are located on cholinergic neurons, whereas the $\beta_2$-adrenoreceptors are located on smooth muscle (90).

### Anticholinergic Agents

An effect of atropine and similar anticholinergic agents on colonic motility has been observed many times and remains controversial (3, 93, 164, 211). The discordant conclusions may be related to differences in methodology. It appears that the inhibitory effect of atropine, if any, is not overwhelming. An inhibitory effect is variably present and, at best, it is incomplete and brief, lasting <30 min. In view of the variability of the reported results and the methodological problems concerned with studies in vivo, it is difficult to accept that any effect at all has been demonstrated. In vitro, the effect of atropine has been examined on the electromyogram of colonic muscle (277): the drug has no effect on the electromyogram, including the spike bursts, which are the electromyographic signals of contractions. Atropine has no influence on the spontaneous contractions of the circular muscle layer of the cat colon in vitro, although the drug does depress spontaneous contractions of the longitudinal muscle layer.

*Polypeptides*

Substance P has been reported to induce powerful contractions of the circular muscle layer of the colon (24). The inferior mesenteric ganglion is now recognized to be a major center for integration of nerve traffic to and from the colon of the guinea pig, and substance P facilitates synaptic transmission along these synaptic pathways to increase colonic motility (177). Substance P is especially potent to excite the muscle of the distal colon of the cat (137). Met-enkephalin stimulates both the proximal and distal cat colon muscle equally. Bradykinin inhibits both layers of the muscle of the colon, but an excitation is seen at high concentrations of the agent in the longitudinal muscle layer in vitro (98). Gastrin heptadecapeptide has little effect on either the longitudinal or the circular layer of human colonic muscle in vitro (27) and in vivo (195). Cholecystokinin stimulates the circular muscle layer of the colon in vivo (134, 239). Angiotensin excites contractions in both longitudinal and circular layers of human colonic muscle in vitro (99). Motilin stimulates contractions of the rabbit rectum (and small intestine), apparently by a direct action on the muscle (1). Neurotensin is a very potent inhibitor of longitudinal muscle of the proximal guinea pig colon, and after washout the relaxation is followed by increased contractions. The peptide acts directly on the muscle (168); the effect of neurotensin has been reported to be excitatory by others (151). Neurotensin increases the activity especially of the proximal colon in the cat (137). Peptide YY inhibits the muscle of the cat colon (186).

*Prostaglandins*

Prostaglandins of the F series excite contraction in both muscle layers of the human colon; prostaglandin E compounds have a differential effect; they contract the longitudinal layer but they relax the circular layer (25). The physiological significance of these agents and their actions is unknown.

*Morphine*

In humans, morphine increases contractions in the left colon in vivo (204, 205); this effect seems to be cholinergically mediated (73). In the cat colon in vitro, at a concentration of 3 $\mu$M, morphine has two effects on the electromyogram (277): it increases the intensity of spike activity, which suggests that it increases the force of contractions, and it prolongs the duration of slow waves. It has no effect on slow-wave frequency. The excitatory effect of morphine in the rat colon may be due either to a direct action on smooth muscle or to a presynaptic inhibition of nonadrenergic inhibitory nerves (122). Some of the effects of morphine on colonic motility are centrally mediated and are related to serotonin release (35).

*$\gamma$-Aminobutyric Acid*

$\gamma$-Aminobutyric acid causes a transient relaxation in both layers of the guinea pig colon. This effect is brought about through the excitation of inhibitory intramural nerves. The GABA has little or no effect on the muscle itself (174). Baclofen, an analogue of GABA, also inhibits the spontaneous contractions of the distal part of the guinea pig colon (201). Both bicuculline, which is an antagonist to some actions of GABA, and tachyphylaxis to GABA reduce motility in the colon of the guinea pig (175).

*Adenosine triphosphate*

There is a large literature that suggests that ATP, ADP, AMP, or adenosine itself may be transmitters of at least some of the nonadrenergic inhibitory nerves in the gut, and some of this work has been done in colonic muscle, where such nerves are readily demonstrated to release ATP. The ATP affects propulsive activity in the rabbit colon (262); it reduces the velocity of propulsion of a balloon in the rabbit colon in vitro and depresses the reflex contractions induced by distension but does not affect responses to transmural stimulation. Evidence suggests that ATP acts on two populations of purinergic receptors located on intrinsic nerves that induce reflex contractions.

*Laxatives*

Many of the agents that are used as laxatives are believed to have that effect because of their ability to alter colonic motility. These are the laxatives commonly classified as contact or irritant laxatives. Little evidence exists, in fact, to support the view that many of these laxatives really do alter colonic motility, except for castor oil or its active principle, ricinoleic acid. Ricinoleic acid seems to have little effect on the amplitude of contractions of colonic muscle in vitro, but it has a pronounced ability to uncouple the electrical slow waves of the colon to induce the formation of extra pacemakers (49, 54).

*Antibiotics*

Several antibiotics have been shown to affect the function of striated and smooth muscle in vitro in small concentrations. In the guinea pig and rabbit colon, clindamycin and trimethoprim depress responses evoked by intramural nerve stimulation; clindamycin has both a prejunctional and a postjunctional action on nerves, and trimethoprim has mainly a postjunctional action on nerves (183).

*Bile Acids*

The secondary bile acid, deoxycholic acid, but not the primary bile acid, glycocholic acid, stimulates colonic motility when infused in vitro into the colonic lumen both in rabbits (96) and in humans (102). This effect is local, i.e., caused by mucosal contact, and is dependent on an intact cholinergic and adrenergic innervation (234).

ANAL SPHINCTERS

*Internal Anal Sphincter*

The internal anal sphincter, a continuation of the circular muscle layer of the rectum, is a thickening of that layer at the level of the dentate line (249, 253). The thickening maintains a tonically contracted state, and this tonic contraction of the internal sphincter is responsible for a part of the closure of the anal canal that is maintained at rest. There is evidence for this in the whole animal from balloon manometry (142); also, it has been shown that the surgical division of the internal anal sphincter with preservation of the striated muscle external anal sphincter weakens but does not abolish the resting force of closure of the anal canal (84, 127). As in other sphincters of the gut, the way in which the tone is maintained by this smooth muscle is not established. It was once thought that the tone is neurogenic, that it is maintained by an excitatory sympathetic innervation; there is, however, little or no evidence for wholly a neurogenic basis for sphincter tone. Much of the tone is myogenic. The internal anal sphincter relaxes in response to rectal distension (80, 230). This relaxation is neurogenic. The reflex response arises from the excitation of mechanoreceptors in the rectal wall. Such receptors seem also to be present in the wall of the sigmoid colon (121, 230). It is not known exactly how far rostrad in the colon these mechanoreceptors can be found in the wall. The pathway of this reflex relaxation of the internal anal sphincter in response to rectal distension has been a matter for considerable investigation. Studies in normal humans (121) have suggested that the reflex pathway involves the spinal cord. Garry (119) observed that simple distensions of a rectal balloon was ineffective in relaxing the sphincter, but that rotation or axial movement of a distended balloon in the rectum caused prompt relaxation in the anal canal in cats that had been anesthetized, decerebrated, decapitated, and cord-transected; the response was not affected by cutting of the pudendal nerves nor by curarization. The effect was, however, abolished by spinal anesthesia, by pelvic nerve section, and by the mucosal application of cocaine; the effect was facilitated by cutting off the lumbar nerves. Garry was cautious in his interpretations of these observations, but he believed that the nerve pathways that induced reflex relaxation of the internal sphincter passed, at least in part, through centers in the spinal cord. Denny-Brown and Robertson (80) examined patients with a variety of neurological lesions using balloons both to distend the rectum and to record responses of the internal sphincter to distension-induced excitation of mechanoreceptors in the wall of the rectum. They concluded that sphincter relaxation is mediated wholly through the intramural plexuses (230). One of the major sources of uncertainty in these studies is related to the technique of recording sphincter muscle function from balloons placed in the anal canal: the fidelity of this technique in distinguishing precisely between the operation of the internal anal sphincter and the external anal sphincter seems questionable.

Various autonomic drugs have been used to answer questions about the mechanisms that produce the tonic contraction and the reflex relaxation of the internal anal sphincter. Garrett et al. (117) used balloon kymography to study the effects of drugs and nerves on the internal anal sphincter in the cat treated with succinylcholine. The drugs were given either intravenously or intra-arterially. The sphincter was observed normally to contract rhythmically at a frequency of 12–36 times/min. Rectal distension by a balloon caused sphincteric relaxation. Resting sphincteric tone was reduced by large doses of pentobarbital. Compression of the urinary bladder and voiding seemed to induce contraction of the sphincter and this effect was blocked by dihydroergotamine. Surgical division of the sympathetic hypogastric nerves caused sphincter tone to fall transiently but it soon returned, and electrical stimulation of the peripheral stump of the severed hypogastric nerves caused contractions that were resistant to atropine and to hexamethonium. Surgical division of the sacral nerves reduced tone permanently, and electrical stimulation of the distal stump of the severed sacral nerve could cause either a contraction or a relaxation; the contractions were not readily antagonized by atropine; the relaxations were resistant to atropine, to hexamethonium, and to adrenergic $\beta$-receptor antagonists. Agents that excited adrenergic α-receptors were excitatory in the sphincter; agents that excite adrenergic β-receptors were inhibitory. Cholinergic agonists were usually excitatory. Sphincteric relaxations induced by rectal distension were unaffected by dihydroergotamine. Propranolol converted the relaxation induced by rectal distension to a dihydroergotamine-sensitive contraction; after treatment with both propranolol and dihydroergotamine, however, sphincteric relaxation in response to rectal distension persisted. Although this study was impressively thorough, questions remain because of the inconsistency of some of the results, because of the general observations that exist as to the physiological significance of experiments in acutely anesthetized animals, and because of the uncertainty that one can selectively follow the behavior of the internal sphincter (as opposed to the external sphincter) by recording from balloons placed in the anal canal.

The study of sphincteric muscle in vitro has overcome many of these objections. Friedmann (105) studied human sphincter muscle in vitro and concluded that stimulation of adrenergic α-receptors induces contraction and that stimulation of adrenergic β-receptors causes inhibition of contraction. He noted poor contractile responses to acetylcholine. Nicotine and other ganglionic stimulants were sometimes excitatory and sometimes inhibitory; this variability was interpreted as representing the consequences of action on adrenergic nerves to release norepinephrine, which could then act on either through α- or β-receptor mechanisms. Parks et al. (207) studied human sphincter muscle in vitro and concluded that adrenergic α-receptors are excitatory and that adrenergic β-receptors are inhibitory in this tissue. They also noted the relative insensitivity of the sphincter muscle to the excitatory action of acetylcholine and that the effects of nicotine are catecholamine mediated. Costa and Furness (66) used isolated innervated preparations of the internal sphincter muscle from the guinea pig in an arrangement that allowed selective stimulation of the colonic, pelvic, and pudendal nerves, as well as the transmural stimulation of intrinsic nerves. They identified 1) cholinergic excitatory nerves arising from the pelvic plexus, 2) adrenergic excitatory nerves supplied from both the pelvic plexuses and the pudendal nerves, and 3) inhibitory nerves descending to the sphincter within the gut wall and arising as well from the pelvic plexus. The guinea pig may not be an appropriate animal model for all mammals, but, in fact, very similar observations were made in a study of the internal anal sphincter of the vervet monkey by Rayner (215).

Bouvier and Gonella (33) studied the sphincter area in cats by recording electromyographic activity in both the longitudinal and the circular muscle layers at rest and in response to intrinsic and extrinsic nerve stimulation. Hypogastric nerve stimulation caused depolarization of the muscle of the internal anal sphincter: this depolarization was due to effects of excitation on adrenergic α-receptors. Parasympathetic nerve stimulation at the second ventral sacral root inhibited spontaneous contraction of the internal sphincter through the action of nonadrenergic, noncholinergic nerves. A similar nonadrenergic neural mechanism was observed to account for the relaxation of the sphincter that was induced by rectal distension. The longitudinal muscle layer of the sphincteric segment behaved quite differently. In this muscle layer, hypogastric nerve stimulation inhibited the muscle by a β-receptor–mediated process, whereas stimulation of the parasympathetic system through the ventral sacral nerve root produced only a cholinergically mediated excitation of the muscle: no nonadrenergic, noncholinergic inhibitory innervation to the longitudinal muscle layer of the sphincteric segment could be demonstrated.

Bouvier and Gonella (32) also examined the spontaneous electromyogram of smooth muscle layers of the anal sphincter both in vitro and in vivo in the cat. They found slow rhythmic variations in the membrane potential of the circular muscle that were accompanied by rhythmic contractions. These variations in membrane potential were myogenic, but they could be modified by various autonomic agents. Norepinephrine raised the frequency of the spontaneous depolarizations by a mechanism that was mediated by adrenergic α-receptors. Acetylcholine had no effect on the depolarizations. In the longitudinal muscle layer, there were spike potentials, each accompanied by contraction, superimposed on long-lasting spontaneous depolarizations. This activity was also myogenic; it was reduced or abolished by norepinephrine through a mechanism mediated by β-receptor activation, and it was enhanced by acetylcholine through excitation of muscarinic receptors. A noncholinergic, nonadrenergic inhibitory innervation of the human internal anal sphincter has been demonstrated by Burleigh (37).

As in other gastrointestinal viscera, the transmitter for the noncholinergic, nonadrenergic inhibitory nerves to the internal anal sphincter has been thought to be ATP or another adenine nucleotide. Crema et al. (68) investigated this idea by studying the internal anal sphincter of the guinea pig in vitro. While both ATP and adenosine were inhibitory, a variety of maneuvers that inhibited the response of the muscle to these agents did not affect the response of the muscle to electrical stimulation of the nonadrenergic, noncholinergic inhibitory nerves. This led to the conclusion that these nerves to not act through an adenine nucleotide-mediated mechanism in the internal anal sphincter.

These studies yield a uniform picture of the innervation of the sphincter. It is apparent that the sphincter has two excitatory innervations, one cholinergic and one adrenergic, and two inhibitory innervations, one adrenergic and the other nonadrenergic. The relative importance of these four different kinds of nerves in the normal physiological operation of the internal anal sphincter, however, remains to be clarified. There appears to be important functions of the adrenergic and cholinergic nerves, and the interactions of these nerves may be quite complex, as discussed by Bouvier and Gonella (33). The two smooth muscle layers in the anal sphincter region are very different from one another. The nonadrenergic, noncholinergic inhibitory nerves may well be responsible for the most important inhibitors of the sphincter, relaxation in defecation: their exact nature in the sphincter, as elsewhere in the gut, remains to be fully described.

Frenckner and Ihre (104) approached the question of the relative importance of the various classes of nerves to the sphincter in determining the resting tonic contraction of the internal sphincter muscle. They studied the intact internal anal sphincter in humans using high spinal anesthesia to block sympathetic outflows and low spinal anesthesia to block parasympathetic outflows from the spinal cord. They found evidence for a tonic excitatory sympathetic discharge from spinal centers to the anal sphincter and they concluded that this accounts for some of the sphincter tone; they found no evidence at all for a tonic parasympathetic discharge to the sphincteric muscle. The study of Frenckner and Ihre (104) also gives evidence for a second point related to the relaxation of the sphincter. They observed relaxations of the internal anal sphincter that occurred in response to distension of the rectum. These relaxations continued during suppression of the parasympathetic supply to the sphincter (by low spinal anesthesia) as well as during suppression of the sympathetic nerve supply (by high spinal anesthesia). From this evidence, it appears that the relaxation of the sphincter caused by rectal distension is neither sympathetic nor parasympathetic.

*External Anal Sphincter*

The external anal sphincter is a ring, or several rings, of striated muscle, constituting several muscle bundles that surround the internal sphincter and lie externally to that sphincter. The several bundles of the external sphincter, however, seem to act together as a single unit. The muscle of the external anal sphincter is a voluntary muscle, like somatic striated muscle. It is usually assumed that the external anal sphincter contributes importantly to anal closure, adding its effect to the tone of the internal anal sphincter to maintain tonic closure of the anal canal. This striated muscle is assumed to maintain a constant state of contraction. Evidence for the existence of such tone in this muscle has been obtained mainly by the recording of the electromyogram of the muscle from electrodes applied as disks to the skin over the musculature of the external sphincter (101). Such evidence suggests that the external anal sphincter maintains a considerable resting tone during waking hours, but the magnitude of this resting tone is greatly reduced during sleep. The magnitude of this tone, indicated by the intensity of electromyographic spike discharges, rises with any maneuver that raises intraabdominal pressure, except for straining at defecation, which reduces magnitude of the tone. These observations have been confirmed in recordings of the electromyogram from needle electrodes inserted in the striated muscle of the sphincter: this method also reveals a continuous discharge of spiking, interpreted as evidence of tone, present at rest in this muscle (8, 103).

There has been some disagreement as to the relative functional importance of the two anal sphincters. Gaston (121) said that the internal sphincter "has nothing to do with sphincteric continence." Hill et al. (142) obtained evidence that the tonic contraction of the internal anal sphincter contributes most of the pressure that is recorded when anal canal pressure is recorded by manometry. Frenckner and Euler (103) anesthetized the pudendal nerves while continuously recording anal canal pressure by manometry and recording the electromyogram of the external anal sphincter. They concluded that the internal sphincter is responsible for ~85% of the recorded pressure in the anal canal at rest, only ~40% of that pressure after sudden rectal distension, and ~65% of that pressure during constant rectal distension. The internal anal sphincter is mainly responsible for continence, they concluded, whereas the external anal sphincter is an important factor in continence only in the event of sudden substantial rectal distension; this is a stimulus that makes the internal anal sphincter relax.

The best current evidence indicates that the external anal sphincter is most important in continence when it is caused to contract as a reflex response to sudden rectal distension (128). This response to rectal distension, together with the induced relaxation of the internal anal sphincter, has been called the inflation reflex (156). In support of this concept, Duthie and Watts (87) observed that the striated muscle of the external anal sphincter contributes importantly to pressure in the anal canal only when a substantial mass is present in the rectum.

The tonic contraction of the external anal sphincter is the result of tonic excitatory neural activation. This conclusion is based on the evidence that the external sphincter and the puborectalis muscle receive only an excitatory innervation. This is a somatic innervation from the second, third, and fourth sacral roots, distributed through the pudendal nerves. No autonomic innervation to this striated muscle has been described. Because the only innervation that is known is an excitatory one, it follows that changes in the level of contraction of the external anal sphincter, including contractions in reflex response to various stimuli, must represent changes in the level of somatic nerve activity in these nerves coming from the sacral segments of the spinal cord. Thus reflexes that involve the external sphincter must be mediated by extrinsic nerves and centers, including probably Onuf's nucleus in the cord (180, 197).

Reflexes that involve the anal sphincters have been studied by Swash (252) and by Pedersen et al. (209). Electrical stimulation of the perianal skin in humans induces reflex contraction of the external anal sphincter, which involves several different reflex mechanisms that exhibit different latencies and represent, probably, different motor pathways of different lengths or connections. Degeneration studies after pudendal neurectomy in monkeys show that there is considerable overlap of the pudendal innervation of the two sides of the external anal sphincter (279). These two duplications in the innervation of the external anal sphincter, one a duplication of reflex pathways and the other a bilateral duplication of the motor innervation, are probably important in contributing to the preservation of function of this sphincter in various neurological diseases.

SOME INTEGRATED COLONIC ACTIVITIES

*Response of the Colon to Eating*

The term *gastrocolic reflex* is widely used, but it is not really appropriate to describe the increased colonic activity that occurs with eating. This is true for three reasons: *1*) the effect is not clearly established as being neural in nature, *2*) the stimulus is not confined to the stomach, and *3*) the response is not restricted to the colon. The term, although convenient, should probably be abandoned.

The fact that eating affects the movements of the colon is evident to laymen and it was first directly studied many decades ago (38, 188). Hertz and Newton (140) reported that mass movements of the colon tend to occur soon after eating. Although this effect seems to be well known, it has not been described with precision, mostly because of the deficiencies of the methods that have been used to observe colonic motility. Both the extent and the magnitude of the response are hard to judge. In most studies of the response, the investigators have examined the distal part of the colon, because it is more accessible to the sensing devices commonly used in vivo, but a recent study that made use of a telemetering capsule makes it clear that both the proximal colon and the distal colon show increased activity in response to eating (194). One of the earliest studies described a response to eating in motility of the cecum (188). A monometric study performed in postoperative patients also showed that the whole length of the colon responds to eating, but the response is most marked in the sigmoid colon (170). The magnitude of the response may be considerable. Measuring magnitudes of responses is difficult with methods that use intraluminal sensing devices to measure contractions. The effect seems to involve an increase both in the frequency of contractions and in the amplitudes of the pressures recorded. Amplitudes of contractions may double (194), but frequency tends to increase less, perhaps only 10%–25%.

The mechanism of the colonic response to eating has been a matter of some conjecture and controversy. Macewen (188) thought that the response was neurally mediated, but more recent investigators have proposed that it may be hormonal. Hertz (139), who seems to have originated the term *gastrocolic reflex*, thought that the major stimulus is the entry of food into the empty stomach; in his report, however, he indicates that he once saw a mass movement in a fasted patient who had only seen the food without eating it. Ruckebusch et al. (227) also have reported increased activity in the colon when food was only presented to a rabbit. These observations raise the possibility that there is a "cephalic phase" in the colonic response to eating. Welch and Plant (272) studied colonic motility in dogs by recording from balloons during feeding. They observed no effect when the food was introduced into the stomach through a gastric fistula. But Connell et al. (61), in a study of the movements of the pelvic colon as observed by balloon manometry, deliberately tried to demonstrate the cephalic phase of the stimulation of colonic motility in eating and failed; they attributed the failure to the unappetizing nature of the meal offered. Ramorino and Cologrande (214) also investigated the cephalic phase in humans; they saw no increase in colonic motion when a large number of human subjects were allowed to see or smell food. Thus the evidence suggests that cephalic phase for the colonic response to eating is either nonexistent or of minor importance.

The existence of a "gastric phase" in the colonic motor response to feeding has slightly more support (116, 146, 216, 227, 243, 250). It is commonly observed that the response begins slowly and persists for an hour or more after the ingestion of food. Because the stomach is normally emptying continuously during eating, so that food is also entering the duodenum, the stimulus cannot be said to be wholly gastric unless gastric emptying is prevented. Gastric distension alone does not excite a colonic response (143, 257). A 1,000-cal meal in humans produces the effect but a 350-cal meal does not (85). Thus the evidence for a distinct and separate gastric phase is not convincing.

Holdstock and Misiewicz (145) postulated an "intestinal phase" in the response of the colon to eating because they found in studies of human subjects that the colonic response does not require the presence of a stomach, the presence of gastric acid, the presence of antral gastrin, or the presence of an intact vagal innervation to the stomach. Furthermore there is a prompt increase in colonic motor activity when food is placed directly into the duodenum (64, 143) and the response occurs in patients with a complete gastrectomy (145). Magnesium sulfate, amino acids, and sodium oleate all initiate prompt increases in colonic contractions when they are infused directly into the duodenum (135, 193). There appear to be several different kinds of receptors that can induce the response. The ingestion of amino acids can inhibit the increases in colonic motility that are induced by ingestion of fat, and by a 1,000-cal meal (21). Thus there is evidence for an intestinal phase in the colonic response to eating, and the evidence suggests that the effect is mediated by stimulation of mucosal chemoreceptors.

There may well be a "colonic phase" in the response as well, because small intestinal motility increases after eating; this causes the entry of chyme into the proximal colon itself.

The neural pathways involved in the transmission of the signals from the chemoreceptive sensors, presumably mainly in the small intestine, to the colon are likewise not entirely clear. In fact, the pathways have not been very thoroughly sought. The effect in humans requires an intact cholinergic innervation at some point in the gastrointestinal tract and to be blocked by naloxone, so that it involves opiate receptors at some point along the pathway (251). The effect of eating on colonic motility persists after vagotomy in humans (59), but it is well known that vagotomy in humans is often far from complete. The effect persists in patients who have had complete transection of the spinal cord (60). The sympathetic innervation can be involved, but an effect of interruption of the splanchnic innervation in humans seems not to have been sought. Studies in experimental animals are scarcely more helpful in revealing pathways. Gregory (130), in a study of Thiry-Vella loops of jejunum in conscious dogs, observed an increase in the motility in such jejunal loops in association with feeding and notices that it occurs also in *1*) sham feeding, *2*) in response to gastric distension by balloon, *3*) in response to mechanical stimulation of the gastric mucosa, and that *4*) vascular denervation of the Thiry-Vella loop abolishes the effect of feeding. However, these observations came from the jejunum; no similar studies have been done in the colon.

It is often assumed that the increased activity of the colon that occurs after eating is caused by the activation of the colonic muscle by increased activity of excitatory cholinergic nerves (244). This assumption is not fully supported by the evidence. There is just as much reason to consider the possibility that the response is caused by an adrenergic mechanism, as suggested by Gregory's data (130) on the effect of perivascular denervation of the jejunum on the jejunal response to feeding. Such a sympathetic neural mechanism would be mediated through stimulation of excitatory $\alpha$-receptors. A good case can also be made that the response is a disinhibition, a transient suspension of a tonic neurogenic inhibition. Such tonic neurogenic inhibition is present in the colon in various animals. Also, the ability of even well-established anticholinergic agents to affect colonic motility is certainly not impressive.

The alternative hypothesis is that the mechanism is hormonal rather than neurally mediated. The most obvious first step to challenge this idea, a cross-circulation experiment, either has not been done or has been widely ignored. The absence of such evidence, however, has not prevented the execution of other, less specific experiments. Gastrin, given in physiological doses in humans and in dogs, increases colonic motor activity (64) and it increases the spike activity in the human rectum and sigmoid (244), but the timing of the colonic response to eating in relation to the timing of gastrin release does not prove that gastrin is solely responsible for the response (244). Furthermore gastrin itself may excite gastrointestinal smooth muscle in part by causing the release of acetylcholine from local intramural stores (268); also atropine can affect the release of both gastrin and CCK (173, 270). Thus attempts to distinguish the putative physiological effects of these and other hormones on the increased colonic contractions after eating from the effects of the colonic innervation in vivo solely through the use of drugs directed at muscarinic receptors are very likely to be futile with the available experimental methods. Hormones and nerves are too closely linked to be an easy matter to study.

The motor response of the colon to eating cannot be fully analyzed until a much more careful and rigorous definition of the whole effect is made. Also, it is no longer satisfactory simply to look for an increase or a decrease in colonic motor activity. Patterns of movements may also be important. These patterns must be fully defined and methods must be developed to allow them to be observed in all kinds of animal preparations.

## Defecation

The complex processes involved in the act of defecation are difficult to understand because of the fact that most of the research on the process of defecation has been performed in humans.

It is evident that the central nervous system is extensively involved in the process. This is clear even superficially from the fact that such a variety of nongastrointestinal actions are involved at least briefly in the act of defecation. Some of the actions are necessary to raise the intra-abdominal pressure. These include the following voluntary actions: the closure of the glottis, the descent of the diaphragm, the contraction of the abdominal wall muscles, and the contraction of muscles of the pelvic floor. Other actions (related to the evacuation of the rectum) include relaxation of the internal and the external anal sphincters and contraction of the muscular wall of the rectum. The nervous centers that are responsible for the integration of these numerous different somatic and visceral movements, which are partly voluntary and partly involuntary, remain to be fully described.

Defecation is normally initiated by the excitation of mechanoreceptors that are located in the anorectal area. These mechanoreceptors can be excited by movements of the rectal mucosa (119) and by rectal distention (230). The exact location of these mechanoreceptors has been a matter of some controversy. Garry (119) thought the mechanoreceptors lie in the mucosa, for he observed that the application of cocaine to the rectal mucosa of the cat abolished all responses to balloon movement in the rectum. This experiment apparently has not been repeated. There is, however, evidence that the receptors are not entirely mucosal in location. In dogs that had a rectal reconstruction operation (in which a total colectomy was modified to preserve a rectum with the seromuscular layers of the rectosigmoid being lined by ileal mucosa) normal defecatory functions return after healing (125). Subsequent general clinical experience has supported the conclusion that rectal mechanoreceptors involved in defecation may not be exclusively mucosal in location. These receptors are either more sensitive or more numerous in the distal rectum than they are when found more proximally in the rectum, because progressively smaller degrees of distention are effective in inducing sphincter relaxation as a stimulating balloon is moved caudad along the rectum (230).

The conflicting evidence about the location of the rectal mucosal mechanoreceptors can be reconciled if the receptors were mucosal (hence accessible to cocaine) but not rectal (hence not removed with the rectal mucosa in the course of ileoanal anastomosis). This would be the case if the receptors were confined to the mucosa in and just above the anal canal. In this location, they would have been exposed to the cocaine in Garry's experiment (119) but might not be fully resected in operations in which the rectal mucosa is stripped. Such a location in the anal canal is suggested by the results of Goligher's survey (127) of continence after a variety of sphincter-sparing operations of the rectum. Goligher observed that an anorectal remnant of at least 6 cm from the anal mucocutaneous junction will usually suffice for perfect defecatory function after rectal resection. Duthie and Gairns (85) examined receptors in the anal canal by applying silver stains to human rectal and anal mucosae to demonstrate the form and distribution of neural structures in the mucosa. In confirmation and extension of earlier studies, they found a profuse innervation of the mucosa in this region, especially in the region of the anal crypts and valves, with both free intraepithelial nerve endings and organized endings. About half of the organized endings were of recognized types, e.g., Golgi-Mazzoni, Krause's, Meissner's, Pacinian, and genital corpuscles. The area containing these structures extends up ~1 cm above the anal valves. The perianal skin contains a less dense distribution of nerves with only peritrichial and some free nerve endings; the more proximal rectal mucosa itself is devoid of nerve endings. The lining of the anal canal is very sensitive to pain, heat, cold, and light touch in humans. Duthie and Gairns (85) proposed that the mucosal receptors of the anal canal are important in continence and defecation. Duthie and Bennett (83) extended this study by plotting the distribution of the sensory area in the anal canal. They found that the sensory zone of the mucosa lies entirely within the high-pressure segment of the anal canal. With rectal distension, the anal canal shortens both by axial retraction of the rectum itself and by relaxation of the internal anal sphincter; this brings the sensory zone of the anal canal more into the rectal vault. The radiographic studies of Phillips and Edwards (210) support this idea. Phillips and Edwards postulated that a flutter-valve mechanism also contributes to the maintenance of closure of the anal canal under the condition of raised intra-abdominal pressure. It seems possible that these anal canal mucosal receptors are the chief source of the rectoanal reflexes that are involved in continence and defecation. Balloon distension of the rectum probably also can move or displace the mucosa of the anal canal to some extent, and such displacement can explain the observation that the sensitivity to rectal distension is more pronounced when the stimulating balloon is placed closer to the anal canal.

When continence is discussed, it is often said that the rectum is empty until the act of defecation is about to occur. This view is not consistent with common clinical experience, because physicians who routinely do digital examination of the anal canal on physical examination usually encounter enough stool at least to check for blood. Also a radiographic study that was directed to the question did not confirm the idea that the rectum is usually empty (131). The rectum was very commonly filled with feces in the absence of the urge to defecate; the study also showed that in some subjects the whole of the left side of the colon from the splenic flexure downward is emptied in defecation. This observation indicates that the reflexes that are involved in defecation also promote a contraction of the muscular wall not only of the rectum itself but also of a long segment of the descending colon as a part of the act of defecation. These wall movements of the distal colon in defecation have not been mapped in more detail, however, so that little more can be said of them.

In any discussion of anal continence, it is usual to speak of sphincteric continence and of rectal continence as though they are two separate functions. *Sphincteric continence* is a term that is usually used to refer to the actions and properties of the two sphincters and of the anal canal in continence. *Rectal continence* is a term that is used to refer to the capacity of the rectum to act as a reservoir for the fecal mass. The ability of the rectum to do so is related to its ability to allow an increase in volume without excitation of defecation. One might assume that, like the gastric fundus, the rectum contains a mechanism for receptive relaxation, but this process seems not be have been much considered.

Defecation may be transiently disturbed in patients who have had cortical injuries or injuries on the spinal cord above the lumbosacral level, but it is often ultimately restored (23). From this, it is generally concluded that the lumbosacral cord alone can sustain the essential reflex mechanisms that are concerned in defecation. Although the conclusion has been amply supported by further observations in patients with cortical injuries, the idea seems not to have been pursued with controlled and objective experimentation in animals. Thus there is insufficient evidence to specify what nerves transmit effective inputs to the postulated "defecation center" in the lumbosacral cord.

*Effect of Emotions on the Colon*

From the studies of Rostad (221–225) and others it is clear that there is an anatomic basis to support the idea that emotions can influence colonic motility. It is widely recognized that anxiety affects colonic motor function. A way to measure or describe such an effect objectively, however, is difficult to identify. The experiments were mainly done in humans, in a setting where the stress is produced by conversation on anxiety-producing topics. Colonic motility was recorded by balloons during such conversations. The experiments that were done were often poorly controlled, and the results of such studies have been to some degree contradictory and unconvincing. The reports are all more than a decade old (4–7, 42, 48, 166), so that such an experimental approach has probably been abandoned. There are other more measurable ways to induce anxiety and stress that have not yet been applied to the question of the possible influence of anxiety and stress on colonic motor function. It has been said that sleep depresses colonic motility and this is taken as evidence for an influence of emotions on colonic motility (34).

## DISORDERS OF COLONIC MOTILITY

*Diverticulosis of the Colon*

Diverticulosis of the colon is a very common clinical entity that is, at least in part, a consequence of disordered colonic motility. The evidence can be summarized in the following observations: there is a thickening caused by hyperplasia of rings of the circular muscle layer adjacent to the diverticula; this thickening long precedes the development of the diverticula; intraluminal pressures recorded in the area of the diverticula are abnormally great when colonic contractions are induced by morphine, by prostigmine, and by eating. Such evidence was generated over a decade ago in a series of well-reviewed studies (17, 203, 278). The thickening of the circular muscle is commonly called hypertrophy, despite the evidence that the ratio of DNA to nitrogen in the thickened circular muscle next to diverticula is not different from that of normal circular or normal longitudinal muscle. Thus the thickening of the rings of the circular muscle layer represents either hyperplasia of the muscle or shortening in the longitudinal axis of the colon due to contraction of the longitudinal muscle (237). There is no explanation as to the immediate cause of the thickening, but there may be one clue in the observation that there is a "plethora of ganglionic tissue" in specimens of the muscular wall that contain diverticula (187). This increase in nerve density could be also a result rather than a cause of the thickening, brought about by retraction of the longitudinal muscle layer. Extensive epidemiological evidence shows that the muscle thickening and the consequent diverticulosis are a result of long-term adherence to a low-residue diet. The pathophysiology to explain such a causal relationship is obscure, and experiments to support it are difficult to design and to execute, because age alone can greatly alter colonic muscle function in independence of dietary practices. The experimental evidence, furthermore, does not support the idea. Carlson and Hoelzel (41), in life-span studies of rats fed diet of varying fiber content, concluded that colonic diverticula form in aging rats as a consequence of a lack of suitable kind and volume of roughage in the diet. The diverticula that they saw were, however, quite unlike those of the human disease in that they were located within or close to the cecum. Furthermore Carlson and Hoetzel did not report muscle thickening, although apparently they did not seek it, not knowing of that feature of the human disease. Dowling et al. (81) fed diets containing large amounts of powdered kaolin to rats; on such a high bulk diet their animals developed an increase in colon weight due mainly to an increase in the thickness of the muscle coats, a change which they attributed to work hypertrophy. Havia and Klossner (136) fed puppies a low-residue diet for 10 mo: no diverticula developed. On manometric and fluoroscopic studies, they observed no abnormalities, nor was muscle thickening found.

*Aganglionosis of the Colon*

Hirschsprung's disease, also called aganglionosis or congenital megacolon, is a well-established example of a motility disorder, localized to the distal colon, that has been recognized for many decades. A neurogenic origin was first proposed only as recently as 1946 (88). The disorder may not be a single nosological entity, however, because some degree of heterogeneity in the disease is evident from epidemiological studies (208). There is heterogeneity especially in the extent of the neurological defect, which is a deficit in intramural ganglion cells. In most patients, the aganglionic segment of the colon extends no further than the anal canal and rectum, but much longer segments have been described that may involve almost the whole of the colon. Furthermore there is a considerable variability in the clinical presentation of the disorder, because some patients may require immediate surgical relief of colonic obstruction in the neonatal period, whereas others who have a similar length of rectum involved may present themselves much later in life with only a history of intractable constipation.

The characteristic barium enema X-ray appearance of the colon in Hirschsprung's disease is well known: there is a narrowed distal segment of the rectum constituting the rectal or rectosigmoid regions that give way sharply to a dilated colon more proximally. Davidson et al. (75) looked for denervation supersensitivity in the distal colon with a triple-lumen nonperfused tube to record intraluminal pressures in response to methacholine. They examined both affected patients and normal control patients. Methacholine relaxed the distal colon in 9 of 20 normal control subjects and it had no effect in the diseased narrowed segment in any of the patients. These workers expected to find denervation supersensitivity in light of the neuropathological lesion. They explained the lack of denervation supersensitivity in the narrow segment on the grounds that the denervation is congenital, not acquired (as it probably is in idiopathic esophageal achalasia where denervation supersensitivity is always found). In one of their six patients, however, who was operated on (with success) because of the clinical presentation and the failure of methacholine to make the distal segment relax, the narrowed distal segment contained intramural ganglia. In studies of the anal sphincteric responses to balloon distension in 10 children with congenital megacolon (229), it was found that the internal anal sphincter failed to relax in response to rectal distension: instead there was a contraction. Lawson and Nixon (182) used a balloon system to record pressures in the anal canal in 24 normal children and in 47 children with congenital megacolon. They observed that the internal anal sphincter is kept closed normally by rhythmic contractions occurring at a frequency of 10–13 cycles/min, and that the sphincter relaxes when there is a sufficient degree of rectal distension. They observed that in Hirschsprung's disease the resting closure pressures in the internal anal sphincter are somewhat raised, with very pronounced rhythmic contractions. Distension of the rectum produced no relaxation of the internal anal sphincter, and in some patients rectal distension raised the base-line pressure and the amplitude of the rhythmic contractions. Similar observations were made by Howard (148). The suggestion of these workers that the abnormal response of the internal anal sphincter to rectal distension could be used as a diagnostic test (182, 229) was repeated by Tobon et al. (261), and the test has now become a commonplace diagnostic maneuver.

The neuropathology of the disease, first completely described by Whitehouse and Kernohan (275), was used to distinguish it from other kinds of idiopathic megacolon by Bodian et al. (30). These authors found an absence of ganglion cells in both the myenteric and the submucous plexuses throughout the narrowed segment and over a length of 1–5 cm into the dilated segment; the plexuses in the aganglionic segments contained numerous coarse and tortuous bundles of unusually dense nerve fibrils. Smith (238) used silver stains in sections cut parallel to the gut wall in two adult cases of Hirschsprung's disease and observed, in the dilated segments above the narrowed zone, a reduced number of ganglion cells (many of them abnormal in appearance), unmyelinated nerve trunks, and a grossly disorganized pattern of nerve bundles. Ehrenpreis et al. (89) used the catecholamine fluorescence technique to examine the intramural nerves in 10 specimens and found that the dilated segment of the colon in Hirschsprung's disease contained normal-appearing basketlike adrenergic networks surrounding ganglion cells; the narrowed segment contained no such structures. In both dilated and normal segments, a small number of adrenergic terminals was found in the submucosa, in the circular muscle layer, and at the interface between the circular muscle layer and the taeniae. Thus it appears that there is adrenergic denervation of the narrowed segment as well as aganglionosis. Bennett et al. (26) suggested that the numbers of adrenergic nerves present in the muscle layers themselves, although sparse, are actually increased. Meier-Ruge (191) applied the cholinesterase stain in Hirschsprung's disease and found a great increase in cholinesterase activity in the abnormal dense and tortuous bundles of nerves in the narrowed segment. He proposed that the sustained contraction of the narrowed segment represents an increased excitatory cholinergic innervation of the muscle that accompanies the aganglionosis, in contrast to the common view that the maintained contraction is a consequence of a cholinergic denervation. Garrett et al. (118) used both catecholamine fluorescence technique and cholinesterase stains to examine nerves in resected specimens. In the circular muscle layer from the aganglionic segment, the number of cholinergic nerves was variable; the cases with the most cholinergic nerves were those with the most severe clinical presentations; those with the fewest such nerves had the mildest clinical presentations. The number of catecholamine-fluorescent nerves was highly variable in the aganglionic segment. In the junctional zone between the ganglionic segment and the aganglionic segment, there was a deficiency of intramuscular nerves. Garrett et al. concluded that the spasm of the contracted segment represents the unopposed action of cholinergic excitatory nerves on the muscle, that the failure of coordinated contraction and relaxation in the narrowed segment is due to the aganglionosis, and that a deficiency in the nerves to the muscle in the junctional region between the dilated and narrowed segments leads to deficient propulsive forces at this level. Subsequent electron-microscopic studies (149, 150) supported the conclusions of previous histochemical studies in revealing a rich supply of intramuscular nerve bundles in the aganglionic segment, without obvious structural abnormality of the constituent axons, and a relative deficiency of these intramuscular nerves at the junction between the ganglionic (dilated) and aganglionic (narrowed) segments. Not surprisingly, other kinds of nerves are abnormal too, as shown by immunocytochemical staining of nerves in resected tissues from patients with Hirschsprung's disease. Larsson et al. (181) and Tsuto et al. (264) have found a deficit or an absence of nerves containing enkephalin, gastrin-releasing peptide, VIP, and substance P. This finding demonstrates the nonselective nature of the denervation in Hirschsprung's disease.

Thus it is clear that there is a considerable degree of heterogeneity in the neuropathology of aganglionosis of the colon. The histology, taken together with the demonstration that the internal anal sphincter fails to relax in Hirschsprung's disease and that internal anal sphincter relaxation in normal subjects in response to rectal distension is nonadrenergic, suggests that at least some of the ganglion cells that are lost may be nonadrenergic inhibitory ganglion cells. Wood (280, 281) has studied a strain of mice with an inherited aganglionic megacolon, which is considered to be a reasonable animal model of the human disease. He suggested that the entity is characterized by an absence of spontaneously active inhibitory neurons from the enteric plexuses. In studies of the development of the anorectal innervation in this same strain of mice, Rothman and Gershon (226) concluded that the denervated segment of the gut is intrinsically abnormal very early in organogenesis, so that it cannot be colonized by the precursors of enteric neurons that migrate from the neural crest in embryonic development. Vaillant et al. (266) also concluded that the constriction in the terminal rectum of the same strain of mice with megacolon is the consequence of a deficit in intrinsic inhibitory neurons; they found normal populations of gut endocrine cells in the aganglionic segment, and this supports the idea that the enteric neurons and the mucosal endocrine cells have different origins. It is thought that the tonically contracted segment that is partially denervated in such mice might represent denervation in the muscle layers. Ligand binding studies by Seidel et al. (232) do not support this idea, so that the obstructing contraction may well be due only to the deficit of inhibitory enteric neurons. This idea was supported physiologically in tissues taken from affected children (178).

### Diarrhea and Constipation

It is commonly held that abnormal patterns or magnitude of colonic motility is a cause in common constipation and diarrhea. It is further commonly believed that diarrhea is a consequence of a hypermotile state, and that constipation is the consequence of hypomotility. Manometric records from the left colon, however, show the opposite to be true: in patients with diarrhea, the number of contractions recorded in the left colon is reduced, whereas the increased numbers of contractions are found in patients who are constipated (58, 163). Although these studies are now quite old, they have not been subsequently extended or elaborated on. Perhaps the most important advance in this matter has been that diarrhea and constipation have been defined quantitatively (62).

### Irritable Colon Syndrome

The *irritable colon syndrome* is a very commonly used diagnostic term, which suggests that a well-defined symptom complex can be blamed on irritability of the colon. That implication is misleading on at least three counts: *1*) the symptom complex has not been carefully defined, *2*) the colon has not convincingly been shown to be involved, and *3*) irritability, an ill-defined concept, has not been demonstrated. Nevertheless many patients and physicians who use the term speak of it as though it applies to a single clinical entity and is a psychosomatic disorder related to stress and to depression (42, 43, 144, 192, 269). This view may be true but it is difficult to substantiate. Most studies supporting the concept of the irritable bowel syndrome as a definite clinical entity have focused on the attempt to find psychological abnormalities in patients who seem to fit this diagnostic category. The observations often seem uncontrolled or poorly controlled, or do not seem objective, but such problems are common in attempts to define psychological abnormalities. Attempts to demonstrate colonic motor abnormalities in such patients have not always been successful. A complete review of the large literature on the topic is beyond the scope of this chapter. The lack of wholly convincing evidence for a colonic motor abnormality in patients considered to have the irritable colon syndrome arises not only from the lack of a clear definition of the syndrome itself but also from the problems that exist with respect to the objective assessment of human colonic motility in vivo. Methods to study colonic motility have recently been refined beyond simple manometry. For example, some reflexes have been examined (274), and the technique of colonic electromyography is used extensively (228). Such new methods have not, however, been fruitful in advancing our understanding of the syndrome, if it exists at all as a solitary, definable clinical entity. The intraluminal perfusion of deoxycholic acid in humans stimulates colonic motility in normal subjects, and Taylor et al. (258) found that patients who seem to have the irritable bowel syndrome are more sensitive to this effect than are normal subjects. A recent attempt to demonstrate abnormalities in urinary epinephrine excretion in patients diagnosed with the syndrome (95) showed a higher excretion in patients in which diarrhea was the dominant symptom (as opposed to those in which pain dominated the clinical picture) than in a control population. The patients with a predominance of diarrhea also showed more evidence for anxiety and neurosis on objective tests for such personality traits than did the control population. The patients with the pain-dominant form of the irritable bowel syndrome did not differ from normal control results in these tests for personality dysfunction.

*Rectal Incontinence*

Rectal incontinence, the abnormal descending perineum syndrome, and rectal prolapse are all debilitating problems that are common in old people and in women after traumatic childbirth. There is recent evidence that these problems are largely a consequence of damage to the innervation of the striated musculature of the pelvic floor, which includes the external anal sphincter (138, 198, 199). This damage may involve the nerves to the puborectalis muscle as well as the nerves to the external anal sphincter (20). In postpartum fecal and urinary incontinence, traumatic damage to the innervation of the pelvic floor muscles is probably the most common cause, as opposed to simple stretch of the musculature of the pelvic floor or incidental surgical division of the anal sphincter (245). Relatively minor damage to the innervation of these muscles can be detected easily and quickly by the measurement of nerve conduction velocity in the pudendal nerves (165).

SUMMARY

The movements of the walls of the colon are organized to produce a pattern of fecal flow that is consistent with three important colonic functions: the conservation of water, the maintenance of an abundant intraluminal colonic bacterial population, and the capacity to control the time and location of the delivery of feces.

The gross patterns of contraction and of flow in the mammalian colon suggest that the colon consists of three segments that can be functionally distinguished. In the proximal part of the colon, the major pattern of contraction is one in which retrograde contraction rings, rhythmic antiperistalsis, function to retain the colonic content in the cecum and ascending colon, where it can be retained and mixed over long periods of time. In an intermediate segment of the colon, the major pattern of contraction consists of contraction rings that divide the fecal mass into separate masses, and that tend to move the feces very slowly antegrade. In the most distal region of the colon, the pattern of contractile main activity is a strong moving contraction ring, oriented to move caudad, that is especially dependent on stimulation of the muscle by the pelvic nerves.

These different patterns of movement of the walls of the colon may be established by differences in control mechanisms of three kinds—myogenic, neurogenic, and hormonal control systems. Myogenic factors, the properties of the smooth muscle itself, account in part for the characteristic contraction patterns in the proximal and intermediate parts of the colon. In these regions, electrical slow waves (pacesetter potentials or electrical control activity) operate in such a way as to establish the frequency and the direction of propagation of rhythmic annular contractions. The influences of the autonomic nerves to the colon have a less clearly defined function in controlling normal patterns of colonic motility in the proximal and middle parts of the colon. There is some evidence to suggest that the pattern of mass movement may be neurogenic, and that mass movement may represent disinhibition, a transient suppression of a tonic neurogenic inhibition. Neurogenic factors may be important in regulating the quantity of contractions rather than the pattern of contractions. Neurogenic factors are clearly most important in the most distal region of the colon, where numerous integrated actions that take place in defecation are clearly a consequence of the effect of nerves that are connected to centers in the central nervous system.

The principal excitatory nerves in the colon are cholinergic, and the principal inhibitory nerves appear to be nonadrenergic. An adrenergic inhibition is also present throughout the colon, and it is directed mainly to the ganglion cells of the intramural plexuses. Hormones may also be involved in the control of colonic motility, and this seems especially likely to be important in the colonic response to eating.

The emotional state is presumed to have an effect on colonic motor function, but this effect remains to be clearly described. Diverticulosis of the colon is a consequence of a disorder of function of colonic smooth muscle, but it is not clear how the muscle disorder is generated. Aganglionosis of the colon is also clearly a colonic motor disorder due to a congenital defect in the development of the innervation of the distal colon, a defect that seems to involve many classes of nerves. A relationship between abnormal colonic motility and the symptoms of diarrhea and constipation is somewhat conjectural. In the irritable colon syndrome, there may be a variety of abnormal functions; this common diagnosis probably encompasses a variety of undefined pathological processes that may involve abnormal nerve function, abnormal muscle function, or abnormal hormonal effects. The complexity of colonic motility and the many remaining obscurities in relation to colonic motor function suggest that more general specific clinical entities involving abnormal motility of the colon remain to be defined.

This work was supported in part by Grants AM 11242 and AM 34986 from the National Institutes of Health.

REFERENCES

1. ADACHI, H., N. TODA, S. HAYASHI, M. NOGUCHI, T. SUZUKI, K. TORIZUKA, H. YAJIMA, AND K. KOYOMA. Mechanism of the excitatory action of motilin on isolated rabbit intestine. *Gastroenterology* 80: 783–788, 1981.
2. ADLER, H. F., A. J. ATKINSON, AND A. C. IVY. A study of motility of the human colon: an explanation of dyssynergia (dyssynergia) of the colon, or of the "unstable colon." *Am. J. Dig. Dis.* 8: 197–202, 1941.
3. ADLER, H. F., A. J. ATKINSON, AND A. C. IVY. The effect of morphine and Dilaudid on the ileum and of morphine, Dilaudid and atropine on the colon of man. *Arch. Intern. Med.* 69: 974–985, 1942.
4. ALMY, T. P., F. K. ABBOT, AND L. E. HINKLE, JR. Alteration in colonic function in man under stress. IV. Hypomotility of the sigmoid colon and its relationship to the mechanism of functional diarrhea. *Gastroenterology* 15: 95–103, 1950.
5. ALMY, T. P., L. E. HINKLE, JR., B. B. BERLE, AND F. KERN, JR. Alterations in colonic function in man under stress. III. Experimental production of sigmoid spasm in patients with spastic constipation. *Gastroenterology* 12: 437–449, 1949.
6. ALMY, T. P., F. KERN, JR., AND M. TULIN. Alterations in colonic function in man under stress. II. Experimental production of sigmoid spasm in healthy persons. *Gastroenterology* 12: 425–436, 1949.
7. ALMY, T. P., AND M. TULIN. Alterations in colonic function in man under stress. I. Experimental production of changes simulating the "irritable colon." *Gastroenterology* 8: 616–626, 1947.
8. ALVA, J., A. I. MENDELOFF, AND M. M. SCHUSTER. Reflex and electromyographic abnormalities associated with fetal incontinence. *Gastroenterology* 53: 101–106, 1967.
9. ANDERSON, P. N., J. MITCHELL, AND D. MAYOR. The uptake of horseradish peroxidase by neuronal elements within the guinea-pig distal colon and its subsequent retrograde transport to the inferior mesenteric ganglion: an in vitro study using an intact neuronal system. *J. Anat.* 130: 153–157, 1980.
10. ANDERSON, P. O., S. R. BLOOM, AND J. JARHUET. Colonic motor and vascular responses to pelvic nerves stimulation and their relation to local peptide release in the cat. *J. Physiol. Lond.* 334: 293–307, 1983.
11. ANSON, B. J., AND W. G. MADDOCK. Ileocecal-appendiceal region. In: *Callander's Surgical Anatomy* (3rd ed.). Philadelphia, PA: Saunders, 1952, chapt. 15, p. 473–479.
12. ANURAS, S. cAMP and calcium in generation of slow waves in cat colon. *Am. J. Physiol.* 242 (*Gastrointest. Liver Physiol.* 5): G124–G127, 1982.
13. ANURAS, S., S. M. CHIEN, AND J. CHRISTENSEN. Metabolic dependence of the electromyogram of the cat colon. *Am. J. Physiol.* 239 (*Gastrointest. Liver Physiol* 2): G173–G176, 1980.
14. ANURAS, S., AND J. CHRISTENSEN. Electrical slow waves of the colon do not extend into the caecum. *Rend. Gastro. Enterol.* 7: 56–59, 1975.
15. ANURAS, S., AND J. CHRISTENSEN. Effects of autonomic drugs on cat colonic muscle. *Am. J. Physiol.* 240 (*Gastrointest. Liver Physiol.* 3): G361–G364, 1981.
16. ANURAS, S., J. CHRISTENSEN, AND D. TEMPLEMAN. Effect of capsaicin on electrical slow waves in the isolated cat colon. *Gut* 18: 666–669, 1977.
17. ARFWIDSSON, S. Pathogenesis of multiple diverticula of the sigmoid colon in diverticular disease. *Acta Chir. Scand. Suppl.* 342: 1–68, 1964.
18. BARCLAY, A. E. Direct x-ray cinematography with a preliminary note on the nature of non-propulsive movements of the large intestine. *Br. J. Radiol.* 8: 652–658, 1935.
19. BARKER, J. D., AND J. CHRISTENSEN. Some effects of quinidine and quinine on the electromyogram of the colon. *Gastroenterology* 65: 773–777, 1973.
20. BARTALO, D. C., J. A. JARRATT, M. G. READ, T. C. DONNELLY, AND N. W. READ. The role of partial denervation of the puborectalis in idiopathic fecal incontinence. *Br. J. Surg.* 70: 664–667, 1983.
21. BATTLE, W. M., S. COHEN, AND W. J. SNAPE, JR. Inhibition of postprandial colonic motility after ingestion of an amino acid mixture. *Dig. Dis. Sci.* 25: 647–652, 1980.
22. BAUMGARTEN, H. G. Uber die verteilung von Catecholaminen im Darm des Menschen. *Z. Zellforsch. Mikrosk. Anat.* 83: 133–146, 1967.
23. BAYLISS, W. M., AND E. H. STARLING. The movements and the innervation of the large intestine. *J. Physiol. Lond.* 26: 107–118, 1900.
24. BENNETT, A. Symposium on colonic function. Pharmacology of colonic muscle. *Gut* 16: 307–311, 1975.
25. BENNETT, A., AND B. FLESHLER. Prostaglandins and the gastrointestinal tract. *Gastroenterology* 59: 790–800, 1970.
26. BENNETT, A., J. R. GARRETT, AND E. R. HOWARD. Adrenergic myenteric nerves in Hirschprung's disease. *Br. Med. J.* 1: 487–489, 1968.
27. BENNETT, A., J. J. MISIEWICZ, AND S. L. WALLER. Analysis of the motor effects of gastrin and pentagastrin on the human alimentary tract in vitro. *Gut* 8: 470–474, 1967.
28. BENNETT, A., AND B. WHITNEY. A pharmacological study of the motility of the human gastrointestinal tract. *Gut* 7: 307–316, 1966.
29. BIANCHI, C., L. BEANI, G. M. FRIGO, AND A. CREMA. Further evidence for the presence of non-adrenergic inhibitory structures in the guinea-pig colon. *Eur. J. Pharmacol.* 4: 51–61, 1968.
30. BODIAN, M., F. D. STEPHENS, AND B. C. H. WARD. Hirschprung's disease and idiopathic megacolon. *Lancet* 1: 6–11, 1949.
31. BORING, E. G. The sensations of the alimentary canal. *Am. J. Psychol.* 26: 1–57, 1915.
32. BOUVIER, M., AND J. GONELLA. Electrical activity from smooth muscles of the anal sphincteric area of the cat. *J. Physiol. Lond.* 310: 445–456, 1981.
33. BOUVIER, M., AND J. GONELLA. Nervous control of the internal anal sphincter of the cat. *J. Physiol. Lond.* 310: 457–469, 1984.
34. BUCKNELL, A., AND B. WHITNEY. A preliminary investigation of the pharmacology of the human isolated taenia coli preparation. *Br. J. Pharmacol.* 23: 164–175, 1964.

35. BUENO, L., AND J. FIORAMONTI. A possible central serotonergic mechanism involved in the effects of morphine on colonic motility in dog. *Eur. J. Pharmacol.* 82: 147-153, 1982.
36. BUENO, L., J. FIORAMONTI, J. FREXINOS, AND Y. RUCKELBUSCH. Colonic myoelectrical activity in diarrhea and constipation. *Hepato-gastroenterology* 27: 381-389, 1980.
37. BURLEIGH, D. E. Non-cholinergic, non-adrenergic inhibitory neurons in human internal anal sphincter muscle. *J. Pharm. Pharmacol.* 35: 258-260, 1983.
38. CANNON, W. B. The movements of the intestines studied by means of the röntgen rays. *Am. J. Physiol.* 6: 251-277, 1902.
39. CAPRILLI, R., AND L. ONORI. Origin, transmission and ionic dependence of colonic electrical slow waves. *Scand. J. Gastroenterol.* 7: 65-74, 1972.
40. CAPURSO, L., C. A. FRIEDMAN, AND A. G. PARKS. Adrenergic fibers in the human intestine. *Gut* 9: 678-682, 1968.
41. CARLSON, A. J., AND F. HOELZEL. Relation of diet to diverticulosis of the colon in rats. *Gastroenterology* 12: 108-115, 1949.
42. CHAUDHARY, N. A., AND S. C. TRUELOVE. Human colonic motility: a comparative study of normal subjects, patients with ulcerative colitis, and patients with the irritable colon syndrome. Resting patterns of motility. II. The effect of prostigmine. III. Effects of emotions. *Gastroenterology* 40: 1-17, 18-26, 27-36, 1961.
43. CHAUDHARY, N. A., AND S. C. TRUELOVE. The irritable colon syndrome: a study of the clinical features, predisposing causes, and prognosis in 130 cases. *Q. J. Med.* 31: 307-322, 1962.
44. CHRISTENSEN, J. The controls of gastrointestinal movements; some old and new views. *N. Engl. J. Med.* 285: 85-98, 1971.
45. CHRISTENSEN, J. Motility of the colon. In: *Physiology of the Gastrointestinal Tract* (1st ed.), edited by L. R. Johnson. New York: Raven, 1981, chapt. 14, p. 445-471.
45a.CHRISTENSEN, J. Motility of the colon. In: *Physiology of the Intestinal Tract* (2nd ed.), edited by L. R. Johnson. New York: Raven, 1987, chapt. 21, p. 665-693.
46. CHRISTENSEN, J., S. ANURAS, AND C. ARTHUR. Influence of intrinsic nerves on electromyogram of cat colon in vitro. *Am. J. Physiol.* 234 (*Endocrinol. Metab. Gastrointest. Physiol.* 3): E641-E647, 1978.
47. CHRISTENSEN, J., S. ANURAS, AND R. L. HAUSER. Migrating spike bursts and electrical slow waves in the cat colon: effect of sectioning. *Gastroenterology* 66: 240-247, 1974.
48. CHRISTENSEN, J., R. CAPRILLI, AND G. F. LUND. Electric slow waves in circular muscle of cat colon. *Am. J. Physiol.* 217: 771-776, 1969.
49. CHRISTENSEN, J., AND B. W. FREEMAN. Circular muscle electromyogram in the cat colon: local effect of sodium ricinoleate. *Gastroenterology* 63: 1011-1015, 1972.
50. CHRISTENSEN, J., AND R. L. HAUSER. Circumferential coupling of electric slow waves in circular muscle of cat colon. *Am. J. Physiol.* 221: 1033-1037, 1971.
51. CHRISTENSEN, J., AND R. L. HAUSER. Longitudinal axial coupling of slow waves in proximal cat colon. *Am. J. Physiol.* 221: 246-250, 1971.
52. CHRISTENSEN, J., G. A. RICK, B. A. ROBISON, M. J. STILES, AND M. A. WIX. Arrangement of the myenteric plexus throughout the gastrointestinal tract of the opossum. *Gastroenterology* 85: 890-899, 1983.
53. CHRISTENSEN, J., M. J. STILES, G. A. RICK, AND J. SUTHERLAND. Comparative anatomy of the myenteric plexus of the distal colon in eight mammals. *Gastroenterology* 86: 706-713, 1984.
54. CHRISTENSEN, J., N. W. WEISBRODT, AND R. L. HAUSER. Electrical slow waves of the proximal colon of the cat in diarrhea. *Gastroenterology* 62: 1167-1173, 1972.
55. CODE, C. F., N. C. HIGHTOWER, JR., AND C. G. MORLOCK. Motility of the alimentary canal in man. Review of recent studies. *Am. J. Med.* 13: 328-351, 1952.
56. COLLMAN, P. I., D. GRUNDY, T. SCRATCHERD, AND R. A. WACH. Vago-vagal reflexes to the colon of the anesthetized ferret. *J. Physiol. Lond.* 352: 395-402, 1984.
57. CONNELL, A. M. The motility of the pelvic colon. I. Motility in normals and in patients with asymptomatic duodenal ulcer. *Gut* 2: 175-186, 1961.
58. CONNELL, A. M. The motility of the pelvic colon. II. Paradoxical motility in diarrhea and constipation. *Gut* 3: 342-348, 1962.
59. CONNELL, A. M. Motor action of the large bowel. In: *Handbook of Physiology. Alimentary Canal. Motility*, edited by C. F. Code. Washington, D.C.: Am. Physiol. Soc., 1968, sect. 6, vol. IV, chapt. 101, p. 2075-2091.
60. CONNELL, A. M., H. FRANKEL, AND L. GUTTMANN. The motility of the pelvic colon following complete lesions of the spinal cord. *Paraplegia* 1: 98-115, 1963.
61. CONNELL, A. M., M. GAAFER, M. A. HASSANEIN, AND M. A. KHAYAL. Motility of the pelvic colon. III. Motility responses in patients with symptoms following amoebic dysentery. *Gut* 5: 443-447, 1964.
62. CONNELL, A. M., C. HILTON, G. IRVINE, J. E. LENNARD-JONES, AND J. J. MISIEWICZ. Variation of bowel habit in two population samples. *Br. Med. J.* 2: 1095-1099, 1965.
63. CONNELL, A. M., J. E. LENNARD-JONES, AND N. MADANAGOPALAN. The distribution of faecal x-ray shadows in subjects without gastro-intestinal disease. *Proc. R. Soc. Med.* 57: 894-895, 1964.
64. CONNELL, A. M., AND C. J. H. LOGAN. The role of gastrin in gastroileocolic responses. *Am. J. Dig. Dis.* 12: 277-284, 1967.
65. CONNORS, N. A., J. M. SULLIVAN, AND K. S. DUBB. An autoradiographic study of the distribution of fibers from the dorsal motor nucleus of the vagus to the digestive tube of the rat. *Acta Anat.* 115: 266-271, 1983.
66. COSTA, M., AND J. B. FURNESS. The innervation of the internal anal sphincter of the guinea-pig. In: *Proc. 4th Int. Symp. Gastrointest. Motil.*, edited by E. E. Daniel. Vancouver, Canada: Mitchell, 1974, p. 681-689.
67. COUTURIER, D., C. ROZE, M. H. COUTURIER-TURPIN, AND C. DEBRAY. Electromyography of the colon in situ: an experimental study in man and in the rabbit. *Gastroenterology* 56: 317-322, 1969.
68. CREMA, A., L. D'ANGELO, G. M. FRIGO, S. LECCHINI, L. ONORI, AND M. TONINI. Effects of desensitization to adenosine 5'-triphosphate and adenosine on non-adrenergic inhibitory responses in the circular muscle of rabbit colon. *Br. J. Pharmacol.* 75: 311-318, 1982.
69. CREMA, A., M. DEL TACCA, G. M. FRIGO, AND S. LECCHINI. Presence of a non-adrenergic inhibitory system in the human colon. *Gut* 9: 633-637, 1968.
70. DALSGAARD, C. J., AND L. G. ELFVIN. Structural studies on the connectivity of the inferior mesenteric ganglion of the guinea pig. *J. Auton. Nerv. Syst.* 5: 265-278, 1982.
71. DALSGAARD, C. J., T. HOKFELT, M. SCHULTZBERG, J. M. LUNDBERG, L. TERENUIS, G. J. DOCKRAY, AND M. GOLDSTEIN. Origin of peptide-containing fibers in the inferior mesenteric ganglion of the guinea pig: immunohistochemical studies with antisera to substance P, enkephalin, vasoactive intestinal polypeptide, cholecystokinin and bombesin. *Neuroscience* 9: 191-211, 1983.
72. DANIEL, E. E. Symposium on colonic function. Electrophysiology of the colon. *Gut* 16: 298-306, 1975.
73. DANIEL, E. E., W. H. SUTHERLAND, AND A. BOGOCH. Effects of morphine and other drugs on motility of the terminal ileum. *Gastroenterology* 36: 510-523, 1959.
74. DARBY, C. F., P. HAMMOND, AND I. TAYLOR. Real time analysis of colonic myoelectrical rhythms in disease. In: *Gastrointestinal Motility in Health and Disease*, edited by H. L. Duthie. Baltimore, MD: University Park, 1978, p. 287-294.
75. DAVIDSON, M., M. H. SLEISENGER, T. P. ALMY, AND S. Z. LEVINE. Studies on distal colonic motility in children; nonpropulsive patterns in normal children. *Pediatrics* 17: 807-818, 1956.

76. DAVIDSON, M., M. H. SLEISENGER, H. STEINBERG, AND T. P. ALMY. Studies of distal colonic motility in children. III. The pathologic physiology of congenital megacolon (Hirschsprung's disease). *Gastroenterology* 29: 803–824, 1955.
77. DE GROAT, W. C., M. KAWATANI, T. HISAMITSU, I. LOWE, C. MORGAN, J. ROPPOLO, A. M. BOOTH, I. NADELHAFT, D. KUO, AND K. THOR. The role of neuropeptides in the sacral anatomic reflex pathways of the cat. *J. Auton. Nerv. Syst.* 7: 339–350, 1983.
78. DE GROAT, W. C., I. NADELHAFT, R. J. MILNE, A. M. BOOTH, C. MORGAN, AND K. THOR. Organization of the sacral parasympathetic reflex pathways to the urinary bladder and large intestine. *J. Auton. Nerv. Syst.* 3: 135–160, 1981.
79. DELLER, D. J., AND A. G. WANGEL. Intestinal motility in man. I. A study combining the use of intraluminal pressure recording and cineradiography. *Gastroenterology* 48: 45–57, 1965.
80. DENNY-BROWN, D., AND E. G. ROBERTSON. An investigation of the nervous control of defecation. *Brain* 58: 256–310, 1935.
81. DOWLING, R. H., E. O. RIECKEN, J. W. LAWS, AND C. C. BOOTH. The intestinal response to high bulk feeding in the rat. *Clin. Sci. Lond.* 32: 1–9, 1967.
82. DURDLE, N. G., Y. J. KINGMA, K. L. BOWES, AND M. M. CHAMBERS. Origin of slow waves in the canine colon. *Gastroenterology* 84: 375–382, 1983.
83. DUTHIE, H. L., AND R. C. BENNETT. The relation of sensation in the anal canal to the functional anal sphincter: a possible factor in anal continence. *Gut* 4: 179–182, 1963.
84. DUTHIE, H. L., AND R. C. BENNETT. Anal sphincteric pressure in fissure in ano. *Surg. Gynecol. Obstet.* 119: 19–21, 1964.
85. DUTHIE, H. L., AND F. W. GAIRNS. Sensory nerve-endings and sensation in the anal region of man. *Br. J. Surg.* 47: 585–595, 1969.
86. DUTHIE, H. L., AND D. KIRK. Electrical activity of human colonic muscles in vitro. *J. Physiol. Lond.* 283: 319–330, 1978.
87. DUTHIE, H. L., AND J. M. WATTS. Contribution of the external anal sphincter to the pressure zone in the anal canal. *Gut* 6: 64–68, 1965.
88. EHRENPREIS, T. Megacolon in the newborn; a clinical and roentgenological study with special regard to the pathogenesis. *Acta Chir. Scand. Suppl.* 112: 1–114, 1946.
89. EHRENPREIS, T., K.-A. NORBERG, AND C. WIRSEN. Sympathetic innervation of the colon in Hirschsprung's disease: a histochemical study. *J. Pediatr. Surg.* 3: 43–49, 1968.
90. EK, B., AND B. LUNDGREN. Characterization of the beta-adrenergic inhibition of motility in cat colon strips. *Eur. J. Pharmacol.* 77: 25–31, 1982.
91. ELLIOTT, T. R., AND E. BARCLAY-SMITH. Antiperistalsis and other muscular activities of the colon. *J. Physiol. Lond.* 31: 272–304, 1904.
92. EL-SHARKAWY, T. Y. Electrical activity of the muscle layers of the canine colon. *J. Physiol. Lond.* 342: 67–83, 1983.
93. ELSOM, K. A., AND J. L. DROSSNER. Intubation studies of the human small intestine. XVII. The effect of atropine and belladonna on the motor activity of the small intestine and colon. *Am. J. Dig. Dis.* 6: 589–593, 1939.
94. EMERY, J. L., AND J. UNDERWOOD. The neurological junction between the appendix and ascending colon. *Gut* 11: 118–120, 1970.
95. ESLER, M. D., AND K. J. GOULSTON. Levels of anxiety in colonic disorders. *N. Engl. J. Med.* 288: 16–20, 1973.
96. FALCONER, J. D., A. N. SMITH, AND M. A. EASTWOOD. The effects of bile acids on colonic motility in the rabbit. *Q. J. Exp. Physiol. Cogn. Med. Sci.* 65: 135–144, 1980.
97. FASTH, S., L. HULTEN, S. NORDGREN, AND I. J. ZEITLIN. Studies on the atropine-resistant sacral parasympathetic vascular and motility responses in the cat colon. *J. Physiol. Lond.* 311: 421–429, 1981.
98. FISHLOCK, D. J. Effect of bradykinin on the human isolated small and large intestine. *Nature Lond.* 212: 1533–1535, 1966.
99. FISHLOCK, D. J., AND A. GUNN. The action of angiotensin on the human colon in vitro. *Br. J. Pharmacol.* 39: 34–39, 1970.
100. FISHLOCK, D. J., AND A. G. PARKS. A study of human colonic muscle in vitro. *Br. Med. J.* 2: 666–667, 1963.
101. FLOYD, W. F., AND E. W. WALLS. Electromyography of the sphincter ani externus in man. *J. Physiol. Lond.* 122: 599–609, 1953.
102. FLYNN, M., P. HAMMOND, C. DARBY, AND I. TAYLOR. Effects of bile acids on human colonic motor function in vitro. *Digestion* 23: 211–216, 1982.
103. FRENCKNER, B., AND C. VON EULER. Influence of pudendal block on the function of the anal sphincters. *Gut* 16: 482–489, 1975.
104. FRENCKNER, B., AND T. IHRE. Influence of autonomic nerves on the internal anal sphincter in man. *Gut* 17: 306–312, 1976.
105. FRIEDMANN, C. A. The action of nicotine and catecholamines on the human internal anal sphincter. *Am. J. Dig. Dis.* 13: 428–431, 1968.
106. FUJITA, T. A fixation muscle system in the human large intestine. *Anat. Rec.* 114: 467–477, 1952.
107. FUKAI, K., AND H. FUKUDA. The intramural pelvic nerves in the colon of dogs. *J. Physiol. Lond.* 354: 89–98, 1984.
108. FURNESS, J. B. The presence of inhibitory nerves in the colon after sympathetic denervation. *Eur. J. Pharmacol.* 6: 349–352, 1968.
109. FURNESS, J. B. An electrophysiological study of the innervation of the smooth muscle of the colon. *J. Physiol. Lond.* 205: 549–562, 1969.
110. FURNESS, J. B. The origin and distribution of adrenergic nerve fibers in the guinea-pig colon. *Histochemie* 21: 295–306, 1970.
111. FURNESS, J. B. An examination of nerve-mediated, hyoscine-resistant excitation of the guinea-pig colon. *J. Physiol. Lond.* 207: 803–821, 1970.
112. FURNESS, J. B., M. COSTA, AND F. ECKENSTEIN. Neurons localized with antibodies against choline acetyltransferase in the enteric nervous system. *Neurosci. Lett.* 40: 105–109, 1983.
113. FURNESS, J. B., M. COSTA, AND J. WALSH. Evidence for and significance of the projection of VIP neurons from the myenteric plexus to the taenia coli in the guinea pig. *Gastroenterology* 80: 1557–1561, 1981.
114. GABELLA, G., AND D. BLUNDELL. Gap junctions of the muscles of the small and large intestine. *Cell Tissue Res.* 219: 469–488, 1981.
115. GAGNON, D. J., G. DEVROEDE, AND S. BELISLE. Excitatory effects of adrenaline upon isolated preparations of human colon. *Gut* 13: 654–657, 1972.
116. GALAPEAUX, E. A., AND A. D. TEMPLETON. The influence of filling the stomach on colon motility in the dog. *Am. J. Physiol.* 119: 312–313, 1937. (Proc. Am. Physiol. Soc. 49th Annu. Meet., Memphis, TN, April 21–24, 1937.)
117. GARRETT, J. R., E. R. HOWARD, AND W. JONES. The internal anal sphincter in the cat: a study of nervous mechanisms affecting tone and reflex activity. *J. Physiol. Lond.* 243: 153–166, 1974.
118. GARRETT, J. R., E. R. HOWARD, AND H. H. NIXON. Autonomic nerves in rectum and colon in Hirschsprung's disease. A cholinesterase and catecholamine histochemical study. *Arch. Dis. Child.* 44: 406–417, 1969.
119. GARRY, R. C. The responses to stimulation of the caudal end of the large bowel in the cat. *J. Physiol. Lond.* 78: 208–224, 1933.
120. GARRY, R. C. The movements of the large intestine. *Physiol. Rev.* 14: 103–132, 1934.
121. GASTON, E. A. Physiological basis for preservation of fecal continence after resection of rectum. *J. Am. Med. Assoc.* 146: 1486–1489, 1951.
122. GILLAN, M. G., AND D. POLLOCK. Acute effects of morphine and opioid peptides on the motility and responses of the rat colon to electrical stimulation. *Br. J. Pharmacol.* 68: 381–392, 1980.
123. GILLESPIE, J. S. Spontaneous mechanical and electrical activ-

ity of stretched and unstretched intestinal smooth muscle cells and their response to sympathetic-nerve stimulation. *J. Physiol. Lond.* 162: 54–75, 1962.
124. GILLESPIE, J. S. The electrical and mechanical responses of intestinal smooth muscle to stimulation of their extrinsic parasympathetic nerves. *J. Physiol. Lond.* 162: 76–92, 1962.
125. GLOTZER, D. J., AND A. N. SHARMA. Experimental total abdominoperineal colectomy with preservation of the sphincters. *Surg. Gynecol. Obstet.* 119: 338–344, 1964.
126. GOLDENBERG, M. M. Analysis of the inhibitory innervation of the isolated gerbil colon. *Arch. Int. Pharmacodyn. Ther.* 175: 347–364, 1968.
127. GOLIGHER, J. C. The functional results after sphincter-saving resections of the rectum. *Ann. R. Coll. Surg. Engl.* 8: 421–439, 1951. (Hunterian Lecture.)
128. GOLIGHER, J. C., AND E. S. R. HUGHES. Sensibility of the rectum and colon; its role in the mechanism of anal continence. *Lancet* 1: 543–548, 1951.
129. GRAMIAK, R., P. ROSS, AND W. W. OLMSTED. Normal motor activity of the human colon: combined radiotelemetric manometry and slow-frame cineroentgenography. *Am. J. Roentgend. Radium Ther. Nucl. Med.* 113: 301–309, 1971.
130. GREGORY, R. A. Some factors influencing the passage of fluid through intestinal loops in dogs. *J. Physiol. Lond.* 111: 119–137, 1950.
131. GRIFFITH, S. G., AND G. BURNSTOCK. Serotonergic neurons in human fetal intestine: an immunohistochemical study. *Gastroenterology* 85: 929–937, 1983.
132. HALLS, J. Bowel content shift during normal defaecation [Summary]. *Proc. R. Soc. Med.* 58: 859–860, 1965.
133. HANSKY, J., AND A. M. CONNELL. Measurement of gastrointestinal transit using radioactive chromium. *Gut* 3: 187–188, 1962.
134. HARVEY, R. F., AND A. E. READ. Effect of cholecystokinin on colonic motility and symptoms in patients with the irritable-bowel syndrome. *Lancet* 1: 1–3, 1973.
135. HARVEY, R. F., AND A. E. READ. Effect of oral magnesium sulphate on colonic motility in patients with the irritable bowel syndrome. *Gut* 14: 983–987, 1973.
136. HAVIA, T., AND J. KLOSSNER. The effect of low-residue diet on the canine colonic wall. *Ann. Chir. Gynaecol.* 60: 132–134, 1971.
137. HELLSTROM, P. M, AND S. ROSELL. Effects of neurotensin, substance P and methionine-enkephalin on colonic motility. *Acta Physiol. Scand.* 113: 147–154, 1981.
138. HENRY, M. M., A. G. PARKER, AND M. SWASH. The pelvic floor musculature in the descending perineum syndrome. *Br. J. Surg.* 69: 470–472, 1982.
139. HERTZ, A. F. The passage of food along the human alimentary canal. *Guy's Hosp. Rep.* 61: 389–427, 1907.
140. HERTZ, A. F., AND A. NEWTON. The normal movements of the colon in man. *J. Physiol. Lond.* 47: 57–65, 1913.
141. HILL, C. J., W. G. OSMAN, AND R. E. REWELL. The caecum of monotremes and marsupials. *Trans. Zool. Soc. Lond.* 28: 185–240, 1954.
142. HILL, J. R., M. L. KELLEY, J. F. SCHLEGEL, AND C. F. CODE. Pressure profile of the rectum and anus of healthy persons. *Dis. Colon Rectum* 3: 203–209, 1960.
143. HINRICHSEN, J., AND A. C. IVY. Studies on the ileocecal sphincter of the dog. *Am. J. Physiol.* 96: 494–507, 1931.
144. HISLOP, I. G. Psychological significance of the irritable colon syndrome. *Gut* 12: 452–457, 1971.
145. HOLDSTOCK, D. J., AND J. J. MISIEWICZ. Factors controlling colonic motility: colonic pressures and transit after meals in patients with total gastrectomy, pernicious anemia and duodenal ulcer. *Gut* 11: 100–110, 1970.
146. HOLDSTOCK, D. J., J. J. MISIEWICZ, T. SMITH, AND E. N. ROWLANDS. Propulsion (mass movement) in the human colon and its relationship to meals and somatic activity. *Gut* 11: 91–99, 1970.
147. HOLZKNECHT, G. Die normale Peristaltik des Colon. *Muench. Med. Wochenschr.* 56: 2401–2403, 1909.
148. HOWARD, E. R. Abnormality of anorectal physiology in Hirschsprung's disease. *Am. J. Dig. Dis.* 13: 432–433, 1968.
149. HOWARD, E. R., AND J. R. GARRETT. Electron microscopy of myenteric nerves in Hirschsprung's disease and in normal bowel. *Gut* 11: 1007–1014, 1970.
150. HOWARD, E. R., AND J. R. GARRETT. Histochemistry and electron microscopy of rectum and colon in Hirschsprung's disease. *Proc. R. Soc. Med.* 63: 1264–1266, 1970.
151. HUIDOBRO-TORO, J. P. Non-neuronal excitatory neurotensin receptors on the taenia coli of the guinea pig: lack of influence on tetrodotoxin and dynorphin. *Neurosci. Lett.* 38: 309–314, 1983.
152. HUIZINGA, J. D., N. E. DIAMANT, AND T. Y. EL-SHARKAWY. Electrical basis of contractions in the muscle layers of the pig colon. *Am. J. Physiol.* 245 (*Gastrointest. Liver Physiol.* 8): G482–G491, 1983.
153. HUIZINGA, J. D., H. STERN, N. E. DIAMANT, AND T. Y. EL-SHARKAWY. The relationship between slow electrical oscillatory activity, spikes, and contractions in human colonic circular muscle (Abstract). *Gastroenterology* 86: 1119, 1984.
154. HUKUHARA, T., AND T. MIYAKA. The intrinsic reflexes in the colon. *Jpn. J. Physiol.* 9: 49–55, 1959.
155. HULTEN, L., AND M. JODAL. Extrinsic nervous controls of colonic motility. *Acta Physiol. Scand. Suppl.* 335: 21–38, 1969.
156. IHRE, T. Studies on anal function in continent and incontinent patients. *Scand. J. Gastroenterol. Suppl.* 25: 1–64, 1974.
157. JESSEN, K. R., J. M. HILLS, M. E. DENNISON, AND R. MIRSKY. Gamma-aminobutyrate as an autonomic neurotransmitter: release and uptake of [$^3$H]gamma-aminobutyrate in guinea pig large intestine and cultured enteric neurons using physiologic methods and electron microscopic autoradiography. *Neuroscience* 10: 1427–1442, 1983.
158. JULÉ, Y. Etude in vitro de l'activité électromyographique du colon proximal et distal du lapin. *J. Physiol. Paris* 88: 305–329, 1974.
159. JULÉ, Y. Modifications de l'activité électrique du colon proximal de lapin in vivo, par stimulation des nerfs vagues et splanchniques. *J. Physiol. Paris* 70: 5–26, 1975.
160. JULÉ, Y. Nerve-mediated descending inhibition in the proximal colon of the rabbit. *J. Physiol. Lond.* 309: 487–498, 1980.
161. KEAST, J. R., J. B. FURNESS, AND M. COSTA. Somatostatin in human enteric nerves. Distribution and characterization. *Cell Tissue Res.* 237: 299–308, 1984.
162. KENT, G. C. *Comparative Anatomy of the Vertebrates*. St. Louis, MO: Mosby, 1965.
163. KERN, F., JR., T. P. ALMY, F. K. ABBOT, AND M. D. BOGDONOFF. The motility of the distal colon in non-specific ulcerative colitis. *Gastroenterology* 19: 492–503, 1951.
164. KERN, F., JR., T. P. ALMY, AND N. J. STOLK. Effects of certain antispasmodic drugs on the intact human colon with special reference to Banthine ($\beta$-diethylaminoethyl xanthene-9-carboxylate methobromine). *Am. J. Med.* 11: 67–74, 1951.
165. KIFF, E. S., AND M. SWASH. Slowed conduction in the pudendal nerves in idiopathic (neurogenic) fecal incontinence. *Br. J. Surg.* 71: 614–616, 1984.
166. KIM, I. C., AND G. J. BARBERO. The pattern of rectosigmoid motility in children. *Gastroenterology* 45: 57–66, 1973.
167. KIRK, D. An electrophysiological study of the smooth muscle of the human colon. *Ann. R. Coll. Surg. Engl.* 63: 393–398, 1981.
168. KITABGI, P., AND J. P. VINCENT. Neurotensin is a potent inhibitor of guinea pig contractile activity. *Eur. J. Pharmacol.* 74: 311–318, 1981.
169. KOBAYASHI, M., T. NAGAI, AND C. L. PROSSER. Electrical interaction between muscle layers of cat intestine. *Am. J. Physiol.* 211: 1281–1291, 1966.
170. KOCK, N. G., L. HULTEN, AND L. LEANDER. A study of the motility in different parts of the human colon. Resting activity, response to feeding and to prostigmine. *Scand. J. Gastroenterol.* 3: 163–169, 1968.

171. KOMURO, T., P. BALUK, AND G. BURNSTOCK. An ultrastructural study of neurons and non-neuronal cells in the myenteric plexus of the rabbit colon. *Neuroscience* 7: 1797–1806, 1982.
172. KOMURO, T., P. BALUK, AND G. BURNSTOCK. An ultrastructural study of nerve profiles in the myenteric plexus of the rabbit colon. *Neuroscience* 7: 295–305, 1982.
173. KONTUREK, S. J., J. TASLER, AND W. OBLULOWICZ. Effect of atropine on pancreatic responses to endogenous and exogenous cholecystokinin. *Am. J. Dig. Dis.* 17: 911–917, 1972.
174. KRANTIS, A., M. COSTA, J. B. FURNESS, AND J. ORBACH. Gamma-aminobutyric acid stimulates intrinsic inhibitory and excitatory nerves in the guinea pig intestine. *Eur. J. Pharmacol.* 67: 461–468, 1980.
175. KRANTIS, A., AND D. I. KERR. The effect of GABA antagonism on propulsive activity of the guinea pig large intestine. *Eur. J. Pharmacol.* 75: 317–319, 1981.
176. KRIER, J., AND D. A. HARTMAN. Electric properties and synaptic connections to neurons in parasympathetic colonic ganglia of the cat. *Am. J. Physiol.* 247 (*Gastrointest. Liver Physiol.* 10): G52–G61, 1984.
177. KRIER, J., AND J. SZURSZEWSKI. Effect of substance P on colonic mechanoreceptors, motility, and sympathetic neurons. *Am. J. Physiol.* 243 (*Gastrointest. Liver Physiol.* 6): G259–G267, 1982.
178. KUBOTA, M., Y. ITO, AND K. IKEDA. Membrane properties and innervation of smooth muscle cells in Hirschsprung's disease. *Am. J. Physiol.* 244 (*Gastrointest. Liver Physiol.* 7): G406–G415, 1983.
179. KUO, D. C., T. HISAMITSU, AND W. C. DE GROAT. A sympathetic projection from sacral paravertebral ganglion to the pelvic nerve and to postganglionic nerves on the surface of the urinary bladder and large intestine of the cat. *J. Comp. Neurol.* 226: 76–86, 1984.
180. KUZUHARA, S., I. KANAZAWA, AND T. NAKANISHI. Topographical localization of the Onuf's nuclear neurons innervating the rectal and vesicle striated sphincter muscles: a retrograde fluorescent double labeling in cat and dog. *Neurosci. Lett.* 16: 125–130, 1980.
181. LARSSON, L. T., G. MALMFORS, AND F. SUNDLER. Peptidergic innervation in Hirschsprung's disease. *Z. Kinderchir.* 38: 301–304, 1983.
182. LAWSON, J. O. N., AND H. H. NIXON. Anal canal pressures in the diagnosis of Hirschsprung's disease. *J. Pediatr. Surg.* 2: 544–552, 1967.
183. LEES, G. M., AND W. H. PERCY. Antibiotic-associated colitis: an in vitro investigation of the effects of antibiotics on intestinal motility. *Br. J. Pharmacol.* 73: 535–547, 1981.
184. LEWIS, F. T. The development of the large intestine. In: *Manual of Human Embryology*, edited by F. Keibel and F. P. Mall. Philadelphia, PA: Lippincott, 1912, vol. 2, p. 393–403.
185. LIPKIN, M., T. ALMY, AND B. M. BELL. Pressure-volume characteristics of the human colon. *J. Clin. Invest.* 41: 1831–1839, 1962.
186. LUNDNBERG, J. M., K. TATEMOTO, L. TERENIUS, P. M. HELLSTROM, V. MUTT, T. HOKFELT, AND B. HAMBERGER. Localization of peptide YY (PYY) in gastrointestinal endocrine cells and effects on intestinal blood flow and motility. *Proc. Natl. Acad. Sci. USA* 79: 4471–4475, 1982.
187. MACBETH, W. A., AND J. H. HAWTHORNE. Intramural ganglia in diverticular disease of the colon. *J. Clin. Pathol. Lond.* 18: 40–42, 1965.
188. MACEWEN, W. The Huxley lecture on the function of the caecum and appendix. *Lancet* 2: 995–1000, 1904.
189. MACKENNA, B. R., AND H. C. MCKIRDY. Peristalsis in the rabbit distal colon. *J. Physiol. Lond.* 220: 33–54, 1972.
190. MANN, C. V., AND J. D. HARDCASTLE. Recent studies of colonic and rectal motor action. *Dis. Colon Rectum* 13: 225–230, 1970.
191. MEIER-RUGE, W. Das Megacolon: seine Diagnose und Pathophysiologie. *Virchows Arch. Abt. A Pathol. Anat.* 344: 67–85, 1968.
192. MENDELOFF, A. I., M. MONK, C. I. SIEGEL, AND A. LILIENFELD. Illness experience and life stresses in patients with irritable colon and with ulcerative colitis. An epidemiologic study of ulcerative colitis and regional enteritis in Baltimore, 1960–1964. *N. Engl. J. Med.* 282: 14–17, 1970.
193. MESHKINPOUR, H., V. P. DINOSO, AND S. H. LORBER. Effect of intraduodenal administration of essential amino acids and sodium oleate on motor activity of the sigmoid colon. *Gastroenterology* 66: 373–377, 1974.
194. MISIEWICZ, J. J., A. M. CONNELL, AND F. A. PONTES. Comparison of the effect of meals and prostigmine on the proximal and distal colon in patients with and without diarrhoea. *Gut* 7: 468–473, 1966.
195. MISIEWICZ, J. J., D. J. HOLDSTOCK, AND S. L. WALLER. Motor responses of the human alimentary tract to 5-hydroxytryptamine in vivo and in vitro. *Gut* 7: 208–216, 1967.
196. MISIEWICZ, J. J., S. L. WALLER, AND M. EISNER. Motor responses of human gastrointestinal tract to 5-hydroxytryptamine in vivo and in vitro. *Gut* 7: 208–216, 1966.
197. NAKAGAWA, S. Onuf's nucleus of the sacral cord in a South American monkey (*Samairi*): its location and bilateral cervical input from area 4. *Brain Res.* 191: 337–344, 1980.
198. NEILL, M. E., A. G. PARKS, AND M. SWASH. Physiological studies of the anal sphincter musculature in fecal incontinence and rectal prolapse. *Br. J. Surg.* 68: 531–536, 1981.
199. NEILL, M. E., AND M. SWASH. Increased motor unit fibre density in the external anal sphincter muscle in ano-rectal incontinence: a single fiber EMG study. *J. Neurol. Neurosurg. Psychiatry* 43: 343–347, 1980.
200. NICKEL, R., A. SCHUMMER, AND E. SIEFERLE. *The Viscera of Domestic Mammals*, translated and revised by W. O. Sack. New York: Springer-Verlag, 1973.
201. ONG, J., AND D. I. KERR. GABAA- and GABAB-receptor-mediated modification of intestinal motility. *Eur. J. Pharmacol.* 86: 9–17, 1982.
202. PACE, J. L. The age of appearance of the haustra of the human colon. *J. Anat.* 109: 75–80, 1971.
203. PAINTER, N. S. Diverticulosis of the colon-fact and speculation. *Am. J. Dig. Dis.* 12: 222–227, 1967.
204. PAINTER, N. S., AND S. C. TRUELOVE. The intraluminal pressure patterns in diverticulosis of the colon. I. Resting patterns of pressure. II. The effect of morphine. *Gut* 5: 201–207, 207–213, 1964.
205. PAINTER, N. S., AND S. C. TRUELOVE. The intraluminal pressure patterns in diverticulosis of the colon. III. The effect of prostigmine. IV. The effect of pethidine and probanthine. *Gut* 5: 365–369, 369–373, 1964.
206. PAINTER, N. S., S. C. TRUELOVE, G. M. ARDAN, AND M. TUCKEY. Segmentation and the localization of intraluminal pressures in the human colon, with special reference to the pathogenesis of colonic diverticula. *Gastroenterology* 49: 169–177, 1965.
207. PARKS, A. G., D. J. FISHLOCK, J. D. H. CAMERON, AND H. MAY. Preliminary investigation of the pharmacology of the human internal anal sphincter. *Gut* 10: 674–677, 1969.
208. PASSARGE, E. The genetics of Hirschsprung's disease. Evidence for heterogeneous etiology and a study of sixty-three families. *N. Engl. J. Med.* 276: 138–143, 1967.
209. PEDERSEN, E., B. KLEMAR, H. D. SCHRODER, AND J. TORRING. Anal sphincter responses after perianal electrical stimulation. *J. Neurol. Neurosurg. Psychiatry* 45: 770–773, 1982.
210. PHILLIPS, S. F., AND D. A. W. EDWARDS. Some aspects of anal continence and defaecation. *Gut* 6: 396–406, 1965.
211. POSEY, E. L., JR., J. A. BARGEN, W. H. DEARING, AND C. F. CODE. The effects of certain so-called antispasmodics on intestinal motility. *Gastroenterology* 11: 344–356, 1948.
212. POSEY, E. L., JR., W. H. DEARING, W. G. SAUER, J. A. BARGEN, AND C. F. CODE. The recording of intestinal motility. *Proc. Staff Meet. Mayo Clin.* 23: 297–304, 1948.
213. RAIFORD, T., AND M. G. MULINOS. The myenteric reflex as exhibited by the exteriorized colon of the dog. *Am. J. Physiol.*

110: 129–136, 1934.
214. RAMORINO, M. L., AND C. COLOGRANDE. Intestinal motility. Preliminary studies with telemetering capsule and synchronized fluorocinematography. *Am. J. Dig. Dis.* 9: 64–71, 1964.
215. RAYNER, V. Observations on the functional internal anal sphincter of the vervet monkey (Abstract). *J. Physiol. Lond.* 213: 27P–28P, 1971.
216. REINKE, D. A., A. H. ROSENBAUM, AND D. R. BENNETT. Patterns of dog gastrointestinal contractile motility monitored in vivo with extraluminal force transducers. *Am. J. Dig. Dis.* 12: 113–141, 1967.
217. RITCHIE, J. A. Movement of segmental constrictions in the human colon. *Gut* 12: 350–355, 1971.
218. RITCHIE, J. A. Mass peristalsis in the human colon after contact with oxyphenisatin. *Gut* 13: 211–219, 1972.
219. RITCHIE, J. A., ARDAN, G. M., AND S. C. TRUELOVE. Motor activity of the sigmoid colon of humans. A combined study by intraluminal pressure recording an cineradiography. *Gastroenterology* 43: 642–668, 1962.
220. ROCKSWALD, G. L., W. E. BRADLEY, AND S. N. CHOU. Innervation of the urethral and external anal sphincters in higher primates. *J. Comp. Neurol.* 193: 521–528, 1980.
221. ROSTAD, H. Colonic motility in the cat. I. Extraluminal strain gage technique. Influence of anesthesia and temperature. *Acta Physiol. Scand.* 89: 79–90, 1973.
222. ROSTAD, H. Colonic motility in the cat. II. Extrinsic nervous control. *Acta Physiol. Scand.* 89: 91–103, 1973.
223. ROSTAD, H. Colonic motility in the cat. III. Influence of hypothalamic and mesencephalic stimulation. *Acta Physiol. Scand.* 89: 104–115, 1973.
224. ROSTAD, H. Colonic motility in the cat. IV. Peripheral pathways mediating the effects induced by hypothalamic and mesencephalic stimulation. *Acta Physiol. Scand.* 89: 154–168, 1973.
225. ROSTAD, H. Colonic motility in the cat. V. Influence of telecephalic stimulation and the peripheral pathways mediating the effects. *Acta Physiol. Scand.* 89: 169–181, 1973.
226. ROTHMAN, T. P., AND M. D. GERSHON. Regionally defective colonization of the terminal bowel by the precursors of enteric neurons in lethal spotted mutant mice. *Neuroscience* 12: 1293–1311, 1984.
227. RUCKEBUSCH, Y., M. L. GRIVEL, AND M. J. FARGEAS. Activité électrique de l'intestin et prise de nourriture conditionelle chez le lapin. *Physiol. & Behav.* 6: 359–365, 1971.
228. SARNA, S., P. LATIMER, D. CAMPBELL, AND W. E. WATERFALL. Effect of stress, meal and neostigmine on rectosigmoid electrical control activity (ECA) in normals and in irritable bowel syndrome patients. *Dig. Dis. Sci.* 27: 582–591, 1982.
229. SCHNAUFER, L., J. L. TALBERT, J. A. HALLER, N. C. R. W. REID, F. TOBON, AND M. M. SCHUSTER. Differential sphincteric studies in the diagnosis of ano-rectal disorders of childhood. *J. Pediatr. Surg.* 2: 538–543, 1967.
230. SCHUSTER, M. M., T. R. HENDRIX, AND A. I. MENDELOFF. The internal anal sphincter response: manometric studies on its normal physiology, neural pathways, and alteration in bowel disorders. *J. Clin. Invest.* 42: 196–207, 1963.
231. SCHUURKES, J. A., AND J. J. TUKKER. The interdigestive colonic motor complex of the dog. *Arch. Int. Pharmacodyn. Ther.* 247: 329–334, 1980.
232. SEIDEL, E. R., J. WOODS, B. E. EIKENBURG, AND L. R. JOHNSON. Muscarinic cholinergic receptors in the piebald mouse model for Hirschsprung's disease. *Gastroenterology* 85: 335–338, 1983.
233. SHEARIN, N. L., K. L. BOWES, AND Y. J. KINGMA. In vitro electrical activity in canine colon. *Gut* 20: 780–786, 1978.
234. SHIFF, S. J., R. D. SOLOWAY, AND W. J. SNAPE, JR. Mechanism of deoxycholic acid stimulation of the rabbit colon. *J. Clin. Invest.* 69: 985–992, 1982.
235. SISSON, S. *The Anatomy of the Domestic Animals* (4th ed.), revised by J. D. Grossman. Philadelphia, PA: Saunders, 1953, p. 972.
236. SJOQUIST, A., P. M. HELLSTROM, M. JODAL, AND O. LUNDGREN. Neurotransmitters involved in the colonic contraction and vasodilatation elicited by activation of the pelvic nerves in the cat. *Gastroenterology* 86: 1481–1487, 1984.
237. SLACK, W. W. Bowel muscle in diverticular disease. *Gut* 7: 668–670, 1967.
238. SMITH, B. Myenteric plexus in Hirschsprung's disease. *Gut* 8: 308–312, 1967.
239. SNAPE, W. J., JR. Effect of calcium on neurohumoral stimulation of feline colonic smooth muscle. *Am. J. Physiol.* 243 (*Gastrointest. Liver Physiol.* 6): G134–G140, 1982.
240. SNAPE, W. J., JR., G. M. CARLSON, AND S. COHEN. Colonic myoelectric activity in the irritable bowel syndrome. *Gastroenterology* 70: 326–330, 1976.
241. SNAPE, W. J., JR., G. M. CARLSON, AND S. COHEN. Human colonic myoelectric activity in response to prostigmine and the gastrointestinal hormones. *Am. J. Dig. Dis.* 22: 881–887, 1977.
242. SNAPE, W. J., JR., G. M. CARLSON, S. A. MATARAZZO, AND S. COHEN. Evidence that abnormal myoelectrical activity produces colonic motor dysfunction in the irritable bowel syndrome. *Gastroenterology* 72: 383–387, 1977.
243. SNAPE, W. J., JR., S. A. MATARAZZO, AND S. COHEN. Effect of eating and gastrointestinal hormones on human colonic myoelectrical and motor activity. *Gastroenterology* 75: 373–378, 1978.
244. SNAPE, W. J., JR., S. H. WRIGHT, W. M. BATTLE, AND S. COHEN. The gastrocolic response: evidence for a neural mechanism. *Gastroenterology* 77: 1235–1240, 1979.
245. SNOOKS, S. J., M. SETCHELL, M. SWASH, AND M. M. HENRY. Injury to innervation of the pelvic floor sphincter musculature in childbirth. *Lancet* 2: 546–550, 1984.
246. SPRIGGS, E. A., C. F. CODE, J. A. BARGEN, R. K. CURTISS, AND N. C. HIGHTOWER, JR. Motility of the pelvic colon and rectum of normal persons and patients with ulcerative colitis. *Gastroenterology* 19: 480–491, 1951.
247. STACH, W. Uber die in der Dickdarmwand azendieren Nerven des Plexus pelvinus und die Grenze der Vagalen und sakralparasympathetischen Innervation. *Z. Mikrosk. Anat. Forsch. Leipz.* 84: 65–90, 1981.
248. STODDARD, C. J., H. L. DUTHIE, R. H. SMALLWOOD, AND D. A. LINKENS. Colonic myoelectrical activity in man: comparison of recording techniques and methods of analysis. *Gut* 20: 476–483, 1979.
249. STONESIFER, G. L., JR., G. P. MURPHY, AND C. R. LOMBARDO. The anatomy of the anorectum. *Am. J. Surg.* 10: 666–671, 1960.
250. SULLIVAN, M. A., S. COHEN, AND W. J. SNAPE, JR. Colonic myoelectrical activity in irritable-bowel syndrome. Effect of eating and anticholinergics. *N. Engl. J. Med.* 298: 878–883, 1978.
251. SUN, E. A., W. J. SNAPE, JR., J. COHEN, AND A. RENNY. The role of opiate receptors and cholinergic neurons in the gastrocolonic response. *Gastroenterology* 82: 689–693, 1982.
252. SWASH, M. Early and late components in the human anal reflex. *J. Neurol. Neurosurg. Psychiatry* 45: 767–769, 1982.
253. SWENSON, O., AND A. H. BILL, JR. Resection of the rectum and rectosigmoid with preservation of the sphincter for benign spastic lesions producing megacolon: an experimental study. *Surgery St. Louis* 24: 212–220, 1948.
254. TAKAKI, M., T. NAYA, AND S. NAKAYAMA. Sympathetic activity in the recto-rectal reflex of the guinea pig. *Pflueger's Arch.* 388: 45–52, 1980.
255. TANIYAMA, K., M. KUSUNOKI, N. SAITO, AND C. TANAKA. Release of gamma-aminobutyric acid from the cat colon. *Science Wash. DC* 217: 1038–1040, 1982.
256. TANIYAMA, K., Y. MIKI, AND C. TANAKA. Presence of gamma-aminobutyric acid and glutamic acid decarboxylase in Auerbach's plexus of cat colon. *Neurosci. Lett.* 29: 53–56, 1982.
257. TANSY, M. J., F. M. KENDALL, AND J. J. MURPHY. The reflex nature of the gastrocolic propulsive response in the dog. *Surg. Gynecol. Obstet.* 135: 404–410, 1972.
258. TAYLOR, I., P. BASU, P. HAMMOND, C. DARBY, AND M. FLYNN.

Effect of bile acid perfusion on colonic motor function in patients with the irritable colon syndrome. *Gut* 21: 843–847, 1980.
259. TAYLOR, I., R. SMALLWOOD, AND H. L. DUTHIE. Myoelectrical activity in the rectosigmoid in man. In: *Proc. 4th Int. Symp. Gastrointest. Motil.*, edited by E. E. Daniel. Vancouver, Canada: Mitchell, 1974, p. 109–119.
260. TEMPLETON, R. D., AND H. LAWSON. Studies in the motor activity of the large intestine. I. Normal motility in the dog, recorded by the tandem balloon method. *Am. J. Physiol.* 96: 667–676, 1931.
261. TOBON, F., N. C. R. W. REID, J. L. TALBERT, AND M. M. SCHUSTER. Nonsurgical test for the diagnosis of Hirschsprung's disease. *N. Engl. J. Med.* 278: 188–194, 1968.
262. TONINI, M., L. ONORI, S. LECCHINI, G. FRIGO, E. PERUCCA, AND A. CREMA. Mode of action of ATP on propulsive activity in rabbit colon. *Eur. J. Pharmacol.* 82: 21–28, 1982.
263. TRUELOVE, S. C. Movements of the large intestine. *Physiol. Rev.* 46: 457–512, 1966.
264. TSUTO, T., H. OKAMURA, K. FUKUI, H. L. OBATA, H. TERUBAYASHI, N. IWAI, S. MAJIMA, N. YANAIHARA, AND Y. IBATA. An immunohistochemical investigation of vasoactive intestinal polypeptide in the colon of patients with Hirschsprung's disease. *Neurosci. Lett.* 34: 57–62, 1982.
265. USTACH, T. J., F. TOBON, T. HAMBRECHT, D. D. BASS, AND M. M. SCHUSTER. Electrophysiological aspects of human sphincter function. *J. Clin. Invest.* 49: 41–48, 1970.
266. VAILLANT, C., A. BULOCK, R. DIMALINE, AND G. J. DOCKRAY. Distribution and development of peptidergic nerves and gut endocrine cells in mice with congenital aganglionic colon, and their normal littermates. *Gastroenterology* 82: 291–300, 1982.
267. VAN MERWYK, A. J., AND H. L. DUTHIE. Characteristics of human colonic smooth muscle in vitro. In: *Gastrointestinal Motility*, edited by J. Christensen. New York: Raven, 1980, p. 473–478.
268. VIZI, S. E., G. BERTACCINI, M. IMPICCIATORI, AND J. KNOLL. Evidence that acetylcholine released by gastrin and related polypeptides contributes to their effect on gastrointestinal motility. *Gastroenterology* 64: 268–277, 1973.
269. WALLER, S. L., AND J. J. MISIEWICZ. Prognosis in the irritable bowel syndrome: a prospective study. *Lancet* 2: 754–756, 1969.
270. WALSH, J. H., R. S. YALOW, AND S. A. BERSON. The effect of atropine on plasma gastrin response to feeding. *Gastroenterology* 60: 16–21, 1971.
271. WANKLING, W. J., B. H. BROWN, C. D. COLLINS, AND H. L. DUTHIE. Basal electrical activity in the anal canal in man. *Gut* 9: 457–460, 1968.
272. WELCH, P. B., AND O. H. PLANT. A graphic study of the muscular activity of the colon, with special reference to its response to feeding. *Am. J. Med. Sci.* 172: 261–268, 1926.
273. WHITE, J. C., M. G. VERLOT, AND O. EHRENTHEIL. Neurogenic disturbances of the colon and their investigation by the colon-metrogram; preliminary report. *Ann. Surg.* 112: 1042–1057, 1940.
274. WHITEHEAD, W. E., B. T. ENGEL, AND M. M. SCHUSTER. Irritable bowel syndrome: physiological and psychological differences between diarrhea-predominant and constipation-predominant patients. *Dig. Dis. Sci.* 25: 404–413, 1980.
275. WHITEHOUSE, F. R., AND J. W. KERNOHAN. Myenteric plexus in congenital megacolon: study of 11 cases. *Arch. Intern. Med.* 82: 75–111, 1948.
276. WIENBECK, M., AND J. CHRISTENSEN. Cationic requirements of colon slow waves in the cat. *Am. J. Physiol.* 220: 513–519, 1971.
277. WIENBECK, M., AND J. CHRISTENSEN. Effects of some drugs on electrical activity of the isolated colon of the cat. *Gastroenterology* 61: 470–478, 1971.
278. WILLIAMS, I. Diverticular disease of the colon: a 1968 view. *Gut* 9: 498–501, 1968.
279. WUNDERLICH, M., AND M. SWASH. The overlapping innervation of the two sides of the external anal sphincter by the pudendal nerves. *J. Neurol. Sci.* 59: 97–109, 1983.
280. WOOD, J. D. Electrical activity of the intestine of mice with hereditary megacolon and absence of enteric ganglion cells. *Am. J. Dig. Dis.* 18: 477–488, 1973.
281. WOOD, J. D. Physiological studies on the large intestine of mice with hereditary megacolon and absence of enteric ganglion cells. In: *Proc. 4th Int. Symp. Gastrointest. Motil.*, edited by E. E. Daniel. Vancouver, Canada: Mitchell, 1974, p. 177–194.
282. YOUMANS, W. B. *Nervous and Neurohumoral Regulation of Intestinal Motility.* New York: Interscience, 1949.

# CHAPTER 25

# Villous motility

WILLIAM A. WOMACK | *Department of Physiology, College of Medicine, University of South Alabama, Mobile, Alabama*

PETER R. KVIETYS

D. NEIL GRANGER | *Department of Physiology and Biophysics, Louisiana State University Medical Center, Shreveport, Louisiana*

## CHAPTER CONTENTS

Anatomical Considerations and Contractile Patterns
Regulation of Villous Motility
   Nervous control
      Parasympathetics
      Sympathetics
      Intrinsic nerves
   Postprandial regulation
      Local factors
      Humoral factors
Physiological Implications of Villous Motility
Conclusions

---

THE FACT THAT INTESTINAL VILLI exhibit spontaneous motility was first noted in 1843 by Lacauchie (36) and Gruby and Delafond (11). Since that time approximately 60 papers dealing with the contractile activity of intestinal villi have appeared in the literature. Table 1 summarizes some of the key contributions to this area. The relatively small number of papers on villous motility presumably results from the technical difficulties inherent in the study of moving microscopic structures. As a result most of the available information regarding villous motility is descriptive in nature. Nonetheless the literature does allow for the development of working hypotheses regarding certain aspects of the regulation and functions of villous motility.

## ANATOMICAL CONSIDERATIONS AND CONTRACTILE PATTERNS

The contractile activity of villi can be attributed to the presence of smooth muscle cells within the lamina propria. The smooth muscle fibers are derived from the muscularis mucosa (57) and are oriented along the longitudinal axis of the villus (12, 57). The muscle fibers are arranged in large bundles near the base of the villus with the number of bundles decreasing gradually toward the tip (12, 57). These muscle bundles form a coarse, loose network surrounding the lacteal (54). Neighboring smooth muscle cells are connected to each other by desmosomes and nexuses (12). Numerous fibroblasts, which contain contractile (actomyosin-like) filaments, have processes in close apposition to smooth muscle cells. It has been suggested that the fibroblasts and smooth muscle cells form an integrated contractile system (12).

The nerve supply of the villus is derived from intrinsic ganglia of the myenteric or submucous plexuses and from extrinsic (sympathetic) ganglia (19). Small nerve fibers have been observed in close apposition to both smooth muscle fibers (12, 53) and fibroblasts (12). Synaptic vesicles of nerve terminals have been noted directly facing fibroblasts (12). However, synaptic contact between nerves and villous smooth muscle cells has not been demonstrated.

Villi have been described as being either fingerlike or leaflike in appearance. Fingerlike villi are slender, cylindrical structures with diameters that remain roughly constant from base to tip, whereas leaflike villi are flat, more two-dimensional structures with widths that vary from base to tip. The preponderance of fingerlike and leaflike villi in different species or within a given species has been attributed to differences in dietary habits (54, 58). However, there is no conclusive evidence to support this contention [Table 2; (58)]. Although the factors that determine villous shape are unknown, it is clear that the contractile patterns of fingerlike and leaflike villi differ.

The motor activity of both fingerlike and leaflike villi is independent of contractions of the outer muscular coat of the intestine (13). In general, movements of leaflike villi are dependent on contractions of the underlying muscularis mucosa, whereas those of fingerlike villi are not (54). In species with leaflike villi, circular contractions of the muscularis mucosa tend to compress and elongate the villi (23). Leaflike villi also exhibit pendular (swaying) movements (54).

Two types of contractile activity have been described in fingerlike villi: pistonlike retractions and pendular movements. These movements can occur in

TABLE 1. *Milestones in Research on Physiology of Villous Contractions*

| Ref. | Year | Contribution |
|---|---|---|
| Lacauchie (36) | 1843 | Observed shortening of villi after death |
| Gruby and Delafond (11) | 1843 | Described shortening, lengthening, and lateral movements of villi in living animals |
| Brücke (2) | 1851 | Described the existence and distribution of visceral smooth muscle in villi; observed contraction of villi when stroking mucosal surface |
| Drasch (6) | 1880 | Described fine nerve fibers in close association with villous smooth muscle fibers |
| Hambleton (13) | 1914 | Observed that villous contractile activity is independent of peristalsis and is increased by nutrients in lumen |
| King and Arnold (20) | 1922 | Described the proximal-to-distal gradient of villous contractile activity along small bowel and effects of extrinsic nerve stimulation on villous motility |
| Kokas (23) | 1930 | Described relationship between shape of villi and contractile patterns |
| Mahler et al. (49) | 1932 | First described villous contractile activity in conscious humans |
| Kokas and Ludány (31, 33) | 1933, 1934 | Provided evidence for humoral control of villous contractions; named humoral mediator *villikinin* |
| Wells and Johnson (62) | 1934 | Observed shortening, lengthening, and lateral movements in isolated villi |
| Kokas and Ludány (35) | 1938 | Demonstrated relationship between villous contractile frequency and nutrient absorption |
| Lee (37) | 1969 | Demonstrated lacteal emptying during villous contraction (villous pump) |
| Nanba et al. (51) | 1970 | Measured contraction frequency of individual villi |
| Güldner et al. (12) | 1972 | Proposed that fibroblasts are part of villous contractile system |

individual villi while their neighbors are quiescent. Pistonlike contractions are the predominant type observed (64). In a given contraction-relaxation cycle, shortening occurs at a much more rapid rate than the subsequent relaxation (51). During a contraction the length of the villus can be reduced by >50% (51). The frequency of pistonlike contractions decreases along the length of the bowel [Fig. 1; (64)]. Quantitative analyses in the small bowel of dogs indicate that the frequency in the duodenum ranges from 3 to 23 contractions/min, whereas that in the ileum ranges from 0 to 8 contractions/min (51, 64). A recent report (64) also indicates that there is an axial gradient of the duration of pistonlike contractions, with the longest duration (2.6 s) in the duodenum and the shortest (1.8 s) in the ileum. Based on the mean data for the rate and duration of pistonlike contractions, it is predicted that villi are in a retracted state for approximately 30%, 13%, and 6% of the time in the duodenum, jejunum, and ileum, respectively (64).

Pendular (side-to-side) movements, without shortening, account for <20% of the contractile activity of fingerlike villi (64). The term *pendular* is misleading for certain species (e.g., dog) in which the movement is characterized as a rapid lateral motion of the entire villus or only the upper portion of the villus. In contrast to the pistonlike contractions, there is no axial gradient of the frequency of pendular movements. However, the occurrence of pendular movements is far greater in the jejunum (0.9/min) than both the duodenum (0.1/min) and ileum (0.4/min) (64).

Although pistonlike and pendular movements are the major physiological contractile patterns, tonic contractions of several or all villi in a microscopic field have also been observed. These tonic villous retractions are often associated with contractions of the underlying muscularis mucosa elicited by intense mechanical, chemical, or neural stimulation (13, 20, 31, 38, 62).

## REGULATION OF VILLOUS MOTILITY

### Nervous Control

PARASYMPATHETICS. The role of parasympathetic (vagus) nerves in the regulation of villous motility has been a subject of controversy. King and co-workers (20, 22) reported that neither vagotomy nor vagal stimulation altered villous activity. Based on these findings, they concluded that vagal fibers did not extend to the villous smooth muscle. Other investigators have offered conflicting evidence regarding the effects of vagal stimulation, which has been noted to either abolish (34, 46) or stimulate (34, 51) villous motility. Womack (63) recently demonstrated that vagotomy causes a mild decrease (20%) in villous contraction frequency. This decrease lasts for ~10 min, after which villous motility returns to control. Vagal stimulation at 5, 10, and 20 Hz causes mild (20%–30%) increases in villous activity. This stimulation is blocked by atropine (1 mg/kg) (63).

The effects of cholinergic agonists and antagonists are unclear (Table 3). Despite reports that atropine completely inhibits (13) or slightly enhances (20) villous motility, most investigators find that this muscarinic blocker does not alter villous motility (16, 22, 27). Acetylcholine, methacholine, carbachol, and choline stimulate villous motility (14, 27, 48). A topical choline chloride concentration of 2 $\mu$g/ml causes a doubling of villous motility, whereas 20 $\mu$g/ml causes a four to fivefold increase (48). King and Robinson (22), however, reported that acetylcholine did not stimulate villous motility. Anticholinesterases (phy-

TABLE 2. *Villous Shape in Relation to Diet*

| Dietary Class | Villous Shape | |
|---|---|---|
| | Fingerlike | Leaflike |
| Herbivorous | Chicken | Gopher |
| | Monkey | Guinea pig |
| | Pigeon | Hamster |
| | Porcupine | Rabbit |
| | Goat | Rat |
| | | Squirrel |
| | | Porcupine |
| Carnivorous | Cat | Mole |
| | Dog | |
| | Eagle | |
| | Fox | |
| Omnivorous | Human | Human* |
| | | Opossum |
| | | Pig |

* Leaflike villi are considered pathologic in humans (54). From King and Arnold (20), Kokas (23), and Sessions et al. (54).

sostigmine and neostigmine) stimulate villous motility (14). Atropine is consistently effective in blocking the responses to cholinergic agonists and anticholinesterases (13, 14, 20, 27).

SYMPATHETICS. Section of the splanchnic or mesenteric (periarterial) sympathetic nerves, either acute or chronic, does not alter villous motility (20, 63). Stimulation of sympathetic nerves to the intestine has been reported to cause a transient increase in villous activity followed by a tonic retraction of the villi, with a resulting loss of rhythmic contractile activity (20, 22, 46, 47). More recent studies indicate, however, that stimulation of sympathetic nerves causes a 30%–50% decrease in villous contraction frequency (51, 63). This inhibition of villous motility is attenuated, but not completely prevented, by $\alpha$-receptor blockade or $\beta$-receptor blockade. A combination of $\alpha$- and $\beta$-blocker is required to completely prevent the inhibition, indicating that both receptor types are involved (63). The $\alpha$-receptor–mediated response is presumably due to an inhibition of acetylcholine release by the enteric nervous system, whereas the $\beta$-receptor causes a direct inhibition of villous smooth muscle (7–9).

The sympathetically mediated increases in villous activity and tonic retractions reported by early investigators (20, 22, 46, 47) are presumably responses to intestinal ischemia and not direct effects of sympathetic stimulation. Although these early investigators neither indicated stimulation frequency nor measured intestinal blood flow, most reported an intense blanching of the intestinal mucosa indicative of a severe reduction in intestinal blood flow (22, 46, 47). It has been shown that cessation of intestinal perfusion results in increased villous activity for 1–3 min followed by total loss of contractile activity (21, 62, 65). Womack (63) did observe a pronounced increase in villous motility during some of the sympathetic stimulations at 20 Hz. This increase, however, followed a 20- to 30-s inhibition of villous activity and was only seen when sympathetic stimulation caused an almost complete cessation of blood flow. It appears, therefore, that the response to sympathetic stimulation is the result of a complex interaction between a $\beta$-receptor–mediated inhibition of villous smooth muscle, an $\alpha$-receptor–mediated inhibition of the enteric nervous system, and a blood flow response. Moderate reductions in intestinal blood flow result in inhibition of villous motility, whereas severe flow reductions cause

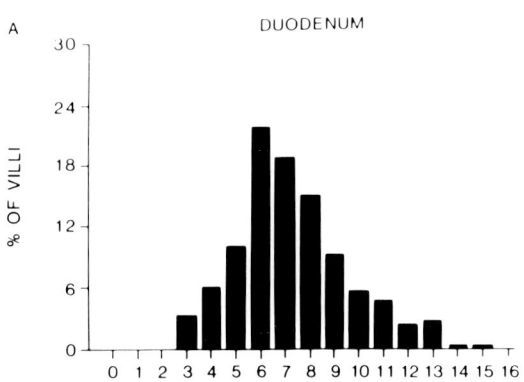
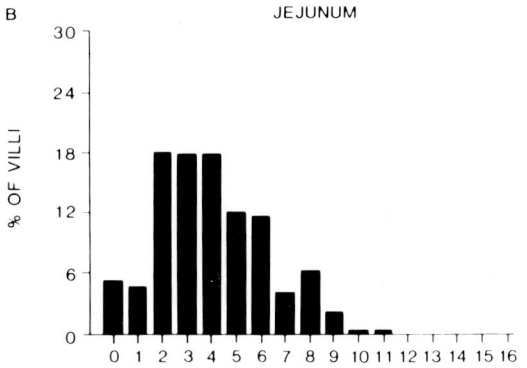
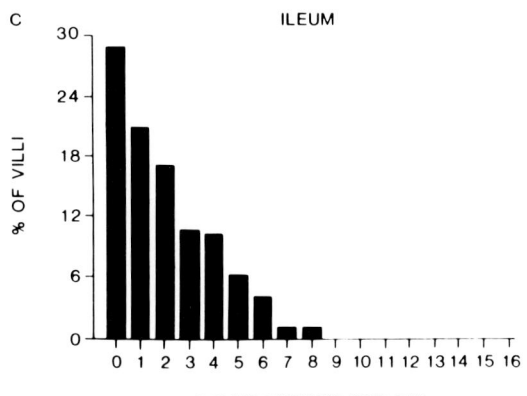

CONTRACTIONS PER MIN

FIG. 1. Frequency distribution of villous contraction rate in dog duodenum, jejunum, and ileum. Mean frequency was highest in duodenum (7.3 ± 0.1), intermediate in jejunum (4.0 ± 0.1), and lowest in ileum (2.0 ± 0.1). [From Womack et al. (64).]

TABLE 3. *Influence of Neuroeffectors and Humoral Factors on Villous Contraction Frequency*

| Substance | Route of Administration | Dose | Villous Motility | Ref. |
|---|---|---|---|---|
| Parasympathetic neuroeffectors | | | | |
| Choline | Intra-arterial | 0.1 µg | ↑ | 48 |
| | Topical | 2 µg/ml | ↑ | 48 |
| | | 20 µg/ml | ↑ | 48 |
| Acetylcholine | Intra-arterial | 10 ng | ↑ | 48 |
| | Intravenous | 50 µg | — | 22 |
| | | 4 µg/kg | ↑ | 14 |
| | Topical | 1 µg/ml | ↑ | 48 |
| | | 10 µg/ml | ↑ | 14 |
| | | 50 µg/ml | ↑ | 27 |
| Methacholine | Intravenous | 4 µg/kg | ↑ | 14 |
| | Topical | 10 µg/ml | ↑ | 14 |
| | | 50 µg/ml | ↑ | 27 |
| Carbachol | Intravenous | 4 µg/kg | ↑ | 14 |
| | Topical | 2.5–5 µg/ml | ↑ | 14 |
| | | 2 µg/ml | ↑ | 48 |
| Atropine | Intravenous | 0.1 mg/kg | ↑ | 20 |
| | | 1 mg/kg | ↓ | 13 |
| | | 1–2 mg/kg | — | 14 |
| | Topical | 10 µg/ml | — | 27 |
| | | 30–40 µg/ml | — | 14 |
| Physostigmine | Intravenous | 50 µg/kg | ↑ | 14 |
| Neostigmine | | 20 µg/kg | ↑ | 14 |
| Sympathetic neuroeffectors | | | | |
| Epinephrine | Intravenous | 50 µg | TR* | 22 |
| | | 4 µg/kg | TR | 14 |
| | Topical | 5–10 µg/ml | ↑ | 14 |
| | | 100 µg/ml | TR | 27 |
| | | 0.2–1000 µg/ml | TR | 20 |
| Norepinephrine | Intravenous | 4 µg/kg | ↑ | 14 |
| | Topical | 10 µg/ml | TR | 27 |
| | | 5–10 µg/ml | ↑ | 14 |
| Phenylephrine | | 10 µg/ml | TR | 27 |
| Isoproterenol | Intravenous | 4 µg/kg | ↓ | 14 |
| | Topical | 10 µg/ml | ↑ | 27 |
| Phentolamine | | 0.5 µg/ml | — | 27 |
| Phenoxybenzamine | Intravenous | 1 mg/kg | — | 14 |
| Tolazoline | | 1–2 mg/kg | ↑ | 14 |
| | Topical | 40–50 µg/ml | — | 14 |
| Propranolol | Intravenous | 0.5–1 mg/kg | ↑ | 14 |
| | Topical | 0.5 µg/ml | — | 27 |
| | | 40–50 µg/ml | — | 14 |
| Humoral factors | | | | |
| Gastrin | Intravenous | 1 µg/kg | ↑ | 18 |
| | Topical | 1–2 µg | ↑ | 18 |
| Pentagastrin | Intravenous | 0.1–1.0 µg/kg | ↓ | 18 |
| | Topical | 1–2 µg | ↓ | 18 |
| Secretin | Intra-arterial | 0.3–1.0 U | ↑ | 52 |
| | Intravenous | ? | — | 33 |
| | | 0.1–0.5 U/kg | ↓ | 18 |
| | Topical | 1 U | — | 18 |
| | Intravenous | 5–10 U/kg | ↑ | 50 |
| Cholecystokinin | | ? | — | 33 |
| | | 0.1–1.0 U/kg | ↓ | 18 |
| | Topical | 0.1–2.0 U | ↓ | 18 |
| Glucagon | Intra-arterial | 0.1–5 µg | ↓ | 17 |
| Enterogastrone | Intravenous | 0.5 mg/kg | ↓ | 18 |
| | Topical | 0.4 µg | ↓ | 18 |
| Gastrointestinal inhibitory polypeptide | Intravenous | 0.1 µg/kg | ↓ | 18 |
| Substance P | Topical | 5 U/kg | ↑ | 43 |
| | | ? | ↓ | 18 |
| | | 5 ng/ml | ↑ | 18 |
| Histamine | Intra-arterial | 0.01–0.5 µg | ↑ | 52 |
| | | 1 µg | ↓ | 52 |
| | Topical | 10 µg/ml | ↑ | 41 |
| | | 100–200 µg/ml | TR | 41 |

TABLE 3—Continued

| Substance | Route of Administration | Dose | Villous Motility | Ref. |
|---|---|---|---|---|
| Serotonin | Intravenous | 2 µg/kg | ↑ | 15 |
|  | Intra-arterial | 10 µg·min$^{-1}$·ml$^{-1}$ | ↑ | 44 |
|  | Intravenous | 10 µg/kg | ↑ | 44 |
|  |  | 2 mg/kg | ↑ | 50 |
|  | Topical | 10 µg/ml | ↑ | 44 |
| Bradykinin | Intra-arterial | 1 µg·min$^{-1}$ml$^{-1}$ | ↓ | 45 |
|  | Intravenous | 7 µg/min | ↓ | 45 |
| Caerulein | Intra-arterial | 2.5–25 pg | ↑ | 17 |
|  | Intravenous | 2.5 ng·kg$^{-1}$·min$^{-1}$ | ↑ | 1 |
|  |  | 25 ng·kg$^{-1}$·min$^{-1}$ | ↓ | 1 |
|  | Topical | 1–5 ng/ml$^1$ | ↑ | 1 |
|  | Intravenous | 0.1–1.0 µg/kg | TR | 18 |
|  | Topical | 0.01–0.3 µg | ↓ | 18 |
| Eledoisin | Intra-arterial | 1 µg·ml$^{-1}$·min$^{-1}$ | ↓ | 45 |
|  | Intravenous | 1.0 µg/kg | ↓ | 18 |
|  | Topical | 0.1 µg | ↑ | 18 |
| Kallidin | Intra-arterial | 1 µg·ml$^{-1}$·min$^{-1}$ | ↓ | 45 |
| Ranatensin | Intravenous | 1–10 µg/kg | TR | 18 |
|  | Topical | 0.2–0.5 µg | TR | 18 |
| Mucosal extract ("villikinin") | Intravenous | 0.1–0.4 ml/kg | – | 15 |
|  |  | 0.5–1.0 ml/kg | ↑ | 15 |
|  |  | 0.1 ml/kg | ↑ | 31 |
|  |  | 1.3 mg/kg | ↑ | 28 |
|  |  | 2.5 mg/kg | ↑ | 28 |
|  |  | 5.0 mg/kg | ↓ | 28 |
|  |  | 0.05 ml/kg | ↓ | 50 |
|  |  | 1 ml/kg | – | 50 |
| Trypsin | Intra-arterial | 10–250 µg | ↓ | 52 |
| Prostaglandin E$_1$ |  | 62–1000 ng | ↓ | 17 |

* TR, tonic retraction with no rhythmic activity.

a transient stimulation of villous activity followed by a loss of rhythmic contractile activity (65).

Epinephrine and norepinephrine have been reported to cause a transient increase in villous motility followed by tonic retraction of all villi similar to that observed with sympathetic nerve stimulation (14, 20, 22, 27). Hooper and Schneider (14) reported that topical epinephrine and norepinephrine produced only an increase in villous motility. The responses to norepinephrine can be prevented by α-receptor blockade and reproduced by α-receptor agonists (14, 22, 27). The responses to β-receptor agonists and antagonists are unclear. Kokas and Gordon (27) reported that epinephrine (in the presence of α-blockade) and isoproterenol both stimulate villous motility. Hooper and Schneider (14), however, found that isoproterenol hydrochloride caused an inhibition of villous motility, whereas epinephrine (in the presence of α-blockade) had no effect. In general, neither α-blockers nor β-blockers, at concentrations that were effective in blocking the actions of norepinephrine and isoproterenol, altered villous motility (14, 27). It is likely that the stimulation of villous motility and tonic villous retractions observed with epinephrine and norepinephrine, like those observed with sympathetic stimulation, are the result of intestinal ischemia rather than a direct effect of the drug on villous smooth muscle.

INTRINSIC NERVES. Ganglion-blocking agents have been used to determine the role of the intrinsic plexuses in controlling villous motility. In dogs, nicotine and ganglion blockers (hexamethonium, tetraethylammonium bromide, tetramethylammonium bromide) produce a biphasic response consisting of a brief stimulation followed by a transient inhibition of villous activity (13, 20, 22, 42). Cocaine and other local anesthetics inhibit movement of dog villi (40). In pigeons, however, neither ganglion blockers (hexamethonium, pentolinium tartrate, and pempidine) nor local anesthetics (cocaine and amethocaine hydrochloride) had any effect on villous activity. The response to nicotine was the same as in the dog, i.e., a brief stimulation followed by transient inhibition (14, 16). It is unclear whether the conflicting results in the literature are entirely due to species differences or whether other experimental factors are involved.

Several groups of investigators have attempted to study villous motility in vitro using isolated villi, strips of intestinal mucosa, or strips of whole intestine. Wells and Johnson (62) reported that isolated villi maintained in warm oxygenated salt solutions continue to contract for many minutes. They noted that the rhythm of contraction is the same in isolated villi as in the living animal, although in vitro contractile activity decreases to very low values after a few minutes. Kokas and Ludany (34) also found that if the intestine was cut out while the villi were very active, the villous contractions continued for ~15 min. King and Arnold (20) were unable to observe villous movements in strips of whole intestine bathed in oxygenated saline, Ringer's, Locke's, or Tyrode's solution. Verzar and McDougall (61) observed that villi cut away from the muscularis mucosae and thus isolated from ganglion cells of the submucous plexus do not contract. Based on this finding, Verzar and McDougall suggested that the villi used by Wells and Johnson (62) may have had intact ganglion cells that stimulated the contractions. Using in vitro strips of mucosa maintained in oxygenated Ringer's solution, Lee (37) did not observe any rhythmic movements of the villi, although he could stimulate them to contract.

*Postprandial Regulation*

LOCAL FACTORS. The observation that chyme stimulates villous motility was first documented by Verzar and Kokas in 1927 (60). They ligated the small intestine of anesthetized dogs and subsequently placed food into the stomach. They noted that the villi above the ligature (which were exposed to chyme) were stimulated, whereas the villi below the ligature were not. Based on these observations, they concluded that the postprandial increase in villous motility is mediated by local factors that depend on the presence of chyme.

Chyme in the intestinal lumen may enhance villous motility via mechanical effects. Mechanical stimulation of the villi with a hair, a pin, or a rapid stream of fluid causes an increase in villous activity. It has been suggested that the enhanced villous motility is mediated by a reflex involving the submucosal plexus because stimulating a villus near its base causes the surrounding villi to contract as well (20). An increase in villous interstitial pressure due to absorption of fluid may also set the villi in motion. Verzar and Kokas (60) noted that villi in a fasting animal are empty and lie flat with little contractile activity. The application of water, Tyrode's, or Ringer's solution causes the villi to swell and to contract more frequently (60). Womack et al. (65) also showed that villous contraction frequency is greater in the presence of fluid absorption (4.4 contractions/min) than in the absence of fluid absorption (1.9 contractions/min). A role for villous swelling in the absorption-induced increase in villous motility is further supported by the observation that conditions that increase interstitial pressure, i.e., plasma dilution, venous pressure elevation, and lymphatic blockage, also cause an increase in villous activity (21, 65).

The chemical composition of chyme also appears to play a role in the postprandial increase in villous motility. In early studies it was reported that application of warmed solutions of glucose, peptone, bile, taurocholic acid, food extracts, water-soluble amino acids, and various organic acids (i.e., cod-liver oil) or spices stimulate villous motility (13, 31). A portion of these effects can be attributed to thermal and me-

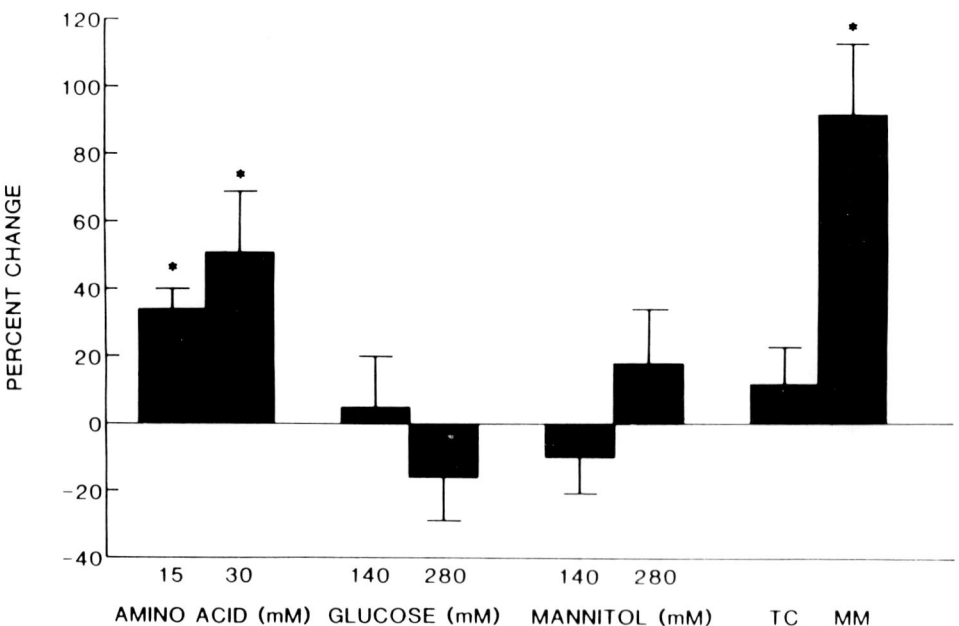

FIG. 2. Percent change in frequency of villous contraction in dog jejunum induced by nutrient solutions. Amino acid solutions (15 and 30 mM) and a micellar oleic acid solution caused significant ($P < 0.05$) increases in contraction frequency. The mixed micellar (MM) solution consisted of 15 mM taurocholic acid, 5 mM monoolein, and 10 mM oleic acid. Taurocholic acid (TC) (15 mM), alone or in combination with monoolein (5 mM), did not increase villous motility. [From Womack et al. (64).]

chanical influences. When mechanical and thermal effects are controlled, amino acid solutions (10 or 20 mM) and a mixed micellar solution of oleic acid (10 mM) increase villous motility, whereas glucose (140 and 280 mM) has no effect [Fig. 2; (64)]. Amino acids cause a 30%–40% increase in contractile frequency, whereas oleic acid causes a doubling of villous motility (64). The precise mechanism by which amino acids and fatty acids stimulate the villi is unknown.

The effects of alterations in luminal pH and osmolality have also been evaluated. Earlier reports on the effect of pH changes are contradictory. Wells and Johnson (62) found that an alkaline medium inhibits villous motility; Verzar and McDougall (61) reported that pH 4.7 inhibits, whereas pH 8.0 stimulates, villous activity. A recent quantitative analysis indicates that changes in pH within the physiological range of the jejunum (5.0–7.4) do not alter villous motility (64). Neither increases (600 mosmol/l) nor decreases (distilled water) in luminal osmolality produce a change in villous activity when compared with isotonic saline (20, 64).

HUMORAL FACTORS. In 1932 Kokas and Ludany (31) provided the first evidence for the involvement of humoral factors in postprandial stimulation of villous motility. They observed that villi, in an isolated autoperfused loop of jejunum, contract at a higher frequency in a fed dog than in a fasted dog. When the artery of a loop of intestine from a fasted dog was perfused by the carotid artery of a fed dog, the villi in the isolated loop began contracting vigorously. When the loop of a fed dog, which had very active villi, was perfused by blood from a fasted dog, villous activity decreased. Instillation of 0.4% hydrochloric acid into the duodenum of a fasted dog increased villous activity 10-fold in an isolated jejunal segment, and an acid extract of duodenal mucosa stimulated villous motility when injected intravenously. Based on these observations, Kokas and Ludany (31) concluded that a peptide called villikinin is released from the duodenal mucosa in response to a meal. Villikinin was presumed to enter the circulation and stimulate villous motility throughout the intestine.

Kokas and co-workers (25, 26, 54) have partially purified and characterized villikinin. Villikinin is a small acidic peptide ($M_r = 1,200$) containing aspartic acid, threonine, serine, glutamic acid, glycine, and alanine residues. It is not hydrolyzed by pepsin or trypsin, is partly hydrolyzed by carboxypeptidase A and B, and is completely inactivated by nagarse, pronase, papain, and leucine aminopeptidase. Villikinin has been extracted from human, canine, bovine, and porcine intestinal mucosa and from human plasma and urine. The effects of these extracts is not species specific, i.e., human villikinin can stimulate dog villi.

The actions of villikinin have been compared with those of other hormones and vasoactive substances (Table 3). The effects of villikinin cannot be attributed to cholecystokinin or secretin because neither of these hormones have significant effects on the villi, and villikinin does not stimulate pancreatic secretion nor gall bladder contraction (33). Villikinin's effect on intestinal villi differs from that of gastrin, pentagastrin, enterogastrone, gastrointestinal inhibitory polypeptide, bradykinin, histamine, and serotonin with respect to onset, duration, magnitude, and/or direction (18). The most potent stimuli of villous motility are villikinin, histamine, serotonin, and substance P. Substance P has many similarities to villikinin, but the action of villikinin can be blocked by hexamethonium, whereas that of substance P cannot (43).

An interesting observation by Kokas and Johnston (29) was that, whereas small amounts of acidic mucosal extract stimulate villous motility, larger amounts inhibit it. Based on this finding, they postulated the existence of a humoral substance that inhibits villous motility. This substance, antivillikinin, is also present in the duodenum and can be recovered from acid extracts of the mucosa. In addition villikinin and antivillikinin can be separated from one another by continuous-flow electrophoresis.

Attempts by other investigators to verify the existence of a villikinin-like substance have been unsuccessful. Hooper and Schneider (15) did not observe an increase in jejunal villous motility in the pigeon after instilling 0.4% hydrochloric acid into the duodenum. Acid extracts of pigeon duodenum, when injected intravenously, did produce a slight increase in villous motility; however, this effect could be blocked by pretreatment with an antihistamine (promethazine). Likewise, Nanba and Hiramatsu (50) found that neither intraduodenal acid nor acid extracts of duodenal mucosa caused an increase in jejunal villous motility in dogs. Womack (63) noted that villous contraction frequency in the jejunum of fed dogs from which the chyme had been removed is no greater than the contraction frequency in fasted dogs. Furthermore perfusion of the duodenum with saline, acidified predigested food (pH 3.0), or 0.4% hydrochloric acid did not increase jejunal villous motility in dogs (63). These data argue against any generalized postprandial increase in villous motility due to humoral or neural factors and indicate that postprandial stimulation of villous motility is mediated by local factors.

PHYSIOLOGICAL IMPLICATIONS OF VILLOUS MOTILITY

Although villous motility was first described over 150 years ago (11), the functional implication(s) of this process remains uncertain. However, it has frequently been suggested that villous movements exert an influence on three physiological processes in the small bowel: lymph flow, blood flow, and nutrient absorption. The concept that villous contractions act as a pump that facilitates the formation and propulsion of intestinal lymph was first proposed by Brücke (2) in 1851. The current version of this concept predicts that, when the villus is in the relaxed state, the higher pressure in the lamina propria opens the intercellular junctions (which function as inlet valves in lymph vessels) and drives interstitial fluid into the central lacteal. When the villus contracts, the intercellular junctions are closed, due to the sudden rise in intralymphatic pressure, and lacteal lymph is ejected into larger lymph vessels in the submucosa. Reflux of lymph into the lacteal during the subsequent villous relaxation is prevented by valves in the larger lymph vessels.

Arguments have been presented both to support and refute the villous pump mechanism. Three lines of evidence have been used to discredit it: 1) lymph formation and propulsion also occur in species with nonretracting leaflike villi (21, 60, 62); 2) even following repetitive retractions of fingerlike villi, the lacteal appears to remain filled (62); and 3) villi do not appear to change in volume during the retraction phase (62). Although pistonlike movements are not seen in leaflike villi, lymphatic pumping may result from the villous compression associated with circular contractions of the muscularis mucosae (54). The argument that the lacteal remains filled after repetitive villous retractions is not supported by the recent work of Lee (37). After injecting mineral oil containing Sudan black B into the central lacteal of dog villi, Lee noted that retractions were always associated with the movement of oil toward the villus base. Finally, inasmuch as the central lacteal accounts for <10% of the total villous volume, it is unlikely that such small volume changes (assuming complete emptying of the lacteal) can be detected by microscopy. Furthermore it is recognized that the compliance of the intestinal interstitium is sufficiently low to allow large changes in interstitial pressure to result from small changes in villous volume. Additional support for the villous pump mechanism is provided by electron-microscope studies of dog jejunal villi, which indicate that the endothelial intercellular junctions of central lacteals are open in the relaxed villus and closed in the contracted villus (3). It has also been noted in histologic specimens that the central lacteals are full of lipid particles when the villus is relaxed, but they are devoid of lipid particles when the villus is contracted (61).

There is also evidence of a relationship between intestinal lymph flow and villous motility. King et al. (21) reported that ligation of major lymph trunks draining a segment of dog intestine led to a significant increase in villous contraction frequency relative to control segments. The contraction frequency returned to a normal level when the lymphatic ligature was removed. These investigators also noted that plasma dilution (reducing plasma oncotic pressure by intravenous saline infusion) led to concomitant increases in intestinal lymph flow and villous contraction frequency. However, the increased lymph flow persisted for a longer period than the enhanced villous motility.

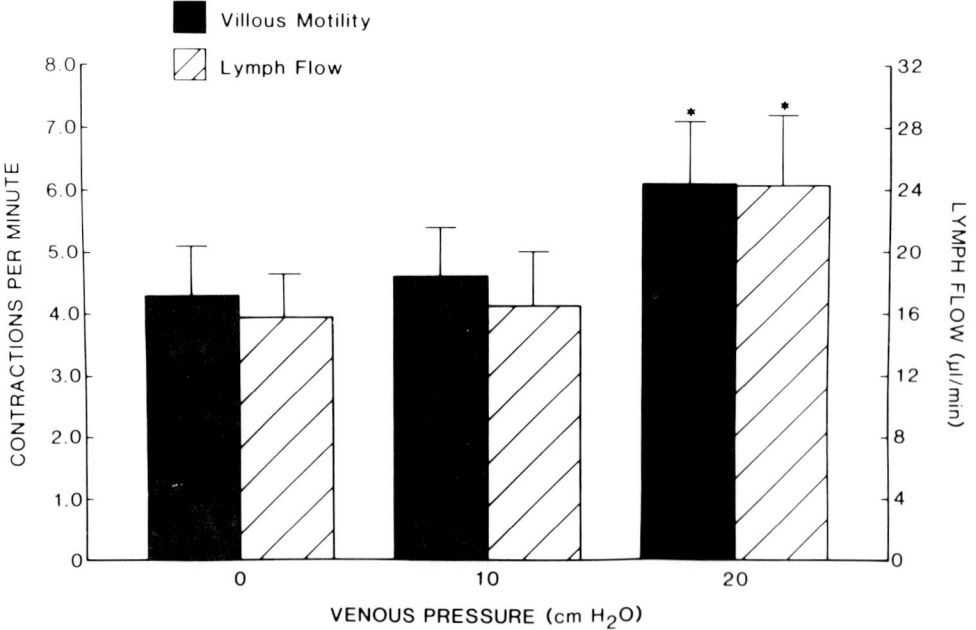

FIG. 3. Effect of venous pressure elevation on villous contraction frequency and lymph flow. A venous pressure elevation of 20 cmH$_2$O caused significant ($P < 0.05$) increases in both parameters. Villous contraction frequency rose 55% ± 14%, whereas lymph flow increased 54% ± 2%. [From Womack et al. (65).]

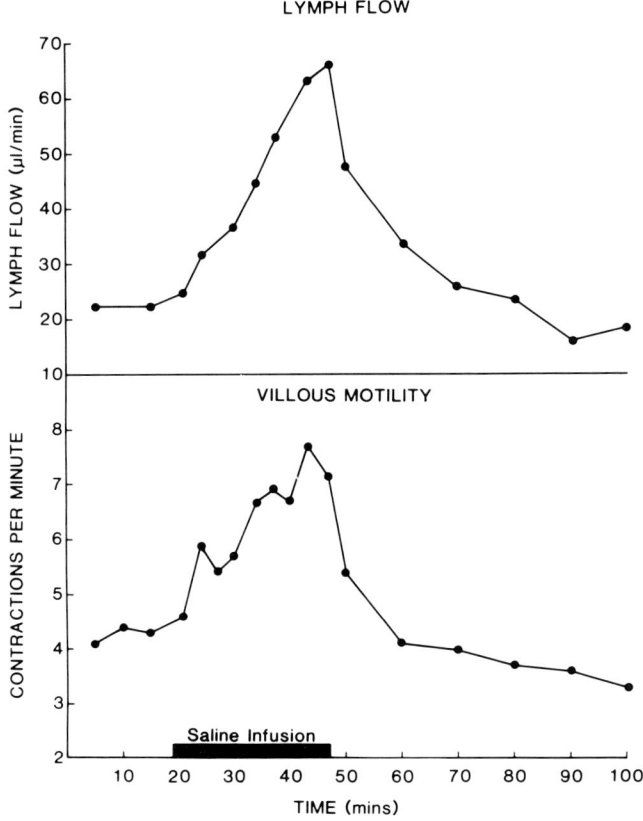

FIG. 4. Representative plasma-dilution experiment. Intravenous saline infusion (2.5 ml·min$^{-1}$·kg$^{-1}$ body wt) resulted in parallel changes in villous motility and lymph flow. [From Womack et al. (65).]

Recent studies in our lab have established a quantitative relationship between villous contraction frequency and lymph flow (65). Venous pressure elevation (Fig. 3) and plasma dilution (Fig. 4) cause parallel increases in lymph flow and villous motility. An excellent positive correlation between villous contraction frequency and lymph flow was observed by Womack et al. [Fig. 5; (65)]. Based on these data and observations by others, the following hypothesis is proposed [Fig. 6; (65)]. Fluid accumulation in the lamina propria leads to an increased interstitial fluid pressure (10, 39). The elevated interstitial pressure increases the driving force for lymphatic filling and elicits a myogenic contraction of smooth muscle fibers in the lamina propria. Consequently the villus retracts and the lacteal is emptied of its contents. An important physiological implication of this scheme is that fluid accumulation into the mucosal interstitium during absorption should elicit villous retraction and thereby facilitate lymphatic removal of absorbed fluid. This contention is supported by the observation that stimulation of net fluid absorption is associated with a 130% increase in villous contraction frequency (65).

Earlier studies on villous motility suggested a possible role for villous contractions in the control of villous blood flow (21, 62). This theory is largely based on the observation that villous retraction tends to squeeze blood out of the capillaries and veins. There is also evidence that alterations in intestinal perfusion pressure and/or blood flow influence villous motility. King et al. (21) found that ligation of the mesenteric artery or vein, or an abrupt fall in blood pressure,

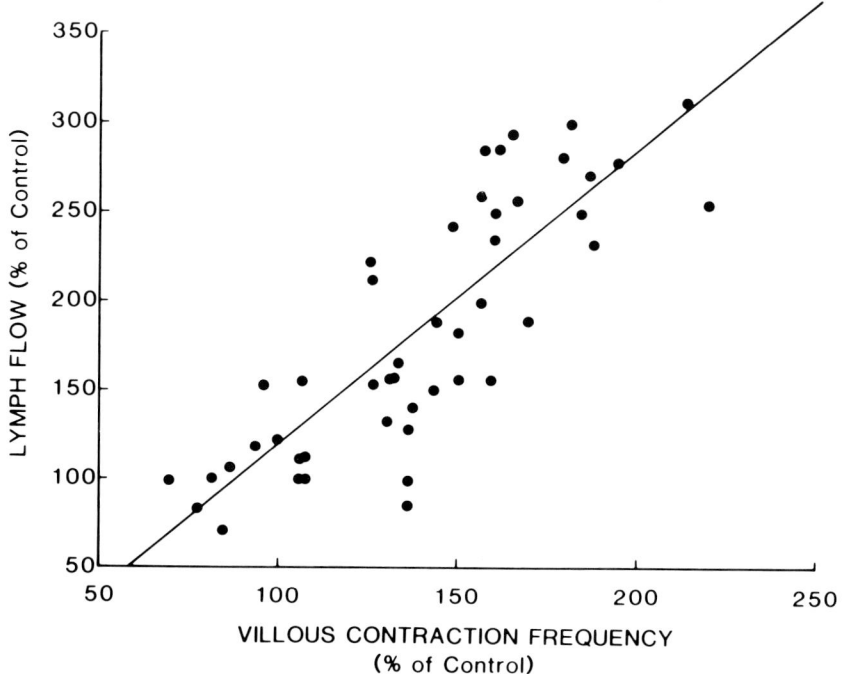

FIG. 5. Relationship between lymph flow (% of control) and villous motility (% of control). Regression analysis yielded statistically significant correlation ($P < 0.001$) with correlation coefficient of 0.83. [From Womack et al. (65).]

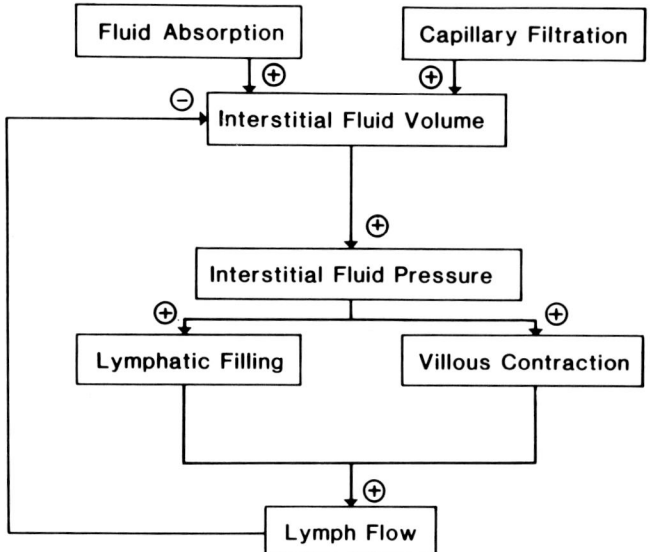

FIG. 6. Proposed mechanism for role of villous motility in lymph propulsion. [From Womack et al. (65).]

causes a transient increase in villous motility followed by a decrease and cessation of activity. They noted that moderate increases or decreases in blood pressure do not alter villous motility. Womack et al. (65) showed that villous motility is independent of arterial pressure and blood flow in the range of 60–120 mmHg (Fig. 7). Only when blood flow is reduced below the level necessary to maintain basal intestinal oxygen uptake (i.e., <50% of control) does villous motility begin to decline. A brief stimulation of villous motility was observed when arterial pressure was reduced to 20 mmHg. However, the enhanced activity usually lasted for only 1–3 min, after which villous activity declined to zero. The fact that villous contraction frequency remained relatively constant, whereas intestinal blood flow fell progressively while local arterial pressure was reduced, indicates that villous motility may not play an important role in the regulation of blood flow. Nonetheless the results indicate that agents or conditions that reduce intestinal blood flow below 50% of control inhibit villous motility, presumably due to a reduction in oxygen delivery (65).

The observation that villous motility is influenced by changes in blood flow only when intestinal oxygenation is compromised supports the view that villous contraction is an energy-consuming process that requires oxygen. The increased intestinal oxygen consumption elicited by acute venous hypertension (55) may be explained by the finding that venous pressure elevation increases villous motility [see Fig. 3; (65)]. More importantly, stimulation of villous motility by fluid absorption and luminal nutrients (64, 65) may contribute to postprandial intestinal hyperemia via increases in oxygen consumption. This possibility is supported by the following observations: 1) many conditions that increase intestinal blood flow postprandially [i.e., fluid absorption and solubilized oleic acid (5, 59)] also stimulate villous motility (64, 65), 2) postprandial intestinal hyperemia occurs primarily in the mucosa (4), and 3) increases in intestinal blood flow (4) and villous motility (63) are limited to areas of the intestine exposed to chyme.

The influence of villous movements on nutrient absorption is an issue characterized by uncertainty and controversy. Many investigators have speculated that villous movements serve as a local stirring apparatus that mixes food with digestive juices and facilitates absorption by keeping the mucosal cells in contact with a relatively constant concentration of nutrients (21, 54, 61). Although one might expect the vigorous villous contractions observed in some species (dog) to significantly stir the aqueous phase immediately surrounding the villus, there is no direct evidence

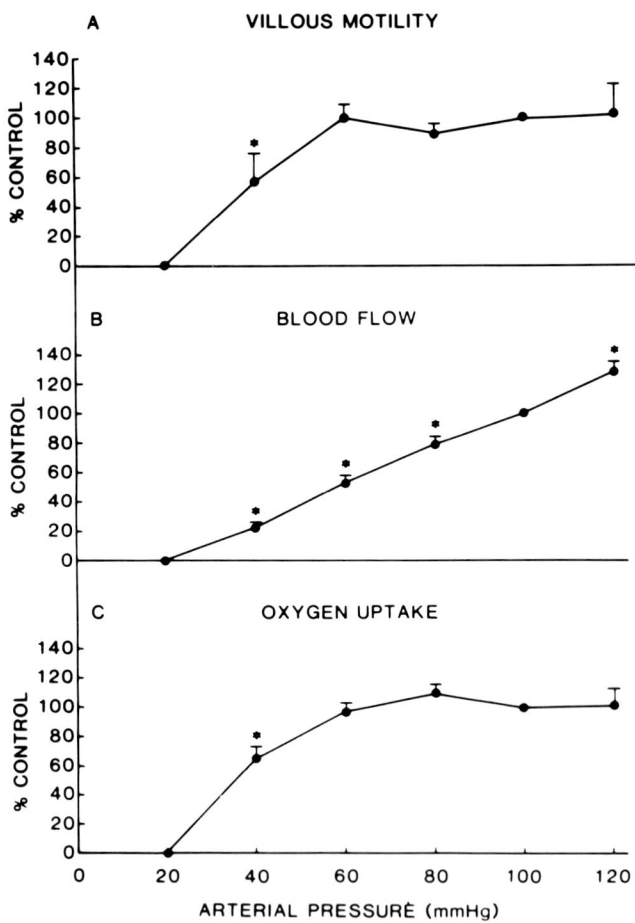

FIG. 7. Response of intestinal villous motility (A), blood flow (B), and oxygen uptake (C) to graded reductions in arterial pressure. Values obtained at 100 mmHg were taken as control, and all other values were expressed as percent of control. Blood flow demonstrated a linear decline as arterial pressure was reduced, and villous motility and oxygen uptake remained at control levels until pressure was reduced to <60 mmHg. *, Significant difference from control ($P < 0.05$). [From Womack et al. (65).]

bearing on this issue. The fact that in vivo estimates of unstirred water-layer resistance in human intestine are larger than in vitro estimates (when villous movements cease) (56) tends to argue against the concept of villous stirring. Even if villous motility does exert a significant stirring effect, it is clear that villous movements are not essential for nutrient absorption, inasmuch as efficient absorption occurs in many species that do not display rhythmic villous contractions.

There are reports that indicate that villous movement exerts a significant influence on glucose (35) and water (37, 38) transport. Kokas and Ludany (35) noted that conditions that increase villous contraction frequency in the dog are associated with enhanced rates of glucose absorption and vice versa. They found that a 3- to 10-fold increase in contraction frequency corresponds to a 13%–31% increase in absorption rate, whereas a 60%–90% reduction in contraction frequency corresponds to a 13%–16% decrease in absorption rate. Lee (37, 38) demonstrated that tonic contraction of dog villi is invariably associated with diminution of water-absorption rate. A variety of substances (including glucose) that inhibit tonic villous contractions also restore fluid-transport rate to a normal level. Unlike the aforementioned studies, Wells and Johnson (62) were unable to demonstrate a correlation between villous motor activity and the rate or direction of net transmucosal fluid movement.

## CONCLUSIONS

Although most of the literature on villous motility is descriptive, there are several tentative conclusions that can be drawn from the available information: *1*) Contractile patterns depend on villous shape; i.e., fingerlike villi exhibit predominantly pistonlike contractions, whereas leaflike villi display little contractile activity. *2*) There is an axial gradient in the frequency and duration of pistonlike contractions from duodenum to ileum. *3*) The parasympathetic and sympathetic nerves exert minimal influence on villous activity. Vagal stimulation causes a mild increase in villous contraction frequency, whereas sympathetic stimulation inhibits villous motility. *4*) Although intramural ganglia may exert a significant influence on basal villous activity, villi do contract following ganglionic blockade. *5*) Villous motility increases significantly following a meal, primarily due to the local effects of chyme. Long-chain fatty acids and amino acids stimulate villous motility at concentrations found in the lumen postprandially. Fluid absorption also enhances villous motility, presumably via changes in interstitial fluid pressure. *6*) The existence and physiological significance of villikinin are questioned. Local factors, rather than villikinin or other humoral substances, appear to play a major role in the postprandial increase in villous contraction frequency. *7*) Villous contractions appear to be important in the formation and propulsion of intestinal lymph (villous pump). The effects of villous motility on mucosal blood flow and nutrient absorption have not been adequately characterized. An improved understanding of the physiological significance of villous motility requires the development of quantitative methods that allow simultaneous measurement of contraction frequency, blood flow, lymph flow, and transport rates in individual villi or small populations of villi.

## REFERENCES

1. ANGELUCCI, L., L. MICOSSI, AND F. CANTALAMESSA. The action of caerulein on the motility of intestinal villi of avians. *Arch. Int. Pharmacodyn.* 196: 89–91, 1972.
2. BRÜCKE, E. Über ein in der darmschleimhaut aufgefundenes muskelsystem. *Sitzungsber. Akad. Wiss. Wien* 6: 214–248, 1851.
3. CASLEY-SMITH, J. R. A fine structural study of variations in protein concentration in lacteals during compression and relaxation. *Lymphology* 12: 59–65, 1979.
4. CHOU, C. C., C. P. HSIEH, Y. M. YU, P. KVIETYS, L. C. YU, R. PITTMAN, AND J. M. DABNEY. Localization of mesenteric hyperemia during digestion in dogs. *Am. J. Physiol.* 230: 583–589, 1976.
5. CHOU, C. C., P. KVIETYS, J. POST, AND S. P. SIT. Constituents of chyme responsible for postprandial intestinal hyperemia. *Am. J. Physiol.* 235 (*Heart Circ. Physiol.* 4): H677–H682, 1978.
6. DRASCH, O. Beiträge zur kenntnis des feineneren baues des dünndarms, im sbesondern über die nerven desselben. *Sitzungsber. Akad. Wiss Wien* 82: 168–198, 1880.
7. EK, B. Studies on mechanisms for beta-adrenergic mediated inhibition of colon motility. *Acta. Physiol. Scand. Suppl.* 546: 1–39, 1985.
8. FURNESS, J. B., AND G. BURNSTOCK. Role of circulating catecholamines in the gastrointestinal tract. In: *Handbook of Physiology. Endocrinology*, edited by H. Blaschko, G. Sayers, and A. D. Smith. Washington, DC: Am. Physiol. Soc., 1975, sect. 7, vol. 6, chapt. 33, p. 515–536.
9. FURNESS, J. B., AND M. COSTA. The adrenergic innervation of the gastrointestinal tract. *Ergeb. Physiol. Biol. Chem. Exp. Pharmacol.* 69: 1–51, 1974.
10. GRANGER, D. N., M. A. PERRY, P. R. KVIETYS, AND A. E. TAYLOR. Capillary and interstitial forces during absorption in the cat small intestine. *Gastroenterology* 88: 267–273, 1984.
11. GRUBY, M., AND M. DELAFOND. Résultats des recherches faites sur l'anatomie et les fonctions des villosités intestinales, l'absorption, la préparation et la composition organique du chyle dans les animaux. *C. R. Acad. Sci.* 16: 1194–1197, 1843.
12. GÜLDNER, F.-H., J. R. WOLFF, AND D. G. KEYSERLINGK. Fibroblasts as a part of the contractile system in duodenal villi of rat. *Z. Zellforsch. Mikrosk. Anat.* 135: 349–360, 1972.
13. HAMBLETON, B. F. Note upon the movements of the intestinal villi. *Am. J. Physiol.* 34: 446–447, 1914.
14. HOOPER, P. A., AND R. SCHNEIDER. The effects of "autonomic drugs" on villous movement in the small intestine of the pigeon. *Br. J. Pharmacol.* 40: 426–436, 1970.
15. HOOPER, P. A., AND R. SCHNEIDER. Evidence against the existence of hormonal control of small intestinal villous movement in the pigeon. *Life Sci.* 9: 1269–1273, 1970.
16. HOOPER, P. A., AND R. SCHNEIDER. The mechanism of small intestinal villous movements in the pigeon. *Life Sci.* 10: 61–66, 1971.

17. IHÁSZ, M., I. KOISS, E. P. NÉMETH, G. FOLLY, AND M. PAPP. Action of caerulein, glucagon or prostaglandin E₁ on the motility of intestinal villi. *Pflueger Arch.* 364: 301–304, 1976.
18. JOYNER, W. L., AND E. KOKAS. Effect of various gastrointestinal hormones and vasoactive substances on villous motility. *Comp. Biochem. Physiol.* 46A: 171–181, 1973.
19. KEAST, J. R., J. B. FURNESS, AND M. COSTA. Origins of peptide and norepinephrine nerves in the mucosa of the guinea pig small intestine. *Gastroenterology* 86: 637–644, 1984.
20. KING, C. E., AND L. ARNOLD. The activities of the intestinal mucosal motor mechanism. *Am. J. Physiol.* 59: 97–121, 1922.
21. KING, C. E., L. ARNOLD, AND J. G. CHURCH. The physiological role of the intestinal mucosal movements. *Am. J. Physiol.* 61: 80–92, 1922.
22. KING, C. E., AND M. H. ROBINSON. The nervous mechanisms of the muscularis mucosae. *Am. J. Physiol.* 143: 325–335, 1945.
23. KOKAS, E. Vergleichend-physiologische untersuchungen über die bewegung der darmzotten. *Plfuegers Arch.* 225: 416–420, 1930.
24. KOKAS, E. Vergleichend-physiologische untersuchungen über die bewegung der darmzotten und die resorption von glykose aus dem darm III. *Z. V. Gl. Physiol.* 26: 74–78, 1938.
25. KOKAS, E. Villikinin. *Prog. Gastroenterol.* 67: 750–752, 1974.
26. KOKAS, E., J. L. DAVIS III, AND W. D. BRUNSON. Separation of villikinin-like substance from intestinal mucosal extract. *Arch. Int. Pharmacodyn. Ther.* 191: 310–317, 1971.
27. KOKAS, E., AND H. GORDON. Adrenergic and cholinergic receptors of intestinal villi in dogs. *J. Pharmacol. Exp. Ther.* 180: 56–61, 1972.
28. KOKAS, E., AND C. L. JOHNSTON, JR. Influence of refined villikinin on motility of intestinal villi. *Am. J. Physiol.* 208: 1196–1202, 1965.
29. KOKAS, E., AND C. L. JOHNSTON, JR. Evidence for an intestinal inhibitor of villous motility. *Arch. Int. Pharmacodyn. Ther.* 160: 211–222, 1966.
30. KOKAS, E., C. L. JOHNSTON, JR., AND E. S. BARROW. Villikinin: Studies of intestinal and plasma villikinin preparations (Abstract). *Federation Proc.* 22: 225, 1963.
31. KOKAS, E., AND G. LUDÁNY. Die hormonale regelung der darmzottenbewegung I. *Pfluegers Arch.* 232: 293, 1933.
32. KOKAS, E., AND G. LUDÁNY. Die wirkung der gewürzmittel auf die bewegung der darmzotten und die glykoseresorption. *Naunyn-Schmiedebergs Arch. Exp. Pathol. Pharmakol.* 169: 140–145, 1933.
33. KOKAS, E., AND G. LUDANY. Die hormonale regelung der darmzottenbewegung II. *Pfluegers Arch.* 234: 182–186, 1934.
34. KOKAS, E., AND G. LUDANY. Weitere untersuchungen über die nervöse beeinflussung der darmzottentätigkeit. *Pfluegers Arch.* 241: 268–271, 1938.
35. KOKAS, E., AND G. LUDÁNY. Relation between the villikinine and the absorption of glucose from the intestine. *Q. J. Exp. Physiol. Cogn. Med. Sci.* 28: 15–22, 1938.
36. LACAUCHIE, M. Memoire sur la structure et le mode d'action des villosites intestinales. *C. R. Acad. Sci.* 16: 1125–1127, 1843.
37. LEE, J. S. A micropuncture study of water transport by dog jejunal villi in vitro. *Am. J. Physiol.* 217: 1528–1533, 1969.
38. LEE, J. S. Contraction of villi and fluid transport in dog jejunal mucosa in vitro. *Am. J. Physiol.* 221: 488–495, 1971.
39. LEE, J. S. Lymph capillary pressure of rat intestinal villi during fluid absorption. *Am. J. Physiol.* 237 (*Endocrinol. Metab. Gastrointest. Physiol.* 5): E301–E307, 1979.
40. LUDÁNY, G. Action de la cocaïne et de quelques succédanés sur la motricité des villosités intestinales. *C. R. Soc. Biol.* 121: 293–295, 1936.
41. LUDÁNY, G., F. FARKAS, AND A. INCZE. Antihistamine und die darmzottenbewegung. *Arch. Int. Pharmacodyn. Ther.* 83: 553–558, 1950.
42. LUDÁNY, G., T. GÁTI, J. RAUSCH, AND J. HIDEG. Ganglienblocker und darmzottenbewegung. *Arch. Int. Pharmacodyn. Ther.* 127: 402–409, 1960.
43. LUDÁNY, G., T. GÁTI, J. RIGÓ, AND H. SZABÓ. Substanz P und die darmzottenbewegung. *Pfluegers Arch.* 270: 499–503, 1960.
44. LUDÁNY, G., T. GÁTI, ST. SZABÓ, AND J. HIDEG. 5-Hydroxytryptamin (enteramin, serotonin) und die darmzottenbewegung. *Arch. Int. Pharmacodyn. Ther.* 118: 62–69, 1959.
45. LUDÁNY, G., M. IHÁSZ, AND J. KARIKA. Polypeptide (bradykinin, kallidin, eledoisin) und die darmzottenbewegung. *Acta Physiol. Hung.* 34: 85–93, 1968.
46. LUDÁNY, G., AND F. JOURDAN. Influences du pneumogastrique et du sympathique sur la motricité des villosités intestinalis. *C. R. Soc. Biol.* 119: 1189–1190, 1935.
47. LUDÁNY, G., AND F. JOURDAN. Die wirkung des vagus, splanchnikus und physiologischer sympatischer erregung auf die darmzottentätigkeit. *Arch. Int. Pharmacodyn. Ther.* 53: 281–287, 1936.
48. LUDÁNY, G., F. OBAL, AND A. SANTHA. Die wirkung des cholins und seiner derivate auf die darmzottenbewegung. *Arch. Int. Pharmacodyn. Ther.* 84: 328–336, 1950.
49. MAHLER, P., W. NONNENBRUCH, AND J. WEISER. Arbeiten über die physiologie und pathologie des dünndarms. I. Beiträge zur physiologie, pharmakologie und pathologie der dünndarmzotten beim hund und beim menschen. *Z. Gesamte Exp. Med.* 85: 71–81, 1932.
50. NANBA, R., AND S. HIRAMATSU. Effect of villikinin on the villus movements of the dog. *Acta Med. Okayama* 27: 91–101, 1973.
51. NANBA, R., S. HIRAMATSU, AND K. MORIMOTO. On the movements of the intestinal villi of the dog. *Jpn. J. Physiol.* 20: 465–471, 1970.
52. NÉMETH, E. P., M. IHÁSZ, G. FOLLY, AND M. PAPP. The action of secretin, trypsin and histamine on the motility of canine intestinal villi. *Am. J. Gastroenterol.* 60: 607–615, 1973.
53. PALAY, S. L., AND L. J. KARLIN. An electron microscopic study of the intestinal villus. I. The fasting animal. *J. Biophys. Biochem. Cytol.* 5: 363–372, 1959.
54. SESSIONS, J. T., JR., S. R. VIEGAS DE ANDRADE, AND E. KOKAS. Intestinal villi: form and motility in relation to function. In: *Progress in Gastroenterology*, edited by G. B. Jerzy Glass. New York: Grune & Stratton, 1968, p. 248–260.
55. SHEPHERD, A. P. Effect of elevated venous pressure on intestinal oxygen extraction. In: *Microcirculation*, edited by J. Grayson and W. Zingg. New York: Plenum, vol. 2, p. 92–93.
56. THOMPSON, A. B. R., AND J. M. DIETSCHY. Intestinal lipid absorption: major extracellular and intracellular events. In: *Physiology of the Gastrointestinal Tract*, edited by L. R. Johnson. New York: Raven, 1981, vol. 1, p. 1147–1220.
57. TRAUTMAN, A. Die muskulatur in den dünndarmzotten der haustiere. *Anat. Anz.* 34: 113–125, 1909.
58. TRIER, J. S., C. L. KRONE, AND M. H. SLEISINGER. Anatomy, embryology and developmental abnormalities of the small intestine and colon. In: *Gastrointestinal Disease: Pathophysiology, Diagnosis, Management*, edited by M. H. Sleisinger and J. S. Fordtran. Philadelphia: Saunders, 1983, p. 780–811.
59. VARRO, V., E. CSERNAY, E. SZARVAS, AND G. BLAHO. Effects of glucose and glycine solution on the circulation of the isolated loop in the dog. *Am. J. Dig. Dis.* 12: 60–64, 1967.
60. VERZAR, F., AND E. KOKAS. Die rolle der darmzotten bei der resorption. *Pfluegers Arch.* 217: 397–412, 1927.
61. VERZAR, F., AND E. J. MCDOUGALL. *Absorption from the Intestine.* New York: Hafner, 1967, p. 53–70.
62. WELLS, H. S., AND R. G. JOHNSON. The intestinal villi and their circulation in relation to absorption and secretion of fluid. *Am. J. Physiol.* 109: 387–402, 1934.
63. WOMACK, W. A. Villous Motility: Regulation and Function. Mobile: Univ. of South Alabama, 1987. PhD dissertation.
64. WOMACK, W. A., J. A. BARROWMAN, W. H. GRAHAM, J. N. BENOIT, P. R. KVIETYS, AND D. N. GRANGER. Quantitative assessment of villous motility. *Am. J. Physiol.* 252 (*Gastrointest. Liver Physiol.* 15): G250–G256, 1987.
65. WOMACK, W. A., P. K. TYGART, D. MAILMAN, P. R. KVIETYS, AND D. N. GRANGER. Villous motility: relationship to lymph flow and blood flow in the dog jejunum. *Gastroenterology*, in press.

CHAPTER 26

# Sphincteric function

MARIA PAPASOVA | Institute of Physiology, Bulgarian Academy of Sciences, Sofia, Bulgaria

CHAPTER CONTENTS

Upper Esophageal Sphincter
Lower Esophageal Sphincter
  Innervation
  Functional characteristics
  Basal tone
  Effect of neurotransmitters on lower esophageal sphincter tone
  Role of humoral and hormonal factors in lower esophageal sphincter regulation
    Prostaglandins
    Peptides
Pyloric Sphincter
  Anatomy and innervation
  Functional characteristics
  Regulation of pyloric sphincter
    Specific features of the smooth muscle
    Neural regulation
    Humoral regulation: peptides and prostaglandins
Ileocecal Sphincter
  Anatomy and innervation
  Functional characteristics
  Regulation of ileocecal sphincter
    Specific features of the smooth muscle
    Neural regulation
    Humoral regulation: peptides and prostaglandins
Anal Sphincter
  Anatomy and innervation
  Internal anal sphincter
    Functional characteristics
    Regulation of anal sphincter
Conclusion

SPHINCTERS PLAY A DEFINITE ROLE in the general functional organization of the gastrointestinal tract. As a rule, they are located between two specialized regions of the tract, preventing the reflux of the content and permitting its propulsion in the distal direction under definite conditions. Gastrointestinal sphincters are morphologically characterized by greater accumulation of the circularly located muscle cells in a definite region, the longitudinal muscle layer being represented to different degrees. There is unanimous opinion that the sphincters of the gastrointestinal tract should manifest definite functional properties: *1*) intraluminal pressure in the sphincter region during rest is always higher compared with the nonsphincter regions of the tract adjacent to it; *2*) in the case of suitable stimulation (inflation of a balloon) proximally to the sphincter, the latter relaxes, and the intraluminal pressure decreases; *3*) in the case of stimulation distal to a sphincter (inflation of a balloon), pressure in the sphincter increases as a result of its contraction (95, 159). The structural organization of the sphincters of the gastrointestinal tract is very diverse. Thus, while the upper esophageal sphincter and the external anal sphincter are formed by striated muscles, the lower esophageal sphincter (LES), the pyloric sphincter (PS), the ileocecal sphincter (ICS) and the internal anal sphincter (IAS) consist of smooth muscle cells, which are characteristic of the entire digestive tract. They are also innervated by vegetative nerves and by the enteric nervous system, which is essentially the same as in the nonsphincter regions of the tract.

Irrespective of the common criteria defining the characteristics of the gastrointestinal sphincters, each one of them has its own specific properties. Above all, a typical feature is the existence of synchrony in the functioning not only between a particular sphincter and its adjacent nonsphincter regions, but also among the different sphincters. Particularly indicative in this respect is the existing coordination between the upper esophageal sphincter (UES), the esophageal body, and the LES, which guarantees the passage of the bolus from the oral cavity through the esophagus into the stomach. At the same time, the LES hampers the reflux of the gastric content into the esophagus. This is the result of the permanent contraction of LES during rest, whereas the esophagus is relaxed. As a result, pressure in the LES zone during rest is higher than in the esophagus and fundus of the stomach (164). The first successful recordings of the LES responses during deglutition were obtained by Burget and Zeller (51). In experiments with dogs they demonstrated LES relaxation during swallowing and distension of the esophagus. Fyke et al. (178) demonstrated for the first time in human subjects the existence of a high-pressure zone between the esophagus and the stomach. Moreover, it has been demonstrated that inflation of the esophageal wall leads to reduced pressure in the sphincter (113, 164), whereas increased pressure in the stomach results in rapid rise of the intraluminal pressure in the sphincter region (113).

The functional state of the LES is of great significance for the correct course of the digestive processes, as well as for the prevention of a number of pathological states both in the digestive tract and in the entire organism. The main physiological function of the LES is to guarantee the transport of the bolus from the esophagus to the stomach and to prevent reflux of the gastric content. This is achieved by its functional state: the LES is closed between the act of swallowing, opens during swallowing, and thus guarantees free passage of the food (90, 139, 178, 193, 216). The functions of the LES as a sphincter have been investigated both experimentally in animals and in clinical practice. There were particularly animated discussions concerning the participation of adjacent structures as well in the closing of LES. However, the studies carried out have not justified the assumption that external compression of the caudal part of the esophagus is the reason for the closing of the sphincter (72, 78). This is supported by the fact that in the case of hernia hiatus, diaphragmatica reflux is observed only when the intrasphincter pressure is reduced (18, 94), as well as by the fact that the reduced intrasphincter pressure is not always accompanied by hernia hiatus diaphragmatica (289). The systematic studies carried out under different experimental setups (in vivo, in situ, and in vitro) give grounds for assuming that the increased pressure in the LES is the result of specific features of the smooth muscles that form the sphincter and that this activity is regulated and modulated by neural and humoral factors.

The question of whether the gastroduodenal junction complies with all criteria for a sphincter is disputable. Nevertheless, the term pyloric sphincter, referring to the gastroduodenal junction, has acquired an ever-growing popularity. Torgerson (384) pointed out that between the pyloric part of the stomach and the duodenum only 25% of the longitudinal muscle layer link these two segments of the gastrointestinal tract. A sulcus is clearly discernible macroscopically between the stomach and the duodenum. X-ray data on PS behavior are controversial. Some researchers claim that the PS is clearly defined radiologically, while others maintain that it is relaxed all the time. It should be taken into consideration that X-ray examinations are performed using contrast matter, which induces contractions when it enters the stomach, hence resulting in propulsion of the gastric content into the duodenum. It is also claimed that the activity of the PS is a component of antral peristalsis (257). On the basis of the existing correlation between the motility of the antrum and PS, the view is supported that the PS functions as a physiological sphincter (217, 307). This assertion is also supported by the fact that increased pressure in the stomach results in PS relaxation before the free hydrochloric acid has reached the necessary stimulatory concentration.

Electrophysiological findings show that PS activity may be triggered by impulses coming from the stomach and from the duodenum. Effect of the duodenum on PS activity is observed also in the case of enhanced duodenal activity occurring either spontaneously or after drug administration. The existence, on the one hand, of synchronous spike activity in PS and the antrum of the stomach is contradictory to the view that the gastroduodenal junction acts as an electrical insulator between the stomach and the duodenum (20). On the other hand, the propagation of the excitatory process from the stomach through the PS into the duodenum and back depends to a great extent on the functional state of the PS itself. The functional state of the duodenum is also very important—it should be at a definite level of excitability, so that the excitation process, which has reached it from the PS, would be able to induce the appearance of spike potentials or contractions, respectively. This evidently can explain the cases where spike activity is recorded from the antrum and PS, but it is not observed in the duodenum.

Regarding the sphincter situated between the lowest part of the ileum and the beginning of the colon, the so-called ileocecal sphincter (ICS), even Elliot in 1904 (153) stated the view that the system controlling the ileocecal junction differs from its adjacent regions. In his opinion, the junction was controlled by a muscle sphincter and not by a mechanical valve. Manometric tests have been used to identify a zone in the ileocecal region having higher intraluminal pressure compared with the adjacent nonsphincter regions (91). Indisputable facts have been obtained to support the view that the ICS regulates the antegrade movement of the ileal content and stops the retrograde movement from the colon (101). According to Alvarez (3), the ileocecal junction resembles in its function the gastroesophageal and especially the gastroduodenal junction, owing to the fact that it separates two adjacent parts of the gastrointestinal tract, which have different motor activities. Agreeing with this characterization, Johanson and Nylander (227) showed that the ileocecal junction guarantees unidirectional movement of the content from the terminal ileum to the colon.

The most distal part of the gastrointestinal tract ends with the IAS and the external anal sphincter. The IAS is a thickening of the most distal part of the circular muscle layer of the large intestine. Musculus sphincter ani externus, which builds up the external anal sphincter, consists of striated muscle and entirely envelops IAS. At the same time, IAS is surrounded by the puborectal part of the muscles of the pelvic fundus (181). This has prompted a number of authors to consider that the state of contraction of the internal and external anal sphincters is maintained and modulated to a great extent by the state of the abdominal pressure. A mechanism of sphincter relaxation in which rectal peristalsis, by increasing the intrarectal pressure, causes passive relaxation of the sphincter has also been proposed. This hypothesis, supported by Edwards (149), does not agree with later findings of a number of researchers. The constantly high pressure in the anal channel is assumed now to result from tonic contraction of the IAS (142, 144, 171). It is assumed that 85% of the pressure in the anal channel is due to the tonic contraction of IAS (172). The IAS is considered to be responsible for the retention of the anal content during rest. The IAS relaxation is observed on sudden stretching of the rectum (182, 183). This results in reduced pressure in the anal channel, whereby the external anal muscle contracts by neural reflex mechanisms. The inhibitory response of the IAS to stretching of the rectum is the result of the rectoanal inhibitory reflex.

The structural and functional relations between the internal and external anal sphincters and the accessory defecation muscles guarantee the effective emptying of the rectum (214). An important role in this complex coordination is attributed to the IAS, which is innervated by complex nerve pathways. The behavior of the anal channel, which results primarily from IAS activity, is the result of the fine balance between the motor and inhibitory mechanisms involved in its innervation.

Sphincter regions in the gastrointestinal tract are key units that guarantee coordination of motility of the different parts of the tract. The maintenance of the complex relations existing between the different sphincters and their adjacent regions, as well as among the sphincters, guarantees effective evacuation of the content from one part of the tract to another. This is the result of equally complex neurohumoral interactions. Intensive research is in progress with a view to revealing the mechanisms underlying the functions of the different sphincters in the gastrointestinal tract. Unfortunately, no generalized surveys on the matter are available. Thus LES physiology is discussed in a number of surveys and books dealing predominantly with the esophageal function (90, 91, 159, 193). Also discussed are PS physiology (150, 238), ICS physiology (298, 400), and IAS and external anal sphincters physiology (80, 362).

A relatively comprehensive discussion of the function of gastrointestinal sphincters is presented in the monograph by Papasova and Lolova (308), as well as in the published abstracts of the Symposium on Physiology and Pathology of the Sphincter Regions of the Digestive System (268), which was held in Tomsk, USSR in 1984.

## UPPER ESOPHAGEAL SPHINCTER

It is generally accepted that there is a high-pressure zone, 2–4 cm wide, between the pharynx and the esophagus. Nevertheless the UES has not been anatomically defined. The UES is believed to consist of cricopharyngeal muscle, which is striated muscle. It has been reported recently that the human esophageal wall is strongly thickened in its proximal part for ~25–30 mm. A characteristic finding is that this muscle thickening is higher in the posterior wall. This thickening is the result of the accumulation of bundles of circularly located muscle fibers. In dogs there is also thickening of the wall of the cranial part of the esophagus for a distance of 10–13 mm (24). The muscle fibers included in the cricopharyngeal muscle originate from the side of the cricoid cartilage, passing from one side to the other. The UES itself consists of cricoid cartilage anteriorly and cricopharyngeus posteriorly. The activity of the cricopharyngeal muscle is controlled by motor nerves whose cell bodies are in the nucleus ambiguus in the medulla. The activity of these neurons is coordinated by the activity of the trigeminal, facial, and hypoglossal nuclei. The mechanisms that determine and regulate the closing and the opening of the UES are not precisely known. There exists an opinion that the closing of the sphincter is passive and that it is the result of the orientation of the muscle fibers and the opening of the sphincter is thought to result from the action of other muscles in the larynx. Another view is that the cricopharyngeal muscle contracts tonically, while the relaxation itself results from the inhibition of the muscle activity (139). This is supported by the continuous spike activity that can be recorded from the cricopharyngeal muscle during rest (9). This occurs in parallel with the increased pressure recorded manometrically in the UES region (11). However, the fact that myotomy of the cricopharyngeal muscle in human subjects is followed only by partial reduction of the pressure in UES does not lend credibility to the assertion that only the cricopharyngeal muscle is responsible for the high pressure in the UES (215). A feasible theory is that the high resting pressure in the UES results from the contraction of the muscle, as well as from the elasticity of the tissues surrounding it (11, 139). Asoh and Goyal (10) found that only ~10 mmHg could be measured in the UES during rest, when muscle activity is totally inhibited. This suggests that these 10 mmHg are the result of passive elastic forces.

## LOWER ESOPHAGEAL SPHINCTER

### Innervation

The extrinsic nerves of the LES are of parasympathetic and sympathetic origin. Parasympathetic fibers originate from the dorsal motor nuclei of the vagus and reach the LES through the cervical vagus, where they join the enteric neurons (195). The sympathetic nerves of the LES originate from cell bodies localized in intermediolateral cell columns $Th_6$ to $Th_{10}$. After passing the greater curvature, their preganglionic axons are connected with the postganglionic nerves in the celiac ganglion. The postganglionic adrenergic fibers originating from the superior cervical and celiac ganglion form synapses with the cells of the myenteric plexus, as well as with the muscle cells.

The role of extrinsic nerves in the attainment of high intraluminal pressure in the LES as well as participation in its relaxation have been the object of many studies and observations. A detailed survey of the problem is presented by Roman and Gonella (343). The observed differences in the functional state of the esophageal body, which is relaxed during rest, and of the LES, which is contracted, are attributed to the neuromuscular specialization of this region (86, 196). It is found that the responses of LES to inflation of a balloon in the esophagus are not disturbed after uni- or bilateral vagotomy (96). The basal LES tone is not changed either (165). In dogs, both cervical and medial thoracic vagotomies reduce the pressure in LES (141, 319), as well as its relaxation induced by inflation of a balloon in the esophagus (96). However, low thoracic vagotomy does not change the sphincter relaxation (72, 96, 116, 264). Lower esophageal sphincter relaxation is observed when the peripheral end of the vagus is stimulated, whereas stimulation of the central end causes contraction (327). Differences are also observed in the responses of different parts of the LES to stimulation of the vagal nerve. The upper part of the LES is characterized by the biphasic response of relaxation, followed by contraction. The contraction occurs after switching off the stimulation. This effect is associated with the proximal part of the sphincter, which possesses smooth-muscle cells that are fundamentally the same as in the wall of the esophageal body (327). The rise in the LES tone during increasing gastric pressure and intense contractions of the gastric wall (88, 131, 275) involves vagal reflex pathways because this effect is reduced or entirely inhibited after vagotomy (131). Disappearance of LES relaxation during swallowing is observed when the vagal nerves are cooled at the cervical level (332). These data, as well as the fact that electrical stimulation of the cervical vagus produces LES relaxation in $93.5 \pm 2.5\%$ of the cases, suggest that vagal innervation is needed for the relaxation of the LES (96). The LES relaxation induced by esophageal stretch in dogs is entirely inhibited by vagosympathetic blockade.

Observations on human subjects after administration of atropine also point to the participation of the cholinergic innervation in the maintenance of resting pressure in the LES. In most cases pressure in the LES after atropine is reduced by 30%–55% (49, 136, 162). This is most probably due to species differences, because in cats atropine reduces the pressure in the LES by up to 60%, whereas no changes are observed in the opossum. In both species atropine antagonizes LES responses to bethanechol (167). After blocking of the adrenergic nerves, DiMarino and Cohen (134) have observed reduction of the resting tone of the LES by $22.5 \pm 5.3\%$ without change in the relaxation during swallowing. These data support the participation of cholinergic mechanisms in maintaining the tone in LES (395). However, after treatment with atropine, the LES still relaxes when the propagating muscle contraction reaches it, indicating that noncholinergic mechanisms are involved in the relaxation.

An important role for the vagal nerves on LES function is attributed to the mechanoreceptors present in the LES wall, namely 1) slowly adapting receptors, which are stimulated by stretching and contraction, and are localized in the muscle layers of the sphincter; 2) rapidly adapting receptors, which are activated only by strong stretching and are localized in the mucosa (270). This problem was further clarified by a very precise study carried out recently by Clerc and Mei (89). This work showed that the slowly adapting receptors located in the LES muscles act as sensors during the opening and closing of the sphincter. There are two types of mucosal receptors that are identified by touching and stretching. Their number is much greater in the esophagus than in other parts of the digestive tract. It is assumed that the role of the mucosal receptors is to inform the central nervous system about the type of food, whereas the muscle receptors inform about the mechanical tension in the wall. The mucosal receptors most probably interact with the muscle receptors during the closing of the sphincter after the passage of the bolus. A particular role is attributed to the mucous receptors in pathological states accompanied with vomiting (89).

Martinson's theory (261–263) is gaining more and more ground recently, namely that there are also nonadrenergic-noncholinergic inhibitory fibers in the cervical vagus, which are responsible for and regulation of LES relaxation (72, 137, 190, 195, 264).

Convincing evidence has also been obtained for the participation of the sympathetic nerves in maintaining the high pressure in LES, although there are species-specific differences here as well. Thus, stimulation of the splanchnic nerve increases the pressure in cat LES but decreases it in opossum LES (80, 167). Section of sympathetic nerves in the opossum does not change LES pressure (166). In intact cats, acetylcholine usually induces LES relaxation, although it may also cause contraction. The relaxation is not antagonized by atropine, it is not potentiated by physostigmine and it is unaffected by hexamethonium (88). (The mechanism of action of acetylcholine will be discussed later.) In cases where the sympathetic nerves are excitatory for the LES, Gonella et al. (191) stressed that sympathetic control over the LES takes place mainly through cholinergic myenteric neurons, which may produce contraction either directly or indirectly through suppression of the inhibitory intrinsic neurons. Contractions of the LES are also induced by stimulation of the perivascular nerves (29).

*Functional Characteristics*

Most researchers assume the existence of a sphincteric mechanism at the boundary between the stomach and the esophagus. However, Fyke et al. (178) were the first to demonstrate the existence of higher intraluminal pressure in the human gastroesophageal junction, compared with adjacent cavities. At the same time, these authors showed that when the pressure in the esophagus increases, the pressure in the sphincter dropped, that is, the sphincter relaxed. The sphincteric function of the gastrointestinal junction was demonstrated later by a number of other researchers as well (164, 216). Using manometric methods, it was demonstrated that the region localized in the most distal part of the esophagus, which is in a state of constant contraction during rest, is 3.07 ± 0.96 cm wide (88, 90). According to others, the zone with higher intraluminal pressure is only 1.2 ± 0.3 cm wide (359), while a third group reports it as 2.7 ± 0.96 cm (252). The zone with maximum intraluminal pressure is localized at a distance of 0.5 cm on both sides of the diaphragmatic hiatus (90, 178). The high-pressure zone has been found in dogs (355), cats (208), monkeys (410), and ruminants (374). The connection between the process of swallowing and the dynamics of the changes in the intrasphincter pressure in these animals are similar to those observed in human subjects. The high-pressure zone comprises a symmetrical region in the upper part of the sphincter. The pressure is higher in its lower part toward the greater curvature of the stomach (403). In the opossum, the high-pressure zone is 1–2 cm wide. According to some authors, the resting pressure does not exceed 50 mmHg (76), being 10 cmH₂O above the pressure in the fundus of the stomach (90), while according to others it is 12–30 mmHg (93, 342). It is difficult to understand the mechanisms underlying the sphincter function of this zone, since the microscopic-anatomical studies have not found specific structural differences. Only a thickening of the wall is found in many species, including humans. Liebermann-Meffert et al. (251) emphasized the existence of a gastroesophageal ring between the esophagus and fundus, resulting from a thickening of the muscles. In their opinion, this thickening was 3 cm wide on the side of the greater curvature of the stomach and 2.3 cm on the side of the lesser curvature. Although three muscle layers are present in the LES [longitudinal, circular, and muscularis mucosa (77)], there is unanimous opinion that the high pressure measured in the region of the gastroesophageal junction is the result of tonic contraction of the circularly situated muscle fibers in this zone (18, 72, 79). Moreover, slow changes in the pressure, having a frequency of 3–4 cycles/min, are also recorded (199) and are associated with the migrating motor complex (MMC) (219, 221). In addition to this, there are also mechanical changes reflecting respiration. The differences in the character of the changes in LES pressure result to a great extent from the kind of recording methods used. Important in this respect are the diameter of the catheter, the exact location of the tip of the catheter, and the depth of respiration. It is almost impossible to identify the LES radiographically, even by using radiopaque material. Relaxation and opening of the LES occurs as soon as the contrast matter is swallowed. However, LES may be identified radiographically in patients with achalasia and abnormal relaxation.

The increased intraluminal pressure in the LES zone is characteristic of the state of rest. The esophageal body is completely relaxed during rest, which is in contrast with the contracted LES. However, the LES relaxes during swallowing. Usually at the beginning of the act of swallowing both the UES and the LES are almost simultaneously opened. Relaxation of the LES is delayed by 2–3 s after the beginning of swallowing and it lasts 5–10 s. This is followed by a contraction of the upper part of the LES (aftercontraction). The aftercontraction is a continuation of the peristaltic wave of the esophageal body and it lasts 7–10 s. The lower part of the LES, however, is not affected by the aftercontraction and gradually the LES returns to resting level (193). The changes taking place in the LES during swallowing and rest are demonstrated by means of electrophysiological studies as well as intraluminal recordings. Chronically implanted electrodes in the LES region reveal two zones that correspond to the manometrically identified zones. During rest, when the sphincter is in a contracted state and increased intraluminal pressure is recorded by means of the manometric method, the electrical activity along the entire length of canine LES is characterized by continuous phasic spikelike activity with a frequency of 1.5–2 cycles/s. At the beginning of swallowing, the electrical activity disappears synchronously with the decrease of the pressure in the LES (8). Anesthesia seems to influence the electrical activity of the LES, because in the anesthetized opossum, interrupted spike activity is recorded from the LES, with or without phasic variations, with a frequency of 20–50 cycles/min and duration 81.2 ± 8.9 ms. When there are spike potentials, the pressure in the LES is higher (10, 265). Correlation is established between interdigestive phasic contraction and LES activity (130, 219; Fig. 1). In human subjects, LES contractions appear during the second and third phases of the gastric interdigestive motor complex and minimally during the first phase. No episodes of gastroesophageal reflux are observed as a result of increased intragastric pressure during interdigestive gastric contractions (130).

*Basal Tone*

The high intraluminal pressure characteristic of the resting state is to a great extent the result of the

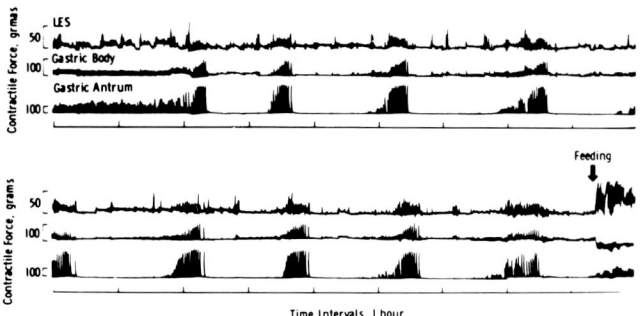

FIG. 1. Changes (18 h) in contractile activity in lower esophageal sphincter and stomach. *Arrow*, feeding. Note significant differences in contractile pattern before and after feeding. In interdigestive state, simultaneous occurrence of contractile episodes are observed at regular intervals. [From Itoh et al. (221).]

specific features of the smooth muscle building up the sphincter (78). Because of this, a basal tone develops in the LES region and is constantly modulated by the nervous system as well as by various humoral and hormonal factors. In the literature, there are many and varied definitions of tone, as well as different opinions about its nature. Relatively very popular is the view that tone is a manifestation of active contraction of the smooth muscle cells and may be characterized as an economic contraction depending on the concentration of intracellular $Ca^{2+}$ and on conservation of energy (290, 348). Because the degree of activation of the contractile proteins depends on the concentration of $Ca^{2+}$, this will determine the level of tone. Depending on whether or not the increased tone is accompanied by action potentials, Rüegg (348) distinguishes two types of tone: *1*) tetanic tone (tonus tetanus), whereby the contraction is associated with the generation of action potentials by the smooth-muscle cells, and *2*) nontetanic tone, which is not connected with action potentials.

Spike potentials in dog LES are recorded only during aftercontraction occurring after the relaxation of the sphincter (8, 206, 276). On the other hand, LES relaxation is not accompanied by changes in the low-amplitude spike activity observed by Thomas and Earlam (378). Although there are data in the literature that continuous spike activity may be observed in opossum, the increase or decrease of the pressure in the sphincter is not always related to changes in the spike activity (11). Asoh and Goyal (10) emphasized that only ~25% of the LES tone of opossum is spike dependent, whereas the spike potential independent component is 55%–75%. Tone that is not connected with spike potentials is also recorded in the LES of cat, opossum, monkey, and human subjects (122, 206, 283, 309). Spontaneous tone is observed in smooth muscle preparations isolated from LES (196), which is not connected with the generation of spike potentials. Furthermore, depolarization of the cell membrane without spike potentials is observed even under the effect of the neurotransmitter's acetylcholine and noradrenaline (122, 190, 191, 310). Under conditions of current clamp, smooth muscle preparations of cat LES have been found to maintain a very well manifested spikefree tone. A linear dependence exists between the degree of depolarization and the degree of tonic tension of the muscle (303, 308, 310). Moreover, in the case of depolarizing current there is a gradual change in the membrane potential, without generation of spike potentials. This shows that the excitability of the sphincter smooth-muscle cells is lower compared with the smooth-muscle cells in the nonsphincter parts of the tract. This is also supported by the fact that under the effect of tetraethylammonium, which is known to inhibit the fast and slow outward $K^+$-currents and to increase the permeability of the cell membrane for $Ca^{2+}$ (202), under conditions of current clamp, the LES smooth muscle responds with phasic contractions. In this case each contraction is preceded by slow depolarization of the cell membrane on which spike potentials are superimposed [Fig. 2; (308)].

The spontaneous tone observed in LES depends on the extracellular $Ca^{2+}$ (165, 305). A direct relationship is observed between LES tone and $Ca^{2+}$ concentration in the extracellular medium. Moreover, tone is abolished by the $Ca^{2+}$ antagonist lanthanum, in concentrations known to inhibit the transmembrane passage of the ions through the cell membrane (391). The fact that $Ca^{2+}$ antagonists of the verapamil-nifedipine group, and especially sodium nitroprusside, influence the basal LES tone both in vivo and in vitro (129, 168, 199, 211, 225, 310, 402), suggests that the basal LES tone is determined by two components: one sensitive to $Ca^{2+}$ antagonists from the verapamil group and

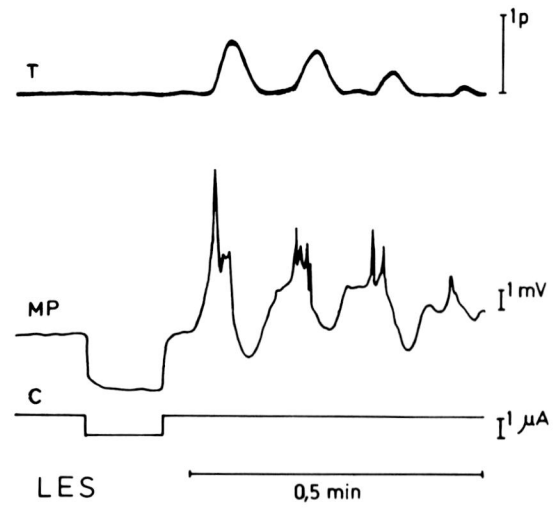

FIG. 2. Increased lower esophageal sphincter (LES) excitability produced by tetraethylammonium (TEA). Effect of inward current. T, tension; MP, membrane potential; C, current. TEA, 5 mmol/l. Recording made by sucrose gap method. [From Papasova and Lolova (308).]

another one sensitive to sodium nitroprusside (308). Both components are eliminated by lanthanum (43). In this connection the question arises about the character of the membrane processes that control entry of $Ca^{2+}$ in the muscle cells forming the LES. In muscle preparations of cat and dog LES it has been demonstrated that outward current injection results in reversible inhibition of the basal tone, which is linearly dependent on the degree of hyperpolarization of the cell membrane (43). These results raise the problem of the dependence of the basal tone of the LES on the membrane potential. It should be borne in mind that the resting potential of the smooth muscle cells forming the LES of opossum is −40 mV (122), while it is −48.5 ± 1.4 mV in cat LES (305). This is lower than the membrane potential of the smooth muscle cells forming the regions adjacent to the LES. The low values of the resting membrane potential of the LES could explain the increased $Ca^{2+}$ conductance in the smooth muscles responsible for the higher tone of the LES muscles (122, 284). Obviously, however, the low potential is not the only reason for the high tone characterizing the LES smooth muscle, because the gradual depolarization of the smooth muscle from the antrum of the stomach leads only to generation of spike potentials and phasic contractions connected with them, whereas the smooth muscle of cat LES responds by a gradual rise in tone (43, 301, 310). The concomitant depolarization, however, does not reach the threshold value needed for the generation of spike potentials. A linear dependence exists between the changes in the tone and the membrane potential over a large range of the voltage-tension curve (Fig. 3). However, in the case of pretreatment of the LES smooth muscle with $Ba^{2+}$ (0.2–0.6 mM) or $Sr^{2+}$, the switching on of depolarizing current and the switching off of hyperpolarizing current result in depolarization on which spike potentials are superimposed. Each group of spike potentials appears on the top of an additional depolarization and precedes a phasic contraction of the muscle. After several stimulations, spontaneous groups of spike potentials appear in a definite rhythm, leading to phasic contractions. These contractions last through the entire period during which the preparation is in the nutrient solution containing $Ba^{2+}$ or $Sr^{2+}$, respectively. The $Ba^{2+}$- and $Sr^{2+}$-induced spike potentials in LES are antagonized by verapamil and D 600. These divalent ions most probably use $Ca^{2+}$-conductance channels, as has been observed in the myometrium (122). The appearance of spike potentials should be associated with the increased inward current and with the fact that it reaches suprathreshold value (398). The fact that neither spike potentials nor phasic contractions are observed spontaneously in the LES smooth muscle suggests the existence of special interrelations of the fast $Ca^{2+}$-dependent inward current and the outward $K^+$ current. This could be explained by the early activa-

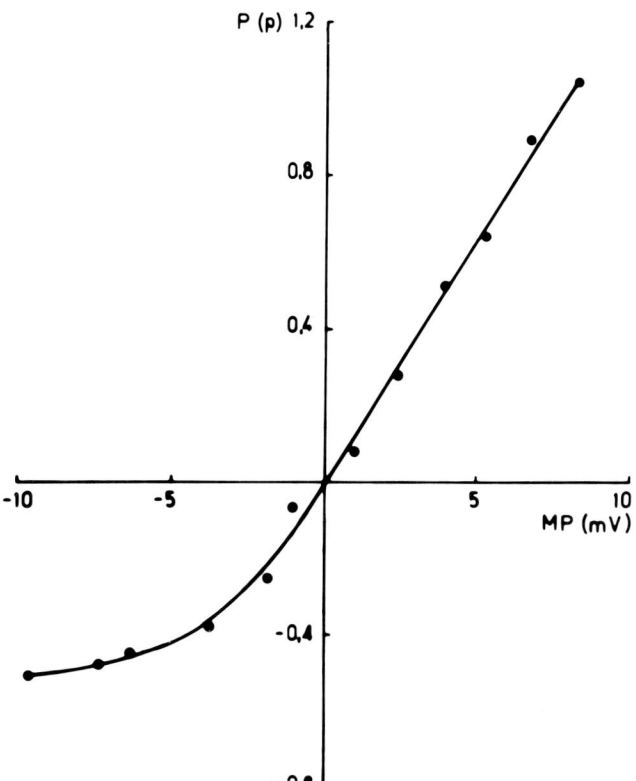

FIG. 3. Dependence between the changes in the tone (P) and membrane potential (MP) of lower esophageal sphincter. Recording made by a sucrose-gap method. [From Papasova and Lolova (308).]

tion of the fast outward current, observed first by Bury and Boev (64) in fundic smooth muscle and later by Milusheva and Bury (274) in the smooth muscle of guinea pig LES, using voltage clamp. Inactivation of the fast inward $Ca^{2+}$ current occurs most probably as a result of early activation of the fast outward $K^+$ current, and this is why spike potentials are not observed spontaneously in the smooth muscle forming the fundus of the stomach and the LES. Regional differences are established in the intracellular $K^+$ concentration in the LES smooth muscle, compared with the esophageal muscle: in the esophagus the $K^+$ concentration is 50 ± 3 meq/kg, in LES it is 38 ± 3 meq/kg, whereas the $Na^+$ concentration is identical (358). The correlation between intra- and extracellular $K^+$ in LES could also explain the specific responses observed in LES in the case of increased extracellular $K^+$. A biphasic response is observed both with respect to the membrane potential and with respect to the contractile process: fast hyperpolarization followed by depolarization precede the relaxation and the contraction of the smooth muscle of cat LES, as well as increased $K^+$ concentration in the nutrient solution. These responses of the LES are not affected by atropine, by adrenoceptor blocking agents or tetrodotoxin (TTX), but they turn into depolarization and contraction after treatment with ouabain. It is assumed that the $Na^+$-$K^+$ pump in the LES smooth muscle functions at a different level of activity compared with the other smooth muscles of the digestive tract (302, 309).Unlike some tonic blood vessels for which it has been shown that prolonged tonic contraction is caused by the functioning of the $Na^+$-$Ca^{2+}$ exchange mechanism (292–294), in the LES smooth muscle a $Na^+$-$Ca^{2+}$ exchange mechanism operates only under extreme conditions and to an insignificant extent (43).

The steep force-length curve (40, 82, 86) also suggests a certain specificity in the organization of the LES smooth muscle. In addition to the specific myogenic properties of the LES smooth muscle, which contribute to the basal tone, LES innervation is also of indisputable significance. It is found that in LES of cats and dogs TTX does not influence (43) and in some cases it may even activate the tone of the sphincter (43, 81). The stimulating effect of TTX could be explained with the existence of noncholinergic-nonadrenergic inhibitory innervation which prevails in the circular muscles of the digestive tract (411).

*Effect of Neurotransmitters on Lower Esophageal Sphincter Tone*

The intrinsic nervous system plays an important role in the total organization and regulation of the digestive tract. The myenteric plexus in the esophagus is well developed, although the submucous plexus is rather scanty (78, 79). However, nerve varicosities in the LES are much more numerous compared with those in the esophageal body of opossum (365) and cat (256). At the same time it is pointed out that there is no difference in the type of varicosities found in the esophageal body and in the LES (365). It is also reported that the density of the smallest dense-core vesicles known to contain norepinephrine (341) is higher in the LES, compared with the adjacent nonsphincter regions. This is in agreement with light microscopic data on the increased number of nerve cells and fibers in the LES (255). Noncholinergic-nonadrenergic innervation plays an essential role in the regulation of the function of gastrointestinal sphincters, the LES included (60). This coincides with the view of Christensen et al. (83) about internal specialization in the innervation of the LES of cat, monkey, and opossum. Muscle strips isolated from the LES demonstrate clearly defined responses to transmural electrical stimulation. Lower esophageal sphincter strips always respond by relaxation and strips from the esophageal body respond by contraction when switching off the stimulation, whereas stomach strips respond by contraction, which lasts during the stimulation (83, 86). The most frequently used terms for the responses observed during electrical stimulation are *on-response* when the stimulation is switched on and *off-response* when it is switched off. The on-response of the LES to stimulation is relaxation (83). This response of the LES is very specific and it is observed only for 1–2 muscle strips. The muscle strips located proximally and distally produce a biphasic response. In proximal strips the on-response is relaxation, whereas the off-response is contraction; in the distal strips, switching on the stimulation leads to contraction and switching off leads to relaxation (Fig. 4). The biphasic response obtained in this case reflects smooth muscle characteristics for the LES and the esophageal body or the LES and stomach in the muscle strip (83). It is proposed to identify the muscle strips of the terminal esophagus as the LES if they respond to electrical stimulation with relaxation (52, 393). Relaxation of the LES during electrical stimulation increases in amplitude when increasing the frequency of the stimulus. For cat LES it reaches maximum at a frequency of 6 Hz (308), whereas in opossum LES the maximum frequency is 5 Hz (119). The amplitude of the relaxation increases in parallel with the increasing duration of the impul-

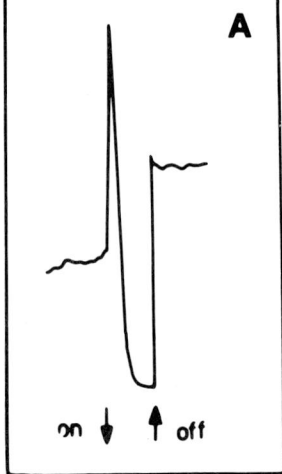
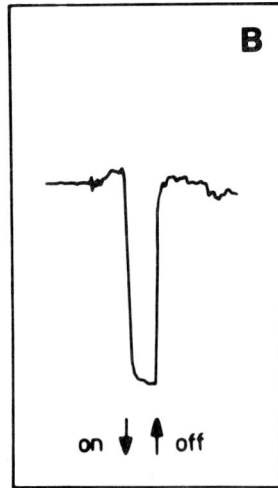
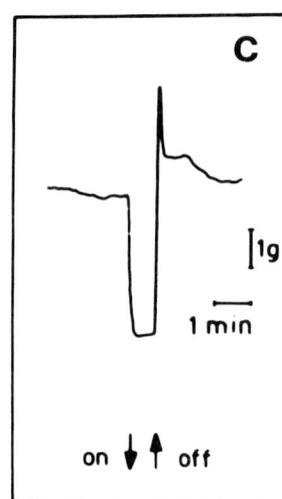

FIG. 4. Response of lower esophageal sphincter (LES) to electrical field stimulation (0.2 ms; 2 Hz; supramaximal current) depending on the place of removal. *A*: removal distally from *B*; *B*: removal from the middle of LES; and *C*: removal proximally from *B*. *Down arrows*, beginning of stimulation; *up arrows*, end of stimulation. [From Velkova et al. (392).]

ses. The differences are significant for impulse durations up to 0.5 ms, after which there are no significant differences in the 0.6–0.9 ms range.

The latency of the off-response of the LES varies exponentially with the temperature of the medium, while the amplitude of the relaxation varies only slightly, deviating sharply in the 20°C–27°C range (127). The nerve structures that produce the LES relaxation are poorly sensitive to changes in the extracellular concentrations of $Ca^{2+}$ and $Mg^{2+}$ (79, 126). Relaxation of the LES does not disappear at $Ca^{2+} = 0$, but it is not observed in the presence of ethylenediaminetetraacetic acid. The off-response of the LES during electrical stimulation occurs as a result of the release of sequestered $Ca^{2+}$ because of the preceding depolarization, and not as a result of the direct influx of $Ca^{2+}$, because it is not affected by verapamil and nifedipin (225). The inhibitory intrinsic neurons in LES manifest slight fatiguability. Relaxation of the LES induced by field electrical stimulation is TTX sensitive (120, 305, 359), but it is not influenced by atropine, phentolamine, or propranolol (305). The preparations taken from cats pretreated with reserpine or 6-OHDA also respond by relaxation to field stimulation. The nonspecific purinergic antagonist quinidine (63) entirely inhibits the electrically induced LES relaxation (155).

Although the identity of the neurotransmitter of the noncholinergic-nonadrenergic innervation is unknown, there is no doubt that the relaxation of LES is mediated by such a transmitter (86, 122, 195, 308, 385). The opinion that ATP is a possible inhibitory neurotransmitter (61, 62) is opposed by the argument that nucleotides are released by various cells as a nonspecific or common agent during processes connected with activation. Some authors consider ATP to be a nonspecific agent accompanying the processes of activation in the cells, rather than a specific, noncholinergic-nonadrenergic inhibitory neurotransmitter (42, 67).

The generally accepted view concerning the activating effect of the parasympathetic neurotransmitter acetylcholine and the inhibitory effect of the adrenergic neurotransmitter norepinephrine on the motility of the gastrointestinal tract proved to be completely invalid with respect to LES. Snape and Cohen (372) stress the existence of excitatory cholinergic receptors and cholinergic nerve fibers in the LES. Data on the effect of acetylcholine on the LES are rather contradictory. It is pointed out that in intact cats acetylcholine usually induces relaxation of the LES, although contraction may also be observed (88, 353). On the other hand, cholinoceptor blocking agents reduce the basal tone of the LES (259). The extremely high sensitivity of the LES smooth muscle to acetylcholine, methacholine, bethanechol, and carbachol, which induce contraction of opossum LES, is emphasized (85, 157). This is associated with the relatively higher concentration of cholinergic receptors in this region of the digestive tract (77). Moreover, in addition to $M_1$ and $M_2$, cholinergic receptors associated with LES relaxation are also present (186). Biphasic effects of acetylcholine are observed in cat LES, depending on the concentration. The threshold concentration of $10^{-11}$ g/ml leads to contraction. Acetylcholine-induced contractions of LES are inhibited by nifedipine (189). Marked relaxation occurs in concentrations above $10^{-6}$–$10^{-5}$ g/ml (155, 392, 393). At the same time, circular strips isolated from the smooth muscle part of the esophagus respond by contraction, irrespective of the concentration. These changes depend on the membrane potential: depolarization precedes the contraction induced by low acetylcholine concentrations. At acetylcholine concentration exceeding $10^{-5}$ g/ml, there is brief depolarization followed by hyperpolarization. These changes in the membrane potential correlate with biphasic contractile response (Fig. 5). The contractile component is not observed when the cholinoceptor antagonist atropine is present, whereas the relaxation is inhibited by $\beta$-adrenoceptor antagonists. Preparations of LES isolated from cats pretreated with reserpine or 6-hydroxydopamine (6-OHDA) respond to acetylcholine only with contraction, irrespective of the concentration (392). Relaxation of the LES occurring under the effect of acetylcholine may be explained in the light of the cholinergic link hypothesis of Burn (57, 58) and Burn and Rand (59). It may also be explained with observations of increased norepinephrine release in the presence of acetylcholine (169). Moreover, it is reported that in smooth muscle preparations of human LES in the presence of hyoscine, the contractile responses to acetylcholine are transformed into relaxation (52). Controversial data are reported about the effects of the adrenergic neurotransmitters. Intravenous injection of epinephrine may stimulate the LES (88), whereas norepinephrine induces spike-dependent contractions (344). It has

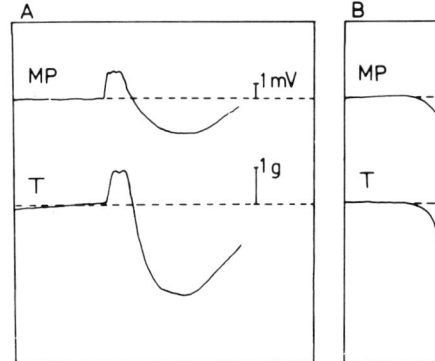
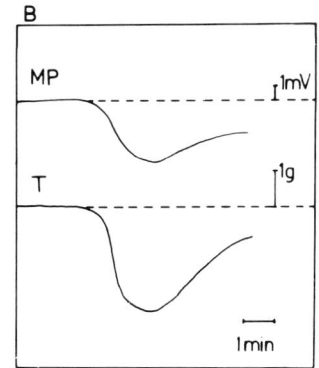

FIG. 5. Relationship between changes in membrane potential (MP) and lower esophageal sphincter pressure in response to acetylcholine (ACh). T, tension. A: ACh $10^{-5}$ g/cm$^3$; B: ACh 15 min after treatment with atropine $10^{-5}$ g/cm$^3$. [From Velkova et al. (392).]

also been found that in vivo the α-adrenergic receptors of opossum are related to the increase of pressure in the LES, while β-adrenergic receptors lead to its reduction (134, 280). However, all studies on LES smooth muscle preparations, irrespective of the species, manifest excitatory effects of epinephrine and norepinephrine that are antagonized by α-adrenoceptor agents (52, 84, 87, 92, 154, 191). The β-adrenergic postsynaptic receptors in the LES are responsible for its relaxation (191, 392). Pharmacophysiological analysis has shown that the α-adrenergic receptors are localized within the LES smooth muscle itself, as well as in the postganglionic neurons, whereas the β-adrenergic receptors are in the sphincteric smooth muscle (198). It is assumed that the excitatory effects of norepinephrine take place mainly through cholinergic mechanisms (191, 192) by means of α-adrenergic receptors on the postganglionic cholinergic terminals (197). Irrespective of the clearly manifested excitatory effect of norepinephrine on LES preparations, it is considered that the physiological role of the sympathetic LES innervation has not been clarified (198). This is apparent from the fact that the basal tone of LES decreases by only 20% when animals are treated with 6-OHDA, while at the same time LES function goes undisturbed. Adrenergic innervation probably only modulates LES contractile activity (198).

Dopamine, one of the norepinephrine precursors, decreases pressure in the LES and increases pressure in the distal part of the esophagus (34, 220, 329, 340). Dopamine induces relaxation of the smooth-muscle preparations, which is antagonized by the specific dopamine antagonists: haloperidol and bulbocapnine (125, 138), but it is not eliminated by TTX. Dopamine receptors are assumed to be localized on the sphincteric muscle itself, because dopamine antagonists do not affect the LES relaxation induced by electrical field stimulation (124, 328). Relaxation of the LES by acetylcholine, involvement of α-adrenergic receptors, as well as the fact that LES relaxation induced by electrical field stimulation or increases in acetylcholine applications on the background of atropine, suggest the existence of complex neurotransmitter relations at the level of the smooth muscle of the LES. These relations are most probably triggered at definite functional states of the sphincter and are involved in the coordination of activity in the LES and the nonsphincteric regions located proximally and distally.

*Role of Humoral and Hormonal Factors in Lower Esophageal Sphincter Regulation*

PROSTAGLANDINS. Biologically active peptides and prostaglandins (PG) play an important role in the modulation and regulation of gastrointestinal motility. Recently published monographs and surveys can be referred to (42, 205, 242, 300, 350, 396). Although there are no specialized structures synthesizing PG and there are no specialized structures for their accumulation, their role for the regulation of a number of functions in the organism is indisputable. Acting as local hormones, also known as autopharmacological agents or autocoids, PG achieve their effect acting directly on the smooth muscle cells (32, 33, 231, 232, 314, 351). There is a generally accepted view of Hedquist (205) about the existence of a PG-mediated feedback-regulation mechanism responsible for the release of norepinephrine by the nerve terminals at the level of the smooth muscles. It is also believed that PG influence the nerve terminal by increasing the permeability for $Ca^{2+}$ and thereby releasing norepinephrine from the synaptic vesicles (404). Convincing data have been reported recently on the modulating effect of PG on cholinergic transmission (203, 204, 226, 229, 286, 314). Acetylcholine release is increased by PG predominantly from group E (31, 151, 324, 325, 357). On the basis of the relations between adrenergic and cholinergic transmission established by Paton and Vizi (313) and Kadleč et al. (229, 230) assume that the effect of PG on cholinergic transmission is indirect: primary inhibition of the norepinephrine release by PG results in increased acetylcholine release by the cholinergic nerve terminals. Regarding the effect of PG on the noncholinergic-nonadrenergic transmission, the data are very scanty and disputable (118, 305). With respect to the LES there is a view that endogenous PG are necessary for maintaining the higher tone characteristic of this sphincter (121, 393). Under in vivo and in vitro conditions, the prostaglandin synthetase inhibitor indomethacin reduces the LES tone in opossum (118), cats, and dogs (43). However, indomethacin does not influence LES relaxation induced by inflation of a balloon localized proximally from the sphincter but does affect LES contraction after deflation of the balloon (121). Species differences are implied in this case, because increase in LES tone after treatment with indomethacin has been observed in human subjects (50). This is in contradiction to the dose-dependent rise in pressure in human LES on infusion of $PGF_{2\alpha}$, reported by Dilawari et al. (133). At the same time, $PGE_1$ does not affect pressure in the sphincter, but it inhibits its responses to pentagastrin. It has been reported that the $PGE_1$-induced decrease of pressure in human LES is greater in the case of venous compared with arterial infusion (370).

With respect to $PGF_{2\alpha}$, Rattan et al. (331) reported three types of changes in opossum LES, namely: in 77% of the cases the response consisted of a rise of the sphincter pressure, in 15% the pressure decreased, and in 8% the response was biphasic. The degree of relaxation of opossum LES under the effect of $PGE_1$ is dose dependent (194, 200). In smooth muscle strips of cat LES, both $PGE_1$ and $PGF_{2\alpha}$ induce a gradual reduction of the LES tone, the maximum being observed on the second minute after treatment. Species differences have also been observed with respect to the effect of the various prostaglandins: in opossum LES, $PGF_{2\alpha}$ always induces contraction, whereas the effect of $PGE_1$ is inconsistent (118).

Noncholinergic-nonadrenergic inhibitory innervation is known to be very well manifested in the sphincteric parts of the digestive tract (60, 176). In the precise work of Daniel et al. (118) it is emphasized that although there is no direct evidence, PG are expected to play an essential role in the release of the noncholinergic-nonadrenergic neurotransmitter. Proof of this must wait until the identity of the neurotransmitter of noncholinergic-nonadrenergic nerves is determined. Some evidence has been obtained supporting a role of PG in the modulation of the release of neurotransmitters from noncholinergic-nonadrenergic nerve terminals. In LES preparations of cats, $PGF_{2\alpha}$ and $PGE_1$ reduce the amplitude of the muscle relaxation induced by electrical field stimulation (Fig. 6). At the same time, a rise in tone is observed. The processes related to the release of the neurotransmitter are much more sensitive to $PGE_1$, because maximum effect is observed from the first minute after the treatment. Thus the inhibition of both on- and off-responses to PG is more pronounced at a stimulus frequency of 2 Hz compared with the effects of stimulation at 5 Hz. The effects of $PGF_{2\alpha}$ and $PGE_1$ are not influenced by adrenergic and cholinergic antagonists. On the background of TTX, however, both $PGF_{2\alpha}$ and $PGE_1$ induce only changes in the tone of the preparation. These data are in support of the assumption made by Daniel et al. (118) that PG influence noncholinergic-nonadrenergic neurotransmission as well. Evidently, PG have not only a direct myogenic effect on the LES smooth muscle, but they also affect the release of the neurotransmitter by the nerve terminals. This is also supported by the ultrastructural changes observed in the intrinsic nerve tissue of LES after treatment with PG (308).

PEPTIDES. Convincing experimental data were obtained during the past decade in support of a modulating role of peptides on the release of neurotransmitters. The particular importance of peptides for the regulation of the intake, digestion, and resorption of the food is well established. However, there is only fragmentary evidence about the effect of specific peptides on the motility of the gastrointestinal tract. This makes it impossible to work out a unifying theory for the role of peptides in this important function of the digestive tract. Data on the participation of peptides in the regulation and modulation of the functions of gastrointestinal sphincters are even fewer and more scanty. Problems related to the effect of peptides on the secretion and motility of the gastrointestinal tract have been presented systematically in the surveys of Papasova and Atanassova (300), Klimov (242), Walsh (396) and Klimov et al. (244).

In view of the significance of the problem, we will review data obtained so far on the effect of peptides on the function of gastrointestinal sphincters, as well as in the coordination of the activity of the sphincters and the nonsphincteric regions adjacent to them. Gastrin and its derivatives are known to induce increased frequency of the pacesetter potentials from the stomach (218, 237, 260), as well as increased percentage of bursts of spike potential groups, that is, disturbance of the MMC (401, 409). This corresponds to the intensified motor function of the stomach, observed after injection of pentagastrin (105, 243), as well as weakening of the duodenal contractile activity (242). At the same time, gastrin I and pentagastrin increase the pressure in the LES (75, 187, 224, 253, 278). Based on the fact that the pressure in the LES increases after infusion of pentagastrin, some authors believe that gastrin is responsible for maintaining high pressure in the LES (74, 75). Such a claim is not sufficiently substantiated in view of the series of other factors pointed out above, which regulate and modulate the pressure in the LES (375). Moreover, it is pointed out that the interaction of gastrin and secretin perhaps determines the sphincter tone during swallowing (97, 399). Pentagastrin has been shown not only to increase the pressure in human LES but also to produce gastrointestinal reflux (315). The effect of gastrin and of its derivatives on LES is explained by release of acetylcholine from cholinergic neurons (125, 253, 295). This is also supported by the fact that there is no correlation between the serum gastrin level and the pressure in the LES.

Cholecystokinin (CCK) has different effects on the various smooth muscles in different parts of the gastrointestinal tract. Whereas CCK manifests an excit-

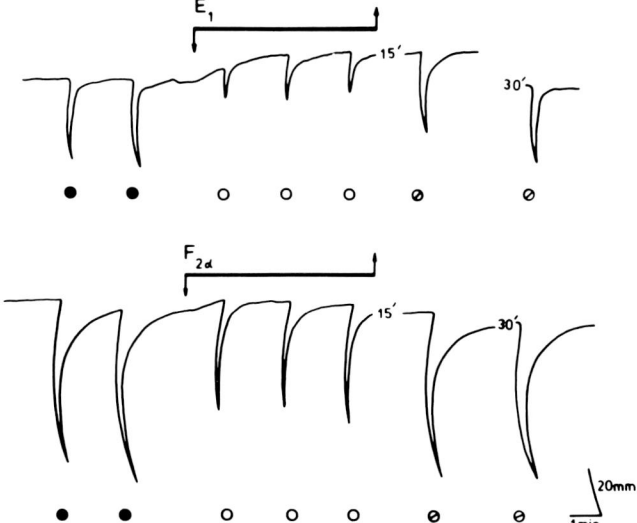

FIG. 6. Effect of PG on the response of lower esophageal sphincter smooth muscle strips to electrical field stimulation (0.2 ms; 2 Hz; supramaximal current) before (●) and after (○) treatment with PG; and after (⊘) washout. Duration of PG treatment is 5 min. [From Papasova and Lolova (308).]

atory effect on isolated smooth muscle preparations from cat and guinea pig fundus (99, 188), the effect on LES preparations is inhibitory (160, 335). Relaxation is observed in human subjects as well (26, 336), whereas in patients with achalasia the effect is excitatory: contraction of the sphincter is observed (135). On the other hand, in the opossum, CCK applied in a dose that evokes relaxation in other species leads to contraction. This pressor effect of CCK is only slightly influenced by TTX (128), whereas the inhibitory effect of CCK on human LES is antagonized by TTX and is transformed into contraction. This is evidence that CCK stimulates the postganglionic inhibitory neurons (26).

Motilin is another of the gastrointestinal peptides that causes LES contraction (249). During the interdigestive state exogenous motilin does not have a significant effect on LES pressure. However, a close correlation is observed between the motilin level in the plasma and the behavior of the sphincter. During the digestive state the plasma motilin level is 35 pg/ml, whereas during the interdigestive state it is 291 ± 96.5 pg/ml, remaining at this level for 20 min and then rapidly decreasing (2). Because atropine blocks the stimulating effect of motilin on the LES, its effect is considered to be due to increased acetylcholine release from the cholinergic nerve terminals (271). It also seems that motilin participates in the synchronization of the LES and stomach activities as the bolus is propelled from the esophagus to the stomach.

Evidence for an essential role for endogenous opioids in gastrointestinal motility is accumulating. The existence of enkephalin-containing interneurons in human and cat LES has been demonstrated (286), while opioid receptors have been identified in opossum LES on the smooth muscle cells themselves and on the myenteric plexus (329). There is evidence that opioids are involved in the LES relaxation (213, 223).

No quantitative differences have been found in the quantity and distribution of vasoactive intestinal peptide (VIP), as determined by specific immunoassay and immunochemistry in the LES and in the adjacent nonsphincteric regions (266). The VIP causes dose-dependent decreases in LES pressure (28, 38, 108, 230, 369). The effect of VIP does not change after treatment with atropine, phentolamine, haloperidol, pyrilamine, methysergide, indomethacin, and TTX, which is in support of the assumed direct action of the peptide on the smooth muscle cells of LES (330). The high doses of Pitressin (8-arginine vasopressin) administered venously predispose toward gastroesophageal reflux soon after the infusion (397).

Bombesin increases LES pressure (338). Intravenous infusion of bombesin in human subjects raises the level of serum gastrin, as well as the pressure in the LES. No correlation is established between the level of serum gastrin and pancreatic polypeptide and the effect of bombesin on LES pressure (107). This effect is assumed to be due to direct influence on the LES smooth muscle cells, as well as indirectly through the postganglionic neurons releasing norepinephrine (285).

Substance P induces a dose-dependent rise in LES pressure and is assumed to be a very important regulator of LES pressure (1). It is also believed that the involvement of substance P as neurotransmitter occurs through a spike-associated enteric neural reflex (340). Somatostatin does not influence LES pressure (36), but it plays a role in the responses of LES to other stimuli (65, 66). It is reported that in normal human subjects somatostatin infusion results in considerable reduction of serum gastrin (201).

The mechanisms determining the effect of peptides on LES activity have not been sufficiently elucidated. Above all, an astonishing fact is that the same peptide has different effects on the sphincter and on its adjacent nonsphincteric regions, because no essential quantitative differences are found with respect to the distribution of the cholinergic, adrenergic nerve terminals and the noncholinergic-nonadrenergic nerve terminals in these parts of the digestive tract (255). Bearing in mind that their effects are to a great extent the result of the modulated release of neurotransmitters, further studies will be necessary in order to reveal the mechanisms of the peptide effects on LES activity.

## PYLORIC SPHINCTER

In spite of the intensive research carried out over the past ten years with the aim of specifying the role of the gastroduodenal junction as a sphincter, there is still no unanimity on the problem as to whether the gastroduodenal junction is a real sphincter. Views on this matter prior to 1968 may be found in the previous edition of the *Handbook of Physiology* on the alimentary canal (150). Modern views on the problem have been presented by Kelly (238) and Papasova and Lolova (308). Nevertheless, a number of problems related to the real sphincter function of the gastroduodenal junction remain unclarified. Based on the specific properties of the gastroduodenal junction and the smooth muscle forming it, we shall use the term *pyloric sphincter* (PS) in this chapter.

### Anatomy and Innervation

The PS is located at the end of the pyloric canal and it is demonstrated as a thickening of the circular muscle layer. Horton (212) described the histological ordering of muscle cells in the PS region. Emphasizing the existence of a connective-tissue barrier—septum—between the stomach and the duodenum, this author has pointed out that in spite of this, part of the longitudinal muscle layer passes above the septum from the stomach to the duodenum. The majority of the longitudinal muscle fibers pass into the transversely located muscle fibers immediately above the septum. It was specified later that only one-quarter of the longitudinal muscle fibers on the side of the lesser curvature pass into the duodenum (384).

The septum, which divides the PS from the duodenum, is considered to consist of connective-tissue barriers extending from the peritoneum to the mucosa (123). However, this tissue does not prevent part of the longitudinal muscle fibers from passing through the barrier to the duodenum. The PS is identified relatively easily in opossum and cat, because a mucous fold is formed immediately above the septum (the fibrous ring) proximal to the thickening of the circular muscle layer. Such a fold does not exist in humans and dogs (6). The PS itself, that is, the thickening of the circular muscle layer, is 3–5 mm wide in the species mentioned. Both sympathetic and parasympathetic nerves innervate PS. Parasympathetic innervation is provided by the nerve branch originating from the ramification of the anterior trunk of the vagal nerves, which go to the liver as the hepatic branch (210). This branch is parallel to the gastroduodenal artery and, before it supplies the PS, it forms branches that project to the head of the pancreas and the proximal duodenum (267).

Sympathetic innervation of the PS, as well as of the stomach and duodenum, is derived entirely by the celiac plexus. The processes originating from the celiac plexus are grouped in the major and minor splanchnic nerves. The intrinsic nervous system of the PS is a continuation of the enteric nervous system in the distal part of the stomach. A characteristic finding is that the ganglion cells in the myenterix plexus (in humans, monkeys, rabbits, guinea pigs, cats, and rats) increase in number in the distal direction along the length of the stomach, reach maximum value in the region of the gastroduodenal junction, and begin to decrease in the distal direction along the duodenum (326). This suggests that specialized activity occurs in this region, although many problems concerning the nervous mechanisms of control of the PS have not been clarified.

*Functional Characteristics*

The sphincteric function of the PS is a disputable matter. One of the fundamental requirements for sphincter function presupposes the existence of a zone with higher luminal pressure compared with the adjacent nonsphincteric regions. In this respect results for the PS are controversial, with two prevailing opinions. One group of researchers reported that it was not possible to record higher pressure in the PS region, therefore they assumed that it was not a real sphincter. It has also been reported that the sphincter is relaxed during rest, and this is supported by endoscopic studies (5, 233, 257). After discovering a high-pressure zone in the region of the gastroduodenal junction, another group of researchers suggested that this was a true sphincter that most probably functioned to prevent reflux of the duodenal content into the stomach (27, 37, 158, 217, 367). The high-pressure zone is not wider than 3–5 mm (338, 405), which corresponds to the microscopically determined dimensions of the PS (6). Pressure in the region of human PS is found to be of the order of $10.2 \pm 1.2$ mmHg (389). The claim that a high-pressure zone exists in the region of the PS is also supported by observations of reflux of biliary acids from the duodenum in cases where reduced sphincteric tone occurs. This results in gastritis and gastric ulcer disease (390). A high-pressure zone has been described both in humans (158, 390) and in dogs (48). Moreover, it has been found that the pressure differs depending on the exact site of insertion of the catheter. When measured by a catheter introduced through the duodenum, it is $8.9 \pm 1.8$ cmH$_2$O and $14.8 \pm 0.9$ cmH$_2$O if the catheter is inserted through the stomach. On the basis of systematic studies on human subjects, Fisher and Cohen (158) concluded that the views of authors who claim that the PS does not possess all properties characteristic of a sphincter should be challenged. Above all, according to them, the sphincteric ring at the end of the gastric antrum is very narrow and therefore it is very difficult to determine the difference in pressure using a balloon or catheter. On the other hand, convincing evidence has been obtained that the administration of hydrochloric acid, olive oil, or hypertonic amino acids in the duodenum leads to increased pressure in PS (48, 106, 158, 217, 389). Increased pressure in the PS in the case of acidification of human and animal duodenum was reported in 1907 by Cannon (68), who stressed that this resulted in delayed evacuation of the gastric content. The amplitude and the frequency of spike potentials generated in the PS region increase when the pressure increases. This response is antagonized by TTX or naloxone (339). It is assumed that this response involves local nerve pathways and opioid receptors (339). Contraction of the PS is also observed in response to mechanical pressure or distension of the duodenum (21, 48, 158). This is in agreement with the closing of the PS observed in human subjects during spontaneous independent contractions of the duodenum (156) and more specifically of the duodenal bulb. This is the reason why regurgitation into the stomach is never observed in normal subjects. In dyspeptic patients and in the case of gastric ulcers this mechanism is disturbed, and regurgitation is a frequent symptom (345). It has been stressed that the PS is not solely a constrictor sphincter but a valve that closes when distended (373).

A justification for disputing the sphincteric function of the gastroduodenal junction is provided by the fact that pacesetter potentials are recorded from the PS region, their frequency being identical to that recorded from the antral part of the stomach, whereby slow waves may be recorded sometimes with the rhythm of slow waves of the duodenum (45, 175). Even Alvarez and Mahoney (4), in 1922, assumed the existence of electrical activity in the gastroduodenal junction when they recorded slow waves in the duodenum with a frequency characteristic of the antrum. It was established later that the electrical activity propagates from the antrum through the PS into the duodenum along electrotonic pathways (117, 175). Electrical activity with frequency of the antral pacesetter potentials has been recorded in human subjects as well (143). On the other hand, Bass et al. (19) did not succeed in recording electrical activity from the anterior wall of canine gastroduodenal junction, which they interpreted as evidence that this zone acts as electrical insulator between the stomach and the duodenum. Such a claim is unjustified, because an electrical link was found not only between the pacesetter potentials of the stomach and the PS on the one hand, but also between the PS and the duodenum on the other (Fig. 7). Furthermore, correlation is observed between the spike activity of the stomach, PS, and duodenum. When their frequency and amplitude are increased, they propagate into the PS but they do not reach the duodenum (Fig. 8). This shows that propagation of the electrical activity is blocked in the PS because of the low excitability of the duodenum (175). When excitation in the stomach is sufficiently high, it will result in the involve-

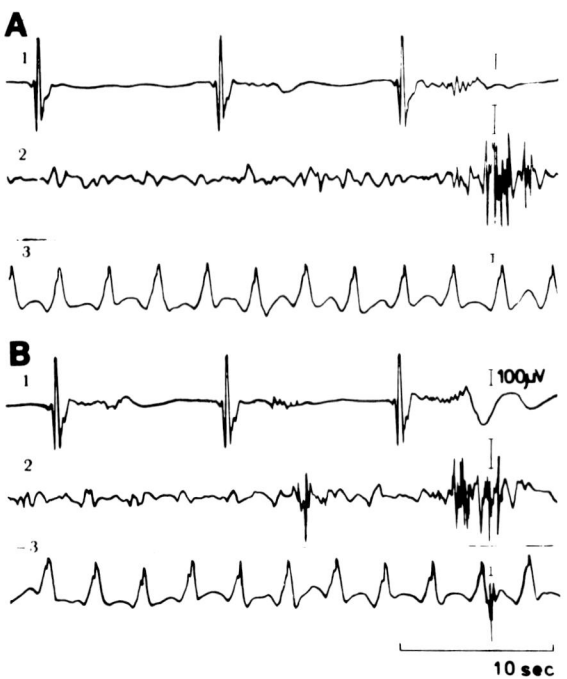

FIG. 8. Coupling between spike activity of stomach and pyloric sphincter (PS). A: spike potentials from stomach spread only in PS; B: spike activity occurs successively in stomach, PS, and duodenum. Designations: 1: electrode implanted in stomach wall; 2: electrode implanted in PS; 3: electrode implanted in duodenum. [From Papasova and Lolova (308).]

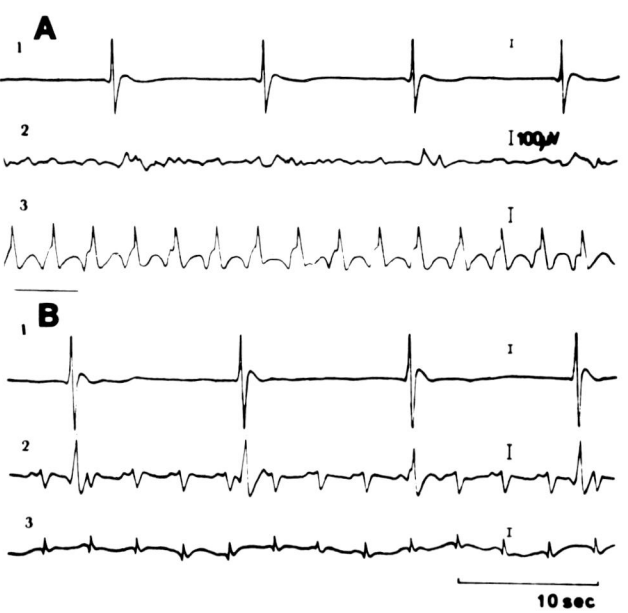

FIG. 7. Coordination between the electrical activity of stomach, pyloric sphincter (PS), and duodenum. A: pacesetter potentials typical of stomach are recorded simultaneously from PS; B: pacesetter potentials typical both of stomach and duodenum are recorded simultaneously from PS. Designations: 1: electrode implanted in stomach wall; 2: electrode implanted in PS; 3: electrode implanted in duodenum. [From Papasova and Lolova (308).]

ment of the duodenum as well, that is, it will lead to the appearance of spike potentials and duodenal contractions. All these observations are consistent with the view that the PS is a transit zone (44) responsible for the electrotonic connection between the stomach and the duodenum (175).

The sequence in the appearance of spike activity in the antrum of the stomach, PS, and duodenum is related to propulsion of the luminal content. Surgical removal of the PS results in lasting disturbances in the coordination between the electrical junction of the stomach and duodenum (12, 14, 387). Moreover, the intrinsic nervous system is essential for achieving coordination between the electrical activities of the stomach and duodenum (13, 15). Horton (212) found that the enteric nervous system was in continuity from the stomach through the PS to the duodenum. When the stomach is transected at the level of incisura angularis and the passage is restored after Billroth II surgery by means of gastrojejunal anastomosis, the removed antral part of the stomach together with the PS manifest electrical activity different from that of the stomach included in the anastomosis. The existence of coordination between the electrical activity of the stomach, PS, and duodenum is often observed with respect to MMC as well.

There is a sequence at the onset of the different MMC phases that occur first in the stomach, then in the PS, and only afterwards in the duodenum (16, 17, 307). Such a coordination between the electrical activity of the antrum, PS, and duodenum is described in the remarkable work of Carlson et al. (70). Using cineradiography, these authors found that the PS contracts almost always with the antrum of the stomach. Two types of waves were differentiated: *1*) ring-like contractions starting from the cardia and reaching the sphincter itself, which were related to propulsion of a small amount of luminal content; and *2*) waves that also start in the cardia, but when these reach the incisura angularis the antrum and the PS suddenly contract. This closure of the PS results in reflux of the luminal content back into the gastric body. At the same time, before the sphincter closes, part of the content is propelled into the duodenum (70).

The PS appears to function in unity with the antral part of the stomach in order to achieve organized emptying of the stomach (228, 241, 320, 367). The PS is considered to play an important role in regulation of the emptying process (25, 233). Removal of the PS affects particularly the evacuation of solid food. This is contrary to the views of Louckes et al. (257), who believe that the PS plays a small role in the regulation of the gastric function. According to these authors, its function consists of prevention of reflux of duodenal content and prevention of mass evacuation of the stomach. In dogs, PS contractions start 1.5 ± 1.4 s after the onset of the contraction of the terminal antrum (152). The movement of the content through the PS is determined by three factors: *1*) driving force, *2*) pressure gradient in the duodenum, and *3*) PS resistance. Evacuation of the content occurs when the pressure in the stomach is higher than that of the duodenum. When the pressure in the duodenum is higher, the PS contracts and prevents reflux of the duodenal content. However, in the case of very high pressure in the duodenum, it is possible for the activity of the sphincter to be coordinated with that of the duodenum, a result of which is that contraction of the PS is in synchrony with the duodenum.

Several minutes after injection of morphine in dogs, intense spike activity is observed, starting in the duodenum, then in the PS, and later in the stomach. Spike potentials in the PS appear in the rhythm of the slow waves characteristic of the duodenum. This antiperistaltic type of propagation of the electrical activity very often precedes vomiting. However, in a state of rest the PS has its own physiological function defined by the high pressure developing in its region, which prevents reflux of the duodenal content into the stomach (367). This is supported by the fact that the PS of starved animals contracts and relaxes with a frequency of 4–6 cycles/min for 2–10 min, after which a state of rest is observed (257) (studies using the inductographic method). These findings correspond to the observed MMC dynamics in the PS (307). The fact that PS preparations contract or generate slow potentials with a frequency of 1 cycle/min in vitro (189, 305) is not contrary to the view of functional unity between the antral part of the stomach and PS. Evidently, the smooth muscle of the PS has its own frequency of slow-potentials generation. The PS may also function in situ as a distinct organ with specific control mechanisms (258).

In the intact organism, the peristaltic wave propagating aborally along the stomach leads to involvement of the PS in the rhythm of generation of pacesetter potentials characteristic of the antrum of the stomach. This makes it possible for the PS to act in unity with the gastric antrum during the process of stomach emptying. However, when the stomach is empty, the PS has its own physiological function, defined by the development of high pressure in its region and preventions of reflux of duodenal content into the stomach (367). This is evidence that the PS manifests its own specific function, different from that of the stomach, irrespective of the coordination between the activity of the antrum and the PS (278, 307, 361).

## Regulation of Pyloric Sphincter

SPECIFIC FEATURES OF THE SMOOTH MUSCLE. Myogenic factors play an important role in the regulation of the gastroduodenal junction. The smooth muscle of the PS of cats and dogs generates slow potentials (in vitro) with a frequency of 1 cycle/min (305), on which spike potentials are superimposed. This change in membrane potential (MP) is followed by contractions. In a medium with $Ca^{2+} = 0$, both the electrical and the contractile activities of the PS are abolished. On gradual increase of the $Ca^{2+}$ concentration in the nutrient solution, maximum changes in the tone of the preparations occur at $Ca^{2+} = 1.5$ mM, and after that concentration the tone decreases sharply. In accordance with the view that extracellular $Ca^{2+}$ carries inward current during the depolarization phase of the spike potential (104), it may be assumed that this inward current is very active in the smooth muscle of the PS, as a result of which maximum contraction is achieved at a relatively low concentration of extracellular $Ca^{2+}$. This is also supported by the fact that tetraethylammonium (TEA) acts at almost ten times lower concentration than the effective concentration for other smooth muscles. Complete blockade occurs at TEA concentration of 0.1–0.3 mM.

Both the spike potentials and the contractions of the PS are $Ca^{2+}$ dependent, because they are not observed after administration of $Ca^{2+}$ antagonists (308). In this respect the smooth muscle of the PS differs from the smooth muscle building up the antral part of the stomach, where 20 mM TEA induce spike potentials with maximum amplitude (377). It is also necessary to point out the higher sensitivity of the PS to bivalent ions ($Ba^{2+}$, $Sr^{2+}$) compared with the sensitivity of the antral smooth muscle. The smooth muscle of the PS manifests specific functions, different from those of the antral muscle. Strips of PS develop higher tension when stretched, as well as higher resistance to stretching (6). The existence of slowly adapting tension receptors in the PS has been reported (41, 110, 269).

NEURAL REGULATION. The vagal and the sympathetic nerves are the motor nerves of the PS. Sympathetic stimulation inhibits the contractions of the antrum and the PS. Reduction of the transpyloric flow is observed (148) to the extent of complete discontinuation (250). The same changes are also observed in the case of infusion of norepinephrine. The vagal nerves innervating the cat PS include both excitatory and inhibitory fibers. The vagovagal excitatory reflex in the PS together with vagovagal relaxation response of the stomach (146) is evoked by stimulation of afferent vagal nerves. The existence of inhibitory nerve fibers in the vagus innervating PS is demonstrated clearly after application of atropine. In the presence of atropine, efferent vagal stimulation causes inhibition of the spontaneous pyloric activity in dogs and this suggests atropine-resistant inhibitory innervation (277).

In intact animals bilateral transthoracic vagotomy leads to changes in the electrical activity of the PS, which are synchronous with those of the antral part of the stomach. The characteristic tachygastria is observed both in the antrum and in the PS in the first 2 wk after the vagotomy (307). This is evidence in support of the view that the PS coordinates its activity with the antrum of the stomach, thus guaranteeing effective evacuation of the gastric content. The intrinsic nervous system occupies an important position in this coordination.

Electron-microscopic studies demonstrate a much higher percentage of purinergic varicosities in the PS, as well as a higher density of dense-core vesicles as compared with the adjacent nonsphincteric regions (255). This is in agreement with the in vitro studies in which electrical field stimulation induces inhibition of the phasic contractions and relaxation of the sphincter, whereas muscle preparations isolated from the antrum and duodenum respond to electrical field stimulation with contractions [Fig. 9; (6, 306)]. According to Schulze et al. (360), muscle from the human pylorus differs from muscle of the antrum and the duodenum by its high base-line tension, its prominent neurogenic relaxation response, and its low level of spontaneous contractile activity.

The amplitude of PS relaxation in the case of field stimulation depends on the frequency of the impulses (Fig. 10). Maximum responses are obtained in the 4–6 Hz range, while the duration of the relaxation reaches its maximum between 16 and 18 Hz. After administration of propranolol, phentolamine, and

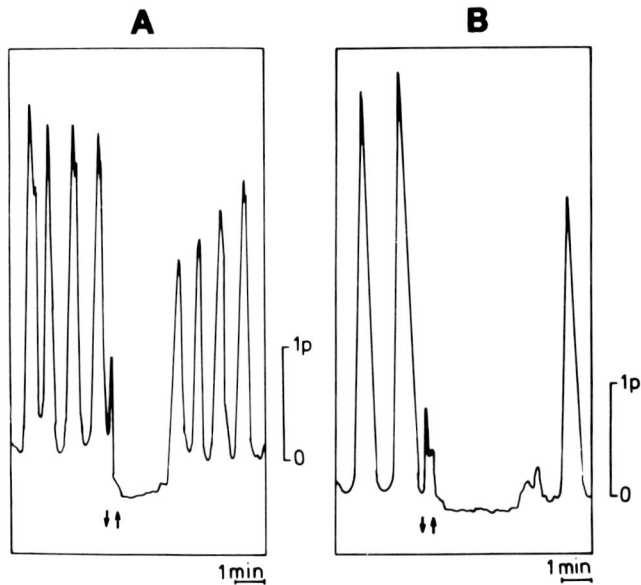

FIG. 9. Effect of frequency of stimulations on pyloric sphincter. $A$: at low frequency (0.5 ms; 2 Hz; supramaximal current); $B$: at high frequency (12 Hz). *Down arrows*, beginning of stimulation; *up arrows*, end of stimulation. [From Papasova et al. (306).]

atropine, the amplitude of PS relaxation during field electrical stimulation increases considerably, especially in the 4–6 Hz range, whereas the duration of the relaxation decreases. Relaxation of the PS in the case of electrical field stimulation is not observed after TTX (306). These observations reveal the PS as a region with marked noncholinergic-nonadrenergic inhibitory innervation, as in LES. In all probability, involvement of the noncholinergic-nonadrenergic inhibitory mechanisms guarantees fast PS relaxation, which ensures evacuation of the gastric content.

HUMORAL REGULATION: PEPTIDES AND PROSTAGLANDINS. Data on the effect of peptides on PS activity are still scanty and very contradictory. Cholecystokinin raises the base-line pressure and increases the frequency of the phasic contractions while decreasing their amplitude in isolated preparations from rat PS (354). Both CCK and secretin stimulate the contractions of smooth muscle preparations isolated from human and opossum PS (158, 161). However, CCK has no effect on canine PS (188). Considerable increase in PS pressure induced by CCK in vivo in human subjects and animals was also reported (217, 412). Whereas the CCK effect on the tonic contraction of the rat PS is mediated through noncholinergic-nonadrenergic pathways, the effect on the phasic contractions is myogenic (354). Substance P increases the tone and the phasic contractions of human and canine PS, this stimulating effect being more pronounced in canine PS (258) as well as in cat PS (147).

Identical effects of bombesin are observed, whereas

secretin, CCK, motilin, and gastric inhibitory polypeptide have no substantial effect (258). While secretin significantly increases the PS pressure in vivo (35, 316), caerulein induces delayed gastric evacuation, due to pylorospasm (376). Local intra-arterial injection of Leu- and Met-encephalin causes contraction of the PS and gastric relaxation in cats. These effects are naloxone sensitive (148). Gastric inhibitory polypeptide results in fast PS dilatation (145). Pressure in PS increases in the case of insulin-induced hypoglycemia as well (317). $PGE_1$ and $PGE_{2\alpha}$ inhibit the contractile activity of PS (188), as well as the spontaneously generated electrical activity (279). This effect is not entirely antagonized by TTX. However, $PGE_1$ and $PGE_{2\alpha}$ totally inhibit the response of PS to transmural electrical stimulation and the spontaneous tone decreases to below the control level [Fig. 11; (393)]. These changes are not observed after application of TTX. It is assumed that PG influence the nonadrenergic-noncholinergic mechanisms of regulation in PS. This is supported by the ultrastructural changes observed in cat PS after treatment with PG (308).

## ILEOCECAL SPHINCTER

### Anatomy and Innervation

The type of connection between the small intestine and the colon manifests a great variety for the different species. In humans, as well as in cats, the terminal part of the ileum intrudes into the colon, so that the muscles of colon ascendens surround it. In dogs, however, the cecum and the ileum are independently connected with the colon. This takes place by means of the ileocolic orifice and the cecocolic orifice. In humans, as well as in cats, a valve (valvula ileococolica or valvula Bauchini) is formed from the mucosa at the site where the ileum joins the colon (288). This has caused a number of researchers to consider for a long time that the ileocecal junction functions on the principle of a valve mechanism. It has been found, however, that the circular muscle layer is strongly thickened at the junction. In humans, the ileocecal sphincter is 4 cm wide (207), in cats it is $1.36 \pm 0.05$ cm on the average (347). Both clinical and experimental studies characterize the ileocecal junction as a sphincter. On the other hand, the term ileocecal sphincter or ileocolic sphincter is used in the literature to denote the ileocecal junction. In this chapter the term ileocecal sphincter (ICS) will be used because of its greater popularity.

Innervation of the ICS is provided by vagal nerves and by sympathetic fibers originating from the superior and inferior mesenteric ganglia. It is characteristic that a nerve plexus from the superior mesenteric ganglia accompanies the ileoceliac artery and penetrates and branches with the artery in the terminal part of the ileum, cecum, appendix, and ICS (272).

The intrinsic nervous system in the ICS region is in direct continuity with the terminal ileum and proximal large bowel. However, it is interesting to note that the innervation of the sphincter is considerably

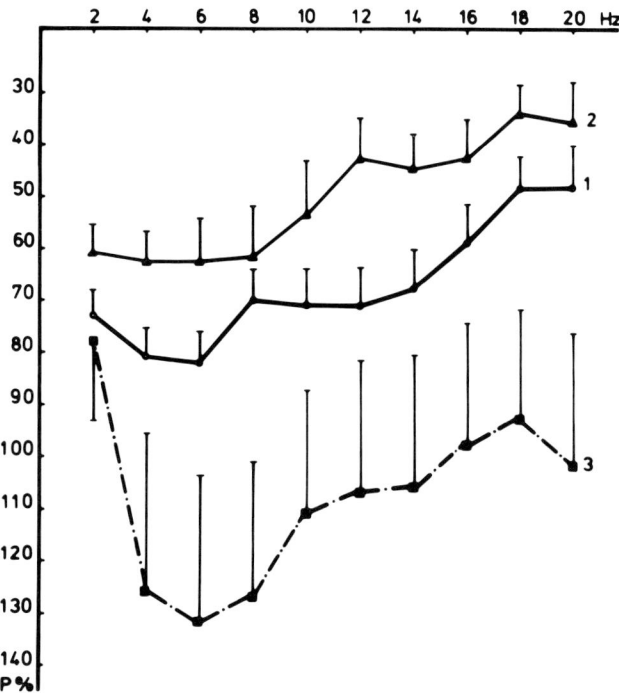

FIG. 10. Dependence of pyloric sphincter relaxation (%) on frequency of electrical field stimulation. Relaxation is expressed in percentage to maximal response ($n = 10$). Designations: *1*: control; *2*: after atropine $10^{-6}$ g/cm$^3$; *3*: after atropine $10^{-6}$ g/cm$^3$, phenoxybenzamine $10^{-5}$ g/cm$^3$, and propranolol $10^{-5}$ g/cm$^3$. [From Papasova et al. (306).]

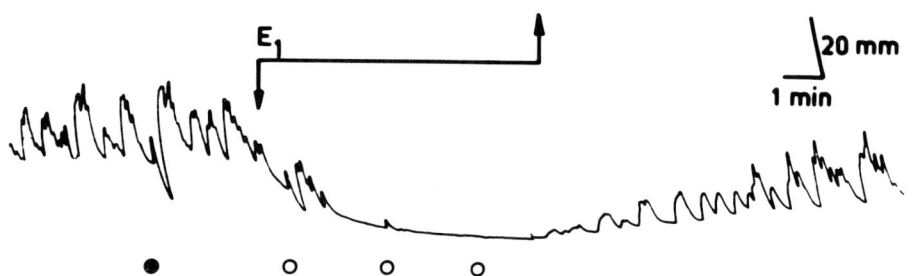

FIG. 11. Effect of prostaglandin (PGE$_1$) on pyloric sphincter smooth-muscle strips to electrical field stimulation (0.2 ms; 2 Hz; supramaximal current) before (●) and after (○) treatment with PGE. Duration of treatment is 5 min. [From Papasova and Lolova (308).]

more dense in the sphincter than in orally and aborally adjacent regions (177, 308). A characteristic finding is that each ganglion of the myenteric plexus contains a greater number of neurons (up to 50). One should also note the great variety and abundance of ganglionic cells in the ileocecal region, with the largest ganglia being located at the base of the sphincter (272). In addition, there are also pseudounipolar neurons, which are identical in their structure to the spinal neurons (245).

*Functional Characteristics*

There is no doubt that in the region of the ileocecal junction the intraluminal pressure is higher compared with the pressure in the ileum and colon located proximally and distally to it. Both in humans and in a number of experimental animals the ICS is found to be closed most of the time, that is, it is in a state of tonic contraction (33, 227, 235). An average resting pressure of 20.3 mmHg is registered in human subjects by means of a perfusion catheter (95), the resting pressure in cats being $12 \pm 0.9$ mmHg (291) and in dogs $66 \pm 2.2$ cmH$_2$O, measured using balloon manometry (236). The increased pressure in the region of the ileocecal junction delays the passage of the content, thus contributing to mucosal absorption in the small intestine (234), at the same time preventing the reflux of the content of the large intestine, which is rich in bacteria (371). Two mechanisms are assumed in connection with the ICS function: namely, a pure valve mechanism that prevents the reflux of the content to the terminal ileum (163) and a sphincter mechanism (184).

The fact that during administration of an enema the ICS is capable of preventing the passage of the content from the large bowel, irrespective of the increased pressure, makes impossible the assumption of a valve mechanism (296). Regarding the question about the extent to which the ICS serves as regulator of the passage of the content from the terminal ileum into the colon, the importance of the pressure difference on both sides of the sphincter is indisputable. Other researchers believe that the combination of the contractions of the terminal ileum and the resistance offered by the ICS to the chyme flow is essential for the passage of intestinal content. At the same time, however, the ICS serves as a barrier and prevents the reflux of content from the colon (400). When the ICS is surgically removed, this mechanism is disturbed and reflux of large intestinal content into the ileum is often observed (371).

Inverse correlations are established between the activity of the ileum and ICS on the one hand and between the colon and ICS on the other. Increasing the pressure in the ileum results in relaxation of the sphincter, whereas increasing the pressure in the colon leads to higher pressure in the ICS (95, 234, 235, 236).

However, while distension of the ileum is paralleled by ICS relaxation in 80% of the cases, distension of the colon produces contraction of the sphincter in 60% of the cases (236). The ileocecal sphincter reflex is a spinal reflex with efferent fibers localized in the major splanchnic and lumbar colonic nerves (297).

Food intake increases the activity of the terminal ileum (102, 103, 207). This is followed by ICS relaxation, which favors the passage of the content to the colon. This is also confirmed by the character of the electrical activity in the ileocecal region. The increase in the slow waves with spike potentials in the ileum after food intake is followed by the appearance of spike potentials in the colon (407, 408). Whereas in dogs the intraluminal pressure in the ICS during fasting has been measured to be $31 \pm 18$ cmH$_2$O, the postprandial pressure decreases to $24 \pm 18$ cmH$_2$O (323). A definite correlation is observed between the LES and ICS during food intake, namely: the pressure in both sphincters decreases and thus the food passes from the esophagus to the stomach, and the content of the small intestine passes into the colon (73).

Considerable difficulties occur in determining the relation between the cyclic motor changes taking place in the gastrointestinal tract, especially in the human ileum and colon, and the functional state in the ICS. Usually this relation is reported to be variable (239). Thus it has been found that in human subjects only 10% of MMCs reach the ICS. This correlates with the observations on the motility of the ileocecal region. It was reported for human subjects that ileal peristalsis reaches the ICS only 1–2 times in 24 h; consequently, the sphincter was relaxed and the ileal content was propelled into the colon only twice a day (321). In dogs 92% of all spike bursts of phase III of the MMC propagate as far as the ICS and 86% pass through the ICS into the proximal colon (322). Probably this is largely the result of methodological difficulties. In this respect it has been found that in dogs most interdigestive myoelectrical complexes propagate to the ICS. During the MMC, the intraluminal pressure in the ICS manifests phasic changes with average frequency of 12 cycles/min for 72% of the time in fasting animals, whereas after feeding this activity increases to 81%. It should be noted that the pressure in the ICS is more pronounced during phase III of the MMC (323).

The ICS differs functionally from the remaining gastrointestinal sphincters. As a rule, the higher pressure distal to the sphincter may result in its opening and passage of the content in the oral direction. Such interactions may be observed both in the PS and in the LES. Thus in the case of functional disturbances there is frequent reflux of duodenal content into the stomach. In this respect the ICS plays the role of complete isolator, which is manifested by the fact that spike activity from the terminal part of the ileum propagates to the colon, whereas the opposite is never observed [Fig. 12; (311, 408)]. In the case of ascending propagation of the excitatory process from the colon, the ICS contracts and stops the passage of the content into the ileum. In muscle strips comprising part of the ileum (the ICS and cecum) isolated from the longitudinal axis of the ileocecal region of the cat, electrical stimulation in the ileal region leads to inhibition of the spontaneous electrical and contractile activity of the cecum. Switching off of the stimulation is followed by a compensatory rise in the frequency and amplitude of the spike potentials, as well as of the associated contractions. No changes in the character of the electrical and contractile activity of the colon are observed during stimulation of the region adjacent to the cecum. Moreover, noncholinergic-nonadrenergic inhibitory mechanisms are involved in the propagation of the excitatory process in the aboral direction from the ileum through the ICS into the cecum. This assumption is justified by the fact that the response of the cecum to stimulation in the ileum is much more pronounced in the presence of atropine, and it is not affected by antagonists of adrenergic receptors and does not occur in the presence of TTX (281). This peculiarity in the propagation of the excitatory process through the ICS can be associated with the structural-functional organization of the plexuses in this part of

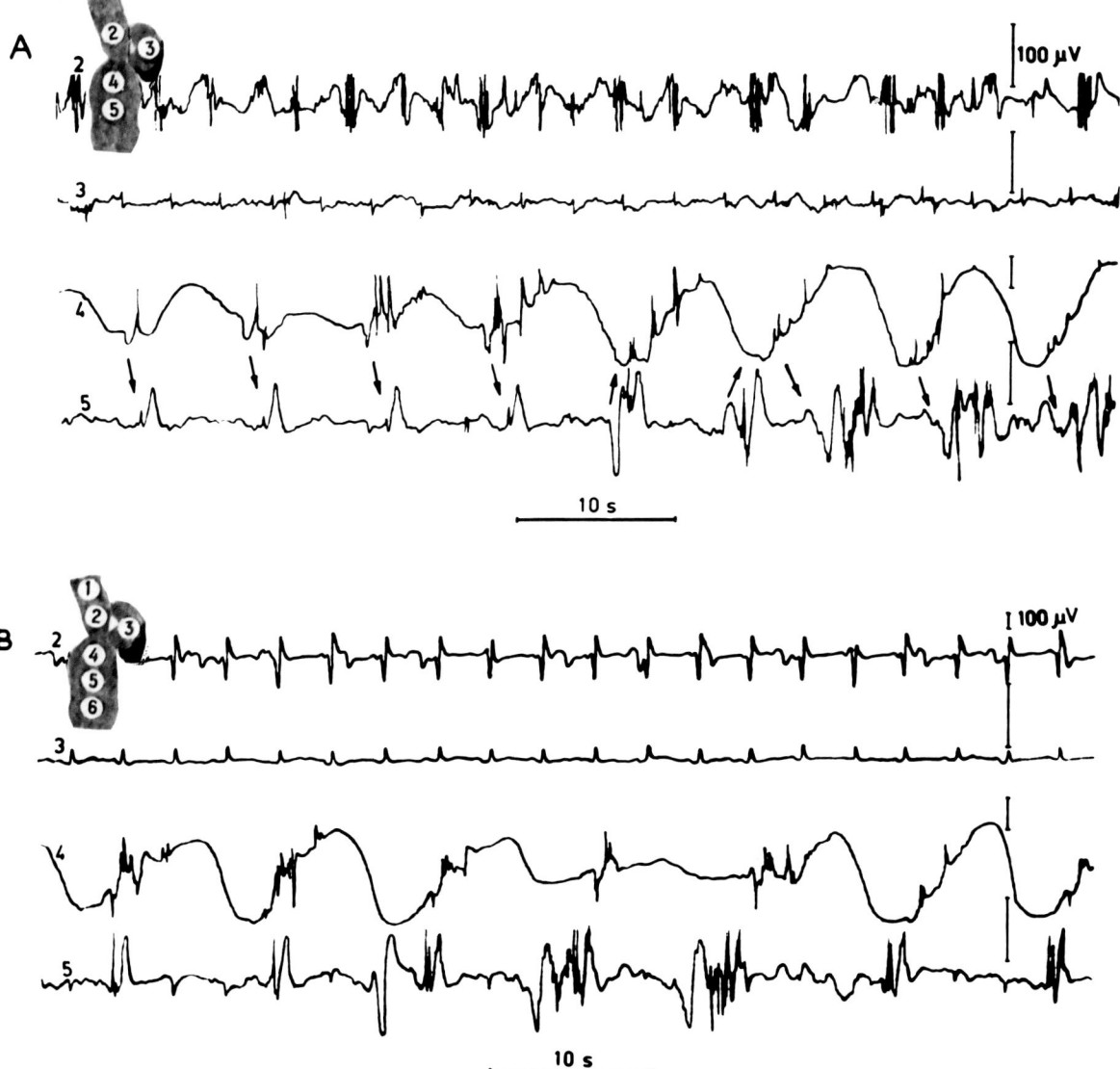

FIG. 12. Specific features in the propagation of the excitatory process in the ileocecal region. A: spike activity propagates from ileum through ileocecal sphincter to colon; B: isolated spike activity in colon. Arrows, direction of propagation of electrical activity. [From Papasova and Mizhorkova (311).]

the gastrointestinal tract. Although the neurons in the submucous layer in the sphincter region do not manifest a different activity compared with that of the ileum (352), it is very likely that there are some specificities in the organization of the myenteric plexus in this region, which cause the failure of the excitatory process to propagate from the colon in the oral direction through the ICS. This justifies the assumption that the ICS is a special barrier between the small and the large intestine (132), which prevents the propagation of the excitatory process in the oral direction from it. Owing to these characteristics of the functional organization of the ICS, reflux of the colonic content into the ileum is impossible. This is important for the organism, because the colonic content is rich in bacteria. An important role in the regulation of this basic and essential function of the ICS should most probably be attributed not only to the vegetative nerves, but also to the intrinsic nervous system located in the wall of the sphincter.

*Regulation of Ileocecal Sphincter*

SPECIFIC FEATURES OF THE SMOOTH MUSCLE. The smooth muscle isolated from ICS manifests spontaneous activity in 50% of the cases: continuous rhythmic changes are recorded in MP with a frequency of 4–6 cycles/min, on which spike potentials are superimposed (Fig. 13). In addition to the tonic changes of the type observed in the LES, part of the preparations manifest spike-dependent phasic contractions as well (311). The phasic contractions are superimposed on the tonic contraction. Whereas the tonic contractions are not connected with spike potentials, phasic contractions appear only with the appearance of spike potentials. The MP of the smooth-muscle cells of the ICS is low (−43 mV) compared with MP of the ileal smooth muscle (−50 mV) (246). The smooth muscle of the ICS is characterized by the high resting pressure maintained during the low degree of stretch, compared

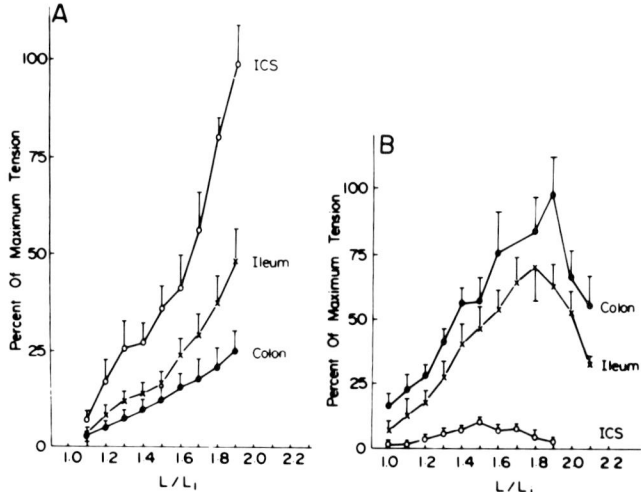

FIG. 14. *A*: length-tension curves for feline circular muscle from ileocecal sphincter (ICS), ileum, and colon. Tension as percent of maximum ICS tension is measured during graded increments of stretch ($L/L_i$). The ICS muscle developed greater tension than adjacent ileum or colon. *B*: active tension as percent of maximum colonic muscle tension in response to acetylcholine (ACh, $10^{-4}$ M) at each increment of stretch ($L/L_i$). Ileum and colon developed greater peak active tension ($P_0$) in response to ACh than ICS. However, ICS peak tension occurred at a lesser degree of stretch. Maximum combined tension due to stretch and stimulation with ACh was similar for each muscle. All responses are normalized for muscle cross-sectional area for studies performed on minimum of 20 muscle strips. [From Cardwell et al. (69).]

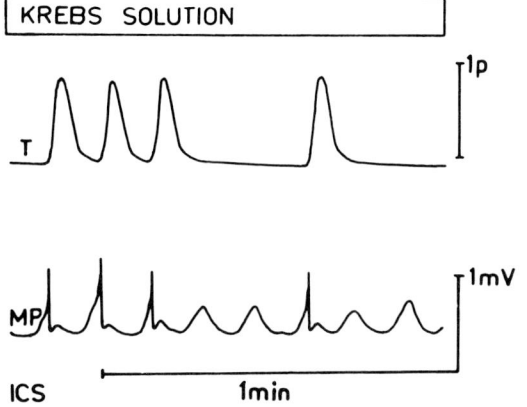

FIG. 13. Spike-dependent phasic contraction of ileocecal sphincter (ICS). Recording made by sucrose-gap method. T, tension; MP, membrane potential. [From Papasova and Lolova (308).]

with the adjacent ileum and colon. Moreover, the different strips manifest a greater resistance to stretching relative to muscle strips from the ileum and colon (100, 101). Resting pressure in the ICS is partially $Ca^{2+}$ dependent: it decreases on reduction of the $Ca^{2+}$ concentration in the nutrient medium, and is totally inhibited at $Ca^{2+} = 0$ with 0.5 mM ethylenediaminetetraacetic acid, as well as by nitroprusside sodium [Fig. 14; (69, 305)]. A linear relation exists between the length of the ICS muscle strips and the recorded tension (101). Under the influence of TEA the excitability of the ICS increases, and each slow depolarization is accompanied by spontaneously discharged spike potentials. Phasic contractions appear at the frequency of the slow depolarizations (304).

After studying the electrical and contractile activity of the ICS smooth muscle, a number of authors believe that the specificity in ICS activity is myogenically determined. There is still insufficient experimental evidence to confirm this view. Further research in this field is needed to specify the role of the myogenic component of the resting pressure characteristic of the ICS.

NEURAL REGULATION. Stimulation of the periarterial nerves increases ICS contraction. When the lumbar colonic nerves are stimulated, the passage of liquids through the ICS stops as a result of the sphincteric contraction. At the same time the ileum and the colon relax. These neural effects are blocked by guanethidine and phenoxybenzamine, and are potentiated by the β-adrenoceptor blocking agent propranolol (296, 297). Pressure in the ICS increases on stimulation of the peripheral end of the greater splanchnic nerve. Severing the sympathetic nerves does not affect the basal tone of the sphincter (346). Obviously, pressure in the ICS results from direct contraction of the sphincter (222) and not from contraction of the intestine on either side of the sphincter.

Another characteristic feature is that sympathetic control of the ICS involves α-adrenergic mechanisms. This is supported by the fact that in the presence of propranolol, the responses of the ICS to stimulation of the sympathetic nerves are potentiated. This is attributed to unmasking of α-adrenergic effects. Contraction of the ICS occurs in response to intravenous administration of adrenergic neurotransmitters. Under in vivo conditions, phenylepinephrine and norepinephrine induce contraction of cat ICS, with this contraction being blocked by phenoxybenzamine and potentiated after propranolol. On the other hand, isoprenaline increases the transsphincter flow (298). Similar effects of adrenergic agents are observed in preparations isolated from cat ICS. It has been reported that the α-adrenergic receptors are much more numerous in the region of the ileocecal junction in monkeys, cats, and guinea pigs (184, 185, 281, 337).

Parasympathetic nerves have a stimulating effect on the ICS (346). Stimulation of the efferent end of the cervical vagal nerve results in discontinuation of the flow of liquids through the ICS (299). Sphincteric contraction occurs also in response to bethanechol (346). However, the opposite effect on the tone is observed when the vagal nerve is stimulated with low stimulation frequency not exceeding 5 Hz (297). The inhibitory effect of parasympathetic stimulation in this case is probably the result of the excitation of the low-threshold nerve fibers in the vagal nerve (261, 262). The dependence of the smooth muscle response of the ICS on the frequency of stimulation is observed in vitro as well. A characteristic finding is that in the case of electrical field stimulation, ICS strips always respond with relaxation at the onset of stimulation (101, 246). The amplitude of the relaxation increases with increasing frequency of stimulation, reaching a maximum at 8–9 Hz (at supramaximal current values and 0.2 ms impulse duration). Two types of responses are observed when the stimulation is switched off, depending on the activity of the preparation prior to the stimulation. In muscle preparations with marked phasic activity, switching off the stimulation results in the appearance of a high-amplitude contraction, followed by a tonic slow contraction (Fig. 15). In the strips manifesting only changes in tone, the off-response consists only of a slow tonic contraction. The fast component of the off-response is not observed in the presence of cholinoceptor blocking agents, which suggests that it is related to the activation of cholinergic neurons in the intrinsic nervous system. The slow tonic component appears to be associated with the α-adrenergic receptors because it is not observed after phenoxybenzamine. The responses of the muscle strips isolated from the ICS to electrical stimulation are TTX sensitive. However, the tone of the ICS preparations is much more sensitive to TTX than the responses to electrical stimulation (101).

The experimental data show that the ICS manifests different responses both to stretch and to electrical stimulation, compared with the ileum and the colon. This is reason to assume the control system in the sphincteric part of the ileocecal region, which is different from the nonsphincteric parts (i.e., the ileum

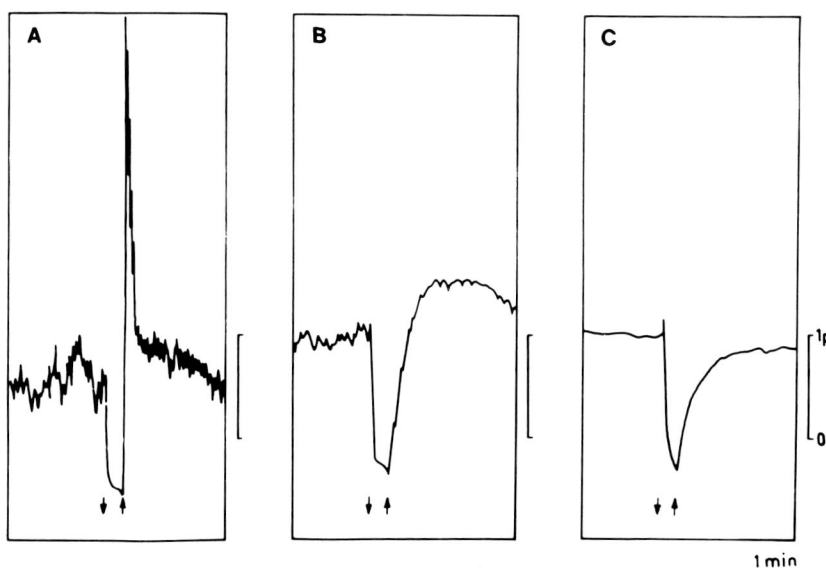

FIG. 15. Mechanisms of conditioning ICS responses to electrical field stimulation. A: control; B: on background of atropine $10^{-6}$ g/cm³; C: on background of atropine $10^{-6}$ g/cm³, phenoxybenzamine $10^{-5}$ g/cm³, and propranolol $10^{-5}$ g/cm³. Down arrows, beginning of stimulation; up arrows, end of stimulation. [From Papasova and Lolova (308).]

and colon) (101). Electron-microscopic studies have shown, however, the existence of the three types of axonal varicosities (cholinergic, adrenergic, and noncholinergic-nonadrenergic) in each of the three parts of the ileocecal region: ileum, ICS, and colon (254). The pronounced relaxation on electrical field stimulation of the ICS results from the activation of both intrinsic noncholinergic-nonadrenergic and extrinsic sympathetic inhibitory mechanisms. Obviously, the possibility of triggering the two mechanisms guarantees ICS relaxation, which is necessary for the passage of the luminal content from the ileum to the colon. On the other hand, the existence of cholinergic and adrenergic excitatory mechanisms guarantees the state of contraction of the ICS during intervening periods (95).

HUMORAL REGULATION: PEPTIDES AND PROSTAGLANDINS. There exist only a few isolated studies on the effects of prostaglandins on the ICS. It has been found that $PGE_1$ does not affect the tone and the spontaneous phasic activity of preparations isolated from cat ICS, whereas $PGF_{2\alpha}$ considerably increases tone. The $PGF_{2\alpha}$-induced rise in the tone is partially myogenically determined, because it is not entirely inhibited by antagonists of the cholinergic and adrenergic receptors and by TTX (393). Whereas $PGE_1$ does not change the responses of smooth-muscle preparations from cat ICS to electrical field stimulation, $PGF_{2\alpha}$ increases both the tone and the amplitude of the LES relaxation induced by this kind of stimulation. Maximum increase in the amplitude of relaxation is observed on the third minute after PG application. Because this effect of $PGF_{2\alpha}$ is not influenced by cholinoceptor and adrenoceptor blocking agents (atropine, propranolol, and phenoxybenzamine), the involvement of the noncholinergic-nonadrenergic neurotransmission must be assumed (308, 393).

There are only a few isolated studies on the effect of peptides on the ICS as well. No activation of cat ileocecal region by pentagastrin is observed (407). However, in human subjects gastrin causes reduction of the pressure in the ICS. Endogenous gastrin also has the same effect, because ICS relaxation is observed following alkalization of the stomach, whereas acidification leads to increase in pressure (73). However, secretin, gastrin, glucagon, and cholecystokinin have no in vitro effects on the ICS (69).

ANAL SPHINCTER

*Anatomy and Innervation*

The sphincter region at the anal end of the digestive tract consists of the combination of smooth and striated muscles that form the two sphincters: the internal anal sphincter (IAS) and the external anal sphincter. The IAS is formed of smooth muscle as a result of the thickening of the circular muscle layer of the most distal part of the rectum. It varies in thickness between 1.5 and 5 mm for a distance of 2.5–3 cm (for the different species). The IAS is surrounded by the external anal sphincter, which is formed of three transversely striated muscle bundles. A characteristic feature is that two bundles envelop the IAS while the third bundle is located distally from it and in fact surrounds the terminal part of the anal channel.

Innervation of the IAS is derived from the autonomic nerves. It receives parasympathetic innervation via the pelvic nerves from the first, second, and third sacral segments of the spine, whereas sympathetic innervation is provided by the hypogastric nerves. The intrinsic nervous system of the IAS is the immediate continuation of the innervation of the rectum. It is reported that the IAS has very few or almost no ganglion cells (22, 23). In fact, the nerve terminals found in the IAS originate from ganglion cells located in the rectal wall.

The external anal sphincter is innervated by the perineal inferior hemorrhoidal branches of the pudendal nerve ($S_2$, $S_3$, $S_4$), as well as by branches from the coccygeal plexus ($S_4$, $S_5$) (80, 362).

*Internal Anal Sphincter*

FUNCTIONAL CHARACTERISTICS. The IAS is almost always in a contracted state, which results in the intraluminal pressure in the sphincter being much higher than that in the rectum (30, 98, 142, 143, 209, 214, 363). The high-pressure zone is 3–7 cm wide (209). The view that the high pressure in the IAS is the result predominantly of mechanical factors maintained by the accessory muscles of the pelvic fundus (149) was disproved to a great extent by the finding that the pressure decreases after surgical section of the IAS (30). Convincing evidence has been obtained in support of the view that the state of constant contraction of the IAS determines the high-pressure state in the anal channel (209). The IAS is responsible for ~85% of the pressure in the anal channel (172). Moreover, during rest the smooth muscle forming the sphincter generates continuous rhythmic low-amplitude contractions (240).

Electrophysiological studies on both human subjects and animals have confirmed the existence of changes in MP with frequency identical to that of the low-amplitude sphincteric contractions. The IAS smooth muscle generates slow rhythmic potentials, referred to as slow waves by analogy with those from the small intestine (250), slow potentials (382), or basic electrical rhythm (111). Unlike the slow waves in the intestine, however, the slow potentials from the IAS induce phasic contractions without being accompanied by spike potentials (46, 282, 379, 406). The in vivo amplitude of the slow potentials is between 200 and 500 μV (240), whereas in vitro it may reach up to 10 mV in studies using the sucrose gap method (380). One should note the inconstancy in the amplitude of the slow potentials, which most frequently follows a waxing and waning pattern (46, 282, 406). The frequency of the slow potentials varies greatly not only for the different species but also for different experimental subjects belonging to the same species. Thus in human subjects some authors report the frequency of the slow potentials to be 20–24 cycles/min (282), others 10–20 cycles/min (240), while others are 14–34 cycles/min (406). The explanation of these differences may be found in the findings reported by Wienbeck and Altaparmacov (406) that the frequency of the slow potentials varies considerably among different healthy subjects, whereas it is relatively constant for each individual subject. The frequency of the IAS slow potentials also depends on the experimental conditions. In awake cats (under chronic experimental conditions) the frequency of the slow potentials is 26–34 cycles/min, whereas under anesthesia it is inconstant and varies between 9 and 30 cycles/min (40).

Slow potentials are recorded during not more than two-thirds of the duration of the study period (111). Recordings using several electrodes spaced at distances of 2–3 cm from one another show that in humans the slow potentials propagate in the oral direction and determine the propagation of the contractile activity in the same direction (240). The same dependence is observed in cats (46), as well as in the IAS musculature isolated in vitro. The frequency of the slow potentials is the highest in the strip isolated from the most distal part of the sphincter and is lowest in the muscle strip immediately next to the anorectal line. This is the basis for assuming the existence of a pacemaker in the IAS in the zone immediately next to the skin (380).

Attempts to associate the electrical activity of the IAS with the tone have come up against difficulties and are not always successful. Above all, a link is not always found between the amplitude and the frequency of the slow potentials, on the one hand, and the pressure in the sphincter, on the other (406). Under in vitro conditions, however, this dependence is found to be clearly manifested. Two types of electrical activity patterns may be recorded in vitro from smooth muscle strips isolated from the IAS. One type observed in humans has a waxing and waning pattern, whereas the other pattern is characterized by the recording of slow potentials having identical amplitude and frequency (Fig. 16). In both cases there is continuous association with the character of the contractions of the IAS smooth muscle strips (380). The fact that the isolated circular muscle strips generate slow potentials supports the view that the slow potential changes characteristic of the IAS are generated in the circular muscle layer (388). Irrespective of the

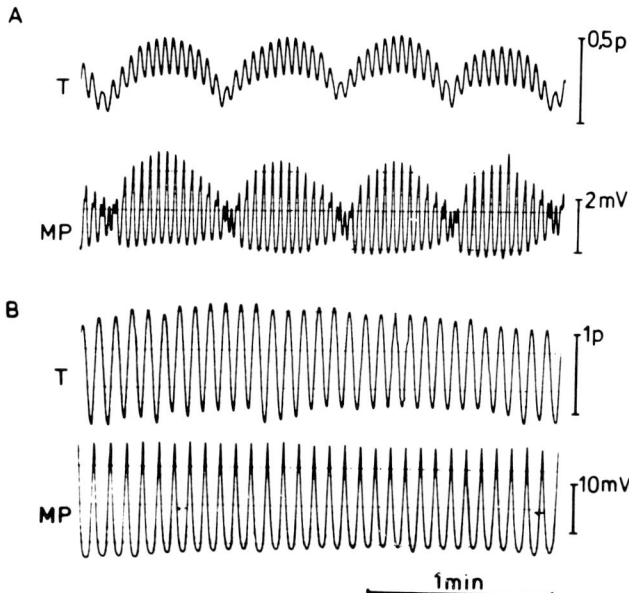

FIG. 16. Spontaneous electric (MP, membrane potential) and contractile (T, tension) activity of smooth muscle strips of cat internal anal sphincter. Recording with single sucrose-gap method. A: waxing and waning pattern type. Every contraction corresponds to slow change of MP; B: MP changes equal in amplitude and duration and concomitant contractions. [From Todorov (379).]

difficulties existing in connection with the precise correlation between the electrical and the contractile activity of the IAS in vivo, there is no doubt that the IAS tone is the active state of the sphincter and that this is maintained by the slow potentials generated by the smooth muscle cells (388). This is also supported by the fact that the amplitude of the slow potentials is decreased or completely inhibited when the pressure in the IAS decreases. This dependence is particularly well manifested in the rectoanal inhibitory reflex. It is known that stretching of the rectum results in IAS relaxation (7, 141, 179, 247, 318). This relaxation of the IAS is preceded by inhibition of the slow potentials (394, 406). The extent of relaxation increases as the volume of the distending balloon is increased (364). The anorectal inhibitory reflex is detected even in newborn babies and it may be used for diagnosing Hirschprung's disease (174, 248). The average pressure in the IAS of children is 47 ± 18 mmHg. When the rectum is distended with 10 ml air, the IAS relaxes. The relaxation continues for 6 s after the distension of the rectum is discontinued, after which the pressure increases to reach the prestimulus level (171). The pressure is 51 ± 18 mmHg in the case of aganglionosis associated with Hirschprung's disease.

The anorectal inhibitory reflex persists after treatment with cholino- and adrenoceptor blocking agents (179, 287, 333), which suggests that it may involve noncholinergic-nonadrenergic neurotransmission (109). Because the IAS relaxation on distension of the rectum is preserved in the case of spinal transection (141, 364), the anorectal inhibitory reflex is considered to be mediated by the enteric nervous system. The spinal cord probably has only a modulating role (170, 173). This is supported by the fact that the reflex is absent in Hirschprung's disease (248, 356). The IAS is responsible for the involuntary retention of the content in the anal channel, whereas the external anal sphincter is responsible for the voluntary retention (366).

REGULATION OF ANAL SPHINCTER. *Specific features of the smooth muscle.* Under in vitro conditions, muscle strips isolated from the cat IAS are spontaneously occurring and continuous phasic contractions are recorded (334, 380). There is a frequency gradient of the contractions from aboral to oral components of the sphincter. The highest frequency is found in muscle strips isolated from the region of the skin zone. This frequency is 20 cycles/min, compared with 13.5 cycles/min for the muscle strips next to the rectum. The frequency of the phasic contractions of muscle strips from the rectum proper is 5 cycles/min. The frequency and the amplitude of the phasic contractions of IAS strips is connected with the slow electrical potentials generated by the muscle. The slow potentials from the IAS are suppressed in $Ca^{2+}$-free solution (46), as well as by $Ca^{2+}$ antagonists (380). The excitability of the IAS smooth muscle depends on availability of $Ca^{2+}$. The tone of the IAS decreases after treatment with the $Ca^{2+}$ antagonist D 600 and is abolished by nitroprusside sodium.

*Neural regulation.* The state of increased tone in the IAS is associated with increased activity in the sympathetic nerves. The hypogastric nerve supplies excitatory innervation to the IAS (362). Severing of the hypogastric nerve in cats results in a temporary decrease in the IAS tone, while the spontaneous activity of the rectum increases (181). Stimulation of the peripheral end of the hypogastric nerve usually raises the IAS tone (362). This is preceded by a slow depolarization of the muscle fiber membranes, which is blocked by guanidine, ergotamine, or phentolamine but is not influenced by the ganglionic blocker hexamethonium (47). The role of the sympathetic nerves in maintaining the IAS tone is also demonstrated by the lasting decrease in the sphincteric tone that occurs after application of 6-OHDA and is accompanied by complete destruction of the adrenergic nerve terminals (180). The stimulating effects of the sympathetic nerves on the IAS were pointed out in the studies of Garry in 1932 (182, 183), in which he found relaxation of the rectum and contraction of the IAS on stimulation of the lumbar sympathetic nerves.

Stimulation of the pelvic nerves causes relaxation of cat and guinea pig IAS (109, 368). In cats, reduction of the IAS tone is observed also after resection of the pelvic nerves. Whereas stimulation of the distal end

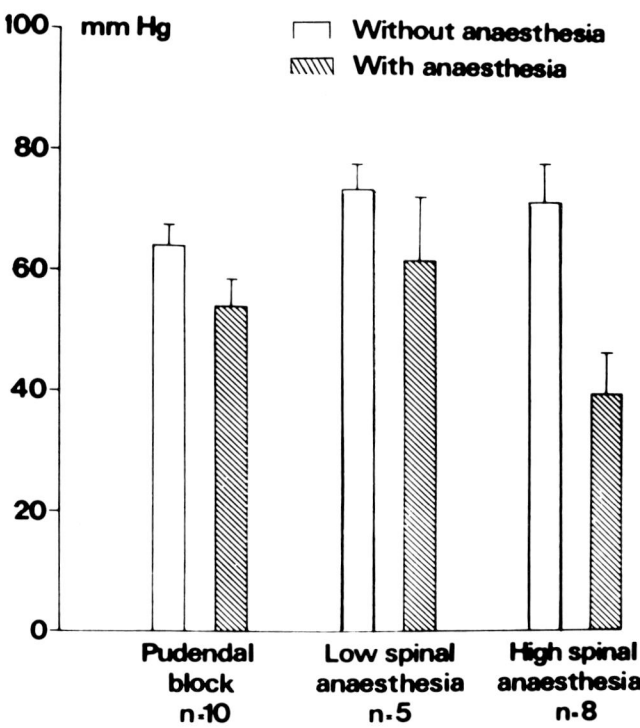

FIG. 17. Maximal anal pressure at rest with and without anesthesia. High spinal anesthesia decreases anal pressure significantly more than low spinal anesthesia or pudendal block. [From Frenckner and Ihre (173).]

of the pelvic nerves evokes contractions of the rectum, the effects on IAS are different. In some cases the IAS tone is increased, and in others the sphincter is relaxed (181). Nevertheless, other authors have reported only relaxation of the IAS under the same conditions (109). The IAS contractions are transformed into relaxation after administration of $\alpha$-adrenoceptor blocking agents, while the contractions of the rectum are inhibited by atropine.

After induction of high spinal anesthesia, the sympathetic innervation of the IAS is inhibited and a decrease in the sphincter tone is observed [Fig. 17; (173)]. This is evidence that the sympathetic nerves are responsible for the high IAS tone during rest. Sympathetic control over the IAS is mediated by $\alpha$-adrenergic mechanisms (181). In addition to the asympathetic nerves, some fibers of sacral origin are also assumed to contribute to the basal tone of the IAS (273). In cats, rats, and guinea pigs the adrenergic innervation is most strongly manifested in the IAS region (109). Very dense adrenergic innervation compared with other parts of the digestive tract has been observed by fluorescent microscopy in the IAS of vervet monkey (334). Bearing in mind that impulses originating from sympathetic nerves raise the IAS tone, most probably the rich adrenergic innervation of IAS determines to a great extent the high tone characteristic of IAS (308).

Exogenously applied norepinephrine and epinephrine induce a very pronounced IAS contraction that is blocked by α-adrenergic antagonists. Intravenous administration of methoxamine in humans, as well as intra-arterial administration of norepinephrine and epinephrine in the vervet monkey (334) and in cats (181), raise the pressure in the IAS, and this is blocked by the α-adrenoceptor blocking agent phentolamine. Norepinephrine and epinephrine also increase the frequency of the slow potentials recorded from IAS. This effect is suppressed by dihydroergotamine and phentolamine (47). Similar effects are also produced by sympathomimetic and sympatholytic agents on smooth muscle preparations isolated from human IAS (21, 38, 55, 56, 312), monkey IAS (334), cat IAS (47, 380), and guinea pig IAS (115).

There are differing views on the existence of β-adrenergic receptors in the muscle of the IAS. In human subjects IAS relaxation in vitro by isoprenaline was reported (55, 312). This relaxation was antagonized by propranolol. On the other hand, a very slight relaxing effect of isoprenaline was found in vervet monkeys (334), and in cats isoprenaline had no effect whatsoever (380).

The data on the influence of parasympathetic innervation on the IAS are controversial. It was reported that stimulation of the sacral nerves produced IAS relaxation, which was atropine resistant and blocked by hexamethonium (180). Stimulation of the second ventral sacral root also results in inhibition of the spontaneous electrical activity of IAS circular muscles (47). Bouvier and Gonella (47) suggested that the sacral preganglionic axons are related to the nonadrenergic-noncholinergic intrinsic neurons that initiate IAS relaxation. Data on the effect of exogenously applied acetylcholine on the IAS are also controversial. It was reported by two different groups that acetylcholine had no effect on the IAS (21, 47). In humans acetylcholine induces contractions only in muscle strips isolated from the upper half of the sphincter, whereas the strips immediately next to the skin zone are unaffected. Acetylcholine induces IAS contraction in cats in vivo. Contractile effects are also observed in muscle strips of monkey IAS (333, 334). Garrett et al. (181) did not find contractile responses in human IAS in response to acetylcholine. Others reported that relaxation occurred in response to the muscarinic agonists bethanechol and acetylcholine (56, 71). Because the action of acetylcholine was blocked by atropine, it was assumed that acetylcholine acts at muscarinic receptors on the muscle of the IAS (312). The effects of acetylcholine and methacholine are transformed into relaxation when the preparations are pretreated with phentolamine. These effects are also blocked by atropine, suggesting some of the actions of acetylcholine are on adrenergic transmission.

Nicotine and high acetylcholine concentrations evoke IAS relaxation in vervet monkeys (334) and in cats [Fig. 18; (383)]. This does not occur in reserpinized animals, it is not affected by propranolol and atropine, but it is abolished by simultaneous application of atropine and hexamethonium or by TTX (Fig. 19). During depolarization of the smooth muscle preparations with $K^+$ (18–20 mM), scorpion venom, or ouabain, the acetylcholine-induced relaxations are transformed into contractions that are blocked by

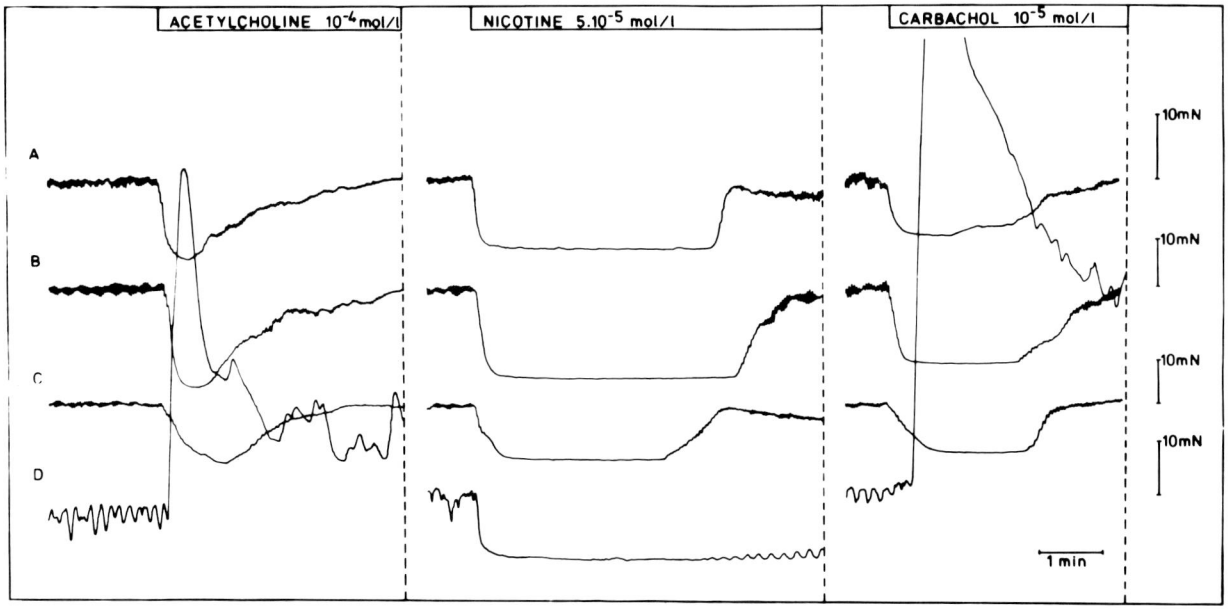

FIG. 18. Effect of acetylcholine, nicotine, and carbachol on the contractile activity of the smooth muscle from cat internal anal sphincter (A, B, and C) and rectum (D). [From Todorov and Papasova (383).]

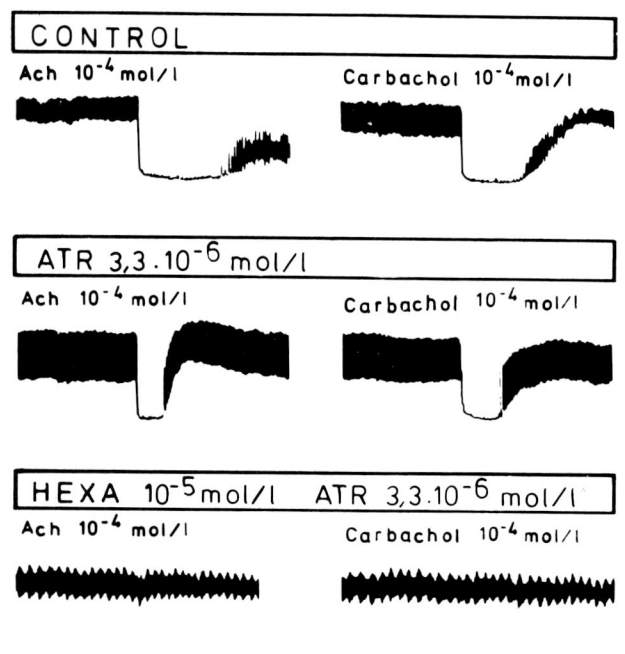

FIG. 19. Character of the acetylcholine (ACh) and carbachol-induced relaxation of internal anal sphincter before and after treatment with atropine and hexamethonium. [From Todorov and Papasova (383).]

adrenoceptor blocking agents. This suggests that activation of nicotinic and muscarinic receptors on noncholineric-nonadrenergic inhibitory neurons leads to the release of noncholinergic-nonadrenergic neurotransmitter, which causes IAS relaxation. Both muscarinic and nicotinic receptors are present on enteric neurons (see chapter by Wood in this *Handbook*).

Acetylcholine may also release norepinephrine; however, the threshold for this is considerably higher than for activation of the noncholinergic-nonadrenergic neurons. It is these differences in threshold that reveal IAS relaxation in response to acetylcholine (383).

The observed differences in the acetylcholine effects on the various animal species suggests species differences in the organization of the processes related to IAS contraction and relaxation. However, it is evident that the inhibitory noncholinergic-nonadrenergic innervation is very well developed and functioning in all species, and this is supported by electron-microscopic observations as well (23). In IAS preparations, in vitro electrical field stimulation results in contraction when the stimulation is switched on, followed by prolonged relaxation (55, 56, 115, 334, 381, 383). The contraction is blocked by $\alpha$-adrenoceptor blocking agents, while the relaxation is blocked by TTX. Blockade of the relaxation response by TTX reflects blockade of nonadrenergic-noncholinergic nerves.

*Humoral Regulation: Peptides.* Studies on the humoral regulation of IAS have been carried out mainly on in vitro preparations. It was reported that $PGF_{2\alpha}$ induced relaxation in human IAS (53, 56).

Substance P always induces contraction in smooth-muscle strips isolated from the IAS, while VIP and bradykinin cause relaxation (39, 54). The assumption that VIP is the noncholinergic-nonadrenergic neurotransmitter remains equivocal. It has been found that pretreatment with the proteolytic enzymes chymotrypsin and carboxypeptidase does not influence IAS relaxation induced by electrical field stimulation (54). This suggests that the inhibitory neurotransmitter is not a peptide.

Caerulein does not change IAS pressure in human subjects in vivo, while on isolated sphincter preparations it leads to a strong reduction of the tone and to a marked relaxation of norepinephrine-contracted preparations (71).

There is no doubt that neural relaxation of the IAS is achieved by noncholinergic-nonadrenergic inhibitory mechanisms, while adrenergic mechanisms participate in guaranteeing the state of contraction, which is characteristic of the IAS during rest. Regarding the cholinergic mechanisms, it has not been determined to what extent their participation is direct, or whether they only modulate the release of adrenergic excitatory and noncholinergic-nonadrenergic inhibitory neurotransmitters. Further studies in this field are necessary, as well as research on the specific features of the IAS smooth muscle and on the effect of the various peptides, in order to decipher the mechanisms responsible for the high intraluminal pressure in the IAS.

The motor function of the IAS and the external anal sphincter, as well as the interactions of the two sphincters, are considered in greater detail in the chapter by Krier in this *Handbook*.

CONCLUSION

Gastrointestinal sphincters play a key role in the general functional organization of the digestive tract. The interactions between the sphincters and the regions located proximally from them, on the one hand, and between the sphincters and the regions located distally from them, on the other hand, are due to the specificity in the structural and functional organization of the intrinsic nervous system, as well as to the relations between it and the different parts of the autonomic and central nervous systems. In some of the sphincters, as can be seen from the observations reviewed in this chapter, many of the mechanisms responsible for these interactions have been clarified. The numerous data accumulated over the past ten years demonstrate the extremely important role of nonadrenergic-noncholinergic inhibitory innervation for the functions of the gastrointestinal sphincters. However, the neurotransmitter responsible for the function of this part of the intrinsic nervous system are not yet identified. This is the main obstacle for understanding the interactions between the different parts of the intrinsic nervous system: cholinergic, adrenergic, and noncholinergic-nonadrenergic. These interactions are among the basic factors defining the functional state of the digestive tract as a whole, being especially responsible for the organization of the basic function of the gastrointestinal sphincters, which is to regulate the evacuation of the content in distal direction and to prevent the reflux of the content in the proximal direction.

Special attention should be devoted to the study of the neurotransmitter relations established in the smooth muscles of the LES and IAS, considering that under definite conditions one neurotransmitter can modulate the release of another neurotransmitter. Our knowledge in this respect is still based on experiments carried out using exogenous neurotransmitters on isolated preparations from the gastrointestinal sphincters. Further detailed and comprehensive studies with accurate quantitative determinations of the released transmitter are needed. The discovery of the factors responsible for and controlling these interactions will most probably make it possible to shed light on the pathological disturbances in sphincteric function observed in clinical practice.

Another essential problem, which is to a great extent of decisive importance in sphincter physiology, concerns the basal tone in gastrointestinal sphincters. Gastrointestinal sphincters are characterized by high intraluminal pressure. A number of aspects of this problem were discussed in the detailed survey of available data on sphincteric function. There are relatively more data for the LES, although the proportional contribution of the myogenic component to the basal tone is not yet clear. No structural differences have been found between the smooth muscles of the sphincter and of the nonsphincter regions of the digestive tract, nevertheless some specific features, revealed recently with respect to the muscle of the gastrointestinal sphincters, suggest that the contributions of myogenic mechanisms to the basal tone is considerable. At the same time, it may be said definitely that the basal tone is an important determinant of the sphincteric behavior produced by neuromuscle interactions. In order to reveal the specific features in the organization of the gastrointestinal sphincters, it is also necessary to study the specificities of the processes taking place at the level of the smooth-muscle cell membrane. Although in the past few years there has been intense research on isolated smooth muscle cells or cell cultures, so far there are no such data on sphincteric smooth muscles. On the other hand, there is considerable knowledge of the specific features of electromechanical coupling in the smooth muscles of the gastrointestinal sphincters. It should be noted that in some sphincters, such as the LES and IAS, the tone is spike independent, whereas in other sphincters (PS, ICS, and IAS) spike-dependent phasic contractions are observed in addition to the changes in the tone. Probably different ionic channels operate at the level of the cell membrane of the sphincter smooth muscle cells, whose gating of these channels defines the character of the muscle activity. Systematic studies are needed in this respect as well (for a detailed review of membrane channels in smooth muscle see the chapter by Bolton in this *Handbook*).

The last ten years are marked by the discovery of a number of peptides with significant regulating and modulating effect on the functions of the digestive tract and more specifically on its motor function. There are only isolated studies in this respect on gastrointestinal sphincters and these are concerned predominantly with the LES. Further studies are necessary in view of the participation of peptides in the modulation of the neurotransmitters release, on the one hand, and the complex neurotransmitter interactions in gastrointestinal sphincters, on the other.

REFERENCES

1. AGGESTRUP, S., AND S. L. JENSEN. Effects of regulatory peptides on the porcine lower oesophageal sphincter. *Regul. Pept.* 4: 155–162, 1982.
2. AIZAWA, K., K. HIWATASHI, I. TAKAHASHI, AND Z. ITOH. Control of motor activity in the lower oesophageal sphincter by motilin. In: *Gastrointestinal Motility*, edited by H. L. Duthie. Trowbridge, UK: Esher, 1978, p. 101–109. (6th Int. Symp. Gastrointest. Motil. Health Dis., Edinburgh, Scotland, Sept. 12–16, 1977.)
3. ALVAREZ, W. C. *An Introduction to Gastro-Enterology.* New York: Harper, 1948.
4. ALVAREZ, W. C., AND L. J. MAHONEY. Action currents in stomach and duodenum. *Am. J. Physiol.* 58: 476–493, 1922.
5. ANDERSON, S., AND M. I. GROSSMAN. Profile of pH, pressure and potential difference at gastroduodenal junction in man. *Gastroenterology* 49: 364–371, 1965.
6. ANURAS, S., A. R. COOKE, AND J. CHRISTENSEN. An inhibitory innervation at the gastroduodenal junction. *J. Clin. Invest.* 54: 529–535, 1974.
7. ARHAN, P., C. FAVERDIN, AND J. THOUVENOT. Ano-rectal motility in sick children. *Scand. J. Gastroenterol.* 7: 309–314, 1972.
8. ARIMORI, M., C. F. CODE, J. F. SCHLEGEL, AND R. E. STURM. Electrical activity of the canine esophagus and gastroesophageal sphincter. *Am. J. Dig. Dis.* 15: 191–201, 1970.
9. ASK, P., AND L. TIBBLING. Effect of time interval between swallows on esophageal peristalsis. *Am. J. Physiol.* 238 (*Gastrointest. Liver Physiol.* 1): G485–G490, 1980.
10. ASOH, R., AND R. K. GOYAL. Electrical activity of the opossum lower esophageal sphincter in vivo. Its role in the basal sphincter pressure. *Gastroenterology* 74: 835–840, 1978.
11. ASOH, R., AND R. K. GOYAL. Manometry and electromyogra-

phy of the upper esophageal sphincter in the opossum. *Gastroenterology* 74: 514–520, 1978.
12. ATANASSOVA, E. The role of the gastroduodenal junction in correlating the spike activities of the gastric and duodenal walls. *C. R. Acad. Bulg. Sci.* 22: 947–949, 1969.
13. ATANASSOVA, E. The role of the intramural nervous system in correlating the spike activity between the stomach and the duodenum. *C. R. Acad. Bulg. Sci.* 22: 1337–1340, 1969.
14. ATANASSOVA, E. Bioelectrical activity of the stomach and duodenum after cutting the gastroduodenal junction. *Bull. Inst. Physiol. Bulg. Acad. Sci.* 13: 211–227, 1970.
15. ATANASSOVA, E. On the mechanism of correlation between the spike activities of the stomach and duodenum. *Bull. Inst. Physiol. Bulg. Acad. Sci.* 13: 229–241, 1970.
16. ATANASSOVA, E. *The Intrinsic Nervous System and Gastro-Intestinal Motility.* Sofia, Bulgaria: Bulgarian Acad. Sci., 1981.
17. ATANASSOVA, E., M. PAPASOVA, AND N. KORTEZOVA. On the character of the electrical activity of the stomach, pyloric sphincter and duodenum of cats. *Acta Physiol. Pharmacol. Bulg.* 8: 34–44, 1982.
18. ATKINSON, N., D. A. W. EDWARDS, A. J. HONOUR, AND E. ROWLANDS. Comparison of cardiac and pyloric sphincters. A manometric study. *Lancet* 2: 918–922, 1957.
19. BASS, P., C. F. CODE, AND E. H. LAMBERT. Motor and electrical activity of the duodenum. *Am. J. Physiol.* 201: 287–291, 1961.
20. BASS, P., C. F. CODE, AND E. H. LAMBERT. Motor and electrical activity of the gastroduodenal junction. *Am. J. Physiol.* 201: 587–592, 1961.
21. BASS, D. D., T. J. USTACH, AND M. M. SCHUSTER. In vitro pharmacologic differentiation of sphincteric and nonsphincteric muscle. *Johns Hopkins Med. J.* 127: 185–191, 1970.
22. BAUMGARTEN, H. G., A. F. HOLSTEIN, AND F. STELZNER. Differences in the innervation of the large intestine and internal anal sphincter in mammals and human. *Virch. Anat. Ges.* 56: 43–47, 1971.
23. BAUMGARTEN, H. G., A. F. HOLSTEIN, AND F. STELZNER. Nervous elements in the human colon of Hirschsprung's disease. *Virchows Arch. A Pathol. Anat.* 358: 113–136, 1973.
24. BAYTINGER, V. F. Functional morphology of the upper esophageal sphincter. In: *Physiology and Pathology of the Sphincter Regions of the Digestive System. Abstracts of the Soviet-Union Symposium,* edited by M. A. Medvedev and V. D. Suhodolo. Tomsk, USSR: Rotprint, 1984, p. 3–4.
25. BECKER, J. M., AND K. A. KELLY. Antral control of canine gastric emptying of solids. *Am. J. Physiol.* 245 (*Gastrointest. Liver Physiol.* 8): G334–G338, 1983.
26. BEHAR, J., AND P. BIANCANI. Effect of cholecystokininoctapeptide on lower esophageal sphincter. *Gastroenterology* 73: 57–61, 1977.
27. BEHAR, J., P. BIANCANI, AND M. P. ZABINSKI. Characterization of feline gastroduodenal function by neural and hormonal stimulation. *Am. J. Physiol.* 236 (*Endocrinol. Metab. Gastrointest. Physiol.* 1): E45–E51, 1979.
28. BEHAR, J., S. FIELD, AND C. MARIN. Effect of glucagon, secretin, and vasoactive intestinal polypeptide on the feline lower esophageal sphincter: mechanisms of action. *Gastroenterology* 77: 1001–1007, 1979.
29. BEHAR, J., M. KERSTEIN, AND P. BIANCANI. Neural control of lower esophageal sphincter (LES) closure (Abstract). *Gastroenterology* 72: 1029, 1977.
30. BENNETT, R. C., AND H. L. DUTHIE. The functional importance of the internal anal sphincter. *Br. J. Surg.* 51: 355–357, 1964.
31. BENNETT, A., K. G. ELEY, AND H. L. STOCKLEY. Modulation by prostaglandins of contractions in guinea-pig ileum. *Prostaglandins* 9: 377–384, 1975.
32. BENNETT, A., AND B. FLESHLER. Prostaglandins and the gastrointestinal tract. *Gastroenterology* 59: 790–800, 1970.
33. BENNETT, A., AND B. WHITNEY. A pharmacological study of the motility of the human gastrointestinal tract. *Gut* 7: 307–316, 1966.
34. BERGES, W., M. WIENBECK, AND G. STROHMEYER. Does dopamine predispose to gastroesophageal reflux? *Z. Gastroenterol.* 17: 681–684, 1979.
35. BERTACCINI, G., M. IMPICCIATORE, AND G. DECARO. Action of caerulein and related substances on the pyloric sphincter of the anaesthetized rat. *Eur. J. Pharmacol.* 22: 320–324, 1973.
36. BERTACCINI, G., AND E. POLI. Failure of somatostatin to inhibit the stimulatory effect of different compounds on the lower esophageal sphincter of the rat. *Farm. Sci.* 39: 273–276, 1984.
37. BIANCANI, P., L. K. LICALIZI, AND R. W. MCCALLUM. Mechanisms of histamine-induced excitation of the cat pylorus. *J. Clin. Invest.* 68: 582–588, 1981.
38. BIANCANI, P., J. H. WALSH, AND J. BEHAR. Vasoactive intestinal polypeptide. A neurotransmitter for lower esophageal sphincter relaxation. *J. Clin. Invest.* 73: 963–967, 1984.
39. BIANCANI, P., J. H. WALSH, C. HILLEMEIER, AND J. BEHAR. Role of VIP and PHI in internal anal sphincter (IAS) relaxation (Abstract). *Dig. Dis. Sci.* 29, Suppl. 10S, 1984.
40. BIANCANI, P., M. P. ZABINSKI, M. D. KERSTEIN, AND J. BEHAR. Comparison of mechanical characteristics of the lower esophageal sphincter (LES) and pyloric sphincter (PS). In: *Gastrointestinal Motility,* edited by H. L. Duthie. Trowbridge, UK: Esher, 1978, p. 547–550. (6th Int. Symp. Gastrointest. Motil. Health Dis., Edinburgh, Scotland, Sept. 12–16, 1977.)
41. BITAR, K., N. MEI, AND M. H. MICHELUCCI. Vagal mechanoreceptors of the lower oesophageal sphincter and the pyloric sphincter in the cat. *J. Physiol. Lond.* 245: 103–104P, 1975.
42. BLOOM, S. R., AND J. M. POLAK. Peptidergic versus purinergic. *Lancet* 1: 94–98, 1978.
43. BONEV, A. On the Basal Tone of Stomach Fundus and Lower Esophageal Sphincter Smooth Muscle (In Vitro Experiments). Sofia, Bulgaria: Bulgarian Acad. Sci., 1984. Dissertation.
44. BORTOFF, A., AND R. S. DAVIS. Myogenic transmission of antral slow waves across the gastroduodenal junction in situ. *Am. J. Physiol.* 215: 889–897, 1968.
45. BORTOFF, A., AND N. WEG. Transmission of electrical activity through the gastroduodenal junction. *Am. J. Physiol.* 208: 531–536, 1965.
46. BOUVIER, M., AND J. GONELLA. Electrical activity from smooth muscle of the anal sphincter area of the cat. *J. Physiol. Lond.* 310: 445–456, 1981.
47. BOUVIER, M., AND J. GONELLA. Nervous control of the internal anal sphincter of the cat. *J. Physiol. Lond.* 310: 457–469, 1981.
48. BRING, B. M., J. F. SCHLEGEL, AND C. F. CODE. The pressure profile of the gastrointestinal junction zone in dogs. *Gut* 6: 163–171, 1965.
49. BROCK-UTNE, J. G., J. RUBIN, J. W. DOWNING, G. E. DIMOPOULOS, M. G. MOSHAL, AND M. NAICKER. The administration of metoclopramide with atropine. A drug interaction effect on the gastroesophageal sphincter in man. *Anesthesia* 31: 1186–1190, 1976.
50. BROWN, F., B. BECK, J. FLETCHER, D. CASTELL, AND C. EASTWOOD. Evidence suggesting prostaglandins mediate lower esophageal sphincter (LES) incompetence associated with inflammation (Abstract). *Gastroenterology* 72: 1033, 1977.
51. BURGET, G. A., AND W. E. ZELLER. A study of the cardia in unanaesthetized dogs. *Proc. Soc. Exp. Biol. Med.* 34: 433–434, 1936.
52. BURLEIGH, D. E. The effects of drugs and electrical field stimulation on the human lower oesophageal sphincter. *Arch. Int. Pharmacodyn.* 240: 169–176, 1979.
53. BURLEIGH, D. E. Non-cholinergic, non-adrenergic inhibitory neurons in human internal anal sphincter muscle. *J. Pharm. Pharmacol.* 35: 258–260, 1983.
54. BURLEIGH, D. E., AND A. D'MELLO. Neural and pharmacologic factors affecting motility of the internal anal sphincter.

*Gastroenterology* 84: 409–417, 1983.
55. BURLEIGH, D. E., A. D'MELLO, AND A. G. PARKS. An in vitro pharmacological investigation of the human internal anal sphincter. *Naunyn-Schmiedebergs Arch. Pharmacol.* 59: (Suppl. 279) R36, 1973.
56. BURLEIGH, D. E., A. D'MELLO, AND A. G. PARKS. Responses of isolated human internal anal sphincter to drugs and electrical field stimulation. *Gastroenterology* 77: 484–490, 1979.
57. BURN, J. H. Release of noradrenaline from the sympathetic postganglionic fibre. *Br. Med. J.* 2: 197–201, 1967.
58. BURN, J. H. The mechanism of the release of noradrenaline. In: *Adrenergic Neurotransmission*, edited by G. E. W. Wolstenholme and M. O'Connor. London: Churchill 1968, p. 16–25.
59. BURN, J. H., AND M. J. RAND. The relation of circulating noradrenaline to the effect of sympathetic stimulation. *J. Physiol. Lond.* 150: 295–305, 1960.
60. BURNSTOCK, G. Purinergic transmission. In: *Handbook of Psychopharmacology*, edited by L. L. Iversen, S. D. Iversen, and S. H. Snyder. New York: Plenum, 1975, vol. 5, p. 131–194.
61. BURNSTOCK, G. Purinergic receptors. *J. Theor. Biol.* 62: 491–503, 1976.
62. BURNSTOCK, G. Past and current evidence for the purinergic nerve hypothesis. In: *Physiological and Regulatory Functions of Adenosine and Adenine Nucleotides*, edited by H. P. Baer and G. I. Drummond. New York: Raven, 1979, p. 3–32.
63. BURNSTOCK, G., AND H. K. WONG. Comparison of the effects of ultraviolet light and purinergic nerve stimulation on the guinea-pig taenia coli. *Br. J. Pharmacol.* 62: 293–303, 1978.
64. BURY, V. A., AND K. BOEV. Studies on the transmembrane ion currents in the smooth-muscle cells of the gastric fundus. *Experientia Basel* 36: 216–218, 1980.
65. BYBEE, D. E., F. C. BROWN, P. GEORGES, D. O. CASTELL, AND J. E. MCGUIGAN. Somatostatin inhibition of lower esophageal sphincter pressure elevation caused by glycine: support for a role of endogenous gastrin in physiologic responses of the sphincter. In: *Gastrointestinal Motility*, edited by H. L. Duthie. Trowbridge, UK: Esher, 1978, p. 585–589. (6th Int. Symp. Gastrointest. Motil. Health Dis., Edinburgh, Scotland, Sept. 12–16, 1977.)
66. BYBEE, D. E., F. C. BROWN, P. GEORGES, D. O. CASTELL, AND J. E. MCGUIGAN. Somatostatin effects on lower esophageal sphincter function. *Am. J. Physiol.* 237 (*Endocrinol. Metab. Gastrointest. Physiol.* 1): E77–E81, 1979.
67. CAMPBELL, G. Autonomic nervous supply to effector tissues. In: *Smooth Muscle*, edited by E. Bülbring, A. F. Brading, A. W. Jones, and T. Tomita. London: Arnold, 1970, p. 451–495.
68. CANNON. W. B. The acid control of the pylorus. *Am. J. Physiol.* 20: 282–322, 1907.
69. CARDWELL, B. A., M. R. RUBIN, W. J. SNAPE, AND S. COHEN. Properties of the cat ileocecal sphincter muscle. *Am. J. Physiol.* 241 (*Gastrointest. Liver Physiol.* 4): G222–G226, 1981.
70. CARLSON, H. L., C. F. CODE, AND R. A. NELSON. Motor activity of the canine gastroduodenal junction: a cineradiographic, pressure and electric study. *Am. J. Dig. Dis.* 11: 155–172, 1966.
71. CARPENEDO, F., A. INFANTINO, M. FLOREANI, AND G. DODI. The relaxing effect of caerulein on isolated human internal anal sphincter. *Eur. J. Pharmacol.* 87: 271–276, 1983.
72. CASTELL, D. O. Lower esophageal sphincter: physiologic and clinical aspects. *Ann. Intern. Med.* 83: 390–401, 1975.
73. CASTELL, D. O., S. COHEN, AND L. D. HARRIS. Response of human ileocecal sphincter to gastrin. *Am. J. Physiol.* 219: 712–715, 1970.
74. CASTELL, D. O., AND L. D. HARRIS. The link between control of gastric acid secretion and control of lower esophageal sphincter strength (Abstract). *Gastroenterology* 56: 1249, 1969.
75. CASTELL, D. O., AND L. D. HARRIS. Hormonal control of gastroesophageal sphincter strength. *N. Engl. J. Med.* 282: 886–895, 1970.
76. CHRISTENSEN, J. Pharmacologic identification of the lower esophageal sphincter. *J. Clin. Invest.* 49: 681–691, 1970.
77. CHRISTENSEN, J. Pharmacology of the esophageal motor function. *Annu. Rev. Pharmacol.* 15: 243–258, 1975.
78. CHRISTENSEN, J. The innervation and motility of the esophagus. In: *The Esophagus*, edited by Leo von der Reis. Basel: Karger, 1978, p. 18–32.
79. CHRISTENSEN, J. Some determinants of the latency of the off response in smooth muscle of the circular layer of opossum esophagus. *Jpn. J. Smooth Muscle Res.* 14: 31–32, 1978.
80. CHRISTENSEN, J. Motility of the colon. In: *Physiology of the Gastrointestinal Tract*, edited by L. R. Johnson. New York: Raven, 1981, vol. I, chapt. 14, p. 445–471.
81. CHRISTENSEN, J. Physiological characteristics of the gastroesophageal junction. *Ital. J. Gastroenterol.* 15: 143–147, 1983.
82. CHRISTENSEN, J., AND J. L. CONKLIN. Studies on the origin of the distinctive mechanics of smooth muscle at the esophagogastric junction. In: *Gastrointestinal Motility*, edited by E. E. Daniel. Vancouver, Canada: Mitchell, 1974, p. 63–71. (4th Int. Symp. Gastrointest. Motil., Banff, Alberta, Canada, Sept. 6–8, 1973.)
83. CHRISTENSEN, J., J. L. CONKLIN, AND B. W. FREEMAN. Physiological specialization at esophagogastric junction in three species. *Am. J. Physiol.* 225: 1265–1270, 1973.
84. CHRISTENSEN, J., AND E. E. DANIEL. Effects of some autonomic drugs on circular esophageal smooth muscle. *J. Pharmacol. Exp. Ther.* 159: 243–249, 1968.
85. CHRISTENSEN, J., AND E. E. DANIEL. Electric and motor effects of autonomic drugs on longitudinal esophageal smooth muscle. *Am. J. Physiol.* 211: 387–393, 1968.
86. CHRISTENSEN, J., B. W. FREEMAN, AND J. K. MILLER. Some physiological characteristics of the esophagogastric junction in the opossum. *Gastroenterology* 64: 1119–1125, 1973.
87. CHRISTENSEN, J., AND G. F. LUND. Atropine excitation of esophageal smooth muscle. *J. Pharmacol. Exp. Ther.* 163: 287–289, 1968.
88. CLARK, C. G., AND J. R. VANE. The cardiac sphincter in the cat. *Gut* 2: 252–262, 1961.
89. CLERC, N., AND N. MEI. Vagal mechanoreceptors located in the lower oesophageal sphincter of the cat. *J. Physiol. Lond.* 336: 487–498, 1983.
90. CODE, C. F., AND J. F. SCHLEGEL. The pressure profile of the gastroesophageal sphincter in man: an improved method of detection. *Proc. Staff Meet. Mayo Clin.* 33: 406–414, 1958.
91. COHEN, B. R., AND B. S. WOLF. Cineradiographic and intraluminal correlations in the pharynx and esophagus. In: *Handbook of Physiology. Alimentary Canal. Motility*, edited by C. F. Code. Washington, DC: Am. Physiol. Soc., 1968, sect. 6, vol. IV, chapt. 91, p. 1841–1860.
92. COHEN, S., AND F. GREEN. Force velocity characteristics of esophageal muscle: effect of acetylcholine and norepinephrine. *Am. J. Physiol.* 226: 1250–1256, 1974.
93. COHEN, S., AND L. D. HARRIS. Lower esophageal sphincter pressure as an index of lower esophageal sphincter strength. *Gastroenterology* 58: 157–162, 1970.
94. COHEN, S., AND L. D. HARRIS. The lower esophageal sphincter. *Gastroenterology* 63: 1066–1073, 1972.
95. COHEN, S., L. D. HARRIS, AND R. LEWITAN. Manometric characteristics of the human ileocecal junctional zone. *Gastroenterology* 54: 72–75, 1968.
96. COHEN, S., J. J. KRAWITZ, AND W. J. SNAPE. Vagal control of lower oesophageal sphincter junction. In: *Gastrointestinal Motility*, edited by H. L. Duthie. Trowbridge, UK: Esher, 1978, p. 101–109. (6th Int. Symp. Gastrointest. Motil. Health Dis., Edinburgh, Scotland, Sept. 12–16, 1977.)
97. COHEN, S., AND W. LIPSHUTZ. Hormonal regulation of human lower esophageal sphincter competence: interaction of gastrin and secretin. *J. Clin. Invest.* 50: 449–454, 1971.
98. COLLINS, C. D., H. L. DUTHIE, T. SHELLEY, AND G. E. WHITTAKER. Force in the anal canal and anal continence. *Gut*

8: 354–360, 1967.
99. COLLINS, S. M., AND J. D. GARDNER. Cholecystokinin-induced contraction of dispersed smooth muscle cells. *Am. J. Physiol.* 243 (*Gastrointest. Liver Physiol.* 6): G497–G504, 1982.
100. CONKLIN, J. L., AND J. CHRISTENSEN. Neuromuscular properties of ileocecal junction. *Federation Proc.* 33: 392, 1974.
101. CONKLIN, J. L., AND J. CHRISTENSEN. Local specialization of the ileocecal junction of the cat and opossum. *Am. J. Physiol.* 228: 1075–1081, 1975.
102. CONNELL, A. M. Motor action of the large bowel. In: *Handbook of Physiology. Alimentary Canal. Motility*, edited by C. F. Code. Washington, DC: Am. Physiol. Soc., 1968, sect. 6, vol. IV, chapt. 101, p. 2075–2091.
103. CONNELL, A. M., AND C. J. LOGAN. The role of gastrin in the gastro ileo colic responses. *Am. J. Dig. Dis.* 12: 277–284, 1967.
104. CONNOR, C., AND C. PROSSER. Comparison of ionic effects on longitudinal and circular muscle of cat jejunum. *Am. J. Physiol.* 226: 1212–1218, 1974.
105. COOKE, A. R., T. E. CHVASTA, AND N. W. WEISBRODT. Effect of pentagastrin on emptying and electrical and motor activity of the dog stomach. *Am. J. Physiol.* 223: 934–938, 1972.
106. COPPOLD, R., K. PHAOSAWASDI, AND R. S. RISHER. Nonadrenergic, noncholinergic pressure responses of the pylorus to duodenal stimuli in man (Abstract). *Clin. Res.* 28: 276A, 1980.
107. CORAZZIARI, E., G. DELLE FAVE, C. POZZESSERE, A. KOHN, L. DE MAGISTRIS, F. ANZINI, AND A. TORSOLI. Effect of bombesin on lower esophageal sphincter pressure in humans. *Gastroenterology* 83: 10–14, 1982.
108. CORUZZI, G., AND G. BERTACCINI. Effect of some vasoactive peptides on the lower esophageal sphincter. *Pharmacol. Res. Commun.* 12: 965–973, 1980.
109. COSTA, M., AND J. B. FURNESS. The innervation of the internal anal sphincter in the guinea-pig. *Rend. R. Gastroenterol.* 5: 47–58, 1973.
110. COTTRELL, D. F., AND A. IGGO. Tension receptors with vagal afferent fibres in the proximal duodenum and pyloric sphincter of sheep. *J. Physiol. Lond.* 354: 457–475, 1984.
111. COUTURIER, D., C. ROSE, M. H. COUTURIER-TURBIN, AND C. DEBRAY. Electromyography of the colon in situ. An experimental study in man and in the rabbit. *Gastroenterology* 56: 317–322, 1969.
112. CRANKSHAW, D. J., R. A. JANIS, AND E. E. DANIEL. The effects of $Ca^{2+}$ antagonists on $Ca^{2+}$ accumulation by subcellular fractions of rat myometrium. *Can. J. Physiol. Pharmacol.* 55: 1028–1032, 1977.
113. CREAMER, B., AND C. PIERCE. Observation on the gastroesophageal junction during swallowing and drinking. *Lancet* 2: 1309–1312, 1957.
114. CREENWOOD, R. K., J. F. SCHLEGEL, C. F. CODE, AND F. H. ELLIS. The effect of sympathectomy, vagotomy and oesophageal interruption on the canine gastroesophageal sphincter. *Thorax* 17: 310–319, 1962.
115. CREMA, A., G. M. FRIGO, S. LECCHINI, L. MANZO, L. ONORI, AND M. TONINI. Purine receptors in the guinea-pig internal anal sphincter. *Br. J. Pharmacol.* 78: 599–603, 1983.
116. CRISPIN, J. S., D. K. MCIVER, AND J. E. LIND. Manometric study of the effect of vagotomy on the gastroesophageal sphincter. *Can. J. Surg.* 10: 299–303, 1977.
117. DANIEL, E. E. The electrical and contractile activity of the pyloric region in dogs and the effects of drugs. *Gastroenterology* 49: 403–418, 1965.
118. DANIEL, E. E., J. CRANKSHAW, AND S. SARNA. Prostaglandins and myogenic control of tension in lower esophageal sphincter in vitro. *Prostaglandins* 17: 629–639, 1979.
119. DANIEL, E. E., J. CRANKSHAW, AND S. SARNA. Prostaglandins and tetrodotoxin-insensitive relaxation of opossum lower esophageal sphincter. *Am. J. Physiol.* 236 (*Endocrinol. Metab. Gastrointest. Physiol.* 2): E153–E172, 1979.
120. DANIEL, E. E., AND V. POSEY-DANIEL. Effects of scorpion venom on structure and function of esophageal lower sphincter (LES) and body circular muscle (BCM) from opossum. *Can. J. Physiol. Pharmacol.* 62: 360–373, 1984.
121. DANIEL, E. E., S. SARNA, W. WATERFALL, AND J. CRANKSHAW. Role of endogenous prostaglandins in regulating the tone of opossum lower esophageal sphincter in vivo. *Prostaglandins* 17: 641–648, 1979.
122. DANIEL, E. E., G. S. TAYLOR, AND M. E. HOLMAN. The myogenic basis of active tension in the lower esophageal sphincter (Abstract). *Gastroenterology* 670: 874, 1976.
123. DAVENPORT, H. W. *The Physiology of the Digestive Tract* (4th ed.). Chicago, IL: Year Book, 1977.
124. DECARLE, D. J., AND J. CHRISTENSEN. Effect of pentagastrin (PG) on opossum esophageal smooth muscle. *Gastroenterology* 70: 876–882, 1976.
125. DECARLE, D. J., AND J. CHRISTENSEN. A dopamine receptor in esophageal smooth muscle of the opossum. *Gastroenterology* 70: 216–219, 1976.
126. DECARLE, D. J., J. CHRISTENSEN, A. C. SZABO, D. C. TEMPLEMAN, AND D. R. MCKINDLEY. Calcium dependence of neuromuscular events in esophageal smooth muscle of the opossum. *Am. J. Physiol.* 232 (*Endocrinol. Metab. Gastrointest. Physiol.* 6): E547–E552, 1977.
127. DECARLE, D. J., D. C. TEMPLEMAN, AND J. CHRISTENSEN. Temperature dependence of responses of esophageal smooth muscle to electrical field stimulation. *Am. J. Physiol.* 232 (*Endocrinol. Metab. Gastrointest. Physiol.* 4): E432–E436, 1977.
128. DENT, J., W. J. DODDS, W. J. HOGAN, R. C. ARNDORFER, AND B. C. TEETER. Effect of cholecystokinin-octapeptide on opossum lower esophageal sphincter. *Am. J. Physiol.* 239 (*Gastrointest. Liver Physiol.* 3): G230–G235, 1980.
129. DENT, J., W. J. DODDS, W. J. HOGAN, J. D. WOOD, AND R. C. ARNDORFER. Depressant effect of sodium nitroprusside on the lower esophageal sphincter of the opossum. *Gastroenterology* 76: 784–789, 1979.
130. DENT, J., W. J. DODDS, T. SEKIGUCHI, W. J. HOGAN, AND R. C. ARNDORFER. Interdigestive phasic contractions of the human lower esophageal sphincter. *Gastroenterology* 84: 453–460, 1983.
131. DIAMANT, N., AND A. AKIN. Effect of gastric contractions on lower esophageal sphincter. *Gastroenterology* 63: 38–44, 1972.
132. DIDIO, L. T. A., AND M. C. ANDERSON. *The "Sphincters" of the Digestive System*. Baltimore, MD: Williams & Wilkins, 1968.
133. DILAWARI, J. B., A. NEWMAN, J. POLEA, AND J. J. MISIEWICZ. Prostaglandins and the cardiac sphincter in man. In: *Gastrointestinal Motility*, edited by E. E. Daniel. Vancouver, Canada: Mitchell, 1974, p. 281–286. (4th Int. Symp. Gastrointest. Motil., Banff, Alberta, Canada, Sept. 6–8, 1973.)
134. DIMARINO, A. J., AND S. COHEN. The adrenergic control of lower esophageal sphincter function: an experimental model of denervation supersensitivity. *J. Clin. Invest.* 52: 2264–2271, 1973.
135. DODDS, W. J., J. DENT, W. J. HOGAN, G. K. PATEL, J. TOOULI, AND R. C. ARNDORFER. Paradoxical lower esophageal sphincter contraction induced by cholecystokinin-octapeptide in patients with achalasia. *Gastroenterology* 80: 327–333, 1981.
136. DODDS, W. J., W. J. HOGAN, W. N. MILLER, J. J. STEF, R. C. ARNDORFER, AND S. D. LYDON. Effect of increased intraabdominal pressure on the lower esophageal sphincter pressure. *Am. J. Dig. Dis.* 20: 298–308, 1975.
137. DODDS, W. J., J. J. STEF, E. T. STEWART, W. J. HOGAN, R. C. ARNDORFER, AND E. B. COHEN. Responses of feline esophagus to cervical vagal stimulation. *Am. J. Physiol.* 235 (*Endocrinol. Metab. Gastrointest. Physiol.* 1): E63–E73, 1978.
138. DOODY, P. T. Adrenergic modulation of vagal inhibitory action: evidence for dopamine receptors (Abstract). *Gastroenterology* 70: 997, 1976.
139. DOTY, R. W. Neural organization of deglutation. In: *Handbook of Physiology. Alimentary Canal. Motility*, edited by C. F. Code. Washington, DC: Am. Physiol. Soc., 1968, sect. 6, vol. IV, chapt. 92, p. 1861–1902.

140. DOZOIS, R. R., K. A. KELLY, AND C. F. CODE. Effect of distal antrectomy on gastric emptying of liquids and solids. *Gastroenterology* 61: 675–681, 1971.
141. DUTHIE, H. L. Dynamic of the rectum and anus. *Clin. Gastroenterol.* 4: 467–477, 1975.
142. DUTHIE, H. L., AND R. C. BENNETT. The relation of sensation in the anal canal to the functional anal sphincter: a possible factor in anal continence. *Gut* 4: 179–182, 1963.
143. DUTHIE, H. L., B. H. BROWN, B. ROBERTSON-DUNN, N. K. KWONG, G. E. WHITTAKER, AND W. WATERFALL. Electrical activity in the gastroduodenal area. Slow waves in the proximal duodenum. A comparison of man and dog. *Am. J. Dig. Dis.* 17: 344–352, 1972.
144. DUTHIE, H. L., AND J. M. WATTS. Contribution of the external anal sphincter to the pressure zone in the anal canal. *Gut* 6: 64–72, 1965.
145. EDIN, R. The vagal control of the pyloric motor function: a physiological and immunohistochemical study in cat and man. *Acta Physiol. Scand. Suppl.* 485: 1–30, 1980.
146. EDIN, R., H. AHLMAN, AND J. KEWENTER. The vagal control of the feline pyloric sphincter. *Acta Physiol. Scand.* 107: 169–174, 1979.
147. EDIN, R., J. LUNDBERG, A. DAHLSTROEM, T. HOEKFELT, L. TERENIUS, AND H. AHLMAN. The peptidergic neural control of the feline pylorus. *Chir. Forum Exp. Klin. Forsch.* 233–237, 1980.
148. EDIN, R., J. LUNDBERG, L. TERENIUS, A. DAHLSTROEM, T. HOEKFELT, J. KEWENTER, AND H. AHLMAN. Evidence for vagal enkephalinergic neural control of the feline pylorus and stomach. *Gastroenterology* 78: 492–497, 1980.
149. EDWARDS, D. A. W. Sphincter mechanism in the gastrointestinal tract. *Am. J. Dig. Dis.* 12: 267–276, 1967.
150. EDWARDS, D. A. W., AND E. N. ROWLAND. Physiology of the gastroduodenal junction. In: *Handbook of Physiology. Alimentary Canal. Motility*, edited by C. F. Code. Washington, DC: Am. Physiol. Soc., 1968, sect. 6, vol. IV, chapt. 97, p. 1985–2000.
151. EHRENPREIS, S., J. GREENBERG, AND E. CONATY. Block of electrical induced contractions of guinea-pig longitudinal muscle by prostaglandin synthetase and receptors inhibitors. *Eur. J. Pharmacol.* 39: 331–340, 1976.
152. EHRLEIN, H. J., P. PROVE, AND W. SCHWEIKER. The function of the pyloric sphincter for regulating gastric emptying and for preventing reflux in dogs. In: *Gastrointestinal Motility*, edited by J. Christensen. New York: Raven, 1980, p. 177–184. (7th Int. Symp. Gastrointest. Motil., Iowa City, Iowa, Sept. 11–14, 1979.)
153. ELLIOTT, T. R. On the innervation of the ileo-colic sphincter. *J. Physiol. Lond.* 31: 157–168, 1904.
154. ELLIS, F. G., B. KAUNTZE, AND J. R. TRONNCE. The innervation of the cardia and lower oesophagus in man. *Br. J. Surg.* 47: 466–472, 1960.
155. EL-SHARKAWY, T. Y., W. W. L. CHAN, AND N. E. DIAMANT. Neural mechanisms of lower esophageal sphincter relaxation. In: *Gastrointestinal Motility*, edited by G. Vantrappen. Herentals: Typoff, 1976, p. 176–180. (5th Int. Symp. Gastrointest. Motil., Lewen, Belgium, Sept. 5–6, 1975.)
156. EYRE-BROOK, I. A., G. E. LINHARDT, R. H. SMALLWOOD, AND A. G. JOHNSON. The timing of pyloric closure in man: studies with impedance electrodes. In: *Gastrointestinal Motility*, edited by C. Roman. Lancaster, England: MTP, 1984, p. 119–120. (9th Int. Symp. Gastrointest. Motil., Aix-en-Provence, France, Sept. 12–16, 1983.)
157. FARRELL, R. L., G. T. ROLING, AND D. O. CASTELL. Stimulation of the incompetent lower esophageal sphincter—a possible advance in therapy of heartburn. *Am. J. Dig. Dis.* 18: 646–650, 1973.
158. FISHER, R. S., AND S. COHEN. Physiological characteristics of human pyloric sphincter. *Gastroenterology* 64: 67–75, 1973.
159. FISHER, R. S., AND S. COHEN. Disorders of the lower esophageal sphincter. *Annu. Rev. Med.* 26: 373–390, 1975.
160. FISHER, R. S., A. J. DIMARINO, AND S. COHEN. Mechanism of cholecystokinin inhibition of lower esophageal sphincter pressure. *Am. J. Physiol.* 228: 1469–1473, 1975.
161. FISHER, R. S., W. LIPSHUTZ, AND S. COHEN. The hormonal regulation of pyloric sphincter function. *J. Clin. Invest.* 52: 1289–1296, 1973.
162. FISHER, R. S., L. S. MALMUD, G. S. ROBERT, AND I. F. LOBIS. The lower esophageal sphincter as a barrier to gastroesophageal reflux. *Gastroenterology* 72: 19–22, 1977.
163. FLEISCHNER, F., AND C. BERNSTEIN. Roentgen-anatomical studies of the normal ileocecal valve. *Radiology* 54: 43–58, 1950.
164. FLESHLER, B., T. R. HENDRIX, P. KRAMER, AND F. J. INGELFINGER. Resistance and reflux function of the lower esophageal sphincter. *J. Appl. Physiol.* 12: 339–343, 1958.
165. FOURNET, J., W. J. SNAPE, AND S. COHEN. Modulation of lower esophageal sphincter relaxation in the opossum. *Am. J. Physiol.* 237 (*Endocrinol. Metab. Gastrointest. Physiol.* 5): E481–E485, 1979.
166. FOURNET, J., W. J. SNAPE, AND S. COHEN. Sympathetic control of lower esophageal sphincter function in the cat. Action of direct cervical and splanchnic nerve stimulation. *J. Clin. Invest.* 63: 562–570, 1979.
167. FOURNET, J., W. J. SNAPE, AND S. COHEN. The cholinergic component of lower esophageal sphincter pressure: a comparison of findings in the opossum and in cat. In: *Gastrointestinal Motility*, edited by J. Christensen. New York: Raven, 1980, p. 11–18. (7th Int. Symp. Gastrointest. Motil., Iowa City, Iowa, Sept. 11–14, 1979.)
168. FOX, J. A., AND E. E. DANIEL. Role of $Ca^{2+}$ in genesis of lower esophageal sphincter tone and other active contractions. *Am. J. Physiol.* 237 (*Endocrinol. Metab. Gastrointest. Physiol.* 2): E163–E171, 1969.
169. FOZARD, J. R., AND E. MUSCHOLL. Atropine-resistant effects of the muscarinic agonists McN-A-343 and AHR 602 on cardiac performance and the release of noradrenaline from sympathetic nerves of the perfused rabbit heart. *Br. J. Pharmacol.* 50: 531–541, 1974.
170. FRENCKNER, B. Function of the anal sphincters in spinal man. *Gut* 16: 638–644, 1975.
171. FRENCKNER, B. Ano-rectal manometry in the diagnosis of Hirschsprung's disease in infants. *Acta Pediatr. Scand.* 67: 187–192, 1978.
172. FRENCHKNER, B., AND C. VON EULER. Influence of pudendal block on the function of the anal sphincters. *Gut* 16: 482–580, 1975.
173. FRENCKNER, B., AND I. IHRE. Influence of autonomic nerves on the internal anal sphincter in man. *Gut* 17: 306–312, 1976.
174. FRENCKNER, B., AND M. L. MOLANDER. Activity of the internal anal sphincter during the first days of life. *Acta Pediatr. Scand.* 69: 73–77, 1980.
175. FUJII, Y. Electrophysiological studies on gastroduodenal junction of the guinea pig. *Am. J. Physiol.* 221: 413–420, 1971.
176. FURNESS, J. B., AND M. COSTA. The nervous release and action of substances which affect intestinal muscle through neither adrenoreceptors nor cholinoreceptors. *Philos. Trans. R. Soc. Lond. B. Biol. Sci.* 265: 123–133, 1973.
177. FURNESS, J. B., AND M. COSTA. Adrenergic innervation of the gastrointestinal tract. *Ergeb. Physiol. Biol. Chem. Exp. Pharmakol.* 69: 1–51, 1974.
178. FYKE, F. E., C. F. CODE, AND J. F. SCHLEGEL. The gastroesophageal sphincter in healthy human being. *Gastroenterology* 86: 135–150, 1956.
179. GARRETT, J. R., AND E. R. HOWARD. Effects of rectal distension on the internal anal sphincter of cats. *J. Physiol. Lond.* 222: 85P–86P, 1972.
180. GARRETT, J. R., AND E. R. HOWARD. Neural control of the internal anal sphincter of cats after chemical sympathectomy with 6-hydroxydopamine. *J. Physiol. Lond.* 247: 25P–26P, 1975.
181. GARRETT, J. R., E. R. HOWARD, AND W. JONES. The internal

anal sphincter in the cat: a study of nervous mechanisms affecting anal sphincter tone and reflex activity. *J. Physiol. Lond.* 243: 153–166, 1974.
182. GARRY, R. C. Observations on the caudal region of the large bowel in the cat. *J. Physiol. Lond.* 74: 14P–15P, 1932.
183. GARRY, R. C. The nervous control of the caudal region of the large bowel in the cat. *J. Physiol. Lond.* 75: 422–431, 1933.
184. GAZET, J. C. The surgical significance of the ileocaecal junction. *Ann. R. Coll. Surg. Engl.* 43: 19–38, 1968.
185. GAZET, J. C., AND R. J. JARRET. The ileocaeco-colic sphincter. Studies in vitro in man, monkey, cat and dog. *Br. J. Surg.* 51: 368–370, 1964.
186. GILBERT, R., S. RATTAN, AND K. GOYAL. Pharmacologic identification activation and antagonism of two muscarine receptor subtypes in the lower esophageal sphincter. *J. Pharmacol. Exp. Ther.* 230: 284–291, 1984.
187. GILES, G. R., M. C. MASON, C. HUMPHRIES, AND C. G. CLARK. Action of gastrin on the lower oesophageal sphincter in man. *Gut* 10: 730–734, 1969.
188. GOLENHOFEN, K., F. E. LÜDTKE, K. MILENOV, AND R. SIEWERT. Excitatory and inhibitory effects on canine pyloric musculature. In: *Gastrointestinal Motility*, edited by J. Christensen. New York: Raven, 1980, p. 203–210. (7th Int. Symp. Gastrointest. Motil., Iowa City, Iowa, Sept. 11–14, 1979.)
189. GOLENHOFEN, K., H. F. WEISER, AND R. SIEWERT. Phasic and tonic types of smooth muscle activity in lower oesophageal sphincter and stomach of the dog. *Acta Hepto-Gastroenterol.* 26: 227–234, 1979.
190. GONELLA, J., J. P. NIEL, AND C. ROMAN. Vagal control of lower oesophageal sphincter motility in the cat. *J. Physiol. Lond.* 273: 647–664, 1977.
191. GONELLA, J., J. P. NIEL, AND C. ROMAN. Sympathetic control of lower oesophageal sphincter motility in the cat. *J. Physiol. Lond.* 287: 177–190, 1979.
192. GONELLA, J., J. P. NIEL, AND C. ROMAN. Mechanism of the noradrenergic motor control on the lower oesophageal sphincter in the cat. *J. Physiol. Lond.* 306: 251–260, 1980.
193. GOYAL, R. K., AND B. W. COBB. Motility of the pharynx, esophagus, and esophageal sphincters. In: *Physiology of the Gastrointestinal Tract*, edited by L. R. Johnson. New York: Raven, 1981, vol. I, chapt. 11, p. 359–391.
194. GOYAL, R. K., AND S. RATTAN. Mechanism of the lower esophageal sphincter relaxation. *J. Clin. Invest.* 52: 337–341, 1973.
195. GOYAL, R. K., AND S. RATTAN. Nature of vagal inhibitory innervation to the lower esophageal sphincter. *J. Clin. Invest.* 55: 1119–1126, 1975.
196. GOYAL, R. K., AND S. RATTAN. Genesis of basal sphincter pressure: effect of tetrodotoxin on lower esophageal sphincter pressure in opossum in vivo. *Gastroenterology* 71: 62–67, 1976.
197. GOYAL, R. K., AND S. RATTAN. Effects of sodium nitroprusside and verapamil on the basal lower esophageal sphincter pressure (Abstract). *Gastroenterology* 74: 1040, 1978.
198. GOYAL, R. K., AND S. RATTAN. Neurohumoral, hormonal and drug receptors for the lower esophageal sphincter. *Gastroenterology* 74: 598–619, 1978.
199. GOYAL, R. K., AND S. RATTAN. Effects of sodium nitroprusside and verapamil on lower esophageal sphincter. *Am. J. Physiol.* 238 (*Gastrointest. Liver Physiol.* 1): G40–G44, 1980.
200. GOYAL, R. K., S. RATTAN., AND T. HERSH. Comparison of the effects of prostaglandins $E_1$, $E_2$ and $A_2$ and of hypovolemic hypotension on the lower esophageal sphincter. *Gastroenterology* 65: 608–612, 1973.
201. GRECO, A. V., A. BIANCO, L. ALTOMONTE, L. D'ACQUARICA, AND G. GHIRLANDA. Effect of somatostatin on lower esophageal sphincter (LES) pressure and serum gastrin in normal and achalasic subjects. *Horm. Metab. Res.* 14: 26–28, 1982.
202. HAEUSLER, G., AND S. THORENS. The effect of tetraethylammonium on contraction, membrane potential and calcium permeability of vascular smooth muscle. In: *Smooth Muscle Pharmacology and Physiology*, edited by M. Worcel and G. Vassort. Paris: INSERM, 1976, vol. 50, p. 363–368.
203. HALL, W. J., P. O'NEILL, AND J. D. SHEEHAN. The role of prostaglandins in cholinergic neurotransmission in the guinea-pig. *Eur. J. Pharmacol.* 34: 39–47, 1975.
204. HARRY, J. D. The action of prostaglandin $E_1$ on the guinea-pig isolated intestine. *Br. J. Pharmacol. Chemother.* 33: 213P–214P, 1968.
205. HEDQUIST, P. Basic mechanism of prostaglandin action on autonomic neurotransmission. *Annu. Rev. Pharmacol.* 17: 259–279, 1977.
206. HELLEMANS, J., AND G. VANTRAPPEN. Electromyographic studies on canine esophageal motility. *Am. J. Dig. Dis.* 12: 1240–1250, 1967.
207. HENDRIX, T. R. The motility of the alimentary canal. In: *Medical Physiology* (13th ed.), edited by V. B. Mountcastle. St. Louis, MO: Mosby, 1974, vol. 2, chapt. 52, p. 1208–1236.
208. HIGGS, B. R., G. SHORTER, AND F. H. ELLIS. A study of the anatomy of the human esophagus with special reference to the gastroesophageal sphincter. *J. Surg. Res.* 5: 503–507, 1965.
209. HILL, J. R., M. M. KELLEY, J. F. SCHLEGEL, AND C. F. CODE. Pressure profile of the rectum and anus of healthy persons. *Dis. Colon Rectum* 3: 203–209, 1960.
210. HOLLINSHEAD, W. H. *Anatomy for Surgeons*. New York: Hoeber, 1956.
211. HONGO, M. Effect of nifedipine on canine lower esophageal sphincter pressure. *Nippon Heikatsukin Gakkai Zasshi* 17: 47–51, 1981.
212. HORTON, B. T. Pyloric musculature with special reference to pyloric block. *Am. J. Anat.* 41: 197–225, 1928.
213. HOWARD, J. M., M. R. BELSHEIM, AND S. N. SALLIVAN. Enkephalin inhibits relaxation of the lower esophageal sphincter. *Br. Med. J.* 285: 1605–1606, 1982.
214. HOWARD, E. R., AND J. R. GARRETT. The intrinsic myenteric innervation of the hind gut and accessory muscles of defecation in the cat. *Z. Zellforsch. Mikrosk. Anat.* 136: 31–44, 1973.
215. HURWITZ, A. L., AND A. DURANCEAU. Upper esophageal sphincter dysfunction. Pathogenesis and treatment. *Am. J. Dig. Dis.* 23: 275–281, 1978.
216. INGELFINGER, F. J. Esophageal motility. *Physiol. Rev.* 38: 533–584, 1958.
217. ISENBERG, J. I., AND A. CSENDES. Effect of octapeptide of cholecystokinin on canine pyloric pressure. *Am. J. Physiol.* 222: 428–431, 1972.
218. ISENBERG, J. I., AND M. I. GROSSMAN. Effect of gastrin and S 15396 on gastric motility in dogs. *Gastroenterology* 56: 450–455, 1969.
219. ITOH, Z., I. AIZAWA, R. HONDA, H. KATSUTOSHI, AND K. HIWATASHI, AND E. F. COUCH. Control of lower esophageal sphincter contractile activity by motilin in conscious dogs. *Am. J. Dig. Dis.* 23: 341–345, 1978.
220. ITOH, Z., I. AIZAWA, AND T. NAKAMURA. Effect of dopamine and its antagonists on contractile activity of the lower esophageal sphincter and the stomach. *Nippon Heikatsukin Gakkai Zasshi* 16: 99–107, 1980.
221. ITOH, Z., R. HONDA, I. AIZAWA, S. TAKEUCH, K. HIWATASHI, AND E. COUCH. Interdigestive motor activity of the lower esophageal sphincter in the conscious dogs. *Am. J. Dig. Dis.* 23: 239–247, 1978.
222. JARRETT, R. J., AND J. C. GAZET. Studies in vivo of the ileocaeco-colic sphincter in the cat and dog. *Gut* 7: 271–275, 1968.
223. JEAN, A., J. P. MIOLAN, AND C. ROMAN. In vitro study of the effect of leu-enkephalin and related drugs on the vagally induced responses of the lower esophageal sphincter. In: *Gastrointestinal Motility*, edited by C. Roman. Lancaster, England: MTP, 1984, p. 29–36. (9th Int. Symp. Gastrointest. Motil., Aix-en-Provence, France, Sept. 12–16, 1983.)
224. JENSEN, D. M., R. W. MCCALLUM, E. CORAZZIARI, J. ELASHOFF, AND J. H. WALSH. Human lower esophageal sphincter

responses to synthetic human gastrins 34 (G-34) and 17 (G-17). *Gastroenterology* 79: 431–438, 1980.
225. JO-ANN, E. T., J. A. FOX, AND E. E. DANIEL. Role of $Ca^{2+}$ in genesis of lower esophageal sphincter tone and other active contractions. *Am. J. Physiol.* 237 (*Endocrinol. Metab. Gastrointest. Physiol.* 2): E163–E171, 1979.
226. JODKE, A., A. RESKAR, AND G. HARTING. On the relation between release of prostaglandins and contractility of rabbit splenic capsular strips. *Naunyn-Schmiedebergs Arch. Pharmacol.* 292: 35–42, 1976.
227. JOHANSON, B., AND M. NYLANDER. Analysis of the ileocaecal emptying mechanism in the rat. *Acta Chir. Scand.* 134: 296–305, 1968.
228. JOHNSON, A. G., C. J. C. KIRK, AND C. S. MARCK. Does pyloric competence depend on antro-duodenal coordination? In: *Gastrointestinal Motility*, edited by E. E. Daniel. Vancouver, Canada: Mitchell, 1974, p. 505–513. (4th Int. Symp. Gastrointest. Motil., Banff, Alberta, Canada, Sept. 6–8, 1973.)
229. KADLEČ, O., K. MAŠEK, AND J. SEFERNA. A modulating role of prostaglandins in contraction of the guinea-pig ileum. *Br. J. Pharmacol.* 51: 565–570, 1974.
230. KADLEČ, O., K. MAŠEK, AND J. SEFERNA. Modulation by prostaglandins of the release of acetylcholine and noradrenaline in guinea-pig isolated ileum. *J. Pharmacol. Exp. Ther.* 204: 635–645, 1978.
231. KADLEČ, O., AND R. RADOMIROV. Effects of prostaglandins $F_{2\alpha}$ and $E_1$ on the longitudinal and circular smooth muscle of the guinea-pig caecum in relation to the concentration of extracellular calcium. *Naunyn-Schmiedebergs Arch. Pharmacol.* 288: 335–343, 1975.
232. KARIM, S. M., AND K. HILLIER. General introduction and some pharmacological actions of prostaglandins. In: *The Prostaglandins*, edited by S. M. Karin. Lancaster, UK: MTP, 1972, p. 1–76.
233. KAYE, M. D., S. J. MEHTA, AND J. P. SHOWALTER. Manometric studies of the human pylorus. *Gastroenterology* 70: 477–480, 1976.
234. KELLEY, M. L., AND J. A. DEWEESE. Effects of eating and intraluminal filling on ileocolonic junctional zone pressures *Am. J. Physiol.* 216: 1491–1495, 1969.
235. KELLEY, M. L., E. A. GORDON, AND J. A. DEWEESE. Pressure studies of the ileocolonic junctional zone of dogs. *Am. J. Physiol.* 209: 333–339, 1965.
236. KELLEY, M. L., E. A. GORDON, AND J. A. DEWEESE. Pressure response of canine ileocolonic junctional zone to intestinal distension. *Am. J. Physiol.* 211: 614–618, 1966.
237. KELLY, K. A. Effect of gastrin on gastric myoelectric activity. *Am. J. Dig. Dis.* 15: 399–405, 1970.
238. KELLY, K. A. Motility of the stomach and gastroduodenal junction. In: *Physiology of the Gastrointestinal Tract*, edited by L. R. Johnson. New York: Raven, 1981, vol. I, chapt. 12, p. 393–410.
239. KERLIN, P., A. ZINSMEISTER, AND S. PHILLIPS. Motor responses to food of the distal colon of healthy humans. *Gastroenterology* 84: 762–771, 1983.
240. KERREMANS, R. Electrical activity and motility of the internal anal sphincter. An "in vivo" electrophysiological study in man. *Acta Gastro-Enterol. Belg.* 21: 465–482, 1968.
241. KING, P. M., R. C. HEADING, AND A. PRYDE. Coordinated motor activity of the human gastroduodenal region. *Dig. Dis. Sci.* 30: 219–225, 1985.
242. KLIMOV, P. K. *Peptides and Gastrointestinal System*. Leningrad, USSR: Nauka, 1983.
243. KLIMOV, P. K., G. M. BARASHKOVA, V. I. BRAGINSKII, V. I. KOTELNIKOVA, E. U. LINAR, N. C. PAVLOVA, E. U. ROZOVA, V. B. TROYZKAYA, V. N. USTINOV, A. A. FOKINA, AND G. I. CHINEIS. Changes in the functions of the stomach, duodenum and gall bladder after synthetic gastrin. *Sechenov Physiol. J. USSR* 58: 579–592, 1972.
244. KLIMOV, P. K., T. MORYANOVICH, E. L. POLYAKOV, I. L. KURANOVA, AND C. I. CHURKINA. Physiological effects of bombesin. *Sechenov Physiol. J. USSR* 71: 145–170, 1985.
245. KOLOSSOV, N. G. *Nervous System of the Gastrointestinal Tract of Vertebrates and Man.* Leningrad, USSR: Nauka, 1968.
246. KUBOTA, M. Electrical and mechanical properties and neuroeffector transmission in the smooth muscle layer of guinea-pig ileocecal junction. *Pfluegers Arch.* 394: 355–361, 1983.
247. LAWSON, J. O. N. Structure and function of the internal anal sphincter. *Proc. R. Soc. Med.* 63, Suppl.: 84–89, 1970.
248. LAWSON, J. O. N., AND H. H. NIXON. Anal canal pressure in the diagnosis of Hirschsprung's disease. *J. Pediatr. Surg.* 2: 544–552, 1967.
249. LEIPSIEN, G., H. R. KOELZ, H. F. WEISER, A. L. BLUM, AND R. SIEWERT. The role of the duodenum in the regulation of lower oesophageal sphincter pressure (LESP) in the dog. In: *Gastrointestinal Motility*, edited by H. L. Duthie. Trowbridge, UK: Esher, 1978, p. 553–561. (6th Int. Symp. Gastrointest. Motil. Health Dis., Edinburgh, Scotland, Sept. 12–16, 1977.)
250. LIDBERG, P., A. DAHLSTOM, AND H. AHLAM. Is 5-HT a mediator in the motor control of the feline pylorus? *Scand. J. Gastroenterol.* 19: 321–328, 1984.
251. LIEBERMANN-MEFFERT, D., M. ALLGOWER, P. SCHMID, A. L. BLUM. Muscular equivalent of the lower esophageal sphincter. *Gastroenterology* 76: 31–38, 1979.
252. LIPSHUTZ, W. H., AND S. COHEN. Physiological determinants of lower esophageal sphincter function. *Gastroenterology* 61: 16–24, 1971.
253. LIPSHUTZ, W. H., A. F. TUCH, AND S. COHEN. A comparison of the site of action of gastrin I on lower esophageal sphincter and antral circular muscle. *Gastroenterology* 64: 454–460, 1971.
254. LOLOVA, I., N. LOLOV, AND M. PAPASOVA. Structure of the myenteric plexus in the sphincters of cat gastrointestinal tract. I. Quantitative assessment of the type of dense-core vesicles. *Acta Physiol. Pharmacol. Bulg.* 6: 60–67, 1980.
255. LOLOVA, I., AND M. PAPASOVA. Comparative quantitative estimation of the granular vesicles in the intramural ganglia of Auerbach's plexus in the nonsphincter and sphincter parts of cat alimentary tract. *Acta Physiol. Pharmacol. Bulg.* 7: 50–59, 1981.
256. LOLOVA, I., I. PETROV, AND M. PAPASOVA. Structure of the myenteric plexus in the sphincters of the cat gastrointestinal tract. VI. Axonal profiles, axonal varicosities, synapses and other membrane differentiations. *Acta Physiol. Pharmacol. Bulg.* 6: 28–38, 1980.
257. LOUCKES, H. S., J. P. QUIGLEY, AND J. KERSEY. Inductograph method for recording muscle activity, especially pyloric sphincter physiology. *Am. J. Physiol.* 199: 301–310, 1960.
258. LÜDTKE, F. E., K. GOLENHOFEN, AND H. D. BECKER. Mechanical activity of isolated human pyloric muscle in comparison with canine pylorus. In: *Gastrointestinal Motility*, edited by C. Roman. Lancaster, England: MTP, 1984, p. 87–94. (9th Int. Symp. Gastrointest. Motil., Aix-en-Provence, France, Sept. 12–16, 1963.)
259. LUND, G. F., AND J. CHRISTENSEN. Electrical stimulation of esophageal smooth muscle and effects of antagonists. *Am. J. Physiol.* 217: 1369–1374, 1969.
260. MARIK, G., AND C. F. CODE. Control of the interdigestive myoelectrical activity in dogs by the vagus nerves and pentagastrin. *Gastroenterology* 68: 387–395, 1975.
261. MARTINSON, J. The effect of efferent vagal nerve fibres on gastric motility. *Acta Physiol. Scand.* 62: 256–262, 1964.
262. MARTINSON, J. Studies on the efferent vagal control of the stomach. *Acta Physiol. Scand.* 65, Suppl. 255: 1–23, 1965.
263. MARTINSON, J., AND A. MUREN. Excitatory and inhibitory effects of vagus stimulation on gastric motility in the cat. *Acta Physiol. Scand.* 57: 309–316, 1963.
264. MATARAZZO, S. A., W. J. SNAPE, J. R. RYAN, AND S. COHEN. Relationship of cervical and abdominal vagal activity to lower esophageal sphincter function. *Gastroenterology* 71: 999–1003, 1976.

265. MAYNARD, D., P. A. THOMAS, AND R. J. EARLAM. Analysis of the electrical activity of the canine gastro-oesophageal sphincter in terms of overlapping pulse sequences. In: *Gastrointestinal Motility*, edited by H. L. Duthie. Trowbridge, UK: Esher, 1978, p. 537–539. (6th Int. Symp. Gastrointest. Motil. Health Dis., Edinburgh, Scotland, Sept. 12–16, 1977).
266. MCGREGOR, G. P., A. E. BISHOP, M. A. BLANK, N. D. CHRISTOFIDES, Y. YIANGOU, J. M. POLAK, AND S. R. BLOOM. Comparative distribution of vasoactive intestinal polypeptide (VIP), substance P and PHI in the enteric sphincters of the cat. *Experientia Basel* 40: 469–471, 1984.
267. MCSWINEY, B. A. Innervation of the stomach. *Physiol. Rev.* 11: 478–505, 1931.
268. MEDVEDEV, M. D., AND V. D. SUHODOLO (editors). *Physiology and Pathology of the Sphincteric Regions of the Digestive System. Abstracts of Soviet-Union Symposium.* Tomsk, USSR: Rotprint, 1984.
269. MEI, N. Mecanorecepteurs vagaux digestifs chez le chat. *Exp. Brain Res.* 11: 502–514, 1970.
270. MEI, N., J. SALDUCCI, H. MONGES, AND F. FARNARIER. Afferent vagal impulses from the lower oesophageal sphincter of the cat. *Rend. R. Gastroenterol.* 4: 65–68, 1972.
271. MEISSNER, A. J., K. L. BOWES, R. ZWICK, AND E. E. DANIEL. Effect of motilin on the lower oesophageal sphincter. *Gut* 17: 925–932, 1976.
272. MELMAN, E. P. *Functional Morphology of the Innervation of the Digestive Organs.* Moscow: Medizina, 1970.
273. MENNIER, P., AND P. MOLLARD. Control of the internal anal sphincter (manometric study with human subjects). *Pfluegers Arch.* 370: 233–239, 1977.
274. MILUSHEVA, E. A., AND V. A. BURY. The role of transmembrane ion currents in the excitability of the smooth muscles of the lower esophageal and pyloric sphincters (Abstract). In: *Proc. 3rd Int. Symp. Physiol. Pharmacol. Smooth Muscle, Varna, Bulgaria.* Sofia, Bulgaria: Bulgarian Acad. Sci., 1982, p. 83.
275. MIOLAN, J. P., AND C. ROMAN. Modification de l'électromyogramme gastrique du chien par stimulation des nerfs extrinséques. *J. Physiol. Paris* 63: 561–576, 1971.
276. MIOLAN, J. P., AND C. ROMAN. Décharge des fibres vagales efférentes destinees au cardia du chien. *J. Physiol. Paris* 66: 171–198, 1973.
277. MIR, S. S., G. R. MASON, AND H. S. ORMSBEE. An inhibitory innervation at the gastroduodenal junction in anaesthetized dogs. *Gastroenterology* 73: 432–434, 1977.
278. MIR, S. S., G. L. TELFORD, G. R. MASON, AND H. S. ORMSBEE. Noncholinergic nonadrenergic inhibitory innervation of the canine pylorus. *Gastroenterology* 76: 1443–1448, 1979.
279. MISHIMA, K., AND H. KURIYAMA. Effects of prostaglandins on electrical and mechanical activities of the guinea-pig stomach. *Jpn. J. Physiol.* 26: 537–548, 1976.
280. MISIEWICZ, J. J., S. L. WALLER, P. P. ANTONEY, AND J. W. GUMMER. Achalasia of the cardia: pharmacology and histopathology of isolated cardiac sphincteric muscle from patients with and without achalasia. *Q. J. Med.* 38: 17–30, 1969.
281. MIZHORKOVA, Z., AND M. PAPASOVA. Excitatory adrenergic receptors in the intestinal and colonic smooth muscle of the ileocaecal region. *Acta Physiol. Pharmacol. Bulg.* 3: 9–17, 1977.
282. MONGES, H., J. SALDUCCI, B. NANDY, F. RANIERI, J. GONELLA, AND M. BOUVIER. The electrical activity of internal anal sphincter: a comparative study in man and in cats. In: *Gastrointestinal Motility*, edited by J. Christensen. New York: Raven, 1980, p. 495–501. (7th Int. Symp. Gastrointest. Motil., Iowa City, Iowa, Sept. 11–14, 1979.)
283. MONGES, H., J. SALDUCCI, AND C. ROMAN. Etude electromyographique de la contraction oesophagienne chez l'homme normal. *Arch. Fr. Mal. Appar. Dig.* 57: 545–550, 1968.
284. MORGAN, K. G., T. G. MUIR, AND J. H. SZURSZEWSKI. The electrical basis for contraction and relaxation in canine fundal smooth muscle. *J. Physiol. Lond.* 311: 475–488, 1981.
285. MUKHOPADHYAY, A. K., AND M. KUNNEMANN. Mechanism of lower esophageal sphincter stimulation by bombesin in the opossum. *Gastroenterology* 76: 1409–1414, 1979.
286. NAKANISHI, H., H. YOSHIDA, AND T. SUZUKI. Inhibitory effects of prostaglandins $E_1$ and $E_2$ on cholinergic transmission in isolated canine tracheal muscle. *Jpn. J. Pharmacol.* 26: 669–674, 1976.
287. NISSAN, S., V. VINOGRAD, A. HADARI, P. MERGUERIAN, O. ZAMIR, O. LERNAU, AND M. HANANI. Physiological and pharmacological studies of the internal anal sphincter in the rat. *J. Pediatr. Surg.* 19: 12–14, 1984.
288. NOZDRACHEV, A. D. *Anatomy of the Cat.* Leningrad, USSR: Nauka, 1973.
289. OLSEN, A. M., J. F. SCHLEGEL, AND W. S. PAYNE. The hypotensive gastroesophageal sphincter. *Mayo Clin. Proc.* 48: 165–172, 1973.
290. ORLOV, R., V. ISAKOV, A. KETKIN, AND I. PLEHANOV. *Regulatory Mechanisms of the Cells of Smooth Muscles and Myocardium.* Leningrad, USSR: Nauka, 1971.
291. OUYANG, A., AND S. COHEN. Multiple 5-hydroxytryptamine receptors on feline ileum and ileocecal sphincter. *Am. J. Physiol.* 244 (*Gastrointest. Liver Physiol.* 7): G426–G434, 1983.
292. OZAKI, H., H. KARAKI, AND N. URAKAWA. Possible role of Na-Ca exchange mechanism in the contractions induced in guinea-pig aorta by potassium free solution and ouabain. *Naunyn-Schmiedebergs Arch. Pharmacol.* 304: 203–209, 1978.
293. OZAKI, H., AND N. URAKAWA. Na-Ca exchange and tension development in guinea-pig aorta. *Naunyn-Schmiedebergs Arch. Pharmacol.* 309: 171–178, 1979.
294. OZAKI, H., AND N. URAKAWA. Involvement of a Na-Ca exchange mechanism in contraction by low Na solution in isolated pig aorta. *Pfluegers Arch.* 390: 107–112, 1981.
295. RADOVAN, W., R. A. GODOY, R. O. DANTAS, U. G. MENEGHELLI, R. B. OLIVEIRA, AND L. E. TRONCON. Lower oesophageal sphincter response to pentagastrin in chagasic patients with megaoesophagus and megacolon. *Gut* 21: 85–90, 1980.
296. PAHLIN, P. E. Extrinsic nervous control of the ileocecal sphincter in the cat. *Acta Physiol. Scand. Suppl.* 426: 1–32, 1975.
297. PAHLIN, P. E., AND J. KEWENTER. Reflexogenic contraction of the ileocecal sphincter in the cat following small or large intestinal distension. *Acta Physiol. Scand.* 95: 126–132, 1975.
298. PAHLIN, P. E., AND J. KEWENTER. Sympathetic nervous control of the cat ileocecal sphincter. *Am. J. Physiol.* 231: 296–305, 1976.
299. PAHLIN, P. E., AND J. KEWENTER. The vagal control of the ileocecal sphincter in the cat. *Acta Physiol. Scand.* 96: 433–442, 1976.
300. PAPASOVA, M., AND E. ATANASSOVA. *Modulatory Role of Some Peptides on the Gastrointestinal Motility.* Sofia, Bulgaria: Bulgarian Acad. Sci., 1983.
301. PAPASOVA, M., AND K. BOEV. The slow potential and its relationship to the gastric smooth muscle contraction. In: *Physiology of Smooth Muscle*, edited by E. Bülbring and M. F. Shuba. New York: Raven, 1976, p. 209–216.
302. PAPASOVA, M., AND K. BOEV. Electromechanical coupling in the phasic and tonic contractions of the gastric smooth muscle. In: *Physiology and Pharmacology of Smooth Muscle*, edited by M. Papasova and E. Atanassova. Sofia: Bulgarian Acad. Sci., 1977, p. 24–31. (1st Int. Symp. Physiol. Pharmacol. Smooth Muscle, Varna, Bulgaria, Sept. 28–30, 1976.)
303. PAPASOVA, M., AND K. BOEV. On the excitation-contraction coupling in the smooth muscles building up the stomach and its sphincters (Abstract). In: *Proc. Int. Symp. Physiol. Pharmacol. Smooth Muscle*, 3rd, Varna, Bulgaria, 1982. Sofia: Bulgarian Acad. Sci., 1982, p. 91.
304. PAPASOVA, M., K. BOEV, A. BONEV, AND E. MILUSHEVA. Relationship between the changes in the membrane potential and the contraction of the smooth muscles of the lower esophageal sphincter and ileocecal sphincter. *Agressologie* 22: 205–208, 1981.

305. PAPASOVA, M., K. BOEV, V. VELKOVA, A. BONEV, E. MAVROVA, N. KORTEZOVA, S. GACHILOVA, AND G. SPASSOV. Electrophysiological properties of the gastrointestinal sphincter smooth muscles (Abstract). In: *Proc. Int. Symp. Physiol. Pharmacol. Smooth Muscle.* 2nd, Varna, Bulgaria, 1979. Sofia: Bulgarian Acad. Sci., 1979, p. 97.
306. PAPASOVA, M., S. GACHILOVA, AND Z. MIZHORKOVA. Analysis of the innervation of the gastroduodenal region. *Acta Physiol. Pharmacol. Bulg.* 7: 3–9, 1981.
307. PAPASOVA, M., N. KORTEZOVA, AND E. ATANASSOVA. Participation of the pyloric sphincter in the coordination of the electrical activity in the stomach and duodenum. In: *Motility of the Digestive Tract*, edited by M. Wienbeck. New York: Raven, 1982, p. 201–206. (8th Int. Symp. Gastrointest. Motil., Köenigstein, FRG, Sept. 7–11, 1981.)
308. PAPASOVA, M., AND I. LOLOVA. *Gastrointestinal Sphincters. Functional-Structural Organization.* Sofia, Bulgaria: Bulgarian Acad. Sci., 1981.
309. PAPASOVA, M., E. MILUSHEVA, A. BONEV, K. BOEV, AND N. KORTEZOVA. On the changes in the membrane potential and the contractile activity of the smooth muscle of the lower esophageal and ileocecal sphincters upon increased $K^+$ in the nutrient solution. *Acta Physiol. Pharmacol. Bulg.* 6: 41–49, 1980.
310. PAPASOVA, M., E. MILUSHEVA, A. BONEV, AND S. GACHILOVA. Specific features in the electrical and contractile activities of the gastrointestinal sphincters. *Acta Physiol. Pharmacol. Bulg.* 6: 19–27, 1980.
311. PAPASOVA, M., AND Z. MIZHORKOVA. Coordination between the electrical activity of the small intestine and the colon in the ileocecal region. *Acta Physiol. Pharmacol. Bulg.* 2: 3–12, 1976.
312. PARKS, A. G., D. J. FISCHLOCK, J. D. H. CAMERON, AND H. MAY. Preliminary investigation of the pharmacology of the human internal anal sphincter. *Gut* 10: 674–677, 1969.
313. PATON, W. D. M., AND E. S. VIZI. The inhibitory action of noradrenaline and adrenaline on acetylcholine output by guinea-pig ileum longitudinal muscle strip. *Br. J. Pharmacol.* 35: 10–28, 1969.
314. PETKOV, B., AND R. RADOMIROV. Interactions of prostaglandin $E_1$ and prostaglandin $F_{2\alpha}$ with the adrenergic and cholinergic transmission in the cat jejunum. In: *Physiology and Pharmacology of Smooth Muscle*, edited by M. Papasova and E. Atanassova. Sofia, Bulgaria: Bulgarian Acad. Sci., 1977, p. 164–170. (1st Int. Symp. Physiol. Pharmacol. Smooth Muscle, Varna, Bulgaria, Sept. 28–30, 1976.)
315. PFLIUKE, F., AND E. LINAR. Effect of pentagastrin on the closing pressure of the inferior esophageal sphincter and gastroesophageal reflux. *Sechenov Physiol. J. USSR* 69: 1050–1052, 1983.
316. PHAOSAWASDI, K., AND R. S. FISHER. Hormonal effects on the pylorus. *Am. J. Physiol.* 243 (*Gastrointest. Liver Physiol.* 5): G330–G335, 1982.
317. PHAOSAWASDI, K., R. GOPPOLD, AND R. S. FISHER. Pyloric pressure response to insulin-induced hypoglycemia in humans. *Am. J. Physiol.* 241 (*Gastrointest. Liver Physiol.* 4): G321–G327, 1981.
318. PORTER, H. N. Megacolon, a physiological study. *Proc. R. Soc. Med.* 54: 224–227, 1961.
319. PRICE, L. M., T. Y. EL-SHARKAWY, H. Y. MUI, AND N. E. DIAMANT. Effect of bilateral cervical vagotomy on balloon-induced lower esophageal sphincter relaxation in the dog. *Gastroenterology* 77: 324–329, 1979.
320. PRÖVE, J., AND H. J. EHRLEIN. Motor function of gastric antrum and pylorus for evacuation of low and high viscosity meals in dogs. *Gut* 23: 150–156, 1982.
321. QUIGLEY, E. M., T. J. BRODY, S. F. PHILLIPS, M. WIENBECK, B. L. TUCKER, AND A. HADDAD. Motility of the terminal ileum and ileocecal sphincter in healthy humans. *Gastroenterology* 87: 857–866, 1984.
322. QUIGLEY, E. M., S. F. PHILLIPS, AND J. DENT. Distinctive patterns of interdigestive motility at the canine ileocolonic junction. *Gastroenterology* 87: 836–844, 1984.
323. QUIGLEY, E. M., S. F. PHILLIPS, J. DENT, AND B. M. TAYLOR. Myoelectric activity and intraluminal pressure of the canine ileocolonic sphincter. *Gastroenterology* 85: 1054–1062, 1983.
324. RADOMIROV, R., V. PETKOV, AND M. DAVIDOFF. Neurotransmitted effect of prostaglandin $F_{2\alpha}$ in isolated cat jejunum. *Methods Find. Exp. Clin. Pharmacol.* 5: 275–279, 1983.
325. RADOMIROV, R., V. PETKOV, AND S. YANEV. Effects of prostaglandin $F_{2\alpha}$ on the contractile responses of guinea-pig ileum to electrical stimulation. *Experientia* 39: 754–755, 1983.
326. RASH, R. M., AND M. D. THOMAS. The intrinsic innervation of the gastro-oesophageal and pyloro-duodenal junctions. *J. Anat.* 96: 389–396, 1962.
327. RATTAN, S., AND R. K. GOYAL. Neural control of the lower esophageal sphincter influence of the vagus nerves. *J. Clin. Invest.* 54: 899–906, 1974.
328. RATTAN, S., AND R. K. GOYAL. Effect of dopamine on the esophageal smooth muscle in vivo. *Gastroenterology* 70: 377–381, 1976.
329. RATTAN, S., AND R. K. GOYAL. Identification and localization of opioid receptors in the opossum lower esophageal sphincter. *J. Pharmacol. Exp. Ther.* 224: 391–397, 1983.
330. RATTAN, S., M. GRADY, AND R. K. GOYAL. Vasoactive intestinal peptide causes peristaltic contractions in the esophageal body. *Life Sci.* 30: 1557–1563, 1982.
331. RATTAN, S., T. HERSH, AND R. K. GOYAL. Effect of prostaglandin $F_{2\alpha}$ and gastrin pentapeptide on the lower esophageal sphincter. *Proc. Soc. Exp. Biol. Med.* 141: 573–575, 1972.
332. RAYAN, J. P., W. J. SNAPE, AND S. COHEN. Influence of vagal cooling on esophageal function. *Am. J. Physiol.* 232 (*Endocrinol. Metab. Gastrointest. Physiol.* 2): E159–E164, 1977.
333. RAYNER, V. Observations on the functional internal anal sphincter of the vervet monkey. *J. Physiol. Lond.* 213: 27P–28P, 1971.
334. RAYNER, V. Characteristics of the internal anal sphincter and the rectum of the vervet monkey. *J. Physiol. Lond.* 286: 383–399, 1979.
335. REHFELD, J. F. Immunochemical studies on cholecystokinin. *J. Biol. Chem.* 253: 4016–4021, 1978.
336. RESIN, H., D. H. STERN, R. A. L. STURDEVANT, AND J. I. ISENBERG. Effect of the C-terminal octapeptide of cholecystokinin on lower esophageal sphincter pressure in man. *Gastroenterology* 64: 946–949, 1973.
337. REYNOLDS, D. G., G. E. DEMAREE, AND M. H. HEIFFER. An excitatory adrenergic $\alpha$-receptor mechanism of terminal guinea-pig ileum. *Proc. Soc. Exp. Biol. Med.* 125: 73–78, 1967.
338. REYNOLDS, J. C., M. R. DUKEHART, A. OUYANG, AND S. COHEN. Bombesin: an interneuron transmitter of the feline lower esophageal sphincter (LES) (Abstract). *Dig. Dis. Sci.* 29, Suppl: 69, 1984.
339. REYNOLDS, J. C., A. OUYANG, AND S. COHEN. Evidence for an opiate-mediated pyloric sphincter reflex. *Am. J. Physiol.* 246 (*Gastrointest. Liver Physiol.* 9): G130–G136, 1984.
340. REYNOLDS, J. C., A. OUYANG, AND S. COHEN. A lower esophageal sphincter reflex involving substance P. *Am. J. Physiol.* 246 (*Gastrointest. Liver Physiol.* 9): G346–G354, 1984.
341. RICHARDS, J. G., AND J. P. TRANZER. The ultrastructural localization of amine storage sites in the central nervous system with the aid of a specific marker 5-hydroxydopamine. *Brain Res.* 17: 463–469, 1970.
342. ROLING, G. T., R. L. FURRELL, AND D. O. CASTELL. Cholinergic response of the lower esophageal sphincter. *Am. J. Physiol.* 222: 967–972, 1972.
343. ROMAN, C., AND J. GONELLA. Extrinsic control of digestive tract motility. In: *Physiology of the Gastrointestinal Tract*, edited by L. R. Johnson. New York: Raven, 1981, vol. I, chapt. 9, p. 289–333.
344. ROMAN, C., J. GONELLA, J. P. NIEL, M. CONDAMIN, AND J. P. MIOLAN. Effets de la stimulation vagale et de l'adrénaline sur la musculeuse lisse du bas oesophage du chat. In: *Smooth*

*Muscle Pharmacology and Physiology*, edited by M. Worcel and G. Vassort. Paris: INSERM, 1976, vol. 50, p. 415–422.

345. ROVELSTAD, R. A. The incompetent pyloric sphincter. Bile and mucosal ulceration. *Am. J. Dig. Dis.* 21: 165–173, 1976.
346. RUBIN, M. R., B. A. CARDWELL, A. OUYANG, W. J. SNAPE, AND S. COHEN. Effect of bethanechol or vagal nerve stimulation on ileocecal sphincter pressure in the cat. *Gastroenterology* 80: 974–979, 1981.
347. RUBIN, M. R., W. J. SNAPE, S. COHEN, AND J. FOURNET. Adrenergic regulation of ileocaecal sphincter function in the cat. *Gastroenterology* 78: 15–21, 1980.
348. RÜEGG, J. G. Smooth muscle tone. *Physiol. Rev.* 51: 201–248, 1971.
349. SAHYOUN, H. A., B. COSTALL, AND R. J. NAYLOR. Catecholamine-induced relaxation and contraction of the lower oesophageal and pyloric sphincters of guinea-pig stomach: modification by domperidone. *J. Pharm. Pharmacol.* 34: 318–324, 1982.
350. SANDERS, K. M. Role of prostaglandins in regulating gastric motility. *Am. J. Physiol.* 247 (*Gastrointest. Liver Physiol.* 10): G117–G126, 1984.
351. SANDERS, K. M., AND G. ROSS. Effects of endogenous prostaglandin E on intestinal motility. *Am. J. Physiol.* 234 (*Endocrinol. Metab. Gastrointest. Physiol.* 2): E204–E208, 1978.
352. SANIN, G. U. Neuronal activity of the submucous plexus of the pyloric and ileocecal sphincters. *Sechenov Physiol. J. USSR* 64: 828–834, 1978.
353. SCHENCK, E. A., AND E. L. FREDERICKSON. Pharmacologic evidence for a cardiac sphincter mechanism in the cat. *Gastroenterology* 40: 75–80, 1961.
354. SCHEURER, U., L. VARGA, E. DRACK, H. R. BUERKI, AND F. HALTER. Mechanism of action of cholecystokinin octapeptide on rat antrum, pylorus and duodenum. *Am. J. Physiol.* 244 (*Gastrointest. Liver Physiol.* 3): G266–G272, 1983.
355. SCHLEGEL, J. E., AND C. F. CODE. Pressure characteristics of the esophagus and its sphincters in dogs. *Am. J. Physiol.* 193: 9–14, 1958.
356. SCHNAUFER, L., J. L. TALBERT, J. A. HALLER, N. C. REID, F. TOBON, AND M. M. SCHUSTER. Differential sphincteric studies in the diagnosis of anorectal disorders of childhood. *J. Pediat. Surg.* 2: 538–543, 1967.
357. SCHULZ, R., AND C. CARTWRIGHT. Sensitization of the smooth muscle by prostaglandin $E_1$ contributes to reversal of drug-induced inhibition of the guinea-pig ileum. *Naunyn-Schmiedebergs Arch. Pharmacol.* 294: 257–260, 1976.
358. SCHULZE, K., J. J. HAJJAR, AND J. CHRISTENSEN. Regional differences in potassium content of smooth muscle from opossum esophagus. *Am. J. Physiol.* 235 (*Endocrinol. Metab. Gastrointest. Physiol.* 6): E709–E713, 1978.
359. SCHULZE, K., W. J. DODDS, J. CHRISTENSEN, AND J. D. WOOD. Esophageal manometry in the opossum. *Am. J. Physiol.* 233 (*Endocrinol. Metab. Gastrointest. Physiol.* 3): E152–E159, 1977.
360. SCHULZE-DELRIEU, K., AND S. S. SHIRAZI. Neuromuscular differentiation of the human pylorus. *Gastroenterology* 84: 287–292, 1983.
361. SCHULZE-DELRIEU, K., AND J. P. WALL. Determinants of flow across isolated gastroduodenal junctions of cats and rabbits. *Am. J. Physiol.* 245 (*Gastrointest. Liver Physiol.* 2): G257–G264, 1983.
362. SCHUSTER, M. M. Motor action of rectum and anal sphincters in continence and defecation. In: *Handbook of Physiology. Alimentary Canal. Motility*, edited by C. F. Code. Washington, DC: Am. Physiol. Soc., 1968, sect. 6, vol. IV, chapt. 103, p. 2121–2146.
363. SCHUSTER, M. M. The riddle of the sphincters. *Gastroenterology* 69: 249–262, 1975.
364. SCHUSTER, M. M., T. R. HENDRIX, AND A. I. MENDELOFF. The internal anal sphincter response: manometric studies of its normal physiology, neural pathways and alteration in bowel disorders. *J. Clin. Invest.* 42: 196–207, 1963.
365. SEELING, L. L., AND R. K. GOYAL. Morphological evaluation of opossum lower esophageal sphincter. *Gastroenterology* 75: 51–58, 1978.
366. SHAFIK, A. A new concept of the anatomy of the anal sphincter mechanism and the physiology of defecation. *Surg. Gastroenterol.* 12: 175–182, 1978.
367. SHEINER, H. L. Gastric motility. In: *Scientific Basis of Gastroenterology*, edited by H. L. Duthie and K. G. Wormsley. London: Churchill Livingstone, 1979, p. 440–460.
368. SHEPHERD, J. J., AND P. G. WRIGHT. The response of the internal anal sphincter in man to stimulation of the presacral nerve. *Am. J. Dig. Dis.* 13: 421–427, 1968.
369. SIEGEL, S. R., F. C. BROWN, D. O. CASTELL, L. F. JOHNSON, AND S. I. SAID. Effects of vasoactive intestinal polypeptide (VIP) on lower esophageal sphincter in awake baboons: comparison with glucagon and secretin. *Dig. Dis. Sci.* 24: 345–349, 1979.
370. SINAR, D. R., J. R. FLETCHER, AND D. O. CASTELL. Prostaglandin $E_1$ effects on resting and cholinergically stimulated lower esophageal sphincter pressure in cats. *Prostaglandins* 21: 581–590, 1981.
371. SINGLETON, A. O., D. C. REDMOND, AND J. E. McMURRAY. Ileocecal resection and small bowel transit and absorption. *Ann. Surg.* 159: 690–694, 1964.
372. SNAPE, W. J., AND S. COHEN. Control of lower esophageal sphincter function: neurohumoral and myogenic factors. In: *The Esophagus*, edited by Leo von der Reis. Basel: Karger, 1978, p. 76–93.
373. STELZNER, F., W. LIERSE, AND M. HENRICH. Die Myoarchitektur des Pylorus. *Langenbecks Arch. Chir.* 354: 237–244, 1981.
374. STEVENS, C. E., AND A. F. SELLERS. Pressure events in bovine esophagus and reticulorumen associated with eructation, deglutition and regurgitation. *Am. J. Physiol.* 199: 598–602, 1960.
375. STURDEVANT, R. A. L. Is gastrin the major regulator of lower esophageal sphincter pressure? *Gastroenterology* 67: 551–553, 1974.
376. SUBISSI, A., AND M. GUELFI. Effects of rociverine and other spasmolytic agents on caerulein-induced delay in gastric emptying in the conscious rat. *Arch. Int. Pharmacodyn.* 257: 130–137, 1982.
377. SZURSZEWSKI, J. H. The effect of tetraethylammonium ion on the action potential of the canine antrum. In: *Smooth Muscle Pharmacology and Physiology*, edited by M. Worcel and G. Vassort. Paris: INSERM, 1976, vol. 50, p. 247–249.
378. THOMAS, P. A., AND R. J. EARLAM. The effect of the gastrointestinal polypeptide hormones on the electrical activity and pressure of the isolated perfused canine gastro-oesophageal sphincter. In: *Gastrointestinal Motility*, edited by E. E. Daniel. Vancouver: Mitchell, 1974, p. 243–249. (4th Int. Symp. Gastrointest. Motil., Banff, Alberta, Canada, Sept. 6–8, 1973.)
379. TODOROV, L. On certain characteristics of the internal anal sphincter of cats. *C. R. Acad. Bulg. Sci.* 35: 1435–1437, 1982.
380. TODOROV, L. Physiological Characteristic of the Nerve Muscle Organization in the Internal Anal Sphincter of the Cat. Sofia, Bulgaria: Bulgarian Acad. Sci., 1984. Dissertation.
381. TODOROV, L., AND M. PAPASOVA. Adrenergic receptors in internal anal sphincter of cat (in vitro study). *C. R. Acad. Bulg. Sci.* 37: 387–389, 1984.
382. TODOROV, L., AND M. PAPASOVA. Modulation of the release of noradrenaline and of noncholinergic, nonadrenergic inhibitory neurotransmitter through presynaptic N-cholinergic receptors by means of depolarizing agents in cat internal anal sphincter. *Acta Physiol. Pharmacol. Bulg.* 10: 42–52, 1984.
383. TODOROV, L., AND M. PAPASOVA. Neurotransmitter interactions in smooth muscle from cat internal anal sphincter. *Acta Physiol. Pharmacol. Bulg.* 10: 3–12, 1984.
384. TORGERSEN, J. The muscular build and movements of the stomach and duodenal bulb. *Acta Radiol. Stockholm Suppl.* 45: 1–191, 1942.
385. TUCH, A., AND S. COHEN. Lower esophageal sphincter relax-

ation: studies on the neurogenic inhibitory mechanism. *J. Clin. Invest.* 52: 14–20, 1973.
386. UDDMAN, R., J. ALUMETS, R. HAKANSON, F. SUNDLER, AND B. WALLES. Peptidergic (enkephalin) innervation of the mammalian esophagus. *Gastroenterology* 78: 732–737, 1980.
387. URSO, S. A., R. FILECCIA, AND M. E. MONTALBANO. Gastric control of duodenal function of the gastroduodenal junction. *Arch. Int. Physiol. Biochim.* 83: 827–835, 1975.
388. USTACH, T. J., F. TOBON, T. HAMBRECHT, D. D. BASS, AND M. M. SCHUSTER. Electrophysiological aspects of human sphincter function. *J. Clin. Invest.* 49: 41–48, 1970.
389. VALENZUELA, J. E., AND C. DEFILIPPI. Pyloric sphincter studies in peptide ulcer patients. *Am. J. Dig. Dis.* 21: 229–232, 1976.
390. VALENZUELA, J. E., C. DEFILIPPI, AND A. CSENDES. Manometric studies on the human pyloric sphincter. Effect of cigarette smoking, metaclopromide, atropine. *Gastroenterology* 70: 481–483, 1976.
391. VAN BREEMEN, C., F. WUYTACK, AND R. CASTEELS. Stimulation of $^{45}Ca$ efflux from smooth muscle cells by metabolic inhibition and high K depolarization. *Pfluegers Arch.* 359: 183–196, 1975.
392. VELKOVA, V., M. PAPASOVA, K. BOEV, AND A. BONEV. Inhibitory action of acetylcholine on the smooth muscle from the lower esophageal sphincter. *Acta Physiol. Pharmacol. Bulg.* 5: 11–19, 1979.
393. VELKOVA, V., M. PAPASOVA, AND R. RADOMIROV. Effects of $PGE_1$ and $PGF_{2\alpha}$ on the responses of gastrointestinal sphincters to field stimulation. *Eur. J. Pharmacol.* 75: 297–303, 1981.
394. VON HOLSCHNEIDER, A. M. Elektromyographische Untersuchungen der musculi sphincter ani externus und internus in Bezug auf die anorektale Manometrie. *Langenbecks Arch. Chir.* 333: 303–316, 1973.
395. WALDECK, F. A new procedure for functional analysis of the lower esophageal sphincter (LES). *Pfluegers Arch.* 335: 74–84, 1972.
396. WALSH, J. H. Gastrointestinal hormones and peptides. In: *Physiology of the Gastrointestinal Tract*, edited by L. R. Johnson. New York: Raven, 1981, vol. I, chapt. 3, p. 59–144.
397. WATANABE, M., C. SUGAWA, T. HATAFUKU, AND S. MORI. Effect of Pitressin (8-arginine vasopressin) on the lower esophageal sphincter in dogs. *Nippon Heikatsukin Gakkai Zasshi* 85: 231–237, 1984.
398. WEIGEL, R. J., J. A. CONNOR, AND C. L. PROSSER. Two roles of calcium during the spike in circular muscle of small intestine in cat. *Am. J. Physiol.* 237 (*Cell Physiol.* 3): C247–C256, 1979.
399. WEISBRODT, N. W. Gastrointestinal motility. In: *Gastrointestinal Physiology I*, edited by A. G. Guyton. Baltimore, MD: University Park, 1974, vol. 4, chapt. 5, p. 139–181.
400. WEISBRODT, N. W. Motility of the small intestine. In: *Physiology of the Gastrointestinal Tract*, edited by L. R. Johnson. New York: Raven, 1981, vol. I, chapt. 13, p. 411–443.
401. WEISBRODT, N. W., E. M. COPELAND, R. W. KEARLEY, E. P. MOORE, AND L. R. JOHNSON. Effects of pentagastrin on electrical activity of small intestine of the dog. *Am. J. Physiol.* 227: 425–429, 1974.
402. WEISER, H. F., G. LEPSIEN, K. GOLENHOFEN, AND R. SIEWERT. Clinical and experimental studies on the effect of nifedipine on smooth muscle of the oesophagus and LES. In: *Gastrointestinal Motility*, edited by H. L. Duthie. Trowbridge, UK: Esher, 1978, p. 565–572. (6th Int. Symp. Gastrointest. Motil. Health Dis., Edinburgh, Scotland, Sept. 12–16, 1977.)
403. WELCH, R. W., AND S. T. DRAKE. Normal lower esophageal sphincter pressure: a comparison of rapid vs. slow pull through techniques. *Gastroenterology* 78: 1446–1451, 1980.
404. WESTFALL, T. C. Local regulation of adrenergic neurotransmission. *Physiol. Rev.* 57: 659–728, 1977.
405. WHITE, C. M., V. POXON, AND J. ALEXANDER-WILLIAMS. A study of motility of normal human gastroduodenal region. *Dig. Dis. Sci.* 26: 609–617, 1981.
406. WIENBECK, M., AND I. ALTAPARMACOV. Is the internal anal sphincter controlled by a myoelectrical mechanism? In: *Gastrointestinal Motility*, edited by J. Christensen. New York: Raven, 1980, p. 487–493. (7th Int. Symp. Gastrointest. Motil., Iowa City, Iowa, Sept. 11–14, 1979.)
407. WIENBECK, M., AND H. JANSSEN. Der Einfluss von Nahrungsaufnahme auf die elektrische Aktivität des Ileokolons. *Z. Gastroenterol.* 11: 717–724, 1973.
408. WIENBECK, M., AND H. JANSSEN. Electrical control mechanisms at the ileo-colic junction. In: *Gastrointestinal Motility*, edited by E. E. Daniel. Vancouver: Mitchell, 1974, p. 97–107. (4th Int. Symp. Gastrointest. Motil., Banff, Alberta, Canada, Sept. 6–8, 1973.)
409. WINGATE, G. L., E. A. PEARCE, M. HUTTON, A. DAND, H. H. THOMPSON, AND E. WUNSCH. Quantitative comparison of the effects of cholecystokinin, secretin and pentagastrin on gastrointestinal myoelectric activity in the conscious fasted dog. *Gut* 19: 593–601, 1978.
410. WINSHIP, D. H., AND F. F. ZBORALSKE. The esophageal propulsive force: esophageal response to acute obstruction. *J. Clin. Invest.* 46: 1391–1401, 1967.
411. WOOD, J. Physiology of the enteric nervous system. In: *Physiology of the Gastrointestinal Tract*, edited by L. R. Johnson. New York: Raven, 1981, vol. I, chapt. 1, p. 1–37.
412. TAMAGISHI, T., AND H. T. DEBAS. Cholecystokinin inhibits gastric emptying by acting on both proximal stomach and pylorus. *Am. J. Physiol.* 234 (*Endocrinol. Metab. Gastrointest. Physiol.* 4): E375–E378, 1978.

CHAPTER 27

# Motor function of anorectum and pelvic floor musculature

JACOB KRIER | *Department of Physiology, Michigan State University, East Lansing, Michigan*

## CHAPTER CONTENTS

Autonomic Innervation
    Lumbar sympathetic innervation to colon, rectum, and internal anal sphincter
    Sacral parasympathetic innervation to colon, rectum, and internal anal sphincter
    Sacral afferent fibers
Somatic Innervation to Skeletal Muscle of Pelvic Floor
    Efferent innervation
    Afferent innervation
Peptides
    Vasoactive intestinal–like peptide
    Enkephalins
    Substance P–like peptide
    Somatostatin-like peptide
Motor Activity of Rectum and Internal Anal Sphincter
    General and historical considerations
    Intraluminal pressure recordings
    Electrical activity of rectum and internal anal sphincter
Motor Activity of Skeletal Muscle of Pelvic Floor
    Electromyography
    Histochemical studies
    Force measurements
Influence of Intrinsic Gastrointestinal Nerves on Motor Activity of Internal Anal Sphincter
    Cholinergic motor neurons
    Noncholinergic, nonadrenergic neurons
    Rectoanal reflexes
    Vesicoanal reflexes
Influence of Lumbar Sympathetic Nerves on Motor Activity of Colon, Rectum, and Internal Anal Sphincter
    Effect of electrical stimulation of lumbar sympathetic nerves
    Effect of interruption of lumbar sympathetic pathways to colon, rectum, and internal anal sphincter
Influence of Sacral Autonomic Nerves on Motor Activity of Internal Anal Sphincter
    Effect of electrical stimulation of sacral parasympathetic nerves
    Cholinergic agonists
Influence of Sacral Autonomic Nerves on Motor Activity of Colon and Rectum
    Effect of electrical stimulation of sacral nerves
    Cholinergic responses
    Noncholinergic, nonadrenergic responses
Influence of Somatic Nerves on Motor Activity of Skeletal Muscle of Pelvic Floor
    Somatic reflexes
    Supraspinal pathways
    Viscerosomatic reflexes
        Effect of colonic-rectal distension
        Micturition
        Electrophysiological studies
        Operant conditioning of viscerosomatic reflexes
    Flexor reflexes
Defecation
    General considerations
    Visceral and somatic afferent fibers
        Sacral visceral afferents
        Sacral somatic afferents
        Lumbar sympathetic afferents
    Sacral parasympathetic efferent fibers
    Relationship between eating and colonic motility
Motor Dysfunction of Colon, Anorectum, and Pelvic Floor Musculature
    Muscle dysfunction
    Neurogenic dysfunctions
        Myenteric plexus
        Lower motor neurons
        Afferent fibers
        Spinal cord
        Supraspinal regions

---

SMOOTH MUSCLE LAYERS of the colon, rectum, and internal anal sphincter and skeletal muscle of the pelvic floor are responsible for the storage, transport, and evacuation of gastrointestinal contents. The two control systems that regulate these activities are the electrical properties of the smooth muscle and the nervous system. Without neural input, the electrical properties of smooth muscle set a basic pattern of contractile activity that is subjected to modulation by intrinsic gastrointestinal nerves and extrinsic autonomic nerves. The intrinsic nerves are located within neural plexuses of the rectum and internal anal sphincter. The extrinsic nerves arise from both sympathetic and parasympathetic divisions of the autonomic nervous system and innervate the muscle layers of the colon, rectum, and internal anal sphincter. Two major autonomic pathways innervate the muscles of the colon, rectum, and internal anal sphincter. The sympathetic outflow arises primarily from lumbar regions of the spinal cord and passes to the smooth muscle via the inferior mesenteric ganglia and lumbar colonic and hypogastric nerves. The parasympathetic outflow passes to smooth muscle via the sacral ventral roots and pelvic nerves. The extrinsic somatic nerves arise from motor neurons in lower lumbar and sacral segments of the spinal cord and provide innervation to the skeletal musculature of the pelvic floor.

Studies of the motor activity of the rectum, internal anal sphincter, and pelvic floor musculature were reviewed in detail nineteen years ago (130, 164, 205) and only briefly since then (29, 54, 57, 206). This chapter summarizes current information about the motor control of the anal canal and rectum. It focuses on anatomical and electrophysiological studies that have provided new information, primarily on central and peripheral organization of autonomic, somatic, and intrinsic neural pathways that regulate defecation and continence. Consequently, it deals with the role of the intrinsic gastrointestinal nerves in the rectum and internal anal sphincter region and the extrinsic autonomic and somatic nerves.

Electrical properties and contractile forces generated by smooth muscle in the rectum and internal anal sphincter and skeletal muscle of the pelvic floor are surveyed. In each section, a summary of past data is presented, followed by a description of more recent observations. The anatomy of pelvic floor musculature is well known (130, 149, 205, 213-215, 220, 246) and is not reviewed in detail.

## AUTONOMIC INNERVATION

### Lumbar Sympathetic Innervation to Colon, Rectum, and Internal Anal Sphincter

The lumbar sympathetic outflow consists of preganglionic fibers arising from neurons located in the autonomic nucleus of the spinal cord [$L_2$–$L_4$ spinal segments (143–145)]. In most mammalian species, preganglionic fibers synapse with neurons in prevertebral ganglia [e.g., inferior mesenteric ganglia, pelvic plexus (40, 80, 138, 143, 148)] and in one species, the guinea pig, in paravertebral ganglia [sacral sympathetic chain (40)].

Postganglionic fibers arising from neurons in the inferior mesenteric ganglia divide into two principal groups: the lumbar colonic nerves and hypogastric nerves. The lumbar colonic nerves form a diffuse network around the inferior mesenteric artery and accompany the artery to the distal colon and rectum. The hypogastric nerves run distally to join the pelvic plexus. Postganglionic fibers that arise from prevertebral and paravertebral ganglia innervate smooth muscle of the rectum, internal anal sphincter, and anal accessory musculature. Adrenergic fibers in the guinea pig hypogastric nerve pass through the pelvic plexus or synapse with neurons located in the pelvic plexus (143). Adrenergic fibers from the sacral sympathetic chain accompany rectal arteries to innervate the internal anal sphincter (40).

Fluorescence and microscopic studies in humans and experimental animals reveal the distribution of adrenergic fibers in the colon, rectum, and internal anal sphincter. Noradrenergic fibers that penetrate the gastrointestinal wall have been identified in the myenteric and submucosal plexus, blood vessels, and external smooth muscle layers (11, 12, 42, 79, 82, 116). Adrenergic varicosities containing small dense-core vesicles typical of adrenergic terminals have been identified in myenteric and submucosal plexuses (124, 175). These varicosities can be destroyed by 6-hydroxydopamine and depleted of transmitter stores with reserpine.

Adrenergic fibers are also distributed to the external muscularis of the colon, rectum, and internal anal sphincter. In most regions of the colon, adrenergic fibers densely innervate circular muscle fibers but sparsely innervate longitudinal muscle fibers. In contrast, in distal colon, rectum, and internal anal sphincter of the cat, longitudinal muscle fibers receive a dense adrenergic innervation (116). In the guinea pig, the density of adrenergic fibers in circular muscle of the rectum and internal anal sphincter is also greater than circular muscle of the colon (41, 42). Higher density of adrenergic innervation to the rectum and internal anal sphincter relative to the colon has also been reported in humans (12, 13) and monkeys (191).

### Sacral Parasympathetic Innervation to Colon, Rectum, and Internal Anal Sphincter

Organization of the sacral parasympathetic outflow was first described in the cat (143, 145). Parasympathetic efferent fibers emerge from the spinal cord usually in the second and third ventral roots, and then pass peripherally via the pelvic nerves. Based upon degeneration experiments, approximately two-thirds (2,200 fibers) of the myelinated fibers are efferent and one-third are afferent. Nonmyelinated efferent axons account for 15% of all sacral ventral root efferents (7, 35) and with the pelvic nerve provide the principal preganglionic innervation to the smooth muscle of the colon and rectum of the cat (46, 47, 137).

Langley and Anderson (143) reported that the peripheral pelvic nerve of the cat is separated into two or three major branches. One of them passes to the surface of the distal colon, and the remainder innervate the urethra and urinary bladder. The branch to the large intestine enters the pelvic plexus. Usually four or five colonic nerve fiber bundles emanate from the pelvic plexus to ascend particularly orad beneath the serosal surface of the colon and between the external smooth muscle layers for considerable distances to mid- and proximal regions of the colon. These anatomical data have been confirmed in cat and dog colon (46, 47, 75, 137).

It is generally assumed that most parasympathetic efferent fibers synapse with neurons in the myenteric plexus. Langley and Anderson (143) reported that in the cat many of the efferent axons terminate in extramural ganglia located on the serosal surface of the distal colon and rectum and along the distribution of colonic nerve fiber bundles. Electrophysiological experiments have confirmed the existence of extramural colonic ganglia and the peripheral arrangement of the sacral parasympathetic pathway to the colon of the cat (Fig. 1). Electrical stimulation of sacral ventral roots or the pelvic nerve elicited contractions of the colon and synaptic inputs to neurons located in colonic parasympathetic ganglia (46, 137). The preganglionic input to neurons in extramural colonic ganglia was carried by nonmyelinated fibers. Synaptic input consisted of excitatory postsynaptic potentials and action potentials mediated by nicotinic receptors (137). Postganglionic neurons in colonic ganglia send their axons to the colon via colonic nerve fiber bundles. Postganglionic parasympathetic axons may provide both phasic and tonic synaptic input to neurons in the myenteric plexus and/or directly innervate colonic smooth muscle, blood vessels, and mucous glands.

The distribution and morphology of parasympathetic preganglionic neurons in the sacral spinal cord that innervate the colon and rectum via the pelvic nerve have been traced using horseradish peroxidase (HRP) techniques (45, 49, 170, 170a). The application of HRP to colonic branches of the pelvic nerve in the cat labeled a dorsal band of neurons at the base of the dorsal horn primarily in lamina V and VI of Rexed (192). This population consisted of 34% of cells in the sacral parasympathetic nucleus when HRP was applied to the main pelvic nerve trunk (Fig. 2). Cells in the dorsal band were shaped like spindles or elongated triangles. Dendrites from dorsal band cells were directed medially from the dorsal horn and laterally to lamina I. A majority of cells in the dorsal band of the nucleus responded by increasing their firing rate, during distension of the colon and rectum, suggesting that some of the cells provide innervation to extrinsic smooth muscle layers (49, 170).

*Sacral Afferent Fibers*

Schofield (201) described the distribution of sacral afferent fibers to the colon of animals including cats. He traced degenerating afferent fibers after sectioning these nerves distal to the sacral dorsal root ganglia. Afferent fibers were distributed to the mucous membrane and external smooth muscle layer and collateral branches of sacral afferents that passed to the ganglion cells of the myenteric plexus. No organized nerve endings have been detected in human rectum (59). Afferent fibers from the colon, rectum, and anal canal of the cat enter the sacral spinal cord in ventral as well as in dorsal roots. Ventral root afferents are primarily nonmyelinated and arise from cells in sacral dorsal root ganglia (7, 35). Afferent fibers in ventral roots were activated by either mechanical, thermal, or chemical stimulation of the anal or rectal mucosa. Neural units that discharged in response to distension were classified as slowly adapting mechanoreceptors (35, 169), as were afferent fibers in sacral dorsal roots that were activated by colonic distension and by spontaneous colonic contractions (68).

The distribution of pelvic nerve afferent projections to the sacral spinal cord has also been shown in experiments using HRP techniques [Fig. 2; (168, 170a)]. In the cat and monkey, afferent fibers in the pelvic nerve project to Lissauer's tract from which collaterals pass medially and laterally in the dorsal horn. Lateral projections terminate in the base of the dorsal horn (lamina V and VI of Rexed) in the region of the sacral autonomic nucleus. Some afferents also project medially in the dorsal commissure.

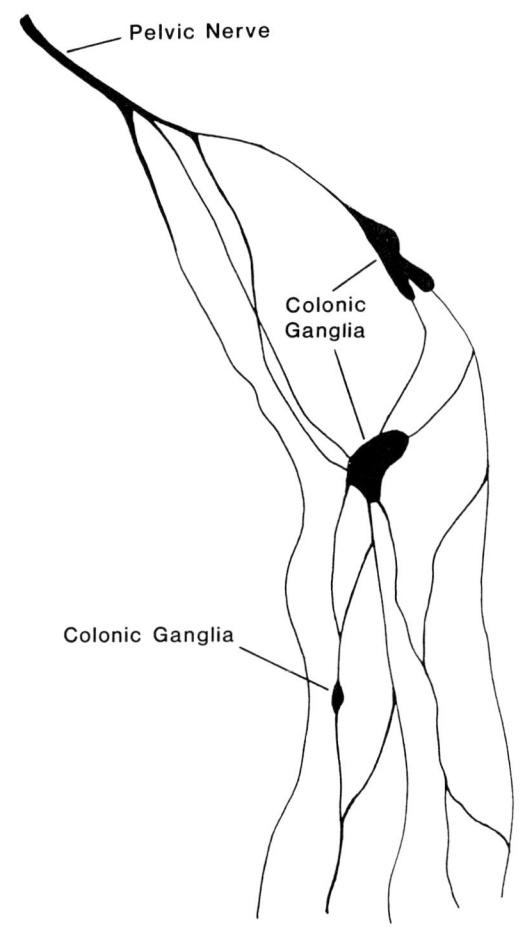

FIG. 1. Sacral parasympathetic innervation to cat colon. Colonic branches of pelvic nerve connect with one or two extramural parasympathetic ganglia. Fiber bundles from ganglia connect ganglia with serosal surface of distal colon and midcolon. [From Krier and Hartman (137).]

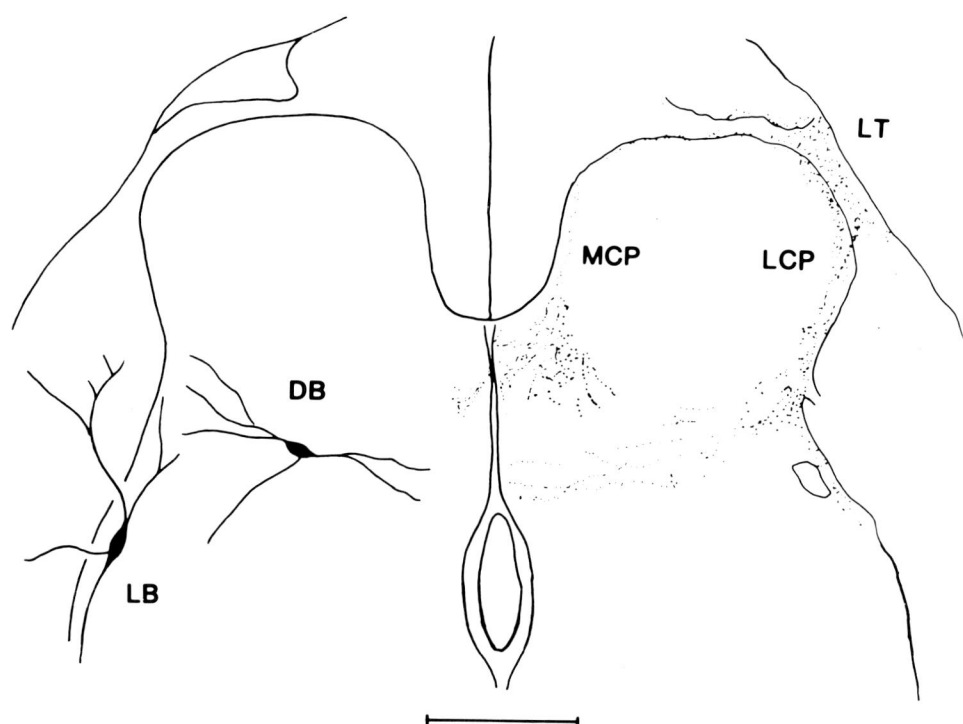

FIG. 2. Relationship between preganglionic neurons in sacral parasympathetic nucleus and pelvic nerve afferents. Neurons in dorsal band (DB) are located primarily in lamina V and VI at base of dorsal horn. Neurons in lateral band (LB) located in lamina VII at lateral border of intermediate gray matter. Preganglionic neurons that innervate colon and rectum are contained within dorsal band. Preganglionic neurons that innervate urinary bladder are contained within lateral band. Visceral afferents are contained in Lissauer's tract (LT) and collateral pathways from Lissauer's tract. LCP, lateral collateral pathway; MCP, medial collateral pathway. Calibration bar, 400 μm. Data based on horseradish peroxidase tracing technique. [From de Groat et al. (49).]

## SOMATIC INNERVATION TO SKELETAL MUSCLE OF PELVIC FLOOR

### Efferent Innervation

The external anal sphincter, puborectalis, and levator ani striated muscles in humans receive motor innervation through the pudendal nerve from motor neurons in the ventral horn of the second and third sacral spinal cord segments (203). One branch of the pudendal nerve, the inferior rectal nerve, innervates the posterior portion of the external anal sphincter, whereas another branch (perineal nerve) innervates the anterior part of the external anal sphincter, puborectalis, levator ani, and other pelvic floor musculature. In the rhesus monkey, pudendal motor fibers innervating the external anal and urethral sphincters arise from the sixth and seventh lumbar spinal cord segments and from the first and second sacral spinal cord segments. In the chimpanzee, pudendal motor fibers that innervate the sphincter arise from the first to fourth sacral segments of the spinal cord (193).

Sherrington (217) first described the pudendal motor outflow to the external anal sphincter of the rhesus monkey. Somatic nerves contained in $L_7$, $S_1$, and $S_2$ ventral roots produced a visible contraction of the external anal sphincter. Symmetrical contractions of the external anal sphincter were obtained using unilateral electrical stimulation, suggesting peripheral crossover of motor fibers. Similarly, unilateral transection of ventral roots did not dilate the anal canal. These observations have been confirmed and extended in the cat and rhesus monkey (21, 251).

The distribution and morphology of pudendal motor neurons that innervate the pelvic floor musculature have been studied in humans, cat, dog, rat, and monkey by chromatolysis, fluorescent dyes, and retrograde transport of HRP (142, 176, 193, 195, 200, 202, 203, 233, 234, 244). The distribution of motoneurons in the ventral horn of the spinal cord has been referred to as Onuf's nucleus or "cell group X" in the nucleus of humans and "cell group Y" in the cat (194). In the rhesus monkey, when HRP was applied to the cut central end of one pudendal nerve, motor neurons were labeled in the ipsilateral spinal cord primarily in the first sacral and seventh lumbar segment (195). The distribution of HRP-reaction product is shown in Figure 3A. Motor neurons were located in the base of the ventral horn. Onuf's nucleus contained medium sized neurons that were considered to be smaller than

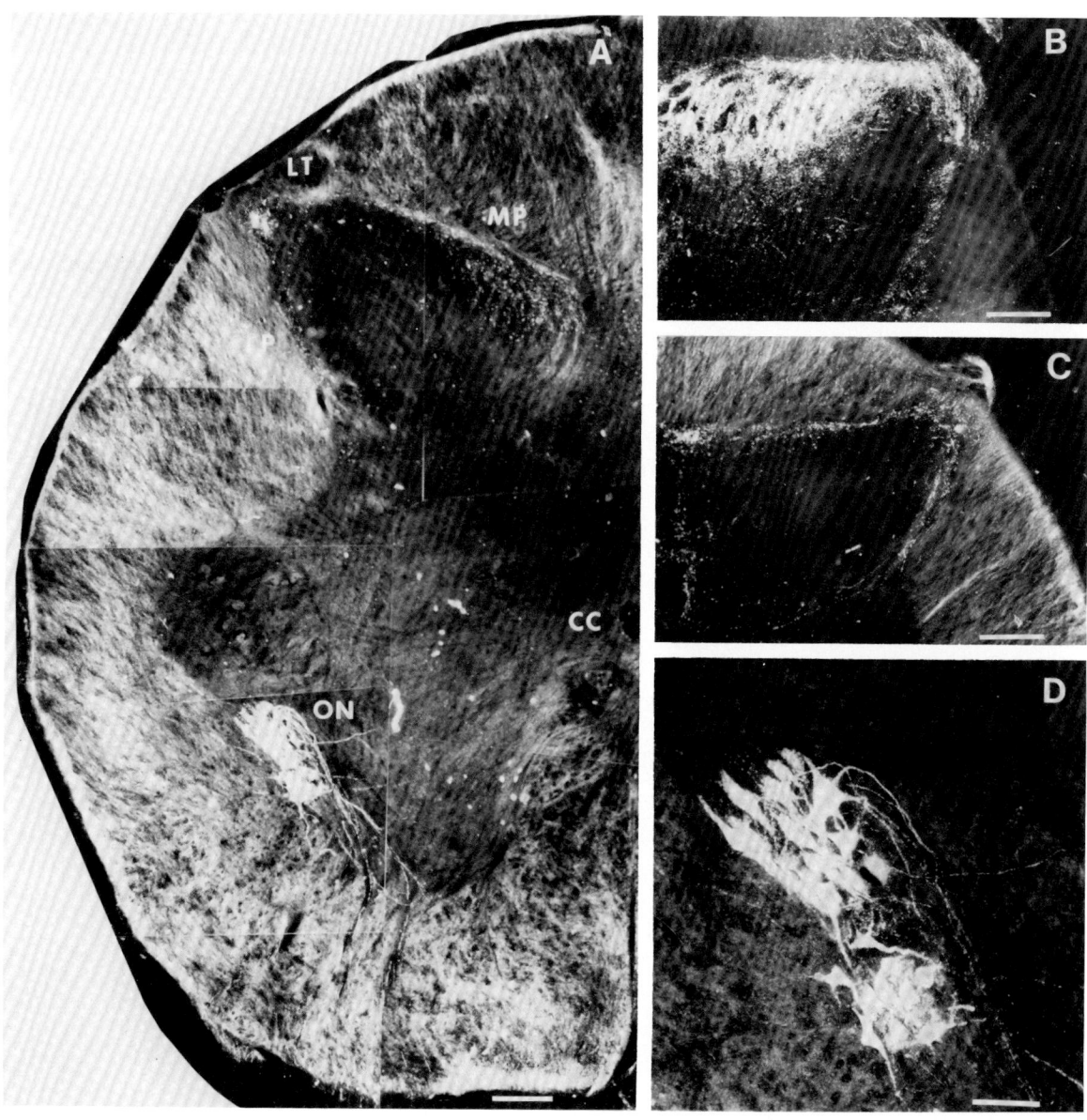

FIG. 3. Dark-field photomicrographs showing relationship between pudendal motor nucleus (Onuf's nucleus) and afferent fibers. A: lumbar ($L_7$) segment; B: sacral spinal cord ($S_1$); and C, D: $S_2$ segment. D shows separation of ON into two parts: dorsolateral and ventromedial. Data obtained from one Rhesus monkey using horseradish peroxidase (HRP) tracing technique; HRP applied to central cut end of one pudendal nerve. ON, neurons in Onuf's nucleus (A, D); LT, afferent fibers in Lissauer's tract (A–C); LP, lateral afferent projections from Lissauer's tract; MP, medial projections from Lissauer's tract; CC, central canal. Bar: A, 200 μm; B, C, 250 μm; D, 80 μm. [From Roppolo et al. (195).]

more laterally located motoneurons. Figure 3D shows topographical division of the nucleus into its dorsolateral and ventromedial parts. The cell bodies of neurons controlling skeletal muscle of the external anal sphincter and levator ani muscles of the cat, dog, and monkey are contained in Onuf's nucleus (142, 195, 202, 252). There is also evidence in humans, rat, cat, and dog for topographical localization of motor neurons (142, 200, 202, 203, 252). In the cat and dog, motor neurons that innervate the external anal sphincter were contained in dorsomedial portions, whereas motoneurons innervating the external urethral sphincters were contained in ventral portions of the nucleus (142, 252).

Anatomical studies have also described descending supraspinal fibers from cortex and brain stem that have been localized in close proximity to dendritic branches of motoneurons in Onuf's nucleus (113, 170,

228). Fibers originating from cortical motor areas (area 4) may be involved in voluntary control of sphincter contractions. Electrical stimulation of cortical areas in humans and monkeys produces contraction of both the external anal sphincter and puborectalis muscle (165, 217).

*Afferent Innervation*

The pudendal nerve contains afferent fibers that innervate skin and skeletal muscle of reproductive organs, perineum, external anal and urethral sphincters, and other pelvic floor musculature (e.g., puborectalis and levator ani). Afferent fibers convey proprioceptive information from skeletal muscle, mechanoreceptor input (tactile and nociceptive), and temperature from the skin and mucosa of the anal canal, skeletal muscle of the pelvic floor, and urinary and genital organs (59). The distribution of afferent fibers in lumbar and sacral spinal cord, dorsal root ganglia, and medulla has been determined in the cat, monkey, and rat by HRP tracing (195, 233, 234). In the rhesus monkey, afferents were localized primarily in the first and sacral dorsal root ganglia, in Lissauer's tract, and in lateral and medial projections (lamina I-IV of Rexed) of the dorsal horn [Fig. 3; (191)]. Lateral afferent projections were dorsal to and in close proximity to the sacral autonomic nucleus. Pudendal somatic afferent fibers overlap considerably with sacral visceral afferents in the pelvic nerve, providing an anatomical basis for viscerosomatic reflexes between the rectum and external anal sphincter during defecation and between the urinary bladder and external urethral sphincter during micturition. Afferent fibers in the pudendal nerve have also been localized within the gracile nuclei of the cat, monkey, and rat (232-234).

## PEPTIDES

A wide variety of peptides have been found in the myenteric and submucosal plexuses of the colon and other regions of the gastrointestinal tract, peripheral autonomic nerves, prevertebral autonomic ganglia, dorsal root ganglia, and lumbar and sacral regions of the spinal cord. The location of these substances in nerve processes and within cell bodies suggests a neuromodulatory or neurotransmitter role. Vasoactive intestinal peptide (VIP), enkephalins, substance P, and somatostatin have been identified by immunocytochemical and biochemical techniques.

*Vasoactive Intestinal-like Peptide*

A network of VIP-like immunoreactive fibers and cell bodies has been found in myenteric and submucosal plexuses of the colon. Immunoreactive fibers have also been found near blood vessels, in association with the muscle layers and with epithelial cells of the mucosa. Fahrenkrug (63) suggested that VIP or a closely related peptide may be involved in regulation of smooth muscle contractile activity, blood flow, and epithelial cell function.

Sphincteric regions of the gastrointestinal tract contain dense accumulations of VIP-immunoreactive material. The occurrence of VIP-immunoreactive nerve terminals in the internal anal sphincter and the ability of VIP to relax the muscle at this site suggest that VIP may regulate smooth muscle contractions of the internal anal sphincter (3a, 18, 19).

Alterations of colonic blood flow during defecation may be mediated by the release of VIP from noncholinergic-nonadrenergic intrinsic nerves. Electrical stimulation of sacral autonomic nerves or rectal distension elicited a vasodilation in the mucosal layer associated with an increase in VIP in venous effluent from the cat colon (64).

The VIP immunoreactivity in the gastrointestinal tract may have an intrinsic origin. The distribution of VIP in the cecum is not changed following abolition of extrinsic mesenteric nerves. Neither vagotomy nor sympathectomy reduced the number of nerve terminals with VIP immunoreactivity (63, 204).

Some of the immunoreactive VIP-like material present in nerve terminals in colon, rectum, and sphincteric region may originate extrinsically. The distribution of VIP-like immunoreactive material closely resembles that of sacral visceral afferent pathways. Vasoactive intestinal peptide is localized primarily in terminals in Lissauer's tract and the dorsal horn (lamina I and V of Rexed) of the sacral spinal cord and also in nerve terminals in the vicinity of the sacral autonomic nucleus (128). Neurons located in sacral dorsal root ganglia also contain VIP-like immunoreactive material. There was reduction in VIP-like material in the sacral dorsal horn after transection of sacral dorsal and ventral roots. This suggests that VIP may be a transmitter in visceral afferent pathways. Sacral visceral afferent fibers innervate the rectum, where they mediate sensation and autonomic reflexes. Some of the VIP nerve processes located in the colon, rectum, and internal anal sphincter may be sensory and may originate from neurons located in sacral dorsal root ganglia.

*Enkephalins*

Enkephalins, endogenous neural pentapeptides with opioid activity, have been detected biochemically and immunocytochemically in the gastrointestinal tract, autonomic ganglia, peripheral autonomic nerves, brain, and spinal cord in a number of animal species. Met- and Leu-enkephalin-immunoreactive cell bodies have been located in the myenteric plexus (119, 187, 204). Using a longitudinal muscle-myenteric plexus preparation of the ileum, one study (220a) reports the synthesis of enkephalins in peripheral gastrointestinal tissue, and another study (159a) reports the release of enkephalins from myenteric neurons in response to electrical stimulation. Both enkephalins and morphine inhibit cholinergic contractions evoked by electrical field stimulation and produce membrane hyperpolarization in neurons of the myenteric plexus. These data strengthen the view that enkephalins play a transmitter or neuromodulator role in the gastrointestinal tract. There are no reports of the distribution of enkephalin-like immunoreactivity in nerve processes and cell bodies of the myenteric plexus in the rectum and internal anal sphincter.

The enkephalinergic system is also present in sacral and lumbar regions of the spinal cord. In the sacral spinal cord of the cat, enkephalin-like terminals have been localized in the superficial layers of the dorsal horn (lamina I and II) and in the sacral autonomic and pudendal motor nuclei. Preganglionic cell bodies containing enkephalin-like material were localized in lateral borders of the intermediate and ventral gray matter of the sacral autonomic nucleus. Preganglionic neurons were demonstrated to synthesize and transport enkephalin or enkephalin-like material to the periphery by way of the sacral ventral roots (8, 94). A similar enkephalinergic distribution has been observed in lumbar preganglionic neurons projecting to the inferior mesenteric ganglion of the guinea pig (43b). Enkephalin-like fibers, thought to arise from lumbar preganglionic neurons, are considered to modulate cholinergic and noncholinergic synaptic transmission by a presynaptic mechanism. Opioids have also been reported to inhibit sympathetic mediated intestinointestinal inhibitory reflexes that are elicited by distension of the gut (152a). The inhibitory actions of opiates are blocked by the administration of naloxone. The physiological role of the enkephalinergic pathway has not been established in lumbar and sacral autonomic pathways to the rectum and internal anal sphincter region.

*Substance P–Like Peptide*

Immunocytochemical techniques reveal that substance P is present in enteric neurons and nerve processes of the gastrointestinal tract as well as in enterochromaffin cells in the intestinal mucosa. Substance P at these sites may serve as a putative neuromodulator substance or function as a locally acting hormone, respectively (249). Substance P depolarizes enteric neurons and increases membrane excitability and enhances motility of the gastrointestinal musculature (249).

Substance P may function as a neurotransmitter in visceral afferent pathways. It has been found in small-diameter sensory neurons in dorsal root ganglia, in superficial layers of the dorsal horn of lumbar regions, and in sacral regions of the spinal cord. The distribution of substance P in the sacral spinal cord closely matches that of visceral afferent fibers in the pelvic nerve labeled by HRP techniques (45a). There is strong evidence that some of the peripheral branches of visceral afferent fibers in lumbar regions release substance P adjacent to neurons in prevertebral autonomic ganglia (43a), where it may mediate noncholinergic slow excitatory synaptic potentials (177). Some of the substance P–containing fibers present in the gut wall may represent branches of primary afferent neurons.

The physiological role of substance P in the regulation of colonic motility and motility of the rectum and internal anal sphincter region is not understood. It may be a transmitter that mediates pain sensation in afferent fibers of visceral nerves.

*Somatostatin-like Peptide*

Somastostatin-like peptide has been localized within enteric neurons and in immunoreactive processes surrounding enteric neurons. It inhibits the release of acetylcholine from intrinsic gastrointestinal nerves during electrical field stimulation and reduces the firing frequency of myenteric neurons (81, 101, 247). Somatostatin has also been localized extrinsic to the gastrointestinal wall. It is present in small-diameter dorsal root ganglion cells and in nerve processes of superficial layers of the dorsal horn of the spinal cord (44). Somatostatin at these sites suggests that it may be involved in sensory pathways. Further, somatostatin has been localized in efferent lumbar sympathetic and sacral parasympathetic pathways (44). It is found in neurons of the inferior mesenteric ganglion (30a) and in those of the sacral parasympathetic nucleus that innervate the colon (44). Its role in motor function of the rectum and anal canal is not established.

## MOTOR ACTIVITY OF RECTUM AND INTERNAL ANAL SPHINCTER

*General and Historical Considerations*

The rectum and internal anal sphincter receive solid material from the distal colon and evacuate colonic contents during defecation. Few quantitative data describe colonic and rectal contractions and those of the pelvic floor skeletal muscle during defecation. Much of the information has been derived from radiological observations of cat and human colon (32, 85, 103, 130, 246). Measurements have been made in humans of the anorectal angle and descent of the pelvic floor during straining and defecation (154, 155). In the cat colon, defecation was associated with a constriction band that progressed aborally causing a marked narrowing of the colonic lumen. These contractions were observed in all regions of the human colon, often involving segments 20–30 cm in length (111), and there is evidence they occur in response to eating (121). Elliott and Barclay-Smith (62) described similar movements in cat decentralized colon during electrical stimulation of sacral parasympathetic fibers in pelvic nerves.

Intraluminal pressures have been recorded with multiple sensors from the human colon during defecation to show propulsive pressure waves occurring at two or more sites. These waves (type IV) were commonly recorded in patients with diarrhea or ulcerative colitis and coincided with defecation (221).

There is little information about contractile patterns of smooth muscle or phasic relationships between electrical potentials generated by smooth muscle cells and contractions in rectum and internal anal sphincter. Current concepts of contractile patterns and electrical activity are based on measurements made in human and cat rectum and sphincteric region. The majority of measurements of contractile activity include intraluminal pressure and force recording in vivo. Electrical activity has primarily been recorded in vivo with extracellular electrodes.

*Intraluminal Pressure Recordings*

Recordings have also been made in vivo in human and cat anal canal to show intraluminal pressure of the resting anal canal and spontaneous pressure waves. These pressures were measured with water-filled catheters or small balloons connected to strain-gauge transducers.

Intraluminal resting pressures recorded in the anal canal are higher than those recorded in the rectum and sigmoid colon (112). Resting pressures in the anal canal are considered to be largely the result of tonic contractile activity in the internal anal sphincter. For example, anal pressures are reduced by division of the internal anal sphincter and not markedly reduced after neuromuscular paralysis of pelvic floor skeletal muscle (73). Wood (249) considered that myogenic mechanisms involving both inherent electrical activity and contractions maintain contractile tone of sphincters in the absence of extrinsic autonomic nerves and circulating hormones.

There are two predominant frequencies of spontaneous pressure waves in the anal canal that are not associated with propulsive movements of the rectal wall during evacuation. Kerremans (129, 130) describes slow sinusoidal pressure waves occurring at a mean frequency of 12 cycles/min with a mean duration of 5 s. Slower spontaneous pressure waves had a mean duration of 33 s and a mean frequency of 2.7 cycles/min. Hancock (104) used balloons and open-tipped catheters to describe rhythmic pressure waves in human anal canal and showed rhythmic slow pressure waves with frequencies from 10 to 20 cycles/min. The frequency of rhythmic slow pressure waves was greater in the distal than in the proximal anal canal. Slower rhythmic pressure waves ranged in frequency from 0.6 to 1.9 cycles/min but occurred in only 5% of normal subjects. Rhythmic contractions in cat anal canal occurred at frequencies ranging from 12 to 36 cycles/min (83, 85).

The motility of the rectum is characterized by spontaneous intraluminal pressure waves of lower frequency and longer duration. In the human rectum, rhythmic pressure waves vary from 3 to 8 cycles/min (3) and from 5 to 10 cycles/min (38). The duration of the pressure waves ranged from 5 to 12 s and their amplitude was <10–20 cmH$_2$O. Kerremans (130) reported spontaneous pressure waves in human rectum occurring regularly at frequencies of 2.2 cycles/min.

*Electrical Activity of Rectum and Internal Anal Sphincter*

Electrical activity has been recorded in vivo from humans (167, 225–227, 241, 245) and cat (24, 25, 131) internal anal sphincter and rectum using extracellular electrodes (e.g., intraluminal suction electrodes, pressure electrodes). In these species, electrical oscillations called slow-wave potentials or basic electrical rhythm have been recorded from the rectum and internal anal sphincteric region. Spike potentials superimposed on slow potentials have been recorded in human rectum but not from internal anal sphincter. In the cat, spike potentials were detected from rectum and longitudinal muscle layer of the sphincter but not from circular muscle of the sphincter (24).

Slow potentials recorded in vivo from internal anal sphincter region in human have a wide frequency range. Weinbeck and Altaparmacov (245) observed frequencies from 14.5 to 30.4 cycles/min, and Monges et al. (167) reported frequencies from 20 to 24 cycles/min. Ustach et al. (235) observed frequencies from 6 to 26 cycles/min (mean 17 cycles/min) in normal volunteers. Kerremans (130, 131) observed two dominant frequencies: one was 18.9 cycles/min and the other was 2.9 cycles/min. The mean duration of the slow potentials was 3.4 s. Wankling et al. (241) recorded two dominant frequencies at mean values of 16.4 and 1.6 cycles/min.

In cats, in vivo slow electrical potentials had frequencies from 15 to 30 cycles/min in one study (131) and from 9 to 34 cycles/min in another (24) in which electrical activity was recorded with pressure electrodes from circular muscle fibers.

The frequency of slow potentials in the rectum is less than that recorded from the sphincteric region. The mean frequency of slow potentials was reported in humans to be 3.8 cycles/min (130). In two other studies, two predominant frequencies in the sigmoid colon and rectum were reported in humans: a fast frequency from 6 to 9 cycles/min and a slow frequency from 2.5 to 4.0 cycles/min (225, 227) associated with rhythmic pressure waves, although the relationship was variable and inconsistent. In another study (226), slow waves occurred at two predominant frequencies when electrical activity was recorded at multiple sites (5–19 cm from the anal verge). Mean values of 7.5 cycles/min and 3.2 cycles/min were reported at distances of 15–19 cm from the anal verge. Mean values of 7.1 cycles/min and 3.2 cycles/min were reported at distances of 5–9 cm from the anal verge (226). This suggests there is no oral-aboral electrical gradient in the rectum. Figure 4 shows representative traces of spontaneous electrical activity recorded in human and cat internal anal sphincter.

Electrical activity of the sphincter and rectum has also been recorded in vitro (15, 24, 140, 141, 151, 153). In the cat the sucrose-gap method was used to record electrical activity from isolated pieces of circular and longitudinal sphincteric muscle. Spontaneous electrical activity was detected in ~75% of muscle strips. In isolated circular muscle, electrical activity consisted of sinusoidal slow potentials with constant amplitude. Since each slow wave potential was in phase with a contraction, they are apparently controlled by this activity. In isolated longitudinal muscle, electrical activity is not continuous but is interrupted by periods of electrical inactivity lasting from 3 s to 7 min.

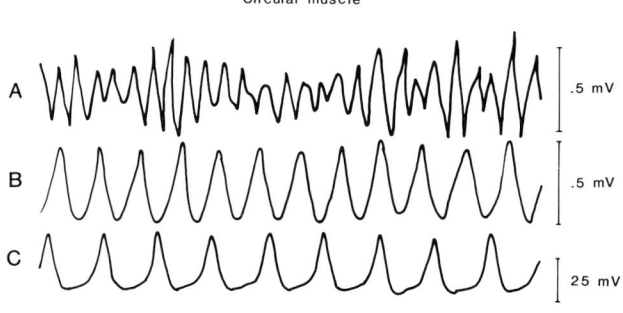
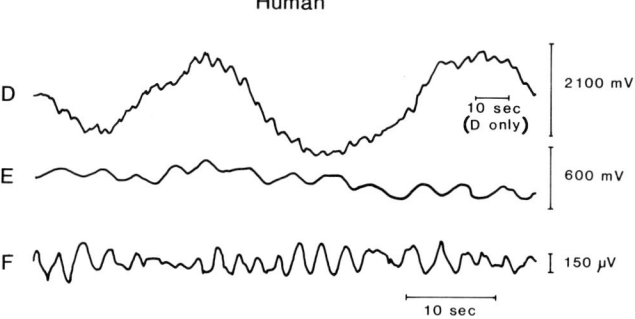

FIG. 4. Electrical activity recorded from smooth muscle of internal anal sphincter in cats (*A–C*) and humans (*D–F*). *A, B, D–F*: tracings obtained in situ with extracellular electrodes. *C*: tracing obtained in vitro with sucrose-gap technique. [*A–C* adapted from Bouvier and Gonella (24). *D, E* adapted from Wankling et al. (241). *F* adapted from Kerremans (130).]

Electrical activity consisted of slow potentials and spike potentials associated with the upstroke of each slow potential. Spontaneous electrical activity in rabbit rectum consisted of slow potentials and transient spike potentials (159).

Intracellular electrical activity of rectum and internal anal sphincter has also been reported (140, 141, 151, 152). Electrical activity was recorded from dog, cat, rabbit, guinea pig, and human. Intracellular recordings were made from circular muscle cells 2 cm from the anal verge. In dog, cat, guinea pig, and human, mean resting potentials for sphincter muscle were similar, exhibiting values of $-52.7$, $-47.0$, $-51.0$, and $-51.5$ mV, respectively. Sphincter muscle of humans exhibited electrical oscillations ranging from 13 to 15 cycles/min (140, 141). Sphincter muscle of dog, cat, and rabbit exhibited electrical oscillations at higher frequencies, ranging from 25 to 34 cycles/min. Rectal smooth muscle strips in all species exhibited electrical oscillations at frequencies <10 cycles/min.

MOTOR ACTIVITY OF SKELETAL MUSCLE OF PELVIC FLOOR

Contractile forces and electrical activity of the skeletal muscle of the pelvic floor have been previously measured in vivo in humans and experimental animals by electromyography, strain gauges, and open and closed manometric techniques. Histochemical techniques have been used to classify skeletal muscle fiber types. Much of the current information on the skeletal muscle in this region is based on these procedures.

*Electromyography*

Electromyographic recording techniques are commonly used to assess skeletal muscle contraction in the pelvic floor (21, 22, 27, 123, 127, 130, 132, 134, 179, 180–183, 188, 230). Surface and bipolar electrodes record extracellular electrical potentials. The majority of studies report recordings of multiunit electrical potentials.

Unlike most other skeletal muscles, the external anal sphincter and puborectalis exhibit continuous electrical activity during electromyographic recording in both humans and experimental animals. Continuous electrical activity recorded during electromyography has been attributed to small-diameter skeletal muscle fibers (21, 22, 70, 130). Muscle units that do not have a spontaneous electrical discharge but exhibit an electrical discharge during reflex or voluntary contractions have been attributed to contractions of large-diameter fibers.

There is some quantitative information about the firing frequency of single motor units from human pelvic floor skeletal muscle. Kawakami (127) described the firing rate of motor units in the skeletal muscle of the external anal sphincter and puborectalis as varying between 2 and 5 cycles/s. Travener and Smiddy (230) reported resting firing rates from 3 to 10 cycles/s for the external anal sphincter and from 3 to 25 cycles/s for the puborectalis. Kerremans (130) reported that spontaneous resting firing rates were low, ranging from 3 to 5 cycles/s. Increases in firing frequencies, ranging from 7 to 14 cycles/s, occurred during reflex or voluntary contraction. In the cat, motor units recorded in the external anal sphincter exhibited resting firing frequencies that ranged from 0.8 to 10.6 Hz (134).

*Histochemical Studies*

Histochemical studies report skeletal muscle fiber types of human external anal sphincter, puborectalis, and levator ani (16, 130, 180). The predominant fibers are small diameter although large and intermediate fibers have also been detected. As in other skeletal muscle, the pelvic floor musculature was classified histochemically into three (130) or two types [type 1 and type 2 (16, 180)] based on differences in energy metabolism. Small-diameter fibers with large amounts of oxidative enzymes and mitochondria that gave strong reactions to succinic dehydrogenase, nadide, nicotinamide-adenine dinucleotide tetrazolium reductase. and ATPase were classified as type 1. In contrast, large-diameter fibers gave a strong reaction to enzymes connected with glycogen metabolism (phosphorylase) and a weaker reaction to oxidative enzymes. These fibers were classified as type II. Fibers of intermediate size that gave an intermediate reaction to both glycolytic and oxidative enzymes have also been detected (130).

*Force Measurements*

Few studies report force measurements in the anal canal of humans and experimental animals (36, 37, 135, 136, 149, 150, 157). Collins and co-workers (36, 37) used strain gauges in humans to assess radial forces during voluntary contractions of pelvic floor musculature and during voluntary increases in intra-abdominal pressure. These studies report relative changes in force from resting base-line levels.

One type of strain-gauge probe has been constructed to measure axial forces in vivo in the anal canal of cats and humans (61, 135, 136, 157). One application of this device in experimental animals has been to measure phasic contractile forces of skeletal muscle of the external anal sphincter in response to electrical stimulation of motor axons in the pudendal nerve (Fig. 5). The contractions were abolished by neuromuscular blocking agents, occurred at short latencies (1–3 ms), and were mediated by low-threshold efferent axons in the pudendal nerve. Contraction times ranged from 45 to 60 ms, and contraction durations ranged from 100 to 160 ms. A comparison of twitch-contraction data with that recorded from other skeletal muscle involved with postural regulation (162) supports earlier views (21, 22) that the skeletal muscle of the external anal sphincter is composed primarily of small-diameter fibers. Another application of the device in humans was to measure the reflex (tactile and nociceptive stimuli applied to anal skin) and voluntary

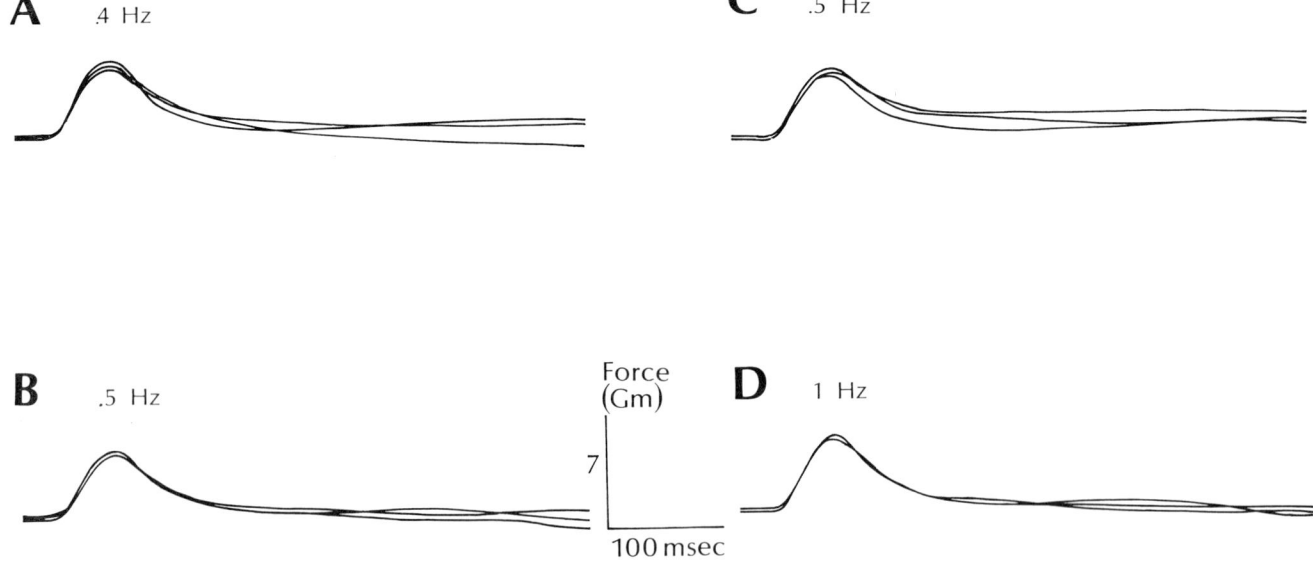

FIG. 5. Phasic isotonic contractions of skeletal muscle of external anal sphincter of cat. Each panel shows superimposed consecutive responses at indicated frequencies of pudendal nerve stimulation. Different decay rates reflect effect of spontaneous contractions of smooth muscle of rectum–internal anal sphincter. [From Krier and Adams (136).]

contraction of the external anal sphincter. The data indicate that there is a direct relationship between external anal sphincter mean maximal force and mean frequency of repetitive voluntary contractions.

## INFLUENCE OF INTRINSIC GASTROINTESTINAL NERVES ON MOTOR ACTIVITY OF INTERNAL ANAL SPHINCTER

As in other regions of the gastrointestinal tract, there are two types of motoneurons in the intrinsic plexuses of the rectum and internal anal sphincter region. The first type is cholinergic neurons that release acetylcholine on muscarinic receptors of the smooth muscle membrane to produce excitation. The second type of neuron has been called noncholinergic, nonadrenergic. The identity of neurotransmitter released from these neurons is not established. Activation of noncholinergic, nonadrenergic neurons inhibits gastrointestinal muscle.

### Cholinergic Motor Neurons

Electrical field stimulation of the myenteric plexus with combined circular and longitudinal muscle strips produced a contraction of smooth muscle and excitatory junctional potentials that was blocked by muscarinic antagonists (40). Excitatory junctional potentials have been demonstrated only in the guinea pig (40).

### Noncholinergic, Nonadrenergic Neurons

Intrinsic noncholinergic, nonadrenergic inhibitory neurons have been demonstrated by a number of investigators in the guinea pig, monkey, rabbit, pig, dog, and human rectum and internal anal sphincter region (2, 18, 29, 30, 40, 43, 83–85, 151, 152). Electrical field stimulation of the myenteric plexus combined circular and longitudinal or isolated circular muscle strips (1–20 Hz) causes the release of a transmitter substance that produces a hyperpolarizing inhibitory junctional potential in smooth muscle cells and a relaxation of spontaneous smooth muscle contractions. These inhibitory responses are present during the administration of muscarinic receptor–blocking agents, adrenergic neuronal blocking agents, and adrenergic $\alpha$- and $\beta$-receptor–blocking agents. In contrast, tetrodotoxin, an agent that selectively blocks sodium channels, abolishes the inhibitory responses. The identity of the transmitter released from axons of the inhibitory neurons is not established. Some studies report that serotonin, ATP, and adenosine may not be the transmitters released from axons of the intrinsic inhibitory neurons (4, 191). Desensitization of smooth muscle receptors to these agents did not alter relaxation of the muscle in response to electrical field stimulation. Other studies suggest that ATP or a related adenine nucleotide may have an inhibitory transmitter function. Electrical field stimulation of nonadrenergic, noncholinergic fibers after [$^3$H]adenosine loading results in the release of tritium. Release of [$^3$H]adenosine was blocked by tetrodotoxin (149, 150). Evidence for VIP as a putative neurotransmitter substance has also been reported. In the rabbit, relaxation of smooth muscle of the internal anal sphincter during electrical field stimulation is partially reduced by treatment of the tissue with a VIP antiserum (18, 19).

Intrinsic inhibitory neurons have nicotinic cholinergic receptors that are activated either by rectal distension or by stimulation of extrinsic sacral autonomic nerves. The inhibitory responses are blocked by the nicotinic antagonist, hexamethonium. Pharmacological evidence in the monkey confirmed the presence of nicotinic cholinergic receptors (191). Acetylcholine, nicotine, and dimethylphenylpiperazinium (DMPP) in the presence of atropine and reserpine produce a relaxation of the internal anal sphincter. The inhibitory actions of the nicotinic agonists were abolished by hexamethonium and by tetrodotoxin.

### Rectoanal Reflexes

Relaxation of the internal anal sphincter occurs during voluntary defecation and in response to distension of the rectum (50, 83–85, 99, 185, 205, 206, 208). This rectoanal response is considered to be mediated, in part, by intrinsic inhibitory neurons of the myenteric plexus, since it is present following destruction of the cauda equina and sacral roots (50, 99, 166, 208, 209). In addition, inhibitory neurons of the rectum and internal anal sphincter region mediate pelvic nerve–induced relaxation of the muscle (25). Meunier and Mollard (166) report that rectoanal reflexes are altered in patients with sacral spinal cord lesions, suggesting the potential for modulation by autonomic nerves. Relaxation of the sphincter does not occur in diseases in which the rectum is aganglionic. Immunohistochemical investigations report a reduction in VIP and substance P-immunoreactive nerve fibers in the aganglionic segment in Hirschsprung's disease (20, 231).

### Vesicoanal Reflexes

Increases in electromyographic activity and elevations in anal canal pressure have been reported during micturition and during distension of the urinary bladder in humans and cats (26, 199). These responses in the cat were considered to be mediated by extrinsic autonomic reflexes involving afferent and efferent fibers in lumbar sympathetic nerves (26), inferior mesenteric ganglion, and lumbar spinal cord.

## INFLUENCE OF LUMBAR SYMPATHETIC NERVES ON MOTOR ACTIVITY OF COLON, RECTUM, AND INTERNAL ANAL SPHINCTER

The physiological role of the lumbar sympathetic nerves in the regulation of motor activity of the muscle of the colon, rectum, and internal anal sphincter during defecation is not precisely understood. Much of our information about this system is based on animal experiments in which lumbar sympathetic nerves were electrically stimulated or acutely transected.

### Effect of Electrical Stimulation of Lumbar Sympathetic Nerves

Langley and Anderson (143–145) were the first to examine the effects of lumbar sympathetic nerves on smooth muscle of the internal anal sphincter and rectum. Contractions of the internal anal sphincter and relaxation of rectal smooth muscle were reported in cats during electrical stimulation of nerve roots arising from the second to fourth lumbar spinal cord segments. In contrast, they observed in the rabbit a relaxation of both the rectum and internal anal sphincter during electrical stimulation of sympathetic nerves. The excitatory responses of the internal anal sphincter and the inhibitory responses of the rectum were mediated by postganglionic fibers, since they were depressed by the administration of nicotine, a ganglionic blocking agent and abolished by section of the nerve trunks running between the inferior mesenteric ganglia and the effector organs.

Sympathetic nerve trunks originating from the inferior mesenteric ganglia (lumbar colonic nerves, hypogastric nerves) mediate contractile responses of the smooth muscle of the internal anal sphincter and relaxation of the smooth muscle of the colon and rectum. The hypogastric nerves have the greatest influence on contractile activity of the internal anal sphincter. The lumbar colonic nerves predominantly influence the extrinsic smooth muscle layers of the colon and rectum (46, 87, 88, 120, 197), although in one study (148), contractile responses of the internal anal sphincter in the dog were reported during activation of lumbar colonic nerves.

The effects of the hypogastric nerves on colonic motor activity are uncertain. In cats, bilateral section of these fibers did not alter spontaneous contractions of the colon (87, 120, 197). Electrical stimulation of the hypogastric nerves resulted in inhibition (86) or it had no effect on the spontaneous or parasympathetic-induced contractions of the colon (120, 197).

The influence of the hypogastric nerves on tone and spontaneous contractions of the internal anal sphincter and rectum has been reported in humans, dog, cat, and monkey (25, 85, 131, 148, 191, 216). In humans, electrical stimulation of efferent axons in the presacral nerve resulted in a relaxation of the rectum and internal anal sphincter. The excitatory and inhibitory responses of the internal anal sphincter and inhibitory responses of the rectum are mediated by the release of norepinephrine from sympathetic nerve terminals. Learmonth and Markowitz (148) stimulated the lumbar sympathetic trunk and the lumbar colonic and hypogastric nerves in dogs and examined the responses of the internal anal sphincter. Contraction was the predominant effect of hypogastric nerve stimulation but was abolished by $\alpha$-adrenergic blockade. The same responses were recorded in cats and monkeys (25, 84, 85, 189). Recording rectal and anal canal pressures in cats demonstrated that hypogastric nerve stimulation produced a contraction of the internal anal sphincter mediated by $\alpha$-adrenergic receptors and that relaxation was mediated by $\beta$-adrenergic receptors (85). Destruction of adrenergic nerve terminals with pretreatment by 6-hydroxydopamine or the administration of dihydroergotamine, an $\alpha$-adrenergic receptor antagonist, abolished the responses (84). Relaxation of the internal anal sphincter in response to stimulation of hypogastric nerves was detected only after $\alpha$-adrenergic receptor blockage.

The influence of the hypogastric nerves on intraluminal pressures in the rectum were predominantly inhibitory and were mediated by $\alpha$- and $\beta$-adrenergic receptors. Bouvier and Gonella (25) confirmed and extended these findings in the cat. Spontaneous electrical activity of circular and longitudinal muscle fibers in the sphincteric region was obtained during electrical stimulation of hypogastric nerves. Electrical stimulation of the hypogastric nerve produced a contraction of circular muscle fibers mediated by $\alpha$-adrenergic receptors. Relaxation of longitudinal smooth muscle was mediated by $\beta$-adrenergic receptors. Neurally evoked contractile responses of the internal anal sphincter were not blocked by hexamethonium. This suggests that fibers in the hypogastric nerve were postganglionic and originated from cell bodies in the inferior mesenteric ganglia. Hypogastric nerve stimulation in the monkey produced contraction of the internal anal sphincter mediated by $\alpha$-adrenergic receptors (191). There were no inhibitory responses during electrical stimulation of hypogastric nerves.

Further confirmation of these results is based on two types of pharmacological experiments performed in cat, dog, monkey, guinea pig, and human. In one preparation in vivo, intraluminal pressure recordings of rectum and anal canal were recorded during intravenous administration of catecholamines. In a second preparation in vitro, tension was recorded in isolated strips of the extrinsic smooth muscle layers of the rectum and internal anal sphincter. Results of these studies are summarized in Table 1. Adrenergic-receptor type was based usually on one concentration of the $\alpha$- or $\beta$-receptor antagonist. In the dog (148) and guinea pig (43) the administration of norepinephrine and epinephrine produced a contraction of the sphinc-

TABLE 1. *Adrenergic Receptor Agonists That Alter Motor Activity of Internal Anal Sphincter*

| Receptor Agonist | Receptor Type | Preparation | Species | Ref. |
|---|---|---|---|---|
| Epinephrine | α, + | In vivo | Dog | 148 |
|  |  | in vitro | Cat | 85, 131, 184 |
| Epinephrine | α, +; β, − | In vitro | Monkey | 191 |
|  |  |  | Human | 74, 178 |
| Norepinephrine | α, +; β, − | In vitro | Monkey | 191 |
|  |  |  | Human | 74 |
|  |  |  | Cat* | 24, 25, 184 |
| Phenylephrine | α, +; β, − | In vitro | Monkey | 191 |
| Norepinephrine | α, + | In vivo | Cat | 84, 85 |
|  |  | in vitro | Guinea pig | 43 |
| Dopamine | α, + | In vitro | Monkey | 191 |
| Isoproterenol | β, − | In vivo | Cat | 85, 184 |
|  |  | in vitro | Human | 178 |

+, Excitatory action; −, inhibitory action. *β-Receptor longitudinal muscle, α-receptor circular muscle.

ter that was mediated by α-adrenergic receptors. In cat internal anal sphincter, circular muscle fibers were excited through α-adrenergic receptors, and longitudinal muscle fibers were inhibited through β-adrenergic receptors (24). In the monkey and in humans, norepinephrine and epinephrine produced a contraction mediated by α-adrenergic receptors and a relaxation mediated by β-adrenergic receptors. Isoproterenol produced relaxation of the internal anal sphincter due to β-adrenergic receptor activation.

*Effect of Interruption of Lumbar Sympathetic Pathways to Colon, Rectum, and Internal Anal Sphincter*

Acute transection of lumbar sympathetic nerves in experimental animals (48, 85–87, 143) or spinal anesthesia in humans (72, 189) enhances colonic and rectal motility but reduces contractile tone in the region of the internal anal sphincter. This suggests that lumbar sympathetic nerves provide a tonic inhibitory input to external smooth muscle layers of the colon and rectum and a tonic excitatory input to smooth muscle of the internal anal sphincter. Langley and Anderson (143) were the first to examine the effects of interruption of lumbar sympathetic nerves to the internal anal sphincter in cats in which they showed that section of the lumbar splanchnic nerves reduced tone of the internal anal sphincter. Similar data were obtained following transection of lumbar sympathetic nerve trunks (e.g., lumbar colonic nerves, hypogastric nerves) originating from the inferior mesenteric ganglia (185).

Frenckner and Ihre (72) measured human resting anal pressures and found that spinal anesthesia at $T_6$–$T_{12}$ spinal cord levels resulted in a reduction in anal canal pressure. These data suggest that sympathetic fibers arising from thoracic and lumbar regions provide a tonic excitatory input to the internal anal sphincter to maintain contractile tone. Further confirmation of these results in humans was reported in a study involving the administration of an α-receptor antagonist and agonist (100a). The infusion of phentolamine resulted in a reduction in tone of internal anal sphincter, whereas the infusion of methoxamine, an α-receptor agonist, results in an increase in tone.

Figure 6 shows the lumbar sympathetic innervation of the internal anal sphincter. Preganglionic fibers from neurons in lumbar spinal cord innervate sympathetic neurons in prevertebral ganglia (e.g., inferior mesenteric). Postganglionic fibers from neurons in prevertebral ganglia travel to the internal anal sphincter via the hypogastric nerves. Norepinephrine release from postganglionic nerves activates postjunctional α-excitatory adrenoceptors and β-inhibitory adrenoceptors located on smooth muscle. Tonic excitatory sympathetic outflow is mediated by α-adrenoceptors. Longitudinal muscle in the cat's anal canal responds to hypogastric nerve stimulation with only β-receptor-mediated relaxation. In contrast, cat circular muscle

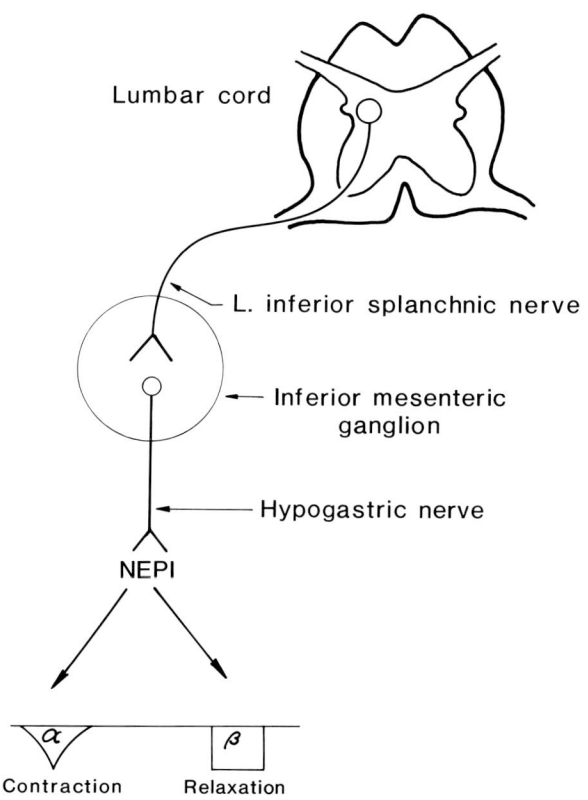

FIG. 6. Schematic representation of lumbar sympathetic innervation of internal anal sphincter. Pathway described based on experiments in cats. Adrenergic receptor types based on experiments in cats and humans. NEPI, norepinephrine. [Adapted from Bouvier and Gonella (25).]

fibers respond with only α-receptor–mediated excitation (25).

## INFLUENCE OF SACRAL AUTONOMIC NERVES ON MOTOR ACTIVITY OF INTERNAL ANAL SPHINCTER

### Effect of Electrical Stimulation of Sacral Parasympathetic Nerves

The effects of electrical stimulation of sacral autonomic nerves on motor activity of the internal anal sphincter have been reported in different animal species (25, 40, 84, 85, 143, 191). Two responses were observed. The first response was a contraction and an excitatory junctional potential that was reduced or abolished after the administration of hexamethonium and atropine (40, 85). These results suggest that some of the efferent fibers in the sacral autonomic nerves that travel to the internal anal sphincter are cholinergic and that acetylcholine is the postganglionic transmitter that acts through muscarinic receptors. The second response was either a relaxation (184), a biphasic response consisting of relaxation during the period of stimulation followed by an aftercontraction (40), or a contractile response following the period of stimulation (191). The relaxation and aftercontractions were abolished by hexamethonium but were not blocked by muscarinic antagonist or adrenoceptor-blocking agents. These results indicate that sphincter relaxation and aftercontractions are mediated by preganglionic cholinergic fibers in the pelvic nerve that synapse with noncholinergic, nonadrenergic inhibitory neurons.

Bouvier and Gonella (25) reported in the cat that sacral autonomic fibers activated noncholinergic, nonadrenergic inhibitory nerves to circular muscle of the sphincter and cholinergic excitatory nerves to longitudinal muscle. Electrical stimulation of autonomic nerves in sacral ventral roots reduced spontaneous electrical activity recorded from circular muscle fibers. The inhibitory response was not blocked by phentolamine, propranolol, and atropine, but was abolished by the administration of hexamethonium. In contrast, sacral ventral root stimulation increased electrical activity recorded from longitudinal muscle of the sphincteric region that was abolished by atropine. In summary, preganglionic fibers in the sacral ventral roots and pelvic nerve inhibit the internal anal sphincter by synaptic activation of intrinsic noncholinergic, nonadrenergic inhibitory nerves and excitatory innervation by activation of cholinergic neurons (Fig. 7).

### Cholinergic Agonists

The effects of cholinergic agonists on contractile activity and tone of the anal canal and internal anal sphincter region have been reported. The administra-

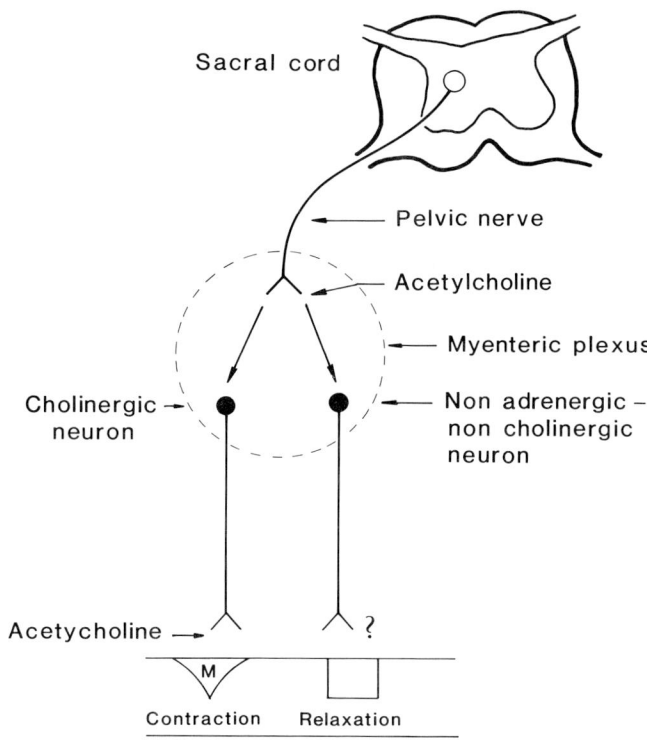

### Internal anal sphincter

FIG. 7. Sacral parasympathetic innervation to internal anal sphincter. Preganglionic fibers that originate from neurons in sacral spinal cord synapse with excitatory cholinergic and inhibitory nonadrenergic, noncholinergic neurons located in rectum-sphincteric region. In cat, cholinergic neurons are considered to provide excitatory innervation mediated by muscarinic receptors. In contrast, circular muscle fibers of sphincter receive only an inhibitory innervation. Transmitter released by noncholinergic, nonadrenergic neurons is not determined. [Adapted from Bouvier and Gonella (24, 25).]

tion of acetylcholine, methacholine chloride, and bethanechol chloride results in either a contraction and/or a relaxation or a biphasic response consisting of a contraction followed by a relaxation (Table 2). Sphincter muscle in the cat may have muscarinic excitatory and inhibitory receptors (25). In isolated longitudinal muscle strips obtained from sphincteric region of cats, contractile responses occurred that were potentiated by anticholinesterase compounds and abolished by muscarinic antagonists. In contrast, in isolated circular muscle fibers of cat, inhibitory responses occurred that were abolished by atropine.

Inhibitory responses by acetylcholine in humans may also be mediated in part by activation of intrinsic inhibitory neurons. In muscle strips of the sphincteric region, the predominant effect of cholinergic agonists is a relaxation that is reduced when the muscle strip is treated with tetrodotoxin (29). These responses are abolished also by the administration of atropine (29).

TABLE 2. *Cholinergic Agonists That Alter Motor Activity of Internal Anal Sphincter*

| Cholinergic Agonist | Response | Preparation | Species | Ref. |
|---|---|---|---|---|
| Acetylcholine, methacholine chloride | +*, − | In vivo | Cat | 83, 85 |
| Acetylcholine Bethanechol chloride | +, longitudinal muscle −, circular muscle | In vitro | Cat | 25 |
| Acetylcholine | −*; +, −, circular muscle; +, longitudinal muscle | In vitro | Cat | 184 |
| Acetylcholine | +, − | In vitro | Monkey | 191 |
| Acetylcholine | −*; +; +, − | In vitro | Human | 29 |
| Acetylcholine | +, − | In vitro | Human | 178 |

+, Excitatory action; −, inhibitory action.  * Predominant action of cholinergic agonist.

## INFLUENCE OF SACRAL AUTONOMIC NERVES ON MOTOR ACTIVITY OF COLON AND RECTUM

### Effect of Electrical Stimulation of Sacral Nerves

Motor and electrical responses of the muscle layers of the colon and rectum to electrical stimulation of efferent axons in sacral parasympathetic nerves have been documented by numerous investigators. Langley and Anderson (143) reported that contraction of the muscle layers was the predominant effect of stimulation of the sacral nerves in vivo. In a few experiments, stimulation of the sacral nerves produced a biphasic response: an initial transient inhibition followed by excitation. Inhibitory effects of pelvic nerve stimulation were confirmed in dog colon. Garry and Gillespie (89) examined the effects of pelvic nerve stimulation in the rabbit colon. They removed the colon and nerves and placed them in an isolated chamber. Electrical stimulation of pelvic nerves at frequencies of 10 Hz for a period of 10 s produced maximal responses. These contractions were maintained for 40–70 s after stimulation. Responses of lower amplitude but similar duration were obtained at lower stimulus frequencies (0.5–5 cycles/s). Electrical stimulation of the pelvic nerves in the rectum of the rabbit in vitro produced a simultaneous increase in tension of both circular and longitudinal muscle layers (159).

The excitatory effects of pelvic nerve stimulation have also been examined in cat colon in vivo. All regions of the colon and rectum contracted during electrical stimulation of the pelvic nerves (65, 120). Pelvic nerve–evoked contractions occurred after a short latency (1–2 s) and were maintained for several minutes after stimulation.

Pharmacological studies provide a partial identification of the transmitters in the sacral parasympathetic pathway to the muscle layers of the colon and rectum. Contractions evoked by electrical stimulation of the sacral ventral roots, pelvic nerve, or sacral spinal cord are depressed or abolished by the administration of competitive ganglionic blocking agents. This indicates that some of the efferent fibers in the pelvic nerve that travel to the colon and rectum are cholinergic (65, 100, 120).

### Cholinergic Responses

Pelvic nerve–evoked contractions are either totally blocked or partially depressed by the administration of atropine, indicating that acetylcholine may be the postganglionic transmitter. In rabbit and guinea pig colon and cat rectum, pelvic nerve stimulation evoked contractions and excitatory junctional potentials that were abolished by atropine (65, 78, 89, 93).

### Noncholinergic, Nonadrenergic Responses

Atropine-resistant contractions of the colon in response to pelvic nerve stimulation have been reported for dog and cat (65, 77, 97, 100, 120, 197). In cat rectum, pelvic nerve stimulation in the presence of atropine evoked a relaxation of the rectum during the period of stimulation and a contraction after the period of stimulation. Atropine-resistant contractions of cat colon and the relaxation and poststimulus contractions of rectum in response to pelvic nerve stimulation are abolished by hexamethonium and not affected by the administration of $\alpha$- and $\beta$-adrenoceptor–blocking agents. This suggests that these responses are mediated by noncholinergic, nonadrenergic fibers. Atropine-resistant relaxation and contractile responses in cat colon are abolished by the administration of naloxone or after desensitization of motor responses by a slowly degradable adenosine triphosphate analogue ($\alpha,\beta$-methylene ATP) (106, 214).

In summary, the majority of these studies were performed in vivo in anesthetized animals with intraluminal pressure recordings obtained from the colon and rectum. Detailed frequency-response relationships have not been provided. Quantitative measurements of intraluminal colonic and rectal pressures during electrical stimulation of the pelvic nerves are also unreported. Nonetheless preganglionic fibers in the pelvic nerve synapse with intrinsic neurons of the intramural plexus. Contractions of the colon and rectum in response to pelvic nerve stimulation are mediated through cholinergic excitatory nerves. Relaxations and delayed excitatory responses to pelvic nerve stimulation are mediated by noncholinergic, nonadrenergic inhibitory nerves. The identity of the transmitter released from the noncholinergic, nonadrenergic nerves is presently unknown.

## INFLUENCE OF SOMATIC NERVES ON MOTOR ACTIVITY OF SKELETAL MUSCLE OF PELVIC FLOOR

A number of reflexes involve skeletal muscle of the external anal sphincter and pelvic floor. These include somatic reflexes mediated by afferent and efferent fibers in the pudendal nerve and viscerosomatic reflexes mediated by afferent fibers in sacral autonomic nerves from the colon and urinary bladder and efferent fibers in the pudendal nerve. A description of these reflexes and their central neural organization are presented here.

### Somatic Reflexes

The anal canal is closed and continence is maintained in part by tonic contractions of skeletal muscle of the external anal sphincter, puborectalis, and levator ani. Phasic contractions of the external anal sphincter muscle have also been reported during distension of the anal canal and reproductive organs and during mechanical stimulation (e.g., touch, nociceptive stimuli) of anal mucosa, perianal skin, and reproductive organs (e.g., glans penis, clitoris) (21, 22, 129, 130, 181, 196, 236). Electromyographic studies have shown that both tonic and phasic contractions of the skeletal muscle of the external anal sphincter are dependent on the integrity of reflex arcs involving somatic afferent and efferent fibers contained in the pudendal nerve, sacral ventral roots, and sacral spinal cord (21, 22). Bilateral transection of the pudendal nerves, local anesthesia of colonic mucosa, or injury to the sacral spinal cord and sacral dorsal roots abolished phasic and tonic contractions and electromyographic electrical activity (21, 22). Pudendal motor reflexes are organized in the sacral spinal cord but occur in humans and experimental animals after transverse section of the spinal cord at cervical, thoracic, and upper lumbar regions (21, 22, 71).

Few studies report spinal interneuronal circuits that organize the somatic motor outflow to the external anal sphincter (134, 153, 161). Mackel (153) reported that 50% of sphincteric motoneurons in the cat (both urethral and external anal sphincters) received weak monosynaptic excitatory inputs during electrical stimulation of low-threshold afferent fibers in sacral dorsal roots and in the pudendal nerve. These responses were considered to be initiated from muscle spindles (34, 180, 241) in the sphincter. There was no evidence for recurrent inhibitory mechanisms in sphincteric motoneurons (153) or disynaptic inhibition in pudendal motoneurons (125).

Segmental somatic reflexes to pudendal motor axons, which innervate the external anal sphincter, were studied in cats with intact spinal cord and in cats with acutely severed spinal cords [$T_{13}$–$L_2$ spinal cord transection (134)]. The reflex discharge pattern of single pudendal motor axons and single motor units was activated reflexly by convergent afferent inputs during distension of the anal canal and reproductive organs and by mechanical stimulation (tactile, nociceptive stimuli) of the mucosa, anal and perianal skin, and skin surrounding reproductive organs. Peak firing frequencies of action potentials during mechanical stimulation of the skin ranged from 8 to 35 Hz. The average firing frequency of action potentials during continuous distension of the anal canal ranged from 4 to 16 Hz. The population of motor units and motor axons studied did not exhibit spontaneous action potential discharges and therefore might represent axonal discharges of phasic motor neurons that innervate sphincteric skeletal muscle. The discharge pattern of one motor unit in skeletal muscle of the external anal sphincter of the cat is shown in Figure 8. Noxious or tactile stimuli were applied to the mucosa of the anal canal. The motor unit initiated peak frequencies of action potentials during the period of stimulation, followed by a decay in the frequency during and after the period of stimulation.

### Supraspinal Pathways

Some of the descending supraspinal pathways to the external anal sphincter mediate voluntary contraction of the external anal sphincter (Figs. 9, 10). Complete spinal cord transection in patients interrupts these pathways and voluntary contraction of the sphincter.

Mackel (153) examined descending supraspinal pathways that control skeletal muscle of anal and urethral sphincters. Descending monosynaptic excitation and polysynaptic inhibition were mediated by fibers in the ventromedial and ventrolateral reticulospinal tracts, respectively. The cells of origin were in the medullary reticular formation in the nucleus reticularis gigantocellularis. Mackel (153) reported that the supraspinal control of the sphincters originated from higher brain centers (i.e., cortex and diencephalon) and that neurons in these areas sent fibers that relayed synaptic input to neurons located in the medullary reticular area. Descending excitatory pathways may be activated during increases in intra-abdominal pressure, which occur during coughing or straining, and function to maintain sphincteric continence. The somatic excitatory reflex pathway to the external anal sphincter is shown in Figure 9.

In animals and humans with an intact spinal cord, continuous tone of EAS is maintained by spinal reflex arcs involving afferent and efferent fibers in pudendal nerve (21, 22, 133). Sphincteric motor neurons receive monosynaptic and polysynaptic inputs (153). Phasic increases in EAS tone occur during stretch of EAS and perineal skeletal muscle and smooth muscle of reproductive organs. Cutaneous afferents originating from receptors in skin and mucosa of anal canal,

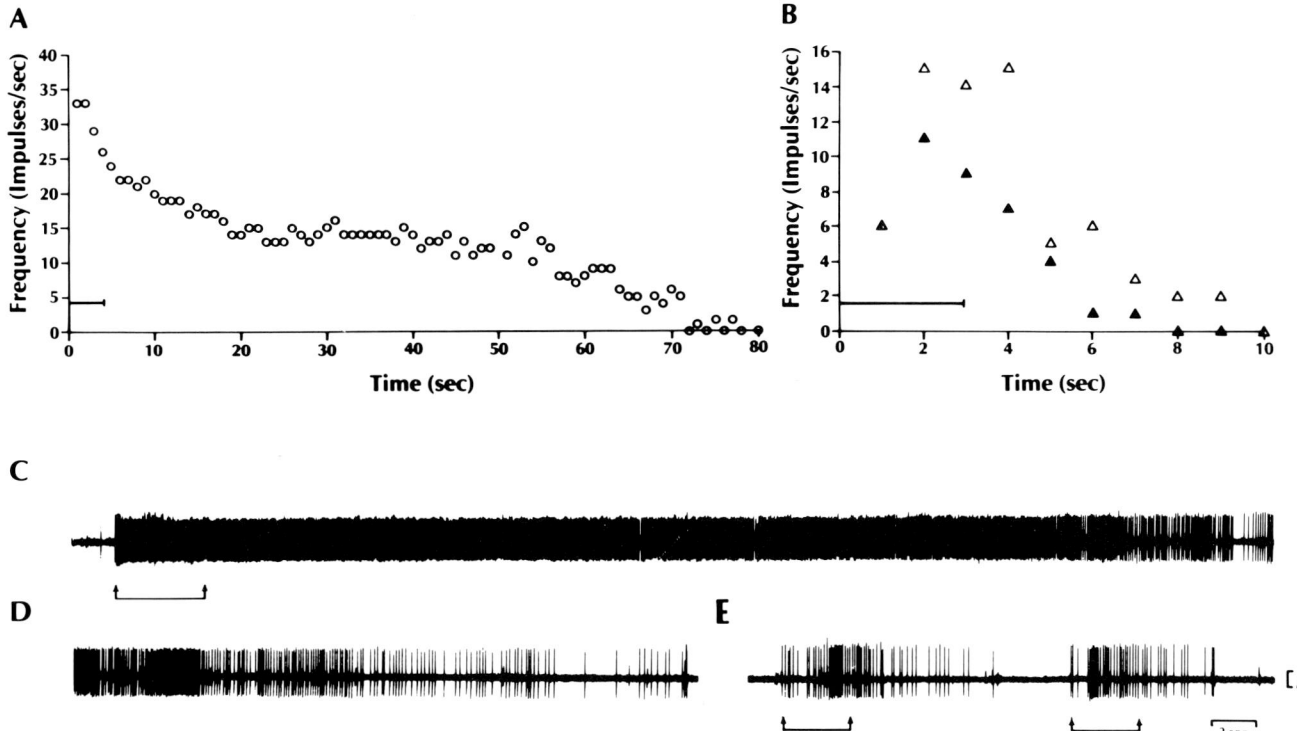

FIG. 8. Discharge pattern of motor unit in skeletal muscle of external anal sphincter of cat in response to noxious stimulus [pinch (A, C, D) and light touch (B, E)] applied to mucosal lining of anal canal by serrated forceps and blunt glass rod (tip diam 2 mm), respectively. A, B: *abscissa*, time in seconds; *ordinate*, frequency expressed in impulses/s. Horizontal bars (A, B) and bar with arrows (C, E), duration of stimulation. Data obtained in cat with acutely severed spinal cord ($L_1$ and $L_2$ transection level). [From Krier (134).]

perineum, and reproductive organs are activated by mechanoreceptors (tactile and nociceptive) and temperature. Afferent fibers in pudendal nerve have also been localized in gracile nuclei in medulla (232–234). Afferent projections from gracile nuclei are not established. Descending supraspinal projections from brain stem and cortex have been localized in close vicinity to pudendal motor neurons (113, 170, 228). Electrical stimulation of cortical motor areas produces contraction of external anal sphincter (165, 217). Electrical stimulation of brain stem sites provide excitatory and inhibitory inputs to pudendal motor neurons (153). Electrical stimulation of motor axons in pudendal nerve elicits phasic contractions of EAS mediated by nicotinic receptors (136). Pathways described are based on electrophysiological and anatomical studies in cats and monkeys and electrophysiological studies in humans.

### Viscerosomatic Reflexes

EFFECT OF COLONIC-RECTAL DISTENSION. Detailed descriptions of reflex contraction and relaxation of the skeletal muscle of the external anal sphincter and puborectalis in response to rectal or rectosigmoid distension in human and colonic distension in experimental animals have been provided by numerous investigators (21, 22, 90, 98, 161, 163, 179, 186, 188, 205, 206, 208). Passive rectal distension or active rectal contraction increases force development and electromyographic activity of skeletal muscle of the pelvic floor followed by a decrease or complete loss of electrical activity. These reflexes occur in humans with transverse lesions of the spinal cord at cervical and thoracic levels (71, 163, 188). Contractions of the external anal sphincter during rectal distension may depend in part on supraspinal mechanisms, since sphincteric contractions were weaker in humans with spinal cord injury (71).

MICTURITION. Contractions of the urinary bladder initiate phasic sphincteric contractions followed by a decrease or loss in electrical activity of the skeletal muscle of the external anal sphincter of humans, dogs, and cats (21, 27, 188, 212). Porter (186) reported in humans that micturition produced a complete loss in continuous electrical activity in skeletal muscle of the external anal sphincter and puborectalis. In patients with rectal resection, micturition still produced a reduction in electrical activity of the sphincter. Bradley (27) reported that human external anal sphincteric muscle contracted after stimulation of the mucosa of the urethra and urinary bladder. In cats and dogs, bladder distension inhibited continuous electrical activity recorded from the external anal sphincter (21, 212).

ELECTROPHYSIOLOGICAL STUDIES. Some of the electrophysiological characteristics of peripheral fibers, spinal interneuronal circuits, and the central organization of viscerosomatic reflexes have been reported (21, 22, 161, 212). In the cat, colonic or urinary bladder distension initiated reflexes mediated by visceral afferent fibers in the pelvic nerve and by motor axons in the pudendal nerve. These reflexes were organized in the sacral spinal cord. In the dog, bladder distension initiated reflexes mediated by afferent fibers in the hypogastric and pelvic nerves and by motor axons in the pudendal nerve (212). McMahon et al. (161) described viscerosomatic reflexes for the cat during distension of the colon and urinary bladder and during electrical stimulation of visceral afferent fibers in the pelvic nerve. Multiunit and single-unit recordings were made from pudendal motor axons that innervate the sphincter and interneurons in the dorsal horn of the sacral spinal cord, respectively. Visceral stimulation elicited reflex somatic discharges on pudendal motor axons at short latencies (5–20 ms). Bladder and colon distension inhibited somatic (pudendal) motor reflexes to the external anal sphincter (Fig. 11). The spinal circuits that organize viscerosomatic reflexes were attributed to a group of gating interneurons that control the pudendal motor outflow to the external anal sphincter (160).

Supraspinal influences on viscerosomatic and somatic reflexes have been reported (161). Electrical stimulation of the raphe nuclei resulted in an inhibition of somatic motor reflexes during electrical stimulation of afferent fibers in the pudendal nerve and inhibition of viscerosomatic reflexes during electrical stimulation of visceral afferent fibers in the pelvic nerve.

OPERANT CONDITIONING OF VISCEROSOMATIC REFLEXES. Reflex contractions of the external anal sphincter in response to rectal distension are respon-

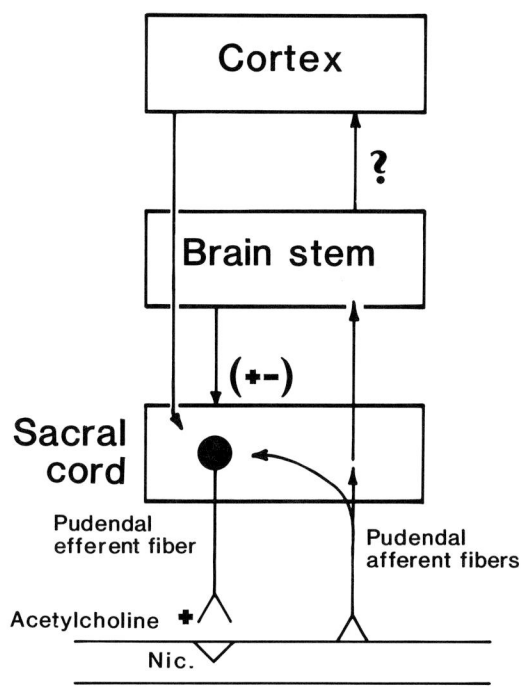

FIG. 9. Diagram of pudendal motor pathway to external anal sphincter (EAS).

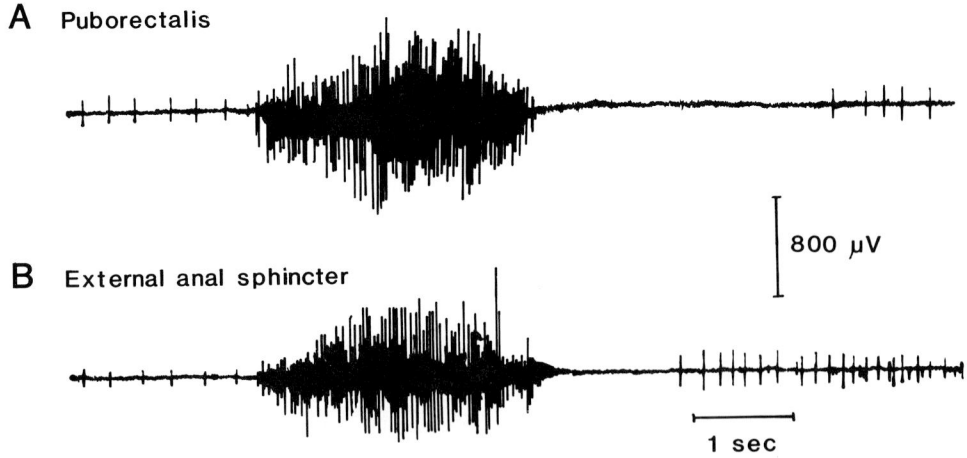

FIG. 10. Electromyographic recordings from human skeletal muscle of pelvic floor. A: puborectalis; B: subcutaneous component of external anal sphincter. Note recruitment of additional motor units during brief voluntary contraction. [Adapted from Kerremans (130).]

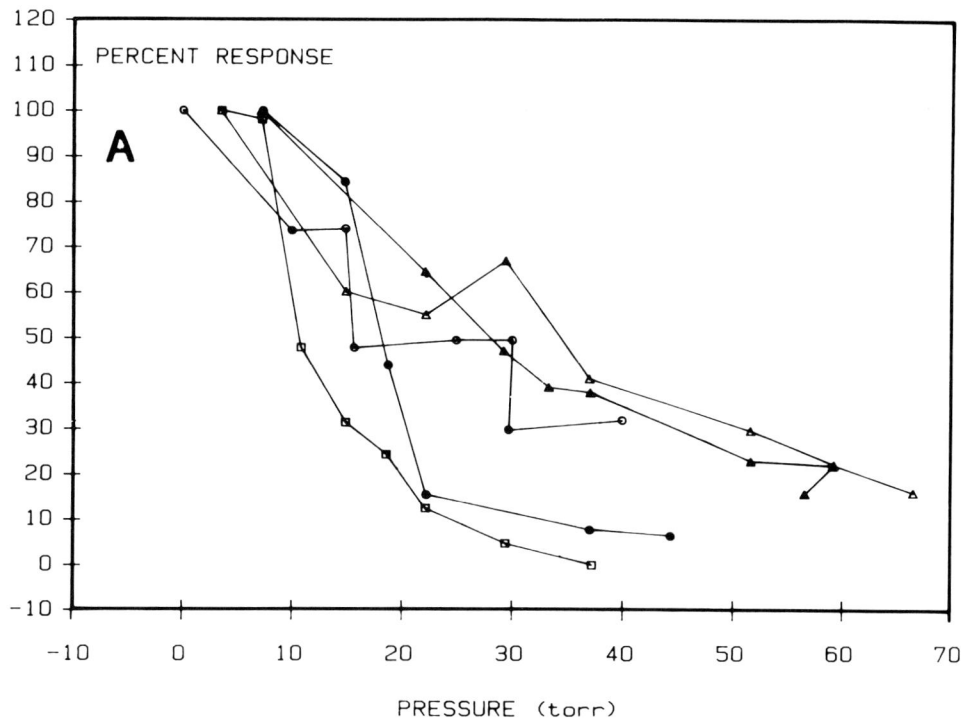

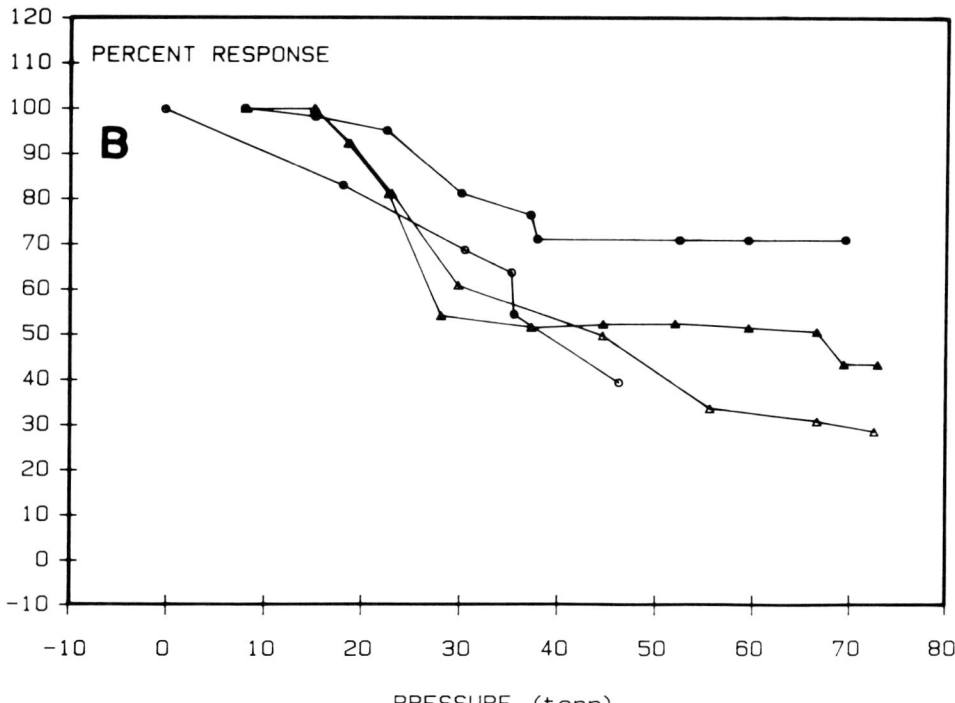

FIG. 11. Effects of intravesical (*A*) and distal intracolonic (*B*) steady-state pressure on synchronous reflex discharges recorded in pudendal nerve branch to external anal sphincter. Afferent fibers in contralateral pudendal nerve were electrically stimulated. *Abscissa*, pressure (Torr); *ordinate*, percent response. *A*: 5 cats; *B*: 4 cats. [○, Data from McMahon et al. (161); □, △, ▲, ●, data from Traxinger and Krier (230a).]

sive to operant conditioning techniques (33, 118, 156, 207, 242). This procedure allows retraining of the external anal sphincter in incontinent persons who have weak or absent external anal sphincter responses. Patients are trained to increase the strength of reflex contractions during visceral sensation induced by rectal distension. Visual display of sphincteric contractions allows the patient voluntarily to correct sphincteric responses. Improved sphincteric contractions have been reported in patients with anorectal surgery but with absence of sensory or motor impairment (33). One study reports improvement of sphincteric contractions in diabetic patients with fecal incontinence (242).

*Flexor Reflexes*

Stimuli (i.e., nociceptive, mechanoreceptive, temperature, and electrical stimulation of afferent fibers in cutaneous and muscle nerves) that evoke flexor reflexes to limb muscles also evoke synchronous reflex discharges on pudendal efferent axons and contractions of external anal and urethral sphincters (126, 161). Nonnoxious and noxious stimuli result, respectively, in contraction of some muscle groups and contraction of a majority of muscle groups associated with withdrawal of the limb. The physiological role of reflex sphincter contractions is uncertain. Jolesy et al. (126) proposed that overactivity of flexor reflexes after injury to the spinal cord may explain excessive contractile activity of the sphincters. It is also possible that these reflexes help maintain sphincter closure during increases in intra-abdominal pressure during exercise.

DEFECATION

*General Considerations*

Defecation occurs by coordinated contractions and relaxations of smooth and skeletal muscles of the colon, rectum, anal sphincters, and pelvic floor. It is a complex act involving the integration of somatic and autonomic reflex mechanisms and is dependent on the participation of neural populations located within the wall of the colon and rectum (enteric nerves) and neuronal populations located at various levels of the neuroaxis (including the spinal cord, brain stem, telencephalon, and diencephalon).

It is generally considered that the primary stimulus of defecation is distension of the rectum. Receptors located in the wall of the rectum are activated, resulting in reflex relaxation of the internal anal sphincter and simultaneous contractions of the external anal sphincter. Rectal distension also generates sensory information that is transmitted via sacral afferent fibers and ascending afferent pathways in the intermediolateral funiculus of the spinal cord (172) to cortical and diencephalic centers. Telencephalic and/or diencephalic centers provide descending input to somatic efferents to elicit appropriate postural adjustments. If the urge to defecate is suppressed, descending inputs to motoneurons in the sacral spinal cord mediate voluntary contractions of the external anal sphincter, puborectalis, and levator ani. Tension in the rectal wall decreases the stimulus for defecation. In contrast, during defecation, inputs to somatic efferents effectively increase intrathoracic and abdominal pressure, which assist evacuation. Increases in intrathoracic and intra-abdominal pressure are mediated by a descent of the diaphragm and closure of the glottis. The assumption of the squatting position also aids in the increase of intra-abdominal pressure.

Descending projections from the brain stem and hypothalamus to preganglionic neurons of the sacral spinal cord facilitate the principal reflexes that underlie defecation. These include activation of parasympathetic efferent fibers in the distal colon and rectum and inhibition of the excitatory input to the external anal sphincter and pelvic floor muscle. Activation of the sacral parasympathetic outflow facilitates excitatory reflexes, which results in smooth muscle contraction and the propulsion of fecal contents. Inhibition of motor input to the external anal sphincter and pelvic floor results in relaxation of the skeletal muscle.

*Visceral and Somatic Afferent Fibers*

Afferent information from the rectum and anal canal is received in the sacral and lumbar regions of the spinal cord. These inputs occur *1)* via the pelvic and pudendal nerve and *2)* via the hypogastric and inferior lumbar splanchnic nerves. Afferent fibers from the anal canal and rectum are involved in the initiation of spinal autonomic and somatic reflex mechanisms and the transmission of visceral and somatic sensation to higher centers in the brain.

SACRAL VISCERAL AFFERENTS. Early investigations in humans of the sacral sensory pathway demonstrate that rectal sensation induced by balloon distension results in a sense of fullness and the desire to defecate. Sensation was often referred to the rectum or sacral spinal cord. Higher pressures produced cramplike or colicky pain (58, 98, 122, 244). Damage to nerve fibers that contain sacral afferent nerves (pelvic nerves, cauda equina, or sacral spinal cord) abolishes rectal sensations. In contrast, rectal sensations are present in patients with bilateral sympathectomy ($T_3$-$L_3$) and bilateral transection of thoracic sympathetic nerves [i.e., greater splanchnic nerves (190)]. These results suggest that integrity of lumbar and thoracic visceral afferent fibers is not essential for transmitting visceral sensation that originates from the rectum.

Studies of selective sacral nerve transection in humans confirm earlier reports (52, 102). Surgical interruption of the sacral nerves bilaterally or section of the pelvic nerves on one side alters rectal sensation and the ability to discriminate fecal quality.

Ascending pathways in the spinal cord are also important in transmitting sacral afferent information from the rectum to supraspinal regions, including the cerebral cortex. Nathan and Smith (172) indicate that the afferent pathways exist in the intermediolateral funiculus of the spinal cord. Disruption of these in the spinal cord abolishes rectal sensation. Frenckner (71) reported that rectal sensation initiated by balloon distension was absent in humans with complete transection of the thoracic and cervical spinal cord.

SACRAL SOMATIC AFFERENTS. Sensory information from the anal canal, perianal skin region, and skeletal muscle of the external anal sphincter is conveyed to the sacral spinal cord via afferent fibers in somatic nerves and sacral dorsal roots (56, 59, 229). Sensory modalities of light touch, pain, and temperature were sensed in the anal canal and perianal skin region in humans.

Two studies report electrophysiological properties of primary afferent fibers in pudendal nerves and sacral dorsal roots of the cat (21, 229). Slowly adapting discharges were recorded in sacral dorsal root fibers during balloon distension of the anal canal. The discharges exhibited a maximum frequency of action potentials that declined to a steady-state level during the distending stimulus (Fig. 12). Contractions of the external anal sphincter produced a transitory pause in the firing frequency. Slowly adapting changes that occurred during distension of the anal canal were considered to be initiated by muscle spindles (34, 180, 240) localized in skeletal muscle of the external anal sphincter. Rapidly adapting discharges were also reported during mechanical stimulation of the skin and during distension and release of distension of the anal canal.

LUMBAR SYMPATHETIC AFFERENTS. Pain associated with distension of the colon in humans may be mediated by sympathetic afferents. Distension of the large intestine of patients with a balloon positioned in the cecum, ascending, transverse colon, and descending colon can elicit a painful response localized around or below the umbilicus. After bilateral transection of sphincter nerves and bilateral sympathectomy, pain in response to distension or electrical stimulation of the colon above the sigmoid was abolished (190).

There are no electrophysiological studies that report properties of visceral afferent fibers in lumbar sympathetic nerves to the rectum and internal anal sphincter. Electrophysiological studies of afferent fi-

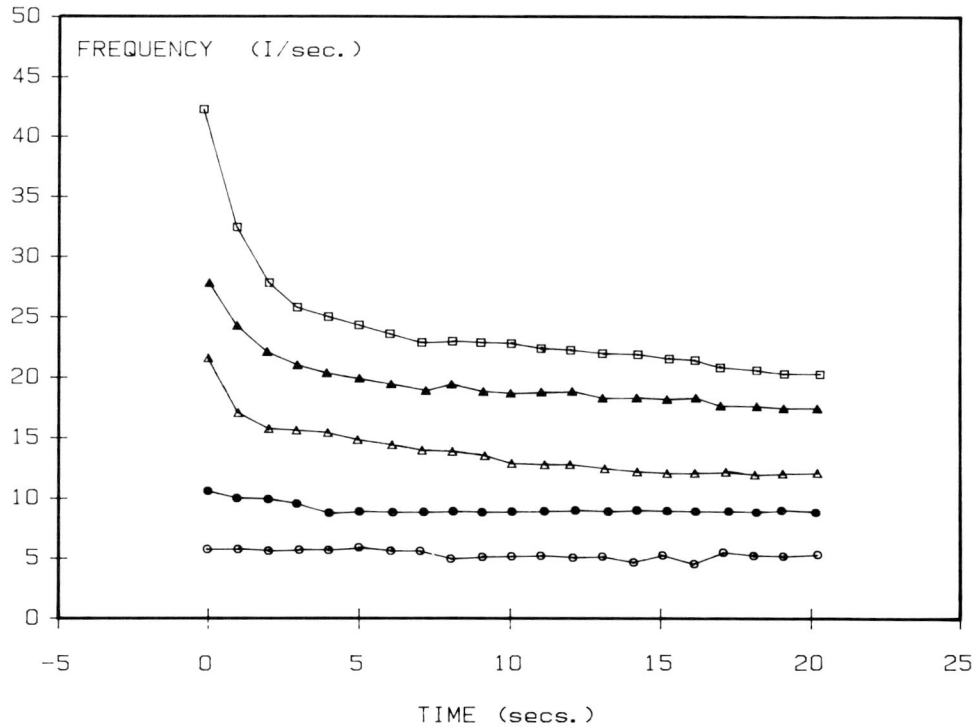

FIG. 12. Discharge pattern of one afferent unit in second sacral dorsal root of cat in response to steady-state pressure in anal canal. *Abscissa*, anal canal pressure; *ordinate*, frequency expressed in impulses/s. Afferent unit was classified as slowly adapting mechanoreceptor considered to be muscle spindle. ○, resting discharge; ●, 10 Torr; △, 20 Torr; ▲, 30 Torr; □, 40 Torr. [Adapted from Todd (229).]

bers in lumbar sympathetic nerves to cat colon have been reported (23, 67, 106).

Floyd, Hick, and Morrison (67) studied electrophysiological properties of primary afferent fibers in lumbar sympathetic nerves. They recorded single afferent unit discharges in inferior lumbar splanchnic and hypogastric nerves. The majority of the units were slowly adapting mechanoreceptors, whose receptive field was located along the vascular branch of the inferior mesenteric artery or confined to the mesentery. The receptors were suggested to be free-branched unmyelinated terminals of the nerves. Spontaneous colonic contractions or contractions evoked by electrical stimulation of the sacral ventral roots were associated with an increase in the discharge rate of the afferent fibers.

Some of the afferent fibers in lumbar sympathetic nerves to the colon have been considered to encode noxious stimulation. The afferent fibers studied were considered similar to polymodal nociceptors in the testes, skin, skeletal muscle, and heart (100). Single afferent units activated by colonic distension were also activated by intra-arterial injection of bradykinin or potassium chloride or partial or complete ischemia produced by occlusion of the superior and inferior mesenteric artery. Single units that were not activated by colonic distension were also not activated by bradykinin or potassium chloride. Colonic distension and the injection of potassium chloride and bradykinin into skin and skeletal muscle have previously been shown to produce pain in humans and pseudoaffective behavior in animals.

### Sacral Parasympathetic Efferent Fibers

Parasympathetic fibers that innervate colon and rectum via the pelvic nerve play an important role in defecation. Earlier studies (62, 143) established that electrical stimulation of sacral ventral roots produced contractions of both longitudinal and circular muscle layers of the colon and rectum, often resulting in defecation. Elliot and Barclay-Smith (62) described a tonic contraction of the distal colon of the cat that moved caudally, resulting in the expulsion of feces. The importance of the sacral parasympathetic pathway has also been demonstrated in studies in which pelvic nerves or sacral ventral roots were sectioned and experimental animals were allowed to recover from the surgical procedure (1, 86). After section of pelvic nerves, most regions of the colon were dilated, and the colon was similar in form to that observed in megacolon. Other investigators noted a dilation of the rectum and anal canal and an accumulation of the feces after sectioning sacral ventral roots (156). In humans, destruction of sacral ventral roots or pelvic nerve (52, 102) leads to fecal incontinence and disturbances in defecation.

Studies performed in the cat suggest that reflex activation of the sacral parasympathetic efferent fibers by distension, electrical stimulation, or frictional stimulation leads to activation of afferent fibers in pelvic nerve and reflex firing in sacral parasympathetic efferent nerves (47, 86, 87, 120). These reflexes enhance motility of the colon and rectum, leading to evacuation of fecal contents. Synchronous parasympathetic reflex discharges recorded on colonic branches of the pelvic nerve occurred at long latencies (range 180–300 ms) and were mediated by nonmyelinated afferent and efferent fibers in the pelvic nerve (47). Parasympathetic reflexes were obtained in decerebrate cats and in cats in which the spinal cords were chronically transected at lower thoracic and upper lumbar regions but were absent after transection of the sacral spinal cord (47, 86, 87). These results indicate that in the cat the sacral parasympathetic reflexes involved with defecation are mediated at a spinal level. Other investigators stress the importance of supraspinal pathway–mediating sacral parasympathetic reflexes to dog colon (76).

### Relationship Between Eating and Colonic Motility

Eating has been associated with increases in colonic motor and electrical activity, sometimes resulting in the urge to defecate (113, 121, 220). Mechanisms underlying these responses are not completely understood. Initially colonic contractions were considered the result of neural reflexes (i.e., gastrocolic reflex), involving afferent and efferent fibers in the vagus nerve (146). This earlier view is no longer tenable because enhanced colonic motility in response to eating occurs in patients with bilateral vagotomy and gastrectomy.

There are conflicting reports regarding the role of the spinal cord in mediating colonic responses during eating. One study reports that injury to and tumors of the spinal cord do not alter colonic responses during eating (39). Another study reports that complete transection of the thoracic cord in patients has been associated with a loss of colonic responses (96) during eating. Patients with peripheral nervous system dysfunction and severe constipation (e.g., those with diabetes mellitus and multiple sclerosis) fail to demonstrate increases in colonic motility after eating (95). These studies suggest that spinal and peripheral autonomic pathways may be important in mediating the colonic responses during eating.

Gastrointestinal hormones (i.e., gastrin, cholecystokinin) have also been considered mediators of this process (55, 173, 220). Exogenous administration of gastrin, pentagastrin, and cholecystokinin enhances colonic motor and electrical activity. The physiological role of these hormones in mediating the colonic responses is not understood.

## MOTOR DYSFUNCTION OF COLON, ANORECTUM, AND PELVIC FLOOR MUSCULATURE

Motor dysfunction can be classified as a failure to eliminate fecal material (i.e., disturbance in colonic rectal transit and defecation) and a failure to store fecal material (i.e., fecal incontinence). Motor dysfunction can result in disorders involving structural damage to smooth and skeletal muscle or in disorders involving nerves (including myenteric plexus, peripheral autonomic and somatic nerves, spinal cord, and supraspinal regions).

### Muscle Dysfunction

Diseases that have been associated with disorders of gastrointestinal smooth muscle [e.g., collagen vascular diseases, amyloidosis (66)]. Diseases of this type can result in dilation of the gastrointestinal tract, constipation, loss of haustra from the colon, and atrophy of circular and longitudinal layers of smooth muscle. One study describes myotonic-type anal contractions of the internal anal sphincter in response to rectal distension in myotonic dystrophy (210).

### Neurogenic Dysfunctions

MYENTERIC PLEXUS. Excessive contractile activity of smooth muscle in an aganglionic segment of the large intestine and failure of the internal anal sphincter to relax reflexly have been attributed to an absence of intrinsic inhibitory neurons (249). In Hirschsprung's disease in which there is outlet obstruction, the aganglionic segment usually involves the entire length of the rectum (117). Proximal colonic segments with a normal myenteric plexus can show enlargement or dilation. Acquired disorders of the myenteric plexus associated with constipation have also been reported in idiopathic megabowel (139).

LOWER MOTOR NEURONS. Motor disturbances due to lesions of lower motor neurons (including pelvic nerve, pudendal nerve, cauda equina, and sacral spinal cord) have been reported (1, 52, 73, 86, 102, 156, 166, 211, 244). Disorders of this type interrupt the efferent limb of spinal autonomic and somatic reflex pathways to smooth and skeletal muscle. Reductions in resting pressures in the anal canal have been reported in humans with meningocele or cauda equina lesions, during lower spinal cord anesthesia (166), and during neuromuscular blockage of the pudendal nerves (73). Damage to sacral parasympathetic nerves in the presence of cauda equina lesions results in a decrease in the compliance of the colon (244). Damage to the pudendal nerve interrupts somatic excitatory reflexes to pelvic floor skeletal muscle, contributing to a weakened pelvic floor and difficulty associated with continence and defecation. In humans with bilateral destruction of the majority of sacral ventral roots ($S_2$–$S_5$), voluntary contraction of the external anal sphincter and reflex contraction of the sphincter in response to rectal distension were diminished or abolished (102). Reflex contractions of the external anal sphincter in response to rectal distension are absent in patients with meningocele (166).

AFFERENT FIBERS. Disorders of sacral visceral and somatic afferent fibers (e.g., tabes dorsalis, sacral spinal cord injury) can result in impairment of sensation from the rectum and anal canal and interruption of somatic reflexes to pelvic floor skeletal musculature. In tabes dorsalis in which there is selective degeneration of afferent fibers, tonic contractile activity of the external anal sphincter is absent, but the efferent somatic pathway is intact, as evidenced by voluntary contractions of the external anal sphincter (206).

SPINAL CORD. In humans, spinal cord injuries and complete spinal cord transection in segments above the lumbosacral outflow have been associated with impairment or loss of rectal sensation, constipation, disturbances in colonic motility and defecation (38, 71, 95, 96, 123, 244), and reduction in resting pressures in the anal canal (243). The compliance of the colon is increased in patients, as evidenced by plots of the relationship between colonic pressure and injected volume. Absence of voluntary contractions of the external anal sphincter has also been reported (71).

SUPRASPINAL REGIONS. Injuries to supraspinal regions have also been associated with disturbances in constipation, micturition and defecation (5, 6, 95) and colonic motility. Lesions of the rostral part of the diencephalon (i.e., septum pellucidum and preoptic regions) produced by aneurysms of the anterior cerebral arteries result in increased frequency of both micturition and defecation (6). Lesions of the anterior medial portion of the frontal lobe of the cortex (including anterior portion of cingulate gyrus) also result in disturbances of both micturition and defecation (5).

I am grateful to Sharon Shaft and Linda Friedsberg for their careful assistance in the preparation of this manuscript. I am also grateful to Dr. Thomas Adams for reviewing the manuscript and replotting some of the figures.

Research was supported in part by a grant from the National Institutes of Health (AM-29920).

## REFERENCES

1. ADAMSON, W. A. D., AND I. AIRD. Megacolon: evidence in favor of a neurogenic origin. *Br. J. Surg.* 20: 220–233, 1932.

2. ADEBANJO, J., N. AMBACHE, AND J. VERNEY. The inhibitory transmission to the internal anal sphincter (Abstract). *Br. J.*

*Pharmacol.* 56: 392P–393P, 1976.
3. ADLER, H. F., A. J. ATKINSON, AND A. C. IVY. A study of the motility of the human colon: an explanation of dysynergia of the colon or of the "unstable colon." *Am. J. Dig. Dis.* 8: 197–202, 1941.
3a. ALUMETS, J., R. HAKANSON, F. SUNDLER, AND R. UDDMAN. VIP innervation of sphincters (Abstract). *Scand. J. Gastroenterol.* 13, Suppl. 49: 6, 1978.
4. ANDERSSON, P. O., S. R. BLOOM, AND J. JÄRHULT. Colonic motor and vascular responses to pelvic nerve stimulation and their relation to local peptide release in the cat. *J. Physiol. Lond.* 334: 293–307, 1983.
5. ANDREW, J., AND P. W. NATHAN. Lesions of the anterior frontal lobes and disturbances of micturition and defecation. *Brain* 87: 233–262, 1964.
6. ANDREW, J., P. W. NATHAN, AND N. C. SPANOS. Disturbances of micturition and defecation due to aneurysms of anterior communicating or anterior cerebral arteries. *J. Neurosurg.* 24: 1–10, 1966.
7. APPLEBAUM, M. E., G. L. CLIFTON, R. E. COGGESHALL, J. D. COULTER, W. H. VANCE, AND W. D. WILLIS. Unmyelinated fibers in the sacral 3 and caudal 1 ventral roots of the cat. *J. Physiol. Lond.* 256: 557–572, 1976.
8. BASBAUM, A. I., AND E. J. GLAZER. Immunoreactive vasoactive intestinal polypeptide is concentrated in the sacral spinal cord: a possible marker for pelvic visceral afferents. *Somatosensory Res.* 1: 69–82, 1983.
9. BASS, D. D., T. J. USTACH, AND M. M. SCHUSTER. In vitro pharmacological differentiation of sphincteric and non-sphincteric muscle. *Johns Hopkins Med. J.* 127: 185–191, 1970.
10. BATTLE, W., W. J. SNAPE, A. ALAVE, S. COHEN, AND S. BAUNSTEIN. Colonic dysfunction in diabetes mellitus. *Gastroenterology* 79: 1217–1221, 1980.
11. BAUMGARTEN, H. G. Uber der Verteilung von catechoeaminen in Darm des Menschen. *Z. Zellforsch. Mikrosk. Anat.* 83: 133–146, 1967.
12. BAUMGARTEN, H. G., A. F. HOLSTEIN, AND F. STELZNER. Unterschiede in der Innervation des Dickdarmes und des Sphincter ani internus bei Säugern und beim Menschen. *Verh. Anat. Ges.* 66: 43–47, 1971.
13. BAUMGARTEN, H. G., A. F. HOLSTEIN, AND F. STELZNER. Nervous elements in the human colon of Hirschsprung's disease. *Virchows Arch. Abt. A Pathol. Anat.* 358: 113–136, 1973.
14. BAYLISS, W. M., AND E. H. STARLING. The movements and innervation of the large intestine. *J. Physiol. Lond.* 26: 107–118, 1900.
15. BEATTIE, D. T., S. P. LIM, AND T. C. MUIR. The accumulation and release of [$^3$H]adenine nucleotides by nerves in the guinea-pig internal anal sphincter (Abstract). *Dig. Dis. Sci.* 30: 759, 1985.
16. BEERSIEK, F., A. G. PARKS, AND M. SWASH. Pathogenesis of ano-rectal incontinence: a histometric study of the anal sphincter musculature. *J. Neurol. Sci.* 42: 111–127, 1979.
17. BENNETT, R. C., AND H. L. DUTHIE. The functional importance of the internal anal sphincter. *Br. J. Surg.* 51: 355–357, 1964.
18. BIANCANI, P., J. WALSH, AND J. BEHAR. VIP: a possible inhibitory transmitter for the internal anal sphincter (Abstract). *Gastroenterology* 86: 1026, 1984.
19. BIANCANI, P., J. WALSH, AND J. BEHAR. Vasoactive intestinal peptide: a neurotransmitter for relaxation of the rabbit internal anal sphincter. *Gastroenterology* 89: 867–874, 1985.
20. BISHOP, A. E., J. M. POLAK, B. D. LAHE, M. D. BRYANT, AND S. R. BLOOM. Abnormalities of the colonic regulatory peptides in Hirschsprung's disease. *Histopathology Oxf.* 5: 679–688, 1981.
21. BISHOP, B. Reflex activity of external anal sphincter of cat. *J. Neurophysiol.* 22: 679–692, 1959.
22. BISHOP, B., R. C. GARRY, T. D. M. ROBERTS, AND J. K. TODD. Control of the external sphincter of the anus of the cat. *J. Physiol. Lond.* 182: 541–558, 1956.
23. BLUMBERG, H., P. HAUPT, W. JÄNIG, AND W. KOHLER. Encoding of visceral noxious stimuli in the discharge patterns of visceral afferents from the colon. *Pfluegers Arch.* 398: 33–40, 1983.
24. BOUVIER, M., AND J. GONELLA. Electrical activity from smooth muscle of the anal sphincter of cat. *J. Physiol. Lond.* 310: 445–456, 1981.
25. BOUVIER, M., AND J. GONELLA. Nervous control of the internal anal sphincter of the cat. *J. Physiol. Lond.* 310: 457–469, 1981.
26. BOUVIER, M., AND J. C. GRIMAUD. Neuronally mediated interactions between urinary bladder and internal anal sphincter motility in the cat. *J. Physiol. Lond.* 346: 461–469, 1984.
27. BRADLEY, W. E. Urethral electromyography. *J. Urol.* 108: 503–564, 1972.
28. BRADLEY, W. E., AND C. T. TEAGUE. Synaptic events in pudendal motor neurons of the cat. *Exp. Neurol.* 56: 237–240, 1977.
29. BURLEIGH, D. E., AND A. D. MELLO. Neural and pharmacologic factors affecting motility of the internal anal sphincter. *Gastroenterology* 84: 409–417, 1983.
30. BURLEIGH, D. E., A. D. MELLO, AND A. G. PARKS. Responses of isolated human internal anal sphincter to drugs and electrical field stimulation. *Gastroenterology* 77: 484–490, 1979.
31. BURNSTOCK, G. Comparative studies of purinergic nerves. *J. Exp. Zool.* 194: 103–134, 1975.
31a. BURNSTOCK, G., T. HÖKFELT, M. D. GERSHON, L. L. IVERSON, H. W. KOSTERLITZ, AND J. H. SZURSZEWSKI. Nonadrenergic, noncholinergic autonomic neurotransmission mechanisms. *Neurosci. Res. Prog. Bull.* 17: 379–519, 1979.
32. CANNON, W. B. The movements of the intestines studied by means of the Röntgen rays. *Am. J. Physiol.* 6: 251–277, 1902.
33. CERULLI, M. A., P. NIKOOMANESH, AND M. M. SCHUSTER. Progress in biofeedback conditioning for fecal incontinence. *Gastroenterology* 76: 742–746, 1979.
34. CHENNELS, M., W. F. FLOYD, AND R. P. GOULD. Muscle spindles in the external sphincter of the cat. *J. Physiol. Lond.* 151: 23P–24P, 1960.
35. CLIFTON, G. L., R. E. COGGESHALL, W. H. VANCE, AND W. D. WILLIS. Receptive fields of unmyelinated ventral root afferent fibres in the cat. *J. Physiol. Lond.* 256: 573–600, 1973.
36. COLLINS, C. D., B. H. BROWN, G. E. WHITTAKER, AND H. L. DUTHIE. New methods of measuring forces in the anal canal. *Gut* 10: 160–163, 1969.
37. COLLINS, C. D., H. L. DUTHIE, T. SHELLEY, AND G. E. WHITTAKER. Forces in the anal canal and anal continence. *Gut* 8: 354–360, 1967.
38. CONNELL, A. M. Significance of the pressure waves of the sigmoid. *Am. J. Dig. Dis.* 10: 481–483, 1965.
39. CONNELL, A. M., H. FRANKEL, AND L. GUTTMENN. The motility of pelvic colon following complete lesions of the spinal cord. *Paraplegia* 1: 98–115, 1963.
40. COSTA, M., AND J. B. FURNESS. The innervation of the internal anal sphincter of the guinea pig. In: *Proc. Fourth Int. Symp. Gastrointest. Motility*, edited by E. E. Daniels, K. Bowes, J. A. L. Gilbert, T. K. Schofield-Schnitka, and G. A. Scott. 1973, p. 681–690.
41. COSTA, M., AND J. B. FURNESS. The origin of the adrenergic fibers which innervate the internal anal sphincter, the rectum and other tissues of the pelvic region of the guinea pig. *Z. Anat. Entwicklungsgesch.* 140: 129–142, 1973.
42. COSTA, M., AND G. GABELLA. Adrenergic innervation of the alimentary canal. *Z. Zellforsch. Mikrosk. Anat.* 122: 357–377, 1971.
43. CREMA, A., G. M. FRIGO, S. LECCHINI, L. MANZO, L. ONORI, AND M. TONINI. Purine receptors in the guinea-pig internal anal sphincter. *Br. J. Pharmacol.* 78: 599–603, 1983.
43a. DALSGAARD, C.-J., T. ELFVIN, L. SKIRBOLE, AND P. EMSON. Substance P-containing primary sensory neurons projecting to the inferior mesenteric ganglion: evidence from combined retrograde tracing and immunohistochemistry. *Neuroscience*

7: 647–652, 1982.
43b. DALSGAARD, C.-J., T. HÖKFELT, L.-G. ELFVIN, AND L. TERENIUS. Enkephalin-containing sympathetic preganglionic neurons projecting to the inferior mesenteric ganglion: evidence from combined retrograde tracing and immunohistochemistry. *Neuroscience* 7: 2039–2050, 1982.
44. DALSGAARD, C.-J., T. HÖKFELT, O. JOHANSSON, AND R. ELDE. Somatostatin immunoreactive cell bodies in the dorsal horn and parasympathetic intermediolateral nucleus of the rat spinal cord. *Neurosci. Lett.* 27: 335–339, 1981.
45. DE GROAT, W. C., A. M. BOOTH, R. J. MILNE, AND J. R. ROPPOLO. Parasympathetic preganglionic neurons in the sacral spinal cord. *J. Auton. Nerv. Syst.* 5: 23–43, 1982.
45a. DE GROAT, W. C., M. KAWATANI, T. HISAMITSU, I. LOWE, C. MORGAN, J. ROPPOLO, A. M. BOOTH, I. NADELHAFT, D. KUO, AND K. THOR. The role of neuropeptides in the sacral autonomic reflex pathways of the cat. *J. Auton. Nerv. Sys.* 7: 339–350, 1983.
46. DE GROAT, W. C., AND J. KRIER. An electrophysiological study of the sacral parasympathetic pathway to the colon of the cat. *J. Physiol. Lond.* 260: 425–445, 1976.
47. DE GROAT, W. C., AND J. KRIER. The sacral parasympathetic reflex pathway regulating colonic motility and defecation in the cat. *J. Physiol. Lond.* 276: 481–500, 1978.
48. DE GROAT, W. C., AND J. KRIER. The central control of the lumbar sympathetic pathway of the large intestine of the cat. *J. Physiol. Lond.* 289: 449–468, 1979.
49. DE GROAT, W. C., I. NADELHAFT, R. J. MILNE, A. M. BOOTH, C. MORGAN, AND K. THOR. Organization of the sacral parasympathetic reflex pathways to the urinary bladder and large intestine. *J. Auton. Nerv. Syst.* 3: 135–160, 1981.
50. DENNY-BROWN, D., AND F. G. ROBERTSON. An investigation of the nervous control of defecation. *Brain* 58: 256–310, 1935.
51. DENT, J., AND B. CHER. A new technique for continuous sphincter pressure measurement. *Gastroenterology* 71: 263–267, 1976.
52. DEVROEDE, G. J., AND J. LAMARCHE. Functional importance of extrinsic parasympathetic innervation to the distal colon and rectum. *Gastroenterology* 66: 273–280, 1974.
53. DIAMANT, N. E., AND L. D. HARRIS. Comparison of objective measurement of anal sphincter strength with anal sphincter pressures and levator ani function. *Gastroenterology* 56: 110–116, 1969.
54. DICKINSON, V. A. Maintenance of anal continence: a review of pelvic floor physiology. *Gut* 19: 1163–1174, 1978.
55. DINOSO, V., H. MESHKINPOUR, AND S. H. LORBER. Motor response of the sigmoid colon and rectum to exogenous cholecystokinin and secretin. *Gastroenterology* 65: 438–444, 1973.
56. DUTHIE, H. L. Anal continence. *Gut* 12: 844–852, 1971.
57. DUTHIE, H. L. Dynamics of the rectum and anus. *Clin. Gastroenterol.* 4: 467–477, 1975.
58. DUTHIE, H. L., AND R. C. BENNETT. The relation of sensation in the anal canal to the functional anal sphincter: a possible factor in anal continence. *Gut* 4: 179–182, 1963.
59. DUTHIE, H. L., AND F. V. GAIRNS. Sensory nerve endings and sensation in the anal region of man. *Br. J. Surg.* 47: 585–595, 1960.
60. DUTHIE, H. L., AND J. M. WATTS. Contributions of external anal sphincter to the pressure zone in the anal canal. *Gut* 6: 64–68, 1965.
61. EHLE, A. L., AND E. L. FOLTZ. A miniature mercury strain gauge for chronic nonobstructive measurement of intestinal motility. *J. Appl. Physiol.* 26: 223–226, 1969.
62. ELLIOTT, J. R., AND E. BARCLAY-SMITH. Anti-peristalsis and other muscular activities of the colon. *J. Physiol. Lond.* 31: 272–304, 1904.
63. FAHRENKRUG, J. Vasoactive intestinal peptide measurement, distribution and putative neurotransmitter function. *Digestion* 19: 149–169, 1979.
64. FAHRENKRUG, J., U. HOGLUND, M. JODAL, J. LUNDGREN, L. OLBE, AND O. B. SCHAFFALITZKY DE MUCKADELL. Nervous release of vasoactive intestinal peptide in the gastrointestinal tract possible physiologic implications. *J. Physiol. Lond.* 284: 291–305, 1978.
65. FASTH, S., L. HULTEN, AND S. NORDGREN. Evidence for a dual pelvic nerve influence on large bowel motility in the cat. *J. Physiol. Lond.* 298: 159–169, 1980.
66. FAULK, D. L., S. ANUROS, AND J. CHRISTENSEN. Chronic intestinal pseudoobstruction. *Gastroenterology* 74: 922–931, 1978.
67. FLOYD, K., U. E. HICK, AND J. F. B. MORRISON. Mechanosensitive afferent units in the hypogastric nerve of the cat. *J. Physiol. Lond.* 259: 457–471, 1976.
68. FLOYD, K., AND G. LAWRENSON. Mechanosensitive afferent units in the cat pelvic nerve (Abstract). *J. Physiol. Lond.* 290: 51P, 1979.
69. FLOYD, K., S. B. MCMAHON, AND J. F. B. MORRISON. Inhibitory interactions between colonic and vesical afferents in the micturition reflex. *J. Physiol. Lond.* 322: 45–52, 1982.
70. FLOYD, W. F., AND F. W. WALLS. Electromyography of the sphincter ani externus in man. *J. Physiol. Lond.* 122: 599–609, 1953.
71. FRENCKNER, B. Function of the anal sphincters in spinal man. *Gut* 16: 482–489, 1975.
72. FRENCKNER, B., AND T. IHRE. Influence of autonomic nerves on the internal anal sphincter in man. *Gut* 17: 306–312, 1976.
73. FRENCKNER, B., AND C. VON EULER. Influence of pudendal block on the function of the anal sphincters. *Gut* 16: 482–489, 1975.
74. FRIEDMANN, C. A. The action of nicotine and catecholamines on the human internal anal sphincter. *Am. J. Dig. Dis.* 13: 428–431, 1968.
75. FUKAI, K., AND H. FUKUDA. The intramural pelvic nerves in the dog. *J. Physiol. Lond.* 354: 89–98, 1984.
76. FUKUDA, H., K. FUKAE, M. YAMANE, AND H. OKADA. Pontine reticular unit responses to pelvic nerve and colonic mechanical stimulation in the dog. *Brain Res.* 207: 59–71, 1981.
77. FULGRAFF, G., AND L. SCHMIDT. Zur frage der humoral verursachten, atropinresistenten kontraktion am palvic-colon-praparat von katzen. *Arch. Exp. Pathol. Pharmakol.* 245: 106–107, 1963.
78. FURNESS, J. B. An examination of nerve mediated hyoscine resistant excitation of the guinea-pig colon. *J. Physiol. Lond.* 207: 803–821, 1970.
79. FURNESS, J. B., AND M. COSTA. The ramifications of adrenergic terminals in the rectum, anal sphincter and anal accessory muscles of the guinea pig. *Z. Anat. Entwicklungsgesch.* 140: 109–128, 1973.
80. FURNESS, J. B., AND M. COSTA. The adrenergic innervation of the gastrointestinal tract. *Ergeb. Physiol. Biol. Chem. Exp. Pharmakol.* 69: 1–52, 1974.
81. FURNESS, J. B., AND M. COSTA. Actions of somatostatin on excitatory and inhibitory nerves in the intestine. *Eur. J. Pharmacol.* 56: 69–74, 1979.
82. GABELLA, G. Innervation of the gastrointestinal tract. *Int. Rev. Cytol.* 59: 129–192, 1979.
83. GARRETT, J. R., AND E. R. HOWARD. Effect of rectal distension on the internal anal sphincter of cats. *J. Physiol. Lond.* 222: 90–91, 1972.
84. GARRETT, J. R., AND E. R. HOWARD. Neural control of the internal anal sphincter of cats after chemical sympathectomy with 6-hydroxydopamine. *J. Physiol. Lond.* 247: 25P–27P, 1975.
85. GARRETT, J. R., E. R. HOWARD, AND W. JONES. The internal anal sphincter of the cat: a study of nervous mechanisms affecting tone and reflex activity. *J. Physiol. Lond.* 243: 153–166, 1974.
86. GARRY, R. C. The nervous control of the caudal region of the large bowel. *J. Physiol. Lond.* 77: 422–431, 1933.
87. GARRY, R. C. The responses to stimulation of the caudal end of the large bowel in the cat. *J. Physiol. Lond.* 78: 208–224, 1933.

88. GARRY, R. C. The movements of the large intestine. *Physiol. Rev.* 14: 103–132, 1934.
89. GARRY, R. C., AND J. S. GILLESPIE. The responses of the musculature of the colon of the rabbit to stimulation in vitro of the parasympathetic and of the sympathetic outflows. *J. Physiol. Lond.* 128: 557–576, 1955.
90. GASTON, E. A. Fecal continence following resections of varius portions of the rectum with preservation of the anal sphincters. *Surg. Gynecol. Obstet.* 81: 669–678, 1948.
91. GASTON, E. A. Physiological basis for preservation of fecal continence after resection of the rectum. *J. Am. Med. Assoc.* 146: 1486–1489, 1951.
92. GERARD, R., P. MINAIRE, J. P. CASTERAN, E. BERARD, AND M. EYSSETTE. Sphincter E.M.G. in spinal cord injured patients. *Paraplegia* 16: 244, 1978.
93. GILLESPIE, J. S. The electrical and mechanical responses of intestinal smooth muscle cells to stimulation of their extrinsic parasympathetic nerves. *J. Physiol. Lond.* 102: 76–92, 1962.
94. GLAZER, E. J., AND A. I. BASBAUM. Leucine enkephalin: localization in and axoplasmic transport by sacral parasympathetic preganglionic neurons. *Science Wash. DC* 208: 1479–1481, 1980.
95. GLICK, M. E., H. MESHKINPOUR, S. HALDEMAN, N. E. BHATIA, AND W. E. BRADLEY. Colonic dysfunction in multiple sclerosis. *Gastroenterology* 83: 1002–1007, 1982.
96. GLICK, M. E., H. MESHKINPOUR, S. HALDEMAN, F. HOEHLER, N. DOWNEY, AND W. E. BRADLEY. Colonic dysfunction in patients with spinal cord injury. *Gastroenterology* 86: 287–294, 1984.
97. GOLDBERG, M. M., AND R. H. BURNS. Atropine-resistance spasm of the dog colon induced by intermittant pelvic nerve stimulation. *Life Sci.* 10: 591–600, 1971.
98. GOLIGHER, J. C., AND E. S. R. HUGHES. Sensibility of the rectum and colon. Its role in the mechanism of anal continence. *Lancet* 1: 543–548, 1951.
99. GOWERS, W. R. The automatic action of the sphincter ani. *Proc. R. Soc. Lond. B Biol. Sci.* 29: 77–84, 1877.
100. GRAY, G. W., L. C. HENDERSHOT, R. M. WHITROCK, AND M. H. SEEVERS. Influence of the parasympathetic nerves and their relation to the action of atropine in the ileum and colon of the dog. *Am. J. Physiol.* 181: 679–687, 1955.
101. GULLERMIN, R. Somatostatin inhibits the release of acetylcholine induced electrically in the myenteric plexus. *Endocrinology* 99: 1653–1654, 1976.
102. GUTENBERG, B., J. KEWENTER, I. PETERSEN, AND B. STENER. Anorectal function after major resections of the sacrum with bilateral and unilateral sacrifice of sacral nerves. *Br. J. Surg.* 63: 546–554, 1976.
103. HALLS, J. Bowel content shifts during normal defecation. *Proc. R. Soc. Med.* 58: 854–860, 1965.
104. HANCOCK, B. D. Measurement of anal pressure and motility. *Gut* 17: 645–651, 1976.
105. HARRIS, L. D., C. S. WINANS, AND C. E. POPE. Determination of yield pressures: a method for measuring anal sphincter competence. *Gastroenterology* 50: 754–760, 1966.
106. HAUPT, P., W. JÄNIG, AND W. KOHLER. Response pattern of visceral afferent fibres, supplying the colon, upon chemical and mechanical stimuli. *Pfluegers Arch.* 398: 41–47, 1983.
107. HAYNES, W. S., AND H. W. READ. Ano-rectal activity in man during rectal infusion of saline: a dynamic assessment of the anal continence mechanism. *J. Physiol. Lond.* 330: 45–56, 1982.
108. HEDLUND, H., L. FÄNDRIKS, D. DELBRO, AND S. FASTH. Blockade of non-cholinergic non-adrenergic colonic contraction in response to pelvic nerve stimulation by large doses of $\alpha,\beta$-methylene ATP acta. *Acta Physiol. Scand.* 119: 451–454, 1983.
109. HEDLUND, H., S. FASTH, AND L. HULTEN. Efferent sympathetic nervous control of rectal motility in the cat. *Acta Physiol. Scand.* 121: 317–324, 1984.
110. HENRIKSEN, F. W., AND B. ANTHONISEN. Measurement of the anal sphincter strength by a simple method for routine use. *Scand. J. Gastroenterol.* 7: 555–558, 1972.
111. HERTZ, A. F., AND A. NEWTON. The normal movements of the colon in man. *J. Physiol. Lond.* 47: 57–65, 1913.
112. HILL, J. R., M. L. KELLY, J. F. SCHLEGAL, AND C. F. CODE. Pressure profile of the rectum and anus of healthy person. *Dis. Colon Rectum* 3: 203–209, 1960.
113. HOLDSTOCK, D. J., J. J. MISIEWICZ, T. SMITH, AND E. N. ROLANDS. Propulsion mass movements in the human colon and its relationship to meals and somatic activity. *Gut* 11: 91–99, 1970.
114. HOLSTEGE, E., AND H. G. J. M. KUYPERS. The anatomy of brainstem pathways to the spinal cord in cat. A labelled amino acid tracing study. In: *Progress in Brain Research. Anatomy of Descending Pathways to the Spinal Cord*, edited by H. G. J. M. Kuypers and G. F. Martin. 1982, vol. 57, p. 146–175.
115. HONDA, C. N., M. RÉTHELYI, AND P. PETRUSZ. Preferential immunohistochemical localization of vasoactive intestinal polypeptide (VIP) in the sacral spinal cord of the cat: light and electron microscopic observations. *J. Neurosci.* 3: 2186–2196, 1983.
116. HOWARD, E. R., AND J. R. GARRETT. The intrinsic myenteric innervation of the hind-gut and accessory muscles of defecation in the cat. *Z. Zellforsch. Microsk. Anat.* 136: 31–44, 1973.
117. HOWARD, E. R., AND H. J. NIXON. Internal anal sphincter. Obervations on development and mechanism of inhibitory responses in premature infants and children with Hirschsprung's disease. *Arch. Dis. Child.* 43: 569–578, 1968.
118. HUBEL, K. A. Voluntary control of gastrointestinal function: operant conditioning and biofeedback. *Gastroenterology* 66: 1085–1090, 1974.
119. HUGHES, J., H. W. KOSTERLITZ, AND T. W. SMITH. The distribution of methionine-enkephalin and leucine-enkephalin in the brain and peripheral tissues. *Br. J. Pharmacol.* 61: 639–647, 1977.
120. HULTEN, L. Extrinsic nervous control of colonic motility and blood flow. *Acta Physiol. Scand. Suppl.* 335: 1–116, 1969.
121. HURST, A. F. The passage of food along the human alimentary canal. *Guy's Hosp. Rep.* 61: 389–397, 1907.
122. HURST, A. F. *The Sensibility of the Alimentary Canal.* London: Oxford Univ. Press, 1911.
123. IHRE, T. Studies of anal function in continent and incontinent patients. *Scand. J. Gastroenterol.* 9, Suppl. 25: 1–64, 1974.
124. JACOBOWITZ, D. Histochemical studies of the autonomic innervation of the gut. *J. Pharmacol. Exp. Ther.* 149: 358–364, 1965.
125. JANKOWSKA, E., Y. PADEL, AND P. ZURZECKI. Cross disynaptic inhibition of sacral motoneurones. *J. Physiol. Lond.* 285: 425–444, 1978.
126. JOLESY, F. A., X. CHENG-TAO, P. W. RUENZEL, AND E. HENNEMAN. Flexor reflex control of the external sphincter of the urethra in paraplegia. *Science Wash. DC* 216: 1243–1245, 1982.
127. KAWAKAMI, M. Electromyographic investigation on the human external sphincter muscle of anus. *Jpn. J. Physiol.* 4: 196–204, 1954.
128. KAWATANI, M., I. P. LOWE, I. NADELHAFT, C. MORGAN, AND W. C. DE GROAT. Vasoactive intestinal polypeptide in visceral afferent pathways to the sacral spinal cord of the cat. *Neurosci. Lett.* 42: 311–316, 1983.
129. KERREMANS, R. Electrical activity and motility of the internal anal sphincter. *Acta Gastro-enterol. Belg.* 31: 465–482, 1968.
130. KERREMANS, R. *Morphological and Physiological Aspects of Anal Continence and Defecation.* Brussels: Arscia, 1969.
131. KERREMANS, R., AND F. PENNINCKX. A study in vivo of adrenergic receptors in the rectum and in the internal anal sphincter of the cat. *Gut* 11: 709–714, 1970.
132. KERREMANS, R., AND N. ROSSELLE. The parameters of the E.M.G. activity of the external anal sphincters and M. puborectalis in normal adult and elderly subjects. *Electromyography* 8: 89–104, 1968.
133. KRIER, J. Sacral motor reflex pathway to the external anal

sphincter of the cat (Abstract). *Federation Proc.* 41: 1745, 1982.
134. KRIER, J. Discharge patterns of pudendal efferent fibers innervating the external anal sphincter of the cat. *J. Physiol. Lond.* 368: 471–480, 1985.
135. KRIER, J., AND T. ADAMS. A method for quantification of contractile forces in the rectum and anal canal (Abstract). *Dig. Dis. Sci.* 27: 660, 1982.
136. KRIER, J., AND T. ADAMS. Quantification of axial forces in rectum-anal canal of the cat. *Am. J. Physiol.* 250 (*Gastrointest. Liver Physiol.* 13): G260–G265, 1986.
137. KRIER, J., AND D. A. HARTMAN. Electrical properties and synaptic connections to neurons in parasympathetic colonic ganglia of the cat. *Am. J. Physiol.* 247 (*Gastrointest. Liver Physiol.* 10): G52–G61, 1984.
138. KRIER, J., P. F. SCHMALZ, AND J. H. SZURSZEWSKI. Central innervation of neurones in the inferior mesenteric ganglion and of the large intestine of the cat. *J. Physiol. Lond.* 332: 125–138, 1982.
139. KRISHNAMURTHY, S., AND M. D. SCHUFFLER. Severe, idiopathic constipation is caused by a distinctive abnormality of the colonic myenteric plexus (Abstract). *Gastroenterology* 84: 1218, 1983.
140. KUBATA, M., AND J. H. SZURSZEWSKI. Mechanical and intracellular electrical activity of canine internal anal sphincter (Abstract). *Federation Proc.* 43, 2579, 1984.
141. KUBATA, M., AND J. H. SZURSZEWSKI. Electrophysiological property of internal anal sphincter of some animals (Abstract). In: *Tenth Int. Symp. Gastrointest. Motility, Rochester, Minnesota, 1985.*
142. KUZUHARA, S., I. KANAYAMA, AND T. NAKANISHI. Topographical localization of the Onuf's nuclear neurons innervating the rectal and vesicle striated sphincter muscles: a retrograde fluorescent double labelling in cat and dog. *Neurosci. Lett.* 16: 125–130, 1980.
143. LANGLEY, J. N., AND H. K. ANDERSON. On the innervation of the pelvic and adjoining viscera. Part I. The lower portion of the intestine. *J. Physiol. Lond.* 18: 67–105, 1895.
144. LANGLEY, J. N., AND H. K. ANDERSON. The innervation of the pelvic and adjoining viscera. Part VI. Histological and physiological observations upon the effects of section of the sacral nerves. *J. Physiol. Lond.* 19: 372–384, 1896.
145. LANGLEY, J. N., AND H. K. ANDERSON. The innervation of the pelvic and adjoining viscera. Part VII. Anatomical observations. *J. Physiol. Lond.* 20: 370–406, 1896.
146. LARSON, L. M., AND I. A. BARGEN. Physiology of the colon. *Arch. Surg.* 27: 1–50, 1933.
147. LAWSON, J. Structure and function of the internal anal sphincter. *Proc. R. Soc. Med.* 53: 84–89, 1970.
148. LEARMONTH, J. R., AND J. MARKOWITZ. Studies on the function of the lumbar sympathetic outflow. I. The relation of the lumbar sympathetic outflow to the sphincter ani internus. *Am. J. Physiol.* 89: 686–691, 1929.
149. LIEBERMAN, W. A new anal tensiometer. *Am. J. Proctol.* 13: 297–301, 1962.
150. LIEBERMAN, W. Objective measurement of external anal sphincter tension. *Am. J. Proctol.* 15: 375–381, 1964.
151. LIM, S. P., AND T. C. MUIR. The electrical basis for the inhibitory response of the guinea pig internal anal sphincter to nerve stimulation and drugs. In: *Gastrointestinal Motility*, edited by C. Roman. Lancaster, UK: MTP, 1983, p. 413–420.
152. LIM, S. P., AND T. C. MUIR. Mechanisms underlying the electrical and mechanical responses of the guinea-pig internal anal sphincter to field stimulation and to drugs. *Br. J. Pharmacol.* 86: 427–437, 1985.
152a. LISANDER, B., AND O. STENQUIST. Extradural fentanyl and postoperative ileus in cats. *Br. J. Anaesth.* 53: 1237, 1983.
153. MACKEL, R. Segmental and descending control of the external urethral and anal sphincters in the cat. *J. Physiol. Lond.* 294: 105–122, 1979.
154. MAHIEU, P., J. PRINGOT, AND P. BODART. Defecography: I. Description of a new procedure and results in normal patients. *Gastrointest. Radiol.* 9: 247–251, 1984.
155. MAHIEU, P., J. PRINGOT, AND P. BODART. Defecography: II. Contribution to the diagnosis of defecation disorders. *Gastrointest. Radiol.* 9: 253–261, 1984.
156. MARZUK, P. Biofeedback for gastrointestinal disorders: a review of the literature. *Ann. Intern. Med.* 103: 240–244, 1985.
157. MAYLE, J. E., T. ADAMS, M. K. PORAYKO, AND D. S. GREENBAUM. Quantification and scoring of external anal sphincter strength and control in humans (Abstract). *Gastroenterology* 88: 1494, 1985.
158. MCFADDEN, G. D. F., J. S. LOUGHRIDGE, AND T. H. MILROY. The nerve control of the distal colon. *Q. J. Exp. Physiol.* 25: 315–327, 1935.
159. MCKIRDY, H. C. Functional relationship of longitudinal and circular layers of the muscularis externa of the rabbit large intestine. *J. Physiol. Lond.* 227: 839–855, 1972.
159a. MCKNIGHT, A. T., R. P. SOSA, J. HUGHES, AND H. W. KOSTERLITZ. Biosynthesis and release of enkephalins. In: *Characteristics and Function of Opioids. Developments in Neuroscience*, edited by J. M. Van Ree and L. Terenius. Amsterdam: North-Holland, 1978, vol. 4.
160. MCMAHON, S. B., AND J. F. B. MORRISON. Two group of spinal interneurons that respond to stimulation of the abdominal viscera of the cat. *J. Physiol. Lond.* 322: 21–34, 1982.
161. MCMAHON, S. B., J. F. B. MORRISON, AND K. SPILLANE. An electrophysiological study of somatic and visceral convergence in the reflex control of the external sphincters. *J. Physiol. Lond.* 328: 379–387, 1982.
162. MCPHEDRAN, A. M., R. M. WUERKER, AND E. HENNEMAN. Properties of motor units in a homogeneous red muscle (soleus) of the cat. *J. Neurophysiol.* 28: 71–84, 1965.
163. MELZAK, J., AND N. H. PORTER. Studies of the reflex activity of the external sphincter ani in spinal man. *Paraplegia* 1: 277–297, 1964.
164. MENDELOFF, A. I. Defecation. In: *Handbook of Physiology. Alimentary Canal, Motility*, edited by C. F. Code. Washington, DC: Am. Physiol. Soc., 1968, sect. 6, vol. IV, chapt. 103, p. 2140–2146.
165. MERTON, P. H. Electrical stimulation through the scalp of pyramidal tract fibres supplying pelvic floor muscles. In: *Coloproctology & the Pelvic Floor: Pathophysiology & Management*, edited by M. M. Henry and M. Swash. London: Butterworth, 1985, p. 125–128.
166. MEUNIER, P., AND P. MOLLARD. Control of the internal anal sphincter (manometric study with human subjects). *Pfluegers Arch.* 370: 233–239, 1977.
167. MONGES, H., J. SALDUCCI, B. NAUDI, F. RANIERE, J. GONELLA, AND M. BOUVIER. Electrical activity of internal anal sphincter. A comparative study in man and cat. In: *Gastrointestinal Motility*, edited by J. M. Christensen. New York: Raven, 1980, p. 495–502.
168. MORGAN, C., I. NADELHAFT, AND W. C. DE GROAT. The distribution of visceral primary afferents from the pelvic nerve to Lissauer's tract and the spinal gray matter and its relationship to the sacral parasympathetic nucleus. *J. Comp. Neurol.* 201: 415–440, 1981.
169. MORRISON, J. F. B. The afferent innervation of the gastrointestinal tract. In: *Nerves and the Gut*, edited by F. P. Brooks and P. W. Evers. Thorofare, NJ: Slack, 1977, p. 297–322.
170. NADELHAFT, I., W. C. DE GROAT, AND C. MORGAN. Location and morphology and parasympathetic preganglionic neurons in the sacral spinal cord of the cat revealed by retrograde axonal transport of horseradish peroxidase. *J. Comp. Neurol.* 193: 265–281, 1980.
170a. NADELHAFT, I., J. ROPPOLO, C. MORGAN, AND W. C. DE GROAT. Parasympathetic preganglionic neurons and visceral primary afferents in monkey spinal cord revealed following application of horseradish peroxidase to pelvic nerve. *J. Comp. Neurol.* 26: 36–52, 1983.
171. NAKAGAWA, S. Onuf's nucleus of the sacral cord in a South

American monkey (*Saimiri*): its location and bilateral cortical input from area 4. *Brain Res.* 191: 337–344, 1980.
172. NATHAN, P. W., AND M. C. SMITH. Spinal pathways subserving defecation and sensation from the large bowel. *J. Neurol. Neurosurg. Psychiatry* 16: 245–256, 1953.
173. NEELY, J. Comparison of the effects of a gastrin extract and a synthetic pentapeptide on gastrointestinal motility in the cat. *Gut* 8: 242–248, 1967.
174. NEIL, M. E., A. G. PARKS, AND M. SWASH. Physiological studies of the anal sphincter musculature in faecal incontinence and rectal prolapse. *Br. J. Surg.* 68: 531–536, 1981.
175. NORBERG, K.-A. Adrenergic innervation of the intestinal wall studied by fluorescence microscopy. *Int. J. Neuropharmacol.* 3: 739–782, 1964.
176. ONUF, B. On the arrangement and function of cell groups of the sacral region of the spinal cord in man. *Arch. Neurol. Psychiatry* 3: 387–411, 1900.
177. OTSUKA, M., AND S. KONISHI. Substance P—the first peptide neurotransmitter. *Trends Neurosci.* 6: 317–320, 1983.
178. PARKS, A. G., D. J. FISHLOCK, J. D. H. CAMERON, AND H. MAY. Preliminary investigation of the pharmacology of the human internal anal sphincter. *Gut* 10: 674–677, 1969.
179. PARKS, A. G., H. PORTER, AND J. MELZAK. Experimental studies of the reflex mechanism controlling the muscles of the pelvic floor. *Dis. Colon Rectum* 5: 401–414, 1962.
180. PARKS, A. G., M. SWASH, AND H. URICH. Sphincter denervation in anorectal incontinence and rectal prolapse. *Gut* 18: 656–665, 1977.
181. PEDERSEN, E. The anal reflex. In: *Coloproctology & the Pelvic Floor, Pathophysiology & Management*, edited by M. M. Henry and M. Swash. London: Butterworth, 1985, p. 104–111.
182. PEDERSEN, E., H. HARVING, B. KLEMAR, AND J. TORRING. Human anal reflexes. *J. Neurol. Neurosurg. Psychiatry* 41: 813–818, 1978.
183. PEDERSEN, E., B. KLEMAR, H. D. SCHRODER, AND J. TORRING. Anal sphincter responses after perianal electrical stimulation. *J. Neurol. Neurosurg. Psychiatry* 45: 770–773, 1982.
184. PENNINCKX, F., R. KERREMANS, AND J. BECKERS. Pharmacological characteristics of the non-striated ano-rectal musculature in cats. *Gut* 13: 393–398, 1973.
185. PENNINCKX, F., AND J. H. MEBIS. The recto-anal reflex in cats and analyzed in vitro. *Scand. J. Gastroenterol.* 17, Suppl. 71: 147–149, 1982.
186. PHILLIPS, S. F., AND D. A. W. EDWARDS. Some aspects of anal continence and defecation. *Gut* 6: 396–406, 1965.
187. POLAK, J. M., S. R. BLOOM, S. N. SULLIVAN, P. FADER, AND A. G. E. PEARSE. Enkephalin-like immunoreactivity in the human gastrointestinal tract. *Lancet* 1: 972–974, 1977.
188. PORTER, N. H. A physiologic study of the pelvic floor and rectal prolapse. *Ann. R. Coll. Surg. Engl.* 31: 379–404, 1962.
189. RANKIN, F. W., AND J. R. LEARMONTH. Section of the sympathetic nerves of the distal part of the colon and rectum in the treatment of Hirschsprung's disease and certain types of constipation. *Ann. Surg.* 92: 710–720, 1930.
190. RAY, B. S., AND C. L. NEIL. Abdominal visceral sensation in man. *Ann. Surg.* 126: 709–724, 1947.
191. RAYNER, V. Characteristics of the internal anal sphincter and the rectum of the vervet monkey. *J. Physiol. Lond.* 286: 383–399, 1979.
192. REXED, B. The cytoarchitectonic organization of the spinal cord. *J. Comp. Neurol.* 96: 415–495, 1952.
193. ROCKSWOLD, G. L., W. E. BRADLEY, AND S. N. CHOU. Innervation of the external urethral and external anal sphincters in higher primates. *J. Comp. Neurol.* 193: 521–528, 1980.
194. ROMANES, G. J. The motor cell columns of the lumbosacral spinal cord of the cat. *J. Comp. Neurol.* 94: 313–363, 1951.
195. ROPPOLO, J. R., I. NADELHAFT, AND W. C. DE GROAT. The organization of pudendal motoneurons and primary afferent projections in the spinal cord of the rhesus monkey revealed by horseradish peroxidase. *J. Comp. Neurol.* 234: 475–488, 1985.
196. ROSSOLINO, S. Der anal reflex, seine physiologie and pathologie. *Neurologisches Centralblatt* 10: 257–259, 1891.
197. ROSTAD, H. Colonic motility in the cat. II. Extrinsic nervous control. *Acta Physiol. Scand.* 89: 79–90, 1973.
198. RUTTER, K. R. P. Electromyographic changes in certain pelvic floor abnormalities. *Proc. R. Soc. Med.* 67: 53–56, 1974.
199. SALDUCCI, J., D. PLANCHE, AND B. NAUDY. Physiological role of the internal anal sphincter and the external anal sphincter during defecation. In: *Motility of the Digestive Tract*, edited by M. Wienbeck. New York: Raven, 1982, p. 513–520.
200. SATO, M., M. MIZUNO, AND A. KONISHI. Localization of motoneurons innervating perianal muscles: a HRP study in the cat. *Brain Res.* 140: 154, 1978.
201. SCHOFIELD, G. C. Anatomy of muscular and neural tissues in the alimentary canal. In: *Handbook of Physiology. Alimentary Canal. Motility*, edited by C. F. Code. Washington, DC: Am. Physiol. Soc., 1968, sect. 6, vol. IV, chapt. 80, p. 1579–1627.
202. SCHRÖDER, H. D. Organization of the motoneurons innervating the pelvic muscles of the male rat. *J. Comp. Neurol.* 192: 567–587, 1980.
203. SCHRÖDER, H. D. Onuf's nucleus X: a morphological study of a human spinal nucleus. *Anat. Embryol.* 162: 443–463, 1981.
204. SCHULTZBERG, M., C. F. DREYGUS, M. D. GERSHON, T. HÖKFELT, R. ELDE, G. NILSSON, S. SAID, AND M. GOLDSTEIN. VIP, enkephalin, substance P, and somatostatin-like immunoreactivity in neurons intrinsic to the intestine: immunohistochemical evidence from organotypic tissue cultures. *Brain Res.* 155: 239–248, 1978.
205. SCHUSTER, M. M. Motor action of rectum and anal sphincters in continence and defecation. In: *Handbook of Physiology. Alimentary Canal. Motility*, edited by C. F. Code. Washington, DC: Am. Physiol. Soc., 1968, sect. 6, vol. IV, chapt. 103, p. 2121–2140.
206. SCHUSTER, M. M. The riddle of the sphincters. *Gastroenterology* 69: 249–262, 1975.
207. SCHUSTER, M. M. Biofeedback treatment of gastrointestinal disorders. *Med. Clin. N. Am.* 61: 907–912, 1977.
208. SCHUSTER, M. M., T. R. HENDRIX, AND A. I. MENDELOFF. The internal anal sphincter response: manometric studies on its normal physiology, neural pathways and alteration in bowel diseases. *J. Clin. Invest.* 42: 196–207, 1963.
209. SCHUSTER, M. M., P. HOOKMAN, J. R. HENDRIX, AND A. J. MENDELOFF. Recordings of internal and external anal sphincteric reflexes. *Bull. Johns Hopkins Hosp.* 116: 70–88, 1965.
210. SCHUSTER, M. M., D. W. TOW, AND D. H. SHERBOURNE. Anal sphincter abnormalities of myotonic dystrophy. *Gastroenterology* 49: 641–648, 1965.
211. SCOTT, H. W., JR., AND J. R. CANTRELL. Colon metrographic studies of the effects of section of the parasympathetic nerve to the colon. *Bull. Johns Hopkins Hosp.* 85: 310–319, 1949.
212. SEMBA, T., H. MISHIMA, AND T. DATE. Studies on a vesicoanal inhibiting reflex. *Jpn. J. Physiol.* 6: 108–111, 1956.
213. SHAFIK, A. A new concept of the anal sphincter mechanism and the physiology of defecation. I. The external anal sphincter: triple loop system. *Invest. Urol.* 12: 412–419, 1975.
214. SHAFIK, A. A new concept of the anatomy of the anal sphincter mechanism and the physiology of defecation. II. Anatomy of the levator ani muscle with special reference to the puborectalis. *Invest. Urol.* 13: 175–182, 1975.
215. SHAFIK, A. A new concept of the anatomy of the anal sphincter mechanism and the physiology of defecation. III. The longitudinal anal muscle: anatomy and role in anal sphincter mechanism. *Invest. Urol.* 13: 271–277, 1976.
216. SHEPARD, J. J., AND P. G. WRIGHT. The response of the internal anal sphincter in man to stimulation of the presacral nerve. *Am. J. Dig. Dis.* 13: 421–427, 1968.
217. SHERRINGTON, C. S. Notes on the arrangement of some motor fibers in the lumbosacral plexus. *J. Physiol. Lond.* 13: 672–675, 1892.
218. SJOQUIST, A., P. M. HELLSTRÖM, M. JODAL, AND O. LUNDGREN. Neurotransmitters involved in the colonic contraction

and vasodilation elicited by activation of the pelvic nerves in the cat. *Gastroenterology* 86: 1481–1487, 1984.
219. SMITH, W. C. The levator ani muscle: its structure in man and its comparative relationships. *Anat. Rec.* 26: 175–203, 1923.
220. SNAPE, W. J., S. MATARAZZO, AND S. COHEN. Effect of eating and gastrointestinal hormones on human colonic myoelectrical and motor activity. *Gastroenterology* 75: 373–378, 1978.
220a.SOSA, R. P., A. T MCKNIGHT, J. HUGHES, AND H. W. KOSTERLITZ. Incorporation of labelled amino acids into the enkephalins. *FEBS Lett.* 84: 135–138.
221. SPRIGGS, E. A., C. F. CODE, J. A. BARGEN, R. K. CURTIS, AND N. C. HIGHTOWER. Motility of the pelvic colon and rectum of normal persons and patients with ulcerative colitis. *Gastroenterology* 19: 480–491, 1951.
222. STELZER, F., H. G. BAUMGARTEN, AND A. F. HOLSTEIN. The significance of the itnernal anal sphincter for continence and supercontinence. *Langenbecks Arch. Chir.* 336: 35–55, 1974.
223. STONESIFER, G. L., G. P. MURPHY, AND C. R. LOMBARDO. The anatomy of the anorectum. *Am. J. Surg.* 100: 666–671, 1960.
224. TAYLOR, B. M., R. W. BEART, AND S. F. PHILLIPS. Longitudinal and radial variations of pressure in the human anal sphincter. *Gastroenterology* 86: 693–697, 1984.
225. TAYLOR, I., H. L. DUTHIE, R. SMALLWOOD, AND P. LINKENS. The effect of stimulation of the myoelectrical activity of the rectosigmoid in man. *Gut* 15: 599–607, 1974.
226. TAYLOR, I., H. L. DUTHIE, R. SMALLWOOD, AND D. LINKENS. Large bowel myoelectrical activity in man. *Gut* 16: 808–814, 1975.
227. TAYLOR, I., R. SMALLWOOD, AND H. L. DUTHIE. Myoelectrical activity of the rectosigmoid in man. *Proc. Fourth Int. Symp. Gastrointestinal Motility, Banff, Canada.* Vancouver, Canada: Mitchell, 1973, p. 111–118.
228. TIGGES, J., S. NAKAGAWA, AND M. TIGGES. Efferents of area 4 in a South American monkey (*Saimiri*) I. Terminations in the spinal cord. *Brain Res.* 171: 1–10, 1979.
229. TODD, J. K. Afferent impulses in the pudendal nerve of the cat. *Q. J. Exp. Physiol. Cogn. Med. Sci.* 49: 258–267, 1964.
230. TRAVENER, D., AND F. G. SMIDDY. An electromyographic study of the normal function of the external anal sphincter and pelvic diaphragm. *Dis. Colon Rectum* 2: 153–160, 1959.
230a.TRAXINGER, D., AND J. KRIER. The effects of colonic distension on pudendal motor reflexes to the external anal sphincter of the cat (Abstract). *Dig. Dis. Sci.* 29: 554, 1984.
231. TSUTO, T., H. OKAMURA, M. FUKUI, H. OBATA, H. TERUBAYASHI, N. IWAI, S. MAYIMA, N. YANARHARA, AND Y. IBATA. An immunohistochemical investigation of vasoactive intestinal polypeptide in the colon of patients with Hirschsprung's disease. *Neurosci. Lett.* 34: 57–62, 1982.
232. UEYAMA, T., H. ARAKAWA, AND N. MIZUNO. Contralateral termination of pudendal nerve fibers in the gracile nucleus of the rat. *Neurosci. Lett.* 62: 113–117, 1985.
233. UEYAMA, T., N. MIZUNO, S. NOMURA, A. KONISHI, K. ITOH, AND H. ARAKAWA. Central distribution of afferent and efferent components of the pudendal nerve of the cat. *J. Comp. Neurol.* 222: 38–46, 1984.
234. UEYAMA, T., N. MIZUNO, O. TAKAHASHI, S. NORMURA, H. ARAKAWA, AND R. MATSUSHIMA. Central distribution of efferent and afferent components of the pudendal nerve in macaque monkeys. *J. Comp. Neurol.* 233: 548–556, 1985.
235. USTACH, T. J., F. TOBON, R. HAMBRECHT, D. D. BASS, AND M. M. SCHUSTER. Electrophysiologic aspects of human sphincter function. *J. Clin. Invest.* 49: 41–48, 1970.
236. VEREECKEN, R. L., J. DE MEIRSMAN, B. PUERS, AND J. VAN MULDERS. Electrophysiological exploration of the sacral conus. *J. Neurol.* 227: 135–144, 1982.
237. VEREECKEN, R. L., AND H. VERDUYN. The electrical activity of the paraurethral and perineal muscles in normal and pathological conditions. *Br. J. Urol.* 42: 457–463, 1970.
238. VODUSEK, M., M. JANKO, AND J. LOKJAR. Direct and reflex reponses in perineal muscles on electrical stimulation. *J. Neurol. Neurosurg. Psychiatry* 46: 67–71, 1983.
239. WALD, A., AND A. K. TUNUGUNTLA. Anorectal sensorimotor dysfunction in fecal incontinence and diabetes mellitus: modification with biofeedback therapy. *N. Engl. J. Med.* 310: 1282–1287, 1984.
240. WALKER, L. B. Neuromuscular spindles in the external anal sphincter of the cat. *Anat. Rec.* 133: 347, 1959.
241. WANKLING, W. J., B. H. BROWN, C. D. COLLINS, AND H. L. DUTHIE. Basal electrical activity in the anal canal in man. *Gut* 9: 457–460, 1968.
242. WEBSTER, W. Aganglionic megacolon in piebald-lethal mice. *Arch. Pathol.* 97: 111–117, 1974.
243. WHEATLEY, I. C., J. K. HARDY, AND J. DENT. Anal pressure studies in spinal patients. *Gut* 18: 488–490, 1977.
244. WHITE, J. C., M. G. VERLOT, AND O. EHRENTHEIL. Neurogenic disturbances of the colon and their investigation with the colonmetrogram. *Ann. Surg.* 112: 1042–1058, 1940.
245. WIENBECK, M., AND I. ALTAPARMACOV. Is the internal anal sphincter controlled by a myoelectrical mechanism? In: *Gastrointestinal Motility*, edited by J. Christensen. New York: Raven, 1980, p. 487–493.
246. WILLIAMS, I. Mass movements (mass peristalsis) and diverticular disease of the colon. *Br. J. Radiol.* 40: 2–14, 1967.
247. WILLIAMS, J. T., AND R. A. NORTH. Inhibition of firing of myenteric neurones by somatostatin. *Brain Res.* 155: 165–168, 1978.
248. WOOD, B. A. Anatomy of the anal sphincters and pelvic floor. In: *Coloproctology & the Pelvic Floor, Pathophysiology & Management*, edited by M. M. Henry and M. Swash. London: Butterworth, 1985, p. 3–21.
249. WOOD, J. D. The physiology of the enteric nervous system. In: *Physiology of the Gastrointestinal Tract* (1st ed.), edited by L. R. Johnson. New York: Raven, 1981, p. 1–37.
250. WOZNIAK, W., AND U. SKOWRONSKA. Comparative anatomy of pelvic plexus in cat, dog, rabbit, macque, and man. *Anat. Anz.* 120: 457–473, 1967.
251. WUNDERLICH, M., AND M. SWASH. The overlapping innervation of the two sides of the external anal sphincter by pudendal nerves. *J. Neurol. Sci.* 59: 97–109, 1983.
252. YAMAMOTO, T., H. SATOMI, H. ISE, H. TAKATAMA, AND K. TAKAHASHI. Sacral spinal innervations of the rectal and vesicle smooth muscles and the sphincteric striated muscles as demonstrated by the horseradish peroxidase method. *Neurosci. Lett.* 7: 41–47, 1978.

# CHAPTER 28

# Motility of the biliary system

WYLIE J. DODDS
WALTER J. HOGAN
JOSEPH E. GEENEN

*Departments of Radiology and Medicine, Medical College of Wisconsin, Milwaukee, Wisconsin*

## CHAPTER CONTENTS

Historical Background
Anatomy of Biliary-Pancreatic Duct System
  Gross structure
    Embryology
    Extrinsic nerves
    Component structures
  Microscopic structure
    Muscle and mucosa
    Innervation
  Species variation
    Anatomical differences
    Functional differences
Methods of Study
  Imaging studies
  Flow measurements
  Manometry
  Electromyography
  Scintigraphy
  Sonography
  Miscellaneous
Pharmacology
Physiology
  Hepatic bile
  Gallbladder
  Cystic duct
  Common duct
  Sphincter of Oddi
    Poiseuille's law
    Humans
    Animals
    Overview
Abnormal Function in Humans
  Gallbladder
    Hyperkinesia
    Hypokinesia
    Treatment
  Sphincter of Oddi
    Biliary sphincter of Oddi dysfunction
    Pancreatic sphincter of Oddi dysfunction
    Treatment
Summary

THIS CHAPTER DEALS WITH the physiology and pathophysiology of biliary tract motor activity with particular attention to the pressure-flow kinetics of bile within the extracanalicular bile duct system. Attention is also given to biliary tract anatomy because function depends on underlying structure. A number of important reviews are included in the bibliography (7, 18, 22, 69, 152, 180).

Delivery of bile into the duodenum involves a series of complex interrelationships among the hepatic secretion of bile and the pressure-flow kinetics of the common duct, cystic duct, gallbladder, and sphincter of Oddi. The standard description for bile transport within the biliary duct system has included consideration of three physiological variables, that is, rate and pressure of hepatic bile production, gallbladder tone, and sphincter of Oddi resistance. For many years, bile secretion was believed to occur at a steady minimal rate during fasting. Earlier workers envisioned that tonic resistance of the sphincter of Oddi prevented common duct emptying and thereby directed all of the hepatic bile into the gallbladder where it was concentrated and stored. Postprandial contraction of the gallbladder associated with sphincter of Oddi relaxation was believed to cause a rapid delivery of bile into the duodenum.

Current information about biliary tract motor function suggests that the traditional notions about its physiology are partially inaccurate. For example, only a portion of the hepatic bile secreted during fasting enters the gallbladder; the remainder passes directly into the duodenum. The cystic duct has characteristics suggestive of a sphincter rather than a passive resistor and thus may modulate gallbladder emptying and filling. Also the biliary duct system is not quiescent during fasting. Contractile activity of the gallbladder and sphincter of Oddi occurs in synchrony with cyclic motor activity of the upper gastrointestinal tract. Last, the sphincter of Oddi exhibits phasic contraction waves as well as a variable tone. A composite picture of integrated biliary dynamics is emerging that shows a more complex system than that originally suspected.

## HISTORICAL BACKGROUND

In 1543 Vesalius observed a membrane near the distal orifice of the common duct and postulated that this structure impeded retrograde bile flow and prevented regurgitation of duodenal contents into the common bile duct. Glisson in 1654 was the first to suspect a sphincter at the distal common duct. More than 200 years later a distal choledochal sphincter was suggested by Rugero Oddi (131), who described bundles of circular muscle fibers at the confluence of the choledochal and pancreatic ducts in various animals. In the early part of this century, investigators such as Boyden, Ivy, Mann, Meltzer, McMaster, Winkelstein, and others (86, 109, 116, 117, 215) published classic landmark studies that investigated gallbladder motor function and its interactions with sphincter of Oddi resistance and bile flow. During the decade from 1920 to 1930, humoral control mechanisms, as opposed to autonomic nerves, were suggested as the main modulators of biliary tract kinetics, particularly gallbladder contraction. Investigators noted that specific food substances, such as fat, when introduced into the duodenum, increased the contractile force of the gallbladder and prompted evacuation of bile. Subsequently, Ivy and Oldberg (86) extracted a substance from hog duodenal mucosa that contracted the canine gallbladder. He called this substance cholecystokinin, meaning gallbladder motion, and its status as a true hormone was confirmed shortly thereafter.

Later advances in experimental design and technology enabled more precise investigation and measurement of biliary tract kinetics. The use of cineradiography, miniaturized high-fidelity manometry, electromyography, isotope techniques, and biochemical identification of hormones and hormone assay dramatically expanded existing information about the motor function of biliary tract structures and its response to physiological stimuli. Presently, manometric pressure and myoelectric activity can be readily monitored concurrently from both the biliary and intestinal tract of animals during intervals of fasting and feeding. By means of such comprehensive studies, a clearer picture is emerging of the interrelationship and integration of biliary tract motor events that deliver bile into the duodenum.

ANATOMY OF BILIARY-PANCREATIC DUCT SYSTEM

*Gross Structure*

The right and left hepatic ducts originate within the liver and transport bile from the hepatocytes. The two main hepatic ducts fuse at the porta hepatis to form the common hepatic duct (Fig. 1). In humans the cystic duct joins the common hepatic duct ~4 cm below the porta hepatis. Below the level of cystic duct entry the main bile duct continues as the common bile duct. The term *common duct* is often used to include both the common bile duct and common hepatic duct. The common duct runs caudad, courses through the posterior portion of the pancreatic head, and enters

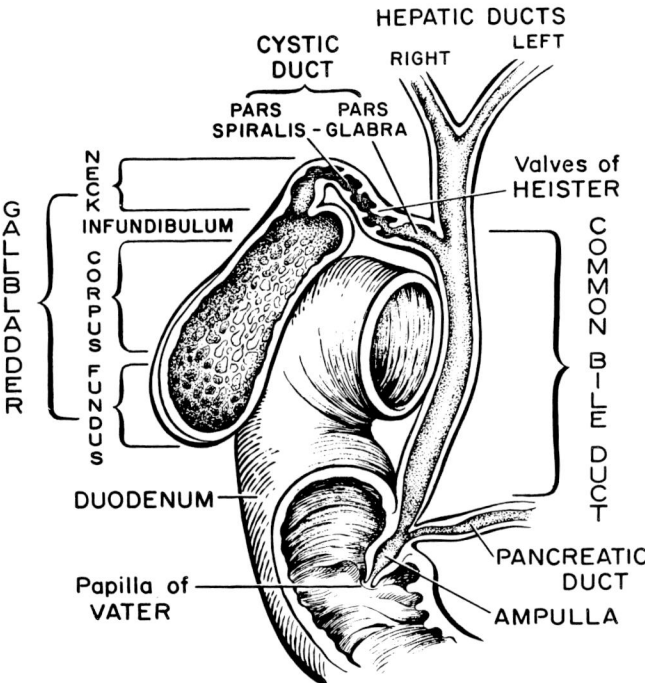

FIG. 1. Gross anatomy of gallbladder and bile ducts. [Adapted from Netter (127a).]

the second portion of the duodenum. The distal common duct and the pancreatic duct generally join to form a common channel, or ampulla, just before they enter the duodenal wall. The common channel drains into the duodenum through a duodenal papilla known as the ampulla of Vater. The length of common duct within the duodenal wall varies from 1 to 3 cm.

EMBRYOLOGY. The gallbladder and bile ducts arise from the caudal portion of a diverticular anlage that originates from the ventral flow of the foregut at a site corresponding to the duodenum (Fig. 2). Boyden (19) confirmed that the muscularis propria of the distal common duct arises de novo from mesenchyme and first appears in the human fetus ~5 wk after the intestinal musculature. The adult pancreas develops from two foregut diverticula, or buds, that sprout in the region of the future duodenum. The pancreatic body and tail develop from a dorsal anlage that is located slightly proximal to the level of the ventral hepatic diverticulum. The ventral pancreatic bud that gives rise to the pancreatic head originates from the gallbladder area of the hepatic diverticulum. During its growth the ventral pancreas, together with the rudimentary common bile duct, rotates dorsally behind the duodenum and fuses with the dorsal pancreas (Fig. 2). The ducts from the dorsal and ventral pancreatic segments generally join. Secretions from the dorsal pancreatic duct of Santorini then flow into the ventral pancreatic duct that subsequently becomes the principal pancreatic duct of Wirsung that drains

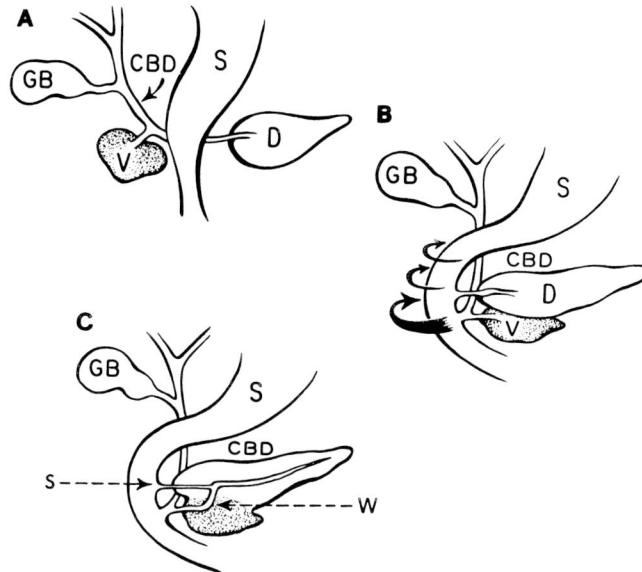

FIG. 2. Embryology of pancreaticobiliary tree. *A*: ventral (V) and dorsal (D) pancreas arise as anlage from duodenum. *B*: biliary and pancreatic anlagen rotate counterclockwise (*arrow*) so ventral pancreas lies posterior to dorsal pancreas. *C*: ventral and dorsal pancreas along with their ducts fuse so duct of Wirsung (W) becomes major pancreatic duct and distal part of duct of Santorini (S) becomes accessory pancreatic duct. GB, gallbladder; CBD common bile duct. [Adapted from Netter (127a).]

through the duodenal papilla of Vater. The duct of Santorini commonly persists as an accessory pancreatic duct that drains into a small papilla located several centimeters proximal to the more prominent papilla of Vater.

EXTRINSIC NERVES. The gallbladder and bile ducts are supplied by both sympathetic and parasympathetic nerves (22). The sympathetic fibers are believed to originate from thoracic spinal segments 7 to 10 and reach the celiac ganglia by way of the splanchnic nerves. The splanchnic nerves supply both motor and sensory fibers. In classic descriptions the parasympathetic innervation of the gallbladder was thought to originate from the left vagus, but it probably arises from both vagal nerves. The vagi supply motor as well as sensory fibers. At the liver hiatus, fibers from both vagal nerves merge into a hepatic plexus that supplies parasympathetic nerves to the extrahepatic bile ducts and gallbladder. Fibers mainly from the anterior (left) vagus supply the gallbladder, whereas the celiac branch of the posterior (right) vagus supplies fibers to the common duct and sphincter of Oddi via the celiac plexus. The majority of sensory nerves from the extrahepatic biliary system are believed to be sympathetic afferent fibers that pass through both splanchnic nerves.

COMPONENT STRUCTURES. *Gallbladder.* The human gallbladder is a thin-walled, pear-shaped sac that nestles along the inferior hepatic surface in a fossa between the right and left lobes of the liver. Anatomically the gallbladder is divided into three parts. The broad inferior portion, or *fundus*, projects beneath the anterior liver margin. The body, or *corpus*, is juxtaposed to the second portion of the duodenum. The funnel-shaped gallbladder neck termed the *infundibulum* (Hartmann's pouch) lies near the free edge of the hepatoduodenal ligament. The infundibulum is a narrow, S-shaped tubular passageway that tapers into the cystic duct. The human gallbladder generally measures 7–10 cm in length and ~3 cm in width. Its average storage capacity is ~20–30 ml. About 350–700 ml of hepatic bile normally enters the gallbladder daily.

*Cystic duct.* The human cystic duct, ~3.5 cm long and 3 mm wide, generally runs parallel to the common hepatic duct before they merge. The mucosa of the proximal cystic duct (pars spiralis) is arranged into 5 to 7 cresentic folds or valves known as the spiral valves of Heister. The valves of Heister arise late in the phylogeny of mammals and exist only in primates (103). The short, distal segment of the cystic duct (pars glabra) has a smooth internal surface, is slightly larger in diameter than the pars spiralis, and joins the common hepatic duct at an acute angle.

*Common duct.* The human common duct is ~10–15 cm long and descends along the free margin of the hepatoduodenal ligament. Distally the common duct tapers as it courses through the pancreatic head. Upon penetration of the duodenal wall, an abrupt narrowing of the duct lumen, known as the notch, may occur.

*Pancreatic duct.* Within the pancreatic head the distal portion of the major pancreatic duct, or duct of Wirsung, travels caudally almost parallel to the distal common duct. The two ducts generally fuse at the level of the common duct notch and become surrounded by a common muscular sheath. The lumina of the two ducts seldom join outside the duodenal wall. After entering the duodenal wall, through a window in its musculature, the pancreatic duct usually joins with the common duct to form a common channel that runs obliquely through the submucosa and opens into the duodenum at the papilla of Vater.

*Sphincter of Oddi.* The term *sphincter of Oddi* defines the terminal portion of the common duct that exhibits a well-defined muscularis propria. This structure came to be known as the sphincter of Oddi because Oddi (131) demonstrated its muscular structure in various animals and was the first to measure its resistance to bile flow. Anatomically the human sphincter of Oddi segment is ~10–15 mm in length and includes zones (Fig. 3) that have been called the *sphincter choledochus, sphincter pancreaticus, ampulla of Vater,* and *sphincter ampullae* (18). The ampulla is a common channel formed by the junction of the pancreatic duct and common bile duct. The sphincter of Oddi segment assumes one of three general config-

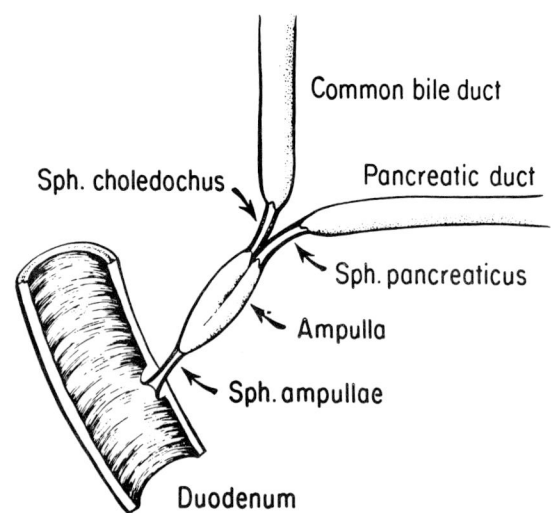

FIG. 3. Schematic anatomical representation of human sphincter of Oddi. Sphincter of Oddi is characterized by muscularis propria distinct from that of duodenum. Boyden observed localized areas of muscle thickening that he termed *sphincter ampullae, sphincter choledochus*, and *sphincter pancreaticus*. Common channel or ampulla is generally present. [Adapted from Boyden (18).]

urations that may be likened in shape to a Y, V, or U. In ~70% of subjects, the ampulla is 4–7 mm in length (Y type). This common channel drains into the duodenum through a single orifice on the duodenal papilla of Vater. In 20% of subjects the common bile duct and pancreatic duct form a diminutive common channel 1–2 mm in length (V type). Last, in 10% of subjects the common duct and pancreatic duct have separate openings on the duodenal papilla (U type).

*Microscopic Structure*

MUSCLE AND MUCOSA. The gallbladder wall has four layers: serosa, perimuscularis, muscularis, and mucosa. The serosa envelopes the entire fundus but covers only the posterior surface of the body and neck. The perimuscularis consists of connective tissue richly supplied with nutrient vessels. The gallbladder muscularis forms a netlike arrangement of longitudinal, transverse, and oblique smooth muscle bundles separated by connective tissue (23, 108). Contraction of the muscle-fiber mesh generates a vector of force directed toward the center of the gallbladder lumen. Unlike the muscularis of the gastrointestinal tract, the thin layer of the gallbladder muscularis is not separated into a muscularis externa and muscularis mucosa. The smooth muscle cells of the gallbladder as well as the cystic duct are small and loose, with few intercellular contacts. This morphology is similar to that of the muscularis mucosa of the intestine, thereby suggesting that the gallbladder mucosa is probably a derivative of intestinal muscularis mucosae (23). A submucosal layer is absent. The gallbladder mucosa consists of numerous elevated folds, or rugae, covered with simple columnar epithelium. True glands are located only in the infundibulum and neck of the gallbladder.

A thin layer of muscle lies beneath the mucosa of the cystic duct. This layer is comprised of longitudinal, oblique, and circular smooth muscle fibers that are present throughout the entire duct but become thicker at its junction with the gallbladder. The muscle layer is arranged as a thin mesh with connective tissue within its interstices. Contraction produces radial narrowing and some shortening of the duct. The muscle fibers also extend into the prominent valvelike mucosal folds of Heister. Debate exists as to whether a localized concentration of the muscle fibers, referred to as the sphincter of Lütkens, is present at the junction of the cystic duct and gallbladder neck. Most workers agree that an anatomical sphincter of Lütkens probably does not exist; rather the entire cystic duct may have sphincterlike properties (167).

The common duct in humans, as well as in species such as the dog, cat, and opossum, contains a few sparse longitudinal muscle fibers that may form a thin layer in the lower half of the duct. Negligible circular smooth muscle is present. In cross section, the duct is comprised of an outer, loose connective tissue layer, a middle subepithelial layer of scattered longitudinal muscle fibers, collagenous connective tissue, and scattered glands. In a few animal species, such as sheep and monkey, a moderate amount of circular smooth muscle is present in the common duct. The inner mucosa layer of the common duct consists of a simple columnar epithelium.

The pancreatic duct has negligible smooth muscle. In some specimens, however, the intraduodenal portion of the duct exhibits a few muscle fibers arranged in a spiral or figure-of-eight configuration (19). The amount of muscle in the terminal pancreatic duct is substantially less than that surrounding the terminal choledochus. Some muscle fibers that lie between the junction of the common duct and pancreatic ducts swing obliquely around the terminal pancreatic duct to decussate near the papilla. The pancreatic duct epithelium consists of a single layer of low columnar cells.

Boyden's (18, 19) dissections, reported initially in 1937, have helped clarify the muscular anatomy of the sphincter of Oddi segment. He referred to thickened zones of muscle at the proximal and distal margins of the human sphincter of Oddi as the sphincter choledochus and sphincter ampullae (Fig. 3). When the pancreatic duct opens separately on the duodenal papilla and an ampulla is absent, the ampullary segment is called the infundibulum and the distal sphincter the sphincter papillae. Boyden divided the sphincter choledochus into a superior portion that encircled the distal common duct (choledochus) just proximal to its entry into the duodenum and an inferior portion that surrounded the submucosal intraduodenal portion of the common duct. The muscle of Boyden's sphincter ampullae surrounds the ampullary duct at the duodenal papilla. The ampullary segment exhibits a sparser arrangement of surrounding muscle fibers than the sphincter zones. In some human specimens an inconstant band of thickened muscle, termed the *sphincter pancreaticus*, is present at the terminus of the pancreatic duct.

Some workers (70, 199, 208) have observed features of sphincter of Oddi muscle anatomy that differ somewhat from those reported in the classic study by Boyden (18). For example, many sphincter of Oddi specimens from humans do not exhibit distinct areas of muscle thickening that correspond to a sphincter choledochus, sphincter ampullae, or sphincter pancreaticus. Importantly regional zones that behave functionally as discrete minisphincters have not been demonstrated within the sphincter of Oddi segment of humans (59).

The mucosa of the sphincter of Oddi segment is comprised of columnar epithelium and contains numerous glands. In all species this mucosa is thrown into numerous longitudinal folds, especially prominent in the distal ampullary segment, that interdigitate to form a spongelike lattice that helps seal the duct lumen (199). Because of the marked redundancy of the sphincter of Oddi mucosa, the sphincter segment has high resistive forces; therefore minimal circular muscle tone can occlude its lumen (23).

INNERVATION. The extrahepatic portion of the biliary duct system has a rich supply of nerves with both sympathetic and parasympathetic components (22). Intrinsic nerve plexuses lie in all three tissue layers of the gallbladder and extrahepatic bile ducts. These plexuses contain numerous groups of cells with features suggesting ganglia. The inner two plexuses, the muscular and mucosal plexuses, are believed to be analogous to Auerbach's and Meissner's plexuses of the gut.

The density of neural components in the gallbladder is not uniform. Nerve fibers and cell bodies are most numerous in the infundibulum. The arrangement of intrinsic nerves in the cystic duct is identical to that of the gallbladder. Histochemical labeling shows that the gallbladder has adrenergic nerves as well as a rich supply of cholinergic nerves. Observations from in vivo as well as in vitro studies indicate that stimulation of postganglionic cholinergic nerves elicit gallbladder contraction (9, 218). Gallbladder contraction evoked by vagal stimulation is blocked by atropine. Adrenergic nerves have also been demonstrated. Stimulation of the right splanchnic nerve causes gallbladder relaxation that is best demonstrated during gallbladder contraction induced by hormones or cholinergic stimuli (152). Sympathetic excitation by an $\alpha$-adrenergic receptor has been demonstrated in some species (138), but the functional implication of this finding is not clear. A recent study shows that immunoreactive peptidergic nerves are present that label with antibodies to vasoactive intestinal polypeptide (VIP). The VIPergic nerve fibers and cell bodies are located within the smooth muscle and subepithelial layers of the gallbladder wall (182). Therefore VIP may represent the neurotransmitter of nonadrenergic, noncholinergic (NANC) nerves that relax the gallbladder (38). Future studies may show that the gallbladder contains additional peptidergic nerves, for example, nerves containing enkephalin, somatostatin, and substance P, as is true elsewhere in the gastrointestinal tract.

A rich ganglionic plexus exists with the sphincter of Oddi (22, 98). The ganglia of the myenteric and submucosal plexuses appear to have a predominance of cholinergic fibers (94). In the cat and dog, postganglionic intramural neurons innervate the sphincter smooth muscle cells (96). Adrenergic nerves are present but are more sparse than cholinergic nerves (94). An adrenergic influence may be exerted by adrenergic nerve fibers acting on cholinergic ganglia; however, some adrenergic fibers may directly innervate smooth muscle cells (97). To our knowledge, studies using immunohistochemical techniques to search for peptidergic nerves have not been reported. In the opossum, neural ganglia are present along the length of the sphincter of Oddi segment but are virtually absent in the common duct and pancreatic ducts (204). The neural ganglia are located mostly on the outer surface of the circular muscle layer and increase in density at the proximal sphincter margin. The high density of ganglion cells in the proximal sphincter segment suggests the possibility of a control center for neural modulation of sphincter function.

Considerable evidence exists that the cholinergic and NANC inhibitory nerves are functionally active (12, 71, 138, 139, 203). Additionally, responses to stimulation of adrenergic and tryptaminergic nerves have been shown in the cat (12). Findings from several studies suggest that vagal stimulation causes an increase in sphincter of Oddi resistance and common duct pressure (198, 213), but these findings have not been confirmed by other studies (80). In one study electrical vagal stimulation decreased sphincter resistance and increased common duct flow (58). The effects of vagotomy on the sphincter of Oddi are inconsistent. Several authors report that vagotomy increases sphincter of Oddi resistance and common duct pressure (142, 213), whereas others have found no effect or an increase in sphincter resistance (58). In the opossum, truncal vagotomy does not affect fasting sphincter of Oddi motor activity but causes a delay in the normal postprandial response of increased phasic contractions (187). Persson (138) concluded that sympathetic stimulation elicited sphincter of Oddi contractions by $\alpha$-receptor stimulation, whereas Ryan (152) suggested that $\beta$-relaxation may occur.

The arrangement of intrinsic innervation of the common duct is comparable to that of the gallbladder and cystic duct, but fewer nerves are present, commensurate with the scanty amount of smooth muscle in the common duct.

*Species Variation*

To better characterize biliary tract motor function, investigators have used various animal species as experimental models. Different types of animals, however, vary in their biliary tract anatomy (19, 69) as well as in their responses to hormonal and pharmacological agents. Therefore findings from one animal species should not be extrapolated uncritically to other animal species.

ANATOMICAL DIFFERENCES. Unlike most animal species, the rat, horse, pigeon, and pocket gopher are without a gallbladder (69). Animals without a gallbladder have a rudimentary sphincter of Oddi musculature and do not have an ampulla (22). The dog has been a popular laboratory animal for investigating the biliary system, but its anatomy is much different from that of humans (18, 19). A duodenal papilla is rudimentary in the dog, and the canine common duct and main pancreatic duct open separately into the duodenum. The posterior wall of the canine duodenum forms a tunnel to enclose the intramural portion of the common duct, but the pancreatic duct lacks this covering. In the dog a delicate band of smooth muscle encircles the distal orifices of the common and pancreatic ducts, respectively, at their entry into the duodenum.

The distal common and pancreatic ducts of the cat join to form a short common channel, or ampulla, that empties into the duodenum (Fig. 4). With respect to function, the most important morphological features appear to be the intramural location of the sphincter of Oddi segment, tapering of the terminal choledochus into a sphincterlike nozzle, a complex musculature, and retrograde-oriented circular mucosal folds within the ampulla. A portion of the distal feline common duct is enclosed in a muscular funnel formed by the circular muscle layer of the posterior duodenal wall. Boyden (18) expressed the view that the terminal common duct of the cat and dog differs from that of humans because the terminal intramural portion of the common duct in these species may be compressed by duodenal contractions. In humans, both the common duct and the pancreatic duct enter the duodenum through a well-defined slit, or window, in the duodenal musculature and are less likely to be compressed by duodenal contractions.

Similar to sphincter of Oddi anatomy in humans, primates such as the chimpanzee and monkey have well-developed zones of circular muscle at the margins of the sphincter of Oddi. The sphincter of Oddi segment of the chimpanzee, however, is more complex

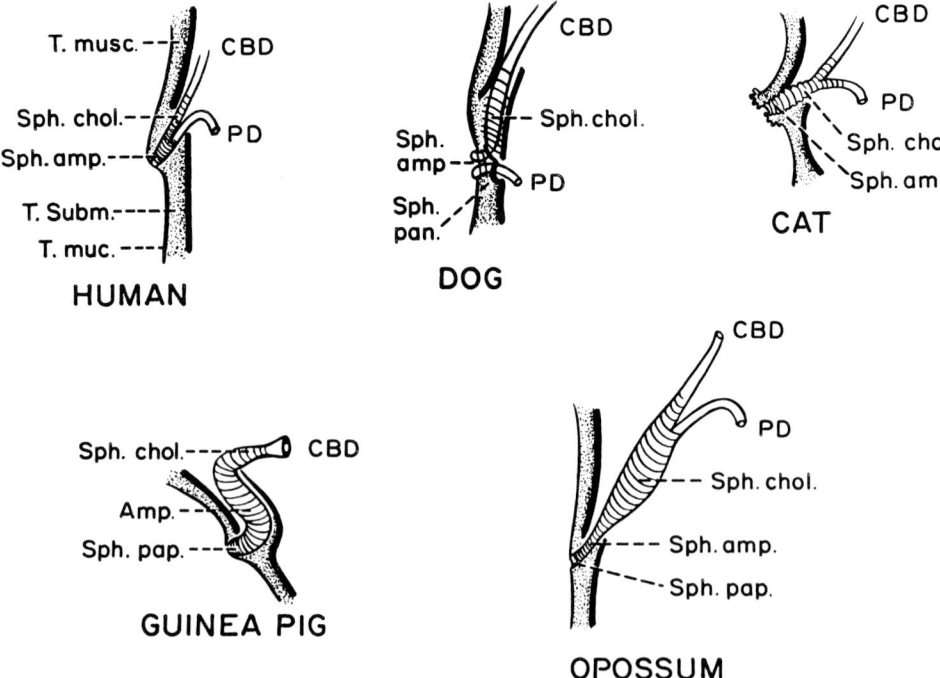

FIG. 4. Species variation in sphincter of Oddi anatomy. CBD, common bile duct; PD, pancreatic duct; T. musc., tunica muscularis; Sph. chol., sphincter choledochus; Sph. amp., sphincter ampullae; Sph. pap., sphincter pancreaticus T. subm., tunica submucosa; T. muc., tunica mucosa. [Adapted from Boyden (18).]

than its counterpart in humans. A striking feature in the chimpanzee is a bulbous sacculation of the terminal pancreatic duct, termed the *pancreatic sinus*, located just proximal to the pancreatic duct–common duct junction. The longitudinal duodenal musculature is incorporated into the sphincter choledochus. The sphincter ampullae is longer in length than the sphincter choledochus, and the duodenal circular musculature becomes continuous with the longitudinal muscle of the ampulla.

In the pig the common duct and pancreatic duct open separately into the duodenum. In contrast, the common and pancreatic ducts of the guinea pig empty at right angles into a large ampulla (23), contained exclusively within the duodenal wall (Fig. 4). Unlike in other rodents, the common and pancreatic ducts of the guinea pig do not join outside the duodenal wall. The intrinsic musculature of the guinea pig sphincter of Oddi is so intertwined with the duodenal circular musculature that the two cannot be clearly separated. In the rabbit, similar to the dog and pig, the common and pancreatic ducts have separate openings into the duodenum (158). The terminal bile duct has a prominent club-shaped ampulla, and the musculature does not mix with that of the duodenum.

The opossum sphincter of Oddi is a large, thick-walled, muscular structure ~3 cm long. Unlike the guinea pig, however, the opossum sphincter of Oddi is largely extraduodenal in location (Fig. 4). At laparotomy, rhythmic peristaltic contractions are observed that propagate caudally along the length of the sphincter segment. These contractions invariably originate at the proximal sphincter margin formed by the junction of the common and pancreatic ducts. The common channel of the sphincter of Oddi segment has parallel walls without an ampullary sacculation. However, its terminal 5 mm forms a narrow nozzle as it passes through the duodenal wall. Duct emptying occurs through a small slitlike orifice without a papilla. The well-developed sphincter musculature consists of a complete inner layer of longitudinal muscle surrounded by a thick layer of circular musculature. These muscle layers are distinctly separate from the muscularis of the duodenum (18). The circular musculature of the sphincter segment is thickest around the terminal sphincter nozzle that corresponds to a high-pressure zone on manometry (204). The muscle layers decrease progressively in thickness toward the proximal sphincter margin and disappear completely just above the junction of the common and pancreatic ducts. These anatomical findings do not suggest a localized choledochal or pancreatic sphincter in the opossum.

In most mammalian species, such as the human, dog, cat, and opossum, smooth muscle fibers are sparse or absent in the common duct. However, in subhuman primates, sheep, guinea pig, and fowl, a moderate amount of longitudinal smooth muscle exists in the subepithelial layer of the common duct. Elastic and collagenous connective tissue elements are located in the duct wall of all species.

FUNCTIONAL DIFFERENCES. In addition to anatomical variations, functional differences in sphincter of Oddi motor function exist among species. For example, phasic contractile activity in the human sphincter of Oddi may propagate cephalad or caudad (205), whereas in the opossum such phasic contractions invariably originate in the proximal sphincter and propagate toward the duodenum (204). Rhythmic, contractile activity is present in the feline and canine sphincter of Oddi but is less forceful than that in humans or the opossum. Spontaneous phasic sphincter contractions are frequently absent in anesthetized primates but may be elicited by excitatory drugs. Cholecystokinin (CCK) inhibits sphincter of Oddi contractile activity in the human, dog, and cat (10, 59) but stimulates contraction in the opossum and rabbit (8, 158, 159). Animals without a gallbladder have negligible sphincter of Oddi tone (110). In contrast to most species, the common bile duct in sheep (21) and fowl (217) exhibits rhythmic peristaltic contractions.

## METHODS OF STUDY

A number of methods have been used for evaluating the physiology and pathophysiology of biliary tract motor function and flow. Some of the most useful methods available are discussed in this section.

### Imaging Studies

Since intravenous cholecystography was developed by Graham and Cole in the 1920s, radiographic imaging has been used widely for studying the gallbladder and biliary tract. Cholecystography utilizes iodinated contrast medium, such as iopanoic acid, that is processed through the liver, similar to bilirubin, and secreted into the hepatic bile as a conjugated glucuronide. In the gallbladder the contrast medium is concentrated, thereby giving dense opacification for imaging (43, 173). Measurement of gallbladder dimensions allows a reasonably accurate estimation of gallbladder volume. In the past this method has been used in humans and dogs to evaluate the effect of pharmacological agents, hormones, and feeding on gallbladder emptying (43). Although cholecystography is still used in the clinical evaluation of patients with suspected gallstones and in animal research, the method is no longer suitable for monitoring gallbladder volume in humans. Cholecystography is cumbersome, depends on hepatic function, and requires considerable radiation.

Cholangiography has generated important information about the kinetics of bile duct flow. Although the bile ducts may be opacified by intravenous cholangiography, most significant observations have accrued via T tube cholangiography, done during laparotomy or postoperatively. Radiomanometry was introduced in Europe in the early 1940s. With this technique, radiographs of the bile ducts were obtained at a low hydrostatic pressure just sufficient to initiate common duct outflow, usually <15 cmH$_2$O, and at a high hydrostatic pressure of 40–50 cmH$_2$O. The general availability of cineradiography since about 1950 enabled rapid imaging of the sphincter of Oddi. Such studies done initially in Europe (24, 73) indicated that the human sphincter of Oddi segment has spontaneous rhythmic contractions that were likened to intervals of systolic contraction separated by intervals of diastolic relaxation (Fig. 5).

Recently a new method called intravital microscopy has been developed for imaging the common bile duct in small anesthetized animals (34). For this method the gallbladder is cannulated and a small amount of sodium fluorescein is injected into the gallbladder bile. The common duct is exposed at laparotomy and placed under a microscope. A laser beam directed at the common duct gives off reflected light from the fluorescein, thereby providing an image of the bile duct. By this method the terminal choledochus of the guinea pig was seen to exhibit spontaneous phasic contractions. This activity may be recorded in real time with a video camera attached to the microscope and run at a frame rate of ~30/s.

*Flow Measurements*

The conventional method for measuring bile duct flow is to drip fluid at a known pressure head into the common duct through a T tube or cystic duct cannula while recording flow with a drop counter. Flow at a given pressure is determined primarily by the resistance of the sphincter of Oddi. The assumption is made that bile duct inflow reflects bile duct outflow. Measurements may be obtained during basal conditions and after the administration of pharmacological agents. Measurement of bile duct flow provides indirect information about the overall resistance of the sphincter but does not evaluate the internal function of the sphincter segment. Findings from flow studies in humans and animals suggest that the sphincter of Oddi functions as both an active and a passive resistor (69). Flow measurements of contrast medium have been obtained during cineradiography to quantitate flow during imaging of sphincter opening and closing (73).

In addition to common duct images, intravital microscopy may also be employed to measure common duct flow. For this purpose, fluorescent beads (10 μm diam) are injected into the gallbladder. Determination of the velocity of bead travel within the common duct and duct diameter enables calculation of the flow rate.

*Manometry*

To study gallbladder contraction, its intraluminal pressure has been recorded, with the cystic duct either patent or occluded, in both anesthetized and awake animals. In humans a few pressure measurements have been made via cystostomy tubes, generally positioned within an abnormal gallbladder. Using these methods, investigators have monitored gallbladder responses to various drugs and hormones and also to electrical stimulation of autonomic nerves.

A new method, based on applied biomechanics, has been developed recently for characterizing gallbladder distensibility and contractility (166). During continuous monitoring of gallbladder pressure, repetitive infusion and withdrawal of fluid from the gallbladder is accomplished with a dual-catheter system and reciprocal infusion pump. The obtained hysteresis loop has both a slope and an area. The mean slope ($\Delta P/\Delta V$, where P is pressure and V is volume) indicates gallbladder "stiffness." The reciprocal of slope represents the mean compliance ($\Delta V/\Delta P$). Loop area represents work performed by the tissue while accommodating to the infused volume. An increase in loop area indicates a decrease in distensibility, usually due to increased muscle contraction. In contrast a decrease in loop area represents a greater ability of the gallbladder to accommodate to an increase in volume. Base-line hysteresis characteristics define the mechanical properties of both the active (smooth muscle) and passive (fibroelastic) elements of the unstimulated gallbladder. Changes of the hysteresis loop in response to drugs or hormones reflect changes in smooth muscle tone. For example, excitatory agents such as pilocarpine and CCK cause smooth muscle contraction, thereby decreasing gallbladder compliance and increasing loop area (Fig. 6A). Atropine does not affect compliance but decreases the loop area, indicating a relaxation of smooth muscle that allows tissue distension with less loss of energy (Fig. 6B). This hysteresis method is more sensitive than conventional methods for detecting changes in gallbladder tone.

Historically pressure measurements from the human bile ducts were obtained initially in patients with an indwelling T tube linked in series with a manometer (69). Often measurements were obtained during laparotomy for biliary tract disease. Initially pressure was monitored visually using a manometer and subsequently by a transducer linked to a polygraph. In this manner, investigators obtained values for steady-state, common duct pressure. In some instances, values for opening, or passage, pressure and closing pressure were obtained by determining the onset or cessation of flow while increasing or decreasing, respectively, the pressure head of a fluid reservoir. Generally opening pressure is a few centimeters of water higher than resting common duct pressure. From measure-

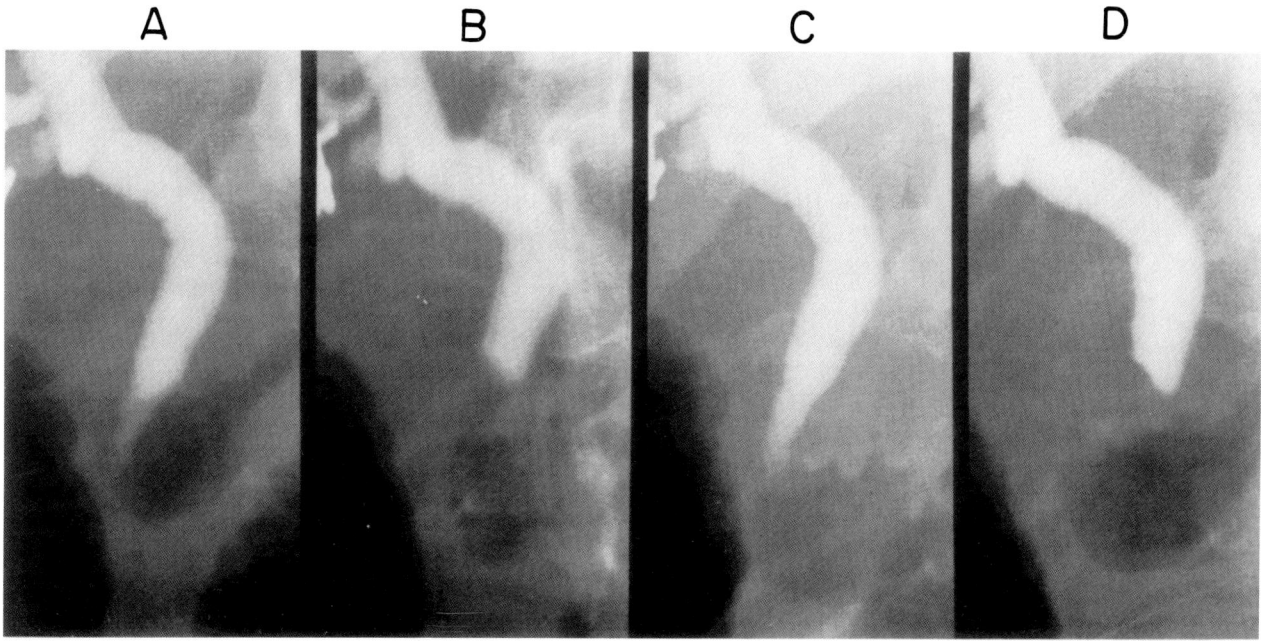

FIG. 5. *A, B, C, D*: sequential radiographic images of common duct and sphincter of Oddi segment. Images taken ~8–10 s apart. Subject was without biliary tract symptoms. Surgical clips from previous cholecystectomy. In *A* and *C*, sphincter segment is relaxed and filled, whereas sphincter is contracted and empty in *B* and *D*.

ments of common duct pressure, inferences were drawn about sphincter of Oddi function. Generally, however, biliary duct manometry through a T tube or cystic duct cannula has suffered from the vagaries of unstandardized methodology, the existence of biliary tract disease, possible effects of anesthesia, and the fact that the sphincter of Oddi segment was not examined directly.

On T-tube manometry, common duct pressure is generally referenced to atmospheric pressure as zero. We have followed this convention unless specified otherwise. When duodenal pressures are known, some workers prefer to reference common duct pressure to intraduodenal pressure to obtain the pressure gradient across the sphincter of Oddi. Because duodenal pressure is usually ~10 cmH$_2$O, a common duct pressure of 15 cmH$_2$O would represent a common duct to duodenal pressure gradient of only ~5 cmH$_2$O. In earlier studies, pressures were measured in centimeters of water, whereas in many recent studies pressures are recorded in millimeters of mercury (1 mmHg = 1.36 cmH$_2$O). These distinctions are important when comparing values from different studies. Recently methods have been described for retrograde positioning of a microtransducer or manometry catheter within the common duct during endoscopy. This method allows monitoring of common duct pressure for several hours or longer (195).

Direct pressure measurements from within the black box of the sphincter of Oddi were not feasible

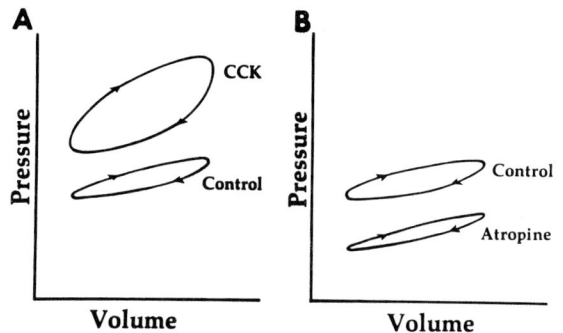

FIG. 6. Hysteresis loops of volume-pressure relationships for baboon gallbladder. *A*: before and after administration of cholecystokinin (CCK). *B*: before and after administration of atropine. [Adapted from Schoetz et al. (166).]

in humans until the development of endoscopic retrograde cholangiopancreatography (ERCP). During ERCP examination, a manometric catheter (~1.7 mm diam) is passed through the biopsy channel of the endoscope and inserted retrograde across the sphincter into the common or pancreatic duct. Accurate recording of sphincter pressure phenomena requires a noncompliant pump for catheter infusion (61). Pressures are obtained directly from within the sphincter of Oddi by incremental withdrawal of the catheter across the sphincter or by stationing one or more recording sites within the sphincter segment for a 10–15 min interval, during which time sphincter motor responses to drugs and hormones may be assessed (59). A second catheter attached to the endoscope monitors concurrent intraduodenal pressure. Improvements in manometric instrumentation and catheter subminiaturization developed for sphincter of Oddi manometry in humans (61) have been refined further for obtaining pressure recordings from the sphincter of Oddi in animals (204). Manometric studies have yielded considerable new information about sphincter of Oddi motor function. Outer catheter diameter must be minimal to avoid an artifactual increase in basal sphincter pressure (56, 204). Well-defined phasic pressure waves in the sphincter, unobserved previously, have been recorded consistently in humans (Fig. 7) and in experimental animals such as the opossum, dog, and cat (25, 35, 59, 170, 204). Studies done during laparotomy indicate that the phasic sphincter contractions persist during anesthesia (55, 134).

*Electromyography*

For electromyography, bipolar or monopolar electrodes are either sutured into the muscularis or closely applied to its surface. This method is suitable for acute in vivo studies (158) or chronic studies in conscious animals with an array of electrodes (79). Earlier studies of myoelectrical recording from the gallbladder of the dog and monkey showed neither electrical control wave activity (slow waves) nor electrical response activity (spike bursts), even during periods of gallbladder contraction (107). However, electromyograms of the gallbladder in conscious sheep exhibit clusters of spike potentials occurring at regular intervals (21). Findings from a recent study in dogs suggest that the canine gallbladder has omnipresent electrical control waves that increase in amplitude in association with phasic gallbladder contractions (113). A myoelectrical equivalent has yet to be demonstrated for slow tonic gallbladder contractions, similar to the lack of an electrical equivalent for tonic contractions elsewhere in the gastrointestinal tract.

Investigators have also used extracellular electrodes to monitor from the common duct of animals. Detectable control waves and electrical response activity have been absent in the bile duct of the dog and opossum. This finding might be expected because the common duct in these species contains negligible smooth muscle. Therefore a similar absence of common duct electrical activity would be expected in humans. On the other hand, some spiking electrical activity has been recorded from the common duct of monkeys and sheep (21), two species that have common duct smooth muscle.

In the late 1950s Japanese investigators (84) began recording myoelectrical activity from the sphincter of Oddi of animal species such as the rabbit. These studies demonstrated that the sphincter of Oddi generated spontaneous, rhythmic, spikelike activity that occurred independently from duodenal myoelectrical activity. Controversy arose about whether or not the rhythmic, sphincter of Oddi electrical activity served

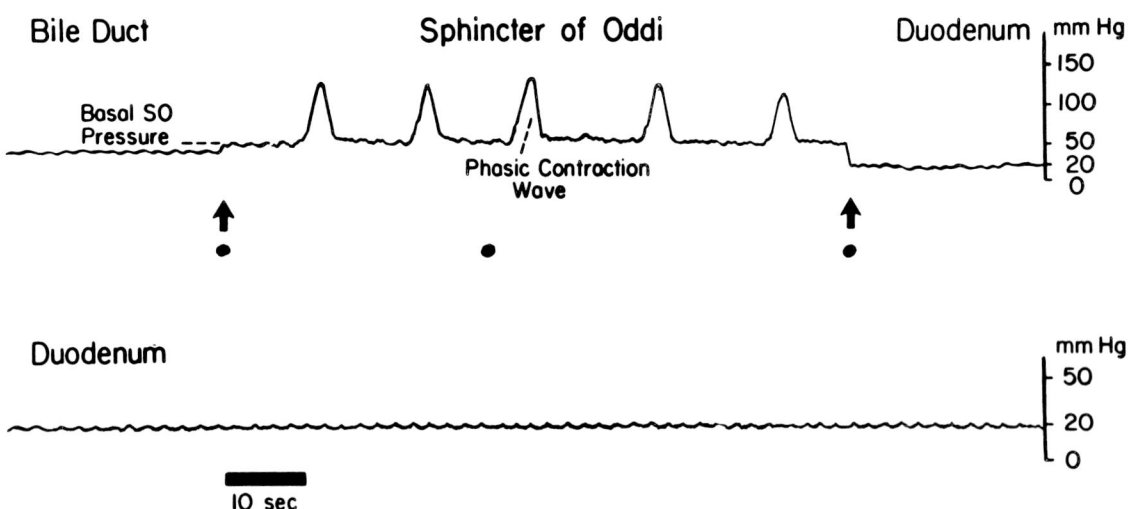

FIG. 7. Manometric recording of station pull-through across sphincter of Oddi (SO) segment. *Upper tracing* from catheter orifice withdrawn across sphincter; *lower tracing* recorded from duodenal catheter taped to endoscope. Each *dot* represents a 2- to 3-mm withdrawal of cannulating catheter. Margins of sphincter segment shown by *arrows*. Small pressure fluctuations caused by respiration. For tracing analysis, pressure may be measured from common bile duct (CBD) as well as from duodenum and CBD-duodenal gradient calculated. Within sphincter, basal (base-line) pressure is only few mmHg greater than common duct pressure. Superimposed on basal SO pressure are phasic pressure waves ~100 mmHg in amplitude. [From Geenen et al. (59). Reprinted with permission of The American Gastroenterological Association, copyright 1980.]

to retard or promote bile flow from the common duct into the duodenum. In 1968 Ono et al. (132) reported the results of myoelectrical recording from the human sphincter of Oddi with electrodes positioned at the time of laparotomy that was done for other reasons. The electrodes were difficult to position because the human sphincter of Oddi is mostly intraduodenal. Notwithstanding, Ono and associates recorded discrete bursts of spikelike activity, attributed to the sphincter, that were clearly not duodenal in origin. They concluded that the sphincter spike activity retarded bile flow. During the past several years investigators have obtained myoelectrical recordings from the sphincter of Oddi of anesthetized opossums (8) and also from awake chronic animals (79). These studies indicate that omnipresent, rhythmic spike bursts occur in the opossum sphincter of Oddi. The rate varies from 1 to 7 bursts/min in the fasted animal. Each burst of electrical activity corresponds to a peristaltic contraction that originates proximally in the sphincter and generally propagates to the sphincter-duodenal junction (Fig. 8). The peristaltic contractions are recorded manometrically as a propagating monophasic pressure wave.

*Scintigraphy*

During the past decade quantitative cholescintigraphy has been developed to image the gallbladder with radioisotope markers. When given intravenously, various $^{99m}$Tc-labeled iminodiacetic acid (IDA) compounds are excreted by the liver into the bile. Within ~30–60 min after its administration, the isotope is cleared through the liver. At this time a portion of the isotope has accumulated in the gallbladder and the remainder has passed into the duodenum. The $^{99m}$Tc gives off 140 keV γ-photons that are ideally suited for imaging and counting by a γ-photon camera. Linkage of the γ-photon camera to a computer allows quantitative cholescintigraphy. By selecting regions of interest over the liver, gallbladder, common bile duct, and small bowel, temporal profiles can be determined for the appearance or disappearance of isotope from these sites (93, 171). After isotope administration the first hour is assigned to monitoring gallbladder filling. Subsequently gallbladder emptying may be measured by giving the subject a meal containing fat or administering cholecystokinin. Computer analysis is used to determine the fraction of liver activity distributed to

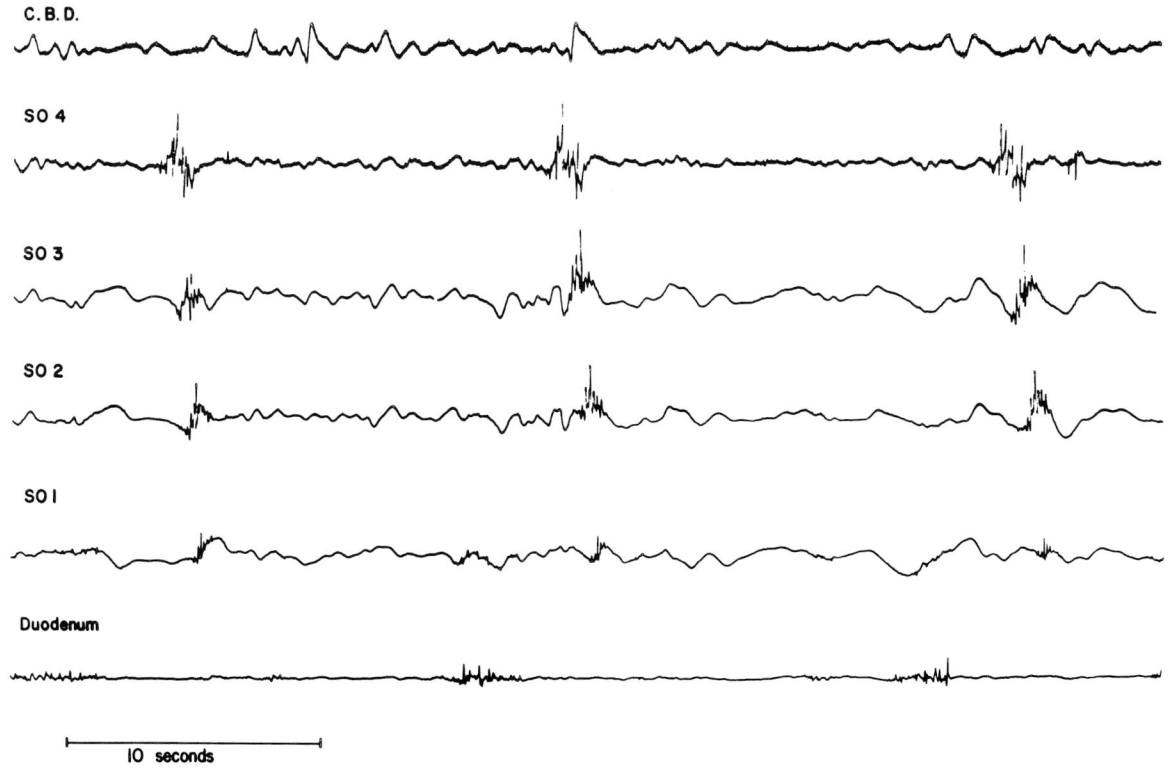

FIG. 8. Recording of electromyographic activity from opossum sphincter of Oddi (SO). One electrode positioned on common bile duct (CBD), four along (SO) segment, and one on duodenum. Tracing shows 3 spontaneous spike-burst sequences originating in proximal sphincter (SO$_4$) and traversing entire SO segment. Two spike bursts, seen in duodenum, occur independently of SO myoelectrical activity.

gallbladder and duodenum, rate of gallbladder filling, and rate of gallbladder emptying.

A major advantage of the isotope method is its noninvasive nature. The short 6-h half-life ($t_{1/2}$) of $^{99m}$Tc causes minimal radiation. The results of quantitative cholescintigraphy have a reproducibility and interobserver error of 5% or less (93). The method measures only changes in count and not gallbladder volume. Although well suited for quantitating rates of gallbladder filling and emptying, the isotope method as used currently gives only semiquantitative information about the kinetics of bile flow through the bile ducts and often does not identify partial duct obstruction. However, the scintigraphy method can be modified to provide time-activity curves of isotope counts over the common duct. When the gallbladder is absent, such time-activity curves may give a reasonable approximation of common duct clearance and assessment for partial sphincter of Oddi obstruction (101, 219).

*Sonography*

Since 1980 investigators (20, 45, 46) have capitalized on the virtues of ultrasound for noninvasive imaging of the gallbladder and major bile ducts. Sonographic imaging does not require the administration of a radioactive marker or contrast agent nor the use of ionizing radiation. Existing evidence indicates that exposure to diagnostic ultrasound is without risk, even during pregnancy. For these reasons sonography represents a powerful new tool for evaluating the biliary tract in humans. For example, the sonographic method allows convenient, frequent sampling of gallbladder volume during intervals of several hours or longer.

Gallbladder volume is determined from sonographic images by obtaining cross-sectional and longitudinal gallbladder images. Subsequently gallbladder volume is closely approximated by a method that calculates volume as the sum of a series of cylinders. Total volume can also be calculated accurately by the ellipsoid method (Fig. 9) from measurements of gallbladder length and diameter (40). Such measurements take only a few minutes to perform using real-time ultrasound, which is generally available in most hospitals. Measurements of gallbladder volume are comparable to those obtained by cholecystography (45).

Because ultrasound readily determines bile duct diameter, the method is used widely to evaluate patients with suspected obstructive jaundice. This promising method, however, has not been fully exploited to investigate changes in common duct caliber during fasting or after a meal. Findings from several recent studies suggest that the normal common duct in cholecystectomized patients generally decreases in diameter after a fatty meal, despite an increase in bile flow (174, 175). This effect is presumably due to the influence of increased levels of circulating CCK that relax

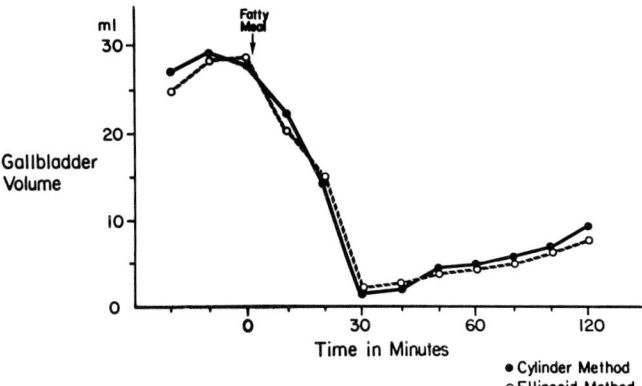

FIG. 9. Measurement of gallbladder volume by sonographic method in single subject. Axial and transverse gallbladder images obtained at 10-min intervals before and after fatty meal. Estimates for gallbladder volume calculated by sums-of-cylinder and ellipsoid methods were comparable. Here gallbladder emptied ~85% of its volume within 30 min after fatty meal (Lipomul, 1.5 ml/kg). During this interval, net emptying rate was ~1 ml/min.

the sphincter of Oddi. In contrast, a fatty meal frequently induces enlargement of the common duct in cholecystectomized patients who have partial duct obstruction. A potential use of ultrasound is for continuous monitoring of bile flow after implantation of pulsed Doppler devices around the common duct in experimental animals.

*Miscellaneous*

Numerous other methods exist for investigating the physiology of biliary tract motor function. Additional in vivo methods include implantation of extraluminal transducers, nerve disruption by vagotomy or sympathectomy, nerve stimulation, and pharmacological dissection employing a battery of appropriate agonists and antagonists. In vitro muscle-bath studies of intact sphincter of Oddi specimens or muscle strips are also helpful.

PHARMACOLOGY

Although the pharmacology of agents that affect biliary tract motor function is discussed extensively in another chapter, a few general comments are warranted here. Cholecystokinin is widely accepted as a naturally occurring enteric hormone that causes physiological gallbladder contraction (152). Release of such a hormone from the proximal small intestine was suggested by observations that food in the duodenum elicited gallbladder contraction, whereas contraction did not occur when food substances were given intravenously.

Subsequently CCK was shown to elicit sphincter of Oddi relaxation in humans (Fig. 10), cats, and dogs (10, 59), whereas it increases sphincter of Oddi con-

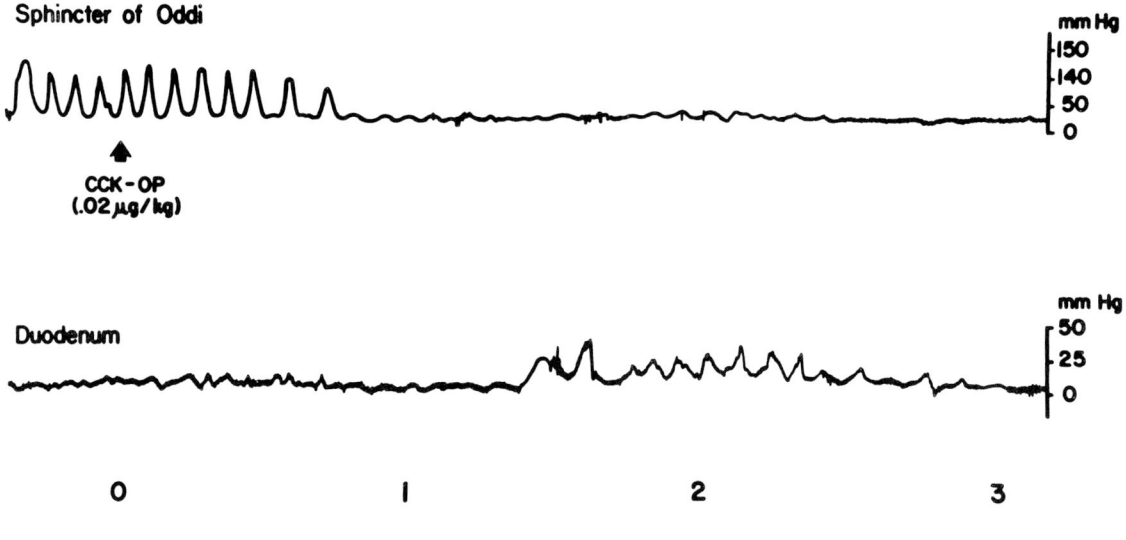

FIG. 10. Effect of cholecystokinin octapeptide (CCK-8) on sphincter of Oddi contractile activity. Pressure recordings obtained at endoscopic retrograde cholangiopancreatography manometry are for sphincter and duodenum. Intravenous administration of CCK-8 associated with prompt inhibition of phasic contractions followed 30 s later by contractile activity in duodenum. CCK-8 also depressed basal sphincter pressure by few mmHg, but this change cannot be appreciated from figure due to high pressure scale used for sphincter tracing. [From Geenen et al. (59). Reprinted with permission of The American Gastroenterological Association, copyright 1980.]

tractile activity in the rabbit, guinea pig, and opossum (8, 158, 159, 204). Cholecystokinin also stimulates pancreatic enzyme secretion and enhances hepatic bile flow. The hormone is present mainly in the mucosa of proximal jejunum and to a lesser extent in the duodenum. Suitable radioimmunoassays for CCK determination are now available (27, 211). The demonstration of a close correlation between changes in serum CCK concentration and changes in gallbladder volume (211) substantiate further the status of CCK as a physiological hormone that regulates gallbladder tone. Recent studies suggest that the effect of CCK on the gallbladder is mediated partially by a direct effect on gallbladder smooth muscle and partially by an indirect effect on postganglionic cholinergic nerves that is antagonized by atropine (10, 68, 218).

Motilin causes gallbladder contraction in laboratory animals, such as the dog, pig, and opossum (183, 190, 194). A similar effect is likely in humans. The gallbladder contraction induced by motilin is antagonized by atropine (194) and is thus likely to be mediated mainly by excitatory cholinergic nerves. Because serum levels of motilin undergo regular fluctuations during fasting, motilin could cause periodic increases in gallbladder tone between meals.

Motilin also increases contractile activity of the sphincter of Oddi, as shown in the cat, opossum, and rabbit (11, 160, 191). At least a portion of motilin's excitatory effect on the sphincter of Oddi is antagonized by atropine, thereby suggesting participation of cholinergic nerves. To our knowledge, motilin's effect on the human sphincter of Oddi has not been investigated.

In all species, cholinergic agonists elicit gallbladder and sphincter of Oddi contraction, thereby indicating the presence of muscarinic smooth muscle receptors. In most species, $\alpha$-adrenergic agonists cause gallbladder and sphincter of Oddi contractions, whereas $\beta$-adrenergic agonists elicit relaxation. The neurotransmitter for inhibitory nerves to the gallbladder and sphincter of Oddi may be VIP (155, 182).

PHYSIOLOGY

The biliary tract is a low-pressure system characterized by slow flow (69). The flow of bile through the bile ducts is entirely passive, determined mainly by the rate of hepatic bile secretion, gallbladder contraction, and sphincter of Oddi motor activity. Factors such as cystic duct resistance, bile viscosity, duodenal contractions, and gravity have an ancillary role.

*Hepatic Bile*

Exclusive of gallbladder contraction, the only active source that generates bile duct flow is hepatic secretion. The human liver secretes up to ~800–1,000 ml of dilute bile daily (215). Variations in bile production are directly related to the quantity of circulating bile acids that are processed by the liver. Hepatic bile has an electrolyte composition similar to that of serum and contains low concentrations of cholesterol, bile acids, phospholipids, and bilirubin. During basal conditions, the pressure gradient between the common duct and duodenum is ~5–8 cmH$_2$O, thereby suggesting that the sphincter of Oddi causes only a modest resistance to common duct outflow. When common duct pressure is increased to >10 cmH$_2$O, net bile secretion decreases (181). After occlusion of the common duct in humans and monkeys, bile duct pressure increases to ~30 cmH$_2$O, then shows no further increase (69). This finding indicates that the normal liver cannot generate net bile outflow against an absolute pressure of >30 cmH$_2$O. Thus the bile duct system is a low-pressure system not only during normal conditions but it also remains at relatively low pressure even when obstructed. Interestingly cirrhotic livers can generate common duct pressures >30 cmH$_2$O, because a reduction in hepatic backflow enhances the net bile outflow (69).

Earlier workers believed that during fasting, tonic contraction of the sphincter of Oddi directed virtually all of the hepatic bile into the gallbladder. Investigation of a baboon model, however, showed that only 35%–50% of the hepatic bile secreted during fasting entered the gallbladder (130). The remainder flowed into the duodenum. An isotope study in humans showed that ~75% of the isotope enters the gallbladder, whereas 25% emptied directly into the duodenum (171). However, it is not established whether the partitioning of hepatic bile between the gallbladder and duodenum occurs as a fixed ratio during fasting or undergoes periodic fluctuations.

Recent evidence reveals that hepatic secretion of bile during fasting is not constant in humans (137, 209) or experimental animals (169, 189) but rather increases and decreases in rhythm with the gastrointestinal migratory motor complex (MMC). The MMC is characterized by a front of intense peristaltic motor activity that generally occurs in the stomach and migrates slowly over the length of the small bowel. At a given location, this band of intense peristaltic contractions, called phase III activity, lasts ~5–10 min. As one phase III activity front dissipates in the distal ileum, a new front usually appears in the stomach or duodenum. Passage of the intense phase III activity is followed by a period of quiescence, termed phase I, that merges into a period of irregular contractions, termed phase II. Phase II culminates in the brief front of phase III activity, and the cycle repeats. In humans, dogs, and opossums, the MMC cycle is ~90 min. The MMC phenomenon is not limited to gastrointestinal motor activity but also encompasses cyclic variations in the secretory activity of the stomach and biliary-pancreatic system. During late phase II of the duodenal MMC, gastric and pancreatic secretions increase in volume and concentration. Concurrently an increase generally occurs in the volume and bile acid concentration of bile entering the duodenum, irrespective of whether or not the gallbladder is present (209).

What is the mechanism(s) that regulates alterations of hepatic bile flow during the MMC cycle? Logical candidates would be some form of neural or hormonal control. Recent work in the dog and opossum, however, suggests that variations in the rate of hepatic flow during fasting are determined by variations in the rate at which bile acids return to the liver (169, 189). Because bile flow and its bile acid concentration are usually greatest during phase II of duodenal MMC cycle (Fig. 11), a large bolus of bile acids is delivered into the small bowel during this period. This bolus of bile is propelled toward the ileum just ahead of the phase III activity front. Consequently bile acids are reabsorbed from the terminal ileum in cyclic fashion, because they are presented to the ileum in cyclic fashion. Thus a large quantity of bile acids are reabsorbed and represented to the liver shortly before the phase III activity terminates in the distal ileum (Fig. 12). The high hepatic concentration of bile acids stimulates bile flow, thereby causing an increase in duodenal bile just before the next phase III front appears in the proximal gastrointestinal tract. As the bile acids are cleared through the liver, serum bile acid concentration falls and bile flow decreases. However, serum bile acids rise again when the bolus of duodenal bile reaches the terminal ileum (Fig. 13). Thus the periodicity of increased and decreased bile flow occurs in rhythm with the MMC cycle. Interruption of the bile acid cycle by aspirating bile from the duodenum dramatically reduces hepatic bile secretion to a constant low value (189). Infusion of bile acids into the duo-

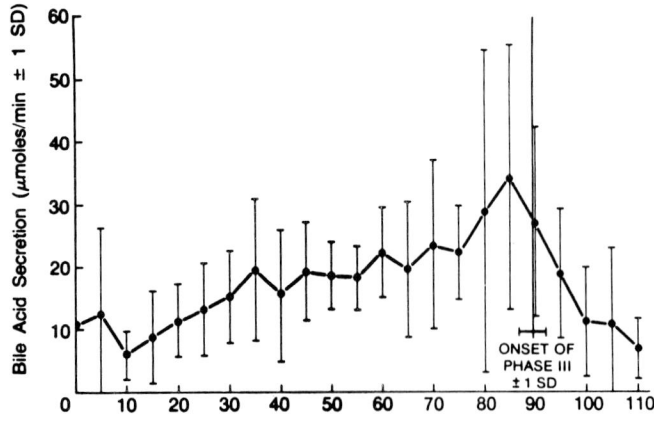

FIG. 11. Hepatic production of bile acids during duodenal migratory motor complex (MMC) cycle in dogs. Data plotted as mean ± 1 SD for 10 MMC cycles. Pooled data indicate that hepatic secretion of bile was generally maximal late in duodenal MMC cycle. [From Scott et al. (170). Reprinted with permission of The American Gastroenterological Association, copyright 1984.]

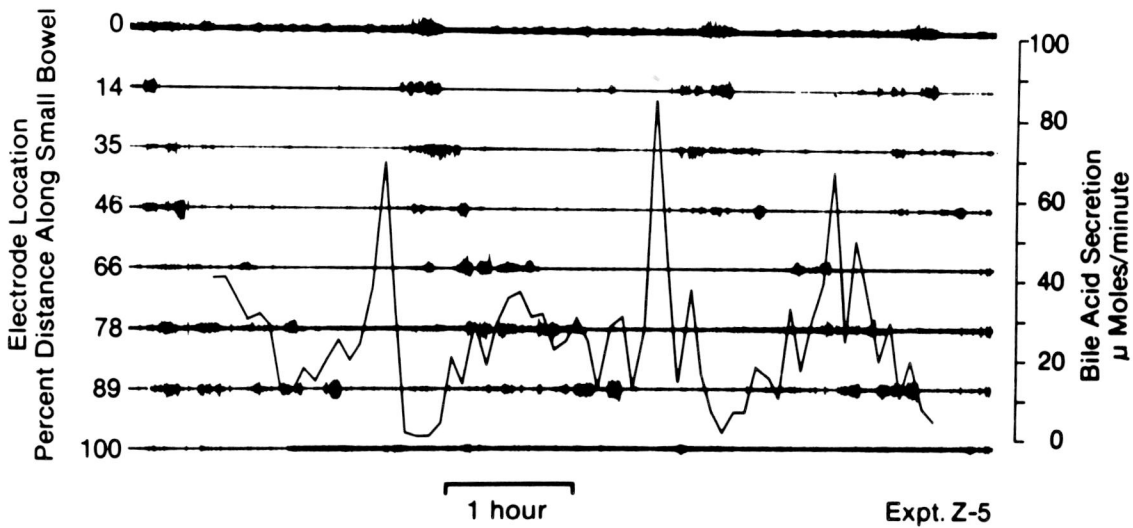

FIG. 12. Example of variations in hepatic secretion of bile acids in fasted dog. Bile acid secretion given in micromoles per minute. Electrodes distributed along entire length of small bowel. Cyclic changes observed in hepatic secretion of bile acid. Volume of bile paralleled bile acid secretion. In this example, peak bile production occurred during phase II of duodenal MMC. [From Scott et al. (170). Reprinted with permission of The American Gastroenterological Association, copyright 1984.]

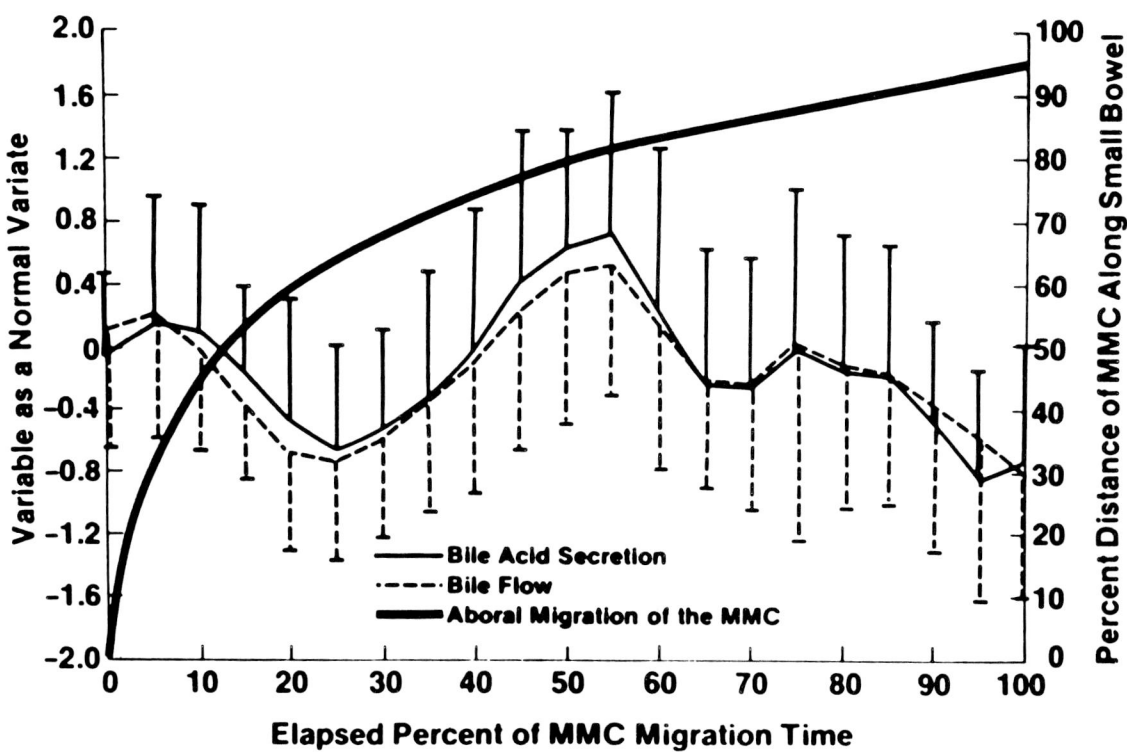

FIG. 13. Graph of common duct bile flow in cholecystectomized dogs. Pooled data obtained from 14 migratory motor complex (MMC) cycles while extrahepatic circulation of bile acids was intact. Bile flow and bile acid secretion plotted against percent migration time of phase III activity through small bowel. *Bold line* indicates position of phase III activity in small bowel. Thus at 50% of migration time, phase III activity has migrated 80% of bowel length. Hepatic bile flow and bile acid secretion become maximal as phase III activity reaches midileum. [From Scott et al. (169).]

denum at a constant rate causes a uniform increase in hepatic bile output. Neither of these manipulations, however, has a major effect on the MMC cycles.

After a meal the volume of bile entering the duodenum increases due to an increased rate of its hepatic secretion as well as gallbladder contraction. In cholecystectomized animals, the hepatic bile flow doubles after a meal (189). The postprandial increase in bile flow is largely bile acid independent and is virtually abolished when the enterohepatic circulation is interrupted by a diverting bile duct fistula. The postprandial increase in bile flow is caused by rapid transit of bile through the small bowel during the fed state, an increase in the enterohepatic circulation of bile acids, and increased circulating levels of CCK as well as secretin that act as hepatic choleretics (88).

Because hepatic bile flow is determined by the rate at which bile acids are processed through the liver, hepatic bile flow is substantially affected by the size of the bile acid pool. During fasting, up to 60% of the total bile acid pool may be sequestered in the gallbladder (119). For this reason the total amount of bile acids is reduced by cholecystectomy or procedures such as sphincterotomy (162). The latter promotes bile runoff into the intestine and thereby diverts hepatic bile from the gallbladder. A reduction in total bile acids is one of several mechanisms whereby cholecystectomy or sphincterotomy may alter mean or peak common duct bile flow during fasting or after a meal.

*Gallbladder*

The major functions of the gallbladder are to concentrate hepatic bile, store bile, and deliver concentrated bile into the duodenum when food leaves the stomach. The average volume of the human gallbladder during fasting ranges from ~15 to 35 ml (45, 46).

Approximately 50%-75% of the hepatic bile secreted during fasting enters the gallbladder (130, 171), whereas minimal bile enters the gallbladder for several hours after a meal. The normal gallbladder concentrates hepatic bile to as little as 10% of its original volume (149). This process is accomplished by the gallbladder mucosa, which extracts electrolytes and water from the dilute hepatic bile. As a result of selective absorption, the gallbladder bile becomes viscous and its nonabsorbable solutes, such as bile acids, cholesterol, and bilirubin, are concentrated even to the point of supersaturation. Precipitation of cholesterol or bile acids is normally prevented more by a proper ratio of cholesterol, bile acids, and phospholipids than by the absolute concentration of these components themselves.

The classic notion is that the normal gallbladder maintains a perpetual net absorption until the gallbladder bile is maximally concentrated. A recent study, however, indicates that the monkey gallbladder exhibits a net secretion after feeding, compared with a net absorption during fasting (184). The postprandial net excretion may be governed by increased circulating levels of secretin and VIP as well as by splanchnic and vagal stimulation. Secretin and adrenergic stimulation are known to increase gallbladder absorption (15, 16), whereas VIP increases secretion. Whether net gallbladder secretion exists in species other than the monkey remains to be determined. Interestingly the gallbladder in the guinea pig, unlike that of other animals, does not concentrate bile (23).

Historically gallbladder contraction was studied mainly by the feeding of a fatty meal or by administration of CCK or its terminal octapeptide, CCK-8. Older studies that quantitated gallbladder volume by cholecystography in humans and dogs showed that the gallbladder generally contracted 30% or more within 30 min after a fatty meal or intravenous CCK (43). In normal subjects a 30-min infusion of CCK-8 at the rate of 60 $ng \cdot kg^{-1} \cdot h^{-1}$ causes a mean reduction in gallbladder volume of 73% (105). Findings from another study suggested that the optimal rate of CCK-8 infusion at 20 $ng \cdot kg^{-1} \cdot h^{-1}$ gave a mean gallbladder emptying of 52%, ~45 min after the onset of the infusion (161).

Studies with $^{99m}Tc$-labeled IDA indicate that during the 30-60 min interval after intravenous administration of isotope, the gallbladder normally fills at a rate of ~2%-3%/min. This percentage is expressed as the percent of maximal counts that accumulate in the gallbladder at 30-60 min. After a basal period of 60-90 min, infusion of CCK at a rate of 0.02 $U \cdot kg^{-1} \cdot min^{-1}$ initiates gallbladder contraction and allows quantitation of its emptying. In normal subjects, gallbladder emptying begins ~5 min after the onset of CCK infusion. The half-emptying time was 12 min. Thus at 30 min after the onset of emptying the gallbladder ejects 75% of its counts (171). Computer plots show that gallbladder emptying occurs as a nearly linear function during an interval of 10-30 min or longer (179). The rate, or slope, of gallbladder emptying during CCK infusion is directly related to the CCK dose. Even after several hours, however, gallbladder emptying was never complete; a minimum of 10% of the isotope counts always remained.

In one sonographic study, mean gallbladder volume in fasted normal subjects averaged ~17 ml (45). After a 420-calorie liquid meal that contained 35% of the calories as fat, the decrease in gallbladder volume averaged 55%, with a rate constant of 0.022. After a 610-calorie breakfast with 44% of the calories as fat, gallbladder emptying averaged 74% (46). The initial rate of emptying to 50% of the fasting volume had a rate constant of 0.022, whereas the rate constant for emptying decreased to 0.009 during the later phase of gallbladder emptying (46). Findings from another sonographic study confirm that after a fatty meal the gallbladder exhibits a period of maximal contraction lasting ~30 min, followed by a period of slower emptying lasting from 30 to 120 min (100). After a regular-sized meal, the gallbladder remained contracted for ~4 h and did not begin to refill until gastric emptying was 87% complete. A recent report suggests that fasting gallbladder volume is greater in males than in females, but the male gallbladder exhibits greater emptying in response to a meal (54).

Although gallbladder emptying may be modulated by the resistance to bile flow at the cystic duct or sphincter of Oddi, the major determinant is contraction of gallbladder smooth muscle. Gallbladder emptying elicited by a meal or exogenous CCK clearly occurs as a slow, steady process that generally requires 30–60 min to achieve a maximal response. The gallbladder is incapable of rapid emptying within a few minutes, as is the case with the urinary bladder. For this reason, rapid-acting bolus doses of CCK are a suboptimal stimulus for testing gallbladder emptying. Sustained physiological gallbladder contraction achieves a prolonged delivery of increased bile flow into the duodenum for 20 min or longer while generating an intraluminal gallbladder pressure that is generally only a few centimeters of water above that in the common duct (57). Indeed the gallbladder seems incapable of increasing its resting intraluminal pressure by more than 10–20 $cmH_2O$. Interestingly the maximal pressure that can be generated by the gallbladder is not appreciably greater than the maximal secretion pressure of the liver.

The only circumstance associated with pronounced increases in intraluminal gallbladder pressure is cystic duct obstruction accompanied by acute cholecystitis (36). When the gallbladder is obstructed, active net secretion associated with inflammation commonly generates intraluminal gallbladder pressures of ~70 mmHg. In one patient a pressure of 200 mmHg was reported (87). In such circumstances indomethacin may reduce gallbladder pressure, thereby suggesting that prostaglandins are involved in the hypersecretion associated with cholecystitis (87).

The slow physiological emptying of the gallbladder is typical of a graded, tonic smooth muscle contraction, such as that occurring in the fundus of the stomach during gastric emptying of liquids. During the postprandial period, low-amplitude tonic contractions have been recorded in the canine gallbladder by a serosal transducer as well as by intraluminal manometry (85, 192). During gallbladder filling its intraluminal pressure is equal to or only a few centimeters of water less than common duct pressure. A minimal pressure gradient, however, may act as a sump that sucks bile into the gallbladder. Some workers, however, suggest that bidirectional flow of bile occurs during gallbladder filling.

Interestingly intermittent rhythmic bursts of spike activity have been recorded from the gallbladder of sheep (21). The rhythmic spike bursts are associated with slow changes in pressure that last 5–10 min. Earlier electromyographic studies of the gallbladder in dogs and monkeys have generally shown negligible electrical activity (107). In some studies from these species, however, electromyographic recordings have shown sporadic, inconsistent clusters of spike-burst activity. In a recent study the canine gallbladder was shown to exhibit omnipresent oscillatory myoelectric activity at a frequency of 18–30 cycles/min (113). During phasic gallbladder contractions the electrical oscillations did not increase in frequency but showed a 5- to 10-fold increase in magnitude without any identifiable spike activity. Therefore a unique type of myoelectric activity exists in the canine gallbladder that exhibits an electrical equivalent of phasic contractions. In the dog model, however, no identifiable alteration of electrical activity was demonstrated in association with tonic gallbladder contraction.

The ability of a fatty meal to elicit gallbladder contraction is an established physiological response that has been well documented in humans and in various animals (69). Proteins entering the duodenum also produce gallbladder contraction, albeit generally less pronounced than that caused by fat. Carbohydrates have only a minimal effect. The gallbladder contraction that follows eating is delayed in the presence of retarded gastric emptying. Therefore the rate of postprandial gallbladder evacuation depends on the rate of gastric emptying as well as the composition and volume of the meal.

Since the classic studies of Ivy, postprandial gallbladder contraction has been attributed to the hormone cholecystokinin (86). This conclusion is based on the observation that 1) CCK contracts the gallbladder, 2) CCK is released by a meal, 3) postprandial gallbladder contraction and relaxation correlate closely with the rise and fall of serum CCK, and 4) proglumide, a CCK antagonist, blocks postprandial gallbladder contraction.

Earlier studies suggested that endogenous CCK was released from the small bowel mucosa when fat or protein entered the duodenal lumen. Recent studies that measure serum CCK levels by radioimmunoassay in normal subjects show that gallbladder contraction induced by intraduodenal infusion of medium-chain triglycerides or intravenous infusion of CCK-33 correlates directly with the level of circulating CCK (53, 105, 111, 211). After intraduodenal administration of fat, serum CCK increased to a peak value at 16 min and the gallbladder contracted maximally at 18 min (211). The initial gallbladder volume of 35 ml decreased 66%. After 18 min, CCK levels began to fall and the gallbladder started to relax. After 45 min the serum CCK concentration fell ~50%. A study by the same workers showed that intravenous infusion of CCK-33 at a rate of 0.6 $\mu g \cdot kg^{-1} \cdot h^{-1}$ for 60 min gave a maximal increase of serum CCK at 8 min after the onset of the infusion (105). Gallbladder contraction became maximal at 10 min when the mean gallbladder volume of 23 ml had decreased 85%. After cessation of hormone infusion, serum CCK fell to control levels within 12 min, with a $t_{1/2}$ of 3.3 min. After 30 min, the gallbladder had refilled completely, with a $t_{1/2}$ of 18 min. Thus the rate of gallbladder filling was substantially slower than its emptying rate, despite the fact that the rate of the CCK rise and fall were comparable. Linear regression analysis showed a significant linear correlation between gallbladder volume and serum CCK concentration both during gallbladder contraction and gallbladder relaxation. The latter finding suggests that falling CCK concentration is sufficient to account for gallbladder relaxation after its postprandial contraction. However, the possibility exists also that inhibitory nerves may have a role. Postprandial gallbladder contraction is blocked by CCK antagonists such as proglumide (188). Findings from a recent study suggest that in addition to CCK, a meal may release non-CCK hormonelike substances that are capable of causing gallbladder contractions (178). The identification and role of such substances awaits further verification.

Recent evidence shows that the gallbladder is not in a persistent state of relaxation during fasting (Fig. 14) but rather contracts and relaxes periodically in rhythm with the gastrointestinal MMC cycle (85, 114, 192). Studies in the opossum indicate that the gallbladder in this species exhibits ~30%–40% contraction during the interval of duodenal phase II activity (192). The MMC-related gallbladder contraction is generally complete just prior to passage of the phase III activity front through the duodenum (Fig. 15). Superimposed on the tonic gallbladder contractions are phasic gallbladder contractions that occur at a rate of ~4–5/min and are linked temporally to phase II–III antral contractions (192). This temporal coupling of phasic gallbladder and antral contractions suggests stimulation by extrinsic excitatory nerves. In the dog, MMC-related phasic gallbladder contractions are generally not superimposed on a tonic contraction but, similar to the opossum, are coupled temporally to antral gastric contractions (114). Force transducers sutured to the gallbladder of sheep show that during fasting the ovine gallbladder exhibits slow phasic contractions, called tonic contractions, that lasted 6–7 min. These contractions occur during phases II and III of the duodenal MMC cycle (150). Superimposed on the slow phasic contractions are rapid rhythmic contractions that occur at a rate of ~6/min and were coordinated with antral contractions. Scintigraphic and sonographic studies in healthy volunteers show that the human gallbladder also undergoes a partial contraction during the latter half of the duodenal MMC cycle (92, 202). A study monitoring radioactive [$^3$H]iminodiacetic acid (HIDA) in the gallbladder of volunteers showed that periodic partial gallbladder emptying occurred concurrent with increases in serum motilin (186).

Gallbladder contractions linked to the gastrointestinal MMC complement the increased rate of hepatic bile flow that generally occurs during late phase II of the duodenal MMC and thereby enhances the delivery of bile into the duodenum, just before the phase III activity front. The periodic gallbladder contractions during fasting empty concentrated viscous bile and enable gallbladder refilling with dilute hepatic bile (191). Thus cyclic changes occur in the concentration of solutes in gallbladder bile. Cyclic contraction and relaxation of the gallbladder during fasting in humans could prevent undue hyperconcentration of bile solutes or rid the gallbladder of any microcalculi that might form between meals, such as during the night.

The control mechanism(s) is not known that elicits gallbladder contraction during fasting and integrates these contractions with the gastrointestinal MMC cycles. A potential candidate is motilin, a hormone produced in the mucosa of the proximal small bowel.

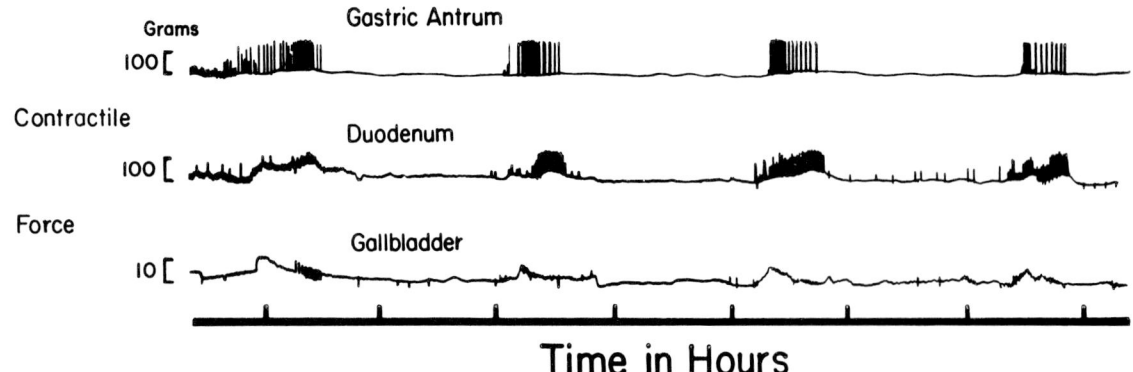

FIG. 14. Periodic contractions of canine gallbladder during fasting. Implanted transducers record motor contractions from gastric antrum, duodenum, and gallbladder. Three complete cycles of migratory motor complex (MMC) seen in antrum and duodenum. Gallbladder contracts during each MMC cycle, just before phase III activity front passes through duodenum. [From Itoh and Takahashi (85).]

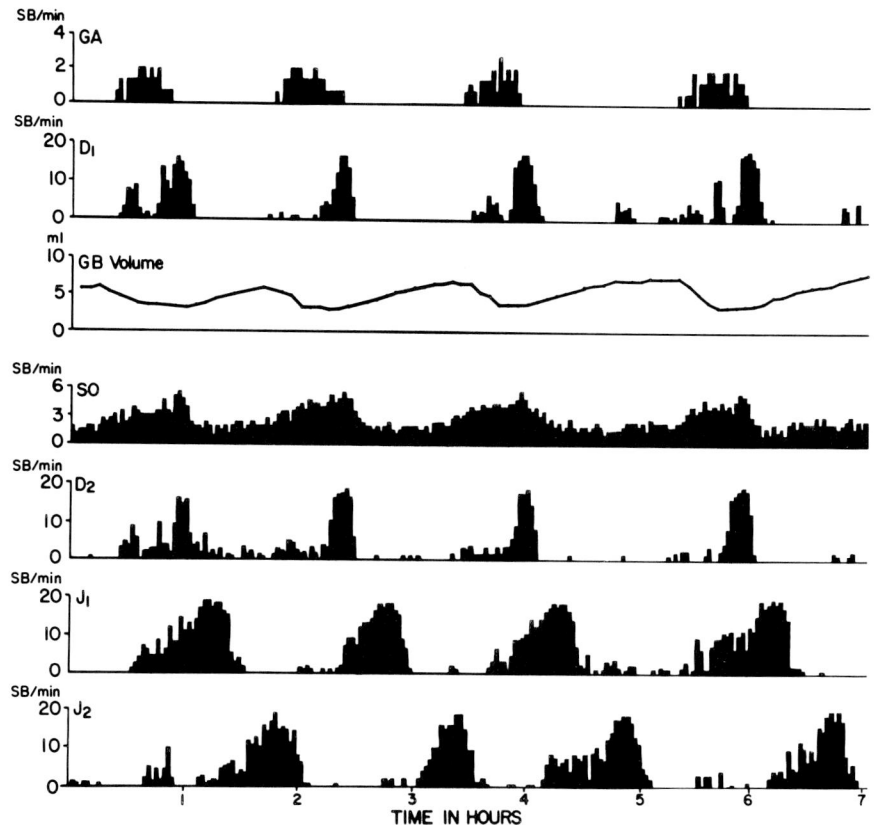

FIG. 15. Relationship between gallbladder (GB) volume and gastrointestinal migrating myoelectrical complex (MMC). Histograms plotted for spike-burst activity in gastric antrum (GA), duodenum (sites $D_1$ and $D_2$), sphincter of Oddi (SO), proximal jejunum ($J_1$), and distal jejunum ($J_2$). Four phase III MMC activity fronts occurred during 7-h recording. Periodic changes in gallbladder volume occurred synchronously with MMC cycles. [From Takahashi et al. (192).]

Serum motilin levels show cyclic changes during MMC cycles, with the peak values corresponding to the occurrence of phase III MMC activity in the duodenum. After a meal, serum motilin concentration decreases for at least several hours. Motilin is a motor hormone that contracts the gallbladder as well as stimulates the stomach and small bowel. Because atropine antagonizes motilin's excitatory effect on biliary tract (194) as well as on gastrointestinal smooth muscle, these effects are believed to be mediated by cholinergic nerves. The gallbladder contractions that occur during the MMC cycle occur concurrent with the rise of motilin during phase II of MMC activity in the duodenum. Whether increases in serum motilin concentration cause periodic gallbladder contraction during fasting remains to be determined.

The role of the autonomic nerves in regulating gallbladder volume is not clear. Vagotomy usually causes an increased fasting volume of the human gallbladder (152). Generally, however, the findings from most studies suggest that vagotomy does not impair gallbladder emptying but rather causes either no change or in some cases enhances gallbladder evacuation elicited by CCK, perhaps by the mechanism of denervation supersensitivity (37, 51, 140). In the opossum, truncal vagotomy significantly diminishes postprandial gallbladder contraction while having no effect on the cyclic changes in gallbladder volume that occur during the fasting MMC cycle (187). On vagal stimulation, gallbladder pressure usually increases, and this effect is partially antagonized by atropine (10). In one study, contraction of the feline gallbladder elicited by vagal stimulation was converted to relaxation by atropine. These findings support the presence of noncholinergic inhibitory nerves. Antral distension in dogs induces immediate gallbladder contraction via an atropine-sensitive, vagovagal, pyloric-cholecystic reflex (39). Such a reflex might mediate the initial phase of postprandial gallbladder contraction prior to an increase in circulating levels of CCK. In another study, vagal stimulation relaxed the guinea pig gallbladder via excitation of nonadrenergic inhibitory nerves (38). These inhibitory nerves are probably peptidergic, and the neurotransmitter might be VIP (182). Although studies of sympathetic innervation have produced inconstant and variable findings, stimulation of sympathetic nerves or intravenous injection of norepinephrine generally relaxes the gallbladder (152). However, splanchnic stimulation contracts the feline gallbladder via adrenergic stimulation that is blocked by phentolamine (10). Such discrepancies do not allow any definite conclusions.

Gallbladder filling after contraction is not simply the reverse of emptying but is affected by a number of factors. These factors include the rate of hepatic bile secretion, sphincter of Oddi function, cystic duct resistance, decreasing serum levels of CCK, and possibly active neural inhibition. The importance of sphincter of Oddi function in gallbladder filling is emphasized by studies that demonstrate that gallbladder filling is diminished by placing a stent across the sphincter segment (197, 210, 216) or by a sphincterotomy (31, 81). Physiological net gallbladder filling in the opossum appears to be linear, whereas one isotope study in humans suggests that gallbladder filling may feature accumulation of common duct bile with abrupt surges into the gallbladder (208).

*Cystic Duct*

As reviewed elsewhere (135, 167), current evidence suggests that the cystic duct is not simply a passive conduit between the gallbladder and common bile duct. The cystic duct has a narrow lumen, prominent intraluminal folds (valves of Heister), and a thin layer of smooth muscle along its length. These features suggest the possibility that the cystic duct may function as a variable resistor that actively regulates flow in and out of the gallbladder. This possibility is supported by observations that common duct and gallbladder pressure often vary independently of one another. A pressure gradient across the cystic duct supports the possibility of a sphincterlike mechanism.

Earlier workers proposed that the spiral valves of Heister favor unidirectional flow into the gallbladder. Subsequent studies indicated that flow across the canine cystic duct is similar in both directions (167). The spiral valves, however, might serve to increase cystic duct resistance in general. Thus a preferential condition could exist whereby flow of dilute hepatic bile into the gallbladder might be favored over the flow of viscous bile out of the gallbladder. The spiral valves might also function as a series of baffles that prevent cystic duct collapse when gallbladder pressure is close to that in the common duct. A leaflike fold between the junction of the cystic duct and common duct directs the flow of bile past the cystic duct orifice toward the sphincter of Oddi. Some resistance to flow at the sphincter of Oddi therefore is necessary to cause a slight back pressure that will promote bile backflow into the cystic duct. When a cannula is placed across the sphincter of Oddi, the gallbladder does not fill (69). Sphincterotomy or cholecystoduodenostomy causes low common duct pressure and rapid bile runoff into the duodenum, thereby resulting in impaired gallbladder filling. This finding has been observed commonly during intravenous cholangiography. In such a circumstance, lack of gallbladder opacification does not indicate cystic duct obstruction.

Although a localized anatomical sphincter of Lütkens has not been substantiated in the cystic duct, the presence of smooth muscle along the entire duct allows for the possibility of sphincter function. Active sphincter function is supported by the observation that cystic duct resistance *1*) varies during changes of ductal flow that are within the physiological range (135) and *2*) increases after the administration of agents, such as epinephrine, morphine, and CCK, that contract smooth muscle (167).

Taken at face value, the finding that CCK contracts the cystic duct as well as the gallbladder appears to be a paradox. Would not cystic duct contraction obstruct gallbladder outflow? Several possibilities militate against this apparent physiological dilemma. First, a difference in sensitivity appears to exist for the gallbladder and cystic duct contraction elicited by CCK (32). Second, an increase in cystic duct resistance during gallbladder contraction might discourage unduly rapid gallbladder emptying and thereby promote a more sustained delivery of bile into the duodenum as well as prevent abrupt common duct distension. In the latter circumstance the cystic duct might function as a brake that prevents rapid common duct distension accompanied by upper abdominal discomfort or pain.

Due to the small diameter of the cystic duct, only a thin layer of muscle is needed to generate a contractile force sufficient to narrow the duct and increase its resistance. According to Poiseuille's law, flow is proportional to the fourth power of the diameter. Therefore small changes in diameter are capable of causing major changes in resistance.

Under simulated physiological conditions, only a small pressure gradient of 1–2 $cmH_2O$ is necessary to initiate flow across the cystic duct in either direction (135). Negligible data are available, however, on pressure measurements from within the cystic duct lumen. Pressure values obtained at the junction of the cystic duct and gallbladder suggest that the canine cystic duct may generate feeble phasic contractile activity as well as a tonic resistance (167). Electromyographic recordings from the cystic duct of sheep demonstrate regular spike bursts that in some instances migrate toward the common duct (21). Manometric recordings made from the human cystic duct during laparotomy suggest the intermittent occurrence of phasic contractions (55). In prairie dogs fed a lithogenic diet, an increase in cystic duct resistance precedes the development of gallstones (141, 143).

*Common Duct*

In most mammalian species, including human, dog, and cat, the common duct has minimal smooth muscle and functions as a passive conduit that exhibits neither electrical nor contractile activity (180). The sparse longitudinal fibers in the human common duct may contribute to duct tone but do not affect bile transport. Common duct flow in humans is determined exclusively by nonductal factors, such as hepatic bile secretion, gallbladder tone, and resistance at the sphincter of Oddi. A few species, such as monkey and sheep, have sufficient common duct smooth muscle to give the potential for an ancillary role in transductal bile flow. The common duct of sheep exhibits spike activity that often propagates toward the sphincter of Oddi (21). In sheep the common duct spike bursts are coordinated with duodenal motor activity and tend to occur ~1 s before spike bursts in the duodenal bulb. This coordination of common duct and duodenal spike-burst activity in sheep might promote delivery of bile into the duodenum just before a duodenal peristaltic contraction.

In humans and most animal species, elastic connective tissue is the main constituent of the common duct wall. Common duct diameter is influenced by the rate of bile flow, intraductal pressure, and bile duct compliance. Because the normal liver may secrete ~800 ml of bile daily, the mean rate of bile flow through the common hepatic duct is roughly 30 ml/h, or 0.5 ml/min. Bile flow through the common duct, however, is not constant. Substantial physiological variations in common duct flow occur both during fasting and after a meal (82, 85). The maximal rate of common duct outflow during fasting, ~1.0 ml/min, may increase to a maximal value of ~2-3 ml/min during postprandial hepatic choleresis and gallbladder contraction. In all circumstances, however, pressure within the common duct remains within a low range of 5-10 $cmH_2O$ above duodenal pressure. In animals without a gallbladder the sphincter of Oddi musculature is rudimentary. In this circumstance bile drains freely into the duodenum, and the common duct to duodenal pressure gradient is only a few centimeters of water (69). During fasting in the opossum and dog, changes in common duct pressure are negligible (170, 196), even though variations occur in hepatic bile secretion and common duct flow (30, 170, 196). Thus common duct pressure is maintained within a narrow physiological range during intestinal MMC cycles. An elevated basal common duct pressure of >15 $cmH_2O$ in humans generally indicates increased sphincter of Oddi resistance, either functional or mechanical.

In humans and experimental animals, the increased common duct flow after a meal is accompanied by only a modest rise of a few centimeters of water in intraductal pressure or no rise at all (63, 69, 136). Intraductal pressure may even decrease during intervals of increased bile flow, if a sufficient decrease occurs in sphincter of Oddi resistance. Cholecystectomy causes either negligible change in fasting common duct pressure or a minimal increase of a few millimeters of mercury (131). With the gallbladder out, postprandial common duct pressure generally decreases 3-4 $cmH_2O$ or shows no change after the meal. After cholecystectomy, however, agents such as morphine that contract the sphincter of Oddi cause an increase in common duct pressure, whereas no change in common duct pressure occurs when the intact gallbladder acts as a reservoir (196). The sensitivity of common duct pressure to agents that contract the sphincter of Oddi has implications about the interpretation of the morphine-prostigmine test, or Nardi test, used to evaluate patients with postcholecystectomy pain syndrome.

Although the differences are generally minimal, the intraluminal pressure in the common duct is generally slightly lower than pressure in the pancreatic duct (30, 59, 136). This slight differential in intraductal pressure discourages the reflux of bile from the common duct into the pancreatic duct when an ampulla is present. In contrast, an increase in common duct ampullary pressure, such as that caused by a small calculus impacted in the distal ampulla, favors bile reflux into the pancreatic duct. This latter circumstance, described by Opie, may cause pancreatitis (89, 133).

Rapid injection of contrast medium into the common duct, such as may occur during overzealous T tube or retrograde cholangiography, commonly causes abrupt duct distension, often accompanied by acute epigastric discomfort (13, 163). Gradual distension of the common duct is frequently unaccompanied by symptoms, such as is often true in patients with painless jaundice caused by a tumor in the head of the pancreas. These observations suggest that sensory stretch receptors in the common duct accommodate to chronic duct dilation.

Sonographic studies that allow precise measurement of common duct diameter, without distortion by magnification, show that the common duct in fasting subjects normally has a diameter of 5 mm or less. Controversy exists about the effect of cholecystectomy on common duct diameter. Some workers believe that cholecystectomy may be accompanied by a modest increase in common duct diameter to 9 or 10 mm in the absence of common duct obstruction or abnormal elasticity. Others suggest that a common duct diameter of >5 mm after cholecystectomy is caused by a loss of duct elasticity due to prior dilation or by a partial obstruction (121). In cholecystectomized patients, a fatty meal normally elicits an increase in hepatic bile flow but does not increase the size of an unobstructed common duct (175). On the contrary, the common duct may decrease in size, allegedly due to a decrease in sphincter of Oddi resistance. In cholecystectomized patients with partial obstruction of the distal common duct, however, a fatty meal often induces an increase in common duct diameter (174, 175). Thus the challenge of a meal may serve as a stress test to unmask subtle partial duct obstruction.

Because the extrahepatic bile ducts are quite compliant, duct dilation can occur with only small increases in intraductal pressure. During slow distension, the viscoelastic common duct elements undergo stress relaxation (176). The normal intraductal pressure of 5-10 $cmH_2O$ above intraduodenal pressure shows a maximal increase of only 10-20 $cmH_2O$ after complete duct obstruction. Such small increases in pressure, however, are generally sufficient to cause substantial bile duct dilation. With distal common duct obstruction, ductal dilation is nearly always more pronounced in the extrahepatic than in the intrahepatic ducts, or the dilation may be limited to the common duct. This phenomenon of preferential dilation of the common duct compared with the intrahepatic ducts may be explained by two factors. First, in contrast to the intrahepatic ducts, the extrahepatic ducts are not buttressed by surrounding liver tissue. Second, consistent with Laplace's law, tension within the common duct wall is greater than that in the walls of the smaller bile ducts, because wall tension is proportional to the luminal radius. Thus for a given pressure, the force for distension is substantially greater in the larger bile ducts than in the smaller ducts. In the presence of obstruction the common duct may reach a diameter of 2 cm or larger. After complete relief of the obstruction, the elasticity of the human common duct usually returns its diameter to a normal or nearly normal size. Occasionally, however, the common duct may remain substantially dilated in the absence of partial obstruction when its elastic fibers are permanently deformed. Due to individual variations of common duct compliance, a correlation has not been found between common duct diameter and common duct pressure in cholecystectomized patients (4).

Several animal studies in the dog and monkey indicate that significant dilation of the common duct occurs within a few hours after acute experimental obstruction of the distal duct (165, 172, 219). The common duct dilation precedes any elevation of the serum bilirubin or alkaline phosphatase. After its complete obstruction, the common duct undergoes rapid dilation during the first 48 h (Fig. 16A) and may continue to dilate before it begins to reach a plateau value within ~4–14 days (145, 219). The biliary duct expands centrifugally away from the ampulla (172). Dilation of the intrahepatic ducts lags behind, and in a dog model it did not occur until 3–6 days after the onset of obstruction (145). In the experimental animal model, release of common duct obstruction is associated with a rapid decrease in common duct diameter followed by a slow decrease during a 4- to 13-wk period (145, 172). In some instances, some residual dilation of the common duct may persist [Fig. 16B; (145, 213)]. These data indicate that common duct dilation generally occurs rapidly due to high duct compliance, whereas the restoration of a dilated duct to a normal

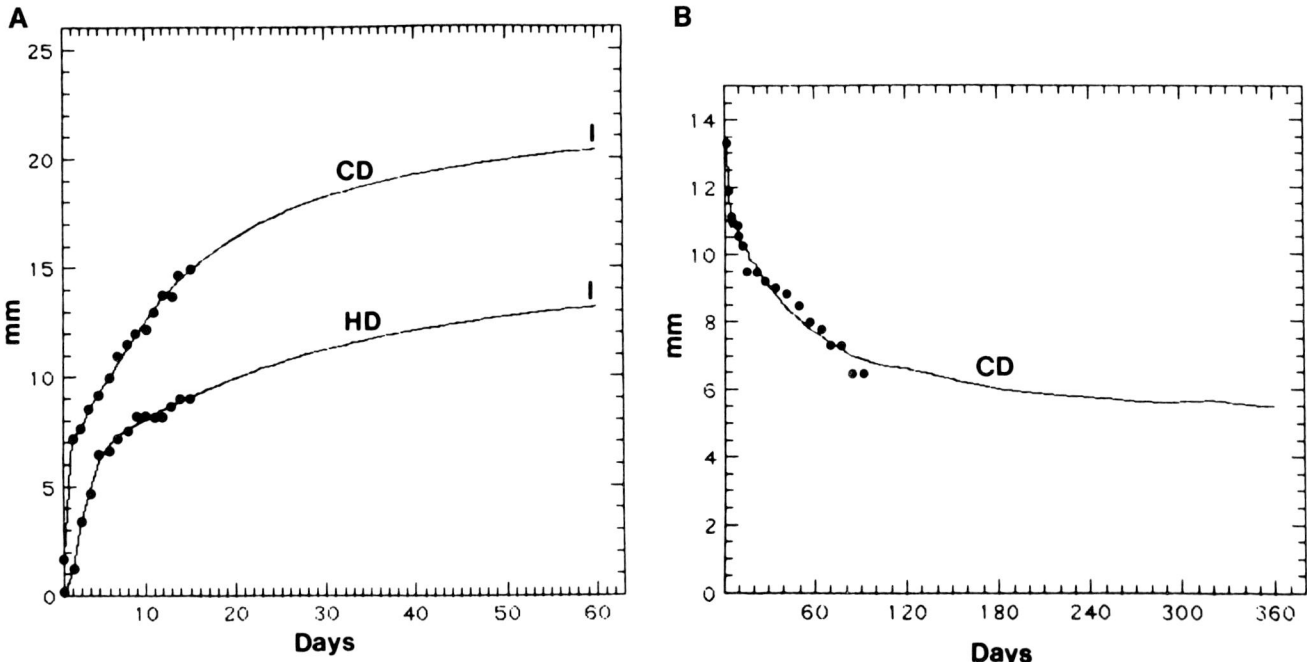

FIG. 16. Bile duct diameter in a model of distal common duct obstruction in dogs. Sonographic measurements obtained of common duct (CD) and hepatic duct (HD). *Dots* represent mean values; *solid lines* are extrapolated curves. A: duct diameter after acute obstruction. CD and HD diameter demonstrated substantial increase within 2 days followed by slower increase that continued for several weeks or longer. B: duct diameter after release of common duct obstruction that was maintained for more than 1 wk. Decrease in common duct diameter slower than rate of dilation and some residual distension remains, 6 mm vs. normal value of 2 mm. If obstruction was released in less than 1 wk, however, common duct returned to normal preobstruction diameter. [From Raptopoulos et al. (145).]

caliber generally occurs slowly or is incomplete because of reversible or nonreversible impairment of common duct elasticity.

*Sphincter of Oddi*

There are three physiological functions of the sphincter of Oddi: *1*) to regulate bile flow into the duodenum, *2*) to divert hepatic bile into the gallbladder, and *3*) to prevent reflux of duodenal contents. Although duodenal motor activity may have an ancillary role in influencing common duct emptying, most workers agree that the sphincter of Oddi functions independently of duodenal contractile or electrical activity (69, 152). The evidence to support this conclusion is fourfold. First, the embryological development of the sphincter of Oddi is entirely separate from that of the duodenal musculature (7, 19). Second, the sphincter of Oddi musculature in many species is distinct from that of the duodenum (94). Third, myoelectrical and contractile activity of the sphincter differ in character and timing from that of the duodenum (204). Last, certain pharmacological agents produce opposite effects in the sphincter and duodenum. For example, in humans, CCK generally causes duodenal contraction while the sphincter of Oddi relaxes (59).

POISEUILLE'S LAW. In a number of earlier studies, Poiseuille's law has been used as a basis for analyzing the kinetics of fluid flow across the sphincter of Oddi (104, 135, 168). For such analyses, the sphincter has been considered a steady-state, direct current (DC)-type resistor that maintains a constant resistance during short time intervals, as opposed to a variable alternating current (AC)-type resistor that undergoes rapid phasic changes in its resistance. For purposes of clarification, a discussion of Poiseuille's law is warranted here.

Poiseuille's law describes the relation between luminal pressure and fluid flow for rigid conduits. The classic equation is

$$P_1 - P_2 = P - \frac{128 \mu L \dot{Q}}{\pi D^4}$$

where $P_1$ is upstream pressure, $P_2$ is downstream pressure, $\mu$ is viscosity, L is conduit length, $\dot{Q}$ is flow, and D is diameter of the conduit.

The Poiseuille's law relationship can also be thought of as the pressure difference across the conduit being proportional to the flow

$$\Delta P \propto \dot{Q}$$

The constant of proportionality is defined as the resistance (R) to flow, wherein

$$\Delta P = R \dot{Q}$$

This latter equation may be written

$$R = \frac{\Delta P}{\dot{Q}} \text{ or } \dot{Q} = \frac{\Delta P}{R}$$

In the case of a rigid tube

$$R = \frac{128 \mu L}{\pi D^4}$$

where D is independent of flow and pressure.

Required conditions for the application of Poiseuille's law include *1*) constant resistance, *2*) laminar flow with a Reynold's number <2,000, *3*) steady flow that is time independent, *4*) constant fluid density, and *5*) negligible turbulence due to end effects. These conditions, however, are rarely met in biological systems. For the sphincter of Oddi the sphincter is not rigid, but rather its resistance varies as a function of flow as the sphincter distends. Additionally, phasic contractions cause rapid variations in sphincter resistance that are time dependent. Last, bile viscosity may vary, depending on whether hepatic bile or concentrated gallbladder bile is moving across the sphincter. In some circumstances, however, the limitations to the application of Poiseuille's law for the analysis of sphincter of Oddi kinetics may be circumvented. For example, the viscosity of common duct bile may be constant during given time intervals. The problem of flow through a nonrigid conduit can be solved by assuming Poiseuille's law holds over some infinitely small length (dx) and pressure change (dP) in a viscoelastic conduit. This assumption yields a differential form of Poiseuille's law, the solution of which indicates that resistance is a power function of flow rate. Application of this type of analysis to the terminal narrowing, or nozzle, of the opossum sphincter of Oddi segment yields predicted values of resistance that correspond closely to the resistance values calculated from experimental data (91).

HUMANS. With the exception of cineradiography, most studies of sphincter of Oddi function in humans have measured resistance across the sphincter, i.e., flow or pressure, rather than measuring activity from the sphincter itself. This circumstance has been prompted by the fact that the human sphincter of Oddi is located largely within the duodenal wall and was generally inaccessible for direct instrumentation. Probably for these reasons the sphincter of Oddi was regarded traditionally solely as a resistor, with a passive component and an active component, that could undergo gradual changes in tone during intervals of minutes to hours. Such changes in tone were believed to regulate bile flow during fasting and after meals (69). However, potential regional variations in sphincter function were ignored, phasic sphincter activity was neglected, and the internal details within the black box of sphincter of Oddi function remained largely unknown.

The recent development of sphincter of Oddi manometry, performed in conjunction with ERCP examination, now allows direct nonsurgical instrumentation of the sphincter in relatively large numbers of subjects. In patients judged to be normal, pull-throughs across the sphincter segment gave a pressure gradient of common duct to duodenum that averaged 12 mmHg and a mean gradient of pancreatic duct to duodenum averaging 15 mmHg (59). These values may have been inflated slightly by the presence of the catheter across the sphincter. Although a trend existed for slightly higher pressure in the pancreatic duct, there was no difference statistically (59). Duodenal pressure averaged ~6 mmHg. Some workers suggest that resting pressure in the pancreatic duct is substantially greater than that in the common duct (25, 35), but the probability exists that pressure in the pancreatic duct was increased artifactually by a catheter infusion rate that was too rapid for the small dimensions of the pancreatic duct.

Pull-throughs at 1- to 2-mm increments demonstrate an identifiable sphincter of Oddi segment that measures ~6 mm long on manometry (see Fig. 7). The specific value given to the base-line sphincter pressure depends on the zero reference. For example, a basal pressure 5 mmHg above that in the common duct might be 15 mmHg above intraduodenal pressure and 25 mmHg above atmospheric pressure. Lack of a standardized zero reference has led to some confusion, but a consensus is emerging to use duodenal pressure as the zero reference. Nevertheless sufficient information should be provided to allow all three assessments.

In a group of subjects judged to be normal, basal pressure within the sphincter segment averaged ~4 mm above the pressure in the common duct (59). This basal sphincter pressure may be partially artifactual, caused by the 1.7-mm catheter stuffing the small sphincter lumen. In some subjects, basal sphincter pressure is isobaric with common duct pressure. During manometry, basal sphincter pressure may remain uniform during a 10- to 15-min interval of continuous monitoring or show slow fluctuations of a few millimeters of mercury. We have never observed abrupt, transient relaxations of basal sphincter of Oddi pressure comparable to the transient relaxations that occur in the lower esophageal sphincter. The fact that agents such as glucagon or atropine cause partial relaxation of the basal sphincter pressure suggests that part of this basal pressure is generated by active contraction of smooth muscle. Findings from sphincter manometry have not identified discrete high-pressure zones at the sphincter margins to correspond with the anatomical choledochal and ampullary sphincters described by Boyden (18).

The most striking feature of manometric tracings from the human sphincter of Oddi is prominent phasic pressure waves that are recorded along the length of the sphincter segment (25, 35, 59). Surprisingly, these phasic pressure waves were not mentioned on the initial reports of direct sphincter of Oddi manometry (126, 147), albeit phasic sphincter contractions had been noted earlier on cineradiographic and electromyographic studies. Possibly the phasic contractions went unobserved on the initial manometric studies because the investigators were not anticipating such contractions or the recordings were greatly dampened by a compliant manometric system. In any case subsequent manometric studies demonstrated rhythmic, phasic contractions along the sphincter of Oddi segment that occurred at an average frequency of ~4/min. These phasic pressure waves were superimposed on a base-line sphincter pressure that was slightly greater than or equal to common duct pressure. The phasic pressure complexes within the sphincter have a peak amplitude that averages ~130 mmHg and a wave duration of ~4–5 s (59). Nonrespiratory phasic waves were not recorded from the common duct. Subsequent studies using three manometric recording orifices, spaced at 2-mm intervals (205), showed that in control subjects an average of 60% of the phasic pressure waves propagated in peristaltic fashion toward the duodenum (Fig. 17). Approximately 14% of the waves propagated retrograde toward the common duct, and 26% were simultaneous.

Limited data are available on electromyography of the human sphincter of Oddi. In the late 1960s, Ono et al. (132) sutured electrodes into the sphincter and duodenal musculature during laparotomy that was done for other reasons. Recordings after surgery showed rhythmic sphincter spike bursts that were independent of duodenal myoelectric activity. Fluid flow through an indwelling T tube was interrupted concurrent with the sphincter spike bursts. In a more recent study, sphincter of Oddi myoelectric activity was recorded in a few subjects by catheter ring electrodes positioned within the sphincter during retrograde ERCP examination (156). The findings reconfirmed that sphincter spike bursts occurred independent of those in the duodenum. Most electromyographic studies of the sphincter of Oddi have been done in experimental animals, particularly in the rabbit and opossum. A consensus exists that fluid flow through the common duct stops concurrent with each phasic sphincter contraction (8, 132, 204). This observation has caused controversy as to whether the phasic sphincter activity enhances or retards common duct emptying.

Cineradiographic studies show that phasic sphincter of Oddi contractions occur at a rate of ~3–5/min when bile duct pressure is kept within the physiological range (73). Virtually all such studies were done on patients with indwelling T tubes that allowed the introduction of contrast medium into the common duct. Rhythmic sphincter of Oddi contractions were observed to result in intervals of sphincter closure and

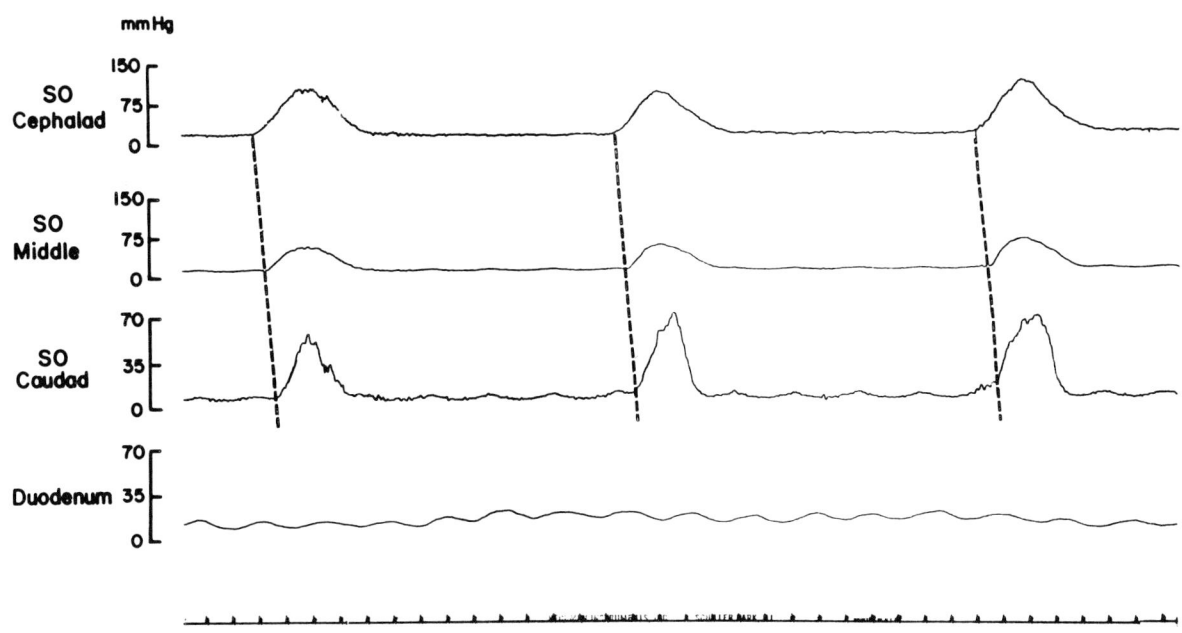

FIG. 17. Multilumen manometric recording from human sphincter of Oddi (SO). Three recording sites spaced at 2-mm intervals located in sphincter, with fourth recording site in duodenum. Three spontaneous peristaltic contraction waves occur that migrate antegrade toward duodenum and traverse entire sphincter segment. Normally ~60% of phasic sphincter contractions migrate antegrade, whereas remainder either migrate retrograde or occur simultaneously at all sites. [From Toouli et al. (205). Reprinted with permission of The American Gastroenterological Association, copyright 1982.]

opening likened to systole and diastole. Caroli et al. (24) called these movements "the dance of the papilla." They categorized sphincter of Oddi phasic contractions into three types: 1) pyloric—the contraction moves caudad and expels ampullary contents into the duodenum; 2) global—simultaneous contraction with parallel edges; and 3) antiperistaltic—the contraction wave moves cephalad. The third was the most frequent type observed. Possibly the prevalence of the different types of contractions might be influenced by the presence of a T tube or the fact that most of the patients had their common duct explorations for stones (205).

Hess (73) obtained cineradiographic recordings concurrent with measurements of common duct pressure and flow of contrast medium into the common duct. His observations were as follows. During sphincter diastole, the upper part of the choledochal sphincter opens from above downward and contrast medium enters the ampulla, or in its absence, the infundibulum. An apparent choledochal sphincter then contracts from above downward, thereby isolating a small portion of contrast medium in the ampulla while the distal sphincter is still closed. Then suddenly the distal sphincter (sphincter ampullae) opens and the systolic volume (~0.5 ml) falls into the duodenum during the opening phase of the distal sphincter. Thereafter, the whole sphincter of Oddi segment contracts again, this time from below upward in an antiperistaltic movement. When this latter contraction is complete, contrast medium is no longer seen in the sphincter segment, and the contracted muscle may produce a convex contour to the distal common duct. This interval is called the closing phase.

These important observations of Hess suggest that a pattern of alternating antegrade and retrograde peristaltic phasic contractions might be expected on sphincter manometry. In our experience, however, this is not the case. The sequences have many variations, often with multiple consecutive antegrade contractions. During ERCP examination we have obtained videotape recordings after retrograde injection of contrast medium into the common duct and withdrawal of the catheter. Our observations are as follows. Phasic contractions in the human sphincter of Oddi propagate antegrade as well as retrograde, or they occur as a simultaneous contraction of the entire sphincter segment. Antegrade contractions start at the proximal sphincter margin. They may propagate incompletely and empty the sphincter partially or traverse the entire sphincter segment and actively sweep all of its contents into the duodenum. Simultaneous sphincter contractions propel its luminal contents either in both directions or mainly retrograde. During some intervals the sphincter segment remains open and contrast medium flows passively into the duodenum. We have not observed convincing evidence of discrete minisphincters at the sphincter margins. However, an incomplete peristaltic sequence in the proximal sphincter segment might be construed as a sphincter choledochus, but this issue is mostly semantic. Manometry has not shown discrete high pressure zones at the sphincter margins. Such zones, however, could be missed because of the short length of the human sphincter segment and perhaps slight axial movement of the sphincter relative to the manometric catheter. Our attempts to obtain good concurrent cine and manometric recordings of sphincter contractions have been unsuccessful because the indwelling catheter obscures imaging of the sphincter lumen.

Cineradiography has been especially informative when combined with concurrent measurements of common duct pressure and flow (13, 157, 163). The opening pressure, or passage pressure, needed to initiate common duct outflow is normally 15 cmH$_2$O or less above atmospheric pressure, i.e., 5–10 cmH$_2$O above intraduodenal pressure. The term *opening pressure* may be somewhat misleading because a low rate of common duct outflow may already exist at the inception of testing. The rate of phasic sphincter contractions, ~3–5/min at physiological duct pressures of 10–12 cmH$_2$O, increases as perfusion pressure and thus flow is increased (73). At excessive ductal pressures of 40–50 cmH$_2$O, sphincter contractions decrease or stop. In this latter circumstance the paralyzed sphincter remains wide open. Transsphincteric flow is then entirely passive, determined solely by the diameter of the sphincter lumen and the fluid pressure head. At common duct flows in the physiological range of >5 ml/min, the rate of phasic sphincter contractions increases linearly with increases in flow, while common duct pressure remains unchanged (73). In the past some studies of sphincter physiology have given misleading results because data were obtained at nonphysiological levels of duct pressure and flow. However, testing with unphysiological levels of common duct flow of up to 20 ml/min may be useful for diagnostic purposes. Whereas substantial nonphysiological increases in common duct flow cause only moderate increases in intraductal pressure when the sphincter of Oddi accommodates normally, intraductal pressure soars in the presence of partial sphincter obstruction (74).

Several informative cine studies have shown that common duct diameter is directly related to intraluminal pressure (13, 163). In some instances common duct diameter during intraductal hypertension of 40–50 cmH$_2$O increased as much as 2.4 times the diameter at passage pressure (163). Patients often experienced vague epigastric fullness or discomfort when the common duct pressure was increased 5–10 cmH$_2$O above passage pressure, and they invariably had upper abdominal pain when duct pressure was increased to 25–50 cmH$_2$O (13). At nonphysiological pressures in the range of 6–35 cmH$_2$O above passage pressure, pancreatic duct reflux is observed in 12%–45% of patients (13, 163). Pancreatic duct reflux occurs during sphincter opening (diastole) in patients with an ampulla. Thus determinant factors of pancreatic duct reflux are sphincter anatomy and elevated common duct pressure.

The control mechanisms that regulate contractile activity of the human sphincter of Oddi remain to be clarified. Early in this century the reciprocal sphincter of Oddi relaxation that occurred during postprandial gallbladder contraction was attributed to contrary autonomic innervation (117). Subsequently the reciprocal relationship of gallbladder contraction and sphincter of Oddi relaxation was explained on a hormonal basis, i.e., the effect of CCK released after eating. The prevalent notion at present is that hormones are the main mechanism that controls sphincter of Oddi function. The probability exists, however, that the nerves also have an important regulatory function. As reviewed elsewhere (152), parasympathomimetic drugs and vagal stimulation cause atropine-sensitive sphincter contractions. In some instances vagal stimulation decreases sphincter contraction. Generally, vagotomy seems to have a negligible effect, albeit some workers report a decrease in sphincter tone. Some workers report that sympathetic stimulation causes sphincter contractions, whereas others have observed relaxation (152). Tests using pharmacological agents and nerve stimulation show that nonadrenergic inhibitory nerves are present in the cat sphincter of Oddi, opossum, and guinea pig (139, 203). To what extent neural influences govern sphincter of Oddi function remains to be determined.

As an alternative to contraction of smooth muscle, an entirely different control mechanism for regulating common duct outflow has been suggested by Tansy and co-workers (199). These investigators propose that changes in vascular engorgement of the sphincter of Oddi mucosa cause substantial changes in luminal resistance and are the major mechanism that regulates flow across the sphincter segment. The mucosa that lines the distal sphincter segment in most species, including humans, is thrown into a spongelike network of folds that seem well suited for modifying transsphincteric flow. These mucosal folds have a supplementary role in regulating transsphincteric flow but cannot account for the high-amplitude, phasic sphincter contractions or the changes in tone caused by certain pharmacological agents.

ANIMALS. In the past, animal models have been useful to study the pressure-flow kinetics of fluid flow across the sphincter of Oddi. Traditionally the dog has been used as the main experimental model, with some studies in the cat, pig, rabbit, guinea pig, and prairie dog, as well as other animal species. During the past decade the opossum has emerged as a useful model for assessing the kinetics of sphincter of Oddi motor activity and transsphincteric movement of fluid. The opossum sphincter of Oddi is useful for these purposes because *1*) its extraduodenal location allows recordings without interference from duodenal motor activity, and *2*) it exhibits spontaneous, rhythmic contractions that are similar in rate and force to those recorded from the human sphincter of Oddi. In these respects the opossum model is exploited for its virtues rather than its limitations. Clearly, however, the opossum sphincter of Oddi differs substantially from that of humans, not only in its longer length but also in its different responses to some hormones, such as CCK, and certain drugs. Nevertheless in this subsection we discuss the opossum sphincter of Oddi at some length because its pressure-flow kinetics have been studied in greater detail than in other laboratory animals, and some extrapolations seem to apply to the human sphincter.

On pull-through manometry, the opossum sphincter of Oddi measures ~3–4 cm in length and has a short high-pressure zone in the terminal 4–5 mm of the sphincter segment (Fig. 18). Proximal to the short high-pressure zone, base-line pressure within the ampulla of the sphincter segment is isobaric with that of the common duct. Convincing evidence was not found to document the presence of functional choledochal or pancreatic sphincters. The terminal high-pressure zone, or sphincter ampullae, had a mean basal pressure of ~20 mmHg and did not exhibit any transit relaxations. Pharmacological testing showed that this high-pressure zone was mostly passive but had a small active component as well. A more recent study of the terminal high-pressure zone, or nozzle, confirms that it acts mainly as a passive, DC-type resistor with viscoelastic properties (91). The opening pressure ranges from 10 to 14 mmHg, whereas closing pressure is a few millimeters of mercury lower.

Prominent phasic pressure complexes were recorded along the length of the sphincter segment, including its terminal high-pressure zone. In anesthetized animals the phasic contractions occurred at the rate of ~3–4/min, and their rate was increased by distension of the sphincter with a balloon or an increase in transsphincteric flow (204). As in the opossum, phasic contractions in the human sphincter of Oddi also persist during anesthesia (55, 134). In opossums the sphincter contractions were maximal in the distal half of the sphincter segment, with amplitudes as high as 200 mmHg. The phasic contraction waves had an average duration of 4–5 s. Contractile activity was not present in the common duct. Studies using multiple recording sites showed that the phasic contractions always started at the proximal sphincter margin and propagated in peristaltic fashion toward the duodenum. Approximately 90% of the peristaltic sequences traversed the entire sphincter segment. Concurrent electromyographic and manometric recordings showed that a spike burst of electrical depolarization immediately preceded the upstroke onset of the peristaltic pressure wave (Fig. 19). In many instances a short ramp or small plateau of low pressure preceded the major upstroke of the peristaltic pressure wave. Direct observations of the opossum sphincter of Oddi at laparotomy indicates that the phasic sphincter contractions sweep small amounts of bile into the duodenum (42).

In studies in vitro the nerve toxin tetrodotoxin did not abolish the phasic pressure waves or electrical spike bursts of the sphincter of Oddi in the opossum or cat (10, 204). The same result was obtained when the sphincter segment was isolated in an in vitro

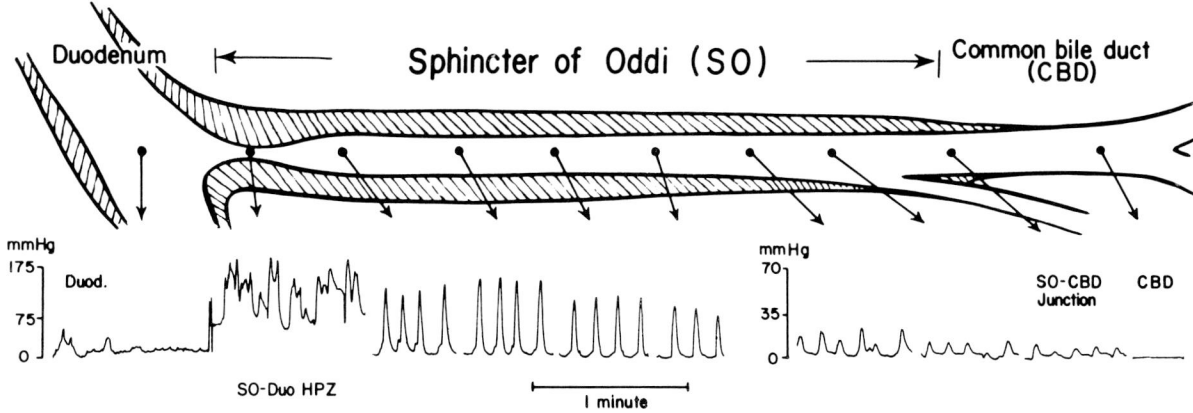

FIG. 18. Station pull-through across opossum sphincter of Oddi (SO). *Sample tracings* shown for sites indicated by *dots*. High-pressure zone (HPZ) seen only in distal SO segment. This HPZ did not exhibit transient relaxations to common duct pressure. Phasic pressure waves occurred along entire sphincter segment but not in common bile duct (CBD). Phasic pressure waves of maximal amplitude occurred in distal half of sphincter. Wave amplitude decreases progressively toward proximal sphincter margin. Contraction waves not recorded in common duct. [From Toouli et al. (204).]

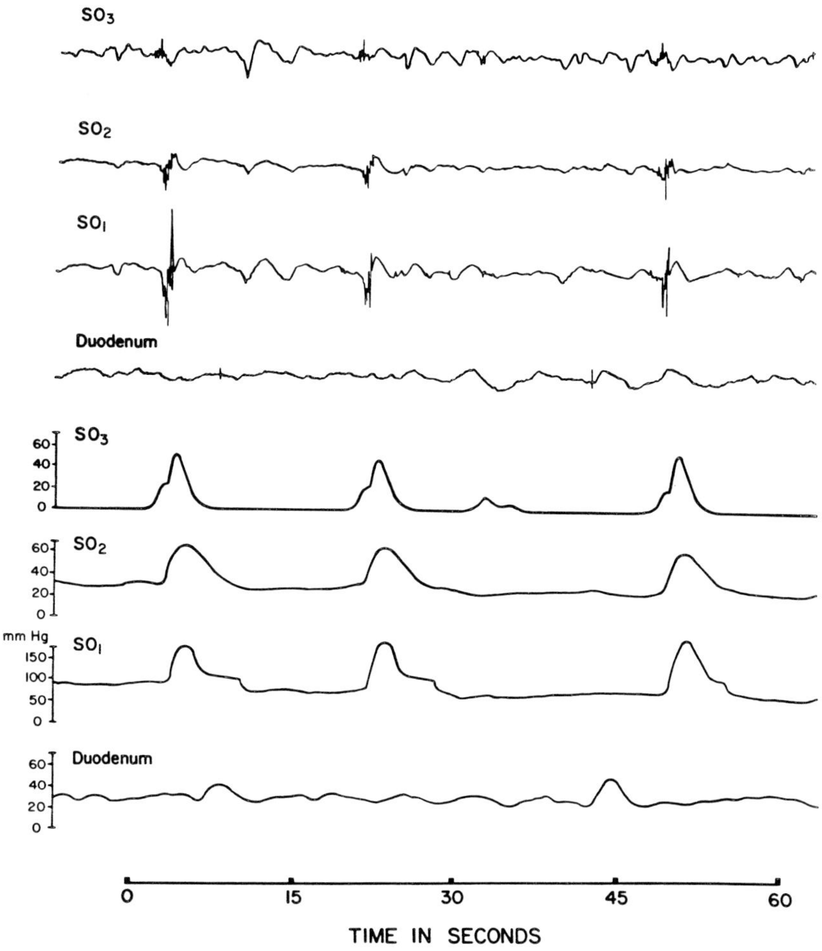

FIG. 19. Concurrent recording of electrical and manometric activity from opossum sphincter of Oddi (SO) and duodenum. Manometric catheter with three orifices spaced at 5-mm intervals was positioned in sphincter so that each recording orifice was at same level as bipolar electrode. Site $SO_3$ located in proximal sphincter. Electrical spike burst occurs at each site immediately before upstroke onset of peristaltic manometric pressure wave. In sequence shown, one of contractions at $SO_3$ does not traverse entire sphincter.

muscle bath (72). These findings indicate that the rhythmic sphincter contractions are myogenic in origin, albeit autonomic nerves, enteric hormones, or both may modulate the rate of sphincter contraction.

After the administration of tetrodotoxin, the phasic pressure waves and underlying spike bursts continue to originate the proximal part of the opossum sphincter of Oddi (72, 204). This observation suggests the presence of a pacemaker in the proximal portion of the sphincter segment. Results from a recent in vitro study provide information about the organization of phasic contractile and electrical activity of the sphincter of Oddi segment. In the study, sphincter specimens were mounted in an organ bath so that regional mechanical and electrical activity were recorded concurrently from four points along the sphincter length (72). In most instances the phasic contractile activity originated in the proximal sphincter and traversed the entire sphincter as a peristaltic sequence (Fig. 20). In some cases caudad propagation of the contractions was incomplete. In about half of the specimens, some phasic contractions originated in the distal part of the sphincter segment and propagated retrograde. Retrograde peristalsis occurred only when antegrade peristalsis failed to traverse the entire sphincter. In vivo, retrograde sphincter contractions rarely occur in the opossum (204) but occur commonly in humans (205).

Muscle rings, sectioned from the sphincter of Oddi segment, exhibited phasic contractions with a proximal-to-distal gradient of inherent contraction rate (Fig. 21). Each contraction was associated with an underlying myoelectric complex. These findings suggest that the pattern of phasic contractile activity in the opossum sphincter of Oddi may be modeled as a linear array of bidirectionally coupled relaxation oscillators. The predominance of antegrade peristalsis in the intact specimens may be explained by a high-frequency oscillator in the proximal sphincter that drives the slower, more distal oscillators. Complete coupling of the regional oscillators yields an antegrade peristaltic sequence that traverses the entire sphincter segment. Retrograde peristalsis may be initiated by an ectopic oscillator in the distal sphincter when antegrade peristalsis fails to propagate the entire sphincter length. In this circumstance ectopic contractions can propagate retrograde when the more-proximal oscillators are not in their absolute refractory period.

The mechanism that controls changes in the rate of

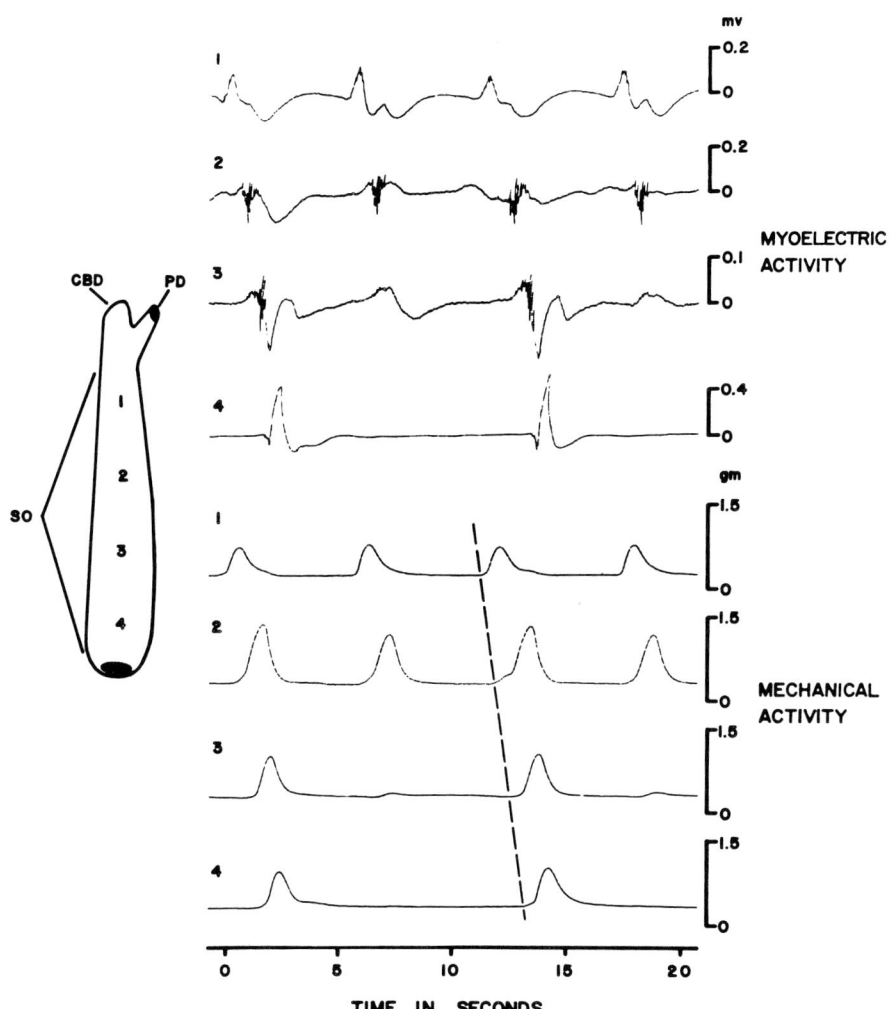

FIG. 20. Myoelectric and contractile activity recorded concurrently from intact sphincter of Oddi (SO) segment in vitro. At regular intervals, phasic contractions originate in proximal SO and propagate antegrade toward duodenum, indicated by *dashed line.* Each phasic contraction was associated with electrical control complex. When control-wave propagation was incomplete, as occurred in alternate sequences, propagation of phasic contraction was incomplete. CBD, common bile duct; PD, papillary duct. [From Helm et al. (72).]

phasic sphincter of Oddi contractions appears to be fundamentally different from the well-established mechanism that determines the rate of phasic contractions in the upper gastrointestinal tract. In the stomach and small bowel, electrical control waves, or slow waves, occur at a constant rate characteristic for a given region in a given species. When the control wave activity is modulated by neurotransmitters or enteric hormones to reach a threshold depolarization, electrical response activity, or spikes, occur that are accompanied by a mechanical contraction. Thus the control waves have a constant rate, but variations in the rate of phasic contractions are determined by the modulation of electromechanical coupling. In contrast, initial evidence suggests that the rate of phasic contractions in the opossum sphincter of Oddi is determined by changes in the rate of a myoelectrical control complex rather than a variation in electromechanical coupling. On extracellular recordings the electrical control complex appears as a triphasic wave that generally exhibits superimposed spikes. Complete coupling exists between the sphincter myoelectrical complex and phasic contractions. Thus changes in the rate of phasic sphincter of Oddi contractions reflect changes in the rate of the underlying electrical control complexes. This activity is generated by an inherent property of sphincter smooth muscle but is undoubtedly modulated in vivo by neurotransmitters, enteric hormones, or both.

In contrast to the observations on the opossum sphincter of Oddi, indirect evidence suggests that the rate of phasic contractions in the canine sphincter may be determined by variable electromechanical coupling to electrical control waves that have a regular frequency of ~18–20/min. This later suggestion is based on the observation (57) that the interval between phasic contractions of the canine sphincter of Oddi has a basic mode of ~3.5 s.

To assess sphincter of Oddi kinetics, cineradiographic sequences were obtained while a drop counter monitored the flow of contrast medium into the common duct, and sphincter contractile activity was re-

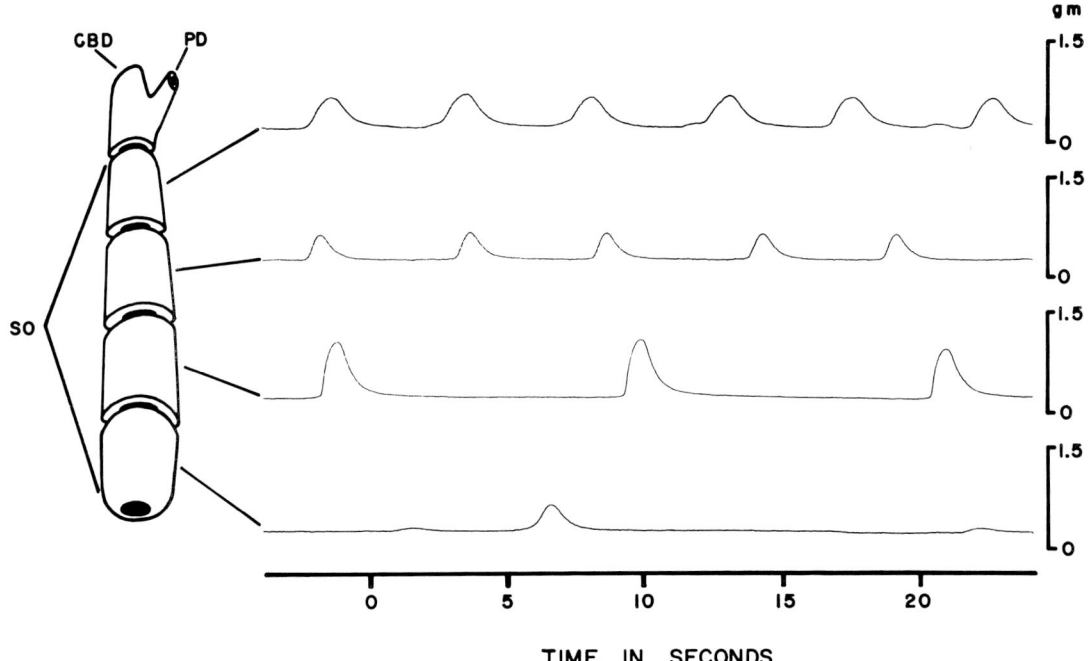

FIG. 21. Contractile activity recorded from muscle rings sectioned from sphincter of Oddi (SO). Rings contract spontaneously at random with respect to one another. Proximal-to-distal gradient of inherent contraction frequencies is evident. CBD, common bile duct; PD, papillary duct. [From Helm et al. (72).]

corded by concurrent intraluminal manometry and electromyography (204). By varying the height of the reservoir of contrast medium, common duct flow was varied from 0.01 to 0.3 ml/min, values that bracket the physiological range in the opossum. Cystic duct ligation simplified the model.

The cineradiographic sequences invariably showed spontaneous, rhythmic peristaltic contractions that started at the proximal margin of the sphincter and generally propagated over its entire length. These peristaltic contractions stripped all of the contrast medium within the sphincter segment into the duodenum. During sphincter peristalsis and emptying, a narrowed nozzlelike segment, 4–5 mm long and 0.5–0.7 mm wide, was observed at the terminus of the sphincter segment. This narrowed segment corresponded to the short high-pressure zone recorded on manometry. The transverse diameter of the distended sphincter segment above the terminal narrowing as well as that of the common duct was ~1.5 mm. During sphincter of Oddi peristalsis, the stroke volume during a complete peristaltic sequence varied from 0 to 0.05 ml, depending on the degree of filling at the onset of peristalsis. When peristalsis was incomplete, only a portion of the sphincter contents was emptied into the duodenum. Retrograde waves were not observed.

Analysis showed a precise correlation between the peristaltic waves imaged on cineradiography, the spike bursts recorded by electromyography, and the pressure recorded on manometry (Fig. 22). During peristalsis, passage of the inverted V-shaped tail of contrast medium by a given sphincter level was coincident with the electrical spike burst and the onset of the manometric pressure wave recorded at that level. Just ahead of the peristaltic wave, pressure within the contrast medium commonly ramped up to 10–20 mmHg as the contraction wave pushed the bolus of contrast through the zone of terminal narrowing. This ramp pressure exceeded the pressure needed to open the narrow nozzle segment. The analysis indicated that reliable, reproducible cross correlations exist between the manifestations of sphincter peristalsis as recorded by the three different modalities of cineradiography, electromyography, and intraluminal manometry. Once the cross correlations are known, the recording of peristalsis by any one of the recording modalities allows an accurate prediction of the findings from the two other types of recording.

Common duct flow occurred entirely as a passive process. During sphincter peristalsis the outflow and inflow of contrast medium into or out of the common duct ceased momentarily for ~6 s (Fig. 23). The 6-s interval is accounted for by the occlusion of the sphincter during the 2 s required for the peristaltic sequence to sweep the sphincter segment plus the 4-s duration of the peristaltic contraction wave. On initial consideration the observation that sphincter peristalsis prevents common duct emptying seems paradoxi-

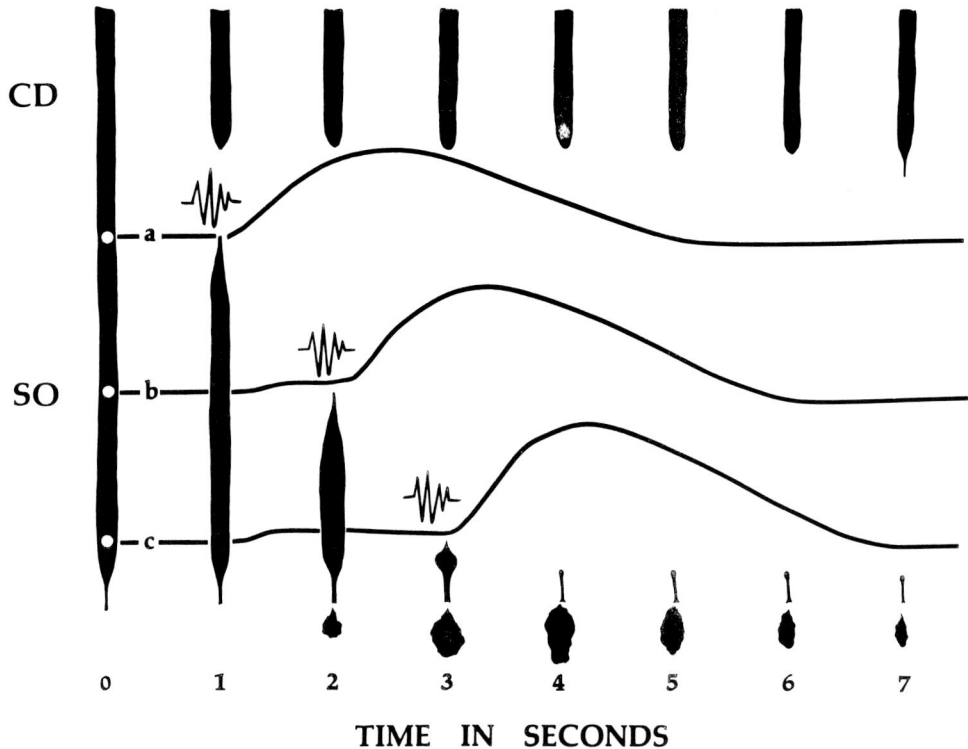

FIG. 22. Relation between sphincter of Oddi (SO) peristaltic sequence recorded by cineradiography, electromyography, and intraluminal manometry. At given sphincter level, spike burst occurs just prior to upstroke onset of peristaltic pressure wave. Onset of contraction pinches off bolus, thereby giving its tail an inverted-V configuration. Passage of tail by a given site corresponds to upstroke of pressure wave. Pressure within bolus, ahead of major manometric pressure complex, ramps up slightly until pressure is reached that overcomes resistance of narrow nozzle. Contrast medium is then pushed into duodenum. Each peristaltic sequence in sphincter interrupts passive bile duct emptying for an interval of ~6 s. CD, common duct.

cal. The temptation exists to conclude that the function of phasic sphincter contractions is to restrain sphincter outflow. To obtain a better understanding of this phenomenon, however, it is useful to consider an analogy with the cardiac cycle. Ventricular systole is the major determinant of cardiac output. During cardiac systole, however, flow of atrial blood into the ventricles stops because intraventricular pressure becomes greater than intra-atrial pressure. Nevertheless we would not conclude that the function of ventricular systole is to obstruct atrial outflow, albeit obstruction of atrial outflow does indeed occur. Considered from a different perspective, cardiac systole empties the ventricles and thereby enables ventricular filling by atrial outflow during ventricular diastole. A similar situation seems to exist for the sphincter of Oddi when the phasic contractions propagate antegrade toward the duodenum. During sphincter peristalsis, passive common duct outflow is arrested because of the high pressure of the sphincter contraction. However, antegrade sphincter peristalsis actively empties the sphincter segment, rendering it empty for passive filling during the ensuing diastole. In the opossum the physiological rates of common duct outflow and sphincter peristalsis are such that virtually all sphincter emptying occurs by active peristalsis. However, when common duct flow is rapid or the interval between peristalsis is long, some sphincter outflow may occur by passive outflow. Passive sphincter outflow is created experimentally when sphincter contractions are abolished by amyl nitrite. Thus sphincter outflow may be active or passive, whereas in the absence of gallbladder contraction, common duct outflow is always passive. In the opossum, modest physiological increases in the rate of sphincter contractions enhance sphincter emptying and therefore enhance bile duct emptying. This circumstance is comparable to the physiological tachycardia that increases cardiac output during exercise. However, overstimulation of the sphincter that results in contraction rates $\leq 10$/min encroaches on sphincter diastole and may prevent its filling. Such a circumstance arrests the flow of bile into the duodenum. An analogous situation exists for the heart when ventricular tachycardia shortens ventricular diastole sufficiently to compromise atrial emptying and thereby cause reduced or absent cardiac output.

Electrodes implanted within the musculature of the

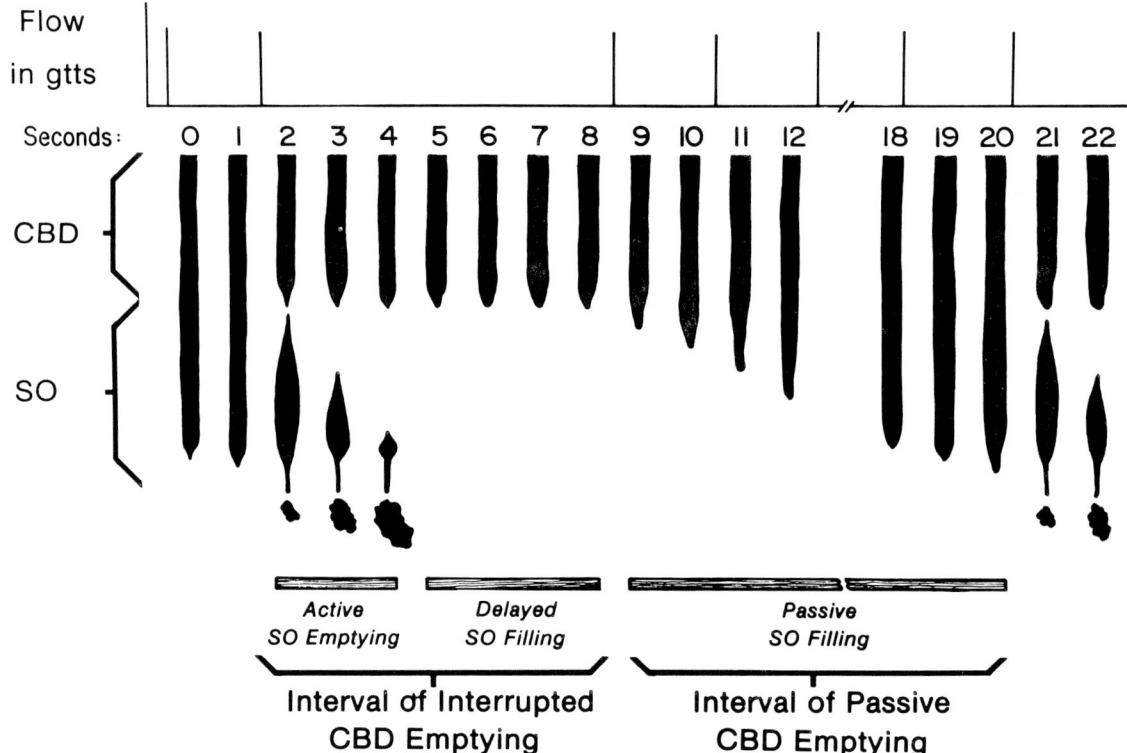

FIG. 23. Bile duct emptying drawn from images of cineradiographic recording. Catheter positioned in proximal common bile duct (CBD) for infusing contrast not shown. Time in seconds given above images of contrast material. In this example, contrast medium flowed into CBD at rate of ~6 drops/min (0.1 ml/min) from reservoir. Before sphincter of Oddi (SO) peristalsis, contrast flowed into CBD, which then emptied passively into SO segment. Drops (gtts) indicate CBD outflow as well as CBD inflow. During 2-s interval, SO peristalsis actively expelled contrast from SO segment into duodenum. Zone of narrowing observed in distal SO segment. During passage of SO contraction wave, SO segment was pinched off from CBD, thereby interrupting passive CBD outflow into SO segment. After SO emptying, short 4-s interval of delayed SO filling persisted until SO contraction was complete. When pressure in SO segment returned to initial value after peristalsis, fluid flow from CBD into SO recommenced, leading to passive SO filling during SO diastole. Cycle repeated itself with onset of next SO peristaltic contraction. [From Toouli et al. (204).]

opossum sphincter of Oddi and upper gastrointestinal tract allow investigation of the relationship of biliary tract and gastrointestinal function in awake chronic animals (Fig. 24). Repeated recordings may be obtained for 8-h intervals or longer. Such studies show a cyclic pattern in the rate of sphincter spike bursts, with a cycle length of 90 min (79). The minimum rate, ~2/min, gradually increases to reach a maximum rate of ~6/min. Each sphincter spike burst represents a peristaltic sequence. The minimum rate of sphincter spike bursts occurs concurrent with the quiescent period of phase I of the duodenal MMC activity (see Fig. 15). During phase II of duodenal MMC activity, the rate of sphincter spike bursts increases gradually and culminates in a 5-min interval of maximal activity concurrent with passage of the phase III activity through the duodenum. Findings in a more recent study in dogs (170) indicate that the canine sphincter of Oddi, similar to that of the opossum, exhibits cyclical changes in its rate of phasic contractions synchronous with the duodenal MMC cycle. During phase I, the mean contraction rate averaged 12/min. This value increased to 15/min during phase II and 22/min during phase III. In the dog, however, the rates of sphincter contractions were about fivefold greater than those of the opossum, and the interval of sphincter diastole was very short, ~2 s. The rate of bile flow across the sphincter was greater during phase II of the duodenal MMC cycle than during phases I or III. However, the specific pressure-flow kinetics of bile flow within the canine sphincter of Oddi segment remain to be evaluated. Variability in sphincter of Oddi contraction rate during fasting has also been shown in the prairie dog (154).

With feeding, the rate of sphincter spike bursts in the opossum increases during a 20-min interval to reach a plateau of ~5 or 6 spike bursts/min that lasts for a minimum of 3 h after a full meal (Fig. 25). Thus

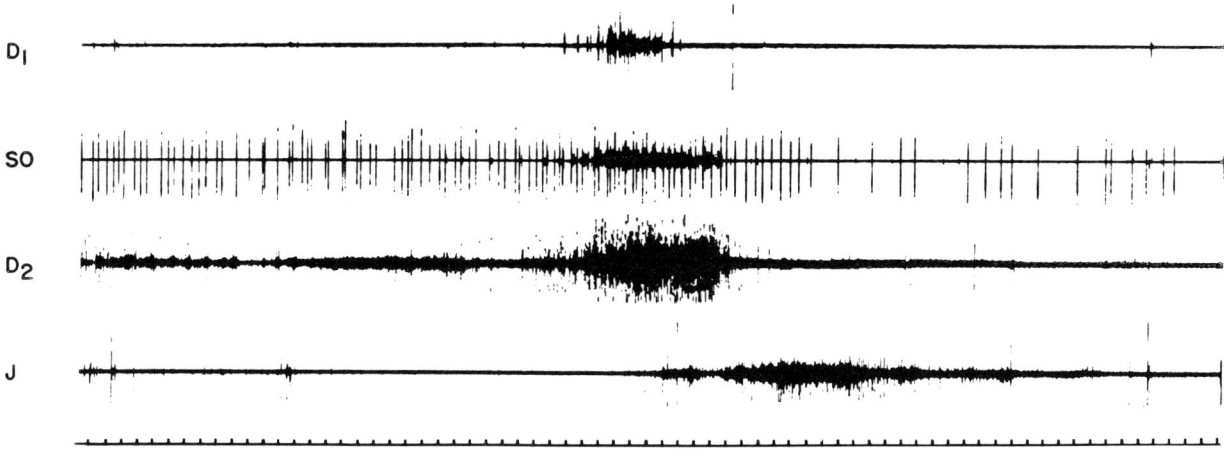

FIG. 24. Myoelectrical spike-burst activity in sphincter of Oddi and gastrointestinal tract of fasted awake opossum. Electrodes positioned on duodenum (sites $D_1$ and $D_2$), sphincter of Oddi (SO), and jejunum (J). Phase III activity of migrating myoelectrical complex (MMC) passes from duodenum to jejunum. Spike-burst activity of sphincter of Oddi is continuous but intensifies and reaches maximal rate concurrent with passage of phase III MMC activity front through duodenum.

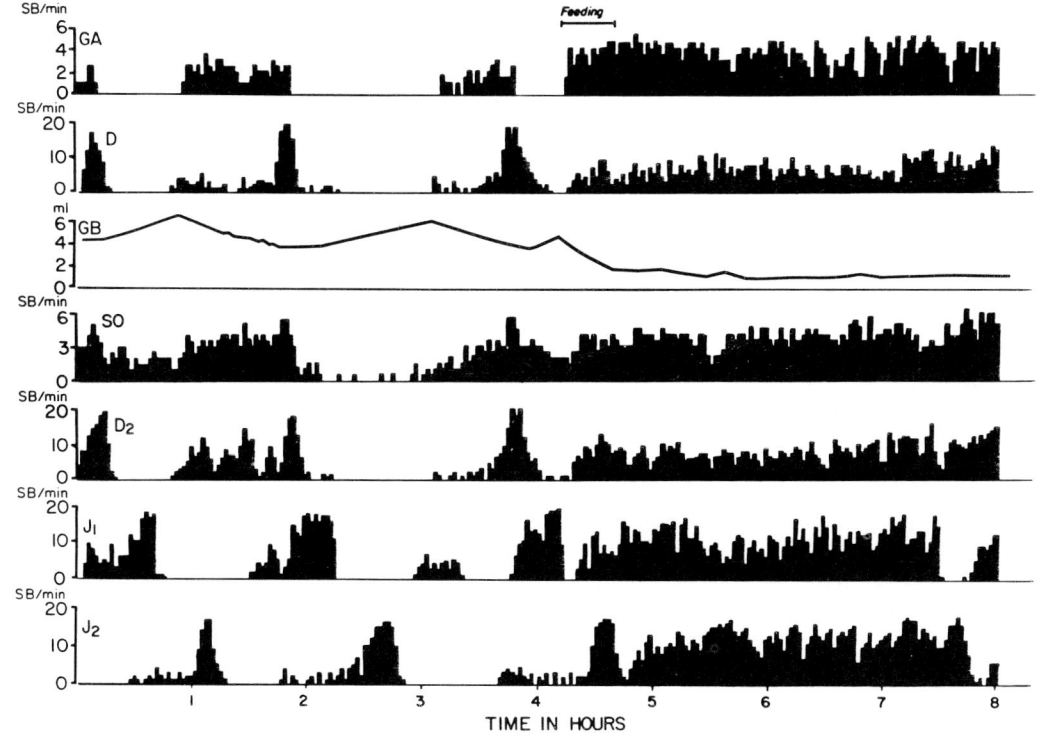

FIG. 25. Effect of feeding on sphincter of Oddi contractile activity and gallbladder volume. Concurrent electrical recordings (spike bursts (SB)/min) obtained from gastric antrum (GA), duodenum (sites $D_1$ and $D_2$), sphincter of Oddi (SO), proximal jejunum ($J_1$), and distal jejunum ($J_2$). Animal was fed after two spontaneous cycles of migratory myoelectric complex during fasting. Feeding abolished fasting pattern of myoelectric activity and elicited continuous feed pattern of spike-burst activity in sphincter of Oddi, stomach, and small bowel. Substantial gallbladder emptying occurred within 40 min after eating, and gallbladder remained contracted for at least several hours. [From Takahashi et al. (192).]

contractile activity in the opossum sphincter of Oddi is coordinated with the patterns of gastrointestinal contractility that occur both during the fasted and fed states. Whether or not a similar coordination exists in humans remains to be determined.

The control mechanisms that alter the rate of spike bursts in the opossum sphincter of Oddi during fasting as well as after feeding and coordinate these changes with the gastrointestinal motor activity are of interest. Potential control mechanisms include changes in transsphincteric bile flow, hormones, and nerves. Diversion of bile flow around the sphincter causes a minimal change in the spike-burst pattern during fasting but no change in the fed pattern (190). Thus, although transsphincteric flow rate may exert some minimal modulation, the basic pattern of sphincter spike-burst rate during fasting and after feeding is determined by other factors. Cyclic increases in serum motilin that peak concurrent with phase III MMC activity in the duodenum (191) might contribute to the cyclic increases of sphincter spike bursts during fasting, whereas CCK could cause the sustained postprandial increase in sphincter spike bursts. At low doses both these hormones excite spike-burst activity in the opossum sphincter of Oddi while having only a minimal effect on basal sphincter tone.

Autonomic nerves undoubtedly have some role in regulating sphincter of Oddi motor activity. In earlier studies (123, 216) electrical or mechanical stimulation of the gallbladder inhibited phasic contractile or electrical activity of the canine or rabbit sphincter of Oddi. Recent studies indicate that distension of the gallbladder or common duct causes a decrease of sphincter of Oddi resistance in the cat and dog (201) and an increase in the rate of phasic sphincter contractions in the prairie dog (122). The inhibitory responses of the feline sphincter of Oddi to proximal distension was blocked by tetrodotoxin and painting the middle portion of the common duct with lidocaine (201). In the dog the cholecysto–sphincter of Oddi reflex appears to be mediated by nerves from the celiac ganglion because the reflex was not blocked by disrupting the middle portion of the common duct (216). Truncal vagotomy delays and suppresses the increased contraction rate of phasic contractions that occur in the opossum sphincter of Oddi after a meal (187).

A recent study with the technique of intravital microscopy demonstrates that the kinetics of flow across the guinea pig sphincter of Oddi differ substantially from those of the opossum or humans (34). In this animal the common duct makes a right angle entry into a large ampulla that is located entirely within the duodenal wall. The ampulla is filled with bile by regular phasic contractions of the distal common duct or choledochus that occur at a rate of 6/min. Retrograde flow from the ampulla is prevented by a flap-valve mechanism. A phasic contraction sweeps the ampulla about once a minute to propel bile into the duodenum.

*Overview*

As shown by studies of both humans and animals, the biliary tract functions as a low-pressure system with slow rates of transductal and transsphincteric flow. Pressure within the common duct is normally only 5–10 cmH$_2$O above that in the duodenum. Common duct flow is solely passive in humans. Two sources generate bile flow: hepatic secretion and gallbladder contraction. These sources are capable of sustaining increased rates of bile outflow for 30 min or longer but can generate only modest increases in intraluminal pressure. Maximal gallbladder contraction pressure is ~15–25 cmH$_2$O. After common duct obstruction, hepatic secretion cannot increase intraductal pressure >20–25 cmH$_2$O above intraduodenal pressure. In normal circumstances small differences in intraluminal pressure between the gallbladder and common duct are sufficient to direct flow either into or out of the gallbladder.

The partition of bile flow within the common bile and cystic ducts is determined by the relative resistances of the cystic duct and sphincter of Oddi. These resistances have active as well as passive components. In humans a small, variable pressure gradient exists across the sphincter segment, but discrete functional minisphincters have not been verified that correspond to the sphincterlike areas of thickened circular muscle that are seen on some histological specimens.

During fasting ~50%–75% of hepatic bile flows into the duodenum, whereas the remainder enters the gallbladder, where it is concentrated and stored. Recent studies in animals and humans, however, indicate that during fasting the gallbladder is not quiescent, but rather it undergoes periodic contractions with partial emptying and refilling in rhythm with the gastrointestinal MMC cycle. These gallbladder contractions may be induced by cyclic increases in circulating motilin, regulated by neural activity, or both. After a meal the gallbladder undergoes a sustained contraction that generally empties 50% or more of gallbladder volume during an interval of 20–30 min or longer. This emptying occurs at a maximal rate of ~2%–3%/min and is characterized by a graded contraction of the gallbladder musculature. Unlike the rapid emptying of the urinary bladder, gallbladder emptying occurs at a slow exponential rate that requires only minimal pressure gradients across the cystic duct and sphincter of Oddi. Substantial evidence exists that postprandial contraction of the gallbladder is mediated by circulating CCK, which is released from the small bowel mucosa when fat or protein enters the duodenal lumen. Concurrent with postprandial contraction of the human gallbladder, a decrease occurs in sphincter of Oddi resistance. This reciprocal relaxation of the human sphincter of Oddi during gallbladder contraction is believed to be elicited by increased circulating levels of endogenous CCK.

Gallbladder filling is accomplished when a minimally negative pressure gradient of a few centimeters of water exists across the cystic duct. This gradient results in a pressure sump that sucks bile into the gallbladder. The slightly negative pressure gradient between the gallbladder and common duct is caused by a combination of gallbladder relaxation and an increase in resistance at the sphincter of Oddi.

In addition to a modest, sustained tonic contraction, the human sphincter of Oddi exhibits prominent rhythmic contractions in fasted subjects. These phasic sphincter contractions appear to account for the common endoscopic observation that bile generally enters the duodenal lumen in rhythmic spurts rather than oozing into the lumen continuously. Findings from the opossum and cat suggest that phasic sphincter of Oddi contractions are elicited by a myogenic oscillator and are modulated by enteric hormones as well as by nerves. The phasic sphincter contractions in humans are decreased or abolished by exogenous CCK, but they have yet to be studied after a meal. We anticipate that release of endogenous CCK after eating would likely inhibit the phasic as well as tonic smooth muscle contractility of the human sphincter of Oddi. In normal subjects the majority of phasic sphincter of Oddi contractions begin in the proximal sphincter and propagate toward the duodenum. Such contraction sequences recorded by manometry undoubtedly correspond to the radiographic images of antegrade peristaltic sequences that rapidly expel sphincter contents into the duodenum. Phasic sphincter contractions that propagate retrograde or occur simultaneously over the length of the sphincter segment expel little, if any, fluid into the duodenum. Sphincter contractions of any type interrupt the passive outflow of the common duct that occurs at a low pressure and cannot enter a segment of higher pressure. Therefore common duct emptying into the sphincter of Oddi segment occurs only during the diastolic interval between phasic sphincter contractions, provided baseline sphincter pressure does not exceed common duct pressure. In fasted opossums, the rate of phasic sphincter of Oddi contractions shows periodic fluctuations that are synchronized with the gastrointestinal MMC cycle. The increased rate of sphincter contraction concurrent with phases II and III of duodenal MMC activity may be elicited by the rising serum levels of motilin that occur during the second half of the duodenal MMC cycle. This possibility needs to be evaluated in humans, albeit such a study will be difficult, because of the existing limitations of long-interval sphincter monitoring in human subjects.

In the past, controversy has existed concerning the function of the phasic sphincter of Oddi contractions (152). Some workers suggest that phasic sphincter contractions retard bile outflow from the common duct (8), whereas others believe that the contractions may act as a peristaltic pump that meters small droplike boluses of bile across the sphincter segment (204). Therefore the physiological role of phasic contractions in the human sphincter of Oddi requires clarification. Several possibilities exist that are not mutually exclusive. First, the antegrade contractions in humans may serve as a peristaltic pump, as in the opossum, that actively expels sphincter contents into the duodenum. The relative rate or percentage of antegrade peristaltic contractions may vary during the MMC cycle and after a meal. Sphincter stroke volume is determined by the degree of sphincter filling at the onset of the peristaltic sequence. In turn, the degree of sphincter filling depends on basal sphincter pressure, the rate of bile flow, common duct pressure, and the interval between phasic sphincter contractions. Second, those sphincter contractions that are simultaneous or retrograde may have an overall effect of retarding common duct emptying and thereby promoting gallbladder filling. Third, the phasic sphincter contractions probably help prevent reflux of duodenal contents into the common duct. Finally, we suggest that phasic sphincter contractions have an important housekeeping role of maintaining the narrow sphincter of Oddi segment free of any sludge, particulate material, or microcalculi that might lodge in the sphincter segment. Small particles could cause significant obstruction within the small confines of the sphincter lumen. Any increase in pressure behind an obstructing particle that was generated solely by hepatic secretion or gallbladder contraction would be modest and likely insufficient to dislodge the particle. Therefore, without some effective mechanism to maintain luminal patency, the sphincter would always be on the brink of obstruction. In contrast, antegrade peristaltic contractions are capable of generating a substantial pressure head behind any particle that transiently occludes the sphincter lumen and thereby eject the particle into the duodenum.

We conclude that the sphincter of Oddi represents a marvelously adaptive structure that has an ejecting as well as occluding function. The major physiological role of the sphincter is to regulate pressure within the biliary system and to prevent reflux. Irrespective of the bile flow rate, pressure within the bile ducts is normally maintained within a narrow physiological range of low pressure that allows hepatic secretion to proceed against negligible hydrostatic resistance. A number of options are available for the sphincter of Oddi to meet its physiological responsibilities. The sphincter may promote common duct outflow by *1)* a decrease in basal tone, *2)* an increase in the rate of antegrade peristaltic contractions accomplished by either an increase in the rate of phasic contractions or the percentage that are antegrade, or *3)* an increase in stroke volume. Conversely the sphincter may retard common duct outflow and consequently promote gallbladder filling by *1)* an increase in its basal tone, *2)* a decrease in the rate of antegrade peristalsis, or *3)* a decrease in stroke volume. Different combinations of changes of these variables are possible. Thus the sphincter of Oddi might adapt to increased postprandial bile outflow by *1*) an increase in the rate of antegrade peristalsis and likely stroke volume, as is the case with the opossum, or *2*) a decrease, or perhaps cessation, of sphincter contractions, as is probably true in humans. The contraction rate of the human sphincter of Oddi probably varies in rhythm with the MMC cycle, as is true with the opossum. We speculate that circulating levels of CCK and motilin modulate changes in the rate of phasic, sphincter contractions while having little effect on the type of contraction. Neural influences appear more likely to affect the propagation direction of the sphincter contractions and probably their rate as well.

ABNORMAL FUNCTION IN HUMANS

As evidenced by the general therapeutic success of cholecystectomy or sphincter bypass procedures, the gallbladder and sphincter of Oddi are not essential for health. However, motor dysfunction of these structures may cause significant clinical symptoms. In many instances abnormalities of motor function are difficult to distinguish from organic disease or congenital aberrations.

*Gallbladder*

Potential abnormalities of gallbladder motor function (dyskinesia) may be characterized by either excessive contraction (hyperkinesia) or by depressed contraction (hypokinesia).

HYPERKINESIA. Primary hyperkinesia of the gallbladder is alleged to exist in some patients with unexplained right upper quadrant pain, who exhibit exaggerated gallbladder contraction in response to CCK. Several reviews of this subject are available (14, 64). Individuals suspected of having symptomatic gallbladder hyperkinesia are generally studied by cholecystokinin cholecystography. To perform this test the gallbladder is opacified by oral cholecystography and the subject given an intravenous bolus injection of CCK-8, e.g., 20 ng/kg. A positive response consists of an exaggerated or abnormal gallbladder contraction accompanied by reproduction of the patient's clinical symptoms (125, 127). The test should be controlled by giving a placebo intravenous injection of saline. An exaggerated contraction features nearly total evacuation of the gallbladder within 5–10 min. Such rapid evacuation may cause abrupt overdistension of the common duct and thus elicit discomfort or pain. Alternately the gallbladder might show an abnormal pattern of contraction by assuming the configuration of a rounded ball, with minimal emptying. Such a ball configuration, likened to a struggling gallbladder, has been assigned to a localized hypercontraction of the gallbladder neck or the proximal cystic duct that would cause obstruction to gallbladder emptying and accompanying pain.

Histological evaluation of gallbladders removed from patients with suspected symptomatic hyperkinesia may show either normal findings or adenomyomatosis, a condition characterized by both muscular and glandular hyperplasia. At present considerable controversy exists about the true existence of gallbladder hyperkinesia, particularly in the absence of adenomyomatosis, and the value of cholecystokinin cholecystography for making such a diagnosis is doubtful (14, 64). Further investigation is needed to resolve this issue.

Increased gallbladder contractility is reported to exist in a minority of patients with gallstones (115), caused possibly by supersensitivity to CCK (128, 200). Enhanced gallbladder emptying after meals would be expected to increase the amount of circulating bile acids. Such enhanced circulation might reduce the bile acid pool by feedback inhibition of bile acid synthesis. Some patients with gallstones demonstrate a decreased bile acid pool that may contribute to bile supersaturated with cholesterol.

HYPOKINESIA. General agreement exists that the major cause for gallstones is "bad bile," i.e., bile with abnormal ratios of cholesterol, bile acids, and phospholipids that may lead to precipitation of cholesterol crystals. Impaired gallbladder contraction, however, may contribute to gallstone formation in some patients (99, 200). Decreased gallbladder contraction might be caused by *1*) a primary abnormality of the gallbladder musculature, *2*) muscle impairment secondary to chronic cholecystitis, *3*) suboptimal hormonal or neural stimulation, or *4*) circulation of an inhibitory substance. Any of these possibilities could result in diminished or absent postprandial gallbladder contraction or impairment of cyclic gallbladder contractions during fasting, or both. Results of studies employing cholecystography or scintigraphy indicate that gallbladder contraction in response to meals or CCK is impaired in a subpopulation of patients with gallstones (17, 49, 99, 105, 144, 171). In some cases the impaired gallbladder contraction may be due to a decreased postprandial release of CCK (105). Independent studies with animal models indicate that a lithogenic diet given to prairie dogs, ground squirrels, or guinea pigs impairs gallbladder contractility prior to the development of gallstones (33, 41, 52).

In some patients, causes of abnormal gallbladder emptying include vagotomy, diabetes, and pregnancy (46, 151, 164). These conditions may lead to gallbladder stasis and an increased incidence of gallstones. Vagotomy and diabetes are believed to compromise gallbladder emptying by interfering with excitatory autonomic innervation (29, 82, 164). In pregnancy, hypotonia of the gallbladder is thought to result from high circulatory levels of female hormones, such as progesterone, that depress the smooth muscle of the gallbladder as well as that of the lower esophageal sphincter and ureters (20, 90). In a guinea pig model, the decreased contractility of gallbladders harvested from pregnant animals was due to an abnormality in the excitation-contraction coupling common to acetylcholine and CCK-8 stimulation (153). During pregnancy the human gallbladder has an abnormally large residual volume and a decreased rate of emptying (20, 46).

Sprue is associated with gallbladder enlargement and impaired postprandial emptying due to impairment of the elaboration and release of CCK by the atrophic intestinal mucosa (106). This abnormality may be reversible after the institution of a gluten-free diet (112). Gallbladder enlargement and stasis also occur in patients on long-term parenteral hyperalimentation (148). This gallbladder stasis is often associated with the development of sludge and even gallstones.

TREATMENT. The most common treatment for patients with symptomatic gallbladder disease is cholecystectomy. This treatment obviously removes the end organ that causes symptoms, irrespective of whether the symptoms are the result of functional or organic gallbladder disease. In evaluating the efficacy of surgical therapy, however, consideration must be given to its placebo effect. Interestingly sphincterotomy in a prairie dog model of gallstone formation inhibits gallstone formation by decreasing gallbladder filling and reducing stasis (81). In selected patients with cholesterol stones, the stones may be dissolved by prolonged treatment with chenodeoxycholic or ursodeoxycholic acid. Gallstones, however, are likely to reform when the treatment is discontinued. Negligible information is available on the efficacy of pharmacological agents that might inhibit or enhance gallbladder contractility in patients with hyperkinetic or hypokinetic gallbladder dysfunction, respectively.

## Sphincter of Oddi

Symptomatic partial obstruction at the sphincter of Oddi may cause clinical symptoms referable to either the biliary or pancreatic tract. Generally symptomatic biliary sphincter of Oddi dysfunction is more common than pancreatic sphincter of Oddi dysfunction. General causes of cryptic partial sphincter of Oddi obstruction consist of congenital anomalies, acquired organic lesions, and abnormal motor function. Significant congenital anomalies include 1) persistence of a ventral pancreas with suboptimal drainage of the dorsal pancreas through the accessory duct of Santorini, 2) a low-lying entry of the sphincter of Oddi into the third portion of the duodenum with loss of its normal oblique course through the duodenal wall, 3) a long ampulla that creates a prominent common channel between the common duct and pancreatic duct, and 4) an anomalous proximal insertion of the common duct on the pancreatic duct. The first three anomalies favor the development of pancreatitis by causing either abnormal drainage of pancreatic juice or reflux of bile into the pancreatic duct. Anomalous insertion of the common duct on the pancreatic duct may result in a stricture of the distal common duct and accompanying cystic dilation of the duct proximally, referred to as a choledochal cyst (2).

Acquired conditions that cause organic sphincter of Oddi narrowing (sphincter of Oddi stenosis) include inflammation, fibrosis, or hyperplastic mucosa (1, 26, 47, 124). These abnormalities may be initiated by pancreatitis, cholangitis, common duct stones, or unknown causes. Frequently organic stenosis may be difficult to distinguish from functional abnormalities of sphincter of Oddi motor function (sphincter of Oddi dyskinesia). Generally histological material is not available for examination. Therefore a useful criteria for the presumptive separation of sphincter stenosis from dyskinesia is the finding that common duct obstruction or an elevated basal sphincter pressure does not decrease (Fig. 26) after the administration of drugs or hormones that normally relax sphincter smooth muscle (75). Partial sphincter obstruction may be expressed clinically as 1) unexplained intermittent or persistent upper abdominal pain, often aggravated by meals, 2) abnormal liver function tests, 3) findings

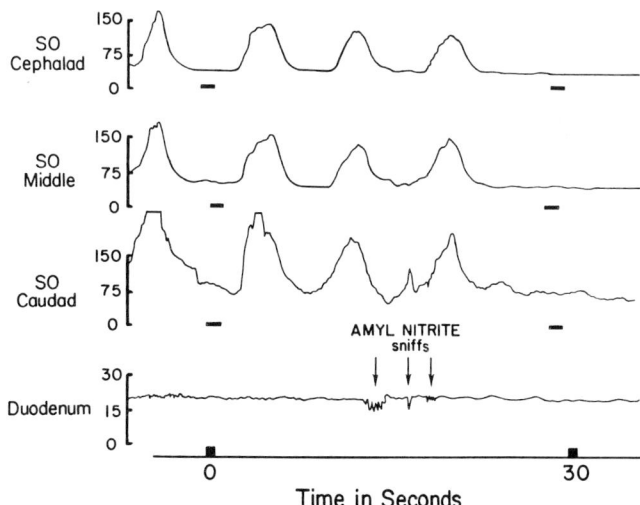

FIG. 26. Manometric recording from patient with sphincter of Oddi (SO) stenosis. Three sphincter recording sites show phasic sphincter contraction superimposed on hypertensive basal sphincter pressure of ~30–45 mmHg above intraduodenal pressure. *Short bars* indicate reference for zero atmosphere pressure. Amyl nitrite inhalation abolished phasic sphincter contractions but had no effect on increased basal sphincter pressure. Failure of smooth muscle relaxant to substantially decrease elevated basal pressure indicates that increased pressure is caused by organic abnormality, such as fibrosis, rather than functional sphincter spasm.

of common duct distension or abnormal emptying on radiological studies, *4)* unexplained pancreatitis, and *5)* abnormal manometric findings.

In the past, symptomatic disorders of sphincter of Oddi motor function, believed to cause partial common duct or pancreatic duct obstruction, have been promulgated rather than supported by firm evidence (95). Alleged clinical entities of sphincter motor dysfunction were often shrouded by mystery and nurtured by excessive speculation that led to considerable controversy. These difficulties were undoubtedly promoted because suitable instrumentation was not available to characterize normal sphincter motor function, let alone abnormalities in its motor function. A confusing array of terms emerged that were often misleading and tended to retard clear analysis of the subject. These terms included *biliary dyskinesia, biliary dyssynergia, sphincter of Oddi spasm, postcholecystectomy syndrome,* and *sphincterisimus.* None of these terms is specific or truly applicable. For example, the term *biliary dyskinesia* had been applied to the gallbladder as well as to the sphincter of Oddi. A priori, sphincter of Oddi motor disorders are not necessarily dyssynergia or spasm. For these reasons, we prefer the term *sphincter of Oddi dyskinesia* because this term localizes the motor abnormality to the sphincter and is broad enough to include different varieties of abnormal sphincter motor function.

In recent years substantial progress has been made in understanding normal and abnormal sphincter of Oddi motor function, albeit much remains to be learned. Characterization of sphincter dyskinesia should not be limited to a single scenario because, like esophageal motility disorders, disordered sphincter of Oddi motor function comprise a spectrum of abnormalities caused by impairment of either sphincter muscle or its innervation. The ensuing discussion of sphincter of Oddi dyskinesia is developed from consideration of the information known currently about normal sphincter motor function and an analysis of potential abnormalities that might occur. Motor abnormalities, either primary or secondary, may involve either the tonic or phasic components of sphincter motor activity, or both.

BILIARY SPHINCTER OF ODDI DYSFUNCTION. Sphincter of Oddi motor abnormalities have been documented most commonly in patients with suspected biliary sphincter of Oddi dysfunction, as opposed to patients with suspected pancreatic sphincter of Oddi dysfunction. In a recent study 14% of patients with the postcholecystectomy syndrome had abnormal findings on sphincter of Oddi manometry (6). The following discussion of abnormal sphincter of Oddi motor function is based on the investigation of patients with biliary tract symptoms.

*Sphincter spasm.* Excessive tonic contraction, or spasm, of the sphincter of Oddi would be expected to impair common duct emptying for two reasons. First, a persistent increase in sphincter tone would prevent bile from flowing passively across the sphincter segment. Second, a sustained increase in base-line sphincter tone would prevent filling of the sphincter segment. Consequently phasic sphincter contractions would not eject bile into the duodenum because the sphincter would always be empty. In our own experience and that of others, most patients with sphincter spasm have normal phasic contractions superimposed on an elevated base-line pressure (3, 65, 115). Basal sphincter of Oddi pressure is considered to be elevated when its value exceeds 25–30 mmHg referenced to duodenal pressure as zero (3). When a high basal sphincter pressure is encountered, the possibility must be considered of an artifact caused by sphincter cannulation. Sphincter spasm following its instrumentation with probes at laparotomy is a well-known phenomenon among surgeons. On operative cholangiograms, the contracted sphincter may produce a meniscus-filling defect in the distal common duct. This filling defect may be misinterpreted as a retained calculus but disappears after the administration of glucagon, which relaxes the sphincter and allows free flow of contrast medium into the common duct (48). Although the possibility always exists that a high basal sphincter pressure recorded on manometry is an iatrogenic artifact, we have observed this finding nearly exclusively in patients with suspected obstructive sphincter of Oddi dysfunction and rarely in any other category of patients. If any doubt exists about whether or not an elevated base-line pressure is a true abnormal finding or an artifact, the manometry may be repeated during another session. Persistent elevation of base-line sphincter of Oddi pressure caused by spasm is reduced substantially by smooth muscle relaxants, such as amyl nitrite inhalation, sublingual nitroglycerin, or intravenous glucagon. Such a reduction in hypertensive sphincter of Oddi pressure distinguishes spasm from stenosis. Findings from recent studies suggest that many patients with suspected biliary sphincter of Oddi dysfunction and documented elevation of sphincter of Oddi pressure benefit from endoscopic sphincteroplasty (62).

*Paradoxical contraction to CCK-8.* In some patients with suspected obstructive sphincter of Oddi dysfunction, CCK-8 causes sphincter contraction instead of its normal response of relaxation (76, 206, 207). The paradoxical sphincter contraction elicited by CCK-8 consists of a substantial increase in basal sphincter pressure accompanied by an increase in the rate of phasic sphincter contractions (Fig. 27). In the 10 patients with paradoxical sphincter contraction whom we have encountered, all exhibited some degree of elevation in basal sphincter pressure and all were suspected of having obstructive sphincter dysfunction. CCK-8 administration reproduced the patient's clinical symptoms in half of the cases. We envision that

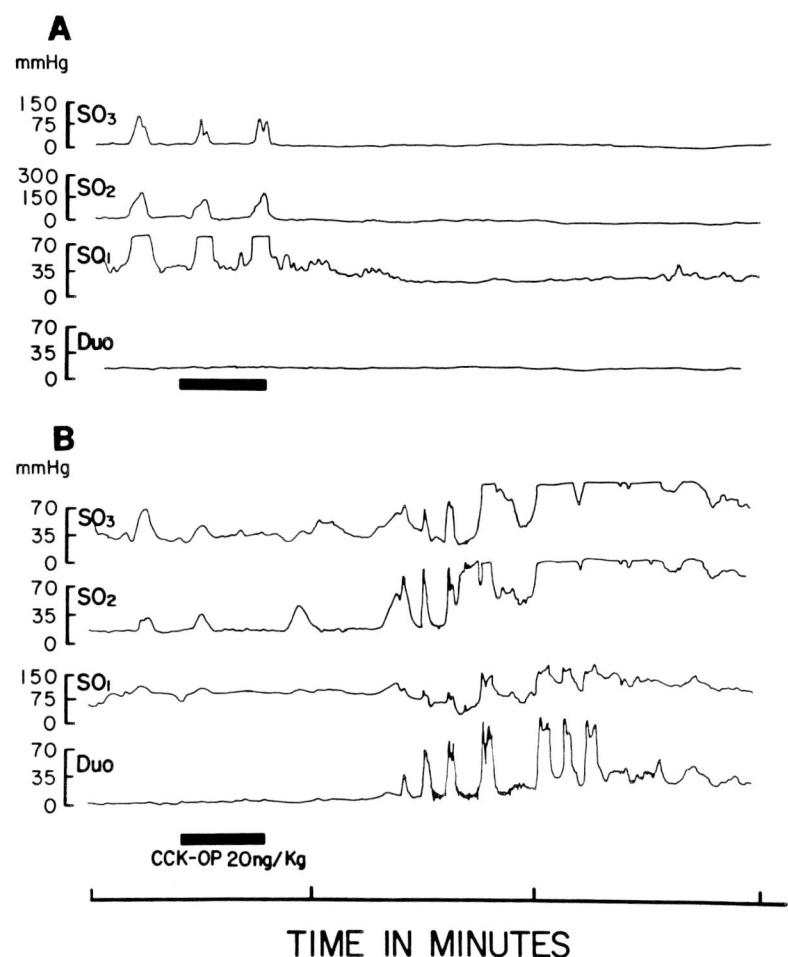

FIG. 27. Manometric recording from human sphincter of Oddi (SO). A: normal response of sphincter of Oddi to cholecystokinin octapeptide (CCK-8), which abolishes phasic contractions and reduces basal SO pressure. B: paradoxical response of sphincter of Oddi to CCK-8 in patient with suspected obstructive sphincter dysfunction. Prior to CCK-8 administration, basal sphincter pressure is elevated. CCK caused paradoxical sphincter contraction consisting of increase in basal pressure and rate of phasic contractions. Concurrent with paradoxical sphincter contraction to CCK-8, patient complained of upper abdominal pain.

the paradoxical sphincter responses to endogenous CCK may occur also in response to endogenous CCK released after meals and thereby cause sphincter obstruction. Sphincter of Oddi obstruction during an interval of increased bile flow would likely lead to duct distension and pain.

A proposed explanation for the paradoxical sphincter contraction elicited by CCK in some patients with suspected obstructive sphincter dysfunction is as follows. Normally, CCK inhibits both tonic and phasic sphincter contractions. By analogy with the cat sphincter of Oddi (10), the effect of CCK on the normal human sphincter is probably mediated by stimulation of inhibitory nerves that override a direct excitatory effect of CCK on sphincter smooth muscle. We propose that in the presence of impaired inhibitory innervation, CCK would cause paradoxical sphincter contraction. Impairment of inhibitory sphincter of Oddi innervation might also account for the elevation in basal sphincter pressure that is present in many of the patients.

*Abnormal propagation of phasic contractions.* Normally ~60% of the phasic sphincter of Oddi contractions propagate antegrade toward the duodenum (206). The remainder either propagate retrograde or occur simultaneously. Thus in normal circumstances the majority of phasic sphincter contractions tend to act as a peristaltic pump that expels sphincter contents into the duodenum. In vitro studies of the opossum sphincter of Oddi suggest that the function of a dominant myogenic pacesetter in the proximal sphincter may occasionally be taken over by an ectopic pacesetter located in the distal sphincter (72). A shifting focus of the dominant pacesetter might account for the variability in propagation direction of phasic contractions in the human sphincter of Oddi. If a distal pacemaker became dominant, the abnormality in sequencing of sphincter phasic contractions could cause clinical symptoms. For example, propagation sequences that were exclusively retrograde could cause common duct stasis and would not expel small particles from the sphincter segment. Of interest is the fact that patients with retained common duct stones demonstrated an aberration in the propagation of their

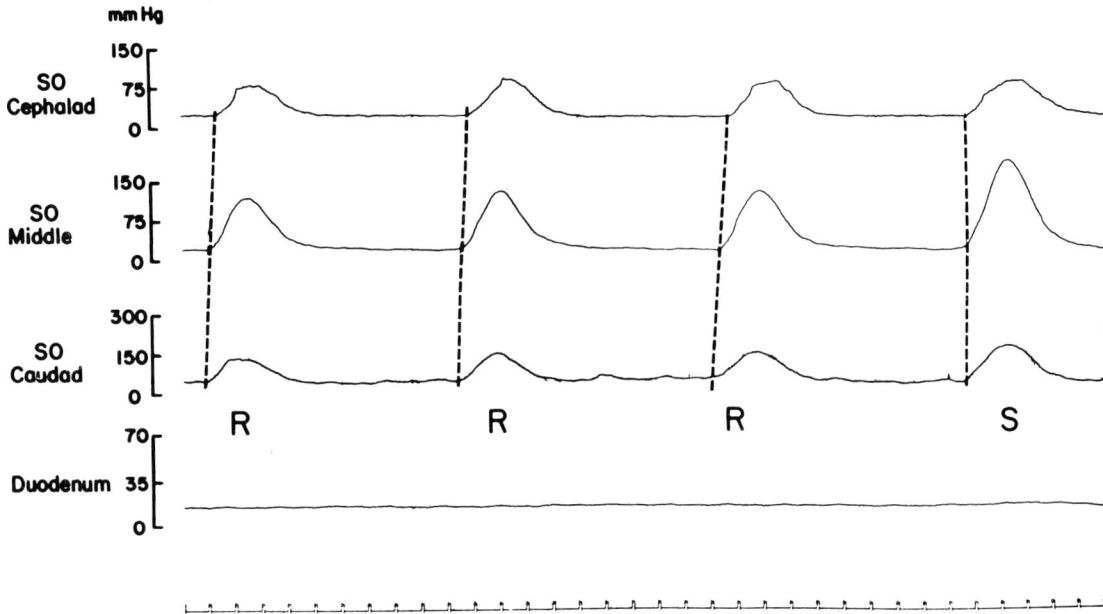

FIG. 28. Manometric recording from human sphincter of Oddi (SO). Phasic sphincter contractions were primarily retrograde in this patient with retained, nonobstructing calculus in common duct. R, retrograde contraction; S, simultaneous contraction. [From Toouli et al. (205). Reprinted with permission of The American Gastroenterological Association, copyright 1982.]

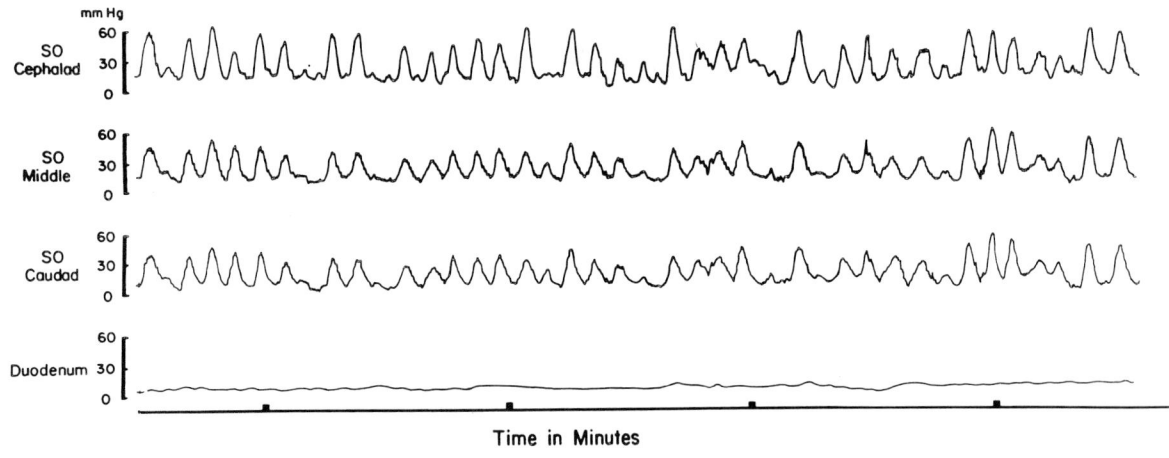

FIG. 29. Manometric recording from the human sphincter of Oddi (SO). Tachyoddia was observed in this patient with suspected obstructive sphincter dysfunction. Rate of phasic sphincter contractions was 10–12/min, compared with normal range of 2–8/min.

phasic sphincter contractions. In contrast to controls, the majority of phasic sphincter contractions in this group of patients propagated retrograde (Fig. 28) and only a small percentage were antegrade (205). It is unclear whether this aberration of motor function preceded the common duct stones or was secondary to their presence. In any case, the prevalence of retrograde sphincter contractions would favor common duct stasis and retention of ductal calculi.

*Tachyoddia.* As suggested by findings from studies (204) in the opossum, an abnormally high rate of phasic contractions in the human sphincter of Oddi, for example, >8/min, or an increase in contraction duration, would be expected to compromise sphincter diastole and thereby cause either transient or persistent common duct obstruction (78, 207). This phenomenon is precisely what occurs in the human sphincter of Oddi after the administration of morphine (75).

Small doses of morphine cause a dramatic increase in the rate of phasic sphincter contraction accompanied by only a minimal increase in the base-line pressure. This morphine-induced tachyoddia is capable of causing complete obstruction of common duct outflow. Large doses of morphine enhance tonic as well as phasic sphincter contraction. During sphincter of Oddi manometry, we have observed unprovoked sphincter tachyoddia in ~20 patients (Fig. 29), most of whom were suspected of having obstructive sphincter dysfunction. The possibility exists that traumatic cannulation of the sphincter might have caused irritability that led to tachyoddia. However, we believe that this possibility was unlikely because the cannulations had gone smoothly. Further, we have not encountered this aberration in patients who were not suspected of having functional sphincter of Oddi obstruction. In the one patient we tested the rapid sphincter contractions were abolished by CCK-8. To what extent sphincter tachyoddia accounts for clinical symptoms in humans remains to be determined.

PANCREATIC SPHINCTER OF ODDI DYSFUNCTION. In patients with recurrent or chronic alcoholic pancreatitis, the sphincter of Oddi generally exhibits normal findings on endoscopic sphincter manometry (35, 129). In contrast, the sphincter of Oddi in a substantial minority of patients with unexplained idiopathic recurrent pancreatitis has elevated basal sphincter pressure (67, 77). In this subgroup of patients the possibility exists that sphincter dysfunction leads to unexplained recurrent pancreatitis. An increase in basal sphincter pressure may also occur when pancreatitis is associated with common duct stones (66).

TREATMENT. The efficacy of medical treatment for sphincter of Oddi dyskinesia has not been systematically evaluated. However, case reports have appeared wherein therapy with long-acting nitrites appears to have relieved symptoms attributed to sphincter of Oddi spasm (5). A moderate amount of evidence suggests that sphincterotomy or sphincteroplasty is an effective therapy for verified sphincter of Oddi stenosis or dyskinesia associated with biliary tract symptoms. However, similar data are not available on the treatment of pancreatic sphincter of Oddi dysfunction. Until recently, sphincterotomy or sphincteroplasty were done at laparotomy (120, 127), but in recent years most sphincterotomies have been accomplished retrograde using a papillotome during duodenal endoscopy. Endoscopic sphincterotomy is extremely effective in the treatment of retained common duct stones (177) and appears to be worthwhile in verified cases of obstructive sphincter dysfunction (62). Mortality from the procedure is ~1% (44, 102). Manometric studies featuring catheter pull-throughs from the common duct into the duodenum establish that sphincterotomy reduces basal sphincter pressure, abolishes the common duct–duodenal pressure gradient, and markedly attenuates phasic sphincter contractions without altering their direction of travel (60, 61, 67). These reductions in pressure have persisted on follow-up studies done 1–2 yr after sphincterotomy (62). However, neither conventional surgical sphincterotomy nor endoscopic sphincterotomy alters the resistance or pressure phenomenon across the pancreatic duct portion of the sphincter of Oddi segment (67, 77). Therefore these therapies are ineffective for treating sphincter hypertension associated with recurrent pancreatitis. In this circumstance the septum between the distal common duct and pancreatic duct needs to be disrupted by a sphincteroplasty or possibly by balloon distension (67, 120). In some patients with pancreas divisum and idiopathic recurrent pancreatitis, surgical sphincterotomy of the accessory papillary papilla has been associated with an improvement in clinical symptoms (146).

SUMMARY

Although considerable information has accrued during the last two decades about the pressure-flow kinetics of the bile duct system, much remains to be learned. In particular the complexities of phasic as well as tonic sphincter of Oddi contractions merit further study and analysis. The sphincter of Oddi segment exhibits a unique function that differs completely from other alimentary tract sphincters, such as the lower esophageal or anal sphincters that maintain a steady tone punctuated by transient relaxations. The message is now clear that the biliary tract structures function in concert with the upper gastrointestinal tract during fasting as well as after a meal.

Although the gallbladder or sphincter of Oddi, as evidenced by cholecystectomy or a sphincter bypass, is not required for health, malfunction of these structures can cause significant clinical symptoms. Increased gallbladder contractility may occasionally cause episodes of upper abdominal pain, whereas primary or secondary abnormalities in gallbladder contraction may contribute to the formation of gallstones. In rare cases, obstructive cystic duct dysfunction may cause pain. When any of these conditions are substantiated, cholecystectomy is a ready solution. Although not yet fully defined, a spectrum of sphincter of Oddi motor abnormalities exists that may cause clinical symptoms. Given sufficient substantiation, a rational treatment for functional sphincter of Oddi obstruction is a myotomy via endoscopic or surgical methods.

This research was supported in part by Public Health Service Grant AM-25731.

## REFERENCES

1. Acosta, J. M., F. Civantos, G. L. Nardi, and B. Castelman. Fibrosis of the papilla of Vater. *Surg. Gynecol. Obstet.* 124: 787–794, 1967.
2. Babbitt, D. P., R. J. Starshak, and A. R. Clemett. Choledochal cyst: a concept of etiology. *Am. J. Roentgenol. Rad. Ther. Nucl. Med.* 119: 57–62, 1973.
3. Bar-Meir, S., J. E. Geenen, W. J. Hogan, W. J. Dodds, E. T. Stewart, and R. C. Arndorfer. Biliary and pancreatic duct pressures measured by ERCP manometry in patients with suspected papillary stenosis. *Dig. Dis. Sci.* 24: 209–213, 1979.
4. Bar-Meir, S., and Z. Halpern. The significance of the diameter of the common bile duct in cholecystectomized patients. *Am. J. Gastroenterol.* 79: 59–60, 1984.
5. Bar-Meir, S., Z. Halpern, and E. Bardan. Nitrate therapy in a patient with papillary dysfunction. *Am. J. Gastroenterol.* 78: 94–95, 1983.
6. Bar-Meir, S., Z. Halpern, E. Bardan, and T. Gilat. Frequency of papillary dysfunction among cholecystectomized patients. *Hepatology Baltimore* 4: 328–330, 1984.
7. Becker, J. M., W. M. Duff, and F. G. Moody. Myoelectric control of gastrointestinal and biliary motility: a review. *Surgery St. Louis* 89: 466–477, 1981.
8. Becker, J. M., F. G. Moody, and A. R. Zinsmeister. Effect of gastrointestinal hormones on the biliary sphincter of the opossum. *Gastroenterology* 82: 1300–1307, 1982.
9. Behar, J., and P. Biancani. Neural control of the feline gallbladder. In: *Gastrointestinal Motility*, edited by J. Christensen. New York: Raven, 1980, p. 97–109.
10. Behar, J., and P. Biancani. Effect of cholecystokinin and the octapeptide of cholecystokinin on the feline sphincter of Oddi and gallbladder. Mechanisms of action. *J. Clin. Invest.* 66: 1231–1239, 1980.
11. Behar, J., and P. Biancani. Effect of motilin on the cat sphincter of Oddi (SO): mechanism of action (Abstract). *Gastroenterology* 84: 1102, 1983.
12. Behar, J., and P. Biancani. Neural control of the sphincter of Oddi. *Gastroenterology* 86: 134–141, 1984.
13. Beneventano, T. C., H. G. Jacobson, E. S. Hurwitt, and C. J. Schein. Cine-cholangiomanometry: physiologic observations. *Am. J. Roentgenol. Radium Ther. Nucl. Med.* 100: 673–679, 1967.
14. Berk, R. N. Cholecystokinin cholecystography in the diagnosis of chronic acalculous cholecystitis and biliary dyskinesia. A critical appraisal. *Gastrointest. Radiol.* 1: 325–330, 1977.
15. Björck, S., H. Ahlman, and A. Dahlström. Effect of extrinsic denervation on the rate of net water transport of the feline gall bladder. *Gut* 25: 603–610, 1984.
16. Björck, S., R. Jansson, and J. Svanvik. Adrenergic influence on concentrating function in the feline gall bladder. *Gut* 23: 1019–1022, 1982.
17. Bobba, V. R., G. T. Krishnamurthy, E. Kingston, F. E. Turner, P. H. Brown, and K. Langrell. Gallbladder dynamics induced by a fatty meal in normal subjects and patients with gallstones. *J. Nucl. Med.* 25: 21–24, 1984.
18. Boyden, E. A. The sphincter of Oddi in man and certain representative mammals. *Surgery St. Louis* 1: 25–37, 1937.
19. Boyden, E. A. The anatomy of the choledochoduodenal junction in man. *Surg. Gynecol. Obstet.* 104: 641–652, 1957.
20. Braverman, D. Z., M. L. Johnson, and F. Kern, Jr. Effects of pregnancy and contraceptive steroids on gallbladder function. *N. Engl. J. Med.* 302: 362–364, 1980.
21. Bueno, L., and F. Praddaude. Electrical activity of the gallbladder and biliary tract in sheep and its relationship with antral and duodenal motility. *Ann. Biol. Anim. Biochim. Biophys.* 19: 1109–1121, 1979.
22. Burnett, W., F. W. Gairns, and P. Bacsich. Some observations on the innervation of the extrahepatic biliary system in man. *Ann. Surg.* 159: 8–26, 1964.
23. Cai, W. Q., and G. Gabella. The musculature of the gallbladder and biliary pathways in the guinea pig. *J. Anat.* 136: 237–250, 1983.
24. Caroli, J., P. Porcher, G. Pequignot, and M. Delattre. Contribution of cineradiography to study of the function of the human biliary tract. *Am. J. Dig. Dis.* 5: 677–696, 1960.
25. Carr-Locke, D. L., and J. A. Gregg. Endoscopic manometry of pancreatic and biliary sphincter zones in man. Basal results in healthy volunteers. *Dig. Dis. Sci.* 26: 7–15, 1981.
26. Cattell, R. B., B. P. Colcock, and J. L. Pollack. Stenosis of the sphincter of Oddi. *N. Engl. J. Med.* 256: 429–435, 1957.
27. Chang, T. M., and W. Y. Chey. Radioimmunoassay of cholecystokinin. *Dig. Dis. Sci.* 28: 456–468, 1983.
28. Chang, V. H., J. J. Cunningham, and J. J. Fromkes. Sonographic measurement of the extrahepatic bile duct before and after retrograde cholangiography. *Am. J. Roentgenol. Radium. Ther. Nucl. Med.* 144: 753–755, 1985.
29. Clave, R. A., and M. R. Gasper. Incidence of gallbladder disease after vagotomy. *Am. J. Surg.* 118: 169–176, 1969.
30. Coelho, J. C., F. G. Moody, and N. Senniger. A new method for correlating pancreatic and biliary duct pressures and sphincter of Oddi electromyography. *Surgery St. Louis* 97: 342–349, 1985.
31. Cohn, M. S., S. I. Schwartz, W. W. Faloon, and J. T. Adams. Effect of sphincteroplasty on gallbladder function and bile composition. *Ann. Surg.* 189: 317–321, 1979.
32. Courtney, D. F., A. S. Clanachan, and G. W. Scott. Cholecystokinin constricts the canine cystic duct. *Gastroenterology* 85: 1154–1159, 1983.
33. Cox, K. L., A. T. W. Cheung, E. M. Walsh, and C. K. Iwahashi-Hosoda. Choledochoduodenal junction (CDJ) dysmotility associated with cholelithiasis and hydrops of the gallbladder (Abstract). *Dig. Dis. Sci.* 30: 765, 1985.
34. Cox, K. L., A. T. W. Cheung, E. M. Walsh, C. K. Iwahashi-Hosoda, and C. L. Lohse. Intravital microscopy: a new in vivo method for quantitating biliary motility (Abstract). *Dig. Dis. Sci.* 30: 766, 1985.
35. Csendes, A., A. Kruse, P. Funch-Jensen, M. J. Oster, J. Ornsholt, and E. Amdrup. Pressure measurements in the biliary and pancreatic duct systems in controls and in patients with gallstones, previous cholecystectomy, or common bile duct stones. *Gastroenterology* 77: 1203–1210, 1979.
36. Csendes, A., and A. Sepulveda. Intraluminal gallbladder pressure measurements in patients with chronic or acute cholecystitis. *Am. J. Surg.* 139: 383–384, 1980.
37. Davison, J. S., and M. Al-Hassani. The role of noncholinergic, nonadrenergic nerves in regulating the distensibility of the guinea pig gallbladder. In: *Gastrointestinal Motility*, edited by J. Christensen. New York: Raven, 1980, p. 89–95.
38. Davison, J. S., and S. Fosel. Interactions between vagus nerve stimulation and pentagastrin or secretin on the guinea pig gallbladder. *Digestion* 13: 251–254, 1975.
39. Debas, H. T., and T. Yamagishi. Evidence for a pylorocholecystic reflex for gallbladder contraction. *Ann. Surg.* 190: 170–175, 1979.
40. Dodds, W. J., W. J. Groh, R. M. A. Darweesh, T. L. Lawson, S. M. A. Kishk, and M. K. Kern. Sonographic measurement of gallbladder volume. *Am. J. Roentgenol. Radium Ther. Nucl. Med.* 145: 1009–1011, 1985.
41. Doty, J. E., H. A. Pitt, S. L. Kuchenbecker, and L. DenBesten. Impaired gallbladder emptying before gallstone formation in the prairie dog. *Gastroenterology* 85: 168–174, 1983.
42. DuBois, F. S., and E. A. Hunt. Peristalsis of the common bile duct in the opossum. *Anat. Rec.* 53: 387–397, 1932.
43. Edholm, P. Gallbladder evacuation in the normal male induced by cholecystokinin. *Acta Radiol.* 53: 257–265, 1960.
44. Escourrou, J., J. A. Cordova, F. Lazorthes, J. Frexinos, and A. Ribet. Early and late complications after endoscopic

sphincterotomy for biliary lithiasis with and without the gall bladder 'in situ'. *Gut* 25: 598–602, 1984.
45. EVERSON, G. T., D. Z. BRAVERMAN, M. L. JOHNSON, AND F. KERN, JR. A critical evaluation of real-time ultrasonography for the study of gallbladder volume and contraction. *Gastroenterology* 79: 40–46, 1980.
46. EVERSON, G. T., C. MCKINLEY, M. LAWSON, M. JOHNSON, AND F. KERN, JR. Gallbladder function in the human female: effect of the ovulatory cycle, pregnancy, and contraceptive steroids. *Gastroenterology* 82: 711–719, 1982.
47. FERRARI, B. T., R. L. O'HALLORAN, W. P. LONGMIRE, JR., AND K. J. LEWIN. Atypical papillary hyperplasia of the pancreatic duct mimicking obstructing pancreatic carcinoma. *N. Engl. J. Med.* 301: 531–532, 1979.
48. FERRUCCI, J. T., JR., J. WITTENBERG, L. B. STONE, AND J. R. DREYFUSS. Hypotonic cholangiography with glucagon. *Radiology* 118: 466–467, 1976.
49. FISHER, R. S., E. ROCK, AND L. S. MALMUD. Cholinergic effects on gallbladder emptying in humans. *Gastroenterology* 89: 716–722, 1985.
50. FISHER, R. S., F. STELZER, E. ROCK, AND L. S. MALMUD. Abnormal gallbladder emptying in patients with gallstones. *Dig. Dis. Sci.* 27: 1019–1024, 1982.
51. FOESEL, S., AND K. F. SEWING. Enhancement of electrically stimulated guinea pig gallbladder contraction by subthreshold concentrations of gastrointestinal hormones in vitro. *Experientia Basel* 34: 205–206, 1978.
52. FRIDHANDLER, T. M., J. S. DAVISON, AND E. A. SHAFFER. Defective gallbladder contractility in the ground squirrel and prairie dog during the early stages of cholesterol gallstone formation. *Gastroenterology* 85: 830–836, 1983.
53. FRIED, G. M., W. D. OGDEN, C. J. FAGAN, I. WIENER, K. INOUE, G. H. GREELEY, JR., AND J. C. THOMPSON. Comparison of cholecystokinin release and gallbladder emptying in men and in women at estrogen and progesterone phases of the menstrual cycle. *Surgery St. Louis* 95: 284–289, 1984.
54. FRIED, G. M., W. D. OGDEN, J. SWIERCZEK, G. H. GREELEY, JR., P. L. RAYFORD, AND J. C. THOMPSON. Release of cholecystokinin in conscious dogs: correlation with simultaneous measurements of gallbladder pressure and pancreatic protein secretion. *Gastroenterology* 85: 1113–1119, 1983.
55. FUNCH-JENSEN, P., P. DIEDERICH, AND K. KRAGLUND. Intraoperative sphincter of Oddi manometry in patients with gallstones. *Scand. J. Gastroenterol.* 19: 931–936, 1984.
56. FUNCH-JENSEN, P., K. KRAGLUND, AND J. C. DJURHUUS. The influence of measuring catheter diameter on direct manometry in the canine sphincter of Oddi. *Scand. J. Gastroenterol.* 19: 926–930, 1984.
57. FUNCH-JENSEN, P., K. KRAGLUND, AND J. C. DJURHUUS. Multimodal contractile activity of the canine sphincter of Oddi. *Eur. Surg. Res.* 16: 312–316, 1984.
58. FUNCH-JENSEN, P., H. STØDKILDE-JØRGENSEN, K. KRAGLUND, AND N. A. LOVGREEN. Biliary manometry in dogs. *Digestion* 22: 89–93, 1981.
59. GEENEN, J. E., W. J. HOGAN, W. J. DODDS, E. T. STEWART, AND R. C. ARNDORFER. Intraluminal pressure recording from the human sphincter of Oddi. *Gastroenterology* 78: 317–324, 1980.
60. GEENEN, J. E., W. J. HOGAN, R. D. SHAFFER, E. T. STEWART, W. J. DODDS, AND R. C. ARNDORFER. Endoscopic electrosurgical papillotomy and manometry in biliary tract disease. *J. Am. Med. Assoc.* 237: 2075–2078, 1977.
61. GEENEN, J. E., W. J. HOGAN, E. T. STEWART, W. J. DODDS, AND R. C. ARNDORFER. ERCP manometry of the sphincter of Oddi. In: *The Papilla Vateri and Its Diseases*, edited by M. Classen et al. Koln, FRG: Witzstrock, 1979, p. 92–98.
62. GEENEN, J., W. HOGAN, J. TOOULI, W. DODDS, AND R. VENU. A prospective randomized study of the efficacy of endoscopic sphincterotomy for patients with presumptive sphincter of Oddi dysfunction (Abstract). *Gastroenterology* 86: 1086, 1984.
63. GILSDORF, R. B. The effect of simulated gallstones on gall-

bladder pressures and bile flow response to eating. *Surg. Gynecol. Obstet.* 138: 161–168, 1974.
64. GOLDBERG, H. I. Cholecystokinin cholecystography. *Semin. Roentgenol.* 11: 175–179, 1976.
65. GREGG, J. A., AND D. L. CARR-LOCKE. Endoscopic pancreatic and biliary manometry in pancreatic, biliary, and papillary disease, and after endoscopic sphincterotomy and surgical sphincteroplasty. *Gut* 25: 1247–1254, 1984.
66. GUELRUD, M., S. MENDOZA, S. VICENT, M. GOMEZ, AND B. VILLALTA. Pressures in the sphincter of Oddi in patients with gallstones, common duct stones, and recurrent pancreatitis. *J. Clin. Gastroenterol.* 5: 37–41, 1983.
67. GUELRUD, M., AND J. H. SIEGEL. Hypertensive pancreatic duct sphincter as a cause of pancreatitis. *Dig. Dis. Sci.* 29: 225–231, 1984.
68. GULLO, L., L. BOLONDI, P. PRIORI, P. CASANOVA, AND G. LABO. Inhibitory effect of atropine on cholecystokinin-induced gallbladder contraction in man. *Digestion* 29: 209–213, 1984.
69. HALLENBECK, G. A. Biliary and pancreatic intraductal pressures. In: *Handbook of Physiology. Alimentary Canal. Secretion*, edited by C. F. Code. Washington, DC: Am. Physiol. Soc., 1967, sect. 6, vol. II, chapt. 57, p. 1007–1025.
70. HAND, B. H. An anatomical study of the choledochoduodenal area. *Br. J. Surg.* 50: 486–494, 1963.
71. HELM, J. F., J. CHRISTENSEN, W. J. DODDS, AND S. SARNA. Intrinsic innervation of the opossum sphincter of Oddi (SO) (Abstract). *Gastroenterology* 84: 1185, 1983.
72. HELM, J. F., W. J. DODDS, J. CHRISTENSEN, AND S. K. SARNA. Control mechanism of spontaneous in vitro contractions of the opossum sphincter of Oddi. *Am. J. Physiol.* 249 (*Gastrointest. Liver Physiol.* 12): G572–G579, 1985.
73. HESS, W. Manometry and radiography in the biliary system during surgery. In: *Endoscopic Sphincterotomy of the Papilla Vateri*, edited by L. Demling and M. Classen. Littleton, MA: PSG, 1978.
74. HESS, W. Physiology of the sphincter of Oddi. In: *Endoscopic Sphincterotomy of the Papilla Vateri*, edited by L. Demling and M. Classen. Littleton, MA: PSG, 1978.
75. HOGAN, W. J., W. J. DODDS, AND J. E. GEENEN. Motor function of the biliary-duct system. In: *A Guide to Gastrointestinal Motility*, edited by J. Christensen, D. L. Wingate, and R. A. Gregory. Bristol, UK: Wright, 1983, p. 157–197.
76. HOGAN, W. J., J. GEENEN, W. J. DODDS, J. TOOULI, R. VENU, AND J. HELM. Paradoxical motor response to cholecystokinin (CCK-OP) in patients with suspected sphincter of Oddi dysfunction (Abstract). *Gastroenterology* 82: 1085, 1982.
77. HOGAN, W. J., J. E. GEENEN, J. KRUIDENIER, R. VENU, J. HELM, W. J. DODDS, AND S. D. WILSON. Ineffectiveness of conventional sphincteroplasty in relieving pancreatic duct sphincter pressure in patients with idiopathic recurrent pancreatitis (Abstract). *Gastroenterology* 84: 1189, 1983.
78. HOGAN, W. J., J. GEENEN, R. VENU, W. J. DODDS, J. HELM, AND J. TOOULI. Abnormally rapid phasic contractions of the human sphincter of Oddi (tachyoddia) (Abstract). *Gastroenterology* 84: 1189, 1983.
79. HONDA, R., J. TOOULI, W. J. DODDS, S. SARNA, W. J. HOGAN, AND Z. ITOH. Relationship of sphincter of Oddi spike bursts to gastrointestinal myoelectric activity in conscious opossums. *J. Clin. Invest.* 69: 770–778, 1982.
80. HOPTON, D., AND T. T. WHITE. Effect of hepatic and celiac vagal stimulation on common bile-duct pressure. *Am. J. Dig. Dis.* 16: 1095–1101, 1971.
81. HUTTON, S. W., C. E. SIEVERT, JR., J. A. VENNES, AND W. C. DUANE. The effect of sphincterotomy on gallstone formation in the prairie dog. *Gastroenterology* 81: 663–667, 1981.
82. IHASZ, M., AND C. A. GRIFFITH. Gallstones after vagotomy. *Am. J. Surg.* 141: 48–50, 1981.
83. INBERG, M. V., AND M. VUORIO. Human gallbladder function after selective gastric and total abdominal vagotomy. *Acta Chir. Scand.* 135: 625–633, 1969.
84. ISHIOKA, T. Electromyographic study of the choledochoduo-

denal junction and duodenal wall muscle. *Tohoku J. Exp. Med.* 70: 73–84, 1959.
85. ITOH, Z., AND I. TAKAHASHI. Periodic contractions of the canine gallbladder during the interdigestive state. *Am. J. Physiol.* 240 (*Gastrointest. Liver Physiol.* 3): G183–G189, 1981.
86. IVY, A. C., AND E. OLDBERG. A hormone mechanism for gallbladder contraction and evacuation. *Am. J. Physiol.* 86: 599–613, 1928.
87. JANSSON, R., E. THORNELL, AND J. SVANVIK. Effects of indomethacin on gallbladder pressure in patients with acute cholecystitis. *Scand. J. Urol. Nephrol.* 75: 51–53, 1983.
88. JONES, R. S., AND M. I. GROSSMAN. Choleretic effects of cholecystokinin, gastrin II, and caerulein in the dog. *Am. J. Physiol.* 219: 1014–1018, 1970.
89. KELLY, T. R., AND P. E. SWANEY. Gallstone pancreatitis: the second time around. *Surgery St. Louis* 92: 571–575, 1982.
90. KERN, F., JR., G. T. EVERSON, B. DEMARK, C. MCKINLEY, R. SHOWALTER, W. ERFLING, D. Z. BRAVERMAN, P. SZCZEPANIK-VAN LEEUWEN, AND P. D. KLEIN. Biliary lipids, bile acids and gallbladder function in the human female. Effects of pregnancy and the ovulatory cycle. *J. Clin. Invest.* 68: 1229–1242, 1981.
91. KERN, M. K., J. H. LINEHAN, W. J. DODDS, I. TAKAHASHI, AND W. J. HOGAN. Mathematical modeling of pressure-flow kinetics of the opossum sphincter of Oddi (Abstract). *Gastroenterology* 86: 1133, 1984.
92. KRAGLUND, K., J. HJERMIND, F. T. JENSEN, H. STØDKILDE-JØRGENSEN, E. OSTER-JØRGENSEN, AND S. A. PEDERSEN. Gallbladder emptying and gastrointestinal cyclic motor activity in humans. *Scand. J. Gastroenterol.* 19: 990–994, 1984.
93. KRISHNAMURTHY, G. T., V. R. BOBBA, AND E. KINGSTON. Radionuclide ejection fraction: a technique for quantitative analysis of motor function of the human gallbladder. *Gastroenterology* 80: 482–490, 1981.
94. KYOSOLA, K. Cholinesterase histochemistry of the innervation of the smooth muscle sphincters around the terminal intramural part of the ductus choledochus in the cat and the dog. *Acta Physiol. Scand.* 90: 278–280, 1974.
95. KYOSOLA, K. Biliary dyskinesia. *Ann. Chir. Gynaecol. Fenn.* 64: 189–194, 1975.
96. KYOSOLA, K. Adrenergic and cholinergic innervation of the supraduodenal common bile duct. *Am. J. Gastroenterol.* 70: 179–183, 1978.
97. KYOSOLA, K. Sympatho-adrenergic neural control of the sphincter of Oddi of the cat and the dog. *Tohoku J. Exp. Med.* 127: 113–117, 1979.
98. MESHKOLA, K., AND L. RECHARDT. The anatomy and innervation of the sphincter of Oddi in the dog and cat. *Am. J. Anat.* 140: 497–521, 1974.
99. LAMORTE, W. W., D. J. SCHOETZ, JR., D. H. BIRKETT, AND L. F. WILLIAMS, JR. The role of the gallbladder in the pathogenesis of cholesterol gallstones. *Gastroenterology* 77: 580–592, 1979.
100. LAWSON, M., G. T. EVERSON, W. KLINGENSMITH, AND F. KERN, JR. Coordination of gastric and gallbladder emptying after ingestion of a regular meal. *Gastroenterology* 85: 866–870, 1983.
101. LEE, R. G., J. A. GREGG, A. M. KOROSHETZ, T. C. HILL, AND M. E. CLOUSE. Sphincter of Oddi stenosis: diagnosis using hepatobiliary scintigraphy and endoscopic manometry. *Radiology* 156: 793–796, 1985.
102. LEESE, T., J. P. NEOPTOLEMOS, AND D. L. CARR-LOCKE. Successes, failures, early complications and their management following endoscopic sphincterotomy: results in 394 consecutive patients from a single centre. *Br. J. Surg.* 72: 215–219, 1985.
103. LICHTENSTEIN, M. E., AND A. C. IVY. The function of the "valves" of Heister. *Surgery St. Louis* 1: 38–52, 1937.
104. LIEDBERG, G., AND M. HALABI. The effect of vagotomy on flow resistance at the choledocho-duodenal junction. *Acta Chir. Scand.* 136: 208–212, 1970.
105. LILJA, P., C. J. FAGAN, I. WIENER, K. INOUE, L. C. WATSON, P. L. RAYFORD, AND J. C. THOMPSON. Infusion of pure cholecystokinin in humans. *Gastroenterology* 83: 256–261, 1982.
106. LOW-BEER, T. S., R. F. HARVEY, E. R. DAVIES, AND A. F. READ. Abnormalities of serum cholecystokinin and gallbladder emptying in celiac disease. *N. Engl. J. Med.* 292: 961–963, 1975.
107. LUDWICK, J. R., AND P. BASS. Contractile and electric activity of the extrahepatic biliary tract and duodenum. *Surg. Gynecol. Obstet.* 124: 536–546, 1967.
108. MACPHERSON, B. R., G. W. SCOTT, J. P. CHANSOURIA, AND A. W. FISHER. The muscle layer of the canine gallbladder and cystic duct. *Acta Anat.* 120: 117–122, 1984.
109. MANN, F. C. A comparative study of the anatomy of the sphincter at the duodenal end of the common bile-duct with special reference to species of animals without a gall-bladder. *Anat. Rec.* 18: 355–360, 1920.
110. MANN, F. C. A study of the tonicity of the sphincter at the duodenal end of the common bile duct. *J. Lab. Clin. Med.* 5: 107–110, 1920.
111. MATON, P. N., A. C. SELDEN, M. L. FITZPATRICK, AND V. S. CHADWICK. Infusion of cholecystokinin octapeptide in man: relation between plasma cholecystokinin concentrations and gallbladder emptying rates. *Eur. J. Clin. Invest.* 14: 37–41, 1984.
112. MATON, P. N., A. C. SELDEN, M. L. FITZPATRICK, AND V. S. CHADWICK. Defective gallbladder emptying and cholecystokinin release in celiac disease. *Gastroenterology* 88: 391–396, 1985.
113. MATSUMOTO, T., S. K. SARNA, AND R. E. CONDON. Gallbladder electrical activity in vivo (Abstract). *Gastroenterology* 88: 1493, 1985.
114. MATSUMOTO, T., S. K. SARNA, R. E. CONDON, AND W. J. DODDS. Gallbladder cyclic motor activity (Abstract). *Gastroenterology* 88: 1493, 1985.
115. MAUDGAL, D. P., R. M. KUPFER, P. L. ZENTLER-MUNRO, AND T. C. NORTHFIELD. Postprandial gallbladder emptying in patients with gall stones. *Br. Med. J.* 280: 141–143, 1980.
116. MCMASTER, P. D., AND R. ELMAN. On the expulsion of bile by the gallbladder and a reciprocal relationship with the sphincter activity. *J. Exp. Med.* 44: 173–198, 1926.
117. MELTZER, S. J. The disturbance of the law of contrary innervation as a pathogenetic factor in the diseases of the bile ducts and the gall bladder. *Am. J. Med. Sci.* 153: 469–477, 1917.
118. MESHKINPOUR, H., M. MOLLOT, G. B. ECKERLING, AND L. BOOKMAN. Bile duct dyskinesia. A clinical and manometric study. *Gastroenterology* 87: 759–762, 1984.
119. MOK, H. Y., K. VON BERGMANN, AND S. M. GRUNDY. Kinetics of the enterohepatic circulation during fasting: biliary lipid secretion and gallbladder storage. *Gastroenterology* 78: 1023–1033, 1980.
120. MOODY, F. G., J. M. BECKER, AND J. R. POTTS. Transduodenal sphincteroplasty and transampullary septectomy for postcholecystectomy pain. *Ann. Surg.* 197: 627–636, 1983.
121. MUELLER, P. R., J. T. FERRUCCI, JR., J. F. SIMEONE, E. VAN SONNENBERG, D. A. HALL, AND J. WITTENBERG. Observations on the distensibility of the common bile duct. *Radiology* 142: 467–472, 1982.
122. MULLER, E. L., M. A. LEWINSKI, AND H. A. PITT. The cholecysto-sphincter of Oddi reflex. *J. Surg. Res.* 36: 377–383, 1984.
123. NAKAYAMA, S., AND H. FUKUDA. Conduction of activity between muscles in the terminal region of the common bile duct and in the neighboring duodenum. *Acta Med. Okayama* 30: 21–35, 1976.
124. NARDI, G. L. Papillitis and stenosis of the sphincter of Oddi. *Surg. Clin. N. Am.* 53: 1149–1160, 1973.
125. NATHAN, M. H., A. NEWMAN, J. MCFARLAND, AND D. J.

MURRAY. Cholecystokinin cholecystography. *Radiology* 93: 1–8, 1969.
126. NEBEL, O. T. Manometric evaluation of the papilla of Vater. *Gastrointest. Endosc.* 21: 126–128, 1975.
127. NESCHIS, M., M. C. KING, AND R. A. MURPHY. Cholecystokinin cholecystography in the diagnosis of acalculous extrahepatic biliary tract disorders. *Am. J. Gastroenterol.* 70: 593–599, 1978.
127a. NETTER, F. H. *The CIBA Collection of Medical Illustrations.* Summit, NJ: Ciba Pharm., 1953, vol. 5, pt. 3.
128. NORTHFIELD, T. C., R. M. KUPFER, D. P. MAUDGAL, P. L. ZENTLER-MUNRO, S. T. MELLER, N. W. GARVIE, AND R. MCCREADY. Gall-bladder sensitivity to cholecystokinin in patients with gall stones. *Br. Med. J.* 280: 143–144, 1980.
129. NOVIS, B. H., P. C. BORNMAN, A. W. GIRDWOOD, AND I. N. MARKS. Endoscopic manometry of the pancreatic duct and sphincter zone in patients with chronic pancreatitis. *Dig. Dis. Sci.* 30: 225–228, 1985.
130. O'BRIEN, J. J., E. A. SHAFFER, L. F. WILLIAMS, JR., D. M. SMALL, J. LYNN, AND J. WITTENBERG. A physiological model to study gallbladder function in primates. *Gastroenterology* 67: 119–125, 1974.
131. ODDI, R. D'une disposition a sphincter de l'ouverture du canal choledogue. *Arch. Ital. Biol.* 8: 317–322, 1887. [Transl. from Italian] *J. Gastroenterol.* 17: 109–111, 1985.
132. ONO, K., N. WATANABE, K. SUZUKI, H. TSUCHIDA, Y. SUGIYAMA, AND M. ABO. Bile flow mechanism in man. *Arch. Surg.* 96: 869–874, 1968.
133. OPIE, E. L. The etiology of acute hemorrhagic pancreatitis. *Johns Hopkins Hosp. Bull.* 12: 182–188, 1901.
134. OSTER, M. J., A. CSENDES, P. FUNCH-JENSEN, AND H. SKJOLDBORG. Intraoperative pressure measurements of the choledochoduodenal junction, common bile duct, cysticocholedochal junction and gallbladder in humans. *Surg. Gynecol. Obstet.* 150: 385–389, 1980.
135. OTTO, W. J., G. W. SCOTT, AND C. M. RODKIEWICZ. A comparison of resistances to flow through the cystic duct and the sphincter of Oddi. *J. Surg. Res.* 27: 68–72, 1979.
136. PARRY, E. W., G. A. HALLENBECK, AND J. H. GRINDLAY. Pressures in the pancreatic and common ducts. *Arch. Surg.* 70: 757–765, 1955.
137. PEETERS, T. L., G. R. VANTRAPPEN, AND J. JANSSENS. Bile acid output and the interdigestive migrating motor complex in normals and in cholecystectomy patients. *Gastroenterology* 79: 678–681, 1980.
138. PERSSON, C. G. Adrenergic, cholecystokinetic and morphine-induced effects on extra-hepatic biliary motility. *Acta Physiol. Scand. Suppl.* 383: 1–32, 1972.
139. PERSSON, C. G. Inhibitory innervation of cat sphincter of Oddi. *Br. J. Pharmacol.* 58: 479–482, 1976.
140. PITT, H. A., J. E. DOTY, AND L. DENBESTEN. Increased intragallbladder pressure response to cholecystectokinin-octapeptide following vagotomy and pyloroplasty. *J. Surg. Res.* 35: 325–331, 1983.
141. PITT, H. A., J. E. DOTY, L. DENBESTEN, AND S. L. KUCHENBECKER. Stasis before gallstone formation: altered gallbladder compliance or cystic duct resistance? *Am. J. Surg.* 143: 144–149, 1982.
142. PITT, H. A., J. E. DOTY, J. J. ROSLYN, AND L. DENBESTEN. The role of altered extrahepatic biliary function in the pathogenesis of gallstones after vagotomy. *Surgery St. Louis* 90: 418–425, 1981.
143. PITT, H. A., J. J. ROSLYN, S. L. KUCHENBECKER, J. E. DOTY, AND L. DENBESTEN. The role of cystic duct resistance in the pathogenesis of cholesterol gallstones. *J. Surg. Res.* 30: 508–514, 1981.
144. POMERANZ, I. S., AND E. A. SHAFFER. Abnormal gallbladder emptying in a subgroup of patients with gallstones. *Gastroenterology* 88: 787–791, 1985.
145. RAPTOPOULOS, V., T. M. FABIAN, W. SILVA, C. J. D'ORSI, A. KARELLAS, C. C. COMPTON, F. J. KROLIKOWSKI, P. DOHERTY, AND E. H. SMITH. The effect of time and cholecystectomy of experimental biliary tree dilatation. *Invest. Radiol.* 20: 276–286, 1985.
146. RICHTER, J. M., R. H. SCHAPIRO, A. G. MULLEY, AND A. L. WARSHAW. Association of pancreas divisum and pancreatitis, and its treatment by sphincteroplasty of the accessory ampulla. *Gastroenterology* 81: 1104–1110, 1981.
147. ROSCH, W., H. KOCH, AND L. DEMLING. Manometric studies during ERCP and endoscopic papillotomy. *Endoscopy* 8: 30–33, 1976.
148. ROSLYN, J. J., H. A. PITT, L. L. MANN, M. E. AMENT, AND L. DENBESTEN. Gallbladder disease in patients on long-term parenteral nutrition. *Gastroenterology* 84: 148–154, 1983.
149. ROUS, P., AND P. D. MCMASTER. The concentrating activity of the gallbladder. *J. Exp. Med.* 34: 47–73, 1921.
150. RUCKEBUSCH, Y., AND G. SOLDANI. Gallbladder motility in sheep: effects of cholecystokinin and related peptides. *J. Vet. Pharm. Ther.* 8: 263–269, 1985.
151. RUDICK, J., AND J. S. HUTCHISON. Evaluation of vagotomy and biliary function by combined oral cholecystography and intravenous cholangiography. *Ann. Surg.* 162: 234–240, 1965.
152. RYAN, J. P. Motility of the gallbladder and biliary tree. In: *Physiology of the Gastrointestinal Tract*, edited by L. R. Johnson. New York: Raven, 1981, p. 473–494.
153. RYAN, J. P. Effect of pregnancy on gallbladder contractility in the guinea pig. *Gastroenterology* 87: 674–678, 1984.
154. RYAN, T., C. A. PELLEGRINI, AND L. W. WAY. Bile kinetics during fasting in the prairie dog (Abstract). *Gastroenterology* 84: 1292, 1983.
155. RYAN, J. P., AND S. RYAVE. Effect of vasoactive intestinal polypeptide on gallbladder smooth muscle in vitro. *Am. J. Physiol.* 234 (*Endocrinol. Metab. Gastrointest. Physiol.* 3): E44–E46, 1978.
156. SALDUCCI, J., B. NAUDI, G. PIN, F. RANIERI, AND H. MONGES. Papilla electromyography: endoluminal recording performed in many by perduodenoscopic cannulation. In: *The Sphincter of Oddi*, edited by J. Delmont. New York: Karger, 1976, p. 77–79. (Proc. Gastroenterol. Symp., 3rd, Nice, Italy.)
157. SALIK, J. O., C. I. SIEGEL, AND A. I. MENDELOFF. Biliary-duodenal dynamics in man. *Radiology* 106: 1–11, 1973.
158. SARLES, J. C., P. DELECOURT, H. CASTELLO, L. GAETA, M. NACCHIERO, J. P. AMOROS, M. A. DEVAUX, AND R. AWAD. Action of gastrointestinal hormones on the myoelectric activity of the sphincter of Oddi in living rabbit. *Regul. Pept.* 2: 113–124, 1981.
159. SARLES, J. C., P. DELECOURT, M. A. DEVAUX, J. P. AMOROS, J. C. GUICHENEY, AND E. WUNSCH. In vivo effect of 13 Leu motilin on the electric activity of the rabbit sphincter of Oddi. *Horm. Metab. Res.* 13: 340–342, 1981.
160. SARLES, J. C., A. MIDEJEAN, AND M. A. DEVAUX. Electromyography of the sphincter of Oddi. *Am. J. Gastroenterol.* 63: 221–231, 1975.
161. SARVA, R. P., D. P. SHREINER, D. VAN THIEL, AND N. YINGVORAPANT. Gallbladder function: methods for measuring filling and emptying. *J. Nucl. Med.* 26: 140–144, 1985.
162. SAUERBRUCH, T., F. STELLAARD, AND G. PAUMGARTNER. Effect of endoscopic sphincterotomy on bile acid pool size and bile lipid composition in man. *Digestion* 27: 87–92, 1983.
163. SCHEIN, C. J., AND T. C. BENEVENTANO. Choledochal dynamics in man. *Surg. Gynecol. Obstet.* 126: 591–596, 1968.
164. SCHEIN, C. J., AND M. L. GLIEDMAN. The influence of vagotomy on the normal and diseased gallbladder. *Digestion* 3: 243–250, 1970.
165. SCHESKE, G. A., P. L. COOPERBERG, M. M. COHEN, AND H. J. BURHENNE. Dynamic changes in the caliber of the major bile ducts related to obstruction. *Radiology* 135: 215–216, 1980.
166. SCHOETZ, D. J., JR., W. W. LAMORTE, W. E. WISE, D. H. BIRKETT, AND L. F. WILLIAMS, JR. Mechanical properties of primate gallbladder: description by a dynamic method. *Am. J.*

Physiol. 241 (Gastrointest. Liver Physiol. 4): G376–G381, 1981.
167. SCOTT, G. W., AND W. J. OTTO. Resistance and sphincter-like properties of the cystic duct. Surg. Gynecol. Obstet. 149: 177–182, 1979.
168. SCOTT, G. W., R. E. SMALLWOOD, AND S. ROWLANDS. Flow through the bile duct after cholecystectomy. Surg. Gynecol. Obstet. 140: 912–918, 1975.
169. SCOTT, R. B., S. M. STRASBERG, T. Y. EL-SHARKAWY, AND N. E. DIAMANT. Regulation of the fasting enterohepatic circulation of bile acids by the migrating myoelectric complex in dogs. J. Clin. Invest. 71: 644–654, 1983.
170. SCOTT, R. B., S. M. STRASBERG, T. Y. EL-SHARKAWY, AND N. E. DIAMANT. Fasting canine biliary secretion and the sphincter of Oddi. Gastroenterology 87: 793–804, 1984.
171. SHAFFER, E. A., P. McORMOND, AND H. DUGGAN. Quantitative cholescintigraphy: assessment of gallbladder filling and emptying and duodenogastric reflux. Gastroenterology 79: 899–906, 1980.
172. SHAWKER, T. H., B. L. JONES, AND M. E. GIRTON. Distal common bile duct obstruction: an experimental study in monkeys. J. Clin. Ultrasound 9: 77–82, 1981.
173. SILVA, G. S. P. A simple method for computing the volume of the human gallbladder. Radiology 52: 94–102, 1949.
174. SIMEONE, J. F., R. J. BUTCH, P. R. MUELLER, E. VAN SONNENBERG, J. T. FERRUCCI, JR., D. A. HALL, D. B. KOPANS, S. L. DAWSON, J. WITTENBERG, AND K. McCARTHY. The bile ducts after a fatty meal: further sonographic observations. Radiology 154: 763–768, 1985.
175. SIMEONE, J. F., P. R. MUELLER, J. T. FERRUCCI, JR., E. VAN SONNENBERG, D. A. HALL, J. WITTENBERG, C. C. NEFF, AND R. C. O'CONNELL. Sonography of the bile ducts after a fatty meal: an aid in detection of obstruction. Radiology 143: 211–215, 1982.
176. SLATER, G., P. I. TARTTER, D. DREILING, A. H. AUFSES, JR., J. RUDICK, D. DELMAN, AND W. BLESSER. Resistance of the canine common bile duct. Bull. NY Acad. Med. 59: 711–720, 1983.
177. SLOTA, T., J. E. GEENEN, W. J. HOGAN, E. T. STEWART, AND W. J. DODDS. The fate of common bile duct (CBD) calculi following endoscopic sphincterotomy (ES): the role of incision length and stone diameter (Abstract). Gastrointest. Endosc. 25: 50, 1979.
178. SOON-SHIONG, P., K. L. COX, G. L. ROSENQUIST, C. IWAHASHI-HOSODA, AND H. CARR. Evidence of a noncholecystokinin stimulant of gallbladder contraction: comparison of fasting serum concentrations in healthy subjects and in patients with gallstones. Am. J. Surg. 149: 163–166, 1985.
179. SPELLMAN, S. J., E. A. SHAFFER, AND L. ROSENTHALL. Gallbladder emptying in response to cholecystokinin. A cholescintigraphic study. Gastroenterology 77: 115–120, 1979.
180. STASIEWICZ, J., AND K. G. WORMSLEY. Functional control of the biliary tract. Acta Hepato-Gastroenterol. 21: 450–468, 1974.
181. STRASBERG, S. M., R. N. REDINGER, D. M. SMALL, AND R. H. EGDAHL. The effect of elevated biliary tract pressure on biliary lipid metabolism and bile flow in nonhuman primates. J. Lab. Clin. Med. 99: 342–353, 1982.
182. SUNDLER, F., J. ALUMETS, R. HÅKANSON, S. INGEMANSSON, J. FAHRENKRUG, AND O. SCHAFFALITZKY DE MUCKADELL. VIP innervation of the gallbladder (Eng. Abstract). Gastroenterology 72: 1375–1377, 1977.
183. SUZUKI, T., I. TAKAHASHI, AND Z. ITOH. Motilin and gallbladder: new dimensions in gastrointestinal physiology. Peptides Fayetteville 2: 229–233, 1981.
184. SVANVIK, J., B. ALLEN, C. PELLEGRINI, R. BERNHOFT, AND L. WAY. Variations in concentrating function of the gallbladder in the conscious monkey. Gastroenterology 86: 919–925, 1984.
185. SVANVIK, J., AND R. JANSSON. An experimental method for studying in vivo gallbladder absorption. Gastroenterology 72: 634–638, 1977.
186. SVENBERG, T., N. D. CHRISTOFIDES, M. L. FITZPATRIC, F. AREOLA-ORTIZ, S. R. BLOOM, AND R. B. WELBOURN. Interdigestive biliary output in man: relationship to fluctuations in plasma motilin and effect of atropine. Gut 23: 1024–1028, 1982.
187. TAKAHASHI, I., W. J. DODDS, W. J. HOGAN, K. BAKER, AND Z. ITOH. Effect of vagotomy on changes in gallbladder volume during fasting and after feeding in the conscious opossum (Abstract). Gastroenterology 86: 1273, 1984.
188. TAKAHASHI, I., W. J. DODDS, W. J. HOGAN, R. LAYMAN, AND Z. ITOH. Effect of proglumide on biliary-tract contractile activity in the opossum (Abstract). Gastroenterology 86: 1274, 1984.
189. TAKAHASHI, I., W. J. DODDS, W. J. HOGAN, AND Z. ITOH. Effect of migrating myoelectric activity on the hepatic secretion of bile in the opossum (Abstract). Gastroenterology 86: 1273, 1984.
190. TAKAHASHI, I., W. J. DODDS, Z. ITOH, W. J. HOGAN, AND M. K. KERN. Influence of transsphincteric fluid flow on spike burst rate of the opossum sphincter of Oddi. Gastroenterology 87: 1292–1298, 1984.
191. TAKAHASHI, I., R. HONDA, W. J. DODDS, S. SARNA, J. TOOULI, Z. ITOH, W. Y. CHEY, W. J. HOGAN, D. GREIFF, AND K. BAKER. Effect of motilin on the opossum upper gastrointestinal tract and sphincter of Oddi. Am. J. Physiol. 245 (Gastrointest. Liver Physiol. 8): G476–G481, 1983.
192. TAKAHASHI, I., M. K. KERN, W. J. DODDS, W. J. HOGAN, S. SARNA, K. H. SOERGEL, AND Z. ITOH. Contraction pattern of opossum gallbladder during fasting and after feeding. Am. J. Physiol. 250 (Gastrointest. Liver Physiol. 13): G227–G235, 1986.
193. TAKAHASHI, I., M. NAKAYA, T. SUZUKI, AND Z. ITOH. Postprandial changes in contractile activity and bile concentration in gallbladder of the dog. Am. J. Physiol. 243 (Gastrointest. Liver Physiol. 6): G365–G371, 1982.
194. TAKAHASHI, I., T. SUZUKI, I. AIZAWA, AND Z. ITOH. Comparison of gallbladder contractions induced by motilin and cholecystokinin in dogs. Gastroenterology 82: 419–424, 1982.
195. TANAKA, M., S. IKEDA, AND F. NAKAYAMA. Continuous measurement of common bile duct pressure with an indwelling microtransducer catheter introduced by duodenoscopy: new diagnostic aid for postcholecystectomy dyskinesia—a preliminary report. Gastrointest. Endosc. 29: 83–88, 1983.
196. TANAKA, M., S. IKEDA, AND F. NAKAYAMA. Change in bile duct pressure responses after cholecystectomy: loss of gallbladder as a pressure reservoir. Gastroenterology 87: 1154–1159, 1984.
197. TANSY, M. F., D. L. INNES, J. S. MARTIN, AND F. M. KENDALL. The role of the intramural common bile duct in the filling of the canine gallbladder. Surg. Gynecol. Obstet. 139: 585–592, 1974.
198. TANSY, M. F., R. C. MACKOWIAK, AND R. B. CHAFFEE. A vagosympathetic pathway capable of influencing common bile duct motility in the dog. Surg. Gynecol. Obstet. 133: 225–236, 1971.
199. TANSY, M. F., L. SALKIN, D. L. INNES, J. S. MARTIN, F. M. KENDALL, AND D. LITWACK. The mucosal lining of the intramural common bile duct as a determinant of ductal opening pressure. Am. J. Dig. Dis. 20: 613–625, 1975.
200. THOMPSON, J. C., G. M. FRIED, W. D. OGDEN, C. J. FAGAN, K. INOUE, I. WIENER, AND L. C. WATSON. Correlation between release of cholecystokinin and contraction of the gallbladder in patients with gallstones. Ann. Surg. 195: 670–676, 1982.
201. THUNE, A., E. THORNELL, AND J. SVANVIK. Flow resistance in the choledocho-duodenal junction is regulated by distending pressure in the biliary tract (Abstract). Gastroenterology 88: 1615, 1985.
202. TOOULI, J., J. DENT, M. BUSHELL, A. WYCHERLEY, AND G. STEVENSON. Gallbladder (GB) emptying in relation to duodenal interdigestive migrating motor contractions (MMC) (Abstract). Gastroenterology 88: 1616, 1985.
203. TOOULI, J., W. J. DODDS, R. HONDA, AND W. J. HOGAN.

Effect of histamine on motor function of opossum sphincter of Oddi. *Am. J. Physiol.* 241 (*Gastrointest. Liver Physiol.* 4): G122–G128, 1981.
204. TOOULI, J., W. J. DODDS, R. HONDA, S. SARNA, W. J. HOGAN, R. A. KOMOROWSKI, J. H. LINEHAN, AND R. C. ARNDORFER. Motor function of the opossum sphincter of Oddi. *J. Clin. Invest.* 71: 208–220, 1983.
205. TOOULI, J., J. E. GEENEN, W. J. HOGAN, W. J. DODDS, AND R. C. ARNDORFER. Sphincter of Oddi motor activity: a comparison between patients with common bile duct stones and controls. *Gastroenterology* 82: 111–117, 1982.
206. TOOULI, J., W. J. HOGAN, J. E. GEENEN, W. J. DODDS, AND R. C. ARNDORFER. Action of cholecystokinin-octapeptide on sphincter of Oddi basal pressure and phasic wave activity in humans. *Surgery St. Louis* 92: 497–503, 1982.
207. TOOULI, J., I. C. ROBERTS-THOMSON, J. DENT, AND J. LEE. Manometric disorders in patients with suspected sphincter of Oddi dysfunction. *Gastroenterology* 88: 1243–1250, 1985.
208. VAN DER LINDEN, W., AND V. KEMPI. Filling of the gallbladder as studied by computer-assisted Tc-99m HIDA scintigraphy: concise communication. *J. Nucl. Med.* 25: 292–298, 1984.
209. VANTRAPPEN, G. The migrating myoelectric complex. In: *Motility of the Digestive Tract*, edited by M. Wienbeck. New York: Raven, 1982, p. 157–167.
210. WHITAKER, L. R. The mechanism of the gall bladder. *Am. J. Physiol.* 78: 411–436, 1926.
211. WIENER, I., K. INOUE, C. J. FAGAN, P. LILJA, L. C. WATSON, AND J. C. THOMPSON. Release of cholecystokinin in man: correlation of blood levels with gallbladder contraction. *Ann. Surg.* 194: 321–327, 1981.
212. WILLIAMS, R. D., J. C. FISH, AND D. D. WILLIAMS. The significance of biliary pressure. *Arch. Surg.* 95: 374–379, 1967.
213. WILLIAMS, R. D., AND T. T. HUANG. The effect of vagotomy on biliary pressure. *Surgery St. Louis* 66: 353–356, 1969.
214. WINKELSTEIN, A. Some observations on the entrance of bile into the duodenum. *Surg. Gynecol. Obstet.* 40: 545–547, 1925.
215. WINKELSTEIN, A., AND P. W. ASCHNER. The mechanism of the flow of bile from the liver into the intestines. *Am. J. Med. Sci.* 171: 104–111, 1926.
216. WYATT, A. P. The relationship of the sphincter of Oddi to the stomach, duodenum and gall-bladder. *J. Physiol. Lond.* 193: 225–243, 1967.
217. YAMASATO, T. Physiological and pharmacological studies on the motility of the bile duct in the chicken. *Jpn. J. Smooth Muscle Res.* 10: 287–297, 1974.
218. YAU, W. M., AND M. L. YOUTHER. Modulation of gallbladder motility by intrinsic cholinergic neurons. *Am. J. Physiol.* 247 (*Gastrointest. Liver Physiol.* 10): G662–G666, 1984.
219. ZEMAN, R. K., K. J. TAYLOR, A. T. ROSENFIELD, A. SCHWARTZ, AND J. A. GOLD. Acute experimental biliary obstruction in the dog: sonographic findings and clinical implications. *Am. J. Roentgenol. Radium Ther. Nucl. Med.* 136: 965–967, 1981.

CHAPTER 29

# Pharmacology of biliary tract

JOSE BEHAR | Department of Medicine, Rhode Island Hospital and Brown
PIERO BIANCANI | University, Providence, Rhode Island

CHAPTER CONTENTS

Anatomic and Physiological Considerations
Pharmacological Considerations
Cholinergic Drugs
Adrenergic Drugs
Autacoids
    Prostaglandins
    Serotonin
    Histamine
Neuropeptides
    Cholecystokinin-gastrin family of peptides
    Gastrin
    Caerulein
    Secretin, vasoactive intestinal polypeptide, glucagon, and gastrointestinal inhibitory polypeptide family
    Somatostatin and bombesin
    Opiates
    Motilin
    Pancreatic polypeptide
    Sex hormones
    Substance P

PHARMACOLOGICAL METHODS have been extensively used as research tools to characterize physiological and pathophysiological processes in the biliary tract and to a lesser extent to develop therapeutic modalities designed to correct its motor disorders. However, an in-depth review of many of these pharmacological studies reveals important shortcomings in the experimental designs of some studies and frequent discrepancies in their results. Moreover, the significance of the studies to human physiology and pharmacology is often unclear because some animal models may not be relevant to humans. This large body of pharmacological data becomes more intelligible, however, when the appropriate anatomic, physiological, and pharmacological considerations are considered. Thus awareness of marked differences among animal species and among experimental methods used in these studies may sometimes allow reconciliation of some of these differences.

Nevertheless the data so far generated by these studies constitute an important first step on which future studies of the gallbladder and sphincter of Oddi should be based to define drug receptors, elucidate the nature of neurotransmitters, employ specific pharmacological methods, and develop drugs capable of correcting their motility disorders.

## ANATOMIC AND PHYSIOLOGICAL CONSIDERATIONS

The biliary tract, more than any other segment of the gastrointestinal tract, exhibits marked anatomic and physiological variations among different animal species. Some species do not contain a gallbladder (176–178); others have gallbladders with varying degrees of contractility (129). Even greater species differences are found in the sphincter of Oddi (110, 111). The choledochal sphincter resistance tends to be weak in animals without a gallbladder; in animals with a gallbladder, the resistance is stronger (129). Generally, however, there appear to be two types of sphincter of Oddi. One type is found in predominantly herbivorous animals that eat for most of the time while awake such as the opossum (93), rabbit, and guinea pig (44). These species have a relatively long sphincter of Oddi that is mostly extraduodenal with a clear peristaltic motor activity that facilitates bile flow through the sphincter (57, 93). This type of sphincter responds to cholecystokinin (CCK) with contraction (142, 236, 262) and contracts weakly or even relaxes in response to the opiate alkaloid morphine [(14); W. J. Dodds, personal communication]. Dubois (93) observed that the infusion of egg yolk and cream meal in the opossum duodenum induced gallbladder contraction and peristalsis of distal ductus choledochus followed by discharge of bile. The other type is found in predominantly carnivorous animals, such as cat, dog, and humans, that eat infrequently but have large meals (45, 46. 96). They have a relatively short sphincter of Oddi with intramural (intraduodenal) and extramural portions. The motor activity of the sphincter of Oddi is characterized by low tonic pressures and forceful phasic contractions that in the cat and human are inversely related to transphincteric bile flow (30, 242). This sphincteric resistance to bile flow facilitates gallbladder filling, because placement of an indwelling cannula in the sphincteric region impedes gallbladder filling (74, 173, 273). In these species, the sphincter relaxes in response to CCK (23, 105, 233) and is very sensitive to the opiate alkaloid morphine, responding with a marked increase in the frequency and force of the phasic contractions. Most of these anatomic and physiological characteristics of the sphincter of Oddi of carnivorous animals are similar to those of the human sphincter of Oddi (33), which in the interdigestive phase exhibits a sustained resistance to the flow of bile; after ingestion of egg yolk, the resistance of the sphincter drops slowly (34). These important differences between herbivorous and carnivorous animals should be considered when experimental results, including responses to drugs, are compared among different species or extrapolated to humans.

The functional consequences of these anatomic and physiological differences, however, are not fully understood at this time. Thus the functional relationship between the sphincter of Oddi more activity, bile flow, and gallbladder filling and storage requires further studies. It is tempting, however, to speculate that in herbivorous animals the sphincter of Oddi propulsive activity may facilitate biliary flow to compensate for a weak CCK release from the low dietary fat content and weak gallbladder contraction; in carnivorous animals, including humans, the sphincter of Oddi behaves like sphincter impeding flow (30, 33, 202) and enabling adequate gallbladder filling of bile to be utilized in the digestive phase (184).

## PHARMACOLOGICAL CONSIDERATIONS

Drugs do not create new physiological functions but only modify existent basal and stimulated physiological processes by increasing or decreasing their activity. Frequently drugs stimulate or antagonize these physiological processes at more than one site and therefore full understanding of a response to a drug can only be obtained by careful physiological and pharmacological analysis. This is particularly true in the biliary tract. If the effect of a drug on bile flow is measured in experimental preparations with the entire biliary tract in vivo, the gallbladder and the sphincter of Oddi may respond in parallel or opposite directions depending on the animal species. Even within the gallbladder or the sphincter of Oddi, a given drug may act on more than one receptor, and therefore the observed response will result from the algebraic sum of the actions of activated receptors. Furthermore, because of differences in receptor affinities and pharmacokinetics, the type of response may also vary with time. Initially the effect on one type of receptor may predominate with high drug concentrations, whereas a second receptor may determine the subsequent event in response to lower concentrations. It is therefore not uncommon to see biphasic responses such as contraction followed by relaxation, or vice versa. Drug actions therefore should be studied continuously over time. Even a monophasic response may involve more than one receptor, because it may result from the activation of two or more receptors. The predominance of one receptor type over others may vary not only from species to species but also from animal to animal, even in the same animal species. Thus individual animals may respond in an unexpected manner because of differences in receptor populations. Only when experimental observations are interpreted in this context apparent contradictions may be resolved and mechanisms of drug actions may be clarified and applied to human physiology and pharmacology. In the interpretation of a drug effect, we also have to pay attention to the experimental conditions, i.e., whether the animals are studied in the conscious (digestive or interdigestive phase) or anesthetized state, whether the experiments are acute or chronic, and whether they are in vivo or in vitro (84). Only when drugs are studied in different experimental preparations can we fully understand their mechanism of action.

If these considerations are taken into account, dose-response studies with specific agonists and antagonists should allow definition of mechanisms of action, sites of action, and receptor types and subtypes of unknown compounds (259). The data obtained from the use of specific agonists and antagonists, however, should also be interpreted with caution. For example, a true antagonist should block a drug effect by competitive mechanisms by binding to receptors without initiating a biological action. Other drugs, however, may antagonize a drug effect by behaving as physiological antagonists, initiating actions that simply oppose those of the agonist being tested or by interfering with the action of the agonist at sites other than its receptor. Moreover a specific antagonist may inhibit the action of an unknown agent by blocking release of the neurotransmitter or by occupying receptors that mediate the action of a substance released by this agent. A typical example is shown with naloxone, which is a specific opiate antagonist that also blocks the effect of motilin on the cat sphincter of Oddi because this effect is mediated by opioid peptides (27).

A selective group of nonspecific blockers can also be useful in defining the site of drug action. One example is the neurotoxin tetrodotoxin (TTX), which is a poison widely used to distinguish between neurally mediated drug effects and those that result from direct action on the smooth muscle (143). Tetrodotoxin blocks axonal propagation of action potentials because it blocks fast sodium channels without affecting smooth muscle function (106). Like other antagonists, TTX can stimulate or inhibit smooth muscle activity indirectly by denervating a predominantly tonic inhibitory or excitatory innervation. An example of this type of indirect effect is shown in Figure 1, which shows that TTX induces a marked increase in sphincter of Oddi motor activity.

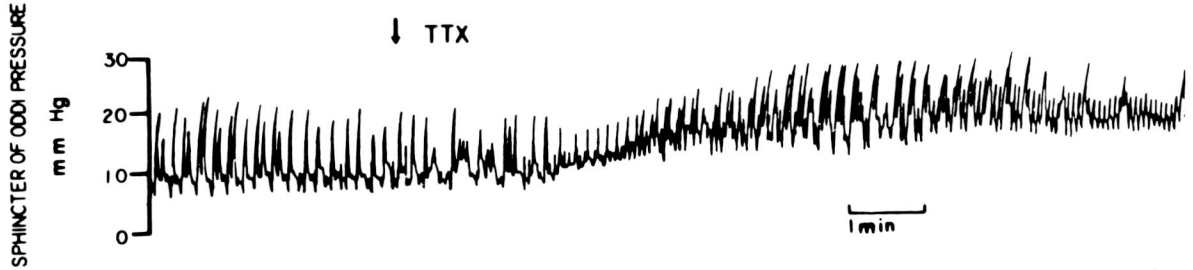

FIG. 1. Effect of tetrodotoxin (TTX) on cat sphincter of Oddi. Marked increase in sphincter of Oddi motor activity is observed after intravenous administration of TTX. [From Behar and Biancani (23).]

TABLE 1. *Effect of Cholinergic and Anticholinergic Drugs on Basal Gallbladder and Sphincter of Oddi Motor Activity*

| | Gallbladder | | | | | | Sphincter of Oddi | | | | | |
|---|---|---|---|---|---|---|---|---|---|---|---|---|
| | Human | Dog | Cat | Guinea pig | Rabbit | Opossum | Human | Dog | Cat | Guinea pig | Rabbit | Opossum |
| Bethanechol | C | C | C | C | C | C | C | C | C | C | C | C |
| Nicotine | * | | C | | | | | | R | | | |
| Atropine | | | R | | | | * | ? | *† | * | * | * |
| Hexamethonium | | | R | | | | | | C‡ | | | |

C, contraction; R, relaxation.　　* No effect.　　† No effect alone.　　‡ Contraction is brief.

Receptor subtypes can be recognized by investigating the structure-activity relationships with analogues of agonists and antagonists. Receptors can be further defined by careful binding studies with radioligands and by isolation and identification of receptors (260). Finally, drug action can be fully understood as the intracellular mechanisms are determined and coupled to receptor activation.

## CHOLINERGIC DRUGS

Cholinergic drugs cause excitation of the gallbladder muscle by direct and indirect actions (Table 1). Muscarinic agonists such as acetylcholine, bethanechol, and carbachol cause gallbladder contraction in all animal species that have been studied [Fig. 2; (23, 82, 155, 175)]. Bethanechol acts directly at receptors located on the smooth muscle because this effect is not prevented by TTX (23). This cholinergic agent, at least in the guinea pig and cat, activates muscarinic receptors because they are specifically blocked by atropine. Muscarinic receptor subtypes, however, are not yet known because no specific $M_1$ or $M_2$ blockers have been used.

Nicotinic receptors of acetylcholine have also been demonstrated in the cat gallbladder in vivo because nicotine causes gallbladder contraction, which is blocked by the ganglionic blocker hexamethonium (23). In contrast, in the in vitro human gallbladder, nicotine has no effect (175). It is not known, however, whether this lack of nicotinic effect is related to spe-

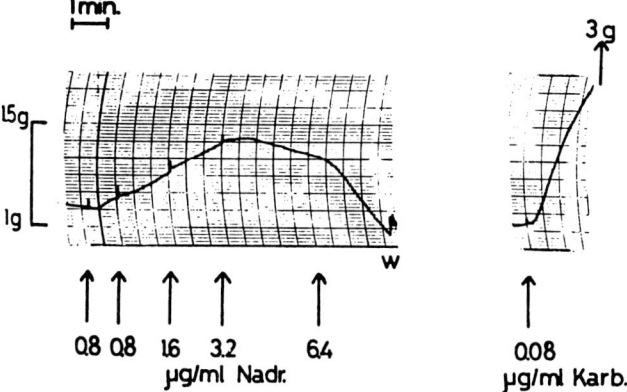

FIG. 2. Carbachol (Karb) causes marked contraction of cat gallbladder strips (*right*) that was of greater magnitude than contraction observed with norepinephrine (Nadr) after propranolol (*left*). [From Persson (207).]

cies differences or to different experimental conditions. Furthermore nicotine does not stimulate nonadrenergic, noncholinergic inhibitory neurons in the gallbladder as it does in other gastrointestinal smooth muscle preparations (23, 218). Not infrequently ganglionic agonists stimulate both excitatory and inhibitory neurons with the combined net effect that results in muscle contraction. The inhibitory action is unmasked only when the excitatory effect is blocked with atropine. In the cat gallbladder, however, nicotine-induced contraction was blocked by atropine, which did not unmask a relaxation (24). The results of these pharmacological studies are consistent with the gallbladder response to electrical stimulation of the cervical vagus nerve (24). In no instance, with vagal stimulation, did various parameters induce relaxation either before or after a dose of atropine that blocks the maximal dose of bethanechol.

In most animal species that have been studied, the gallbladder is innervated by the vagus nerves, particularly by the right vagus (152), which appears to synapse with intramural postganglionic cholinergic neurons. Pharmacological studies have presented evidence for the existence of excitatory intramural postganglionic cholinergic neurons in the guinea pig and cat gallbladder. First, compounds that inhibit the breakdown of acetylcholinesterase, such as physostigmine and edrophonium, cause gallbladder contraction in the guinea pig and cat; this contraction is prevented by pretreatment with atropine (284; J. Behar, unpublished observations). Second, effective doses of atropine reduce basal gallbladder pressures in cats (23). Third, electrical stimulation of the cervical vagus or splanchnic nerves or direct stimulation of gallbladder muscle strips cause contraction, which is antagonized by atropine and TTX (25, 282, 284). Tetrodotoxin also blocks the acetylcholine release by the guinea pig gallbladder muscle strips (282). Fourth, several peptides such as CCK (23) and neurotransmitters such as $\gamma$-aminobutyric acid (232) have been shown to contract the gallbladder through cholinergic neurons or with a concomittant release of acetylcholine. These effects are antagonized by atropine and TTX. These findings also suggest that the intramural cholinergic neurons participate in the vagal excitatory pathway and that they contribute to the genesis of basal gallbladder muscle tone.

Cholinergic drugs affect the sphincter of Oddi in a variety of species. Muscarinic agonists such as acetylcholine, bethanechol, or pilocarpine cause sphincter of Oddi contraction in human, dog, cat, opossum, and guinea pig (23, 33, 80, 83, 185). This contraction is characterized by a pronounced elevation of tone followed by an increase in the frequency and force of phasic contractions. These responses are not affected by complete neural block with TTX, and thus they are mediated by receptors located directly on the sphincter of Oddi smooth muscle (23). As for the gallbladder, these receptors have not yet been characterized as either $M_1$ or $M_2$. Unlike the gallbladder, nicotinic receptors mediate relaxation of the cat sphincter of Oddi through inhibitory neuron (210). Nicotine causes dose-dependent relaxation, which is blocked by hexamethonium and TTX (23). Nicotine-induced relaxation is mediated by specific nicotinic receptors as it is not affected by atropine, adrenergic, or histamine antagonists (J. Behar and P. Biancani, unpublished observations).

Cholinergic muscarinic antagonists do not affect basal sphincter of Oddi motor activity in the cat (26, 28). Atropine has no effect unless it is given in combination with the serotonin antagonist methysergide. The simultaneous administration of both antagonists markedly decreases tonic pressures and the frequency and force of phasic contractions. Atropine has no effect on the sphincter of Oddi of human, opossum, guinea pig, or rabbit (33, 62). Conflicting results have been observed in the dog sphincter of Oddi shortly after atropine. When pressures are determined over a long period of time, however, the relaxation is brief even though the anticholinergic effect persists (148, 185). Nicotinic antagonists such as hexamethonium cause a dose-related increase in tonic pressures and in the frequency and force of phasic contractions in the cat sphincter of Oddi (26). This is a transient response even though the antagonism to nicotine persists after the excitatory response has ceased. It does not appear to be the result of the systemic effect of hexamethonium because the fall in arterial blood pressure also persists. Most likely it may result from a transient imbalance between excitatory and inhibitory pathways. This assumption is consistent with the observation that pretreatment with atropine and methysergide or naloxone, which antagonize the excitatory pathway, prevents sphincter of Oddi excitation induced by hexamethonium (J. Behar and P. Biancani, unpublished observations).

ADRENERGIC DRUGS

In humans, cats, and guinea pigs, sympathetic fibers from the thoracic spinal cord pass to the gallbladder through the splanchnic nerves and celiac plexus and mix with parasympathetic fibers from the vagi and the right phrenic nerve to form the anterior and posterior hepatic plexuses. Neural fibers enter the gallbladder from both plexuses. The gallbladder wall contains a ganglionated nerve plexus located at the outer surface of the muscle coat and a second nerve plexus containing adrenergic and cholinergic nerve fibers without ganglia present in the lamina propria between the mucosa and the muscle coat (64, 189).

Bainbridge and Dale (16), as early as 1905, stated that "gallbladder relaxation was the invariable result of faradising the right splanchnic nerve," and numerous studies have shown that stimulation of sympathetic nerves or exogenous norepinephrine produce gallbladder relaxation (17, 207, 209, 273). The gallbladder has to be contracted with CCK or vagal stimulation, however, to obtain a consistent relaxation (204). Others have reported that norepinephrine causes contraction and isoproterenol causes relaxation of the guinea pig gallbladder strips (92, 142, 195). Epinephrine, a mixed adrenergic agonist, contracted or relaxed these muscle strips (Table 2). When more specific adrenergic agonists such as phenylephrine and isoproterenol are used, the isolated guinea pig gallbladder shows the existence of excitatory $\alpha$-adrenergic

TABLE 2. *Effect of Adrenergic Agonists and Blockers on Biliary Tract Motor Function*

| | Gallbladder | | | | | | Sphincter of Oddi | | | | |
|---|---|---|---|---|---|---|---|---|---|---|---|
| | Human | Dog | Cat | Opossum | Guinea pig | Rabbit | Human | Dog | Cat | Guinea pig | Rabbit |
| Phenylephrine | | | C | | C | | | | C | | C |
| Norepinephrine | | | R | | C | | | R | C/R* | R/C† | C/R |
| Epinephrine | | | R | | C/R | | | R | C/R* | | R |
| Isoproterenol | R | R | R | R | R | | | | R | R | R |
| Phentolamine | | | ‡ | | | | | | ‡ | | |
| Propranolol | | | ‡ | | | | | | ‡ | | |

C, contraction; R, relaxation; C/R, contraction followed by relaxation; R/C, relaxation followed by contraction.  * Conflicting results in cat.  † Depends on dose of norepinephrine.  ‡ No effect.

receptors and inhibitory β-adrenergic receptors (92, 155–157). Human gallbladder preparations in vitro are also relaxed by stimulation of β-receptors with isoproterenol and terbutaline (Table 2), and this effect was prevented by propranolol (207). In other animal species, however, conflicting evidence has also been presented. For instance, although epinephrine relaxes the isolated monkey gallbladder (221), the response in vivo to epinephrine has been reported to be unpredictable (238). This wealth of contradictory data could be explained by accounting for varying proportions of excitatory α-receptors and inhibitory β-receptors in preparations from different animal species.

Similar conflicting observations have been made in the cat gallbladder. Mixed adrenergic agonists such as norepinephrine and epinephrine cause gallbladder relaxation through β-adrenergic receptors and contraction through α-adrenergic receptors. Figure 3 shows that the relaxation mediated by β-receptors is prevalent, although sometimes cat gallbladder strips respond to norepinephrine with contraction (207). The relaxation is changed to contraction in the presence of β-adrenergic receptor blockers (Fig. 2), while the contraction is blocked by α-adrenergic antagonists. α-Adrenergic receptors are located directly on the cat gallbladder smooth muscle, because the effect of phenylephrine, a relatively pure α-adrenergic agonist, is not blocked by the neural blocker TTX (23). Its action is blocked by the α-receptor antagonist phentolamine. β-Adrenergic agonists such as isoproterenol and terbutaline relax the gallbladder also by direct action on the smooth muscle and are blocked by the α-antagonist propranolol. Neither phentolamine nor propranolol affect basal gallbladder motor function in the cat (23), suggesting that adrenergic neurons do not play a role in maintaining gallbladder tone. The gallbladder, however, responds to splanchnic nerve stimulation, but the type of response appears to depend on its physiological conditions. The resting cat gallbladder responds with contraction to electrical stimulation of the splanchnic nerves (24). This response is blocked by a combination of hexamethonium and atropine or by phentolamine, suggesting that preganglionic nerve fibers synapse with postganglionic adrenergic neurons.

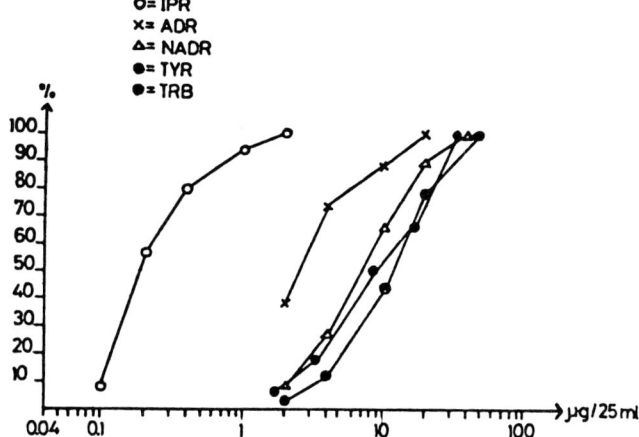

FIG. 3. Cumulative dose-response curves of isoprenaline (IPR), epinephrine (ADR), norepinephrine (NADR), tyramine (TYR), and terbutaline (TRB) obtained on isolated cat gallbladder strips. These catecholamines cause gallbladder relaxation expressed as percent from base line. [From Persson (207).]

In the same animal species, other studies have suggested that the splanchnic nerve may modulate the effects of CCK or vagal stimulation (204). Stimulation of the right splanchnic nerve inhibits the gallbladder contraction induced by CCK and vagal stimulation. Furthermore norepinephrine and epinephrine reduced by 40%–60% the gallbladder contraction induced by transmural stimulation in the guinea pig but did not affect the contraction induced by acetylcholine. Phentolamine blocked the catecholamine-induced inhibition, whereas atropine blocked the contractile response to transmural stimulation (158). These findings suggest the existence of presynaptic α-adrenergic receptors in the postganglionic cholinergic neurons that inhibit acetylcholine release.

The sphincter of Oddi of cat, dog, rabbit, and guinea pig contains adrenergic axons, identified by fluorescence histochemical methods (191). The number of axons and the fluorescence intensity are not affected by vagotomy, suggesting that the adrenergic fibers in the sphincter of Oddi derive from the sympathetic plexus and ganglia, with negligible contribution from the vagus (152). These data confirm previous findings by Baumgarten and Lange (19) showing adrenergic nerves in the gallbladder and sphincter of Oddi of the cat. Furthermore in the same animal species stimulation of the splanchnic nerves caused sphincter of Oddi contraction (204).

The isolated cat sphincter of Oddi also responds to exogenously administered adrenergic amines epinephrine and norepinephrine and to tyramine, which releases endogenous adrenergic amines (162, 206, 209), with an increase in tone and phasic activity and increased resistance to flow. These effects are blocked by phenoxybenzamine. Furthermore the response to tyramine is abolished after treatment with reserpine, which causes depletion of catecholamine stores. These data suggest the presence of catecholamine-containing neurons that may have an excitatory effect on the cat sphincter of Oddi. However, some of the effects of tyramine may also be explained by its ability to release serotonin (146), which has been shown to occur in the sphincter of Oddi (26). The adrenergic-induced contraction is mediated by $\alpha$-receptors while $\beta$-receptors mediate inhibition, as isoproterenol and the $\beta_2$-agonist terbutaline cause relaxation of the sphincter of Oddi (209). Other studies have reported, however, that in the in vivo cat and dog the phasic contractions of the sphincter of Oddi are inhibited by exogenous epinephrine and norepinephrine (49). Similar conflicting observations have been made in the rabbit and guinea pig choledochoduodenal junction, which could have resulted from the use of mixed agonists such as epinephrine and norepinephrine. One study showed that norepinephrine excites and isoproterenol inhibits the phasic contractions of the rabbit sphincter of Oddi (191), whereas other studies performed in vitro and in vivo have failed to confirm these observations (278, 280). In these studies, the mixed adrenergic agonists epinephrine and norepinephrine and the pure $\beta$-agonist isoproterenol produce inhibition of phasic contractions, whereas the relatively pure $\alpha$-adrenergic agonist phenylephrine caused excitation. In the guinea pig the sphincter of Oddi relaxed in response to low doses of norepinephrine and isoproterenol and was blocked by either phentolamine or propranolol. In contrast, high doses of norepinephrine produced a sphincter of Oddi contraction (195), which was blocked by phentolamine. Proper interpretation of these results requires additional pharmacological studies.

As in the gallbladder, $\alpha$-receptors appear to be mostly excitatory and $\beta$-receptors are inhibitory (209), with $\alpha$-receptors being prevalent in most animal species, as demonstrated by the sphincter of Oddi response to the mixed adrenergic agonist norepinephrine.

AUTACOIDS

*Prostaglandins*

Prostaglandins are a naturally occurring family of unsaturated hydroxy fatty acids, synthesized from arachidonic acid, that are widely distributed and extremely active in the gastrointestinal tract. The concentration of free arachidonic acid is low, and it is thus generally believed that endogenous biosynthesis of prostaglandins and related compounds depends on release of arachidonic acid from cellular phospholipid stores. Once released, arachidonic acid is rapidly metabolized in a stepwise manner leading to formation of various prostaglandins, leukotrienes, and intermediate products (120, 276).

Responses to prostaglandins in the gastrointestinal tract vary widely with species, location, type of muscle, and the particular prostaglandin (Table 3). In general longitudinal muscle, from stomach to colon, is contracted by prostaglandins of the E (PGE) and F (PGF) family, while circular muscle is relaxed by PGE and contracted by PGF (31, 32).

The effect of prostaglandins in the biliary tree has been studied by examining the effect of PGE and PGF. A possible physiological role of prostaglandins has been assessed by inhibiting their synthesis with indomethacin, a blocker of the enzyme prostaglandin synthetase, which promotes prostaglandin synthesis from arachidonic acid, or by employing agents that

TABLE 3. *Effect of Autacoids on Biliary Tract Motor Activity*

| | Gallbladder | | | | Sphincter of Oddi | | | | | |
|---|---|---|---|---|---|---|---|---|---|---|
| | Human | Baboon | Guinea pig | Rabbit | Baboon | Cat | Dog | Opossum | Guinea pig | Rabbit |
| Prostaglandins | | | | | | | | | | |
| PGE$_1$ | C | | C | | | | | | | |
| PGE$_2$ | C | | C | | | | R | | R | C/R |
| PGF$_{2\alpha}$ | C | | C | | | | | | R | |
| Serotonin | | | C | | | C/R | | | | |
| Histamine | | | | | | | | | | |
| H$_1$ | C | C | C | C | | | | R and C* | | |
| H$_2$ | R | R | R | | R | | | † | | |

C, contraction; R, relaxation; C/R, contraction followed by relaxation.    * H$_1$ receptors mediate relaxation in basal conditions and contraction after denervation with tetrodotoxin.    † No effect.

block the effect of prostaglandins in some experimental preparations.

Prostaglandins may participate in the genesis of gallbladder muscle contraction. In the guinea pig, the isolated gallbladder is capable of synthesizing $PGE_2$ and $PGF_{2\alpha}$, with the amount of $PGE_2$ being greater than $PGF_{2\alpha}$ (196). The prostaglandin precursor arachidonic acid induces the contraction of gallbladder muscle strips, and this effect is prevented by pretreatment with indomethacin at low concentrations (0.5 µg/kg). This inhibition is specific because indomethacin does not appreciably affect the contractions produced by acetylcholine, the octapeptide of CCK (CCK-8), and $PGE_2$ (12, 194). The specificity of the arachidonic acid effect is supported by the actions of SC19220, a prostaglandin antagonist that blocks the effect of arachidonic acid and $PGE_2$ but does not affect the responses to acetylcholine and CCK-8. The physiological role of prostaglandins in gallbladder muscle contraction is further supported by the finding that pretreatment with indomethacin enhanced the gallbladder contractile response to $PGE_1$, $PGE_2$, and $PGF_{2\alpha}$ and that the application of exogenous prostaglandins potentiates the gallbladder response to acetylcholine and transmural stimulation (196). Even more significant results were obtained from the simultaneous measurement of the rates of prostaglandin synthesis and the magnitude of the gallbladder contractile response to transmural stimulation. The guinea pig gallbladder muscle is capable of prostaglandin synthesis during muscle contraction, and indomethacin inhibits both prostaglandin synthesis and the gallbladder contractile response (194). Additional support for a physiological role of endogenous prostaglandins in the contraction of gallbladder muscle was also obtained from pharmacological studies with adrenergic drugs. Endogenous prostaglandins may mediate α-adrenergic receptor stimulation with norepinephrine because the contractile response was blocked by indomethacin even after the muscle tone was restored by the addition of exogenous prostaglandins (279).

These investigations in the guinea pig gallbladder have been extended to the human gallbladder (147). They have examined the effect of exogenous prostaglandins on gallbladder muscle and assess the pathophysiological role of endogenous prostaglandins in the abnormal motor response of the inflamed gallbladder. Despite the variable degree of inflammatory involvement, all gallbladder muscle strips exhibit normal tone and spontaneous rhythmic contractions at the rate of 2–3/min. This intrinsic activity appears to depend on the rate of prostaglandin synthesis because it is reduced or abolished by indomethacin (147). Muscle strips with mild chronic inflammatory involvement respond to exogenous prostaglandins with greater contractions than do strips with severe chronic inflammation. Furthermore strips from acutely inflamed gallbladders did not respond to prostaglandins at all but responded to acetylcholine partially. The failure of the severely inflamed gallbladder strips to respond to prostaglandins could reflect increased prostaglandin release from these severely inflamed tissues; it could also result from the alterations of receptor sites or to the intrinsic inability of the muscle to respond, because the response of the muscle strips to acetylcholine was also reduced.

All these findings consistently support the view that prostaglandins are implicated in the maintenance of basal gallbladder tone and in mediating the contractile response to transmural stimulation. A major unresolved issue that has not been examined further is the discrepancy between the effects of indomethacin on gallbladder contraction induced by acetylcholine and by the neurotransmitter released during transmural stimulation that has been shown to be cholinergic (194). Indomethacin blocks the gallbladder response to transmural stimulation at concentrations that inhibit prostaglandin synthesis and arachidonic acid–induced contraction; it does not antagonize the effects of acetylcholine. This discrepancy cannot be explained at this time unless the nature of the neurotransmitter is noncholinergic, in disagreement with most studies on this subject.

It is also conceivable that smooth muscle contraction in response to some neutrotransmitters is mediated by autacoids that are not generated through the cyclooxygenase cycle and therefore are indomethacin insensitive. Leukotrienes (LT) have been shown to be powerful excitatory compounds of guinea pig gallbladder muscle strips (119, 122, 285). These studies have shown that $LTC_4$, $LTD_4$, and $LTE_4$ cause powerful gallbladder contraction and are antagonized by FPL-55712. However, their role in the genesis of basal or stimulated gallbladder contraction has not been evaluated.

In contrast to the gallbladder, a physiological role of prostaglandins has not been established for the sphincter of Oddi. Although PGE and PGF exert pronounced pharmacological effects (Table 3), basal and stimulated sphincter of Oddi motor activity of the guinea pig and rabbit are not affected by indomethacin (179, 194). In both animal species, $PGE_1$ causes relaxation with a concomitant decrease in the myoelectrical activity, whereas, $PGF_{2\alpha}$ produces an increase in the frequency of phasic contractions and spike bursts (10, 179, 195). Similar effects were observed when they were tested in the dog sphincter of Oddi in vivo (193). Only minimal differences have been observed with $PGE_2$, which perhaps can be accounted by species differences. Prostaglandin $E_2$ causes relaxation in the guinea pig and dog sphincter of Oddi, whereas in the rabbit it induces a slight biphasic response with an initial contraction followed by relaxation. None of these studies, however, has attempted to assess the mechanism of action of prostaglandins in the sphincter of Oddi in any of the animal species studied. It has been suggested, however, that in addition to their possible myogenic effect, $PGE_1$ may cause sphincter of Oddi relaxation by inhibiting presynaptic transmission (141).

### Serotonin

Ample evidence has been presented supporting serotonin as a neurotransmitter in the gastrointestinal tract (77, 107, 108). Its exact physiological role, however, has not yet been established. Serotonergic neurons may activate smooth muscles directly or act as interneurons in the myenteric plexus (51, 52, 223). Serotonin can be released by pharmacological and vagal stimulation (59–61).

In the guinea pig, serotonin produced gallbladder contraction that is unaffected by atropine (Table 3), suggesting that this action is not mediated by cholinergic neurons (14). In the cat sphincter of Oddi, serotonin appears to be a neurotransmitter in the excitatory neural pathway. In this sphincter, as in the opossum and cat lower esophageal sphincter (219; J. Behar and P. Biancani, unpublished observations), exogenous serotonin stimulates three different receptors resulting in a biphasic response, characterized by a brief but sharp contraction followed by a more prolonged relaxation [Table 3; (26)]. The excitatory effect results from stimulation of cholinergic neurons and from direct action on the circular smooth muscle fibers. The relaxation is mediated by nonadrenergic, noncholinergic postganglionic inhibitory neurons because it is blocked only by TTX. Thus, exogenous serotonin simultaneously activates three receptors, two excitatory and one inhibitory. Atropine or the serotonin antagonist methysergide each reduces the excitatory response by ~50%; the combination of these two antagonists blocks completely the sphincter of Oddi contraction in response to serotonin. Furthermore, serotonin may play a physiological role by participating in the excitatory pathway, which may contribute to the genesis of basal sphincter of Oddi motor activity. The combination of atropine and methysergide in doses that effectively block maximal doses of serotonin decreases basal tonic pressures and abolishes phasic contractions; in addition, pharmacological studies suggest that serotonin is released by the action of exogenous enkephalin because these serotonin antagonists also block the effects of the opioid peptide (28).

In contrast, neither atropine nor methysergide alone has any effect on sphincter of Oddi relaxation caused by serotonin. Paradoxically, TTX enhances the sphincter of Oddi contraction in response to serotonin even though it blocks the cholinergic component. This is due to a simultaneous blockade of serotonin stimulation of inhibitory neurons and excitatory cholinergic neurons. The inhibitory effect of serotonin cannot be blocked by 5-methoxy-$N,N$-dimethyltryptamine, another antagonist of serotonin known to block neural receptors of serotonin (109). It is thus conceivable that this inhibitory receptor may be nonspecific or that it may have affinity for other selective serotonin antagonists. Thus additional studies are needed with other serotonin antagonists (117) to determine the specificity of the neural inhibitory receptor and its physiological role on the sphincter of Oddi motor function.

In the guinea pig sphincter of Oddi, serotonin causes contraction that is blocked by atropine and antagonized by morphine (14). Morphine seems to inhibit the sphincter of Oddi response to serotonin and transmural stimulation by reducing acetylcholine release.

### Histamine

Histamine has been shown to affect the gastrointestinal motor function by stimulating smooth muscle cells and neurons through $H_1$ and $H_2$ receptors. It is widely distributed throughout the gastrointestinal tract, stored in mast cells, APUD cells, and other still unrecognized sites. Many physiological roles have been sought for this autacoid because of its marked motor effects but none has been established.

Histamine causes a marked gallbladder contraction in all animal species including humans. This response is the result of the activation of excitatory $H_1$ and inhibitory $H_2$ receptors. These different histamine receptors have been defined by using selective $H_1$ and $H_2$ histamine agonists and antagonists. On administration of histamine, a nonselective agonist, the gallbladder responds with contraction, reflecting the prevalence of $H_1$ receptors (Table 3).

Excitatory $H_1$ and inhibitory $H_2$ effects have been observed in the human gallbladder in vitro, because the histamine-induced contraction is abolished by the $H_1$ antagonist mepyramine (175). The sensitivity of the muscle strips depended on the degree of inflammatory involvement (160). Stimulation of $H_1$ receptors with the selective agonist 2-pyridylethylamine also causes contraction in the guinea pig gallbladder muscle strips, which is greater than the maximum contraction induced by histamine. Conversely, $H_2$ receptors mediate gallbladder smooth muscle relaxation in vitro in this animal species (103, 126, 271). These observations also have been reproduced in other animal species irrespective of the experimental conditions. In awake baboons, intravenous infusions of histamine caused a dose-dependent increase in gallbladder pressures that was antagonized by the $H_1$ blocker diphenhydramine hydrochloride and was significantly enhanced by the $H_2$ blocker metiamide (239). In addition, the selective $H_1$ agonist 2-pyridylethylamine resulted in gallbladder contraction, whereas dimaprit, a selective $H_2$ agonist, resulted in gallbladder relaxation. All these studies uniformly suggest that $H_1$ receptors mediate gallbladder contraction, whereas $H_2$ receptors mediate relaxation, which is consistent with most of the results obtained elsewhere in the gastrointestinal tract except for sphincteric structures (36, 220). Although the receptor sites have not been determined for the gallbladder, it is conceivable that, as in other gastrointestinal nonsphincteric structures, $H_1$ receptors may be present at the smooth muscle and $H_2$ receptors may be present at nonadrenergic, noncholinergic, inhibitory neurons.

Despite these detailed pharmacological studies, however, there is little evidence supporting a physiological role of histamine in the gallbladder motor function or of the presence of histamine-containing cells of functional importance. Neither $H_1$ nor $H_2$ receptor blockers have been shown to affect basal gallbladder motor function. So far the only indirect and fairly weak evidence is the finding that blockade of $H_2$ receptors with cimetidine augmented the contractile effect of caerulein and CCK in the isolated gallbladder muscle strips (247, 271). These findings suggest that CCK and its analogues could stimulate the release of histamine from histaminergic cells that become apparent only when the $H_2$ inhibitory effects are eliminated.

The effect of histamine on the sphincter of Oddi has not been as extensively studied as on the gallbladder (Table 3). In the anesthetized opossum, intravenous histamine depressed the frequency and force of the phasic contractions (243, 261). This inhibitory effect was reproduced by the selective $H_1$ agonist 2-pyridylethylamine and blocked by the correspondent $H_1$ antagonist pyrylamine. This effect was also blocked by TTX, but it was not antagonized by cholinergic and adrenergic blockers such as atropine, hexamethonium, phentolamine, and propranolol. It was also not blocked by the selective $H_2$ antagonist metiamide. After TTX, histamine or 2-pyridylethylamine caused an increased frequency and amplitude of the sphincter of Oddi contractions, which also was blocked by pyrylamine (261). These data indicate that the opossum sphincter of Oddi has two $H_1$ receptors, one inhibitory at the noncholinergic, nonadrenergic inhibitory neurons, the other excitatory at the sphincteric smooth muscle. The opossum sphincter of Oddi does not seem to contain $H_2$ receptors. In contrast, the sphincter of Oddi of the unsedated baboon has exclusive inhibitory $H_2$ receptors (153). It is not affected by the specific $H_1$ agonist 2-pyridylethylamine, but it is relaxed during an intravenous infusion of the specific $H_2$ agonist dimaprit. Thus, the actions of histamine in this animal species are similar to those of CCK, producing gallbladder contraction and sphincter of Oddi relaxation.

### NEUROPEPTIDES

*Cholecystokinin-Gastrin Family of Peptides*

Cholecystokinin is a major participant in the hormonal control of biliary tract motor function. Cells containing CCK have been identified by immunohistochemical methods in the mucosa of mammalian duodenum and jejunum (56, 215). Ultrastructural studies reveal that these cells are the intestinal I cells in the human intestine (55, 56). Moreover, CCK-33 and CCK-8 have been extracted from this segment (90, 192), and physiological studies reveal that these two peptides are released into the circulation (186). Orally administered fatty or mixed meals, intraduodenal fatty acids, or amino acids caused gallbladder contraction, sphincter of Oddi relaxation, and increased biliary flow into the duodenum (15, 63, 161). Gallbladder-emptying studies using a radionuclide ($^{131}$I-labeled iopanoic acid) as marker have shown that fatty meals or constant intravenous infusions of CCK produce complete gallbladder evacuation (97). Circulating levels of CCK-like immunoreactivity increased significantly during these physiological events (131, 161, 181). Similar correlations between duodenal release of CCK, its immunoreactive blood levels, and gallbladder contraction has been demonstrated in humans (274). Gel-filtration studies have identified three major forms of CCK bioactivity: an abundant form that eluted with CCK-33, a smaller form that eluted with CCK-8, and an intermediate form that eluted between them. Constant intravenous infusions of CCK-33 or CCK-8, which increased the circulating levels of CCK-like immunoreactivity to levels similar to those measured after the infusion of intraduodenal fat, causes gallbladder contraction and sphincter of Oddi relaxation in humans and in most animal species (144, 182, 222). Specific CCK-gastrin antagonists such as proglumide and dibutyryl cGMP blocked the actions of both endogenous and exogenous CCK (104). Thus a physiological role of CCK on biliary tract motor function is well established.

In the guinea pig and rabbit, CCK causes gallbladder contraction (Table 4) by stimulating excitatory receptors present in the smooth muscle exclusively (7, 137, 281). This effect of CCK has been studied in gallbladder preparations in vivo and in vitro and is unaffected by complete denervation with TTX or by blocking cholinergic neurons with atropine. In the cat (23), dog (256, 258), and human (180), CCK contracts the gallbladder by stimulating both smooth muscle and cholinergic neurons, resulting in an increase in gallbladder pressures and in reduction in gallbladder size and emptying of bile. In humans, CCK-8 causes a dose-dependent contraction of the gallbladder (254) and atropine shifts the CCK dose-response curve to the right, blocking the effect of lower doses (115). These findings suggest that the response of the human gallbladder to CCK is largely dependent on cholinergic innervation. The cat gallbladder response to CCK is reduced by 50% after pretreatment with atropine and hexamethonium or TTX (23). Figures 4 and 5 show the gallbladder response to CCK-8 in control conditions and after TTX. Figure 5 clearly shows that the gallbladder is still capable of contracting in response to CCK after denervation with TTX. Both antagonists also reduce basal gallbladder pressures, but these pressure changes do not influence the magnitude of the pressure response to agonists that act directly on its smooth muscle. For instance, although TTX reduces resting gallbladder pressure, it does not affect the increase in pressure in response to bethanechol; isoproterenol, which also reduces basal gallbladder pressures, does not affect the response to CCK or bethanechol (23).

The octapeptide of CCK and CCK-33 are potent stimuli of biliary tract motor function. Threshold doses of CCK-33 as low as 0.06 Ivy dog units/ml (1 µg/CCK-33 = 3 Ivy dog units) can cause gallbladder contraction in the rabbit, and 0.04 Ivy dog units/ml can cause contraction in humans; CCK-8 doses as low as 0.25 ng/ml in the cat and 0.05–0.025 ng/kg in the opossum can also cause contraction of the gallbladder.

By using a series of CCK analogues, it has been shown that the cholecystokinetic potency of the peptide molecule resides in the seven amino acids of the COOH-terminal chain with a sulfuric acid ($HSO_3$) radical on the tyrosine residue in position 7. Thus, most changes in this COOH-terminal chain produced marked reductions in its potency and receptor affinity, as shown by bioassays and radioligand studies. It has also been suggested that CCK-8 was more potent than CCK-33 per molar basis; more recent studies, however, have shown that this is incorrect. If the concentration of the CCK analogues is corrected for loss of peptide as measured by radioimmunoassay, CCK-8 was not more potent than longer analogues such as CCK-33 and CCK-39 (245). Without this correction, there is a significant loss of up to 10-fold difference between CCK-33 and CCK-39 from the bath. The longer peptides will bind to the bath surfaces unless albumin is used. Thus the potency of CCK-7, CCK-8, and CCK-33 is similar per molar basis.

Ondetti et al. (201) studied in great detail the structure-activity relationships of CCK analogues on the guinea pig gallbladder in vitro and in vivo. A marked reduction in cholecystokinetic potency of both preparations was demonstrated when the sulfuric radical was removed or its position changed, when aspartic acid was replaced by alanine, or when aspartic acid or methionine replaced tyrosine, which was then displaced to position 8. Because of the importance of the presence of the sulfuric radical in the tyrosine position 7, it was found that the shortest analogue with biological activity is the COOH terminus heptapeptide (CCK-7). Removal of the sulfuric acid residue reduces the potency of the CCK molecule by a factor of 150 in causing contraction of the guinea pig gallbladder both in vivo and in vitro (201). Even a transfer of the sulfuric acid residue from the tyrosine hydroxyl to the aromatic ring (sulfonated CCK-8 compared with the sulfated CCK-8) resulted in a fall in potency by a factor of 30. Changes in the distance of the tyrosine residue from the COOH-terminus caused a 200-fold reduction in potency of these molecules.

Similar studies also were performed in the cat gallbladder in vivo (29). Removal of the sulfuric acid radical from CCK-7 caused an 80-fold drop in potency

TABLE 4. *Effect of Neuropeptides on Biliary Tract Motor Function*

|  | Gallbladder | Sphincter of Oddi |
|---|---|---|
| Cholecystokinin | C | R[a] or C[b] |
| Caerulein | C | R |
| Gastrin | C | C/R |
| Secretin | R | R |
| Glucagon | R[c] | R |
| Vasoactive intestinal polypeptide | R | R |
| Opiates |  |  |
|   Morphine | [d] | C |
|   Enkephalins | [d] | C/R |
|   Dynorphin | [d] | C/R |
| Motilin | [e] | C |
| Substance P | C | C |
| Somatostatin | [f] | [f] |
| Bombesin | [f] | [f] |
| Pancreatic polypeptide | R | C |

C, contraction; R, relaxation; C/R, contraction followed by relaxation. [a] In human, dog, and cat. [b] In opossum, guinea pig, and rabbit. [c] In vivo. [d] No effect. [e] No effect in most animal species. [f] No direct effect.

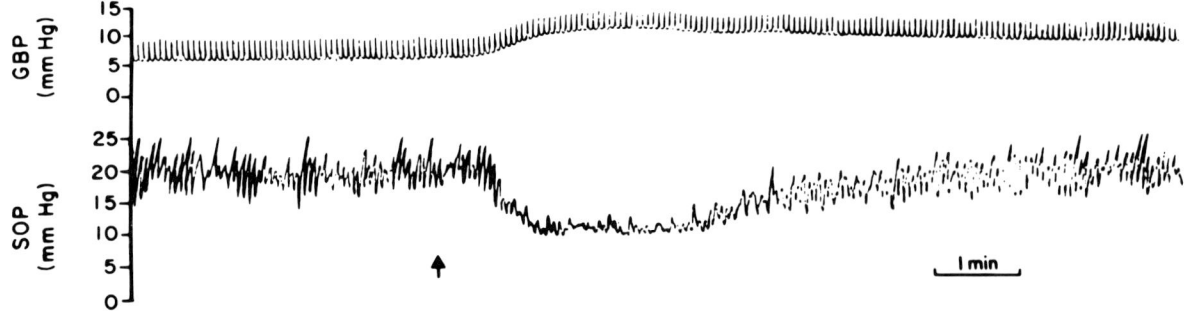

FIG. 4. Effect of octapeptide of cholecystokinin (OP-CCK) on cat gallbladder (GBP) and sphincter of Oddi pressures (SOP). OP-CCK causes gallbladder contraction and sphincter of Oddi relaxation. *Arrow* indicates timing of OP-CCK administration. [From Behar and Biancani (23).]

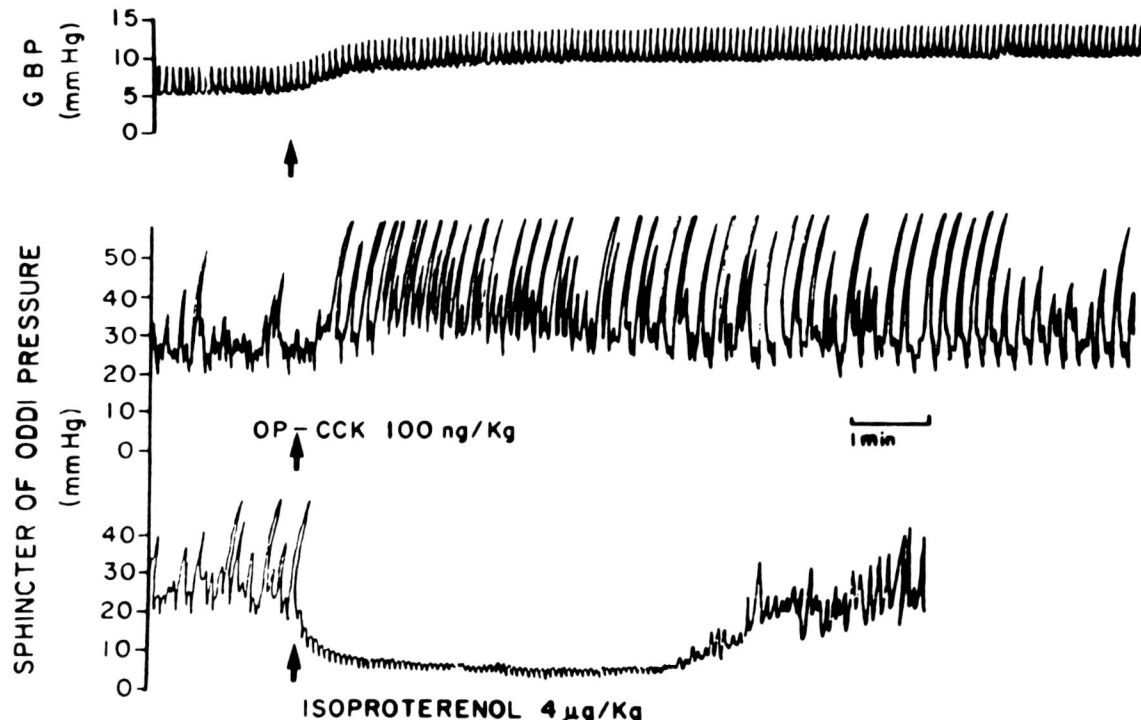

FIG. 5. Effect of octapeptide of cholecystokinin (OP-CCK) on cat gallbladder (GBP) and sphincter of Oddi pressures after denervation with tetrodotoxin. OP-CCK causes gallbladder and sphincter of Oddi contraction. In contrast, isoproterenol is still capable of causing sphincter of Oddi relaxation. [From Behar and Biancani (23).]

when compared with the effects of sulfated CCK-7. The fall in cholecystokinetic activity was mainly due to absence of stimulation of the cholinergic neurons. Whereas TTX and atropine reduced the gallbladder response to sulfated CCK-7 by 50%, they did not affect the weaker response to desulfated CCK-7. These findings suggest that the latter activates the smooth muscle receptors exclusively. Moreover the length of the COOH-terminal amino acid chain of CCK is important because the gallbladder did not respond at all to shorter fractions of CCK, CCK-3, and CCK-2. The reduced potency of desulfated and shorter CCK analogues is the result of decreased binding to CCK receptors as shown by their weaker antagonism to the radioligand $^{121}$I-labeled CCK-33 to gallbladder smooth muscle receptors (248). In contrast to mammalian gallbladders, the coho salmon gallbladder seems to be the exception because CCK-33, CCK-8, and gastrin II are equipotent, suggesting that its CCK receptor cannot distinguish between agonists that differ in the location of a sulfated tyrosyl residue at position 6 and 7 from the COOH terminus (269).

Exogenous CCK (Fig. 4) or intraduodenal infusions of fats and amino acids causes sphincter of Oddi relaxation in the dog, cat, pig, and human [Table 4; (23, 105, 145, 163, 165, 263)]. Figures 6 and 7 show that CCK-8 abolishes the phasic contractions of the human sphincter of Oddi. In other animal species such as the opossum (20, 263), rabbit (235, 236), and guinea pig (142), exogenous CCK caused contraction with increases in the frequency and force of the phasic contractions. Intraduodenal infusions of fatty meals in the opossum also causes increased sphincter of Oddi motor activity and discharge of bile into the duodenum. These findings suggest that the increase in sphincter of Oddi motor activity, presumably the result of CCK release, facilitates the passage of bile (93).

The mechanisms by which CCK affects the sphincter of Oddi also seem to vary with the animal species. In the cat, sphincter of Oddi relaxation in response to CCK is due to stimulation of the nonadrenergic, noncholinergic, postganglionic inhibitory neurons (23). This CCK action is not blocked by any adrenergic and cholinergic antagonists and is only blocked by TTX (Fig. 5). Complete neural block with TTX unmasks an excitatory receptor at the smooth muscle that causes sphincter of Oddi contraction characterized by an increase in tonic pressures and in the force and frequency of the phasic contractions. In the opossum, the CCK-induced contractions are the result of direct action on the smooth muscle because the sphincter of Oddi response is unaffected by TTX (264).

The sphincter of Oddi, like the gallbladder, is extremely sensitive to CCK. In the cat biliary tract the same doses from 5 to 100 μg/kg that cause gallbladder contraction also relax the sphincter of Oddi (23).

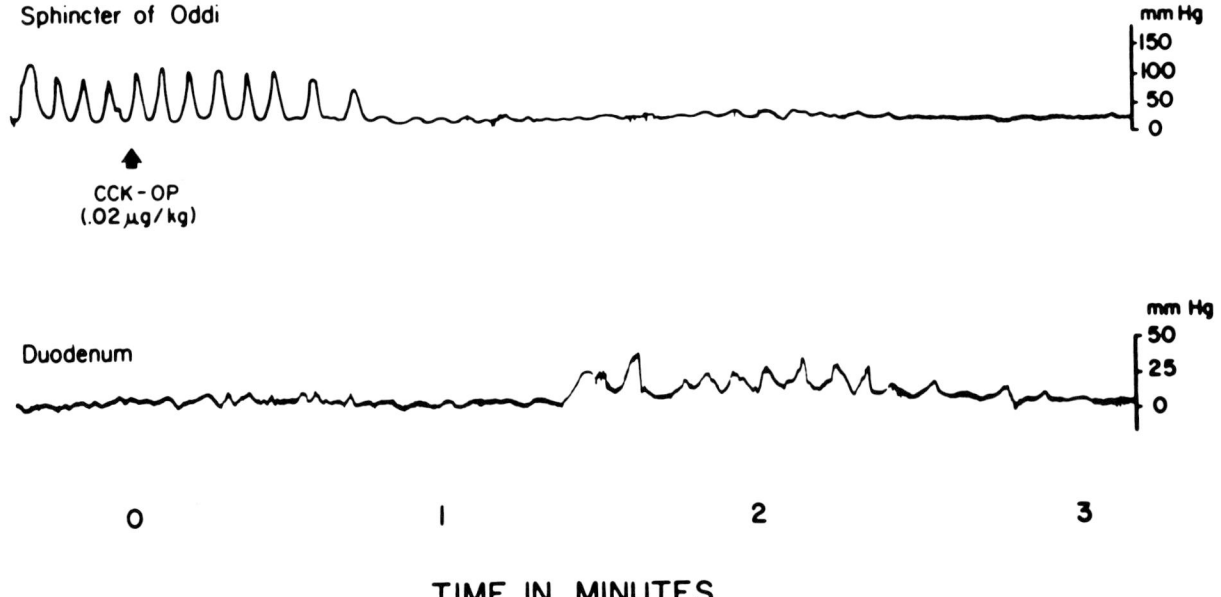

FIG. 6. Effect of octapeptide of cholecystokinin (CCK-OP) on human sphincter of Oddi and duodenum in vivo. [From Geenan et al. (105). Copyright 1980 by the American Gastroenterological Association.]

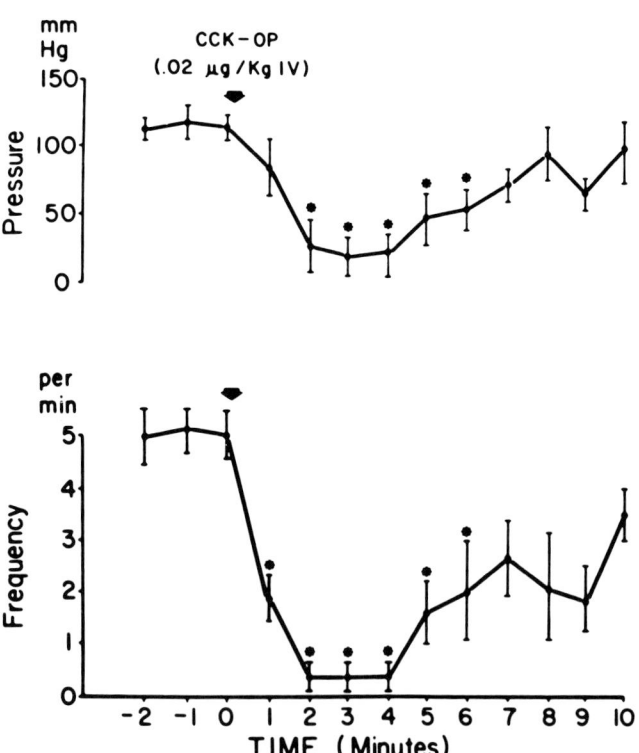

FIG. 7. Effect of octapeptide of cholecystokinin (CCK-OP) on amplitude (pressure) and frequency of phasic contractions of human sphincter of Oddi in vivo. *Asterisks* indicate that changes were statistically significant from base line. [From Geenan et al. (105). Copyright 1980 by the American Gastroenterological Association.]

Pharmacological studies performed with CCK analogues to determine structure-activity relationships revealed that receptors at the postganglionic, nonadrenergic, noncholinergic inhibitory neurons are markedly different from those at the postganglionic cholinergic neurons of the gallbladder (29). Removal of the sulfuric acid radical by using desulfated CCK-7 or by shortening the length of the CCK peptide chain by using CCK-3 and CCK-2 reduced significantly the potency of these analogues, but they could still fully relax the sphincter when sufficiently high doses were used. The doses of desulfated CCK-7 required to fully relax the sphincter of Oddi in vivo was five times higher than those of sulfated CCK-7. For shorter COOH-terminal fractions of CCK-3 and CCK-2, the doses required were 1,000–2,000 times higher than the maximal dose of sulfated CCK-7. The dose of CCK-3 needed to induce sphincter of Oddi relaxation was 10–80 nmol/kg, and for CCK-2 20–160 nmol/kg were required. However, unlike sulfated CCK-7, these analogues had little or no effect on the myogenic CCK excitatory receptor. After denervation with TTX, the sphincter of Oddi responded with contraction to sulfated CCK-7 but did not at all to CCK-3 or CCK-2.

A better understanding of CCK-receptor interaction and specificity has become possible with the use of specific CCK antagonists. Three types of CCK receptor antagonists have been described: *1*) derivatives of amino acids such as proglumide, a derivative of glutaramic acid, and benzotript, a derivative of triptophan (70, 87, 118); *2*) derivatives of cyclic nucleotides such as dibutyryl cGMP (18); and, 3) CCK fractions such as the N-acetyl CCK-26–32-NH$_2$, the N-acetyl CCK-26–32, and the CCK-26–32-NH$_2$, which are COOH-terminal CCK molecules minus the phenylalanine residue (104). In addition, Jensen et al. (136) reported that CCK-3 and CCK-2 could act also as antagonists in the pancreatic acini.

Although most of these studies have been carried out in the pancreatic acini (18, 118), a few studies with the CCK antagonists have been carried out in the guinea pig gallbladder and ileum (86, 277). These antagonists, and particularly dibutyryl cGMP, are effective blockers of CCK actions on the guinea pig gallbladder smooth muscle in vitro and on the guinea pig ileomyenteric plexus. The mechanism of action of these antagonists is reversible competitive binding to CCK receptors and thus preventing binding to CCK molecules (73, 86). This has been shown in the pancreatic acinar cells by using dibutyryl cGMP, which inhibits the binding of the radioligand $^{125}$I-labeled CCK to cell surface receptors, blocking the action of CCK on calcium transport and amylase secretion (234). Dibutyryl cGMP does not require the butyryl moiety because 8-bromocyclic nucleotides also inhibit the action of CCK (18). In the pancreas, dibutyryl cGMP acts like an agonist-antagonist because it is also capable of increasing pancreatic enzyme secretion. There is no correlation, however, between its ability to stimulate enzyme secretion and its ability to antagonize the effect of CCK. Both compounds also seem to share some antigenic properties because cyclic nucleotide derivatives inhibit the binding of $^{125}$I-labeled CCK to antibodies specific for the biologically active COOH-terminal region of CCK. Thus certain cyclic nucleotide derivatives possess a conformational structure that resembles that of the biologically active portion of CCK.

In the cat biliary tract, the amino acid derivatives and the nucleotide derivatives act as CCK antagonists (29). The CCK fractions CCK-3 and CCK-2, however, do not block the actions of CCK. This failure to antagonize CCK-8 may be related to the experimental conditions in which they were administered as bolus doses in preparations in vivo. Their agonist effects are rather brief, probably because they are rapidly degraded (89). Their antagonistic actions may be more effective in vitro where the concentrations may remain stable over a longer period of time. Furthermore other CCK analogues that have been used as CCK antagonists, like the CCK-26–32 analogues, have not been used in the biliary tract. Proglumide and dibutyryl cGMP, however, act as competitive antagonists, blocking the action of CCK-8 both in the gallbladder and in the sphincter of Oddi, preventing contraction of the gallbladder and relaxation of the sphincter of Oddi. In the gallbladder, proglumide appears to act as an exclusive antagonist, shifting the dose-response curve of CCK-8 to the right. The sphincter of Oddi shows similar displacement of the dose-response curves but requires higher doses of proglumide than does the gallbladder. Whereas 10 mg·kg$^{-1}$·min$^{-1}$ is sufficient to block CCK in the gallbladder, twice as much (up to 20 mg·kg$^{-1}$·min$^{-1}$) was necessary for a similar effect in the sphincter of Oddi. As shown in the pancreatic acini, dibutyryl cGMP acts as an agonist-antagonist. It caused a brief contraction of the gallbladder and relaxation of the sphincter of Oddi, with persistent antagonism after pressures had returned to base-line levels. As with proglumide, the sphincter of Oddi requires higher doses of dibutyryl cGMP to block CCK than those needed for the gallbladder.

The cellular mechanism of action of CCK in the gallbladder has not been established. It has been suggested that CCK causes muscle contraction by increasing the influx of calcium, probably through receptor-operated channels (13). Calcium will in turn stimulate cGMP. It has been shown that CCK increases the intracellular level of cGMP (8); however, this finding has not been confirmed (11). More recent studies have presented evidence that CCK utilizes calcium from both extracellular sources and intracellular stores (224). Moreover, the hypothesis that CCK, like other peptides (244), causes muscle contraction by increasing the synthesis of prostaglandin was tested by blocking its effect by pretreatment with the prostaglandin synthesis inhibitor indomethacin. These studies did not support this hypothesis (12, 196).

### Gastrin

Gastrin-containing cells, or G cells, have been identified in the antral and duodenal mucosa (112). The major molecular structure is a 17–amino acid residue (G-17) having an identical COOH-terminal pentapeptide sequence with CCK. In the gastrointestinal tract, it behaves exclusively as a hormone, because it is released during the digestive phase and stimulated by proteins, amino acids, calcium, and antral alkalinization (272). Like CCK, the tyrosine residue is sulfated but is present in position 6 instead of position 7 (91).

Although gastrin is a powerful stimulus of smooth muscle contraction in vitro and in vivo in a variety of tissues (190), it is a weak agonist of the gallbladder muscle (9). In the cat gallbladder, synthetic human gastrin I was ~1,000 times less potent than CCK-8, and the maximal dose of gastrin caused a contraction that was 66% of that caused by a maximal dose of CCK-8 in vitro (71). These studies, however, did not compare the actual concentrations of CCK-8 and gastrin I determined by radioimmunoassay, as has been done comparing CCK-8 with CCK (245). Nevertheless, they seem to confirm the assumption that gastrin I is weaker than CCK-8, because the former behaves in the gallbladder like an agonist-antagonist. Increasing the background of gastrin by gradually increasing its concentration inhibited the expected greater response to a maximal dose of CCK-8; the total response to these two hormones never exceeded the maximal response to CCK-8 alone, suggesting that they share common receptors, as one would expect from their structural similarities (71). In contrast, the addition of acetylcholine to the bath caused a further increase in gallbladder contraction after it had contracted in response to maximal doses of both gastrin I and CCK-8. These results suggest that the factor limiting further gallbladder contraction is the number of CCK-gastrin receptors and that the muscle was still capable of having a further contraction in response to different agonists.

Studies on the structure-activity relationships of gastrin indicate that the sulfuric radical in position 6 for gastrin I is not as important as the sulfuric radical in position 7 for CCK to induce gallbladder contraction. Sulfated and nonsulfated G-17 were equipotent in the dog gallbladder in vivo (267). In other species such as rabbit and guinea pig gallbladder, the sulfated G-17 was slightly more potent than the nonsulfated G-17 (6). Likewise, in the cat gallbladder in vitro the sulfated residue did not appear to be as critical for determining biological potency because desulfated G-17 was only 10 times less potent than was the sulfated form (72). In contrast, pentagastrin with a shorter nonsulfated molecule had no effect on basal gallbladder pressures in the cat (22) and guinea pig in vivo (85) and on human gallbladder strips (175). In the guinea pig, however, it only potentiated the contraction evoked by vagal stimulation.

Although it is weaker than CCK, the plasma concentration of sulfated gastrin is higher than that of CCK (9) and might therefore contribute to the overall endogenous CCK activity. It is doubtful that sulfated gastrins participate in the hormonal control of the biliary tract, at least by themselves. This conclusion is based on the finding that the concentration required to cause gallbladder contraction far exceeds the gastrin concentrations required for its major physiological effect, the stimulation of gastric acid secretion.

Gastrin has not been studied in the sphincter of Oddi as extensively as in the gallbladder. Gastrin mimics the action of CCK on the sphincter of Oddi with marked differences in some animal species (Table 4). Lin and Spray (168) observed that pentagastrin decreased the resistance of directly perfused choledochus of the conscious dog. Subsequent studies showed that gastrin and the COOH-terminal tetra- and tripeptide of gastrin were also effective (163). Similar observations were made in the sphincter of Oddi of the anesthetized guinea pig, where human gastrin I was 0.025–0.1 as active as CCK in causing relaxation (4). In vitro, however, Toouli and Watts (264) found that gastrin I stimulated the circular muscle of the canine sphincter. In other animal species, even though the experiments were performed in vivo, the sphincter response to gastrin was also quite different. The response of the human sphincter of Oddi is one of exclusive contraction (105). This hormone, however, produced vigorous retching, which may have prevented the detection of a subsequent relaxation. Gastrin also caused an increase in spike-burst activity in the rabbit sphincter of Oddi (236), and pentagastrin had a similar effect in the opossum (20). A biphasic response after pentagastrin is seen in the cat sphincter of Oddi (22). It responds with initial contraction followed by a more prolonged relaxation. The relaxation is neurally mediated, whereas the contraction is due to direct action on the smooth muscle because it is not blocked by complete denervation with TTX. Like CCK, pentagastrin relaxes this sphincter by stimulating noncholinergic, nonadrenergic inhibitory nerves. Only TTX blocks this inhibition.

*Caerulein*

Caerulein is a natural sulfated decapeptide, an analogue of CCK, possessing the same COOH-terminal peptide and amino acid residues such as the tyrosyl 0-sulfate residue. This peptide has a powerful excitatory action on the gallbladder of several animal species (Table 4). It produces a dose-dependent gallbladder contraction in the guinea pig, rabbit, dog, cat, and human (35, 266). Of all these animal species, however, the in vitro rabbit gallbladder appears to be the preparation most sensitive to caerulein. On a molar basis, this peptide was found to be 16 times more potent than CCK (267).

The location of the caerulein receptor has not been elucidated completely. The spasmogenic effect of caerulein on the dog gallbladder is atropine resistant (35). In the guinea pig gallbladder, the action of caerulein is not blocked by atropine, hexamethonium, dibenamine, and mepyramine, suggesting it may act directly on the gallbladder smooth muscle. Tetrodotoxin, however, was not used to determine conclusively whether its action is neurally mediated. In humans, however, with ultrasonography as the method of assessing the gallbladder contraction, atropine significantly reduces the gallbladder response to caerulein (180); this finding suggests that cholinergic neurons are involved in the gallbladder response to caerulein. As with CCK, removal of a sulfate residue deprived this peptide of most of its potency (100, 139).

The action of caerulein also has been studied in the guinea pig and rabbit sphincter of Oddi (Table 4). In contrast to the reported effects of CCK on the guinea pig sphincter of Oddi, caerulein caused relaxation. This effect was particularly striking after the sphincter was contracted with morphine (4, 35). These findings are also in conflict with other studies that have reported that morphine causes relaxation of the guinea pig sphincter of Oddi by antagonizing the release of acetylcholine. These discrepant results between CCK and caerulein in the same animal species cannot be explained at the present time. Caerulein, like CCK and gastrin, causes an increase in the spike-burst activity in the rabbit sphincter of Oddi (236).

*Secretin, Vasoactive Intestinal Polypeptide, Glucagon, and Gastrointestinal Inhibitory Polypeptide Family*

The family of peptides that includes secretin, vasoactive intestinal polypeptide (VIP), glucagon, and gastrointestinal inhibitory polypeptide (GIP) shares a large number of amino acids in their 27 residues, with VIP having the greatest number of unique residues (192). These structural differences may explain the greater potency of VIP motor function on the biliary tract.

Secretin is present in the S cells of the duodenum and jejunum (214), and its major biological action in the biliary tract is to increase biliary output. The increase in biliary secretion is achieved by stimulating the ductular and gallbladder epithelial secretion of water and bicarbonate and is not the result of its actions on gallbladder motor function, which is rather weak (134, 140). Duodenal acidification, a major stimulus for secretin release, however, causes gallbladder contraction. It is difficult to accept that this effect is mediated by secretin alone, which in pharmacological doses has either no effect or produces a weak gallbladder relaxation (Table 4). Gallbladder contraction in response to duodenal acidification may be mediated by release of CCK or other peptides or even by a neural reflex.

Most in vivo studies have shown that exogenous secretin alone either has no cholecystokinetic effect or decreases gallbladder pressures in the guinea pig, cat, and opossum (135, 225, 268). In dogs with chronic gallbladder and gastric fistulas, increasing doses of secretin has no effect on gallbladder motility (249). However, when given with CCK, secretin shifts the CCK dose-response curve to the left, suggesting that it enhances the CCK action on gallbladder motility. Lin and Spray (169) made similar observations in conscious dogs, with secretin potentiating the cholecystokinetic action of CCK. They also found that natural and synthetic secretin preparations increase intragallbladder pressure. Chowdhury et al. (71) confirmed these results in the cat gallbladder in vitro showing that secretin potentiates the effect of CCK. It also enhances the gallbladder contraction evoked by vagal stimulation (85). In the anesthetized cat and opossum, secretin alone was unable to cause gallbladder contraction in vivo (J. Behar, unpublished observations; W. J. Dodds, personal communication). Only very high doses of natural secretin, 8–16 clinical units, had a slight relaxing effect on basal cat gallbladder pressures. These observations have been confirmed in gallbladder preparations in vitro. The doses of secretin that act alone or enhance the action of CCK far exceed those required for the stimulation of pancreatic exocrine secretion, a known physiological effect of secretin. However, its participation in the hormonal control of gallbladder motor activity cannot be completely ruled out because it may interact with other duodenal hormones and neural reflexes during physiological events.

In contrast to secretin, VIP is a potent inhibitor of basal and CCK-stimulated gallbladder pressures [Table 4; (231)]. Continuous intravenous infusion of VIP causes gallbladder relaxation in the cat (133) or a dose-dependent rightward shift of the gallbladder pressure-volume relationships in the opossum (226). In addition, dose-response studies with intra-arterial bolus injections of VIP as low as 0.1–1 $\mu$g/kg caused relaxation of the cat gallbladder (J. Behar and P. Biancani, unpublished observations). Maximal doses of VIP (1 $\mu$g/kg) completely relax the gallbladder because it cannot be augmented by the addition of isoproterenol. In contrast, Feeley et al. (101) found that VIP was a weak inhibitory agonist to guinea pig gallbladder muscle strips and had no effect on human gallbladder strips. These findings appear to be the exception because most studies performed in a variety of species including guinea pig, rabbit, dog, cat, opossum, and pig have shown that VIP is a potent inhibitor of basal and CCK-stimulated gallbladder contraction (211) in vitro or in vivo (3, 133, 171, 226, 229, 275).

The inhibitory action of VIP is direct on the gallbladder muscle because it is unaltered by complete denervation with TTX or by any cholinergic, adrenergic, histaminergic, or serotonergic antagonist tested (J. Behar and P. Biancani, unpublished observations). These findings suggest that VIP is a possible candidate as a neurotransmitter of the noncholinergic, nonadrenergic inhibitory neurons that may mediate gallbladder relaxation during the interdigestive period when the gallbladder fills with bile. This possibility is supported by the finding that VIP is present in the neuronal bodies of the guinea pig myenteric plexus of the gallbladder, as shown by immunocytochemistry and radioimmunoassay techniques (64, 255). Furthermore, peptide histidine isoleucine (PHI)-like immunoreactivity was also found in the gallbladder wall, and like VIP it relaxes the guinea pig gallbladder in vitro (48, 283). A nonadrenergic, noncholinergic, inhibitory pathway, however, has not been demonstrated conclusively in the gallbladder. Some evidence has been presented to support its existence in the guinea pig gallbladder (5). Transmural stimulation of the isolated gallbladder produced a biphasic response consisting of contraction followed by relaxation. Both responses were blocked by atropine and TTX (284). These results, however, do not clearly indicate whether the relaxation is simply rebound response or the result of the stimulation of specific neurons because the antagonists were not able to dissociate the contraction from the relaxation. Neurally mediated relaxation has been demonstrated in the cat gallbladder by stimulating the sympathetic innervation through the right splanchnic nerve, which synapses with postganglionic adrenergic neurons. This relaxation can only be demonstrated when the gallbladder pressure is elevated after CCK (204). Nonadrenergic, noncholinergic inhibitory neurons did not mediate this response.

Glucagon, another member of the secretin family of hormones, does not appear to have any excitatory or inhibitory effect on the human or guinea pig gallbladder in vitro (65). In the canine gallbladder in vivo, however, subcutaneous or intravenous administration of glucagon causes relaxation (164). Similar observations have been made in vivo in the cat (J. Behar and P. Biancani, unpublished observations). Also in humans an increase in gallbladder size has been shown after glucagon administration (69). In contrast to the results of these studies in which bolus doses were used, continuous intravenous infusion of a wide range of concentrations of glucagon (1–20 $\mu g \cdot kg^{-1} \cdot h^{-1}$) had no effect on basal gallbladder motor activity in the cat (134). These last observations indicate that the glucagon concentrations required for gallbladder relaxation in vivo far exceeds those required to induce glycogenesis, a physiological effect of this hormone. Thus this hormone by itself is unlikely to play a physiological role in the control of gallbladder motor activity.

Finally, another member of the secretin family of gut hormones, GIP, has been reported to have no effect on the gallbladder motor function in most animal species when synthetic GIP is used (134).

In the sphincter of Oddi, this family of peptides also causes relaxation, resulting in a reduction in tonic pressures and in the frequency and force of the phasic contractions in all species studied. Natural secretin at high doses either has no effect or inhibits motor activity. High doses of secretin have no effect in the opossum (20, 263), and rabbit (236), whereas in the dog, cat, and human they cause a depression of tonic pressures and frequency and the force of phasic contractions (164, 169; J. Behar and P. Biancani, unpublished observations). The inhibitory action of secretin in the cat sphincter of Oddi is not modified by any antagonist that was used, including TTX, indicating that this action is direct on the smooth muscle. In humans, relaxation of the sphincter of Oddi is preceded by a brief contraction (105). The doses needed, however, far exceed those required to stimulate pancreatic exocrine secretion, which is its major physiological effect (114). This conclusion is supported by the results obtained with intravenous infusions that resulted in plasma secretin concentrations within postprandial levels; the concentrations had no effect on the sphincter of Oddi (66). A contribution to the control of this sphincter motor function, however, cannot be entirely excluded because it may participate in conjunction with other duodenal peptides and neural reflexes.

Like it relative secretin, glucagon in very high doses causes decrease in the sphincter of Oddi motor activity in human, dog, cat, rabbit, and opossum (105, 123, 168, 236; J. Behar, unpublished observations). It decreases tonic pressures and the frequency and force of the phasic contractions. However, as in the gallbladder, the doses of glucagon required to relax the sphincter of Oddi far exceeds the doses known to induce physiological effects. The mechanism of action of glucagon on the sphincter of Oddi motor function has not been worked out.

Vasoactive intestinal polypeptide is another potent inhibitor of sphincter of Oddi motor activity. Doses as low as 0.05 $\mu g/kg$ inhibit the cat sphincter tonic pressures and force of phasic activity (J. Behar and P. Biancani, unpublished observations). Like secretin, VIP relaxes the sphincter of Oddi by direct action on the smooth muscle because TTX, hexamethonium, or propranolol do not alter the magnitude of the inhibitory response. In contrast to the gallbladder, the cat sphincter of Oddi appears to have a predominant nonadrenergic, noncholinergic inhibitory pathway as suggested by its response to electrical stimulation of the cervical vagus in vivo, to field stimulation of muscle strips in vitro (J. Behar and P. Biancani, unpublished observations), or to pharmacological stimulation with a variety of drugs such as CCK, serotonin, and some opioid peptides (26, 28). Vasoactive intestinal polypeptide is being considered a candidate neurotransmitter of this inhibitory pathway because its actions are unaffected by TTX. This hypothesis is supported by the finding that VIP has been demonstrated in the guinea pig sphincter of Oddi by immunocytochemistry and radioimmunoassay techniques (64).

*Somatostatin and Bombesin*

Somatostatin is a peptide that is widely distributed in the gastrointestinal tract and has been identified throughout the pancreas, stomach, and intestine in endocrine-like cells or D cells (94, 174) and throughout the myenteric plexus in cell bodies and nerve endings (78). Somatostatin has a wide spectrum of gastrointestinal effects, but two of its most important actions are inhibition of release of gastrointestinal hormones and antagonism of their peripheral effects (241).

Somatostatin has been studied in the biliary tract, in part because of the high incidence of gallstones in patients with somatostatin-secreting tumors of the pancreas (149). Conflicting results, however, have been reported on the effect of somatostatin on gallbladder motility, suggesting that its actions may be species dependent. Furthermore its physiological role has not been established, and, at least in the guinea pig, this peptide has been found only in the mucosa and not in the neurons or nerve endings (64). In pharmacological doses, somatostatin not only blocks gallbladder contraction induced by CCK and carbachol (81, 154, 270) but also reduces basal gallbladder pressures in the fistula dog and conscious pig (3, 170). In the in vivo and in vitro guinea pig gallbladder (212), somatostatin also blocks gallbladder contraction during intraduodenal infusion of fat, which is presumably caused by release of endogenous CCK, but fails to antagonize the contraction in response to exogenous CCK or acetylcholine. Likewise, somatostatin blocks gallbladder contraction elicited by duodenal acidification in the anesthetized cat (38). Somewhat different results were obtained in the pig and human gallbladders, where somatostatin blocks the effects of both exogenous and endogenous CCK. The pig gallbladder contraction in response to exogenous and endogenous CCK was prevented by pretreatment with somatostatin (41). In humans, somatostatin antagonizes the gallbladder response to exogenous CCK as assessed by sonography and blocks the release of immunoreactive CCK in response to intraduodenal infusion of olive oil (237).

Thus somatostatin influences gallbladder motor function by blocking CCK release in response to physiological stimuli and, as some studies suggest, the peripheral action of this hormone on the gallbladder. These inhibitory effects may interfere with gallbladder emptying during the digestive phase and may perhaps contribute to gallstone formation in patients with somastinomas. Unfortunately, no studies are available on direct or indirect effects of somatostatin on motor activity of the sphincter of Oddi, which may also contribute to the pathogenesis of gallstone formation (170). It is possible that high circulating levels of somatostatin blocking the release of CCK may prevent the sphincter of Oddi relaxation during the digestive phase impeding bile flow.

Bombesin, like somatostatin, affects the biliary tract predominantly through indirect mechanisms (132). Although bombesin-immunoreactive nerves have been demonstrated in the guinea pig sphincter of Oddi, it is likely that its pharmacological actions are mediated by CCK (132). Intravenous bombesin elicits gallbladder contraction and decreases pressure in the choledocho-duodenal junction (98). This effect always took place after a latency period of 5–10 min. The action of bombesin is unaffected by antrectomy, suggesting that gastrin plays no role in it (132). Similar results were observed in humans, in whom intravenous bombesin increases gallbladder emptying (75, 76). This peptide also increases spike-burst activity of the rabbit sphincter of Oddi in vivo similar to the effects of CCK and gastrin in this animal species (236).

Bombesin also is virtually ineffective in isolated gallbladder preparations. Its weak contractile effect in vitro, however, is independent of CCK release because it is not blocked by the CCK antagonist dibutyryl cGMP (212). Furthermore, the bombesin mammalian counterpart gastrin-releasing peptide (GRP) stimulates gallbladder contraction in the isolated gallbladder (183).

*Opiates*

Pharmacological studies both in vivo and in vitro have demonstrated the existence of multiple opiate receptors in the central nervous system and gastrointestinal tract. These studies are significant because of the opiates' therapeutic potential and important analgesic and motor effects throughout the gastrointestinal tract. Their importance has been enhanced by the discovery of endogenous opioid peptides both in the central nervous system and in the neural plexi of the gastrointestinal tract (124, 125). Using two independent techniques of immunocytochemistry and radioimmunoassay, Polak et al. (213) demonstrated the presence of Met-enkephalin immunoreactivity both in the special endocrine type cells of the APUD series and in the nerve fibers of the myenteric plexus. The largest amount of Met-enkephalin was detected in the antrum and the upper small intestine, which presumably includes the sphincter of Oddi. Opioid peptides were also found in the myenteric plexus of the gallbladder and bile ducts in humans (213) and in cats (37). Release of opiate-like material has been demonstrated after electrical stimulation of the myenteric plexus of the guinea pig ileum (217, 240). In addition, the specific opiate antagonist naloxone alters certain physiological processes, suggesting that opioid peptides participate in the control mechanism of these functions. A potential physiological role of opioids has been shown in the cat pylorus (95) and sphincter of Oddi (26) and in the control of intestinal peristalsis and peristaltic reflex of the colon in the guinea pig (113, 150).

The action of opiates on the gallbladder has been investigated in a variety of animal species with different in vitro and in vivo preparations. One study showed that intravenous infusions of Met-enkephalins caused contraction in the cat gallbladder, which was antagonized by naloxone (37). Other studies performed in several animal species, however, have failed to confirm this finding. Opiate alkaloids (morphine) and peptides (Met-enkephalins, dynorphin 1–13, and β-endorphin) have no effect in either guinea pig (14) or cat gallbladder pressures (28) in basal conditions in vivo or during transmural electrical stimulation in vitro (203). Morphine, however, caused a significant inhibition of the gallbladder emptying rates in humans (230). This effect could also be explained by the known stimulatory effects of opiate alkaloids on the sphincter of Oddi, which could antagonize the gallbladder emptying induced by CCK. Thus despite the presence of immunoreactive Met-enkephalin nerves in the guinea pig gallbladder wall (64), opiates seem to have little or no effect on gallbladder motor function.

In the sphincter of Oddi, morphine has a marked stimulatory effect, increasing both tonic pressures and force and frequency of the phasic contractions. This effect has been demonstrated in most animal species; the magnitude of the response, however, varies considerably from species to species. A pronounced excitatory effect has been shown in the sphincter of Oddi of human (83, 88, 130), dog (148, 173), and cat (28, 208), which are extremely sensitive to morphine, whereas the opossum sphincter of Oddi is relatively insensitive (W. J. Dodds, personal communication). In the cat sphincter of Oddi in vitro, however, morphine is totally ineffective (205). In the dog, one study showed that the sphincter of Oddi has a dual response to morphine (138) consisting of a greater excitatory response at smaller doses (0.1 mg/kg) than that at higher doses (1 mg/kg). This response is thought to be due to a combination of stimulatory and inhibitory activity with inhibition occurring at higher doses, although the exact mechanism responsible for these results has not been completely elucidated. Development of tolerance or tachyphylaxis to morphine should be considered as another possible explanation for the inhibition observed with higher doses. Because morphine and Demerol have no effect on basal gallbladder motor function of any animal species studied, the increase in intraductal pressures caused by these alkaloids results from their action on the sphincter of Oddi. Thus the increase in choledochal pressures induced by a small intravenous dose of morphine sulfate in humans that was quickly reversed by naloxone can only be interpreted by sphincter of Oddi contraction and decreased transphincteric bile flow (88). In contrast, in the guinea pig sphincter of Oddi in vitro, morphine inhibits the spontaneous phasic contractions as well as those induced by transmural stimulation but did not block the phasic contractions caused by acetylcholine. The phasic contractions were also suppressed by atropine and TTX. These findings suggest that morphine and TTX inhibit the phasic contractions of the sphincter of Oddi by blocking acetylcholine release (14), whereas atropine has the same effect by blocking muscarinic receptors.

Although it has been shown that morphine stimulates the gastrointestinal motor function by central and/or local mechanisms (58, 250), only local mechanisms have been demonstrated in the sphincter of Oddi. No studies have been performed using intrathecal or intraventricular morphine with simultaneous measurement of a sphincter of Oddi or gallbladder motor function (58, 251). Intravenous or intra-arterial morphine causes a marked increase in tonic pressure and amplitude and frequency of phasic contractions of the sphincter of Oddi. Morphine, as in other preparations, stimulates the sphincter of Oddi through $\mu$-receptors. The peptide morphiceptin, a $\mu$-ligand, has similar excitatory effects (67). In the cat sphincter of Oddi, both $\mu$-agonists are easily blocked by relatively low doses of naloxone (40 $\mu$g/kg). These $\mu$-receptors appear to be localized in the neuronal bodies of the myenteric plexus because they are blocked by relatively small doses (12 $\mu$g/kg) of TTX. The neurons involved are cholinergic, because the actions of the $\mu$-agonists are also blocked by atropine in doses that are effective against the maximal dose of bethanechol (208).

In addition to $\mu$-receptors, the sphincter of Oddi has $\delta$- and $\kappa$-opiate receptors. In the cat, the sphincter of Oddi responds in a biphasic fashion to the relatively pure $\delta$-agonists Met- and Leu-enkephalin (28). Low doses of these enkephalins (0.5–8 $\mu$g/kg) administered intra-arterially cause an initial contraction followed by a more prolonged relaxation (Fig. 8). Complete antagonism of the excitatory response requires larger doses of naloxone, ~16 times those required to block the actions of morphine, a $\mu$-agonist. This is consistent with the view that the receptors activated by enkephalins are $\delta$-receptors. They also seem to be present on different neurons because atropine only partially blocks their excitatory effect. Atropine (30 $\mu$g/kg) completely antagonizes the action of a maximal dose of morphine or bethanechol but only decreases the excitatory effect of enkephalin by 50%. The remaining 50% is blocked by the addition of a specific serotonin antagonist, methysergide. The inhibitory effect of enkephalin, however, is unaffected. These data suggest that enkephalins activate $\delta$-receptors present on serotonergic neurons releasing serotonin, which, as previously discussed, would in turn stimulate cholinergic neurons and the smooth muscle of the sphincter of Oddi. Opiates have been shown to stimulate the release of intestinal serotonin (61). These observations, however, do not exclude the existence of separate $\delta$-receptors on cholinergic and on serotonergic neurons. The enkephalin-induced inhibition is also mediated by $\delta$-receptors (J. Behar and P Biancani, unpublished observations). When the sphincter of Oddi motor activity is maintained by a constant infusion of bethanechol, large doses of naloxone (up to 400 $\mu$g/kg) are needed to block this enkephalin effect. This relaxation induced by enkephalins is not antagonized by adrenergic (propranolol) or cholinergic (hexamethonium) antagonists but is blocked by TTX. Thus enkephalins activate receptors on postganglionic nonadrenergic, noncholinergic inhibitory neurons. In the guinea pig, Met-enkephalin inhibited dose dependently the sphincter of Oddi contraction induced by transmural stimulation (203).

Dynorphin 1–13 produces sphincter of Oddi contraction followed by relaxation in the cat (J. Behar and P. Biancani, unpublished observations). Pharmacological analysis of these actions indicates that dynorphin may activate excitatory $\mu$-receptors at cholinergic neurons because this effect is blocked by relatively small doses of naloxone (40 $\mu$g/kg) similar to those required to antagonize morphine by atropine and TTX. After treatment with atropine, dynorphin 1–13 causes relaxation exclusively which is antagonized by intermediate doses of naloxone (160 $\mu$g/kg). This finding would suggest that dynorphin activates opiate receptors that are neither $\mu$- or $\delta$- and possibly κ-receptors. Like δ-receptors, the site of κ-receptors is at the nonadrenergic, noncholinergic inhibitory neurons because the inhibitory effects of dynorphin are only antagonized by TTX. In the guinea pig, dynorphin 1–13 causes a dose-dependent sphincter of Oddi relaxation similar to the effects of enkephalins and β-endorphin (203).

Naloxone appears to be a specific opiate antagonist in the cat sphincter of Oddi. It does not antagonize a variety of other agonists such as bethanechol, phenylephrine, serotonin, histamine, substance P, and gastrin (J. Behar, unpublished observations). It does antagonize motilin because this peptide may stimulate the sphincter of Oddi by activating opioid neurons (27). Naloxone causes a dose-dependent relaxation of the cat sphincter of Oddi (Fig. 9). This effect is neurally mediated because it is abolished by TTX and is produced as a result of its antagonism against the tonic effect of opioid neurons (25, 28). Naloxone-induced relaxation does not seem to be due to stimulation of the inhibitory pathway. Drugs that activate this pathway, such as CCK, are capable of relaxing bethanechol-stimulated sphincter of Oddi motor activity, whereas naloxone is not. The inhibitory effect is indirect and is produced by blocking the tonic excitatory activity of opioid neurons and thus enhancing the tonic action of the postganglionic, noncholinergic, and nonadrenergic inhibitory fibers.

### Motilin

Motilin is a decosapeptide containing 22 amino acids that has been shown to act in the gastrointestinal tract exclusively as a hormone. Duodenal acidification appears to be its most important stimulus, inducing a prompt increase in plasma motilin (188). This hormone has been localized mainly in the proximal small intestine in humans and in other animal species. By

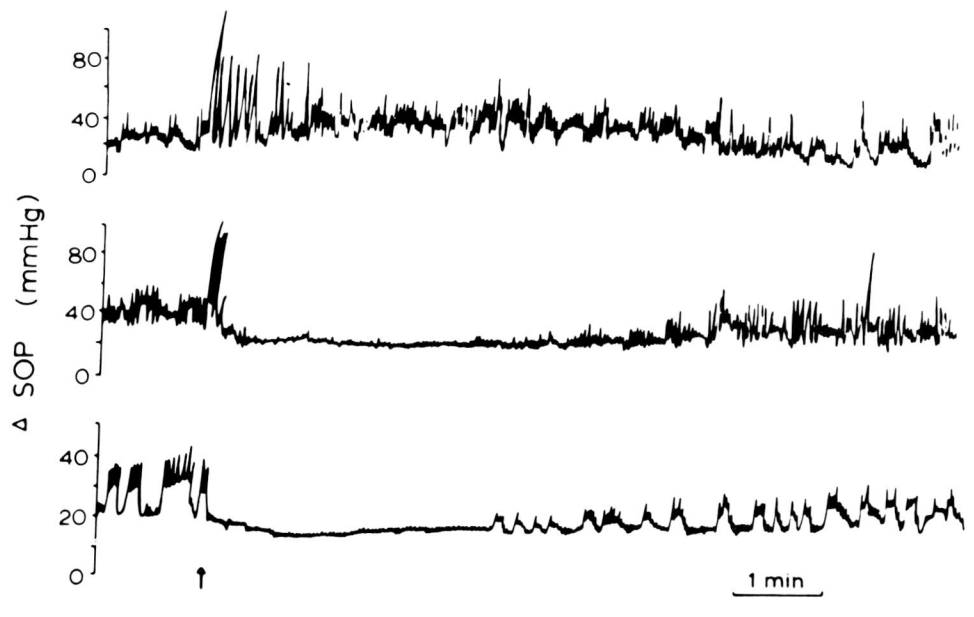

FIG. 8. Cat sphincter of Oddi responses to an intra-arterial dose of Met-enkephalin. Biphasic response (middle) of contraction followed by relaxation was most common. SOP, sphincter of Oddi pressure. [From Behar and Biancani (27). Copyright 1984 by the American Gastroenterological Association.]

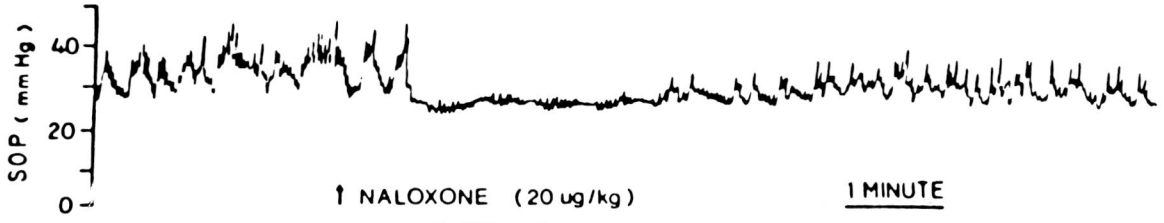

FIG. 9. Effect of naloxone on cat sphincter of Oddi in vivo. This opiate antagonist causes relaxation with decrease in tonic pressures and abolition of phasic contractions. SOP, sphincter of Oddi pressure. [From Behar and Biancani (24).]

radioimmunoassay techniques, it has been demonstrated in the endocrine M cells of the antrum, duodenum, and proximal jejunum (42). It has not been detected in neural structures of the gastrointestinal tract. Its most important action is an excitatory motor effect (50). Fluctuations of serum motilin correlate with the phases of the interdigestive migrating motor complex (128, 212). Before phase III of the migrating motor complex, high circulating levels are observed with a gradual decrease throughout the other phases and during the digestive period (128, 212).

Motilin causes contraction of the gallbladder and the sphincter of Oddi. In the conscious pig (3) and dog (40, 258) or in decerebrated dogs (197), motilin produces a typical motor complex or a dose-dependent increase in gallbladder pressures. The excitatory effect on the canine gallbladder muscle takes place toward the end of phase II of the interdigestive state and depends on vagal tone being enhanced by increased vagal activity and largely diminished or abolished after vagotomy or treatment with atropine (256, 258). It is conceivable that the vagal tone is increased during the interdigestive state because constant infusions of motilin induce transient contractions of the gallbladder during the interdigestive but not during the digestive period. In the interdigestive state of a conscious animal, the gallbladder response to motilin is not dose dependent (256). In humans during fasting, an association between endogenous plasma motilin concentrations and spontaneous gallbladder emptying has been observed. Plasma motilin concentrations were found to invariably rise before the onset of gallbladder concentrations (127, 166). In contrast, 13-norleucine motilin, a synthetic analogue, or the natural motilin had no effect on in vitro gallbladder strips from rabbit, guinea pig, rat, and human but contracted strips from antrum and proximal small bowel (216, 252).

The sphincter of Oddi, however, is more sensitive than the gallbladder, at least in anesthetized animals. For instance in the cat, the sphincter of Oddi responds to intra-arterial administration of as little as 32 ng/kg of motilin, whereas the gallbladder does not respond to doses of up to 1 $\mu$g/kg (27). It has been shown that motilin causes sphincter of Oddi contraction characterized by an increase in frequency and force of phasic contractions in a variety of animal species such as cat, dog, opossum, and rabbit (27, 236, 257). It modifies the dog and cat sphincter of Oddi motor activity by peripheral actions because extrinsic denervation, particularly vagotomy, does not alter its effects.

The local mechanisms of action of motilin has not been entirely worked out and in some animal species is still controversial. In the dog most studies suggest that motilin acts in the gastrointestinal tract exclusively through cholinergic mechanisms because it is completely antagonized by adequate doses of atropine. Other studies have suggested that motilin may act through noncholinergic mechanisms and even perhaps directly on the smooth muscle of the sphincter of Oddi. Neya et al. (198) studied the effect of motilin on flow through the sphincter of Oddi into the duodenal lumen in decerebrated dogs and found that this hormone decreases flow significantly. This effect was not antagonized by extrinsic denervation, which consisted of vagotomy or splanchnicectomy, and by atropine. Thus it was suggested that this effect was direct on the muscle. It is conceivable, however, that motilin may act through noncholinergic intrinsic neural mechanisms because the sphincter of Oddi was not completely denervated with a neurotoxin such as TTX. In the cat, motilin causes sphincter of Oddi contraction characterized by a slight increase in tonic pressures and marked increase in the frequency and amplitude of phasic contractions (26). Motilin also decreases sphincter of Oddi flow, and this effect is dose dependent with a maximal dose of 128 ng/kg (27). In the cat, as in other species, the effect of motilin is not affected by extrinsic denervation or by use of maximal doses of the ganglionic blocker hexamethonium but is antagonized by TTX, indicating that it is mediated exclusively by neural mechanisms (26). Motilin is also antagonized partially by atropine or by methysergide. It is entirely antagonized by the combination of atropine and methysergide or by the specific opiate antagonist naloxone. These findings suggest that the effect of motilin is mediated through endogenous opiates, which in turn stimulate serotonergic and cholinergic neurons (27). In the opossum motilin also causes excitation, increasing the frequency of the phasic contractions that could, in part, explain the increase in the frequency and force of the phasic contractions associated with the duodenal phase of the migrating motor complex (257). Atropine antagonizes the migrating motor complex as well as the effects of motilin, suggesting that this hormone may contribute to the genesis of the phase III of the migrating motor complex in the sphincter of Oddi by stimulating cholinergic neurons.

These pharmacological studies indicate that motilin could play a physiological role in the sphincter of Oddi in several animal species. Increasing serum levels of motilin during the interdigestive phase may stimulate the cat sphincter of Oddi motor activity, decrease transphincteric flow, and divert bile toward the gallbladder. In the opossum, motilin may increase phasic activity and facilitate flow. Motilin could also be one of the non-CCK peptides found in the human serum that causes gallbladder contraction (79). These conclusions are entirely speculative at this point.

*Pancreatic Polypeptide*

Pancreatic polypeptide (PP) is a newly recognized 36–amino acid peptide that is released in response to intraduodenal fat in a pattern that parallels that observed for CCK (102). Its release is under neurohormonal control. Pharmacological doses of CCK, caerulein, pentagastrin, and bombesin cause an increase in the circulating levels of PP-like immunoreactivity in several animal species including humans (21, 116, 172, 222, 265). Likewise, infusion of caerulein, a natural analogue of CCK, causes a significant rise in serum PP (1, 265). In contrast, somatostatin and atropine inhibit its release. Furthermore, endogenous CCK and exogenous infusion of CCK at rates that mimic physiological plasma levels stimulate PP release (172). These findings may be physiologically significant because PP affects the biliary tract motor function. Its biological effects, however, differ a great deal depending on the species of PP used. Although one major biological action of bovine PP is on the dog pancreas, it also relaxes the gallbladder and contracts the sphincter of Oddi (167, 171). Porcine PP also causes a dose-dependent decrease in gallbladder pressures in the conscious pig (2). By relaxing the gallbladder, physiological infusions of bovine PP promotes gallbladder storage of bile in humans (39). However, PP had no effect on muscle strips from human or rabbit gallbladders (137, 216).

These actions of PP are directly opposite to the actions of CCK. Thus it is tempting to speculate that PP may participate in either modulating the actions of CCK or as part of a negative feedback mechanism opposing the physiological action of CCK. Attempts to determine the antagonistic effect of endogenous PP to CCK or CCK-like peptides (caerulein) have failed mainly because of lack of specific PP antagonists. These studies are required to establish a possible physiological role of PP.

*Sex Hormones*

Pregnancy and sex hormones are known to affect the mechanical and electrical properties of gastrointestinal smooth muscle (43, 53, 54, 151, 187). There is substantial evidence that sex hormones affect the gallbladder motor function adversely and thereby contribute to the pathogenesis of gallstone formation. First, there is a disproportionate incidence of gallstones in females during their reproductive years. This discrepancy gradually decreases toward a 1:1 ratio in the last decades of life. Second, pregnancy increases the fasting gallbladder volume and its residual volumes because of a decrease in emptying rates (47). These abnormalities are found to be present in every trimester of pregnancy; they increase linearly during the first two, without further increase in the third. These changes are transient because they disappear in the postpartum period. Third, similar but controversial evidence has been presented during the luteal phase of the menstrual cycle. Gallbladder emptying was found to be impaired in the luteal phase of the menstrual cycle (200). Others have found, however, that elevated progesterone levels associated with the luteal phase do not affect gallbladder volumes or emptying during the ingestion of regular and liquid meals or during the intraduodenal infusion of amino acids (99). Furthermore women taking contraceptive steroids seem to have normal gallbladder volumes and emptying rates after a liquid meal (47). These discrepancies could be reconciled if estrogen-progesterone ratios are taken into account because it is known that these hormones exert independent but opposite effects (228). In addition, gallbladders from female subjects may be less sensitive to progesterone than male gallbladder because they have already been exposed to low-level effects of this hormone. This becomes apparent when experimental studies are performed with male guinea pigs.

The experimental work has been carried out mostly in the guinea pig gallbladder and strongly implicates progesterone in the motor changes observed in the gallbladder during pregnancy. The magnitude of the gallbladder response to a maximal dose of acetylcholine and CCK-8 is significantly reduced after progesterone treatment. However, the sensitivity to these agonists, defined as the response to the $ED_{50}$, or when the control and pregnant data was normalized, was not affected. Moreover the gallbladder muscle strips response to extracellular potassium chloride was no different from that of control muscle strips. The effect of progesterone is more clearly observed when its effects are tested against male gallbladder muscle strips. Figures 10 and 11 show that progesterone pretreatment produced a rightward shift in the acetylcholine and CCK-8, with a decrease in maximal contractile response and sensitivity to these two agonists (227). In contrast, estrogen pretreatment increases the sen-

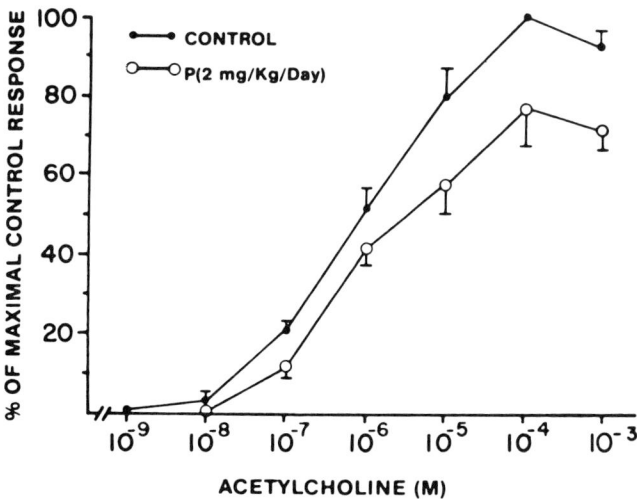

FIG. 10. Effect of progesterone (P) pretreatment (2 mg·kg$^{-1}$·day$^{-1}$) on in vitro contractile response of male guinea pig gallbladder smooth muscle to acetylcholine stimulation. [From Ryan and Pellecchia (227). Copyright 1982 by the American Gastroenterological Association.]

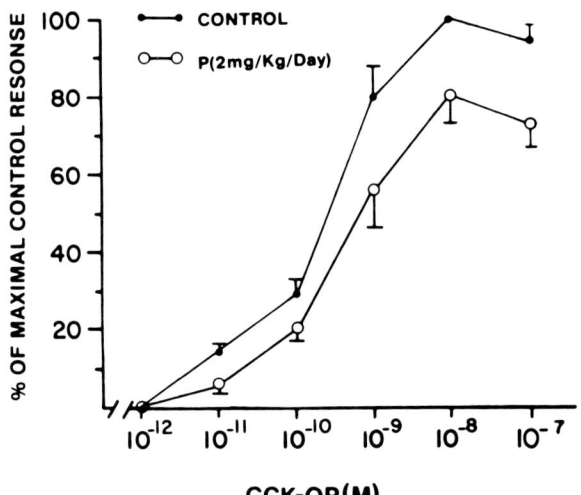

FIG. 11. Effect of progesterone (P) pretreatment (2 mg·kg$^{-1}$·day$^{-1}$) on in vitro contractile response of male guinea pig gallbladder smooth muscle to octapeptide of cholecystokinin (CCK-OP) stimulation. [From Ryan and Pellecchia (227). Copyright 1982 by the American Gastroenterological Association.]

sitivity to acetylcholine without affecting the amplitude of maximal response and antagonizes the effect of progesterone (228). These findings suggest that pregnancy through progesterone affects one step of the excitation-contraction coupling common to both acetylcholine and CCK-8. Progesterone could alter the receptor-operated calcium channel or the mechanisms of utilization of intracellular calcium stores. Voltage-operated calcium channels and the ability of the muscle to contract appear to be intact because of the unchanged response to potassium chloride.

No studies are available on the effects of pregnancy or sex hormones on sphincter of Oddi motor activity.

*Substance P*

Substance P (SP) is an 11-amino acid peptide that is chemically similar to tachykinins such as phylasaemin and eledoisin in which four or five COOH-terminal of each peptide are identical (253). Immunoreactive SP has a widespread distribution in several mammalian species with a highest concentration in the duodenum (199). Most of the immunoreactive SP has been demonstrated in nerves but some is also present in endocrine-like cells of duodenal and colonic mucosa (enterochromaffin cells) (253). Neurons containing SP also have been demonstrated in the cat gallbladder wall, around the ganglia, and a few in contact with smooth muscle cells. Considerable evidence has been accumulated that SP may function as a neurotransmitter or as a neuromodulator of synaptic transmission of the peripheral autonomic system (121). This peptide causes marked smooth muscle contraction in the lower esophageal sphincter, esophageal muscularis mucosa, antrum, and small and large intestine. These actions are mediated partly by cholinergic neurons because the smooth muscle contraction is partly blocked by atropine.

Intravenous doses of SP produces strong gallbladder contraction in several animal species studied (159). It also contracts dog gallbladder in vivo (246) and rabbit and guinea pig gallbladder strips in vitro (159). In the cat biliary tract, SP causes intense but brief gallbladder contraction that is partly blocked by atropine or TTX and completely antagonized by SP tachyphylaxis (J. Behar and P. Biancani, unpublished observations). Substance P tachyphylaxis does not affect basal gallbladder pressures nor does it alter the effect of other agonists such as CCK or physostigmine, suggesting that SP does not participate in the neurohormonal control of the gallbladder motor function (68).

In the sphincter of Oddi of several animal species, Lembeck and Juan (159) observed that SP caused sphincteric relaxation. A more recent study in the cat, however, found that SP causes marked contraction characterized mainly by an increase in tonic pressures (J. Behar, unpublished observations). As in the gallbladder, the excitatory effect of this peptide is partly blocked by atropine and TTX, suggesting that its actions are mediated by cholinergic neurons in addition to a direct effect on the sphincter of Oddi muscle. Substance P tachyphylaxis does not affect basal sphincter of Oddi motor activity or its response to bethanechol and serotonin. Further studies are needed, however, to determine whether it alters the effect of opiates (morphine and enkephalins) or motilin to determine whether it participates in the excitatory pathways.

REFERENCES

1. Adrian, T. E., H. S. Besterman, T. J. C. Cooke, S. R. Bloom, A. J. Barnes, R. C. G. Russell, and R. G. Faber. Mechanism of pancreatic polypeptide release in man. *Lancet* 1: 161–163, 1977.
2. Adrian, T. E., P. Mitchenere, G. Sagor, and S. R. Bloom. Effect of pancreatic polypeptide on gallbladder pressure and hepatic bile secretion. *Am. J. Physiol.* 243 (*Gastrointest. Liver Physiol.* 6): G204–G207, 1982.
3. Adrian, T. E., P. Mitchenere, G. Sagor, N. D. Christofides, and S. R. Bloom. Effect of motilin and other gut hormones on gallbladder pressure. *Regul. Peptide Suppl.* 1: S1, 1980.
4. Agosti, A., P. Mantovani, and L. Mori. Action of caerulein and related substances on the sphincter of Oddi. *Naunyn-Schmiedebergs Arch. Pharmacol.* 268: 114–118, 1971.
5. Al-Hassani, M. H., and J. S. Davison. The role of non-cholinergic, non-adrenergic inhibitory neurons in the regulation of the guinea-pig gall-bladder (Abstract). *J. Physiol. Lond.* 292: 48P, 1979.
6. Amer, M. S. Studies with cholecystokinin. II. Cholecystoki-

netic potency of porcine gastrins I and II and related peptides in three systems. *Endocrinology* 84: 1277–1281, 1969.
7. AMER, M. S. Studies with cholecystokinin in vitro. III. Mechanism of the effect on the isolated rabbit gallbladder strips. *J. Pharmacol. Exp. Ther.* 183: 527–534, 1972.
8. AMER, M. S. Cyclic guanosine 3′,5′-monophosphate and gallbladder contraction. *Gastroenterology* 67: 333–337, 1974.
9. ANDERSEN, B. N. Measurement and occurrence of sulfated gastrins. *Scand. J. Clin. Lab. Invest.* 168: 5–24, 1984.
10. ANDERSSON, K. E., R. ANDERSSON, P. HEDNER, AND C. G. A. PERSSON. Analogous effects of cholecystokinin and prostaglandin $E_2$ on mechanical activity and tissue levels of cAMP in biliary smooth muscle. *Acta Physiol. Scand.* 89: 571–579, 1973.
11. ANDERSSON, K. E., R. ANDERSSON, P. HEDNER, AND C. G. A. PERSSON. Interrelations between cyclic AMP, cyclic GMP, and contraction in guinea pig gallbladder stimulated by cholecystokinin. *Life Sci.* 20: 73, 1977.
12. ANDERSSON, K. E., P. HEDNER, AND C. G. A. PERSSON. Differentiation of the contractile effects of prostaglandin $E_2$ and the C-terminal octapeptide of cholecystokinin in isolated guinea-pig gallbladder. *Acta Physiol. Scand.* 90: 657–663, 1974.
13. ANDERSSON, K. E., P. HEDNER, AND C. G. A. PERSSON. Effects of lanthanum and calcium antagonists on contractile responses of isolated guinea pig gallbladder. *Acta Physiol. Scand.* 91: 16A, 1974.
14. ASAOKA, H., AND M. OOUCHI. Effects of morphine on the guinea pig biliary tract. *Eur. J. Pharmacol.* 80: 311–316, 1982.
15. ASHKIN, J. R., D. T. LYON, S. D. SHULL, C. I. WAGNER, AND R. D. SOLOWAY. Factors affecting delivery of bile to the duodenum in man. *Gastroenterology* 74: 560–565, 1978.
16. BAINBRIDGE, F. A., AND H. H. DALE. The contractile mechanism of the gallbladder and its extrinsic nervous control. *J. Physiol. Lond.* 33: 138–155, 1905.
17. BANFIELD, W. J. Physiology of the gallbladder. *Gastroenterology* 69: 770–777, 1975.
18. BARLAS, N., R. T. JENSEN, M. C. BEINFELD, AND J. D. GARDNER. Cyclic nucleotide antagonists of cholecystokinin: structural requirements for interaction with the cholecystokinin receptor. *Am. J. Physiol.* 242 (*Gastrointest. Liver Physiol.* 5): G161–G167, 1982.
19. BAUMGARTEN, H. G., AND W. LANGE. Extrinsic adrenergic innervation of the extrahepatic biliary system in guinea pigs, cats, and rhesus monkeys. *Z. Zellforsch. Mikrosk. Anat.* 100: 606–615, 1969.
20. BECKER, J. M., F. G. MOODY, AND A. R. ZINSMEISTER. Effect of gastrointestinal hormones on the biliary sphincter of the opossum. *Gastroenterology* 82: 1300–1307, 1982.
21. BEGLINGER, C., F. MEYER, W. HACK, AND K. GYR. The release of pancreatic polypeptide by exogenous CCK in man and dog. *Digestion* 22: 225–228, 1981.
22. BEHAR, J. Effect of pentagastrin on the feline sphincter of Oddi: evidence for a PG inhibitory receptor. *Gastroenterology* 78: 1139, 1980.
23. BEHAR, J., AND P. BIANCANI. Effect of cholecystokinin and the octapeptide of cholecystokinin on the feline sphincter of Oddi and gallbladder. *J. Clin. Invest.* 66: 1231–1239, 1980.
24. BEHAR, J., AND P. BIANCANI. Neural control of the feline gallbladder. In: *Gastrointestinal Motility*, edited by J. Christensen. New York: Raven, 1980, p. 97–109.
25. BEHAR, J., AND P. BIANCANI. Effect of naloxone on the cat sphincter of Oddi (SO): evidence for a physiological role of opioid peptides in the regulation of the sphincter of Oddi. In: *Motility of the Digestive Tract*, edited by M. Weinbeck. New York: Raven, 1982, p. 397–403.
26. BEHAR, J., AND P. BIANCANI. Neural control of the sphincter of Oddi: a physiological role of 5-hydroxytryptamine in the regulation of basal sphincter of Oddi motor activity in the cat. *J. Clin. Invest.* 72: 551–559, 1983.
27. BEHAR, J., AND P. BIANCANI. Effect of motilin on the cat sphincter of Oddi: mechanisms of action. *Gastroenterology* 84: 1102, 1983.
28. BEHAR, J., AND P. BIANCANI. Neural control of the sphincter of Oddi: physiologic role of enkephalins on the regulation of basal sphincter of Oddi motor activity in the cat. *Gastroenterology* 86: 134–141, 1984.
29. BEHAR, J., AND P. BIANCANI. Pharmacological characterization of excitatory and inhibitory cholecystokinin receptors of the cat gallbladder and sphincter of Oddi. *Dig. Dis. Sci.* 29: 8, 1984.
30. BEHAR, J., AND P. BIANCANI. Role of cat sphincter of Oddi motor activity on trans-sphincteric flow (TSF). *Gastroenterology* 88: 1320, 1985.
31. BENNETT, A., J. G. MURRAY, AND J. G. WYLLIE. Occurrence of prostaglandin $E_2$ in the human stomach, and a study of its effects on human isolated gastric muscle. *Br. J. Pharmacol.* 32: 339–349, 1968.
32. BENNETT, A., AND J. POSNER. Studies on prostaglandin antagonists. *Br. J. Pharmacol.* 42: 584–594, 1971.
33. BERGH, G. S. The effect of food upon the sphincter of Oddi in human subjects. *Am. J. Dig. Dis.* 9: 40–43, 1942.
34. BERGH, G. S., AND J. A. LAYNE. A demonstration of the independent contraction of the sphincter of the common bile duct in human subjects. *Am. J. Physiol.* 128: 690–694, 1940.
35. BERTACCINI, G., G. DE CARO, R. ENDEAN, V. ERSPAMER, AND M. IMPICCIATORE. The actions of caerulein on the smooth muscle of the gastrointestinal tract and the gall bladder. *Br. J. Pharmacol.* 34: 291–310, 1968.
36. BIANCANI, P., L. K. LICALZI, AND R. W. MCCALLUM. Mechanism of histamine-induced excitation of the cat pylorus. *J. Clin. Invest.* 68: 582–588, 1981.
37. BJORCK, S., J. M. LUNDBERG, L. JIVEGARD, AND J. SVANIK. Substance-P, enkephalin, and VIP in the feline gallbladder: distribution of immunoreactivity and functional effects by exogenous administration. In: *Mechanisms of Gastrointestinal Motility and Secretion*, edited by A. Bennet and G. P. Velo. New York: Plenum, 1984, p. 159–175.
38. BJORCK, S., AND J. SVANIK. The influence of somatostatin on gallbladder response to intraduodenal acid and autonomic nerve stimulation in the cat. *Scand. J. Gastroenterol.* 19: 173–177, 1984.
39. BJORNSSON, O. G., T. E. ADRIAN, J. DAWSON, R. F. MCCLOY, G. R. GREENBERG, S. R. BLOOM, AND V. S. CHADWICK. Effects of gastrointestinal hormones on fasting gallbladder storage patterns in man. *Eur. J. Clin. Invest.* 9: 293–300, 1979.
40. BLOOM, S. R., T. E. ADRIAN, P. MITCHENERE, G. R. SAGOR, AND N. D. CHRISTOFIDES. Motilin-induced gallbladder contraction—a new mechanism. *Gastroenterology* 80: 1113, 1981.
41. BLOOM, S. R., S. N. JOFFE, AND J. M. POLAK. Effect of somatostatin on pancreatic and biliary function. *Gut* 16: 836–837, 1975.
42. BLOOM, S. R., P. MITZNEGG, AND M. G. BRYANT. Measurement of human plasma motilin. *Scand. J. Gastroenterol.* 11: 47–52, 1976.
43. BORTOFF, A., E. MORELLO, AND P. MISTRETTA. Effects of progesterone and 17-OH progesterone on intestinal slow wave propagation. In: *Gastrointestinal Motility*, edited by J. Christensen. New York: Raven, 1980, p. 387–393.
44. BOYDEN, E. A. The sphincter of Oddi in man and certain representative mammals. *Surgery St. Louis* 1: 25–37, 1937.
45. BOYDEN, E. A. The choledochoduodenal junction in the cat. *Surgery St. Louis* 41: 773–786, 1957.
46. BOYDEN, E. A. The anatomy of the choledochoduodenal junction in man. *Surg. Gynecol. Obstet.* 104: 641–652, 1957.
47. BRAVERMAN, D. Z., M. L. JOHNSON, AND F. KERN. Effects of pregnancy and contraceptive steroids on gallbladder function. *N. Engl. J. Med.* 302: 362–364, 1980.
48. BRENNAN, L. J., T. A. MCLOUGHLIN, V. MUTT, K. TATEMOTO, AND J. R. WOOD. Effects on PHI, a newly isolated peptide, on gallbladder function in the guinea pig (Abstract). *J. Physiol. Lond.* 329: 71P, 1982.
49. BROUGHTON, A. C., D. C. SECORD, AND G. W. SCOTT. Effects

of adrenergic stimulation on the choledochoduodenal sphincter mechanism. *Pharmacology* 15: 152–161, 1977.
50. BROWN, J. C., V. MUTT, AND J. R. DRYBURGH. The further purification of motilin, a gastric motor activity stimulating polypeptide from the mucosa of the small intestine of hogs. *Can. J. Physiol. Pharmacol.* 49: 399–405, 1971.
51. BROWNLEE, G., AND E. S. JOHNSON. The site of the 5-hydroxytryptamine receptor on the intramural nervous plexus of the guinea-pig isolated ileum. *Br. J. Pharmacol.* 21: 306–322, 1963.
52. BROWNLEE, G., AND E. S. JOHNSON. The release of acetylcholine from the isolated ileum of the guinea-pig induced by 5-hydroxytryptamine and dimethylphenylpiperazinium. *Br. J. Pharmacol.* 24: 689–700, 1965.
53. BRUCE, L. A., AND F. M. BEHSUDI. Differential inhibition of regional gastrointestinal tissues. *Life Sci.* 25: 729–734, 1979.
54. BRUCE, L. A., AND F. M. BEHSUDI. Differential inhibition of regional gastrointestinal tissue to progesterone in the rat. *Life Sci.* 27: 427–438, 1980.
55. BUCHAN, A. M. J., J. M. POLAK, E. SOLCIA, C. CAPELLA, D. HUDSON, AND A. G. E. PEARSE. Electron immunohistochemical evidence for the human intestinal I cell as the source of CCK. *Gut* 19: 403–407, 1978.
56. BUFFA, R., E. SOLCIA, AND V. L. W. GO. Immunohistochemical identification of the cholecystokinin cell in the intestinal mucosa. *Gastroenterology* 70: 528–532, 1976.
57. BURGET, G. E., AND R. J. BROCKLEHURST. The bile-expelling mechanism in the guinea pig. *Am. J. Physiol.* 83: 578–588, 1928.
58. BURKS, T. F. Central sites of action of gastrointestinal drugs. *Gastroenterology* 74: 322–324, 1978.
59. BURKS, T. F., AND J. P. LONG. Catecholamine-induced release of 5-hydroxytryptamine from perfused vasculature of isolated dog intestine. *J. Pharm. Sci.* 55: 1383–1386, 1966.
60. BURKS, T. F., AND J. P. LONG. Release of 5-hydroxytryptamine from isolated dog intestine by nicotine. *Br. J. Pharmacol.* 30: 229–239, 1967.
61. BURKS, T. F., AND J. P. LONG. Release of intestinal 5-hydroxytryptamine by morphine and related agents. *J. Pharmacol. Exp. Ther.* 156: 267–276, 1967.
62. BUTSCH, W. L., J. M. MCGOWAN, AND W. WALTERS. Clinical studies on the influence of certain drugs in relation to biliary pain and to the variations in intraductal pressure. *Surg. Gynecol. Obstet.* 63: 451–456, 1936.
63. BYRNES, D. J., T. BORODY, G. DASKALOPOULOS, M. BOYLE, AND I. BENN. Cholecystokinin and gallbladder contraction: effect of CCK infusion. *Peptides* 2: 259–262, 1981.
64. CAI, W., AND G. GABELLA. Innervation of the gallbladder and biliary pathways in the guinea pig. *J. Anat.* 136: 97–109, 1983.
65. CAMERON, A. J., S. F. PHILLIPS, AND W. H. J. SUMMERSKILL. Effect of cholecystokinin, gastrin, secretin and glucagon on human gallbladder muscle in vitro. *Proc. Soc. Exp. Biol. Med.* 131: 149–154, 1969.
66. CARR-LOCKE, D. L., J. A. GREGG, AND W. Y. CHEY. Effect of exogenous secretin on pancreatic and biliary ductal and sphincteric pressures in man demonstrated by endoscopic manometry and correlation with plasma secretin levels. *Dig. Dis. Sci.* 30: 909–917, 1985.
67. CHANG, K. J., A. KILLIAN, E. HAZUM, AND P. CUATRECASAS. Morphiceptin: a potent and specific agonist for morphine receptors. *Science Wash. DC* 212: 75–77, 1981.
68. CHANG, R. S., V. J. LOTTI, AND T. B. CHEN. Further evidence that substance P partly mediates the action of cholecystokinin octapeptide (CCK-8) on the guinea pig ileum but not gall bladder: studies with a substance P antagonist. *Neurosci. Lett.* 46: 71–75, 1984.
69. CHERNISH, S. M., R. E. MILLER, B. D. ROSENAK, AND N. E. SCHOLZ. Effect of glucagon on size of visualized human gallbladder before and after a fat meal. *Gastroenterology* 62: 1218–1226, 1972.
70. CHIODO, L. A., AND B. S. BUNNEY. Proglumide: selective antagonism of excitatory effects of cholecystokinin in central nervous system. *Science Wash. DC* 219: 1449–1451, 1983.
71. CHOWDHURY, J. R., J. M. BERKOWITZ, M. PRAISSMAN, AND J. W. FARA. Interaction between octapeptide-cholecystokinin, gastrin, and secretin, on cat gallbladder in vitro. *Am. J. Physiol.* 229: 1311–1315, 1975.
72. CHOWDHURY, J. R., J. M. BERKOWITZ, M. PRAISSMAN, AND J. W. FARA. Effect of sulfated and non-sulfated gastrin and octapeptide-cholecystokinin on cat gall bladder in vitro. *Experientia* 32: 1173–1175, 1976.
73. COLLINS, S. M., S. ABDELMOUMENE, R. T. JENSEN, AND J. D. GARDNER. Reversal of cholecystokinin-induced persistent stimulation of pancreatic enzyme secretion by dibutyryl cyclic GMP. *Am. J. Physiol.* 240 (*Gastrointest. Liver Physiol.* 3): G466–G471, 1981.
74. COPHER, G. H., S. KODAMA, AND E. A. GRAHAM. The filling and emptying of the gallbladder. *J. Exp. Med.* 44: 65–73, 1926.
75. CORAZZIARI, E., F. I. HABIB, G. F. DELLE FAVE, P. MELCHIORRI, A. TORSOLI, AND R. CARRATU. Gastrointestinal and gallbladder motor effects of bombesin in man. *Mater. Med. Pol.* 9: 139–143, 1977.
76. CORAZZIARI, E., A. TORSOLI, P. MELCHIORRI, AND G. F. DELLE FAVE. Effect of bombesin on human gallbladder emptying. *Rend. Gastroenterol.* 6: 227, 1974.
77. COSTA, M., AND J. B. FURNESS. The sites of action of 5-hydroxytryptamine in nerve-muscle preparations from the guinea-pig small intestine and colon. *Br. J. Pharmacol.* 65: 237–248, 1979.
78. COSTA, M., Y. PATEL, J. B. FURNESS, AND A. ARIMURA. Evidence that some intrinsic neurons of the intestine contain somatostatin. *Neurosci. Lett.* 6: 215–222, 1977.
79. COX, K. L., G. L. ROSENQUIST, AND C. K. IWAHASHI-HOSODA. Noncholecystokinin peptides in human serum which cause gallbladder contraction. *Life Sci.* 31: 3023–3029, 1982.
80. CREMA, A., G. BENZI, G. M. FRIGO, AND F. BERTE. The responses of the terminal bile duct to morphine and morphine-like drugs. *J. Pharmacol. Exp. Ther.* 149: 373–378, 1965.
81. CREUTZFELDT, W., P. G. LANKISCH, AND U. R. FOLSCH. Hemmung der sekretin- und cholecystokinin-pankreozymin-induzierten saft-und enzymasekretion des pankreas und der gallenblasenkontraktion beim menschen durch somatostatin. *Dtsch. Med. Wochenschr.* 100: 1135–1138, 1975.
82. CROSSLEY, A. W. A., AND J. S. GILLESPIE. The effect of an inhibitory factor from the bovine retractor penis on the gastrointestinal tract and gallbladder of the guinea-pig. *Br. J. Pharmacol.* 78: 213–220, 1983.
83. CURRERI, A. R., AND J. W. GALE. Effect of analgesics and antispasmodics on common duct pressures. *Ann. Surg.* 132: 348–361, 1950.
84. DANIEL, E. E., J. E. T. FOX, J. JURY, AND S. M. COLLINS. Sites and mechanisms of actions of neuro-peptides on gut motility differ in vivo and in vitro. *Gastroenterology* 82: 1039, 1982.
85. DAVISON, J. S., AND S. FOSEL. Interactions between vagus nerve stimulation and pentagastrin or secretin on the guinea pig gallbladder. *Digestion* 13: 251–254, 1975.
86. DAVISON, J. S., AND S. A. NAJAFI-FARASHAH. Dibutyryl cyclic GMP, a competitive inhibitor of cholecystokinin/pancreozymin and related peptides in the gallbladder and ileum. *Can. J. Physiol. Pharmacol.* 59: 1100–1104, 1981.
87. DAVISON, J. S., AND S. A. NAJAFI-FARASHAH. Proglumide: a specific antagonist to the actions of cholecystokinin-like peptides in guinea-pig gallbladder and ileum. *Pharmacol. Physiol.* 10: 409–410, 1982.
88. DEDRICK, D. F., W. W. TANNER, AND F. L. BUSHKIN. Common bile duct pressure during enflurane anesthesia. *Arch. Surg.* 115: 820–822, 1980.
89. DESCHODT-LANCKMAN, M., N. D. BUI, D. KOULISCHER, P. PAROUTAUD, AND A. STROSBERG. Cholecystokinin octa- and tetrapeptide degradation by synaptic membranes. II. Solubilization and separation of membrane-bound CCK-8 cleaving

enzymes. *Peptides* 4: 71-78, 1983.
90. DOCKRAY, G. J. Immunoreactive component resembling cholecystokinin octapeptide in intestine. *Nature Lond.* 270: 357-361, 1977.
91. DOCKRAY, G. J., J. F. REHFELD, AND J. H. WALSH. Naming gastrin and cholecystokinin peptides. In: *Gastrins and the Vagus*, edited by J. F. Rehfeld and E. Amdrup. London: Academic, 1979, p. 95-97.
92. DOGGRELL, S. A., AND G. W. SCOTT. The occurrence of postsynaptic alpha and beta-adrenoceptors in the guinea-pig gall bladder. *Br. J. Pharmacol.* 71: 185-189, 1980.
93. DUBOIS, F. S., AND E. A. HUNT. Peristalsis of the common bile duct in the opossum. *Anat. Rec.* 53: 387-397, 1932.
94. DUBOIS, M. P. Immunoreactive somatostatin is present in discrete cells of the endocrine pancreas. *Proc. Natl. Acad. Sci. USA* 72: 1340-1343, 1975.
95. EDIN, R., J. LUNDBERG, L. TERENIUS, A. DAHLSTROM, T. HÖKFELT, J. KEWENTER, AND H. AHLMAN. Evidence for vagal enkephalinergic neural control of the feline pylorus. *Gastroenterology* 78: 492-497, 1980.
96. EICHHORN, E. P., AND E. A. BOYDEN. The choledochoduodenal junction in the dog. A restudy of Oddi's sphincter. *Am. J. Anat.* 97: 431-460, 1955.
97. ENGLERT, E., AND V. S. CHIN. Quantitation of human biliary evacuation with a radioisotope technique. *Gastroenterology* 50: 506-508, 1966.
98. ERSPAMER, V., G. IMPROTA, P. MELCHIORRI, AND N. SOPRANZI. Evidence of cholecystokinin release by bombesin in the dog. *Br. J. Pharmacol.* 52: 227-232, 1974.
99. EVERSON, G. T., C. MCKINLEY, M. LAWSON, M. JOHNSON, AND F. KERN. Gallbladder function in the human female: effect of the ovulatory cycle, pregnancy, and contraceptive steroids. *Gastroenterology* 82: 711-719, 1982.
100. FARA, J. W., AND S. M. ERDE. Comparison of in vivo and in vitro responses to sulfated and non-sulfated ceruletide. *Eur. J. Pharmacol.* 47: 359-363, 1978.
101. FEELEY, T. M., A. S. CLANACHAN, AND G. W. SCOTT. The effects of vasoactive intestinal polypeptide on the motility of human and guinea pig gallbladder. *Can. J. Physiol. Pharmacol.* 62: 356-359, 1984.
102. FRIED, G. M., W. D. OGDEN, C. J. FAGAN, K. INOUE, G. GREELEY, AND J. C. THOMPSON. Plasma concentrations of cholecystokinin in patients with duodenal ulcer disease. *Surgery St. Louis* 95: 27-33, 1984.
103. GADACZ, T. R. Effect of an H-2 antagonist on gallbladder contraction. *J. Surg. Res.* 25: 334-341, 1978.
104. GARDNER, J. D., M. KNIGHT, V. E. SUTLIFF, C. A. TAMMINGA, AND R. T. JENSEN. Derivatives of CCK-(26-32) as cholecystokinin receptor antagonists in guinea pig pancreatic acini. *Am. J. Physiol.* 246 (*Gastrointest. Liver Physiol.* 9): G292-G295, 1984.
105. GEENEN, J. E., W. J. HOGAN, W. J. DODDS, E. T. STEWART, AND R. C. ARNDORFER. Intraluminal pressure recordings from the human sphincter of Oddi. *Gastroenterology* 78: 317-324, 1980.
106. GERSHON, M. D. Effects of tetrodotoxin on innervated smooth muscle preparations. *Br. J. Pharmacol. Chemother.* 29: 259-279, 1967.
107. GERSHON, M. D. Putative neurotransmitters: serotonin. *Neurosci. Res. Program Bull.* 17: 414-424, 1979.
108. GERSHON, M. D., AND S. M. ERDE. The nervous system of the gut. *Gastroenterology* 80: 1571-1594, 1981.
109. GESSNER, P. K. Pharmacological studies of 5-methoxy-N,N-dimethyltryptamine, LSD, and other hallucinogens. In: *Psychosomatic Drugs*, edited by D. H. Efron. New York: Raven, 1969, p. 105-122.
110. GORHAM, F. W., AND A. C. IVY. Evolutionary contributions to the general function of the gallbladder. *Am. J. Digest. Dis.* 4: 792-796, 1938.
111. GORHAM, F. W., AND A. C. IVY. General function of the gallbladder from the evolutionary standpoint. *Zoo. Ser. Field Museum Natl. Hist.* 22: 159-213, 1938.
112. GREIDER, M. H., V. STEINBERG, AND J. E. MCGUIGAN. Electron microscopic identification of the gastrin cell of the human antral mucosa by means of immunocytochemistry. *Gastroenterology* 63: 572-582, 1972.
113. GRIDER, J. R., AND G. M. MAKHLOUF. Regulation of intestinal peristalsis by intramural opioid neurons. *Gastroenterology* 86: 1099, 1984.
114. GROSSMAN, M. I. Candidate hormones of the gut. I. Introduction. *Gastroenterology* 67: 730-731, 1974.
115. GULLO, L., L. BOLONDI, P. PRIORI, P. CASANOVA, AND G. LABO. Inhibitory effect of atropine on cholecystokinin-induced gallbladder contraction in man. *Digestion* 29: 209-213, 1984.
116. GUZMAN, S., J. LONOVICS, K. E. HEJTMANCIK, P. L. RAYFORD, AND J. L. THOMPSON. Hormone-stimulated release of pancreatic polypeptide before and after vagotomy in dogs. *Gastroenterology* 76: 1147, 1979.
117. GYERMEK, L. 5-Hydroxytryptamine antagonists. *Pharmacol. Rev.* 13: 399-439, 1961.
118. HAHNE, W. F., R. T. JENSEN, G. F. LEMP, AND J. D. GARDNER. Proglumide and benzotript: members of a different class of cholecystokinin receptor antagonists. *Proc. Natl. Acad. Sci. USA* 78: 6304-6308, 1981.
119. HEDQVIST, P., S. DAHLEN, L. GUSTAFSSON, S. HAMMARSTROM, AND B. SAMUELSSON. Biological profile of leukotrienes $C_4$ and $D_4$. *Acta Physiol. Scand.* 110: 331-333, 1980.
120. HINMAN, J. W. Prostaglandins. *Annu. Rev. Biochem.* 41: 161-178, 1972.
121. HÖKFELT, T., O. JOHANSSON, A. LJUNGDAHL, J. M. LUNDBERG, AND M. SCHULTZBERG. Peptidergic neurons. *Nature Lond.* 284: 515-521, 1980.
122. HOLME, G., G. BRUNET, H. PIECHUTA, P. MASSON, Y. GIRARD, AND J. ROKACH. The activity of synthetic leukotriene C-1 on guinea pig trachea and ileum. *Prostaglandins* 20: 717-728, 1980.
123. HONDA, R., J. TOOULI, W. J. DODDS, W. J. HOGAN, J. GEENEN, AND Z. ITOH. Effect of enteric hormones on sphincter of Oddi and gastrointestinal myoelectric activity in fasted conscious opossums. *Gastroenterology* 84: 1-9, 1983.
124. HUGHES, J. Isolation of an endogenous compound from the brain with pharmacological properties similar to morphine. *Brain Res.* 88: 295-308, 1975.
125. HUGHES, J., H. W. KOSTERLITZ, AND T. W. SMITH. The distribution of methionine-enkephalin and leucine-enkephalin in the brain and peripheral tissues. *Br. J. Pharmacol.* 61: 639-647, 1977.
126. IMPICCIATORE, M. Occurrence of H1- and H2-histamine receptors in the guinea pig gallbladder in situ. *Br. J. Pharmacol.* 64: 219-222, 1978.
127. ITOH, Z., I. TAKAHASHI, AND T. SUZUKI. Contractile patterns of the gallbladder between meals in the dog. In: *Motility of the Digestive Tract*, edited by M. Weinbeck. New York: Raven, 1982, p. 405-413.
128. ITOH, Z., S. TAKEUCHI, I. AIZAWA, K. MORI, T. TAMINATO, Y. SEINO, H. IMURA, AND N. YANAIHARA. Changes in plasma motilin concentration and gastrointestinal contractile activity in conscious dogs. *Dig. Dis. Sci.* 23: 929-935, 1978.
129. IVY, A. C. The physiology of the gallbladder. *Physiol. Rev.* 14: 1-102, 1934.
130. JACOBSSON, B., J. KEWENTER, AND N. G. KOCK. Action of codeine and some other antitussive drugs on choledochal pressure and duodenal activity: a study in cholecystectomized patients. *Acta Chir. Scand.* 122: 407-413, 1961.
131. JANSEN, J. B., AND C. B. LAMERS. Radioimmunoassay of cholecystokinin in human tissue and plasma. *Clin. Chim. Acta* 131: 305-316, 1983.
132. JANSEN, J. B., AND C. B. LAMERS. Effect of bombesin on plasma cholecystokinin in normal persons and gastrectomized patients measured by sequence-specific radioimmunoassays. *Surgery St. Louis* 96: 55-60, 1984.
133. JANSSON, R., G. STEEN, AND J. SVANVIK. Effects of intrave-

nous vasoactive intestinal peptide (VIP) on gallbladder function in the cat. *Gastroenterology* 75: 47–50, 1978.

134. JANSSON, R., G. STEEN, AND J. SVANVIK. A comparison of glucagon, gastric inhibitory peptide, and secretin on gallbladder function, formation of bile, and pancreatic secretion in the cat. *Scand. J. Gastroenterol.* 13: 919–925, 1978.

135. JANSSON, R., AND J. SVANVIK. Effects of intravenous secretin and cholecystokinin on gallbladder net water absorption and motility in the cat. *Gastroenterology* 72: 639–643, 1977.

136. JENSEN, R. T., S. W. JONES, AND J. D. GARDNER. COOH-terminal fragments of cholecystokinin: a new class of cholecystokinin receptor antagonists. *Biochim. Biophys. Acta* 757: 250–258, 1983.

137. JOHNSON, A. G., C. E. MARSHALL, AND I. A. WILSON. Effects of some drugs and peptide hormones on the responsiveness of the rabbit isolated gallbladder to cholecystokinin. *J. Physiol. Lond.* 332: 415–425, 1982.

138. JOHNSON, E. E. Morphine: a dual effect at the canine choledochoduodenal junction. *J. Pharmacol. Exp. Ther.* 219: 274–280, 1981.

139. JOHNSON, L. R., G. F. STENING, AND M. I. GROSSMAN. Effect of sulfation on the gastrointestinal actions of caerulein. *Gastroenterology* 58: 208–216, 1970.

140. JONES, R. S., R. E. GEIST, AND A. D. HALL. The choleretic effects of glucagon and secretin in the dog. *Gastroenterology* 60: 64–68, 1971.

141. KADLEC, O., K. MASEK, AND I. SEFERNA. Modulation by prostaglandins of the release of acetylcholine and noradrenaline in guinea pig isolated ileum. *J. Pharmacol. Exp. Ther.* 205: 635–645, 1978.

142. KAMATA, M. Electrical and mechanical properties of smooth muscle cells of the guinea pig biliary system. *Jpn. J. Physiol.* 30: 179–204, 1980.

143. KAO, C. Y. Pharmacology of tetrodotoxin and satitoxin. *Federation Proc.* 31: 1117–1123, 1972.

144. KERSTENS, P. J., C. B. LAMERS, J. B. JANSEN, A. J. DEJONG, M. HESSELS, AND J. C. HAFKENSCHEID. Physiological plasma concentrations of cholecystokinin stimulate pancreatic enzyme secretion and gallbladder contraction in man. *Life Sci.* 36: 565–569, 1985.

145. KIMURA, M., S. KOBAYASHI, AND I. KIMURA. Evidence that relaxation of hog biliary muscle is mediated by the interaction between the protein inhibitor of cyclic AMP dependent protein kinase and cholecystokinin C-terminal peptides. *Biochem. Pharmacol.* 32: 795–798, 1983.

146. KOELLE, G. B. Neurohormonal transmission and the autonomic nervous system. In: *The Pharmacological Basis of Therapeutics* (5th ed.), edited by L. S. Goodman and A. Gilman. New York: Macmillan, 1975, chapt. 21, p. 404–444.

147. KOTWALL, C. A., A. S. CLANACHAN, H. P. BAER, AND G. W. SCOTT. Effects of prostaglandins on motility of gallbladders removed from patients with gallstones. *Arch. Surg.* 119: 709–712, 1984.

148. KOZOLI, D. D., AND H. NECHELES. A study of the mechanics of bile flow. III. Responses to pharmacological stimuli. *Surg. Gynecol. Obstet.* 74: 961–967, 1942.

149. KREJS, G. J., L. ORCI, J. M. CONLON, M. RAVAZZOLA, G. R. DAVIS, P. RASKIN, S. M. COLLINS, D. M. MCCARTHY, D. BAETENS, A. RUBENSTEIN, T. A. M. ALDOR, AND R. H. UNGER. Somatostatinoma syndrome. *N. Engl. J. Med.* 301: 285–292, 1979.

150. KROMER, W., AND W. PRETZLAFF. In vitro evidence for the participation of intestinal opioids in the control of peristalsis in the guinea pig small intestine. *Naunyn-Schmiedebergs Arch. Pharmacol.* 309: 153–157, 1979.

151. KUMAR, D. In vitro inhibitory effect of progesterone on extrauterine human smooth muscle. *Am. J. Obstet. Gynecol.* 84: 1300–1304, 1962.

152. KYOSOLA, K., AND L. RECHARDT. The anatomy and innervation of the sphincter of Oddi in the dog and cat. *Am. J. Anat.* 140: 497–521, 1974.

153. LAMORTE, W. W., J. M. GACA, W. E. WISE, D. H. BIRKETT, AND L. F. WILLIAMS. Choledochal sphincter relaxation in response to histamine in the primate. *J. Surg. Res.* 28: 373–378, 1980.

154. LANKISCH, P. G., R. ARNOLD, AND W. CREUTZFELDT. Wirkung von Somatostatin auf die betzolstumulierte Pancreas-Sekretion und Gallenblasenkontraktion des Menschen. *Dtsch. Med. Wochenschr.* 36: 1798, 1975.

155. LEE, W. H., AND M. FUJIWARA. Pharmacometrics of guinea-pig's gallbladder in vitro. *J. Formosan. Med. Assoc.* 70: 687–696, 1971.

156. LEE, W. H., AND M. FUJIWARA. Adrenoreceptors in the guinea pig's gallbladder. *Jpn. J. Pharmacol.* 22: 271–273, 1972.

157. LEE, W. H., AND M. FUJIWARA. Quantitative studies of adrenoceptors in guinea-pig gallbladders. *Jpn. J. Pharmacol.* 23: 586–588, 1973.

158. LEE, W. H., AND M. FUJIWARA. Mechanism of action of catecholamines on the electrically-stimulated, isolated guinea-pig gallbladder. *Arzneim. Forsch.* 27: 1149–1153, 1977.

159. LEMBECK, F., AND H. JUAN. Comparative actions of peptides on the gallbladder and the sphincter of Oddi. *Adv. Exp. Med. Biol.* 21: 337–346, 1972.

160. LENNON, F., T. M. FEELEY, A. S. CLANACHAN, AND G. W. SCOTT. Effects of histamine receptor stimulation on diseased gallbladder and cystic duct. *Gastroenterology* 87: 257–262, 1984.

161. LIDDLE, R. A., I. D. GOLDFINE, M. S. ROSEN, R. A. TAPLITZ, AND J. A. WILLIAMS. Cholecystokinin bioactivity in human plasma. Molecular forms, responses to feeding, and relationship to gallbladder contraction. *J. Clin. Invest.* 75: 1144–1152, 1985.

162. LIEDBERG, G., AND C. G. A. PERSSON. Adrenoceptors in the cat choledochoduodenal junction studied in situ. *Br. J. Pharmacol.* 39: 619–626, 1970.

163. LIN, T. M. Hepatic, cholecystokinetic, and choledochal actions of cholecystokinin, secretin, caerulein and gastrin-like peptides (Abstract). In: *Proc. Int. Congr. Physiol. Sci., 25th, Munich, 1971*, vol. 9, p. 1877.

164. LIN, T. M. Actions of secretin, glucagon, cholecystokinin, and endogenously released secretin and cholecystokinin on gallbladder, choledochus, and bile flow in dogs. *Federation Proc.* 33: 391, 1974.

165. LIN, T. M. Actions of gastrointestinal hormones and related peptides on the motor function of the biliary tract. *Gastroenterology* 69: 1006–1022, 1975.

166. LIN, T. M., AND R. E. CHANCE. Spectrum of gastrointestinal actions of bovine PP. In: *Gut Hormones*, edited by S. R. Bloom. Edinburgh: Churchill Livingstone, 1978, p. 242–246.

167. LIN, T. M., T. C. EVANS, C. J. SHAAR, AND R. E. CHANCE. Physiological versus pharmacological actions of bovine pancreatic polypeptide on the pancreas, stomach, gallbladder, choledochal sphincter and intestine of dogs. In: *Gut Peptides: Secretion, Function and Clinical Aspects*, edited by A. Miyoshi. Amsterdam: Elsevier, 1979, p. 175–181.

168. LIN, T. M., AND G. F. SPRAY. Effect of pentagastrin, cholecystokinin, caerulein and glucagon on the choledochal resistance and bile flow of conscious dog. *Gastroenterology* 56: 1178, 1969.

169. LIN, T. M., AND G. F. SPRAY. Choledochal, hepatic, and cholecystokinin action of secretin, potentiation by cholecystokinin. *Gastroenterology* 60: 783, 1971.

170. LIN, T. M., G. F. SPRAY, AND R. H. TUFT. Actions of somatostatin (SS) on choledochal sphincter (CS), gallbladder (GB), and bile flow (BF) in dog. *Federation Proc.* 36: 557, 1977.

171. LONOVICS, J., P. DEVITT, P. L. RAYFORD, AND J. C. THOMPSON. Actions of VIP, somatostatin, and pancreatic polypeptide on gallbladder tension and CCK-stimulated gallbladder. *Surg. Forum* 30: 407, 1979.

172. LONOVICS, J., S. GUZMAN, P. DEVITT, K. E. HEJTMANCIK, R. L. SUDDITH, P. L. RAYFORD, AND J. C. THOMPSON. Release of pancreatic polypeptide in humans by infusion of cholecys-

tokinin. *Gastroenterology* 79: 817–822, 1980.
173. LUETH, H. C. Studies on the flow of bile into the duodenum and the existence of a sphincter of Oddi. *Am. J. Physiol.* 99: 237–252, 1931.
174. LUFT, R., S. EFENDIC, T. HÖKFELT, O. JOHANSSON, AND A. ARIMURA. Immunohistochemical evidence for the localization of somatostatin-like immunoreactivity in a cell population of the pancreatic islets. *Med. Biol.* 52: 428–430, 1974.
175. MACK, A. J., AND J. K. TODD. A study of human gall bladder muscle in vitro. *Gut* 9: 546–549, 1968.
176. MANN, F. C. A study of the tonicity of the sphincter at the duodenal end of the common bile duct (with special reference to animals without a gallbladder). *J. Lab. Clin. Med.* 5: 107–110, 1919.
177. MANN, F. C. A comparative study of the anatomy of the sphincter at the duodenal end of the common bile-duct with special reference to species of animals without a gallbladder. *Anat. Rec.* 18: 355–360, 1920.
178. MANN, F. C., J. P. FOSTER, AND S. D. BRIMHALL. The relation of the common bile duct to the pancreatic duct in common domestic and laboratory animals. *J. Lab. Clin. Med.* 5: 203–206, 1920.
179. MARTINEZ, E., AND J. C. SARLES. Effect of prostaglandins $E_1$, $E_2$, and $F_{2\alpha}$ on the electric activity of the sphincter of Oddi in living rabbit. *Eur. Surg. Res.* 15: 322–327, 1983.
180. MARZIO, L., A. M. DIGIAMMARCO, M. NERI, F. CUCCURULLO, AND P. MALFERTHEINER. Atropine antagonizes cholecystokinin and cerulein-induced gallbladder evacuation in man: a real-time ultrasonographic study. *Am. J. Gastroenterol.* 80: 1–4, 1985.
181. MATON, P. N., A. C. SELDEN, AND V. S. CHADWICK. Large and small forms of cholecystokinin in human plasma: measurement using high pressure liquid chromatography and radio-immunoassay. *Regul. Peptide* 4: 251–260, 1982.
182. MATON, P. N., A. C. SELDEN, M. L. FITZPATRICK, AND V. S. CHADWICK. Infusion of cholecystokinin octapeptide in man: relation between plasma cholecystokinin concentrations and gallbladder emptying rates. *Eur. J. Clin. Invest.* 14: 37–41, 1984.
183. MCDONALD, T. J. Non-amphibian bombesin-like peptides. In: *Gut Hormones*, edited by S. R. Bloom and J. M. Polak. London: Churchill Livingstone, 1981.
184. MCMASTER, P. D., AND R. ELMAN. On the expulsion of bile by the gallbladder: and a reciprocal relationship with the sphincter activity. *J. Exp. Med.* 44: 173–198, 1926.
185. MENGUY, R. B., G. A. HALLENBECK, J. L. BOLLMAN, AND J. H. GRINDLAY. Intraductal pressures and sphincteric resistance in canine pancreatic and biliary ducts after various stimuli. *Surg. Gynecol. Obstet.* 106: 306–320, 1958.
186. MEYER, J. H., AND R. S. JONES. Canine pancreatic responses to intestinally perfused fat and products of fat digestion. *Am. J. Physiol.* 226: 1178–1187, 1974.
187. MILENOV, K., AND L. KAZAKOV. Influence of ovarian hormones on electromyograms of uterus, stomach, and intestines in dogs. *Endocrinol. Exp.* 7: 163–170, 1970.
188. MITZNEGG, P., S. R. BLOOM, N. CHRISTOFIDES, H. BESTERMAN, W. DOMSCHKE, S. DOMSCHKE, E. WUNSCH, AND L. DEMLING. Release of motilin in man. *Scand. J. Gastroenterol.* (Suppl. 11), 39: 53–56, 1976.
189. MIYAZAKI, T., AND M. ONDA. The adrenergic and cholinergic innervation of gallbladder and extrahepatic biliary duct system in the cat and human. *Nippon Shokakibyo Gakkai Zasshi* 77: 935–948, 1980.
190. MORGAN, K. G., P. F. SCHMALZ, V. L. GO, AND J. H. SZURSZEWSKI. Electrical and mechanical effects of molecular variants of CCK on antral smooth muscle. *Am. J. Physiol.* 235 (*Endocrinol. Metab. Gastrointest. Physiol.* 4): E324–E329, 1978.
191. MORI, J., H. AZUMA, AND M. FUJIWARA. Adrenergic innervation and receptors in the sphincter of Oddi. *Eur. J. Pharmacol.* 14: 365–373, 1971.
192. MUTT, V., AND E. JORPES. Hormonal polypeptides of the upper intestine. *Biochem. J.* 125: 57P–58P, 1971.
193. NAKANO, J., R. E. MCCLOY, A. C. GIN, AND S. K. NAKANO. Effect of prostaglandins $E_1$, $E_2$, and $F_{2\alpha}$, and pentagastrin on the gallbladder pressure in dogs. *Eur. J. Pharmacol.* 30: 107–112, 1975.
194. NAKATA, K., K. ASHIDA, K. NAKAZAWA, AND M. FUJIWARA. Effects of indomethacin on prostaglandin synthesis and on contractile response of the guinea pig gallbladder. *Pharmacology* 23: 95–101, 1981.
195. NAKATA, K., AND K. KURAHASHI. Effects of C-terminal octapeptide of cholecystokinin and prostaglandins on adrenergic functions in the guinea-pig gallbladder and sphincter of Oddi. *Jpn. J. Pharmacol.* 31: 77–83, 1981.
196. NAKATA, K., Y. OSUMI, AND M. FUJIWARA. Prostaglandins and the contractility of the guinea pig biliary system. *Pharmacology* 22: 24–30, 1981.
197. NAKAYAMA, S., M. MIZUTANI, T. NEYA, AND M. TAKAKI. Effect of motilin on gallbladder and gastroduodenal motility in dogs. *Ital. J. Gastroenterol.* 13: 6, 1981.
198. NEYA, T., M. MIZUTANI, M. TAKAKI, AND S. NAKAYAMA. Effect of motilin on the sphincter of Oddi in the dog. *Acta Med. Okayama* 35: 417–420, 1981.
199. NILSSON, G., AND E. BRODIN. Tissue distribution of substance-P like immunoreactivity in dog, cat, rat, and mouse. In: *Substance P*, edited by U. S. von Euler and B. Pernow. New York: Raven, 1977, p. 49–57. (Nobel Symp. Ser. no. 37.)
200. NILSSON, S., AND S. STATTIN. Gallbladder emptying during the normal menstrual cycle. *Acta Chir. Scand.* 133: 648–652, 1967.
201. ONDETTI, M. A., B. RUBIN, S. L. ENGEL, J. PLUSCEC, AND J. T. SHEEHAN. Cholecystokinin-pancreozymin: recent developments. *Dig. Dis.* 15: 149–156, 1970.
202. ONO, K., N. WATANABE, K. SUZUKI, H. TSUCHIDA, Y. SUGIYAMA, AND M. ABO. Bile flow mechanism in man. *Arch. Surg.* 96: 869–874, 1968.
203. OOUCHI, M., H. ASAOKA, T. MITSUTAKE, AND M. MIYAGAWA. Endogenous opioid peptide effects on the guinea-pig biliary tract. *Peptides* 4: 125–127, 1983.
204. PALLIN, B., AND S. SKOGLUND. Neural and humoral control of the gallbladder emptying mechanism in the cat. *Acta Physiol. Scand.* 60: 358–362, 1964.
205. PERSSON, C. G. A. The action of morphine on the cat choledochoduodenal tract. *Acta Pharmacol. Toxicol.* 30: 321–329, 1971.
206. PERSSON, C. G. A. Adrenoceptor functions in the cat choledochoduodenal junction in vitro. *Br. J. Pharmacol.* 42: 447–461, 1971.
207. PERSSON, C. G. A. Adrenoceptors in the gallbladder. *Acta Pharmacol. Toxicol.* 31: 177–185, 1972.
208. PERSSON, C. G. A. Adrenergic, cholecystokinetic and morphine-induced effects on extra-hepatic biliary motility. *Acta Physiol. Scand.* 383: 1–32, 1972.
209. PERSSON, C. G. A. Dual effects on the sphincter and gallbladder contraction induced by stimulation of the right great splanchnic nerve. *Acta Physiol. Scand.* 87: 334–343, 1973.
210. PERSSON, C. G. A. Inhibitory innervation of cat sphincter of Oddi. *Br. J. Pharmacol.* 58: 479–482, 1976.
211. PIPER, P. J., S. I. SAID, AND J. R. VANE. Effects on smooth muscle preparations of unidentified vasoactive peptides from intestine and lung. *Nature Lond.* 225: 1144–1146, 1970.
212. POITRAS, P., T. YAMADA, AND J. H. WALSH. Absence of effect of somatostatin on the guinea pig gallbladder. *Can. J. Physiol. Pharmacol.* 58: 179–182, 1980.
213. POLAK, J. M., S. R. BLOOM, S. N. SULLIVAN, P. FACER, AND A. G. PEARSE. Enkephalin-like immunoreactivity in the human gastrointestinal tract. *Lancet* 1: 972–974, 1977.
214. POLAK, J. M., I. COULLING, S. BLOOM, AND A. G. E. PEARSE. Immunofluorescent localization of secretin and enteroglucagon in human intestinal mucosa. *Scand. J. Gastroenterol.* 6: 739–744, 1971.
215. POLAK, J. M., A. G. E. PEARSE, S. R. BLOOM, A. M. J.

Buchan, P. L. Rayford, and J. C. Thompson. Identification of cholecystokinin-secreting cells. *Lancet* 2: 1016–1021, 1975.
216. Pomeranz, I. S., J. S. Davison, and E. A. Shaffer. In vitro effects of pancreatic polypeptide and motilin on contractility of human gallbladder. *Dig. Dis. Sci.* 28: 539–544, 1983.
217. Puig, M. M., P. Gascon, G. L. Craviso, and J. M. Musacchio. Endogenous opiate receptor ligand: electrically induced release in the guinea pig ileum. *Science Wash. DC* 195: 419–420, 1977.
218. Rattan, S., and R. K. Goyal. Effect of nicotine on the lower esophageal sphincter: studies on the mechanism of action. *Gastroenterology* 69: 154–159, 1975.
219. Rattan, S., and R. K. Goyal. Effects of 5-hydroxytryptamine on the lower esophageal sphincter—evidence for multiple sites of action. *J. Clin. Invest.* 59: 125–133, 1977.
220. Rattan, S., and R. K. Goyal. Effects of histamine on the lower esophageal sphincter in vivo: evidence for actions at three different sites. *J. Pharmacol. Exp. Ther.* 204: 334–342, 1978.
221. Ravdin, I. S., and J. L. Morrison. Gallbladder function. The contractile function of the gallbladder. *Arch. Surg.* 222: 810, 1931.
222. Regan, P. T., V. L. W. Go, and E. P. Dimagno. Comparison of the effects of cholecystokinin and cholecystokinin octapeptide on pancreatic secretion, gallbladder contraction, and plasma pancreatic polypeptide in man. *J. Lab. Clin. Med.* 96: 743–748, 1980.
223. Rocha, E., M. Silva, J. R. Valle, and Z. P. Picarelli. A pharmacological analysis of the mode of action of serotonin (5-hydroxytryptamine) upon the guinea-pig ileum. *Br. J. Pharmacol.* 8: 378–388, 1953.
224. Ryan, J. P. Calcium and gallbladder smooth muscle contraction in the guinea pig: effect of pregnancy. *Gastroenterology* 89: 1279–1285, 1985.
225. Ryan, J., and S. Cohen. Interaction of gastrin I, secretin, and cholecystokinin on gallbladder smooth muscle. *Am. J. Physiol.* 230: 553–556, 1976.
226. Ryan, J., and S. Cohen. Effect of vasoactive intestinal polypeptide on basal and cholecystokinin-induced gallbladder pressure. *Gastroenterology* 73: 870–872, 1977.
227. Ryan, J., and D. Pellecchia. Effect of progesterone pretreatment on guinea pig gallbladder motility in vitro. *Gastroenterology* 83: 81–83, 1982.
228. Ryan, J., and D. Pellecchia. Effect of ovarian hormone pretreatment on gallbladder motility in vitro. *Life Sci.* 31: 1445–1449, 1982.
229. Ryan, J. P., and S. Ryave. Effect of vasoactive intestinal polypeptide on gallbladder smooth muscle in vitro. *Am. J. Physiol.* 234 (*Endocrinol. Metab. Gastrointest. Physiol.* 3): E44–E46, 1978.
230. Sacchetti, G., L. Roncoroni, V. Mandelli, F. Rocca, and E. Magni. Effect of analgesic agents on emptying of the gallbladder in man. *Eur. J. Clin. Pharmacol.* 10: 127–131, 1976.
231. Said, S. I., and G. M. Makhlouf. Vasoactive intestinal polypeptide: spectrum of biological activity. In: *Endocrinology of the Gut*, edited by W. Y. Chey and F. P. Brooks. Thorofare, NJ: Slack, 1974, p. 83–87.
232. Saito, N., K. Taniyama, and C. Tanaka. ³H-ACh release from guinea pig gallbladder evoked by GABA through the bicuculline-sensitive GABA receptor. *Naunyn Schmiedebergs Arch. Pharmacol.* 326: 45–48, 1984.
233. Sandblom, P., W. L. Voegtlin, and A. C. Ivy. The effect of cholecystokinin on the choledochoduodenal mechanism (sphincter of Oddi). *Am. J. Physiol.* 93: 175–180, 1935.
234. Sankaran, H., I. D. Goldfine, A. Bailey, V. Licko, and J. A. Williams. Relationship of cholecystokinin receptor binding to regulation of biological functions in pancreatic acini. *Am. J. Physiol.* 242 (*Gastrointest. Liver Physiol.* 5): G250–G257, 1982.
235. Sarles, J. C., J. M. Bidart, M. A. Devaux, C. Echinard, and C. Castagnini. Action of cholecystokinin and caerulein on the rabbit sphincter of Oddi. *Digestion* 14: 415–423, 1976.
236. Sarles, J. C., P. Delecourt, M. A. Devaux, J. P. Amoros, J. C. Guicheney, and E. Wunsch. In vivo effect of 13 Leu motilin on the electric activity of the rabbit sphincter of Oddi. *Horm. Metab. Res.* 13: 340–342, 1981.
237. Schlegel, W., S. Raptis, R. F. Harvey, J. M. Oliver, and E. F. Pfeiffer. Inhibition of cholecystokinin-pancreozymin release by somatostatin. *Lancet* 2: 166–168, 1977.
238. Schoetz, D. J., D. H. Birkett, and L. F. Williams. Gallbladder motor function in the intact primate: autonomic pharmacology. *J. Surg. Res.* 24: 513, 1978.
239. Schoetz, D. J., W. E. Wise, W. W. Lamorte, D. H. Birkett, and L. F. Williams. Histamine receptors in primate gallbladder. *Dig. Dis. Sci.* 28: 353–358, 1983.
240. Schultz, R., M. Wuster, R. Simantov, S. Snyder, and A. Herz. Electrically stimulated release of opiate-like material from the myenteric plexus of the guinea pig ileum. *Eur. J. Pharmacol.* 41: 347–348, 1977.
241. Schusdziarra, V., D. Rouiller, V. Harris, and R. H. Unger. Gastric and pancreatic release of somatostatin-like immunoreactivity during the gastric phase of a meal. *Diabetes* 28: 658–663, 1979.
242. Scott, G. W., D. O. Ferris, G. A. Hallenbeck, E. S. Judd, and E. J. Baldes. Resistance to flow through the common bile duct in man. *Bull. Soc. Intern. Chir.* 22: 509–516, 1963.
243. Shaw, B. W., J. M. Becker, and F. G. Moody. Histaminergic responses of biliary sphincter in opossum. *Surg. Forum* 30: 400–402, 1979.
244. Shio, H., J. Shaw, and P. Ramwell. Relation of cyclic AMP to the release and actions of prostaglandins. *Ann. NY Acad. Sci.* 185: 327–335, 1971.
245. Solomon, T. E., T. Yamada, J. Elashoff, J. Wood, and C. Beglinger. Bioactivity of cholecystokinin analogues: CCK-8 is not more potent than CCK-33. *Am. J. Physiol.* 247 (*Gastrointest. Liver Physiol.* 10): G105–G111, 1984.
246. Starke, K., F. Lembeck, W. Lorenz, and U. Weiss. Gallen- und pankreas secretion unter substanz P und einem physalaminderivat. *Naunyn Schmiedebergs Arch. Pharmacol.* 260: 269, 1968.
247. Stasiewicz, J., W. Szaaj, and A. Gabryelewicz. Motor interaction between cimetidine and cholecystokinin-related peptides in the gallbladder. *Pol. J. Pharmacol. Pharm.* 32: 643–646, 1980.
248. Steigerwalt, R. W., I. D. Goldfine, and J. A. Williams. Characterization of cholecystokinin receptors on bovine gallbladder membranes. *Am. J. Physiol.* 247 (*Gastrointest. Liver Physiol.* 10): G709–G714, 1984.
249. Stening, G. F., and M. I. Grossman. Potentiation of cholecystokinetic action of cholecystokinin by secretin. *Clin. Res.* 17: 528, 1969.
250. Stewart, J. J., N. W. Weisbrodt, and T. F. Burks. Intestinal stimulant response after intraventricular morphine in the conscious cat. *Proc. West. Pharmacol. Soc.* 20: 399–403, 1977.
251. Stewart, J. J., N. W. Weisbrodt, and T. F. Burks. Central and peripheral actions of morphine on intestinal transit. *J. Pharmacol. Exp. Ther.* 205: 547–555, 1978.
252. Strunz, U., W. Domschke, P. Mitznegg, S. Domschke, E. Schubert, E. Wunsch, E. Jaeger, and L. Demling. Analysis of the motor effects of 13-norleucine motilin on the rabbit, guinea pig, rat, and human alimentary tract in vitro. *Gastroenterology* 68: 1485–1491, 1975.
253. Studer, R. O., H. Trazeciak, and W. Lergier. Substance P from horse intestine: its isolation, structure, and synthesis. In: *Substance P*, edited by U. S. von Euler and B. Pernow. New York: Raven, 1977, p. 15–18. (Nobel Symp. Ser. no. 37.)
254. Sturdevant, R. A. L., D. H. Stern, H. Resin, and J. I. Isenberg. Effect of graded doses of octapeptide of cholecystokinin on gallbladder size in man. *Gastroenterology* 64: 452–456, 1973.
255. Sundler, F., J. Alumets, R. Hakenson, S. Ingemansson,

J. FAHRENKRUG, AND O. SCHAFFALITZKY DE MUCKADELL. VIP innervation of the gallbladder. *Gastroenterology* 72: 1375–1377, 1977.
256. SUZUKI, T., I. TAKAHASHI, AND Z. ITOH. Motilin and gallbladder: new dimensions in gastrointestinal physiology. *Peptides* 2: 229–233, 1981.
257. TAKAHASHI, I., R. HONDA, W. J. DODDS, S. SARNA, J. TOOULI, Z. ITOH, W. Y. CHEY, W. J. HOGAN, D. GREIFF, AND K. BAKER. Effect of motilin on the opossum upper gastrointestinal tract and sphincter of Oddi. *Am. J. Physiol.* 245 (*Gastrointest. Liver Physiol.* 8): G476–G481, 1983.
258. TAKAHASHI, I., T. SUZUKI, I. AIZAWA, AND Z. ITOH. Comparison of gallbladder contractions induced by motilin and cholecystokinin in dogs. *Gastroenterology* 82: 419–424, 1982.
259. TALLARIDA, R. J., AND L. S. JACOB. The dose-response relation. In: *The Dose-Response Relation in Pharmacology*, edited by R. J. Tallarida and L. S. Jacob. New York: Springer-Verlag, 1979, chapt. 1, p. 1–17.
260. TALLARIDA, R. J., AND L. S. JACOB. Drug binding and drug effect. In: *The Dose-Response Relation in Pharmacology*, edited by R. J. Tallarida and L. S. Jacob. New York: Springer-Verlag, 1979, chapt. 5, p. 111–136.
261. TOOULI, J., W. J. DODDS, R. HONDA, AND W. J. HOGAN. Effect of histamine on motor function of opossum sphincter of Oddi. *Am. J. Physiol.* 241 (*Gastrointest. Liver. Physiol.* 4): G122–G128, 1981.
262. TOOULI, J., W. J. DODDS, R. HONDA, S. SARNA, W. J. HOGAN, R. A. KOMAROWSKI, J. H. LINEHAN, AND R. C. ARNDORFER. Motor function of the opossum sphincter of Oddi. *J. Clin. Invest.* 71: 208–220, 1983.
263. TOOULI, J., W. J. HOGAN, J. E. GEENEN, W. J. DODDS, AND R. C. ARNDORFER. Action of cholecystokinin-octapeptide on sphincter of Oddi basal pressure and phasic wave activity in humans. *Surgery St. Louis* 92: 497–503, 1982.
264. TOOULI, J., AND J. M. WATTS. Actions of cholecystokinin/pancreozymin, secretin, and gastrin on extra-hepatic biliary tract motility in vitro. *Ann. Surg.* 175: 439–447, 1972.
265. TSUDA, K., Y. SEINO, H. SAKURAI, S. SEINO, J. TAKEMURA, H. KUZUYA, H. ADACHI, AND H. IMURA. Cerulein-induced pancreatic polypeptide secretion. Its inhibition by atropine and its possible role in regulating gallbladder relaxation. *Am. J. Gastroenterol.* 74: 355–358, 1980.
266. TURNER, F. E., G. T. KRISHNAMURTHY, V. R. BOBBA, AND K. LANGRELL. A new scintigraphic technique for cholecystokinin gallbladder dose-response study: validation in rabbits. *J. Clin. Pharmacol.* 24: 84–88, 1984.
267. VAGNE, M., AND M. I. GROSSMAN. Cholecystokinetic potency of gastrointestinal hormones and related peptides. *Am. J. Physiol.* 215: 881–884, 1968.
268. VAGNE, M., AND V. TROITSKAJA. Effects of secretin, glucagon, and VIP on gallbladder contraction. *Digestion* 14: 62–67, 1976.
269. VIGNA, S. R., AND A. GORBMAN. Effects of cholecystokinin, gastrin, and related peptides on coho salmon gallbladder contractions in vitro. *Am. J. Physiol.* 232 (*Endocrinol. Metab. Gastrointest. Physiol.* 1): E485–E491, 1977.
270. VON KLEIST, D., M. ZSCHIEDRICH, D. STOPIK, AND K. E. HAMPEL. Das Verhalten der secretin-pankreozymin-stimulaierten Sekretion des Pankreas, der Gallenblasenkontraktion und der Cholerese unter Somatostatin. *Dtsch. Z. Verdau. Stoffwechselkr.* 41: 219, 1981.
271. WALDMAN, D. B., A. M. ZFASS, AND G. M. MAKHLOUF. Stimulatory (H1) and inhibitory (H2) histamine receptors in gallbladder muscle. *Gastroenterology* 72: 932–936, 1977.
272. WALSH, J. H., AND M. I. GROSSMAN. Medical progress: gastrin. *N. Engl. J. Med.* 292: 1324–1332, 1975.
273. WHITAKER, L. R. The mechanism of the gallbladder. *Am. J. Physiol.* 78: 411–436, 1926.
274. WIENER, I., K. INOVE, C. J. FAGAN, P. LILJA, L. C. WATSON, AND J. C. THOMPSON. Release of cholecystokinin in man. Correlation of blood levels with gallbladder contraction. *Ann. Surg.* 194: 321–327, 1981.
275. WILLIAMS, R. D., AND T. T. HUANG. New techniques for experimental repeated long-term measurement of biliary pressure. *Surgery St. Louis* 65: 454–456, 1969.
276. WILSON, D. E. Prostaglandins and the gastrointestinal tract. *Prostaglandins* 4: 281–293, 1972.
277. YAJIMA, H., Y. KAI, H. OGAWA, M. KUBOTA, AND Y. MORI. Structure-activity relationships of gastrointestinal hormones: motilin, GIP, and CCK-PZ. *Gastroenterology* 72: 793–796, 1977.
278. YAMADA, K., AND M. IIZUKA. Enhancement of the contraction of the isolated duodenum and Oddi's sphincter of rabbits by alpha adrenergic agents. *Nippon Heikatsukin Gakkai Zasshi* 19: 115–122, 1983.
279. YAMAMOTO, F. Contribution of prostaglandin to the contraction induced by catecholamines in the isolated gallbladder of the guinea-pig. *Gastroenterol. Jpn.* 15: 433–438, 1980.
280. YANAURA, S., AND S. ISHIKAWA. Adrenoreceptors and autonomic nerve control mechanisms in the biliary tract. *Folia Pharmacol. Jpn.* 71: 39–51, 1975.
281. YAU, W. M., G. M. MAKHLOUF, L. E. EDWARDS, AND J. T. FARRAR. Mode of action of cholecystokinin and related peptides on gallbladder muscle. *Gastroenterology* 65: 451–456, 1973.
282. YAU, W. M., AND M. L. YOUTHER. Modulation of gallbladder motility by intrinsic cholinergic neurons. *Am. J. Physiol.* 247 (*Gastrointest. Liver Physiol.* 10): G662–G666, 1984.
283. YIANGOU, Y., N. D. CHRISTOFIDES, J. GU, P. J. PIPER, J. M. POLAK, AND S. R. BLOOM. PHI-like immunoreactivity in the GB and in vitro effect of porcine PHI on smooth muscle of the GB. *FEBS Lett.* 175: 307–312, 1984.
284. YOSHIDA, M., AND S. ISHIURA. Transmural electrical stimulation-induced relaxation of the guinea pig gallbladder. *J. Pharmacobiodyn.* 4: 751–758, 1981.
285. YUSKO, P., R. A. HALL, AND A. W. FORD-HUTCHINSON. Contraction of guinea pig gallbladder strips by leukotrienes and other agonists. *Prostaglandins* 25: 397–403, 1983.

# CHAPTER 30

# Parasite infections and gastrointestinal motility

GILBERT A. CASTRO | *Department of Physiology and Cell Biology, Medical School, University of Texas Health Science Center, Houston, Texas*

CHAPTER CONTENTS

Parasite-Induced Alterations
   Esophagus
   Stomach
   Small intestine
      Manometric measurements
      Transit measurements
      Myoelectric measurements
      In vitro measurements of altered responsiveness
   Cecum, colon, and rectum
Basis for Motility Changes
   Parasite-derived substances
   Gastrointestinal hormone imbalances
   Inflammation
Summary

ANIMAL PARASITES (protozoans and helminths) alter properties of smooth muscle in the hollow organs of the gastrointestinal (GI) tract. Alterations in structure are evident primarily from the histological examination of muscle layers. Alterations in function are reflected in measurements of intraluminal pressure, gastric emptying, intestinal transit, and myoelectric activity in intact hosts and in measurements of contractile and fluid-propelling properties of isolated tissue. Although each method of measurement offers certain advantages, electromyography has proved to be uniquely valuable in studies of the pathogenesis of infection. This sensitive method of measurement provides not only quantifiable indices of motility, but it allows a single host to be monitored throughout the course of infection, i.e., in close relationship to the life cycles of the parasites.

Parasite-induced alterations are interpreted generally to be a component in the pathogenesis of disease or an adaptive response involved either in resistance to infection (38, 44, 52) or in compensation for defects in digestion, absorption, and secretion (17). Most investigations of motility in parasitized hosts are rationalized or justified on the basis of one or both of these possibilities, and they represent a relatively recent pursuit in parasitology. Because new fields usually evolve through an early descriptive phase, it is not unexpected that most publications in this area describe the nature of alterations in motility rather than their physiological basis or regulatory processes. Accordingly this chapter is weighted heavily toward descriptive accounts of motility changes.

## PARASITE-INDUCED ALTERATIONS

### Esophagus

American trypanosomiasis or Chagas' disease is a rare example not only of the influence of parasites on esophageal function but of a parasitic infection in which the basis for altered smooth muscle responses is evident. In this disease the protozoan *Trypanosoma cruzi* causes destruction of myenteric ganglion cells resulting, in extreme cases, in autonomic denervation throughout the length of the digestive tract (41).

A manifestation of severe nerve destruction is megaesophagus. This condition is associated with impaired peristalsis (9) as well as a decrease in the basal lower esophageal sphincter (LES) pressure. Padovan et al. (61), using intraluminally positioned water-filled tubes to transmit luminal pressures to external transducers, measured basal LES pressures of 15.16 ± 1.53 mmHg (mean ± SE) in 14 patients with megaesophagus and 20.27 ± 1.16 mmHg in 15 control patients. Pressure in the gastric fundus served as the zero reference.

The LES pressure is believed to be regulated by postganglionic cholinergic nerves and by the hormone gastrin, both of which act to increase contractility. Although gastrin purportedly acts via cholinergic neurons (61), there is evidence that the hormone stimulates the LES directly (37, 86). In patients with intrinsic denervation of the LES there was lower sensitivity to gastrin as compared with normal individuals (controls). Although the maximal contraction of esophageal sphincter between control (42.54 ± 3.94 mmHg, $n = 15$) and Chagasic (35.40 ± 6.17 mmHg, $n = 11$) patients in response to gastrin was similar, the dose of gastrin pentapeptide causing half-maximal contraction was significantly greater in the latter group (172

± 71 ng/kg) as compared with the former (35 ± 6 ng/kg). In this experiment pentagastrin was given intravenously in 30-s injections. Successive injections of 25–500 ng/kg were given in one day and were separated by intervals sufficient to allow the LES pressure to return to basal levels. These results indicate that denervation of the LES in Chagas' disease results in loss of vagal activity to LES muscle fibers, thereby decreasing responsiveness to pentagastrin.

Surgically acquired control specimens of LES responded to field stimulation with electrical pulses of 0.5 ms in duration by relaxation, whereas tissue from Chagasic patients was relatively nonresponsive (34). Stimulation with pulses of greater duration caused contractions in infected tissue, apparently through direct action on the LES muscle because contractions were insensitive to tetrodotoxin. Supersensitivity of the LES due to denervation was indicated from its response to carbachol. The $ED_{50}$ (dose required for 50% of maximum response) for Chagasic tissue was $2.4 \pm 0.4 \times 10^{-7}$ M and for normal tissue was $20.0 \pm 5.0 \times 10^{-7}$ M. Morphological findings of greater numbers of gap junctions between smooth muscle cells from Chagasic patients was offered as an explanation for the heightened response to carbachol, as opposed to the possibility that the supersensitivity was due to an increase in the number of end organ receptors for neurotransmitter. It was reasoned that the increase in gap junctions should increase cell coupling and require less stimulation to produce a contractile response (34).

## Stomach

Tracings of myoelectric activity of the abomasum and jejunum of sheep infected concurrently with two parasitic nematodes, *Trichostrongylus axei* and *Chabertia ovina*, revealed alterations in motility patterns (Fig. 1). A decrease in contractile activity of the stomach that propagated from the abomasum to the duodenum was associated with diarrhea (11).

A coccidian (protozoan) *Eimeria magna*, which inhabits the epithelial cells of the rabbit distal small intestine, causes gastric hypomotility. This parasite is seldom fatal and infection usually lasts for ~2 wk. Gastric disturbances were detected in association with anorexia and were most evident during the fifth day of infection. Alterations in gastric motility, assessed by measuring myoelectric activity, consisted of a reduction in the mean frequency of spike burst activity. This was accompanied by a reduction in the frequency of small bowel contractions, an increase in transit time, and an increase in net serosa-to-mucosa movement of fluid (33). It was implied that gastric changes are a consequence of disturbances at the primary site of infection, the small intestine, and that the influence on the stomach is probably mediated through nerves. Also it was suggested that gastric stasis, due to hypomotility, may be the cause of decreased food intake (33).

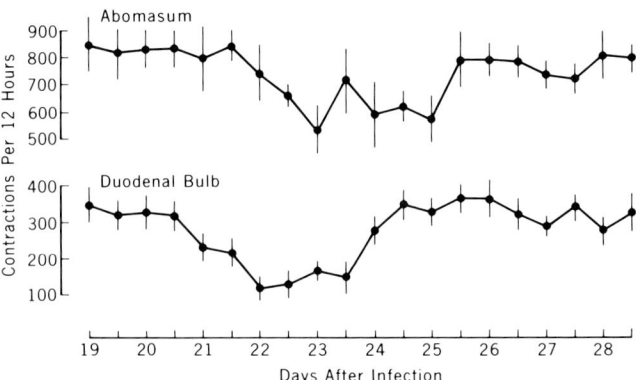

FIG. 1. Alterations in contractile activity of stomach and antroduodenal junction of sheep infected with *Trichostrongylus axei* and *Chabertia ovina*. [From Buéno et al. (11).]

*Eimeria nieschulzi*, an intraepithelial protozoan that predominantly inhabits the upper and middle regions of the small intestine of rats, increases intestinal transit during its 2-wk stay in that organ. During the same period it causes reflux of intestinal contents into the stomach. This was concluded from the appearance of a $^{51}Cr$ marker in the stomach after its injection into the duodenum via an enterocutaneous catheter (28).

Abomasal motility in sheep infected with the stomach roundworm *Haemonchus contortus* was investigated by electromyography (10). Animals were infected initially with $25 \times 10^3$ $L_3$ (third stage) larvae and a second time, 39 days after the first injection, with a similar dose of worms. The pathogenesis of infection was described over the initial 8-wk period (Fig. 2).

Spike bursts superimposed on slow waves with a mean frequency of 3.36/min characterized the electrical activity in the antral part of the abomasum before infection. Activity was organized into cycles lasting an average of 84 min with interposed 10- to 15-min periods of quiescence. Infection did not affect the frequency or the amplitude of antral spike bursts when they occurred, but it did reduce the duration of the cycle to <55 min. This occurred between days 9 and 16 after primary infection. Reinfection also shortened the cycle time. The major disturbance in gastric motor activity preceded the emergence of larvae from the gastric mucosa. This was interpreted as supporting the view that larval stages rather than adult worms damage the abomasal mucosa (10).

## Small Intestine

In considering GI parasitism, the small intestine without doubt has been studied more extensively than other organs of the alimentary canal. Nevertheless the total number of studies in small and collective results are too inconclusive to support the formation of general parasitological-physiological tenets. Various studies of motility employing an array of techniques are described next.

MANOMETRIC MEASUREMENTS. In human Chagas' disease, manometric techniques were used to detect alterations in motility patterns of the duodenum and jejunum (58). Intraluminal pressures were monitored by means of water-filled, multilumen polyvinyl catheters passed via the nostrils into preselected positions in the intestine. Recordings were obtained from infected and uninfected patients after a 10-h fast.

Pressure recordings were analyzed to identify the migrating motor complexes from which the duration and propagation velocity of the activity fronts (phase III of the migrating motor complex) and the frequency of contractions in the activity fronts were calculated. Patients who had circulating antibodies to *Trypanosoma cruzi* but displayed no radiological abnormalities or clinical manifestations had motility patterns indistinguishable from uninfected, seronegative individuals. In contrast, seropositive patients with megaesophagus, megacolon, and electrocardiogram abnormalities were characterized by having disturbances in motility. Electrocardiogram alterations develop from injury resulting from the predilection of the parasite for cardiac muscle. These patients displayed abnormal jejunal contractile patterns when compared with controls on the basis of propagation velocity and duration of the activity front. The duration of the activity front ranged from 3.1–5.6 min (mean 4.6 min) in control patients and 3.0–22.3 min (mean 6.5 min) in Chagasic patients. Fasting jejunal motility patterns showing the migrating motor complex are illustrated in Figure 3. The velocity of propagation of the migrating motor complex, summarized in Figure 4, was lower in Chagasic patients with megacolon and megaesophagus. The frequency of migrating motor complexes and the frequency of contractions in the activity front of the complex were not significantly altered by infection. Contraction frequencies ranged from 10.5 to 12.0/min in control subjects and 11.0 to 11.7/min in infected patients.

In summary the duration of the activity front and propagation velocity of the migrating motor complex are abnormal in *Trypanosoma cruzi*–infected patients displaying clinical manifestations of disease. These

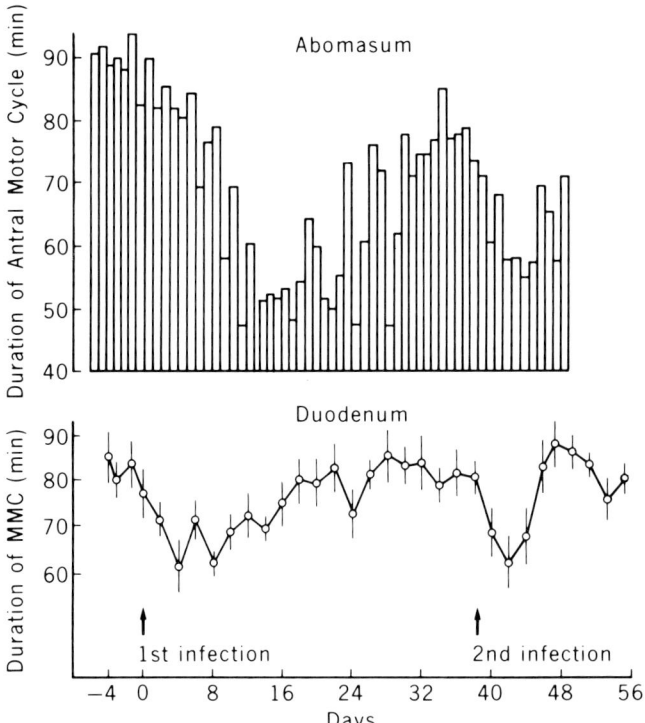

FIG. 2. Duration of motor complex in antral part of abomasum and migrating myoelectric complex (MMC) in the duodenum of sheep infected with $2.5 \times 10^3$ $L_3$ larvae of *Haemonchus contortus*. [From Bueno et al. (10). Reproduced with permission by Cambridge University Press, Copyright 1982.]

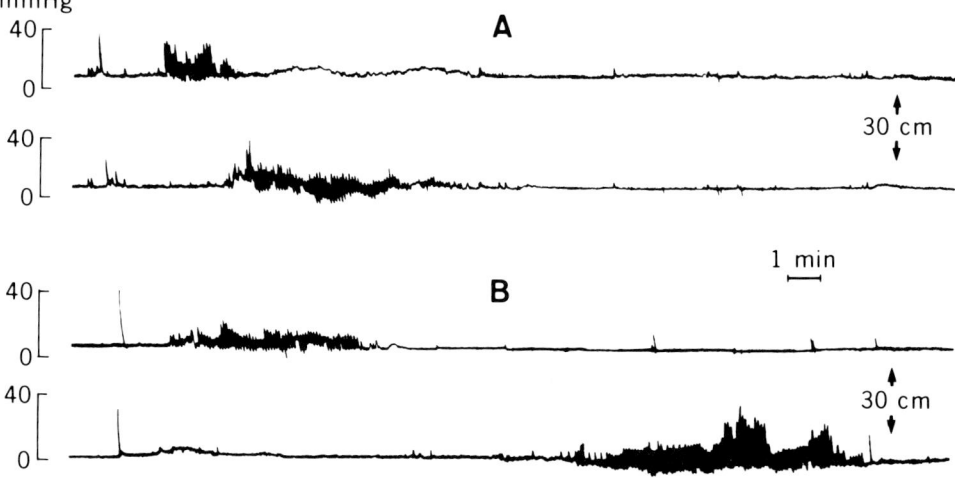

FIG. 3. Pressure recordings of migrating motor complex in jejunum from fasted control patient (A) and patient with Chagas' disease (B) determined by manometry. Open-tip catheters were 30 cm apart. Note slower propagation in infected patient. [From Oliveira et al. (58).]

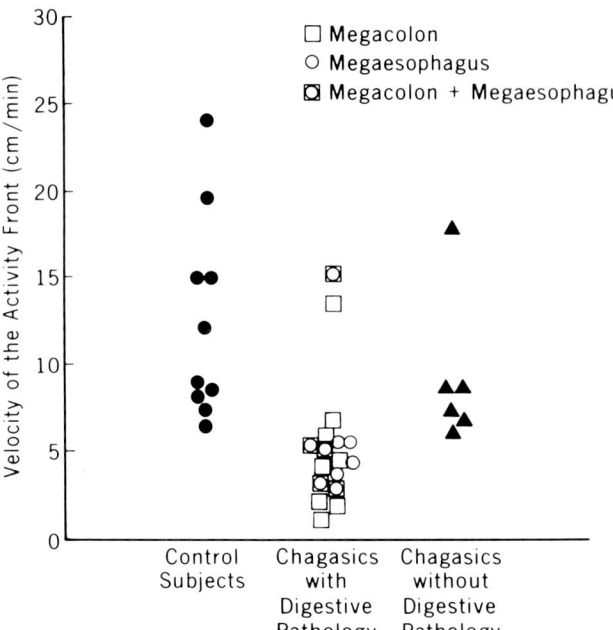

FIG. 4. Velocity of propagation of migrating motor complex in jejunum from control patients and its reduction in patients with Chagas' disease relative to megaorgan pathology. *Open squares*, megacolon; *open circles*, megaesophagus; *open circle in square*, megacolon and megaesophagus. [From Oliveira et al. (58).]

manifestations are associated with intrinsic denervation of the GI tract (42). From this relationship it is suggested that abnormal motility patterns are due to intrinsic denervation caused by the parasite (58).

In the guinea pig–*Trichinella spiralis* system, hosts sensitized by infection to antigens of this nematode have been challenged specifically to determine the effect on intestinal intraluminal pressure changes. The intraluminal administration of antigens derived from sonicated $L_1$ (infective, first stage) larvae was followed by an increase in luminal pressure. This was detected through use of a water-filled, open-tipped polyethylene catheter placed intraluminally through a laparotomy in anesthetized animals (59). This observation indicates that the host immune response may be important in modulating motility (see *Inflammation*, p. 1148).

TRANSIT MEASUREMENTS. The role of intestinal motility in host-parasite associations was investigated by testing whether the strong natural resistance in mice to the dwarf tapeworm *Hymenolepis nana*, which anchors by its scolex to the small bowel mucosa, was due to a relatively short intestinal transient time (43). The intensity of infection in mice given a standardized dose of tapeworm eggs was measured and compared with that in mice treated with either opium or morphine to increase transit time. Transit time was measured by following the movement through the small intestine and colon of an intragastrically administered dose of carbon ink in aqueous solution.

Results revealed that within 30 min after oral administration the ink had reached the colon of control mice but had progressed only 5–7 in. from the stomach in drug-treated hosts. The fasted versus fed states purportedly had no differential influence on transit. Significantly more worms became established and began development in drug-treated as compared with untreated hosts. Thus the data supported the hypothesis that resistance was related to rapid transit (43).

This hypothesis was extended in an attempt to explain why the nematode parasite *Trichinella spiralis* localizes primarily in the aboral half of the small bowel of young mice and in the oral half in old mice (44). To test whether intestinal motility influenced worm localization, experiments were designed to examine small bowel transit time, which was known to be shorter in young mice as compared with old ones. Transit time was determined from the movement of ink through the GI tract after its intragastric administration. Several results were obtained. First, transit time in young mice was confirmed to be less than that in old mice. Second, morphine sulfate administered before inoculation with ink dramatically increased transit time. Third, treatment of young mice with morphine before inoculation with $L_1$ *Trichinella spiralis* larvae reversed the natural worm localization pattern; i.e., 95% of the administered larvae became localized in the proximal half of the small bowel.

These findings, in the absence of age-related resistance to infection, indicate that the localization of *Trichinella spiralis* in the intestine is influenced by intestinal transit time (44). The conclusion is based on the unsupported assumption that gastric emptying was not altered by drug treatment.

Although it was concluded that intestinal transit can influence parasite establishment in the host, it is also quite clear that established parasites can influence intestinal transit. This was demonstrated in the mouse infected with *Trichinella spiralis*. By visually following the movement of intragastrically administered, undigestible chromatography beads, it was determined that intestinal transit time was decreased 5 days after infection with $L_1$ larvae (Fig. 5). Antiinflammatory steroids administered to mice during the course of infection prevented the worm-induced change in transit time. These results suggest that primary infection causes more rapid movement of material through the small intestine and that this is dependent on the local inflammatory reaction (74).

Rats infected with *Trichinella spiralis* for 3–5 days also have a shorter transit time as compared with uninfected hosts. The nonabsorbable marker $^{51}$Cr was placed directly into the duodenum of infected rats by a surgically implanted duodenocutaneous catheter and was propelled through the intestine at a greater velocity than it was in uninfected rats (18). Endpoints for

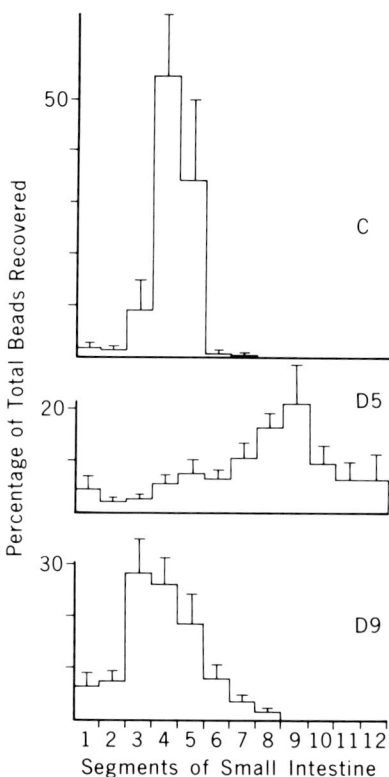

FIG. 5. Transit of chromatography beads through small intestine of mice 15 min after intragastric administration of marker. Segment 1 is duodenum and segment 12 is ileum. C, D5, and D9 represent, respectively, uninfected mice, mice infected for 5 days with *Trichinella spiralis*, and mice infected for 9 days with *T. spiralis*. [From Sukhdeo and Croll (74).]

measurement were the moving front of radioactivity and the amount of radioactivity traversing the midpoint of the small bowel (Fig. 6). Clearly this enhanced movement of $^{51}$Cr through the intestine during the first week of infection occurs at a time when mucosal myeloperoxidase levels (a marker for myeloid or acute inflammatory cells) are abnormally high, intestinal brush-border enzyme activity (i.e., disaccharidase activity) is significantly reduced, and the net serosa-to-mucosa flux of fluid in the intestine is enhanced (19, 69). Collectively the physiological responses indicate that increased transit in this infection is associated with inflammation (17) and enhanced intestinal secretion.

An analogous experiment but focused on secondary infection was performed. In contrast to the observation in primary infection, secondarily infected rats did not express alterations in motility when examined within the first hour (66) or 3–5 days after a second inoculum (20). These findings suggest that factors that regulate motility, as reflected in transit time, in the previously infected host are unaffected by a challenge infection. However, such a notion is dispelled by results of myoelectric measurements discussed in the next section.

Intestinal transit in rats infected with the roundworm *Nippostrongylus brasiliensis* purportedly is enhanced in some regions and slowed in others after feeding (76). This presents a difficulty in drawing conclusions from measurements of transit, if transit is examined only in a single region. In addition to regional differences it is necessary when determining physiological significance of parasite-induced changes to consider that transit time varies during the course of infection. As a working premise, regional differences are assumed to be less important than the average change in gut transit time in assessing the consequences of infection on motility during a given period. Transit time was measured in nippostrongylosis by following the transit of $^{51}$Cr through the small bowel at various times during infection (29). It is evident from results in Figure 7 and Table 1 that transit time is decreased to a significant degree at day 8 postinfection. These results have been cautiously interpreted in relation to the expulsion of the parasite from the intestine of the infected host (29). It has been suggested that prostaglandins released during worm-induced damage may contribute to increased gut motility.

MYOELECTRIC MEASUREMENTS. Electromyography has been used to examine the motility patterns in sheep harboring the two nematodes *Trichostrongylus axei* and *Chabertia ovina*. Electrodes implanted in the seromuscular surface of the jejunum were used to detect alterations in myoelectric activity. These disturbances were evident in the disappearance of the normal interdigestive migrating myoelectric complex (MMC). This characteristic complex was replaced by a pattern of random spiking. The altered jejunal pattern had its onset ~22 days postinfection and was accompanied by diarrhea (11).

Duodenal myoelectric patterns have been measured in sheep during both primary and secondary infections with the stomach roundworm *Haemonchus contortus* (33). Duodenal electromyograms of uninfected hosts exhibited patterns of slow waves and spike bursts that changed after infection. The mean duration of the MMC was ~79 min with a frequency of ~18/day. Infection caused an increase in the MMC frequency to ~23/day, thereby shortening the duration of each cycle. The change was evident 4–12 days after primary infection (see Fig. 2) and was correlated in the same sheep with a rise in duodenal and abomasal pH and an increase in net duodenal fluid secretion (10). Secondary infection caused a more precipitous decrease in the duration of the MMC and a faster return to preinfection level.

Dogs infected with hookworms, as evident by the passage of eggs in diarrheic stools, reportedly had a disrupted MMC. Both slow-wave frequency of the jejunum as well as spiking patterns were abnormal as compared with patterns in uninfected dogs (Fig. 8).

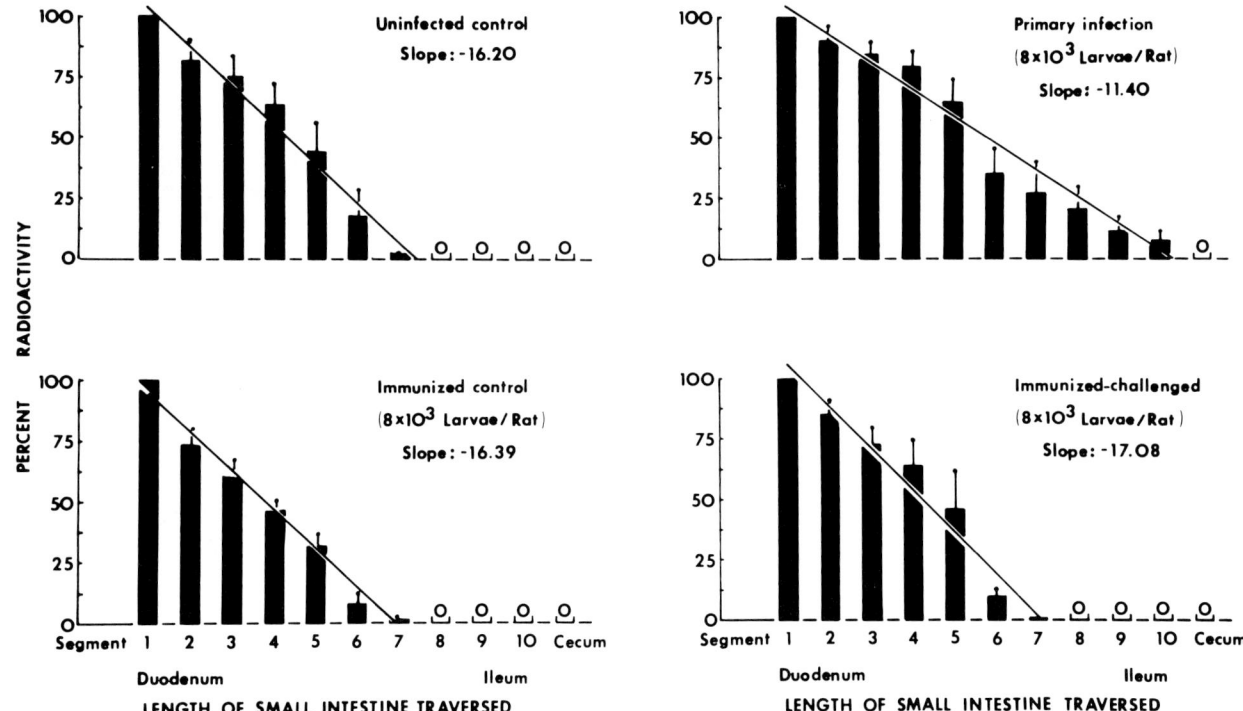

FIG. 6. Transit of $^{51}$Cr through rat small intestine before infection with *Trichinella spiralis* (*uninfected control*), 3–5 days after primary infection (*primary infection*), 30 days after primary infection (*immunized control*), and 3–5 days after reinfection (*immunized-challenged*). Percentage (mean ± SE) of radioactivity passing through or present in successive equal-length segments of small intestine during 15-min period after intraduodenal administration of marker is plotted as function of gut length. Slope of regression of percent radioactivity on gut length for primary infection is significantly different from other three groups. [From Castro et al. (18).]

Interestingly the dogs had not been experimentally infected but had acquired a natural infection. Alterations in motility were due to the adult parasites in the intestine because administration of an antihelminthic resulted in the disappearance of eggs from the feces, an alleviation of diarrhea, and a return of the myoelectric pattern to that observed in uninfected dogs (83).

Other evidence stemming from experimental cases of canine trichinosis clearly established that the dog reacts strongly toward enteric helminths and that this reaction involves a smooth muscle response (68). Small bowel myoelectric activity was monitored during fasted and fed states in unanesthetized dogs during the intestinal phase of primary and secondary trichinosis. After the ingestion of $5$–$30 \times 10^3$ larvae/kg body wt, dogs were monitored daily. Additionally several dogs were monitored after a challenge dose of $2 \times 10^4$ larvae/kg body wt given 6 wk after the initial infection.

Clinical signs of the host response to *Trichinella* included the failure of animals to eat and the development of diarrhea. Also observed was a rise in circulating eosinophils and the appearance of circulating antibodies to the parasite.

Alterations in motility patterns characterized by specific relationships between slow waves and spiking activity, as shown in Figure 9B, were detected as early as 18 h after administering the infective dose of *Trichinella spiralis*. Changes in motility were expressed maximally 3–4 days postinfection when dogs were markedly diarrheic. Myoelectric changes induced by the parasite, as evident in the fasted state, included a decrease in amplitude and disruption of the slow-wave pattern, an intense complex of spikes migrating in an aboral direction, and a disruption of the MMC. The rapidly migrating spike complex is equivalent to the migrating action potential complex (MAPC) described by Mathias et al. (50). Motility patterns measured 11–15 days postinfection were comparable to those in uninfected hosts (Fig. 9A). In short the fasted pattern was changed by infection to one resembling the fed pattern in uninfected hosts with the addition of MAPC. Secondary infection failed to produce a significant deviation from the control pattern (Fig. 10) or to elicit visible signs of disease.

The *Trichinella*-rat system has been examined also with emphasis on parasite-induced myoelectric changes (63). Rats that were monitored 2–12 days after infection with $7 \times 10^3$ L$_1$ larvae displayed several alterations in the normal myoelectric pattern. Altered contractile activity was expressed 2–12 days postinfection and was characterized by a significant reduction in mean slow-wave frequency from 37/min to

~33/min, a reduction in spiking activity and a reduction in the mean frequency of MMC (Fig. 11). The pattern of the parasite-induced change in electrical activity is summarized in Figure 12.

An unusual infection-induced qualitative change in electrical activity occurred that was designated a MAPC. The MAPC activity is defined as an action potential discharge, $\geq 2.5$ s in duration, that occurs at an electrode site and propagates in an aboral direction to at least two consecutive electrode sites (50). The most striking feature of the MAPC is the rapidity with which it propagates. Whereas the MMC propagates in an aboral direction in minutes, the MAPC propagates in seconds (Fig. 13). The MAPC activity occurred only

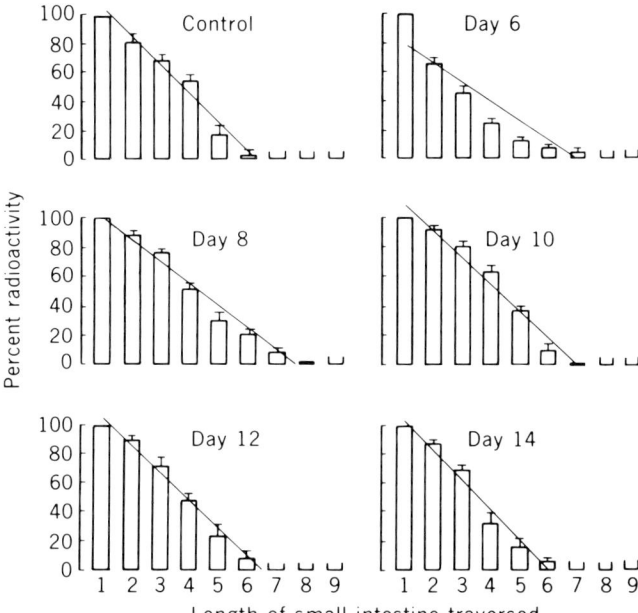

FIG. 7. Percentage (mean ± SE) of $^{51}$Cr passing through given segment (segment 1, duodenum; segment 9, ileum) of small intestine of rats during 15-min period immediately after its intraduodenal administration by an enterocutaneous catheter. Values are for uninfected (control) rats and rats at various times during infection with Nippostrongylus brasiliensis. Only at day 8 is transit increased over control value. Regression equations and statistical analysis of slopes are given in Table 1. [From Farmer (29).]

in infected rats; this presented 2 days postinfection and had the greatest frequency 2–6 days postinfection.

Both qualitative and quantitative myoelectric changes occurred in rats that were reinfected (62). Changes in myoelectric activity caused by a challenge injection included a rapidly induced decrease in intestinal slow-wave frequency, enhanced spiking activity (Table 2), and a disruption of the MMC. A tracing of myoelectric activity before and after challenge is illustrated in Figure 14. These observations of altered motility by electromyographic analysis coupled with results of transit studies, which failed to reveal significant effects of a secondary infection in the rat (20, 66), emphasize the value of employing more than one technique to study motility.

Changes in electrical parameters were inducible in previously infected rats by challenge with live larvae but not with dead worms or worm antigens administered intraduodenally (Fig. 15). Infection of Trichinella-sensitized hosts with the intestinal protozoan Eimeria nieschulzi was without effect on myoelectric parameters. These results indicate that altered intestinal contractile activity in the Trichinella-sensitized host is part of an anamnestic response. These alterations that are induced rapidly after challenge may represent the in vivo equivalent of the anaphylactically mediated intestinal smooth muscle contraction elicited in vitro in the Schultz-Dale assay (24, 62). The latter is described in Inflammation, p. 1148.

Results of only a single study are available on the effects of protozoan parasites on small intestinal myoelectric activity. This involves coccidiosis in the rabbit (33). Intestinal motility was examined by electromyographic techniques 6 days before and 18 days after inoculation with $1 \times 10^5$ oocysts of Eimeria magna, an intraepithelial parasite of the distal small intestine. The effect of infection on complexes of slow waves and spike bursts is shown in Figure 16. During the preinfection, control period myoelectric activity was organized in a MMC. Five days postinfection jejunoileal activity was represented by a series of spike bursts. Spike bursts resembling MAPC were observed that often propagated over the entire length of the small intestine at a velocity of 10 cm/s. Spiking activity was strongly inhibited on days 8–12 postinfection.

TABLE 1. Regression Statistics of Transit Time in Rats Infected With Nippostrongylus brasiliensis Larvae

| Group | n | Regression Coefficient* | Regression Equation† | Groups Compared‡ | F | P |
|---|---|---|---|---|---|---|
| 1. Control | 14 | −20.05 | $y = 124 − 20.05x$ | 1 vs. 2 | 3.900 | NS |
| 2. Day 6 | 7 | −13.32 | $y = 92 − 13.32x$ | 1 vs. 3 | 7.985 | <0.025 |
| 3. Day 8 | 11 | −15.11 | $y = 116 − 15.11x$ | 1 vs. 4 | 0.966 | NS |
| 4. Day 10 | 9 | −17.86 | $y = 127 − 17.86x$ | 1 vs. 5 | 0.060 | NS |
| 5. Day 12 | 10 | −19.55 | $y = 125 − 19.55x$ | 1 vs. 6 | 0.053 | NS |
| 6. Day 14 | 10 | −20.62 | $y = 124 − 20.62x$ | | | |

* Values indicate that the slope of the line was significant. † Regression equation represents y (percentage of radioactivity) as a function of x (length of intestine traversed). ‡ Regression coefficients were compared for significant differences by analysis of variance. NS, no significance ($P > 0.05$) between groups compared. [From Farmer (29).]

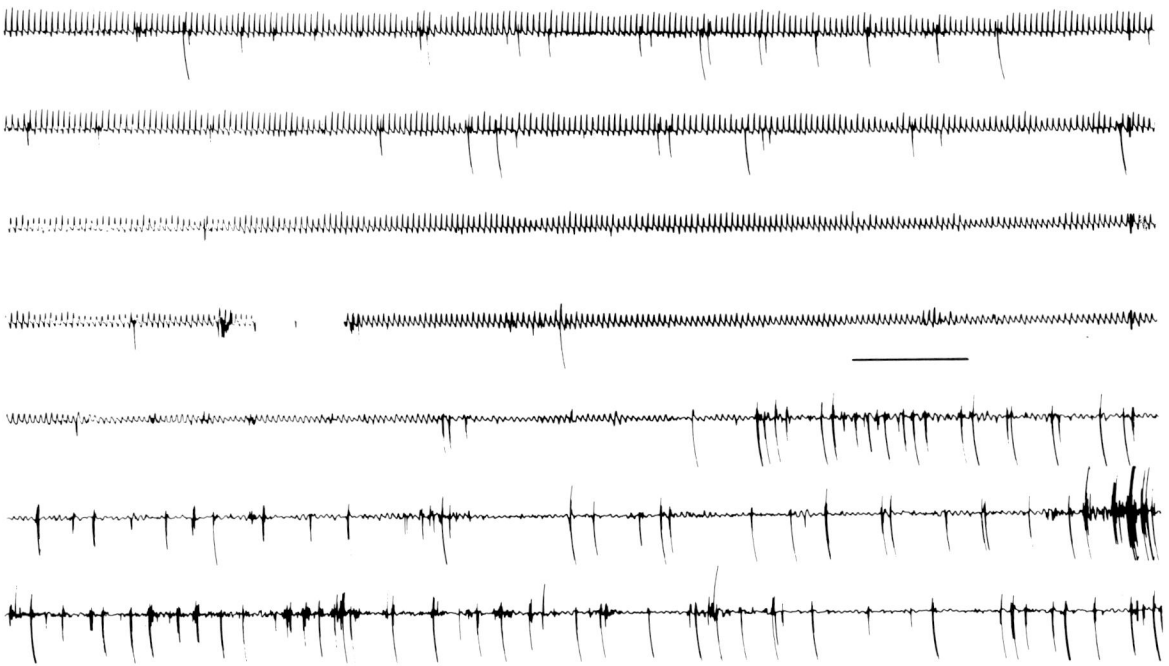

FIG. 8. Electromyograph tracing of dog infected with hookworms. Recording is continuous (*left* to *right*) from single electrode site in small intestine. Note unstable nature of spiking pattern as well as diminution of slow-wave amplitude. Normal migrating myoelectric complexes were not evident until dog was treated to eliminate parasites. *Horizontal bar*, 1-min interval.

IN VITRO MEASUREMENTS OF ALTERED RESPONSIVENESS. *Propulsion.* The propulsive behavior of isolated small intestine from parasitized hosts has been measured in vitro (1) by a method described recently by Weems and Weisbrodt (81). In this procedure separate tubes are inserted into both the oral and aboral ends of an isolated gut segment. The cannulated segment is placed in an organ bath containing an appropriate buffer solution. Both ends of the segment are connected to a glass port that in turn is connected to a propulsive evaluation system. This system requires hydrostatistic work to effect fluid ejection. Pressures exerted at both the oral and aboral ends of the segment are monitored continuously by means of a pressure transducer. In general, propulsion is measured as changes in pressure and volume flow.

Experiments were conducted to characterize the fluid-propelling behavior of jejunal segments from guinea pigs and to determine if *Trichinella spiralis* infection alters this behavior (1). Jejunal segments were obtained from control guinea pigs and guinea pigs infected 10 days previously with 2,000 larvae. Segments from control animals simultaneously ejected nearly equal volumes of fluid from each end in a spontaneous and rhythmic pattern. The average complex interval was 120 s, complex duration was 33 s, maximal aboral flow was 0.40 ml/s, and peak oral and aboral pressures were 23.7 and 24.3 cmH$_2$O, respectively. Significant changes were caused by infection. Infected segments had a complex interval of 98 s with a duration of 15 s. There was a net aboral ejection of fluid with a maximum pressure development of 46 cmH$_2$O and maximum flow rate of 0.55 ml/s. The maximal oral pressure was 29 cmH$_2$O. It was subsequently demonstrated that propulsive changes occur also at 20 days but not 30 or 60 days postinfection. Attempts to detect changes at 7 days postinfection were not successful. These results led to the conclusion that *Trichinella spiralis* infection induces a new pattern of propulsive behavior in jejunal segments initiated by 10 days postinfection and lasting as long as the parasite is present in the small intestine (2). This method of measuring motility may prove useful in evaluating relationships between contractile patterns and fluid movement in the intestine that may be important in the development of diarrhea in infected hosts.

*Length-tension relationships.* The physiological responses of smooth muscle to parasite-derived stimuli may be related to alterations at the level of the muscle per se. Compelling evidence is derived from work by Farmer and co-workers (30, 31, 32). As is noted in a subsequent section of this chapter, several helminth infections are associated with morphological changes

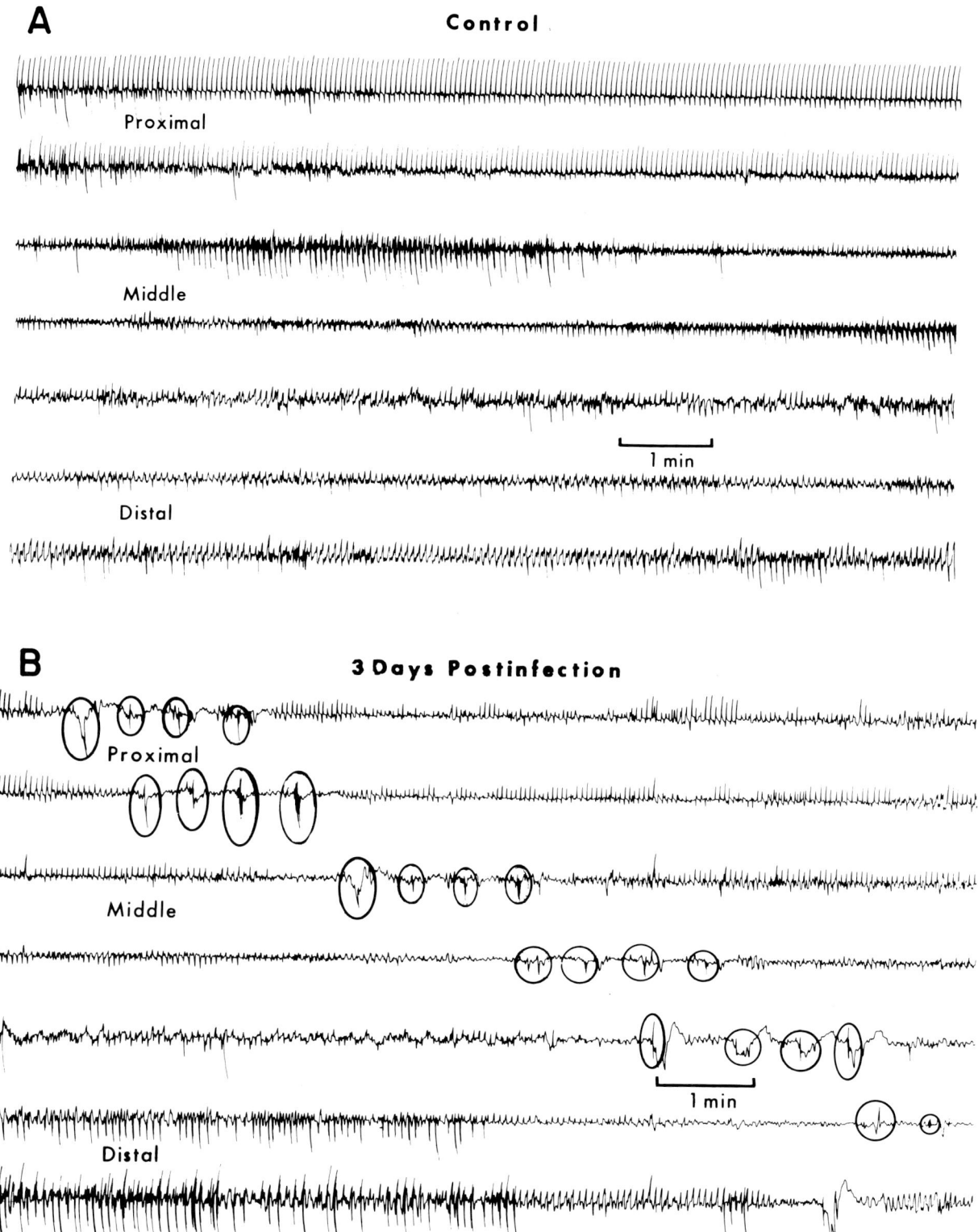

FIG. 9. Recording of myoelectric activity from fasted dogs at seven sites on small intestine before (A) and 3 days after inoculation (B) with $2 \times 10^4$ *Trichinella spiralis* larvae/kg body wt. Note rapid movement of complex of spike potentials (*circled*) down the bowel. [From Schanbacher et al. (68).]

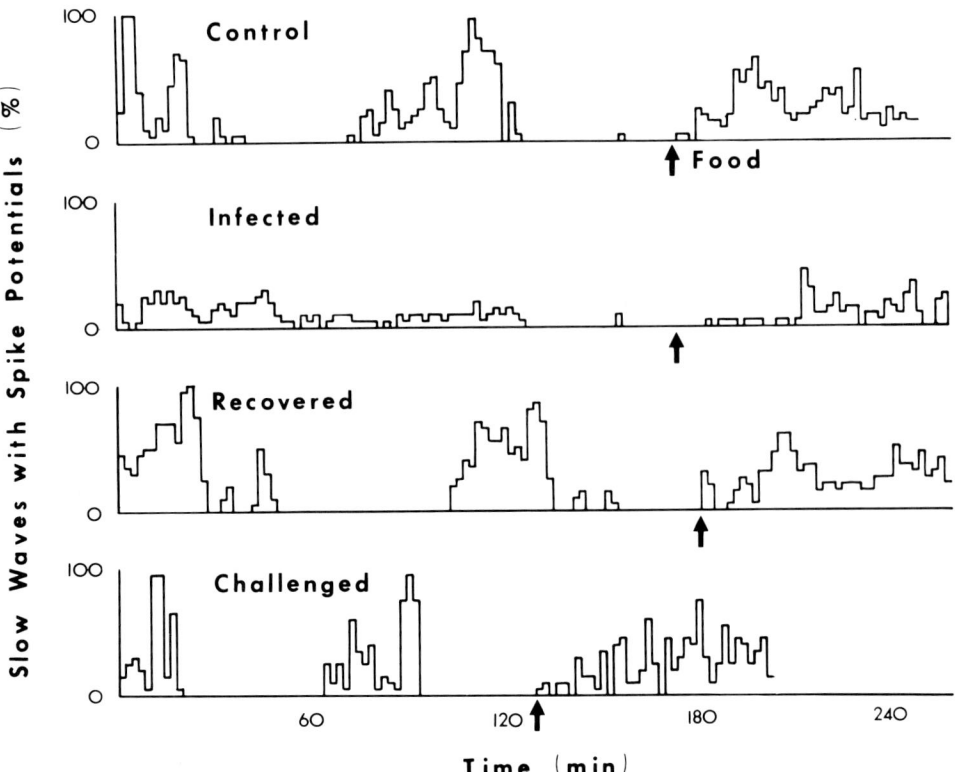

FIG. 10. Electrical spike activity in proximal small intestine of dog before infection with *Trichinella spiralis* (*control*), 3 days after primary inoculum of larvae (*infected*), 11 days postprimary inoculation (*recovered*), and 3 days after a secondary infection (*challenged*). Challenge infection was given 6 wk after primary inoculation. Percentage of slow waves with superimposed spikes for consecutive 2-min intervals are plotted as function of time. [From Schanbacher et al. (68).]

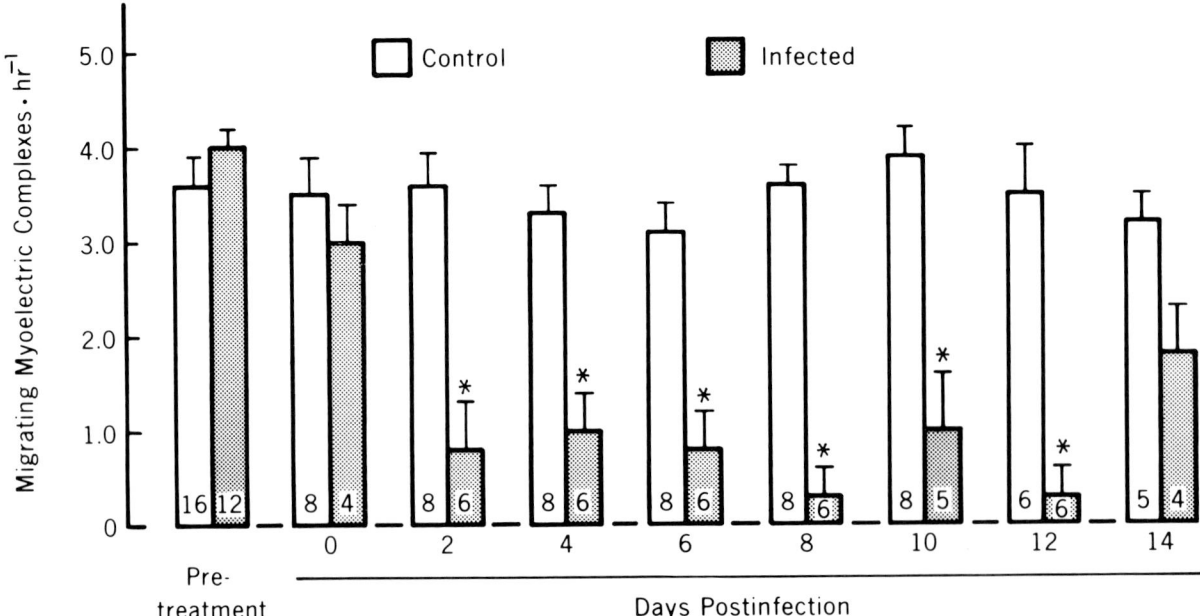

FIG. 11. Frequency of migrating myoelectric complexes recorded in proximal small intestine before (*open bars*) and after (*shaded bars*) infection with *Trichinella spiralis* in rats. Values are means ± SE for number of recordings designated at base of the bars. Values for each animal were established by examining 60 min of myoelectric tracing. *Asterisk*, significant difference as compared with respective control values. [From Palmer et al. (63).]

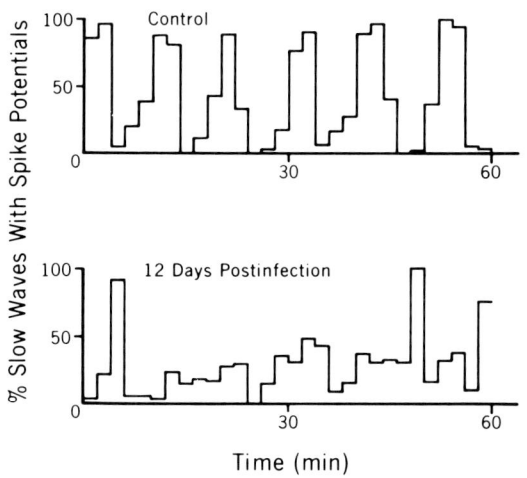

FIG. 12. Histogram of fasted myoelectric pattern in rat in uninfected (*control*) state and 12 days after inoculation with infective *Trichinella spiralis* larvae. Infection disrupted normal phasic pattern of activity. [From Palmer et al. (63).]

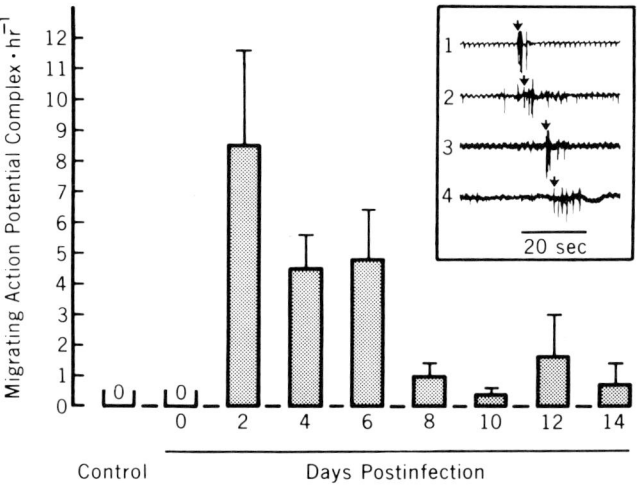

FIG. 13. Migrating action potential complexes (MAPC) in 1-hr interval from six rats infected with *Trichinella spiralis*. MAPC (*inset*) did not occur in uninfected control rats. Values are means ± SE. [From Palmer et al. (63).]

TABLE 2. *Small Intestinal Myoelectric Activity in Rats After Infection With* Trichinella spiralis

| Myoelectric Parameter | Uninfected | Infected[a] | | |
|---|---|---|---|---|
| | | Primary | Secondary | |
| | | | Prechallenge[b] | Postchallenge |
| n | 8 | 4 | 6 | 6 |
| Slow-wave frequency, cycles/min[c] | 36.3 ± 0.6 | 36.1 ± 0.7 | 36.9 ± 0.6 | 33.2 ± 0.3[d] |
| Slow waves with spike potentials/min, % | 32.9–39.8[e] | 32.0[f] | 38.4[f] | 53.7[f,g] |

[a] Data obtained 0–15 min after infection. [b] Rats previously immunized by infection but allowed to recover before secondary infection. [c] Data are means ± SE. [d] Significantly different ($P < 0.05$) as compared with all other groups. [e] Data are 95% confidence intervals. [f] Data are means. [g] Significantly different ($P < 0.05$) as compared with uninfected groups. [From Palmer and Castro (62).]

in intestinal smooth muscle (see *Inflammation*, p. 1148). One such infection is nippostrongylosis in the rat, which is associated with an increase in smooth muscle mass (75). In rats infected with *N. brasiliensis*, functional alterations occur (Fig. 17). The maximum response to both serotonin and acetylcholine (ACh) is increased, whereas the sensitivity to serotonin is reduced (30, 31). The subsensitivity to serotonin was speculated to be due to elevated levels of serotonin during infection and to the possible development of tachyphylaxis (32). The specificity of the subsensitivity to serotonin is believed to be due to some alteration in serotonin receptors as a adaptive response to chronic stimulation by excessive amounts of mast cell–derived serotonin in the *Nippostrongylus*-infected rat.

The increased maximum responsiveness to agonists was measured as an approximately twofold increase in tension developed per cross-sectional area of isolated tissue (Fig. 18), indicative of an increased contractile capacity. Increased maximum responsiveness was considered due to hypertrophic alterations (31), based on dramatic increases in cross-sectional areas of gut segments.

The mechanism underlying the enhanced contractility may be due to an increased number of available agonist receptors (30). However, this was not supported by experiments on receptor characteristics. Collins and Fox (22), using the muscarinic ligand quinuclidinyl benzilate (QNB) and Scatchard analysis to study QNB binding to isolated smooth muscle cells, observed no significant difference in receptor number or affinity for QNB between cells from control rats and rats infected with *N. brasiliensis*.

Other results supported the conclusion that increased contractility of smooth muscle from infected rats is associated with the influx of extracellular $Ca^{2+}$, whereas contractility of muscle from uninfected hosts is largely independent of extracellular $Ca^{2+}$. Removal of $Ca^{2+}$ from the solution bathing infected muscle reduce a carbachol-induced tension of isometric contraction by 80%; a value of 7% was obtained for control tissue. Also the addition of the $Ca^{2+}$ channel blocker nitrendipine to the bath in the presence of $Ca^{2+}$ reduced carbachol-stimulated tension development by 25% in the muscle from infected rats as compared with uninfected rats. The channel blocker was without effect on agonist-stimulated tension development in control rats (35).

Another possibility to explain increased contractility in the infected rat is that the number of contractile elements per cross-sectional area was increased by infection. An increase in actomyosin levels per milli-

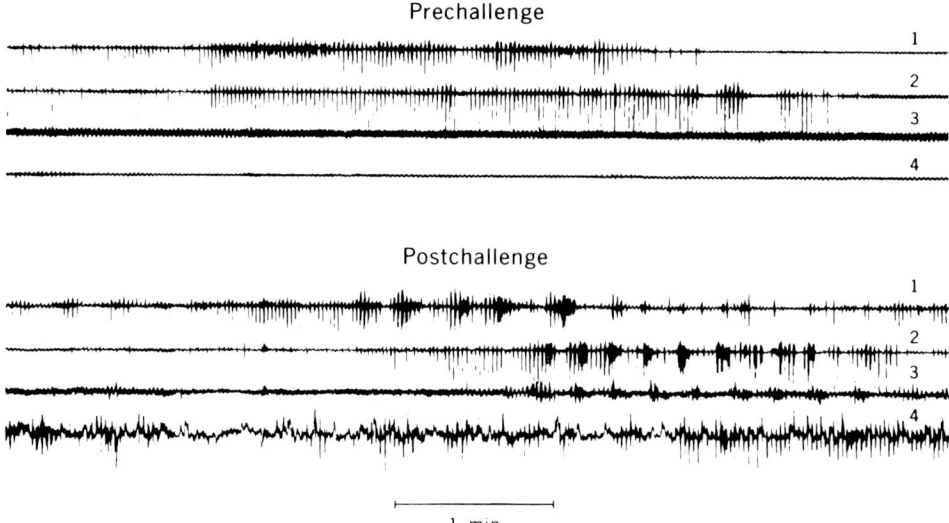

FIG. 14. Electromyograph recorded from four electrodes in proximal small intestine before and 6–12 min after intraduodenal challenge of rat immune to *Trichinella spiralis*. Challenge was with live larvae. [From Palmer and Castro (62).]

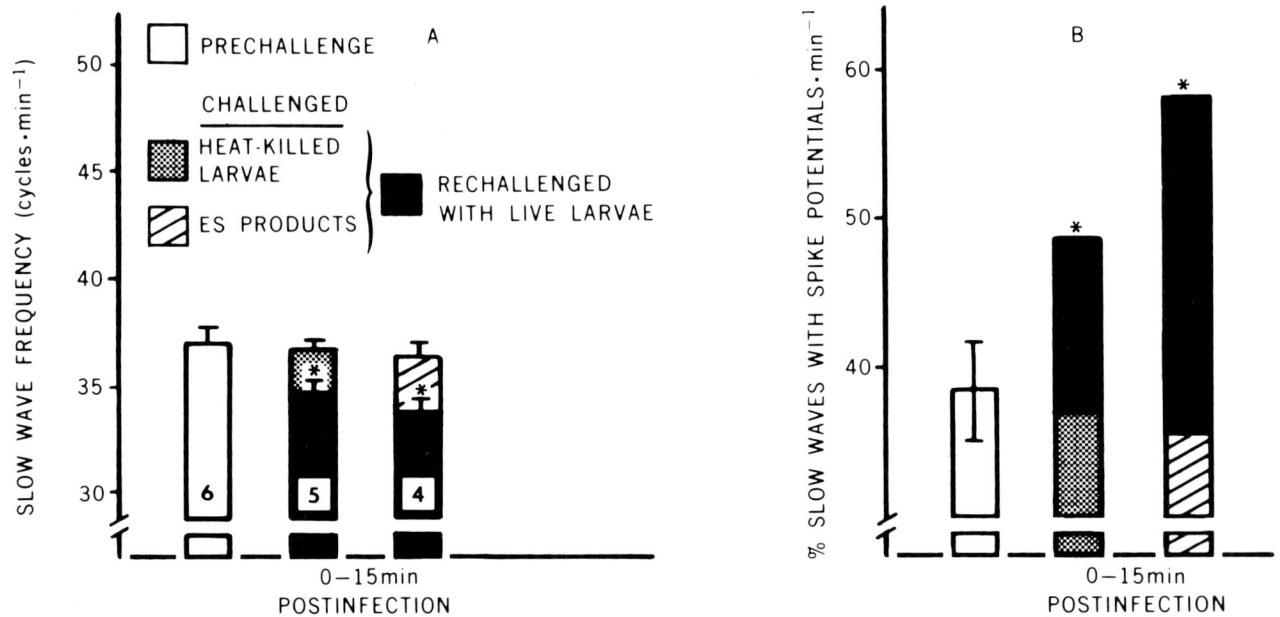

FIG. 15. Slow wave and spiking activity in small intestine of rats immune to *Trichinella spiralis* and challenged with heat-killed larvae on excretory-secretory (ES) antigens and then rechallenged 90 min later with live larvae. All agents were administered intraduodenally. *A*: values are means ± SE. Asterisk indicates significant difference caused by rechallenge with live larvae compared with prechallenged state. *B*: values are means and 95% confidence interval for prechallenge group and means for other groups. Means excluded from 95% confidence interval are significantly different from prechallenge group. Only live larvae induced myoelectric changes. [From Palmer and Castro (62).]

gram isolated small intestinal smooth muscle has been observed in rats infected with *Trichinella spiralis* (7).

In the *Nippostrongylus*-rat model the contractile responsiveness of vascular smooth muscle to agonists, measured as a pressor response in hindleg vessels, is enhanced. Maximum responsiveness of both gut and vascular smooth muscle occurred 14 days after inoculation of the host with infective larvae. Because the

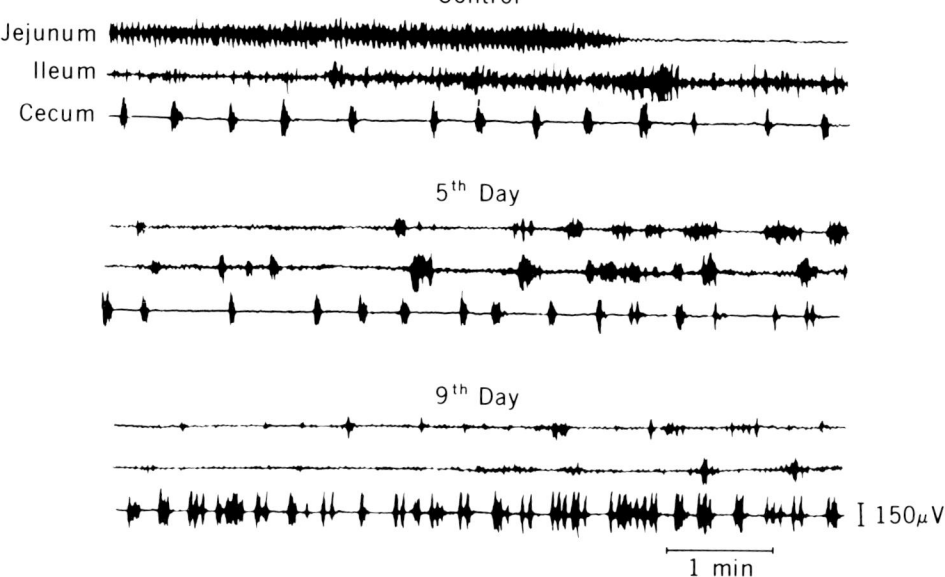

FIG. 16. Electromyogram of jejunum, ileum, and cecum of rabbit infected with *Eimeria magna*. On ninth day after inoculation with oocysts, spiking activity of small intestine was inhibited and frequency of spike bursts in cecum increased. [From Fioramonti et al. (33).]

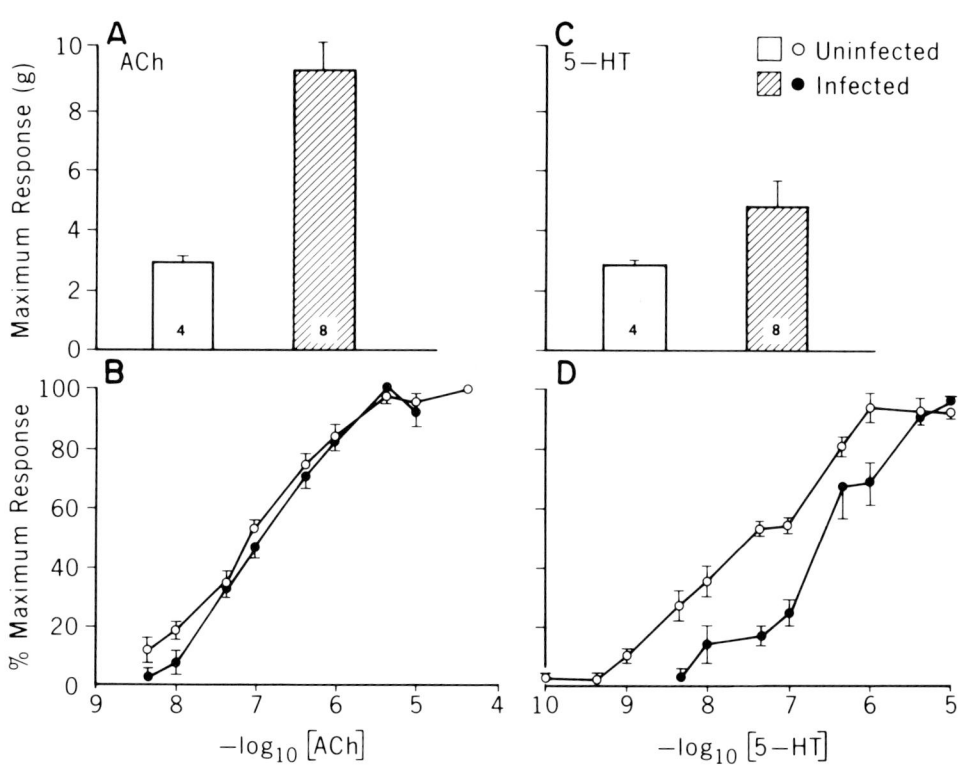

FIG. 17. Maximum (*A* and *C*) and graded responses (*B* and *D*) to acetylcholine (ACh) and serotonin (5–HT) of isolated small intestinal segments from uninfected (*open bar, open circle*) rats and rats infected (*hatched bar, filled circle*) with *Nippostrongylus brasiliensis*. Segments were standardized for length and for region of intestine. Values are means ± SE. Number of animals per group are given at base of the bars. [From Farmer and Laniyonu (32).]

parasite had no contact with the vasculature, there must be a systemic mechanism involved. Furthermore the responses in the two tissues might be related to the immune reaction involved in adult worm expulsion. This was supported when treatment of infected hosts with betamethasone inhibited both worm expulsion and the elevated responsiveness of gut smooth muscle (31).

*Cecum, Colon, and Rectum*

Manometric methods were used to investigate the influence of pentagastrin on the motility of the sigmoid colon and rectum of humans with Chagas' disease. The intravenously administered hormone had a stimulating effect on the motility of uninfected patients and in parasitized patients without the megacolon syndrome. In Chagasic patients with megacolon, pentagastrin had little or no stimulatory effect on motility (Fig. 19). The absence of response to the hormone was believed to result from the malfunctioning of myenteric nerves due to their destruction by *Trypanosoma cruzi*. The implication is that effects of gastrin are neurally mediated (55).

The influence of parasites on the myoelectric activity of the lower GI tract (i.e., cecum and colon) has not been studied extensively. Altered myoelectric patterns have been observed in horses with strongyle infections (12). In general there was hypomotility in the ileocolic region characterized in electromyographs by a decrease in spiking activity. Horses often expressed this change in association with diarrhea.

Hypermotility of the cecum characterized the basic change in rabbits infected with the small intestinal

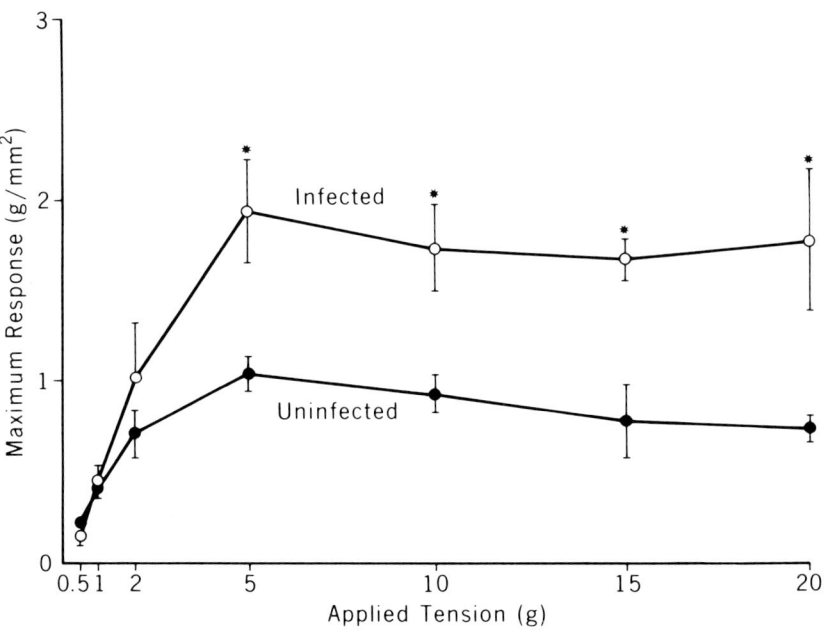

FIG. 18. Relationship between applied tension and maximum developed tension, expressed as function of cross-sectional area of smooth muscle in response to acetylcholine. Tension was measured in 2-cm long small intestinal segments taken 20 cm from pylorus. Segments were from uninfected rats and rats infected with *Nippostrongylus brasiliensis*. Values are means ± SE for 3–5 observations per point. *Asterisk* indicates significant difference as compared with respective control (uninfected) values. [From Farmer et al. (31).]

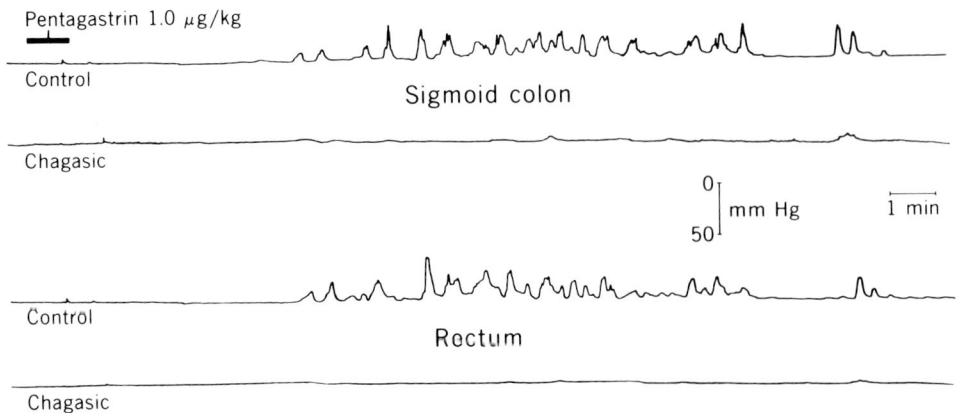

FIG. 19. Pressure changes in sigmoid colon and reaction of control and Chagasic patients with megacolon after intravenous administration of pentagastrin. [From Meneghelli et al. (55).]

parasite *Eimera magna* (33). Electromyograms of the normal cecum consisted of spike bursts of ~3 s duration with a mean frequency of 2.3/min. Changes caused by coccidiosis were expressed 8–9 days postinfection. The duration of the spike bursts lasted only ~1.5 s and the frequency of bursts increased to ~4.6/min (see Fig. 16).

BASIS FOR MOTILITY CHANGES

Direct invasion of the GI smooth muscle by parasites would be a rare event. Thus it can be surmised that changes in function are due directly to stimuli from parasites in the lumen or mucosa of the alimentary canal or indirectly to alterations in the neural, endocrine, or paracrine signals that normally control or regulate smooth muscle function.

*Parasite-Derived Substances*

Although there is little evidence to support the suspicion that parasite-derived substances directly influence smooth muscle cells, the potential for such dictates the need to consider pertinent biochemical and metabolic aspects of parasites. Catabolic processes in parasites result in low-molecular-weight and macromolecular metabolites that are excreted or secreted into the microenvironment. Most enteric parasites are facultative anaerobes whose metabolic energy production is based on fermentation reactions (67). Thus organic acids are predictable excretory products of their energy-producing pathways. An array of such acids have been identified in fluids in which parasites have been maintained in vitro (8). In addition to fermentation acids, ammonia, urea, aliphatic amines, amino acids, and a variety of poorly characterized proteinaceous macromolecules are excretory-secretory (ES) products of parasite metabolism (82).

Influences of parasite-derived fermentation and putrefaction products on host physiology have not been determined. Macromolecular ES products may be enzymes, antienzymes, or so-called toxins. The ES products that might be toxic to the parasitized host have not been examined in relation to their effects on GI motility, although toxic products from parasites have been described. Regardless of their pharmacological or physiological effects these macromolecules are important because of their antigenicity.

The protozoan *Entamoeba histolytica* produces a substance regarded as cytotoxic and possessive of cathepsin B proteinase-like activity (39, 48, 53). A positive correlation has been made between strain virulence and proteinase activity in amebic lysates. Enterotoxic activity of crude lysates of *Entamoeba histolytica* has been demonstrated through its action as a secretagogue in ileal loops of rabbits (49) and when added in vitro to the serosal surface of rat and rabbit colon and ileum (54). A potential mediator of fluid secretion was identified as serotonin. Although serotonin occurs in lysates of the ameba it is not known to be secreted during infection. Because fluid movement in the intestine can influence motility (80), the secretory action of parasite-derived substances must be considered as a possible means through which enteric organisms alter motility patterns.

Megaesophagus and megacolon in Chagas' disease result from destruction of ganglionic nerve cells postulated to be due to toxins from the parasitic amastigote tissue stage (42). A factor in cell-free extracts of *Trypanosoma cruzi* was demonstrated to be toxic for mammalian red blood cells and vero cells in vitro (57). However, this effect alone is not sufficient to label the factor a true toxin in the pharmacological sense or implicate it in the pathogenesis of infection.

Larval worms presumably penetrate and migrate through host tissues aided by secreted enzymes (73). Adult worms may also secrete enzymes that function in extracorporal digestion (73, 77). The nematodes *Nematodirus battus*, *Nippostrongylus brasiliensis*, and *Necator americanus*, parasites of lambs, rats, and humans, respectively, secrete large amounts of acetylcholinesterase (45, 85). The production and release of this enzyme have potentially interesting implications in regard to cholinergic control of smooth muscle contractility. However, no evidence is available that would suggest that acetylcholinesterase derived from these worms affects neural regulation of smooth muscle function.

*Gastrointestinal Hormone Imbalances*

The specific pathways through which parasites alter smooth muscle structure and function are not well known. Broad amplification of motility responses to parasites localized in a specific region of the GI tract implies modulation by neural or humoral control mechanisms. Circulating levels of GI hormones, several of which are known to influence GI motility, are altered during various parasitic infections. *Trichinella* infection in dogs interferes with the normal release of secretin and cholecystokinin (CCK) in response to secretagogues (26, 27). In rats with nippostrongylosis, plasma CCK is reduced and secretin is elevated (60). Inflammation of the gastric mucosa of sheep (3) and intestinal mucosa of pigs (78) is associated with hypergastrinemia. Rats infected with the liver stage of the tapeworm *Taenia taeniaeformis* (23) have plasma gastrin levels 20 times greater than normal. Patients with Chagas' disease also have elevated plasma gastrin (79). Thus far no parasitological studies have been performed in an attempt to relate alterations in smooth muscle function to altered levels of GI hormones.

## Inflammation

Local inflammation in the GI tract resulting from parasitism may be responsible for inducing changes in smooth muscle structure and function. An increase in smooth muscle mass as a result of parasitism was first described about three decades ago in rats infected with the nematode *Nippostrongylus brasiliensis*. A marked thickening of the muscularis externa in the small intestine was attributed to hypertrophy of the longitudinal smooth muscle layer (75). Analogous observations have been made in other host-parasite systems. For example, primary infection with the nematode *Trichinella spiralis* in both guinea pigs and rats is characterized in part by a gross thickening of small intestinal smooth muscle layers. This is evident within 1 wk after oral inoculation of hosts with infective ($L_1$) larvae (18, 47, 69). The response in guinea pigs has been attributed to changes in the longitudinal muscle layer and may be accelerated in its expression after a secondary infection (47). Total mass of the small intestine smooth muscle increases also in rats infected with the acanthocephalan (thorny-headed worm) *Moniliformis dubius* (25), in horses infected with *Parascaris equorum* (21), and in pigs harboring *Ascaris suum* (72). The dramatic alteration occurring in *Ascaris*-infected pigs is shown in Figure 20.

Smooth muscle changes in the *Ascaris* and acanthocephalan infections were interpreted as adaptive responses aimed either at expelling worms from the gut or moving chyme through the intestinal lumen stenosed with adult worms. Experimental support comes from the induction of marked hypertrophy of intestinal smooth muscle in rats and guinea pigs as a result of stenosis produced through surgical means (36).

Although the stenosis hypothesis may explain increased intestinal smooth muscle mass resulting from infection with large lumen-dwelling parasites, an alternate hypothesis is required to explain changes caused by almost microscopic organisms such as *Trichinella spiralis* and *Nippostrongylus brasiliensis*. A possible explanation hinges on relationships between smooth muscle changes and local inflammation (16). Inference of a possible relationship between growth of smooth muscle and inflammation in the gut are based on descriptions of a similar relationship involving vascular smooth muscle. Smooth muscle proliferation in arterial wall occurs after damage to vascular endothelium caused by infections, immunological reactions, or trauma (56, 64, 70). Presumably smooth muscle proliferation in these cases is stimulated by plasma components and by factors released from platelets (84). Possibly inflammation caused by parasites leads to the release of similar factors from the microcirculation or from extravascular components that stimulate intestinal smooth muscle proliferation.

Inflammation induced by parasites may result from nonspecific stimuli (71) such as traumatic damage to or lysis of mucosal tissue and through the release of histolytic or cytolytic enzymes (73). In late primary infection and during secondary infection, immunological reactions may intervene to modulate smooth muscle responses (16, 17). Substances released by inflammatory cells or immunologically competent cells, e.g.,

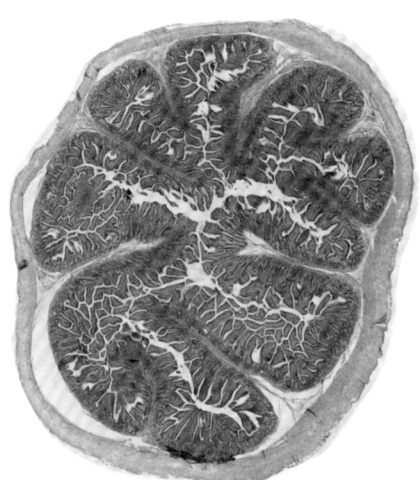
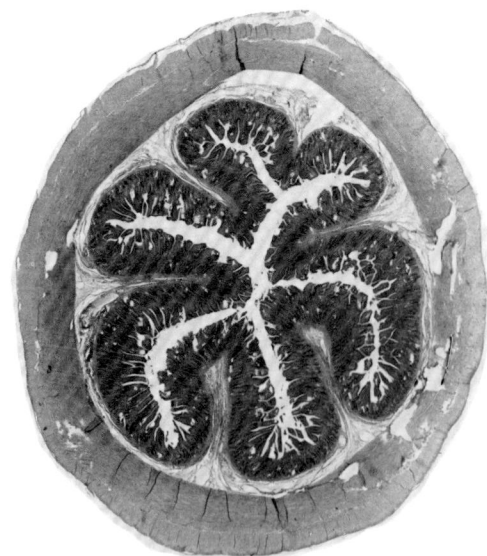

FIG. 20. Transverse section of middle jejunum of noninfected pig (*left*) and pig harboring 49 adult *Ascaris suis* (*right*). Pigs were infected at 3 wk of age and were killed 8 wk later. Infection was induced by oral inoculation with 15-day-old *Ascaris* recovered from infected rabbits. This method of infection prevented extraintestinal stages of parasite from developing. Changes caused by infection were generalized and not restricted to area of worm localization in intestine. [From Stephenson et al. (72).]

T and B lymphocytes, macrophages, and mast cells, are likely candidates as factors that modulate smooth muscle physiology either directly or via neural mechanisms. Agents involved may include ACh, substance P, serotonin, vasoactive intestinal peptide, histamine, prostaglandins, and leukotrienes (4, 13).

The accelerated increase in smooth muscle mass in secondary as compared with primary trichinosis in guinea pigs (47) suggests involvement of an immunological response in mediating this change. The immune expulsion of *Nippostrongylus brasiliensis* implicates the influence of immunological responses on smooth muscle structure. Expulsion of this nematode from the rat small intestine in a primary infection is associated with increased responsiveness of intestinal smooth muscle to agonists and electrical stimulation (30, 31). An example of the potential influence that immunologically competent cells have on intestinal smooth muscle function is demonstrated in the Schultz-Dale reaction (24). This reaction results in a rapid, dose-dependent contractile response of isolated intestinal segments taken from immunized animals when challenged in vitro with the sensitizing antigen. The reaction is based on the release of potent agonists of smooth muscle contractile activity released from mast cells (4, 46) after the interaction of membrane-bound homocytotropic antibodies with antigen. The Schultz-Dale response is immunologically specific and reflects immediate hypersensitivity of the target tissue detected in vitro. The possible occurrence of smooth muscle anaphylaxis in vivo was suggested from the altered myoelectric activity in conscious rats sensitized by primary infection to *Trichinella spiralis* and challenged by reinfection (62). The challenge infected elicited, within minutes, changes in the myoelectric pattern that proved to be stimulus specific and anamnestic in nature.

## SUMMARY

Evidence from roentgenological examinations (65) and from measurements of intraluminal pressure changes, transit time, and myoelectric activity indicate that enteric parasites perturb normal patterns of GI motility. The significance of these perturbations in the host-parasite relationship remains speculative.

Almost invariably parasite-induced changes in motility are assessed in relationship to the pathogenesis of infection, particularly in relationship to diarrhea. However, the suggestion has been made that changes in smooth muscle contractions play little or no role in causing diarrhea (6). These opposing views will likely be reconciled as the functional alterations associated with parasitism are viewed in an integrated fashion by more investigators. For example, Mathias et al. (51), studying the role of enterotoxins in bacterial pathogenicity, suggested that changes in contractile patterns alone may be inadequate to cause diarrhea. However, propulsive forces may be a contributing factor when they occur in conjunction with secretion and enteropooling of fluid. This view is clearly supportive of the unification theory of motility of Weems (80), which attempts to interrelate intestinal wall motions, propulsive forces, and fluid movement. Adherence to such a theory for an explanation of host-parasite interactions would seem compelling since relatively few conclusive precepts can be derived from the collection of studies described in this chapter. Also it should be evident that enteric parasite infections are almost universally associated with disturbances in digestion, absorption, and secretion, all of which can influence the content of fluid in the gut lumen.

Important in the interpretation of results is the fact that motility patterns in the GI tract vary considerably with the feeding state. Because sick hosts tend to decrease food intake, it is important to dissect motility changes due directly to parasitism from those caused indirectly by altered patterns of feeding.

Some changes in motility can be envisioned as beneficial to the host, i.e., adaptive in nature. Alterations similar to the MAPC in rats with trichinosis occur in ligated loops of rabbit ileum exposed to invasive strains of the bacterium *Escherichia coli* (14, 15), invasive and noninvasive strains of *Shigella dysenteriae*, and enterotoxin from *S. dysenteriae*, *Clostridium perfringens*, and *Vibrio cholerae* (40, 50). Possibly the MAPC represents a host defense reaction aimed at clearing noxious agents from the lumen, a hypothesis that has prevailed in parasitology for many years, i.e., that natural and acquired resistance to infection may be effected through changes in peristalsis (38, 43, 44, 52). The hypothesis rests more on conclusions derived from loose associations rather than on definitive evidence. Supportive of the hypothesis is the work involving increased intensity of *Hymenolepis nana* infections in mice treated with opium or morphine to increase transit time (43) and the proximal relocalization of *Trichinella spiralis* from the distal small intestine in morphine-treated young mice (44). In secondary murine trichinosis there is a close temporal association between motility changes induced by infective larvae and immune rejection of the parasite from its gut habitat (63). An attempt has been made to examine effects of an inhibitor of small intestinal peristalsis on immune expulsion of *Trichinella spiralis* (5). Treatment of rats with oxyphenonium bromide, an agent described as causing hypomotility, failed to prevent worm rejection, leading to the conclusion that motility has no significant role in effecting worm rejection. Conclusions of a cause-effect relationship between drug treatment and effects on parasite development made without a thorough examination of the simultaneous effect on motility are subject to question and should be challenged. Such challenges should lead to the design of experiments that will provide clearer results necessary to better understand the role of altered GI motility in the host-parasite relationship.

This work was supported in part by NIH (NIAID) Grant AI-11361.

REFERENCES

1. ALIZADEH, H., G. A. CASTRO, AND W. A. WEEMS. Intestinal jejunal propulsion in the guinea pig during parasitism with *Trichinella spiralis*. *Gastroenterology* 93: 784–790, 1987.
2. ALIZADEH, H., G. A. CASTRO, AND W. A. WEEMS. Onset and duration of intrinsic jejunal propulsive behavior induced by primary *Trichinella spiralis* infection (Abstract). *Gastroenterology* 90: 1324, 1986.
3. ANDERSON, N., J. HANSKY, AND D. A. TICHEN. Effects of a series of infections of *Ostertagia circumcincta* on gastric secretion of sheep. *Parasitology* 72: 1–12, 1976.
4. BACH, M. K. Mediators of anaphylaxis and inflammation. *Annu. Rev. Microbiol.* 36: 371–413, 1982.
5. BELL, R. G., D. D. MCGREGOR, AND L. S. ADAMS. Studies on the inhibition of rapid expulsion of *Trichinella spiralis* in rats. *Int. Arch. Allergy Appl. Immunol.* 69: 73–80, 1982.
6. BINDER, H. J., AND M. DONOWITZ. Clinical trends and topics: a new look at laxative action. *Gastroenterology* 69: 1001–1005, 1975.
7. BOWERS, R. L., G. A. CASTRO, AND N. W. WEISBRODT. Alterations in intestinal smooth muscle of the rat induced by *Trichinella spiralis* (Abstract). *Gastroenterology* 90: 1353, 1986.
8. BRAND, T. VON. Carbohydrates II: metabolism of carbohydrates. In: *Biochemistry of Parasites*, edited by T. von Brand. New York: Academic, 1966, p. 79–156.
9. BRASIL, A. A peristalsis of the esophagus. *Rev. Bras. Gastroenterol.* 7: 21–31, 1965.
10. BUENO, L., A. DAKKAK, AND J. FIORAMONTI. Gastro-duodenal motor and transit disturbances associated with *Haemonchus contortus* infection in sheep. *Parasitology* 84: 367–374, 1982.
11. BUÉNO, L., P. DORCHIES, AND Y. RUCKEBUSCH. Analyse électromyographique perturbations motrices liées aus strongyloses gastrointestinales chez les ovins. *C. R. Seances Soc. Biol. Fil.* 169: 1627–1632, 1975.
12. BUENO, L., Y. RUCKEBUSCH, AND P. DORCHIES. Disturbances of digestive motility in horses associated with strongyle infection. *Vet. Parasitol.* 5: 253–260, 1979.
13. BURKS, T. F. Actions of drugs on gastrointestinal motility. In: *Physiology of the Gastrointestinal Tract* (1st ed.), edited by L. R. Johnson. New York: Raven, 1981, p. 495–516.
14. BURNS, T. W., J. R. MATHIAS, G. M. CARLSON, J. L. MARTIN, AND R. P. SHIELDS. Effect of toxigenic *Escherichia coli* on myoelectric activity of small intestine. *Am. J. Physiol.* 235 (*Endocrinol. Metab. Gastrointest. Physiol.* 4): E311–E315, 1978.
15. BURNS, T. W., J. R. MATHIAS, J. L. MARTIN, G. M. CARLSON, AND R. P. SHIELDS. Alteration of myoelectric activity of small intestine by invasive *Escherichia coli*. *Am. J. Physiol.* 238 (*Gastrointest. Liver Physiol.* 1): G57–G62, 1980.
16. CASTRO, G. A. Spatial and temporal integration of host responses to intestinal stages of *Trichinella spiralis*: retro- and prospective views. In: *Biochemistry of Parasites and Host-Parasite Relationships*, edited by H. Van den Bossche. Amsterdam: North-Holland, 1976, p. 343–358.
17. CASTRO, G. A. Immunological regulation of epithelial function. *Am. J. Physiol.* 243 (*Gastrointest. Liver Physiol.* 6): G321–G329, 1982.
18. CASTRO, G. A., F. BADIAL-ACEVES, J. W. SMITH, S. J. DUDRICK, AND N. W. WEISBRODT. Altered small bowel propulsion associated with parasitism. *Gastroenterology* 71: 620–625, 1976.
19. CASTRO, G. A., J. J. HESSEL, AND G. WHALEN. Altered intestinal fluid movement in response to *Trichinella spiralis* in immunized rats. *Parasite Immunol. Oxf.* 1: 259–266, 1979.
20. CASTRO, G. A., C. A. POST, AND S. A. ROY. Intestinal motility during the enteric phase of trichinosis in immunized rats. *J. Parasitol.* 63: 713–719, 1977.
21. CLAYTON, H. M., AND J. L. DUNCAN. Experimental *Parascaris equorum* infection of foals. *Rev. Vet. Sci.* 23: 109–114, 1977.
22. COLLINS, S. M., AND A. E. FOX. Gut inflammation alters calcium handling properties of intestinal smooth muscle (Abstract). *Gastroenterology* 86: 1052, 1984.
23. COOK, R. W., J. F. WILLIAMS, AND L. LICHTENBERGER. Hypergastric gastropathy in the rat due to *Taenia taeniformis* infection: parabiotic transfer and hypergastrinemia. *Gastroenterology* 80: 728–734, 1981.
24. COULSON, E. J. The Schultz-Dale technique. *J. Allergy* 24: 458–473, 1953.
25. CROMPTON, D. W. T., AND A. SINGHUI. Intestinal responses of rats to *Moniliformis* (Acanthocephala) (Abstract). *Parasitology* 84: IXX, 1982.
26. DEMBINSKI, A. B., L. R. JOHNSON, AND G. A. CASTRO. Influence of enteric parasitism on hormone-regulated pancreatic secretion in dogs. *Am. J. Physiol.* 237 (*Regulatory Integrative Comp. Physiol.* 6): R232–R238, 1979.
27. DEMBINSKI, A. B., L. R. JOHNSON, AND G. A. CASTRO. Influence of parasitism on secretin-inhibited gastric secretion. *Am. J. Trop. Med. Hyg.* 28: 854–859, 1979.
28. DUSZYNSKI, D. W., S. A. ROY, J. STEWART, AND G. A. CASTRO. Intestinal transit time during infection with *Eimeria nieschulzi* in rats. *J. Protozool.* 25: 370–374, 1978.
29. FARMER, S. G. Propulsive activity of the rat small intestine during infection with nematode *Nippostrongylus brasiliensis*. *Parasite Immunol. Oxf.* 3: 227–234, 1981.
30. FARMER, S. G. Changes in responsiveness of intestinal smooth muscle to agonists in rats infected with *Nippostrongylus brasiliensis* (Abstract). *Br. J. Pharmacol.* 74: 199P, 1981.
31. FARMER, S. G., J. M. BROWN, AND D. POLLOCK. Increased responsiveness to intestinal and vascular smooth muscle to agonists in rats infected with *Nippostrongylus brasiliensis*. *Arch. Int. Pharmacodyn. Ther.* 263: 217–227, 1983.
32. FARMER, S. G., AND A. A. LANIYONU. Effects of p-chlorophenylaline on the sensitivity of rat intestine to agonists and on intestinal 5-hydroxytryptamine during *Nippostrongylus brasiliensis* infection. *Br. J. Pharmacol.* 82: 883–889, 1984.
33. FIORAMONTI, J., J. M. SORRAING, D. LICOIS, AND L. BUENO. Intestinal motor and transit disturbances associated with experimental coccidiosis (*Eimeria magna*) in the rabbit. *Ann. Rech. Vet.* 12: 413–420, 1981.
34. FOX, J. E. T., E. E. DANIEL, C. R. DEFARIA, J. M. REZENDEZ, L. RASSI, J. DERENZENDEZ, JR., AND V. P. DANIEL. Relationship of functional changes to structural changes in megaesophagus of Chagas' disease. In: *Gastrointestinal Motility*, edited by C. Roman. Lancaster, UK: MTP, 1983, p. 51–58.
35. FOX-ROBICHAUD, A. E., AND S. M. COLLINS. Altered utilization of $Ca^{++}$ by smooth muscle from inflamed gut (Abstract). *Gastroenterology* 88: 1386, 1985.
36. GABELLA, G. Hypertrophy of intestinal smooth muscle. *Cell Tissue Res.* 163: 199–214, 1975.
37. GOYAL, R. K. Does gastrin act via cholinergic neurons to maintain lower-esophageal sphincter pressure (Letter to the editor)? *N. Engl. J. Med.* 291: 849–850, 1974.
38. HUNINNEN, A. V. Studies on the life history and host-parasite relation of *Hymenolepis fraterna* (*H. nana* var. *fraterna* Stiles) in white mice. *Am. J. Hyg.* 22: 414–443, 1935.
39. JARUMILINTA, R., AND F. KRADOLFER. The toxic effect of *Entamoeba histolytica* on leucocytes. *Ann. Trop. Med. Parasitol.* 58: 375–381, 1964.
40. JUSTUS, P. G., J. R. MATHIAS, J. L. MARTIN, G. M. CARLSON, R. P. SHIELD, AND S. B. FORMAL. Myoelectric activity in the small intestine in response to *Clostridium perfringens* A enterotoxin: correlation with histological findings in an in vivo rabbit model. *Gastroenterology* 80: 902–906, 1981.

41. KOBERLE, F. Chagas' disease and Chagas' syndrome. The pathology of American trypanosomiasis. *Adv. Parasitol.* 6: 63–116, 1968.
42. KOBERLE, F. The causation and importance of nervous lesions in American Trypanosomiasis. *Bull. WHO* 42: 739–743, 1970.
43. LARSH, J. E. The relationship in mice of intestinal emptying time and natural resistance to *Hymenolepis*. *J. Parasitol.* 33: 79–84, 1947.
44. LARSH, J. E., AND J. R. HENDRICKS. The probable explanation for the difference in the localization of adult *Trichinella spiralis* in young and old mice. *J. Parasitol.* 35: 101–106, 1949.
45. LEE, D. L., AND J. MARTIN. Changes in *Nematodirus battus* associated with the development of immunity to this nematode in lambs. In: *Biochemistry of Parasites and Host-Parasite Relationships*, edited by H. Van den Bossche. Amsterdam: North-Holland, 1976, p. 311–318.
46. LEID, R. W., AND J. F. WILLIAMS. Helminth parasites and the host inflammatory system. In: *Chemical Zoology*, edited by M. Florkin and B. T. Scheer. New York: Academic, 1979, vol. XI, p. 229–271.
47. LIN, T. M., AND L. J. OLSON. Pathophysiology of reinfection with *Trichinella spiralis* in guinea pigs during the intestinal phase. *J. Parasitol.* 56: 529–539, 1970.
48. LUSHBAUGH, W. B., A. F. HOFBAUER, AND F. E. PITTMAN. Proteinase activities of *Entamoeba histolytica* cytotoxin. *Gastroenterology* 87: 17–27, 1984.
49. LUSHBAUGH, W. B., A. B. KAIRALLA, J. R. CANTEY, A. F. HOFBAUER, AND F. E. PITTMAN. Isolation of cytotoxin-enterotoxin from *Entamoeba histolytica*. *J. Infect. Dis.* 139: 9–17, 1979.
50. MATHIAS, J. R., G. M. CARLSON, G. BERTIGER, J. L. MARTIN, AND S. COHEN. Migrating action potential complex of cholera: a possible prostaglandin-induced response. *Am. J. Physiol.* 232 (*Endocrinol. Metab. Gastrointest. Physiol.* 1): E529–E534, 1977.
51. MATHIAS, J. R., G. M. CARLSON, J. L. MARTIN, R. P. SCHIELDS, AND S. FORMAL. *Shigella dysenteriase* I enterotoxin: proposed role in pathogenesis of shigellosis. *Am. J. Physiol.* 239 (*Gastrointest. Liver Physiol.* 2): G382–G386, 1980.
52. MCCOY, O. R. Rapid loss of *Trichinella* larvae fed to immune rats and its bearing on the mechanism of immunity. *Am. J. Hyg.* 32: 105–116, 1940.
53. MCGOWAN, K., C. F. DENEKE, G. M. THORNE, AND S. L. GORBACH. *Entamoeba histolytica* cytotoxin: purification, characterization, strain virulence and protease activity. *J. Infect. Dis.* 146: 616–625, 1982.
54. MCGOWEN, K., A. KANE, N. ASARKOF, J. WICKS, V. GUERINA, J. KELLUM, S. BARON, A. R. GINTZLER, AND M. DONOWITZ. *Entamoeba histolytica* causes intestinal secretion: role of serotonin. *Science Wash. DC* 221: 762–764, 1983.
55. MENEGHELLI, U. G., R. A. GODOY, R. B. OLIVEIRA, J. C. M. SANTOS, JR., AND R. O. DANTAS. Effect of pentagastrin on the motor activity of the dilated and nondilated sigmoid and rectum in Chagas' disease. *Digestion* 27: 152–158, 1983.
56. MINICK, C. R., G. E. MURPHY, AND W. G. CAMPBELL. Experimental induction of athero-arterio-sclerosis by synergy of allergic injury to arteries and lipid-rich diet. I. Effect of repeated injections of horse serum in rabbits fed a dietary cholesterol supplement. *J. Exp. Med.* 124: 635–652, 1966.
57. O'DALY, J. A., AND P. M. ASO. *Trypanosoma cruzi, Lieshnania donovani* and *L. mexicana*: extract factor that lyses mammalian cells. *Exp. Parasitol.* 47: 222–231, 1979.
58. OLIVEIRA, R. B., U. G. MENEGHELLI, R. A. DEGODOY, R. O. DANTAS, AND W. PODOVAN. Abnormalities of interdigestive motility of the small intestine in patients with Chagas' disease. *Dig. Dis. Sci.* 28: 294–299, 1983.
59. OLSON, L. J. In vivo responses of small intestine of guinea pigs following challenge with sonicated *Trichinella spiralis* larvae. *Program, American Society of Parasitologists, 42nd Annual Meeting, Tucson, Arizona, August 21–25, 1967*, p. 41.
60. OVINGTON, K. S., A. J. BACARESE-HAMILTON, AND S. R. BLOOM. *Nippostrongylus brasiliensis*: changes in plasma levels of gastrointestinal hormones in the infected rat. *Exp. Parasitol.* 60: 276–284, 1986.
61. PADOVAN, W., R. A. GODOY, R. A. DANTAS, U. G. MENEGHELLI, R. B. OLIVEIRA, AND L. E. A. TRONCON. Lower oesophageal sphincter response to pentagastrin in Chagasic patients with megaoesophagus and megacolon. *Gut* 21: 85–90, 1980.
62. PALMER, J. M., AND G. A. CASTRO. Anamnestic stimulus-specific myoelectric responses associated with intestinal immunity in the rat. *Am. J. Physiol.* 250 (*Gastrointest. Liver Physiol.* 13): G266–G273, 1986.
63. PALMER, J. M., N. W. WEISBRODT, AND G. A. CASTRO. *Trichinella spiralis*: intestinal myoelectric activity during enteric infection in the rat. *Exp. Parasitol.* 57: 132–141, 1984.
64. PESONEN, E. Coronary wall thickening in children. *Atherosclerosis* 20: 173–187, 1974.
65. REEDER, N. M., AND L. C. HAMILTON. Radiologic diagnosis of tropical diseases of the gastrointestinal tract. *Radiol. Clin. N. Am.* 7: 57–81, 1969.
66. RUSSELL, D. A., AND G. A. CASTRO. Physiological characterization of a biphasic immune response to *Trichinella spiralis* in the rat. *J. Infect. Dis.* 139: 304–312, 1979.
67. SAZ, H. J. Facultative anaerobiosis in the invertebrates: pathways and control systems. *Am. Zool.* 11: 125–135, 1971.
68. SCHANBACHER, L. M., J. K. NATIONS, N. W. WEISBRODT, AND G. A. CASTRO. Intestinal myoelectric activity in parasitized dogs. *Am. J. Physiol.* 234 (*Regulatory Integrative Comp. Physiol.* 3): R188–R195, 1978.
69. SMITH, J. W., AND G. A. CASTRO. Relation of peroxidase activity in gut mucosa to inflammation. *Am. J. Physiol.* 234 (*Regulatory Integrative Comp. Physiol.* 3): R72–R79, 1978.
70. SPAET, T. H., M. B. STEMMERMAN, S. J. VEITH, AND I. LEJNIECKS. Intimal injury and regrowth in the rabbit aorta. *Circ. Res.* 36: 58–70, 1975.
71. SPRINZ, H. Morphological response of intestinal mucosa to enteric bacteria and its implication in sprue and Asiatic cholera. *Federation Proc.* 21: 57–64, 1962.
72. STEPHENSON, L. S., W. G. POND, M. C. NEISHEIM, L. T. KROCK, AND D. W. T. CROMPTON. *Ascaris suum*: nutrient absorption, growth and intestinal pathology in young pigs experimentally infected with 15-day-old larvae. *Exp. Parasitol.* 49: 15–25, 1980.
73. STIRWALT, M. A. Skin penetration mechanisms of helminths. In: *Biology of Parasites*, edited by E. J. L. Soulsby. New York: Academic, 1966, p. 41–59.
74. SUKHDEO, M. V. K., AND N. A. CROLL. Gut propulsion in mice infected with *Trichinella spiralis*. *J. Parasitol.* 67: 906–910, 1981.
75. SYMONS, L. E. A. Pathology of infection of the rat with *Nippostrongylus myris* (Yokagawa). I. Changes in water content, dry weight and tissues of the small intestine. *Aust. J. Biol. Sci.* 10: 374–383, 1957.
76. SYMONS, L. E. A. Digestion and absorption of maltose in rats infected by the nematode *Nippostrongylus brasiliensis*. *Exp. Parasitol.* 18: 12–24, 1966.
77. THORSON, R. E. The stimulation of acquired immunity in dogs by injection of extracts of the esophagus of adult hookworms. *J. Parasitol.* 42: 501–504, 1956.
78. TICHEN, D. A. The role of hormones in the reactions of the host to enteric parasites. In: *Parasites–Their World and Ours*, edited by D. F. Mettrick and S. S. Desser. Amsterdam: Biomedical, 1982, p. 245–247.
79. TRONCON, L. E. A., R. B. OLIVEIRA, U. G. MENEGHELLI, R. O. DANTAS, AND R. A. GODOY. Fasting and food-stimulated plasma gastrin levels in chronic Chagas' disease. *Digestion* 29: 171–176, 1984.
80. WEEMS, W. A. Intestinal wall motion, propulsion, and fluid movement: trends toward a unified theory. *Am. J. Physiol.* 243 (*Gastrointest. Liver Physiol.* 6): G177–G188, 1982.
81. WEEMS, W. A., AND N. W. WEISBRODT. Comparison of colonic and ileal propulsive capabilities under conditions requiring hydrostatic work. *Am. J. Physiol.* 246 (*Gastrointest. Liver Physiol.* 9): G587–G593, 1984.

82. WEINSTEIN, P. P. Excretory mechanisms and excretory products of nematodes. In: *Host Influence on Parasite Physiology*, edited by L. A. Stauber. New Brunswick, NJ: Rutgers Univ. Press, 1960, p. 65-92.
83. WEISBRODT, N. W., AND G. A. CASTRO. Intestinal myoelectric activity of the dog during hookworm infection (Abstract). *Federation Proc.* 36: 595, 1977.
84. WOLINSKY, H. A new look at atherosclerosis. *Cardiovasc. Med.* 1: 41-54, 1976.
85. YEATES, R. A., AND B. M. OGILVIE. Nematode acetylcholinesterases. In: *Biochemistry of Parasites and Host-Parasite Relationships*, edited by H. Van den Bossche. Amsterdam, North-Holland, 1976, p. 307-310.
86. ZWICK, R., K. L. BOWES, E. E. DANIEL, AND S. K. SARNA. Mechanism of action of pentagastrin on the lower esophageal sphincter. *J. Clin. Invest.* 57: 1644-1651, 1976.

CHAPTER 31

# Alterations of small intestine motility by bacteria and their enterotoxins

JOHN R. MATHIAS | Veterans Administration Medical Center and Department of
MARY H. CLENCH | Medicine, University of Florida, Gainesville, Florida

CHAPTER CONTENTS

Historical Background and Animal Model
Migrating Action-Potential Complex (MAPC)
   Cholera toxin
   Choleragen and choleragenoid
   Historical background of MAPC
   Association of MAPC with prostaglandins
   Relationship of enteric nervous system with MAPC
   MAPC in vitro
   Other substances that stimulate MAPC
      *Escherichia coli* and its enterotoxin
      *Salmonella*
      Castor oil and ricinoleic acid
      Vasoactive intestinal peptide
      Bile salts
   Control mechanisms of MAPC
   Questions for the future
Repetitive Bursts of Action Potentials
   Invasive *Escherichia coli*
   *Shigella dysenteriae* 1 and purified enterotoxin from strain 60R
   *Clostridium perfringens* A enterotoxin
   *Clostridium difficile*
   Heat-stable toxins from *Escherichia coli*
   *Campylobacter jejuni*
   Summary
Bacterial Overgrowth of Small Intestine
   Mechanisms of diarrhea
      Brush-border injury
      Mucosal injury
      Bile acids
      Hydroxylation of fat
      Motility
      Metabolic products from bacteria
   Questions for the future
Summary

CERTAIN BACTERIA and their enterotoxins that induce diarrhea have emerged over the past two decades as unique and physiologically important biologic probes to investigate cellular mechanisms. Understanding these cellular mechanisms has led to the discovery that these biologic substances act via specific receptors on the membranes of cells. Intracellular secondary and tertiary messengers are thus formed and induce characteristic intracellular and organ responses (75, 157, 159). These biologic probes are important pharmacologic tools and have allowed us to begin understanding the secretory physiology (157) and alterations of motor function of the gastrointestinal tract (145). Understanding these mechanisms has also led to more effective therapy for a major clinical problem, diarrhea. Most diarrheal diseases are caused by infectious microorganisms or their associated enterotoxins, and they constitute the largest cause of human mortality and morbidity on a worldwide scale (91, 95, 190, 208).

It is generally accepted that these organisms alter cellular function and subsequently cause disease by two mechanisms. They may produce heat-labile (57, 179) or heat-stable (58, 94) toxins that bind to enterocyte receptors and induce changes in secretion, absorption, and/or motility, or they may directly invade the enterocyte and/or produce cytotoxic products that cause an inflammatory process (10, 85). Diarrhea is not only a significant cause of self-limited disease but also a major cause of death, especially in Third-World countries.

The effects of bacteria and their enterotoxins on alterations in intestinal muscle contractions is a relatively new field of research. A review by Grady and Keusch in 1971 (85) did not mention the interplay of motility in diarrheogenic states. In a 1973 review Banwell and Sherr (10) noted that the effects of bacteria and their enterotoxins on motility needed to be studied and indicated that such research could provide important new understanding of the mechanisms of experimentally induced diarrhea.

Until the early 1970s diarrhea was considered to be solely a secretory phenomenon (9, 28, 29, 57, 121, 165). Secretion of water and electrolytes by the enterocyte and impairment of sodium absorption by cholera toxin, for example, were considered to be secondary to the activation of intracellular adenylate cyclase, which increased cAMP (178, 179). The resultant secretory process was initiated by binding toxin to monosialoganglioside ($G_{M1}$) receptors on the enterocyte membrane (103) and activation of the cAMP-protein kinase A system (74, 76, 99). Cholera toxin has also been shown to antagonize the hydrolysis of cGMP, which in turn interferes with the shutoff of cAMP production (30, 31). The secretory process seemed relatively simple with secretion of electrolytes and concomitant movement of water into the lumen by the enterocyte resulting in diarrhea by a single mechanism. How the intraluminal contents moved within the lumen was not considered, and diarrhea was referred to as an open-pipe phenomenon; that is, it was believed to involve only passive movement of fluid through the lumen of the intestine.

The concept of diarrhea has since undergone considerable change. It is now clear that diarrhea involves more than just active secretion of electrolytes and the movement of water into the lumen of the intestine; alterations in motility and malabsorption are also important (145). In this chapter an attempt is made to balance the former exclusive emphasis on the importance of secretion by alterations only within the enterocyte with a discussion of the motor changes that occur during experimentally induced diarrhea; what is currently known about the mechanism or mechanisms of the interaction between enteric nerves and circular smooth muscle of the intestine is also summarized.

In 1976 Mathias et al. (138) observed in the small intestine of an anesthetized animal model a myoelectric response secondary to live *Vibrio cholerae* and its purified enterotoxin choleragen. This alteration in myoelectric activity was the first of two complexes (25, 138) that were found to be caused by certain bacteria or their enterotoxins (25).

## HISTORICAL BACKGROUND AND ANIMAL MODEL

The investigation of the effect of diarrheogenic bacteria and their enterotoxins began in 1894 when Metchnikoff (154) demonstrated secretion in the rabbit intestine infected with cholera. Sanarelli (176) also used the rabbit intestine in further studies in 1921. Later the rabbit intestine was shown to provide consistent results in research on secretion by Dee and Chatterjee in 1953 (45) and by Dutta and Habbu in 1955 (51). Although the intestine of other mammalian species such as the rat, cat, mouse, guinea pig, and dog responds to cholera toxin (173), the reliable and consistent manner in which the rabbit intestine responds has led to a preference for this animal as the model for investigating secretion. As a result the New Zealand White rabbit has become the animal model of choice in the investigation of secretory diarrhea. This rabbit model was also used to investigate the effects of bacteria and their enterotoxins on motility, to correlate what had already been described regarding secretion with what was being learned about altered neuromuscular responses (45, 51). In addition the anesthetized state was selected to eliminate background activity, e.g., the migrating myoelectric complex (MMC) described by Szurszewski (196), and the fed-state activity (148) that normally occurs in unanesthetized animals. In retrospect this decision was fortuitous because the stimulated responses might otherwise have been obscured by normal ongoing motor activity.

The model was an in vivo, 15-cm ligated segment or loop of ileum (Fig. 1) in a New Zealand White rabbit anesthetized with sodium pentobarbital. Initial anesthetization was through an ear vein, and additional anesthetic was administered, as needed, through a catheter placed in the external jugular vein (138). Each animal also received a tracheostomy. The distal ileum was isolated through a midline abdominal incision. Four silver–silver chloride monopolar electrodes (149) were sewn onto the serosa of the loop at 2.5-cm intervals (138). A large-bore catheter (ID, 0.187 in.; OD, 0.250 in.) was inserted at the distal end of the loop for outflow of luminal contents, and a second large-bore catheter was inserted above the proximal ligature to allow outflow from the remaining small intestine. For injection or infusion of the test substance a small-bore catheter (ID, 0.030 in.; OD, 0.048 in.) was placed within the lumen at the proximal end of the ligated loop and secured with a purse-string suture.

Each electrode was connected to a rectilinear physiological recorder through AC couplers. Myoelectric activity was recorded at a sensitivity of 0.5 mV/cm, a time constant of 1.0 s, a high-frequency filter cutoff of 22 Hz, and a paper speed of 2.5 mm/s. A recording made under control conditions is shown in Figure 2.

## MIGRATING ACTION-POTENTIAL COMPLEX (MAPC)

The migrating action-potential complex (MAPC) is a single moving ring contraction that was found ini-

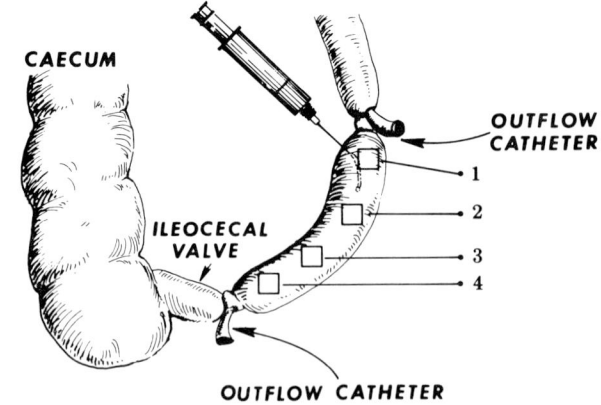

FIG. 1. Schematic of 12-cm distal ileal loop model. Four monopolar silver–silver chloride electrodes (No. 1–4) are placed 2.5 cm apart on ileal loop. Small catheter is inserted proximally for administration of test material. Larger catheters are inserted distally for outflow of luminal contents from proximal ileum and from loop. [Adapted from Mathias et al. (138).]

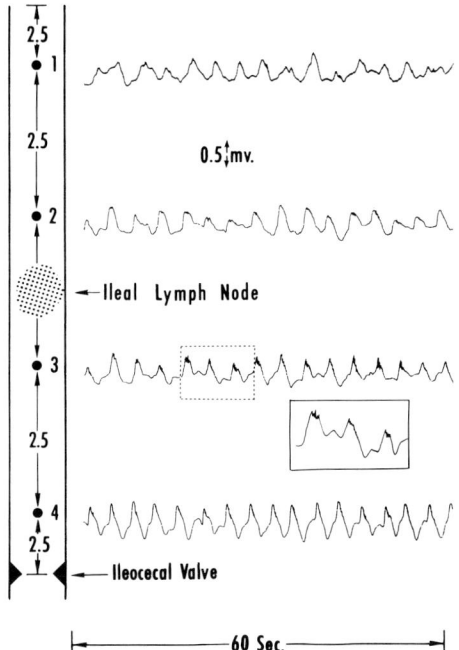

FIG. 2. Control tracing from distal ileal segment. Electrode placement is illustrated on the *left*. Time and sensitivity calibrations are also shown. Slow-wave rhythm is illustrated on all four electrode sites. There is brief action potential activity on lead three; it is also shown in enlarged enclosure. [From Burns et al. (24).]

tially in loops provoked by *Vibrio cholerae* (Calcutta strain), the whole-cell lysate of *V. cholerae*, or its purified enterotoxin choleragen (138). The MAPC was defined as spike-potential activity that occurred for >2.5 s on a single-electrode recording site and that migrated over at least three consecutive electrode-recording sites (Fig. 3). The MAPC shown in Figure 3 migrated over all four electrode sites. In other studies the MAPC has been shown to traverse the entire small intestine (142), cross the ileocecal sphincter (162), and traverse the colon (J. R. Mathias, unpublished observations). The mean propagation velocity of the MAPC was ~1.0 cm/s, the onset time of altered motor activity was ~3.5 h after injection of the provocative substance, and the activity reached a plateau level of ~8–10 complexes/h [Fig. 4; (138)]. Substantial fluid movement from the distal outflow catheter occurred only during MAPC activity. Although the MAPC has since been found to occur under many different circumstances, the basic study of it occurred with the biologic probe *V. cholerae* or choleragen in the rabbit model.

## Cholera Toxin

The purified enterotoxin from *V. cholerae* is a heat-labile enterotoxin that is ~84,000 daltons (Da) and is composed of three dissimilar peptides: $A_1$ and $A_2$ (active) and B (binding) (76, 103). The $A_1$ (23,500 Da) is linked to the $A_2$ (5,500 Da) by a single disulfide bond. Five identical B subunits ($B_5$, 11,000 Da each) are bound in a noncovalent ring structure (choleragenoid) and consist of the component of the protein that binds to $G_{M1}$ receptors on epithelial cell surfaces (203). After binding, the $A_2$ protein penetrates the cell membrane and dissociates from the $A_1$ protein, allowing the $A_1$ protein to enter the cytosol of the cell. The $A_1$ peptide is the active stimulatory unit of the toxin and activates adenylate cyclase through a cascade of reactions (74, 99). Adenylate cyclase is activated irreversibly by catalyzing the ADP ribosylation of the $\alpha$-subunit of the stimulatory guanine nucleotide–binding regulatory component ($G_s$) of the hormone-dependent adenylate cyclase system (30). In the presence of $G_s$, NAD, GTP, and a cytosolic factor, ADP-ribosylation factor (ARF), induce ADP ribosylation of $G_s$ by the $A_1$ protein (ADP ribosyltransferase) and form a ternary complex that activates adenylate cyclase (116). This cascade of reactions results in activation of the adenylate cyclase–cAMP system and the subsequent activation of protein kinase A. Choleragenoid, however, is inactive in stimulating the secretory apparatus of the intact cell (102) or in disrupted cells (76).

Similar toxins associated with other infectious organisms, such as enterotoxigenic *Escherichia coli*, may exert a choleralike illness. The proposed mechanism is also adenylate cyclase activation by a similar heat-labile enterotoxin, which in turn alters intracellular 3′,5′-cAMP (121, 178, 179) and causes secretion, much as does cholera toxin.

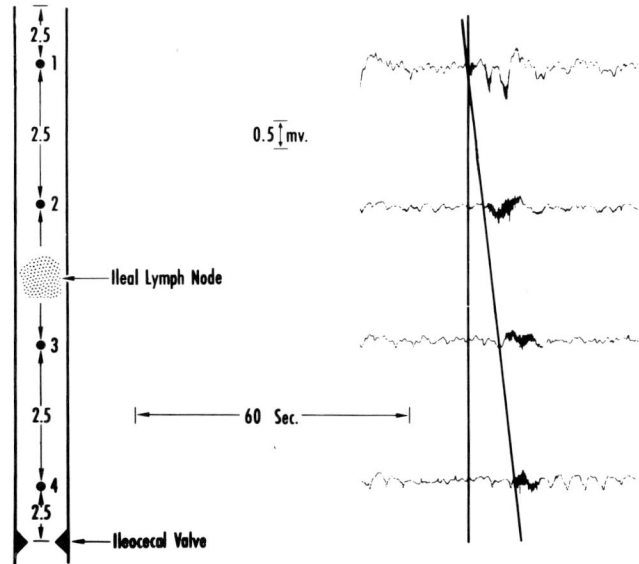

FIG. 3. Migrating action-potential complex (MAPC). Electrode placement is illustrated on the *left*. Time and sensitivity calibrations are also shown. Slope of line as compared with vertical reference line represents propagation velocity of MAPC. Propagation velocity of this complex was 0.85 cm/s. [From Mathias et al. (138).]

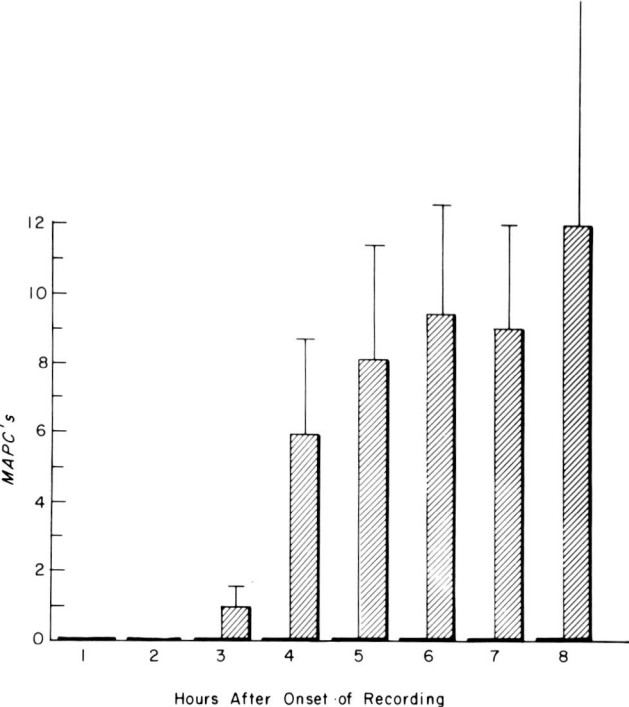

FIG. 4. Onset time of migrating action-potential complex (MAPC) activity for 8-h recording period. *Abscissa*, mean number of MAPC/h. *Solid bars*, controls (saline); *hatched bars*, cholera-infected loops. Results are expressed as mean ± SE. [From Mathias et al. (138).]

*Choleragen and Choleragenoid*

The MAPC occurs secondary to live *V. cholerae* and its purified enterotoxin choleragen (138). The aforementioned changes (i.e., $B_5$ binding to $G_{M1}$ receptors and the activation of adenylate cyclase by $A_1$) account for the classic hypothesis of the active secretion of chloride and bicarbonate and the passive movement of water from the crypt cells of the enterocyte with impairment of sodium absorption.

In contrast, choleragenoid, which consists of only the bound five B subunits of the holotoxin (61, 62), binds to the $G_{M1}$ receptors of the enterocyte (104, 158) but fails to activate the adenylate cyclase–cAMP system and thus does not cause active secretion. However, unlike choleragen ($A_1$, $A_2$, $B_5$), choleragenoid has been shown to alter motility of the small intestine in a manner similar to that of choleragen but without causing active secretion (183). Recombinant strains of *V. cholerae* (Inaba) that do not produce an enterotoxin ($A^-B^-$) or that make only the B subunits ($A^-B^+$) have failed to induce MAPC activity (130). The classic strain of Inaba ($A^+B^+$), however, induced MAPC activity as previously shown with choleragen and the Calcutta strain of *V. cholerae* (138). The effects of choleragenoid on the neuromuscular function require further investigation. This differentiation between secretion and motility is an important observation on the interaction of the two processes: both may be activated by the same disease (the enterotoxin), but they most probably operate through separate and independent intracellular mechanisms (144). This fact discloses an important aspect of the relationship between motility and secretion; that is, although motility and secretion do exist together, they may be mediated by different second messengers or different pathways, or both. Future investigation with choleragenoid will be important in defining how the message is transmitted from the enterocyte to sensory nerve and subsequently to circular muscle.

*Historical Background of MAPC*

Although researchers may often think they have been the first to observe a specific biological event, they find only too soon that they are merely using a more sophisticated technique to make the same observation made by some earlier scientist. This is certainly true of the MAPC. Although the electrical characteristics of a single moving ring contraction (the MAPC) were not described until 1976 (138), the mechanical equivalent of the MAPC (i.e., the single moving ring contraction) was first observed at least as early as 1872 in asphyxiated animals (105) and was studied under more physiological conditions in 1906–1907 by Meltzer and Auer (153). These authors described the moving contraction as the peristaltic rush.

In 1924 Alvarez and Mahoney (4) used kymographs to record the peristaltic rush in rabbit small intestine. Alvarez and Taylor (5) observed that this motor event occurred under physiological conditions and in intestine it was provoked by several different purgatives, especially castor oil (see CASTOR OIL AND RICINOLEIC ACID, p. 1162). The acceptance and recognition of the peristaltic rush then went essentially unnoticed until recent years. The importance of this complex cannot be stated more emphatically than Alvarez and Mahoney (4) did in their classic paper of 1924:

> As soon as physiologists began to study the movements of the intestine with the animal opened under salt solution, they observed that there are two main types of activity. In the first place, there are small localized rhythmic contractions which do not seem to forward the intestinal contents to any great extent but which knead those contents; mix them with the digestive juices, and spread them again and again over the absorbing surface of the mucous membrane. Then, from time to time, there appear larger waves which usually run from one end of the bowel to the other and which serve to carry the food on its way from the stomach to the rectum. They have been called by different writers peristaltic rushes, diastaltic waves, rollbewegungen and schubbewegungen. On account of their important function in health and disease, these waves must always be of the greatest interest to the physiologist, the physician and the surgeon, and it is

In 1976 Mathias and co-workers (136, 137) reported that the cyclooxygenase inhibitors ASA and indomethacin had a significant effect on the MAPC induced by cholera toxin. Indomethacin and ASA not only altered the propagation velocity of the MAPC by increasing the velocity in a dose-related fashion (Fig. 5) but at higher doses indomethacin also actually eliminated the MAPC altogether. In addition, as the propagation velocity became faster, the output from the distal catheter diminished; when the MAPC was completely eliminated, the output from the ileal loop ceased (Fig. 6). These observations suggested that prostaglandins were involved with the motor response but were not necessary for the secretory process. When prostaglandin $F_{2\alpha}$ ($PGF_{2\alpha}$) was infused into the ileal loop, the MAPC was reproduced in a manner similar to that with cholera toxin–induced MAPC activity. Indomethacin did not affect $PGF_{2\alpha}$-induced MAPC activity (Fig. 7). These results indicated that $PGF_{2\alpha}$ may be involved in the motor response of cholera toxin–induced disease and that the response of cyclooxygenase inhibitors was not just a nonspecific

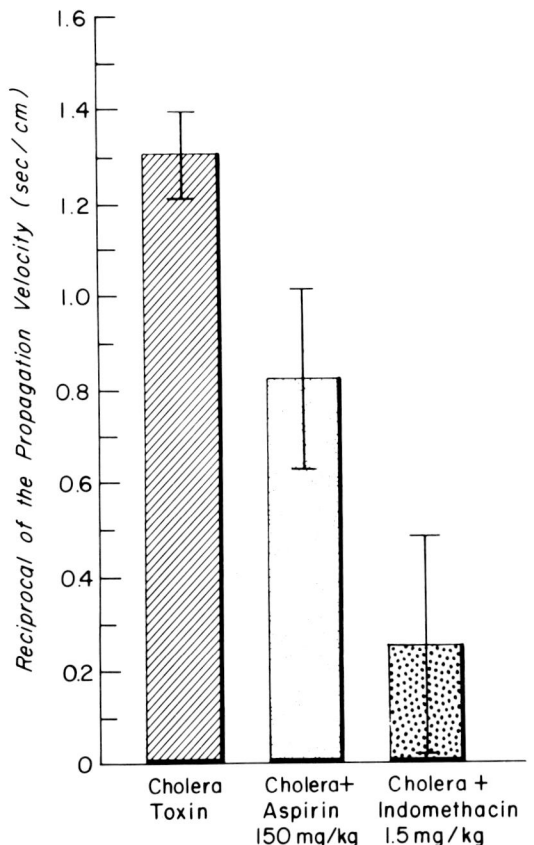

FIG. 5. Effect of cyclooxygenase inhibitors [aspirin (acetylsalicylic acid) and indomethacin] on propagation velocity of migrating action-potential complex. *Hatched bar*, cholera-infected loops; *clear bar*, cholera-infected loops treated with aspirin; and *dotted bar*, cholera-infected loops treated with indomethacin. Results are expressed as mean ± SE.

unfortunate that as yet we know so little about their origin and their mode of propagation.

### Association of MAPC With Prostaglandins

In the early 1970s cholera toxin–induced secretion was thought to occur via a second messenger, which in turn activated the adenylate cyclase–cAMP system. Cyclooxygenase inhibitors, such as acetylsalicylic acid (ASA) or indomethacin, were shown to alter cholera toxin–induced secretion; this fact suggested that prostaglandins were actively involved in the mediation of secretion (59, 110, 202). However, Boyle and Gardner (19) demonstrated that cholera toxin and prostaglandins had separate receptors on rat thymocytes, and Kimberg et al. (121) showed that prostaglandins had a secretory summation effect, through mechanisms other than cholera toxin–induced secretion. Thus cholera toxin was thought to induce its secretory events by direct stimulation of the enterocyte (later shown to occur by the binding of the toxin to $G_{M1}$ receptors) and was independent of prostaglandins.

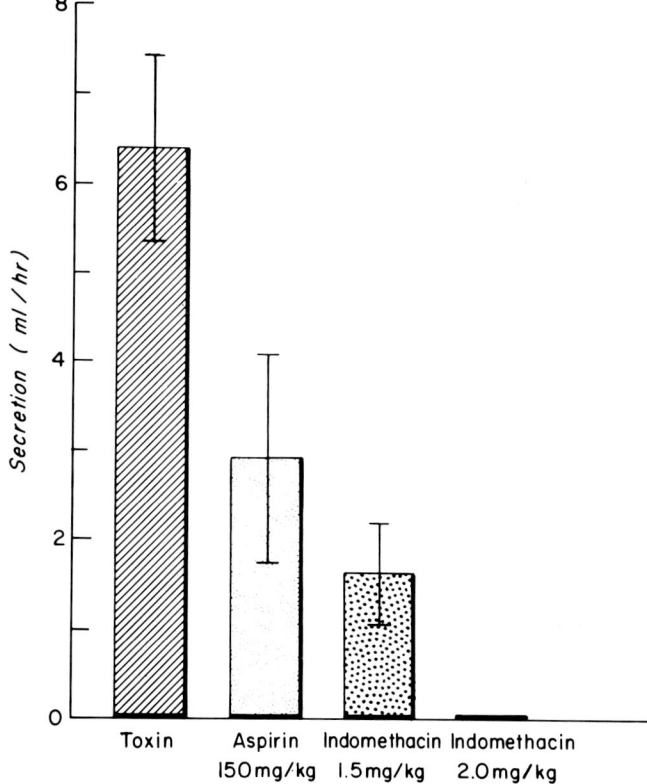

FIG. 6. Effect of cyclooxygenase inhibitors [aspirin (acetylsalicylic acid) and indomethacin] on fluid output from distal ileal catheter. *Hatched bar*, cholera-infected loops; *clear bar*, cholera-infected loops treated with aspirin; *dotted bar*, cholera-infected loops treated with low-dose indomethacin; and *solid bar*, cholera-infected loops treated with high-dose indomethacin. High-dose indomethacin inhibited all migrating action-potential complex activity. Results are expressed as mean ± SE.

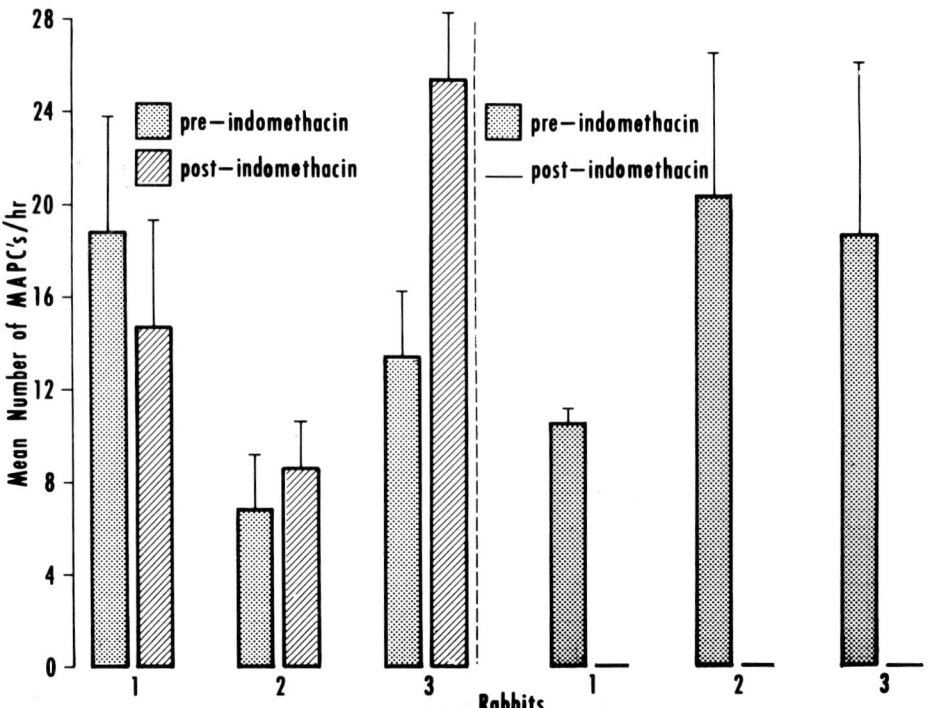

FIG. 7. Effect of cyclooxygenase inhibitor, indomethacin, on prostaglandin $F_{2\alpha}$–infused ileal loops and on cholera-infected ileal loops. Results are from ileal loops in three rabbits exposed to prostaglandin $F_{2\alpha}$ (*left*) and three rabbits exposed to cholera toxin (*right*), before and after treatment with indomethacin (2.0 mg/kg IV). Results are expressed as mean ± SE.

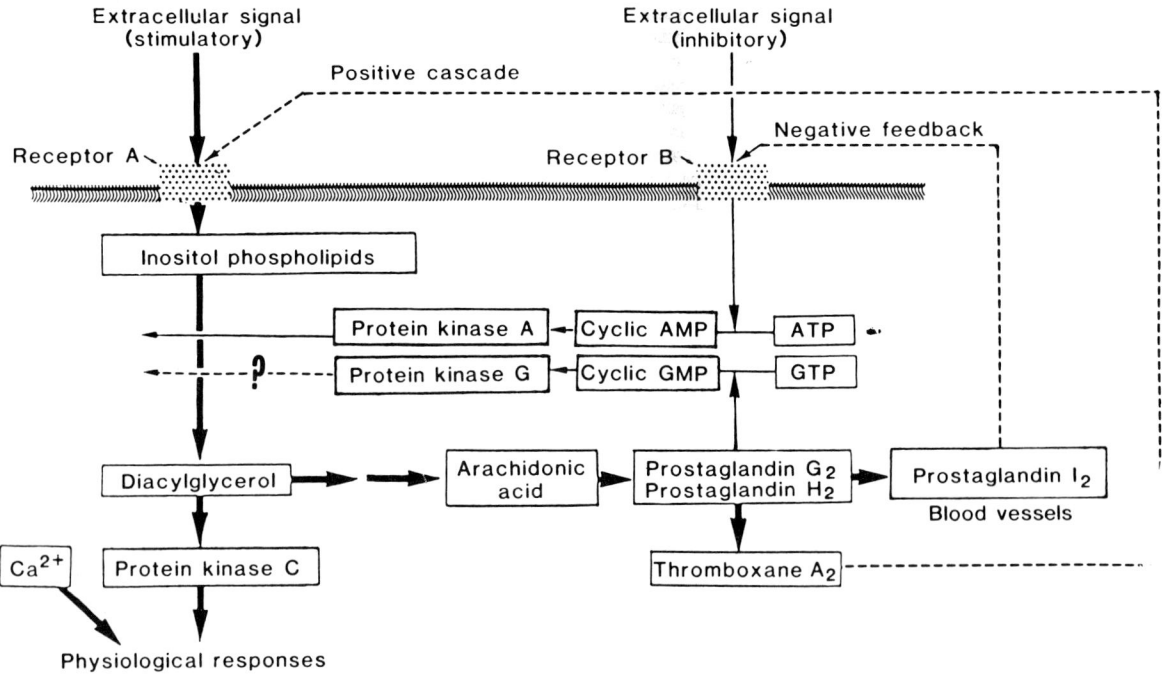

FIG. 8. Theoretical cascade and feedback control of cellular functions. Cascade involves interaction of protein kinases A, G, and C with inositol phospholipids, which results in the mobilization of calcium and formation of prostinoids. This schema was developed from platelet model but may be applicable for activities occurring at epithelial cell of small intestine. [From Nishizuka (160). Copyright 1984, by the American Association for the Advancement of Science.]

effect on the cell membrane but that it directly affected the enzyme that was converting arachidonic acid to prostaglandins (136). These observations are important for understanding the interplay of this pathway with the protein kinase C system, a major cellular mechanism for signal transduction and mobilization of intracellular calcium (Fig. 8). At present, preliminary information regarding the motor events of the small intestine that are stimulated directly through the protein kinase C pathway suggests another type of myoelectric pattern. Phorbol esters, which activate the protein kinase C system, have been shown to induce luminal secretion (210) and also to induce retrograde migrating myoelectric activity (44).

TABLE 1. *Effect of Neuroantagonists on Cholera-Induced Secretion and Motility*

| | Secretion Activity | Motility Activity |
|---|---|---|
| Sensory receptor antagonist | | |
| Lidocaine hydrochloride | Inhibited | Inhibited |
| Neural axon poison | | |
| Tetrodotoxin | Inhibited | Inhibited |
| Ganglionic antagonists | | |
| Trimethaphan camsylate | | Inhibited |
| Hexamethonium | Inhibited | |
| Muscarinic receptor antagonists | | |
| Atropine | Inhibited | |
| Scopolamine hydrobromide | | Reduced* |

* $P < 0.01$ compared with control values.

Prostaglandins are found abundantly within the gastrointestinal tract. Arachidonic acid may be converted to 11-hydroperoxyeicosatetraenoic acid (11-HPETE) by the enzyme cyclooxygenase. The main primary eicosanoids from the 11-HPETE cascade of the gastrointestinal tract are $PGE_2$, $PGF_{2\alpha}$, $PGI_2$, and thromboxane $B_2$ [see Fig. 8; (185)]. Synthesis of 12-hydroxy eicosatetraenoic acid (12-HETE) also occurs (98). Interestingly the main site of prostaglandin synthesis is in the lamina propria (185) where the sensory mucosal receptors of the submucosal plexus are located [see Fig. 10; (41)]. Prostaglandins may indeed be the tertiary messenger for neurosensory stimulation (paracrine) of an intrinsic reflex arc of the enteric nervous system.

Because the contractile event, i.e., circular muscle contraction, is at a distance far beyond what is occurring at the enterocyte level, it is evident that the muscular response is mediated through neuropathways perhaps triggered by excitatory neuropeptides such as $PGF_{2\alpha}$. Mathias et al. (136) have shown that the MAPC is abolished by certain neuroantagonists.

*Relationship of Enteric Nervous System With MAPC*

Mathias et al. (137) have shown that MAPC activity is mediated by an intrinsic reflex arc of the enteric nervous system. Lidocaine hydrochloride (a sensory-receptor antagonist), tetrodotoxin (a neural-axon poi-

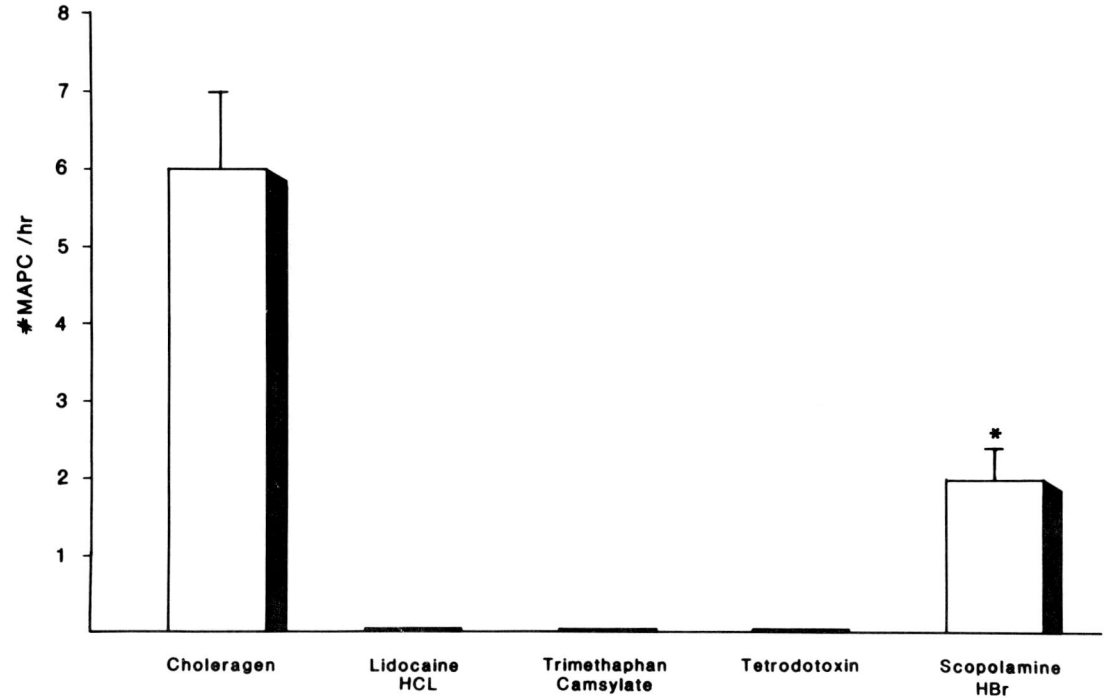

FIG. 9. Effects of specific neuroantagonists on migrating action–potential complex (MAPC) activity. Results are from cholera-infected loops after peak MAPC activity and are expressed as mean ± SE. *Asterisk*, $P < 0.02$ compared with choleragen.

son), and trimethaphan camsylate (a ganglionic antagonist) all inhibited MAPC activity. Scopolamine hydrobromide, a muscarinic-receptor antagonist, significantly reduced but did not completely inhibit MAPC activity (Table 1; Fig. 9). This finding suggests that there is an alternative postganglionic excitatory neural pathway that is not cholinergic and excitatory (Fig. 10), but the transmitter of the pathway has not been defined.

Cassuto and co-workers (32–35) have demonstrated that these same neural antagonists inhibit cholera toxin–induced secretion. The initial event consists of the toxin-activated, adenylate cyclase–dependent mechanism within the enterocyte, but these investigators showed that there is also stimulation of sensory mucosal receptors of the submucosal plexus neurons (32, 36). These neurons then may cause continued secretion by stimulating neuropeptide or neurotransmitter (serotonin) release from the enterochromaffin cells or by stimulating the crypt cells through a submucosal reflex arc (Fig. 10, *small open circles*). The submucosa is rich with nicotinic and muscarinic receptors (35, 41, 156, 200, 207, 213). Thus the inhibition of fluid secretion by atropine or hexamethonium may be possible by inhibiting these receptors within the mucosa or submucosal plexus, respectively. The afore-

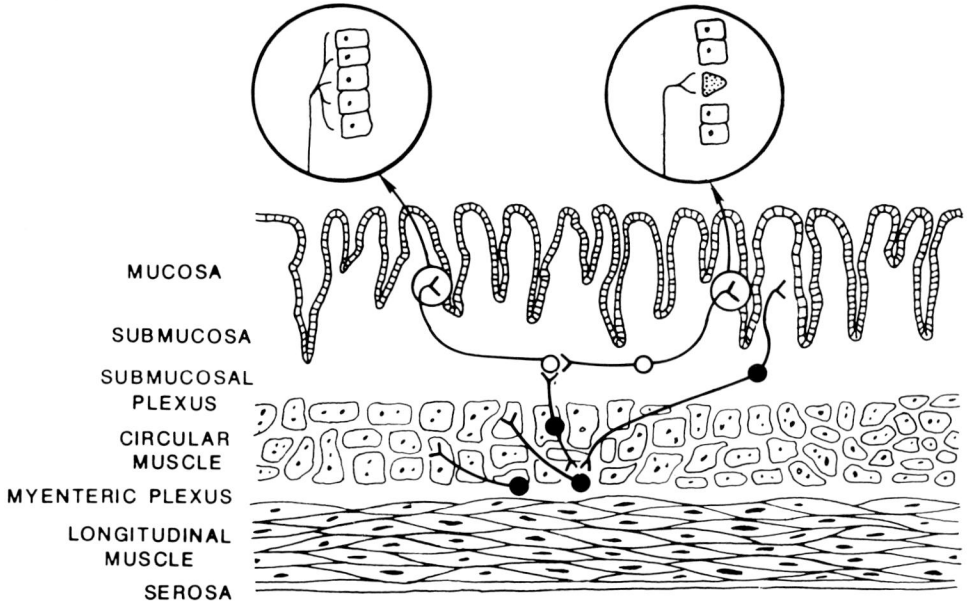

FIG. 10. Schematic of possible neural reflex arcs of enteric nervous system, which may provide an explanation for secretory-motor events of cholera toxin–induced disease (see Table 1). *Enlarged areas*, enterocytes (*left*) and enterocytes with an enterochromaffin cell (*right*); *small open circles*, submucosal reflex arc; and *small closed circles*, intrinsic reflex arc involving myenteric plexus.

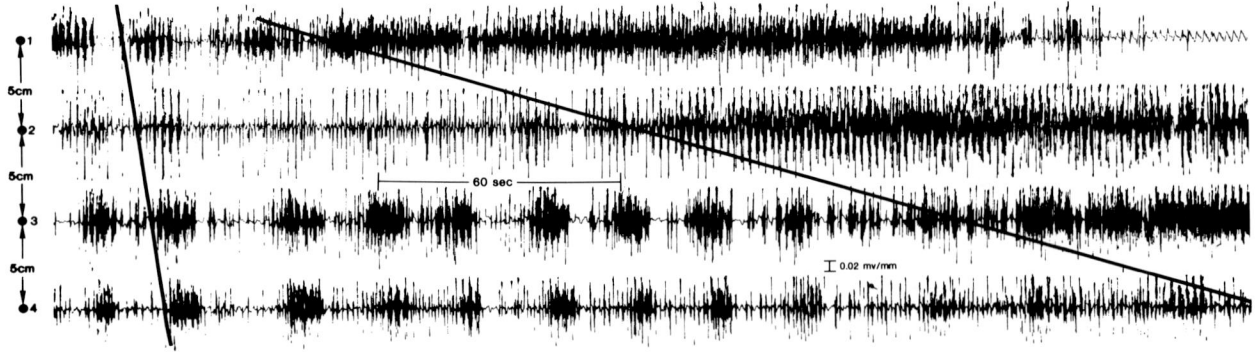

FIG. 11. Effect of 6-hydroxydopamine on activity front of migrating myoelectric complex (MMC). Electrode placement is illustrated on the *left*, and time and sensitivity calibrations are also indicated. Migrating action-potential complexes (MAPC) are shown preceding activity front of MMC. Propagation velocity of MAPC (sloped line on the *left*) was 0.84 cm/s; propagation velocity of MMC (sloped line on the *right*) was 3.65 cm/min. [From Mathias et al. (141).]

mentioned effects of these neural antagonists on secretion and motility (Table 1) indicate an important interaction of nerve function in toxin-induced diseases.

These ideas contradict the current and classic concept of cholera-induced secretion. An alternative hypothesis may involve the interplay of the protein kinase A and G systems with the inositol triphosphate–protein kinase C system (160) and the processes that activate the prostaglandin pathways and/or the mobilization of intracellular calcium. These kinase pathways provide provocative models for further investigation (see Fig. 8).

One point is incontrovertible: more is involved than just the activation of adenylate cyclase. The neural tube (68) with all of its neurons, axons, dendrites, and neurotransmitters is intimately involved in the process of diarrhea, which in turn involves secretion, alterations in motility, and malabsorption.

The MAPC may also be intimately related to the MMC. Juorio and Gabella (111) demonstrated that administration of 6-hydroxydopamine at a dose of 35 mg/kg destroyed at least 75% of the varicosities containing the neurotransmitter norepinephrine. Mathias et al. (141) have shown in an unanesthetized rat model that administration of 6-hydroxydopamine at the same dose unmasked or allowed expression of the MAPC from the MMC (Fig. 11). These observations suggest that the MAPC may not be just a provoked motor complex but may be a basic physiological event in gastrointestinal tract motility, responding to a variety of stimuli and resulting in increased clearance of luminal contents.

In the same rat model Piñeiro-Carrero et al. (167) found that reserpine, a substance that depletes the endogenous stores of catecholamines as well as serotonin, produced similar results, i.e., apparently unmasked the MAPC from the MMC. Reserpine also, however, disrupted the MMC. Previous studies with 5,6- and 5,7-dihydroxytryptamine, false neurotransmitters that destroy serotonergic neurons (69), also disrupted the MMC (166). These studies indicate that serotonin, in addition to norepinephrine, appears to be an important control mechanism of the MAPC as well as being a major neurotransmitter of enteric nerve function (68, 212).

## MAPC in Vitro

Koch et al. (124) have also shown that the MAPC occurs in rabbit ileal loops stimulated with cholera toxin in an in vitro bath system. The extrinsic nerves and blood vessels were severed at the mesenteric border of ileal segments that had been infected with cholera toxin; the loop was removed and placed over a 15-cm plastic fenestrated mandrel and then immersed in an in vitro bath. The lumen of the mandrel was perfused with Krebs solution gassed with 97% oxygen and 3% carbon dioxide, which maintained the pH at 7.4–7.5. Control loops treated with saline showed only slow-wave activity with intermittent short bursts of action potentials. Loops exposed to cholera toxin showed MAPC activity in a manner similar to that seen in the in vivo–infected rabbit model. The frequency, duration, and propagation velocity of action-potential activity were similar to the MAPC activity that occurred in vivo; however, 25% of the MAPC in vitro propagated in an orad direction, whereas all of the MAPC in vivo had propagated in an aborad direction. These studies demonstrated that the MAPC occurred independent of the central nervous system or circulating hormonal stimulation. These studies also suggested that the central nervous system may have modulated MAPC activity by controlling the direction of propagation but that it was not essential for the autonomy of MAPC activity.

In contrast the MMC, the cyclic activity front of slow propagating ring contractions, has been found in denervated, devascularized jejunal segments transplanted in the distal ileum (1, 177). However, the MMC has not been shown to occur in an in vitro bath independent of the central nervous system or circulating hormonal control. Under appropriate stimulatory conditions the MMC may occur in vitro. This possibility is a challenge for future investigations because it could help define the control mechanisms and the site of origin for both the MMC and the MAPC—important motor complexes in the movement of luminal contents in health and disease.

## Other Substances That Stimulate MAPC

ESCHERICHIA COLI AND ITS ENTEROTOXIN. Toxigenic *E. coli* and its whole-cell lysate have also stimulated MAPC activity similar to that produced by choleragen (24). The strain of *E. coli* used was H-10407, a type known to produce a heat-labile enterotoxin and to induce an active secretory response similar to that of choleragen, which is also heat sensitive (92, 93, 172, 174). Heating the *E. coli* toxin to 100°C for 30 min also eliminated all MAPC activity.

SALMONELLA. Weisberg et al. (211) demonstrated that *Salmonella typhimurium* induced MAPC activity in the early phases of infection. Often the complexes were split and disorganized. These observations of the early stages may have important implications in that during the (later) acute stage of salmonellosis the organism is cleared from the intestine. During the early phase of the infection an enterotoxin is produced that probably stimulates the adenylate cyclase–cAMP system. Weisberg et al. (211) also showed that at 24 h, invasion of the organism occurs and that the pattern of motor activity changes to one that is less well organized. These changes are similar to those of *Shigella dysenteriae* (139) and *Campylobacter jejuni* infection (188). Thus far preliminary studies by others have suggested the presence of a purified toxin for *C. jejuni*; the anesthetized rabbit model should provide a useful biological assay for the presence of enterotoxins produced by this bacterium and others.

CASTOR OIL AND RICINOLEIC ACID. Castor oil and its active ingredient, ricinoleic acid, have also been shown to induce MAPC activity (142). In addition, chronic experiments were conducted with electrodes placed on the duodenum, jejunum, and ileum to assess the distance over which the MAPC migrated. When an MAPC began in the duodenum, 1 ml of sulfobromophthalein was injected into the lumen of the duodenum. The luminal contents were then tested with sodium hydroxide for color change. The individual MAPC induced by ricinoleic acid was seen to migrate down the entire length of the small intestine, ejecting luminal contents from the outflow catheter placed at the distal ileum. The fluid tested usually changed to a burgundy color (positive for sulfobromophthalein) after each MAPC had migrated the length of the bowel, thus demonstrating the extent to which the MAPC may move luminal contents and the short time involved (<1 min was required for luminal fluid to traverse the entire small intestine of a rabbit) (142).

Ouyang et al. (162), also using ricinoleic acid, showed that the MAPC crosses the ileocecal valve and traverses the colon. These findings were similar to those of J. R. Mathias (unpublished observations) in initial experiments with cholera toxin in unligated preparations. Thus a single MAPC may traverse the entire intestinal tract within a short period of time, propelling the luminal contents aborally.

More recently the MAPC has been shown in humans given castor oil through a jejunal tube or by mouth (42). The characteristics of the MAPC in humans were similar to those of the rabbit model treated with ricinoleic acid or castor oil (142).

VASOACTIVE INTESTINAL PEPTIDE. Sninsky et al. (189) have shown that vasoactive intestinal peptide (VIP), when placed into the lumen of the intestine, also induced MAPC activity. Portal and systemic vein VIP levels were measured hourly during infusion experiments; that no significant increase in systemic VIP occurred further supports the hypothesis that the peptide has a direct effect on the enterocyte. Portal vein VIP levels rose significantly as expected; however, the liver has been shown to inactivate VIP completely (52). The adenylate cyclase–cAMP system is also known to be induced by VIP as well as by cholera toxin (125, 126), and receptors for VIP have been found on the membranes of intestinal epithelial cells in both the rat (126) and the guinea pig (12). Many gastrointestinal peptides, including VIP, have been shown to occur within the lumen of the intestine (155). The function of these peptides remains unclear. These peptides remain technically difficult to quantify because of the presence of luminal proteases.

Mathias et al. (147) used a semiconductor recording probe to study upper gastrointestinal tract motor function in two human subjects with diarrhea secondary to tumors that secreted VIP. Rectal tubes were placed in these subjects to collect high volume output. In each subject, as the motor equivalent of the MAPC (single moving ring contractions) was seen on the recording of the proximal end of the small bowel, within 1–2 min there was outflow from the rectal catheters (J. R. Mathias, unpublished observations). These observations further indicate that the MAPC occurs in human subjects (146) and is intimately involved with the movement of luminal fluid in diarrheic conditions.

BILE SALTS. Bile salts have been reported to induce MAPC activity in the proximal end of the colon of the rabbit (187); Figure 12 shows colonic MAPC activity secondary to 16 mM deoxycholic acid. In contrast to the effect of neural antagonists on the MAPC (Table 1), the ganglionic blocker trimethaphan camsylate did not inhibit MAPC activity; this was despite an inhibitory effect of the sensory antagonist procaine and the muscarinic antagonist atropine. In addition the $\alpha$-adrenergic antagonist phentolamine blocked MAPC activity; the $\beta$-adrenergic antagonist propranolol reduced but did not completely inhibit the MAPC. These data suggest that, compared with the small intestine, the colon may have alternative neural control mechanisms (181).

## Control Mechanisms of MAPC

The MAPC, or its motor equivalent the peristaltic rush, has emerged as an important motor complex of the intestine (138, 145). The MAPC appears to have an undefined relationship to the activation of the adenylate cyclase–cAMP system. Previous studies indicate that $PGF_{2\alpha}$ may be one of the predominant neuropeptides (see Fig. 7) that stimulates neurosensory receptors in the mucosa-submucosal plexus (137). Organization of MAPC activity appears neural dependent, most likely within the myenteric plexus ganglia. Certainly the motor complex is mediated by an intrinsic reflex arc of the enteric nervous system (144). The MAPC also appears to be under inhibitory control by the adrenergic nervous system (124, 141). Chronic studies with unanesthetized rats treated with 6-hydroxydopamine, a false neurotransmitter that destroys the neural varicosities containing the neurotransmitter norepinephrine, showed that the MAPC may be intimately associated with (perhaps a component of) the MMC (Fig. 11). These studies suggest that the MAPC is not just a provoked motor response but that it may have important functions under normal physiological conditions (141).

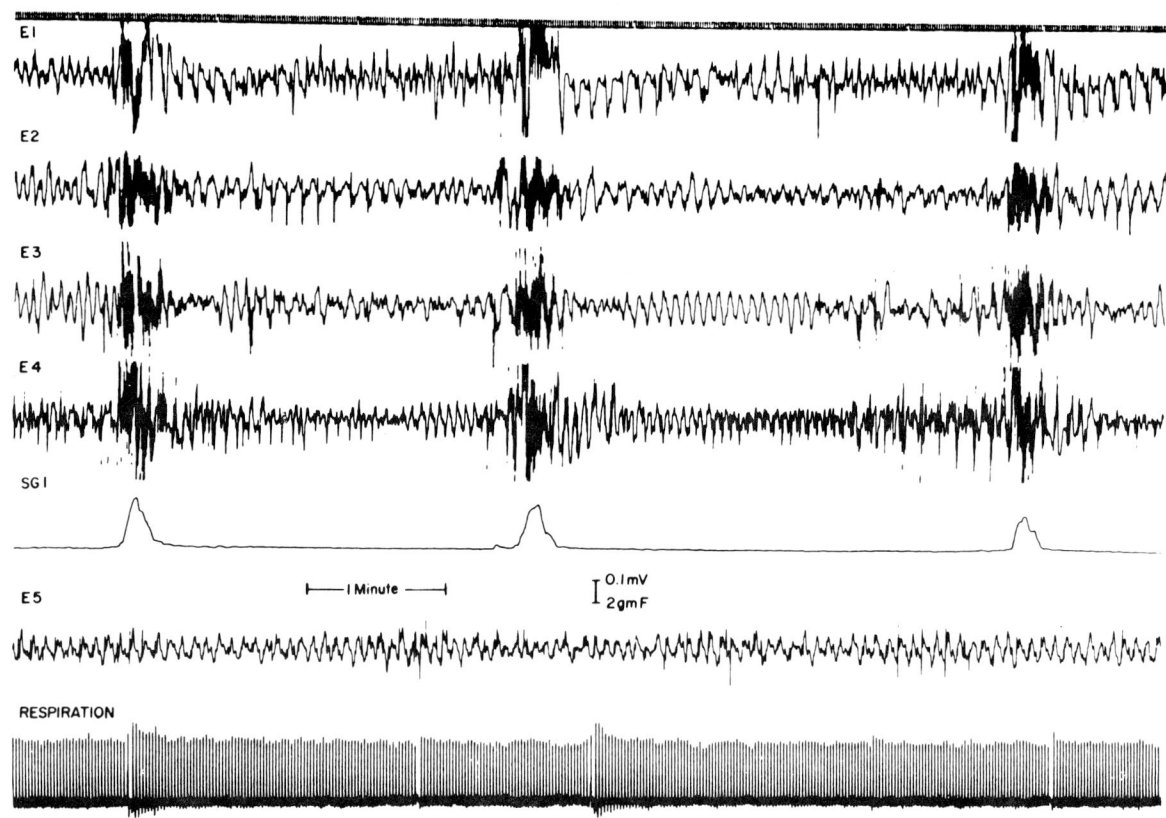

FIG. 12. Migrating action-potential complexes observed in rabbit colon secondary to deoxycholic acid. Electrode placement is shown schematically on the *left*: E1–E4 are on ascending colonic loop and E5 is distal to loop. Strain gauge 1 (SG-1) is located between E2 and E3. Respiration is indicated on *bottom tracing*, and time and sensitivity calibrations are also shown. [From Shiff et al. (181).]

## Questions for the Future

Many questions remain key to understanding the mechanisms of the MAPC. First, how are the neurosensory receptors stimulated in the mucosa-submucosal plexus and by what substances? Is $PGF_{2\alpha}$ the main neuropeptide (paracrine) responsible for activating the sensory neurons of the enteric nervous system that results in the MAPC? Second, what is responsible for the lag time (e.g., the ~3.5 h always experienced between introduction of cholera toxin and the onset of the first MAPC)? Does the lag time represent the period necessary for programming the myenteric plexus neurons? Third, where is the autonomy of the MAPC? Does the autonomy rest within the nerves of the plexus, the nervelike cells such as the interstitial cells of Cajal, or the circular muscle itself? The myenteric plexus neurons are most likely the center of control for the MAPC. If so, what type of nerves? Certainly cellular techniques involving neurophysiology will be required for many of the answers to these questions. This much is clear right now—the MAPC is a complex distinct from the MMC, and each of these complexes has its own function in the gut. The final and most important question is: What functions do each of these motor complexes perform and under what circumstances? The time of Boldyreff (17), Meltzer and Auer (153), and Alvarez and Mahoney (4) must not be forgotten. These early physiologists made important observations simply by watching; there is no reason to believe that researchers today cannot do much the same by thoughtful application of modern technology.

## REPETITIVE BURSTS OF ACTION POTENTIALS

The second myoelectric complex found in association with bacteria was called repetitive bursts of action potentials (RBAP) (25). This complex was defined as action potential activity >1.5 s in duration that occurred on at least three successive slow waves on the same recording site. This complex was originally described as secondary to invasive *E. coli* (Fig. 13).

### Invasive Escherichia coli

Strains 4608-58 and TD 213 CL of invasive *E. coli* have been used to assess changes in myoelectric activity (25). These strains of *E. coli* produce neither heat-labile nor heat-stable toxins and, when placed in rabbit ileum, invade the mucosa within 7 h (50). The average onset time of altered motor activity is 4.2 h. Tissue samples taken from ileum infected with invasive *E. coli* and examined by microscopy with hematoxylin- and eosin-staining techniques showed acute inflammation at the time of peak alteration in RBAP activity (25). The epithelial cells were also damaged, with sloughing and necrosis of the villous tips. Heat treatment of the whole-cell lysate from these strains of *E. coli* abolished all RBAP activity. These studies suggested that alterations in the integrity of the mucosa were essential for RBAP activity to occur (25). Later studies performed with heat-stable toxin from *E. coli* showed that this may not always be the case (143).

### Shigella dysenteriae 1 and Purified Enterotoxin From Strain 60R

The bacterium *Shigella dysenteriae* 1 also invades the mucosa of the small intestine and colon. In addition the organism produces a number of toxic substances, heretofore called shiga toxin. Shiga toxin (the whole-cell lysate of *S. dysenteriae* 1) causes paralysis and death when injected into the host (54) and is cytotoxic in monolayer cultures of mammalian cells (119).

Gemski et al. (67) first suggested that shiga toxin may be important in enhancing the invasive characteristics of the bacterium. In general the RBAP is a myoelectric complex that usually does not propagate. Mathias et al. (139) suggested that it induces stasis and thus promotes the proliferation and subsequent invasion of bacteria. The RBAP may well represent another virulent factor of invasive organisms (143).

Mathias et al. (139) investigated the effects of two strains of *S. dysenteriae*: 3818-T, an invader and toxin producer, and 3818-O, which does not invade but which does produce the heat-labile cytolytic enterotoxin (206). Mathias et al. (139) also studied the whole-cell lysate of *S. dysenteriae* (shiga toxin) prepared by the method of van Heyningen and Gladstone (204). In the rabbit model both strains of *Shigella* (3818-T and 3818-O) and shiga toxin significantly altered motor activity of the small intestine and all produced RBAP activity, which indicated the importance of the toxin in affecting motor function.

O'Brien et al. (161) have isolated a purified protein (*Shigella* enterotoxin) from the whole-cell lysate (shiga toxin) of *S. dysenteriae* strain 60R. Shiga toxin most likely contains several components that can induce specific cellular events such as secretion, tissue injury, or altered motility. When the purified enterotoxin from strain 60R was placed into rabbit intestinal loops, motility was not altered. Instead the enterotoxin caused mild fluid accumulation and moderate-to-severe inflammation of the mucosa (55). In contrast the whole-cell lysate from strain 60R induced RBAP activity similar to that caused by the shiga toxin from *S. dysenteriae* 1. These data suggested that a motor-altering substance was present within the whole-cell lysate (shiga toxin). As discussed under the heading Clostridium difficile, p. 1165, these findings are similar to those caused by *Clostridium difficile* and have importance in understanding the mechanisms of cytotoxin-induced disease (114).

### Clostridium perfringens A Enterotoxin

*Clostridium perfringens*, the most common cause of food-borne diarrhea in the United States (131), is characterized clinically by moderate-to-severe abdominal pain with mild diarrhea (85). In contrast to *Shigella* or invasive *E. coli*, *C. perfringens* does not invade the mucosa but does produce *C. perfringens* A enterotoxin, which induces fluid secretion and tissue injury in an animal model (150) as well as in humans (53, 192, 195).

In investigating the effects of *C. perfringens* A enterotoxin in the rabbit model, Justus et al. (114) found the toxin primarily induced RBAP activity. Thus although earlier studies had suggested that tissue injury and invasion were responsible for RBAP activity, this investigation indicated that the complex may be mediated by a cytotoxin.

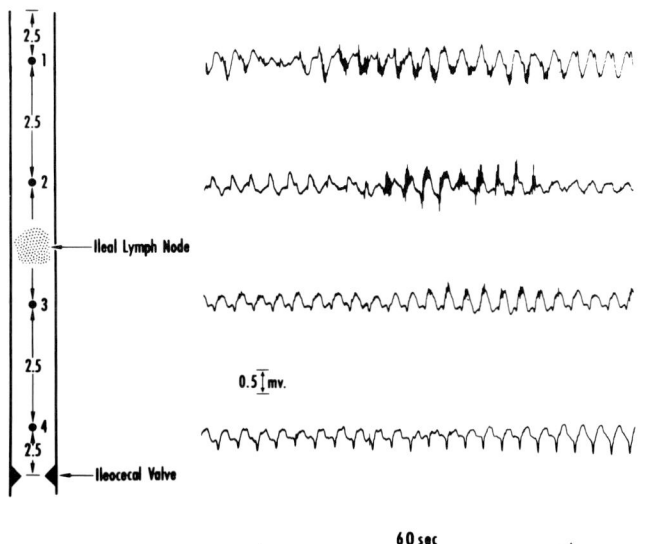

FIG. 13. Repetitive bursts of action potentials (RBAP). Electrode placement is illustrated schematically on the *left*, and time and sensitivity calibrations are also shown. Action potential activity >1.5 s in duration, occurring over at least three successive slow waves on single recording site, is shown on electrode 1. RBAP activity may propagate short distances, as shown in this instance, but it usually does not.

## Clostridium difficile

The bacterium responsible for pseudomembranous enterocolitis, C. difficile (11), produces two purified proteins, both of which Taylor and co-workers (198, 199) have isolated: a heat-labile protein that has a $M_r$ of 240,000 and causes in vitro cell damage in tissue culture (i.e., a cytotoxin) (198) and a protein that is also heat labile but causes only minimal changes in vitro (i.e., an enterotoxin) (199). However, when the enterotoxin (toxin A) is placed into the intestine of the host in vivo, florid cell damage to the mucosa occurs. The cytotoxin (toxin B) on the other hand induces only mild secretion (113). Surprisingly, in the rabbit model the enterotoxin and the cytotoxin induced cell injury and secretion, respectively, but did not alter myoelectric activity (Fig. 14). However, the whole-cell lysate induced RBAP activity (114). The lysate was then separated into high- and low-molecular-weight fractions. The high-molecular-weight fractions (>50,000) induced RBAP activity. These studies suggest that a substance from C. difficile, not the known enterotoxin or cytotoxin, induces motility alterations independent of the cellular events caused by these two toxins. The high-molecular-weight fraction (protein?) has not been identified; possibly this substance has its effect through the activation of the guanylate cyclase–cGMP system (see Fig. 8).

Percy and Christensen (164) described the effects of certain antibiotics on the muscularis mucosa. They demonstrated that antibiotics associated with pseudomembranous enterocolitis cause relaxation of the muscularis mucosa. In contrast, antibiotics such as vancomycin, used to treat the disease, had no effect in altering the muscularis mucosa. Their studies indicated that the effects of certain antibiotics on this muscle layer may encourage the overgrowth of bacteria by decreasing villous movement and allowing bacterial adherence. This effect on the muscularis mucosa is another mechanism by which bacteria or their toxins, or both, may induce disease of the small intestine.

### Heat-Stable Toxins From Escherichia coli

Perhaps the best understanding of the mechanisms of RBAP activity has come from investigation of the heat-stable toxins from E. coli. The toxins have been shown to induce active secretion and disease in human subjects (2, 109). The toxins are low-molecular-weight proteins, usually ranging from 2,000 to 5,000 $M_r$ (191).

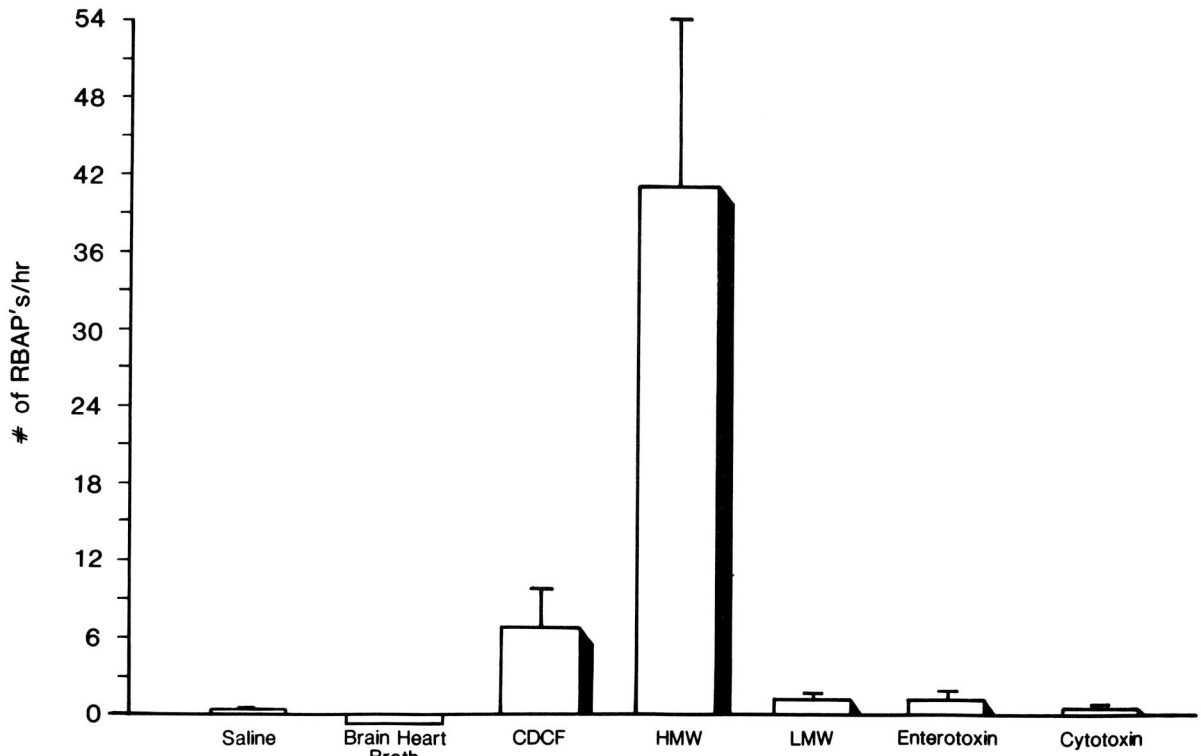

FIG. 14. Effects of products from *Clostridium difficile* on myoelectric activity in rabbit ileum. Controls, saline; control media, brain-heart broth; CDCF, *C. difficile* culture filtrate; HMW, high-molecular-weight fraction from *C. difficile* (>50,000 $M_r$); LMW, low-molecular-weight fraction from *C. difficile* (<50,000 $M_r$). Results are expressed as mean ± SE. [From Justus et al. (113). Copyright 1982 by The American Gastroenterological Association.]

They produce their secretory response by stimulating receptors for the guanylate cyclase–cGMP system, resulting in an increase in intracellular cGMP (50, 70, 72, 107).

Two types of heat-stable toxin have been identified from *E. coli*. The first, heat-stable a ($ST_a$), induces active secretion in the suckling mouse (70). It is this toxin that acts through cGMP. The other type, heat-stable b ($ST_b$), causes an active secretory process in the piglet by an unknown mechanism (22, 71, 87, 118).

Using $ST_a$ [from strain 18D, serotype 042:K86:H37, originally isolated from an infant with watery diarrhea (72)], Mathias et al. (143) investigated its effects on myoelectric activity in the rabbit model. Strain 18D produces only $ST_a$. The $ST_a$ primarily induced RBAP activity (Fig. 15), its maximum effect being at a 10-mg dose (800 mouse units) administered intraluminally as a 1-ml bolus (143). When the toxin was inactivated with 1 mM dithiothreitol and placed in the ileal loop, no RBAP activity was observed (Fig. 16). These studies indicated that $ST_a$ altered motility through the activation of cGMP.

As mentioned, $PGF_{2\alpha}$ induced MAPC activity in a manner similar to that of cholera toxin. Thus other prostaglandins may mediate the motor response of the RBAP. Consequently the effects of $PGE_2$ were investigated in the rabbit model (144). The preliminary data suggest that $PGE_2$ induces RBAP activity in a manner similar to that of $ST_a$. Therefore prostaglandins may serve as local neurotransmitters (paracrine) in stimulating the enteric nervous system. Other questions, however, remain. *1*) In addition to prostaglandins are there other local transmitters that stimulate altered motor activity (RBAP)? *2*) How is the sensory information organized and interpreted at the myenteric plexus ganglia? *3*) What postganglionic neural fibers are involved in the RBAP, a nonpropagating motor complex? *4*) Does $ST_b$ cause altered motor activity in humans (and the piglet)?

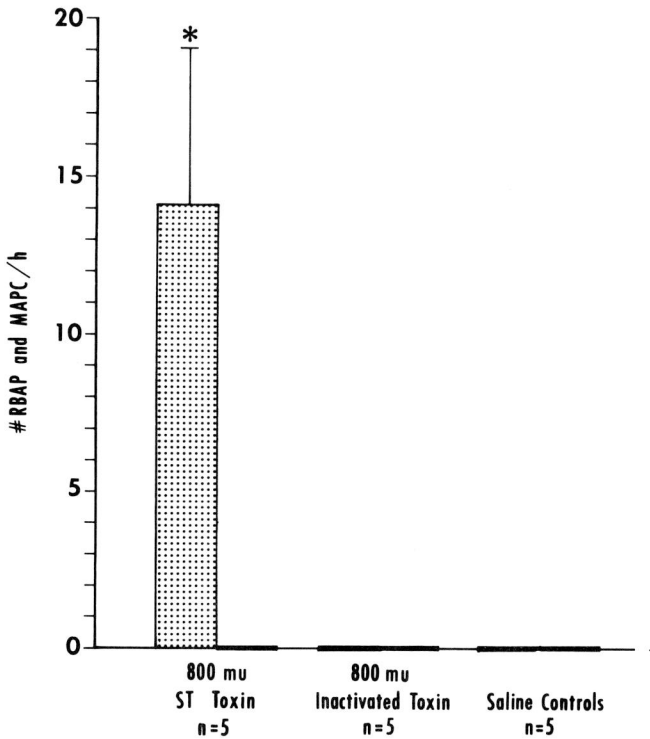

FIG. 16. Effects on repetitive bursts of action potential (RBAP) activity of $ST_a$ inactivated by dithiothreitol. *Stippled bars*, RBAP; *solid bars*, migrating action-potential complexes (MAPC). Results are of active $ST_a$ (ST toxin); inactivated $ST_a$ (inactivated toxin), and saline controls and are expressed as mean ± SE. Asterisk, $P < 0.03$. [From Mathias et al. (143).]

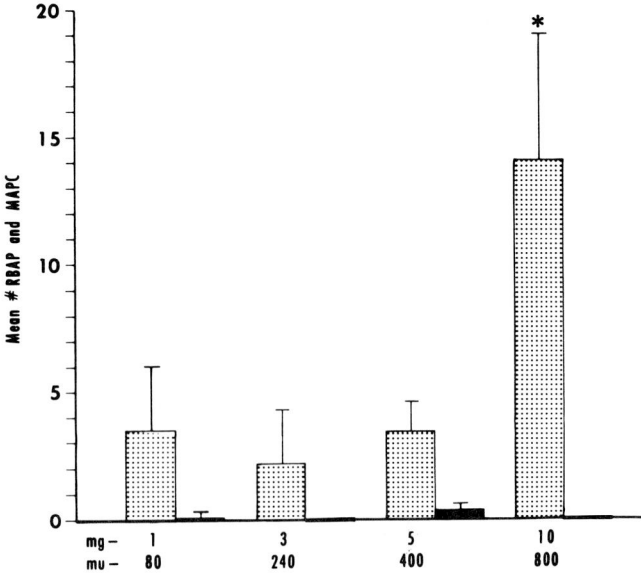

FIG. 15. Effects of heat-stable toxin ($ST_a$) from *Escherichia coli*. *Stippled bars*, repetitive bursts of action potentials (RBAP); *solid bars*, migrating action-potential complexes (MAPC). mu, Mouse units; asterisk, $P < 0.05$. Results are expressed as mean ± SE. [From Mathias et al. (143).]

### Campylobacter jejuni

*Campylobacter jejuni* is a bacterium that causes abdominal pain and bloody diarrhea (14, 15, 48, 184). The mechanism for the pathogenicity of *C. jejuni* remains unknown. The evidence for invasion is circumstantial but probable, because patients have bloody diarrhea and white cells in the stool. The search for a toxin, as in *Shigella*, has been met with frustration; there are conflicting reports on the presence of a toxin contributing to the pathophysiology of the disease (26, 56, 134, 171).

Sninsky et al. (188) investigated the motor effects of *C. jejuni* in the rabbit model. *Campylobacter jejuni* induced RBAP activity similar to that of invasive *E. coli*, *S. dysenteriae*, and $ST_a$ from *E. coli*. The whole-cell lysate of *C. jejuni* also induced alterations in myoelectric activity similar to those caused by the live organism (188). These studies indicate that *C. jejuni* produces a toxin, most likely a substance that activates the guanylate cyclase–cGMP system; these studies also support the validity of the anesthetized rabbit model as an excellent assay system for detecting the presence of biologically active substances. The identification of a motor-altering substance (a toxin) is forthcoming for *C. jejuni* and perhaps for other bacteria with unidentified mechanisms of pathophysiology. Whether the toxin or toxins will be shown to act through one of the three kinase systems (see Fig. 8) may well provide important information for further understanding of diarrheal disorders.

*Summary*

The RBAP, generally a nonpropagating motor complex (25), appears to be stimulated by substances, such as *E. coli* $ST_a$ and *C. perfringens* A enterotoxin, that have their effect through the guanylate cyclase–cGMP system (90). Other bacteria seem to produce a substance that stimulates RBAP activity independent of either their purified enterotoxin or cytotoxin (113). The RBAP may be another virulent factor of bacteria that results in stasis, thus enhancing proliferation of the organism, with invasion into the cell wall (139). Preliminary evidence suggests that $PGE_2$ and perhaps other local neurotransmitters/peptides may also initiate RBAP activity through an intrinsic reflex arc of the enteric nervous system.

## BACTERIAL OVERGROWTH OF SMALL INTESTINE

The bacterial overgrowth syndrome (13, 47, 78, 81, 108, 123, 182) commonly causes nutrient malabsorption (27), steatorrhea (44), brush-border injury (73), enterocyte injury (201), or altered motor function of the small intestine (112), or a combination of these disorders. Although bacterial contamination of the small intestine has been extensively investigated, the underlying cause of most cases remains unexplained. Known mechanisms contributing to the development of overgrowth include anatomical alterations such as ileal or jejunal diverticula or morphological changes secondary to surgery (140). Motility may be altered because these surgical procedures (e.g., hemigastrectomy) usually also include a vagotomy (21, 88). Bacterial overgrowth is also commonly associated with scleroderma of the intestine (175) and diabetes mellitus (77), which are often associated with neuropathy of the intestine secondary to the small vessel vasculitis associated with scleroderma and diabetes. Finally, overgrowth has been found in some patients with idiopathic intestinal pseudo-obstruction (163, 205).

This observation again underscores the importance of effective motility of the intestine.

Under normal conditions in fasting human subjects the concentration of bacteria in the small intestine does not exceed $10^5$ organisms/ml in duodenal or jejunal aspirates. Usually the organisms are Gram-positive (staphylococci, streptococci, lactobacilli), and none are anaerobic; fungi may also be seen (49, 97). In the ileum the concentration of bacteria increases to levels of $10^7$–$10^8$ and includes both aerobes and anaerobes (123). In the colon, however, a striking increase in numbers of bacteria occurs, to $10^{10}$–$10^{11}$; more importantly, anaerobic and coliform bacteria predominate (49, 77, 79, 80, 97, 117, 163).

Three factors have been proposed to cause bacterial overgrowth in the small intestine: *1*) lack of gastric acid, such as in chronic gastritis with achlorhydria, *2*) lack of an effective clearing mechanism (impaired motility), and *3*) a defect in the mucin layer containing immunoglobulins.

Bacteria increase in number in direct proportion as the pH of the stomach increases toward alkalinity (49, 86, 133). Anaerobic bacteria also increase in the small intestine of patients with achlorhydria of unknown cause (49, 86, 180) or secondary to gastric surgery (89) that includes a vagotomy. The importance of acid has been emphasized by these studies, but it must be remembered that a vagotomy not only changes acid production in itself but also alters motor function of the small intestine.

The MMC has been proposed as a clearing mechanism of the intestine in the fasted state (40). Although the MMC has been called the intestinal housekeeper, its true function remains unknown. Studies by Vantrappen et al. (205) suggested that in some patients with intestinal pseudo-obstruction, bacterial overgrowth was a common finding. These studies indicated a close association with motility and the development of overgrowth.

Although there have been few studies of the mechanism of intestinal mucin in the bacterial overgrowth syndrome, the mucin layer may provide important clues to the cause of this problem (127–129, 193). The absence of or decrease in immunoglobulins seems an immediate consideration, but studies in patients with hypogammaglobulinemia, especially secretory immunoglobulin A deficiency, showed no difference in intestinal flora (20). Mucin is a complex substance consisting of several sugars and protein (glycoproteins) (3, 63). A defect in these glycoproteins may occur, creating a favorable environment for overgrowth of bacteria to develop spontaneously, or perhaps the bacteria themselves can produce substances that damage this protective layer (64, 127, 194). Indications that mucin may be one of the more important factors in overgrowth come from studies of patients with malnutrition (84, 186) or with chronic or acute diarrhea (37, 79) and from studies of elderly patients. Sudden unexplained deterioration of geriatric patients has been shown to occur secondary to overgrowth (101, 151, 170). Their nutritional balance may already be compromised, thus providing the right environment for bacterial overgrowth.

*Mechanisms of Diarrhea*

BRUSH-BORDER INJURY. In bacterial overgrowth of the small intestine the concentration of brush-border enzymes has been shown to be decreased (73). Thus carbohydrate substrate may not be metabolized properly because of insufficient disaccharidases. The sugars may then be fermented by overgrowth of bacteria in the intestine or may pass on into the colon where they are fermented by the colonic bacteria and produce alcohols and volatile fatty acids (38, 169). How these two substances may contribute to diarrheal stools is poorly understood. Alcohol has been shown to stimulate intestinal motor activity in a manner similar to that of cholera toxin or ricinoleic acid (135); higher concentrations of alcohol may even contribute to the mucosal injury that develops (135). Diminished uptake of sugars has also been shown, probably related in part to the damaged brush border (73, 169). Not only is the brush border acutely injured by bacterial overgrowth but the injury also may require an indefinite period of time to heal after appropriate antibiotic and medical therapy (112, 123).

MUCOSAL INJURY. Besides the brush-border injury, mucosal damage is also apparent in animals (16, 83) and in humans (6) with diarrhea. The lesion is patchy in distribution and consists of a nonspecific flattening of the villous tips (122). The cause of this enterocyte injury remains unknown. The bacteria themselves may injure the mucosa by direct invasion or by means of the toxins (cytotoxins) produced by many bacteria. Toxic products of bacterial metabolism may also account for tissue injury. Bacteria deconjugate bile salts that have been shown to damage tissue (43, 122, 132), and they ferment carbohydrate, producing alcohols, volatile fatty acids, and proteases such as elastase, and they also cause hydroxylation of fatty acids (73), resulting in compounds similar to ricinoleic acid. A promising focus for future investigation involves the effect of the many by-products that come from the metabolism of various malabsorbed substrates on the intestine. Little information exists on the subject.

BILE ACIDS. Bile acids conjugated with glucuronide or sulfate are nontoxic substances that convert fat-soluble substances to a water-miscible phase. This micellar phase is readily absorbed by the enterocyte. If bile acids become deconjugated by bacterial enzymes during bacterial overgrowth, micelles fail to form and the enterocyte may be injured (43, 96, 122, 132), and nutrient substances then are not absorbed (23, 82, 120, 168, 182, 209). Deconjugated bile salts also may stimulate motility of the intestine as has been shown in the proximal fusiform colon of the rabbit (187). Diarrhea induced by deconjugated bile salts has been referred to as choleretic diarrhea. The salts may not only affect the small intestine but may also act as powerful secretagogues of the ascending colon (100). Thus the action of bacteria on bile salts is an important factor in the diarrhea caused by the overgrowth syndrome.

HYDROXYLATION OF FAT. Bacteria may similarly affect fatty acids that are malabsorbed because of tissue injury or because of the deconjugation of bile salts and consequent failure to form micelles. Bacteria may hydroxylate fatty acids, producing potent secretagogues similar to ricinoleic acid (7, 8). Ricinoleic acid, a $C_{18}$-hydroxy fatty acid that is the active ingredient of castor oil (18, 60), causes secretion of water and electrolytes from the small intestine (8, 39) and colon (65). Ricinoleic acid also induces formation of single ring contractions (MAPC) in a manner similar to that of cholera toxin (142), thus altering motility. Ricinoleic acid may also actually damage the villous tips, producing extravasation of fluid and protein from injured mucosa (66).

MOTILITY. Motility may have a dual function in the bacterial overgrowth syndrome. In some patients with overgrowth defined by a [$^{14}$C]glycocholate breath test, the etiologic mechanism may be the absence of motor function (i.e., loss of the intestinal housekeeper of the MMC) (196). Studies of the bacterial overgrowth syndrome in rats that had either surgically created self-emptying blind loops (the surgical control) or self-filling blind loops show that the rats with the self-filling blind loops consistently produced bacterial overgrowth (46, 73, 202). Using the same rat model, Justus et al. (112) demonstrated that bacteria or their products, or both, alter motor function; both MAPC and RBAP were seen. Figure 17 illustrates the number of MAPC/h in anesthetized control rats that had not had surgery, in rats with self-emptying (surgical controls) or self-filling blind loops, and in rats with self-filling loops but that were treated with chloramphenicol, an especially effective antibiotic for reducing numbers of aerobic and anaerobic organisms (73). There was no MAPC observed in the control rats or rats with self-emptying blind loops (112). However, there were 12.8 ± 4.3 (mean ± SE) MAPC/h in the rats with self-filling blind loops. Chloramphenicol significantly reduced MAPC activity to 2.0 ± 1.1 MAPC/h ($P < 0.01$). The RBAP activity occurring in this model was described as the percentage of slow waves occupied with action potentials. There was also RBAP activity present in the rats with self-filling blind loops, in contrast with a lack of RBAP activity in the controls or rats with self-emptying blind loops (Fig. 18).

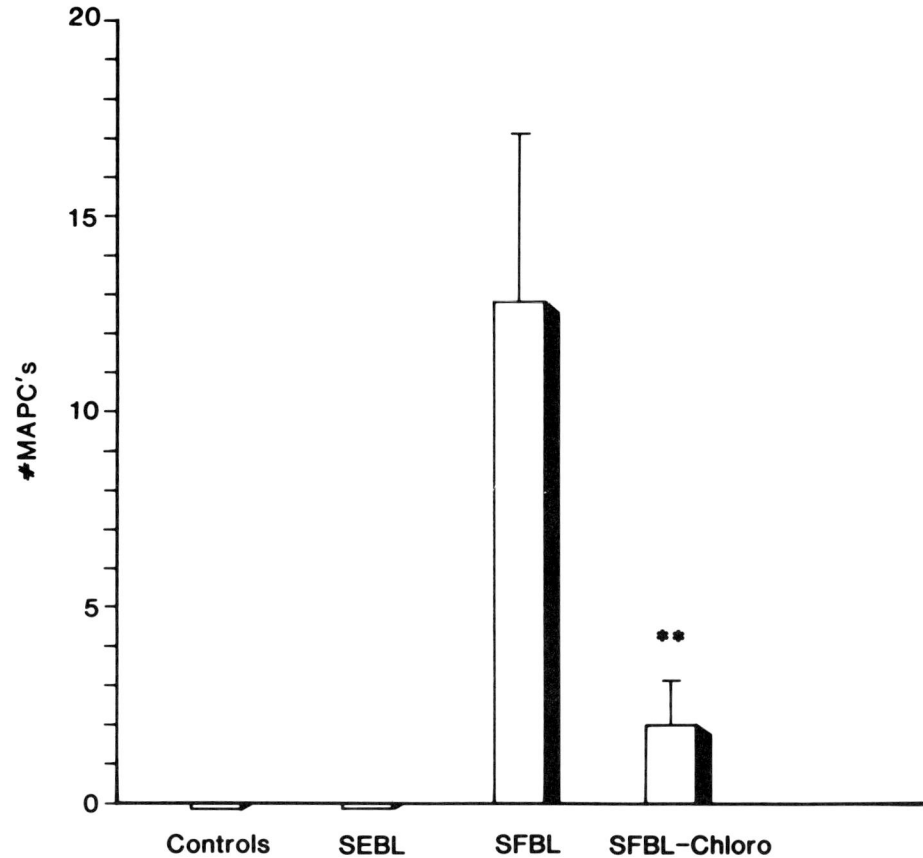

FIG. 17. Number of migrating action-potential complexes (MAPC) per hour in control, self-emptying blind loop rats (SEBL), self-filling blind loop rats (SFBL), and SFBL rats treated with chloramphenicol (SFBL-Chloro) in the experimental bacterial overgrowth syndrome. Results are expressed as mean ± SE. *Double asterisk*, $P < 0.01$ compared with SFBL rats. [From Justus et al. (112).]

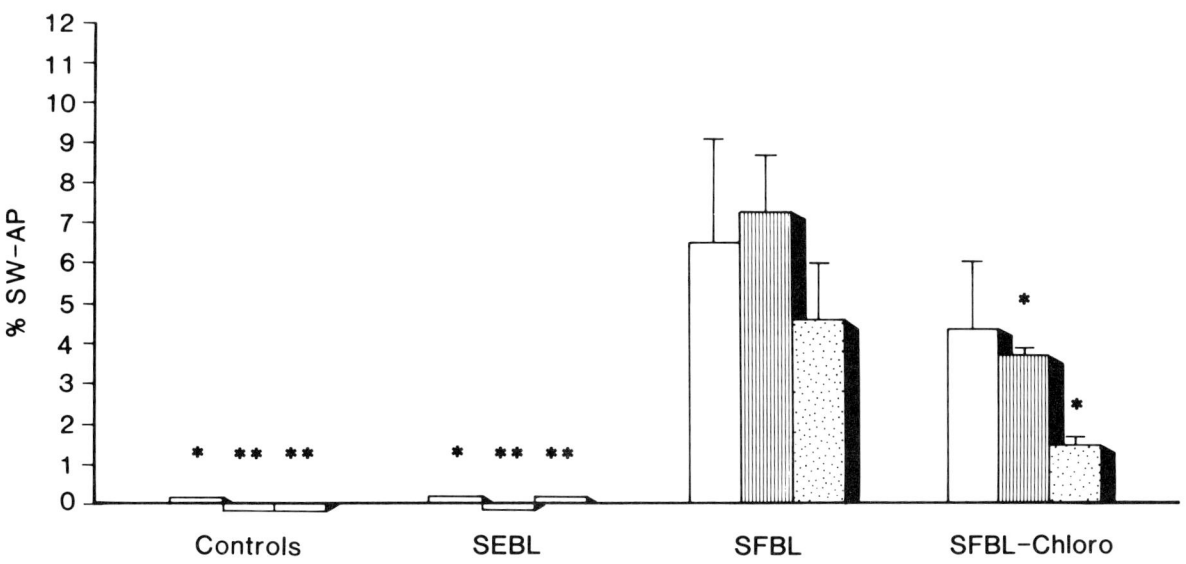

FIG. 18. Repetitive bursts of action-potential activity expressed as slow waves occupied by action potentials (% SW-AP) in control rats, self-emptying blind loop rats (SEBL), self-filling blind loop rats (SFBL), and SFBL rats treated with chloramphenicol (SFBL-Chloro) in experimental bacterial overgrowth syndrome. *Open bar*, sections proximal (afferent) to loop; *stippled bar*, sections distal (efferent) to loop; *striped bar*, blind loop itself. Results are expressed as mean ± SE. *Asterisk*, $P < 0.05$; *double asterisk*, $P < 0.01$ compared with SFBL rats. [From Justus et al. (112).]

Chloramphenicol-treated rats with self-filling loops had significantly fewer RBAP in the blind loop and efferent intestine ($P < 0.05$). In separate experiments both self-emptying and self-filling blind loops were prepared in rats (112). The blind loop was excised 2 wk after surgery. Myoelectric activity was recorded in controls, in rats with self-filling blind loops, and in rats at 2, 7, and 21 days after the blind loop was excised. Figure 19 shows the number of MAPC/h; MAPC activity significantly decreased at 2 and 7 days and had disappeared by day 21. Gnotobiotic rats with self-filling blind loops had no MAPC activity. Figure 20 also shows the effect of excision of the blind loop on RBAP, which were significantly decreased on days 2, 7, and 21. In contrast to the elimination of MAPC activity by day 21, the RBAP remained, which suggests the persistence of mucosal injury. Prior observations of nutrient absorption have shown that a lengthy time period may be necessary to reverse completely the damage to the mucosa and submucosa after overgrowth is eliminated (73, 201).

More recent studies by Justus et al. (115) have shown that soon (1 wk) after a blind loop was created, MAPC frequency was higher than it was 3 wk later. This corresponded with high bacterial counts for *E. coli* at 1 wk, but at 3 wk *Bacteroides* appeared in greater numbers, corresponding to an increase in RBAP. These studies suggest that *Bacteroides* sp. may be the primary agent causing tissue injury in the overgrowth syndrome (115).

METABOLIC PRODUCTS FROM BACTERIA. Of the mechanisms of bacterial overgrowth that have been studied, the contribution of bacterial metabolic products remains the most speculative. A few of these products have been mentioned: deconjugated bile salts, hydroxy fatty acids, alcohols and volatile fatty acids fermented from carbohydrates, and even enterotoxins and cytotoxins from certain bacteria. The metabolic by-products of bacteria are probably numerous, and these substances may interact, causing secretion, impaired absorption, maldigestion, and altered motility that results in the clinical response of diarrhea in the bacterial overgrowth syndrome. Over the next decade substances may well be found that act specifically on nerve receptors (e.g., neurotransmitters). McGowen et al. (152) identified the neurotransmitter serotonin in the whole-cell lysate of *Entamoeba histolytica*. This finding not only is provocative but also provides insight for the future identification of related substances that are known transmitters of nerve function.

## Questions for the Future

The mechanisms of diarrhea of the bacterial overgrowth syndrome are as multifactorial as are their

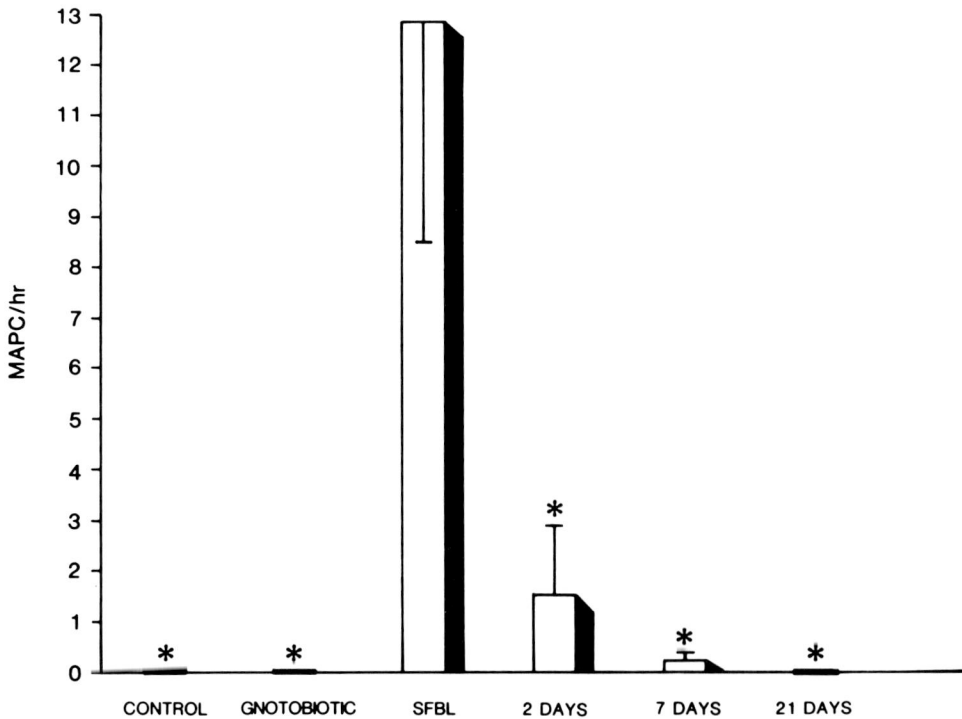

FIG. 19. Number of migrating action-potential complexes (MAPC) per hour in control rats, gnotobiotic rats, self-filling blind loop rats (SFBL), and SFBL rats 2, 7, and 21 days after the loops were surgically removed. Results are expressed as mean ± SE. Asterisk, $P < 0.05$ compared with SFBL rats. [From Justus et al. (112).]

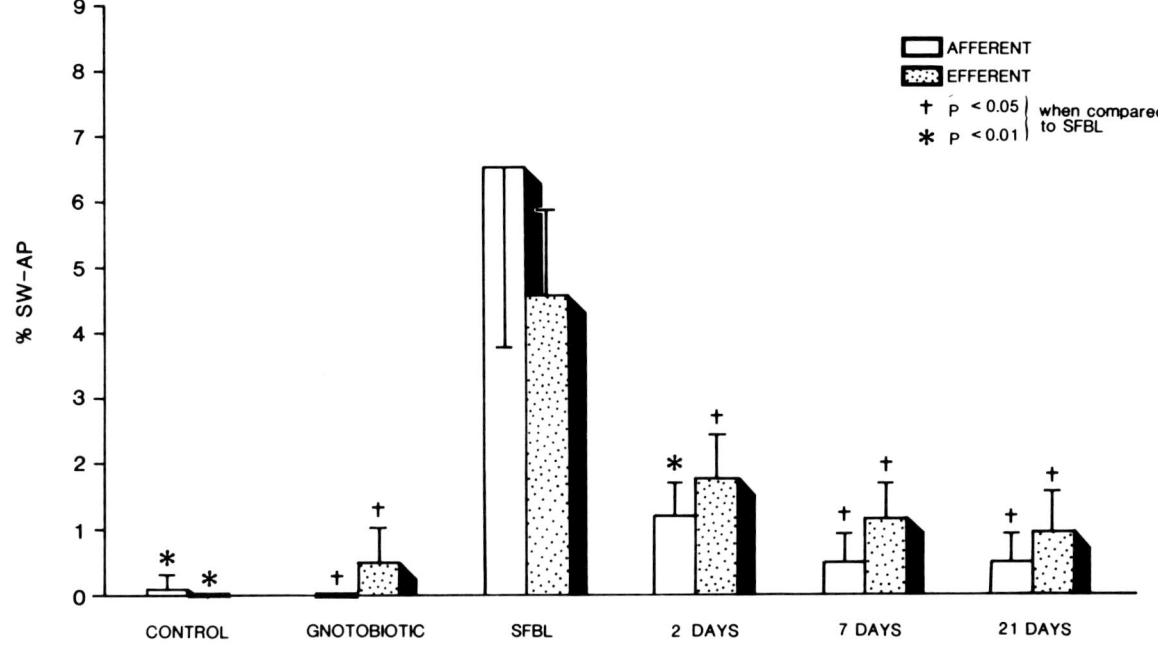

FIG. 20. Repetitive bursts of action potential activity expressed as slow waves occupied by action potentials (% SW-AP) in afferent (*open bars*) and efferent (*stippled bars*) sections of the jejunum of control rats, gnotobiotic rats, self-filling blind loop (SFBL) rats, and SFBL rats 2, 7, and 21 days after loops were surgically removed. Results are expressed as mean ± SE. [From Justus et al. (112).]

causes. However, if the mysteries of this disorder can be solved, there will be a clearer understanding of secretion, absorption, digestion, and motility. Investigators tend to consider only their own specific area of interest or discipline in their research projects, but clearly this is one disease in which multiple mechanisms of the alimentary canal are disrupted and each provides a major contribution to the disease. A multidisciplinary approach will be necessary for its full understanding.

## SUMMARY

Diarrhea is more than just the secretion of chloride and bicarbonate, with passive flow of water and malabsorption of sodium from the enterocyte alone. With evidence that has emerged within the last 10 years, the following concept of secretory diarrheas can be proposed.

Without doubt the usual initial event is when substances such as enterotoxins or cytotoxins attach to receptors on the enterocyte membrane and activate the intracellular "machinery" within the enterocyte. Activation of second messengers within the cell (e.g., cAMP or cGMP) causes the initial secretory event (9, 28, 29, 57, 121, 165, 178, 179). Cassuto (32) has shown that cholera-induced secretion may be inhibited by neural antagonists (see Table 1), which suggests that the intrinsic nerve pathways of the enteric nervous system provide important interaction in sustaining an ongoing secretory process (see Fig. 9).

Hubel (106) has demonstrated that norepinephrine is an active secretagogue, and Cassuto et al. (35) have shown that serotonin also induces active secretion. Cooke (41) has shown that a neural reflex arc present in the mucosa-submucosa is antagonized by lidocaine, atropine, and hexamethonium. This intrinsic nerve plexus may well be contributing to ongoing secretion by stimulating the crypt cells to secrete.

Alterations in motility that occur from bacterial toxins clearly exist (136–143). These alterations may be ongoing events but most probably are mediated by cellular mechanisms that are separate from secretion (e.g., as in cholera-induced activity). Stimulation of both secretion and MAPC activity occurs with choleragen, the holotoxin from *V. cholerae*. However, only the MAPC occurs with choleragenoid, the $B_5$ subunits of the holotoxin (183). Both toxins bind to $G_{M1}$ receptors on the enterocyte membrane, but each results in separate events. Motility alterations are also inhibited by certain neural antagonists (see Table 1).

It is possible that besides activation of the classic second messengers (e.g., cAMP or cGMP) that alter secretion within the enterocyte, additional second messengers are produced, such as calcium/calmodulin, protein kinase C, prostaglandins, or other undefined pathways. Stimulation of afferent sensory dendrites of the mucosa-submucosal plexus neurons may occur by either the release of neurotransmitters from the enterochromaffin cells or from tertiary messengers as a result of activation of various kinases (see Fig. 8). The activation of these sensory neurons could conceivably communicate directly with other submucosal neurons to induce continued secretion through the crypt cells. More probable, however, is the communication of the mucosa-submucosal neurons with the ganglia of the myenteric plexus, which in turn provides the means for additional stimulation of efferent pathways to the submucosal nerves. Because $PGF_{2\alpha}$ and $PGE_{2\alpha}$ have been shown to alter motor activity in a manner similar to that of choleragen or *E. coli* $ST_a$, respectively, and because intracellular second messengers are an important part in the phosphatidylinositol system, an important pathway for membrane signal transduction, there is the intriguing possibility that these substances may be intimately involved in the process of diarrhea as neurosensory messengers. How the kinase pathways interact with one another in this process remains to be assessed. The question provides provocative thought for experimental research over the next decade. One point appears clear: in the mechanism of diarrhea, the enterocyte no longer stands alone. Nerves with their dendrites, axons, and neurotransmitters are important in altering motility of the small intestine and sustaining or inhibiting secretion.

Solving the mechanisms of diarrhea and certainly of the idiopathic form of bacterial overgrowth of the small intestine will require the unselfish collaborative efforts of multiple disciplines.

We thank Anne Crawford for typing the manuscript and Alice Cullu for editorial advice. We also wish to recognize the persons who have made contributions to this laboratory: Dr. Gerald M. Carlson, Dr. Theodore W. Burns, Dr. Kenneth L. Koch, Dr. Peter G. Justus, Dr. Charles A. Sninsky, Dr. Augustin Fernandez, Dr. Victor M. Piñeiro-Carrero, Dr. Christopher D. Lind, Joanne L. Martin, and Richard H. Davis.

This research was supported by funds from the Veterans Administration.

Present address of J. R. Mathias and M. H. Clench: Division of Gastroenterology, Department of Internal Medicine, G64, University of Texas Medical Branch, Galveston, TX 77550.

## REFERENCES

1. AEBERHARD, P. F., L. D. MAGNENAT, AND W. A. ZIMMERMANN. Nervous control of migrating myoelectric complex of the small bowel. *Am. J. Physiol.* 238 (*Gastrointest. Liver Physiol.* 1): G102–G108, 1980.
2. ALDERETE, J. F., AND D. C. ROBERTSON. Purification and chemical characterization of the heat-stable enterotoxin produced by porcine strains of enterotoxigenic *Escherichia coli*. *Infect. Immun.* 19: 1021–1030, 1978.
3. ALLEN, A. Structure and function of gastrointestinal mucus. In: *Physiology of the Gastrointestinal Tract* (1st ed.), edited by L. R. Johnson. New York: Raven, 1981, vol. 1, chapt. 21, p. 617–639.
4. ALVAREZ, W. C., AND L. J. MAHONEY. Peristaltic rush in the rabbit. *Am. J. Physiol.* 69: 211–225, 1924.
5. ALVAREZ, W. C., AND F. B. TAYLOR. Changes in rhythmicity, irritability and tone in the purged intestine. *J. Pharmacol. Exp. Ther.* 10: 365–377, 1917.
6. AMENT, M. E., S. S. SHIMODA, D. R. SAUNDERS, AND C. E. RUBIN. Pathogenesis of steatorrhea in three cases of small intestinal stasis syndrome. *Gastroenterology* 63: 728–747, 1972.
7. AMMON, H. V., AND S. F. PHILLIPS. Inhibition of ileal water absorption by intraluminal fatty acids. Influence of chain length, hydroxylation and conjugation of fatty acids. *J. Clin. Invest.* 53: 205–210, 1974.
8. AMMON, H. V., P. J. THOMAS, AND S. F. PHILLIPS. Effects of oleic and ricinoleic acids on net jejunal water and electrolyte movement. *J. Clin. Invest.* 53: 374–379, 1974.
9. BANWELL, J. G., N. F. PIERCE, R. C. MITRA, K. L. BRIGHAM, G. J. CARANASOS, R. I. KEIMOWITZ, D. S. FEDSON, J. THOMAS, S. L. GORBACH, R. B. SACK, AND A. MONDAL. Intestinal fluid and electrolyte transport in human cholera. *J. Clin. Invest.* 49: 183–195, 1970.
10. BANWELL, J. G., AND H. SHERR. Effect of bacterial enterotoxin on the gastrointestinal tract. *Gastroenterology* 65: 467–497, 1973.
11. BARTLETT, J. G., N. MOON, T. W. CHANG, N. TAYLOR, AND A. B. ONDERDONK. Role of *Clostridium difficile* in antibiotic-associated pseudomembranous colitis. *Gastroenterology* 75: 778–782, 1978.
12. BINDER, H. J., G. F. LEMP, AND J. D. GARDNER. Receptors for vasoactive intestinal peptide and secretin on small intestinal epithelial cells. *Am. J. Physiol.* 238 (*Gastrointest. Liver Physiol.* 1): G190–G196, 1980.
13. BJØRNEKLETT, A. Small bowel bacterial overgrowth syndrome. *Scand. J. Gastroenterol. Suppl.* 85: 83–93, 1983.
14. BLASER, M. J., AND L. B. RELLER. Campylobacter enteritis. *N. Engl. J. Med.* 305: 1444–1452, 1981.
15. BLASER, M. J., J. G. WELLS, R. A. FELDMAN, R. A. POLLARD, AND J. R. ALLEN. Campylobacter enteritis in the United States. A multicenter study. *Ann. Intern. Med.* 98: 360–365, 1983.
16. BLOCH, R., H. MENGE, H. LORENZ-MEYER, H. G. STOCKERT, AND E. O. RIECKEN. Functional, biochemical and morphological alterations in the intestines of rats with an experimental blind-loop syndrome. *Res. Exp. Med.* 166: 67–78, 1975.
17. BOLDYREFF, V. Periodic wave phenomena in the secretory function of the digestive tract [in Russian]. *Gaz. Hop. Botkine* 34: 1529–1542, 1902.
18. BONNYCASTLE, D. D. Cathartics and laxatives. In: *Drill's Pharmacology in Medicine*, edited by J. R. DiPalma. New York: McGraw-Hill, 1971, p. 911–975.
19. BOYLE, J. M., AND J. D. GARDNER. Sequence of events mediating the effect of cholera toxin on rat thymocytes. *J. Clin. Invest.* 53: 1149–1158, 1974.
20. BROWN, W. R., D. C. SAVAGE, R. S. DUBOIS, M. H. ALP, A. MALLORY, AND F. KERN, JR. Intestinal microflora of immunoglobulin-deficient and normal human subjects. *Gastroenterology* 62: 1143–1152, 1972.
21. BROWNING, G. G., K. A. BUCHAN, AND C. MACKAY. The effect of vagotomy and drainage on the small bowel flora. *Gut* 15: 139–142, 1974.
22. BURGESS, M. N., R. J. BYWATER, C. M. COWLEY, N. A. MULLAN, AND P. M. NEWSOME. Biological evaluation of a methanol-soluble, heat-stable *Escherichia coli* enterotoxin in infant mice, pigs, rabbits, and calves. *Infect. Immunol.* 21: 526–531, 1978.
23. BURKE, V., M. GRACEY, J. THOMAS, AND A. MALAJCZUK. Inhibition of intestinal uptake of amino acids by unconjugated bile salt. *Aust. J. Exp. Biol. Med. Sci.* 54: 391–402, 1976.
24. BURNS, T. W., J. R. MATHIAS, G. M. CARLSON, J. L. MARTIN, AND R. P. SHIELDS. Effect of toxigenic *Escherichia coli* on myoelectric activity of small intestine. *Am. J. Physiol.* 235 (*Endocrinol. Metab. Gastrointest. Physiol.* 4): E311–E315, 1978.

25. BURNS, T. W., J. R. MATHIAS, J. L. MARTIN, G. M. CARLSON, AND R. P. SHIELDS. Alteration of myoelectric activity of small intestine by invasive *Escherichia coli. Am. J. Physiol.* 238 (*Gastrointest. Liver Physiol.* 1): G57–G62, 1980.
26. BUTZLER, J. P., AND M. B. SKIRROW. *Campylobacter* enteritis. *Clin. Gastroenterol.* 8: 737–765, 1979.
27. CAMERON, D. G., G. M. WATSON, AND L. J. WITTS. The experimental production of macrocytic anemia by operations on the intestinal tract. *Blood* 4: 803–815, 1949.
28. CARPENTER, C. C. J., JR. Cholera enterotoxin—recent investigations yield insights into transport processes. *Am. J. Med.* 50: 1–7, 1971.
29. CARPENTER, C. C. J., JR., R. B. SACK, J. C. FEELEY, AND R. W. STEENBERG. Site and characteristics of electrolyte loss and effect of intraluminal glucose in experimental canine cholera. *J. Clin. Invest.* 47: 1210–1220, 1968.
30. CASSEL, D., AND T. PFEUFFER. Mechanism of cholera toxin action: covalent modification of the guanyl nucleotide-binding protein of the adenylate cyclase system. *Proc. Natl. Acad. Sci. USA* 75: 2669–2673, 1978.
31. CASSEL, D., AND Z. SELINGER. Mechanism of adenylate cyclase activation by cholera toxin: inhibition of GTP hydrolysis at the regulatory site. *Proc. Natl. Acad. Sci. USA* 74: 3307–3311, 1977.
32. CASSUTO, J. Nervous mechanisms in cholera secretion. An experimental study in cats and rats. Göteburg, Sweden: Univ. of Göteburg, 1981. PhD thesis.
33. CASSUTO, J., M. JODAL, AND O. LUNDGREN. The effect of nicotinic and muscarinic receptor blockade on cholera toxin induced intestinal secretion in rats and cats. *Acta Physiol. Scand.* 114: 573–577, 1982.
34. CASSUTO, J., M. JODAL, R. TUTTLE, AND O. LUNDGREN. On the role of intramural nerves in the pathogenesis of cholera toxin–induced intestinal secretion. *Scand. J. Gastroenterol.* 16: 377–384, 1981.
35. CASSUTO, J., M. JODAL, R. TUTTLE, AND O. LUNDGREN. 5-Hydroxytryptamine and cholera secretion. Physiological and pharmacological studies in cats and rats. *Scand. J. Gastroenterol.* 17: 695–703, 1982.
36. CASSUTO, J., A. SIEWERT, M. JODAL, AND O. LUNDGREN. The involvement of intramural nerves in cholera toxin induced intestinal secretion. *Acta Physiol. Scand.* 117: 195–202, 1983.
37. CHALLACOMBE, D. N., J. M. RICHARDSON, B. ROWE, AND C. M. ANDERSON. Bacterial microflora of the upper gastrointestinal tract in infants with protracted diarrhoea. *Arch. Dis. Child.* 49: 270–277, 1974.
38. CHERNOV, A. J., W. F. DOE, AND D. GOMPERTZ. Intrajejunal volatile fatty acids in the stagnant loop syndrome. *Gut* 13: 103–106, 1972.
39. CLINE, W. S., V. LORENZSONN, L. BENZ, P. BASS, AND W. A. OLSEN. The effects of sodium ricinoleate on small intestinal function and structure. *J. Clin. Invest.* 58: 380–390, 1976.
40. CODE, C. F., AND J. A. MARLETTE. The interdigestive myoelectric complex of the stomach and small bowel of dogs. *J. Physiol. Lond.* 246: 289–309, 1975.
41. COOKE, H. J. Neurobiology of the intestinal mucosa. *Gastroenterology* 90: 1057–1081, 1986.
42. COREMANS, G., S. CHAUSSADE, J. JANSSENS, AND G. VANTRAPPEN. Migrating action-potential complexes (MAPC), a motility pattern associated with diarrhea in man (Abstract). *Dig. Dis. Sci.* 30: 765, 1985.
43. DAVIS, R. H., E. Y. EAKER, G. B. BIXLER, M. H. CLENCH, AND J. R. MATHIAS. Phorbol esters induce unique myoelectric activity in rabbit ileum (Abstract). *Clin. Res.* 34: 438A, 1986.
44. DAWSON, A. M., AND K. J. ISSELBACHER. Studies on lipid metabolism in the small intestine with observations on the role of bile salts. *J. Clin. Invest.* 39: 730–740, 1960.
45. DEE, S. N., AND D. N. CHATTERJEE. An experimental study of the mechanism of action of *Vibrio cholerae* on the intestinal mucous membrane. *J. Pathol. Bacteriol.* 66: 559–562, 1953.
46. DONALDSON, R. M., JR. Studies on the pathogenesis of steatorrhea in the blind loop syndrome. *J. Clin. Invest.* 44: 1815–1825, 1965.
47. DONALDSON, R. M., JR. Small bowel bacterial overgrowth. *Adv. Intern. Med.* 16: 191–212, 1970.
48. DRAKE, A. A., M. J. GILCHRIST, J. A. WASHINGTON II, K. A. HUIZENGA, AND R. E. VAN SCOY. Diarrhea due to *Campylobacter fetus* subspecies *jejuni*: a clinical review of 63 cases. *Mayo Clin. Proc.* 56: 414–423, 1981.
49. DRASAR, B. S., M. SHINER, AND G. M. MCLEOD. Studies on the intestinal flora. I. The bacterial flora of the gastrointestinal tract in healthy and achlorhydric persons. *Gastroenterology* 56: 71–79, 1969.
50. DUPONT, H. L., S. B. FORMAL, R. B. HORNICK, M. J. SNYDER, J. P. LIBONATI, D. G. SHEAHAN, E. H. LABREC, AND J. P. KALAS. Pathogenesis of *Escherichia coli* diarrhea. *N. Engl. J. Med.* 285: 1–9, 1971.
51. DUTTA, N. K., AND M. K. HABBU. Experimental cholera in infant rabbits: a method for chemotherapeutic investigation. *Br. J. Pharmacol.* 10: 153–159, 1955.
52. EBEID, A. M., J. ESCOURROU, P. B. SOETERS, P. MURRAY, AND J. E. FISCHER. Hepatic inactivation of vasoactive intestinal peptide in man and dog. *Ann. Surg.* 188: 28–33, 1978.
53. ENDERS, G. L., JR., AND C. L. DUNCAN. Preparative polyacrylamide gel electrophoresis purification of *Clostridium perfringens* enterotoxin. *Infect. Immun.* 17: 425–429, 1977.
54. ENGLEY, F. B., JR. The neurotoxin of *Shigella dysenteriae* (Shiga). *Bacteriol Rev.* 16: 153–178, 1952.
55. FERNANDEZ, A., C. A. SNINSKY, A. D. O'BRIEN, M. H. CLENCH, AND J. R. MATHIAS. Purified *Shigella* enterotoxin does not alter intestinal motility. *Infect. Immun.* 43: 477–481, 1984.
56. FERNANDEZ, H., U. F. NETO, F. FERNANDES, P. M. DE ALMEIDA, AND L. R. TRABULSI. Culture supernatants of *Campylobacter jejuni* induce a secretory response in jejunal segments of adult rats. *Infect. Immun.* 40: 429–431, 1983.
57. FIELD, M. Intestinal secretion: effect of cyclic AMP and its role in cholera. *N. Engl. J. Med.* 284: 1137–1144, 1971.
58. FIELD, M., L. H. GRAF, JR., W. J. LAIRD, AND P. L. SMITH. Heat-stable enterotoxin of *Escherichia coli*: in vitro effects on guanylate cyclase activity, cyclic GMP concentration, and ion transport in small intestine. *Proc. Natl. Acad. Sci. USA* 75: 2800–2804, 1978.
59. FINCK, A. D., AND R. L. KATZ. Prevention of cholera-induced intestinal secretion in the cat by aspirin. *Nature Lond.* 238: 273–274, 1972.
60. FINGEL, E. Cathartics and laxatives. In: *Pharmacological Basis of Therapeutics*, edited by L. S. Goodman and A. Gilman. New York: Macmillan, 1970, p. 1020–1024.
61. FINKELSTEIN, R. A., K. FUJITA, AND J. J. LOSPALLUTO. Procholeragenoid: an aggreveted intermediate in the formation of choleragenoid. *J. Immunol.* 107: 1043–1051, 1971.
62. FINKELSTEIN, R. A., AND J. J. LOSPALLUTO. Production of highly purified choleragen and choleragenoid. *J. Infect. Dis.* 121, Suppl.: S63–S70, 1970.
63. FLOREY, H. W. The secretion and function of intestinal mucus. *Gastroenterology* 43: 326–329, 1962.
64. FOSTNER, J. F. Intestinal mucins in health and disease. *Digestion* 17: 234–263, 1978.
65. GAGINELLA, T. S., V. S. CHADWICK, J. C. DEBONGNIE, J. C. LEWIS, AND S. F. PHILLIPS. Perfusion of rabbit colon with ricinoleic acid: dose-related mucosal injury, fluid secretion, and increased permeability. *Gastroenterology* 73: 95–101, 1977.
66. GAGINELLA, T. S., AND S. F. PHILLIPS. Ricinoleic acid (castor oil) alters intestinal surface structure: a scanning electronmicroscopic study. *Mayo Clin. Proc.* 51: 6–12, 1976.
67. GEMSKI, P., JR., A. TAKEUCHI, O. WASHINGTON, AND S. B. FORMAL. Shigellosis due to *Shigella dysenteriae*. I. Relative importance of mucosal invasion versus toxin production in pathogenesis. *J. Infect. Dis.* 126: 523–530, 1972.
68. GERSHON, M. D., AND S. M. ERDE. The nervous system of the gut. *Gastroenterology* 80: 1571–1594, 1981.

69. GERSHON, M. D., D. L. SHERMAN, AND C. F. DREYFUS. Effect of indolic neurotoxins on enteric serotonergic neurons. *J. Comp. Neurol.* 190: 581–596, 1980.
70. GIANNELLA, R. A. Suckling mouse model for detection of heat-stable *Escherichia coli* exterotoxin: characteristics of the model. *Infect. Immun.* 14: 95–99, 1976.
71. GIANNELLA, R. A. Pathogenesis of acute bacterial diarrheal disorders. *Annu. Rev. Med.* 32: 341–357, 1981.
72. GIANNELLA, R. A., AND K. W. DRAKE. Effect of purified *Escherichia coli* heat-stable enterotoxin on intestinal cyclic nucleotide metabolism and fluid secretion. *Infect. Immun.* 24: 19–23, 1979.
73. GIANNELLA, R. A., W. R. ROUT, AND P. P. TOSKES. Jejunal brush border injury and impaired sugar and amino acid uptake in the blind loop syndrome. *Gastroenterology* 67: 965–974, 1974.
74. GILL, D. M. Multiple roles of erythrocyte supernatant in the activation of adenylate cyclase by *Vibrio cholerae* toxin in vitro. *J. Infect. Dis.* 133, Suppl: S55–S63, 1976.
75. GILL, D. M. Mechanism of action of cholera toxin. In: *Advances in Cyclic Nucleotide Research*, edited by P. Greengard and G. A. Robison. New York: Raven, 1977, vol. 8, p. 85–118.
76. GILL, D. M., AND C. A. KING. The mechanism of action of cholera toxin in pigeon erythrocyte lysates. *J. Biol. Chem.* 250: 6424–6432, 1975.
77. GOLDSTEIN, F., C. W. WIRTS, AND O. D. KOWLESSAR. Diabetic diarrhea and steatorrhea. Microbiologic and clinical observations. *Ann. Intern. Med.* 72: 215–218, 1970.
78. GORBACH, S. L. Intestinal microflora. *Gastroenterology* 60: 1110–1129, 1971.
79. GORBACH, S. L., G. NEALE, R. LEVITAN, AND G. W. HEPNER. Alterations in human intestinal microflora during experimental diarrhoea. *Gut* 11: 1–6, 1970.
80. GORBACH, S. L., A. G. PLAUT, L. NAHAS, L. WEINSTEIN, G. SPANKNEBEL, AND R. LEVITAN. Studies of intestinal microflora. II. Microorganisms of the small intestine and their relations to oral and fecal flora. *Gastroenterology* 53: 856–867, 1967.
81. GRACEY, M. Intestinal absorption in the "contaminated small-bowel syndrome." *Gut* 12: 403–410, 1971.
82. GRACEY, M., V. BURKE, AND A. OSHIN. Reversible inhibition of intestinal active sugar transport by deconjugated bile salts in vitro. *Biochim. Biophys. Acta* 225: 308–314, 1971.
83. GRACEY, M., J. PAPADIMITRIOU, AND G. BOWER. Ultrastructural changes in the small intestines of rats with self-filling blind loops. *Gastroenterology* 67: 646–651, 1974.
84. GRACEY, M., SUHARJONO, SUNOTO, AND D. E. STONE. Microbial contamination of the gut: another feature of malnutrition. *Am. J. Clin. Nutr.* 26: 1170–1174, 1973.
85. GRADY, G. F., AND G. T. KEUSCH. Pathogenesis of bacterial diarrheas. *N. Engl. J. Med.* 285: 831–841, 891–900, 1971.
86. GRAY, J. D., AND M. SHINER. Influence of gastric pH on gastric and jejunal flora. *Gut* 8: 74–81, 1967.
87. GREENBERG, R. N., AND R. L. GUERRANT. *E. coli* heat-stable enterotoxin. *Pharmacol. Ther.* 13: 507–531, 1981.
88. GREENLEE, H. B., S. M. GELBART, A. J. DEORIO, D. S. FRANCESCATTI, J. PAEZ, AND G. F. REINHARDT. The influence of gastric surgery on the intestinal flora. *Am. J. Clin. Nutr.* 30: 1826–1833, 1977.
89. GREENLEE, H. B., R. VIVIT, J. PAEZ, AND A. DIETZ. Bacterial flora of the jejunum following peptic ulcer surgery. *Arch. Surg.* 102: 260–265, 1971.
90. GUERRANT, R. L. Pathophysiology of the enterotoxic and viral diseases. In: *Diarrhea and Malnutrition*, edited by L. C. Chen and N. S. Scrimshaw. New York: Plenum, 1983, p. 23–43.
91. GUERRANT, R. L. Microbial toxins and diarrhoeal diseases: introduction and overview. In: *Microbial Toxins and Diarrhoeal Disease*, edited by D. Evered and J. Whelan. London: Pitman, 1985, p. 1–13. (CIBA Found. Symp. 112.)
92. GUERRANT, R. L., C. C. CARPENTER, AND N. F. PIERCE. Experimental *E. coli* diarrhea: effects of viable bacteria and enterotoxin. *Trans. Assoc. Am. Physicians* 86: 111–120, 1973.
93. GUERRANT, R. L., U. GANGULY, A. G. P. CASPER, E. J. MOORE, N. F. PIERCE, AND C. C. J. CARPENTER. Effect of *Escherichia coli* on fluid transport across canine small bowel. Mechanism and time-course with enterotoxin and whole bacterial cells. *J. Clin. Invest.* 52: 1707–1714, 1973.
94. GUERRANT, R. L., J. M. HUGHES, B. CHANG, D. C. ROBERTSON, AND F. MURAD. Activation of intestinal guanylate cyclase by heat-stable enterotoxin of *Escherichia coli*: studies of tissue specificity, potential receptors and intermediates. *J. Infect. Dis.* 142: 220–228, 1980.
95. GUERRANT, R. L., L. V. KIRCHOFF, D. S. SHIELDS, M. K. NATIONS, J. LESLIE, M. A. DE SOUSA, J. G. ARAUJO, L. L. CORREIA, K. T. SAVER, K. E. MCCLELLAND, F. L. TROWBRIDGE, AND J. M. HUGHES. Prospective study of diarrheal illness in northeastern Brazil: patterns of disease, nutritional impact, etiologies and risk factors. *J. Infect. Dis.* 148: 986–987, 1983.
96. HAJJAR, J. J., R. N. KHURI, AND A. B. BIKHAZI. Effect of bile salts on amino acid transport by rabbit intestine. *Am. J. Physiol.* 299: 518–523, 1975.
97. HAMILTON, J. D., N. H. DYER, A. M. DAWSON, F. W. O'GRADY, A. VINCE, J. C. B. FENTON, AND D. L. MOLLIN. Assessment and significance of bacterial overgrowth in the small bowel. *Q. J. Med.* 39: 265–285, 1970.
98. HAWKEY, C. J., AND D. S. RAMPTON. Prostaglandins and the gastrointestinal mucosa: are they important in its function, disease or treatment? *Gastroenterology* 89: 1162–1188, 1985.
99. HEWLETT, E. L., R. L. GUERRANT, D. J. EVANS, JR., AND W. G. GREENOUGH III. Toxins of *Vibrio cholerae* and *Escherichia coli* stimulate adenylate in rat fat cells. *Nature Lond.* 249: 371–373, 1974.
100. HOFMANN, A. F., AND J. R. POLEY. Role of bile acid malabsorption in pathogenesis of diarrhea and steatorrhea in patients with ileal resection. I. Response to cholestyramine or replacement of dietary long chain triglyceride by medium chain triglyceride. *Gastroenterology* 62: 918–934, 1972.
101. HOLDEN, R. J., P. MILLS, L. CRAIG, J. D. SLEIGH, I. MACKENZIE, W. WATSON, G. WATKINSON, AND G. CREAN. Bacterial contamination of the small bowel in the elderly (Letter to the editor). *Lancet* 1: 502–503, 1978.
102. HOLMGREN, J. Comparison of the tissue receptors for *Vibrio cholerae* and *Escherichia coli* enterotoxins by means of gangliosides and natural cholera toxoid. *Infect. Immun.* 8: 851–859, 1973.
103. HOLMGREN, J., AND I. LÖNNROTH. Structure and function of enterotoxins and their receptors. In: *Cholera and Related Diarrheas*, edited by O. Ouchterlony and J. Holmgren. Basel: Karger, 1980, p. 88–109. (Proc. 43rd Nobel Symp.)
104. HOLMGREN, J., I. LÖNNROTH, J. MÅNSSON, AND L. SVENNERHOLM. Interaction of cholera toxin and membrane $G_{M1}$ ganglioside of small intestine. *Proc. Natl. Acad. Sci. USA* 72: 2520–2524, 1975.
105. HOUCKGEEST, VAN B. Untersuchungen über Peristaltik des Magens und Darmkanals. *Pfluegers Arch. Gesamte Physiol. Menschen Tiere* 6: 266–302, 1872.
106. HUBEL, K. A. The effects of electrical field stimulation and tetrodotoxin on ion transport by the isolated rabbit ileum. *J. Clin. Invest.* 62: 1039–1047, 1978.
107. HUGHES, J. M., F. MURAD, B. CHANG, AND R. L. GUERRANT. Role of cyclic GMP in the action of heat-stable enterotoxin of *Eschericia coli*. *Nature Lond.* 271: 755–756, 1978.
108. ISAACS, P. E., AND Y. S. KIM. The contaminated small bowel syndrome. *Am. J. Med.* 67: 1049–1057, 1979.
109. JACKS, T. M., AND B. J. WU. Biochemical properties of *Escherichia coli* low-molecular-weight, heat-stable enterotoxin. *Infect. Immun.* 9: 342–347, 1974.
110. JACOBY, H. I., AND C. H. MARSHALL. Antagonism of cholera enterotoxin by anti-inflammatory agents in the rat. *Nature Lond.* 235: 163–165, 1972.

111. JUORIO, A. V., AND G. GABELLA. Noradrenaline in the guinea pig alimentary canal: regional distribution and sensitivity to denervation and reserpine. *J. Neurochem.* 22: 851–858, 1974.
112. JUSTUS, P. G., A. FERNANDEZ, J. L. MARTIN, C. E. KING, P. P. TOSKES, AND J. R. MATHIAS. Altered myoelectric activity in the experimental blind loop syndrome. *J. Clin. Invest.* 72: 1064–1071, 1983.
113. JUSTUS, P. G., J. L. MARTIN, D. A. GOLDBERG, N. S. TAYLOR, J. G. BARTLETT, R. W. ALEXANDER, AND J. R. MATHIAS. Myoelectric effects of *Clostridium difficile*: motility-altering factors distinct from its cytotoxin and enterotoxin in rabbits. *Gastroenterology* 83: 836–843, 1982.
114. JUSTUS, P. G., J. R. MATHIAS, J. L. MARTIN, G. M. CARLSON, R. P. SHIELDS, AND S. B. FORMAL. Myoelectric activity in the small intestine in response to *Clostridium perfringens* A enterotoxin: correlation with histologic findings in an in vivo rabbit model. *Gastroenterology* 80: 902–906, 1981.
115. JUSTUS, P. G., L. E. MCHERRON, AND T. T. WARD. Altered motility and duration of bacterial overgrowth in experimental blind loop syndrome. *Dig. Dis. Sci.* 29: 643–648, 1984.
116. KAHN, R. A., AND A. G. GILMAN. Purification of a protein cofactor required for ADP-ribosylation of the stimulatory regulatory component of adenylate cyclase by cholera toxin. *J. Biol. Chem.* 259: 6228–6234, 1984.
117. KALSER, M. H., R. COHEN, I. ARTEAGA, E. YAWN, L. MAYORAL, W. R. HOFFERT, AND D. FRAZIER. Normal viral and bacterial flora of the human small and large intestine. *N. Engl. J. Med.* 274: 500–505, 558–563, 1966.
118. KENNEDY, D. J., R. N. GREENBERG, J. A. DUNN, R. ABERNATHY, J. S. RYERSE, AND R. L. GUERRANT. Effects of *Escherichia coli* heat-stable enterotoxin $ST_b$ on intestines of mice, rats, rabbits and piglets. *Infect. Immun.* 46: 639–643, 1984.
119. KEUSCH, G. T., AND S. T. DONTA. Classification of enterotoxins on the basis of activity in cell culture. *J. Infect. Dis.* 131: 58–63, 1975.
120. KIM, Y. S., AND W. SPRITZ. Metabolism of hydroxy-fatty acids in dogs with steatorrhea secondary to experimentally produced intestinal blind loops. *J. Lipid Res.* 9: 487–491, 1968.
121. KIMBERG, D. V., M. FIELD, J. JOHNSON, A. HENDERSON, AND E. GERSHON. Stimulation of intestinal mucosal adenyl cyclase by cholera enterotoxin and prostaglandins. *J. Clin. Invest.* 50: 1218–1230, 1971.
122. KING, C. E., AND P. P. TOSKES. Malabsorption following gastric resection. In: *Postgastrectomy Syndromes*, edited by F. L. Bushkin and E. R. Woodward. Philadelphia, PA: Saunders, 1976, p. 129–146. (Major Problems in Clinical Surgery, vol. 20.)
123. KING, C. E., AND P. P. TOSKES. Small intestine bacterial overgrowth. *Gastroenterology* 76: 1035–1055, 1979.
124. KOCH, K. L., J. L. MARTIN, AND J. R. MATHIAS. Migrating action-potential complexes in vitro in cholera-exposed rabbit ileum. *Am. J. Physiol.* 244 (*Gastrointest. Liver Physiol.* 7): G291–G294, 1983.
125. KREJS, G. J., R. M. BARKLEY, N. W. READ, AND J. S. FORDTRAN. Intestinal secretion induced by vasoactive intestinal polypeptide. A comparison with cholera toxin in the canine jejunum in vivo. *J. Clin. Invest.* 61: 1337–1345, 1978.
126. LABURTHE, M., J. C. PRIETO, B. AMIRANOFF, C. DUPONT, D. HUI BON HOA, AND G. ROSSELIN. Interaction of vasoactive intestinal peptide with isolated intestinal epithelial cells from rat. 2. Characterization and structural requirements of the stimulatory effect of vasoactive intestinal peptide on production of adenosine 3':5'-monophosphate. *Eur. J. Biochem.* 96: 239–248, 1979.
127. LAMONT, J. T. Structure and function of gastrointestinal mucus. *Viewpoints Gastrointest. Dis.* 17: 1–4, 1985.
128. LAMONT, J. T., B. S. TURNER, D. DIBENEDETTO, R. HANDIN, AND A. I. SCHAFER. Arachidonic acid stimulates mucin secretion in prairie dog gallbladder. *Am. J. Physiol.* 245 (*Gastrointest. Liver Physiol.* 8): G92–G98, 1983.
129. LAMONT, J. T., AND A. VENTOLA. Stimulation of colonic glycoprotein synthesis by dibutyryl cyclic AMP and theophylline. *Gastroenterology* 72: 82–86, 1977.
130. LIND, C. D., R. H. DAVIS, R. L. GUERRANT, J. B. KAPER, AND J. R. MATHIAS. Effects of *Vibrio cholerae*, with and without enterotoxin production, on myoelectric activity of rabbit ileum in vivo (Abstract). *Dig. Dis. Sci.* 32: 918, 1988.
131. LOEWENSTEIN, M. Epidemiology of *Clostridium perfringens* food poisoning. *N. Engl. J. Med.* 286: 1026–1028, 1972.
132. LOW-BEER, T. S., R. E. SCHNEIDER, AND W. O. DOBBINS. Morphological changes of the small intestinal mucosa of guinea pig and hamster following incubation in vitro and perfusion in vivo with unconjugated bile salts. *Gut* 11: 486–492, 1970.
133. MAFFEI, H. V., AND F. J. NÓBREGA. Gastric pH and microflora of normal and diarrhoeic infants. *Gut* 16: 719–726, 1975.
134. MANNINEN, K. I., J. F. PRESCOTT, AND I. R. DOHOO. Pathogenecity of *Campylobacter jejuni* isolates from animals and humans. *Infect. Immun.* 38: 46–52, 1982.
135. MARTIN, J. L., P. G. JUSTUS, AND J. R. MATHIAS. Altered motility of the small intestine in response to ethanol (ETOH): an explanation for the diarrhea associated with consumption of alcohol (Abstract). *Gastroenterology* 78: 1218, 1980.
136. MATHIAS, J. R., G. M. CARLSON, G. BERTIGER, J. L. MARTIN, AND S. COHEN. Migrating action potential complex of cholera: a possible prostaglandin-induced response. *Am. J. Physiol.* 232 (*Endocrinol. Metab. Gastrointest. Physiol.* 1): E529–E534, 1977.
137. MATHIAS, J. R., G. M. CARLSON, A. J. DIMARINO, G. BERTIGER, AND S. COHEN. The effect of cholera toxin on ileal myoelectric activity: a neural-hormonal mechanism. In: *Proc. Fifth Int. Symp. Gastrointest. Motil.*, edited by G. Vantrappen. Herentals, Belgium: Typoff, 1976, p. 219–226.
138. MATHIAS, J. R., G. M. CARLSON, A. J. DIMARINO, G. BERTIGER, H. E. MORTON, AND S. COHEN. Intestinal myoelectric activity in response to live *Vibrio cholerae* and cholera enterotoxin. *J. Clin. Invest.* 58: 91–96, 1976.
139. MATHIAS, J. R., G. M. CARLSON, J. L. MARTIN, R. P. SHIELDS, AND S. FORMAL. *Shigella dysenteriae* I enterotoxin: proposed role in pathogenesis of shigellosis. *Am. J. Physiol.* 239 (*Gastrointest. Liver Physiol.* 2): G382–G386, 1980.
140. MATHIAS, J. R., AND M. H. CLENCH. Review: pathophysiology of diarrhea caused by bacterial overgrowth of the small intestine. *Am. J. Med. Sci.* 289: 243–248, 1985.
141. MATHIAS, J. R., M. H. CLENCH, R. H. DAVIS, C. A. SNINSKY, AND V. M. PIÑEIRO-CARRERO. Migrating action potential complex: unmasked by 6-hydroxydopamine. *Am. J. Physiol.* 249 (*Gastrointest. Liver Physiol.* 12): G416–G421, 1985.
142. MATHIAS, J. R., J. L. MARTIN, T. W. BURNS, G. M. CARLSON, AND R. P. SHIELDS. Ricinoleic acid effect on the electrical activity of the small intestine in rabbits. *J. Clin. Invest.* 61: 640–644, 1978.
143. MATHIAS, J. R., J. NOGUEIRA, J. L. MARTIN, G. M. CARLSON, AND R. A. GIANNELLA. *Escherichia coli* heat-stable toxin: its effect on motility of the small intestine. *Am. J. Physiol.* 242 (*Gastrointest. Liver Physiol.* 5): G360–G363, 1982.
144. MATHIAS, J. R., AND C. A. SNINSKY. Motor effects of enterotoxins and laxatives. In: *Intestinal Absorption and Secretion*, edited by E. Skadhauge and K. Heintze. Lancaster, UK: MTP, 1984, p. 161–169. (Falk Symp. Ser. no. 36.)
145. MATHIAS, J. R., AND C. A. SNINSKY. Motility of the small intestine: a look ahead. *Am. J. Physiol.* 248 (*Gastrointest. Liver Physiol.* 11): G495–G500, 1985.
146. MATHIAS, J. R., C. A. SNINSKY, J. L. MARTIN, AND A. FERNANDEZ. The migrating action potential complex in a human subject: a case of surreptitious laxative abuse diagnosed by recording probe (Abstract). *Clin. Res.* 31: 286A, 1983.
147. MATHIAS, J. R., C. A. SNINSKY, H. D. MILLAR, M. H. CLENCH, AND R. H. DAVIS. Development of an improved multi-pressure-sensor probe for recording muscle contraction in human intestine. *Dig. Dis. Sci.* 30: 119–123, 1985.

148. McCoy, E. J., AND R. D. Baker. Effect of feeding on electrical activity of dog's small intestine. *Am. J. Physiol.* 214: 1291–1295, 1968.
149. McCoy, E. J., AND P. Bass. Chronic electrical activity of gastroduodenal area: effects of food and certain catecholamines. *Am. J. Physiol.* 205: 439–445, 1963.
150. McDonel, J. L., AND C. L. Duncan. Histopathological effect of *Clostridium perfringens* enterotoxin in the rabbit ileum. *Infect. Immun.* 12: 1214–1218, 1975.
151. McEvoy, A., J. Dutton, AND O. F. James. Bacterial contamination of the small intestine is an important cause of occult malabsorption in the elderly. *Br. Med. J.* 287: 789–793, 1983.
152. McGowen, K., A. Kane, N. Asarkof, J. Wicks, V. Guerina, J. Kellum, S. Baron, A. R. Gintzler, AND M. Donowitz. *Entamoeba histolytica* causes intestinal secretion: role of serotonin. *Science Wash. DC* 221: 760–764, 1983.
153. Meltzer, S. J., AND J. Auer. Peristaltic rush. *Am. J. Physiol.* 20: 259–281, 1907.
154. Metchnikoff, E. Recherches sur le choléra et les vibrions. Mem. 4th. Sur l' immunité et la réceptivité vis-à-vis de choléra intestinal. *Ann. Inst. Pasteur Paris* 8: 529–589, 1894.
155. Miller, L. J., AND V. L. W. Go. Radioimmunoassay of cholecystokinin and gastric inhibitory peptide. In: *Gastrointestinal Hormones*, edited by G. B. J. Glass. New York: Raven, 1980, p. 863–864.
156. Moriarty, K. J., N. B. Higgs, M. Woodford, AND L. A. Turnberg. Is cholera toxin-induced intestinal secretion mediated via a neurogenic mechanism (Abstract). *Gut* 26: A111, 1985.
157. Moss, J., D. L. Burns, J. A. Hsia, E. L. Hewlett, R. L. Guerrant, AND M. Vaughan. Cyclic nucleotides: mediators of bacterial toxin action in disease. *Ann. Intern. Med.* 101: 653–666, 1984.
158. Moss, J., P. H. Fishman, R. L. Richards, C. R. Alving, M. Vaughan, AND R. O. Brady. Choleragen-mediated release of trapped glucose from liposomes containing ganglioside $G_{M1}$. *Proc. Natl. Acad. Sci. USA* 73: 3480–3483, 1976.
159. Moss, J., AND M. Vaughan. Activation of adenylate cyclase by choleragen. *Annu. Rev. Biochem.* 48: 581–600, 1979.
160. Nishizuka, V. Turnover of inositol phospholipids and signal transduction. *Science Wash. DC* 225: 1365–1370, 1984.
161. O'Brien, A. D., G. D. LaVeck, D. E. Griffin, AND M. R. Thompson. Characterization of *Shigella dysenteriae* 1 (Shiga) toxin purified by anti-Shiga toxin affinity chromatography. *Infect. Immun.* 30: 170–179, 1980.
162. Ouyang, A., W. J. Snape, Jr., AND S. Cohen. Myoelectric properties of the cat ileocecal sphincter. *Am. J. Physiol.* 240 (*Gastrointest. Liver Physiol.* 3): G450–G458, 1981.
163. Pearson, A. J., A. Brzechya-Ajdukiewicz, AND C. F. McCarthy. Intestinal pseudo-obstruction with bacterial overgrowth in the small intestine. *Am. J. Dig. Dis.* 14: 200–205, 1969.
164. Percy, W. H., AND J. Christensen. Antibiotic depression of evoked and spontaneous responses of opossum distal colonic muscularis mucosae in vitro: a factor in antibiotic-associated colitis? *Gastroenterology* 88: 964–970, 1985.
165. Pierce, N. F., W. B. Greenough III, AND C. C. Carpenter, Jr. *Vibrio cholerae* enterotoxin and its mode of action. *Bacteriol. Rev.* 35: 1–13, 1971.
166. Piñeiro-Carrero, V. M., M. H. Clench, R. H. Davis, J. M. Andres, AND J. R. Mathias. Alterations of the migrating myoelectric complex after destruction of enteric serotonergic neurons by 5,7,-dihydroxytryptamine (Abstract). *Gastroenterology* 88: 1540, 1985.
167. Piñeiro Carrero, V. M., M. H. Clench, R. H. Davis, J. M. Andres, AND J. R. Mathias. Myoelectric activity of the small intestine: depletion of catecholamines and serotonin within the myenteric plexus by reserpine (Abstract). *Gastroenterology* 88: 1540, 1985.
168. Pope, J. L., T. M. Parkinson, AND J. A. Olson. Action of bile salts on the metabolism and transport of water-soluble nutrients by perfused rat jejunum in vitro. *Biochim. Biophys. Acta* 130: 218–232, 1966.
169. Prizont, R., J. S. Whitehead, AND Y. S. Kim. Short chain fatty acids in rats with jejunal blind loops. I. Analysis of SCFA in small intestine, cecum, feces, and plasma. *Gastroenterology* 69: 1254–1264, 1975.
170. Roberts, S. H., O. James, AND E. H. Jarvis. Bacterial overgrowth syndrome without "blind loop"; a cause for malnutrition in the elderly. *Lancet* 2: 1193–1195, 1977.
171. Ruiz-Palacios, G. M., J. Torres, N. I. Torres, E. Escamilla, B. R. Ruiz-Palacios, AND J. Tamayo. Cholera-like enterotoxin produced by *Campylobacter jejuni*. Characterization and clinical significance. *Lancet* 2: 250–253, 1983.
172. Sack, R. B. Human diarrheal disease caused by enterotoxigenic *Escherichia coli*. *Annu. Rev. Microbiol.* 29: 333–353, 1975.
173. Sack, R. B., AND C. C. Carpenter. Experimental canine cholera. I. Development of the model. *J. Infect. Dis.* 119: 138–149, 1969.
174. Sack, R. B., S. L. Gorbach, J. G. Banwell, B. Jacobs, B. D. Chatterjee, AND R. C. Mitra. Enterotoxigenic *Escherichia coli* isolated from patients with severe cholera-like disease. *J. Infect. Dis.* 123: 378–385, 1971.
175. Salen, G., F. Goldstein, AND C. W. Wirts. Malabsorption in intestinal scleroderma. Relation to bacterial flora and treatment with antibiotics. *Ann. Intern. Med.* 64: 834–841, 1966.
176. Sanarelli, G. De la pathogénie du choléra. Le "choléra intestinal" des jeunes animaux. *Ann. Inst. Pasteur Paris* 35: 745–796, 1921.
177. Sarr, M. G., AND K. A. Kelly. Myoelectric activity of the autotransplanted canine jejunum. *Gastroenterology* 81: 303–310, 1981.
178. Schafer, D. E., W. D. Lust, B. Sircar, AND N. D. Goldberg. Elevated concentration of adenosine $3':5'$-cyclic monophosphate in intestinal mucosa after treatment with cholera toxin. *Proc. Natl. Acad. Sci. USA* 67: 851–856, 1970.
179. Sharp, G. W., AND S. Hynie. Stimulation of intestinal adenyl cyclase by cholera toxin. *Nature Lond.* 229: 266–269, 1971.
180. Sherwood, W. C., F. Goldstein, F. I. Haurani, AND C. W. Wirts. Studies on the small-intestinal bacterial flora and of intestinal absorption in pernicious anemia. *Am. J. Dig. Dis.* 9: 416–425, 1964.
181. Shiff, S. J., R. D. Soloway, AND W. J. Snape, Jr. Mechanism of deoxycholic acid stimulation of the rabbit colon. *J. Clin. Invest.* 69: 985–992, 1982.
182. Shimoda, S. S., T. K. O'Brien, AND D. R. Saunders. Fat absorption after infusing bile salts into the human small intestine. *Gastroenterology* 67: 7–18, 1974.
183. Sinar, D. R., L. G. Charles, AND T. W. Burns. Migrating action-potential complex activity in absence of fluid production is produced by B subunit of cholera enterotoxin. *Am. J. Physiol.* 242 (*Gastrointest. Liver Physiol.* 5): G47–G51, 1982.
184. Skirrow, M. B. *Campylobacter* enteritis: a 'new' disease. *Br. Med. J.* 2: 9–11, 1977.
185. Smith, G. S., G. Warburst, AND L. A. Turnberg. Synthesis and degradation of prostaglandin $E_2$ in the epithelium and subepithelial layers of the rat intestine. *Biochim. Biophys. Acta* 713: 684–687, 1982.
186. Smyth, P. M. Changes in intestinal bacterial flora and role of infection in kwashiorkor. *Lancet* 2: 724–727, 1958.
187. Snape, W. J., Jr., S. Shiff, AND S. Cohen. Effect of deoxycholic acid on colonic motility in the rabbit. *Am. J. Physiol.* 238 (*Gastrointest. Liver Physiol.* 1): G321–G325, 1980.
188. Sninsky, C. A., R. Ramphal, D. J. Gaskins, D. A. Goldberg, AND J. R. Mathias. Alterations of myoelectric activity associated with *Campylobacter jejuni* and its cell-free filtrate in the small intestine of rabbits. *Gastroenterology* 89: 337–344, 1985.
189. Sninsky, C. A., M. M. Wolfe, J. L. Martin, B. A. Howe, T. M. O'Dorisio, J. E. McGuigan, AND J. R. Mathias.

Myoelectric effects of vasoactive intestinal peptide on rabbit small intestine. *Am. J. Physiol.* 244 (*Gastrointest. Liver Physiol.* 7): G46–G51, 1983.

190. SNYDER, J. D., AND M. H. MERSON. The magnitude of the global problem of acute diarrhoeal disease: a review of active surveillance data. *Bull. WHO* 60: 605–613, 1982.
191. STAPLES, S. J., S. E. ASHER, AND R. A. GIANNELLA. Purification and characterization of heat-stable enterotoxin produced by a strain of *E. coli* pathogenic for man. *J. Biol. Chem.* 255: 4716–4721, 1980.
192. STARK, L., AND C. L. DUNCAN. Biologic characteristics of *Clostridium perfringens* type A enterotoxin. *Infect. Immun.* 4: 89–96, 1971.
193. STARKEY, B. J., D. SNARY, AND A. ALLEN. Characterization of gastric mucoproteins isolated by equilibrium density-gradient centrifugation in caesium chloride. *Biochem. J.* 141: 633–639, 1974.
194. STROMBECK, D. R., AND D. HARROLD. Binding of cholera toxin to mucins and inhibition by gastric mucin. *Infect. Immun.* 10: 1266–1272, 1974.
195. STRONG, D. H., C. L. DUNCAN, AND G. PERRA. *Clostridium perfringens* type A food poisoning. II. Response of the rabbit ileum as an indication of enteropathogenicity of strains of *Clostridium perfringens* in human beings. *Infect. Immun.* 3: 171–178, 1971.
196. SZURSZEWSKI, J. H. A migrating electric complex of the canine small intestine. *Am. J. Physiol.* 217: 1757–1763, 1969.
197. TABAQCHALI, S. The pathophysiological role of small intestinal bacterial flora. *Scand. J. Gastroenterol. Suppl.* 6: 139–163, 1970.
198. TAYLOR, N. S., AND J. G. BARTLETT. Partial purification and characterization of a cytotoxin from *Clostridium difficile*. *Rev. Infect. Dis.* 1: 379–385, 1979.
199. TAYLOR, N. S., G. M. THORNE, AND J. G. BARTLETT. Comparison of two toxins produced by *Clostridium difficile*. *Infect. Immun.* 34: 1036–1043, 1981.
200. TIEN, X. Y., R. WAHAWISAN, L. J. WALLACE, AND T. S. GAGINELLA. Intestinal epithelial cells and musculature contain different muscarinic binding sites. *Life Sci.* 36: 1949–1955, 1985.
201. TOSKES, P. P., R. A. GIANNELLA, H. R. JERVIS, W. R. ROUT, AND A. TAKEUCHI. Small intestinal mucosal injury in the experimental blind loop syndrome. Light- and electron-microscopic and histochemical studies. *Gastroenterology* 68: 1193–1203, 1975.
202. VANE, J. R. Inhibition of prostaglandin synthesis as a mechanism of action for aspirin-like drugs. *Nature New Biol.* 231: 232–235, 1971.
203. VAN HEYNINGEN, W. E., C. C. J. CARPENTER, N. F. PIERCE, AND W. B. GREENOUGH III. Deactivation of cholera toxin by ganglioside. *J. Infect. Dis.* 124: 415–418, 1971.
204. VAN HEYNINGEN, W. E., AND G. P. GLADSTONE. The neurotoxin of *Shigella shigae*; production, purification and properties of the toxin. *Br. J. Exp. Pathol.* 34: 202–216, 1953.
205. VANTRAPPEN, G., J. JANSSENS, J. HELLMANS, AND Y. CHOOS. The interdigestive motor complex of normal subjects and patients with bacterial overgrowth of the small intestine. *J. Clin. Invest.* 59: 1158–1166, 1977.
206. VICARI, G., A. L. OLITZKI, AND Z. OLITZKI. The action of the thermolabile toxin of *Shigella dysenteriae* on cells cultivated in vitro. *Br. J. Exp. Pathol.* 41: 179–189, 1960.
207. WAHAWISAN, R., L. J. WALLACE, AND T. S. GAGINELLA. Muscarinic receptors on rat ileal villus and crypt cells. *J. Pharm. Pharmacol.* 38: 150–153, 1986.
208. WALSH, J. A., AND K. S. WARREN. Selective primary health care. *N. Engl. J. Med.* 301: 967–974, 1979.
209. WANITSCHKE, R., AND H. V. AMMON. Effects of dihydroxy bile acids and hydroxy fatty acids on the absorption of oleic acid in the human jejunum. *J. Clin. Invest.* 61: 178–186, 1978.
210. WEIKEL, C. S., J. J. SANDO, AND R. L. GUERRANT. C-kinase activators stimulate intestinal secretion in vivo (Abstract). *Clin. Res.* 33: 327A, 1985.
211. WEISBERG, P. B., G. M. CARLSON, AND S. COHEN. Effect of *Salmonella typhimurium* on myoelectrical activity in the rabbit ileum. *Gastroenterology* 74: 47–51, 1978.
212. WOOD, J. D., AND C. J. MAYER. Serotonergic activation of tonic-type enteric neurons in guinea pig small bowel. *J. Neurophysiol.* 42: 582–593, 1979.
213. WU, Z. C., S. D. KISSLINGER, AND T. S. GAGINELLA. Functional evidence for the presence of cholinergic nerve endings in the colonic mucosa of the rat. *J. Pharmacol. Exp. Ther.* 221: 664–669, 1981.

CHAPTER 32

# Motor and myoelectric activity associated with vomiting, regurgitation, and nausea

IVAN M. LANG
SUSHIL K. SARNA

*Departments of Surgery and Physiology, Medical College of Wisconsin, and Surgical Research Service, Zablocki Veterans Administration Medical Center, Milwaukee, Wisconsin*

## CHAPTER CONTENTS

Digestive Tract Motor and Myoelectric Activity Associated With Vomiting
  Motor events
    Esophagus and its sphincters
    Proximal stomach
    Antrum and small intestine
    Colon and gallbladder
  Myoelectric events
    Antrum and small intestine
    Independence from retching and vomitus expulsion
    Functions of retrograde giant contraction
  Neural control
    Sensory receptors and afferent pathways
    Central integration
    Efferent innervation
  Neuropharmacology
    Dopaminergic receptors
    Opiate receptors
    Cholinergic receptors
    Adrenergic receptors
    Serotonergic receptors
    Nonadrenergic-noncholinergic receptors
    Peptidergic receptors
Digestive Tract Motor Activity Associated With Regurgitation
Nausea and Prodromal Signs of Vomiting
  Nausea
    Sensory mechanisms of gastrointestinal tract
    Gastrointestinal correlates of nausea
  Prodromal signs of vomiting
Conclusions

---

*It is remarkable how little has been written about the behavior of the bowel during the act of vomiting. One can read for days about the roles played by the medulla, the vagi, the pharyngeal sensitive points, the esophagus, the abdominal muscles, and the stomach, but only here and there will one find a brief reference to the bowel.*
                                    W. C. Alvarez (10)

THIS STATEMENT IN 1925 could have been written today. Because of the lack of research investigations and the inadequacies of older recording techniques, the existence of significant motor events of the small intestine occurring in association with vomiting was not widely known even 50 years (40) after such activity was first graphically recorded by Alvarez (10). By the 1970s, however, reliable techniques for recording gastrointestinal myoelectric (130) and contractile (14) activity from awake animals had been developed, and a better understanding of this role of the digestive tract in vomiting and related phenomena had begun to emerge. Although evidence for the importance of the gastrointestinal tract in vomiting has been documented for over 100 years (94, 100, 103, 132), we are just beginning to understand these events.

## DIGESTIVE TRACT MOTOR AND MYOELECTRIC ACTIVITY ASSOCIATED WITH VOMITING

In many studies of the role of the digestive tract in vomiting, investigators limited their viewpoint to vomitus expulsion and concluded that the digestive tract played little role in vomiting (21, 40). However, vomitus expulsion is only the culmination of numerous physiological events. This chapter considers vomiting not just vomitus expulsion but all of the autonomic, somatomotor, and behavioral responses stereotypically associated with vomitus expulsion: i.e., the responses that always occur in the same temporal sequence regardless of the emetic stimulus.

### Motor Events

ESOPHAGUS AND ITS SPHINCTERS. Direct visualization of the esophagus in dogs revealed in 1881 that retrograde contractions did not occur in the esophagus during vomiting (88). Rather the esophagus filled and emptied with gastric contents at each retch until finally the esophageal contents were released into the oral cavity during vomitus expulsion [Fig. 1; (58)]. These findings were later confirmed in the cat (109), dog (82), and human (82) with radiographic tech-

1180   HANDBOOK OF PHYSIOLOGY ~ THE GASTROINTESTINAL SYSTEM I

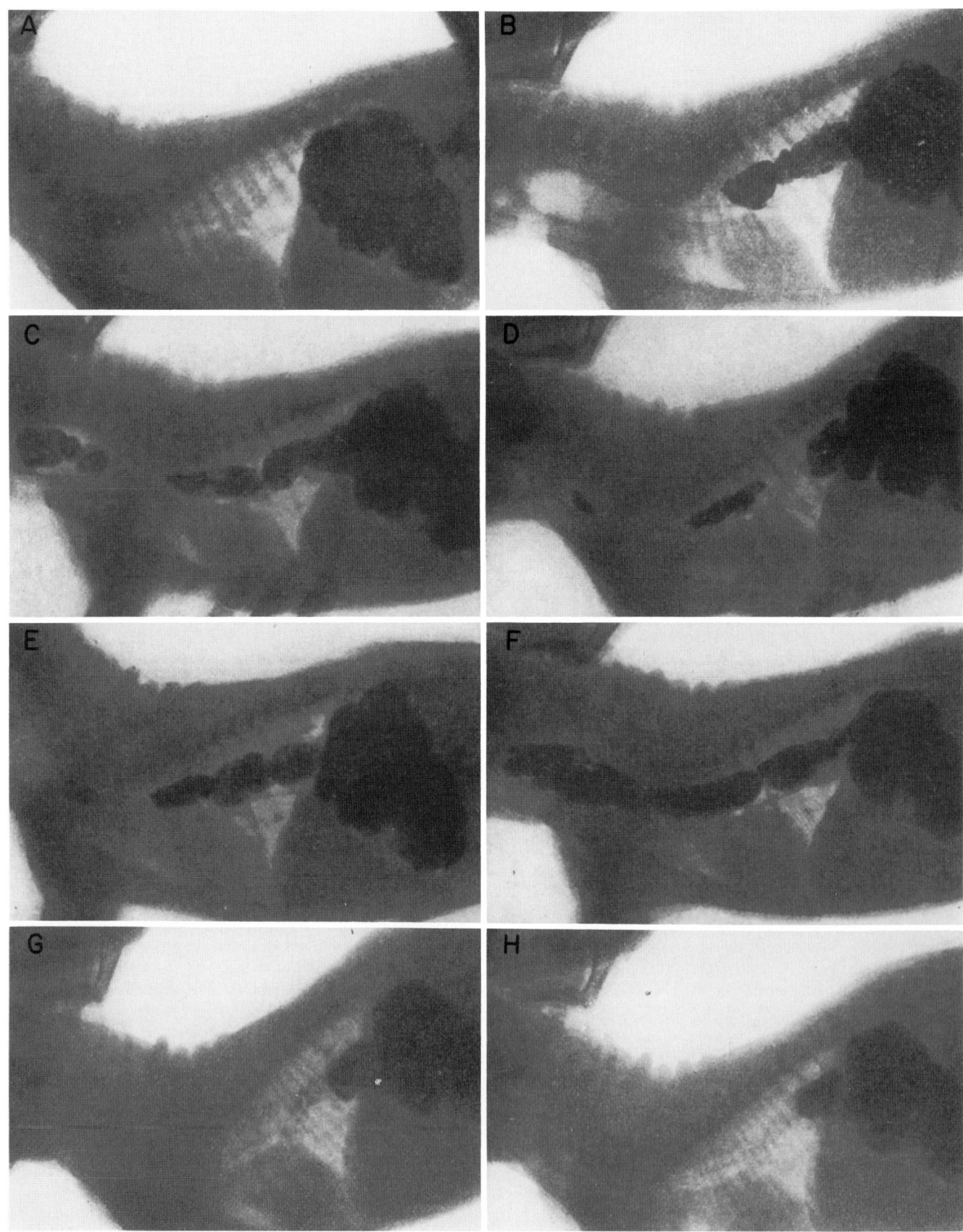

niques. The free flow of luminal contents between stomach and esophagus was aided by dilation of the cardia and gastroesophageal junction, which remained open during the entire retching episode and formed a funnel between the stomach and the esophagus [Fig. 2; (34, 58, 62, 82, 109, 131)]. In 1983 Derbyshire and Ferguson (34) found, and Smith and Brizzee (109) later confirmed, that the dilation of the gastroesophageal junction actually occurred prior to retching. By radiographically observing the movement of metal markers sutured to the diaphragm and cardia of dogs, Johnson and Laws (62) found that the gastroesophageal junction dilated as much as 1 min before retching and that the hiatus and cardia rose into the thoracic cavity by 3 and 4.5 cm, respectively. This resulted in elimination of the abdominal esophagus and produced a transient hiatal hernia of the cardia (Fig. 3). Furthermore, metal markers sutured to the submucosa rose 7 cm, and at this level of the esophagus the lumen became constricted. A similar elevation of the cardia (84) and esophageal constriction (109) were observed by others in cats. Direct recording of esophageal contractile activity indicated that most of the longitudinal contraction occurred in the skeletal muscle portion of the esophagus (120). Thus prior to vomiting the longitudinal muscle of the esophagus contracts, pulling open a relaxed gastroesophageal junction, which forms a funnel allowing free flow of gastric contents to the esophagus.

The difference in physiological events between retching and vomitus expulsion that allows oral evacuation of gastric contents is attributed to the respiratory rather than the gastrointestinal musculature. During retching, both diaphragmatic dome and crura muscular fibers contract, but during vomitus expulsion only the dome fibers contract (93a). The relaxed hiatus allows oral reflux of gastric contents in response to increased abdominal pressure caused by contraction of the diaphragmatic dome and abdominal muscles. After vomitus expulsion, the remaining esophageal contents are swept into the stomach by secondary peristaltic contractions that are followed by closure of the lower esophageal sphincter and return of the cardia to its usual position (82, 109).

PROXIMAL STOMACH. Radiographic studies in humans (82), cats (25, 100, 109), and dogs (58) revealed that spontaneous contractions of the proximal stomach ceased and the proximal stomach dilated before or at the onset of retching. No retrograde contraction or other type of strong contraction of the proximal stomach was observed during each retch or during vomitus expulsion; therefore all investigators con-

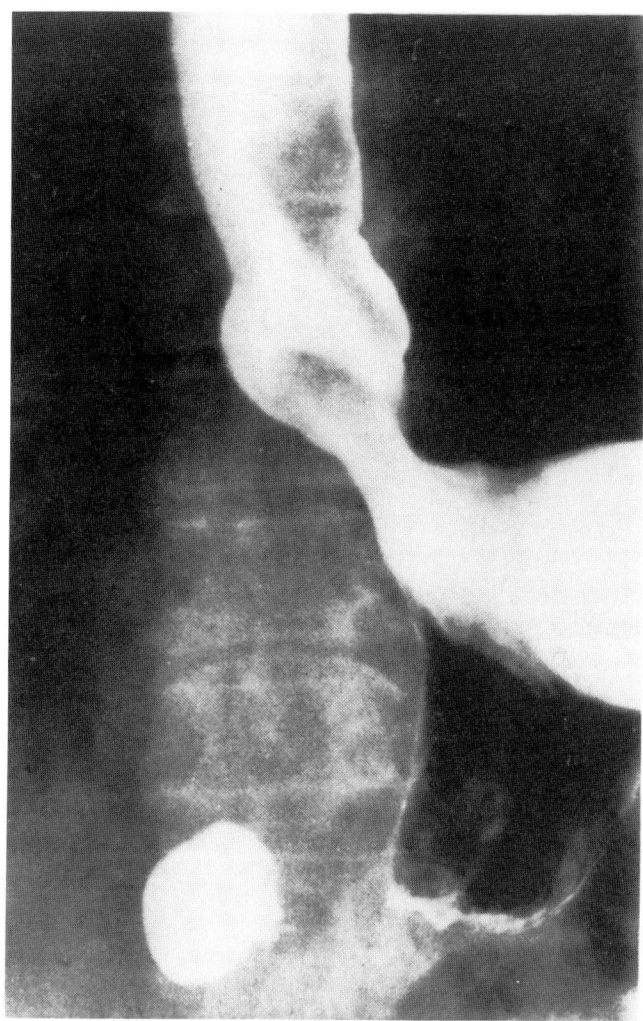

FIG. 2. Radiograph of the stomach and esophagus of a woman in supine position during vomitus expulsion of barium. Cardia and gastroesophageal junction are elevated and dilated, forming a funnel between the stomach and esophagus. [From Lundsen and Holden (82).]

FIG. 1. Consecutive radiographs of abdomen, thorax, and neck of a dog before, during, and after retching and vomitus expulsion. Prior to initiation of vomiting by apomorphine (1.5 mg/kg), 1.2-kg dog was fed 50 g of finely ground meat with 10 g of contrast material. A: contrast material filled the stomach but was not displaced during prodromal signs of vomiting. B: 60 s later the first retch occurred, which propelled the gastric contents into lower third of esophagus as gastroesophageal junction widened. Time between each radiograph from B to G was 3–5 s. C: contrast material moved to cervical esophagus but expulsion to oral cavity did not occur. D: at end of the retch, contents of esophagus returned to the stomach as gastroesophageal junction remained dilated. E: next retch propelled gastric contents back into esophagus. F: esophagus became filled with contrast material, and expulsion to oral cavity occurred between F and G. G: after vomitus expulsion, dilated gastroesophageal junction and cardia remained filled with contrast material. H: 6 s later the stomach contour had not yet returned to control state. [From Hesse (58).]

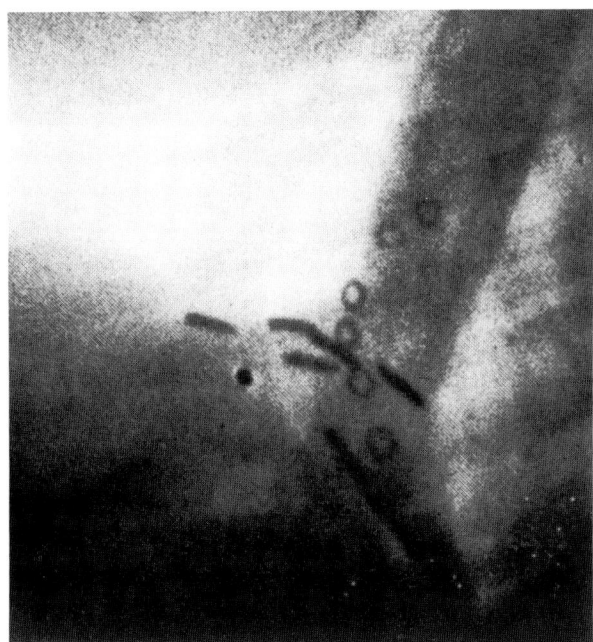

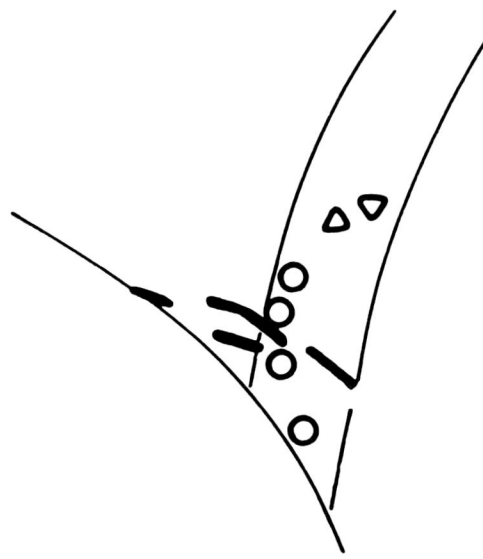

FIG. 3. Radiograph (*top*) and diagram (*bottom*) of gastroesophageal region of a dog with metal markers sewn on hiatus and gastroesophageal junction just prior to retching and vomiting. Six metal bars were sewn on upper surface of crura of the diaphragm, forming a ring around the esophageal hiatus. Four metal rings were sewn on seromuscular layer of cardia in a line around the circumference. Two metal triangles were sewn on submucosa of the most distal centimeter of esophagus after separation of the overlying seromuscular layer. This radiograph was taken 1 min after apomorphine administration (2 mg iv) but before onset of retching or vomitus expulsion. Markers of submucosa and cardia have risen in the thoracic cavity, but markers of the hiatus have not. [From Johnson and Laws (62).]

cluded that motor activity of the proximal stomach did not aid in the retropulsion of gastric contents (25, 58, 82, 100, 109).

Relaxation of the proximal stomach during vomiting was graphically recorded with balloon manometry in the awake dog (3, 76, 77) and decerebrate cat [Fig. 4; (4, 5)]. These studies found that the tone of the proximal stomach decreased ~2 min before vomitus expulsion and lasted ~20 min. In addition, doses of emetic agents just below the level that initiated vomiting still reduced gastric tone (3, 4, 77).

ANTRUM AND SMALL INTESTINE. The role of the antrum and small intestine during vomiting has been disputed for ~100 years. Even as late as 1978 (40), the consensus of many gastroenterologists was that motor activity of the small intestine played little role in emesis and that no retrograde contraction occurred during any part of the vomiting process. It is now well established, however, that prior to vomiting a single giant contraction begins in the small intestine and propagates retrogradely through the gastric antrum. Evidence for this retrograde giant contraction (RGC) has been found in humans (33, 82, 118), dogs (6, 12, 29, 38, 39, 42, 58, 71, 115), and cats (10, 12, 100, 109, 115) with many different techniques, including radiography (33, 42, 58, 82, 100, 109), fluoroscopy (29, 38), direct kymographic recording of contractile activity (10), manometry (12, 83, 101, 118), and mechanoelectrical transduction (6, 38, 39, 71). This contraction is called a giant contraction because its amplitude and duration are ~1.5 and 3 times larger than the peak contractions of the migrating motor complex (6, 71). The failure of other investigators to observe or record the RGC prior to vomiting can be attributed to differences in techniques. In all known investigations of the gastrointestinal motor responses during vomiting in which the RGC was never observed, contractile activity had been recorded from either transected segments of the small intestine (47–50, 66, 108) or intestinal segments whose walls had been physically disrupted by the injection of contrast material (87). These techniques may have altered responses of the segments under study by damaging the enteric nervous system or severing enteric neural pathways (67a).

Recent characterization of the gastrointestinal motor events accompanying spontaneous episodes of vomiting in the dog has revealed four distinct motor patterns, referred to collectively as the gastrointestinal motor correlates of vomiting (71). These patterns occur in the following order (Fig. 5): *1*) a large-amplitude contraction of the small intestine that begins ~170 cm from the pylorus and travels retrogradely at ~8 cm/s to the gastric antrum, the RGC; *2*) a period of decreased contractile activity of the small intestine both orad and aborad to the propagating RGC that begins and ends at the same times as the RGC, the peri-RGC inhibitory period; *3*) a series of moderate-amplitude phasic contractions that occur after the RGC at all levels of the small intestine and last longest in the small intestine below the point of initiation of RGC, the post-RGC phasic contractions; and *4*) a period of decreased contractile activity of the upper

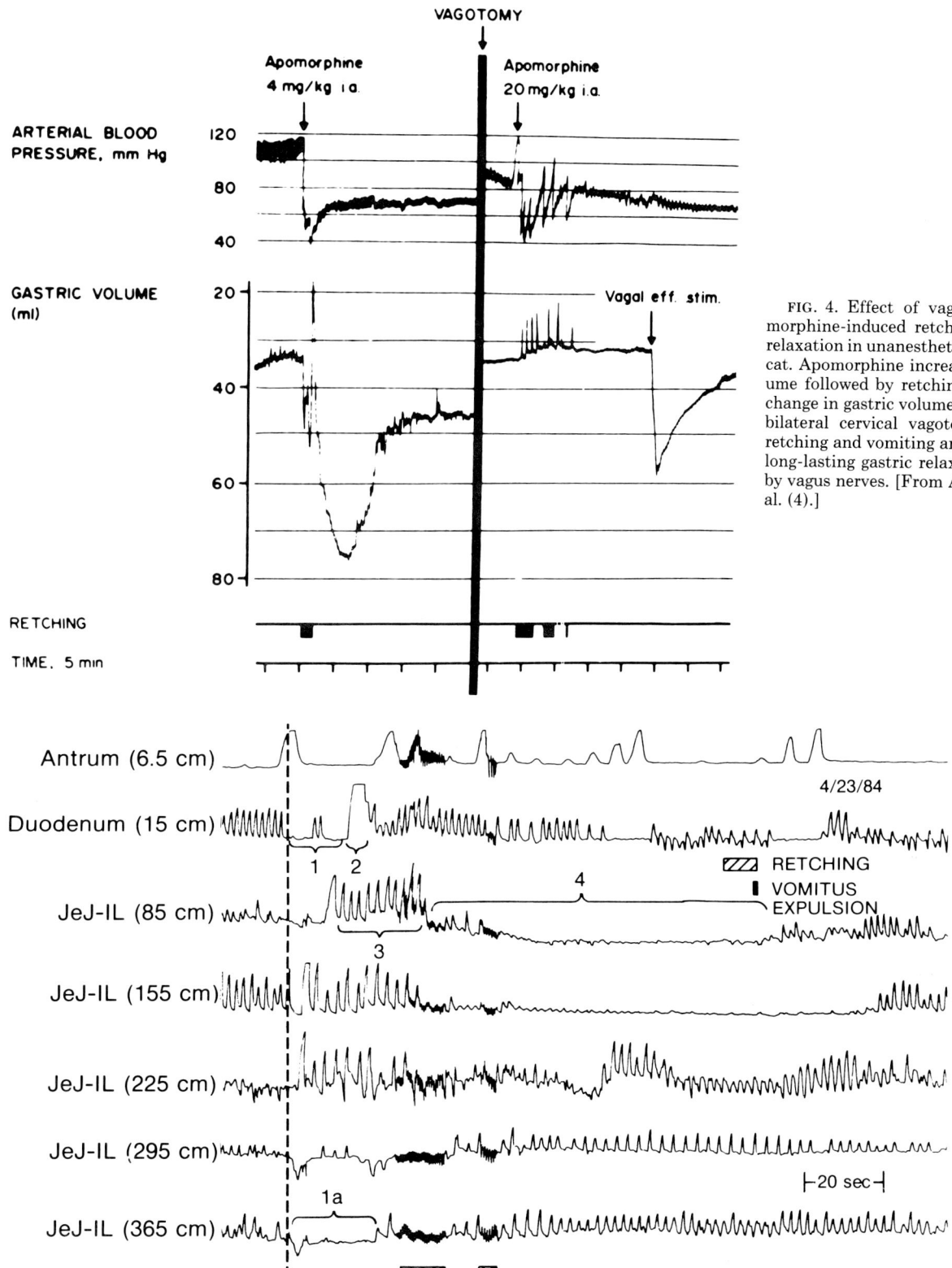

FIG. 4. Effect of vagotomy on apomorphine-induced retching and gastric relaxation in unanesthetized decerebrate cat. Apomorphine increased gastric volume followed by retching, but only the change in gastric volume was blocked by bilateral cervical vagotomy. Therefore retching and vomiting are preceded by a long-lasting gastric relaxation mediated by vagus nerves. [From Abrahamsson et al. (4).]

FIG. 5. Gastrointestinal motor correlates of vomiting in the dog. This emetic episode occurred spontaneously. Numbers in parentheses indicate position in gastrointestinal tract of strain-gauge force transducers from the pylorus. *Broken vertical line*, time of first observation of gastrointestinal motor correlates of vomiting. Numbers on chart identify the 4 different motor responses comprising gastrointestinal motor correlates of vomiting: *1* and *1a*, peri–retrograde giant contraction (RGC) inhibitory period of small intestine; *2*, RGC; *3*, post-RGC phasic contractions; and *4*, post-RGC inhibitory period. [From Lang et al. (71). Copyright 1986 by The American Gastroenterological Association.]

small intestine lasting only 1–5 min, the post-RGC inhibitory period.

The RGC has also been referred to as the retrograde peristaltic contraction [RPC (71)], retroperistaltism (38), reverse peristalsis (10, 38, 39, 42, 109), or antiperistalsis (6, 12, 29, 66, 87, 101); however, as others have cautioned (11, 59, 128), the term *peristalsis* can be misleading. According to Bayliss and Starling (17), peristalsis consists of a contraction preceded by inhibition where both contraction and inhibition propagate along the bowel. The RGC probably does not represent such a contraction because the inhibition of the small intestine during propagation of the RGC (peri-RGC inhibitory period) occurs simultaneously at all levels (71). In addition this inhibition is independent of the RGC because pharmacological blockade of the RGC by atropine does not block the peri-RGC inhibitory period (71). The use of the term *peristaltic* to refer to the RGC therefore may be confusing and misleading.

The RGC is one of the strongest contractions recorded from the small intestine. The RGC amplitude is greatest in the duodenum (170% of peak contractions of phase III activity of migrating motor complex), and the amplitude decreases progressively in the aboral direction until its point of initiation, where the amplitude is ~125% of phase III contractions. The RGC of the gastric antrum is about the same amplitude (105%) as phase III antral contractions [Table 1; (71)].

The gastrointestinal motor correlates of vomiting that occur during spontaneous emetic episodes do not differ qualitatively from those that occur during vomiting activated by low or moderate doses of the emetic apomorphine [Fig. 6; (70, 71)]: i.e., doses of apomorphine (2.5–15 µg/kg iv) that caused three or fewer vomits. When more than one vomit occurred, however, the second or third vomit may not be preceded by an RGC or the other gastrointestinal motor correlates of vomiting. At high doses of apomorphine (10 mg sc) neither vomiting nor its gastrointestinal motor correlates may occur (38).

Specific components of the gastrointestinal motor correlates of vomiting activated by different emetic agents and different doses were compared quantitatively (71). The magnitude of the RGC at different levels of the gastrointestinal tract and the starting point of the RGC in the small intestine were not significantly different whether activated by apomorphine, luminal irritation, or spontaneously (Table 2). In addition these variables did not differ at doses of apomorphine ranging from 2.5 to 10 µg/kg (Table 1). This all-or-none nature of the RGC suggested that emetic agents did not directly control the gastrointestinal correlates of vomiting but simply triggered a set of responses whose attributes were determined by other factors. Although the magnitude of the RGC and its starting point do not depend on the dose of emetic agent, the probability of activating the gastrointestinal correlates of vomiting and the number of vomits do increase with the dose (71).

The peri-RGC inhibitory period (12, 29, 47–50, 71, 83), the post-RGC phasic contractions (12, 38, 47–50, 66, 71, 83, 101), and the post-RGC inhibitory period (49, 50, 71) have been observed by various investigators over the past 60 years, but these components of the gastrointestinal motor correlates of vomiting have not yet been fully characterized or quantified.

Using radiographic (25, 82) or fluoroscopic (33, 58) techniques, some early investigators described a strong stationary contraction of the pylorus or antrum during retching that formed a barrier between the proximal stomach and the duodenum but did not observe the RGC. These early investigators probably did not observe the RGC because of its rapid velocity in the small intestine (6, 71) and mistook the long-duration antral (6, 38, 39, 71) and pyloric (38, 39) component of the RGC as a stationary contraction. In their attempt to determine the role of the gastrointestinal tract during the somatomotor phase of vomiting, i.e., retching and vomitus expulsion, many observations were made at the start of the retching movement, a time when the RGC had already traversed the small intestine (6, 38, 39, 71) and the antrum was still

TABLE 1. *Lack of Relationship Between Apomorphine Dose and Magnitude of RGC Variables*

| RGC Variable | Apomorphine Dose, µg/kg iv | | | | |
|---|---|---|---|---|---|
| | 2.5 | 5.0 | 7.5 | 10.0 | $P(F)$ |
| Starting point, cm from pylorus | 170 ± 20 | 177 ± 17 | 171 ± 14 | 182 ± 18 | NS |
| Velocity to antrum, cm/s | 8.2 ± 0.8 | 9.2 ± 1.1 | 9.3 ± 1.1 | 8.6 ± 1.2 | NS |
| Velocity to duodenum, cm/s | 10.6 ± 0.6 | 11.8 ± 0.9 | 10.9 ± 1.2 | 10.5 ± 1.7 | NS |
| Magnitude, % of phase III contractile height | | | | | |
| Gastric antrum | 104 ± 6 | 107 ± 6 | 107 ± 4 | 105 ± 5 | NS |
| Duodenum | 177 ± 7 | 172 ± 8 | 180 ± 10 | 171 ± 10 | NS |
| Jejunum, 0%–19% | 159 ± 5 | 159 ± 5 | 157 ± 5 | 161 ± 5 | NS |
| Jejunum, 20%–39% | 156 ± 15 | 153 ± 13 | 155 ± 18 | 156 ± 10 | NS |
| Jejunum, 40%–65% | 122 ± 10 | 118 ± 16 | 126 ± 5 | 122 ± 9 | NS |

Values are means ± SE for 5 animals. RGC, retrograde giant contraction; $P(F)$, probability of a difference in variables due to dose of apomorphine by one-way analysis of variance; NS, not statistically significant. [From Lang et al. (71). Copyright 1986 by The American Gastroenterological Association.]

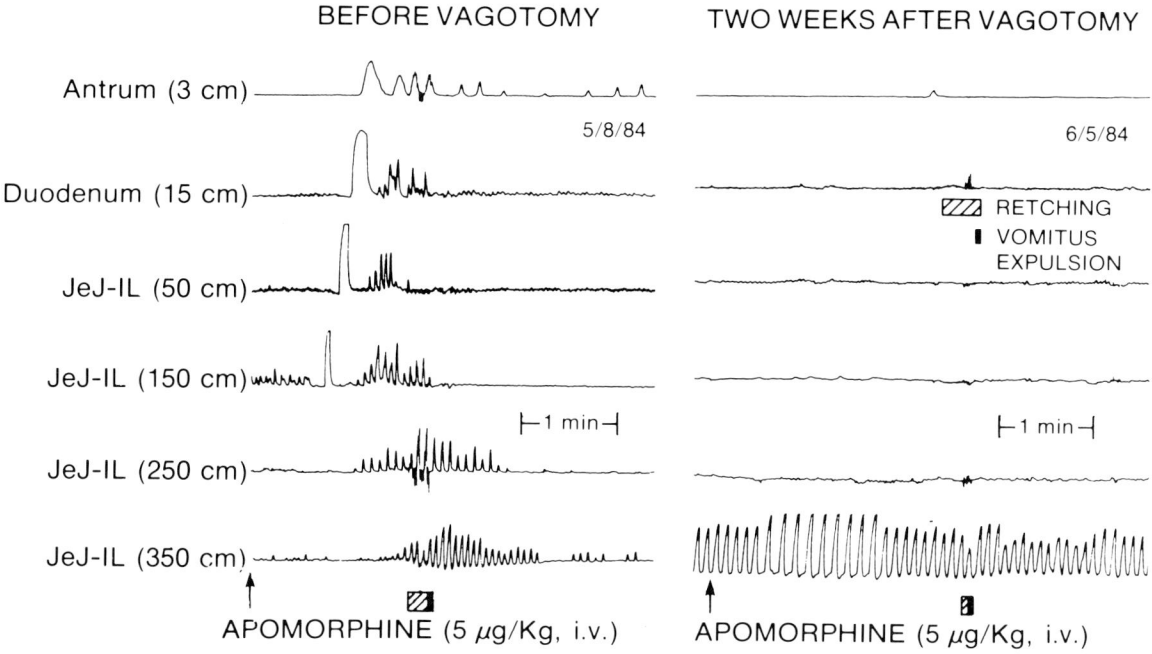

FIG. 6. Effect of supradiaphragmatic vagotomy on gastrointestinal motor correlates of vomiting activated by apomorphine. Vagotomy blocked gastrointestinal motor correlates of vomiting but not retching or vomitus expulsion. [From Lang et al. (71). Copyright 1986 by The American Gastroenterological Association.]

TABLE 2. *Characteristics of RGC Activated Under Different Conditions*

| RGC Variable | Spontaneous RGC | | Apomorphine (5 µg/kg) | | Luminal Stimulation, No vomit | $P(F)$ |
|---|---|---|---|---|---|---|
| | No Vomit | Vomit | No Vomit | Vomit | | |
| Starting point, cm from pylorus | 173 ± 21 | 168 ± 22 | 180 ± 17 | 171 ± 14 | 182 ± 16 | NS |
| Velocity to antrum, cm/s | 15.3 ± 2.1[1] | 7.9 ± 0.6[2] | 9.6 ± 1.0[2] | 8.7 ± 0.8[2] | 16.1 ± 1.2[1] | <0.01 |
| Velocity to duodenum, cm/s | 25.5 ± 4.3[1] | 11.2 ± 1.0[2] | 12.3 ± 1.6[2] | 11.4 ± 0.4[2] | 27.0 ± 4.3[1] | <0.01 |
| Magnitude, % of phase III contractile height | | | | | | |
| Gastric antrum | 107 ± 13 | 106 ± 13 | 108 ± 6 | 107 ± 5 | 102 ± 9 | NS |
| Duodenum | 172 ± 15 | 170 ± 9 | 169 ± 5 | 173 ± 8 | 170 ± 6 | NS |
| Jejunum, 0%–19% | 164 ± 11 | 154 ± 8 | 161 ± 4 | 156 ± 6 | 148 ± 14 | NS |
| Jejunum, 20%–39% | 157 ± 16 | 152 ± 7 | 150 ± 5 | 155 ± 10 | 139 ± 6 | NS |
| Jejunum, 40%–65% | 129 ± 13 | 126 ± 15 | 122 ± 13 | 119 ± 14 | 125 ± 6 | NS |

Values are means ± SE for 5 animals. RGC, retrograde giant contraction; $P(F)$, probability of a difference in variable due to experimental conditions by analysis of variance; NS, no statistically significant difference; [1] and [2], values with the same superscript were not significantly different by the Newman-Keuls multiple-comparison test but those with different superscripts were significantly different. [From Lang et al. (71). Copyright 1986 by The American Gastroenterological Association.]

contracted by the RGC (38,71). In addition the RGC may occur prior to the first of a series of vomits only (70, 71).

COLON AND GALLBLADDER. Few studies of the motor responses from colon or gallbladder associated with vomiting have been reported, and some of these reports are contradictory. In 1917 Alvarez (9) noted numerous clinical examples of vomitus expulsion of colonic contents, but these findings do not necessarily indicate the activation of specific motor responses of the colon. To the contrary, Weitz and Vollers (131) observed no change in colonic tone during vomiting in humans. Some investigators (72, 99) have recorded transient increases in colonic pressure during retching episodes using balloon manometry in anesthetized dogs, but these changes may have been due to the increased intra-abdominal pressure generated by retching (84).

Bile-stained vomitus is a common observation (9, 101, 135) that was noted as early as 1893 by Hirsch (60). Using radiographic techniques in humans, Sosman et al. (110) observed gallbladder contraction during vomiting, but under similar conditions Levine (79) found gallbladder relaxation. Perhaps both responses occur in association with vomiting, because Ohasi (99)

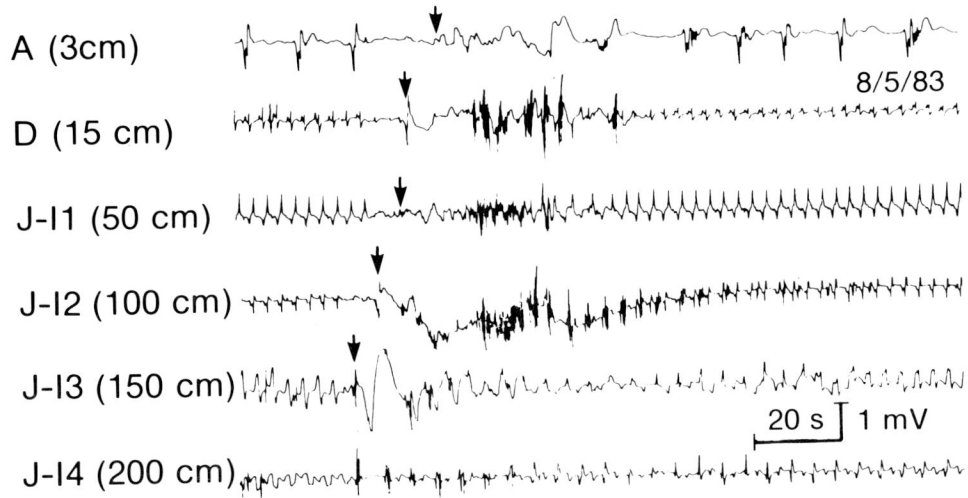

FIG. 7. Myoelectric responses associated with gastrointestinal motor correlates of vomiting. These responses occurred spontaneously and were not followed by retching or vomitus expulsion. Arrows, occurrences of the RGC potential (i.e., myoelectric correlate of RGC). Cycling of electrical control activity (ECA) in small intestine is disrupted before and after RGC potential. A, antrum; D, duodenum; and J-I, jejunoileum. [From Lang et al. (70).]

observed gallbladder contraction just prior to retching and gallbladder relaxation during and after retching in anesthetized dogs.

*Myoelectric Events*

ANTRUM AND SMALL INTESTINE. The myoelectric activity of the digestive tract associated with vomiting so far has been recorded only from the gastric antrum and small intestine of animals. Two distinct changes in gastrointestinal electrical control activity (ECA) of dogs occur in association with vomiting: *1*) slowing of ECA frequency (70) and *2*) partial or complete loss of ECA cycling (29, 70, 75, 85, 93) referred to as ECA disruption [Fig. 7; (70)]. The slowing of ECA frequency preceded ECA disruption; furthermore, whereas ECA disruption occurred only in the gastric antrum and upper half of the small intestine, the slowing of ECA frequency occurred primarily in the lower half of the small intestine [Fig. 8; (70)]. The ECA frequency of the lower half of the small intestine slowed a maximum of ~4 cycles/min, and the duration of this slowing increased aborad from 1 min in the jejunum to ~6 min in the ileum (70). The slowing of ECA frequency of the gastric antrum lasted ~1 min. The ECA disruption began at about the middle of the small intestine and propagated orad to the duodenum at ~15 cm/s. The duration of ECA disruption in the middle of the small intestine was ~6 s and increased orad to ~20 s in the duodenum. During the interval of ECA disruption of the small intestine, the base-line electrical activity sometimes fluctuated widely (70, 85).

These changes in ECA organization are the same in both spontaneous and pharmacologically induced vomiting (70). Qualitatively similar changes in ECA were reported in the cat (113, 114, 129, 130). The differences between cat and dog are that in the cat the ECA disruption began at more aborad sites, the ECA

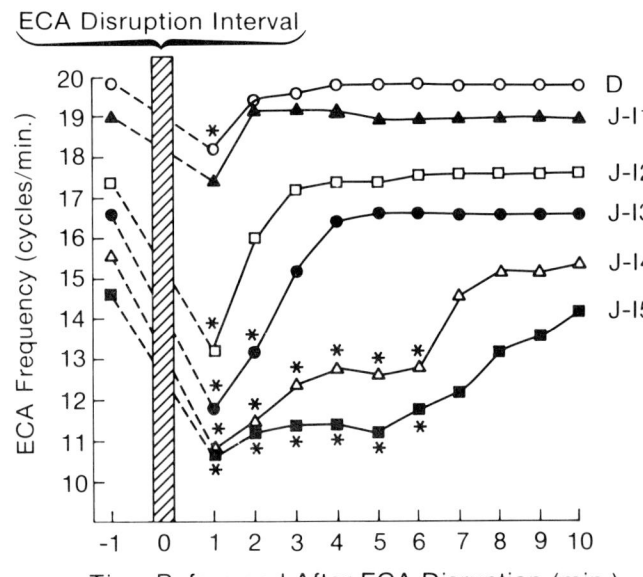

FIG. 8. Changes in ECA frequency in association with spontaneous occurrences of gastrointestinal motor correlates of vomiting. ECA frequency of lower jejunum and ileum slows ~4 cycles/min, and this slowing lasts longer at more distal sites. D, duodenum at 15 cm from pylorus; J-I, jejunoileum at 75 ± 5 cm (J-I1), 125 ± 5 cm (J-I2), 165 ± 5 cm (J-I3), 220 ± 5 cm (J-I4), and 285 ± 10 cm (J-I5) from pylorus. [From Lang et al. (70).]

frequency slowing lasted longer, and the duration of ECA slowing was the same at all sites. The slowing of ECA frequency and ECA disruption are probably not controlled by the same mechanism, because *1*) low doses of the emetic apomorphine initiated only the slowing of ECA frequency and *2*) the only intestinal myoelectric response associated with vomiting not blocked by prior administration of atropine was slowing of ECA frequency (70).

The RGC occurs only during the interval of ECA

disruption (70). The significance of this disruption in ECA cycling may be to eliminate the myogenic mechanisms that normally control the caudad propagation of phasic contractions in preparation for the orad propagation of the RGC (70, 85). The myoelectric correlate of the RGC in dogs consists of one or a few oscillations in electrical potential lasting <1 s (70, 85) that occur at the upstroke of the RGC [Fig. 9; (70)]. This correlation was accomplished by recording these electrical and contractile activities simultaneously from the same locations (70). A similar myoelectric activity was found in cats, except that the burst of electrical potentials lasted longer, i.e., ~2–5 s (113, 130). The duration and amplitude of usual phasic contractions of the small intestine are related to the number and frequency of potentials in a burst of electrical response activity (ERA) (13). Such a correlation does not exist for the RGC. The duration and amplitude of the RGC are much larger than those of the usual phasic contractions, and yet the electrical activity associated with this contraction is of much shorter duration and lower frequency than the activity associated with the usual phasic contractions. This lack of correlation between the magnitude of electrical and contractile activities makes it difficult to identify the RGC from recordings of electrical activity only. This uncertainty of identifying the RGC from electrical recordings only may account for the variety of myoelectric events during the RGC described in studies where contractile activity was not recorded simultaneously (8, 75, 91, 93).

In contrast to the RGC, the post-RGC phasic contractions occur only during the period of ECA frequency slowing (70) after ECA disruption has ended (Fig. 9). These contractions are associated with regular ECA cycles and are superimposed with bursts of ERA like the usual phasic contractions. Because these contractions are controlled in time and space by ECA, the maximum frequency of the post-RGC phasic contractions is slower than that of the usual phasic contractions.

In comparison with the small intestine, the myoelectric changes in the gastric antrum associated with RGC and post-RGC phasic contractions are less well defined. One reason for this is the irregular appearance of these changes (70, 75, 85, 91, 93). Although the RGC and post-RGC phasic contractions of the gastric antrum are quite similar to the corresponding contractile activity of the small intestine, the associated myoelectric events differ markedly. In the gastric antrum both the RGC and subsequent phasic contractions occur during an interval of ECA disruption (70) but are associated with random fluctuations in electrical activity [Fig. 9; (70, 85)], which some investigators have referred to as tachyarrhythmia (75).

No studies have been reported on the changes in myoelectric activity of the human gastric antrum and small intestine during vomiting. The main reason perhaps is that no satisfactory method is available to record myoelectric activity during vomiting. Intraluminal recording devices are unsatisfactory because they may be dislodged during retching and vomiting and may pose a hazard to the subject. Cutaneous recordings are possible (2, 43, 52, 111, 112), but the information obtainable by this method is limited because the signal-to-noise ratio is low, and only composite signals from the antrum are recordable.

*Independence From Retching and Vomitus Expulsion*

In 1917 Alvarez (9) hypothesized, based on anecdotal clinical findings, that the gastrointestinal motor

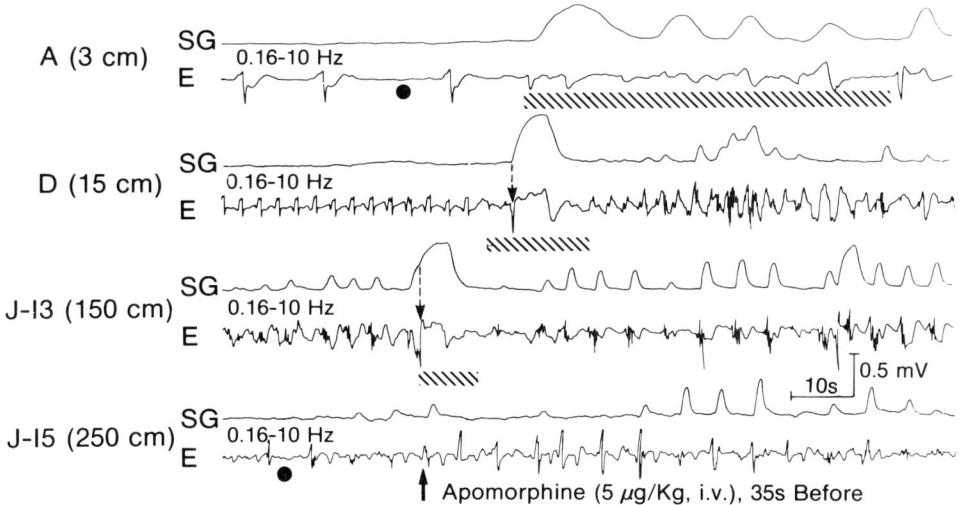

FIG. 9. Simultaneous recording of myoelectric (E) and contractile (SG) activities of gastrointestinal tract from same sites during gastrointestinal motor correlates of vomiting activated by apomorphine. *Hatched bars*, period of ECA disruption; *filled circles*, initiation of ECA frequency slowing; and *vertical arrows*, occurrences of RGC potential at upstroke of RGC. [From Lang et al. (70).]

correlates of vomiting may occur in other situations, e.g., nausea or regurgitation, and therefore represented a phenomenon independent of retching and vomitus expulsion. Evidence for this theory was presented in 1926 by Babsky (12). Using balloon manometry through fistulas of the gastrointestinal tract, he found that low doses of the emetic agents apomorphine (given subcutaneously) or cupric sulfate (oral administration) initiated the gastrointestinal motor correlates of vomiting in awake dogs or decerebrate cats without causing retching, vomiting, or regurgitation. These findings have been corroborated by a number of investigators using a variety of recording methods (3, 4, 39, 47, 71, 77). Similar results were found with other agents administered intravenously [carbachol (38) or pentagastrin (38)] or intraluminally [hydrochloric acid (38), vinegar (71), or hypertonic saline (71)]. In addition, Lang et al. (71) observed spontaneous occurrences of these contractile events in dogs (Fig. 10) and found that they did not differ qualitatively or quantitatively from the gastrointestinal motor correlates of spontaneous or chemically induced vomiting (Table 2). Therefore, as first theorized by Alvarez (9), the gastrointestinal motor correlates of vomiting represent a phenomenon that is independent of vomitus expulsion.

*Functions of Retrograde Giant Contraction*

The large amplitude and rapid orad propagation of the RGC indicate that it should be very effective in orad propulsion of intraluminal contents of the small intestine into the stomach. This has been confirmed by observing fluoroscopically the return of a barium meal from the small intestine simultaneous with the orad propagation of the RGC recorded by extraluminal strain-gauge force transducers [Fig. 11; (38)]. The motor function of the RGC when it occurs in association with vomiting may therefore be to retropel the contents of the small intestine into the stomach in preparation for their oral expulsion by the somatomotor responses. This would certainly be useful if vomiting were initiated by an undesirable or toxic substance in the small intestine. In situations where there is no undesirable substance in the small intestine (e.g., motion sickness) the RGC may serve to bring up small intestinal (48) or pancreaticobiliary secretions (9, 60, 101, 135) into the stomach. These secretions may dilute or buffer the contents of the stomach to prevent damage of the esophageal mucosa during vomitus expulsion.

Spontaneous occurrences of the gastrointestinal motor correlates of vomiting without retching or vomitus expulsion are infrequent (71), but intragastric administration of nontoxic doses of irritant solutions predictably initiate these motor events [e.g., hydrochloric acid (38), vinegar (71), hypertonic saline (71), and cupric sulfate (12)]. In these situations the RGC may also function to dilute or buffer gastric contents.

*Neural Control*

Few studies of the neural pathways controlling the digestive tract motor activity associated with vomiting have been published, but all available evidence indicates that the sensory receptors and afferent pathways mediating the digestive tract and somatomotor correlates of vomiting are the same. That is, stimulation of sensory receptors of the gastrointestinal mucosa (6, 12, 38, 71, 75, 78) or chemoreceptive trigger zone (CTZ) (70, 71), which initiates the gastrointestinal correlates of vomiting without retching and vomitus expulsion, also initiates retching and vomitus expulsion at higher levels of stimulation. On the other hand, the efferent pathways mediating control of various somatomotor and autonomic correlates of vomiting may differ.

SENSORY RECEPTORS AND AFFERENT PATHWAYS. The digestive tract not only functions as a motor element in the vomiting reflex but also contains sensory elements that form an important source of emetic signals. The precise nature or location of these receptors has not been determined, but evidence indicates that both mechano- and chemoreceptors from abdominal sources may provide sensory input to the vomiting center. Mechanoreceptors activated by pinching the seromuscular layer (10), rubbing the mucosa (81, 135), distension (45, 47, 56), or occlusion (6, 107) have been found in the stomach (10, 45), jejunum (6, 47, 56), and ileum (107). The location of these receptors in the gut

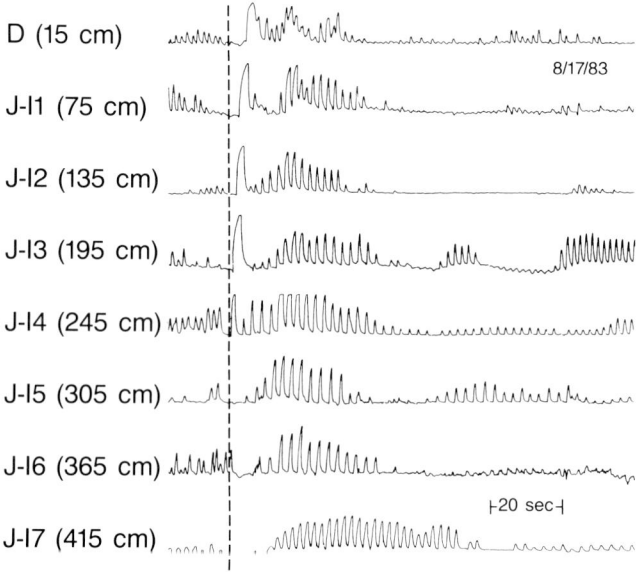

FIG. 10. Spontaneous occurrence of gastrointestinal motor correlates of vomiting without subsequent retching or vomitus expulsion. *Broken vertical line*, first observed occurrence of gastrointestinal motor correlates of vomiting.

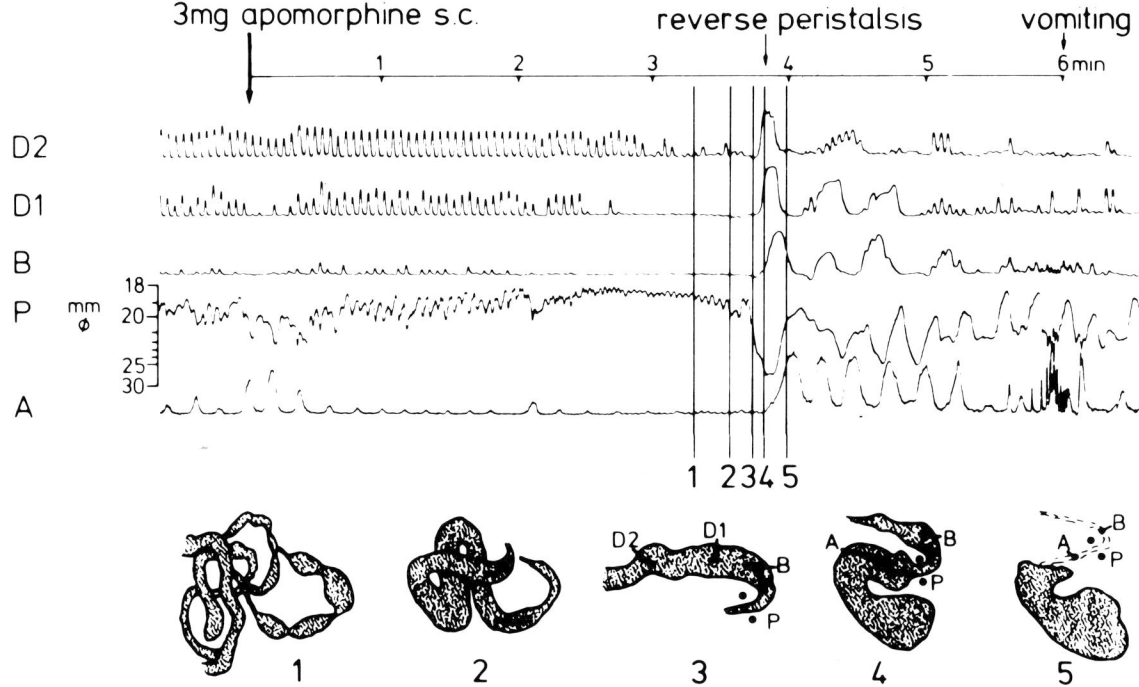

FIG. 11. Recording of gastrointestinal motor correlates of vomiting simultaneously with radiographic observations of movement of intraluminal contrast material after apomorphine administration. *Top*: motor activity of stomach and duodenum recorded with strain-gauge force transducers and diameter of pylorus measured with induction coil. *Bottom*: distribution of contrast material in stomach and small intestine. A, antrum; P, pylorus; B, duodenal bulb; D1, proximal duodenum; and D2, distal duodenum. Numbers of radiographic images (*bottom*) correspond with numbered time marks on chart recording (*top*) and indicate when each image was taken relative to RGC. RGC was observed to empty contents of upper small intestine into proximal stomach. [From Ehrlein (38). Reprinted from *Scand. J. Gastroenterol.* by permission of Norwegian University Press, Oslo.]

wall or the type of mechanical stimuli most effective in exciting these receptors is unknown, but differences are evident. Although pinching the seromuscular layer of the fundus (10) was an effective stimulus, fundic distension (45) was not.

The chemoreceptors have a similar distribution; they have been found in the stomach (6, 12, 69, 75, 100, 101, 124, 125), duodenum (55, 69, 135), and jejunum (47). These receptors are probably located within the mucosa, and they respond to a variety of chemical irritants, including hydrochloric acid (47, 55), cupric sulfate (12, 55, 69, 75, 100, 101, 124, 125), vinegar (71), hypertonic saline (71), potassium antimonyltartrate (tartar emetic) (55, 100, 101), syrup of ipecac (101, 135), mustard (90), and mercuric chloride (55). Regardless of the type of receptor, the proximal duodenum may be more sensitive to emetic stimuli than the stomach (81, 135).

Both vagus and splanchnic nerves carry afferent fibers from gastrointestinal receptors that project to the vomiting center, but the receptive fields of these nerves differ. The stomach receptors for vomiting project primarily through the vagus nerves, because either chemical (90) or mechanical (45) stimulation of the stomach that induced vomiting was blocked by vagotomy but not by splanchnicectomy. In addition centripetal electrical stimulation of either the gastric branches of the vagus nerves (90) or the abdominal vagal trunks (90, 125) activated vomiting. The receptors of the lower small intestine that mediate vomiting project primarily through the splanchnic nerves, because vomiting activated by ileal obstruction (107) was blocked by spinal cord transection at $C_7$–$T_1$ but not by vagotomy. The vomiting caused by emetic stimuli not confined to a particular level of the digestive tract, as during oral (55, 124), intragastric (55), or intraperitoneal administration (16, 122), was blocked only after both vagus and splanchnic nerves were cut. However, the vagus nerves may provide a greater or more significant afferent input, because thoracic truncal vagotomy increased the threshold for initiation of vomiting more than splanchnicectomy (16, 124).

Abdominal receptors also mediate vomiting initiated by peritonitis or X irradiation, but the nature or location of these receptors is unknown (16, 18b, 22, 122). On the other hand, although abdominal receptors mediate vomiting activated in a number of different ways, these receptors probably are not involved in motion-induced vomiting. Wang et al. (126) found that abdominal vagotomy and sympathectomy did not consistently affect the sensitivity of dogs to swing-induced vomiting.

In contrast to receptors in the abdomen, vomiting-related receptors of the thorax may be either excitatory or inhibitory. Hatcher and Weiss (54) reported that low cervical cord transection or excision of the stellate ganglia sometimes blocked the emetic action of cardiac glycosides. More specifically, denervation of the heart either blocked vomiting (41) or greatly increased (36) the threshold for initiating vomiting by cardiac glycosides. Electrical stimulation of the right cardiac nerve caused gastric relaxation and vomiting (5). Activation of these cardiac receptors may account for the nausea and vomiting that sometimes occur after coronary occlusion (119) or with vasovagal syncope (97).

Although cardiac receptors activate vomiting, pulmonary receptors may inhibit it. Zabara et al. (139) found that centripetal electrical stimulation of the cervical vagal trunk that caused hyperventilation also blocked emesis induced by stimulation of the abdominal vagus nerves or fine nerve bundles of the cervical vagus nerves. Also respiratory maneuvers that tended to decrease or stop activation of pulmonary afferent fibers enhanced the sensitivity to motion sickness (80). Therefore pulmonary vagal afferent fibers may inhibit retching and vomiting and thereby coordinate respiratory movements during emesis.

Vomiting can also be initiated by stimulation of central sensory systems. These systems mediate the vomiting of motion sickness, space-adaptation syndrome, and sickness due to foul odors. In addition, one area of the dorsal medulla is specialized to sense vascular constituents. This area, the CTZ (123, 125), is probably located within the area postrema (19, 23, 26, 123), which is devoid of a blood-brain barrier (65, 133) and is sensitive to many different chemical agents (26). The central mechanisms by which these sensory systems initiate vomiting are reviewed in the chapter by Carpenter in this *Handbook*.

The gastrointestinal motor correlates of vomiting precede vomiting induced by stimulation of the CTZ (6, 12, 29, 39, 70, 71, 91, 93, 113, 129, 130) or vestibular system (118), and it is assumed, but not proved, that these gastrointestinal events accompany vomiting activated from other sensory systems as well.

CENTRAL INTEGRATION. The autonomic, somatomotor, and behavioral responses associated with vomiting occur in a well-coordinated manner independent of the sensory systems that provided the initiating stimulus. To account for this coordination of responses, a central pattern generator referred to as the vomiting center has been proposed (20, 44, 53, 71, 123). Many studies have attempted to define the nuclear regions that comprise this pattern generator (see the chapter by Carpenter in this *Handbook*), but none has directly examined the role of these nuclei in the generation of the digestive tract motor activity associated with vomiting. Recent studies suggest that the vomiting center may be compartmentalized with regard to its control of the gastrointestinal and somatomotor systems. Based on the findings that *1*) the gastrointestinal motor correlates of vomiting always precede vomiting and *2*) the gastrointestinal motor correlates of vomiting can occur without retching and vomitus expulsion, it was suggested that the vomiting center may consist of two functionally distinct parts that are activated sequentially: one controlling the gastrointestinal responses and the other controlling the somatomotor responses [Fig. 12; (71)].

EFFERENT INNERVATION. The efferent pathway from the central pattern generator that controls the gastrointestinal correlates of vomiting projects to the abdomen through the vagus nerves only. In 1947 Gregory (48) found that in awake dogs the changes in motor activity of Thiry-Vella loops of jejunum that preceded vomiting were eliminated after thoracic vagotomy but not after bilateral abdominal sympathectomy. Similarly the gastric relaxation that preceded

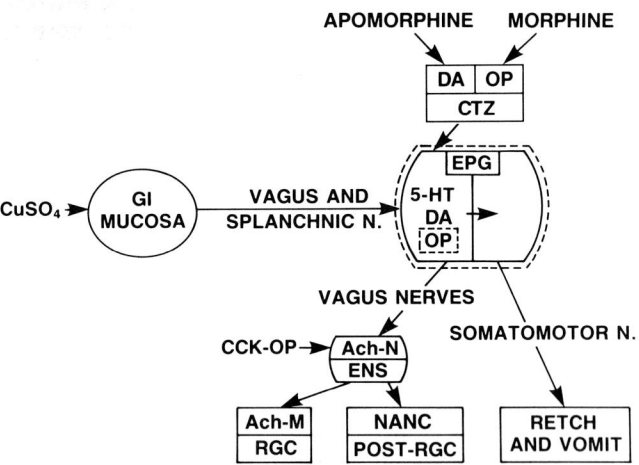

FIG. 12. Mechanisms involved in initiation of gastrointestinal motor correlates of vomiting. DA, dopaminergic receptor; CTZ, chemoreceptive trigger zone; EPG, emetic pattern generator; ACh, acetylcholine; OP, opioid receptor; 5-HT, serotonergic receptor; CCK-OP, cholecystokinin octapeptide; N, nicotinic receptor; M, muscarinic receptor; NANC, nonadrenergic-noncholinergic receptor; RGC, retrograde giant contraction. Stimulation of receptors in CTZ or gastrointestinal mucosa activates the EPG, which consists of 2 functionally distinct parts that are activated sequentially and always in the same order. At low stimulus intensities, only gastrointestinal responses are activated; at high stimulus intensities, retching and vomitus expulsion occur and are always preceded by gastrointestinal responses. All gastrointestinal motor correlates of vomiting are mediated by vagus nerves. Neurotransmitters mediating responses at each level of neuraxis are depicted. Opioid receptor of EPG is inhibitory, and *dotted line* around EPG shows blood-brain barrier.

vomiting was blocked by vagotomy [see Fig. 4; (3, 4)]. These results obtained with balloon manometry were later confirmed with more reliable techniques, such as recording contractile activity with extraluminal strain-gauge force transducers [see Fig. 6; (70, 71)]. These vagal efferents project to the intestinal wall through the mesenteric nerves (47, 67a), but the pathway from the anterior and posterior vagal trunks to the mesenteric nerves is unknown.

The role of the enteric nervous system or the prevertebral ganglia in the expression and coordination of these gastrointestinal responses associated with vomiting is incompletely understood. Recent evidence in dogs suggests that these peripheral neural elements control some of these functions. Lang et al. (68) reported that high doses (50–200 ng/kg) of cholecystokinin octapeptide (CCK-OP) initiated the gastrointestinal motor correlates of vomiting by a peripheral mechanism. That is, CCK-OP activated a series of motor and myoelectric events with characteristics like those associated with vomiting. Most notably CCK-OP activated a single giant contraction that occurred in an all-or-none fashion at the same locations and magnitudes as the RGC associated with vomiting. Although the gastrointestinal motor events associated with vomiting are initiated by the central nervous system through the vagus nerves, vagotomy and splanchnicectomy did not block the responses to CCK-OP. These results plus the observations that CCK-OP did not usually initiate vomiting (26, 68) or its prodromal signs (68) and did not readily cross the blood-brain barrier in dogs (140) indicated that CCK-OP activated the gastrointestinal motor correlates of vomiting by a peripheral neural mechanism. Therefore peripheral neural elements can generate the gastrointestinal motor correlates of vomiting, but under physiological conditions the central nervous system may be required to initiate and coordinate these contractions.

The enteric nervous system may also participate in both the initiation and propagation of the RGC. Circumferential myotomy of the proximal jejunum blocked the RGC initiated by apomorphine from occurring for ~25 cm aboral of the myotomy but did not block the RGC at more orad or aboral sites. In addition, the RGC above the myotomy began before the RGC in the aboral portions of the jejunum ended (67a). Therefore the myenteric plexus may project or facilitate initiation of the RGC at aboral sites and may participate in the control of the retrograde propagation of the RGC. The loss of these functions of the myenteric plexus may explain the inability of investigators to record an RGC in short Thiry-Vella loops of the jejunum (47, 93).

*Neuropharmacology*

DOPAMINERGIC RECEPTORS. Perhaps the most studied receptors involved in the initiation of vomiting and its digestive tract motor correlates are dopaminergic receptors. Apomorphine, the dopaminergic agonist used most often, initiates vomiting (20, 26, 37) and its gastrointestinal correlates (3, 4, 6, 12, 25, 29, 33, 38, 39, 42, 47–50, 58, 62, 66, 70, 71, 76, 77, 91, 93, 98, 101, 108, 113) by activating the CTZ (104, 123, 125). These receptors are probably $D_2$ dopaminergic receptors, because apomorphine-induced responses were blocked by domperidone (39, 76, 77, 91) and sulpiride [Fig. 12; (73, 104)]. Domperidone does not readily cross the blood-brain barrier (67, 96); therefore it is unlikely that it affects receptors within the vomiting center. There are some indications, however, that a second set of dopaminergic receptors that mediate vomiting and its gastrointestinal motor correlates is located within the vomiting center. Dopamine antagonists that readily cross the blood-brain barrier, i.e., haloperidol (69, 77), sulpiride (73), or pimozide (77), blocked vomiting and its gastrointestinal motor correlates initiated by mechanisms other than stimulation of dopaminergic receptors of the CTZ, e.g., cupric sulfate–induced vomiting (Fig. 12). It is unlikely that peripheral dopaminergic receptors mediate the gastrointestinal motor correlates of vomiting, because domperidone did not block these motor events when initiated by morphine (77) or cupric sulfate (69).

The dopamine antagonist metoclopramide is widely used as an antiemetic for chemotherapy-induced emesis (106). However, because *1*) the mechanism of initiation of this form of emesis is unknown (8), *2*) metoclopramide readily crosses the blood-brain barrier (28, 116), and *3*) metoclopramide may not be selective for dopaminergic receptors (18, 64, 105), the mechanism by which metoclopramide blocks chemotherapy-induced emesis is unknown.

OPIATE RECEPTORS. It has long been known that morphine initiates vomiting, but the prior occurrence of its gastrointestinal motor correlates was found more recently (76, 113, 129, 130). These excitatory opiate receptors, which were activated by δ-agonists (18a) and antagonized by naloxone (18a, 76, 113), are located within the CTZ [Fig. 12; (127)]. Like dopaminergic receptors, however, a second set of opiate receptors within the vomiting center may also be involved in the control of vomiting and its gastrointestinal motor correlates. The μ-agonist fentanyl or κ-agonists blocked vomiting and its gastrointestinal motor correlates (18a, 69, 76) induced by agents that acted at the CTZ, i.e., apomorphine (18a, 69, 76) and morphine (76), as well as agents that acted elsewhere, e.g., cupric sulfate [Fig. 12; (69)]. In addition the κ-receptor antagonist MR2266 blocked the antiemetic effects of morphine and κ-agonists (18a).

These results have been interpreted to indicate the existence of inhibitory μ- or κ-receptors in the vomiting center (69, 76). The failure of fentanyl to stimulate vomiting and its gastrointestinal motor correlates (69,

76) was attributed to its ability to freely cross the blood-brain barrier (31) and activate the inhibitory receptors of the vomiting center before activation of excitatory receptors of the CTZ. This suggestion is consistent with the prior findings that high doses of morphine were less effective in inducing vomiting than low doses (127) and that naloxone increased the sensitivity of dogs to vomiting initiated by other stimuli (69). It is unlikely that peripheral opiate receptors have a role in the control of the gastrointestinal correlates of vomiting, because naloxone did not block these motor events when activated by apomorphine (69, 76).

CHOLINERGIC RECEPTORS. No studies have been reported concerning the role of central cholinergic receptors in the control of the digestive tract motor correlates of vomiting; however, much evidence indicates that central cholinergic receptors mediate retching and vomitus expulsion associated with motion sickness (21, 27). On the other hand, peripheral cholinergic receptors have been reported to mediate some of the gastrointestinal motor correlates of vomiting. The muscarinic cholinergic antagonist atropine blocked the RGC (69–71) and its myoelectric correlates (70, 113, 129) but not vomiting or the other gastrointestinal motor or myoelectric correlates of vomiting [Fig. 12; (69–71, 113, 129)]. The nicotinic cholinergic antagonist hexamethonium blocked all gastrointestinal correlates of vomiting but not retching or vomitus expulsion [Fig. 12; (69, 91)]. Because most of the nicotinic and muscarinic cholinergic antagonists used do not readily cross the blood-brain barrier and because retching and vomitus expulsion were not blocked, these cholinergic receptors were probably located peripherally. These results suggest that the neural input originating from the vagus nerves that controls initiation of the gastrointestinal motor correlates of vomiting synapses on the enteric ganglia before innervating the gastrointestinal musculature.

ADRENERGIC RECEPTORS. Central adrenergic receptors play a role in the control of vomiting and its gastrointestinal motor correlates, but the specific location and the type of receptors are unknown. Epinephrine (85, 102, 113, 114, 129), levarterenol bitartrate (85), or clonidine (67b) injected intravenously or intracerebroventricularly initiated vomiting and its gastrointestinal motor correlates, but the prior administration of propranolol (91), phentolamine (91, 113), phenoxybenzamine (91), or guanethidine (4) did not block the gastrointestinal or somatomotor effects of the CTZ stimulants apomorphine and morphine. All of these adrenergic antagonists except phenoxybenzamine readily cross the blood-brain barrier, and therefore this excitatory adrenergic receptor may not form a part of the obligatory central pathway for activation of vomiting and its gastrointestinal motor correlates. Rather, these adrenergic receptors may mediate an afferent pathway to the vomiting center other than that from the CTZ, or a modulatory synapse in the vomiting center or one of its afferent systems. Consistent with this theory is the finding that ablation of the CTZ did not block the emetic effects of epinephrine (102).

SEROTONERGIC RECEPTORS. Evidence suggests a role for central serotonergic receptors in the control of vomiting and its gastrointestinal motor correlates. Lang et al. (69) reported that the serotonergic [5-hydroxytryptamine (5-HT)] antagonists 1-(1-naphthyl)piperazine and methysergide maleate blocked vomiting and its gastrointestinal motor correlates activated by stimulation of the CTZ with apomorphine or by stimulation of the gastrointestinal mucosa with cupric sulfate (Fig. 12). A similar blockade of vomiting initiated by apomorphine was found by Dhawan and Gupta (35) with lysergic acid diethylamide (LSD-25), but similar doses of LSD-25 did not block vomiting initiated by stimulation of cardiac vagal afferent fibers with cardiac glycosides or veratrum alkaloids. These results indicated that central serotonergic receptors mediated vomiting and its gastrointestinal correlates initiated by stimulation of receptors in the CTZ and the gastrointestinal tract but not in the heart.

Some investigators have suggested a role for peripheral serotonergic receptors in the initiation of the gastrointestinal correlates of vomiting (91), but these results have not been corroborated (69). In addition the selective 5-HT M-receptor antagonist MDL7222 blocked cytotoxin-induced vomiting in ferrets (90a), but the location of this receptor and the mechanism of cytotoxin-induced vomiting are unknown.

NONADRENERGIC-NONCHOLINERGIC RECEPTORS. A number of gastrointestinal excitatory and inhibitory responses associated with vomiting persist after the administration of cholinergic and adrenergic receptor antagonists. Such resistance to blockade in other motor events has been ascribed to the existence of nonadrenergic-noncholinergic (NANC) receptors (15, 24). In particular, of the gastrointestinal correlates of vomiting, the muscarinic antagonist atropine blocked only the RGC (70, 71) and its myoelectric correlates (70, 113). The peri-RGC inhibitory period (70, 71), the post-RGC phasic contractions (70, 71), the slowing of gastrointestinal ECA frequency (70), and gastric relaxation (4) initiated by apomorphine in association with vomiting were not blocked by prior administration of atropine. In addition, none of the gastrointestinal motor or myoelectric correlates of vomiting was blocked by $\alpha$-adrenergic (91, 113) or $\beta$-adrenergic (91) antagonists or blockade of the release of endogenous adrenergic agents (4). A number of agents have been proposed as the NANC neurotransmitter, including purine nucleotides, opiate peptides, vasoactive intestinal peptide, substance P, somatostatin, neurotensin, and serotonin (15, 23). Evidence cited above indicated that neither opiate peptides nor serotonin served this function, and Lefebvre and Willems (76) concluded that ATP may not be the NANC neurotransmitter of the stomach. They found that the gastric relaxatory effects of ATP but not apomorphine were blocked by theophylline. The role of other putative neurotransmitters in the control of the gastrointestinal correlates of vomiting has not been examined, and it is not known whether all of the NANC-mediated gastrointestinal responses are mediated by the same neurotransmitter.

PEPTIDERGIC RECEPTORS. Many different peptides can initiate vomiting (see the chapter by Carpenter in this *Handbook*), but the role of the gastrointestinal tract in these responses has been examined only for CCK-OP and pentagastrin. Ehrlein (38) found in dogs that pentagastrin infusion initiated the gastrointestinal motor correlates of vomiting without activating retching and vomitus expulsion. He concluded that these motor events were secondary to increased gastric acid secretion because intravenous administration of other gastric acid stimulants and intragastric administration of hydrochloric acid caused similar effects. A central site of action of pentagastrin, however, cannot be excluded, because the vagus nerves were intact and because gastrin causes emesis and stimulates neurons of the area postrema, the anatomical correlate of the CTZ (26, 27). Although the intravenous administration of CCK-OP only rarely initiated vomiting, Lang et al. (68) found that bolus injections of high doses of CCK-OP always initiated many of the gastrointestinal motor and myoelectric correlates of vomiting. Some differences in the timing of these events compared with those activated by apomorphine were noted but were attributed to differences in the site of action of these agents. Unlike apomorphine, CCK-OP activated the gastrointestinal motor correlates of vomiting at a peripheral site, because neither vagotomy nor splanchnicectomy blocked these responses (Fig. 12). The physiological role of these CCK-OP receptors is unknown; however, they probably do not form part of the obligatory neural pathway for initiation of the gastrointestinal motor correlates of vomiting, because the specific CCK antagonist proglumide did not block the gastrointestinal responses induced by apomorphine. These effects of CCK-OP may not represent the specific ability to initiate the gastrointestinal motor correlates of vomiting but the general ability of CCK-OP to evoke acetylcholine release from nerve endings at specific sites (7, 92, 95).

## DIGESTIVE TRACT MOTOR ACTIVITY ASSOCIATED WITH REGURGITATION

The term *regurgitation* as used here refers to the return of gastrointestinal contents to the oral cavity without the initiation of retching movements or the forceful contraction of abdominal or expiratory muscles (10, 71). The somatomotor correlates of vomiting (i.e., contractions of abdominal and respiratory muscles during retching and vomitus expulsion) provide the force for expulsion of the vomitus, but the mechanisms that provide the force for expulsion of gastric contents during regurgitation are unknown.

In 1925 Alvarez (10) reported that regurgitation in anesthetized cats stimulated by pinching the fundus was accompanied by the gastrointestinal motor correlates of vomiting. More than 60 years later, using unanesthetized dogs, Lang et al. (71) found that spontaneous episodes of regurgitation were also preceded by the gastrointestinal motor correlates of vomiting and that these motor events were qualitatively similar to those that occur prior to vomiting.

## NAUSEA AND PRODROMAL SIGNS OF VOMITING

### Nausea

In humans, nausea has been defined as an unpleasant feeling vaguely referred to the epigastrium and duodenum that often culminates in vomiting. This discomfort felt by people experiencing nausea may vary in duration from a few minutes to several hours, may vary in intensity, may occur in waves, and may be accompanied by pain (1, 63, 89, 134, 135). Although such widely ranging subjective experiences are difficult to quantitate, subjective scales adopted from accepted measures of pain have successfully established three indices of nausea (89). Such measures of nausea or other methods of categorizing these sensations, however, have not yet been applied to the study of the role of the digestive tract in nausea.

SENSORY MECHANISMS OF GASTROINTESTINAL TRACT. Mechanical (61, 63, 78, 82, 135) or chemical (1, 57, 63, 135) stimulation of the mucosa of the proximal duodenum elicited feelings of nausea that were not evident when the same stimuli were applied to the stomach or other regions of the small intestine. Although mechanical stimulation of the duodenum can elicit feelings of nausea, no specific motor pattern of the duodenum or other area of the gastrointestinal tract has been found to cause nausea. Some investigators (51, 63) have suggested that the gastrointestinal correlates of vomiting, the RGC in particular, caused nausea by stimulating duodenal receptors, but this is unlikely because the gastrointestinal correlates of vomiting last only minutes, whereas nausea can last for hours.

Several investigators have reported dysrhythmias in gastric antral ECA in patients with chronic nausea and vomiting (32, 52, 117, 121, 136–138) or in normal individuals subjected to nauseating stimuli (111, 112). Because gastrectomy (32, 137) of the affected region in these patients blocked nausea and vomiting, it was suggested (32, 137) that these gastric antral dysrhythmias may cause nausea and vomiting. However, gastric dysrhythmias in these patients (32, 138) did not always occur concomitantly with the feeling of nausea, and normal subjects (86) experienced gastric dysrhythmias without nausea. These findings are not consistent with the hypothesis that gastric dysrhythmias cause nausea. These gastrectomies may have been successful because of the removal of sensory receptors or neural pathways initiating nausea, but the dysrhythmias may be an effect of nausea rather than its cause.

GASTROINTESTINAL CORRELATES OF NAUSEA. The reflux of duodenal catheters or balloons to the stomach during episodes of nausea has been reported (1, 63, 78), but no specific contractile event, including the RGC, has been found to accompany the feeling of nausea. Sustained contractions of the duodenum (1), migrating motor complexes (118), and gastric antral dysrhythmias (32, 52, 111, 112, 117, 121, 136–139) have been associated with periods of nausea, but their relationship to this subjective experience is unknown. The only consistent change in gastrointestinal contractility associated with nausea is a decrease in spontaneous contractile activity of the stomach [Fig. 13; (134)]. This change in contractile activity was not specific to nausea, however, because similar changes occurred when the nauseating stimuli (i.e., caloric vestibular stimulation or swinging) had not elicited the feelings of nausea. Understanding of the relationship between specific motor events of the digestive tract and nausea will remain confused until this wide range of sensations is categorized and quantified. These sensations may be quantifiable in physiological terms, because it is well known that they are accompanied by a wide variety of autonomic correlates, including changes in heart rate (134), skin resistance (118, 134), gastric secretion (30, 134), gastric mucosal blood flow (134), pupillary diameter (27), skin blood flow (27), and respiration (27). Nausea can also be quantified in subjective terms with appropriate subjective scales (89).

*Prodromal Signs of Vomiting*

The feeling of nausea cannot be defined in animals, but animals exhibit characteristic autonomic and behavioral responses like yawning, licking of the lips or nose, salivation, dilation of the pupils, and changes in respiratory rhythm and heart rate just prior to vomiting (21, 47). These responses have been referred to as the prodromal signs of vomiting (21). Each animal may not experience all of these responses, and the magnitude of these responses may differ with each

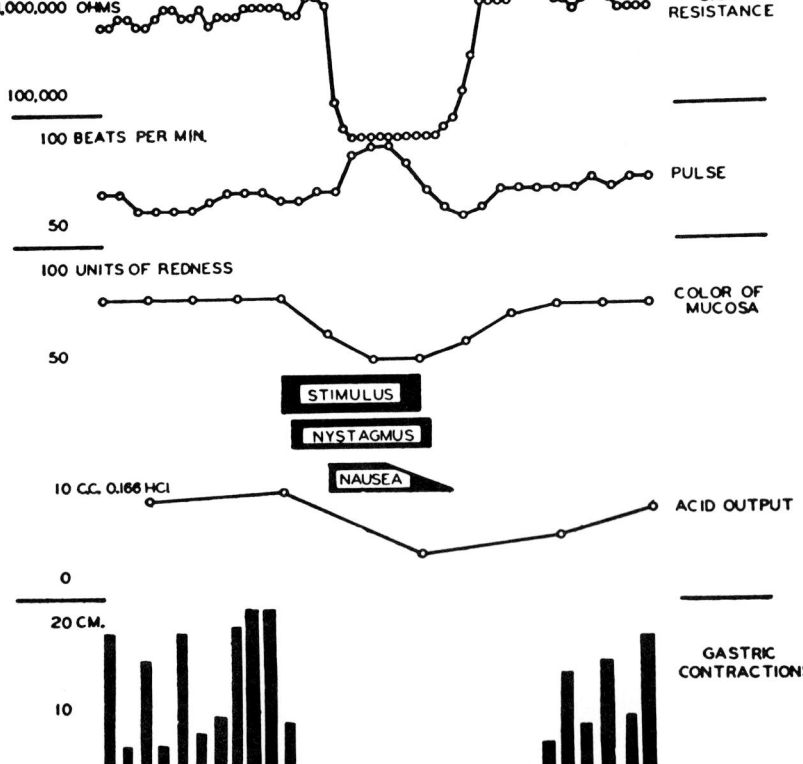

FIG. 13. Changes in autonomic functions associated with nausea induced by caloric stimulation of vestibular apparatus in subject with gastric fistula. Nausea was accompanied by decreased skin resistance, increased heart rate, blanching of gastric mucosa, decreased gastric acid secretion, and decreased gastric contractile activity. [From Wolf (134).]

vomit. Probably the most reliable indices of the prodromal signs of vomiting are an increase in heart rate and a change in respiratory rhythm. The prodromal signs of vomiting begin before but may occur during the gastrointestinal motor correlates of vomiting (71). In contrast to nausea in humans, the prodromal signs of vomiting are brief and always bear a fixed temporal relationship with vomiting. After experiencing the prodromal signs of vomiting, however, animals do not always progress to the gastrointestinal motor correlates of vomiting or to retching and vomitus expulsion.

CONCLUSIONS

The role of the digestive tract in vomiting has been debated for many years. Even as late as 1978, a significant role for the small intestine in this process was questioned (40). However, it is now well established that prior to vomitus expulsion a giant contraction moves retrogradely from the small intestine to the stomach. Although this contraction does not function to expel gastric contents, it effectively returns intestinal contents to the stomach in preparation for oral expulsion during vomiting or regurgitation. In addition, this RGC may occur without oral expulsion of gastric contents. Based on these and other recent findings, the most important function of the RGC may be to buffer or dilute gastric contents with transported intestinal or pancreaticobiliary secretions.

The initiation and propagation of the RGC are controlled by a complex interrelationship of central, peripheral, and enteric nervous systems. This is quite unlike the control of peristalsis in the esophageal skeletal muscle, which requires the central nervous system for both functions, or the esophageal smooth muscle, which does not require the central nervous system for either function.

It is generally accepted that the motive force for expulsion of gastric contents during vomiting is provided by abdominal pressure generated by contractions of abdominal and respiratory muscles. Although the RGC does not participate in this gastric evacuation, it should not be concluded that the digestive tract plays no role in vomitus expulsion. Evidence indicates that the esophagus shortens longitudinally and that the lower esophageal sphincter relaxes prior to and during vomitus explusion. It is unlikely that vomitus expulsion could occur without these motor events. In addition, during regurgitation the expulsion of gastric contents occurs without strong contractions of the abdominal and expiratory muscles. Therefore the mechanisms of oral reflux of gastric contents may involve a complex coordination of gastrointestinal and respiratory muscles rather than a domination of one system over the other.

The role of digestive tract motor activity in nausea remains unknown. Mechanical and chemical stimulation of the gut may cause nausea, but no specific change in digestive tract motor activity has yet been associated with nausea. Myoelectric dysrhythmias of the gastric antrum have been associated with periods of nausea, but a cause-and-effect relationship has not been established.

We thank Mary Farrar for her excellent secretarial assistance and Jeffrey Marvig for his dedicated technical support.

This work was supported in part by grants from the Veterans Administration (5120-02P) and National Institutes of Health (AM-32346).

REFERENCES

1. ABBOTT, F. K., M. MACK, AND S. WOLF. The relations of sustained contraction of the duodenum to nausea and vomiting. *Gastroenterology* 20: 238–248, 1952.
2. ABELL, T. L., AND J.-R. MALAGELADA. Glucagon-evoked gastric dysrhythmias in humans shown by an improved electrogastrographic technique. *Gastroenterology* 88: 1932–1940, 1985.
3. ABRAHAMSSON, H. Studies on the inhibitory nervous control of gastric motility. *Acta Physiol. Scand. Suppl.* 390: 1–38, 1973.
4. ABRAHAMSSON, H., G. JANSSEN, AND J. MARTINSON. Vagal relaxation of the stomach induced by apomorphine in the cat. *Acta Physiol. Scand.* 88: 296–302, 1973.
5. ABRAHAMSSON, H., AND P. THORÉN. Vomiting and reflex vagal relaxation of the stomach elicited from heart receptors in the cat. *Acta Physiol. Scand.* 88: 433–439, 1973.
6. AIZAWA, I., K. NEGISHI, T. SUZUKI, AND Z. ITOH. Gastrointestinal contractile activity associated with vomiting in the dog. In: *Gastrointestinal Motility*, edited by C. Roman. Lancaster, UK: MTP, 1984, p. 159–164.
7. AKASU, T., M. TSURUSAKI, AND M. ARIYOSHI. Presynaptic effect of cholecystokinin octapeptide on neuromuscular transmission in the frog. *Neurosci. Lett.* 67: 329–333, 1986.
8. AKWARI, O. E. The gastrointestinal tract in chemotherapy-induced emesis. A final common pathway. *Drugs* 25, Suppl. 1: 18–34, 1983.
9. ALVAREZ, W. C. The syndrome of mild reverse peristalsis. *J. Am. Med. Assoc.* 64: 2018–2024, 1917.
10. ALVAREZ, W. C. Reverse peristalsis in the bowel, a precursor of vomiting. *J. Am. Med. Assoc.* 85: 1051–1054, 1925.
11. ALVAREZ, W. C. *An Introduction to Gastro-enterology* (4th ed.). New York: Hoeber, 1948.
12. BABSKY, F. Zür Frage des Mechanismus des reflecktorischen Brechaktes. *Pfluegers Arch. Gesamte Physiol. Menschen Tiere* 215: 692–698, 1926.
13. BASS, P., C. F. CODE, AND E. H. LAMBERT. Motor and electric activity of the duodenum. *Am. J. Physiol.* 201: 287–291, 1961.
14. BASS, P., AND N. S. WILEY. Contractile force transducers for recording muscle activity in unanesthetized animals. *J. Appl. Physiol.* 32: 561–562, 1972.
15. BAUER, V., AND O. MATUSAK. The non-adrenergic non-cholinergic innervation and transmission in the small intestine. *Arch. Int. Pharmacodyn. Ther.* 280, Suppl.: 137–163, 1986.
16. BAYLISS, M. Studies on the mechanism of vomiting produced by staphylococcus enterotoxin. *J. Exp. Med.* 72: 669–684, 1940.
17. BAYLISS, W. M., AND E. H. STARLING. The movements and innervation of the small intestine. *J. Physiol. Lond.* 24: 99–143, 1899.
18. BIRTLEY, R. D. N., AND M. W. BAINES. The effect of metoclopramide on some isolated intestinal preparations. *Postgrad.*

*Med. J. Suppl.* 4: 13–18, 1973.
18a. BLANQUAERT, J.-P., R. A. LEFEBVRE, AND J. L. WILLEMS. Emetic and antiemetic effects of opioids in the dog. *Eur. J. Pharmacol.* 128: 143–150, 1986.
18b. BORISON, H. L. Site of emetic action of x-radiation in the cat. *J. Comp. Neurol.* 107: 439–453, 1957.
19. BORISON, H. L., AND K. R. BRIZZEE. Morphology of emetic chemoreceptor trigger zone in cat medulla oblongata. *Proc. Soc. Exp. Biol. Med.* 77: 38–42, 1951.
20. BORISON, H. L., AND S. C. WANG. Functional localization of central coordinating mechanism for emesis in cat. *J. Neurophysiol.* 12: 305–313, 1949.
21. BORISON, H. L., AND S. C. WANG. Physiology and pharmacology of vomiting. *Pharmacol. Rev.* 5: 193–230, 1953.
22. BRIZZEE, K. R. Effect of localized brain stem lesions and supradiaphragmatic vagotomy on x-irradiation emesis in the monkey. *Am. J. Physiol.* 187: 567–570, 1956.
23. BRIZZEE, K. R., AND L. M. NEAL. A reevaluation of the cellular morphology of the area postrema in view of recent evidence for a chemoreceptor function. *J. Comp. Neurol.* 100: 41–62, 1954.
24. BURNSTOCK, G., T. HÖKFELT, M. D. GERSHON, L. L. IVERSON, H. W. KOSTERLITZ, AND J. H. SZURSZEWSKI. Nonadrenergic, non-cholinergic autonomic neurotransmission mechanisms. *Neurosci. Res. Program Bull.* 17: 379–519, 1979.
25. CANNON, W. B. The movements of the stomach studied by means of Roentgen rays. *Am. J. Physiol.* 1: 359–382, 1898.
26. CARPENTER, D. O., D. B. BRIGGS, AND N. STROMINGER. Behavioral and electrophysiological studies of peptide-induced emesis in dogs. *Federation Proc.* 43: 2952–2954, 1984.
27. CHINN, H. I., AND P. K. SMITH. Motion sickness. *Pharmacol. Rev.* 7: 33–83, 1955.
28. COCHLIN, D. L. Dystonic reaction due to metoclopramide and phenothiazines resembling tetanus. *Br. J. Clin. Pract.* 28: 201–202, 1974.
29. CODE, C. F., J. H. STEINBACH, J. F. SCHLEGEL, J. R. AMBERG, AND G. A. HOLLENBECK. Pyloric and duodenal motor contributions to duodenogastric reflex. *Scand. J. Gastroenterol. Suppl.* 92: 13–16, 1984.
30. COHEN, M. M., H. T. DEBAS, I. B. HOLUBITSKY, AND R. C. HARRISON. Effect of nausea on human gastric secretory responses. *Dig. Dis. Sci.* 16: 156–159, 1971.
31. COSTELLO, D. J., AND H. L. BORISON. Naloxone antagonizes narcotic self-blockade of emesis in the cat. *J. Pharmacol. Exp. Ther.* 203: 222–230, 1977.
32. CUCCHIARA, S., J. JANSSENS, G. VANTRAPPEN, K. GEBOES, AND P. CECCATELLI. Gastric electrical dysrhythmias (tachygastria and tachyarrhythmia) in a girl with chronic intractable vomiting. *J. Pediatr.* 108: 264–267, 1986.
33. CZYHLARZ, E. V., AND A. SELKA. Das röntgenologische Verhalten des Magens bei gastrischen Krisen und beim Brechakte. *Wien Klin. Wochenschr.* 26: 842–843, 1913.
34. DERBYSHIRE, A. J., AND J. K. W. FERGUSON. Studies on the vomiting reflex in cats and dogs. *Am. J. Physiol.* 123: 52–53, 1938.
35. DHAWAN, B. N., AND G. P. GUPTA. Antiemetic activity of D-lysergic acid diethylamide. *J. Pharmacol. Exp. Ther.* 133: 137–139, 1961.
36. DRESBACK, M., AND K. C. WADDELL. The emetic action of digitalis bodies and strophanthidin in cats with denervated heart. *J. Pharmacol. Exp. Ther.* 34: 43–64, 1928.
37. EGGLESTON, G., AND R. A. HATCHER. The seat of the emetic action of apomorphine. *J. Pharmacol. Exp. Ther.* 3: 551–580, 1912.
38. EHRLEIN, H. J. Retroperistaltism and duodenogastric reflux in dogs. *Scand. J. Gastroenterol. Suppl.* 67: 29–32, 1981.
39. EHRLEIN, H. J. Inhibition of reverse peristalsis of the intestine by domperidone. *Scand. J. Gastroenterol. Suppl.* 67: 199–200, 1981.
40. FELDMAN, M., AND J. S. FORDTRAN. Vomiting. In: *Gastrointestinal Disease: Pathophysiology, Diagnoses and Management*, edited by M. Sleisenger and J. S. Fordtran. Philadelphia, PA: Saunders, 1978, p. 200–216.
41. FUKUDA, T., AND T. KUSHIYAKI. The cardiac reflex as the cause of digitalis emesis. *Kyushu Mem. Med. Sci.* 2: 137–144, 1951.
42. GARDINER, J. P. Vomiting and pregnancy. *J. Am. Med. Assoc.* 91: 1937–1941, 1928.
43. GELDOF, H., E. J. VAN DER SCHEE, AND J. L. GRASHUIS. Electrogastrographic characteristics of interdigestive migrating complex in humans. *Am. J. Physiol.* 250 (*Gastrointest. Liver Physiol.* 13): G165–G171, 1986.
44. GIANNUZZI, G. Untersuchungen über die Organe, welche an dem brechakt theilnehmen, und über die physiologische Wirkung des tartanus stibiatis. *Zentralbl. Med. Wiss.* 1: 1–4, 1865.
45. GOLDBERG, S. C. The afferent paths of nerves involved in the vomiting reflex induced by distension of an isolated pyloric pouch. *Am. J. Physiol.* 99: 156–159, 1931.
46. GOYAL, R. K., AND B. W. COBB. Motility of the pharynx, esophagus, and the esophageal sphincters. In: *Physiology of the Gastrointestinal Tract* (1st ed.), edited by L. R. Johnson. New York: Raven, 1981, p. 372.
47. GREGORY, R. A. Changes in intestinal tone and motility associated with nausea and vomiting. *J. Physiol. Lond.* 105: 58–65, 1946.
48. GREGORY, R. A. Nervous pathways of intestinal reflexes associated with nausea and vomiting. *J. Physiol. Lond.* 106: 95–103, 1947.
49. GRUBER, C. M., AND J. T. BRUNDAGE. Actions of apomorphine hydrochloride upon the small intestine in unanesthetized dogs. *Proc. Soc. Exp. Biol. Med.* 32: 863–865, 1935.
50. GRUBER, C. M., V. G. HAURY, AND M. E. DRAKE. Action of apomorphine hydrochloride on the intact intestine in unanesthetized dogs. *Proc. Soc. Exp. Biol. Med.* 42: 193–197, 1939.
51. GUYTON, A. C. *Textbook of Medical Physiology*. Philadelphia, PA: Saunders, 1896, p. 803–804.
52. HAMILTON, J. W., B. E. BELLAHSENE, M. REICHELDERFER, J. G. WEBSTER, AND P. BASS. Human electrogastrograms. Comparison of surface and mucosal recordings. *Dig. Dis. Sci.* 31: 33–39, 1986.
53. HATCHER, R. A. The mechanism of vomiting. *Physiol. Rev.* 4: 479–504, 1924.
54. HATCHER, R. A., AND S. WEISS. The seat of the emetic action of digitalis bodies. *Arch. Intern. Med.* 29: 690–704, 1922.
55. HATCHER, R. A., AND S. WEISS. Studies on vomiting. *J. Pharmacol. Exp. Ther.* 22: 139–193, 1923.
56. HERRIN, R. C., AND W. J. MEEK. Distension as a factor in intestinal obstruction. *Arch. Intern. Med.* 51: 152–168, 1933.
57. HERTZ, A. F., F. COOK, AND E. G. SCHLESINGER. The sensibility of the stomach and intestines in man. *J. Physiol. Lond.* 37: 481–490, 1908.
58. HESSE, O. Zur Kenntnes des Brechaktes. Nach Röntgenversuchen an Hunden. *Pfluegers Arch. Gesamte Physiol.* 152: 1–22, 1913.
59. HIGHTOWER, N. C. Motor action of the small bowel. In: *Handbook of Physiology. Alimentary Canal*, edited by C. F. Code. Washington, DC: Am. Physiol. Soc., 1968, sect. 6, vol. IV, chapt. 98, p. 2001–2024.
60. HIRSCH, A. Weitere Beiträge zur motorischen Funktion des Magens nach Versuchen an Hunden mit Darmfisteln. *Zentralbl. Klin. Med.* 14: 377–383, 1893.
61. IVY, A. C., AND D. A. VLOEDMAN. The small intestine in hunger. *Am. J. Physiol.* 72: 99–106, 1925.
62. JOHNSON, H. D., AND J. W. LAWS. The cardia in swallowing, eructation and vomiting. *Lancet* 2: 1268–1273, 1966.
63. KEETON, R. W. Nausea and related sensation elicited by duodenal stimulation. *Arch. Intern. Med.* 35: 687–697, 1925.
64. KILBRINGER, H., R. KRUEL, I. PFEUFFER-FRIEDERICH, AND I. WASSLER. The effect of metoclopramide on acetylcholine release and on smooth muscle response in the isolated guinea-

pig ileum. *Naunyn-Schmiedeberg's Arch. Pharmacol.* 319: 231–238, 1982.
65. KLARA, P. M., AND K. R. BRIZZIE. The ultrastructural morphology of the squirrel monkey area postrema. *Cell Tissue Res.* 160: 315–326, 1975.
66. KRATINOFF, A. G., AND A. L. SACH. Beiträge zur Physiologie des Erbrechans. I. Mitteilung. Über den Innervationsmechanismus der Brechbeiwegungen des Darmes unter dem Einfluss des Apomorphins. *Pfluegers Arch. Gesamte Physiol. Menschen Tiere* 216: 754–764, 1927.
67. LADURON, P. M., AND J. E. LEYSEN. Domperidone, a specific in vitro dopamine antagonist, devoid of in vivo central dopaminergic activity. *Biochem. Pharmacol.* 28: 2161–2165, 1979.
67a. LANG, I. M., J. MARVIG, AND S. K. SARNA. The role of the enteric nervous system in the initiation and propagation of the gastrointestinal motor correlates of vomiting (Abstract). *Dig. Dis. Sci.* 32: 918, 1987.
67b. LANG, I. M., J. MARVIG, AND S. K. SARNA. Activation of the GI motor correlates of vomiting by stimulation of central $\alpha_2$-adrenergic receptors (Abstract). *Gastroenterology* 92: 1490, 1987.
68. LANG, I. M., J. MARVIG, AND S. K. SARNA. Comparison of gastrointestinal responses to CCK-8 and associated with vomiting. *Am. J. Physiol.* 254 (*Gastrointest. Liver Physiol.* 17): G254–G263, 1988.
69. LANG, I. M., J. MARVIG, S. K. SARNA, AND R. E. CONDON. Mechanism of initiation of the gastrointestinal motor correlates of vomiting activated by luminal irritation (Abstract). *Gastroenterology* 91: 1059, 1986.
70. LANG, I. M., J. MARVIG, S. K. SARNA, AND R. E. CONDON. The gastrointestinal myoelectric correlates of vomiting in the dog. *Am. J. Physiol. (Gastrointest. Liver Physiol.* 14) 251: G830–G838, 1986.
71. LANG, I. M., S. K. SARNA, AND R. E. CONDON. Gastrointestinal motor correlates of vomiting in the dog: quantification and characterization as an independent phenomenon. *Gastroenterology* 90: 40–47, 1986.
72. LARSIN, L. M., AND J. A. BARGEN. Action of cathartics on isolated dog's colon. Motor activity. *Arch. Surg.* 27: 1130–1145, 1933.
73. LAVILLE, C., AND J. MARGARIT. Activité antiémétique du sulpiride vis-à-vis des divers poisons émétisants chez le chien. *C. R. Seances Soc. Biol. Fil.* 162: 869–874, 1968.
74. LEAKE, C. D. The action of morphine on the vomiting center in the dog. *J. Pharmacol. Exp. Ther.* 20: 359–364, 1923.
75. LEE, K. Y., H. J. PARK, AND W. Y. CHEY. Studies on mechanisms of retching and vomiting in dogs. Effect of peripheral dopamine blocker on myoelectric changes in antrum and upper small intestine. *Dig. Dis. Sci.* 30: 22–28, 1985.
76. LEFEBVRE, R. A., AND J. L. WILLEMS. Gastric relaxation by apomorphine and ATP in the conscious dog. *J. Pharm. Pharmacol.* 31: 561–563, 1979.
77. LEFEBVRE, R. A., J. L. WILLEMS, AND M. G. BOGAERT. Gastric relaxation and vomiting by apomorphine, morphine, and fentanyl in the conscious dog. *Eur. J. Pharmacol.* 69: 139–145, 1981.
78. LEHMAN, E. P., AND H. V. GIBSON. Observations in a case of jejunal fistula. *J. Am. Med. Assoc.* 82: 1918–1920, 1924.
79. LEVINE, G. The study of gall-bladder contractions as an aid in the Roentgen diagnosis of gall-bladder disease. *Am. J. Roentgenol.* 26: 87–91, 1931.
80. LIPARA, J. G., J. FLETCHER, W. BROWN, AND G. COHEN. Effects of various respiratory maneuvers in the physiologic response to angular acceleration. *Aerosp. Med.* 40: 976–980, 1969.
81. LUCKHARDT, A. B., H. T. PHILLIPS, AND A. J. CARLSON. Contributions to the physiology of the stomach: LI. The control of the pylorus. *Am. J. Physiol.* 50: 57–60, 1919.
82. LUNDSEN, K., AND W. S. HOLDEN. The act of vomiting in man. *Gut* 10: 173–179, 1969.
83. MATHUR, P. D., J. H. GRINDLAY, AND F. C. MANN. Observations on duodenal motility in dogs, with special reference to activity during vomiting. *Gastroenterology* 10: 866–879, 1948.
84. MCCARTHY, L. E., H. L. BORISON, P. K. SPIEGEL, AND R. M. FRIEDLANDER. Vomiting: radiographic and oscillographic correlates in the decerebrate cat. *Gastroenterology* 67: 1126–1130, 1974.
85. MCCOY, E. J., AND P. BASS. Chronic electrical activity of gastroduodenal area: effects of food and certain catecholamines. *Am. J. Physiol.* 205: 439–445, 1963.
86. MCINTYRE, J. A., M. DEITEL, M. BAIDA, AND S. JALIL. The human electrogastrogram at operation: a preliminary report. *Can. J. Surg.* 12: 275–284, 1969.
87. MECRAY, P. M., JR. A study of the movements of the duodenum with special reference to antiperistalsis. *Am. J. Dig. Dis.* 8: 76–82, 1941.
88. MELLINGER, C. Beitrage zur Kenntnis des Erbrechens. *Pfluegers Arch. Gesamte Physiol. Menschen Tiere* 24: 232–245, 1881.
89. MELZACK, R., Z. ROSBERGER, M. L. HOLLINGSWORTH, AND M. THIRLWELL. New approaches to measuring nausea. *Can. Med. Assoc. J.* 133: 755–761, 1985.
90. MILLER, F. R. On gastric sensation. *J. Physiol. Lond.* 41: 409–415, 1910.
90a. MINER, W. D., AND G. J. SANGER. Inhibition of cisplatin-induced vomiting by selective 5-hydroxytryptamine M-receptor antagonism. *Br. J. Pharmacol.* 88: 497–499, 1986.
91. MIOLAN, J. P., A. M. LAJARD, P. REGA, AND C. ROMAN. Vagal control of gastrointestinal tract during vomiting. In: *Gastrointestinal Motility,* edited by C. Roman. Lancaster, UK: MTP, 1984, p. 167–176.
92. MO, N., AND N. J. DUN. Cholecystokinin octapeptide depolarizes guinea-pig inferior mesenteric ganglion cells and facilitates nicotinic transmission. *Neurosci. Lett.* 64: 263–268, 1986.
93. MONGES, H., J. SALDUCCI, AND B. NANDY. Electrical activity of the gastrointestinal tract in dog during vomiting. In: *Proc. Int. Symp. GI Motility,* 3rd, edited by E. E. Daniel. Vancouver, Canada: Mitchell, 1974, p. 479–488.
93a. MONGES, H., J. SALDUCCI, AND B. NANDY. Dissociation between the electrical activity of the diaphragmatic dome and crura muscular fibers during esophageal distension, vomiting, and eructation. An electromyographic study in the dog. *J. Physiol. Paris* 74: 541–554, 1978.
94. MÜLLER, J. Handbuch der physiologie des Menschen. Koblenz, Germany: Hölscher, 1834, vol. I, pt. 2.
95. NGU, M. D. Activation of enteric nerve pathway in the guinea-pig duodenum by cholecystokinin-octapeptide and pentagastrin. *J. Physiol. Lond.* 364: 31–44, 1985.
96. NIEMEGEERS, C. J. E., K. H. L. SCHELLEKENS, AND P. A. J. JANSSEN. The antiemetic effects of domperidone, a novel potent gastrokinetic. *Arch. Int. Pharmacodyn. Ther.* 244: 130–140, 1980.
97. ÖBERG, B., AND P. THORÉN. Increased activity in left ventricular receptors during hemorrhage in ulceration of caval veins in the cat. A possible cause of the vaso-vagal reaction. *Acta Physiol. Scand.* 88: 164–173, 1972.
98. OHASI, K. On the movement of the stomach and the jejunum during nausea and vomiting. *J. Physiol. Soc. Jpn.* 30: 736–750, 1968.
99. OHASI, K. On the movements of the colon and gallbladder during nausea and vomiting. *J. Physiol. Soc. Jpn.* 30: 771–778, 1968.
100. OPENCHOWSKI, V. Über die nervösen Virrechtungen des Magens. *Zentralbl. Physiol.* 3: 1–10, 1889.
101. OPPENHEIMER, M. J., AND F. C. MANN. Role of the small intestine during emesis. *Am. J. Dig. Dis.* 8: 86–89, 1941.
102. PENG, T. M. Locus of emetic action of epinephrine and dopa in dogs. *J. Pharmacol. Exp. Ther.* 139: 345–349, 1963.
103. POENSGEN, E. Die motorischen Verichtungen des menschlechen Magens und ihre Störungen mit Ausschluss der Lehre vom Erbrechen. Strassburg: 1882.

104. REINA, G., C. SACCHI, AND G. AGUGGINI. Analysis of antiemetic effects of sulpiride isomers in dogs. In: *Sulpiride and other Benzamides*, edited by P. F. Spano, M. Trabucchi, G. V. Corsini, and G. L. Gessa. Milan: Italian Brain Found., 1979, p. 83–89.
105. SANGER, G. J. Mechanism by which metoclopramide can increase gastrointestinal motility. In: *Mechanisms of Gastrointestinal Motility and Secretion*, edited by A. Bennett and G. Velo. New York: Plenum, 1984, p. 303–324.
106. SCHULZE-DELRIEU, K. Metoclopramide. *New Engl. J. Med.* 305: 28–33, 1981.
107. SHARMA, R. N., P. C. DUBEY, K. S. DIXIT, AND K. P. BHARGAVA. Neural pathways of emesis associated with experimental intestinal obstruction in dogs. *Indian J. Med. Res.* 60: 291–295, 1972.
108. SLAUGHTER, D., AND E. G. GROSS. The effect of apomorphine on the movement of the small intestine in unanesthetized dogs. *J. Pharmacol. Exp. Ther.* 63: 289–291, 1938.
109. SMITH, C. C., AND K. R. BRIZZIE. Cineradiographic analysis of vomiting in the cat. I. Lower esophagus, stomach, and small intestine. *Gastroenterology* 40: 654–664, 1961.
110. SOSMAN, M. C., L. R. WHITAKER, AND P. J. EDSON. Clinical and experimental cholecystography. *Am. J. Roentgenol.* 14: 495–503, 1925.
111. STERN, R. M., K. L. KOCH, H. W. LEIBOVITZ, I. M. LINDBLAD, C. L. SHUPERT, AND W. R. STEWART. Tachygastria and motion sickness. *Aviat. Space Environ. Med.* 56: 1074–1077, 1985.
112. STERN, R. M., K. L. KOCH, W. R. STEWART, AND I. M. LINDBLAD. Spectral analysis of tachygastria recorded during motion sickness. *Gastroenterology* 92: 92–97, 1987.
113. STEWART, J. J., T. F. BURKS, AND N. W. WEISBRODT. Intestinal myoelectric activity after activation of central emetic mechanism. *Am. J. Physiol.* 233 (*Endocrinol. Metab. Gastrointest. Physiol.* 3): E131–E137, 1977.
114. STEWART, J. J., N. W. WEISBRODT, AND T. F. BURKS. Centrally mediated intestinal stimulation of morphine. *J. Pharmacol. Exp. Ther.* 202: 174–181, 1977.
115. TANAKA, K. Studien über die Bewegung des operierten Magendarmes von Hund und Katze nach Beobachtung und Kinemetrographie am Koiwaischen Bauchfenster. II. Über die Bewegung des opierten Magens und Dünndarmes. *Z. Jpn. Chir. Ges.* 36: 122–125, 1935.
116. TANSY, D., J. D. PARKES, AND C. D. MARSDEN. Metoclopramide and pimozide in Parkinson's disease and levodopa-induced dyskinesias. *J. Neurol. Neurosurg. Psychiatry* 38: 331–335, 1975.
117. TELANDER, R. L., K. G. MORGAN, D. L. KREULEN, P. F. SCHMALZ, K. A. KELLY, AND J. H. SZURSZEWSKI. Human gastric atony with tachygastria and gastric retention. *Gastroenterology* 75: 497–501, 1978.
118. THOMPSON, B. G., AND J.-R. MALAGELADA. Vomiting and the small intestine. *Dig. Dis. Sci.* 27: 1121–1125, 1982.
119. THORÉN, P. Left ventricular receptor activated by severe asphyxia and by coronary artery occlusion. *Acta Physiol. Scand.* 85: 455–463, 1972.
120. TORRANCE, H. B. Studies on the mechanisms of gastro-esophageal regurgitation. *J. R. Coll. Surg. Edinb.* 4: 54–62, 1958.
121. VANTRAPPEN, G., E. SCHIPPERS, J. JANSSENS, AND M. VANDEWEED. What is the mechanical correlate of gastric dysrhythmia? (Abstract). *Gastroenterology* 84: 1288, 1984.
122. WALTON, F. E., R. M. MOORE, AND E. A. GRAHAM. The nerve pathways in vomiting of peritonitis. *Arch. Surg.* 22: 829–837, 1931.
123. WANG, S. C., AND H. L. BORISON. The vomiting center: a critical experimental analysis. *Arch. Neurol. Psychiatry* 63: 928–941, 1950.
124. WANG, S. C., AND H. L. BORISON. Copper sulphate emesis: a study of afferent pathways from the gastrointestinal tract. *Am. J. Physiol.* 164: 520–526, 1951.
125. WANG, S. C., AND H. L. BORISON. A new concept of organization of the central emetic mechanism: recent studies on the sites of action of apomorphine, copper sulfate, and cardiac glycosides. *Gastroenterology* 22: 1–11, 1952.
126. WANG, S. C., H. I. CHINN, AND A. A. RENZI. Experimental motion sickness in dogs. Role of abdominal visceral afferents. *Am. J. Physiol.* 10: 578–580, 1957.
127. WANG, S. C., AND V. V. GLAVIANO. Locus of emetic action of morphine and hyderzine in dogs. *J. Pharmacol. Exp. Ther.* 111: 329–334, 1954.
128. WEISBRODT, N. W. Motility of the small intestine. In: *Physiology of the Gastrointestinal Tract*, edited by L. R. Johnson. New York: Raven, 1981, p. 441–493.
129. WEISBRODT, N. W., AND T. F. BURKS. Central nervous control of intestinal motility. In: *Proc. Int. Symp. GI, 3rd*, edited by E. E. Daniel. Vancouver, Canada: Mitchell, 1974, p. 649–656.
130. WEISBRODT, N. W., AND J. CHRISTENSEN. Electrical activity of the cat duodenum in fasting and vomiting. *Gastroenterology* 63: 1004–1010, 1972.
131. WEITZ, W., AND W. VOLLERS. Beitrag zur Kenntnis des Brechmechanism. *Z. Gesamte Exp. Med.* 54: 152–160, 1927.
132. WEPFER, J. J. Quoted by Brinton, W. In: *Cyclopedia of Anatomy and Physiology*. London: Churchill, 1859, vol. 5, p. 317.
133. WISLOKI, G. B., AND T. J. PUTNAM. Note on the anatomy of the area postrema. *Anat. Rev.* 19: 281–287, 1920.
134. WOLF, S. The relation of gastric function to nausea in man. *J. Clin. Invest.* 22: 877–882, 1943.
135. WOLF, S. Studies on nausea. Effect of ipecac and other emetics on the human stomach and duodenum. *Gastroenterology* 12: 212–218, 1949.
136. YOU, C. H., AND W. Y. CHEY. Study of electromechanical activity of the stomach in humans and in dogs with particular attention to tachygastria. *Gastroenterology* 86: 1460–1468, 1984.
137. YOU, C. H., W. Y. CHEY, K. Y. LESS, R. MENGUY, AND A. BORTOFF. Gastric and small intestinal myoelectric dysrhythmia associated with chronic intractable nausea and vomiting. *Ann. Intern. Med.* 95: 449–451, 1981.
138. YOU, C. H., K. Y. LEE, W. Y. CHEY, AND R. MENGUY. Electrogastrographic study of patients with unexplained nausea, bloating and vomiting. *Gastroenterology* 79: 311–314, 1980.
139. ZABARA, J., R. B. CHAFFEE, JR., AND M. TANSY. Neuroinhibition in the regulation of emesis. *Space Life Sci.* 3: 282–292, 1972.
140. ZHU, X.-G., G. A. GREELEY, JR., B. G. LEWIS, P. LILYA, AND J. C. THOMPSON. Blood-CSF barrier to CCK and effect of centrally administered bombesin on release of brain CCK. *J. Neurosci. Res.* 15: 393–402, 1986.

# CHAPTER 33

# Adaptation to surgical perturbations

MARIA PAPASOVA  
ELENA ATANASSOVA

*Institute of Physiology, Bulgarian Academy of Sciences, Sofia, Bulgaria*

CHAPTER CONTENTS

Postoperative Paresis (Ileus)
Esophagus
Stomach
  Resection
  Vagotomy
    Truncal vagotomy
    Selective vagotomy
    Vagotomy combined with drainage operations
Small Intestine
  Transection
  Resection
  Vagotomy
Large Intestine
Conclusions

---

THE DIFFERENT TYPES of surgical interventions undertaken in connection with diseases of the gastrointestinal tract result in grave structural and functional disturbances. However, because of the adaptability of the system, the function of the organ subjected to surgical intervention is gradually restored, and in some cases even complete recovery is observed. Normal interactions between the different organs in the digestive system as a whole are also restored.

The two most frequent surgical interventions used in gastrointestinal surgery that may lead to changes in the motility of the gastrointestinal tract are different types of resections and vagotomies.

A century ago, Billroth introduced two methods for radical treatment of gastric ulcer disease, namely, resection of the antral part of the stomach with restoration of the food passage by directly joining the gastric remnant with the duodenum [Billroth-I (B-I) in 1881] and resection of the antral part of the stomach with anterior gastroenteroanastomosis [Billroth-II (B-II) in 1885]. These two operations, together with the gastroenterostomy performed by Wölfler, marked a new stage in the history of surgery. The operations became part of the daily clinical practice of all surgical clinics since then, and their skillful execution has brought relief to many suffering patients.

Gastroenterostomy was preferred in the first quarter of the century and was subsequently replaced by gastric resections on account of the high ulcer-recurrence rate (129). Although it is admitted that B-I is more physiological, because it restores anatomical relationships between the stomach and the small intestine, it creates technical difficulties in performing the gastroduodenal anastomosis in cases with adhesions and changes in the region of the gastroduodenal junction. Frequent application widens the indications for the operation and, because greater resection is needed in cases of considerable changes in the wall, especially in gastric cancer, B-II is preferred, because it gives better chances for a more reliable performance of the gastroenteroanastomosis. Many surgeons have introduced modifications to consolidate the anastomosis and improve the conditions of gastric emptying (e.g., Krönlein in 1887, Roux in 1893, Reichel in 1908, Polya in 1911, and Balfour in 1927). However, the modifications of Hoffmeister (in 1903) and Finsterer (in 1911) proved to be most suitable. Suturing of an intestinal loop higher than the anastomosis prevents to a great extent the penetration of food from the gastric remnant into the afferent loop near the anastomosis. The main characteristic feature of the B-II operation is the closing of the proximal part of the duodenum as a stump. Blind suturing of the duodenum offers two possibilities to surgeons, i.e., to perform a sound anastomosis and to perform, if necessary, extensive resection or total gastrectomy, in accordance with the requirements for radical intervention (211). The B-II operation proved particularly suitable in the case of total gastrectomy.

Surgeons devote more attention to the operation technique and to clinical data than to the problems of the postoperative functions of the gastrointestinal tract. In connection with the character of digestion after resection, the question arises as to how the remaining part of the stomach is adapted to undertake the motor function of the antral part of the stomach that is removed by the operation.

The changes in the functions of the digestive tract, which follow gastric resections, are tolerated relatively easily by many patients. The adaptation to the new digestive conditions and the compensation of the disturbed functions are so complete that the majority of the patients subjected to antral resection feel practically healthy and fit to work for many years, provided they observe a suitable diet and life-style. The Russian surgeon Feodorov has pointed out that the positive results obtained after the application of various methods prove not the perfection of the method but the enormous adaptability of the digestive tract.

Viewed from another angle, however, subtotal gastrectomy produces direct mortality in ~4% of the cases, the recurrent ulcer rate is ~1.5%, and postcibal symptoms appear in ~10% of the patients (129). This means that in those patients the adaptation is incomplete and insufficient; as a result of such maladaptation, the patients suffer from various dyspeptic and dystrophic disturbances, which make them ill again. These patients feel discomfort after eating, they lose weight, and their working ability is decreased compared with the period before the operation. Evidently in these patients the removal of the antral part of the stomach was not followed by compensatory adaptation in digestion at the expense of duodenal and small intestinal digestion. Intestinal digestion is disorganized, because the undigested food passes directly into the small intestine. In the case of B-II, the blind suturing of the duodenum excludes the direct participation of the hepatopancreatoduodenal system, with its great compensatory possibilities, in the digestive processes. Numerous examinations of patients have demonstrated a sharp decrease in the hepatic and pancreatic functions. As a result, considerable disturbances in digestion and absorption of the nutrients, as well as disturbances in the metabolism of all substances, have been observed.

Postoperative disturbances in the motor activity of the gastrointestinal tract can be divided into three main types: enterogastric reflux, fast gastric emptying, and delayed gastric emptying (31, 131). Patients with duodenogastric reflux complain of pain, feeling of distension, and bile vomiting (3). This is considered to be caused by blockage of the afferent loop, whereby bile and pancreatic secretions are collected in it. At a certain moment, they are rapidly evacuated from the loop, which results in vomiting, i.e., in afferent loop syndrome. The existence of bile leads to delayed evacuation of the gastric content, which creates a feeling of discomfort in the patients.

The group of disturbances resulting in fast gastric emptying comprises the dumping syndrome and diarrhea. It is believed that the gastric content, because of the small volume of the gastric remnant, leaves the stomach very rapidly. Because it is mechanically coarse and insufficiently permeated by gastric juice, it strongly distends the intestinal wall. Gastrointestinal hormones and peptides are, evidently, released from the distended muscle wall (30). The induced powerful peristaltic waves propel the content to the end of the small intestine within ~25–50 min, in some cases in only ~15 min instead of 2 h, which is the normal transit time (162, 163). (There are several other complex and interconnected causes for the dumping syndrome, whose discussion would be irrelevant here.) The patients complain of nausea, palpitations, vomiting, diarrhea, weight loss, etc. Usually their working ability is impaired as well.

After resection, the gastric stasis is manifested through vomiting, heaviness, and discomfort accompanied by gastric dilatation and bezoars (49). The cause for this state is the narrowing of the gastroenteroanastomosis (49).

In the 1940s surgeons accepted the method proposed by Dragstedt—truncal vagotomy—in their search for a more physiological method for surgical treatment of gastric and duodenal ulcer. The application of vagotomy in surgical practice has had a varied course over the years, which is to a great extent the result of various postvagotomy complications. Most of these complications are related to grave disturbances in the motor evacuatory function of the gastrointestinal tract. Even the pioneers in this field report a sharp decrease in gastric motility after severing of the cervical vagal nerves (58) and a strong delay in its evacuating ability (51). Special attention is devoted in detailed surveys published later to the strong inhibition of the tone, of the contractions, and of the evacuating capacity of the stomach with the development of dilatation after truncal vagotomy (5, 6, 145, 153). Systematic studies performed with modern methods have made it possible to specify the changes in the gastric motor activity during different postoperative stages and to explain the mechanism of some of the undesirable complications observed in clinical practice. At the same time, it has been demonstrated that gradual restoration of gastrointestinal motility occurs in a large part of the cases (53, 147, 195). However, this view is not fully shared by all researchers; some authors claim that complete restoration of the gastrointestinal motility does not occur after truncal vagotomy (238).

The severe disturbances in the motor evacuatory function of the stomach observed during the early postoperative period and manifested as a sense of heaviness, belching, nausea, and vomiting, especially the late functional disturbances in the motor and secretory function of the stomach, brought to the fore the need to seek new solutions to the problem. In this respect, selective vagotomy has been proposed instead of truncal vagotomy, thus avoiding the denervation of the other viscera in the abdomen, as well as proximal stomach vagotomy with which the innervation of the antrum and of pylorus sphincter (PS) is preserved intact. In a high percentage of the cases, however, gastric stasis appears, and drainage operations become necessary (92).

After vagotomy, the direct mortality is ~1%, the

recurrent ulcer rate is 5%, and among the other late results diarrhea is observed in 4% of the patients (129). Because truncal vagotomy after Dragstedt procedure results in 10.6% of recurrent ulcer rate (89), truncal vagotomy is combined with resection of the antral part of the stomach. After introduction of selective vagotomy, it is also recommended to add resection of the distal part of the stomach (104).

Thus gastric resection still continues to be a viable method in surgical practice for radical treatment of gastric and duodenal ulcer, gastric cancer, gastric polyposis, etc. To diminish the late postoperative consequences, many surgeons have tried to throw light on the mechanism of the disturbances obtained. The literature on this subject is discussed elsewhere.

The purpose of this chapter is to discuss the changes that take place in the motor function of the stomach and intestines after resection of the stomach, resection of the intestines, truncal and selective vagotomies, as well as vagotomy combined with drainage operations. We present here the experimental and clinical observations on the adaptation of the motor function of the gastrointestinal tract during various periods after surgery.

## POSTOPERATIVE PARESIS (ILEUS)

Abdominal surgery results in inhibition of the motility of the gastrointestinal tract, i.e., in the postoperative paresis or physiological ileus. Several basic factors influence gastrointestinal motility during abdominal surgery: *1*) mechanical trauma, *2*) drugs administered before and after the operation, and *3*) anesthesia. The state of the gastric and intestinal contractile activity may be assessed as a sum of the intestinal responses to these factors (242).

Even Cannon and Murphy (52) have described, using X-ray and manometric tests, a secondary period of inhibition of the gastrointestinal motility after surgery. It consists of a "silent period" followed by irregular and prolonged but low activity lasting 12–24 h. On the next day after the operation, there are still no peristaltic waves and no flatus; the stomach remains inactive for 18–24 h. There is physiological ileus after every abdominal operation (26, 252). Gastric motility is usually restored after 24 h, although 36–48 h are needed after intestinal anastomosis (176). The large intestine is still inactive even on days 2 and 3 after surgery (252). Large intestinal inertia may last up to 5 days (176); accumulated gases increase the volume of the large intestine. The distension of its walls makes passage of flatus impossible for 24–48 h (252). The small intestine, however, manifests motility early. The contrast medium passes, and the gases move rapidly (208). By measuring the intraluminal pressure in the small intestine it has been found that the duodenal motor activity is restored 2 h after closing of the stomach in all patients (57). Complexes of rhythmic activity (phase 3) appear, whereby pressure of 50 mmHg is created. Gastric activity appears after the duodenal activity is already stabilized. Gastric motility appears 9 h after truncal vagotomy and pyloroplasty in the form of isolated contractions. Duodenal migrating myoelectrical complexes (MMC) are observed before MMC from the stomach. In the case of partial gastrectomy, the duodenal complexes are not related to those of the stomach. The length of the duodenal complexes and their duration vary for different patients, but they are longer than in healthy people, the fact that is reported in dogs as well (23, 199).

The disturbances in gastric motility and the delay in its restoration, compared with duodenal motility, are associated with disturbances in the pacesetter potentials (PPs). The following terms are used by various authors: slow potential, basic electrical rhythm (BER), electrical control activity (ECA), and slow wave (SW) (77). It has been found that during abdominal surgery PPs have a frequency of 2.7 cycles/min for 15–180 min, after which time the rhythm becomes irregular; it is pointed out that spike activity is absent at that time (214). The irregularity of the PP rhythm of the stomach, jejunum, ileum, and colon is considered to be the main reason for postoperative paresis (78).

However, the studies of other authors on the electrical activity of the small and large intestines have shown that the appearance of the clinical symptoms of restoration of the intestinal passage is preceded by bursts of spike activity (258). During day 1, only slow waves are recorded from the small and large intestines (Fig. 1). They are characteristic of the state of intestinal paresis. On day 2, small groups of spike potentials (SP) usually appear in the small intestine, followed by SP in the large intestine on the same day or on the next day. They are followed by peristaltic sounds. The bursts of larger groups of SP precede the appearance of flatus and the defecation during days 3 and 4. The administration of stimulants of intestinal motility also results in increased amplitude of the slow waves from the gut and in appearance of SP. Thus the character of the spike activity may be used for assessing the changes in the dynamics of the functional state of the small and large intestines. The appearance of spike activity is of great diagnostic significance and it may have prognostic significance as well (258).

It has been shown in experiments on animals that anesthesia per se influences gastrointestinal motility. Ethyl ether anesthesia completely inhibits the motility of the gastrointestinal tract in rats (46). Pentobarbital anesthesia is followed by inhibition of the motility for ~60 min in dogs, whereas in sheep the inhibition lasts 40 min (47). Laparotomy stops the intestinal activity in both species mentioned above, although the discontinuation lasts less long in dogs (90 min). Incision of the pertioneum results in disappearance of intestinal motility for 1 h in dogs and for 6 h in sheep (47).

Clamping of the small intestine causes a stop that lasts ≤5 min after the removal of the clamp. The secondary period of inhibition of the gastrointestinal motility lasts between 6 h after colonic resection and 24 h after transection of the small intestine, but after 3–6 h of transient activity. Inhibition after abdominal surgery in sheep lasts 48–72 h.

No MMC activity fronts have been observed on postoperative days 1 and 2 (174). However, the activity is slightly reduced between days 3 and 6, and after day 7 MMC are manifested with a pronounced phase 3. Spike potentials are observed in other experiments on dogs after transection and anastomosis, but they are not organized in MMC (55). The MMC occur on postoperative day 2, but the intervals between phase 3 decrease. The percentage of the spike activity increases during subsequent days; there is some activity, but this does not mean that the intestine is functioning normally (55).

The experimental investigations are in agreement with the classic notion about ileus, based on clinical observations. While the stomach and the large intestine are inactive, the small intestine manifests a certain activity; consequently, the small intestine is more resistant to surgical intervention.

## ESOPHAGUS

Anatomically and functionally the esophagus consists of three defined parts: upper esophageal sphinc-

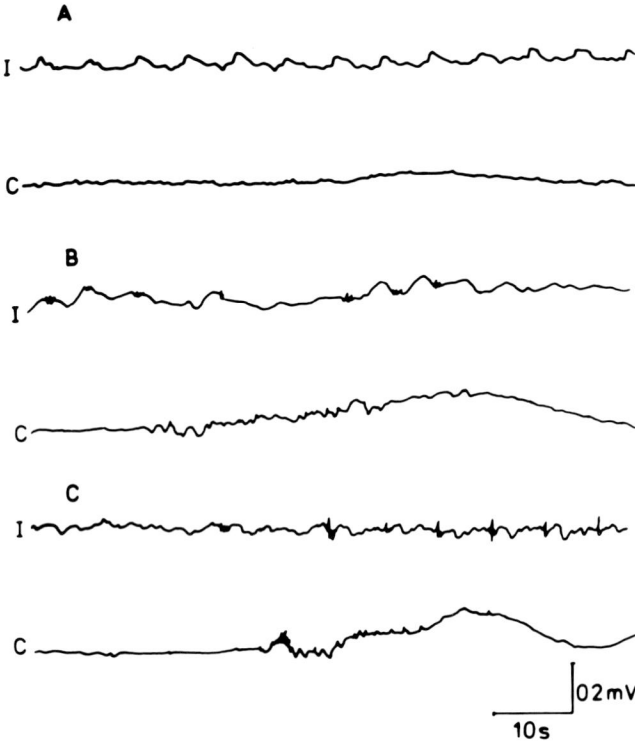

FIG. 1. Electrical activity of muscle wall of small (I) and large (C) intestine in patient in early postoperative period. *A*: day 1; *B*: day 2; *C*: day 5 after surgery. [From Zlatarski et al. (258).]

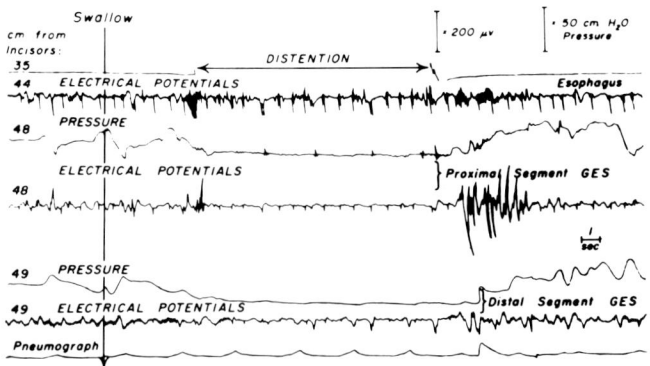

FIG. 2. Changes in pressure and electrical potentials of gastroesophageal sphincter (GES) during balloon distension of esophagus. [From Arimori et al. (10).]

ter, body, and lower esophageal sphincter. The upper two-thirds of the human esophageal body are composed of striated muscle, whereas the lower one-third consists of smooth muscle. The two types of muscles are represented differently in the various species, the correlation in cats being the same as in humans, whereas in dogs the esophageal body is made up of striated muscle.

Esophageal peristalsis is a complicated process of propagating contractile activity, determined by extrinsic and intrinsic nerve mechanisms and possibly by myogenic mechanisms as well (see the chapter by Goyal and Paterson in this *Handbook*). While the upper and lower sphincters, which are located proximally and distally from the esophageal body, are in contracted state during rest, the body is flaccid. Swallowing results in contraction of the esophageal wall, i.e., in primary peristalsis, because of which the propulsion of the bolus to the stomach takes place (Fig. 2). An intraluminal bolus is necessary for the normal propagation of the peristaltic wave in the cervical part of canine esophagus, whereas central mechanisms without bolus produce peristaltic contraction only at the level of the thoracic esophagus (122). Moreover the esophageal contraction is much more frequently peristaltic when a solid bolus is swallowed than when a liquid bolus is swallowed (240).

Deviation of the swallowed bolus at the cervical level by means of a cannula or esophagostomy eliminates the entire peristaltic activity at the level of the bolus deviation (110, 148).

In the case of esophageal transection, the swallow effect depends on the level of the transection. The transection with anastomosis muscle-to-muscle contact in the region of the esophageal striated muscles does not impede the propagation of the primary peristalsis (56, 123). This suggests that at the level of the striated muscles primary peristalsis is centrally regulated. Esophageal transection and bolus deviation at the thoracic level in the dog, as well as at all levels in the rabbit, opossum, and rhesus monkey, do not eliminate primary peristalsis below the level of deviation

(121). The differences observed in various species after esophageal transection are related to the anatomical organization of the esophagus and more specifically to the extent to which striated or smooth muscles are represented in the esophageal wall. If the transection is made at the level of the esophageal smooth muscles, the propagation of the peristaltic wave during swallowing is disturbed (123). These data suggest that the intrinsic elements in the wall of the smooth muscle part of the esophagus are involved in primary peristalsis (121). In the monkey and opossum with intact extrinsic nerves, the secondary peristaltic wave passes through the transection.

The effect of vagotomy on primary and secondary peristalsis of the esophagus is different. Bilateral cervical vagotomy leads to inhibition of esophageal responses to stimuli in the pharynx, connected with the act of swallowing, as well as to the intraluminal distension of the esophagus (56, 67, 118, 181, 200, 244). However, in the smooth muscle part of the esophagus, vagotomy does not result in paralysis, and the ability to perform peristaltic contraction under the influence of liquids and intraluminal distension of a balloon in the esophagus is preserved (48, 82). This correlates with the observation that after subdiaphragmatic vagotomy above lower esophageal sphincter (LES), the sphincter continues to relax as a result of intraluminal distension (68, 143, 160, 194). The relaxation of LES in response to swallowing, however, is reduced or totally inhibited [Fig. 3; (10, 35, 86, 143)]. Evidently, intact vagal nerves at the thoracic level are needed for primary peristalsis in the smooth muscle part of the esophagus, as well as for LES relaxation during swallowing (67, 84, 209). Reynolds et al. (200) have pointed out that complete aperistalsis may be observed in the smooth muscle part of the esophagus several hours after bilateral vagotomy, after which the peristalsis is restored for a different period of time. Obviously a nonvagal central pathway is involved after the vagotomy or, most probably, an intrinsic mechanism operates in the smooth muscle part of the esophagus and guarantees peristalsis in this part of the esophagus (200).

In addition to primary and secondary esophageal peristalsis, defined for the first time in 1899 by Meltzer (165), Cannon (50) observed esophageal peristalsis upon intraluminal balloon inflation after vagotomy, which he referred to as "tertiary peristalsis." This peristalsis of the esophagus apparently results from the activation of intrinsic nerves and myogenic mechanisms (204, 205); therefore it is suggested that it be called "autonomous" rather than "tertiary" (203).

The changes observed in esophageal peristalsis after transection and vagotomy are the result of experimental manipulations. However, they may also occur after surgical intervention in the esophagus or in the esophageal region, and they may explain the possible complications observed.

## STOMACH

### Resection

Evacuation of the gastric content from the stomach, which is reduced in volume after resection of its antral part, is known to occur within minutes. In the first 30 min after feeding, the patients have the feeling of distension in the stomach, borborygmi, heaviness, desire to lie down, sweating and palpitations, and finally a watery diarrhea (112). The rapid evacuation nevertheless depends on the resection method. It has been observed that the food is retained longer in the gastric remnant of patients after B-I. One of the reasons for this is the fixing of the gastric remnant in both the esophageal hiatus and the duodenum. In this way, the location of the gastric remnant is close to that of the stomach before the operation. In the case of B-II, the gastric remnant is fixed only in the esophageal hiatus. Anastomosis with the small intestine shapes the gastric remnant as a funnel directed almost vertically, and this facilitates food evacuation (245). In addition to the more favorable position of the gastric remnant, contractions of the gastroduodenal anastomosis are observed in patients after B-I; the contractions guarantee rhythmic evacuation of the contrast material (X-ray examination) in 59 of 67 patients (88%). As a result of the rhythmic evacuation, in 48% of the patients, gastric remnant emptying lasts for >1 h. In the case of B-II, in 15 of 56 patients studied (17%), the evacuation was rhythmic; however, in 41 patients (73%) it was continuous (169). Importance is attributed to the regulatory role of the gastroduodenal anastomosis, which manifests pyloric-like contractions to the regulatory role of the duodenum in the case of pronounced passage through it and to the existence of antiperistaltic waves in the duodenum.

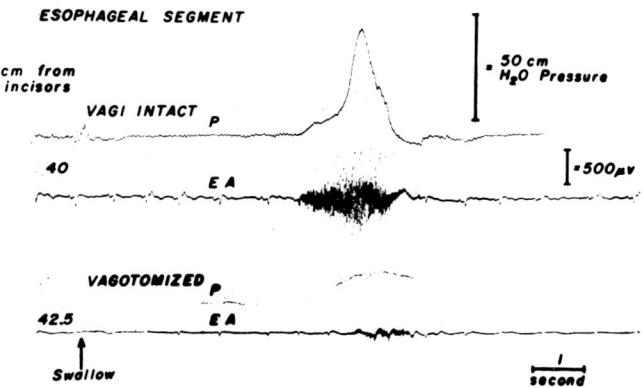

FIG. 3. Simultaneous detection of electrical activity (EA) and intraluminal pressure (P) of vagally innervated and vagally denervated portions of dog esophagus during swallowing. In vagotomized segment, pressure increase was feeble and electrical activity much lower than in vagally intact segment. Exact temporal association between electrical activity and pressure changes was also abolished. [From Arimori et al. (10).]

Not only the evacuation velocity but also the type of the surgical method is important for the frequency and severity of the postresection complications. Thus at the same gastric emptying rate (30 min) complications are observed in 32% of the patients after B-I, whereas after B-II complications appear in 52% of the cases (169). Nevertheless, when the two methods are compared, food retention in the gastric remnants for more than 5 h occurs more frequently after B-I than after B-II (233).

Comparison of the food evacuation velocity in healthy people and in patients with subtotal gastrectomy has shown that in healthy people gastric emptying has a linear pattern and an average velocity of 27.96% of gastric content per hour. Three phases in the emptying of the gastric remnant are distinguished in subtotal gastrectomy: 1) initial phase, characterized by precipitous emptying of 15%–65% of the gastric content; 2) delayed emptying for 20–30 min; and 3) smooth nonlinear curve of the emptying. Approximately 5%–15% of the gastric remnant content is emptied in ~2 h (151). The evacuation velocity of solid foods in patients with subtotal gastrectomy is more variable than the evacuation velocity of liquids (151).

The evacuation of the gastric remnant content in patients with B-II procedure starts before the end of the meal (191). The so-called lag phase, i.e., the time between the end of feeding and the beginning of the evacuation, which for healthy patients is 4.6 min for porridge and 22.2 min for pancake, disappears for semisolid foods after gastric resection and is reduced for solid foods to ~6.5 min. The fact that there exists a lag phase for solid foods is in favor of the antrumlike function of the gastric remnant. The evacuation phase for solid foods in patients after B-II surgery is greatly reduced, but there is a statistically significant difference between the emptying time of solid and semisolid foods (191).

The difference in the emptying of liquids and solids (radiopaque spheres) in healthy dogs has been demonstrated in experimental work (88). The difference in the evacuation disappears after distal antrectomy. It is believed that distal antrectomy perceptibly accelerates the emptying of the gastric remnants and disturbs the ability of the stomach to distinguish between liquids and solids. No retropulsion of the plastic spheres is observed after antrectomy, although the usual role of the terminal antral contraction is to push the finely ground particles through the pylorus, whereby the larger particles return under pressure, i.e., retropulsion takes place, and they are further ground (54). After antrectomy, when grinding of the particles becomes impossible, the discriminating capacity of the antropyloric region is also lost (155).

After the operation, the evacuating function of the proximal gastric remnant is particularly accelerated during the first 6 mo (192). In only 3 of 61 patients observed, evacuation lasted for >1 h. Between postoperative months 6 and 12, the emptying is delayed, in the 30- to 60-min range for the majority of the patients. More than 1 yr after the operation, the evacuation in 49 of 61 patients takes 30–60 min or >60 min (192).

Evacuation of liquids and solids has been studied with double-isotope technique after stomach bypass operation in cases of obesity, when a pouch measuring ≦100 ml in volume is made from the proximal stomach (114, 115). The emptying of solids is initially faster, then it becomes delayed. Evacuation of liquids is generally faster, as in healthy people. No dependence is established between the size of the stomach in the case of gastroduodenostomy and the evacuation velocity for liquids and solids.

Hypotonic stomach is discovered in the course of the preliminary examination of the patients before the operation. However, resection of the stomach wall is followed by a gradual rise in the tone of the muscle wall of the gastric remnant (192, 245). Parallel with this, the appearance of contractile activity in the muscle wall is also noted. Rhythmic activity with wave duration of ~20 s is recorded with the electrographic method invented by Sobakin (192, 227). Manometric tests have also demonstrated quite strong contractions, with a frequency of ~3 contractions/min, which are typical of the antrum of intact stomach (191). Most probably these changes are responsible for the improved emptying of the gastric remnant. Rhythmic evacuation of the gastric remnant is observed in patients after B-I; continuous evacuation was found only in 7 of 74 patients (245). The gradual increase in the tone of the gastric remnant wall restores the possibility to contain the food mass and to prevent its precipitous evacuation into the intestine (192).

Adaptive changes are also observed in experimental studies on dogs and cats with resection of two-thirds of the stomach, by chronically implanted electrodes on the muscle wall of the gastric remnant. The rhythm of the fundic slow waves changes from 1.5–2 cycles/min in healthy dogs to ~4 cycles/min in dogs with resected stomach, as it is in the corpus and antrum of the stomach (Fig. 4). Spike potentials burst with the higher amplitude PPs and form the phases of the myoelectric complexes (17). Five months after the resection, the slow sinusoidal waves of the fundus change their configuration to plateau-type action potential, similar to the configuration of PPs from the in vitro experiments on the corpus and antrum of the stomach (16). This determines the change in the type of the fundic contractile activity from predominantly tonic to predominantly phasic in the gastric remnant (16), such as it is in the corpus and the antrum of the stomach. The changes in the electrical and contractile activity of the muscle wall of the gastric remnant have proved to be related to deep structural changes. Histological studies demonstrate hypertrophy and hyperplasia of the smooth muscle cells, which explains the

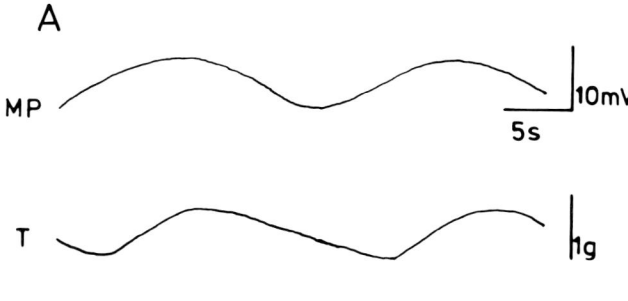

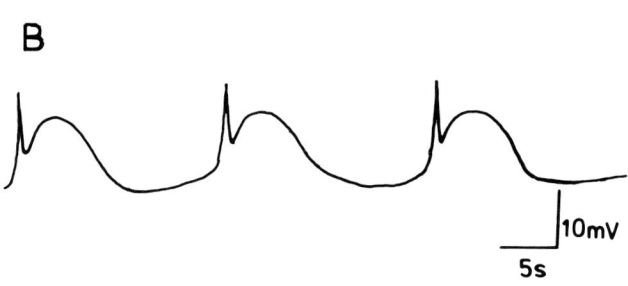

FIG. 4. Slow potential changes from fundic muscle wall before and after Billroth I gastrectomy. A: sinusoidal slow waves from smooth muscle cell of intact fundus in cat. B: spontaneous electrical activity of single smooth muscle cell from gastric remnant after functional loading: configuration of action potential–type plateau. MP, electrical activity; T, contractile activity of smooth muscle strip. [From Bayguinov and Atanassova (29).]

increased wall thickness of the gastric remnant and the general increase in its volume (19). Microelectrode studies of the postsynaptic responses of the smooth muscle cells have demonstrated a gradual increase in the excitatory responses of the smooth muscle cells of the stomach residue, so that nerve transmission becomes predominantly excitatory toward the end of the sixth month after gastric resection (29). This is connected with structural changes in the myenteric plexus (Fig. 5).

All these changes take place faster and more completely if part of the pacemaker region of the stomach, which is located in the oral one-third of the corpus, is included in the gastric remnant. This is achieved when the resection line passes at a distance of 1 or 1.5 cm distally from the boundary between the fundus and the corpus. This boundary is located far more distally from the one described in most anatomy textbooks; it is approximately at the level of the entry of the short gastric arteries into the stomach. This localization is supported by the fact that slow waves with frequency characteristics of the fundus, i.e. ~2 cycles/min, are still recorded in this region (16).

In cases of more extensive resection, when the gastric remnant is made only from the fundus, slow waves continue to be recorded but in a relatively slow rhythm. Frequencies of ~3–4 cycles/min are found only during the ninth month after the resection (16).

Differences in the recovery processes occur also depending on the type of restoration of the food passage. The PPs rhythm of ~4 cycles/min is established faster in cases of anastomosis B-I and especially in B-I Maki procedure (19, 154). When the passage is restored with B-II Polya-Reichel procedure, changes in the PPs rhythm take place, although with slightly more delay (19). This difference may be due to the degree of functional loading. In the case of B-I Maki, the muscle wall of the gastric remnant is expected to overcome the greater resistance of the preserved pylorus, hence the more developed adaptation.

Resection of the proximal part of the stomach is performed in the case of cancer in the region of the cardia, whereby the gastric remnant comprises the antral part of the stomach. The muscle wall of the distal gastric remnant manifests rhythmic activity, although with delayed rhythm of 1.8–2.2 cycles/min. Food evacuation is accelerated and is of the continuous type (192). Such a reduced PP frequency in the stomach is observed in humans after gastric transection, which is in agreement with experimental findings in dogs subjected to gastric transections. Stomach wall transection results in drop of PP frequency in the distal segment of the stomach (13, 168, 236, 247). After removal of the pacemaker region of the stomach, the proper rhythm of the distal gastric segment, which is slower, becomes apparent. Modeling of the gastric PPs has led to the conclusion that the disturbance in the evacuation may be the result of loss of phase locking of the control waves in the distal segment (216).

Accelerated emptying of the content of the gastric remnant from the distal part of the stomach is observed both in humans (192) and in dogs (255). The

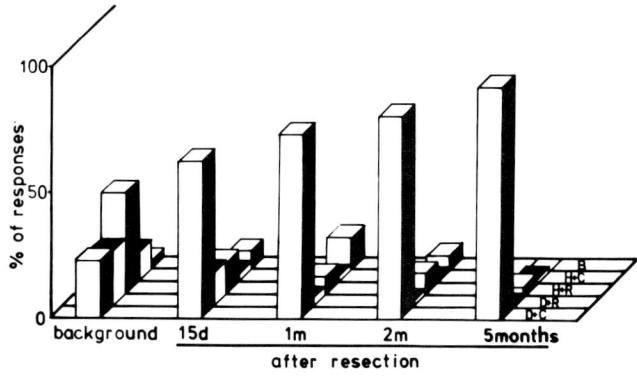

FIG. 5. Dynamics of changes in nerve transmission of gastric remnant after subtotal gastrectomy. D + C, depolarization and contraction of smooth muscle strip; D + R, depolarization and relaxation; H + R, hyperpolarization and relaxation; H + C, hyperpolarization and contraction; B, biphasic responses. [From Atanassova et al. (18).]

emptying corresponds to the changes in the electrical activity. Stomach transection also leads to dissociation of the spike activity between its two segments (13). Moreover the spike activity of the part of the stomach distal to the transection considerably exceeds the spike activity of the proximal segment. This could be explained by the assumption that the distal part of the stomach is subordinate and driven by the gastric region located proximally to it. When it is liberated from the influence of the proximal stomach and of the intrinsic nervous system in that region after transection, the distal part of the stomach manifests substantially increased spike activity (14). Disturbance of the steplike subordination of the intrinsic nervous system, which exists in intact organs, results after transection in more pronounced and independent spike activity of the distal part (14).

The rhythmic pattern of gastric content emptying is associated with normal function of PS. However, in radical gastric resections the PS is removed. In such cases the sphincteric role is played to a greater extent by the anastomosis. The anastomosis is believed to produce rhythmic contractions that regulate the evacuation (169). The evacuatory function in the distal gastric remnant can be explained by the fact that the PS is considered to be the terminal part of the pyloric antrum, and that it contracts in the same rhythm as the pyloric antrum (188). Additionally, the emptying function can be influenced by ability of the distal part of the gastric remnant to contract in the rhythm of the corpus and antrum (19, 29). This is a manifestation of the adaptation of the muscle wall of the gastric remnant to the increased requirements imposed by the effect of distension of the wall by the relatively greater food volume.

Based on experimental work in dogs, hemigastrectomy is recommended to preserve PS function. In this procedure, the antral mucosa is removed to ensure the elimination of the gastrin phase in the production of gastric juice (138). Food evacuation proceeds much more slowly after this kind of operation.

In the case of gastric ulcer along the lesser curvature, an excision in the form of a thin tongue that comprises the ulcer can be performed in order to preserve the PS (81). The pylorus may be preserved if 1 or 1.5 cm of the antrum is left in the antrectomy. The gastric remnant is connected to the remaining part of the antrum. In such patients, the evacuation is delayed, and dumping syndrome does not develop (154). This observation may be explained to a certain extent by the following experimental studies.

With an intact gastroduodenal junction, there is sequencing between the spike activities of the stomach and duodenum (11, 12). The percentage of PPs that evoke SP, with respect to the total number of PPs throughout the experiment, is 36.3% for the stomach, which is close to that of the duodenum, i.e., 30.0% (12, 14). Section of the gastroduodenal junction results in dissociation of the gastric and duodenal spike activities, with the spike activity of the duodenum considerably increased; 48% of the duodenal slow waves have SP, compared with 34% PPs with SP in the stomach, i.e., the duodenal SP after pyloric transection exceed those of the stomach by 50% (Fig. 6). Other authors also report more pronounced spike activity of the small intestine after removal of the gastroduodenal junction (28, 41, 55, 57). Moreover the values for the dogs operated according to the B-I or B-II are similar, 45.56% and 52%, respectively (12, 14). The dogs suffer from diarrhea and weight loss, although their stomach has not been reduced in volume. Increased spike activity is observed when the dogs are hungry, i.e., without the influence of coarse and undigested food in the small intestine, as is the case in gastric resection after feeding. In the case of pyloric section, the intrinsic nervous system of the duodenum is liberated from the controlling influence of the gastric intrinsic nervous system, and the spike activity of the small intestine increases apparently as a result of the greater release of acetylcholine.

The antral part of the stomach plays a regulating role for the motility of the small intestine. In the case of transection at the level of incisura angularis, the spike activity of the duodenum bursts in the rhythm of the delayed PPs from the antral part of the stomach. When at the end of week 1 after surgery the rhythm of PPs below the transection becomes equal to that above the anastomosis because of the regeneration of the gastric smooth muscle cells (20), the duodenal SP burst in the unified rhythm of PPs. For this reason, in the B-I Maki operation the PS does not simply regulate the evacuation from the gastric remnant, but the remaining part of the muscle wall of the antral part of the stomach has a controlling influence on the motility of the small intestine. Moreover the control is in the form of a braking action on intestinal motility.

An enormous number of resections have been per-

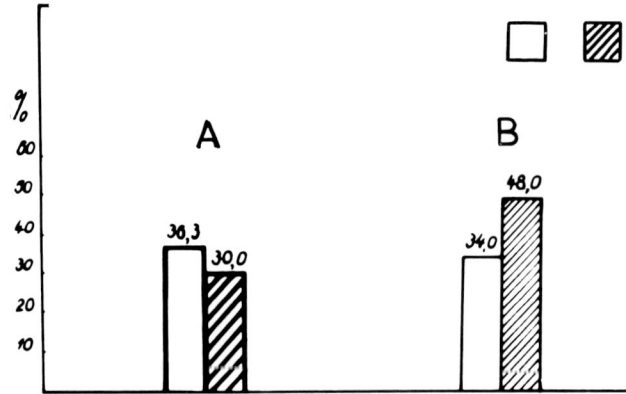

FIG. 6. Percentage correlation of slow waves with spike potentials to total number of slow waves in stomach (*A*) and duodenum (*B*) with intact (*open bars*) and transected (*hatched bars*) gastroduodenal junction. [From Atanassova (14).]

formed. The initial high mortality rate is no longer a grave problem, because it has been reduced to 1% (135). However, undesirable side effects resulting from the anatomical and functional changes imposed by the surgeon, in addition to ulcer recurrence, necessitate a second intervention, called reconstructive surgery, in ~10% of the patients. Conversion of B-II to B-I is recommended especially to correct various phenomena during dumping, diarrhea, and gastroesophageal reflux (44, 135). In patients with very significant weight loss and diarrhea, the operation has usually good effect, because it restores the anatomical relationships. The results are similar for jeujunogastroplasty (211). Enteroanastomosis is recommended in patients with retrocolic gastrectomy (Fig. 7). In other cases, Roux loops are applied (124, 134, 135), construction of a reservoir from the jejunum (221) or jejunal interposition (134, 135, 198).

The first experiments with reversed segments were made by Halsted in 1887 (108). After this operation, the transit time is increased (149) and the patients gain weight and tolerate carbohydrates to a certain extent (166). The reversal of the loop is not without risk, because it may be followed by ischemia of the loop with perforation or stricture. Gastric stasis was the reason for the surgery in 15 of 173 patients (134). In all cases, although Kelly has reported excellent or very good results in 108 of 173 patients (134), it is recommended to subject the patients to conservative therapy for 1 yr in advance, because the result of the reconstructive surgery is difficult to predict (44).

In addition, propagation of duodenal PPs in the oral direction toward the pyloris has been induced experimentally by means of duodenal electrical pacing (1, 31), thus achieving a 25% delay of gastric emptying (133, 175). This method, however, has not been applied in humans (31).

## Vagotomy

TRUNCAL VAGOTOMY. There is unanimous agreement that the contractions of the stomach wall are connected with the myogenic generation of PPs. As they propagate along the stomach wall, the PPs synchronize the activity of the smooth muscle cells of the stomach wall, and thereby lock the contractions to the temporal and spatial characteristics of the PPs (189). It is also evident that the myogenically generated electrical activity of the stomach is continuously modulated by nervous and humoral factors (14, 65, 184, 185).

Disturbances in the electrical activity and motility of the stomach occur even on day 1 after truncal vagotomy. Incoordination between the electrical activity of the antrum and of the corpus of the stomach is observed (Fig. 8). While PPs with frequency characteristic of the stomach (4.5–5 cycles/min in dogs) are generated from the corpus of the stomach, groups of high-frequency PPs are recorded from the antral region. These changes usually last until after postoperative day 5 (132), or according to some authors, even until the end of postoperative wk 2 (186).

Disorganization of the gastric electrical activity after truncal vagotomy was observed for the first time by Nelsen et al. (180) and Hegglin et al. (109). It was later reported by several researchers working on this problem (1, 144, 180, 186). These changes are much more manifested after truncal vagotomy than after selective vagotomy (144, 232).

No incoordination in the gastric electrical activity

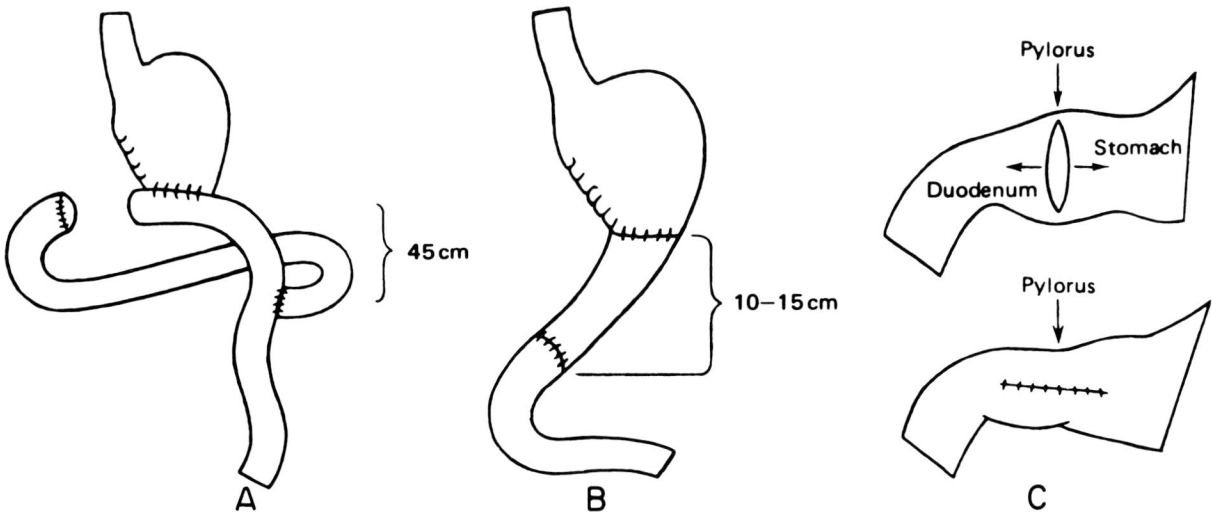

FIG. 7. Reconstructive gastric operations employed. *A*: Roux gastrojejunostomy; *B*: jejunal interposition; *C*: pyloric reconstruction. [From Kelly et al. (131), by permission of the publishers, Butterworth and Co., copyright 1981.]

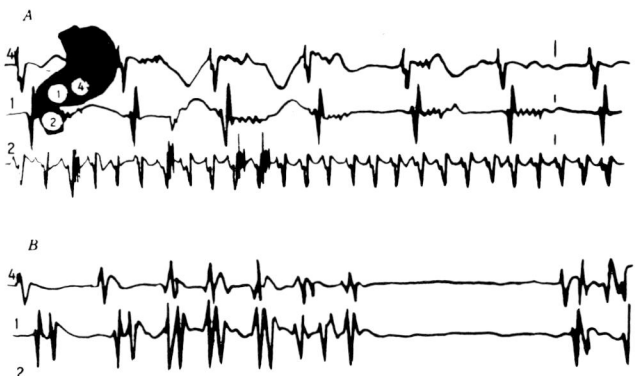

FIG. 8. Disturbance of unified character of pacesetter potential rhythm of the antrum. *A*: before; *B*: after thoracic vagotomy. *Upper left corner*, position of electrodes; calibration 200 μV. [From Papasova and Atanassova (185).]

and motility after vagotomy has been observed in either acute experiments (38, 177, 178) or immediately after the vagotomy (M. Papasova and E. Atanassova, unpublished observations). The same frequency PPs are recorded from the body and the antrum of the stomach. However, bursts of high-frequency PPs are observed from time to time in the antral recording during day 1 after the vagotomy. A characteristic finding is that these potentials are dysrhythmic and have different amplitudes (tachygastria). At the same time, the electrical activity of the corpus of the stomach is characterized by rhythmic PPs with frequencies typical of the stomach of intact animals. The rhythm of PPs generated in the antrum is restored on appearance of SP; i.e., slow potentials whose rhythm is identical to that of the stomach corpus are recorded. However, the appearance of SP is preceded by a prolonged pause (132). The percentage of PPs from the antrum of the stomach, accompanied by SP, is also reduced (Table 1). The appearance of SP in the corpus of the stomach leads most frequently to elimination of the incoordination between the electrical activity of the corpus and the antrum. After feeding, the unified rhythm of PPs along the entire length of the stomach is also restored with the appearance of SP.

Carbachol induces the appearance of SP, with parallel regulation of the rhythm of PPs generated in the antrum, which become identical in frequency to those generated in the corpus of the stomach (186).

Truncal vagotomy leads to changes in the adaptability of the stomach. The responses of the gastric electrical activity to water instillation in the stomach itself are temporarily disturbed; they are strongly reduced or altogether absent when oil is introduced and disturbed also in cases of insulin-induced hypoglycemia (132).

Disorganization of the gastric electrical activity after truncal vagotomy lasts 1–2 wk. In some animals, it may appear sporadically but seldom in fasting animals (132, 186). Simultaneous recording of the contractions of the stomach wall by means of force transducers demonstrates that the stomach wall practically does not contract at all during the appearance of tachygastria in the antrum of the stomach (Fig. 9). When the rhythm of the antral PPs is switched to that of PPs from the corpus of the stomach, which usually happens when SP propagate from the body to the antrum, the first PP is followed by a high-amplitude contraction (187). Single high-amplitude contractions during the first postvagotomy days on the background of suppressed gastric activity are also reported in studies on the character of the intraluminal pressure in the stomach after transthoracic vagotomy (31, 161). It is characteristic that food intake during the early postvagotomy period results in the appearance of chaotic motility, three to four times weaker than in intact animals (161).

The changes observed in the gastric motility after vagotomy undergo a definite evolution and depend above all on the character of the vagotomy. They are most severe and last longest after bilateral truncal vagotomy. The lack of receptive relaxation is one of the main disturbances characterizing this vagotomy (142, 228). In the case of intact vagal nerves in humans, the fundus is filled and emptied almost linearly. The fundus is filled for no more than 6 s, which is a manifestation of receptive relaxation. This ability of the stomach is lost after vagotomy, and the stomach is filled with food for at least 9 s (223). Adaptation of both the fundus and the antrum of the stomach takes

TABLE 1. *Effect of Transthoracic Vagotomy on Gastric Electrical Activity in Fasting Dogs*

| Dog | Mean Frequency of PP, cycles/min | | Mean Corporal Propagation Time, s | | Mean Antral Propagation Time, s | | Mean Percentage of Antral PP With Action Potentials | |
|---|---|---|---|---|---|---|---|---|
| | Before vagotomy | After vagotomy | Before vagotomy | After vagotomy | Before vagotomy | After vagotomy | Before vagotomy | After vagotomy |
| 1 | 5.5 | 5.4 | 6.9 ± 0.3 | 8.3 ± 0.4 | 2.7 | 3.3 | 29 ± 6 | 25 ± 6 |
| 2 | 5.7 | 5.8 | 9.4 | 10.5 ± 0.3 | 1.1 | 1.4 | 23 ± 9 | 15 ± 5 |
| 3 | 5.3 | 5.2 | 7.7 | 8.6 ± 0.2 | 2.0 | 2.4 | 37 ± 11 | 32 ± 9 |
| 4 | 5.3 | 5.8 | 5.9 | 7.9 | 3.2 | 3.8 | 31 ± 8 | 15 ± 5 |
| 5 | 5.4 | 5.2 | 9.5 ± 0.2 | 10.5 ± 0.3 | 2.2 | 3.0 | 11 ± 4 | 2 ± 1 |
| Grand mean | 5.4 | 5.5 | 7.9 | 9.2 | 2.2 | 2.8 | 26 | 18 |

PP, pacesetter potential. [From Kelly and Code (132).]

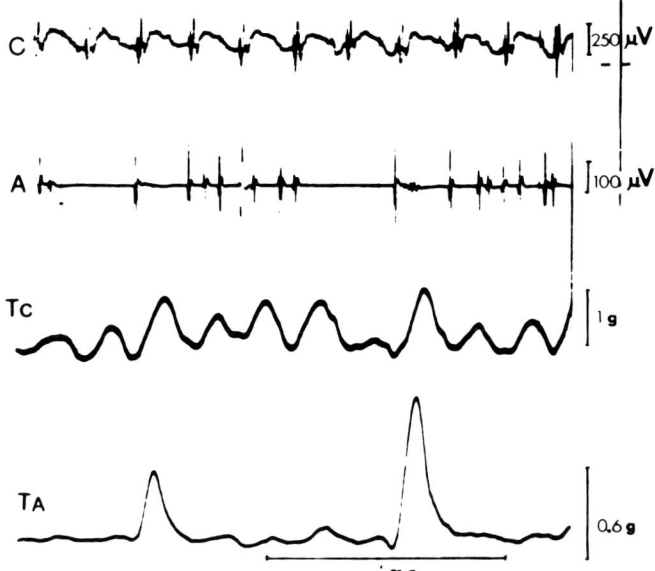

FIG. 9. Lack of coordination between electrical and contractile activities of corpus (C) and antrum (A) of dog stomach after bilateral transthoracic vagotomy. Tc and Ta, contractile activity in corpus and antrum, respectively. [From Papasova and Atanassova (186).]

much longer (229). The loss of receptive relaxation and the disturbed accommodation after truncal vagotomy are expressed by a feeling of stomach distension in ~25% of the patients (130). However, the plastic tone of the stomach antrum is unchanged (37) or raised (120). Lower sensitivity of the antral part of the stomach to mechanical stimulation is also noted (161). According to other researchers, the intragastric pressure may be increased even after vagotomy (53, 193). These findings contradict the observations of some authors, who report reduction of the gastric tone and strong decrease in the contractility of gastric muscles (60, 93, 237, 249).

The early motor evacuatory disturbances observed during the first 5–10 days after surgical intervention may be eliminated by means of ganglionic blockers (161). This is the reason for questioning the cause of the disturbances as resulting from activation of the intrinsic nervous system after severing of the extrinsic nerves and, more specifically, activation of the noncholinergic, nonadrenergic inhibitory neurons of the stomach (158, 159). Severing of the efferent fibers to the inhibitory neurons explains the lack of receptive relaxation in the vagotomied stomach. There is no doubt that the evacuating ability of the stomach is strongly changed after truncal vagotomy (24, 25, 224, 241). This is usually manifested by delayed gastric emptying (83, 116, 122, 156, 196), more frequent after a solid meal (119), whereas liquids and liquid food components are evacuated very fast (130). This is largely the result of the increased intragastric pressure (130), which is particularly pronounced when truncal vagotomy is combined with pyloroplasty; this suggests that pyloroplasty additionally contributes to the ab-

normally early emptying of liquids from the stomach after truncal vagotomy (4, 64, 97, 98, 170). In the case of vagotomy with pyloroplasty named after the method of Heineke-Miculicz (pyloroplasty at 3.5 cm and 7 cm), irrespective of the type and volume of the food, 51%–60% of the gastric content passes into the duodenum in the very first 10 min (111). The evacuation of hypertonic glucose solution is particularly fast, whereas the emptying of hypotonic NaCl solution is almost the same as before the vagotomy (106). Rapid evacuation of liquids after truncal vagotomy may lead to dumping and diarrhea. Postoperative dumping is observed in ~20% and diarrhea in 30% of the operated patients. Diarrhea is a frequent postoperative complication; it occurs sporadically, starts suddenly, and is characterized by loss of great amounts of fluids. The main factor causing diarrhea is the rapid evacuation of liquids (150). Thus, in the case of truncal vagotomy with pyloroplasty, this is particularly pronounced during postoperative weeks 1–4 and decreases gradually in postoperative weeks 4–8, so that evacuation becomes normal between postoperative years 1 and 3 (72). Other authors, however, report fast early evacuation of solid food as well (70).

Evacuation of the gastric content is considered to take place at the expense of the tonic component of the gastric motility, which, according to some authors, does not change after vagotomy (183). The character of the dynamics of the stomach evacuation capacity is considered in detail in the monographic work of Matrossova et al. (161) based on extensive experimental material. According to these observations, gastric emptying after truncal vagotomy is periodically sharply intensified, then it becomes weaker again, until finally chyme release from the stomach stops completely. When the evacuation of the content starts, gastric emptying is much faster than in healthy animals. A characteristic feature is that it has a cyclic course, each 20–50-min cycle of fast emptying followed by a cycle of sharply delayed evacuation, which lasts 70–120 min. During month 1 after vagotomy, the duration of the evacuatory process sharply increases, then during subsequent months it becomes gradually shorter. In dogs subjected to truncal vagotomy with pyloroplasty or gastrojejunostomy, the duration of the gastric content emptying is close to that in healthy animals.

Systematic studies on the character of the gastric electrical activity and motility during different posttruncal vagotomy stages demonstrate, according to some authors, gradual improvement of the activity without complete restoration. According to Tetyaeva (238), four phases of restoration of the gastric motility after truncal vagotomy may be observed, i.e., phase 1, during which gastric motility is strongly inhibited; phases 2 and 3, with progressive intensification of gastric motility (even to the extent that the motility may become continuous); and phase 4 (1 yr after vagotomy), when symptoms of periodicity in gastric motility appear. Tetyaeva (238) maintains that phase 4 is the result of the restitution of the inhibitory functions of the regenerated vagal nerves. The impossibility of complete recovery of gastric motility after truncal vagotomy is claimed by other authors as well (61, 235). There are data, however, according to which complete recovery of gastric motility occurs at different postvagotomy periods (147, 195). It is worth noting that according to Matrossova et al. (161) disturbances in the motility are not always accompanied by disturbances in the evacuatory activity of the stomach.

After studying the character of the electrical activity of the dog stomach between days 1 and 150 after truncal vagotomy, Marik and Code (157) emphasized the irregularity of the cycle periods after vagotomy. In their opinion, MMC phase 1 is significantly changed and phase 3 of the complex is especially strongly reduced. Most often a postprandial activity pattern takes its place. Systematic studies of the gastric electrical activity during 6 mo after truncal vagotomy demonstrate a certain tendency toward restoration of the different MMC phases, although their duration remains different compared with prevagotomy values (22). Intensification of the spike activity is observed toward the end of week 1 after vagotomy, when the incoordination between the electrical activity of the antrum and the corpus of the stomach begins to decrease. In fact, the intensification of the spike activity precedes the surmounting of the incoordination. The percentage of PPs accompanied by SP increases, so that the gastric electrical activity becomes typical of phase 2 of MMC (Fig. 10). At the beginning of month

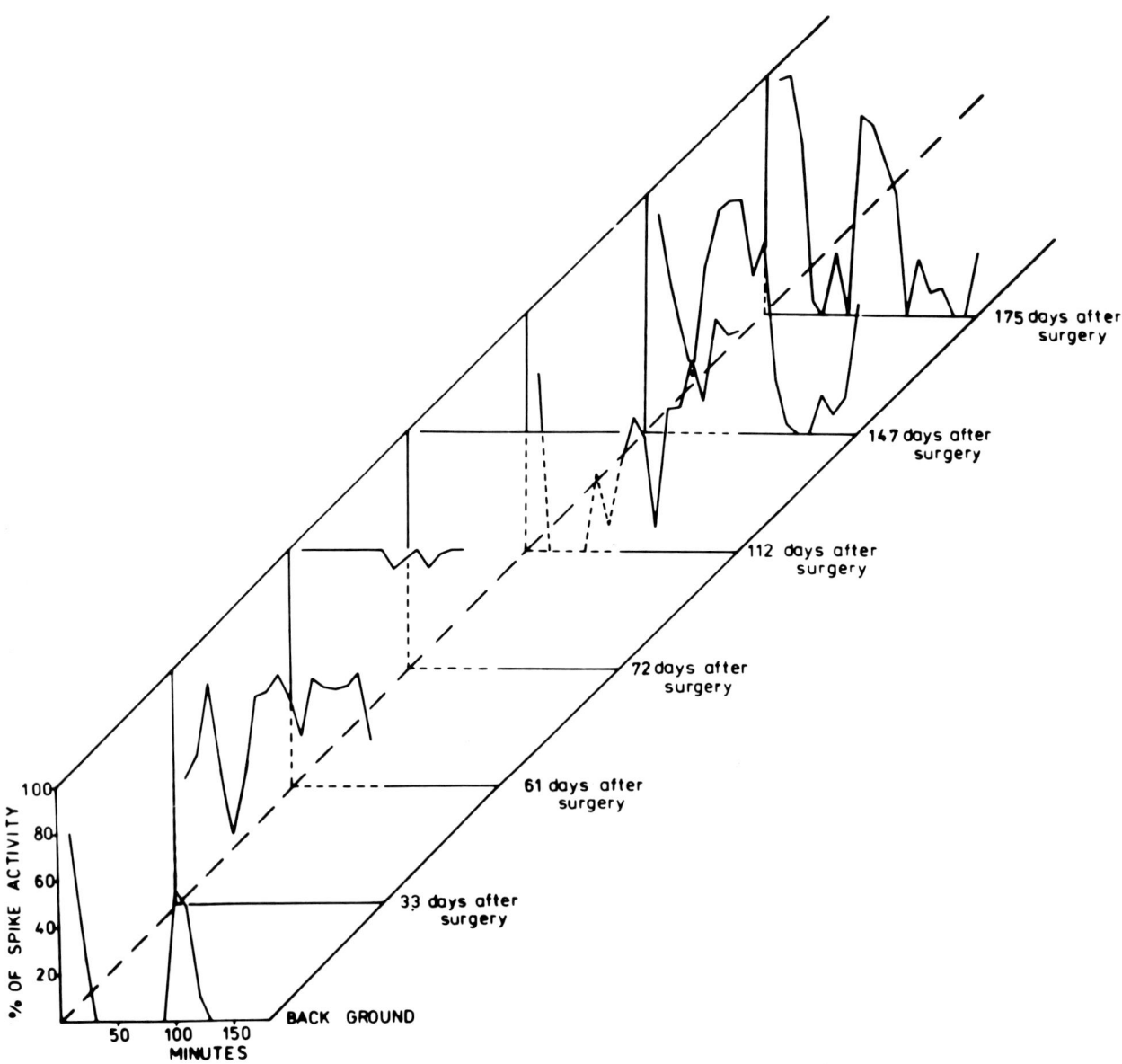

FIG. 10. Dynamics of changes in phases of migrating myoelectrical complexes in stomach at different periods after vagotomy. [From Atanassova (14).]

2 after vagotomy, SPs are recorded throughout the duration of the experiment (5–6 h). However, the characteristic dynamics of the MMC is disturbed: phase 3 is prolonged and phase 1 is absent. Spike activity begins to decrease during month 3 after vagotomy, and toward the end of this month it is possible to observe brief periods during which only PPs are recorded. This tendency is intensified during month 5, whereas myoelectrical complexes with the four characteristic phases appear during month 6, although their duration is not identical to that before the vagotomy. Phase 1 is shortened at the expense of phase 4, which is longer (14). These data correlate with the findings of Matrossova et al. (161) who claim that the periodic activity of the digestive tract is preserved in most dogs subjected to truncal vagotomy, although sometimes recurrences with disturbances may occur. Disturbances are observed also in the electrical activity of the stomach, which may be manifested by appearance of ectopic pacemakers: PPs are generated in the antrum and propagate in the oral direction to the corpus. Nausea and vomiting in humans are most probably the manifestation of this phenomenon. However, the gradual restoration of the different MMC phases and the restoration of the periodic character of the gastric motility suggest that the intrinsic nervous system undertakes the function of regulator of the gastric electrical activity and motility (14, 185) without compensating for this function completely. At the same time, it guarantees the propagation of peristaltic waves along the entire stomach (161).

The early manifestations of incoordination between the electrical activity and the motility of the antrum and of the corpus of the stomach immediately after the vagotomy are most probably the result of disturbances in the interactions between the different neurotransmitters, which function in the neural circuits that generate normal gastric motility. This is supported by the observed normalization of the gastric electrical activity and motility after injection of carbachol. Disturbance of the neurohumoral equilibrium after transthoracic vagotomy is not to be excluded, since it results in the appearance of disorganization between the electrical activity of the antrum and stomach. One should bear in mind Sanders' view [(212); see the chapter by Sanders and Publicover in this *Handbook*] that tachygastria is the result of increased release of prostaglandins. However, further studies are needed to determine the level of prostaglandins during postvagotomy tachygastria. In discussing the problem, one should consider Daniel's opinion (76) about the disturbed balance between the neurotransmitters at the expense of norepinephrine after the vagotomy. Acetylcholine release is increased during week 2 after vagotomy, which leads to increased spike activity and to overcoming of incoordination. Later the intensified spike activity and the absence of phase 1 in MMC may also be associated with the intensified acetylcholine release. Most probably there is a general restoration of the balance between neurotransmitters, which corresponds to the observed tendency toward MMC stabilization. This process, however, is not complete; therefore even after month 6 after vagotomy the different MMC phases are not yet identical in their duration to prevagotomy values. This hypothesis requires systematic studies at the level of the different neurotransmitters. The process is probably much more complex, and it is presumably connected with the release not only of classic neurotransmitters (33, 96) but also of a number of peptides, which recently were identified together with the neurotransmitters in the nerve terminals and which have a definite regulatory influence on gastric electrical activity and motility.

SELECTIVE VAGOTOMY. Different types of selective vagotomy have been proposed to eliminate the complications observed after truncal vagotomy in the therapy of ulcer disease. The aim of selective vagotomy is to preserve the vagal innervation of the remaining organs in the abdominal cavity, as well as of the antrum and PS. Two methods are most popular: *1*) selective vagotomy, whereby the vagal branches innervating the other viscera are preserved intact, and *2*) proximal stomach vagotomy (PSV). Different names are used in the literature for PSV, e.g., parietal cell vagotomy, selective vagotomy of parietal cell mass (7, 8), highly selective vagotomy (176), highly selective proximal vagotomy (117), proximal gastric vagotomy (101, 139, 254), etc.

Griffith and Harkins (103) were the first to report selective vagotomy, whereas Amdrup and Jensen (8) first reported proximal vagotomy without pyloroplasty. Later they reported delayed evacuation of solid food (9) —this finding was shared by other authors (32, 107) —while the evacuation of liquids is accelerated in the first 10 min after the vagotomy (63, 62, 248). Many of the symptoms observed after truncal vagotomy are characteristic of selective vagotomy as well. Disturbances after PSV are relatively transient. Normal gastric emptying is preserved much better after PSV, compared with the other types of vagotomy (107, 137). A definite type of dynamics is observed in this process during different postoperative periods. In month 3 after PSV, the velocity of gastric evacuation is increased during the first 5 min after food intake. This is still apparent in months 6 and 12 after vagotomy, while the rest of the food is evacuated more regularly (100). A particularly important fact is the preservation of the exponential dynamics of gastric emptying (71), because this process is much closer to the process in the stomach of control healthy individuals (116). This agrees with observations on the character of the gastric motility in humans after PSV (228). The basal pressure with which the faster emptying of liquids may be associated is increased (Fig. 11). This could explain to an extent the complaints of discomfort reported by patients after meals (228).

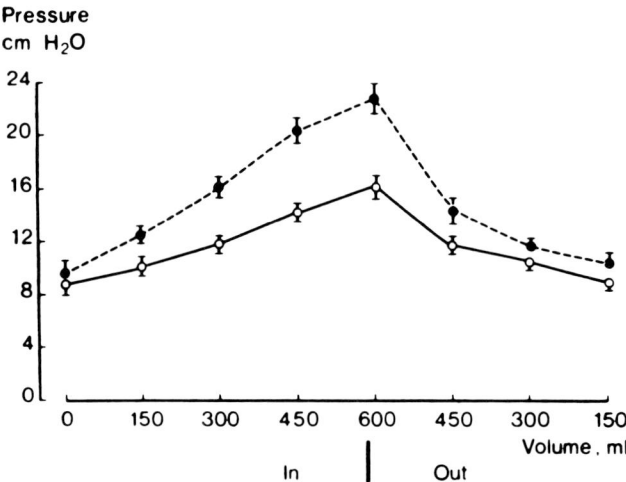

FIG. 11. Intragastric basal pressure of different volumes before (*solid line*) and after (*dotted line*) proximal gastric vagotomy (PGV). Balloon volumes are given along the *x*-axis. Curves represent mean values with *vertical bars* indicating ± SEM; *P* values given for significant differences between values before and after PGV. [From Stadaas (228).]

When extraluminal gastric contractions are recorded with implanted strain gauges after food intake, it is found that, although antral motility is strongly reduced after truncal vagotomy, it is unchanged after PSV (246). The electrical activity of canine stomach after PSV is not changed (1). In humans, however, although the shape of PPs is preserved, their amplitude is markedly reduced (231). Comparative studies of the changes after different types of vagotomy (truncal vagotomy, PSV) demonstrate that the propagation velocity of PPs is very slightly reduced after PSV (144). No changes are observed in the coordination between the antral and the duodenal electrical activities (1). This could also explain the fact that the motor and evacuating functions of the antrum are relatively well preserved (39).

The hypothesis of Wilbur and Kelly (254) is quite feasible. They assumed that the vagally innervated proximal stomach regulates the evacuation of liquids, whereas the vagally innervated antrum regulates the evacuation of solid food, which takes place by means of the terminal antral contraction. The preservation of the latter in the case of PSV guarantees, in their opinion, the normal emptying of solid food. Other authors also reported normal evacuation of solid food after PSV (43, 125, 256). However, the problem needs further clarification, because some researchers have found delayed evacuation of solid foods after PSV (32, 107). The delay in solid food evacuation is manifested immediately after PSV, but it is restored several weeks or months later. It is particularly important that, although after truncal vagotomy and selective vagotomy in dogs 80% of the postprandial motility of the antral part of the stomach is inhibited, after PSV the inhibition of the motility is only 42% (134).

The existing contradictions concerning the character of the evacuation of different types of food after PSV are probably due to the fact that the studies have been performed during different postvagotomy stages and that some of the observations have been made on humans vagotomized for ulcer treatment. The postvagotomy character of the gastric motility is largely determined by its state before the operation. If it was weakened before the operation, prerequisites are created for the occurrence of stasis after the surgery, with all its consequences (161). Systematic investigations in this field, involving following up of the dynamics in the changes of the gastric motility and evacuating activity, are needed for the accurate determination of the adaptive capacities of the stomach after PSV. Available data give support to the assumption that these processes after PSV have a more favorable course, but they occur faster compared with findings after truncal vagotomy. The preserved antral and PS innervation indisputably favors the more correct evacuating capacity of the stomach. This is also favored by the preserved normal interrelations between the electrical activity and motility of the antrum and duodenum after PSV.

Application of PSV in surgical practice for over 15 yr has demonstrated several advantages of PSV over truncal and selective vagotomies, i.e., *1*) gastric emptying is almost normal or it is rapidly normalized after surgical intervention; *2*) the inhibitory effect on acid secretion mediated via epigastric antral nerves is preserved; *3*) the pyloric function is preserved, which reduces gastric reflux; and *4*) duodenal innervation is preserved, which permits normal release of hormones (127). Many of the complications observed after truncal and selective vagotomies are avoided. There are far fewer incidents of dumping (94, 218, 230) and diarrhea (218). Following up the condition of 137 patients treated with highly selective vagotomy (HSV), truncal vagotomy, and selective vagotomy with pyloroplasty, Stoddard et al. (230) emphasized that best results have been obtained after HSV (83%), compared with the results after truncal vagotomy with pyloroplasty (64%). The ulcer recurrence rate was 8.8% in the case of HSV and 9.4% after truncal vagotomy with pyloroplasty. Ulcer recurrence rate seems to be a quite frequent complication after PSV: according to Storey et al. (234), in the fifth postoperative year it occurs in 16.1% of 93 patients. The same researchers postulate that despite the numerous advantages of PSV, it should be applied cautiously. One should also bear in mind that the local responses of the antrum to food also change after vagotomy, and this is associated with disturbances in the release of gastrin (79, 80). The preservation of the antral innervation after PSV also ensures the normal release of gastrin, whose role in the regulation of gastric motility is indisputable.

VAGOTOMY COMBINED WITH DRAINAGE OPERATIONS. Late changes in the evacuating capacity of the stomach are among the most severe postvagotomy disturbances that may lead to dilatation of the stomach (predominantly in the corpus) due to retention of gastric content. This may result in the secondary development of pylorospasm (225). The concomitant symptoms such as bloating, nausea, and vomiting are particularly severe and unpleasant. Dumping with or without diarrhea frequently occurs as a consequence of selective vagotomy or truncal vagotomy. It is difficult to associate the diarrhea only with the fast emptying of the stomach. The disturbed nervous regulation of the small intestine also plays some role in the episodic character of diarrheas. The fact that diarrheas are very frequent in the case of truncal vagotomy, where the vagal innervation of the small intestine is severed, compared with selective vagotomy also supports the role of the nervous regulation (136). To facilitate gastric emptying after truncal and selective vagotomies, it is proposed to combine these vagotomies with various additional operations of the stomach, i.e., vagotomy with draining operations (pyloroplasty, gastroduodenostomy, gastrojejunostomy), as well as with various types of gastric resection. The choice of a procedure additional to the vagotomy is a controversial issue. Some authors believe that drainage operations should be undertaken as routine operations for the treatment of duodenal ulcer by means of vagotomy (92). Above all, a reduction in the stasis and a much better restoration of the motor evacuatory function of the stomach are reported (41, 42, 91, 182, 224). No disturbances have been found in the evacuation of solid meals (164). However, other authors report that the dumping syndrome occurs twice as frequently in the case of selective vagotomy with pyloroplasty than in the case of PSV only (62, 90). Selective vagotomy together with suprapyloric antrectomy is recommended as a suitable operation in ulcer disease (102). Kelly and Kennedy (134) stress that the combination of PSV with drainage operations maintains an effective pyloric pump, which is rapidly restored after the operation. According to Kalbasi et al. (128), in patients subjected to PSV and antrectomy, the evacuation of a solid meal is delayed only during month 1 after the operation; later it does not differ from the evacuation in healthy control patients. However, some authors report abnormal gastric evacuation (152) and the appearance of severe diarrheas (139, 202). Particularly indicative is the comparison made by Hoffmann et al. (113) with respect to complications after truncal vagotomy with drainage (TVD), selective vagotomy with drainage (SVD), and PSV without drainage. In 233 patients, 5 yr after the operation, complications after TVD, SVD, and PSV were as follows. Ulcer recurrence rates: 13.6%, 19.8%, and 30.4%, respectively; diarrhea: 4.9%, 6.3%, and 1.9%; pain and dyspepsia: 3.6% 6.3%, and 3.8%; nausea and vomiting: 0%, 1.6%, and 0.6%.

In fact, for the three types of vagotomy only the ulcer recurrence rate is higher after PSV. On the other hand, the fast gastric emptying and the concomitant diarrhea after vagotomy with pyloroplasty may result not so much from the vagotomy as from the increased evacuation after the drainage operation itself (25).

Observations and the results of the studies on the character of the gastric motility after vagotomies, combined with various additional operations, concern predominantly humans. There is no doubt that the character of the disturbances depends not only on the surgical technique applied but also on the preoperative state and the damage to the functions of the stomach and the state of the gastrointestinal tract as a whole. The choice of additional surgical intervention in the treatment of ulcer disease by vagotomy depends very much on the above factors, and therefore concrete decisions should be made for each individual case (161, 182).

SMALL INTESTINE

Surgical interventions in the small intestine are most frequently associated with disturbed intactness of the intestinal wall. Therefore it is necessary for the specialist to be well familiar with the disturbances in intestinal motility that occur after transection.

*Transection*

As early as in 1939 Douglas and Mann (86) reported reduced rhythm of the contractions of intestinal segments in the aboral direction. Moreover the contractile frequency of each intestinal loop decreased as a function of the distance between the loop and the pylorus. It was described later that transection of the small intestine results in decreased frequency of the slow waves below the transection (21, 28, 36, 66, 141, 171). However, the slow-wave propagation velocity below the transection of the small intestine increases. The increased conduction velocity of the contractile waves may be associated with the greater propagation velocity of slow waves and could account for the fast transit of intestinal content observed after the operation (83).

Duodenal transection results not only in reduced slow-wave frequency but also in increased spike activity of the muscle wall of the distal duodenal segment [Fig. 12; (23, 27)]. This is caused by periods of independent spike activity of the distal segment of the small intestine. Phase 3 of MMC for the intestinal segment below the transection is longer than the normal phase, phase 2, i.e., the phase of irregular spike activity, is even more prolonged (23, 199), while the resting phase (phase 1) is almost completely absent in some cases. The dissociation of the spike activity is most pronounced at the end of month 1 after the operation. A tendency toward reduction of the dissociation between the spike activity of the two intestinal segments starts in month 2 after surgery and is well manifested during month 3 (14, 15). These data sup-

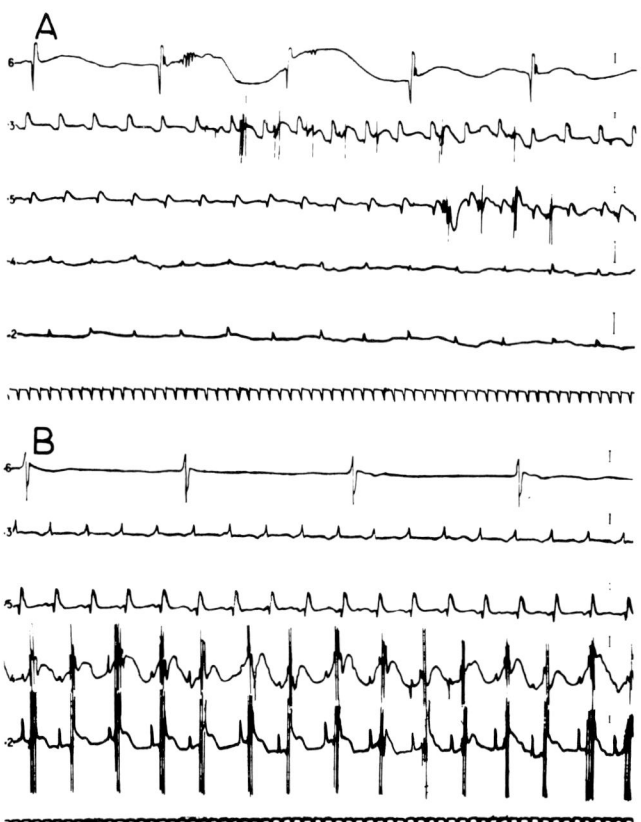

FIG. 12. Dissociation of spike activity of 2 duodenal segments after transection. *A*: spreading of groups of spike potentials from stomach in proximal duodenum to transection site; *B*: spike activity of distal duodenal segment in quiescent state of stomach and of proximal duodenum. *Trace 1*, stomach; *traces 2 and 3*, above transection; *traces 4 and 5*, below transection. Time in seconds. [From Atanassova et al. (23).]

port the notion of steplike subordination of the different parts of the intrinsic nervous system in the aboral direction along the digestive tract (14, 15).

Because the distal segment of the small intestine is liberated from the inhibitory influence of the upper part, the spike activity of the intestinal segment below the transection increases. This is manifested by the decrease or absence of phase 1 of MMC (23, 213). The decrease of the spike activity during months 2 and 3 after the resection, as well as the propagation of SP groups through the anastomosis, follows the regeneration of the intrinsic nervous system, whereby the steplike subordination is restored (23). This agrees with the observations on the propagation of segmental contractions from the proximal to the distal segments of severed small intestine in sheep and dogs (105).

The notion of steplike subordination of the intrinsic nervous system is in agreement with the view of Sarna et al. (217) about MMC, the electrical slow waves, as a phenomenon of the myogenic oscillators. The link between the relaxing oscillators is that the proximal oscillators drive the distal ones (Fig. 13). When there is coupling of all oscillators, a typical MMC is manifested from the stomach to the ileocolic sphincter. Uncoupling of some of the distal oscillators (severing of the intestinal wall) results in the appearance of independent spike activity for this oscillator (257). This is why phase 3 of MMC increases considerably in the distal segments.

*Resection*

The first successful massive resection of the small intestine was performed by Koeberle in 1881 (140). Half of the small intestine may be removed without great problems for normal digestion (243). In some clinical cases, it is necessary to remove as much as 70% of the small intestine.

Diarrhea, steatorrhea, hypoglycemia, anemia, and weight loss are observed after resection of the small intestine. This is called the short bowel syndrome. Maldigestion and malabsorption of all components of the food result from the fact that the contact of the content with the mucosa of the small intestine is short because of reduced transit time. When the jejunum is removed, the ileum may take over part of its absorptive function. However, the loss of the ileum involves even more severe consequences, because this is where resorption of bile salts and vitamin $B_{12}$ takes place (243). The changes are usually smaller when the resection of 4 cm from the ileum is made, but extensive resection of ~60 cm from the ileum leads to excretion of a considerable part of the fats, proteins, sodium, potassium, and water. There is correlation between the velocity of the intestinal passage and the amount of fats excreted (179). Resection of <100 cm of the ileum results in considerable diarrhea with moderate steatorrhea. It is believed that the bile salts enter the colon and that they not only retain water there but also cause the secretion of more water, which also contributes to the development of diarrhea (243).

For prognostic purposes, it is particularly important to preserve the ileocolic sphincter, which, in addition to delaying the passage to the colon, prevents the reflux of bacteria from the large intestine to the ileum (172, 243).

Weight loss of ≤54% is reported in experimental observations on dogs with massive intestinal resection

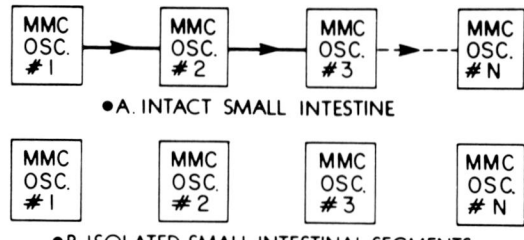

FIG. 13. Model of migrating myoelectrical complexes (MMC). Each segment of small intestine behaves like an independent MMC relaxation oscillator. Oscillators are coupled by intrinsic cholinergic neurons. [From Sarna et al. (215).]

(85%), which the animals partly compensate at a later stage. The animals eat more, the food consumed increases from 40% to 300%, but body fats are greatly reduced and some animals reach cachexia (75). X-ray investigations have revealed greatly increased dimensions of the remaining small intestine in all animals, as well as a very accelerated passage of contrast medium.

The increased loading caused by the ingredients found in the intestinal lumen is a possible stimulus for the jejunum mucosa that is hypertrophied. The intestinal villi become longer (87, 226). This may be the result of gastrin release, which more than doubles after massive resection. [Gastrin is known to be a trophic hormone for the intestinal mucosa (34, 253)]. The levels of pancreatic polypeptide increase three times, enteroglucagon twice, and motilin four times after large resections (34). Cell proliferation may be influenced also by other regulatory peptides such as enteroglucagon (210). The observed adaptive changes after intestinal resection appear to be primarily humorally mediated (34).

Operations to reverse a segment or to create a circular loop are performed to delay the rate of luminsal passage and in fact to increase the absorption of nutrients (75). The construction of a new sphincter along the small intestine is performed experimentally also (219, 220). It is believed that with the removal of the longitudinal muscle layer at a distance of 1 cm, the nerve plexus belonging to it is also removed. Freed from the inhibitory innervation, the circular layer becomes more active and behaves like a sphincter. With the narrowing of the lumen of the new sphincter, the mucosa is folded in the intestinal lumen, especially if the removal of the longitudinal muscle is ~4 cm. A ring of the longitudinal muscle may be removed by deep seromuscular diathermy (73).

Retrograde electrical pacing of experimentally resected intestine also delays the intestinal passage (31, 70). As a result, dogs gain weight, and the amounts of nitrogen and fats in the feces are reduced. Absorption of glucose, water, and electrolytes is improved (146).

*Vagotomy*

Most authors are unanimous that vagotomy does not disturb essentially the motility of the small intestine (206, 207, 250). Transit time after PSV and selective vagotomy is very close to normal, compared with patients who have been subjected to truncal vagotomy and selective vagotomy with pyloroplasty. No changes are observed in the frequency of the slow waves generated by the smooth muscle of the wall of the small intestine (99, 186, 201). Certain changes are observed, however, in the character of the interdigestive MMC (Fig. 14). Even during week 2 after vagotomy, phase 1 of MMC becomes shorter, whereas phase 2 is prolonged. At the beginning of month 2, phase 1 lasts only 10–15 min, whereas its prevagotomy duration is 40–60 min. Between postoperative months 3 and 4, the dynamics in the distribution of the different MMC phases (and especially their duration) approach, although do not reach, the values recorded before the operation (14). These data oppose the view that vagotomy has a slight or no effect on the fasting motility pattern of the duodenum (250). On the other hand, Matrossova et al. (161) have found sporadic appearance of a rhythm with reduced frequency of 10–11 cycles/min in canine small intestine after vagotomy, whereas the frequency in the controls is 18–20 cycles/min. These contractions are characterized by increased average amplitude. The tone of the small intestine also increases during the recording of this rhythm. At the same time, accelerated passage of the small intestinal content is also observed. This prompted Matrossova et al. (161) to associate this rhythm with the frequently occurring diarrheas after vagotomy. Sharp decrease of the transit time of the small intestinal content is observed with the X-ray method (167) as well as with radioisotope methods (241). However, the observed disturbances in the character of MMC and more specifically the shortening to complete inhibition of phase 1 of MMC, with prevalence of the active phases between postoperative day 15 and the end of month 4, are probably among the factors contributing to the severe diarrheas occurring after truncal vagotomy and selective vagotomy. The SP determine the contraction amplitude of the gastric and intestinal wall. The prevalence of the active MMC phases 2, 3, and 4 is indisputably connected with the decrease of the transit time of the intestinal content. However, the changes in MMC begin to decrease, and between months 3 and 4, the MMC dynamics resembles dynamics before the vagotomy. Another indicative finding is that in patients with postvagotomy diarrhea the duration of the feeding pattern is reduced (239). Probably both the accelerated gastric emptying and the changed character of the intestinal electrical activity and motility contribute to the occurrence of diarrheas after vagotomy. Their combination with duodenal receptor insensitivity is the cause for this severe postvagotomy complication (239).

LARGE INTESTINE

The large intestine is subjected to surgical intervention in cases of obstruction and benign or malignant tumors on its wall. In these diseases, it is usually necessary to perform transection of the colon with excision of the affected section or of the neoplasm and restoration by means of anastomosis or colostomy. However, the colonic motility after such interventions has been insufficiently studied.

In cases of experimental colonic obstruction in monkeys, the increase in the electrical and contractile activity is observed above the obstruction (95). Such

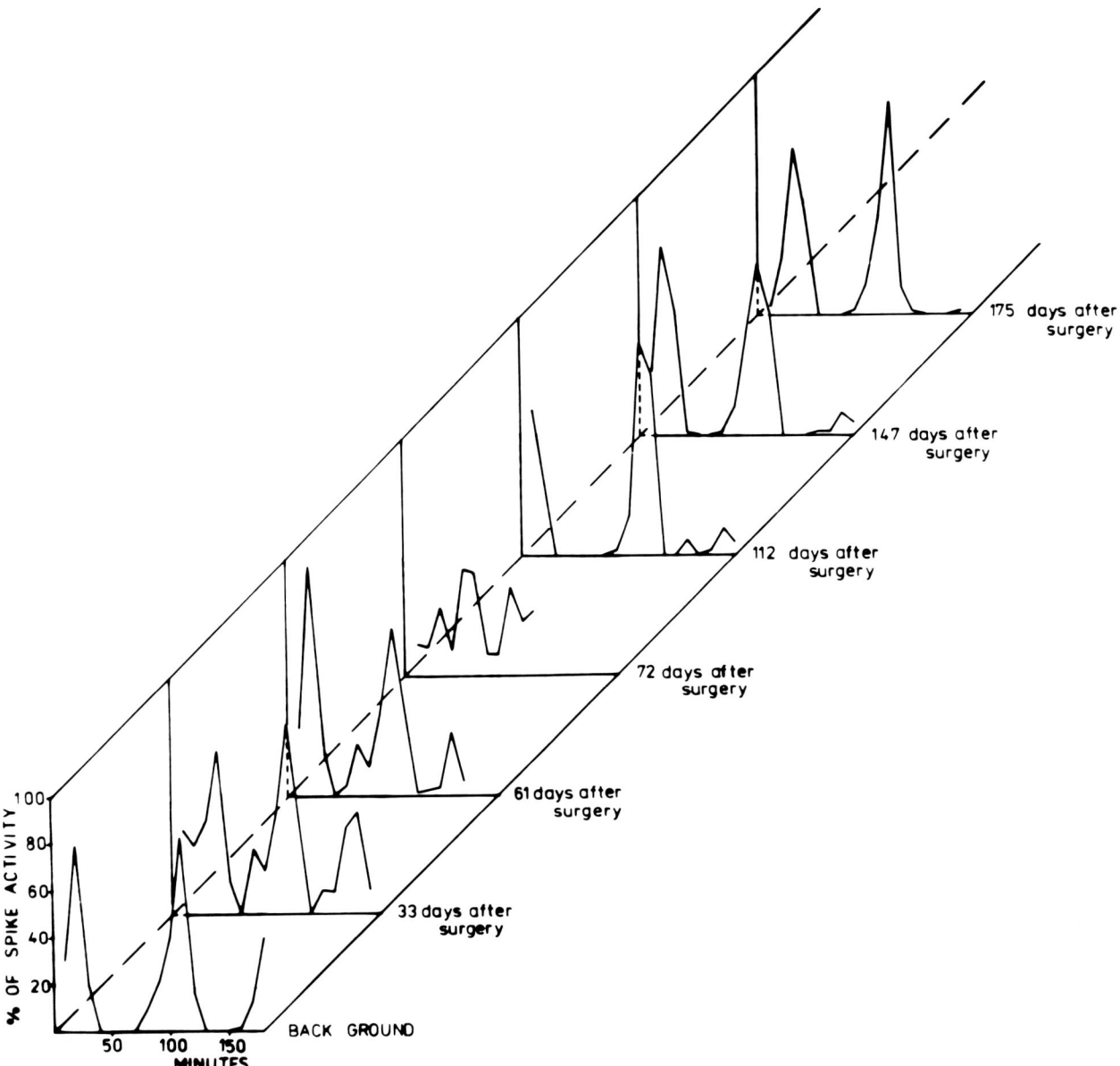

FIG. 14. Dynamics of changes in phases of migrating myoelectrical complexes of small intestine at different periods after vagotomy. [from Atanassova (14).]

changes demonstrate increased duration of the groups of SP, as well as increased SP frequency and amplitude above the obstruction, whereas the electrical activity is suppressed below the ligature (E. Atanassova, G. Zlatarski, and C. Christov, unpublished observations). Antiperistaltic propagation of spike activity from the colon to the terminal ileum is observed on day 3 of the experimental ileus (Figs. 15, 16). Removal of the obstruction is followed on day 2 by spreading of the spike activity along the large intestine.

Total excision of the colon (proctocolectomy) is necessary when the pathological process is generated along the entire length of the large intestine. The Kock's reservoir is made from the terminal ileum that is opened into the rectum (190). It has been demonstrated experimentally that this reservoir behaves like a capacitance organ: while the ileum responds with contraction to stretching with a 30-ml volume, it is necessary to stretch its wall with a volume of 322 ml (balloon) to induce constriction of the reservoir (197). However, this reservoir is not capable of being completely emptied, which distinguishes it from the rectum (74)

CONCLUSIONS

The adaptive and recuperative capacities of mammalian species are remarkable. These capacities are expressed by the observed dynamics in the changes of

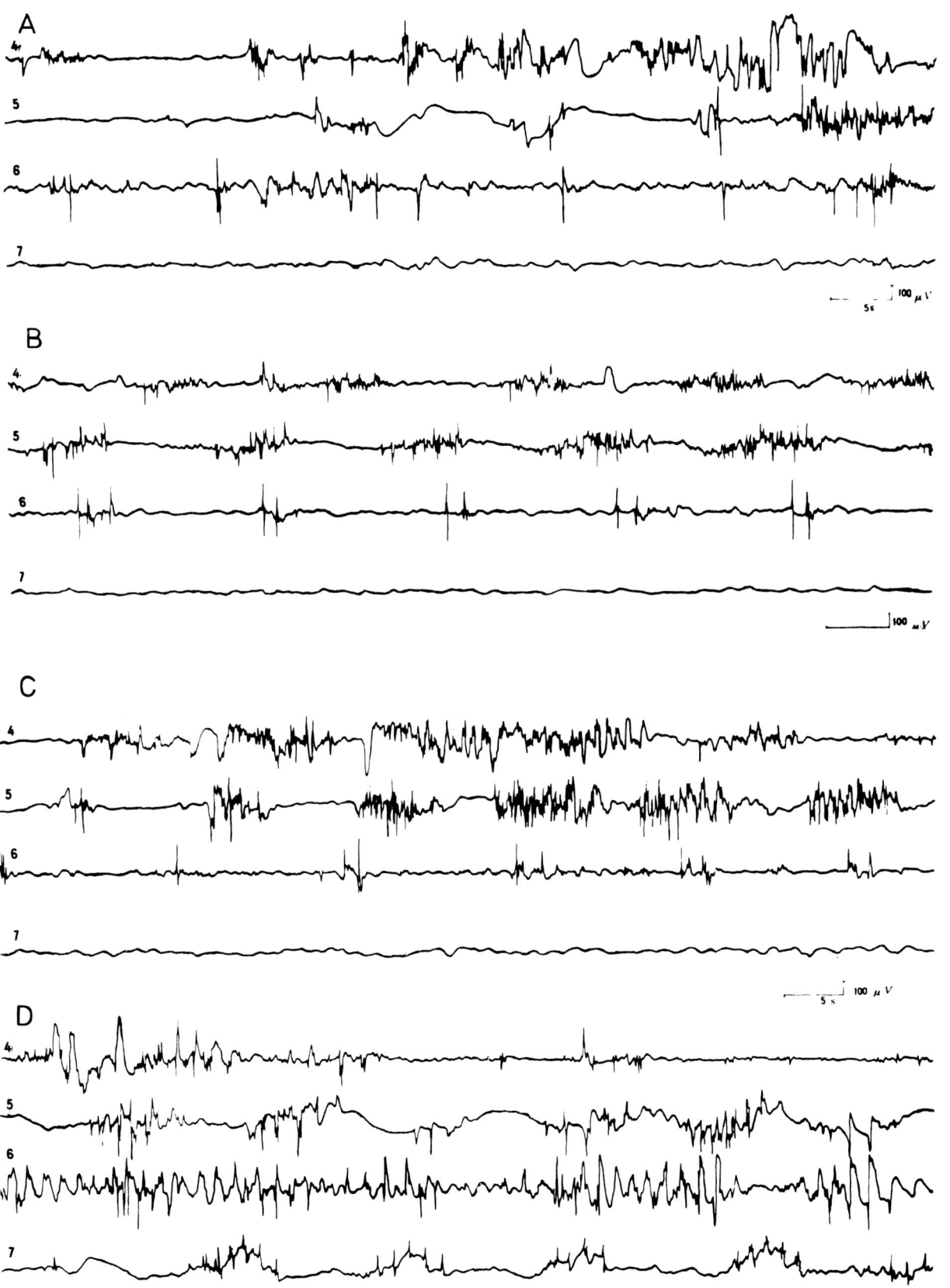

FIG. 15. Electrical activity of dog colonic muscle wall in experimental obstruction. *A*: 24 h after making of a ligature between electrodes (small numbers) 6 and 7; *B*: 48 h later; *C*: 72 h later; *D*: 24 h after removing ligature. (Data from E. Atanassova, G. Zlatarski, and C. Christov, unpublished observations.)

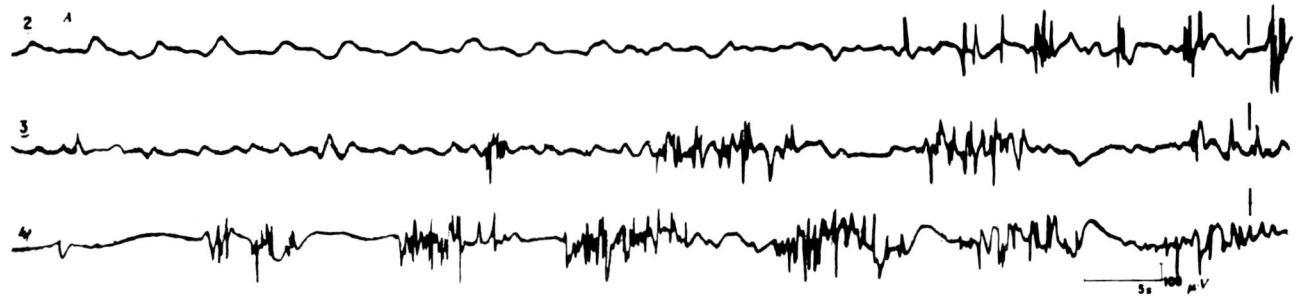

FIG. 16. Antiperistaltic spreading of spike activity from transverse colon to ileum during experimental obstruction. *Trace 2*, ileum; *trace 3*, proximal colon; *trace 4*, transverse colon. (Data from E. Atanassova, G. Zlatarski, and C. Christov, unpublished observations.)

the gastrointestinal motility after surgical interventions, whereby the different regions of the digestive tract manifest different recuperative capacities. Although the motility of the small intestine is restored within the first 2 h after abdominal surgical intervention, a considerably longer period is needed to restore the motility of the stomach and large intestine. The disturbances in the various regions of the digestive tract caused by resection, vagotomy, or their simultaneous application are not identical in severity and duration. The experimental models created in this respect have made it possible to trace the dynamic changes in gastric and intestinal motility. There is also considerable clinical evidence on the objective and subjective findings after gastrectomy and vagotomy necessitated by various diseases. Unfortunately, however, in clinical practice it is not always possible to trace the dynamics of the changes taking place in the motility of the digestive tract. On the other hand, these disturbances are to a great extent complicated by the influence of the main disease that has necessitated the surgical intervention. This compels the surgeon even more to be very familiar with the physiology of the digestive tract, so that possible disturbances can be predicted and on this basis the most suitable surgical intervention can be applied.

Although there are relatively more data, both experimental and clinical, on the disturbances in gastric motility after various surgical interventions, data concerning the small intestine are insufficient and contradictory. The data on the motility of the large intestine after surgical intervention are also scanty. Further studies in this field are necessary, with various experimental models of the types of operations applied in surgical practice. Such studies will make it possible to reveal some unknown aspects of the regulation mechanisms of the motor function of the gastrointestinal tract, and they will also guide surgeons to choose the type of surgical intervention that causes minimal damage to the normal functioning of the digestive tract. To achieve this goal, both the surgeon and the gastroenterologist should not only be familiar with the physiology of the gastrointestinal tract but they should also adopt a physiological way of thinking.

REFERENCES

1. AEBERHARD, P., AND B. S. BEDI. Effects of proximal gastric vagotomy (PGV) followed by total vagotomy (TV) on postprandial and fasting myoelectrical activity of the canine stomach and duodenum. *Gut* 18: 515–523, 1977.
2. AKWARI, O. E., K. A. KELLY, J. H. STEINBACH, AND C. F. CODE. Electric pacing of the intact and transected canine small intestine and its computer model. *Am. J. Physiol.* 229: 1188–1197, 1975.
3. ALEXANDER-WILLIAMS, J. Duodenogastric reflux after gastric operations. *Br. J. Surg.* 68: 685–687, 1981.
4. ALEXANDER-WILLIAMS, J., I. A. DONOVAN, I. F. GUNN, A. BROWN, AND L. K. HARDING. The effect of the vagotomy on gastric emptying. *Proc. R. Soc. Med.* 66: 1102–1103, 1973.
5. ALVAREZ, W. C. Sixty years of vagotomy; a review of some 200 articles. *Gastroenterology* 10: 413–441, 1948.
6. ALVAREZ, W. C. *An Introduction to Gastroenterology.* New York: Hoeber, 1948.
7. AMDRUP, B. E., AND C. A. GRIFFITH. Selective vagotomy of the parietal cell mass; part I: with preservation of the innervated antrum and pylorus. *Ann. Surg.* 170: 207–215, 1969.
8. AMDRUP, B. E., AND H. E. JENSEN. Selective vagotomy on the parietal cell mass preserving innervation of the undrained antrum. A preliminary report of results in patients with duodenal ulcer. *Gastroenterology* 59: 522–527, 1970.
9. AMDRUP, B. E., H. E. JENSEN, D. JOHNSTON, B. F. WALKER, AND J. C. GOLIGHER. Clinical results of parietal cell vagotomy (highly selective vagotomy) two to four years after operation. *Ann. Surg.* 179: 279–284, 1974.
10. ARIMORI, M., C. F. CODE, J. F. SCHLEGEL, AND R. E. STRUM. Electrical activity of the canine esophagus and gastroesophageal sphincter. *Am. J. Dig. Dis.* 15: 191–208, 1970.
11. ATANASSOVA, E. The role of the gastroduodenal junction in correlating the spike activities of the gastric and duodenal walls. *C. R. Acad. Bulg. Sci.* 22: 947–949, 1969.
12. ATANASSOVA, E. Bioelectrical activity of the stomach and duodenum after cutting the gastroduodenal junction. *Bull. Inst. Physiol.* 13: 211–227, 1970.
13. ATANASSOVA, E. Bioelectrical activity of the stomach and duodenum after section of the stomach at the level of incisura angularis. *Bull. Inst. Physiol. Sofia* 13: 243–250, 1970.
14. ATANASSOVA, E. *The Intrinsic Nervous System and Gastrointestinal Motility.* Sofia, Bulgaria: Bulgarian Acad. Sci., 1981.
15. ATANASSOVA, E. Control of the myoelectric complex of the stomach and small intestines by the intrinsic nervous system.

In: *Advances in Physiological Sciences. Nutrition, Digestion and Metabolism*, edited by T. Gati, L. G. Szollar, and G. Ungvary. Oxford, UK: Pergamon, 1981, vol. 12, p. 287–298. (28th Int. Congr. Physiol. Sci., Budapest, July 13–19, 1980.)

16. ATANASSOVA, E., AND O. BAYGUINOV. Changes in the character of electrical and contractile activities of the isolated fundus with functional loading (Billroth I). *J. Physiol. Paris* 78: 326–330, 1982.
17. ATANASSOVA, E., AND O. BAYGUINOV. Spike activity of the muscle wall of the stomach after gastric resection. *Acta Physiol. Pharmacol. Bulg.* 10(3): 63–69, 1984.
18. ATANASSOVA, E., O. BAYGUINOV, AND I. LOLOVA. Changes in the innervation of the fundus after subtotal gastrectomy. In: *Gastrointestinal Motility*, edited by C. Roman. Lancaster, UK: MTP, 1984, p. 103–111. (9th Int. Symp. Gastrointest. Motil., Aix-en-Provence, France, Sept. 12–16, 1983.)
19. ATANASSOVA, E., Z. JURUKOVA, AND E. DRAGANOVA. Transformation of the slow potential rhythm of the fundus of the stomach after functional loading following Billroth I gastrectomy. In: *Gastrointestinal Motility in Health and Disease*, edited by H. L. Duthie. Lancaster, UK: MTP, 1978, p. 495–505. (6th Int. Symp. Gastrointest. Motil., Edinburgh, Sept. 12–16, 1977.)
20. ATANASSOVA, E., Z. JURUKOVA, AND J. ZACHEVA. Regeneration of the smooth muscle cells—a structural basis for restoration of the slow potential rhythm in the distal part of the stomach after transection. *J. Physiol. Paris* 68: 291–304, 1974.
21. ATANASSOVA, E., AND N. KORTEZOVA. On the role of the intrinsic nervous system in the small bowel slow bioelectrical activity. *Bull. Inst. Physiol. Sofia* 16: 135–150, 1974.
22. ATANASSOVA, E., N. KORTEZOVA, I. LOLOVA, AND I. PETROV. Changes in the myoelectric complex of the stomach and small bowel under the influence of the intrinsic nervous system. *Acta Physiol. Pharmacol. Bulg.* 6(3): 11–18, 1980.
23. ATANASSOVA, E., I. A. SOLOVIOVA, M. PAPASOVA, AND N. KORTEZOVA. Character of the spike activity on both sides of duodenal transection depending on the regeneration of the intrinsic nervous system. *Acta Physiol. Pharmacol. Bulg.* 4(2): 3–12, 1978.
24. AUNE, S. Intragastric pressure after vagotomy in man. *Scand. J. Gastroenterol.* 4: 447–452, 1969.
25. AYLETT, P., C. WASTELL, AND I. WISE. Gastric secretion and emptying before and after vagotomy and pyloroplasty with and without continuous infusion of peptavlon pentagastrin. *Am. J. Dig. Dis.* 14: 245–252, 1969.
26. BAKER, L. W., AND D. R. WEBSTER. Postoperative intestinal motility. An experimental study on dogs. *Br. J. Surg.* 55: 374–378, 1968.
27. BASS, P., G. W. GULLIECKSON, AND H. OKUDA. Electrical and motor activity of the surgically altered gastroduodenal junction of the dog. *Jpn. J. Smooth Muscle Res.* 14, Suppl.: 29–30, 1978.
28. BASS, P., AND J. WILEY. Electrical and extraluminal contractile force activity of the duodenum of the dog. *Am. J. Dig. Dis.* 10: 183–200, 1965.
29. BAYGUINOV, O., AND E. ATANASSOVA. Changes in the character of the postsynaptic potentials of the fundic smooth muscle cells after functional loading. *Acta Physiol. Pharmacol. Bulg.* 7(1): 3–10, 1981.
30. BECKER, H. D. Dumping syndrome and hormones. In: *Gastric and Gastroduodenal Motility*, edited by L. M. A. Akkermans, A. G. Johnson, and N. W. Read. New York: Praeger, 1984, vol. 4, p. 263–281. (Surgical Sci. Ser.)
31. BECKER, J. M. Electrical pacing for post-surgical disorders of gastric motility. In: *Gastric and Gastroduodenal Motility*, edited by L. M. A. Akkermans, A. G. Johnson, and N. W. Read. New York: Praeger, 1984, vol. 4, p. 318–326. (Surgical Sci. Ser.)
32. BEGER, H. G., M. MEVES, AND R. BITTNER. Magenentleerung nach Vagotomie. *Z. Gastroenterol.* 17: 531–537, 1979.
33. BENNETT, A., AND H. STOCKLEY. The intrinsic innervation of the human alimentary tract and its relation to function. *Gut* 16: 443–453, 1975.
34. BESTERMAN, A. S., T. E. ADRIAN, C. N. MALLINSON, N. D. CHRISTOFIDES, D. L. SARSON, A. PERA, L. LOCUBARDO, R. MODIGLIANI, AND S. R. BLOOM. Gut hormone release after intestinal resection. *Gut* 23: 854–861, 1982.
35. BINDER, H. J., D. L. BLOOM, H. STERN, G. B. SOLITARE, W. R. THAYER, H. M. SPIRO, AND E. R. POINDEXTER. The effect of cervical vagotomy on esophageal function in the monkey. *Surgery St. Louis* 64: 1075–1083, 1968.
36. BOGACH, P. G. On the frequency of the rhythmic contractions of the small bowel. *Bull. Exp. Biol. Med. Engl. Transl. Byull. Eksp. Biol. Med.* 4: 6–12, 1959.
37. BOGACH, P. G., AND S. D. GROISMAN. Tonometric studies on the vagotomized stomach. *Sechenov Physiol. J. USSR Engl. Transl. Fiziol. Zh. SSSR Im. I. M. Sechenova* 54: 467–471, 1968.
38. BOGACH, P. G., S. D. GROISMAN, R. A. LOUKAZKIY, A. I. NOVOSSELOVA, AND E. A. PLOTKIN. Influence of the vagotomy on the electrical reactions of dog stomach. *Sechenov Physiol. J. USSR Engl. Transl. Fiziol. Zh. SSSR Im. I. M. Sechenova* 60: 251–254, 1974.
39. BONE, J., O. BRANDSBORG, M. BRANDSBORG, N. A. LOVGREEN, AND K. MIKKELSEN. Gastroduodenostomy in dogs with and without parietal cell vagotomy. Effect upon gastric emptying and motility, Heidenhein pouch acid secretion and serum gastrin concentration. *Digestion* 15: 9–17, 1977.
40. BORTOLOTTI, M., G. BERSANI, A. LONGANESI, T. CALLETTI, S. FOSCHI, AND G. LABO. Modification of the interdigestive migrating motor complex (IMMC) in patients with partial gastrectomy and gastrojejunostomy. In: *Gastrointestinal Motility*, edited by C. Roman. Lancaster, UK: MTP, 1984, p. 297–299. (9th Int. Symp. Gastrointest. Motil., Aix-en-Provence, France, Sept. 12–16, 1983.)
41. BORTOLOTTI, M., G. LABO, C. SERANTONI, AND P. CIANI. Effect of highly selective vagotomy on gastric motor activity of duodenal ulcer patients. *Digestion* 17: 108–120, 1978.
42. BRANDSBORG, O., M. BRANDSBORG, N. A. LOVEGREEN, K. MIKKELSEN, B. MOLLER, M. ROKKJAER, AND B. E. AMDRUP. Influence of parietal cell vagotomy and selective gastric vagotomy on gastric emptying rate and serum gastrin concentration. *Gastroenterology* 72: 212–214, 1977.
43. BRUCE, G., M. D. WILLBUR, AND K. A. KELLY. Effect of proximal gastric and truncal vagotomy on canine gastric electric activity, motility and emptying. *Ann. Surg.* 178: 295–303, 1973.
44. BUCHAN, R., C. G. CLARK, AND R. W. M. DOWNIE. Conversion to Billroth-I anastomosis or entero-anastomosis for postgastrectomy states. *Br. J. Surg.* 52: 651–657, 1965.
45. BUCKLER, K. G. Effects of gastric surgery upon gastric emptying in cases of peptic ulceration. *Gut* 8: 137–147, 1967.
46. BUENO, L., J.-P. FERRÉ, AND Y. RUCKEBUSCH. Effect of anesthesia and surgical procedures on intestinal myoelectric activity in rats. *Am. J. Dig. Dis.* 23: 690–696, 1978.
47. BUENO, L., J. FIORAMONTI, AND Y. RUCKEBUSCH. Postoperative intestinal motility in dogs and sheep. *Am. J. Dig. Dis.* 23: 682–690, 1978.
48. BURGESS, J. N., J. F. SCHLEGEL, AND F. H. ELLIS, JR. Effect of denervation on feline esophageal function and morphology. *J. Surg. Res.* 12: 24–33, 1972.
49. CAIN, G. D., P. MOORE, AND M. PATTERSON. Bezoars—a complication of the postgastrectomy state. *Am. J. Dig. Dis.* 13: 801–809, 1968.
50. CANNON, W. B. Esophageal peristalsis after bilateral vagotomy. *Am. J. Physiol.* 19: 436–444, 1904.
51. CANNON, W. B. *The Mechanical Factors of Digestion*. London: Arnold, 1911.
52. CANNON, W. B., AND F. T. MURPHY. The movement of the stomach and intestine in some surgical conditions. *Ann. Surg.* 43: 512–536, 1906.
53. CARLSON, A. J. *The Control of Hunger in Health and Disease*. Chicago, IL: Univ. of Chicago Press, 1916.
54. CARLSON, H. C., C. F. CODE, AND R. A. NELSON. Motor action of the canine gastroduodenal junction: a cineradiographic, pressure and electric study. *Am. J. Dig. Dis.* 11: 155–172, 1966.

55. CARMICHAEL, M. J., N. W. WEISBRODT, AND E. M. COPELAND. Effect of abdominal surgery on intestinal myoelectric activity in the dog. *Am. J. Surg.* 133: 34–38, 1977.
56. CARVETH, S. W., J. F. SCHLEGEL, AND C. F. CODE. Esophageal motility after vagotomy, phrenicotomy, myotomy and myomectomy in dogs. *Surg. Gynecol. Obstet.* 114: 31–42, 1962.
57. CATCHPOLE, B. N., AND H. L. DUTHIE. Postoperative gastrointestinal complexes. In: *Gastrointestinal Motility in Health and Disease*, edited by H. L. Duthie. Lancaster, UK: MTP, 1978, p. 33–41. (6th Int. Symp. Gastrointest. Motil., Edinburgh, Sept. 12–16, 1977.)
58. CHASHKOV, A. M. One Year and Seven Months Life of a Dog after Bilateral Cervical Transection of the Vagus Nerves [in Russian]. St. Petersburg, 1902. PhD thesis.
59. CHERNIAKEVICH, S. A. Influence of vagotomy with pyloroplasty on the motor-emptying function of the stomach. In: *Surgery of Gastric and Duodenal Ulcers*. Moscow: Medicina, 1973, vol. 8, p. 112–119.
60. CHOCHOLAC, J. L'influence de la vagotomie sur le tonus, le péristaltisme et l'evacuation gastriques. *Acta Gastro-Enterol. Belg.* 29: 1–83, 1966.
61. CLARKE, J. S., E. H. STORER, AND L. R. DRAGSTEDT. The effect of vagotomy on the physiology of the stomach in patients with peptic ulcer. *J. Clin. Invest.* 26: 784–795, 1947.
62. CLARKE, R. J., AND J. ALEXANDER-WILLIAMS. The effect of preserving antral innervation and of a pyloroplasty on gastric emptying after vagotomy in man. *Gut* 14: 300–307, 1973.
63. CLARKE, R. J., AND J. A. WILLIAMS. Prevention of "dumping" by retaining antral innervation. *Surg. Forum* 23: 329–331, 1972.
64. COBB, J. S., S. BANK, I. N. MARKS, AND J. H. LOUW. Gastric emptying after vagotomy and pyloroplasty. *Am. J. Dig. Dis.* 16: 207–215, 1971.
65. CODE, C. F., AND J. MARLETT. The interdigestive myoelectric complex of the stomach and small bowel of dog. *J. Physiol. London* 246: 289–310, 1975.
66. CODE, C. F., AND J. H. SZURSZEWSKI. The effect of duodenal and mid small bowel transection on the frequency gradient of the pacesetter potential in the canine small intestine. *J. Physiol. London* 207: 281–289, 1970.
67. COHEN, S., J. J. KRAVITZ, AND W. J. SNAPE, JR. Vagal control of lower oesophageal sphincter function. In: *Gastrointestinal Motility in Health and Disease*, edited by H. L. Duthie. Lancaster, UK: MTP, 1978, p. 505–510. (6th Int. Symp. Gastrointest. Motil., Edinburgh, Sept. 12–16, 1977.)
68. COHEN, S., J. RYAN, S. MATARAZZO, AND J. W. SNAPE. Nervous control of the esophageal motor activity. In: *Nerves and the Gut*, edited by F. P. Brooks and P. W. Evers. Thorofare, NJ: Slack, 1977, p. 207–222.
69. COLLINE, J., K. A. KELLY, AND S. F. PHILLIPS. Increased canine jejunal absorption of water, glucose, and sodium with intestinal pacing. *Am. J. Dig. Dis.* 23: 1121–1124, 1978.
70. COLMER, M. R., G. M. OWEN, AND R. SHIELDS. Pattern of gastric emptying after vagotomy and pyloroplasty. *Br. Med. J.* 2: 448–450, 1973.
71. COOK, A. R. Control of gastric emptying and motility. *Gastroenterology* 68: 804–816, 1975.
72. COWLEY, D. J., P. VERNON, P. JONES, T. GLLAS, AND A. G. COX. Gastric emptying of solid meals after truncal vagotomy and pyloroplasty in human subjects. *Gut* 13: 176–181, 1972.
73. CRANLEY, B., AND S. T. D. MACKELVEY. The Kock ileostomy reservoir: an experimental study of methods of improving valve stability and competence. *Br. J. Surg.* 68: 545–550, 1981.
74. CRANLEY, B., AND S. T. D. MACKELVEY. The pelvic ileal reservoir: an experimental assessment of its function compared with that of normal rectum. *Br. J. Surg.* 69: 465–469, 1982.
75. CUTHBERTSON, E. M., R. S. GILFILLIAN, H. J. BURHENNE, AND M. J. MACKBY. Massive small bowel resection in the beagle including laboratory data in severe undernutrition. *Surgery St. Louis* 68: 698–705, 1970.
76. DANIEL, E. E. On the effect of transthoracic vagotomy. *Gastroenterology* 57: 109–110, 1969.
77. DANIEL, E. E., W. H. SUTHERLAND, AND A. BOGOCH. Effects of morphine and other drugs on motility of the terminal ileum. *Gastroenterology* 36: 570–575, 1959.
78. DAUCHEL, J., J. C. SHANG, J. KAHELHOFFER, R. ELOY, AND J. F. GRENIER. Gastrointestinal myoelectrical activity during the postoperative period in man. *Digestion* 14: 293–303, 1976.
79. DEBAS, H., J. WALSH, AND M. GROSSMAN. After vagotomy atropine suppresses gastrin release by food. *Gastroenterology* 70: 1082–1084, 1976.
80. DE CASTELLA, H., AND W. T. IRVINE. The role of the vagus in the antral responses to food. *Br. J. Surg.* 54: 828–831, 1967.
81. DE MIGUEL, J. Pylorectomy and prepyloric antrectomy for gastric ulcer. *Br. J. Surg.* 66: 48–50, 1979.
82. DIAMANT, N. E., AND T. Y. EL-SHARKAWY. Neural control of esophageal peristalsis, a conceptual analysis. *Gastroenterology* 72: 546–556, 1974.
83. DIAMANT, N. E., K. HALL, H. MUI, AND T. Y. EL-SHARKAWY. Vagal control of the feeding motor pattern in the lower esophageal sphincter, stomach and small intestine of dogs. In: *Gastrointestinal Motility*, edited by J. Christensen. New York: Raven, 1980, p. 365–370. (7th Int. Symp. Gastrointest. Motil., Iowa City, Iowa, Sept. 11–14, 1979.)
84. DIAMANT, N. E., H. MUI, T. Y. EL-SHARKAWY, AND K. HALL. The vagus controls the lower esophageal sphincter and gastric components of the migrating motor complex in the dog (Abstract). *Gastroenterology* 76: 1122, 1979.
85. DIAMANT, N. E., J. WONG, AND L. CHEN. Effects of transection on small intestinal slow-wave propagation velocity. *Am. J. Physiol.* 225: 1497–1500, 1973.
86. DOUGLAS, D. M., AND F. C. MANN. An experimental study of the rhythmic contractions in the small intestine of the dog. *Am. J. Dig. Dis.* 6: 318–322, 1939.
87. DOWLING, R. H., AND C. C. BOOTH. Structural and functional changes following small intestinal resection in the rat. *Clin. Sci. London* 32: 139–149, 1967.
88. DOZOIS, R. R., K. A. KELLY, AND C. F. CODE. Effect of distal antrectomy on gastric emptying of liquids and solids. *Gastroenterology* 61: 675–681, 1971.
89. EDWARDS, L. W., W. H. EDWARDS, J. L. SAWYERS, W. G. GOBBEL, J. L. HERRINGTON, AND H. W. SCOTT. The surgical treatment of duodenal ulcer by vagotomy and antral resection. *J. Surg.* 105: 352–357, 1963.
90. EMÅS, S., AND M. FERNSTRÖM. Prospective randomized trial of selective vagotomy with pyloroplasty and selective proximal vagotomy with and without pyloroplasty in the treatment of duodenal, pyloric and prepyloric ulcers. *Am. J. Surg.* 149: 236–243, 1985.
91. EVERETT, M. T., AND C. A. GRIFFITH. The effects of selective vagotomy plus suprapyloric antrectomy upon gastric motility and Heidenhain pouch secretion. *Ann. Surg.* 171: 36–45, 1970.
92. FEGGETTER, G. Y., AND R. PRINGLE. The relationship between the severity of duodenal ulceration and the results of bilateral vagotomy and gastrojejunostomy. *Br. J. Surg.* 52: 691–693, 1965.
93. FRANK-KAMENEZKIY, L. S. *On the Motor Innervation of the Stomach and Duodenum*. Moscow: Medgis, 1948.
94. FRASER, A. G., P. W. BRUNT, AND N. A. MATHESON. A comparison of highly selective vagotomy with truncal vagotomy and pyloroplasty—one surgeon's results after 5 years. *Br. J. Surg.* 70: 485–488, 1983.
95. FRASER, J. D., R. F. CONDON, W. J. SCHULTE, J. J. DECOSSE, AND V. E. COWLES. Bowel activity after primary resection for colonic obstruction. *Br. J. Surg.* 68: 113–116, 1981.
96. GABELLA, G. Synapses in the rat stomach and small intestine. *Experientia Basel* 26: 619–620, 1970.
97. GEORGE, J. D., A. M. CONNEL, AND T. KENNEDY. Gastric emptying in patients with postvagotomy diarrhea (Abstract). *Gut* 9: 732, 1968.
98. GEORGE, J. D., AND J. MAGOWAN. Diarrhea after total and

selective vagotomy. *Am. J. Dig. Dis.* 16: 635–640, 1971.
99. GIDDA, J. S., AND R. K. GOYAL. Influence of vagus nerves on electrical activity of opossum small intestine. *Am. J. Physiol.* 239 (*Gastrointest. Liver Physiol.* 2): G406–G410, 1980.
100. GLEYSTEEN, J. J., AND J. H. KALBFLEISCH. Progression of changes in gastric emptying of hypertonic liquids after proximal gastric vagotomy: an experimental study. *Dig. Dis. Sci.* 26: 119–124, 1981.
101. GRASSI, G. The technique of proximal selective vagotomy. *Chir. Gastroenterol. Engl. Ed.* 5: 399–405, 1971.
102. GRIFFITH, C. A. Selective vagotomy plus suprapyloric antrectomy with and without pylorotomy for duodenal ulcer. *Ann. Surg.* 179: 516–518, 1974.
103. GRIFFITH, C. A., AND H. N. HARKINS. Partial gastric vagotomy; an experimental study. *Gastroenterology* 32: 96–102, 1957.
104. GRIFFITH, C. A., L. S. STAVNEY, T. KATO, AND H. N. HARKINS. Selective gastric vagotomy combined with hemigastrectomy and Billroth I anastomosis. *Am. J. Surg.* 105: 361–369, 1963.
105. GRIVEL, M. L., AND Y. RUCKEBUSCH. The propagation of segmental contractions along the small intestine. *J. Physiol. Lond.* 227: 611–625, 1972.
106. HALL, W. N., AND R. C. READ. Effect of vagotomy on gastric emptying. *Am. J. Dig. Dis.* 15: 1047–1053, 1970.
107. HALLENBECK, G. A., AND J. J. GLEYSTEEN. Proximal gastric vagotomy without "drainage"; an experimental study. *Ann. Surg.* 179: 608–617, 1974.
108. HALSTED, W. S. Circular suture of the intestine—an experimental study. *Am. J. Med. Sci.* 94: 436–461, 1887.
109. HEGGLIN, J., F. LARGIADER, AND I. BABOTAI. Elektromyographische Studien am Magen vor und nach Vagotomie. *Helv. Chir. Acta* 35: 274–281, 1968.
110. HELLEMANS, J., J. JANSSENS, G. VANTRAPPEN, W. PELEMANS, AND P. VALEMBOIS. The role of a bolus in the peristaltic contraction of the esophagus. In: *Gastrointestinal Motility*, edited by E. E. Daniel. Vancouver: Mitchell, 1974, p. 573–584. (4th Int. Symp. Gastrointest. Motil., Banff, Alberta, Canada, Sept. 6–8, 1973.)
111. HINDER, R. A., AND C. G. BREMNER. Relative role of pyloroplasty size, truncal vagotomy and milk meal volume in canine gastric emptying. *Dig. Dis. Sci.* 23: 210–216, 1978.
112. HOBSLEY, M. Dumping and diarrhea. *Br. J. Surg.* 68: 681–684, 1981.
113. HOFFMANN, J., H. E. JANSEN, S. SCHULZE, P. E. POULSEN, AND J. CHRISTENSEN. Prospective controlled vagotomy trial for duodenal ulcer: results after five years. *Br. J. Surg.* 71: 582–585, 1984.
114. HOROWITZ, M., P. J. COLLINS, B. E. CHATTERTON, P. E. HARDING, J. MACWATTS, AND D. J. C. SHEARMAN. Gastric emptying after gastroplasty for morbid obesity. *Br. J. Surg.* 71: 435–437, 1984.
115. HOROWITZ, M., D. J. COOK, P. J. COLLINS, P. E. HARDING, M. J. HOOPER, J. E. WALSH, AND D. J. C. SHEARMAN. Measurement of gastric emptying after gastric bypass surgery using radionuclides. *Br. J. Surg.* 69: 655–657, 1982.
116. HOWLETT, P. J., H. J. SHEINER, D. C. BARBER, A. S. WARD, C. A. PEREZ-AVIBA, AND H. L. DUTHIE. Gastric emptying in control subjects and patients with duodenal ulcer before and after vagotomy. *Gut* 17: 542–550, 1976.
117. IMPERATI, L., C. NATALE, AND F. MARINACCIO. Acid-fundic selective vagotomy of the stomach without drainage in the treatment of duodenal ulcer: technique and results. *Br. J. Surg.* 59: 602–605, 1972.
118. INGELFINGER, F. J. Esophageal motility. *Physiol. Rev.* 38: 533–584, 1958.
119. INTERONE, C. V., J. E. DEL FINADO, B. MILLER, C. T. BOMBECK, AND L. M. NYHYS. Parietal cell vagotomy. *Arch. Surg.* 102: 43–44, 1971.
120. JAHNBERG, T. Gastric adaptive relaxation. Effect of vagal activation and vagotomy. An experimental study in dogs and in man. *Scand. J. Gastroenterol. Suppl.* 46: 1–36, 1977.

121. JANSSENS, J. *The Peristaltic Mechanism of the Esophagus.* Leuven, Belgium: ACCO, 1978.
122. JANSSENS, J., P. VALEMBOIS, G. VANTRAPPEN, G. HELLEMANS, AND W. PELLEMANS. Is the primary peristaltic contraction of the canine esophagus bolus dependent? *Gastroenterology* 65: 750–756, 1973.
123. JANSSENS, J., I. DE WEVER, G. VANTRAPPEN, AND G. HELLEMANS. Peristalsis in smooth muscle esophagus after transection and bolus deviation. *Gastroenterology* 71: 1004–1009, 1976.
124. JOHNSON, A. G. Surgical treatment of gastric motility disorders and enterogastric reflux. In: *Gastric and Gastroduodenal Motility*, edited by L. M. A. Akkermans, A. G. Johnson, and N. W. Read. New York: Praeger, 1984, vol. 4, p. 314–317. (Surgical Sci. Ser.)
125. JOHNSTON, D. Highly selective vagotomy. *Gut* 15: 748–757, 1974.
126. JOHNSTON, D., AND A. R. WILKINSON. Highly selective vagotomy without drainage procedure in the treatment of duodenal ulcer. *Br. J. Surg.* 57: 289–296, 1970.
127. JORDAN, P. H., JR. Current status of parietal cell vagotomy. *Ann. Surg.* 184: 659–667, 1976.
128. KALBASI, H., F. R. HUDSEN, A. HERRING, S. MOSS, H. I. GLASS, AND J. SPENCER. Gastric emptying following vagotomy and antrectomy and proximal gastric vagotomy. *Gut* 16: 509–513, 1975.
129. KAY, A. W. The physiological basis of surgery for duodenal ulcer. *Acta Gastro-Enterol. Belg.* 26: 193–201, 1963.
130. KELLY, K. A. Effect of gastric surgery on gastric motility and emptying. In: *Gastric and Gastroduodenal Motility*, edited by L. M. A. Akkermans, A. G. Johnson, and N. W. Read. New York: Praeger, 1984, vol. 4, p. 241–262. (Surgical Sci. Ser.)
131. KELLY, K. A., J. M. BECKER, AND J. A. VAN HEERDEN. Reconstructive gastric surgery. *Br. J. Surg.* 68: 687–691, 1981.
132. KELLY, K. A., AND C. F. CODE. Effect of transthoracic vagotomy on canine gastric electrical activity. *Gastroenterology* 57: 51–58, 1969.
133. KELLY, K. A., AND C. F. CODE. Duodenal gastric reflux and slowed gastric emptying by electrical pacing of the canine duodenal pacesetter potential. *Gastroenterology* 72: 429–433, 1977.
134. KELLY, M., AND T. KENNEDY. Motility changes in the antrum after proximal gastric vagotomy. *Br. J. Surg.* 63: 215–220, 1975.
135. KENNEDY, T. The failures of gastric surgery. *Br. J. Surg.* 68: 674–677, 1981.
136. KENNEDY, T., A. M. CONNELL, A. H. G. LOVE, K. D. MACRAE, AND A. E. F. SPENCER. Selective or truncal vagotomy? Five-year results of a double-blind, randomized, controlled trial. *Br. J. Surg.* 60: 944–948, 1973.
137. KILBY, J. O., AND C. A. GRIFFITH. Selective and total vagotomy with suprapyloric antrectomy; a comparative study of gastric secretion and emptying in dogs. *Surgery St. Louis* 69: 702–707, 1971.
138. KILLEN, D. A., AND P. N. SYMBAS. Effect of preservation of pyloric sphincter during antrectomy and postoperative emptying. *Am. J. Surg.* 104: 836–840, 1962.
139. KLEMPA, I., E. HOLLE, W. BRUCKNER, K. H. WELSH, H. HANDLE, AND A. VON WOLF. The effect of selective proximal vagotomy and pyloroplasty on gastric secretion and motility in the dog. *Arch. Surg.* 103: 713–719, 1971.
140. KOEBERLE, H. Resection de deux mètres d'intestin grêle. *Bull. Acad. Med.* 10: 128–132, 1881.
141. KORTEZOVA, N. Changes in the frequency of the slow waves from the small intestine upon partial and full transverse section. *C. R. Acad. Bulg. Sci.* 26: 977–980, 1973.
142. KÖSTER, N., AND P. MADSON. The intragastric pressure before and immediately after truncal vagotomy. *Scand. J. Gastroenterol.* 5: 381–383, 1970.
143. KRAVITZ, J. J., W. J. SNAPE, JR., AND S. COHEN. Effect of thoracic vagotomy and vagal stimulation on esophageal function. *Am. J. Physiol.* 234 (*Endocrinol. Metab. Gastrointest.*

*Physiol.* 3): E359–E364, 1978.
144. KUWASHIMA, T. Effects of various types of vagotomy on electrical and contractile activities of the canine stomach. *Gastroenterol. Jpn.* 9: 407–421, 1974.
145. LATARJET, M. A. Resection des nerfs de l'estomac. Technique opératoire. Résultats cliniques. *Bull. Acad. Med.* 87: 681–691, 1922.
146. LAYZELL, T., AND J. COLLIN. Retrograde electrical pacing of the small intestine—a new treatment for the short bowel syndrome. *Br. J. Surg.* 68: 711–713, 1981.
147. LEBEDEV, N. N. About the physiological mechanisms of the periodical activity of the digestive tract. In: *Proc. Sci. Conf. Physiol. Pathol. of Cortico-Visceral Relationship and Functional Systems of the Organism.* Moscow: Medicina, 1965, vol. 1, p. 561–564.
148. LONGHI, E. H., AND P. H. JORDAN, JR. Necessity of a bolus for propagation of primary peristalsis in the canine esophagus. *Am. J. Physiol.* 220: 609–612, 1971.
149. LUDWICK, J., J. WILEY, AND P. BASS. Extraluminal contractile force and electrical activity of reversed canine duodenum. *Gastroenterology* 54: 41–51, 1968.
150. LUDWICK, J., J. WILEY, AND P. BASS. Gastric emptying following Finney pyloroplasty and vagotomy. *Am. J. Dig. Dis.* 15: 347–352, 1970.
151. MACGREGOR, I. L., P. MARTIN, AND J. H. MEYLER. Gastric emptying of solid food in normal man and after subtotal gastrectomy and truncal vagotomy with pyloroplasty. *Gastroenterology* 72: 206–211, 1977.
152. MCKELVEY, S. T. D. Gastric incontinence and post-vagotomy diarrhoea. *Br. J. Surg.* 57: 741–747, 1970.
153. MCSWINEY, B. A. Innervation of the stomach. *Physiol. Rev.* 11: 478–514, 1931.
154. MAKI, T., T. SHIRATORI, T. HATAFUKI, AND K. SUGAWARA. Pylorus preserving gastrectomy as an improved operation for gastric ulcer. *Surgery St. Louis* 61: 838–845, 1967.
155. MALAGELADA, J. R. Physiologic basis and clinical significance of gastric emptying disorders. *Dig. Dis. Sci.* 24: 657–661, 1979.
156. MALAGELADA, J. R., W. D. W. REES, L. MAZZOTTA, AND V. L. W. GO. Gastric motor abnormalities in diabetic and postvagotomy gastroparesis: effect of metaclopramide and betanechol. *Gastroenterology* 78: 286–293, 1980.
157. MARIK, F., AND C. F. CODE. Control of the interdigestive myoelectric activity in dogs by the vagus nerves and pentagastrin. *Gastroenterology* 69: 387–395, 1975.
158. MARTINSON, J. The effect of graded stimulation of efferent vagal nerve fibres on gastric motility. *Acta Physiol. Scand.* 62: 256–262, 1964.
159. MARTINSON, J. Vagal relaxation of the stomach. Experimental re-investigation of the concept of the transmission mechanism. *Acta Physiol. Scand.* 64: 453–462, 1965.
160. MATARAZZO, S. A., W. J. SNAPE, J. P. RYAN, AND S. COHEN. Relationship of cervical and abdominal vagal activity to lower esophageal sphincter function. *Gastroenterology* 71: 999–1003, 1976.
161. MATROSSOVA, E. M., A. A. KURYGIN, AND S. D. GROISMAN. *Vagotomy (Consequences and their Mechanisms).* Leningrad: Nauka, 1981.
162. MATTSON, O., AND G. PERMON. Small intestinal transit time studied in patients with dumping syndrome. *Acta Chir. Scand.* 124: 326–332, 1962.
163. MATTSON, O., G. PERMON, AND H. LAGERLOF. The small intestine transit time with a physiological contrast medium. *Acta Radiol.* 54: 332–344, 1960.
164. MAYER, E. A., J. B. THOMSON, D. JEHN, T. REEDY, J. ELASHOFF, C. DEVENY, AND J. H. MEYER. Gastric emptying and sieving of solid food and pancreatic and biliary secretions after solid meals in patients with nonresective ulcer surgery. *Gastroenterology* 87: 1264–1271, 1984.
165. MELTZER, S. T. On the causes of the orderly progress of the peristaltic movement in the esophagus. *Am. J. Physiol.* 2: 226–272, 1899.
166. MENDOZA, C. B., G. W. EASLEY, AND W. H. GERWIG. Jejunal interposition as remedial operation for severe dumping syndrome. *Am. J. Surg.* 125: 318–323, 1973.
167. MIALARET, J., AND G. EDELMAN. Accidents et sequelles de la vagotomie. *Acta Gastro-Enterol. Belg.* 26: 148–162, 1963.
168. MILENOV, K. Electrical and motor activities of the stomach after partial resections of the small and big curvature. *Bull. Inst. Physiol. Sofia* 11: 79–96, 1968.
169. MILKOV, G., AND P. ELENKOV. Motor-evacuative functions of resected stomach and their role in the development of postresection complications. *Chirurgia Buchar.* 3: 213–218, 1977.
170. MILLAR, J. W., G. P. MACLOUGHLIN, I. B. MACLEOD, AND R. C. HEADING. The effect of vagotomy on gastric emptying of solid and liquid components of a meal. In: *Gastrointestinal Motility in Health and Disease*, edited by H. L. Duthie. Lancaster: MTP, 1978, p. 215–222. (6th Int. Symp. Gastrointest. Motil., Edinburgh, Sept. 12–16, 1977.)
171. MILTON, G., AND A. SMITH. Pacemaking area of the duodenum. *J. Physiol. London* 132: 100–114, 1956.
172. MITCHELL, A., R. M. WATKINS, AND J. COLLIN. Surgical treatment of the short bowel syndrome. *Br. J. Surg.* 71: 329–333, 1984.
173. MORDOVZEV, A. I. On the central nervous mechanisms of the contractile activity of the stomach. In: *Gastrointestinal System Activity and Its Regulation in Health and Disease.* Moscow: Medgis, 1961, p. 214–221.
174. MORRIS, I. R., C. F. DARBY, H. P. HAMMOND, AND I. TAYLOR. Changes in small bowel myoelectrical activity following laparotomy. *Br. J. Surg.* 70: 547–548, 1983.
175. MUNK, J. F., AND A. G. JOHNSON. Effect of duodenal and antral pacing on pyloric reflux in the cat. In: *Gastrointestinal Motility*, edited by J. Christensen. New York: Raven, 1980, p. 173–176. (7th Int. Symp. Gastrointest. Motil., Iowa City, Iowa, Sept. 11–14, 1979.)
176. NACHLAS, M. M., M. T. YOUMIS, C. P. RODA, AND J. G. WITYK. Gastrointestinal motility studies as a guide of postoperative management. *Ann. Surg.* 175: 510–522, 1972.
177. NAGAOKA, K. Electromyographic study on the mechanism of delayed gastric emptying after vagotomy in dogs. *J. Exp. Med.* 95: 1–13, 1968.
178. NANA, A., C. MIRION, E. NEUMANN, AND M. NANA. Gastrointestinal and biliary biopotentials following various forms of vagotomy. *Digestion* 4: 269–280, 1971.
179. NEAL, D. E., N. S. WILLIAMS, M. C. J. BARKER, AND R. F. C. J. KING. The effect of resection of the distal ileum on gastric emptying, small bowel transit and absorption after proctocolectomy. *Br. J. Surg.* 71: 666–670, 1984.
180. NELSEN, T. S., E. H. EIGENBRODT, L. A. KEOSHIAN, C. BUNKER, AND L. JOHNSON. Alterations in muscular and electrical activity of the stomach following vagotomy. *Arch. Surg.* 94: 821–836, 1967.
181. NINOMIYA, I., H. IRISAWA, AND G. WOOLLEY. Intestinal mechanoreceptor reflex effects on sympathetic nerve activity to intestine and kidney. *Am. J. Physiol.* 227: 684–691, 1974.
182. PANZIREV, U. M., AND A. A. GRINBERG. *Vagotomy in Case of Complicated Duodenal Ulcers.* Moscow: Medicina, 1979.
183. PANZIREV, U. M., A. A. GRINBERG, AND C. A. CHERNIAKEVICH. Motor-evacuatory function of the stomach after surgical intervention with vagotomy. In: *Electrical Activity of the Smooth Muscles and Motor Function of Gastrointestinal Tract*, edited by P. G. Bogach. Kiev: University Press, 1970, p. 205–206.
184. PAPASOVA, M. Nervous mechanism of regulation of the gastrointestinal tract bioelectrical activity. In: *Contemporary Tendencies in Neurophysiology*, edited by E. M. Kreps. Leningrad: Nauka, 1977, p. 234–247.
185. PAPASOVA, M., AND E. ATANASSOVA. Changes in the bioelectric activity of the stomach after bilateral transthoracal vagotomy. *Bull. Inst. Physiol. Sofia* 14: 121–133, 1972.
186. PAPASOVA, M., AND E. ATANASSOVA. Electrical activity of the stomach. Nervous control. *Scand. J. Gastroenterol.* 96: 45–53, 1984.
187. PAPASOVA, M., E. ATANASSOVA, AND K. BOEV. Modulation of

the gastric electrical pattern under the influence of nerve impulses. In: *Proc. 5th Int. Symp. Gastrointest. Motil.*, edited by G. Vantrappen. Herentals, Belgium: Typoff, 1976, p. 164–168.
188. PAPASOVA, M., N. KORTEZOVA, AND E. ATANASSOVA. Participation of the pyloric sphincter in the coordination of the electrical activity in the stomach and duodenum. In: *Motility of the Digestive Tract*, edited by M. Wienbeck. New York: Raven, 1982, p. 201–206. (8th Int. Symp. Gastrointest. Motil., Königstein, FRG, Sept. 7–11, 1981.)
189. PAPASOVA, M. P., T. NAGAI, AND C. L. PROSSER. Two-component slow waves in smooth muscle of cat stomach. *Am. J. Physiol.* 214: 695–702, 1968.
190. PARKS, A. G., R. J. NICHOLLS, AND P. BELLIVEAR. Proctocolectomy with ileal reservoir and anal anastomosis. *Br. J. Surg.* 67: 533–538, 1980.
191. PASMA, F. G., L. M. A. AKKERMANS, H. Y. OEI, A. J. P. M. SMOUT, AND P. WITTEBOL. Gastric emptying in asymptomatic partial gastrectomy (B-II) patients. In: *Gastrointestinal Motility*, edited by C. Roman. Lancaster, UK: MTP, 1984, p. 143–148. (9th Int. Symp. Gastrointest. Motil., Aix-en-Provence, France, Sept. 12–16, 1983.)
192. PECHATNIKOVA, E. A., AND N. N. KUZNETSOV. *Physiological Aspects of Gastrectomy*. Leningrad: Medicina, 1969.
193. PERRET, C. E., AND F. H. HESSER. Studies on gastric motility in the cat. I. Effect of supradiaphragmatic vagotomy, cervical cord transection, sympathosplanchnicectomy and posterior root ganglionectomy. *Gastroenterology* 38: 218–230, 1960.
194. PRICE, L. M., T. Y. EL-SHARKAWY, H. Y. MUI, AND N. D. DIAMANT. Effect of bilateral cervical vagotomy on balloon-induced lower esophageal sphincter relaxation in dog. *Gastroenterology* 77: 324–329, 1979.
195. QUIGLEY, J. P. Motor physiology of the stomach, the pylorus and the duodenum. *Arch. Surg.* 44: 414–437, 1943.
196. QUIGLEY, J. P., AND H. LOUCKES. The effects of complete vagotomy on the pyloric sphincter and the gastric evacuation mechanism. *Gastroenterology* 19: 533–542, 1951.
197. RABAN, M. Y., J. P. PERCY, AND A. G. PARKS. Ileal pelvic reservoir: a correlation between motor patterns and clinical behaviour. *Br. J. Surg.* 69: 391–395, 1982.
198. RAMUS, N. Y., R. C. N. WILLIAMSON, AND D. JOHNSTON. The use of jejunal interposition for intractable symptoms complicating peptic ulcer surgery. *Br. J. Surg.* 69: 265–268, 1982.
199. REMINGTON, M., J.-R. MALAGELADA, A. ZINSMEISTER, AND C. R. FLEMING. Abnormalities in gastrointestinal motor activity in patients with short bowels: effect of a synthetic opiate. *Gastroenterology* 85: 629–636, 1983.
200. REYNOLDS, R. P., T. Y. EL-SHARKAWY, AND N. E. DIAMANT. Esophageal peristalsis in cat: the role of central innervation assessed by transient vagal blockade. *Can. J. Physiol. Pharmacol.* 63: 122–130, 1985.
201. REVERDIN, N., M. R. HUTTON, A. LING, H. H. THOMSON, D. L. WINGATE, N. CHRISTOFIDES, T. E. ADRIAN, AND S. R. BLOOM. Vagotomy and the motor response to feeding. In: *Gastrointestinal Motility*, edited by J. Christensen. New York: Raven, 1980, p. 359–364. (7th Int. Symp. Gastrointest. Motil., Iowa City, Iowa, Sept. 11–14, 1979.)
202. RITCHIE, J. A. Pain from distension of the pelvic colon by inflating a balloon in the irritable colon syndrome. *Gut* 14: 125–132, 1973.
203. ROMAN, C., AND J. GONELLA. Extrinsic control of digestive tract motility. In: *Physiology of Gastrointestinal Tract*, edited by L. R. Johnson. New York: Raven, 1981, p. 289–333.
204. ROMAN, C., AND L. TIEFFENBACH. Motricité de l'oesophage à musculeuse lisse après bivagotomie. Étude électromyographique. *J. Physiol. Paris* 63: 733–762, 1971.
205. ROMAN, C., AND L. TIEFFENBACH. Enregistrement de l'activité unitaire des fibres motrices vagales destinées à l'oesophage du babouin. *J. Physiol. Paris* 64: 479–506, 1972.
206. ROSE, B., B. W. WATSON, AND A. W. KAY. Studies on the effect of vagotomy on small intestinal motility using radiotelemetring capsule. *Gut* 4: 77–81, 1963.
207. ROTH, H. P., AND A. J. BEAMS. The effect of vagotomy on the motility of the small intestine. *Gastroenterology* 36: 452–458, 1959.
208. ROTHNIE, N. G., R. A. KEMP HARPER, AND B. N. CATCHPOLE. Early postoperative gastrointestinal activity. *Lancet* 2: 64–67, 1963.
209. RYAN, J. P., W. J. SNAPE, JR., AND S. COHEN. Influence of vagal cooling on esophageal function. *Am. J. Physiol.* 232 (*Endocrinol. Metab. Gastrointest. Physiol.* 2): E159–E164, 1977.
210. SAGOR, G. R., M. A. CHATEL, D. J. O'SHAUGHNESSY, M. Y. T. AL-MUKHTAR, N. A. WRIGHT, AND S. R. BLOOM. Influence of somatostatin and bombesin on plasma enteroglucagon and cell proliferation after intestinal resection in the rat. *Gut* 26: 89–95, 1985.
211. SAHAROV, E. I., AND A. E. SAHAROV. *Jejunogastroplasty in Diseases of the Resected Stomach*. Moscow: Medicina, 1970.
212. SANDERS, K. M. Role of prostaglandins in regulating gastric motility. *Am. J. Physiol.* 247 (*Gastrointest. Liver Physiol.* 10): G117–G126, 1984.
213. SARR, M. C., AND K. A. KELLY. Myoelectric activity of the autotransplanted canine jejunoileum. *Gastroenterology* 81: 303–311, 1981.
214. SARNA, S. K., K. L. BOWES, AND E. E. DANIEL. Postoperative gastric electrical control activity (ECA) in man. In: *Gastrointestinal Motility*, edited by E. E. Daniel. Vancouver, Canada: Mitchell, 1974, p. 73–83. (4th Int. Symp. Gastrointest. Motil., Banff, Alberta, Canada, Sept. 6–8, 1973.)
215. SARNA, S. K., E. CONDON, AND V. COWLES. Enteric mechanisms of initiation of migrating myoelectric complexes in dog. *Gastroenterology* 84: 814–822, 1983.
216. SARNA, S. K., E. E. DANIEL, AND Y. J. KINGMA. Effects of partial cuts on gastric electrical control activity and its computer model. *Am. J. Physiol.* 223: 332–340, 1972.
217. SARNA, S., P. NORTHCOTT, AND L. BELBECK. Mechanism of cycling of migrating myoelectrical complexes: effect of morphine. *Am. J. Physiol.* 242 (*Gastrointest. Liver Physiol.* 5): G588–G595, 1982.
218. SAWYERS, J. L., J. L. HERRINGTON, AND P. D. BURNEY. Proximal gastric vagotomy compared with vagotomy and antrectomy and selective vagotomy and pyloroplasty. *Ann. Surg.* 186: 510–517, 1977.
219. SCILLER, W. R., L. I. A. DIDIO, AND M. C. ANDERSON. Production of artificial sphincters. Ablation of the longitudinal layer of intestine. *Arch. Surg.* 95: 436–442, 1967.
220. SCHILLER, W. R., C. SURIYAPA, J. H. W. MUTCHLER, AND M. C. ANDERSON. Surgical alteration of intestinal motility. *Am. J. Surg.* 125: 122–128, 1973.
221. SELF, J. B. A gastric reconstruction. *Br. J. Surg.* 55: 602–604, 1968.
222. SHAHIDULLAH, M., T. L. KENNEDY, AND T. G. PARKS. The vagus, the duodenal brake and gastric emptying. *Gut* 16: 331–336, 1975.
223. SHEINER, H. J., M. F. QUINLAN, AND I. J. THOMPSON. Gastric motility and emptying in normal and postvagotomy subjects. *Gut* 21: 753–759, 1980.
224. SHIINOR, E., AND C. A. GRIFFITH. Selective and total vagotomy without drainage: a comparative study of gastric secretion and motility in dogs. *Ann. Surg.* 169: 326–335, 1969.
225. SHIRATORI, T. Electromyographic studies on the mechanism of pylorospasm following vagotomy. *Jpn. J. Smooth Muscle Res.* 6: 141–146, 1970.
226. SKALA, I., AND V. KONRADOVA. Hypertrophy of the small intestine after its partial resection. Ultrastructure of the intestinal epithelium. *Am. J. Dig. Dis.* 14: 182–189, 1969.
227. SOBAKIN, M. A., J. P. SMIRNOV, AND L. N. MISHIN. Electrogastrography. *Trans. Bio-Med. Electronics* 9: 129–132, 1962.
228. STADAAS, J. O. Intragastric pressure/volume relationship before and after proximal vagotomy. *Scand. J. Gastroenterol.* 10: 1–6, 1975.
229. STADAAS, J. O., E. SCHRUMPF, AND J. F. W. HAFFNER. The

effect of gastric distension on gastric motility and serum gastrin in acutely vagotomized pigs. *Scand. J. Gastroenterol.* 9: 127–131, 1974.
230. STODDARD, C. J., A. G. JOHNSON, AND H. L. DUTHIE. The four to eight year results of the Sheffield trial of selective duodenal ulcer surgery—highly selective or truncal vagotomy? *Br. J. Surg.* 71: 779–782, 1984.
231. STODDARD, C. J., R. SMALLWOOD, B. H. BROWN, AND H. L. DUTHIE. The immediate and delayed effects of different types of vagotomy on human gastric myoelectrical activity. *Gut* 16: 165–170, 1975.
232. STODDARD, C. J., W. E. WATERFALL, B. H. BOWN, AND H. L. DUTHIE. The effects of varying the extent of the vagotomy on the myoelectrical and motor activity of the stomach. *Gut* 14: 657–664, 1973.
233. STORDY, S. N. The steak and barium meal. A method for evaluating gastric emptying after partial gastrectomy. *Am. J. Dig. Dis.* 14: 463–469, 1969.
234. STOREY, D. W., P. B. BOULOS, M. W. N. WARD, AND C. G. CLARK. Proximal gastric vagotomy after five years. *Gut* 22: 702–704, 1981.
235. STROUKOV, M. V. Changes in the motor function of the stomach and duodenum after bilateral vagotomy. *Vest. Chir.* 69: 38–43, 1949.
236. SUGAWARA, K. An electromyographic study on the motility of canine stomach after transection and end-to-end anastomosis. *Tohoku J. Exp. Med.* 84: 113–121, 1964.
237. SUGAWARA, K., J. ISAKA, E. R. WOODWARD, AND L. R. DRAGSTEDT. The short-term effect of vagotomy on gastric motility. *Arch. Surg.* 99: 1–5, 1969.
238. TETYAEVA, M. E. *Evolution of the Vagus Function in the Activity of the Gastrointestinal Tract.* Moscow: Acad. Sci. USSR, 1960.
239. THOMPSON, D. G., H. D. RITCHIE, AND D. L. WINGATE. Patterns of small intestinal motility in duodenal ulcer patients before and after vagotomy. *Gut* 23: 517–524, 1982.
240. TIEFFENBACH, L., AND C. ROMAN. Rôle de l'innervation extrinsèque vagale dans la motricité de l'oesophage à musculeuse lisse: étude électromyographique chez le chat et le babouin. *J. Physiol. Paris* 64: 193–226, 1972.
241. TINKER, J., N. KOCAK, T. JONES, H. GLASS, AND H. G. COX. Supersensitivity and gastric emptying after vagotomy. *Gut* 11: 502–505, 1970.
242. TINKLER, L. F. Surgery and intestinal motility. *Br. J. Surg.* 52: 140–152, 1965.
243. URBAN, E. Metabolic consequences of small bowel resection. *Gastroenterology* 77: 572–579, 1979.
244. VANTRAPPEN, G., AND H. HELLEMANS. *Diseases of the Esophagus.* New York: Springer-Verlag, 1974.
245. VITKIN, S. F. Motor functions of the stomach after resection. *Ann. Surg.* 111: 27–48, 1940.
246. WALKER, G. D., J. J. STEWART, AND P. BASS. The effect of parietal cell truncal vagotomy on gastric and duodenal contractile activity of the unanesthetized dog. *Ann. Surg.* 179: 853–858, 1974.
247. WEBER, J., AND S. KOHATSU. Pacemaker localisation and electrical conduction patterns in the canine stomach. *Gastroenterology* 59: 717–726, 1970.
248. WEDDLE, C. O., A. C. SPRINGFIELD, AND H. S. ORMSBEE. Parietal cell vagotomy and gastric emptying of liquids in the dog. *Arch. Surg.* 108: 83–86, 1973.
249. WENBERG, J. A. Vagotomy and pyloroplasty for the surgical treatment of duodenal ulcer. In: *Surgery of the Stomach and Duodenum,* edited by H. N. Harkins and L. M. Nyhus. Boston, MA: Little, Brown, 1962, p. 473–486.
250. WEISBRODT, N. W., E. M. COPELAND, E. P. MOORE, R. W. KEARLEY, AND L. R. JOHNSON. Effect of vagotomy on electrical activity on the small intestine of the dog. *Am. J. Physiol.* 228: 650–654, 1975.
251. WEISBRODT, N. W., E. M. COPELAND, P. J. THOR, AND N. S. J. DUDRICK. Small bowel motility during intravenous hyperalimentation in the dog (Abstract). *Gastroenterology* 68: 1011, 1975.
252. WELLS, C., K. RAWLINSON, L. TINCKLER, H. JONES, AND J. SAUNDERS. Ileus and postoperative motility. *Lancet* 2: 136–137, 1961.
253. WESER, E. Intestinal adaptation after small bowel resection. *Gastroenterology* 77: 575–577, 1975.
254. WILBUR, B. G. AND K. A. KELLY. Effect of proximal, complete gastric and truncal vagotomy on canine gastric electric activity, motility and emptying. *Ann. Surg.* 178: 295–303, 1973.
255. WILBUR, B. G., K. A. KELLY, AND C. F. CODE. Effect of gastric fundectomy on canine gastric electrical and motor activity. *Am. J. Physiol.* 226: 1445–1449, 1974.
256. WILKINSON, A. R., AND D. JOHNSTON. Effect of truncal selective and highly selective vagotomy on gastric emptying and intestinal transit of a food—barium meal in man. *Ann. Surg.* 178: 190–193, 1973.
257. WINGATE, D. L. Complex clocks. *Dig. Dis. Sci.* 28: 1133–1140, 1983.
258. ZLATARSKI, G., E. ATANASSOVA, AND C. CHRISTOV. Electromyographic studies of the intestinal tract in emergency abdominal surgery. *Chirurgia Buchar.* 34: 241–245, 1981.

CHAPTER 34

# Gastrointestinal motor functions in ruminants

YVES RUCKEBUSCH | Department of Physiology, National Veterinary School, Toulouse, France

CHAPTER CONTENTS

Mammalian Herbivore Stomach
  Morphological adaptation to bulky food
    Anatomy
      Physical breakdown of solid digesta
      Diversion of liquid digesta
  Functional adaptation to fermentation
  Functional adaptation to absorption
  Retention time and food propulsion
Forestomach Motility
  Cyclical contractions of reticulorumen
    Measurement
    Mechanical activity
    Electrical activity
  Events associated with rumination
    Mechanism of regurgitation
    Nervous control of rumination
    Hormonal influences
  Events associated with eructation
  Cyclical activity of omasum
  Reticular groove mechanisms
  Nervous control of forestomach motility
    Intrinsic contractions
    Extrinsic contractions
    Gastric centers
    Visceral sensory mechanisms
Stomach Motility
  Motor patterns of activity
  Duodenal brake mechanism
  Control of gastric emptying
    Milk-fed animals
    Adult ruminants
Small Intestine Motility
  Periodic activity
  Mixing versus propelling activity
  Motor function of duodenal bulb
  Pancreaticobiliary secretions
  Nervous control
  5-Hydroxytryptamine
Large Intestine Motility
  Functional organization
  Cecal motility patterns
  Pelleted feces formation
  Neural influences
Pharmacological Considerations
  Drugs affecting forestomach motility
  Drugs affecting gastroduodenal junction
  Perspectives

MICROBIAL DEGRADATION of the structural carbohydrates of plants is vital to digestion in mammalian herbivores and has been of great evolutionary advantage in enabling some species to occupy nutritional niches free of competitors (131). Where microbial fermentation takes place in the stomach, a voluminous "fermentation vat" is differentiated, hence the term *forestomach* or *foregut fermenters*. This provides a gastric capacity to hold food for fermentation that, according to Hungate (116), may be in line between the cardia and the pylorus or can be set off in a blind sac or diverticulum where a portion of the gastric contents is stored for a longer time. As a consequence of the detour of the gastric contents via the forestomach blind sacs and their passage through small apertures between different compartments (ostium reticulo-omasicum and ostium omaso-abomasicum), there is an increase in the transit time of solid digesta from cardia to pylorus. An esophageal or reticular groove, the sulcus reticuli, allows a direct passage of liquid digesta from the cardia toward the abomasum in the neonate until the time of weaning (i.e., before weaning).

The early interest in the studies of the ruminant gastrointestinal motor functions has been directed to the changes in rumen motility patterns in relation to fermentative processes, methanogenesis, rumination, and food propulsion (29, 32, 47, 48, 73, 106, 107, 120, 157, 198, 213, 227, 234). Major advances in the appreciation of the role of ruminal microbes (bacteria, protozoa, anaerobic fungi) in mediating digestion of nutrients by the ruminant have been made. Fermentation manipulations (2, 100, 242) to increase the efficiency with which feed nutrients are utilized by the host animal have been improved (222).

In addition to the progress in ruminant surgery (49, 98) and laboratory techniques (25, 69), the utilization of the sheep as a laboratory animal (101) has revealed three other interesting aspects of the ruminant species in gastroenterology: *1*) the cyclical contractions of the rumen under the rigid control of the vagus nerves represent a unique model in terms of nervous control of motility; *2*) the true stomach of the adult ruminant, the abomasum, behaves as the stomach of other species with the advantage of a constant delivery of digestive contents through the gastroduodenum regardless of feeding or other behaviors; and *3*) the abomasum of the preruminant receives directly the milk or the milk substitutes that bypass the rumen. The motor patterns involved in gastric emptying, digesta propulsion, and digesta retropulsion (dietary sensitivities of the lamb or calf) are comparable to those of monogastric species. In addition, well-patterned functional secretory activities develop postnatally in the neonatal ruminant, which is considered to be immature in terms of its ability to secrete acid and pepsin (186).

MAMMALIAN HERBIVORE STOMACH

It was believed that the forestomach (reticulorumen and omasum) represented esophageal diverticula and that only the last compartment, the abomasum, developed from the gastric spindle that supplies the entire stomach of other species. This idea has as its basis the fact that there is an extension of an esophageal type of epithelium throughout the rumen, reticulum, and omasum (59).

Detailed embryological studies show that all four parts of the ruminant stomach are of gastric origin, an interpretation that is confirmed by the adult topography, the attachments of the omenta, and the source and ramification of the gastric nerves and vessels. Figure 1 shows the parts of the spindle from which the different compartments originate. The rumen and reticulum enlarge from the fundic region facing the cardia, the omasum from the lesser curvature at a more distal level, and the abomasum from the terminal section, mainly the aspect corresponding to the greater curvature of the simple stomach. The channel along which milk passes to the abomasum in the sucking neonates thus follows the lesser curvature. With further comparison between unichamber and multichamber stomach, the homologies proposed for certain of the smaller divisions of the stomach appear to be more speculative with regard to the different types of stomachs (249).

Although the abomasum dominates abdominal topography at birth, extending from one flank to the other and from the diaphragm almost to the pelvic inlet, the picture is different only a few weeks later. The topography can hardly be distinguished from that seen in the adult at 2 mo.

The reticulum and rumen increase in weight by a factor of 15 during the first 2 mo. They contain very little ingesta during the first 2 or 3 wk, but when the animal first shows a serious interest in solid food, they gain in volume very quickly. In 2-wk-old lambs the reticulorumen holds less than half the content of the abomasum; it contains an equal volume 1 wk later and almost 20 times as much after 2 mo (250). This latter value is approximately the adult ratio, and the volume of the rumen thereafter maintains a steady relationship to the abomasal volume and to the body weight. The forms assumed by the rumen and reticulum clearly depend on the arrangement of smooth muscle bundles in tracts that can be homologized with the simpler pattern of the fibers of the simple-chambered organ (Fig. 2). The bundles continue into the pillars or inflections of the walls, i.e., the cranial pillar that separates the dorsal and ventral sac and the atrium ruminis as inflections involved in the individualization of the caudal blind sacs.

*Morphological Adaptation to Bulky Food*

ANATOMY. In forestomach fermenters, an increase in stomach cross-sectional diameter is obtained by either taenia, haustra, or semilunar folds (138). The relative size of the gastric compartments in which the total stomach represents 100% is given in Table 1 for Artiodactyla and other herbivores. The Artiodactyla groups include Nonruminantia: Hippopotamidae (hippopotamuses) and Tayassuidae (peccaries), and the Ruminantia: Pecora, Tragulina, and Tylopoda (Fig. 3). Fermentation in well-developed forestomachs has been identified in Potoroinae (rat-kangaroos), Macropodinae (kangaroos and wallabies), Colobidae (leaf monkeys), and Bradypodidae (tree sloths). An exception is the Sirenia, in which the capacity of the duodenal ampulla that follows the stomach is nearly equal to that of the total stomach (161).

The complex mechanism that slows the passage of food in kangaroo or leaf monkeys consists of longitudinal muscular bands or taenia and dilations or haustra; these structures are found in omnivorous-like pigs or herbivorous-like equids or the rabbits, which are hindgut fermenters.

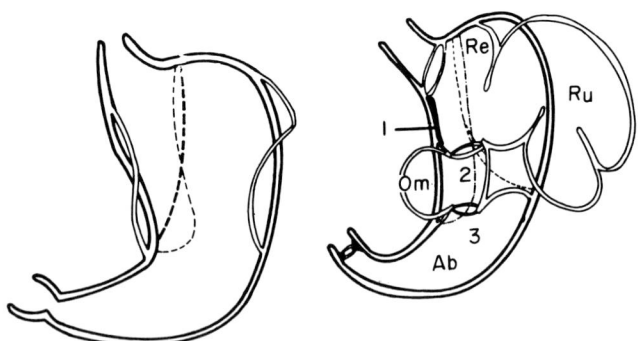

FIG. 1. Expansion of simple stomach into multichambered stomach in ruminant herbivore (associated with specialized motor function, fermentation, and absorption). Esophageal groove (*1*) directs sucked liquid from cardia toward abomasum. Groove is bound by 2 fleshy lips that run spirally; the one that lies caudally at upper right end of groove passes left to gain cranial aspect about reticuloomasal orifice (*2*). Relative infrequency with which the abomasal contents reflux through wide omaso-abomasal opening (*3*) depends on development of abomasal plicae, which rise abruptly around margin of opening and act like a ball valve to close orifice when pressure within abomasum rises. Re, reticulum; Ru, rumen; Om, omasum; Ab, abomasum. [From Dyce (59).]

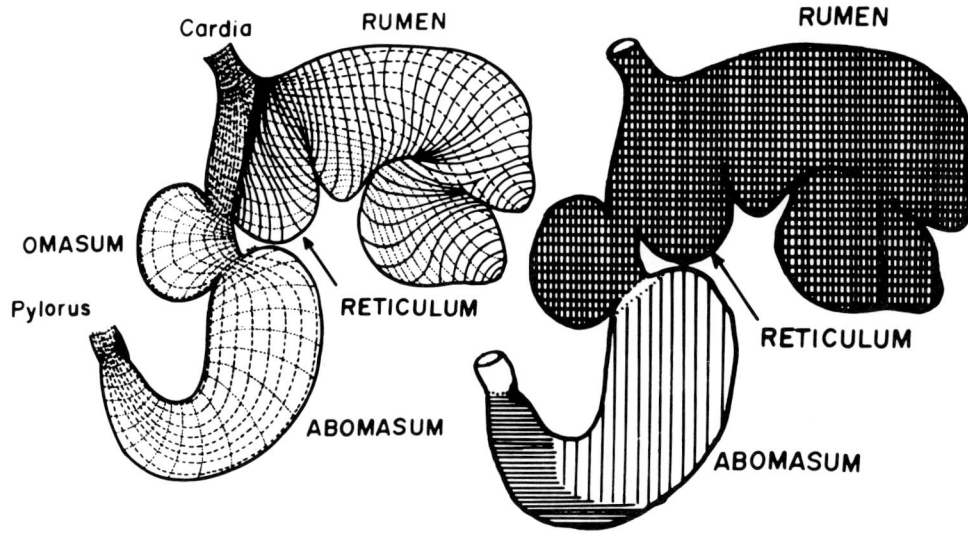

FIG. 2. Arrangement of smooth muscle bundles in adult ruminant stomach. Reticulum and rumen, which together are known as reticulorumen, hold on average 84% of total capacity. Nonglandular mucosa covers dorsal sac and ventral sac of rumen, reticulum, and omasum (*cross-hatching*). Cardiac gland region (*open areas*) is near omaso-abomasal opening. Fundic glands (*vertical lines*) and pyloric glands (*horizontal lines*) involve whole abomasum.

TABLE 1. *Relative Volume of Different Stomach Segments in Herbivores*

| | Segment | Volume, % |
|---|---|---|
| Pecora (ruminants with horns and antlers) | Reticulorumen | 88 |
| | Omasum | 6 |
| | Abomasum | 6 |
| Tragulina (chevrotains) | Reticulorumen | 95 |
| | Abomasum | 5 |
| Tylopoda (camellike mammals) | Reticulorumen | 89 |
| | Tubiform forestomach | 9 |
| | Hind stomach | 2 |
| Hippopotamidae (hippopotamus and pygmy hippopotamus) | Blind sacs and vestibulum | 42 |
| | Connecting compartment | 52 |
| | Hind stomach | 6 |
| Tayassuidae | Blind sac | 40 |
| | Gastric pouch | 45 |
| | Hind stomach | 15 |
| Macropodinae (true kangaroos) | Sacciform forestomach | 31 |
| | Tubiform forestomach | 60 |
| | Hind stomach | 9 |
| Colobidae (leaf monkeys) | Saccus gastricus and praesaccus | 73 |
| | Tubus gastricus | 24 |
| | Pars pylorica | 3 |
| Sirenia (sea cow) | Stomach | 32 |
| | Cardiac gland | 9 |
| | Duodenal ampulla | 47 |
| | Pyloric blind sacs | 12 |

[From Langer (131).]

Extensive transverse folds, which probably function like valves connecting compartments such as the hind stomach and the forestomach, act to regulate digesta transit in the Hippopotamidae. The rumen is in open connection with the reticulum in both the Pecora and Tragulina.

PHYSICAL BREAKDOWN OF SOLID DIGESTA. Coarse particles are retained until they are able to leave the forestomach (i.e., the reticulorumen) in a finely divided form. The reduction in particle size results in part from mastication, when food is eaten, and from rumination in the Pecora, Tragulina, and Tylopoda or merycism in some kangaroos. Both processes reduce the size of food particles that have already been swallowed. Chewing of the cud is related to the reticulorumen motor function differentiation and to its functional adaptation; the time spent ruminating is reduced from 8 to 2 h/day by grinding of roughage before feeding (160, 165, 179, 233). Comparative studies of comminution of feed during eating and rumination show that rumination is the more important process (181). Particle size reduction due to eating in sheep ranges from 12% to 15% of the dry matter intake, irrespective of food type, whereas rumination reduces 12%–16% of fresh and 27%–39% of hay dietary dry matter (233).

DIVERSION OF LIQUID DIGESTA. A well-developed feature in the reticulum (the sulcus reticuli) of Ruminantia functions, in sucking animals, to bypass the rumen and direct liquid digesta toward the abomasum. The reticular groove, described earlier by Flourens (74) as being able to push digesta into the cardia during regurgitation, is stimulated to contract as part of a complex response in which the opening of cardia and reticulo-omasal orifice is coordinated so that milk runs

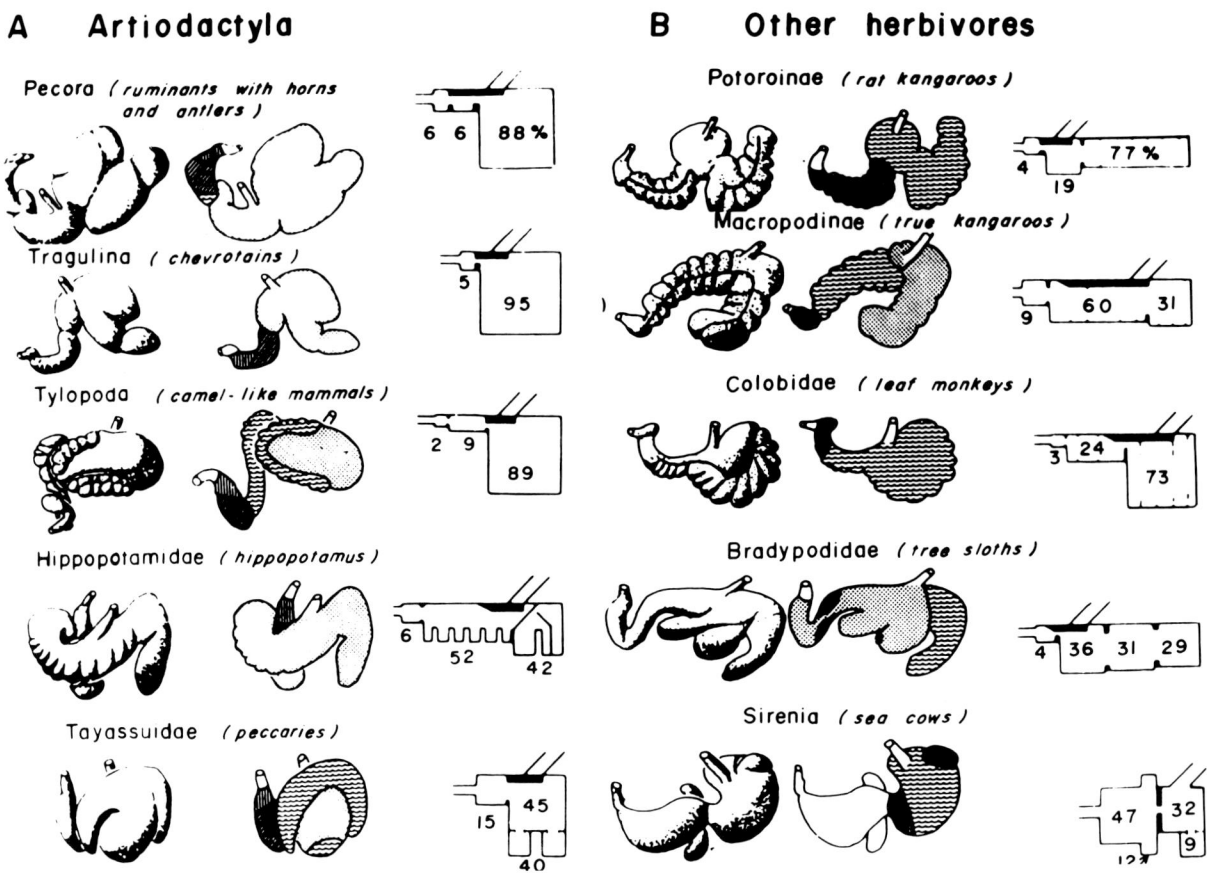

FIG. 3. Gastric form and relative volumes indicated as percentages of stomach regions in herbivores [Artiodactyla (A)] and others (B). Gastric groove is represented schematically (*horizontal filled bar*) and apertures between gastric regions are also represented. *Dotted structures*, semilunar folds. Esophagus comes in from *top right*, and duodenum points to *left*. Hatched areas correspond to HCl-producing fundic glands and pyloric glands. [Adapted from Langer (131).]

through the omasum to the abomasum (Fig. 4). Closure of the reticular groove is the result of a reflex in which the afferent nerve endings are situated in the mouth and pharynx. This was demonstrated by Wester in 1926 (see ref. 227) in studies in which he had created a rumen fistula large enough to allow him to put his hand inside the reticulorumen to feel the behavior of the esophageal groove. He noted that the groove closed when the calf drank milk but that closure did not occur if milk was given through a tube introduced into the cervical esophagus via the nasal canal and moreover that closure occurred in sham-fed calves when they drank milk even though the milk did not reach the stomach (183). Anesthesia of the buccal and pharyngeal mucosa, by swabbing the mouth with a solution of cocaine, inhibited the closure of the groove when the calf subsequently drank milk. Large doses of atropine similarly inhibit closure of the groove (163). Closure of the groove in response to swallowing fluid from the mouth is an inborn reflex and can be demonstrated in the lamb near full term and in the newborn animal when it first sucks (55). Normally the responsiveness of the reflex diminishes with age, the responses to milk and water being similar until weaning. However, age by itself is not necessarily associated with a loss of response to sucked milk (90). The response seems to depend on whether the animal retains a delight in taking milk, and the shift from the sucking pattern of behavior to a thirst pattern of behavior appears to be an outward sign of whether the groove will respond (126, 258). In the adult, water seldom evokes the reflex when it is drunk, and attempts to sensitize the reflex by withholding water do not influence the result (251).

*Functional Adaptation to Fermentation*

The symbiotic association with microorganisms enables the host to live on high-fiber diets (125, 239, 255). The regulatory systems developed are a large fermentation vessel (136), gathering and selection of substrate, maceration and mixing of food (86), temperature control, pH control through the buffering action of saliva (121, 256), provision of extra nutrients

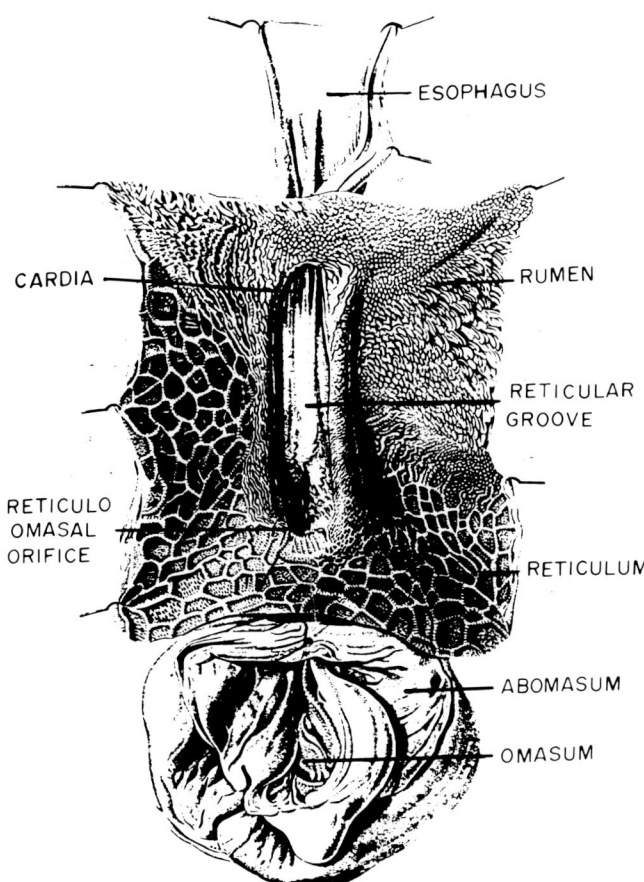

FIG. 4. The illustration by Flourens of the esophageal (reticular) groove in sheep, which he claimed to close on food lying within and to force it into thoracic esophagus. Colin disproved its role in regurgitation after tying the lips together with a wire in a steer, and Wester showed the opening and closing to be in relation with biphasic or triphasic contraction of reticulum. [From Flourens (74).]

(e.g., urea and phosphates in the saliva), anaerobiosis (10, 43), and removal of inhibitory soluble products and indigestible solids. The animal can regulate the activities of the rumen microorganisms only by varying these facilities. The microorganisms are controlled by the limitations of their growth physiology and competition between species (116, 242).

There are no gross differences between uninoculated gnotobiotic lambs and conventional lambs in the weights of the reticulorumen plus contents and the cecum plus contents relative to body weight (138). However, the weight of the empty reticulorumen is very low, with an apparent lack of musculature and muscular tone in the rumen walls. The intact rumen at postmortem examination is a flaccid sac resembling an oval, fluid-filled plastic bag. The position of the rumen pillars is less obvious from the outside and has less effect in maintaining the rumen shape after death, in accordance with the thinness of the wall and the small size of the papillae. Despite the hypoplasia of the musculature of the rumen, gnotobiotic lambs are able to consume 0.8–1.5 kg of solid feed per day over a 5-wk period compared with 1.1 kg/day for conventional lambs. The inoculation of gnotobiotic animals with rumen bacteria resulted in development of the papillae, production of volatile fatty acids, and increase in weight of the parotid salivary glands (138).

Among wild ruminants, those that live in dense vegetation select fruit and succulent leaves and hence possess a high rate of fermentation. These ruminants present *1*) a profusely papillated mucosa, which provides a huge surface area for absorption of the volatile fatty acids (156); *2*) large parotid glands relative to body weight, which can produce an abundant flow of alkaline saliva to buffer rumen acidity (126); and *3*) a reduced cellulosis with a rapid transit of food so that the digestive part of the diet escapes microbial attack in the rumen (143, 155). In contrast, ruminants that have access only to roughage diet possess an enlarged forestomach with little papillary development and slow but complete cellulolysis encouraged by a long retention time of the food (41, 86, 253).

*Functional Adaptation to Absorption*

The glandular areas of the unichambered stomach (cardiac, oxyntic or fundic, and pyloric) are situated caudally, lying between the capacious nonglandular gastric compartments and the duodenum in foregut fermenters.

Absorption of organic products of fermentative digestion (4, 8, 9, 232) takes place in the omasum and reticulorumen of the Pecora across the squamous epithelium that lines the entire forestomach. The epithelial surface of the rumen is increased by papillae up to 13-fold in the goat and 21-fold in cattle (110).

The development of papillae varies, according to seasonal and biotic influences (156), in the roe deer and fallow deer. In several East African ruminants, the major increase in rumen surface area arises from the presence of papillae in the atrium ruminis. Increases in surface area of over 3 and 4 times have been detected in Tragulina and Hippopotamidae, respectively (110). Morphological changes in ruminal epithelium occur with changes in the quality of food. An increase in density and changes in shape of papillae occur within 2 wk after better quality food becomes available at the start of the rainy season in East Africa. Substances such as ammonia and volatile fatty acids that are subject to absorption (88, 211) then stimulate papillary development and epithelial growth (73) and blood circulation (204). Similar changes, characterized by increased mitosis, have been shown to be stimulated by butyrate, propionate, and acetate (65, 200).

Among Tylopoda, four species of camelids (llama, alpaca, guanaco, and vicuna) live in an extensive Andean zone, often at 14,000–18,000 ft above sea level where the pastures consist of fibrous and woody grasses. These animals effectively utilize this poor quality roughage at altitudes where cattle and sheep cannot graze.

As in the first compartment (equivalent to the rumen) both glandular and stratified squamous epithelia are found in the second compartment (homologue of the reticulum). The continuation of the ventricular groove is lined by stratified squamous epithelium. The course of the groove is defined by a single lip. This muscular lip extends along the lesser curvature to the orifice of the tubular passage to the third compartment, considered as the homologue of the abomasum. It has been suggested that the sacculated glands elaborate mucus, whereas others believed that they produce digestive juices and they function as accessory salivary glands that buffer the volatile fatty acid produced. Electron-microscopic investigation has indicated that this mucosa may be adapted for absorption and active transport as well as mucus production. According to Vallenas et al. (235) the New World camelid stomach, via its sacculated area, is very efficient in neutralizing the volatile fatty acids produced by bacterial fermentation. As one explanation for this finding they suggest that the secretion of the glandular epithelium has a buffering capacity. Under this circumstance, saccular eversion would deliver buffer to the bulk of the ingesta in the compartmental lumen.

*Retention Time and Food Propulsion*

The suborder Ruminantia comprises 176 species ranging in weight from ~1 kg in the mouse deer (*Tragulus javanicus*) to 1,000 kg in a large bull giraffe (*Giraffa camelopardalis*). A physiological mechanism of filtering at the sphincteric-like reticulo-omasal orifice has been suggested to selectively retain within the reticulorumen the larger food particles and thus ensure prolonged exposure to fermentation. Mean values of retention time of markers and lignin are given in Table 2. Solid matter is retained in the rumen until it is reduced to a size that will enable it to pass readily through the reticulo-omasal orifice (Fig. 5) and omasum to the lower gut. Breakdown of solids is achieved by a combination of primary and secondary chewing (eating and rumination), microbial attack, and attrition during churning by rumen contractions (181). The more digestible fibrous particles break down quickly and are retained for only a few hours; the more refractory ones may be retained for days. As a result the time fibrous particles are retained in the rumen tends to be matched by the time needed for most of the potentially digestible constituents to be degraded. As it is progressively broken down, fibrous food may be regarded as cascading through a series of pools, each having definable particle size and retention time, until it is reduced to a size small enough to flow unimpeded to the abomasum (83). In sheep, most

TABLE 2. *Observation and Prediction of Mean Retention Time of Markers in Gastrointestinal Tract of a Sheep*

| | $^{51}$Cr-Labeled EDTA | | Lignin | |
|---|---|---|---|---|
| | Observed | Predicted | Observed | Predicted |
| Reticulorumen | 6.8 | 17.5 | 9.6 | 16.9 |
| Abomasum | 1.2 | | 2.8 | |
| Cecum/proximal colon | 17.5 | 7.0 | 17.1 | 10.9 |
| Transit through omasum, small intestine, and distal large intestine | 11.9 | 8.9 | 13.7 | 10.5 |
| Total mean retention time | 37.4 | 33.4 | 43.2 | 38.3 |

Values are in hours. [From Faichney (69).]

abomasal particles will pass through a 0.6-mm sieve. If a sheep is given a hay diet that has been ground to this size, it flows so rapidly through the rumen that dry matter digestibility is reduced by up to 9% and food intake increases. This mechanism of filtering has been mainly studied in the domestic ruminants, and similar anatomy would suggest that it is also present in at least some of the other bovids and probably the cervids, giraffids, and antilocaprids. The tragulids have little (*Hyemoschus*) or no (*Tragulus*) omasal tissue or any apparent constriction to the reticulum and so probably lack the mechanism. The camelids have an apparently analogous constriction between the second and third compartments of the stomach, but it is not known whether an analogous function exists (103).

However, such structure or function is not known to occur in any other foregut fermenter, with passage of digesta from the fermentative to the acidic part of the stomach being little if at all impeded. In addition the particle size of the food retained in the cattle reticulorumen for fermentation is far lower that that able to flow through the relaxed reticulo-omasal orifice, as studied with endoscopy (146). A possible explanation is that some particles remain trapped within the fibrous mass of ingesta that is retained in the center of the rumen (217).

The distinction between grazing (cattle, buffalo) and browsing (goat, roe deer) ruminants is based on more or less developed rumen size, pillars, omasum, and retention time (111). The distinctive characteristics of the browsers, i.e., selective feeders, are not only well-developed salivary glands to compensate a high fermentation rate but also a shorter retention time by absence of trapping particles of critical size.

FORESTOMACH MOTILITY

Motility of the reticulorumen is involved in the retention and mixing of the ingesta so that the con-

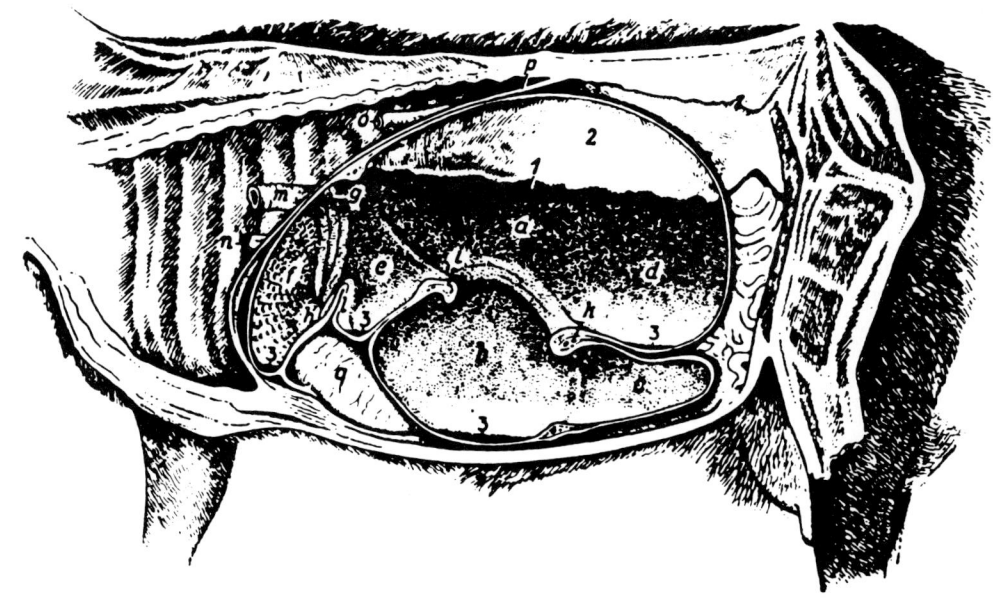

FIG. 5. Topography of thoracic and abdominal organs of a goat. Left lung has been removed and reticulum and rumen have been opened. Reticulum lies against costal part of the diaphragm. Its ventral relations are sternal part of diaphragm, caudal end of sternum, and xiphoid cartilage. Rumen is divided into dorsal and ventral sacs. *a*, Rumen dorsal sac; *b*, rumen ventral sac; *c*, ventral blind sac; *d*, dorsal blind sac; *e*, atrium; *f*, reticulum; *g*, cardia; *h*, esophageal groove; *i*, cranial pillar; *k*, caudal pillar of rumen; *l*, reticuloruminal fold; *m*, esophagus; *n*, vena cava caudalis; *o*, aorta; *p*, diaphragm; *1*, level of solid material; *2*, gas pouch; *3*, sediment (small particles). [From Grau (78).]

tents can undergo a relatively slow process of microbial digestion followed by absorption. Some of the contents must be regurgitated, reinsalivated, and reswallowed while large amounts of gas produced in the rumen (1 liter·min$^{-1}$·500 kg$^{-1}$ body wt) must be eructated. Finally, the contents must leave the reticulorumen in an orderly and controlled fashion through the omasum before they reach the abomasum. Such events are accomplished by coordinated cyclical contractions of the different chambers of the stomach occurring every 50–70 s, i.e., 1,440 times/day. These contractions (extrinsic contractions) are dependent on bursts of efferent (motor) nerve impulses traveling in the vagal nerves and are essential to the maintenance of fermentation as a vigorous and continuous process. In the absence of vagal nerves, the smooth muscle of the reticulorumen walls undergoes low-amplitude contractions (intrinsic contractions), and stagnation with accumulation of feed and gas occurs until the animal dies (112, 198). That the paralysis it not by itself the immediate cause of death is indicated by the fact that animals survive for several months if fed through an abomasal fistula (170, 171).

*Cyclical Contractions of Reticulorumen*

MEASUREMENT. The methods used for examining the extrinsic contractions of the reticulorumen are direct internal palpation through a fistula (74, 180), recording of pressure changes that accompany movements (119, 227), fluoroscopic examination after radiopaque meals (48, 259), and measurement of electrical activity of the smooth muscle wall (188). Measurement of outflow through the reticulo-omasal orifice (18, 65) is suitable for quantitative appreciation of the propulsion of contents toward the abomasum. The palpation through a fistula in the left paralumbar fossa was used by Flourens (74), who carried out the first experimental investigation of the ovine ruminant stomach some 150 years ago. This method was later used in fistulated steers to disprove the hypothesis that the reticular groove had a prehensile capacity for regurgitation and in cows to establish the sequential contraction of the reticulum, dorsal ruminal sac, and ventral ruminal sac at intervals of ~1 min. These cycles were variously termed *primary cycle movements, A sequences,* or *mixing contractions* to distinguish them from sequential contractions restricted to the dorsal and ventral ruminal sacs that occur more irregularly and are termed "secondary cycle movements," "B sequences," or "belching contractions" (204).

Pressure recordings of the ovine reticulorumen were initially obtained by insertion of inflated balloons through an esophageal fistula (113, 125, 153). Modifications of the technique were widely used later by introducing the balloon nasally for recording of reticulum movements in conscious animals, e.g., during eating (26, 75) and by fixing the balloons into the rumen through a rumen fistula (Fig. 6). More recently the technique has been refined either by the use of

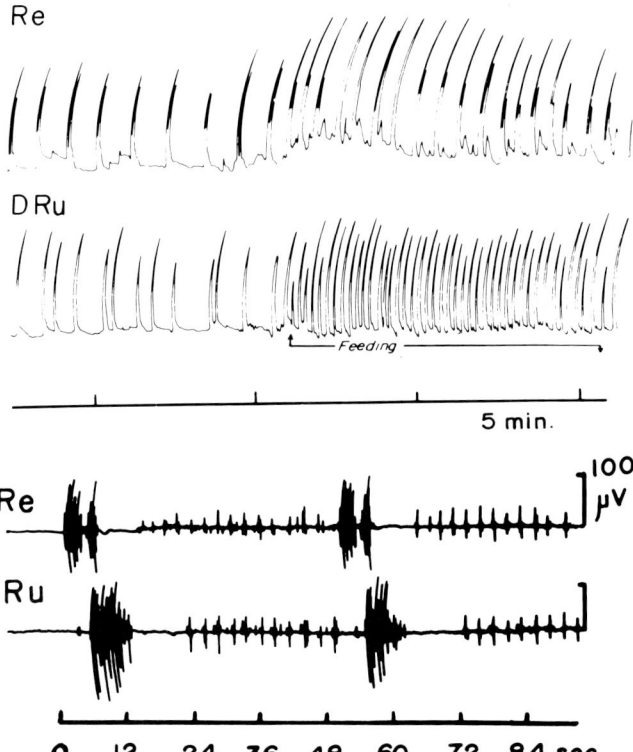

FIG. 6. Typical record showing pressure registered simultaneously in reticulum (Re) and dorsal rumen sac (DRu) in a sheep fasted 18 h and while receiving oats for 10 min. Lightly inflated balloons, inserted through a rumen fistula, are connected to tambours writing on kymograph. *Bottom*: electromyogram showing normal biphasic reticulum contractions spread backward over anterior sac of rumen with a lag of ~5 s. Regular small group discharges correspond to intrinsic motility.

electronic pressure-sensing devices (Fig. 7) or by fixing strain-gauge transducers on the forestomach wall. The reticulum and different regions of the rumen have been partially exteriorized through the original skin incision and have been used to observe, film, and record kymographically the sequences of contractions. Partial exteriorization of the reticulum requires costal resection thoracotomy (101), and that of the rumen involves a laparotomy designed to place and retain part of the wall of the dorsal or ventral sac in a subcutaneous position (128, 154).

Fluoroscopy, not conveniently applicable to large ruminants nor suitable for continuous observation, has been successfully used with small ruminants (sheep, goats, and calves) (48, 227, 259). Endoscopic observation of digesta transfer from the reticulorumen to omasum has been conducted in conscious, standing cattle in a fed state (146) to study how the reticulo-omasal orifice (10 mm) blocks the passage of small-size particles (2–4 mm) from entering the omasum.

Electromyographic recordings from pairs of insulated nichrome wires (1.2-mm diam, 120-cm long) inserted 2 mm apart into the muscle of different parts of the reticulorumen, have been used to monitor mechanical events [Fig. 6; (188)]. The insulation is burned from the wire near to the tip, and the end of the wire is inserted through the serosa and muscular layers by using a needle as a trocar. After removal of the needle, the free end is knotted at the limit of the insulation to complete a loop with the main wire and is then cut short to avoid any antenna-like action. Electrical activity is recorded after 4 days, when insulation and fixation are achieved by proliferation of the serosa after surgery, and for periods of 2–3 mo. The electrodes are directly connected to AC amplifiers with a time constant of 0.1 s corresponding to a low-frequency cutoff of 0.5 Hz. The total impedance measured between these electrodes (~10 times lower than that of classic Ag/AgCl serosal electrodes) allows a high level of the recorded signal, and the small diameter of the electrodes reduces tissue reactions and peritoneal adhesions.

Measurements of the reticulorumen outflow have been obtained directly from omasal fistulas (214) or, after transection of the omaso-abomasal junction, from the external part of a reentrant cannula fixed in each chamber at the site of transection. Reticulorumen outflow is recorded directly, and the contents are returned manually to the abomasum. This technique, which has obvious limitations for long-term studies and also disrupts the continuity of the tract, shows that the absence of contents in the aborad part of the junction enhances the propulsive activity of the orad part (172). Alternative approaches included a rigid cannula fitted with a side arm in the omasal orifice (172), a nylon sleeve attached to the omaso-abomasal orifice (64), and a reentrant omaso-abomasal preparation later used for the small intestine (99, 114). Quantitative estimates of normograde and retrograde flow of digesta in the duodenum have been measured by an electromagnetic flowmeter probe placed around the connecting tube of a reentrant duodenal cannula (206) or around the serosa (39).

Indigestible reference substances, i.e., markers, can be used for the measurement of digesta outflow past the reticulorumen and thus the evaluation of the turnover rate of liquid rumen digesta in relation with motility (11, 209). Polyethylene glycol has been considered a good marker for the liquid phase (210), i.e., nonabsorbable, not affecting or being affected by the microbial population, physically similar to the material it is to mark, and easily estimated in digesta samples. Because the digesta of the reticulorumen consist of a liquid and of a particulate phase, a single marker could not be used to measure the flow of whole digesta and its constituents. Chromium sesquioxide, though often used in the past, has been shown to be unsatisfactory for this purpose (68). The simultaneous use of two markers, $^{51}$Cr-labeled ethylenediamine-tetraacetate to mark the liquid phase and lignin to mark the particulate phase (Table 2), when administered

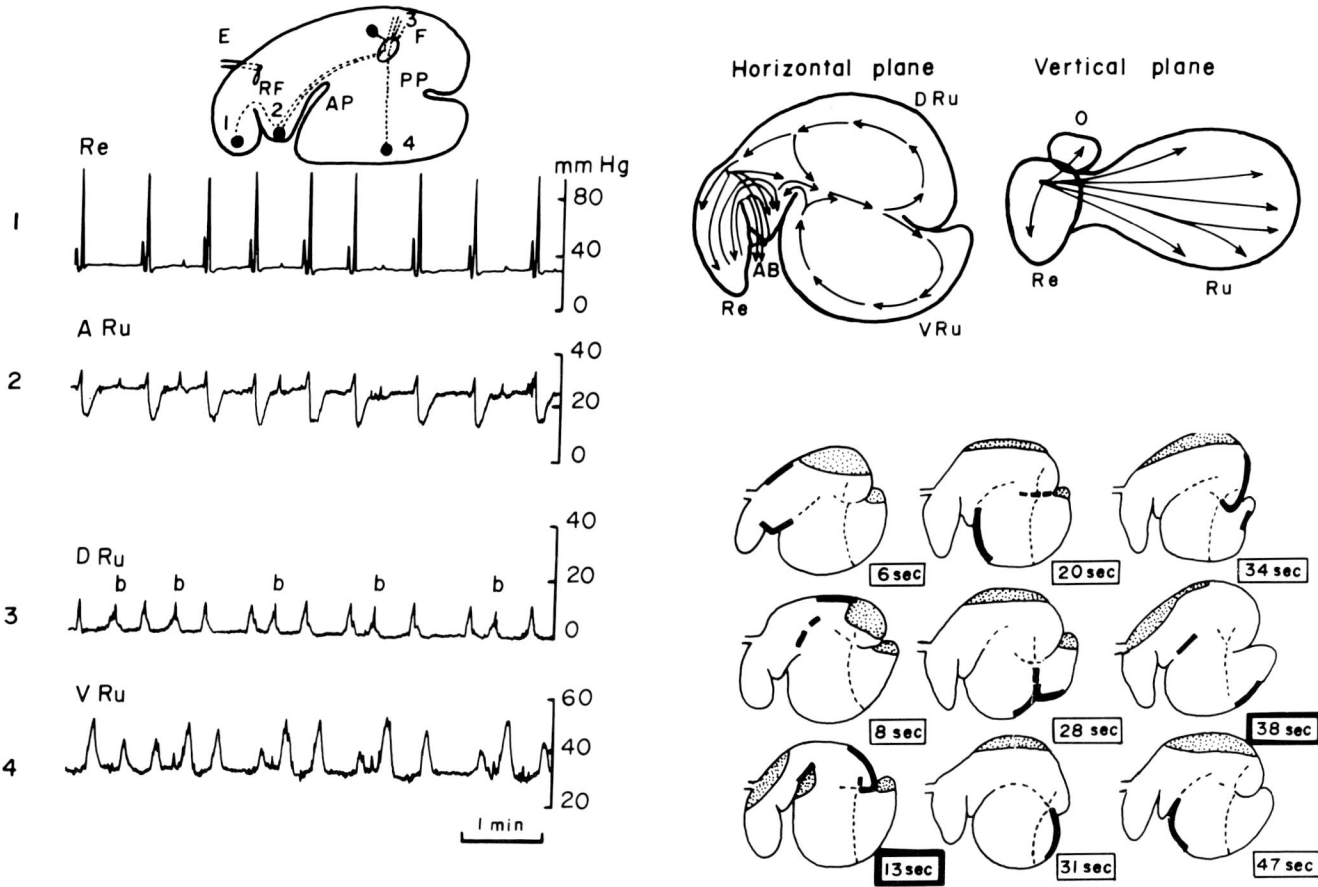

FIG. 7. *Left*, diagram of bovine reticulorumen showing 4 recording points and typical pressure patterns. *1*, Reticulum; *2*, anterior rumen sac; *3*, dorsal rumen; *4*, ventral rumen sac. AP, anterior pillar; F, fistula; E, esophagus; PP, posterior pillar; RF, reticuloruminal fold. Note belching contractions (*b*) of rumen and hydrostatic pressure changes in anterior rumen sac. [From Reid and Cornwall (181).] *Right*, drawing summarizing movement of digesta in ovine reticulorumen as seen radiographically in horizontal and vertical planes. *Arrows* indicate direction of movement [From Waghorn and Reid (247)] and main contraction sequences as indicated by radiography. Time in seconds indicates interval after reticular movement, and contracting region of reticulorumen wall is indicated by a *heavy line*. Gas bubble (*stippled*), is brought over cardiac orifice at 13 s and during eructation sequence at 38 s. [From Wyburn (259).]

continuously, is more accurate to measure digesta flow.

The measurement of mean retention time in the reticulorumen involves the sampling of all or part of the digesta present in or leaving the rumen. As the integral of a time function, it can be calculated (as can the fractional outflow rate, which is the reciprocal of mean retention time) from the curve of concentration versus time if a steady state exists during the measurement. The equation for such a curve takes the form $C(t) = C(0)\exp(-kt)$, where C is the concentration of marker, $t$ is the time after dosing, and k is the fraction of the marker pool that flows out per unit of time (67, 69, 70).

MECHANICAL ACTIVITY. A direct inspection of the forestomach through an open fistula (8 × 12 cm) in cattle shows that a biphasic contraction of the reticulum occurs to propel the digesta distally over the reticuloruminal fold into the dorsal sac of the rumen. During this time the reticuloruminal fold actually drops to facilitate the distal movement of digesta out of the reticulum. The reticular groove then stretches open, in conjunction with the opening of the reticulo-omasal orifice, and the finer digesta are propelled forward by a wave of contraction of the ventral and cranial sacs of the rumen and are spiraled into the open funnel-like reticular groove and reticulo-omasal orifice. Immediately on completion of this sequence, the reticular groove folds and remains closed until the next contraction sequence begins (181). The corresponding pressure changes obtained from transducers placed at different locations in the reticulorumen reflect contractions and relaxations of these compartments. However, in the records from the reticulum and anterior sac of the rumen, decrements of pressure, which might otherwise be attributed to relaxations, are associated with hydrostatic changes due to passive movements of the floors of these compartments (Fig. 7).

The primary cycle movement recognized in the bovine reticulorumen (i.e., the mixing contraction or sequence A) is initiated by a sharp contraction of both the reticulum and the reticuloruminal fold, is primarily concerned with the circulation of the contents within the organ as a whole, and takes 25–30 s to complete. The secondary cycle (i.e., the belching contraction, the extraruminal contraction (181), or sequence B) appears to start posteriorly and is associated with the transfer of gas bubbles cranially to the cardia. It is composed of two main groups of contractions that cause an increase in pressure of the posterior dorsal and then the ventral blind sacs followed by a ruminal contraction identical to that of sequence A. During the primary cycle movement, a second phase of contraction of the reticulum starts within 3 s after the first phase, before its full relaxation, peaks at a pressure of 80 mmHg, and is followed by the contraction for 15 s of the dorsal rumen sac. A simultaneous contraction of the anterior, posterior, and ventral rumen sacs then occurs during which the anterior pillar contracts downward to form a low ridge between the anterior and ventral sacs of the rumen until the following cycle (247). This pattern results in a series of ingesta fluxes constituting, as seen radiographically in sheep (259), a cycle of digesta outflow from the reticulum to the anterior ruminal sac and the dorsal ruminal sac, from the anterior ruminal sac back into the reticulum, and finally from the dorsal sac to the ventral sac and from the posterior ventral region forward over the anterior pillar (Fig. 7).

Partial exteriorization of the reticulorumen can be obtained in the anesthetized sheep by a simple cut in the skin over the region of the stomach to be exteriorized, followed by splitting the several muscle and tissue layers of the body wall to create an opening through which the rumen is brought up through the opening in the body wall and stitched to the edges to form adhesions with the skin during healing. When the stomach contracts, it pulls the skin with it, and the lateral regions of the rumen tend to herniate when relaxed. The reticulorumen motility is especially well defined with local or smooth muscle tone changes and sequential contractions and exhibits variation in almost every dimension, i.e., absolute frequency of sequences, relative frequency of sequences A and B, degree of tonic activity, magnitude and duration of the contractions of individual regions, and time of onset of the contractions of the different regions of the rumen relative to the start of a sequence.

Basically two extreme states of motility may be recognized. That present in the animal fasted until the contents of the stomach are freely liquid displays a low frequency of contractions, a low proportion of sequence B, and a simultaneous response of the whole rumen. That present in a feeding sheep is characterized by a high frequency of coordinated sequences, as many as 3/min, a high ratio of sequence B to sequence A, a high level of tonic activity, and strong rumen contractions, with those of the ventral regions being vigorous, prolonged, and polyphasic (180).

ELECTRICAL ACTIVITY. Each contraction of the reticulorumen is associated in sheep with a large group discharge of spike potentials (188), showing a primary reticulorumen cycle rhythm of 0.80 ± 0.07/min in the sheep at rest (Fig. 8). At times, low-amplitude, regular, small-group discharges are registered at a frequency of 20–30/min on the reticulum and ~15/min on the rumen. This pattern of activity may be preceded by

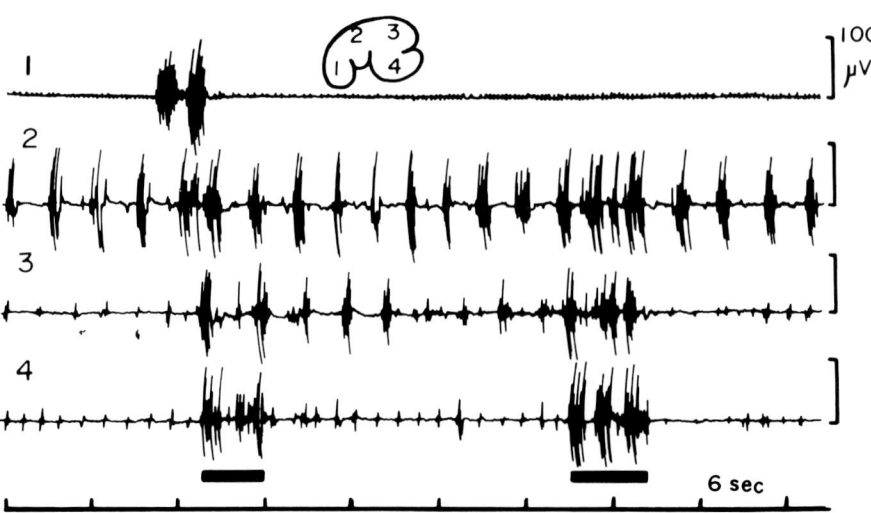

FIG. 8. Intrinsic electrical activity of ovine rumen during impaction. Slow-wave–like activity at frequency of 18–20/min is superimposed with clustered burst spike potentials (*bars*) at time of contractions.

slow waves and corresponds to local intrinsic electrical activity, the only activity present in the chronically vagotomized reticulorumen (79, 198).

The mixing cycle (reticulorumen contractions) occurs as group discharge propagating along the anterior and posterior portions of the dorsal sac of the rumen and spreading along the ventral sac to reach the posterior ventral sac in 24 s. In the belching cycle (rumen contractions), no more than 8 s is required to bring the gas bubble over the cardiac orifice. The electrical activity of the reticulorumen wall not associated with extrinsic contractions consists of irregular bursts of activity in the reticulum and slow waves with superimposed regular small-group discharges in the rumen. Two situations (rumen impaction and reticulorumen distension by gas or bloat) considerably enhance this intrinsic activity.

Transient ruminal stasis is a common pathophysiological state observed after overingestion of grain in sheep (ruminal acidosis) (50). The abolition of motility that occurs at the earliest stage may be regarded as a self-curing maneuver because this situation will lead to some reduction in fermentation rate. The large group discharge of spike potentials disappears at the expense of the intrinsic activity that consists of slow waves (18–20/min) with superimposed spike potentials. Note that at the time of the extrinsic contractions, the frequency of these spike potentials increases (Fig. 8), suggesting a balance between the central and local regulatory mechanisms of reticulorumen activity.

The distension of the reticulorumen by insufflation of air above 10 mmHg in the ruminal dorsal sac induces a continuous discharge of intrinsic electrical activity in the reticulum and increases the duration and sometimes also the frequency of the small group discharges in the ruminal dorsal sac. The increased response is maintained over a prolonged distension, whereas the rumen exhibits rapidly propagated contractions (Fig. 9). Such isolated, coordinated ruminal contractions suggest that the regulation of the primary cycle movement by the vagus nerves as a vagovagal reflex (see EXTRINSIC CONTRACTIONS, p. 1247) is more strict than the regulation of the secondary cycle movement, which can be elicited after partial vagotomy (112).

Comparative studies of reticulorumen motility patterns in small and large ruminants indicate that the contractions of the posterior dorsal (Dp) caudal sac of the rumen can occur independently of those of the dorsal sac (D) (60, 61) and that the contractions of

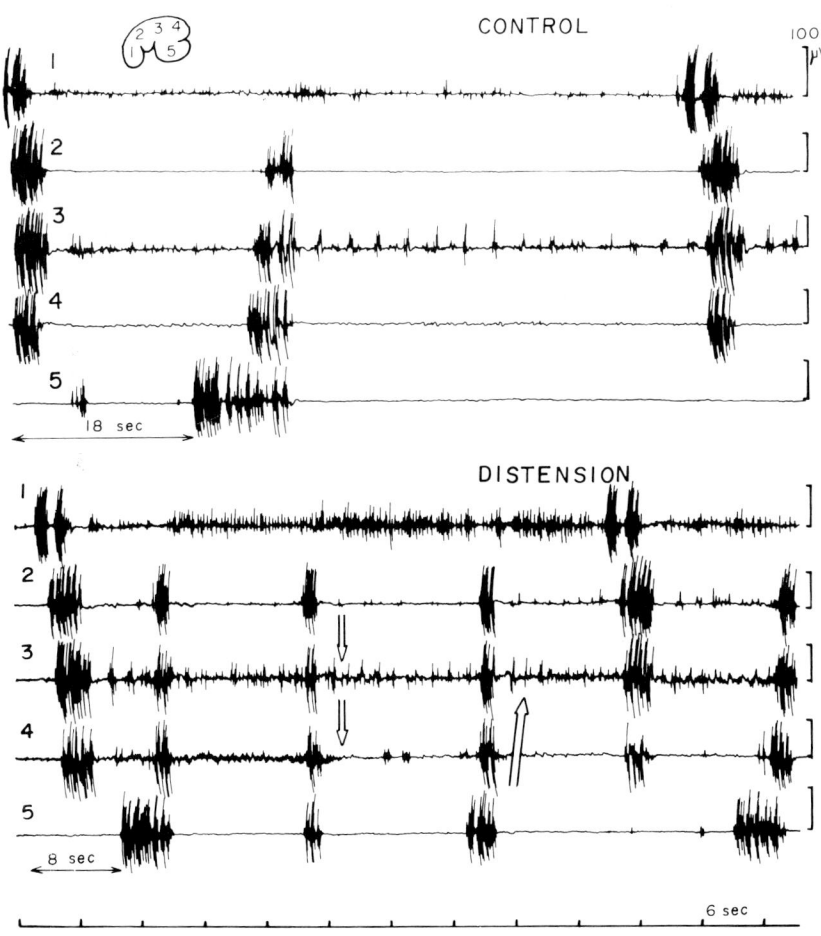

FIG. 9. Stimulation by distension of local intrinsic activity and ruminal contractions. *Top*: normal biphasic reticular contraction (*1*) spreading over the rumen (*2, 3, 4*), and followed within 18 s by a backward contraction of the rumen starting on the posterior ventral sac (*5*). Local intrinsic activity as group discharges at 3-s intervals on the dorsal sac of the rumen (*3*). *Bottom*: distension by air at mean pressure of 10 mmHg is accompanied by a backward contraction of rumen starting within 6 s on the posterior ventral sac (*5*) and followed by to-and-fro contractions of rumen (*arrows*). Intrinsic activity is increased at both reticular (*1*) and ruminal levels (*3*).

TABLE 3. *Reticulorumen Motility Patterns Associated With Ruminating Behavior*

| Diet: Chaffed Lucerne | Cattle | Sheep | Observations |
|---|---|---|---|
| Intake, % body wt | 1.13 | 2.12 | 2.12 in sheep receiving pelleted lucerne |
| Time spent eating/ruminating, min/day | 231/350 | 207/516 | 87/254 in sheep receiving pelleted lucerne |
| Ruminal contractions during eating versus ruminating, cycles/min | 2.3/1.5 | 2.6/1.6 | 3.5/1.6 in sheep receiving pelleted lucerne |

[From Waghorn and Reid (247).]

TABLE 4. *Reticulorumen Patterns Associated With Loss of Vigilance Comprising Drowsiness, Slow-Wave Sleep, and Deep Sleep*

| Diet: Hay | Nonlactating Cow | Sheep | Goat |
|---|---|---|---|
| Increase in cycle duration during slow-wave sleep/deep sleep versus drowsiness, s | 7/42 | 44/55 | 19/31 |
| Increase in cycle duration during rumination and slow-wave sleep, s | 32 | 37 | 26 |
| Percentage of secondary cycles during slow-wave sleep and drowsiness | 51/7 | 49/21 | 46/6 |

the posterior ventral sac (Vp), which can be split into two or three responses at different levels of magnitude ($Vp_1$-$Vp_2$; $Vp_1$-$Vp_{2a}$-$Vp_{2b}$), occur in addition to or in place of the ventral sac (V). Finally, in the fed state, the majority of cycles correspond to the following six sequences in domestic ruminants: RD or RDV; RD, DV or RDV, DV; RDVp, DV or RDV-Vp, DV, where R represents reticulum and D and V main dorsal or ventral sac of rumen (Fig. 14). Less frequent combinations (3%–5%) include the contraction of Vp instead of the ventral sac (198). Beyond these variations, it is of interest to mention that the cyclical contractions of the reticulorumen at very short intervals (~12 s) in the alpaca and guanaco occur in groups of about six separated by periods of quiescence (102, 236), suggesting a different central nervous control of motility (235).

*Events Associated With Rumination*

Cattle on a diet of lucerne chaff spend ~350 min/day in rumination, involving regurgitation of ingesta (corresponding to 1.13% of body wt) (51, 158) to the mouth for further mastication. The intake in sheep is even greater (2.12% of body wt), and the time spent ruminating reaches 516 min/day (52, 53, 247). Rumination occurs also as a behavioral state depending on the coarseness of digesta and can be associated with drowsiness or even light sleep (Tables 3 and 4). Regurgitation of liquid material occurs as an event superimposed on the sequential contractions of the reticulorumen, or more precisely at the beginning of a reticulorumen cycle. A preliminary contraction of the reticulum, termed extracontraction, happens just before the regular reticular contractions and floods the cardia with ingesta that are carried orally by esophageal antiperistalsis at a higher velocity of propagation than that which occurs during swallowing (Fig. 10).

MECHANISM OF REGURGITATION. In regurgitation, which principally involves floating coarse material (grass or hay), the driving force is an inspiratory effort against a closed glottis, hence the aspiration of ingesta from the reticulorumen through the open cardia. The first event occurring at this time is a long-lasting extracontraction of the reticulum, immediately followed by the normal biphasic reticular contraction. The triphasic reticulum contraction (213) is in association with both the inspiratory effort at the origin of the negative pressure produced in the thoracic esophagus (which causes the transfer of stomach contents into the esophagus) and the antiperistaltic esophageal contraction (which carries the regurgitated material to the mouth). The aspiration resulting from the short-lasting negative pressure in the thoracic

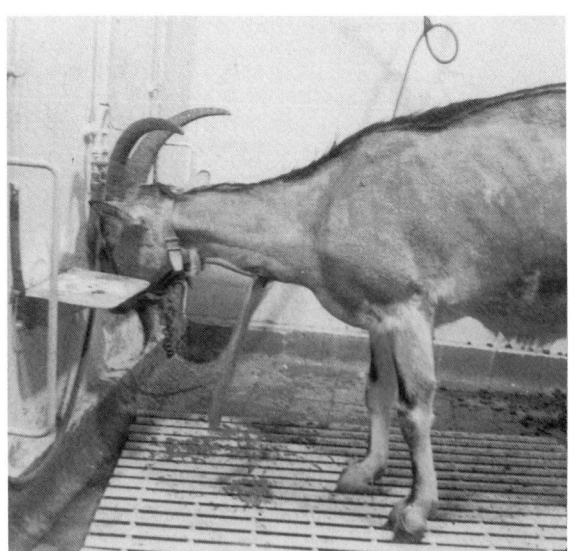

FIG. 10. Goat fitted with esophageal cannula. Illustration of force at which digesta are propelled by antiperistalsis from rumen during rumination. Cannula was open within 1 s after visible inspiratory effort that signals a regurgitation. Average volume (~200 ml) was ejected in toto through cannula within 2 s.

esophagus occurs at the end of the extrareticular contraction that floods the cardia with liquid ingesta, thus moving the coarse contents from the rumen into the thoracic esophagus.

Electromyographic (228) and fluoroscopic studies show that influx of digesta into the esophagus occurs when the lower esophageal sphincter, already relaxed after swallowing the previously masticated bolus (Fig. 11), becomes actively opened (95). Then an antiperistaltic wave passes over the esophagus at more than twice the rate of those recorded during deglutition (24,

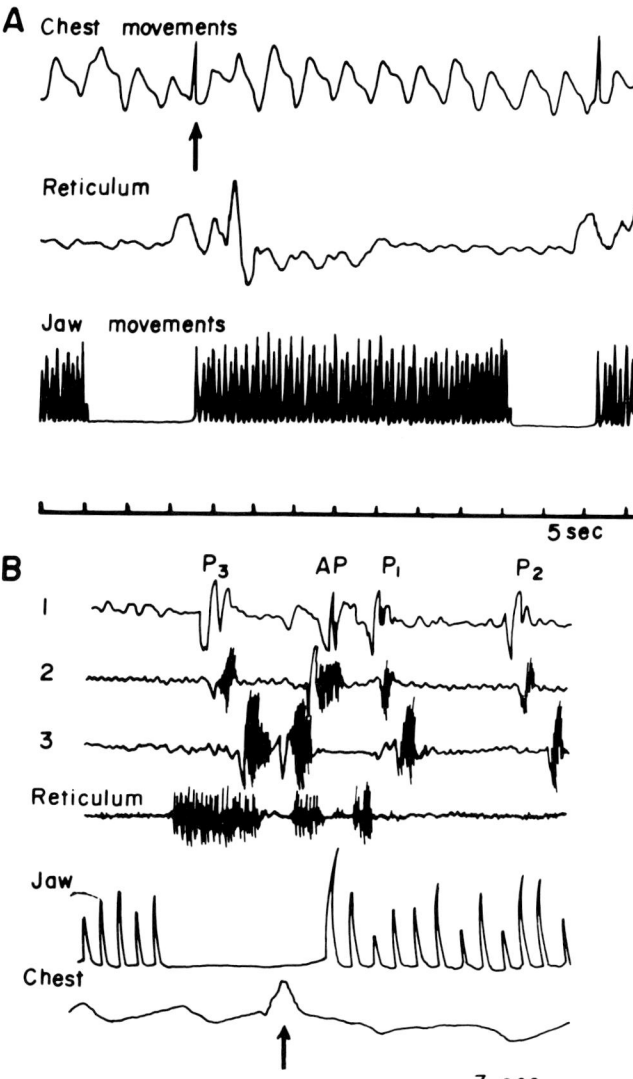

FIG. 11. Events on esophagus, reticulum, jaw, and chest associated with regurgitation. A: inspiratory effort occurs (arrows) toward end of extracontraction of reticulum and is followed in less than 1 s by chewing. B: esophageal electromyograms are recorded from electrodes placed at equal distance on esophagus, near glottis (1), at the entry of chest (2) and close to cardia (3) and reticulum. Regurgitation of digesta (AP) is followed by swallowing first the excess liquid on 2 occasions ($P_1$ and $P_2$) and then the bolus ($P_3$).

257). Because the negative intrathoracic esophageal pressure can reach 40 mmHg at the time of regurgitation and the reticular contraction is accompanied by only a 5–6 mmHg rise of pressure at the base of the reticulum, aspiration may be considered as the primary force moving digesta into the esophagus (212). The act of regurgitation thus comprises a series of events occurring reflexly and in an orderly fashion (103). Attempts to prevent the regurgitated bolus from passing toward the mouth (e.g., by pressing the neck with the hand to occlude the cervical esophagus or by derivation of the bolus) stop the occurrence of the masticatory movements. This suggests that if the sequence is interrupted at any point, the "program" is not terminated. However, it remains unclear whether this is a centrally controlled phenomenon rather than the result of removing the reflex stimuli. For example, esophageal wall distension performed on standing conscious sheep by inflating a rubber balloon at different levels inside the cervical and thoracic esophagus is always followed by a conspicuous increase of parotid saliva secretion (126) and frequently induces the onset of chewing movements, whatever the level of the esophageal distension. This response persists after atropine but is suppressed by midcervical anesthetic blockade of vagal conduction, suggesting that the masticatory response to esophageal distension is a reflex mechanism whose afferent pathway from the distal part lies in the vagal trunk. Such a reflex may participate early in the initiation of chewing movements during rumination prior to the arrival of the regurgitated bolus into the mouth (16). It is also unlikely that the first stage of rumination is a controlled variation of emesis seen in other species. In animals with simple stomachs, vomiting is accompanied by contraction of the duodenum and pyloric sphincter, relaxation of the whole stomach, and the action of the "abdominal press" (see the chapter by Lang and Sarna in this Handbook). None of these occurs during rumination. On the other hand the sheep can eject or vomit abomasal contents into its reticulorumen under conditions that stimulate emesis in other species, e.g., abomasal torsion, duodenal obstruction, or apomorphine (63). Ruminants also eject digesta from the mouth, i.e., in cases of reticulitis, functional stenosis of the reticulo-omasal orifice or of the pylorus, and after the injection of alkaloid extracts from *Veratrum viride*. In these instances the ejection of contents is associated with a drop in intratracheal pressure and marked rise in intraruminal pressure (up to 90 mmHg in the sheep and 200 mmHg in the cow), suggesting a concomitant role of the abdominal press not seen in rumination.

NERVOUS CONTROL OF RUMINATION. The synchronous interplay of an extracontraction of the reticulum with an inspiratory effort and the opening or relaxation of the lower esophageal sphincter suggests coordination at a central level by a "ruminating center." This center, which is located in the brain stem and associated with the rostral hypothalamic area (3), is distinct from the "gastric centers" responsible for producing the extrinsic reticulorumen movements.

The inherent drive for rumination occurs as early as 5 days after birth in camels and is present in preruminant lambs or calves maintained on a milk diet as "pseudorumination." The term is used to designate a ruminating-like activity with irregular regurgitation of little solid material and only 3–10 masticatory movements, after which the material is swallowed. Pseudorumination can reach high levels as an alternative to rumination in adult sheep by feeding them long versus chopped silage (46) or in calves after complete isolation of the rumen from the reticulum. The liquid contents of the reticulum limit the possibilities of rumination, and the amount of time spent in pseudorumination can be doubled by mechanical stimulation of the rumen wall by using inert (plastic) particles (170).

Because the time spent ruminating is related to the coarseness of food (see Tables 3 and 4), it is probable that pseudorumination is the expression of the inability to ruminate. Such cases are the lack of contents (e.g., when the rumen is separated from the reticulum) or the absence of tactile stimuli in the region of the cardia (e.g., long silage that remains as a fibrous mass in the center of the rumen).

The afferent arms of the reflex(es) involved in the extrareticular contraction, inspiratory effort, dilation of the cardia, antiperistaltic contraction of the esophagus, and intense salivation during chewing (27) are not well defined. However, regurgitation and thus the sequence of events can be initiated by mechanical stimulation (friction) of three specific sensitive areas, the cardia, the reticuloruminal fold, and the reticuloomasal orifice (118). Rumination (as a type of behavior) can be evoked or enhanced in several ways. In sheep fitted with a reentrant cannula in the duodenum, the resulting physical stimulation or slight distension of the abomasum due to the resistance to digesta flow may be the cause of the excess rumination recorded, pari passu, during 3 wk, (i.e., 369–496 min/day instead of 278–343 min/day) (178).

Factors that induce satiety, such as gastrinlike peptides (85), when administered centrally or peripherally, may also enhance the occurrence of rumination. The COOH-terminal octapeptide of cholecystokinin (CCK-8), which has been identified in sheep brain as a satiety factor, is effective in reducing feeding that is replaced by rumination. The fact that effects of CCK-like peptides are antagonized by enkephalins is theoretically consistent with the successive involvement of a neuropeptidergic and an enkephalinergic (192) pathway in the transfer at fixed times of feeding with rumination.

The role of higher nervous influences in the control of rumination has been observed indirectly. At weaning, when the rumen enlarges for the digestion of cellulose, there is a marked increase in drowsiness or somnolence at the expense of sleep time. Such a change in the transition to the ruminant state may imply some causal relationships between the process of rumination and sleep other than a facilitation of slow-wave sleep by the monotony of chewing the cud (189). Orbitofrontal lobectomy has been shown to increase the duration of rumination; conversely animals appear to become drowsy when they ruminate, with an increased response to painful electrical stimuli (42). Finally, conditioning the sequence of reflexes, which involves extracontraction, inspiratory effort, and antiperistalsis, has been obtained by association of an intermittent light stimulation as the conditioned stimulus, with the gentle brushing (2.5 min) of the cardia as the unconditioned stimulus. When six daily

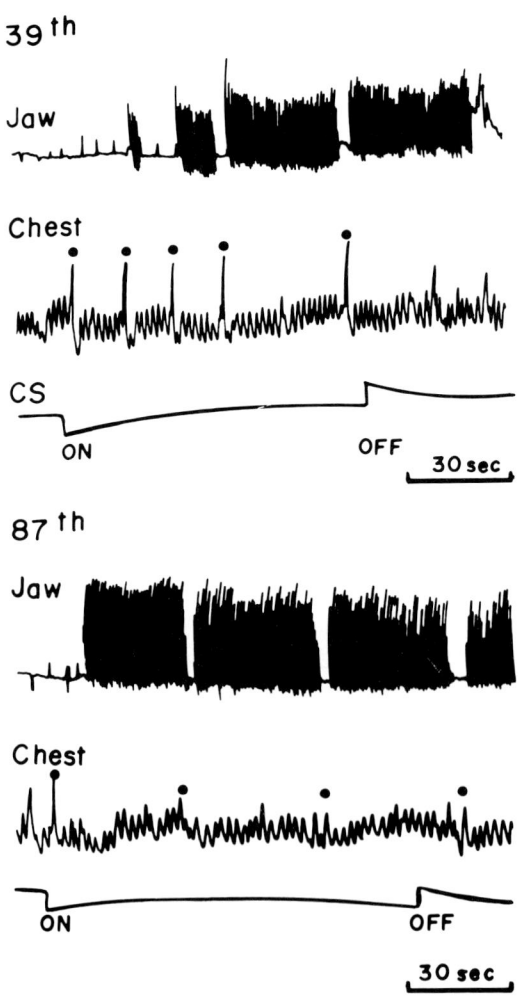

FIG. 12. Conditioned regurgitation in a goat. *Top*: inspiratory efforts followed by regurgitation occurred 15 s after emission of conditioned stimulus (CS) after 39 associations. *Bottom*: latency becomes very short and regurgitation was seen immediately after 87 associations. [From Ruckebusch (187).]

combinations of flashes at 8/s were applied before and during the cardia orifice stimulation, a progressive stabilization of the conditioned reflex occurred after 40 and 80 associations (Fig. 12). A negative conditioned reflex able to stop the masticatory movements can be obtained by the association of the end of the unconditioned stimulus with disturbances such as pinching the tail or an ear and the word "stop." The verbal order alone induces an immediate arrest of the chewing movements followed by the deglutition of the bolus (187).

HORMONAL INFLUENCES. Evidence for a hormonal control of rumination can be obtained by measuring the time elapsed between a morning meal and the first period of rumination that occurs in sheep within 1.2–2 h. Triggering factors can be assessed by the measurement of extrareticular contractions induced in conscious sheep at rest or even during feeding.

More than 25 years ago it was found that rumination evoked by stroking the interior wall of the reticulum can be mimicked in sheep by an injection (bolus) of epinephrine at doses of 0.5–2 µg/kg (122). A transient relaxation of the reticulorumen and a marked salivary secretion (215) appear to facilitate the occurrence of regurgitation and mastication. In sheep the intravenous and intracerebroventricular administration of naloxone at doses of 0.1 mg/kg and 10 µg/kg, respectively, reduces the latency of regurgitation caused by the injection of epinephrine and other biogenic amines such as dopamine (Fig. 13). Because the regurgitation due to epinephrine and dopamine can be obtained regularly after naloxone pretreatment in sheep receiving only concentrates or when eating, the involvement of an inhibitory opioid system in the central control of rumination, more precisely in the occurrence of the extra contractions required for regurgitation, is likely (192). Such a central opioidergic control of rumination may be at the origin of the lack of rumination observed in stressed animals subsequent to the release of endogenous opioid peptides. Rumination induced by milking in dairy cows could be a consequence of the reduced release of endorphins during the milk letdown (3).

It has been suggested that insulin hypoglycemia may act as a triggering factor for the ruminating center, although the ruminant differs from other mammals in that little glucose is absorbed from the digestive tract and plasma glucose concentration is only about one-half that of nonruminants. In addition the ruminant central nervous system is unusually resistant to the deleterious effects of severe hypoglycemia caused by insulin (0.5–2 IU/kg). Only the initiation of chewing movements after the injection of insulin has been ascertained (19), and neither the deficit of metabolizable glucose in the central nervous system obtained by the administration of 2-deoxy-D-glucose nor the hyperglycemia with hypoinsulinemia induced by ad-

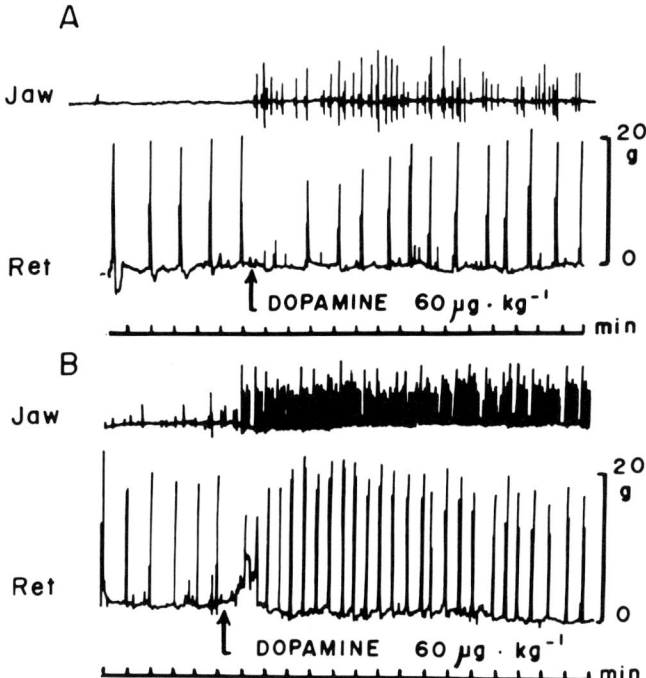

FIG. 13. Effects of intravenous administration (bolus) of dopamine before (A) and within 5 min after (B) injection of naloxone on reticular (Ret) contractions in sheep. Lower jaw movements are recorded by balloon fixed on halter. Injection of dopamine induces transient inhibition of reticular contractions but increases salivary flow, resulting in frequent swallowing movements. Dopamine at same dosage after naloxone pretreatment was able to induce rumination.

renergic-receptor agonists such as clonidine, xylazine, or CCK-8 has major effects on the time spent ruminating (85).

*Events Associated With Eructation*

Coordinated gastric and esophageal reactions lead to the frequent eructation of the gases (mainly carbon dioxide and methane) produced as by-products of fermentive digestion. Eructation in ruminants most commonly occurs after a contraction of the rumen that spreads in a cranial direction over its dorsal sac (252). Such contractions can be stimulated reflexly in decerebrate preparations by insufflation of gas into the rumen (182) and have been identified by displacing gas cranially towards the cardia from a caudal and dorsal position in the rumen. After each of these contractions, there is passage of gas into and along the esophagus; some may escape directly into the atmosphere, but most passes into the respiratory tract (48). Passage of gas into the esophagus is followed by passive distension of the caudal thoracic esophagus for periods of 0.5–2.8 s, at the end of which there is electromyographic evidence of esophageal contraction. Movements of the diaphragm observed radiographically during ventilation cease at the end of expiration or become more shallow during the period of esophageal distension. This results in a varying degree of interruption of the rhythm of ventilation; the first inspiration marks a return of ventilation to its former character, being deeper than normal (103).

Analogous with the extracontraction of the reticulum associated with regurgitation, the contraction of the rumen involved in eructation has also been termed extracontraction (252). The measurement of eructated gas by means of a tracheal cannula (28) has proved to be more accurate than that obtained with a face mask. Because nearly all the eructated gas is found in the cranial part of the transected trachea (48), the values agree closely with those obtained by aspirating the gas directly from the rumen (45). The mean volume of a single eructation in the sheep varies from 140 to 180 ml. The usual values found in cattle are 15–20 liters/h, corresponding to 15–20 eructations (Fig. 14).

Eructation occurs in association with several different forms of esophageal activity (257). Pressure increases that occur in the esophagus are referred to as the filling phase, an eructation contraction, and clearing contractions. The filling phase refers to an initial, long-lasting (>1 s in some eructations), relatively low pressure increase (~15 mmHg). The eructation contraction occurs commonly at the end of, but never independently of, the filling phase and leads to a relatively short (0.2–0.3 s), markedly varying pressure increase (up to 68 mmHg). Clearing contractions apply to caudally progressing esophageal contractions that occur independently of buccopharyngeal movements of swallowing after eructations (24).

Eructation is closely associated with a secondary cycle movement in cattle (Fig. 15), whereas in sheep it can occur at any point in the cyclical reticuloruminal movements, e.g., after a primary cycle. When eructation is associated with a rumen contraction (secondary cycle), the fall in pressure in the esophagus coincides with the peak of the contraction, and the antiperistaltic wave occurs as it is ending. In addition the time of eructation coincides with the end of the more or less prolonged contraction of the rumen posterior ventral sac.

Antiperistaltic contractions similar in amplitude and rate of progression to those occurring during eructation can usually be initiated by a rapid injection of 40–70 ml of gas (air, $CO_2$, or $N_2$) into the esophagus. This is effective whether the gas is injected into the posterior thoracic esophagus or the anterior cervical esophagus. The antiperistalsis always starts at the cardia regardless of where the injections are made. The time spent in injecting the gas is less than 1 s and antiperistalsis usually follows in less than 1 s after the injection (257). By examination of the neck during the injection of gas into the anterior cervical esophagus, the gas is seen to move down through the cervical esophagus before its expulsion by an antiperistaltic contraction (24, 184).

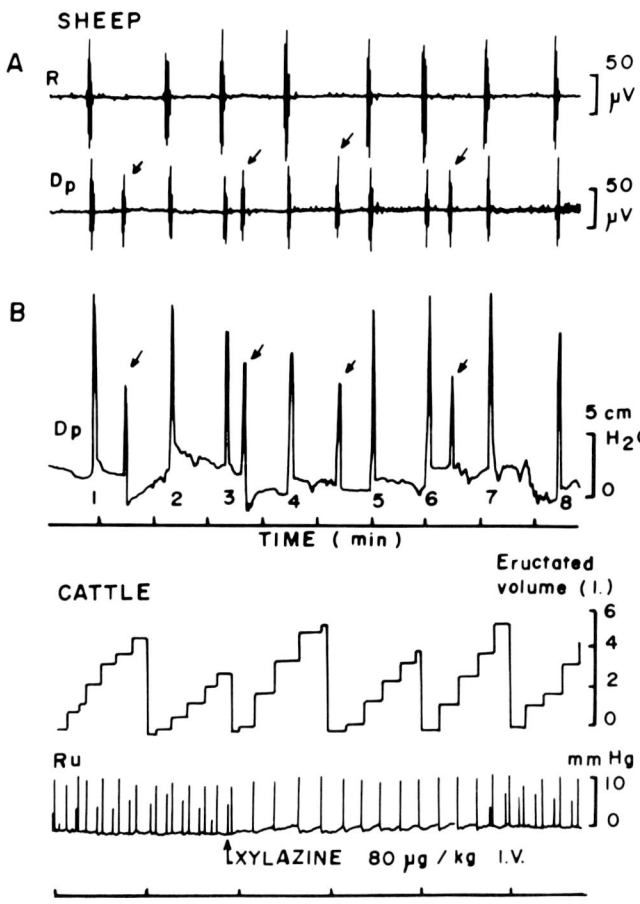

FIG. 14. In sheep, electromyogram (A) of reticulum (R) and posterior dorsal sac (Dp) of rumen in conjunction with recording (B) of intraruminal pressure. 1–8, Primary cycle movements. Secondary contraction of rumen (↗) may occur immediately after a primary contraction (3) or much later (4) [From Ruckebusch and Tomov (198).] In cattle, measurement of volume of eructated gas passing into trachea cannula, inserted into trachea near larynx and connected to a spirometer. Transient blockade of primary reticulorumen cycles is obtained by an $\alpha_2$-adrenergic receptor agonist xylazine. Each secondary contraction of rumen (Ru) is accompanied by elimination of 200–500 ml of gas.

Insufflation of the rumen with gas has increased the incidence of secondary rumen contractions in conscious (196) and in decerebrate sheep (182). The occurrence of reticulum contractions has an inhibitory effect on secondary rumen contractions, especially those of the ventral sac and the ventral blind sac that usually end a secondary cycle, allowing the new primary rumen cycle to occur in its normal and usual sequence. According to Louvier et al. (137), an increase in resting intraruminal pressure below 10 mmHg resulted in a linear increase in primary contraction (sequence A) frequency. Resting intraruminal pressures exceeding 10 mmHg had a suppressing effect on primary contraction frequency. This suppression of contraction frequency was greater when the insuf-

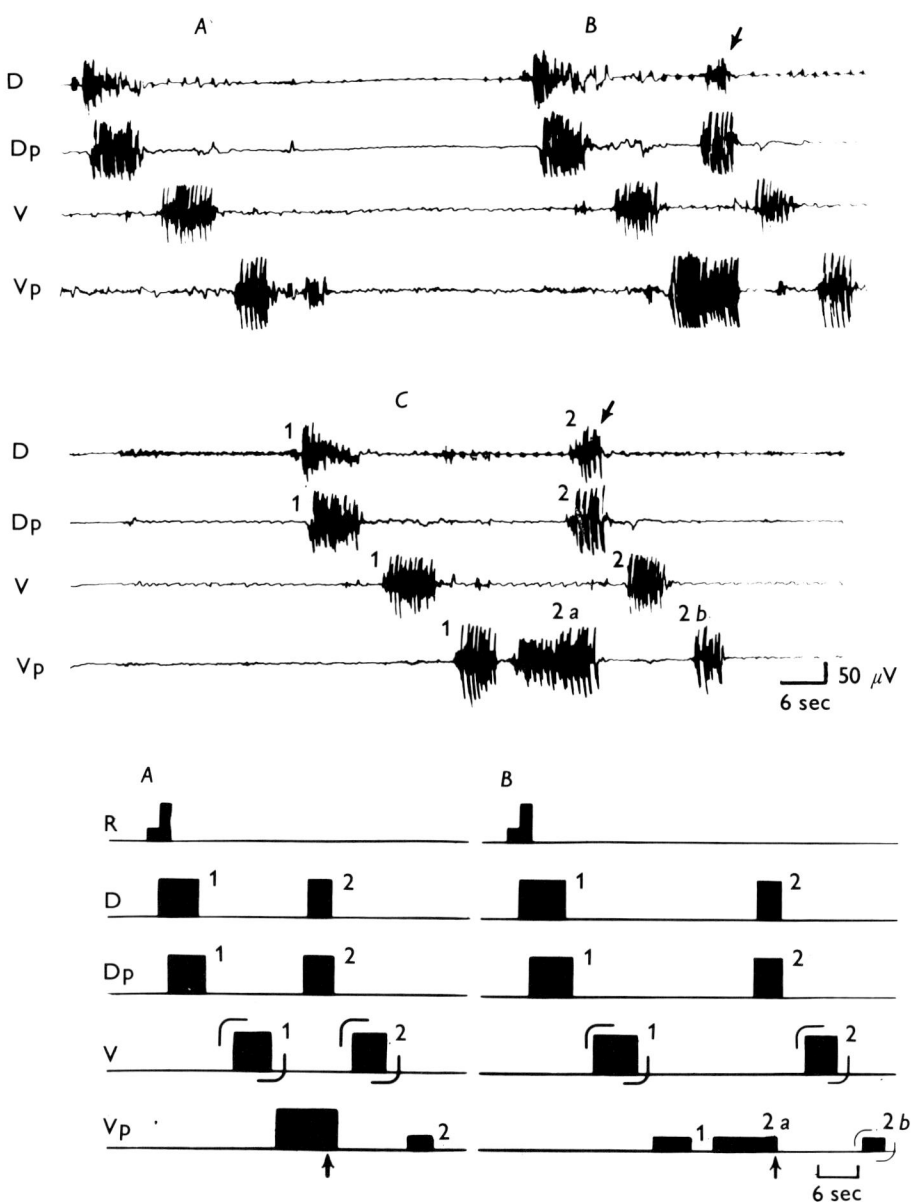

FIG. 15. *Top*, electromyographic responses of ruminal wall for primary cycle of movement (*A*) and for primary cycle followed by secondary cycle of movement (*B* and *C*). *Bottom*, diagrammatic representation of strength of each contraction and orderly sequence of 2 primary cycles followed more or less rapidly by secondary cycle. *Top*, *A*, single cycle involves dorsal (D) and posterior dorsal sac (Dp) of rumen followed by ventral (V) and posterior ventral sac (Vp). *B*, double cycle with short time interval between primary and secondary eructative (✓) ruminal contractions. *C*, time interval between primary (*1*) and secondary (*2*) contractions of rumen is longer because of an additional contraction of posterior ventral sac ($V_{p_2}$ split into $V_{p_{2a}}$ and $V_{p_{2b}}$). *Bottom*: eructation (↑) occurs ~28 s after reticular (R) contraction in *A* but much later (42 s) in *B* because of sustained weak contraction of Vp. Some contractions of ventral sac of rumen are missing and indicated by ⌒. [From Ruckebusch and Tomov (198).]

flating gas contained no $CO_2$. Secondary contraction (sequence B) frequency is found to increase linearly with all gases and pressure levels tested. However, the presence of $CO_2$ in the insufflating gas mixture resulted in a lower frequency of secondary contractions (137).

The effect of a 42-h fast on the composition of eructated rumen gases (ml/100 ml) consisted of a reduction in the $CO_2$ content from 51.3 ± 3.4 to 9.9 ± 5.1 ml/100 ml and of the ratio of $CO_2/CH_4$ from 1.7 (pH 6.5) to 0.34 (pH 7.5). The $CH_4$ content, which increases to 53.0 ± 2.9 ml/100 ml 12 h after a meal, fell to 27.7 ± 3.3 ml/100 ml.

The unitary activity of sensory vagal neurons recorded from the nodose ganglion of anesthetized sheep during eructation originates from the lower esophageal sphincter where numerous mechanoreceptors are located (71). This activity is spontaneous, consisting of tonic discharges due to a slight longitudinal tension that are inhibited before the passage of the bolus. The lack of inhibition may be the cause of transient free-gas bloating observed 60 min postprandially in cattle on a high-fermentable diet when the gas bubble is close to the cardia but unable to fill the esophagus (259). Frothy bloat, a major cause of death of stocker cattle grazed on winter wheat pastures, is not accompanied by major changes in reticulorumen motility, so it has been hypothesized that unknown substances of the rumen fluid may influence the circular muscle layer of the ruminant lower esophageal sphincter, which contracts in a tetanic manner when exposed to the wheat pasture rumen fluid. The lower esophageal sphincter also contracts spasmodically in the presence of 5-HT (5-hydroxytryptamine, serotonin), and a possible role for 5-HT receptors in the regulation of lower esophageal sphincter tone has been assessed by the use of antagonists to alleviate excessive gas accumulation (194).

*Cyclical Activity of Omasum*

The omasum is a compact organ containing numerous leaves of epithelium that originate from its greater curvature (221). Omasal motor function has been mainly studied in sheep or goats by radiologic examination (175), manometric studies (62, 166), and electromyography (188).

In cattle, movements of the omasal leaves have not been detected, even after vagal stimulation, which may explain the high proportion of dry matter of the ingesta trapped in the interlaminar spaces of the omasum. Contractions of the reticulo-omasal orifice and of the omasal groove occur at each ruminoreticular cycle (213), but those of the omasal body may be absent for periods of two to five reticulorumen cycles. In sheep the contraction of the omasal body is cyclical (21) and is obviously timed by the onset of reticular contractions.

The contractions of the omasal body cease in a regular manner when a reticulorumen cycle starts (Fig. 16), and the omasal contractions are prolonged during sleep. Such interactions are present but less pronounced in cattle because a strong contractile response of the omasum coincides with the reticulorumen inhibition induced by pentagastrin (Fig. 17). The inhibitory-like effect of the onset of reticular contraction on the omasal activity also is demonstrated during feeding when the duration of omasal contractions are strongly reduced concurrently with an increase in the frequency of reticular contractions. The duration of group discharges of the omasal body is reduced from $30 \pm 7$ to $10 \pm 3$ s when the frequency of contraction of the reticulum is increased (Table 5). In addition, at the end of a rumination period, the two or three last cycles show longer intervals between reticular contractions and subsequently prolonged contractions of the omasal body. The significance of this phenomenon was described by Laplace (132) in terms of a short paroxysm involved in the emptying of materials stored in the omasal body.

The cyclical activity of the omasal groove and most of the omasal body is far slower than a rhythmical activity of 6- to 8-s intervals recorded from the omasal canal near the reticulo-omasal orifice. This interval probably is related to the spontaneous closing and opening movements of this orifice (162, 188). This activity seems to fuse into a more prolonged contraction that spreads over the omasal body along the free

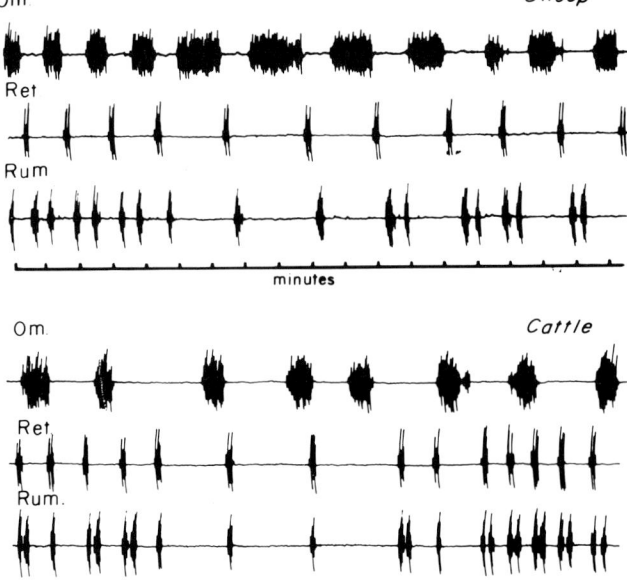

FIG. 16. *Tracing* showing that cyclical contractions of omasal body (Om) occurred at same rate as reticulorumen (Ret-Rum) contractions in sheep. This is not the case in cattle during slower rate of reticulorumen contractions during deep sleep (~7 min).

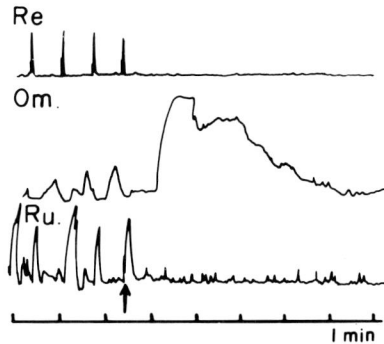

FIG. 17. Motility of omasum (Om) and reticulum (Re) in cattle. Pressure changes recorded from small balloon inserted near middle part of greater curvature of bovine omasum, reticulum, and rumen (Rm). *Arrow*, intravenous injection of pentagastrin (1 µg/kg), which transiently blocks reticulorumen contractions and increases omasal pressure.

border of the omasal leaves (Fig. 18). However, the reticulo-omasal orifice plays an all-or-none role in the transfer of digesta related to the reticuloruminal cycles. In addition the critical size of particles remaining in the rumen is far smaller than that permitted by the reticulo-omasal orifice because of their entrapment in the mass of fibrous diet.

Local anesthesia of the vagus nerves in sheep is accompanied by tachycardia followed by the arrest of reticular contractions for 10–15 min and dilation of the reticulo-omasal orifice. Surprisingly the movements of the omasal body persists. Neither the rhythmic movements nor the mean diameter of the reticulo-omasal orifice seems to be modified by local anesthesia. When general anesthesia was used to study the extent that vagal innervation was involved in the motility of the omasum, the frequency of contractions of the omasal body at first increased despite a complete cessation of reticular contractions and then decreased before the reticular contractions reappeared. The strength of the omasal contractions increased so that the mean level of activity remained unchanged (Fig. 19).

One of the most striking features is that the activity of the omasal body, which is not suppressed either by local or general anesthesia as is the cyclic motility of the reticulorumen, appears to be mostly intrinsic and locally controlled by the nature and volume of contents. The closure of the reticulo-omasal orifice after vagotomy, which is followed by emptying of the omasum, must be interpreted as due to an intrinsic motility of the omasum until all the contents are squeezed out. Such motility disappears as soon as the ingesta are allowed to flow between the leaves by artificially opening the reticulo-omasal orifice (112, 163).

TABLE 5. *Relationship Between Omasal Body Motility Index and Eating and Ruminating*

|  | Rest | Eating* | Ruminating* |
|---|---|---|---|
| Motility index, %/min | 54.5 ± 8.7 | 54.7 ± 3.6 | 67.3 ± 7.02† |
| Number of cycles/min | 1.02 ± 0.05 | 1.4 ± 0.09 | 0.99 ± 0.07 |
| Duration of contraction, s | 34.8 ± 5.4 | 24.2 ± 4.8 | 37.5 ± 3.4 |

* Values are means ± SD for 48 h for a sheep on hay.
† Indicates a correlation with rumination significant at $P < 0.05$.
[From Bueno and Ruckebusch (21).]

### Reticular Groove Mechanisms

When young mammals suck their dams a behavior pattern that is quite different from that seen during drinking to relieve thirst is evoked. Closure of the esophageal groove, a component of sucking behavior, ensures that milk is channeled directly to the abomasum instead of entering the forestomach. When the sucking animals start to eat solid food the forestomach

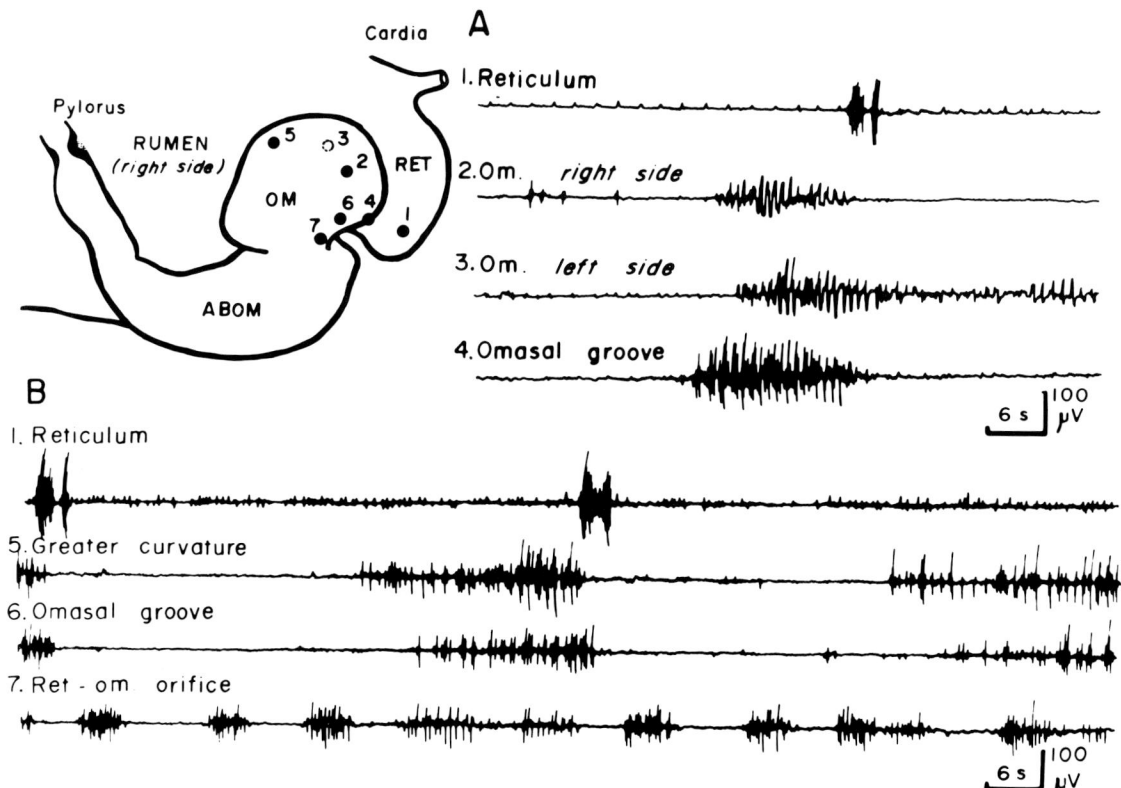

FIG. 18. Electrical activity of omasal wall (right and left sides, omasal groove, and greater curvature) in relation to contraction of reticulum (*A*) and reticulo-omasal orifice (*B*). [From Ruckebusch (188).]

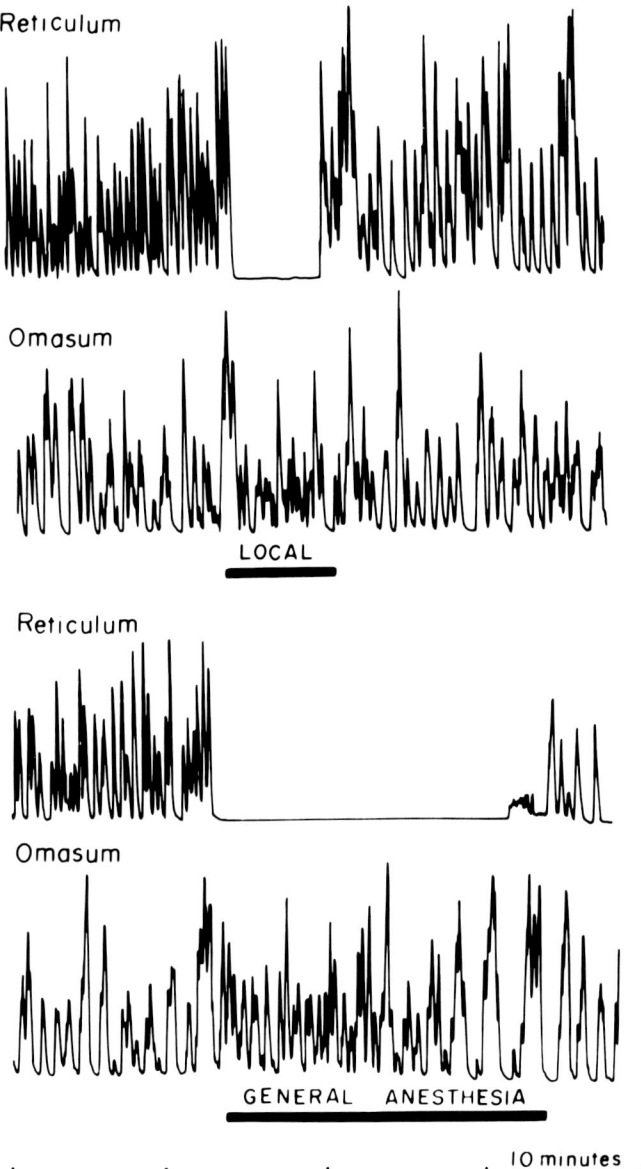

FIG. 19. Motility of reticulum and omasal body under local anesthesia of vagus nerves (*top*) and general anesthesia (*bottom*). Omasal contractions persist in both cases despite arrest of reticular contractions. Arrest of activity of reticulum during 20 min first increases frequency then strength of omasal contractions without changing mean level of activity. [(From Bueno and Ruckebusch (21).]

rapidly develops and assumes its function as a fermentation chamber (249, 250). A lamb normally loses it sucking behavior soon after being separated from its mother, but if it is trained to suck milk or other fluids from a bottle or pail, sucking can be retained well into adult life (125, 169).

Evidence for the reflex character of reticular groove contractions has been obtained by Comline and Titchen (30) in decerebrate preparations of young lambs and calves. The efferent limb of the reflex consists of cholinergic parasympathetic fibers distributed to the esophageal groove mainly in the dorsal abdominal vagus nerve but also, to some extent, in the ventral abdominal vagus nerve. Both the reflex response of the reticular groove and its contraction on peripheral stimulation of the vagus are annulled by the intravenous administration of atropine (31). The introduction of water into the posterior mouth cavity and mechanical stimulation of this region are effective sensory stimuli in decerebrate preparations. The majority of the afferent nerve fibers concerned in mediating these responses are contained in the cranial laryngeal nerves, because stimulation of its central end evokes both swallowing and esophageal groove contraction. In conscious sheep the closure is a function of the route taken by the milk. When barium sulfate mixed with warm water to form 350 ml of a 15% suspension is drunk from a trough by a lamb, a right lateral radiograph taken 20 min after trough feeding shows barium in the caudal part of the abomasum, which is vigorously contracting, and in the duodenal bulb. When barium is injected through a catheter into the esophagus of a lamb standing quietly, the barium passes to the reticulum and anterior rumen (168).

The properties of the reflex demonstrable in decerebrate preparations are summation of inadequate stimuli, fatigue, reflex latency, afterdischarge, and inhibition. This inhibition is both peripheral and central. The peripheral inhibition appears to be an effect of epinephrine on the musculature of the esophageal groove or its release after stimulation of the peripheral end of a splanchnic nerve. The central inhibition is produced by stimulation of the central end of an abomasal branch of the ventral abdominal vagus nerve (144) or of the glossopharyngeal nerve. Abomasal stretch or distension inhibits the reflex contraction of the reticular groove; this effect is mediated by the abomasal branch of the ventral vagus nerve, stimulation of which also produces inhibition (162).

Inhibition of ruminoreticular contractions associated with closure of the reticular groove during sucking was first reported by Schalk and Amadon in 1928 (see ref. 227) in three unweaned calves and also in an adult cow when licking salt. During the sucking of milk (or water), reticulum contractions are decreased in frequency. After sucking (or after introduction of fluid directly into the abomasum), reticulum contractions are slower, whereas rumen and omasum contractions are more fully suppressed. It can be postulated that the inhibitory response to sucking has two phases: a cephalic phase dependent on the eagerness of sucking, which mainly influences the strength of the contractions of the forestomach, and an abomasal phase dependent on the degree of distension of the abomasum, which mainly affects the frequency of contractions (Fig. 20). These results have been obtained in a 12-mo-old bull fitted with a rumen cannula while

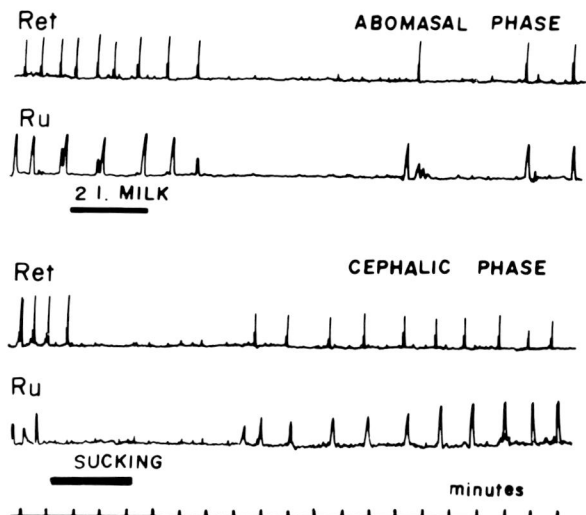

FIG. 20. Responses of an adult bull to the introduction of 2 liters of warm milk into abomasum by a tube inserted through reticulo-omasal orifice (*top*) and the sucking of 2 liters of milk (*bottom*). Bars indicate duration of these procedures.

sucking 2 liters of milk from a watering can and when 2 liters of milk were introduced into the abomasum through the reticulo-omasal orifice. The inhibition of the cephalic phase is therefore mainly inotropic in nature, whereas that of the abomasal phase is mainly chronotropic (127).

The reticular groove reflex is an all-or-none response in both fed calves and lambs (168). Copper salt in sheep (251) and sodium salts in calves (183) are able to favor the closure of the groove. This has been studied by using polyethylene glycol 4,000 as a marker (21) in animals fitted with rumen fistulas and measuring the proportion of ingested liquid food found in the rumen after a meal.

The reflex progressively disappears with age. A very small proportion (<10%) of the skim milk, suspension of soybean oil and meal, or solution of fish protein concentrate used as liquid food instead of milk is recovered in the rumen of young calves. In older calves the proportion of liquid food recovered in the rumen is much higher, except when access to water is withheld during the night (90).

### Nervous Control of Forestomach Motility

The frequency, amplitude, and form of the cyclical contractions of the reticuloruminal smooth muscle coat are centrally controlled (93) and therefore disappear after section of the vagus nerves (Fig. 21). In fact the ability of the reticulorumen to contract rhythmically once a minute is the result of a vagovagal reflex system mediated by gastric centers in the brain stem outside the blood-brain barrier (227). The role of the central nervous system is to achieve the integration of activity from separated regions to order their sequential contractile activity and to control the frequency, amplitude, and form of the extrinsic contractions. The gastric centers do not appear to have a spontaneous rhythmicity but require an overall excitatory drive to be provided by inputs coming from other parts of the central nervous system and from the periphery (94, 225), mainly from the alimentary tract itself. Situations that have general effects on the central nervous system (e.g., sleep, hyperthermia) or that alter conditions within the gut (e.g., distension, pH) will therefore affect motility (50). Each left and right vagus nerve divides in the thorax into a dorsal and ventral branch. The two dorsal branches unite to form a dorsal vagal trunk with a predominance of right vagal fibers. Likewise the two ventral branches form a ventral vagal trunk with a predominance of left vagal fibers. The dorsal trunk innervates all regions of the reticulorumen, whereas the ventral trunk supplies the reticulum but little of the rumen (91, 159). The vagi provide pathways for afferent and efferent fibers in the ratio of 9:1, respectively (185). In chronically denervated sheep, extrinsic contractions of nor-

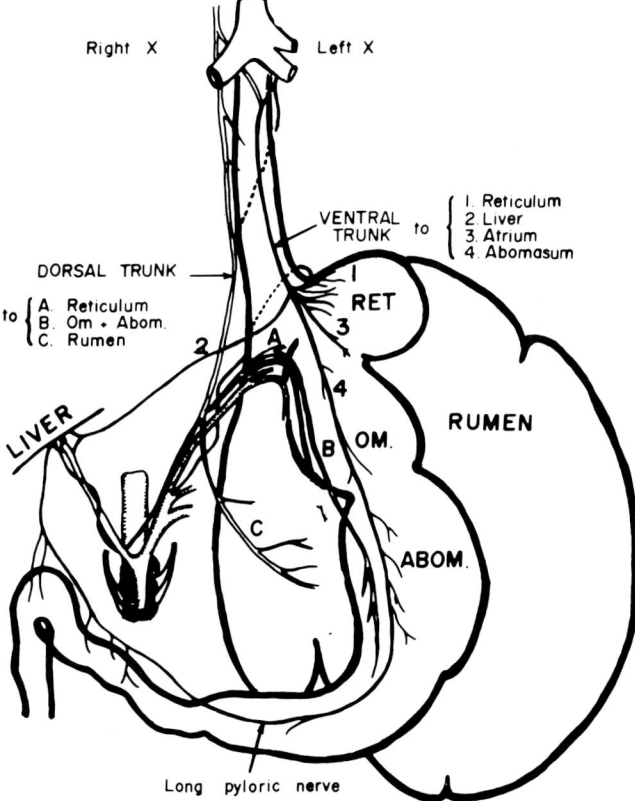

FIG. 21. Termination of dorsal and ventral trunks in the goat, showing their origin from right and left vagus nerves. After section of dorsal vagal trunk, which has 3 branches *A*, *B*, and *C*, reticular cyclical activity persists, whereas dorsal sac of the rumen shows small group discharges later grouped in regular series. Section of ventral vagal trunk (branches *1, 2, 3, 4*) alters activity of reticulum. [Adapted from Coulouma (36).]

mal amplitude and frequency require the presence of not less than half of the total vagal supply (54). After bilateral vagotomy, the sequential contractions of the reticulorumen are transformed in systolic low-amplitude movements (Fig. 22).

INTRINSIC CONTRACTIONS. Two separate mechanisms exist for the production of intrinsic contractions: myogenic contractions that are attributable to the rhythmic contractility of the muscle cells and neurogenic contractions that require the involvement of the neurons of the myenteric plexus (105).

Evidence exists for neurogenic intrinsic activity in the reticulorumen. In halothane-anesthetized sheep, reticuloruminal tension receptor activities recorded by the single afferent vagal fiber technique (133) exhibited during the interval between extrinsic contractions phasic discharges of action potentials at a rate of ~10 cycles/min for the reticulum and 12 cycles/min for the dorsal sac of the rumen. Neither the phasic discharges of these tension receptors nor the frequency of efferent vagal discharges responsible for extrinsic contractions are affected by the administration of anticholinesterases, ganglionic blockers, or muscarinic blockers.

In contrast the amplitudes of the extrinsic contractions are enhanced with neostigmine and are reduced or abolished by the blockers. This suggests that the intrinsic contractions are myogenic in nature or at least not dependent on any tonically active neuronal mechanism with a cholinergic synapse either at a ganglionic or at a postganglionic site (134). The existence and properties of intrinsic myogenic contractions inferred from the characteristics of the resting discharges of reticular and ruminal tension receptors appear to have as their counterparts in conscious sheep the slow-wave activity recorded from electrodes placed in the muscle layers of the reticulorumen (188). Additional counterparts are probably the large spike group discharges of the reticulum and of the dorsal and ventral ruminal sacs that appear after section of the vagal dorsal trunk. Such group discharges are enhanced by an anticholinesterase (eserine) and, conversely, are abolished by cholinergic blockers (hexamethonium, atropine). These group discharges might thus represent intrinsic neurogenic contractions involving cholinergic pathways and the myenteric plexus. These intrinsic contractions are accelerated by increasing ruminal volume (198) and are inhibited by acidifying the ruminal contents (80).

The extent to which intrinsic neurogenic contractions may play a role in the normal conscious animal remains in doubt. They tended to increase in circumstances where the extrinsic contractions were abolished (e.g., during the later stages of a pyrogen-induced inhibition), whereas the central nervous system depression was still present. In this case, the intrinsic contractions were exaggerated until the extrinsic contractions returned (134). Because the magnitude of the intrinsic contractions reflexly influences the rate

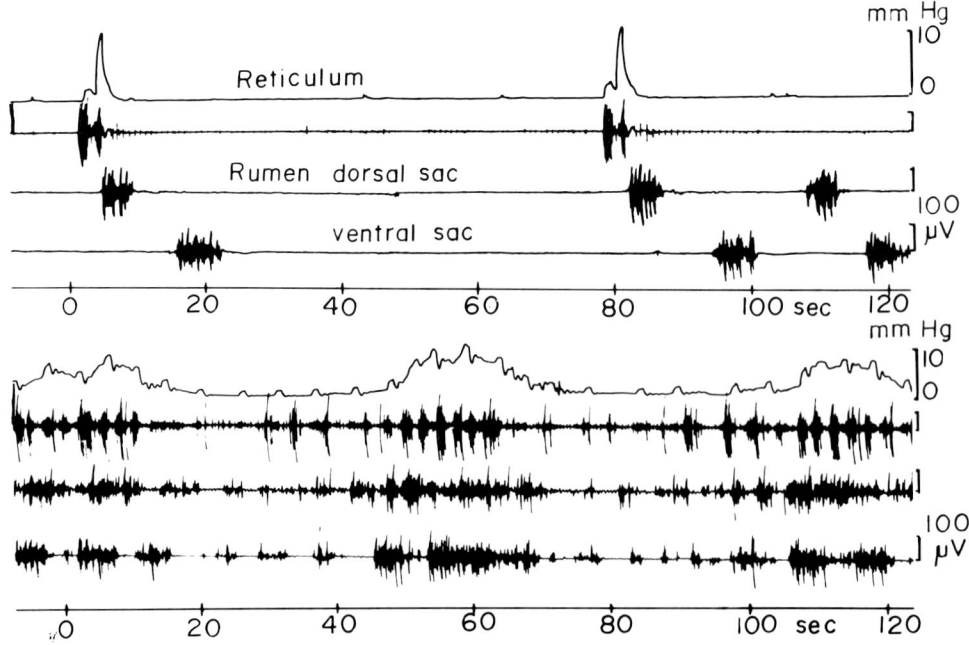

FIG. 22. Extrinsic (*top traces*) versus intrinsic (*bottom traces*) motor activity of reticulum (intraluminal pressure and electrical activity) and dorsal sac and ventral sac of rumen as seen 12 days after cervical vagotomy. [From Ruckebusch and Tomov (198), ©1972, with permission from Pergamon Press, Ltd.]

and amplitude of the extrinsic contractions, any factor that affects intrinsic contractions will have consequential effects on extrinsic contractions. A moderate increase in intrinsic contractions has a reflexly excitatory effect on extrinsic contractions, but those factors that lead to a large increase in intrinsic contractions (i.e., drugs producing sustained contractures) have a reflexly depressing effect on extrinsic contractions (244, 245).

The reticuloruminal intrinsic motility has been found to develop within 1–2 wk after vagotomy (54, 79, 198) such that strong contractions affect the whole reticulorumen within 20 s at intervals of 80–120 s. This rhythmic motility pattern is evidently organized through the enteric nervous system, which can be studied during several weeks when sheep are maintained by continuous gastric infusion of a complete liquid diet (170, 171). In long-term vagotomized sheep, when the rumen volume (~4 liters) is permanently filled with 2–2.5 liters of a solution of volatile fatty acids buffered to pH 5.0 with $NaHCO_3$, the frequency of intrinsic contractions varies with the degree of intraluminal pressure (e.g., from 4.5 to 5 contractions per 10 min in the standing animal to 8.5–9.5 during recumbency). Accordingly the transient distension of the dorsal sac of the rumen obtained by the insufflation of air (2 liters), which is rapidly eructated, reduces by half the duration of the quiescent periods between the contractions (Fig. 23).

The final common motor pathway of the reticuloruminal enteric nervous system seems to be cholinergic, as suggested by enhancement of the rhythmic activity by cholinomimetic agents (Fig. 23). Among the growing number of compounds implicated as possible enteric nervous system neurotransmitters or modulators of the small or large intestine, only 5-HT or its precursor 5-hydroxytryptophan (5-HTP) and prostaglandins were found able to strongly stimulate the frequency of ruminal contractions during 2–3 h (Fig. 23) at dosages that did not affect significantly the motor activity of the abomasum. An increased frequency of shallow contractions was also found as a rebound effect after the inhibition as a result of histamine or morphine infusion. Equimolar infusions of several peptides, including secretin and pentagastrin, were without effect on the frequency of ruminal contractions.

EXTRINSIC CONTRACTIONS. Electrical stimulation of a vagal branch peripheral to a cold block or to a nerve section led to a reticular contraction and, in the case of the dorsal trunk, to a ruminal contraction. The duration, form, and amplitude of the evoked contractions were proportional to the duration of the pattern and the intensity of the stimulation. The ruminal contractions developed and decayed slightly later than the reticular contractions, presumably because of the polysynaptic nature of the efferent pathways (134).

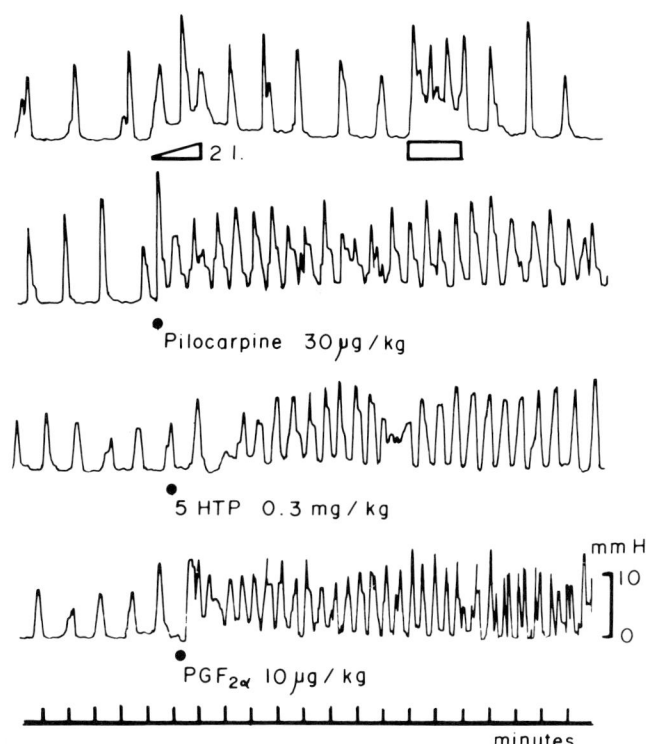

FIG. 23. Intrinsic motor activity of rumen (intraluminal pressure) recorded 6 wk after thoracic vagotomy in a sheep maintained at constant body weight by intragastric infusion of complete liquid diet (see refs. 170 and 171). From top to bottom, increased frequency of intrinsic contractions after progressive or sudden distension during 2 min and cholinergic, serotonergic, or prostaglandin stimulation obtained by intravenous injection of pilocarpine, 5-hydroxytryptophan (5-HTP), or prostaglandin $F_{2\alpha}$ ($PGF_{2\alpha}$). (From Y. Ruckebusch and C. H. Malbert, unpublished observations.)

In halothane-anesthetized sheep in which primary cycle movements are present, Iggo and Leek (118) were able to record various patterns of nervous discharges in individual efferent vagal fibers innervating different parts of the reticulorumen. In all cases, each cyclical burst of nervous activity had a fixed temporal relationship when the peak of the reticular contraction was used as the reference point. Similar unitary discharges were obtained by Dussardier (57) in conscious sheep by recording the unitary activity of the diaphragmatic muscle reinnervated by efferent vagal fibers that had grown from the central end of a cut vagus nerve into the sutured peripheral stump of a cut phrenic nerve.

The efferent vagal pathways responsible for the extrinsic contractions involved cholinergic ganglionic and postganglionic transmission. Efferent gastric vagal discharges recordable in the preganglionic axons in the cervical region failed to evoke extrinsic contractions after the administration of tetraethylammonium chloride or atropine. Conversely the administration of neostigmine led to an enhancement of the amplitude and duration of the extrinsic contractions. Neither cholinergic blockers nor the anticholinesterase changed the resting interval between the cyclical bursts of efferent discharges. Neither chronic splanchnic denervation in conscious sheep (54) nor acute splanchnic denervation in the halothane anesthetized sheep (93) had any detectable effect on extrinsic contractions. Moreover, splanchnic denervation did not appear to affect the intrinsic neurogenic movements seen in the chronically vagotomized sheep (79).

GASTRIC CENTERS. The term *gastric centers* is used to denote the bilateral areas of the brain stem responsible for producing the extrinsic movements (117) of the forestomach via discharges in the gastric vagal efferent nerve fibers. Early studies of the location of gastric centers involved direct intramedullary stimulation (3), focal electrolytic lesions, and unitary activity recording (12) as well as cellular degeneration after nerve section and/or rumenotomy [Fig. 24; (56, 58, 220)]. Splitting the brain medially between 0 and 7 mm rostral to the obex cut the commissural connections responsible for synchronizing the efferent activity patterns of the motoneurons confined to each dorsal vagal motor nucleus. Consequently the frequency of contractions was increased as each center produced its own motor activity (93).

The mechanism controlling the frequency of extrinsic contractions is partly known. On the basis of microelectrode studies, each medullary pattern generator is considered to consist of a neuronal network modulating the reticular and ruminal motor neuronal activity. According to Leek and Harding (134), neurons that did not fulfill the criteria for motoneurons are considered to be type A interneurons with close functional proximity to motoneurons. Another kind of interneuronal activity (type B) is characterized by a progressively increased discharge after a reticular contraction that reaches a peak prior to the onset of the next contraction. These rate circuit interneurons are maintained in an inhibited state by type C interneurons as shown by the single efferent fiber technique (118).

The cell bodies located in the dorsal vagal motor nucleus corresponding to type A interneurons are thus considered to display an amplitude activity on the vagal motoneurons steady tonic discharge (inotropic regulation). The threshold activity that ceased at the onset of the reticular contraction is modulated by type B and C interneurons acting by both excitation and inhibition of type A interneurons during quiescence between primary cycle contractions (Fig. 25). The discharge of type B and C interneurons as time elapsed after the previous primary cycle contractions is considered to form the basis of a rate circuit (chronotropic regulation) in which afferent inputs are integrated cumulatively until a central excitatory state is attained.

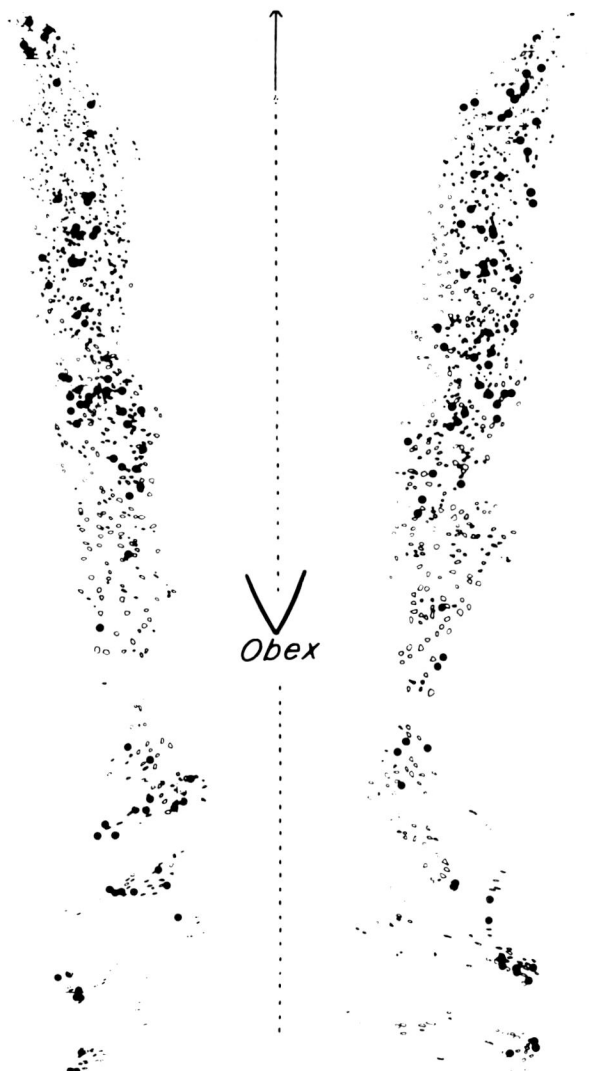

FIG. 24. Gastric centers in medulla. On each side, region relative to obex extends laterally from 1 to 3 mm, caudally 2 mm, and rostrally 4 mm. *Black dots*, retrograde cellular degeneration 16 days after rumenectomy in lamb. [Adapted from Szabo and Dussardier (220).]

Among the excitatory influences (chronotropic regulation), distension of the reticulum alters the frequency of contractions by acting on the rate circuit. Three other reflexogenic areas involved in the chronotropic control are the cardia, the reticulo-omasal orifice, and the reticuloruminal fold.

VISCERAL SENSORY MECHANISMS. Classic reflex studies have shown that the mouth, esophagus, forestomach, abomasum, and duodenum are important reflexogenic areas for effects on reticuloruminal motility (71), salivation (123), and food intake (88).

Mechanical stimulation of the oral mucous membranes excited reticuloruminal motility. Receptors with afferent pathways mainly in the second and third branches of the trigeminal nerves are considered to be tonically active because primary cycle motility is reduced by trigeminal nerve section (17). During chewing, augmentation of this tonic activity is responsible for the reflexly enhanced forestomach motility. Chemical stimulation through the taste mechanism does not appear to be involved.

Distension of the terminal esophagus, cardia, reticulo-omasal orifice, and reticulum reflexly enhances primary cycle motility (24). Distension of the dorsal ruminal sac enhances secondary cycle motility (137). Manual distension of the reticulum, especially the reticuloruminal orifice (226), is an effective means of promoting primary cycle contractions. Manually stretching the cardia, reticular groove, reticulo-omasal orifice, reticuloruminal fold, and cranial ruminal pillar

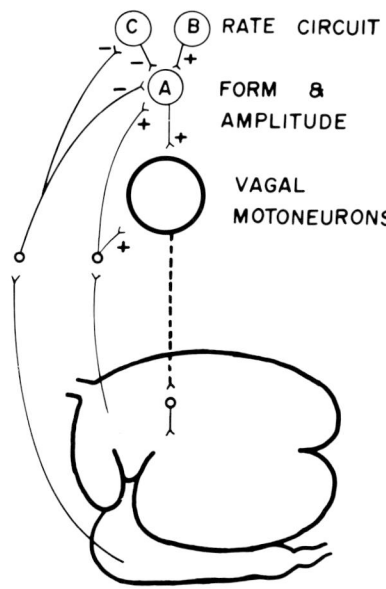

FIG. 25. Functional organization of gastric centers. Neuronal network with type B and C interneurons may constitute rate circuit responsible for chronotropic regulation of extrinsic movements. Another network with type A interneurons is involved in inotropic (amplitude) regulation of cyclic movements of reticulum through early vagal discharges and of rumen through later vagal discharges. Rate and amplitude circuits are inhibited by abomasal distension. Amplitude circuit and vagal motoneurons are stimulated by reticular distension. Strong net excitatory drive on rate and amplitude circuits arises from central nervous system. [Adapted from Leek and Harding (134).]

is a potent stimulus for parotid salivation (176) in conscious (121) and anesthetized (84) sheep.

The presence of coarse fibers in the forestomach favors rumination. Conversely, rumination is virtually eliminated by finely grinding the food (76). Squeezing the reticuloruminal fold and scratching the ruminal mucosa readily induce rumination (7, 124).

Acidification of the reticuloruminal contents reflexly inhibits forestomach motility. The potency of an acid is not dependent on its pH but is closely related to its titratable acidity or to its undissociated concentration (37). Acidification of the abomasum is a potent stimulus for primary cycle motility through a vagovagal reflex (118), whereas distension of the abomasum and of the duodenum inhibited primary cycle motility (226).

At least three distinct types of visceral sensory receptors have been demonstrated electrophysiologically: 1) epithelial (mucosal) receptors near the basement membrane of the lining epithelium, 2) tension receptors in the muscle layers, and 3) serosal receptors in the serosa (see the chapter by Grundy and Scratcherd in this Handbook; Fig. 26). There is evidence also of visceral thermoreceptors, and the mesenteries contain classic Pacinian corpuscles. The epithelial and tension receptors project via the vagi. The serosal receptors project via the splanchnic nerves.

The epithelial receptors in sheep were first described in the abomasum and the duodenum (113) and later in the reticulorumen (94). They are rapidly adapting mechanoreceptors that are also excited by certain chemicals. As mechanoreceptors they give a typical rapidly adapting on-off response to a maintained moderate mechanical stimulus; the repeated movement of fibrous digesta across the luminal epithelium can be expected to excite them. Excitation of epithelial receptors in the reticulorumen acts as an inhibitory input to the gastric centers and reflexly reduces primary cycle motility (94). They appear to have no reflex effect on salivation and in triggering rumination. It is possible that they maintain a tonic inhibitory effect on the gastric centers because selective vagal deafferentation in conscious sheep has been shown to result in an increased rate of primary cycle contractions (72).

A role for the epithelial receptors on the basis of their chemosensitive properties is obvious in the inhibition of reticuloruminal motility evoked experi-

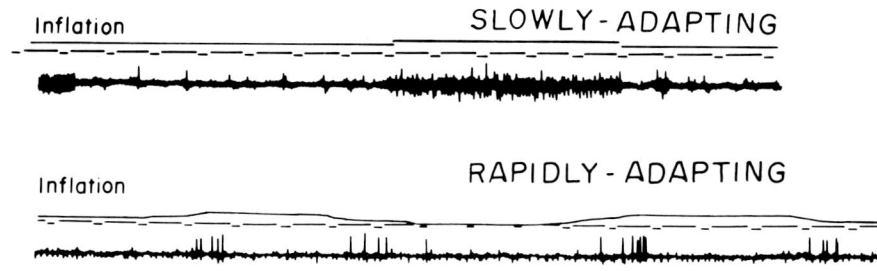

FIG. 26. Responses of mechanoreceptors. Tension receptor gives a steady (slowly adapting) discharge throughout period of distension (horizontal bar). Discharges occur only at times of inflation and of deflation for epithelial receptors. (From E. C. Crichlow, unpublished observations).

mentally by the intraruminal infusion of acids or during the ruminal acidosis of the grain engorgement syndrome. The abomasal epithelial receptors may have a physiological role as monitors of abomasal acid secretion, and experimentally their activation would account for the reflex enhancement of primary cycle motility arising from abomasal acidification (226). Experimentally the regulation of gastric emptying based on the results of infusing acids and alkali into the calf's duodenum (15) is consistent with duodenal epithelial-receptor activation (35).

Tension receptors are slowly adapting mechanoreceptors situated in the muscle layers in series with the smooth muscle cells. In the reticulorumen the tension receptors are innervated by finely myelinated nerve fibers with conduction velocities more than 10 times faster than the unmyelinated nerve fibers. Receptive fields of single afferent fibers may possess diameters of 5–20 mm. When an intrinsic or extrinsic contraction occurs, there is a large discharge that resembles that of the Golgi tendon organs in skeletal muscle. The discharge rate of a tension receptor is thus a composite feature reflecting the passive tension due to distension and the active tension developed by intrinsic and extrinsic contractions.

In the reticulorumen, tension receptors are densely located around the cardia, the reticulo-omasal orifice, the margins of the reticular groove, the reticulum, the reticuloruminal fold, the cranial pillar, and the longitudinal pillars (133). Tension receptor fields can be found in the floor of the omasal canal. They are plentiful in the terminal regions of the esophagus and are particularly abundant in the pyloric region. Recently, Cottrell and Iggo (35) described their behavior in the circular muscle of the sheep's duodenum.

The roles of tension receptors may be at the esophageal level to elicit secondary contractions in the event of the swallowed bolus falling behind the primary contractions. In the forestomach, tension receptors of the reticulum and the reticuloruminal fold provide an excitatory input to the gastric centers, leading to an increase in the rate, duration, and amplitude of the primary cycle contractions. Tension developed during the early phases of the primary cycle contraction provides a reflex feedback to influence the vagally evoked later phases of the contraction. Feeding, which passively distends the reticulorumen with ingesta and accumulation of gases, enhances motility presumably by tension receptor activation, although some degree of reflex inhibition arising from epithelial receptors may also occur, which would modify the expected enhancement. Pyrogen production during febrile disease may inhibit the intrinsic contractions and hence reduce the excitatory input from tension receptors to the gastric centers (240).

The tension receptors around the reticular groove, reticuloruminal fold, and cranial pillar excite parotid salivary gland secretion (176). In the cranial ruminal sac, tension receptors facilitate secondary cycle contractions that in concert with the activation of other receptors (probably tension receptors) around the reticular groove lead to eructation. In the reticulorumen, tension receptors probably signal "rumen fill" to the appetite control centers and modify the release of growth hormone (225).

In the abomasum, tension receptors with afferent vagal pathways reflexly inhibit reticuloruminal motility (118), and this may provide a mechanism for regulating abomasal filling. Similarly, tension receptors in the duodenum are presumably responsible for the inhibition of reticuloruminal motility that occurs during duodenal distension (35, 196).

To summarize, the extrinsic contractions of the forestomach are essential for mixing and aboral propulsion of the contents, for eructation, and for rumination. They are the consequence of central nervous system activity, reflexly modified by sensory inputs largely from the alimentary tract itself. Any clinical situations or drug programs that affect either the general level of central nervous system activity or the gut contents will modify extrinsic contractions.

Full control of ruminant nutrition can now be achieved by the supply of energy as a liquid diet into the forestomach and of protein into the abomasum for several months. The slow but strong and rhythmic contractions of the rumen developed in chronically vagotomized sheep, which are infused with volatile fatty acids at levels of estimated energy requirement and with bicarbonate to compensate for the reduced secretion of saliva in animals not eating or ruminating solid food, reflect the general level of enteric nervous system activity. This activity, which is not helpful for propulsion, is principally regulated by the degree of reticuloruminal distension. The rate of the intrinsic contractions is similarly stimulated by cholinergic or serotonergic agonists and by prostaglandins, at variance with the effects in the vagally intact animal.

STOMACH MOTILITY

The abomasum lies in the lower right part of the abdominal cavity, partly covered by the edge of the rib cage. The fundic part commences in the xiphoid region and extends backward under the right costal arch where its cannulation is relatively easy (129). Construction of fundic pouches (149) is more difficult than construction of antral pouches (150) because of the large folds or rugae corresponding to 85% of the area of the fundic mucosa. Several methods of making innervated fundic pouches in the ruminant have been described (108), the simplest being a semicircular line of interrupted, overlapping, through-and-through sutures placed through both layers of the unopened abomasal wall. This line starts and ends at the greater curvature, and it isolates the pouch while leaving a lumen of ~5 cm at the lesser curvature for digesta to pass through to the pylorus.

The abomasum is the only part of the stomach that secretes digestive juices. The secretion from the fundic area is similar to that of dogs in that it contains pepsin and hydrochloric acid; it is a watery fluid with two major variable constituents, $H^+$ and $Na^+$, that exchange with each other. The pH from sheep feeding ad libitum varies between 1.05 and 1.32. After an overnight fast, the sight of food (148) and the abomasal distension (104) increase the acid output from 10 to 60 mEq $H^+$/liter. Fluid collected from innervated antral pouches is slightly alkaline and contains visible strands of mucus and clumps of epithelial cells (151, 152). When its pH is adjusted to 2, its peptic activity is much less than that of fundic juice (99). The total amount of fluid secreted by the abomasum varies considerably with the level of feeding and the diet (109).

Ratios of flow from abomasum to flow from the reticulorumen are the highest during high levels of feeding and for grass harvested at early maturity. For a mean ruminal retention time of ~10–14 h and a reticulorumen outflow of 5, 7, and 10 liters/day, the abomasal digesta outflow is 6, 8, and 13 liters/day in sheep receiving straw. On a diet of grass, the reticulorumen outflow can reach 11–12 liters/day and the abomasal outflow 15–20 liters/day (96, 99).

*Motor Patterns of Activity*

It is frequently stated that the gastric emptying of a fully fed ruminant is a continuous process. This conception has been disproved by the measurement of the abomasal outflow of digesta (114) and the presence of cyclical changes in the magnitude and frequency of the contractions of the pyloric antrum in sheep. The fundic motor activity consists of permanent shallow contractions in contrast to the antral motor activity, which is inhibited at the occurrence of a period of regular contractions on the antroduodenal junction (Fig. 27). This occurs 18–20 times/day. Because of the continuous supply of contents through the reticulo-omasal orifice, it is likely that cyclical periods of high pressures at the level of the gastroduodenal junction and their subsequent phases of quiescence correspond to periods of no delivery of chyme to the duodenum.

The electrical activity of the pyloric antrum is characterized by regular slow waves at a frequency of 6.5 ± 0.8/min with almost continuous bursts of spike potentials of 2-s duration. These bursts of spike potentials are occasionally coupled with spike potentials on the duodenal bulb area that, in sheep, did not show slow waves over the first 10 cm beyond the pylorus. The typical spiking activity of the antrum also shows changes in its magnitude with quiescence at 5–10 cm before the pylorus at the onset of maximal activity on the duodenal bulb. When recording electrodes are placed at short intervals, it is obvious that the pattern of antral spiking activity is influenced by strong bursts

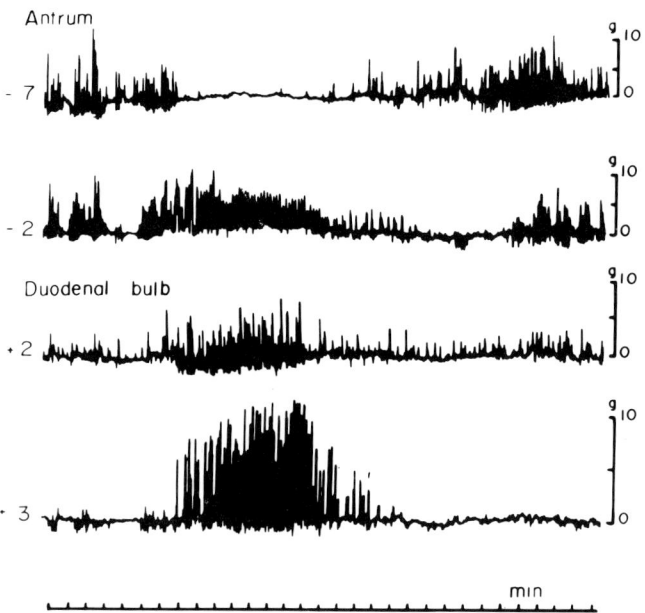

FIG. 27. Mechanical activity of pyloric antrum in sheep recorded from curved strain-gauge force transducers fixed on the antrum at 7 and 2 cm before pylorus and duodenal bulb and 2 and 3 cm beyond pylorus.

of spike potentials of 5-s duration that originate either on the antroduodenal junction or at 10 mm from the junction and by a series of spike potentials also initiated at different sites (Fig. 28).

The manner in which digesta pass to the duodenum was studied in sheep and goats by Singleton (206) in 1961. Using an electromagnetic flow meter, he measured the passage of material through the exteriorized first part of the duodenum.

The flow into the duodenum usually occurs in gushes as great as 30–40 ml at a time. A series of gushes of this magnitude may occur within 10–15 min followed by a period of rest in which nothing or only insignificant trickles of food are passed to the duodenum. The mean value per hour for a sheep weighing 40 kg is ~400 ml. In this pioneering work it was also observed that 40% of the material flowing to the duodenum returned to the abomasum in goats, whereas in sheep only 10% moved in an antiperistaltic direction. Correction of the measurements for antiperistaltic flow showed that goats weighing ~33 kg passed from 10 to 15 liters of abomasal contents to the duodenum per 24 h, whereas sheep weighing ~65 kg passed 11–12 liters. Such differences between sheep and goats also are observed regarding feeding behavior (77) and motility (189).

In cattle the motility pattern of the abomasal antrum and the proximal part of the duodenum was studied by electromyography, and special attention was paid to retrograde motility. Although on the abomasum 81.1% of the slow waves were followed by spikes, 48.8% of these spikes passed aborally to the

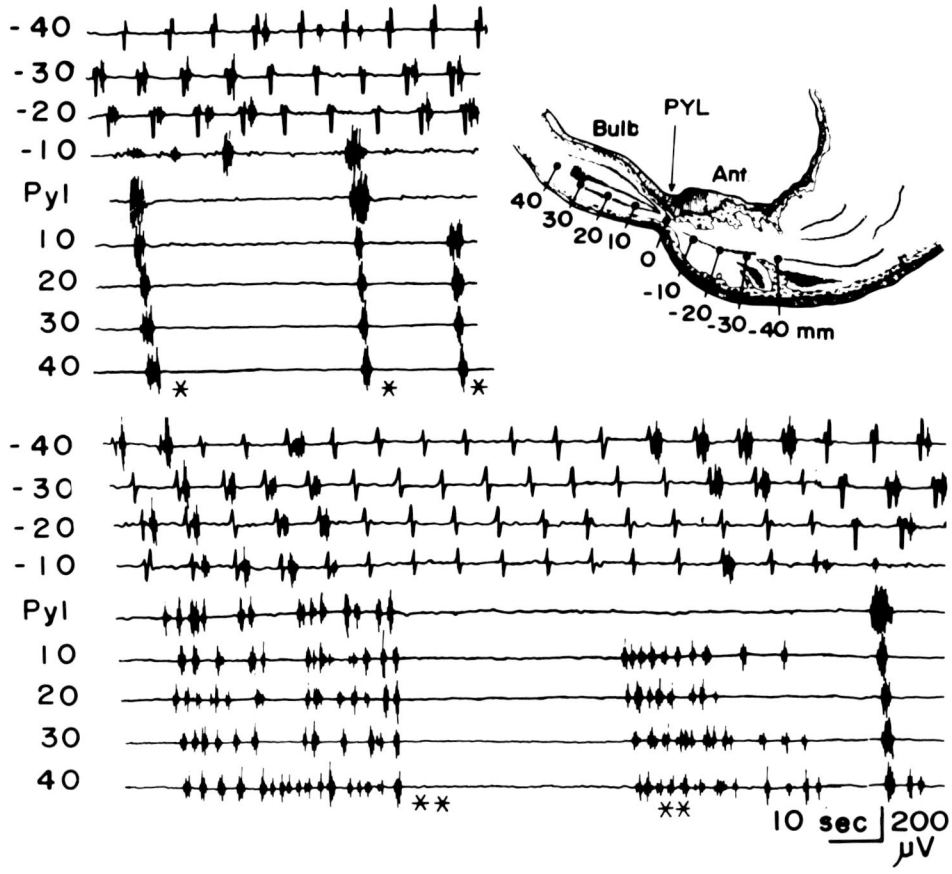

FIG. 28. Electrical activity recorded from pairs of electrodes fixed at 10-mm intervals on gastroduodenal junction in sheep showing propulsive waves (*) and continuous spiking activity (**) commencing at pylorus (PYL) or duodenal bulb (Bulb). Ant, pyloric antrum.

duodenal bulb. On the duodenum, peristaltic activity, local antegrade, and local retrograde motility were recorded as shown in Figure 29. The starting point of peristaltic contractions was mostly found on the antrum (70%), whereas most of the retrograde contractions (25%) started at the level of the entrance of the ductus choledocus (167). The retrograde motility occurring during the period of irregular spiking activity may run over long or short distances and favor the backflow of bile, thus increasing the neutralizing capacity of the most proximal part of the duodenum. In ruminants the pancreatic duct joins the common bile duct and a mixture of bile and pancreatic juice flows into the duodenum at more than 25–30 cm from the pylorus. The delivery of acidic chyme through the pylorus at pH 3 makes the ruminant gastroduodenal junction a unique example of a sphincteric function separating digestive contents of similar acidity (196).

*Duodenal Brake Mechanism*

The flow of food through the abomasum and the secretion of abomasal juice are integrated so that the volume and acidity of the abomasal contents, although varying, are maintained fairly constant. Integration of passage of digesta to and from the abomasum with gastric secretion (150) is as follows: *1*) the strength and frequency of reticular contractions are reduced if the abomasal content is increased, and the flow of digesta to the omasum that occurs after every reticular contraction thus decreases, and *2*) the outflow from the abomasum to the duodenum, which is influenced by the quantities of material in the recipient organ, is reduced by the fatty acid content of the material entering the duodenum (164). In addition the secretion of acid in the abomasum is inhibited if the pH of the contents falls in the region of pH 2 and if acid is introduced into the duodenum (81).

The continuous delivery of contents through the pylorus in the adult ruminant is rhythmic because of the initiation of the migrating myoelectric complexes (MMCs) on the duodenal bulb (193, 195). Stimulation of duodenal motor activity via distension, acid, and serotoninergic mechanisms (190), which increased the frequency of MMCs, resulted in corresponding transient inhibition of the antral motor activity (Fig. 30).

In contrast the inhibition of the motor activity of the antrum, whatever its origin, resulted in a higher frequency of the duodenal cyclic motor events. The motor profile of the antroduodenal junction thus corresponds to interactions that fulfill the homeostasis of gastric emptying functions, with the first part of the duodenum as an extremely sensitive and rapid braking mechanism. Because most of the factors involved in the control of the transfer of chyme through the pylorus are of duodenal origin, the term duodenal brake seems relevant. Because of the continuous gastric secretion and delivery of acidic chyme, the pH of the duodenal contents of the bulb, measured by means of glass electrodes placed in the lumen through a T-cannula at equal distance from the pylorus and the entrance of the pancreaticobiliary secretions, was 2.8 to 3.2 during the periods of irregular spiking activity (ISA). During the development of a period of regular spiking activity (RSA) or phase III and its subsequent period of quiescence, duodenal chyme flow was reduced and its pH rose by 2–3 units (Fig. 31). These cyclical pH changes lasted only 15 min in sheep and correspond to antral inhibition, during and after the development of a phase III pattern of the MMCs. Absence of dilution and transit of both duodenal and pancreaticobiliary secretions could account for the pH changes. Furthermore in sheep the pH will remain acidic when the flow of chyme or gastric emptying is accelerated by agents, such as acetylcholine, that stimulate gastric peristalsis in excess of duodenal motor activity. In contrast, a rise in pH occurs after giving drugs, such as opiates, that impede abomasal emptying by preferentially enhancing duodenal peristalsis or after mechanical obstruction to the gastric outflow. A major pitfall in the duodenal pH measurement as an

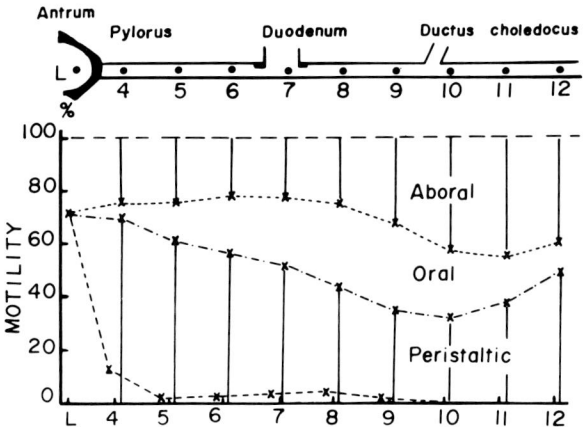

FIG. 29. Percentages of propulsive (peristaltic) and aboral or oral locally propagated activity along duodenum in cattle. [From Ooms and Oyaert (167).]

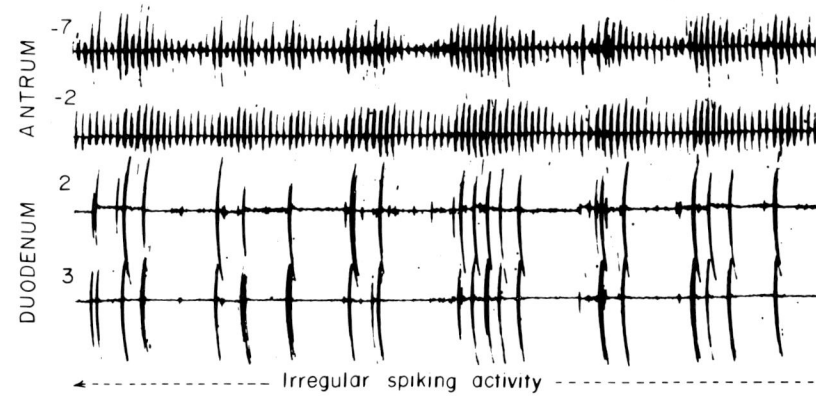

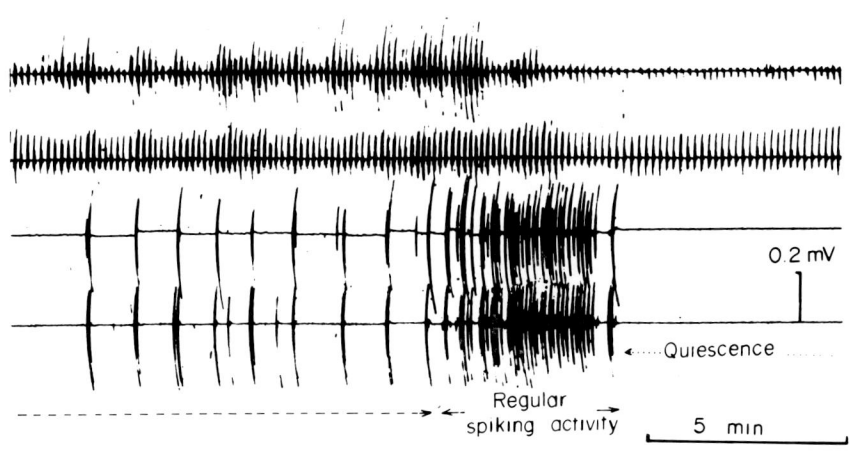

FIG. 30. Electromyography of ovine gastroduodenal area from electrodes fixed 2 cm apart on pylorus, antrum (−7 cm), and duodenum (3 cm). *Tracings* are consecutive. *Top*: irregular spiking activity showing spike bursts of antrum at frequency of 6.5/min. Magnitude of spike bursts waxes and wanes with activity on duodenum. *Bottom*: cyclical period of regular spiking activity followed by quiescence.

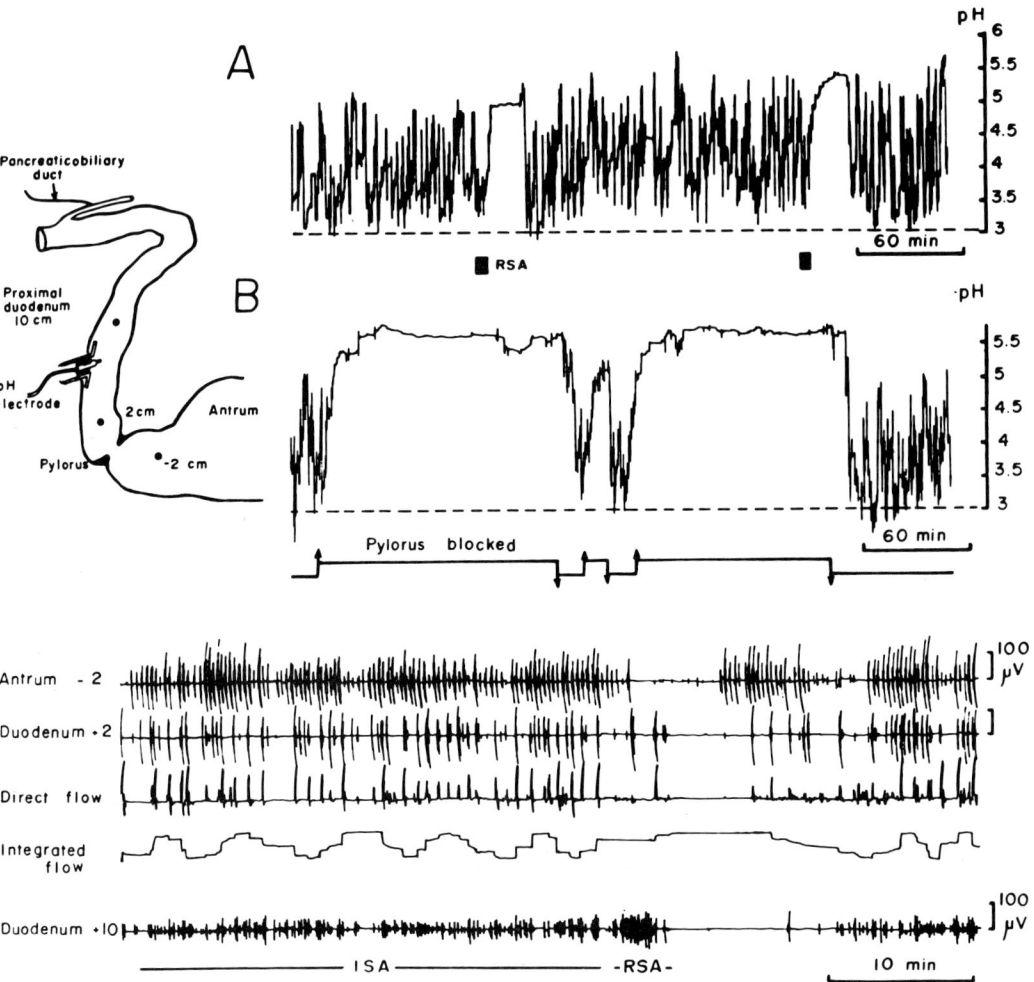

FIG. 31. Changes in intraduodenal pH over time in sheep as measured by pH electrode inserted through cannula placed ~7 cm from pylorus. Prolonged periods of relatively high, stable pH indicating myoelectrical quiescence follows cyclical phase of regular spiking activity (RSA) indicated as a *bar*. *Trace A* is suggestive of fairly high delivery rate of acid from abomasum to duodenum with mean pH of 4.1. *Trace B* was obtained by obstructing transpyloric outflow with a balloon of a Foley catheter inserted via duodenal cannula. Rise of 2.5 pH units within 6 min occurred that remained stable until cessation of occlusion. *Bottom*: changes in abomasal outflow as measured by electromagnetic probe at 7 cm from pylorus in cattle. Note absence of flow at the time of RSA phase.

indication of transpyloric digesta flow resulting from the antroduodenal motor interactions is represented by concomitant antisecretory effects.

The inhibition of abomasal motility in response to the osmotic environment of the duodenum depends to varying degrees on a neural mechanism called the enterogastric inhibitory reflex. The vagus is a component of this reflex arc, since the inhibitory effect is partially abolished if both vagi are severed, whereas section of sympathetic nerve has no effect. Thus the information of the enterogastric inhibitory reflex seems to travel from duodenum to brain and back to the stomach with both afferents and efferents in the vagi; the vagal inhibition is mediated by efferent noncholinergic, nonadrenergic nerves. A variety of duodenal receptors other than osmoreceptors, i.e., $H^+$ receptors and mechanoreceptors (35), may be involved also in the reflex inhibition of abomasal motility.

The inhibition of abomasal motility in response to fat in the duodenum is not completely removed after vagotomy and involves the forestomach motility and the normal patterns of feeding (238) and rumination. In sheep the initial period of feeding is abbreviated by a duodenal infusion of 100 ml of peanut oil. It is sometimes reduced to one-half of that observed in control animals. This reduced period of feeding was usually succeeded by a period of rumination, but thereafter there was only desultory eating with short periods of rumination and long periods of inactivity. Intensive feeding commonly resumed 3–4 h after the infusion ended (230).

In an attempt to determine the region of the intestine sensitive to the fatty acid emulsion, it was found that oleic or linoleic emulsions pumped into a cannula beyond the drainage of bile have only slightly less inhibitory effects than similar infusions given through a cannula just beyond the pylorus (164).

*Control of Gastric Emptying*

MILK-FED ANIMALS. Excitatory and inhibitory effects of gastric motility and emptying originating in the duodenum have been demonstrated by infusion with hypotonic, hypertonic, and acid solutions. These actions are not limited to simple molecules because direct introduction of milk and milk fat into the intestine caused profound slowing of gastric emptying and reduction in gastric secretion (6). Secretin and glucagon infusions reduced the electrical spiking activity of the abomasum and inhibited emptying and acid secretion (13, 14). Cholecystokinin also inhibited gastric emptying but was dissimilar in that acid secretion was stimulated. By reducing antral motility, the inhibitory effect of CCK on gastric motility would contribute to the associated slowing in gastric emptying in the calf. In addition, because secretin and pancreatic glucagon are increased in the plasma after duodenal infusion of HCl, they are candidates for the physiological mediation of the gastric inhibition in the calf that results from duodenal acidification (15). Finally, insulin stimulated the secretion of acid and increased the gastric emptying, despite an initial inhibitory effect at higher doses. So strong was the later stimulation of abomasal motility after insulin infusion that virtually no meal remained in the abomasum at 45 min. The marked stimulation of motor activity in the body and antral regions of the abomasum, which became evident 25–30 min after the commencement of the administration of insulin, is compatible with the course of events that led to lowered blood glucose and vagal excitation (147). The initial inhibitory effect on gastric emptying of insulin at high doses may possibly be because of the release of small amounts of glucagon during the stimulation of the secretion of acid by insulin (147).

Two major factors affect the well-controlled pattern of abomasal emptying in milk-fed animals, i.e., unweaned ruminants (186): *1*) the amount of milk intake and *2*) the modalities of feeding, i.e., teat versus bucket feeding. Intakes of 2 kg of milk do not appreciably affect the cyclical pattern of abomasal motility because an outflow of 2.8 kg during 6 h is accompanied by a total of six MMCs. The pattern of cumulative digesta flow through the proximal duodenum registered by an electromagnetic flow probe inserted into a reentrant duodenal cannula, after the animal was fed 2 kg of milk, presents six periodic interruptions in flow that probably correspond to the phases of quiescence of the MMCs.

When 6 kg of milk are given, there are considerable increases in rates of gastric outflow, indicating a disturbance of the mechanisms regulating digesta movement. For the first 3 h after the 6-kg intake, no periodic interruption in flow could be seen, and the rate of emptying, by slope calculation, was more rapid, corresponding to an outflow of 3.5 kg. This apparent upset in gastric outflow was thus related to a notable change in the frequency of myoelectric activity at the antrum and pylorus, suggesting a feeding pattern of activity. From 3 to 6 h after the 6-kg intake, the pattern of digesta flow presents again periodic interruptions corresponding to the quiescent phases of MMCs. An outflow of 2.5 kg during 3 h was accompanied by 4–5 MMCs (207).

Concurrent recordings of digesta flow and electrical activity (Fig. 32) show that the period of high rate of abomasal emptying is related to the presence of strong spike bursts in the proximal duodenum and that the number of such propulsive waves is directly related to the amount of fluid propelled (40). The aforementioned results suggest that the main factor involved in the regulation of the gastric outflow of milk is the amount ingested, which in turn stimulates the antro-duodenal motor activity to cause an increase in the number of propulsive waves, an increase in frequency of MMCs and, if necessary, obliteration of the phases of quiescence (208).

Secretory and motor responses can be affected by the modalities of feeding, i.e., teat versus bucket feeding. Raw whole milk when taken from a nipple by a calf is transformed into large curd particles and whey with a watery appearance, whereas direct administration in the abomasum results in small curd particles and milky whey, suggesting an incomplete coagulation. Teat feeding appears to increase both salivary and gastric secretion compared with bucket feeding the same amount of milk (258). The pH values measured continuously within the pylorus are increased by 30%–50% for ~2 h after raw milk is sucked from a nipple, even if the gastric acid secretion is stimulated by pentagastrin infusion. No changes occur when the same amount of milk is taken from a bucket or when a solution of casein or soya protein is sucked from a nipple. The area below the pH curve after sucking corresponds to ~10 g of sodium bicarbonate, i.e., approximately the secretion of 0.8 liter of saliva compared with nil after drinking. The abomasal motor responses are markedly different after bucket feeding. There is an overall uniform and long-lasting increased spiking activity on the antrum and the duodenal bulb without changes within the fundus. In contrast, teat feeding induces a transient inhibition of the spiking activity of the fundus followed by the occurrence of several propulsive waves across the pylorus during the period of high pH and finally a pattern of activity at a slightly higher level than before feeding.

These results suggest that the motor functions of the abomasum in the milk-fed animals may depend on the amount of oral nutrients and on the way they reach the stomach (5, 66). Intense salivary secretion

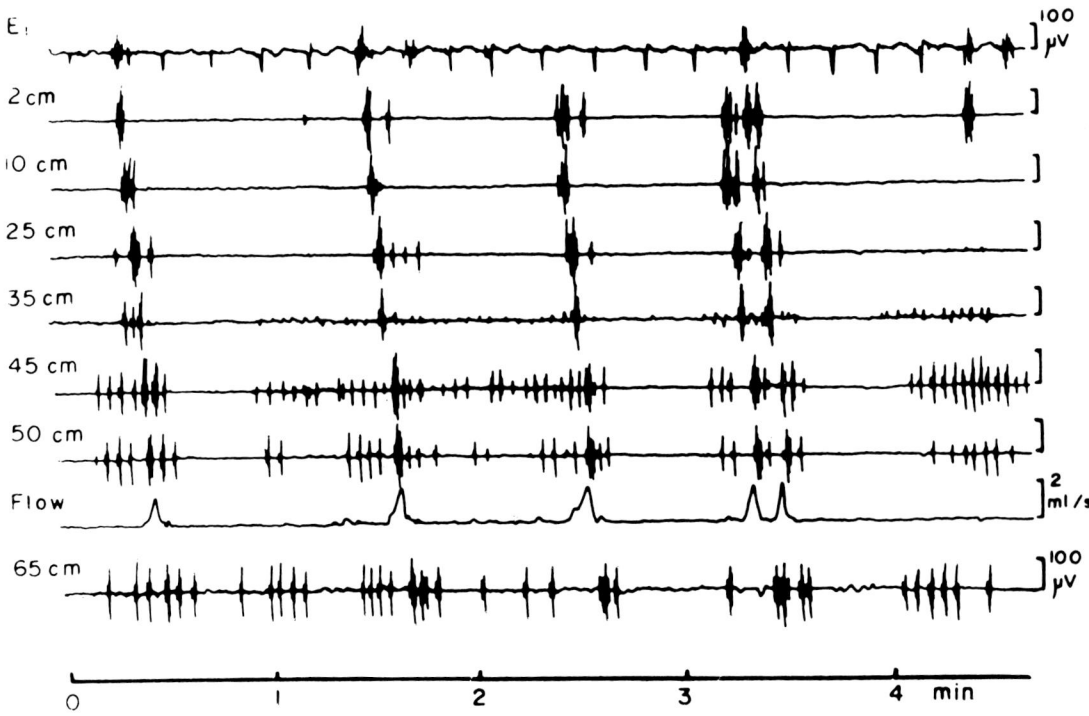

FIG. 32. Duodenal myoelectrical activity from 8 electrode sites placed 2 cm orad to pylorus ($E_1$) and along duodenum, indicative of postprandial propulsive waves in the calf. Flow probe was fixed around duodenum 65 cm aborad to pylorus. Four propulsive waves are seen propagating away from pylorus where their corresponding spike bursts differed by a higher amplitude and longer duration from the others at sites 45 and 65 cm from pylorus. [Adapted from Dardillat (39).]

is elicited by sucking, as by feeding (174), and hence well-buffered contents flowed through the pylorus. This can be part of the mechanisms of duodenal origin that facilitate gastric emptying (147).

ADULT RUMINANTS. The fact that antral peristalsis is stimulated in response to the distension of the gastric wall and that receptors send impulses over afferent fibers to the brain, which in turn relays impulses back to the stomach by way of the vagi to stimulate contraction, is apparently masked in adult ruminants by the continuous delivery of reticulorumen contents to the abomasum.

The gastrogastric reflex, along with any myogenic contractile activity that might be elicited directly in response to muscle stretch, provides the excitation required to empty the stomach of its contents after feeding or drinking in monogastric species; however, these are inoperative in adult ruminants. One of the major factors influencing the rate of delivery of liquid reticulorumen contents into the abomasum and thus the passage of digesta through the abomasum is the level of dietary intake (89). Long-term studies of the motor activity of the abomasum in sheep fed ad libitum compared with intake restricted to 25%–85% of the voluntary intake show a linear relationship between the abomasal volume and emptying with the level of food intake. The magnitude of antral spiking activity increases and the length of the quiescent period decreases with increases in food intake and abomasal outflow (81). Because the duodenal frequency of MMCs was unaffected by the level of food intake, the rate of gastric evacuation varies directly with the level of spiking activity, an effect probably related to the volume of contents and thus the degree of distension of the stomach. The frequency and the number of propulsive waves in the duodenum during the prolonged irregular spiking activity phases also increase with the level of food intake, suggesting that the abomasum behaves mostly as a reservoir of liquid contents accommodating upward or downward changes in volume by variations in the magnitude of the antral contractions. The relatively steady composition of the gastric liquid contents delivered into the duodenal bulb favors the concept that the capacity of the duodenum to handle the volume of chyme is the main factor regulating antral motility and gastric outflow.

In adult ruminants, ingested water is delivered into the reticulorumen, except in very dehydrated animals. In this case, water is directed toward the abomasum. A sheep weighing 60 kg with no access to water can drink 10% of its body weight within 2 min, resulting in gastric overload. The motor responses corresponding to the emptying of 2 liters of water consist of an increase by 200%–300% of the antral spiking activity, the triggering of a RSA-like phase of activity on the duodenum without antral inhibition, and the occurrence of a high number of duodenal propulsive waves during 45–60 min (Fig. 33). This observation further suggests the concept that the ability of increased gastric emptying by quantitative changes in its motor activity generously exceeds the usual requirements.

To summarize, the abomasal outflow in the adult ruminant seems closely controlled by a complex local nervous network in which the most obvious manifestation of the interaction between the stomach and the intestine is an inhibition of antral myoelectrical activity that coincides with the cyclical development during 3–4 min of maximal spiking activity on the duodenal bulb (196). A similar antral inhibition is seen when the proximal duodenum develops continuous maximal spiking activity in response to moderate distension. Once the duodenum empties, propulsive waves are seen on both the antrum and duodenal bulbs. Such an activity is effective as long as the volume of the gastric fundus is kept constant. The effect of the propulsive waves propagated aborally at a high velocity on the proximal duodenum is the transfer of chyme beyond the duodenal flexure, avoiding any further distension of the duodenal bulb. The emptiness of the duodenal bulb reservoir in turn stimulates the motor activity of the fundus. Conversely a delay in gastric emptying reflexly inhibits the reticulorumen delivery of contents to the abomasum, hence the forestomach fullness and anorexia.

Conceivably in such a context the role of hormones (85, 229) is difficult to assess. For example, it is well documented that anorexia in sheep infected by nematodes coincides with high plasma levels of CCK (219). It is likely that CCK exerts its satiety action peripherally, probably in the upper gastrointestinal tract, by

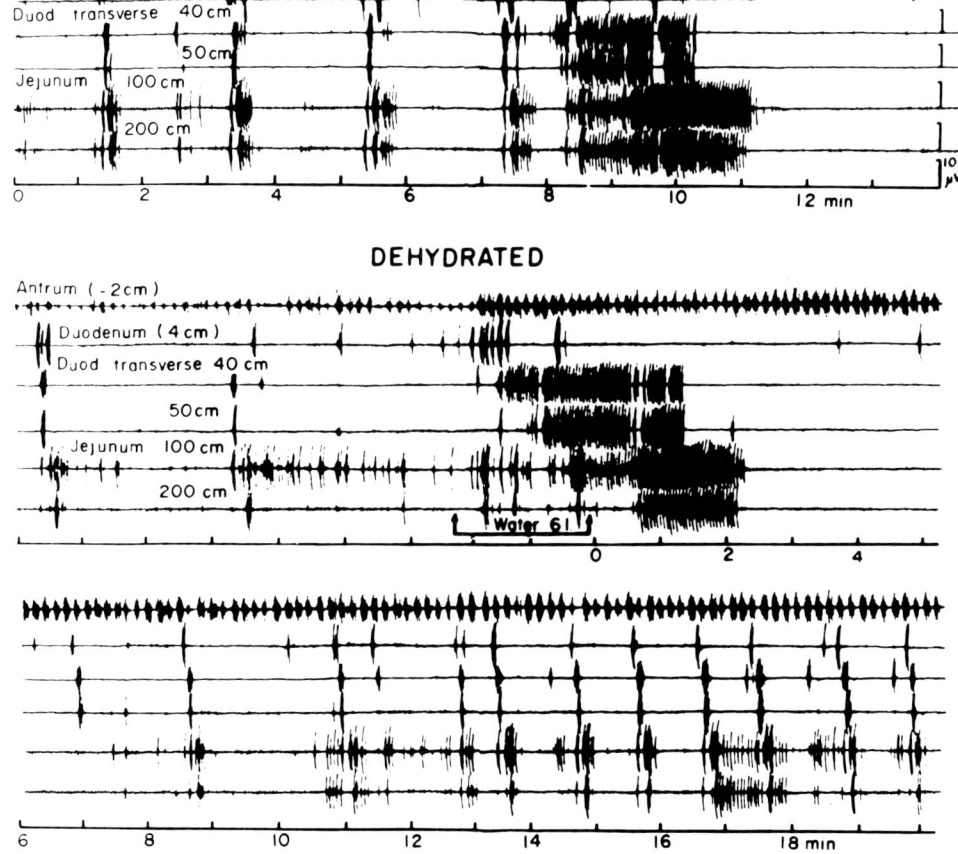

FIG. 33. Relationship between antroduodenal myoelectrical activity and fluid propulsion in a 60-kg sheep. *Top traces* show end of a phase of irregular spiking activity with propulsive waves at 2-min intervals and regular spiking activity (RSA) followed by quiescence on both antrum and duodenum in a fully fed sheep. *Middle traces* are from a dehydrated animal without access to water for 72 h. Drinking increases antral spike activity and triggers occurrence of an RSA-like activity phase with propulsive waves at less than 1-min intervals corresponding to propulsion of water along upper part of small intestine. *Bottom traces* show persistence of these patterns 6 to 18 min after drinking.

delaying abomasal emptying and then the reticulorumen contents outflow, which inhibits food intake.

Responses in sheep to duodenal acidification are graded according to the amount of acid introduced (23) but do not lead to neutralization of duodenal contents that are still about pH 4.5 in the region caudal to the point of entry of the pancreaticobiliary duct (Fig. 31). The threshold pH for the operation of the duodenal secretion mechanisms still has to be determined, and thus the biological significance of the reduction of gastric emptying in calves (147) or food intake in sheep (85) during the infusion of secretin at $0.5 \text{ U} \cdot \text{kg}^{-1} \cdot \text{h}^{-1}$ is difficult to assess.

The release of gastrin and pancreatic polypeptide has been demonstrated in calves after stimulation of the vagus and splanchnic nerves (1). In sheep, direct evidence of vagal control of gastrin release has been obtained, and both gastrin and pancreatic polypeptide levels in the blood rose after insulin hypoglycemia (229). However, the inhibitory effects of the reticuloruminal contractions (Fig. 17) of infusion of gastrin (87) and the short-lived stimulation preceding a long-lasting inhibition of the antroduodenal motor activity (194) are probably pharmacological responses because no such abnormal motor patterns are seen in sheep with high plasma levels of gastrin infected by nematodes.

The blood concentration of somatostatin rises in lambs after suckling and in adult sheep after provision of fresh food, and immunization against somatostatin has been tested as a potential means of stimulating food intake. The inhibition of antral motility induced by the administration of exogenous somatostatin (194) is in agreement with the decrease in all postomasal gut tissues observed after a 6-day infusion (70).

Finally, it has been demonstrated that the inhibition (i.e., the opening) of the reticulo-omasal orifice during sucking (see Fig. 20, lower part, for the concomitant inhibition of reticular contractions) can be produced by the infusion of vasoactive intestinal peptide (VIP). The effects are observed by close intra-arterial infusion of VIP at concentrations not exceeding those found in effluent blood from the orifice region during vagal stimulation (229). The possible role of VIP as a neurotransmitter released by the stimulation of the vagus nerves and by sucking emphasizes the importance of synergism between hormonal and nervous controls in the regulation of gastrointestinal function. Furthermore it is possible, although not demonstrated, that, as recently shown for the gastric fundus in the rat (135), VIP rather than ATP is the neurotransmitter involved in the nonadrenergic, noncholinergic vagal inhibition.

## SMALL INTESTINE MOTILITY

The ruminant small intestine is a highly specialized structure adapted to propel continuously large amounts of liquid chyme (96, 114) over distances of 20 m in sheep and 40 m in cattle. The electrical basis for the occurrence of intestinal contractions of the circular muscle as a moving ring has been elucidated as slow waves present all the time at any location of the small intestine at a rhythm that is fixed for a given segment of the bowel. If spike potentials are superimposed on the slow waves, then the bowel wall contracts. This was identified in the thick-walled small intestine of fasted dogs as an electric complex characterized by a front of intense spiking activity, in which each slow wave has superimposed spike potentials, and that migrates down the entire small bowel, indicates that the occurrence of spike potentials was organized in a periodic manner with the subsequent phase I, slow waves; phase II, some slow waves with spike potentials; and phase III, each slow wave with spike potentials. From an electromyographic viewpoint, phases I, II, and III were more appropriately called no spiking activity (NSA), ISA, and RSA, respectively. Such cyclical activity in which phases I, II, and III last 10, 80, and 5 min, respectively, persists only as long as a dog is fasting and as long as the contents to be propelled do not exceed 20-30 ml/h. Feeding disrupts the recurrence of these MMCs and changes the interdigestive MMCs or fasted pattern into a pattern of continuous activity resembling phase II (ISA) and termed the fed pattern associated with the propulsion of 100-150 ml/h of contents along an intestine 2-3 m long. The nature of this cyclical pattern of motor activity suggests a propulsive activity restricted to the digestive secretions and debris because the pattern of MMCs apparently disappears after a large meal in monogastric species or in milk-fed preruminants.

### Periodic Activity

Unlike in dogs where the volume of duodenojejunal contents is scanty, the vertically positioned duodenum in sheep is continuously flooded by liquid chyme with a percentage of dry matter not exceeding 4%. The passage of digesta (~300 ml/h) from the pylorus to the ileum, i.e., along 25 m in a sheep, is assumed regardless of feeding by the regular repetition and propagation along the thin-walled intestine (115, 177) of the RSA phase preceded by a long period of ISA and followed by a short period of quiescence (NSA). The part of the MMCs during which spike potentials are regularly superimposed on consecutive slow waves for 4-6 min (phase III or RSA phase) is initiated near the pylorus (193) and propagated in a caudad direction at a high velocity. As shown in Figure 34, the longer the small intestine the higher the velocity of propagation of the RSA phases among the ruminant species. The RSA phase thus takes approximately the same time to propagate along the small intestine of a goat and a cow.

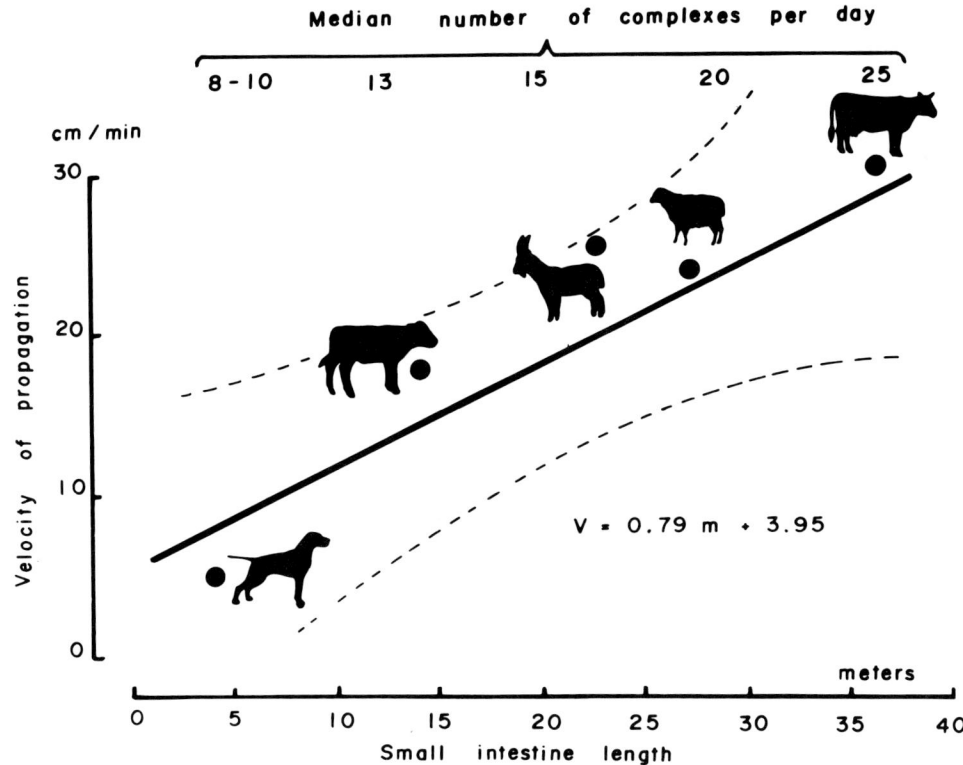

FIG. 34. Relationship between the velocity of propagation of myoelectric complexes (regular spiking activity phases) and length of small intestine. Median daily number of jejunal complexes is high in ruminants and low in carnivores because of obliterating effect of feeding in latter species.

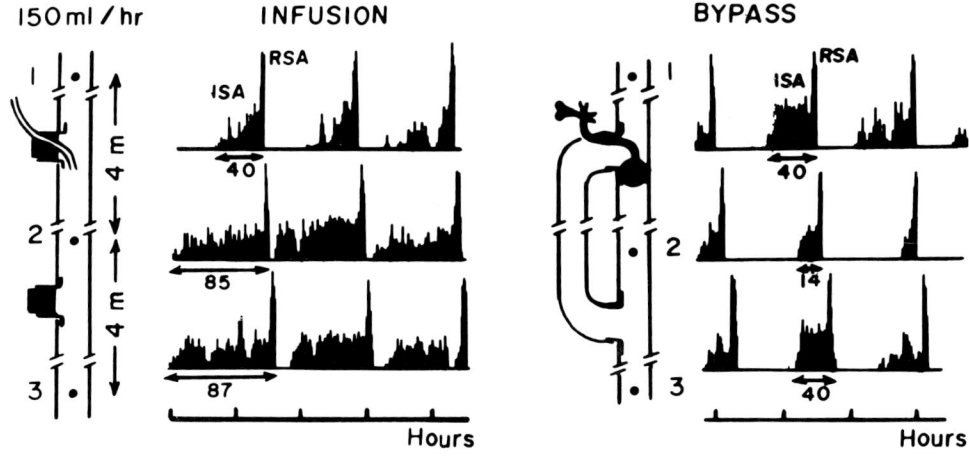

FIG. 35. Effect of digestive bulk on pattern of mitigating myoelectric complexes in a sheep fitted with 2 cannulas at an interval of 4 m on jejunum. Electrode sites were 2 m orad and aborad to each cannula. Flow bypass of segment of 4 m markedly reduced duration of phase of irregular spiking activity (ISA) at site 2 and to a much lesser extent at site 3. Duration of ISA was doubled at both sites 2 and 3 after infusion of 150 ml/h of contents. RSA, regular spiking activity.

Another characteristic of the periodic motor activity associated with a high propulsive activity over long distances is the tendency to react to excessive loading in several ways. These include the increase of the ISA phase at the expense of the NSA phase especially on the middle jejunum and an increase in their velocity of propagation. On a normal regimen of hay, offered ad libitum, with a mean food intake of ~600 g/day, the mean duodenal flow of digesta does not exceed 292 ± 67 ml/h in a sheep weighing 40 kg (178). Concomitantly the intestinal motility exhibits from 12 to 14 complexes per day with a mean duration of

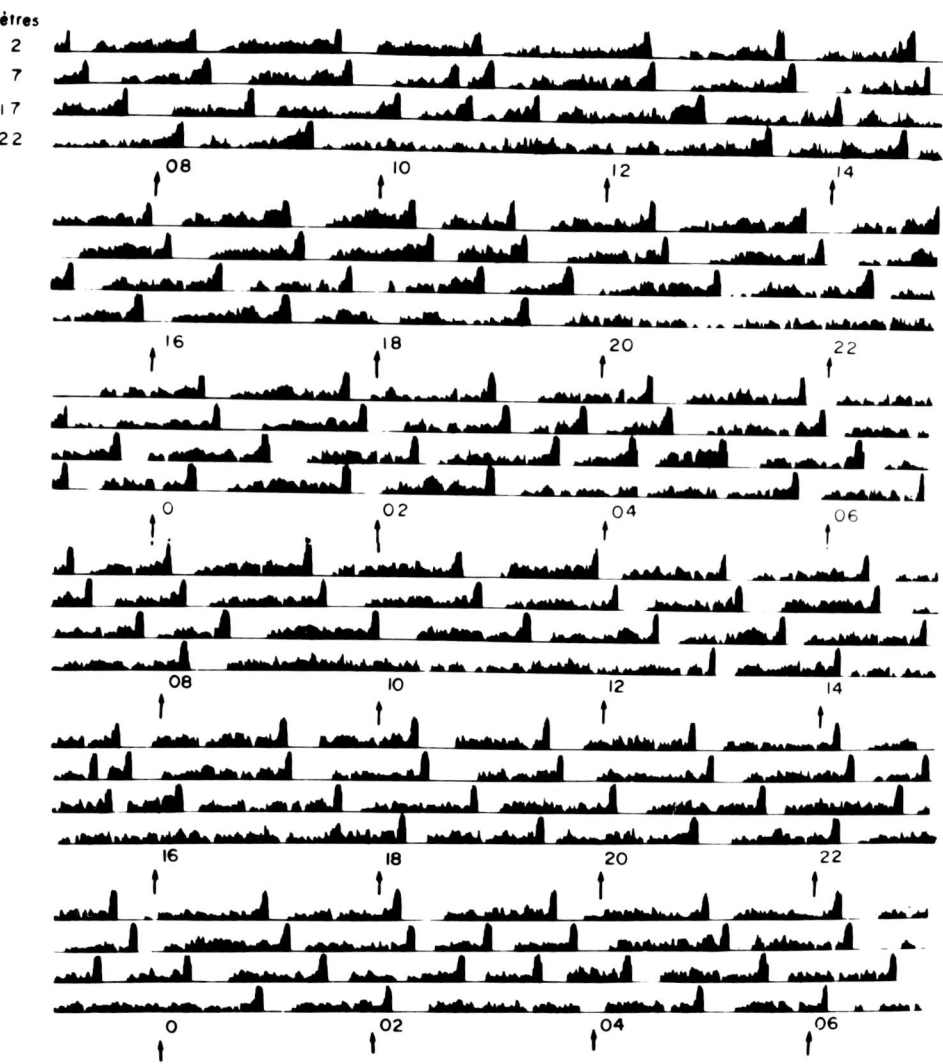

FIG. 36. Integrated record of electrical spiking activity during 48 h in sheep fed a normal diet of hay. Electrode sites at 2, 7, 17, and 22 m from pylorus. Number of mitigating myoelectric complexes is 36.8% less in ileum than in duodenum (12 vs. 19).

50 min and 5 min for the phases of ISA and RSA, respectively. The complexes are propagated from the duodenum to the ileum at a mean velocity of 19 cm/min, with the highest value occurring at the proximal part of the small intestine. The transit time is ~140 min, with only seven complexes reaching the ileum. When the mean food intake is 1,200 g (33), the mean duration of the ISA and RSA phases of the complex is increased to 85 and 7.5 min, respectively. An equal number of MMCs is seen propagated from the duodenum to the ileum at a mean velocity of 34 cm/min, hence a reduction of transit time to ~100 min.

The concept that the propulsion along the small intestine is directly mediated by the pattern of MMCs is also based on the fact that the duration of the ISA phase is directly related to the volume of luminal contents (Fig. 35). Furthermore, ontogenetic development of the motor function in ruminants shows a very early pattern of nonpropagated cyclical motor events during prenatal life that resembles the pattern of MMCs only a few days before birth (199). This coincides with an increased retention of amniotic fluid in the gut lumen and is recorded as an increase by 20% of the slow-wave frequency and by 40% of associated spike potentials in the fetal lamb (191). In ruminants the main function of the MMCs, which are omnipresent and fade out near the ileum (Fig. 36), thus seems to command via the level of ISA the rate of passage of digesta in front of the intestinal segment occluded by the RSA phase. This is similar to what is seen for digestive secretions and debris during the interdigestive period in dogs with a thick-walled intestine, in pigs maintained on numerous daily meals, and in the fetal lamb just prior to birth.

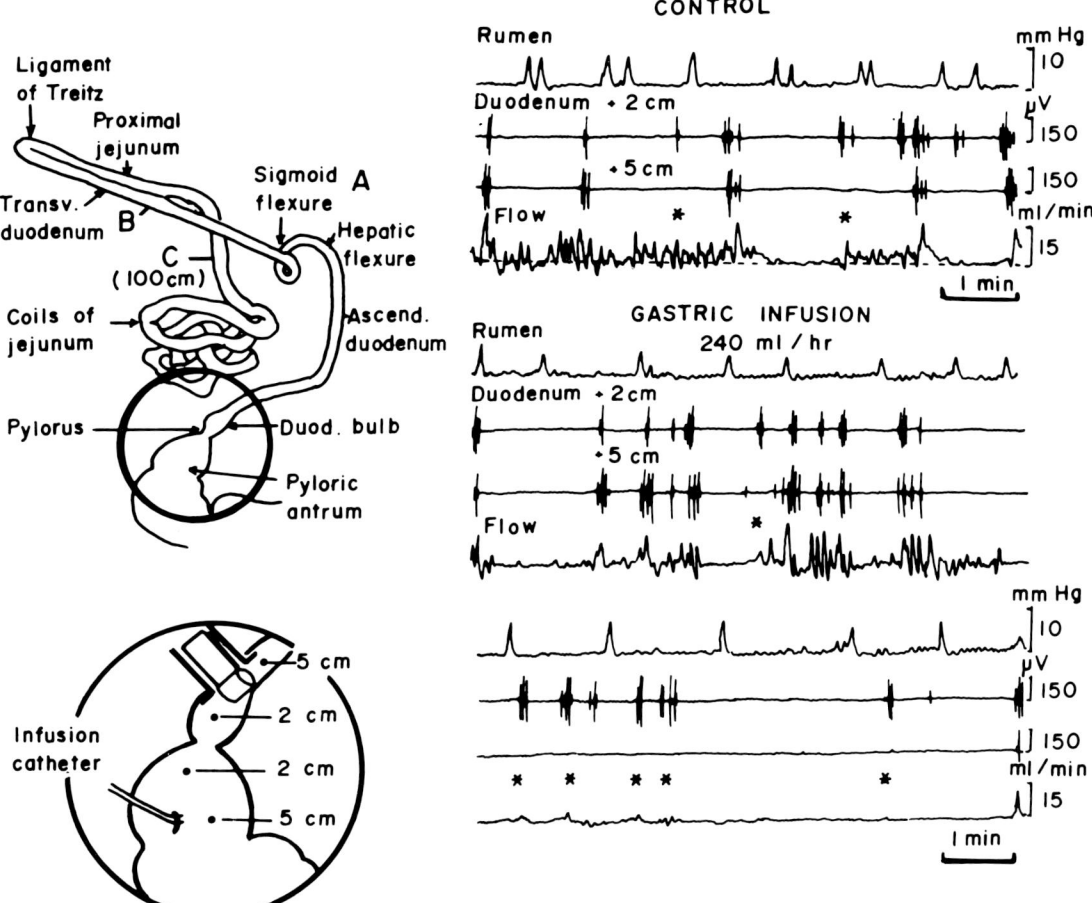

FIG. 37. Radiographic anatomy of proximal duodenum in vertical position until hepatic flexure (*A*), transverse duodenum (*B*), and jejunum (*C*). *Insert* shows position of flow probe inserted in a T-shaped cannula on duodenal bulb and the catheter required to infuse a protein solution at a fixed rate of 240 ml/h. Duodenal spiking activity associated with propulsion of fluids as gushes is characterized by bursts of spike potentials propagated along duodenal bulb. In hay-fed sheep (control) and during gastric infusion, no flow was recorded when bursts of spike potentials remained localized to duodenal bulb (*asterisks*).

*Mixing Versus Propelling Activity*

Simultaneous radiocinematographic and electromyographic studies in fully fed sheep show that propulsion is absent during quiescence (phase I or NSA) and almost nullified during phase III or RSA. Propulsive contractions are spread over distances of 40–60 cm during phase II or ISA. The activity front (phase III or RSA) is composed of a series of consecutive peristaltic contractions passing rapidly along the 10–20 cm of bowel displaying the RSA phase with a progression velocity much faster in the duodenum (40 cm/min) than in the jejunum (30 cm/min) and ileum (20 cm/min). The efficiency of this periodic pattern as a propelling system can be reinforced by an increased velocity of propagation of the MMCs along the intestine and/or the increase of the ISA phase at the expense of the NSA phase.

The part of the pattern of MMCs that behaves as a mixing system is that of the multiple rings of contractions developed during the RSA phase. This activity has a tendency to increase in duration when the luminal contents are decreased, whereas the ISA phase is almost reduced to nil. Such a physiological situation is realized in ruminants during the perinatal period when comparisons are made between the pattern of MMCs the day before birth in the fetal lamb, when the amniotic fluid is not propelled down the large intestine, and the pattern of MMCs of the 5- to 10-day-old suckling neonate. The mixing activity is characterized in the fetus by a higher percentage of orally propagated contractions (10% vs. 3%) and a lower velocity of propagation of the RSA phase (1.9 cm/min vs. 4–12 cm/min). No major changes in the duration of the spiking activity that occupies ~50% of the recording time are observed, but it should be men-

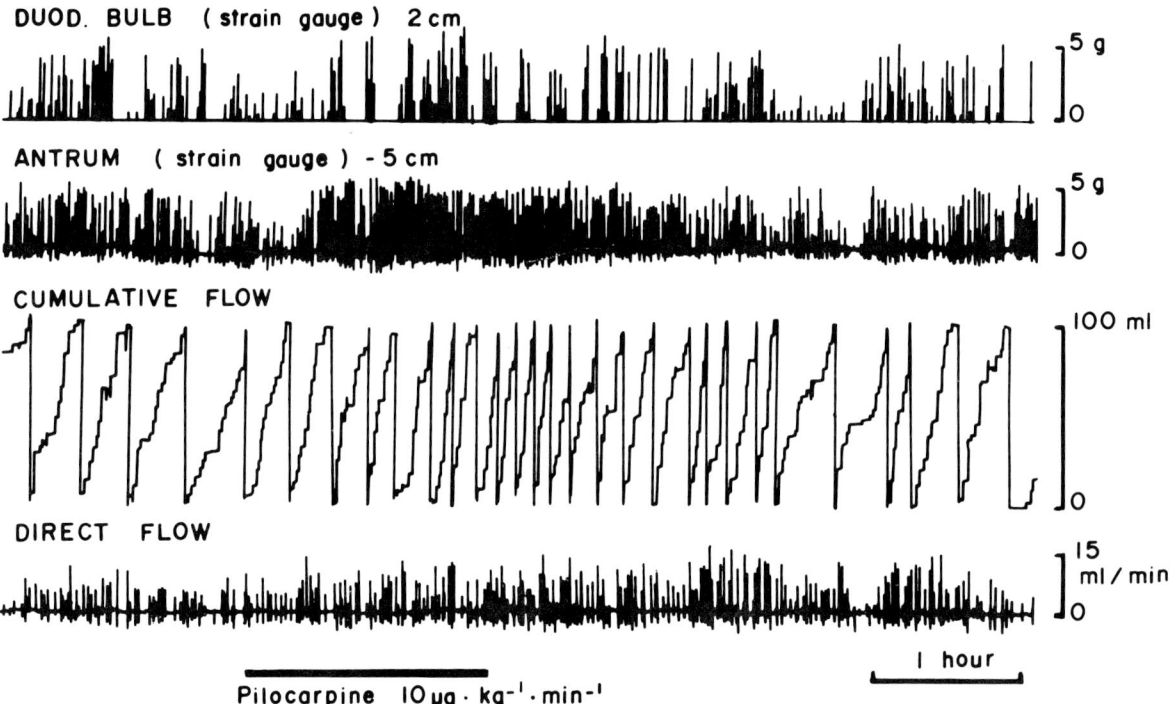

FIG. 38. Changes in flow of digesta along proximal duodenum induced by cholinergic stimulation of antroduodenal junction in a sheep under continuous abomasal infusion of a casein solution at a fixed rate of 240 ml/h. Note high rate of flow associated with duodenal bulb stimulation. Duod. bulb, duodenal bulb.

tioned that the length of the small intestine is only 8.9 m in the fetus versus 11–12 m 1 wk after birth (191).

### Motor Function of Duodenal Bulb

The common use of reentrant duodenal cannulas in sheep (88, 96, 114), calves (14, 147, 207), or cows (34, 243, 246) has shown that low pressure beyond the pylorus due to sampling stimulates the gastric outflow otherwise strongly reduced by the cannulation system. Such inconveniences are now avoided by flowmetry, which uses ringlike probes inserted into single T-shaped cannulas (177, 178). In sheep fed once daily, the mean flow rate of digesta at the postpyloric level increases by 30% when fed the same ration 3 times daily. This was due to an enhanced salivary and gastric secretion because the dry matter intake and pyloric outflow were similar.

The flow of digesta evaluated by a flowmeter just beyond the duodenal bulb (Fig. 37) occurs as gushes of 6–20 ml every 0.5–1.2 min separated by periods of no flow during the phases of antroduodenal quiescence. The increased flow of digesta corresponding to a same amount of food given 3 times daily resulted in gushes of greater volume rather than higher frequency and in a lower percentage of contractions localized to the duodenal bulb. This indicates that the duodenal bulb accommodates the increased gastric outflow by little or no variation of the frequency of contractions but by their aboral propagation.

When sheep are totally nourished by ruminal volatile fatty acids and abomasal casein infusion at the constant rate of 240 ml/h (171), continuous measurement of the duodenal flow shows periods of low flow, especially at night during sleep (189). Conversely, nonpropagation of duodenal bulb contractions reflects the decrease in flow rate of digesta (Fig. 37). In this model of liquid digesta infused at a constant rate in the stomach, the resulting pressure gradient between the antrum and the duodenal bulb seems to be the major factor in determining the transpyloric flow rate of digesta. Prerequisites for this are the relaxed state and low resting tone of the ovine pyloric sphincter.

The continuous manometric study of the pyloric activity by changes in fiberoptic light transmission and sleeve pressure shows that the pylorus closes as a functional appendage of the terminal antrum and in association with the duodenal bulb contractions (195) (Fig. 38). More precisely these closures of the pyloric sphincter may favor the one-way clearance through the gastroduodenal junction. Accordingly the infusion of cholinomimetic agents at very low dosages, which stimulates the antrum more intensively than the duodenal bulb contractile activity (196), is accompanied by an increased volume of liquid digesta propelled through the duodenal bulb.

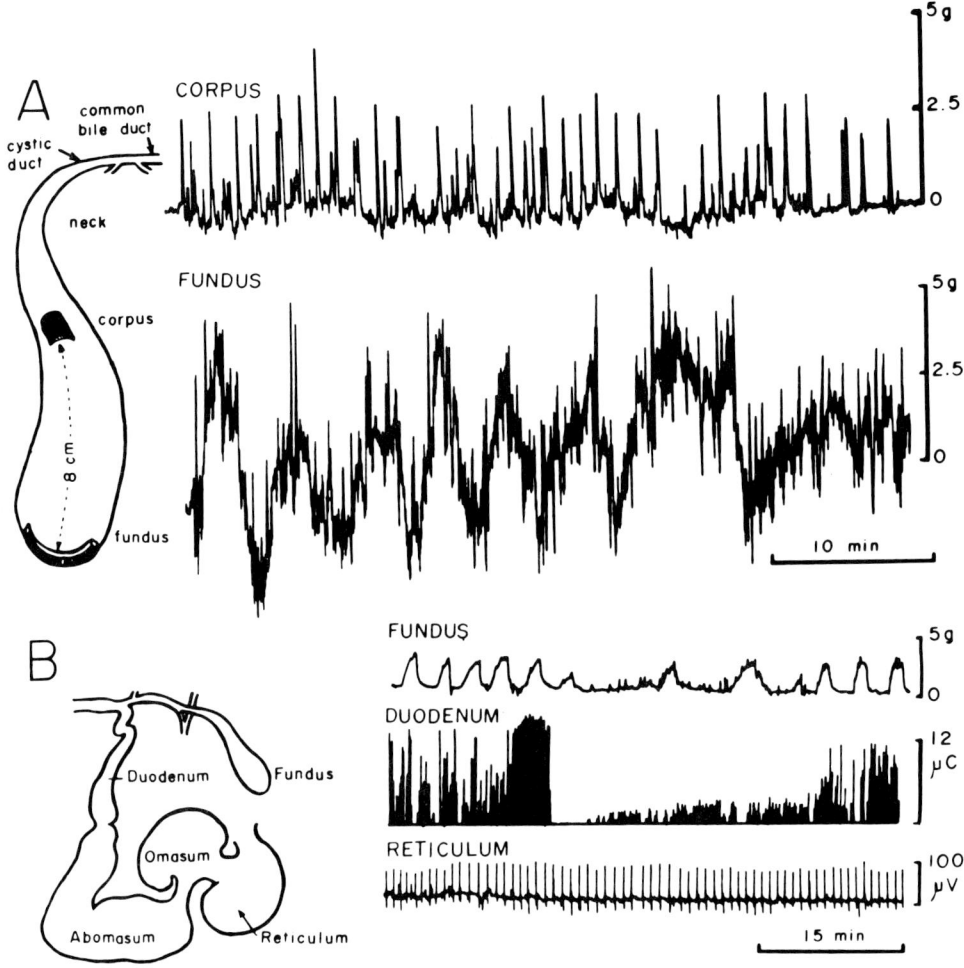

FIG. 39. *A*: diagram of ovine gallbladder with strain-gauge force transducers sewn on fundus and corpus at 8 cm from short cystic duct and common bile duct. Note cyclical changes in smooth muscle tone. *B*: nichrome wires were fixed on reticulum and transverse duodenum 20 cm beyond bile duct. Changes in fundus and corpus tone (direct record) occurred during phases of irregular and regular spiking activity of transverse duodenum (integrated record) and ceased during phase of quiescence.

*Pancreaticobiliary Secretions*

Collections from chronic duodenal and pancreatic fistulas in the sheep have shown that 10 liters of mixed bile and pancreatic juice enter the duodenum each day (97). As in dogs the gut motility may act as a triggering factor for the rhythmic and tonic contractions of the gallbladder (23). The tonic contractions of the fundus occur at an hourly frequency of 8–10, except during the periods of quiescence of the MMCs (Fig. 39*B*). There exists also a relation between the rhythmic contractions of the gallbladder and the propulsive waves propagated along the proximal duodenum (Fig. 39*A*). The process of eating in fasted sheep or even the sight of oats after an overnight fast increases the frequency of reticular contractions and both rhythmic and tonic contractions of the gallbladder, thus suggesting the importance of a neural pathway for gallbladder motility. The excitatory effects on gallbladder and antroduodenal motility are mimicked by pilocarpine and blocked by atropine. However, CCK-8 and caerulein elicit motor responses of the gallbladder in a dose-related manner without antroduodenal stimulation, whereas pentagastrin induces gallbladder motor responses with concomitant stimulation of the antroduodenal area. Therefore feeding may act to trigger gallbladder motor activity through a mechanism related to the increased antroduodenal activity, but direct effects of CCK-8 and caerulein confirm that gallbladder motor function also may be mediated through specific receptor sites (197).

The rate of secretion of pancreatic juice for adult sheep averages 3.1 ml/15 min (142). The volume of juice secreted is briefly increased by vagal stimulation, whereas greater responses are obtained by the injection of pilocarpine or secretin. It seems that the pH of solutions introduced into the duodenum more readily influences the quantity of juice secreted and its amylase content because stimulating effect of such solutions is reduced as the H⁺ concentration of the solution decreases (142, 201-203).

*Nervous Control*

Several observations indicate that extrinsic nerves have only a regulatory function because the pattern of MMCs persists after section of the splanchnic and/or vagus nerves. The daily number of MMCs decreases from 18 to 13 after splanchnectomy and rises from 18 to 25 after total extrinsic denervation. The permissive role of the vagus nerves is partially shown by the reduction in duration of the ISA phase after vagotomy and the slower velocity of propagation (Fig. 40). In a recent study using radiography and electromyography in conscious sheep before and after total thoracic vagotomy (81), it was found that vagotomy does not prevent the migration of the MMCs but reduces the rate of propagation of the RSA phase from 40.5 to 16.7 cm/min in the duodenum (Table 6). Furthermore, duodenal infusion of 0.5-3 mmol HCl (0.035-0.1 M HCl), which induces premature duodenal RSA phases within 1-7 min when infused at 20 min after a natural RSA phase, was not active after vagotomy. Thus the role of the vagus nerves is to contribute to the regulation of the frequency and propagation of the MMCs in sheep. Duodenal acidification is not essential nor is it the normal stimulus for initiation of RSA phases, but duodenal infusion of HCl or hyperosmolar NaCl can trigger a premature duodenal RSA phase via the vagus nerves.

*5-Hydroxytryptamine*

It has been demonstrated that several agents such as motilin, morphine, bovine pancreatic polypeptide, and somatostatin can initiate phase III-like activity prematurely (Table 7). However, such compounds do not reset the enteric basic biological clock controlling the cycles of MMCs at a faster rhythm as was recently observed by using lysergic acid derivatives administered either locally or by the systemic route (190).

The increment in daily number of MMCs is consistent with the hypothesis that 5-HT neurotransmission plays a major role in the physiological organization of the ultradian timing of the cycles of MMCs acting locally via the enteric nervous system and/or the smooth muscle cells (Fig. 41). When the period of RSA of the cycle of MMCs on the duodenal bulb is considered as the indicator for the timing of cyclic events in the sheep, it is obvious that the effect is more pronounced at this site. This is in agreement with the antroduodenal origin of MMCs in the ovine species (193) and the high concentrations of neurotransmitters at this level (254). Comparison of the effects of methysergide in the ovine model with other species indicates a rather specific response in the ruminant species, which always exhibit an enhancement of the cyclic motor activity instead of only an increased activity, e.g., as in dogs. A possible explanation is that the activity of the duodenal bulb reservoir, which has a vertical configuration, is permanently triggered by volume distension in ruminants, hence a low threshold of excitability. Another peculi-

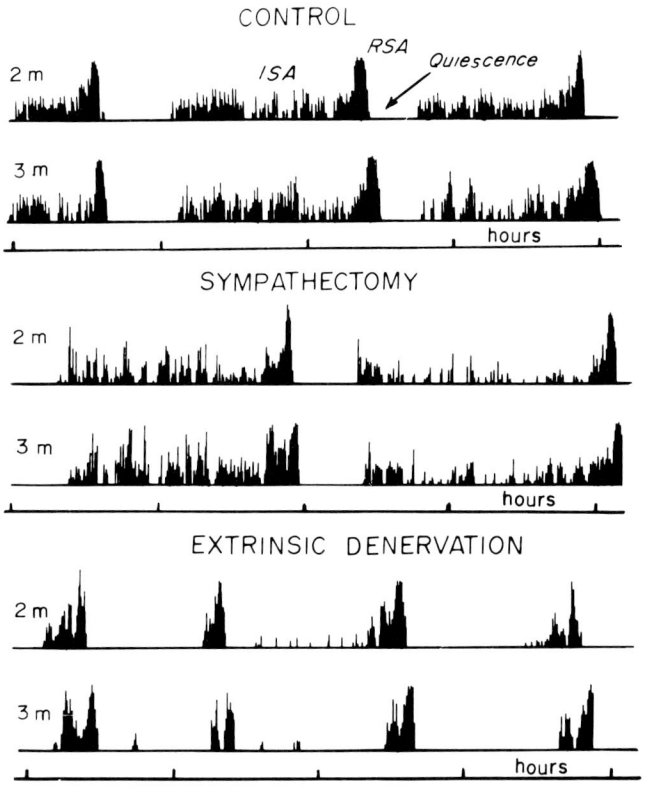

FIG. 40. Influence of splanchnic nerve section and additional bilateral vagotomy of phases of irregular spiking activity (ISA) and regular spiking activity (RSA) of cyclic motor events of ovine jejunum. Note reduced ISA after total denervation due to a functional stenosis of pylorus. *Tracings* are integrated records of electrical activity at 2 and 3 m from pylorus.

TABLE 6. *Influence of Vagotomy on Migrating Myoelectric Complexes in Sheep*

| | Time Between Consecutive RSA Phases, min | | | Rate of Propagation of RSA, cm/min | |
|---|---|---|---|---|---|
| | Control | 24 h after vagotomy | 1 wk after vagotomy | Control | 1 wk after vagotomy |
| Duodenum | 98.4 ± 6.8 | 23.4 ± 1.8 | 60.1 ± 3.1 | 40.5 ± 7.2 | 16.7 ± 0.1 |
| Jejunum | 68.9 ± 3.7 | 38.5 ± 3.9 | 63.4 ± 4.4 | 27.3 ± 4.1 | 16.6 ± 0.8 |
| Terminal ileum | 109.8 ± 6.1 | 64.2 ± 5.7 | 82.7 ± 11.1 | 21.4 ± 1.1 | 13.7 ± 0.7 |

RSA, regular spiking activity. [From Gregory et al. (82).]

TABLE 7. *Initiation of Phase III–Like Activities Propagated Along Proximal Duodenum in Sheep*

| Initiator | Dosage | Effect |
|---|---|---|
| Duodenal bulb acidification | 1 mmol HCl | Phase III blocked by atropine or prevented by local anesthesia |
| Duodenal hyperosmolarity | 5 ml NaCl, 30% | Propagated phase III not prevented by atropine |
| Serotonergic stimulation | | |
| 5-Hydroxytryptophan | 0.1 mg/kg iv | Series of phase III reinforced by methysergide pretreatment |
| 5-Hydroxytryptamine | 3 µg/kg iv | Long-lasting, dose-dependent phase III–like activity |
| Lysergic acid derivatives (methysergide, ergonovine) | Parenteral and enteral routes, 50 µg/kg | Reset at a faster rhythm of myoelectric motor complex pattern for 4–8 h |
| Opioid stimulation | | |
| Morphine | 0.1 mg/kg iv | Phase III followed by long-lasting quiescence |
| Trimebutine | 1 mg/kg iv | Short phase III |
| κ-Receptor agonists (ketazocine, U 50488) | 0.1 mg/kg iv | Long-lasting phase III without inhibition of the forestomach |
| Adrenergic and other triggering factors | | |
| $\alpha_2$-Receptor antagonists (tolazoline, idazoxan) | 1 mg/kg iv | Short phase III on the antrum and proximal duodenum |
| Dopamine | 0.3 mg/kg iv | Phase III slowly propagated |
| Isoprenaline (under cholinergic stimulation by bethanechol, carbachol, pilocarpine) | 1 µg/kg iv | Phase III–like activity evoked after inhibition during 4–5 min |
| Histamine (after chlorpheniramine pretreatment) | 30 µg/kg iv | Short-lasting phase III–like activity, restricted to the duodenum |
| Antibiotics (erythromycin, lincomycin, spiramycine) | Therapeutic doses, iv | Nonpropagated phase III |
| Hormonal and hormonelike peptide stimulants† | | |
| Somatostatin | 2.5 µg/kg iv | Duodenal stimulation accompanied by antral inhibition |
| Motilin | 10 µg/kg iv | Phase III on the mid-jejunum |
| Glucagon | 30 µg/kg iv | Stimulation of the pyloric segment |

iv, Intravenous.   * Reset at lower rhythm of pattern of migrating myoelectric complexes for 18–24 h was found for the 5-HT$_2$ antagonists ketanserin and ritanserin (0.1 mg/kg).   † Major site of activity of substances of the gastrin group, bombesin and prostaglandins, was found to be the antrum and not the duodenum.

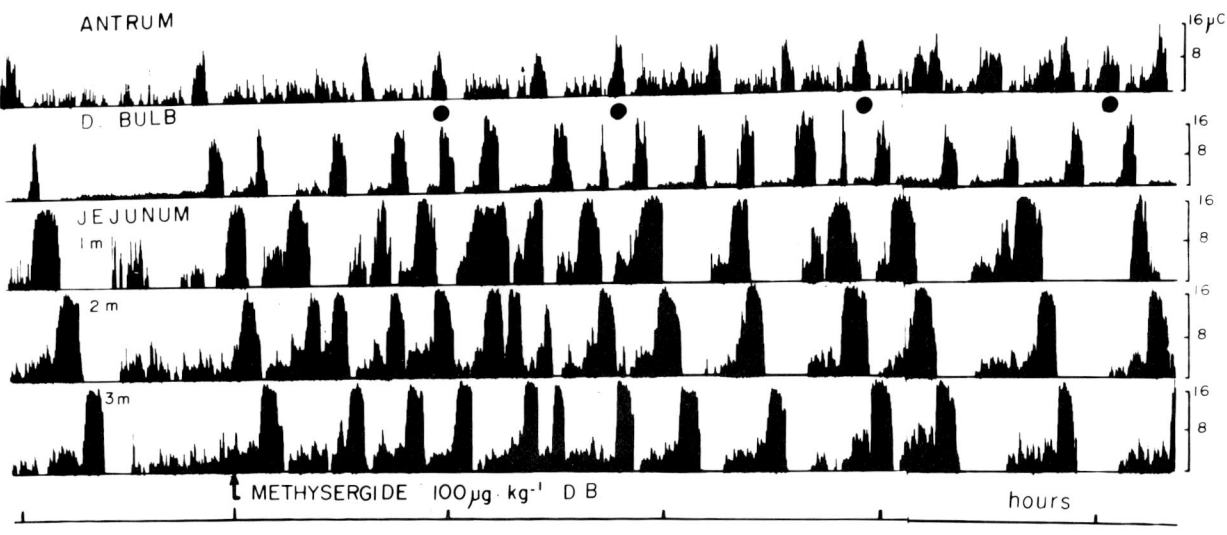

FIG. 41. Increment of frequency of migrating myoelectric complexes on ovine proximal small intestine after intraduodenal administration of methysergide. *Tracings* are integrated records of electrical spike activity from 1 electrode on pyloric antrum 4 cm proximal to pylorus, 1 electrode on duodenal bulb 4 cm distal to pylorus, and 3 electrodes on the jejunum at 1 m-intervals. Dots correspond to expected pattern of migrating myoelectric complexes without treatment. Effect is more pronounced at site of administration (duodenal bulb) where 11 more regular spiking activity phases are recorded than at antrum and jejunum (7–9 phase III).

arity of the ruminant small intestine, considered as a very efficient propulsive system compared with the dog, is the relatively low motor responses to the infusion of several gastrointestinal hormones. For example, there is circumstantial evidence that motilin is involved as the cause or the consequence in the initiation of MMCs because the plasma level of endogenous motilin changes cyclically in accordance with MMCs. In sheep the effects of the infusion of 10–100 times higher doses of motilin than required in dogs to initiate an RSA-like activity are only a transient increase in the magnitude of spiking activity.

The digestive upsets in ruminants associated with an obstruction of the upper part of the gastrointestinal tract are due to a variety of causes, such as intestinal intussusception, abomasal displacement, or vagal nerve damage, and are rapidly dramatic (92). The signs of a jejunal ligation occur within 10–30 min and consist of retropropulsive motor activity and oral dilation of the small bowel, despite the occurrence of propulsive-like waves during 2–3 h. A reduction in fluid space and subsequent dehydration, but without loss in body weight, result from the movement of water into the gastrointestinal tract. These data are consistent with the large amount of digesta that the enteric canal has to propel in herbivores and a high degree of distensibility of its thin wall.

LARGE INTESTINE MOTILITY

The large intestine is a versatile organ with different homeostatic functions, i.e., electrolyte and fluid balance. It is also a potential site for absorption of nutrients and a major harbor for billions of microorganisms. The distal bowel acts as a temporary store for excreta until controlled elimination is convenient.

The cecocolic segment, which occupies 41% of the whole digestive tract in monogastric herbivores such as the horse or the rabbit, represents only 10%–15% in the ruminant animal and is comprised of the cecum, proximal colon, centripetal and centrifugal coils of the spiral colon, distal colon, and rectum (Fig. 42).

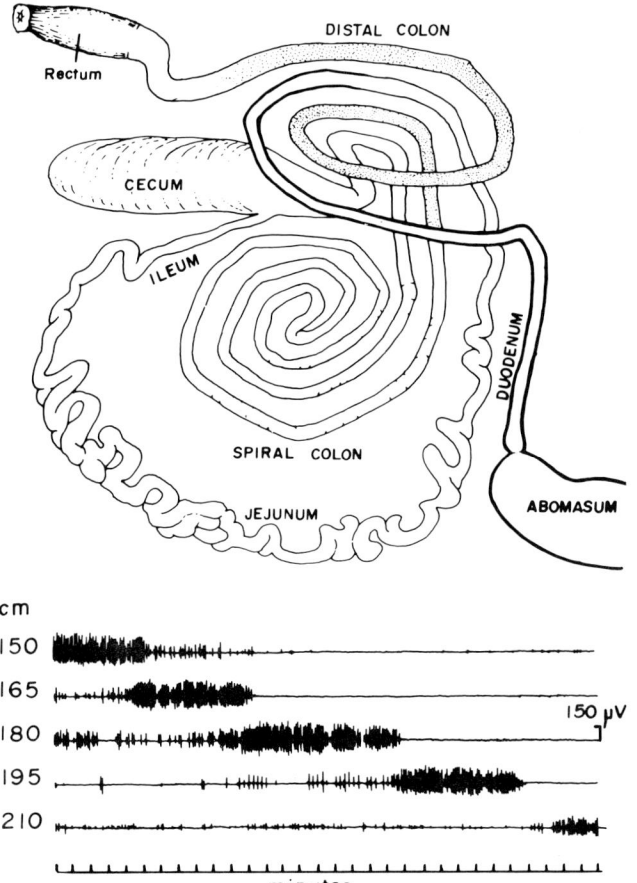

FIG. 42. *Top*, schematic representation of bovine gastrointestinal tract showing spiral colon, which is the equivalent of human transverse colon, and relatively large cecum. Fermentation of ingested cellulose that has passed intraruminal degradation occurs in both organs. *Bottom*, propagation at low velocity (2.1 ± 0.4 cm/min) of a period of spiking activity lasting 6 min along 5 electrode sites at 15-cm intervals on spiral colon of the cow. First electrode was 150 cm from the ileocecal valve. Such a migrating spike burst pattern occurs from 8 to 10 times/day.

### Functional Organization

The prime functions of the colon are reabsorption of electrolytes and water and microbial digestion, both of which depend to a large degree on delayed colonic transit. Despite the efficiency of forestomach diges-

TABLE 8. *Contribution to Oxidative Metabolism of Ruminal and Cecal Production of Volatile Fatty Acids in Sheep*

| Diet | Dry Matter | | Volatile Fatty Acids | | | Percentage of Expired $CO_2$ Derived From Acetate | | |
|---|---|---|---|---|---|---|---|---|
| | Intake, g/day | Digestibility, % | Production rate, moles/day | | Percent from cecum | Rumen | Cecum | Percent from cecum |
| | | | Rumen | Cecum | | | | |
| Fresh, white clover | 385 | 84.0 | 2.1 | 0.2 | 8.6 | 33.2 | 4.3 | 11.5 |
| Lucerne, chopped | 420 | 53.6 | 1.5 | 0.3 | 16.8 | 45.0 | 7.7 | 14.7 |
| Lucerne, pellets | 540 | 71.3 | 3.6 | 0.4 | 9.1 | 49.9 | 4.8 | 8.8 |
| | 1,080 | 71.3 | 6.8 | 0.9 | 12.0 | 45.8 | 8.1 | 15.8 |

[From Ulyatt et al. (234).]

tion, as much as 15% of the soluble carbohydrate still reaches the colon under conditions of high grain feeding and as much as 30% of the cellulose in diets of high fiber (242).

In sheep the cecum is a blind sac 25–35 cm in length and 5–7 cm in diameter and is continuous with the proximal colon at the ileal orifice. The cecum and first region of the proximal colon thus act as a single compartment, which may contain in excess of 1,000 g of digesta. This compartment is effective in delaying the passage of digesta and is the main site of fermentative digestion in the large intestine. The amount of volatile fatty acids produced in the ovine cecum may reach 0.9 mol/day versus 6.8 mol/day in the rumen (Table 8).

The contribution of acetate produced in the cecum to oxidative metabolism assessed by measuring the output of $^{14}CO_2$ in expired air during an infusion of sodium [$^{14}C$]acetate into the rumen or cecum represents 8.8%–15.8% of acetate production. More than 10% of methane production may occur in the cecum of sheep fed lucerne. This indicates that the cecum makes a significant contribution to fermentative digestion and energy requirements in ruminants particularly when they are fed diets of low nutritive value.

The secretions of the mucosa have not been studied except for their rates, which are in the order of 20–180 ml/day for cecal pouch preparation (141) and 100–400 ml/day for spiral colon. The secretion rates are increased during distension with air (233). From 95% to 99% of the volatile fatty acids produced in the hind gut and present as anions are absorbed primarily by simple diffusion (64). Bicarbonate accumulates in the lumen in proportion to the amount of volatile fatty acids absorbed. This accumulation in the cecum severely inhibits the motility (218). Compared with rumen epithelium (73), cecal epithelium has been shown to oxidize less total volatile fatty acids and has a greater preference to acetate, a lower oxygen uptake, and a lower preference for butyrate (47). Approximately 90% of water entering the cecum is normally absorbed. Studies based on ratios of dry matter to water indicate that water is absorbed along the whole length of the organ, with the centripetal coils of the spiral colon probably being the most efficient size. This ability, one of the main physiological functions of the organ, is vital to the water economy of ruminants in arid regions.

Because no great variation in the anatomy of the large intestine appears to exist between small and large ruminants, the formation of pellets in sheep or goats and of soft feces in cattle must be related to some functional aspect of a colonic segment. The mucosa of the large intestine of sheep typically lacks villi, although some longitudinal folding occurs in the spiral colon and in the rectum. The lamina propria, which varies in thickness, is approximately twice as deep in the centripetal coils of the spiral colon as in the other regions of the large intestine. The distribution of goblet cells closely follows their thickness, with the greatest numbers in the spiral colon. This phenomenon is probably related to an increased requirement for mucus to act as a lubricant because the spiral colon is the site of the formation of pellets. The retention time of digesta in the spiral colon averages ~20 h in sheep instead of 8 h in cattle. Accordingly, radiographic and electromyographic (188) studies suggest that the dominant activity of the ovine spiral colon is "segmentation," i.e., the division of the lumen into fairly uniform segments by narrow ring contractions, these contractions propelling contents over only short distances and in both directions. In contrast, the major pattern of activity of the spiral colon in cattle is represented by periods of contractions lasting 5–6 min and migrating slowly along the whole organ on 8–10 occasions per day (Fig. 42).

Of interest is the fact that in other species like the rabbit, which also produces pellets as hard feces, the motor profile of the site of pellet production, i.e., the proximal haustrated colon, consists, like in the ovine spiral colon, of localized short bursts of spike potentials occurring during ~90% of the recording time so that the activity seems continuous. In contrast the unpropagated contractions of the oral part of the proximal colon are decreased during the production of soft feces with higher water content in the rabbit, a phenomenon that could be induced by the infusion of prostaglandins and conversely blocked by inhibitors of their synthesis (173).

The most important conclusion from these studies is that cecocolonic contents flow in response to a pressure gradient caused by propagated contractions, hence the term *phasic activity*, recorded as bursts of spike potentials lasting more than 5 s. The effect of much of the segmenting activity recorded as spike potential bursts lasting 4–5 s and presumably tonic in nature is to retard rather than accelerate passage of contents.

*Cecal Motility Patterns*

The flow of digesta, past a cannula placed in the terminal ileum, to the cecum and proximal colon appears as gushes of 70 ml for a single propagated contraction and 80–90 ml flowing in 10 min for a series of short contractions. Such flows are followed by a period of quiescence varying from 30 to 300 min. Estimated flows of ileal contents are ~6–8.5 liters/day in cattle (233).

Regular coordinated contractions (peristaltic and antiperistaltic) are the predominant form of activity in the cecum and usually occur at a frequency of 3–7/10 min in cattle (Table 9). Radiologic observations show that the majority of these contractions originate either at the blind pole of the cecum or at the ileocecal junction, with the peristaltic contractions initiated at the blind pole often being associated with an antiperistaltic wave of contraction initiated at the ileocecal

TABLE 9. *Duration of Spike Bursts on Cecum and Colon*

|  | Sheep | | Cow | |
|---|---|---|---|---|
|  | Duration, s | Frequency, per min | Duration, s | Frequency, per min |
| Cecum | 5.9 ± 1.5 | 1.0 ± 0.2 | 10.4 ± 2.0* | 1.2 ± 0.3 |
| Proximal colon | 5.6 ± 1.1 | 1.3 ± 0.2 | 9.8 ± 1.3* | 1.4 ± 0.4 |
| Spiral colon | 3.9 ± 0.3 | 14.6 ± 0.8 | 3.8 ± 1.0 | 7.0 ± 0.6* |
| Distal colon |  |  |  |  |
| Bursts of spike potentials, <5 s | 3.2 ± 0.8 | 14.2 ± 0.9 | 0 | 0 |
| Bursts of spike potentials, >5 s | 7.1 ± 1.6 | 4.8 ± 0.5 | 8.1 ± 1.9 | 5.7 ± 0.5* |

Number of sheep, 20; number of cows, 20. \*$P < 0.05$.

junction. Contractions that originate at the junction travel toward the pole and are followed by a wave of contraction that returns from the pole and may travel some distance along the proximal colon. Single peristaltic contractions, originating either at the junction or as a continuation of a cecal contraction, travel along the proximal colon often as far as the spiral colon. The antiperistaltic contractions that occur in the proximal colon result in the flow of digesta back to the cecum. Linked to the occurrence of an RSA phase of MMCs on the ileum is a series of 4–12 intense contractions lasting ~2 min in sheep and 6 min in cattle that occurs at irregular intervals (30–240 min) and results in evacuation of contents from the cecum.

Such total contractions of the cecum result in almost complete evacuation of contents to the proximal colon and a rush of digesta reaching the spiral colon. Then a phase of hyperactivity resembling a migrating spike burst is propagated along the whole spiral colon in cattle (Fig. 42).

Radiologic observations have also shown that when contrast medium passes from the ileum through the ileocecal valve, it is rapidly dispersed throughout the digesta in the cecum and the proximal colon, indicating that the regular coordinated contractions result in extensive mixing of the digesta (141). However, kinetic studies (i.e., constant volume, inflow, and outflow) using markers have led to the conclusion that the cecum and proximal colon do not act as an ideal compartment in ruminants because of the pulsatile nature of the inflow of digesta from the ileum and the intermittent outflow of digesta from the cecum (68). Nevertheless, monitoring cecal motility over a prolonged period thus reveals a complex pattern of motility with at least localized contractions, presumably tonic in nature; regular coordinated contractions that appeared to result in mixing of the cecal contents; and, at long intervals, trains of two to five very strong contractions, often associated with transfer of the cecal contents to the spiral colon (Fig. 43).

*Pelleted Feces Formation*

The nearly continuous spiking activity of the ovine spiral colon consists of unpropagated bursts of spike potentials developed at a high rate of 10–15/min (Fig. 43). This activity is transiently reduced by the two to five strong contractions propagated from the cecum along the proximal colon and associated with transfer of contents. The localized spiking activity of the spiral colon results in segmentative contractions and in dehydration. The fact that plastic beads (5-mm diam) introduced sequentially through a cannula in the proximal end of the spiral colon are recovered in essentially the same order suggests that these segmentative contractions are not associated with mixing of digesta. It

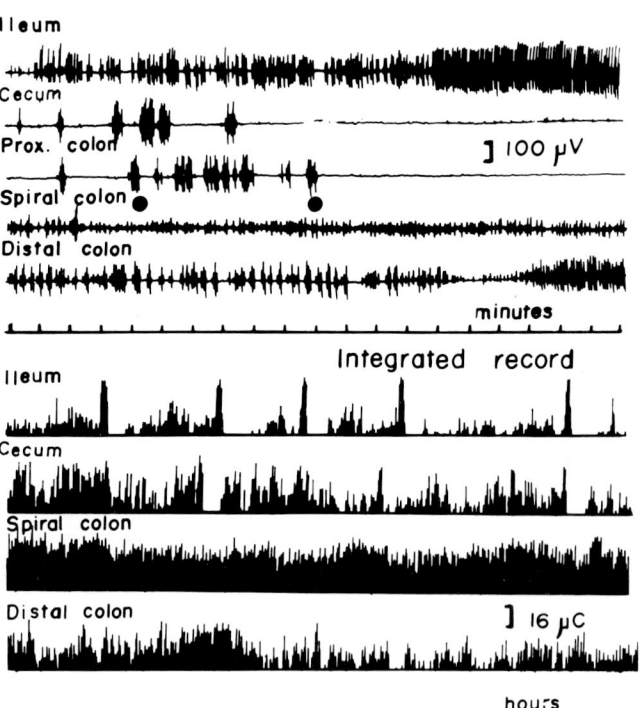

FIG. 43. Electrical activity of ovine large intestine. *Top*, direct record of propagated contractions from cecum toward proximal colon (*filled circles*) occurring ~5 min before presence of a phase of regular spiking activity on terminal ileum. Trains of 2–5 strong contractions faded out at level of spiral colon. *Bottom*, integrated record showing pattern of activity of migrating myoelectric complexes on ileum and continuous spiking activity of spiral colon involved in pellet formation in small ruminants.

is likely that the presence of mucus, which is stimulated by contact between the goblet cells and contents, facilitates the progressive closure of the lumen at one site and thus the separation of fecal pellets. The fecal pellets in sheep have a round shape, in contrast to those spindled shape in the rat. The reason may be that pellet formation in rat proceeds from retropulsion-propulsion contractile waves in the transverse colon and not from progressive closure of the lumen.

The absence of pelleted feces in cattle may be related to a lower activity of the spiral colon, which occupies 25% of the recording time. In addition the mean frequency of contractions is about half that seen in sheep (Fig. 44). However, the propagation at a velocity of ~2 cm/min from the proximal to the distal part of the colon of periods of spiking activity lasting 6 min and followed by a period of quiescence remains the functional characteristic of the bovine colonic motility. The propulsion of a large volume of digesta by this kind of mass action contraction is likely because their daily number corresponds approximately to the number of defecations. It is noteworthy that molded feces can be obtained in cattle when this pattern of activity is blocked transiently after the use of atropine.

*Neural Influences*

There are conflicting opinions on the effect of feeding on the cecal motility of ruminants. Feeding sheep once a day has been reported to have little effect, except an increase in the frequency and amplitude of the contractions by 20%–30% from 15 to 20 min after the onset of feeding. This response is present, although diminished, in sham-fed animals. Evidence for the presence of a "gastrocolic reflex" in sheep also is based on the fact that proximal colonic activity may be doubled during the first 10 min after feeding (233). Presumably as a result of increased or abnormal cecal fermentation, feeding grain results in a decreased colonic activity in sheep and cattle, whereas the infusion of volatile fatty acids, especially butyric acid, inhibits motility. This effect is considered as the causative factor in pathological conditions of cecal dilatation (218).

The duality of spiking activity of the colon, i.e., bursts of spike potentials of long and short duration, is common to other species. Spike bursts of long duration are characterized by their oral and aboral propagation. Spike bursts lasting <5 s remained localized. The third pattern of activity, the migrating spike burst, is only seen in cattle. Each segment of the large intestine exhibits its own characteristics of spiking activity because the cecum, the proximal colon, and the distal colon present mainly propagated spike bursts, and localized activity largely predominated on the spiral colon. Finally, differences in the motility patterns between sheep and cattle are in accordance

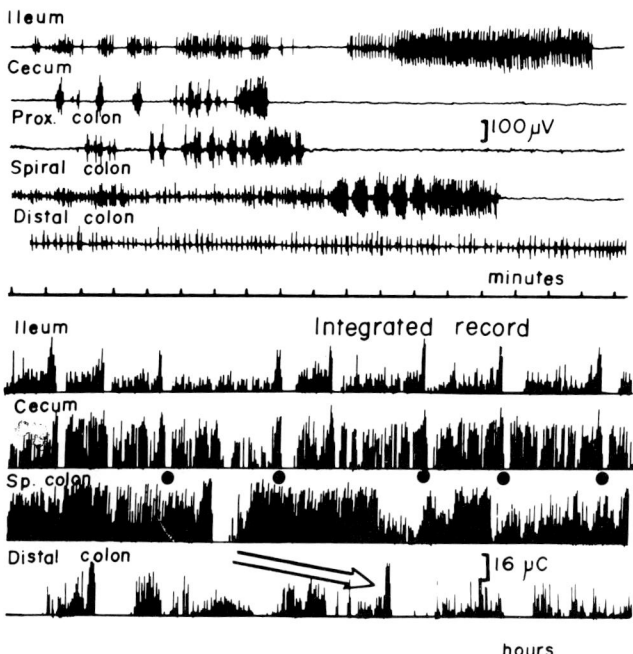

FIG. 44. Electrical activity of bovine large intestine. *Top*, direct record of contractions propagated from cecum through spiral colon. *Bottom*, integrated record showing ileal pattern of activity of migrating myoelectric complexes and high values of activity on cecum (*filled circles*) corresponding to phases of regular spiking activity of ileum. *Arrow*, aboral migration of a 6-min period of hyperactivity that slowly propagated from 8 to 10 times/day from spiral colon to distal colon.

with the differences in colonic transit time between these species. The relatively high level of localized spiking activity observed in the ovine spiral colon (85% of recording time vs. 25% in cattle) could explain a prolonged storage function in sheep and the formation of pellets. In contrast the specific spike burst activity of the bovine spiral colon, which migrates at a velocity nearly 10 times lower than that seen in the jejunum, may be related to the propulsion toward the rectum of very large amounts of residual digesta.

There is much evidence that the spinal cord is the source of tonic neural inhibition of colonic motility via the hypogastric plexus in ruminants as in other species. The intrathecal administration of $\alpha_2$-adrenergic receptor blockers and lumbosacral anesthesia is accompanied by an increased activity of the bovine spiral colon (Y. Ruckebusch, unpublished observations). In addition, reflex contractions of the rectum are markedly decreased and defecation is impeded, probably by augmentation of the anal sphincter tone during epidural anesthesia.

PHARMACOLOGICAL CONSIDERATIONS

Two pharmacological aspects are emphasized: the cyclical reticuloruminal contractions and the cyclical motor events of the gastroduodenal junction. The raison d'être of considerations related to the forestomach is that gastric motor disturbances in ruminants, e.g., reticulorumen stasis or bloating, involve primarily the activity of the gastric centers because the reticuloruminal extrinsic contractions are caused by coordinated nervous activity emanating from gastric centers and passing down vagal motor nerve fibers. Hypomotility, defined as a lower frequency and/or magnitude of extrinsic contractions, could be simply the result of an inhibition of the activity of the centers or of their motor pathways, e.g., hypomotility induced by general anesthetics, central nervous system–depressant drugs, febrile diseases (240), or reticuloruminal stasis, subsequent to the administration of ganglion-blocking and parasympatholytic drugs such as tetraethylammonium and atropine (38).

A reduction in the net excitatory drive to the gastric centers from the rumen (176) and/or an increased inhibitory input from the gastroduodenal function represent other possibilities leading to hypomotility and reticuloruminal stasis. The absence of production of volatile fatty acids by the fermenting mass of food (171, 217) may reduce the amount of afferent stimuli to the gastric centers, hence their lower activity (20). Reflex inhibition of the extrinsic contractions resulting from afferent inhibitory stimuli initiated in the duodenum and in the rumen itself by spasmogenic agents such as 5-HT, substance P (245), angiotensin, and bradykinin in vitro is commonly recorded in conscious animals (244).

A complicated situation can result from the temporal association of opposite effects on the different parts of the forestomach, e.g., the infusion of gastrin reduces the rate and amplitude of reticulorumen contractions but stimulates the contraction of the omasal body (Fig. 17). The effects on the rate of reticular contractions seem of central origin, whereas those on the amplitude of reticular contractions and the omasum are of peripheral origin. A more complicated situation is due to the dissimilar influences of the extrinsic nerves on the reticulum < rumen < omasum (91). This explains the persistence of omasal body contractions under general anesthesia (Fig. 19) and also the possible blockade of the reticular contractions after the intracerebroventricular administration of several regulatory peptides without inhibition of the occurrence of the secondary ruminal contractions. Conversely the secondary ruminal contractions may be inhibited peripherally without changes in the reticuloruminal primary cycles, e.g., during the hypocalcemia induced in cattle by infusion of EDTA (22, 38).

The raison d'être of considerations related to the ruminant gastroduodenal junction is that the cyclical activity of this area is at the origin of MCCs without prandial disruption. Of importance also is the control of gastric emptying linked to the negative feedback control on the antral motor activity and if necessary on reticuloruminal contractions exerted by the duodenal bulb acting as a brake.

## Drugs Affecting Forestomach Motility

The existence of a central opioid inhibitory system of the reticulorumen cyclical activity is based on several observations. These include increased rumen motility after naloxone (139), competitive antagonism by nalorphine, bloating after the ingestion by cattle of poppy bulbs, enhancement by opiate antagonists of the extracontractions of the reticulum induced by epinephrine, as demonstrated by rumination at a lower threshold dosage and shorter latency (192), and potentiation of the central inhibitory effects of fentanyl on bovine ruminal motility by antihistamines. The latter effect approximates that noted in human abusers of pentazocine who experience a heroin-like euphoria after ingestion of tripelennamine.

The concept of multiple forms of opioid receptors is supported by the comparative effects of different classes of agonists. The intravenous administration of the $\mu$-opioid agonists evokes a blockade of the frequency of reticular contractions and stimulates the duodenum. Similar effects are recorded after the administration of enkephalins considered as mixed $\mu$- and $\delta$-opioid agonists. Despite a stimulation of the duodenal bulb motor activity, reticular contractions are enhanced in amplitude and in frequency by the $\kappa$ agonist ethylketazocin (192), indicating that the opioid effects on reticular motility are of central origin rather than the consequence of duodenal stimulation. The inhibitory effects of the opioid $\mu$- and $\delta$-agonists on the reticulum are prevented by naloxone but not by the quaternary parent compound methylnaloxone that blocked the duodenal stimulation. This further suggests that reticulorumen inhibition by $\mu$- and $\delta$-opioid agonists is centrally mediated in contrast to the peripheral effects on the duodenum.

Different biogenic amines seem to act as central neurotransmitters involved in the control of reticuloruminal motor functions and associated behaviors. Oral activities such as wool biting in sheep and compulsive chewing movements in cattle were described after the administration of apomorphine, a dopamine agonist. They probably are, like the internal vomiting observed in sheep with very high doses of apomorphine (63), the result of direct stimulation of dopamine receptors in the central nervous system. Dopamine antagonists like sulpiride increase chewing movements with an increased rumination time of 30%–60%, whereas metoclopramide increases the ratio of secondary to primary ruminal contractions. In contrast, domperidone blocks the peripheral inhibitory effects of dopamine (140).

In contrast to the effects of 5-HT on the reticulorumen contractions that involve a stimulation of intramural cholinergic neurons (223) in addition to a direct myogenic effect, the $\alpha_2$-adrenoceptor agonists xylazine or clonidine suppress the reticular contractions in a dose-dependent manner (232). This centrally mediated effect does not modify the occurrence of secondary ruminal contractions. Tolazoline and to a lesser extent yohimbine behave as specific and competitive antagonists (Fig. 45).

Despite different mechanisms for synthesis and replacement after synaptic release, specific peptides frequently coexist with monoamine transmitters, e.g., substance P and 5-HT, acetylcholine and VIP. The functional significance of this coexistence lies in the fact that the peptide amplifies the effects caused by the classic transmitters. Such disposition has also been found in the ruminal stomach (254) with inhibition of the extrinsic contraction after the central or peripheral administration of gastrin and of the other peptides (pentagastrin, CCK-8, caerulein) that share a similar amino acid sequence.

The inhibitory effects of central infusion of pentagastrin on motility are only slightly more pronounced than those after subcutaneous administration of similar dosages (87), suggesting a peripherally mediated effect. Accordingly the effects are partly blocked by quaternary narcotic antagonists like naloxone methobromide or levallorphan methyliodide that do not reach the gastric centers to any large extent (Fig. 46). Among other endogenous neuropeptides, thyrotropin-releasing hormone and neurotensin have opposite long-lasting effects on the reticulorumen motor function, e.g., thyrotropin-releasing hormone administered either centrally or peripherally prevents the hypomotility due to the infusion of neurotensin. However, additional studies are required to discern the mechanisms involved in such inhibitory effects because hyperthermia, hyperglycemia, and/or release of prostaglandin $E_2$ can be the cause of such effects.

From a practical viewpoint, centrally mediated alteration in the timing of extrinsic contractions, e.g., by anesthetics or $\alpha_2$-agonists, can be relieved by spe-

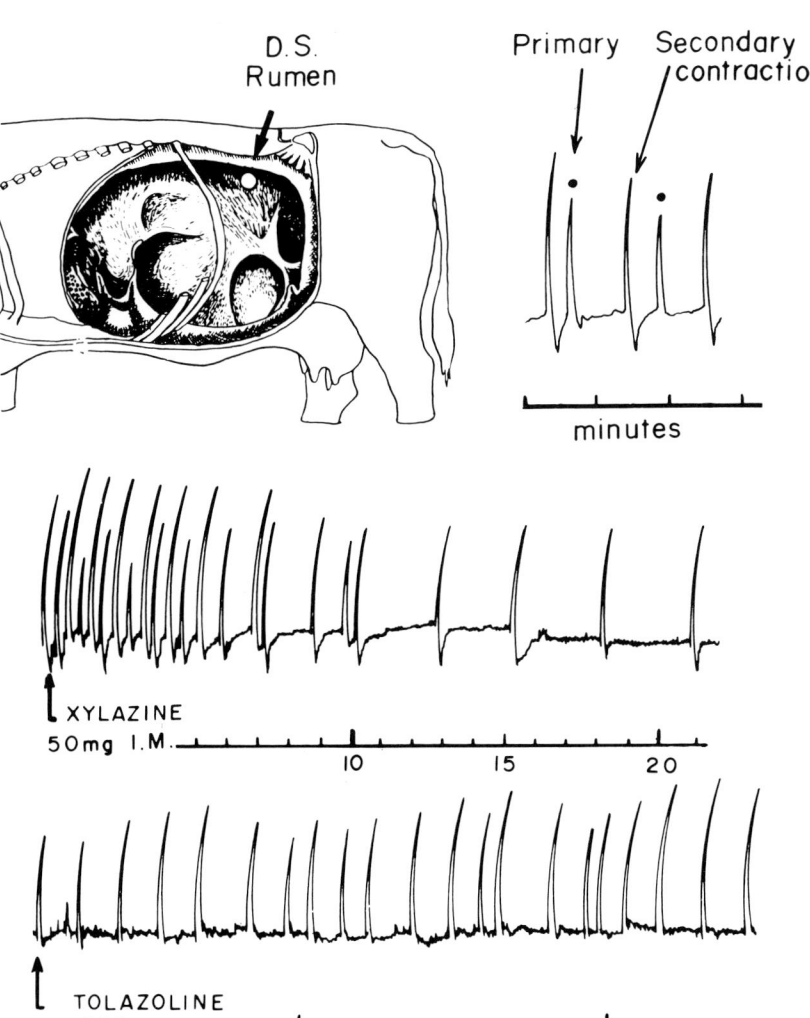

FIG. 45. Blockade within 6–7 min of primary ruminal contractions after intramuscular injection of xylazine (0.08 mg/kg) in cattle (see Fig. 14). Contractions that persisted after xylazine correspond to secondary contractions of dorsal sac rumen (D. S. rumen). Primary contractions reappear after injection of the $\alpha_2$-adrenoceptor antagonist tolazoline at a dosage ratio of 5:1.

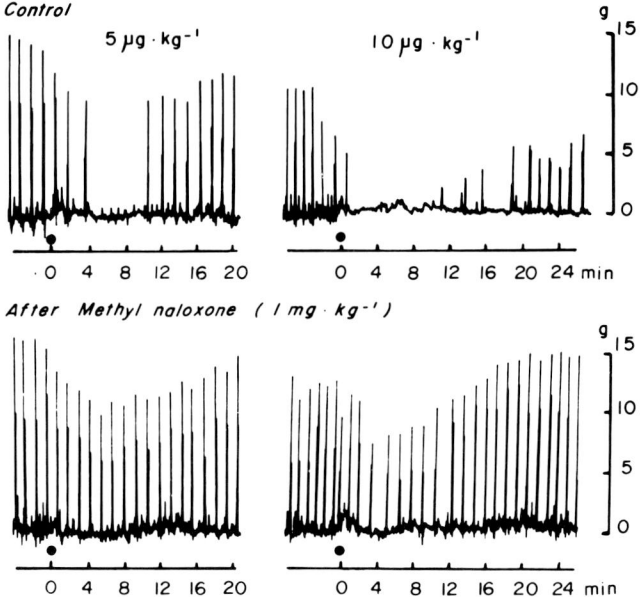

FIG. 46. Inhibition of rate and amplitude of reticular contractions measured by strain gauges in sheep after subcutaneous administration of pentagastrin at 2 different dosages. Effects of central origin (see Fig. 25) but outside blood-brain barrier are prevented by intravenous methylnaloxone.

cific antagonists. For example, the peripheral effects of atropine with blockade of the esophageal groove reflex in milk-fed animals or blockade of primary and secondary movement cycles with stasis and bloating in the adult ruminant can be prevented by pretreatment with cholinergic agents. The interplay between central and peripheral effects of exogenous and endogenous opioids or between biogenic amines and neuropeptides and the species-specific differences in responsiveness between sheep and cattle [e.g., in the reflex inhibition of forestomach motility via the stimulation of the gastroduodenal function (194)] have yet to be defined.

*Drugs Affecting Gastroduodenal Junction*

The primary control of motility of the abomasum is of myogenic origin. Receptors (mechano-, chemo-, and osmoreceptors), neurons, and hormones influence stomach motility by a direct action on the muscles or by influences on the release of neurotransmitters and hormones. The receptive function of the proximal part (fundus) is obviously less well delineated in ruminants than is the cyclical activity of the distal part (antrum).

A major characteristic of the motor responses of the junction is an inhibition of antral contractions during stimulation of the duodenal bulb. Such effects can be the result of different sensitivities between the antrum and the duodenum as is the case for substance P, a histamine and acetylcholine releaser more active, like bombesin and prostaglandins, on the antrum than on the duodenum. As recently shown in the isolated canine antrum, the myogenic effects of substance P are atropine sensitive, especially for the longitudinal smooth muscle (145). In the conscious sheep, antral but not duodenal effects of substance P were prevented by atropine pretreatment (Fig. 47).

Other mechanisms involve reflex inhibition of the antrum, e.g., morphine and other opiate analgesics that are notorious for causing gastric retention. Initial contractions of the duodenum, resembling a phase of RSA induced by morphine injection in dogs, are followed by a long-lasting period of duodenal inhibition concomitant with antral inhibition. In sheep, morphine and to a lesser extent loperamide, a synthetic opiate administered by the systemic route, induce similar effects, e.g., a long-lasting inhibition of the antrum accompanied by stimulation and then an inhibition of the duodenal bulb activity. Nalorphine, a partial opiate antagonist, which has only stimulatory effects on the duodenal bulb, inhibits the antrum without impairment of forestomach motility (Fig. 48).

In sheep, bethanechol (0.01 mg/kg), a parasympathomimetic drug with a relatively selective action on the gastroduodenal area and urinary bladder, and pilocarpine (0.05 mg/kg) are equipotent stimulating agents, with less marked effects on the duodenum than on the antrum. In contrast, centrally long-acting cholinomimetic agents such as 4-aminopyridine, known to potentiate release of prejunctional stores of acetylcholine, have strong stimulatory effects on the duodenal bulb, hence the concomitant inhibition of the antral activity. This is not the case for cisapride, which facilitates the peripheral release of cholinergic neurotransmitter from intramural cholinergic nerves and exerts excitatory effects on the whole junction. The cholinergic action of metoclopramide, which has revolutionized the therapy of gastric retention, is ascribed to either a facilitation of acetylcholine release or to gastric smooth muscle sensitization to acetylcholine. In sheep, metoclopramide (0.5 mg/kg) has an equipotent stimulatory effect on the fundus, antrum, and duodenal bulb and is able to antagonize the inhibitory effects of dopamine and its metabolic precursor, L-dopa, on the fundus and antrum (194).

Anticholinergics such as atropine, diphemanil methylsulfate, and hyoscine change the myoelectrical activity to modify the motor profile into a nonpropulsive pattern by inhibiting both antral and duodenal activity. This inhibition is more marked on the antrum than on the duodenum. The fact that the synthetic opiate loperamide, which supposedly acts peripherally on the enteric nervous system and does not reach the gastric centers, has marked inhibitory effects on the frequency of reticular contractions, as does morphine, suggests the importance of the duodenal bulb as a "reflexogenic area" for both the antrum and reticulum and possibly the pylorus (193).

Among the gut hormones that alter gastric empty-

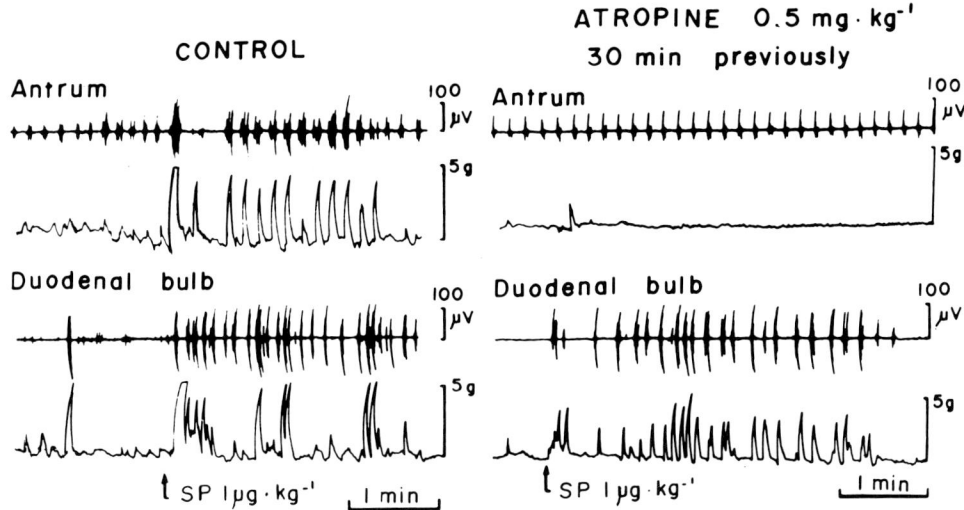

FIG. 47. Blockade of motor effects of substance P (SP) on electrical and mechanical activities of ovine gastroduodenal junction 2 cm from pylorus. Stimulation induced by intravenous SP was equipotent on antrum and duodenal bulb. Atropine pretreatment prevented SP-induced stimulation of antrum (and pylorus, not shown) but not of bulb. [From Ruckebusch and Merritt (196).]

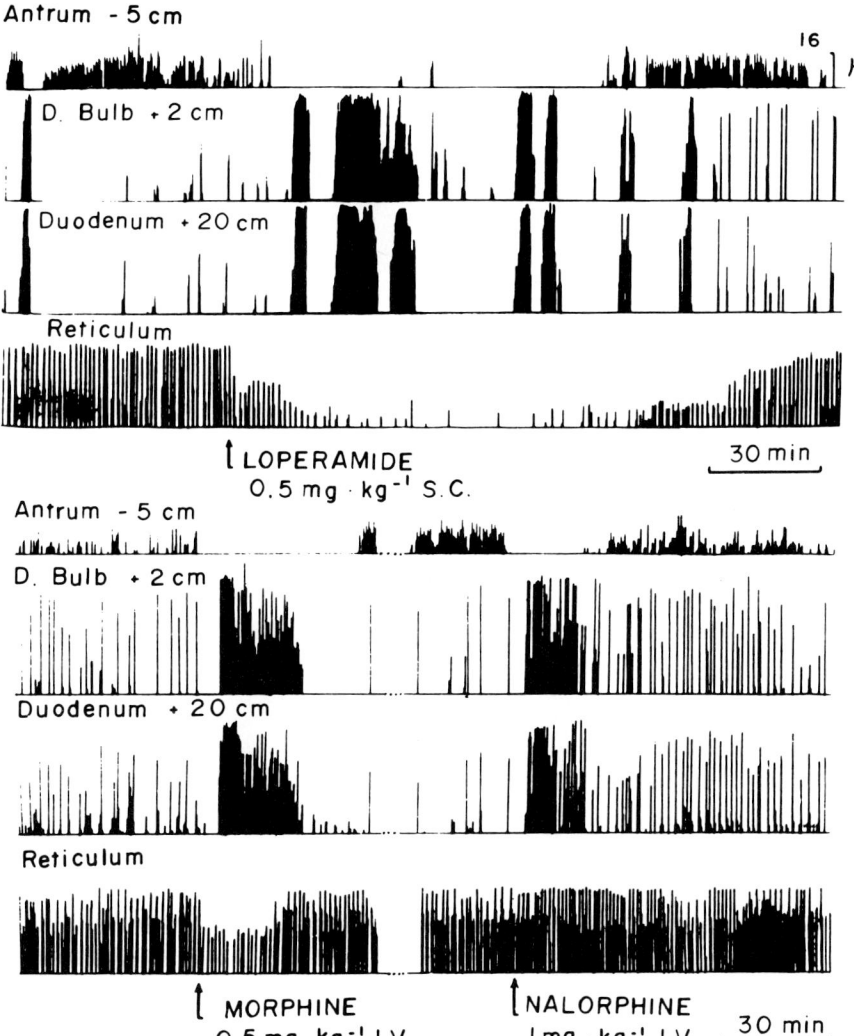

FIG. 48. Integrated record of electrical activity of ovine gastroduodenal junction 5 cm proximal and 2 cm distal to the pylorus, the proximal duodenum (20 cm), and reticulum. Top. Stimulation of duodenum by the synthetic opiate loperamide and morphine or nalorphine was accompanied by inhibition of antral activity. Bottom. Nalorphine did not inhibit amplitude and/or frequency of reticular contractions, and its stimulatory effects on duodenum were not followed by inhibition as for morphine. D. Bulb, duodenal bulb; S.C., subcutaneous; I.V., intravenous. [From Ruckebusch and Merritt (196).]

ing, somatostatin was found to function as an endogenous inhibitor of the secretory and motor effects exerted by bombesin. Its release is suspected to be involved in the feedback control of abomasal emptying in calves (14). In adult ruminants, somatostatin, infused at the doses of 2.5 and 5 $\mu g \cdot kg^{-1} \cdot min^{-1}$ during 20 min, stimulates the duodenal bulb in a manner similar to morphine, with parallel antral inhibition as occurs in dogs (224), whereas gastrin and the gastrin-releasing peptide bombesin have stronger stimulatory effects on the antrum than on the duodenal bulb.

The physiological significance of 5-HT is still unknown because it can act as a neurotransmitter within the enteric nervous system, by directly stimulating vascular and digestive smooth muscle, or as a hormone. Intraluminal acid can release 5-HT from the duodenum, and its level in plasma reaches a peak by 60 min after a meal in calves (14). In addition, 5-HT can reset the cyclic motor events of the gastroduodenal junction to a faster rhythm.

The systemic administration of 5-HT, and its precursor 5-HTP, increases the cyclical activity of the duodenal bulb in a dose-related fashion (0.25–1 mg/kg) (190). An inhibition of the antral motor activity occurs at the time of maximal excitation on the duodenal bulb, hence recordings resemble those of MMCs occurring at the short intervals of 40 min instead of 120 min (Fig. 49).

Different attempts have been made to antagonize this antroduodenal interplay provoked by 5-HTP. The 5-HT antagonists that are active peripherally fall by and large into two categories: those effective in opposing the effects of 5-HT on smooth muscle, such as metergoline (1 mg/kg), which can partially block both the excitatory and inhibitory effects of 5-HTP; and those that at low doses preferentially block the effects of 5-HT on the enteric nervous system, such as methysergide (0.05 mg/kg), which resets the cyclical pattern at a faster rhythm (190).

A final comment concerns the adrenergic supply (216) to the gastroduodenal junction. $\alpha_2$-Adrenergic receptor agonists (clonidine, xylazine, or detomidine)

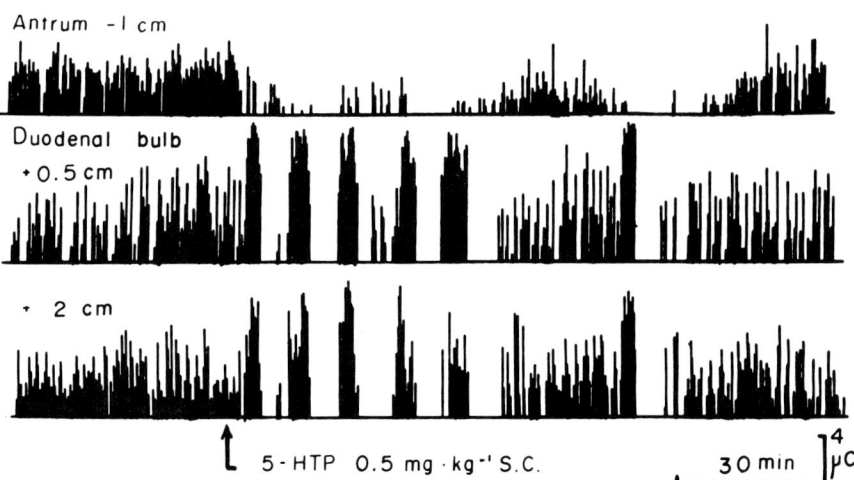
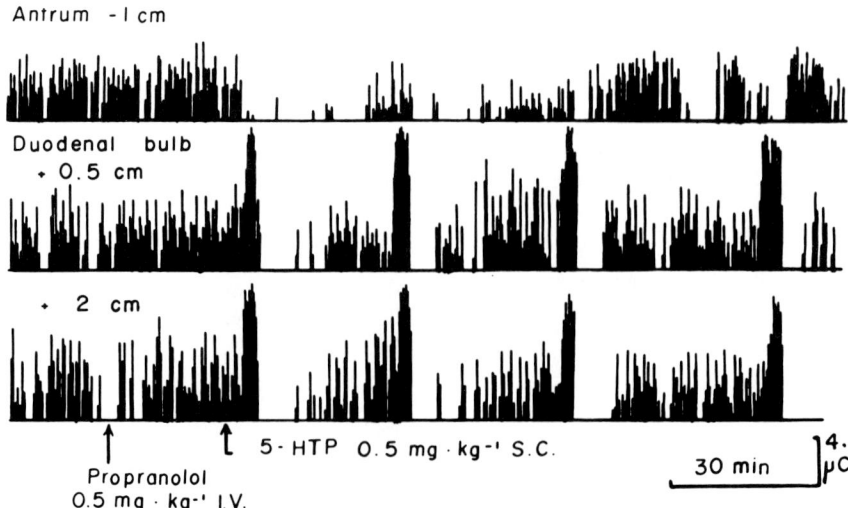

FIG. 49. Comparative effects of 5-hydroxytryptophan (5-HTP) on ovine myoelectrical activity of gastroduodenal junction (integrated record). Occurrence of the regular spiking activity–like phases at short intervals (*top*) is partly prevented by propranolol administration (*bottom*). S.C., subcutaneous; I.V., intravenous.

have been shown to alter gastric emptying in several species. In sheep the $\alpha_2$-blocking agents (yohimbine, idazoxan, tolazoline) instantaneously counteracted the atony of the junction induced by $\alpha_2$-agonists, with more pronounced effects on the duodenal bulb than on the antrum. It also appears that $\beta$-adrenergic agonists relax the gastroduodenal junction, whereas the antagonists, like some opiate antagonists, have protective effects against the 5-HT–induced hyperkinesia (Fig. 49).

*Perspectives*

Because the daily intake of feed is a major factor limiting production in livestock ruminants, emphasis has been placed on the means to chemically modify voluntary food intake. The types of regulation involved in voluntary food intake are *1*) the gastrointestinal fill (51, 52, 76, 165), hence the attempts to modify this peripheral factor by changes in reticulorumen smooth muscle tone, and *2*) humoral feedback signals, especially metabolites (160, 164) and brain and gut hormones such as CCK (44), hence a way of food intake stimulation by use of specific antagonists, e.g., CCK antibodies.

A recent histochemical study of the ovine ruminant stomach (254) shows that the cholinergic nerve supply was more dense in the reticulum than in the rumen dorsal sac or the omasum and pylorus. This is in contrast with the absence of basic differences in the adrenergic supply of the myenteric ganglia. The presence of 5-HT in mucosal cells of every digestive segment of the fetal lamb has not been found in the adult, where 5-HT was demonstrated only in the abomasum and antrum pyloricum (Fig. 50). The VIP immunoreactivity is located in the nervous tissue, especially of the inner circular muscle of the reticulum, omasum, and abomasum. A VIPergic innervation is also evidenced in the well-developed muscularis mucosae of the reticular groove, the omasum, and the wall of the larger intramural blood vessels. Although the immunocytochemical reaction against substance P is not as pronounced as for VIP, substance P immunoreactive fibers were mainly localized in the circular muscle layers.

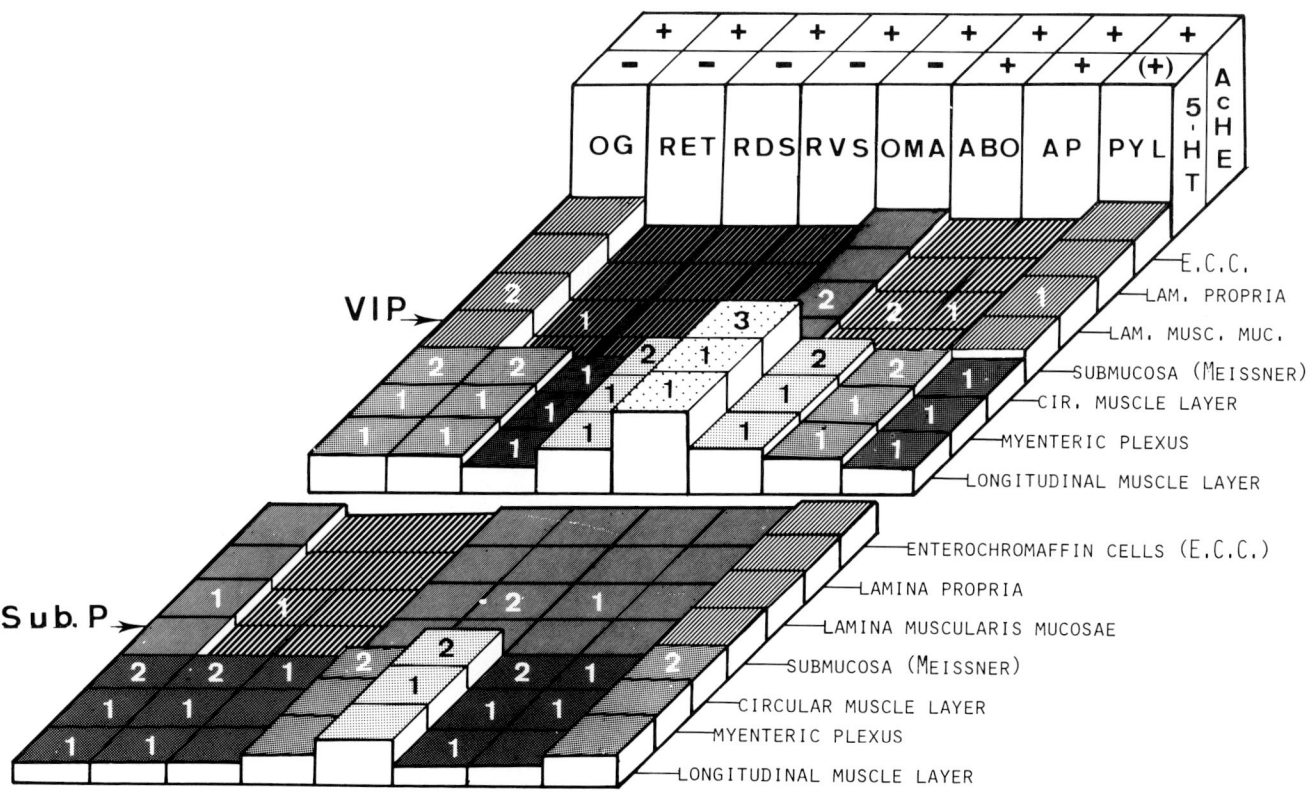

FIG. 50. Presence of hydroxytryptamine (5-HT) and acetylcholinesterase (ACHE) in different parts of ovine forestomach and stomach. Difference in height of the blocks and the numbers 1–3 are directly related to content in vasoactive intestinal peptide (VIP) and in substance P of the different layers determined by radioimmunoassays (blocks) and by immunochemistry (numbers). OG, oesophageal groove; RET, reticulum; RDS, rumen dorsal sac; RVS, rumen ventral sac; OMA, omasum; ABO, abomasum; AP, pyloric antrum; PYL, pylorus. [From Weyns et al. (254)].

These data suggest that 5-HT and regulatory peptides function within the context of the autonomic nervous system. Conceivably the intramural peptidergic neurons can mediate or modulate the response(s) to the extrinsic nerve impulse flow according to local needs and in addition to the local reflex mechanisms evoked through the myenteric plexus (229). In mucosa-free strips of rumen, 5-HT increased the muscle tone through a receptor-linked $Ca^{2+}$ channel. The changes that were resistant to verapamil and methoxyverapamil were suppressed by sodium nitroprusside and $5\text{-HT}_2$ antagonists (ketanserin or ritanserin). The long-lasting reduction in smooth muscle tone obtained by ritanserin and the concomitant relaxation of the lower esophageal sphincter have been found useful in the alleviation of postprandial gas accumulation or the prevention of chronic bloating. This reduced ruminal smooth muscle tone can also favor overeating because the meal size is no longer limited by reticulorumen distension (76).

Among the humoral feedback signals involved in controlling feeding and associated motor functions, the increased blood concentrations of volatile fatty acids produced in the rumen have been considered as factors controlling the meal size and motility. However, in the majority of the trials, spontaneous food intake was only affected by unphysiological levels that also could raise blood osmolality. An increase of plasma insulin levels occurs in ruminants during feeding as rapidly as that seen in other species but without motility changes; this suggests a possible role in the long-term control of the energy balance and body weight. The involvement of CCK as a satiety signal in ruminants is based on the reduced food intake without major motility changes after its infusion into the ovine lateral cerebral ventricles (44) or systematically (85). However, despite an increase of intake in satiated sheep during the infusion of CCK antibodies, the release of CCK into the cerebrospinal fluid in response to a meal has yet to be demonstrated.

Reliable assays to clarify the role of brain peptides in satiety and gastrointestinal motility are needed to gain insight in the mechanisms of hyperphagia induced by a variety of agents, such as opioids or benzodiazepines. For example, there is some evidence that opiate agonists mediate the CCK-induced inhibition of food intake and reticulorumen motility, because naloxone abolished these effects. The elfazepam-induced feeding response also is suppressed by naloxone, hence the possibility that benzodiazepines may override the central control of feeding and motility patterns by the release of endogenous opioid peptides.

REFERENCES

1. ADRIAN, T. E., S. R. BLOOM, AND A. V. EDWARDS. Neuroendocrine responses to stimulation of the vagus nerves in conscious calves. *J. Physiol. Lond.* 344: 25–35, 1983.
2. AMMERMAN, C. B., AND R. D. GOODRICH. Advances in mineral nutrition in ruminants. *J. Anim. Sci.* 57, Suppl. 2: 519–533, 1983.
3. ANDERSSON, B., R. KITCHELL, AND N. PERSSON. A study of rumination induced by milking in the goat. *Acta Physiol. Scand.* 44: 92–102, 1958.
4. ANNISON, E. F., K. J. HILL, AND D. LEWIS. Studies on the portal blood of sheep. 2. Absorption of volatile fatty acids from the rumen of the sheep. *Biochem. J.* 66: 592–599, 1957.
5. ASAI, T. Developmental processes of reticulo-rumen motility in calves. *Jpn. J. Vet. Sci.* 35: 239–252, 1973.
6. ASH, R. W. Abomasal secretion and emptying in suckled calves. *J. Physiol. Lond.* 172: 425–438, 1964.
7. BAE, D. H., J. G. WELCH, AND A. M. SMITH. Forage intake and rumination by sheep. *J. Anim. Sci.* 49: 1292–1299, 1979.
8. BARCROFT, J., R. A. MCANALLY, AND A. T. PHILLIPSON. Absorption of volatile acids from the alimentary tract of the sheep and other animals. *J. Exp. Biol.* 20: 120–129, 1944.
9. BAUCHOP, T. Foregut fermentation. In: *Microbial Ecology of the Gut*, edited by R. T. J. Clark and T. Bauchop. New York: Academic, 1977, p. 223–250.
10. BAUCHOP, T. Rumen anaerobe fungi of cattle and sheep. *Appl. Environ. Microbiol.* 38: 148–158, 1979.
11. BAUMAN, D. E., C. L. DAVIS, R. A. FROBISCH, AND D. S. SACHAN. Evaluation of polyethylene glycol method in determining rumen fluid volume in dairy cows fed different diets. *J. Dairy Sci.* 54: 928–930, 1971.
12. BEGHELLI, V., G. BORGATTI, AND P. L. PARMEGGIANI. On the role of the dorsal nucleus of the vagus in the reflex activity of the reticulum. *Arch. Ital. Biol.* 101: 365–384, 1963.
13. BELL, F. R., A. R. GREEN, J. A. H. WASS, AND D. E. WEBBER. Intestinal control of gastric function in the calf: the relationship of neural and endocrine factors. *J. Physiol. Lond.* 321: 603–610, 1981.
14. BELL, F. R., AND M. L. GRIVEL. The effect of duodenal infusion on the electromyogram of gastric muscle during activation and inhibition of gastric emptying. *J. Physiol. Lond.* 248: 377–391, 1975.
15. BELL, F. R., S. H. HOLBROOKE, AND D. A. TITCHEN. A radiological study of gastric (abomasal) emptying and acid secretion in the milk-fed calf. *J. Physiol. Lond.* 282: 51–57, 1977.
16. BOIVIN, R., J. BOST, AND F. E. PERALTA. Oesophageal stimulation of chewing movements in sheep. *Ann. Rech. Vet.* 16: 227–235, 1985.
17. BORGATTI, G., AND R. MATSCHER. Voies et signification du réflexe oral du réseau. *Arch. Ital. Biol.* 96: 38–57, 1958.
18. BOST, J., H. VERINE, AND B. MATRAT. Particularités du transit réticulo-omasal chez le mouton. *C. R. Seances Soc. Biol. Fil.* 159: 2410–2415, 1965.
19. BOWEN, J. M. Effects of insulin hypoglycemia on gastrointestinal motility in the sheep. *Am. J. Vet. Res.* 23: 948–954, 1962.
20. BROWNLEE, A. The development of rumen papillae in cattle fed on different diets. *Br. Vet. J.* 112: 369–375, 1956.
21. BUENO, L., AND Y. RUCKEBUSCH. The cyclic motility of the omasum and its control in sheep. *J. Physiol. Lond.* 238: 295–312, 1974.
22. BÜRGIN, H. The role of calcium in the mechanical performance of cattle ruminal muscle. *J. Vet. Pharm. Ther.* 2: 305–311, 1979.
23. CAPLE, I. W., AND T. J. HEATH. Regulation of output of electrolytes in bile and pancreatic juice in sheep. *Aust. J. Biol. Sci.* 25: 155–165, 1972.
24. CARR, D. H., P. C. SCOTT, AND D. A. TITCHEN. Manometric and electromyographic observations of the esophagus of sheep in eructation, regurgitation and swallowing. *Q. J. Exp. Physiol.* 68: 661–674, 1983.
25. CHURCH, D. C. *The Ruminant Animal. Digestive Physiology and Nutrition.* New York: Simon & Schuster, 1988, p. 14–201.

26. CIRIO, A., T. BOIVIN, AND J. BOST. Stimulation prandiale de la motricité réticulaire chez le mouton: phase céphalique et réflexe oral. *Ann. Rech. Vet.* 12: 291–302, 1981.
27. CLARK, R., AND K. E. WEISS. Reflex salivation in sheep and goats initiated by mechanical stimulation of the cardiac area of the fore stomachs. *J. S. Afr. Vet. Med. Assoc.* 23: 163–165, 1952.
28. COLVIN, H. W., P. T. CUPPS, AND H. H. COLE. Dietary influences on eructation and related phenomena in cattle. *J. Dairy Sci.* 41: 1565–1579, 1958.
29. COMLINE, R. S., I. A. SILVER, AND D. H. STEVEN. Physiological anatomy of the ruminant stomach. In: *Handbook of Physiology. Alimentary Canal. Bile; Digestion; Ruminal Physiology*, edited by C. F. Code. Washington, DC: Am. Physiol. Soc., 1968, sect. 6, vol. V, p. 2647–2671.
30. COMLINE, R. S., AND D. A. TITCHEN. Reflex contractions of the oesophageal groove in young ruminants. *J. Physiol. Lond.* 115: 210–226, 1951.
31. COMLINE, R. S., AND D. A. TITCHEN. Reflex contractions of the reticulum and rumen and parotid salivary secretion. *J. Physiol. Lond.* 139: 24P, 1957.
32. COMLINE, R. S., AND D. A. TITCHEN. Nervous control of the ruminant stomach. In: *Digestive Physiology and Nutrition of the Ruminant*, edited by D. Lewis. London: Butterworths, 1961, p. 10–22.
33. COOMBE, J. B., AND R. N. B. KAY. Passage of digesta through the large intestine of sheep: retention times in the small and large intestines. *Br. J. Nutr.* 19: 325–338, 1965.
34. CONNOR, H. G., A. D. MCGILLARD, AND C. F. HUFFMAN. Bovine re-entrant duodenal fistula studies. *J. Anim. Sci.* 16: 692–697, 1957.
35. COTTRELL, D. F., AND A. IGGO. Tension receptors with vagal afferent fibres in the proximal duodenum and pyloric sphincter of sheep. *J. Physiol. Lond.* 354: 454–475, 1984.
36. COULOUMA, P. La terminaison des Nerfs Pneumogastriques et ses Variations. Etude d'Anatomie Descriptive Comparée chez l'Homme et dans la Série des Vertébrés. Lille, France: Université de Lille, 1936. PhD thesis.
37. CRICHLOW, E. C., AND B. G. LEEK. The importance of pH in relation to the acid-excitation of epithelial receptors in the reticulorumen of sheep. *J. Physiol. Lond.* 310: 60P–61P, 1981.
38. DANIEL, R. C. W. Motility of the rumen and abomasum during hypocalcaemia. *Can. J. Comp. Med.* 47: 276–280, 1983.
39. DARDILLAT, C. Analyse électromyographique et débitmétrique du transit alimentaire chez le veau nouveau-né. *J. Physiol. Paris* 73: 925–944, 1977.
40. DARDILLAT, C., AND Y. RUCKEBUSCH. Aspects fonctionnels de la jonction gastro-duodénale chez le veau nouveau-né. *Ann. Rech. Vet.* 4: 31–56, 1973.
41. DEAN, R. E., T. THORNE, AND T. D. MOORE. Passage of alfalfa through the digestive tract of elk. *J. Wild. Manage.* 44: 272–273, 1980.
42. DEDASHEV, I. P. Conditioned reflexes of motor activity in the reticulum and rumen of sheep. *Setchenov. J. Physiol.* 45: 104–108, 1959.
43. DEHORITY, B. A. Carbon dioxide requirement of various species of rumen bacteria. *J. Bacteriol.* 105: 70–76, 1971.
44. DELLA-FERA, M. A., C. A. BAILE, B. S. SHNEIDER, AND J. A. GRINKER. Cholecystokinin antibody injected in cerebral ventricles stimulates feeding in sheep. *Science Wash. DC* 212: 687–689, 1981.
45. DEMEYER, D. I., AND C. J. NEVEL. Methanogenesis, an integrated part of carbohydrate fermentation, and its control. In: *Digestion and Metabolism in the Ruminant*, edited by I. W. McDonald and A. C. I. Warner. Armidale, Australia: Univ. New Engl. Publ. Unit, 1975, p. 366–382.
46. DESWYSEN, A. G., AND H. J. EHRLEIN. Silage intake, rumination and pseudo-rumination activity in sheep studied by radiography and jaw movement recordings. *Br. J. Nutr.* 46: 327–335, 1981.
47. DOBSON, A., AND A. T. PHILLIPSON. Absorption from the ruminant forestomach. In: *Handbook of Physiology. Alimentary Canal. Bile; Digestion; Ruminal Physiology*, edited by C. F. Code. Washington, DC: Am. Physiol. Soc., 1968, sect. 6, vol. V, p. 2761–2774.
48. DOUGHERTY, R. W. Physiology of eructation in ruminants. In: *Handbook of Physiology. Alimentary Canal. Bile; Digestion; Ruminal Physiology*, edited by C. F. Code. Washington, DC: Am. Physiol. Soc., 1968, sect. 6, vol. V, p. 2695–2698.
49. DOUGHERTY, R. W. *Experimental Surgery in Farm Animals*. Ames: Iowa State Univ. Press, 1981.
50. DOUGHERTY, R. W., J. L. RILEY, AND H. M. COOK. Changes in motility and pH in the digestive tract of experimentally overfed sheep. *Am. J. Vet. Res.* 36: 827–829, 1975.
51. DUCKWORTH, J. E., AND D. W. SHIRLAW. A study of factors affecting feed intake and the eating behaviour of cattle. *Anim. Behav.* 6: 147–154, 1958.
52. DULPHY, J. P., AND G. BECHET. Influence du stade de végétation et de l'espèce végétale sur le comportement alimentaire et mérycique de moutons recevant des fourrages verts hachés. *Ann. Zootech. Paris* 25: 505–519, 1976.
53. DULPHY, J. P., B. MICHALET-DOREAU, AND C. DEMARQUILLY. Etude comparée des quantités ingérées et du comportement alimentaire et mérycique d'ovins et de bovins recevant des ensilages d'herbe réalisés selon différentes techniques. *Ann. Zootech. Paris* 33: 291–320, 1984.
54. DUNCAN, D. L. The effects of vagotomy and splanchnotomy on gastric motility in the sheep. *J. Physiol. Lond.* 119: 157–169, 1953.
55. DUNCAN, D. L., AND A. T. PHILLIPSON. The development of the motor responses in the stomach of the foetal sheep. *J. Exp. Biol.* 28: 32–40, 1951.
56. DUSSARDIER, M. Contrôle nerveux du rhythme gastrique des ruminants. *J. Physiol. Paris* 47: 170–173, 1955.
57. DUSSARDIER, M. Réinnervation d'un muscle strié par des fibres préganglionnaires parasympathiques. Application à l'enregistrement de l'activité des fibres efférentes vagales chez l'animal éveillé. *Ann. Biol. Anim. Biochim. Biophys.* 3: 405–425, 1963.
58. DUSSARDIER, M., J. FLINOIS, AND J. P. ROUSSEAU. Localisation des centres bulbaires qui commandent la motricité gastrique. *J. Physiol. Paris* 52: 90–91, 1960.
59. DYCE, K. M. Some remarks upon the functional anatomy of the ruminant stomach. *Tijdschr. Diergeneeskd.* 93: 1334–1344, 1968.
60. DZIUK, H. E. Eructation, regurgitation and reticuloruminal contraction in the American bison. *Am. J. Physiol.* 208: 343–346, 1965.
61. DZIUK, H. E., B. A. FASHINGBAER, AND J. L. IDSTROM. Ruminoreticular pressure patterns in fistulated white-tailed deer. *Am. J. Vet. Res.* 24: 772–782, 1963.
62. EHRLEIN, H. J. Untersuchungen über die Motorik des Labmagens der Ziege unter besonderer Berücksichtigung des Pylorus. *Zentralbl. Veterinaermed. Reihe A* 17: 481–497, 1970.
63. EILER, H., W. A. LYKE, AND R. JOHNSON. Internal vomiting in the ruminant: effect of apomorphine on ruminal pH In sheep. *Am. J. Vet. Res.* 42: 202–204, 1981.
64. ENGELHARDT, W. V., AND J. R. S. HALES. Partition of capillary blood flow in rumen, reticulum, and omasum of sheep. *Am. J. Physiol.* 232 (*Endocrinol. Metab. Gastrointest. Physiol.* 1): E53–E56, 1977.
65. ENGELHARDT, W. V., AND R. HAUFFE. Role of the omasum in absorption and secretion of water and electrolytes in sheep and goats. In: *Digestion and Metabolism in the Ruminant*, edited by I. W. McDonald and A. C. I. Warner. Armidale, Australia: Univ. New Engl. Publ. Unit, 1975, p. 216–230.
66. EVANS, L., AND F. A. SPURRELL. Technique for the direct injection of materials into the ruminant abomasum. *J. Appl. Physiol.* 22: 1030–1037, 1967.
67. FAICHNEY, G. J. The use of markers to measure digesta flow from the stomach of sheep fed once daily. *J. Agric. Sci.* 94: 313–318, 1980.

68. FAICHNEY, G. J. Measurement in sheep of the quantity and composition of rumen digesta and of the fractional outflow rates of digesta constituents. *Aust. J. Agric. Res.* 31: 1129–1137, 1980.
69. FAICHNEY, G. J. Marker techniques for the study of gastrointestinal tract function in ruminants. In: *Techniques in Digestive Physiology*, edited by L. H. Heywood and D. A. Titchen. County Clare, Ireland: Elsevier, 1982, vol. 211, p. 33–36.
70. FAICHNEY, G. J., AND T. N. BARRY. Intravenous somatostatin infusion affects gastrointestinal tract function in sheep. *Can. J. Anim. Sci.* 64: 93–94, 1984.
71. FALEMPIN, M., N. MEI, AND J. P. ROUSSEAU. Vagal mechanoreceptors of the inferior thoracic oesophagus, the lower oesophageal sphincter and the stomach in sheep. *Pfluegers Arch.* 373: 25–30, 1978.
72. FALEMPIN, M., AND J. P. ROUSSEAU. Vagal digestive deafferentation in sheep. *Ann. Rech. Vet.* 10: 186–188, 1979.
73. FELL, B. F., AND T. E. C. WEEKES. Food intake as a mediator of adaptation in the ruminal epithelium. In: *Digestion and Metabolism in the Ruminant*, edited by I. C. McDonald and A. C. I. Warner. Armidale, Australia: Univ. New Engl. Publ. Unit, 1975, p. 101–118.
74. FLOURENS, P. Expériences sur le mécanisme de la rumination. *C.R. Acad. Sci. Paris Mém.* 12: 531–550, 1844.
75. FORBES, J. M., J. A. WRIGHT, AND A. BANNISTER. A note on rate of eating in sheep. *Anim. Prod.* 15: 211–214, 1972.
76. FREER, M., AND R. C. CAMPLING. Factors affecting the voluntary intake of food by cows. 7. The behaviour and reticular motility of cows given diets, dried grass, concentrates and ground pelleted hay. *Br. J. Nutr.* 19: 195–207, 1965.
77. GEOFFROY, F. Etude comparée du comportement alimentaire et mérycique de deux petits ruminants: la chèvre et le mouton. *Ann. Zootech. Paris* 23: 63–73, 1974.
78. GRAU, H. Zur Funktion der Vormägen, besonders des Netzmagens der Wiederkäuer. *Berl. Muench. Tieraerztl. Wochenschr.* 68: 271–275, 1955.
79. GREGORY, P. C. Forestomach motility in the chronically vagotomized sheep. *J. Physiol. Lond.* 328: 431–447, 1980.
80. GREGORY, P. C. Control of intrinsic reticulo-ruminal motility in the vagotomized sheep. *J. Physiol. Lond.* 346: 379–393, 1984.
81. GREGORY, P. C., S. J. MILLER, AND A. C. BREWER. The relationship between food intake and abomasal emptying and small intestinal transit time in sheep. *Br. J. Nutr.* 53: 373–380, 1985.
82. GREGORY, P. C., D. V. RAYNER, AND C. WENHAM. Initiation of migrating myoelectric complex in sheep by duodenal acidification and hyperosmolarity: role of vagus nerves. *J. Physiol. Lond.* 355: 509–521, 1984.
83. GRENET, E. Taille et structure des particules végétales au niveau du feuillet et des fèces chez les bovins. *Ann. Biol. Anim. Biochim. Biophys.* 10: 643–657, 1970.
84. GROVUM, W. L. Factors affecting the voluntary intake of food by sheep. 2. The role of distension and tactile input from compartments of the stomach. *Br. J. Nutr.* 42: 425–436, 1979.
85. GROVUM, W. L. Factors affecting the voluntary intake of food by sheep. 3. The effect of intravenous infusions of gastrin, cholecystokinin and secretin on motility of the reticulo-rumen and intake. *Br. J. Nutr.* 45: 183–201, 1981.
86. GROVUM, W. L. Integration of digestion and digesta kinetics with control of feed intake—a physiological framework for a model of rumen function. In: *Proc. Symp. Herbivore Nutrition in Sub-Tropics and Tropics*, edited by F. M. C. Gilchrist and R. I. Mackie. Pretoria, South Africa: Science, 1984, p. 244–268.
87. GROVUM, W. L., AND H. W. CHAPMAN. Pentagastrin in the circulation acts directly on the brain to depress motility of the stomach in sheep. *Regul. Pept.* 5: 35–42, 1982.
88. GROVUM, W. L., AND G. D. PHILLIPS. Factors affecting the voluntary intake of food by sheep. 1. The role of distension, flow-rate of digesta and propulsive motility in the intestine. *Br. J. Nutr.* 40: 323–336, 1978.
89. GROVUM, W. L., AND V. J. WILLIAMS. Rate of passage of digesta in sheep. 6. The effect of level of food intake on mathematical predictions of the kinetics of digesta in the reticulorumen and intestines. *Br. J. Nutr.* 38: 425–436, 1977.
90. GUILHERMET, R., C. M. MATHIEU, AND R. TOULLEC. Transit des aliments liquides au niveau de la gouttière oesophagienne chez le veau préruminant et ruminant. *Ann. Zootech. Paris* 24: 69–79, 1975.
91. HABEL, R. E. A study of the innervation of the ruminant stomach. *Cornell Vet.* 46: 555–633, 1956.
92. HAMMOND, P. B., H. E. DZIUK, E. A. USENIK, AND C. E. STEVENS. Experimental intestinal obstruction in calves. *J. Comp. Pathol. Ther.* 74: 210–222, 1964.
93. HARDING, R., AND B. F. LEEK. The locations and activities of medullary neurones associated with ruminant forestomach motility. *J. Physiol. Lond.* 219: 587–610, 1971.
94. HARDING, R., AND B. F. LEEK. The effect of peripheral and central nervous influences on gastric centre neuronal activity in sheep. *J. Physiol. Lond.* 225: 309–338, 1972.
95. HARDING, R., AND D. A. TITCHEN. Oesophageal and diaphragmatic activity during sucking in lambs. *J. Physiol. Lond.* 321: 317–329, 1981.
96. HARRIS, L. E., AND A. T. PHILLIPSON. The measurement of the flow of food to the duodenum of the sheep. *Anim. Prod.* 4: 97–116, 1962.
97. HARRISON, F. A. Bile secretion in the sheep. *J. Physiol. Lond.* 162: 212–224, 1962.
98. HARRISON, F. A. Advances in the application of experimental surgery in digestive physiology. In: *Digestive Physiology and Metabolism in Ruminants*, edited by Y. Ruckebusch and P. Thivend. Lancaster, UK: MTP, 1980, p. 829–840.
99. HARRISON, F. A., AND K. J. HILL. Digestive secretions and the flow of digesta along the duodenum of the sheep. *J. Physiol. Lond.* 162: 225–243, 1962.
100. HARTNELL, G. F., AND L. D. SATTER. Determination of rumen fill, retention time and ruminal turnover rates of ingesta at different stages of lactation in dairy cows. *J. Anim. Sci.* 48: 381–392, 1979.
101. HECKER, J. F. *The Sheep as an Experimental Animal.* London: Academic, 1983, p. 34–134
102. HELLER, R., P. C. GREGORY, AND W. V. ENGELHARDT. Pattern of motility and flow of digesta in the forestomach of the Llama (*Lama guanacoe f. glama*). *J. Comp. Physiol. Biochem. Syst. Environ. Physiol.* 154: 529–533, 1984.
103. HEYWOOD, L. H., AND A. K. W. WOOD. Thoracic oesophageal motor activity during eructation in sheep. *Q. J. Exp. Physiol.* 70: 603–613, 1985.
104. HILL, K. J. Continuous gastric secretion in the ruminant. *Q. J. Exp. Physiol.* 40: 32–39, 1955.
105. HILL, K. J. Nervous structures in the reticulo-ruminal epithelium of the lamb and kid. *Q. J. Exp. Physiol.* 44: 222–238, 1959.
106. HILL, K. J. Abomasal secretory function in the sheep. In: *Physiology of Digestion in the Ruminant*, edited by R. W. Dougherty. Washington, DC: Butterworth, 1965, p. 221–230.
107. HILL, K. J. Abomasal function. In: *Handbook of Physiology. Alimentary Canal. Bile; Digestion; Ruminal Physiology*, edited by C. F. Code. Washington, DC: Am. Physiol. Soc., 1968, sect. 6, Vol. V, p. 2747–2759.
108. HILL, K. J., AND R. A. GREGORY. The preparation of gastric pouches in the ruminant. *Vet. Rec.* 63: 647–652, 1951.
109. HODGSON, J. The development of solid food intake in calves. 5. The relationship between liquid and solid food intake. *Anim. Prod.* 13: 593–597, 1971.
110. HOFFMANN, R. R., AND B. SCHNOOR. *Die funktionelle Morphologie des Wiederkäuer-Magens.* Stuttgart, FRG: Ferdinand Enke, 1982, p. 1–170.
111. HOFFMANN, R. R., AND D. R. M. STEWART. Grazers or browsers: a classification based on the stomach structure and feeding habit of East African ruminants. *Mammalia* 36: 226–240, 1972.

112. HOFLUND, S. Untersuchungen über Störungen in den Funktionen der Wiederkäuermagen, durch Schädigungen des N. vagus Verursacht. *Svensk. Vet. Dskrift. Suppl.* 45: 1–59, 1940.
113. HOFMEYER, C. F. B., AND H. C. VOSS. Oesophageal fistulation of sheep. *J. S. Afr. Vet. Med. Assoc.* 35: 579–582, 1964.
114. HOGAN, J. P., AND A. T. PHILLIPSON. The rate of flow of digesta and their removal along the digestive tract of the sheep. *Br. J. Nutr.* 14: 147–155, 1960.
115. HOPCROFT, S. C., AND A. W. BANKS. The production of an isolated loop of upper small intestine in the sheep. *Exp. Med. Surg.* 23: 203–206, 1965.
116. HUNGATE, R. E. Ruminal fermentation. In: *Handbook of Physiology. Alimentary Canal. Bile; Digestion; Ruminal Physiology*, edited by C. F. Code. Washington, DC: Am. Physiol. Soc., 1968, vol. V, chapt. 130, p. 2725–2745.
117. IGGO, A. Central nervous control of gastric movements in sheep and goats. *J. Physiol. Lond.* 131: 248–256, 1956.
118. IGGO, A., AND B. F. LEEK. An electrophysiological study of vagal efferent units associated with gastric movements in sheep. *J. Physiol. Lond.* 191: 177–204, 1967.
119. ITABISASHI, T. Relations between periodic potential fluctuations and intragastric pressure in goats. *Natl. Inst. Animal Health Qt. Yatb.* 4: 115–124, 1964.
120. ITABISASHI, T. Potential changes that accompany movement of the ruminant stomach. In: *Physiology of Digestion and Metabolism in the Ruminant*, edited by A. T. Phillipson. Newcastle upon Tyne, UK: Oriel, 1970, p. 42–51.
121. KAY, R. N. B. Continuous and reflex secretion by the parotid gland in ruminants. *J. Physiol. Lond.* 144: 463–475, 1958.
122. KAY, R. N. B. Rumination in sheep caused by injection of adrenaline. *Nature Lond.* 183: 552–553, 1959.
123. KAY, R. N. B. The rate of flow and composition of various salivary secretions in sheep and calves. *J. Physiol. Lond.* 150: 515–537, 1960.
124. KAY, R. N. B., W. V. ENGELHARDT, AND R. G. WHITE. The digestive physiology of wild ruminants. In: *Digestive Physiology and Metabolism in Ruminants*, edited by Y. Ruckebusch and P. Thivend. Lancaster, UK: MTP, 1980, p. 743–761.
125. KAY, R. N. B., AND E. D. GOODALL. The intake, digestibility and retention time of roughage diets by red deer (*Cervus elaphus*) and sheep. *Proc. Nutr. Soc.* 35: 98A, 1976.
126. KAY, R. N. B., AND A. T. PHILLIPSON. Response of the salivary glands to distension of the oesophagus and rumen. *J. Physiol. Lond.* 148: 507–523, 1959.
127. KAY, R. N. B., AND Y. RUCKEBUSCH. Movements of the stomach compartments of a young bull during sucking. *Br. J. Nutr.* 26: 301–309, 1971.
128. KOMAREK, R. J., AND E. C. LEFFEL. Gas-tight cannula for rumen fistula. *J. Anim. Sci.* 20: 782–784, 1961.
129. KONDOS, A. C. A new method for cannulation of the abomasum in sheep. *Aust. Vet. J.* 43: 149–151, 1967.
130. LANGER, P. Stomach evolution in the Artiodactyla. *Mammalia* 38: 295–314, 1974.
131. LANGER, P. Comparative anatomy of the stomach in mammalian herbivores. *Q. J. Exp. Physiol.* 69: 615–625, 1984.
132. LAPLACE, J. P. Omaso-abomasal motility and feeding behavior in sheep: a new concept. *Physiol. Behav.* 5: 61–65, 1970.
133. LEEK, B. F. Reticulo-ruminal mechanoreceptors in sheep. *J. Physiol. Lond.* 202: 585–609, 1969.
134. LEEK, B. F., AND R. HARDING. Sensory nervous receptors in the ruminant stomach and the reflex control of reticuloruminal motility. In: *Digestion and Metabolism in the Ruminant*, edited by I. W. McDonald and A. C. I. Warner. Armidale, Australia: Univ. of New Engl. Publ. Unit, 1975, p. 60–76.
135. LEFEBVRE, R. A. Study on the possible neurotransmitter of the non-adrenergic non-cholinergic innervation of the rat gastric fundus. *Arch. Int. Pharmacodyn. Ther.* 280, Suppl. 2: 110–136, 1986.
136. LENG, R. A. Formation and production of volatile fatty acids in the rumen. In: *Physiology of Digestion and Metabolism in the Ruminant*, edited by A. T. Phillipson. Aberdeen, UK: Oriel, 1970, p. 406–421.
137. LOUVIER, J. A., H. W. COLVIN, JR., G. ISHIZAKI, G. A. IWAMOTO, AND H. R. PARKER. Effect of rumen insufflation on ruminal contraction rate in sheep. *J. Anim. Sci.* 48: 934–940, 1979.
138. LYSONS, R. J., AND T. J. L. ALEXANDER. The gnotobiotic ruminant and in vivo studies of defined bacterial populations. In: *Digestion and Metabolism in the Ruminant*, edited by I. W. McDonald and A. C. I. Warner. Armidale, Australia: Univ. of New Engl. Publ. Unit, 1975, p. 180–204.
139. MAAS, C. L. Opiate antagonists stimulate ruminal motility of conscious goats. *Eur. J. Pharmacol.* 77: 71–74, 1982.
140. MAAS, C. L., C. T. M. VAN DUIN, AND A. S. J. P. A. M. VAN MIERT. Modification by domperidone of dopamine- and apomorphine-induced inhibition of extrinsic ruminal contraction in goat. *J. Vet. Pharm. Ther.* 5: 191–194, 1982.
141. MACRAE, J. C., C. S. W. REID, D. W. DELLOW, AND R. S. WYBURN. Caecal cannulation in the sheep. *Res. Vet. Sci.* 14: 78–85, 1973.
142. MAGEE, D. F. An investigation into the internal secretion of the pancreas in sheep. *J. Physiol. Lond.* 158: 132–143, 1961.
143. MALOIY, G. M. O., AND R. N. B. KAY. A comparison of digestion in red deer and sheep under controlled conditions. *Q. J. Exp. Physiol.* 56: 257–266, 1971.
144. MATSCHER, R., AND V. BEGHELLI. L'influenza dell'attivita abomasale sui prestomaci. Inibizione dell'atrio e del sacco ventrale del rumine per stimulazione elletrica del N. abomasale. *Arch. Sci. Biol.* 42: 251–262, 1958.
145. MAYER, E. A., G. VAN DEVENTER, J. ELASHOFF, S. KHAWAJA, AND J. H. WALSH. Characterization of substance P effects on canine antral muscle. *Am. J. Physiol.* 251 (*Gastrointest. Liver Physiol.* 14): G140–G146, 1986.
146. MCBRIDE, B. W., R. BERZINS, L. P. MILLIGAN, AND B. V. TURNER. Development of a technique for gastrointestinal endoscopy of domestic ruminants. *Can. J. Anim. Sci.* 63: 349–354, 1983.
147. MCLEAY, L. M., AND F. R. BELL. Effect of cholecystokinin, secretin, glucagon, and insulin on gastric emptying and acid secretion in the calf. *Am. J. Vet. Res.* 41: 1590–1594, 1981.
148. MCLEAY, L. M., AND D. A. TITCHEN. Abomasal secretory responses to teasing with food and feeding in the sheep. *J. Physiol. Lond.* 206: 605–628, 1970.
149. MCLEAY, L. M., AND D. A. TITCHEN. Effects of the amount and type of food eaten on secretion from fundic abomasal pouches of sheep. *Br. J. Nutr.* 32: 375–387, 1974.
150. MCLEAY, L. M., AND D. A. TITCHEN. Gastric, antral and fundic pouch secretion in sheep. *J. Physiol. Lond.* 248: 595–612, 1975.
151. MCLEAY, L. M., AND D. A. TITCHEN. Acid and pepsin secretion of separated gastric pouches during perfusion of antral pouches with cholinergic stimulating and blocking agents and lignocaine. *J. Physiol. Lond.* 264: 215–227, 1977.
152. MCLEAY, L. M., AND D. A. TITCHEN. Inhibition of hydrochloric acid and pepsin secretion from gastric pouches by antral pouch acidification in sheep. *J. Physiol. Lond.* 273: 707–716, 1977.
153. MCMANUS, W. R., G. W. ARNOLD, AND F. J. HAMILTON. Improved techniques in oesophageal fistulation of sheep. *Aust. Vet. J.* 38: 275–281, 1962.
154. MENDEL, V. E. Pneumatic and semipneumatic plugs for large-diameter rumen fistulas in cattle. *J. Dairy Sci.* 44: 679–686, 1961.
155. MILNE, J. A. Comparative digestive physiology and metabolism of the red deer and the sheep. *Proc. N. Z. Soc. Anim. Prod.* 40: 151–157, 1980.
156. MILNE, J. A., J. C. MACRAE, A. M. SPENCE, AND S. WILSON. A comparison of the voluntary intake and digestion of a range of forages at different times of the year by the sheep and the red deer (*Cervus elaphus*). *Br. J. Nutr.* 40: 347–357, 1978.

157. MOIR, R. Ruminant digestion and evolution. In: *Handbook of Physiology. Alimentary Canal. Bile; Digestion; Ruminal Physiology*, edited by C. F. Code. Washington, DC: Am. Physiol. Soc., 1968, sect. 6, vol. V, p. 2673-2694.
158. MORGAN, C. A., AND R. C. CAMPLING. Chewing behaviour of hay-fed cows given supplements of whole barley and oat grains. *J. Agric. Sci. Camb.* 91: 415-418, 1978.
159. MORRISON, A. R., AND R. E. HABEL. A quantitative study of the distribution of vagal nerve endings in the myenteric plexus of the ruminant stomach. *J. Comp. Neurol.* 122: 297-309, 1964.
160. MURPHY, C. A., AND J. M. NICOLETTI. Potential reduction of forage and rumen digesta particle size by microbial action. *J. Dairy Sci.* 67: 1221-1226, 1984.
161. MURRAY, R. M., H. MARSH, G. E. HEINSOHN, AND A. V. SPAIN. The role of the midgut caecum and large intestine in the digestion of sea grasses by the dugong (Mammalia:Sirenia). *Comp. Biochem. Physiol.* 56: 7-10, 1978.
162. NEWHOOK, J. D., AND D. A. TITCHEN. Effects of stimulation of efferent fibres of the vagus on the reticulo-omasal orifice of the sheep. *J. Physiol. Lond.* 222: 407-418, 1972.
163. NEWHOOK, J. C., AND D. A. TITCHEN. Effects of vagotomy, atropine, hexamethonium and adrenaline on the destination in the stomach of liquids sucked by milk-fed lambs and calves. *J. Physiol. Lond.* 237: 415-430, 1974.
164. NICHOLSON, R., AND S. A. OMER. The inhibitory effect of intestinal infusions of unsaturated long-chain fatty acids on forestomach motility of sheep. *Br. J. Nutr.* 50: 141-149, 1983.
165. NORDIN, M. Voluntary food intake and digestion by the lesser mousedeer. *J. Wild. Manage.* 42: 185-187, 1978.
166. OGHA, A., Y. OTA, AND Y. NAKAZATO. The movement of the stomach of the sheep with special reference to the omasal movement. *Jpn. J. Vet. Sci.* 27: 151-160, 1965.
167. OOMS, L., AND W. OYAERT. Electromyographic study of the abomasal antrum and proximal duodenum in cattle. *Zentralbl. Veterinaermed. Reihe A* 25: 464-473, 1978.
168. ORSKOV, E. R., AND D. BENZIE. Studies on the esophageal groove reflex in sheep and on the potential use of the groove to prevent the fermentation of food in the rumen. *Br. J. Nutr.* 23: 415-420, 1969.
169. ORSKOV, E. R., D. BENZIE, AND R. N. B. KAY. The effect of feeding procedure on closure of the oesophageal groove in young sheep. *Br. J. Nutr.* 24: 785-795, 1970.
170. ORSKOV, E. R., D. A. GRUBB, G. WENHAM, AND W. CORRIGALL. The sustenance of growing and fattening ruminants by intragastric infusion of volatile fatty acids and protein. *Br. J. Nutr.* 41: 533-558, 1979.
171. ORSKOV, E. R., N. A. MACLEOD, R. N. B. KAY, AND P. C. GREGORY. Method and validation of intragastric nutrition. *Can. J. Anim. Sci.* 64: 138-139, 1984.
172. OYAERT, W., AND J. H. BOUCKAERT. A study of the passage of fluid through the sheep's omasum. *Res. Vet. Sci.* 2: 41-52, 1961.
173. PAIRET, M., T. BOUYSSOU, AND Y. RUCKEBUSCH. Colonic formation of soft feces in rabbits: a role for endogenous prostaglandins. *Am. J. Physiol.* 250 (*Gastrointest. Liver Physiol.* 13): G302-G308, 1986.
174. PATTERSON, J., P. BRIGHTLING, AND D. A. TITCHEN. Beta-adrenergic effects on composition of parotid salivary secretion of sheep on feeding. *Q. J. Exp. Physiol.* 67: 57-67, 1982.
175. PHILLIPSON, A. T. The movements of the pouches of the stomach of the sheep. *Q. J. Exp. Physiol.* 29: 395-415, 1939.
176. PHILLIPSON, A. T., AND C. S. W. REID. Distension of the rumen and salivary secretion. *Nature Lond.* 181: 1722-1723, 1958.
177. PONCET, C., AND M. IVAN. Effects of duodenal cannulation in sheep on the pattern of gastrointestinal motility and digestive flow. *Nutr. Reprod. Dev.* 24: 887-902, 1984.
178. PONCET, C., M. IVAN, AND M. LEVEILLE. Electromagnetic measurements of duodenal digesta flow in cannulated sheep. *Reprod. Nutr. Dev.* 22: 651-660, 1982.
179. QUIN, J. I., AND J. G. VAN DER WATH. Studies on the alimentary tract of Merino sheep in South Africa. V. The motility of the rumen under various conditions. *Onderstepoort J. Vet. Sci. Anim. Ind.* 11: 361-382, 1938.
180. REID, C. S. W. Diet and motility of the forestomachs of the sheep. *Proc. N. Z. Soc. Anim. Prod.* 23: 169-188, 1963.
181. REID, C. S. W., AND J. B. CORNWALL. The mechanical activity of the reticulo-rumen of cattle. *Proc. N. Z. Soc. Anim. Prod.* 19: 23-35, 1959.
182. REID, C. S. W., AND D. A. TITCHEN. Reflex stimulation of movements of the rumen in decerebrate sheep. *J. Physiol. Lond.* 181: 432-448, 1965.
183. RIEK, R. F. The influence of sodium salts on the closure of the oesophageal groove in calves. *Aust. Vet. J.* 30: 29-37, 1954.
184. ROMAN, C. Contrôle nerveux du péristaltisme oesophagien. *J. Physiol. Paris* 58: 79-108, 1966.
185. ROUSSEAU, J. P. Electrophysiological study of vagal afferent and efferent units in conscious sheep. *Q. J. Exp. Physiol.* 69: 627-637, 1984.
186. ROY, J. H. B. Factors affecting susceptibility of calves to disease. *J. Dairy Sci.* 63: 650-664, 1980.
187. RUCKEBUSCH, Y. Liaisons réflexes conditionnelles chez les ruminants. II. Rumination. *Bull. Acad. Vet. Fr.* 36: 99-107, 1963.
188. RUCKEBUSCH, Y. The electrical activity of the digestive tract of the sheep as an indication of the mechanical events in various regions. *J. Physiol. Lond.* 210: 857-882, 1970.
189. RUCKEBUSCH, Y. Motility of the ruminant stomach associated with states of sleep. In: *Digestion and Metabolism in the Ruminant*, edited by I. W. McDonald and A. C. I. Warner. Armidale, Australia: Univ. New Engl. Publ. Unit, 1975, p. 77-90.
190. RUCKEBUSCH, Y. Enhancement of the cyclic motor activity of the ovine small intestine by lysergic acid derivatives. *Gastroenterology* 87: 1049-1055, 1984.
191. RUCKEBUSCH, Y. Development of digestive motor patterns during perinatal life: mechanism and significance. *J. Pediatr. Gastroenterol. Nutr.* 5: 523-536, 1986.
192. RUCKEBUSCH, Y., T. BARDON, AND M. PAIRET. Opioid control of the ruminant stomach motility: Functional importance of $\mu$, $\kappa$ and $\delta$ receptors. *Life Sci.* 35: 1731-1738, 1984.
193. RUCKEBUSCH, Y., AND L. BUENO. Origin of migrating myoelectric complex in sheep. *Am. J. Physiol.* 233 (*Endocrinol. Metab. Gastrointest. Physiol.* 2): E484-E487, 1977.
194. RUCKEBUSCH, Y., C. DARDILLAT, AND P. GUILLOTEAU. Development of digestive function in the newborn ruminant. *Ann. Rech. Vet.* 14: 360-374, 1983.
195. RUCKEBUSCH, Y., AND C. H. MALBERT. Physiological characteristics of ovine pyloric sphincter. *Am. J. Physiol.* 251 (*Gastrointest. Liver Physiol.* 14): G804-G814, 1986.
196. RUCKEBUSCH, Y., AND A. M. MERRITT. Pharmacology of the ruminant gastroduodenal junction. *J. Vet. Pharm. Ther.* 8: 339-351, 1985.
197. RUCKEBUSCH, Y., AND G. SOLDANI. Gallbladder motility in sheep: effects of cholecystokinin and related peptides. *J. Vet. Pharm. Ther.* 8: 263-269, 1985.
198. RUCKEBUSCH, Y., AND T. TOMOV. The sequential contractions of the rumen associated with eructation in sheep. *J. Physiol. Lond.* 235: 447-458, 1973.
199. RUCKEBUSCH, Y., C. H. TSIAMITAS, AND L. BUENO. The intrinsic electrical activity of the ruminant stomach. *Life Sci.* 11: 55-64, 1972.
200. SAKATA, T., AND H. TAMATE. Rumen epithelium cell proliferation accelerated by propionate and acetate. *J. Dairy Sci.* 62: 49-52, 1979.
201. SCOTT, D. Factors influencing the secretion and absorption of calcium and magnesium in the small intestine of the sheep. *Q. J. Exp. Physiol.* 50: 312-318, 1965.
202. SCOTT, D. The effects of sodium depletion and potassium supplements upon electrical potentials in the rumen of the

sheep. *Q. J. Exp. Physiol.* 51: 60–69, 1966.
203. SELLERS, A. F., AND A. DOBSON. Studies on reticulo-rumen sodium and potassium concentrations and electrical potentials in sheep. *Res. Vet. Sci.* 1: 95–102, 1960.
204. SELLERS, A. F., AND C. E. STEVENS. Motor functions of the ruminant forestomach. *Physiol. Rev.* 46: 634–661, 1966.
205. SELLERS, A. F., C. E. STEVENS, A. DOBSON, AND F. D. MCLEOD. Arterial blood flow to the ruminant stomach. *Am. J. Physiol.* 207: 371–377, 1964.
206. SINGLETON, A. G. The electromagnetic measurement of the flow of digesta through the duodenum of the goat and the sheep. *J. Physiol. Lond.* 155: 134–147, 1961.
207. SISSONS, J. W. Effect of feed intake on digesta flow and myoelectric activity in the gastrointestinal tract of the preruminant calf. *J. Dairy Sci.* 50: 387–395, 1983.
208. SISSONS, J. W., AND R. H. SMITH. Effect of duodenal cannulation, abomasal emptying and secretion in the pre-ruminant calf. *J. Physiol. Lond.* 322: 409–417, 1982.
209. SISSONS, J. W., S. M. THURSTON, AND R. H. SMITH. Reticular myoelectric activity and turnover of rumen digesta in the growing steer. *Can. J. Anim. Sci.* 64: 70–71, 1984.
210. SPERBER, I., S. HYDEN, AND J. ECKMAN. The use of polyethylene glycol as a reference substance in the study of ruminant digestion. *K. Lantbrukshogsk. Ann.* 20: 337–344, 1953.
211. STEVENS, C. E. Transport of sodium and chloride by the isolated rumen epithelium. *Am. J. Physiol.* 206: 1099–1105, 1964.
212. STEVENS, C. E., AND A. F. SELLERS. Studies of the reflex control of the ruminant stomach with special reference to the eructation reflex. *Am. J. Vet. Res.* 20: 461–482, 1959.
213. STEVENS, C. E., AND A. F. SELLERS. Rumination. In: *Handbook of Physiology. Alimentary Canal. Bile; Digestion; Ruminal Physiology*, edited by C. F. Code. Washington, DC: Am. Physiol. Soc., 1968, sect. 6, vol. V, p. 2699–2704.
214. STEVENS, C. E., A. F. SELLERS, AND F. A. SPURRELL. Function of the bovine omasum in ingesta transfer. *Am. J. Physiol.* 198: 449–455, 1960.
215. STEWART, W. E., AND D. G. STEWART. Technique for cannulation of parotid salivary duct of sheep. *J. Appl. Physiol.* 16: 203–209, 1961.
216. STOYANOV, I. N., Y. B. LOUKANOV, P. V. VASSILEVA, AND V. I. VASSILEV. Comparative studies of the alpha and beta adrenergic receptors in the longitudinal and circular smooth muscle layers of the simple and complex stomach. *Gen. Pharmacol.* 7: 399–404, 1976.
217. SUTTON, J. D. Carbohydrate fermentation in the rumen—variations on a theme. *Proc. Nutr. Soc.* 38: 275–281, 1979.
218. SVENDSEN, P. Experimental studies on gastrointestinal atony in ruminants. In: *Digestion and Metabolism in the Ruminant*, edited by I. W. McDonald and A. C. I. Warner. Armidale, Australia: Univ. New Engl. Publ. Unit, 1975, p. 563–575.
219. SYMONS, L. E. A., AND D. R. HENNESSEY. Cholecystokinin and anorexia in sheep infected by the intestinal nematode *Trichostrongylus colubriformis*. *Int. J. Parasitol.* 11: 55–58, 1981.
220. SZABO, T., AND M. DUSSARDIER. Les noyaux d'origine du nerf vague chez le mouton. *Z. Zellforsch. Mikrosk. Anat.* 63: 247–276, 1964.
221. TADMOR, A., AND H. NEWMARK. An abdominal approach for producing permanent omasal fistulae in the ox and sheep. *Aust. Vet. J.* 48: 408–415, 1972.
222. TAMATE, H., A. D. MCGILLARD, N. I. JACOBSON, AND R. GETTY. Effect of various dietaries on the anatomical development of the stomach in the calf. *J. Dairy Sci.* 45: 408–420, 1962.
223. TANEIKE, T. 5-Hydroxytryptamine potentiates contraction mediated by the intramural cholinergic nerves in the longitudinal smooth muscle of the ruminant forestomach. *J. Vet. Pharm. Ther.* 2: 59–68, 1979.
224. TANSY, M. F., J. S. MARTIN, W. E. LANDIN, AND F. M. KENDALL. Species difference in GI motor response to somatostatin. *J. Pharm. Sci.* 68: 1107–1113, 1979.
225. TINDAL, J. S., L. A. BLAKE, A. D. SIMMONDS, I. C. HART, AND H. MIZUNO. Control of growth hormone release in goats: effects of vagal cooling, feeding and artificial distension of the rumen. *Horm. Metab. Res.* 14: 425–429, 1982.
226. TITCHEN, D. A. The production of rumen and reticulum contractions in decerebrate preparations of sheep and goats. *J. Physiol. Lond.* 151: 139–153, 1960.
227. TITCHEN, D. A. Nervous control of motility of the forestomach of ruminants. In: *Handbook of Physiology. Alimentary Canal. Bile; Digestion; Ruminal Physiology*, edited by C. F. Code. Washington, DC: Am. Physiol. Soc., 1968, sect. 6, vol. V, p. 2705–2724.
228. TITCHEN, D. A. Diaphragmatic and oesophageal activity in regurgitation in sheep: an electromyographic study. *J. Physiol. Lond.* 292: 381–390, 1979.
229. TITCHEN, D. A. Gastrointestinal peptide hormone distribution, release and action in ruminants. In: *Control of Digestion and Metabolism in Ruminants*, edited by L. P. Milligan, W. L. Grovum, and A. Dobson. Englewood Cliffs, NJ: Prentice-Hall, 1986, p. 498–515.
230. TITCHEN, D. A., C. S. W. REID, AND P. VLIEG. Effects of intraduodenal infusions of fat on the food intake of sheep. *Proc. N. Z. Soc. Anim. Prod.* 26: 36–51, 1966.
231. TOUTAIN, P. L., M. R. ZINGONI, AND Y. RUCKEBUSCH. Assessment of alpha 2 adrenergic antagonists on the central nervous system using reticular contraction in sheep as a model. *J. Pharmacol. Exp. Ther.* 223: 215–218, 1982.
232. TSUDA, T. Studies on absorption from the rumen. 2. Absorption of several organic substances from the miniature rumen of the goat. *Tohoku J. Agric. Res.* 7: 241–256, 1956.
233. ULYATT, M. J., D. W. DELLOW, A. JOHN, C. S. W. REID, AND G. C. WAGHORN. Contribution of chewing during eating and rumination to the clearance of digesta from the ruminoreticulum. In: *Control of Digestion and Metabolism in Ruminants*, edited by L. P. Milligan, W. L. Grovum, and A. Dobson. Englewood Cliffs, NJ: Prentice-Hall, 1986, p. 498–515.
234. ULYATT, M. J., D. W. DELLOW, C. S. W. REID, AND T. BAUCHOP. Structure and function of the large intestine of ruminants. In: *Digestion and Metabolism in the Ruminant*, edited by I. W. McDonald and A. C. I. Warner. Armidale, Australia: Univ. New Engl. Publ. Unit, 1975, p. 119–133.
235. VALLENAS, A., J. F. CUMMINGS, AND J. F. MUNNELL. A gross study of the compartmentalized stomach of two new-world camelids, the llama and guanaco. *J. Morphol.* 134: 399–423, 1971.
236. VALLENAS, A. P., AND C. E. STEVENS. Motility of the llama and guanaco stomach. *Am. J. Physiol.* 220: 275–282, 1971.
237. VANDEPLASSCHE, G., W. OYAERT, AND A. HOUVENAGHEL. The influence of prostaglandins on in vitro motility of the fundus and the pyloric sphincter of the bovine abomasum. *Arch. Int. Pharmacodyn. Ther.* 260: 306–310, 1982.
238. VANDERMEERSCHEN-DOIZE, F., AND R. PAQUAY. Effects of continuous long-term intravenous infusion of long-chain fatty acids on feeding behaviour and blood components of adult sheep. *Appetite* 5: 137–146, 1984.
239. VAN LENNEP, E. W. The glands of the digestive system in the one-humped camel, *Camelus dromedarius* L. *Acta Morphol. Neerl. Scand.* 1: 286–292, 1958.
240. VAN MIERT, A. S. J. P. A. M., L. E. VAN DER WAL-KOMPROE, AND C. T. M. VAN DUIN. Effects of antipyretic agents on fever and ruminal stasis induced by endotoxin in conscious goats. *Arch. Int. Pharmacodyn. Ther.* 225: 39–50, 1977.
241. VAN MIERT, A. S. J. P. A. M., AND F. VAN VUGT. The effect of dopamine on gastric adrenergic receptors in the goat. *Zentralbl. Veterinaermed. Reihe A* 21: 96–104, 1974.
242. VAN SOEST, P. J. *Nutritional Ecology of the Ruminant.* Corvallis, Oregon: O & B Books, 1982.
243. VAN'T KLOOSTER, A. T., A. KEMP, J. H. GEURINK, AND P. A.

M. ROGERS. Studies on the amount and composition of digesta flowing through the duodenum of dairy cows. 1. Rate of flow of digesta measured direct and estimated indirect by the indicator dilution technique. *Neth. J. Agric. Sci.* 20: 314–324, 1972.

244. VEENENDAAL, G. H., F. M. A. WOUTERSEN-VAN NIJNANTEN, AND A. S. J. P. A. M. VAN MIERT. Responses of goat ruminal musculature to bradykinin and serotonin in vitro and in vivo. *Am. J. Vet. Res.* 41: 479–483, 1980.

245. VEENENDAAL, G. H., F. M. A. WOUTERSEN-VAN NIJMANTEN, AND A. S. J. P. A. M. VAN MIERT. Responses of goat ruminal musculature to substance P in vitro and in vivo. *Vet. Res. Commun.* 5: 363–367, 1982.

246. VLAMINCK, K., C. VAN DEN HENDE, W. OYAERT, AND E. MUYLLE. Studies on abomasal emptying in cattle. 1. Correlation between abomasal emptying, electromyographic activity and pressure changes in the abomasum. *Zentralbl. Veterinaermed. Reihe A* 31: 561–566, 1984.

247. WAGHORN, G. C., AND C. S. W. REID. Rumen motility in sheep and cattle as affected by feeds and feeding. *Proc. N. Z. Soc. Anim. Prod.* 37: 176–181, 1977.

248. WARDROP, I. D., AND J. B. COOMBE. The development of rumen function in the lamb. *Aust. J. Agric. Res.* 12: 661–680, 1961.

249. WARNER, E. D. The organogenesis and early histogenesis of the bovine stomach. *Am. J. Anat.* 102: 33–64, 1958.

250. WARNER, R. G., W. P. FLATT, AND J. K. LOOSLI. Dietary factors influencing the development of the ruminant stomach. *Agric. Food Chem.* 4: 788–792, 1956.

251. WATSON, R. Studies on deglutition in sheep. 1. Observations on the course taken by liquids through the stomach of the sheep at various ages from birth to maturity. *Bull. Council Sci. Industr. Res.* 180: 1–94, 1944.

252. WEISS, K. E. Physiological studies on eructation in ruminants. *Onderstepoort J. Vet. Res.* 26: 251–283, 1953.

253. WESTRA, R., AND R. J. HUDSON. Digestive function of Wapiti calves. *J. Wild. Manage.* 45: 148–155, 1981.

254. WEYNS, A., L. A. OOMS, A. VEHHOFSTAD, T. PEETERS, L. VAN NASSAUW, AND P. KREDIET. Neurotransmitters/neuromodulators of the ruminant stomach: a histochemical, radioimmunological, immunocytochemical and functional approach. In: *The Ruminant Stomach*, edited by L. A. Ooms, A. Degryse, and R. Marsboom. Beerse, Belgium: Janssen Foundation, 1985, vol. 1, p. 53–117.

255. WEYRETER, H., AND W. V. ENGELHARDT. Adaptation of Heidschnucken, Merino and Blackhead sheep to a fibrous roughage diet of poor quality. *Can. J. Anim. Sci.* 64, Suppl. 1: 152–153, 1984.

256. WILSON, A. D. The influence of diet on the development of parotid salivation and the rumen of the lamb. *Aust. J. Agr. Res.* 14: 226–238, 1963.

257. WINSHIP, D. H., F. F. ZBORALSKE, W. N. WEBBER, AND K. H. SOERGEL. Esophagus in rumination. *Am. J. Physiol.* 207: 1189–1194, 1964.

258. WISE, G. H., AND G. W. ANDERSON. Factors affecting the passage of liquids into the rumen of the dairy calf. 1. Method of administering liquids: drinking from open pail versus sucking through a rubber nipple. *J. Dairy Sci.* 22: 697–705, 1939.

259. WYBURN, R. S. The mixing and propulsion of the stomach contents of ruminants. In: *Digestive Physiology and Metabolism of Ruminants*, edited by Y. Ruckebusch and P. Thivend. Lancaster, UK: MTP, 1980, p. 35–51.

# CHAPTER 35

# Avian gastrointestinal motor function

GARY E. DUKE | *Department of Veterinary Biology, College of Veterinary Medicine, University of Minnesota, St. Paul, Minnesota*

---

## CHAPTER CONTENTS

Gross Anatomy
    Mouth and pharynx
    Esophagus and crop
    Glandular stomach
    Muscular stomach
    Small intestine
    Ceca, rectum, and cloaca
    Liver and pancreas
Methods of Study of Motility in Birds
Prehension and Swallowing
Motility of Esophagus and Crop
Motility of Stomach and Duodenum
    Motility patterns: fowl
    Regulation of motility: fowl
    Motility patterns: raptors
    Regulation of motility: raptors
Motility of Ileum, Ceca, and Rectum
    Ileum
    Ceca
    Rectum
Passage Rate

---

THE DIGESTIVE SYSTEM, like other avian systems, shows adaptations associated with flight (50). In the oral area, the teeth and heavy jaw bones and muscles of reptiles and mammals have been replaced by a much lighter beak, jaw bones, and jaw muscles in birds. Because birds do not chew food, the esophagus is large in diameter to accommodate larger food items. The heavy muscular stomach (gizzard) for mechanical digestion and the glandular stomach (proventriculus) (Fig. 1) are located within the main mass of the avian body, which is suspended below the wings during flight. Less modification is evident in the avian small intestine and rectum; however, a cloaca is present, like in reptiles.

For more information on histology of the gastrointestinal tract in domestic species, see Calhoun (17); for more details on morphological and histological variations between species, see Ziswiler and Farner (100) and McLelland (70).

## GROSS ANATOMY

### Mouth and Pharynx

The tongue and beak are important in food manipulation and exhibit many interesting adaptations in birds (70). There is no sharp distinction between the mouth and the pharynx, and there is no soft palate in most birds. The hard palate communicates with the nasal cavities via a median slit.

Salivary glands are present and, in general, they are poorly developed in species that ingest aquatic food and well developed in those eating dry food. The glands of some species (e.g., house sparrow) contain appreciable amounts of amylase, whereas others, such as the chicken and turkey, do not (61). Secretion of saliva is increased by feeding and by parasympathetic stimulation (19).

The taste buds of birds vary in location and number among species, but they are mostly located on the back of the palate, around the glottis, and on the tongue.

### Esophagus and Crop

The esophagus of most birds is relatively long; it has outer longitudinal and inner circular muscles and numerous mucous glands to help lubricate the passage of food. The crop is an enlargement of the esophagus and serves to store food for subsequent passage to the stomach. Early investigators (77, 84) considered the crop to be a part of the stomach and believed it to be analogous to the mammalian cardia. The two structures are similar histologically. The size and shape of crops vary between species. The crops of pigeons consist of two large pouches; gallinaceous birds (e.g., chickens) have a single pouch, whereas the crops of hawks are spindle shaped (Fig. 1). A crop is not present in owls (Fig. 1).

The crops of several species, especially doves and pigeons, produce crop "milk," and during the breeding season the proliferation of the crop epithelium and its sloughing are induced by prolactin. These birds regurgitate the sloughed material to feed their young.

### Glandular Stomach

The glandular stomach is a fusiform organ (Fig. 1) that also varies in size between species. It is relatively small in graminivorous species but may be quite large and distensible in carnivores that ingest large food items; in such species it has a storage function. In most species, however, food passes rapidly through the glandular stomach and is held in the muscular stomach, where action of the gastric secretions occurs. The primary function of the glandular stomach is the production and release of pepsinogen, HCl, and mucus. Both acid and pepsinogen are secreted from the same cell, the chief cell. Pepsinogen granules increase in number in chief cells during fasting and decrease immediately after feeding.

Both inner circular and outer longitudinal smooth muscle layers are present in the glandular stomach.

*Muscular Stomach*

This organ is complex in most species and consists of two pairs of opposing muscles (Fig. 1) termed *thin* and *thick muscle pairs* (48). In chickens, the thin and thick muscles are 1–3 mm and 6–9 mm in thickness, respectively. All four muscles consist virtually entirely of circular smooth muscle arising from a central aponeurosis. A more simple muscular stomach found in raptors (birds of prey) (Fig. 1) and in heronlike birds has both inner circular and outer longitudinal muscle layers. The main functions of both types of muscular stomachs are mechanical digestion and serving as the site of preliminary proteolysis.

The muscular stomach has an inner lining called koilin that is thick and coarse in graminivores to aid in mechanical digestion. The koilin is formed by secretion of protein (96) from simple tubular glands and by entrapment of sloughed cells and cellular debris (50). It has a greenish or brownish color due to bile pigments refluxed from the duodenum. This lining is periodically sloughed in some species.

There are several variations in this general anatom-

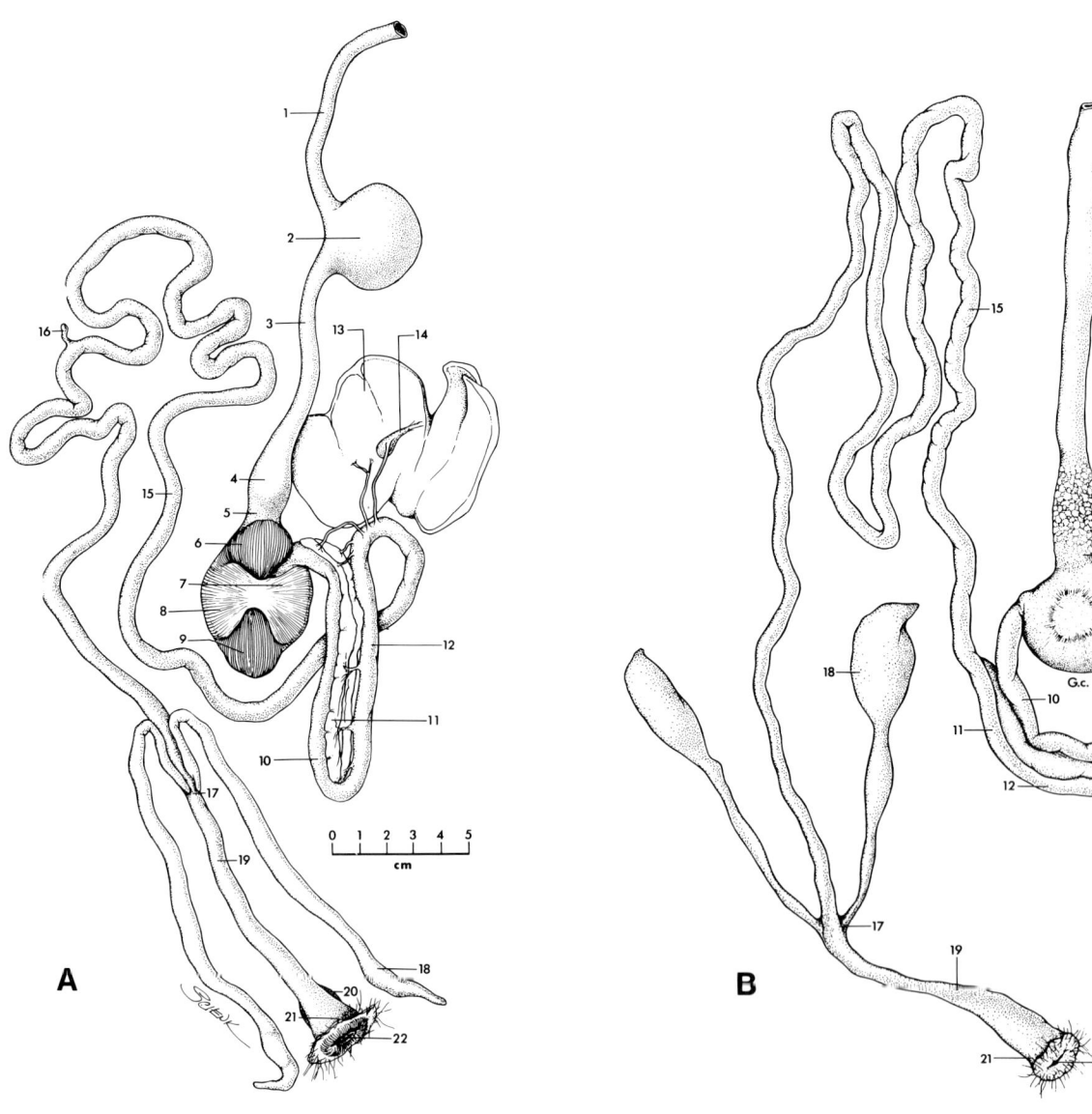

ical scheme for the glandular and muscular stomachs (70). Most notable is the presence of a third chamber, aborad to the muscular stomach, called the pyloric stomach in several species of aquatic birds. This chamber contains feathers or projecting mucosal processes that apparently serve as a filter to prevent larger portions of the chyme from leaving the muscular stomach.

The muscular stomach is served by extrinsic fibers from both the vagus and the sympathetic systems (9, 16, 71, 73). The vagus contains both pre- and postganglionic cholinergic excitatory fibers. There are also nonadrenergic inhibitory fibers in the vagus, which are apparently of sympathetic origin, but they appear to be associated only with ganglion cells or blood vessels (6–8, 10, 11). Because a longitudinal muscle layer in the muscular stomach is almost absent, the myenteric plexus is grossly visible just under the transparent serosa. A plexus comparable to Meissners' in mammals is absent in birds (11).

## Small Intestine

Because there is no histological differentiation within the lower small intestine, the avian small intestine is divided into only the duodenal loop and the ileum (Fig. 1). Some authors refer to the upper and lower ileum as corresponding to the jejunum and ileum in mammals and use the remnant of the attachment of the yolk stalk (Meckel's diverticulum) (Fig. 1) as a boundary point. The small intestine tends to be longer in herbivores and graminivores than in carnivores.

The wall of the small intestine consists, as in mammals, of the mucosa, inner circular muscle, outer longitudinal muscle, and serosa. There is a submucosal nerve plexus serving blood vessels and glands and a myenteric nerve plexus between the two muscle layers to serve those muscles. The myenteric system of the duodenum is intimately associated with that of the muscular stomach and glandular stomach.

The mucosa of the small intestine has Lieberkühn's crypts and, although Brunner's glands are absent in the chicken (17), tubular glands similar to Brunner's glands of mammals may be present in some species (100). Carnivorous birds have well-developed, fingerlike villi, whereas the villi in herbivores are flattened and leaflike (100). An extensive extrinsic innervation of the intestine exists, including pre- and postganglionic cholinergic fibers that may be vagal or symphathetic in origin (13, 49).

The small intestine is the principal site of chemical digestion involving enzymes of both intestinal and pancreatic origins. It also secretes hormones that are primarily involved in regulation of gastric and intestinal actions. Additionally most nutrient absorption occurs in the small intestine.

## Ceca, Rectum, and Cloaca

Ceca, when present, originate at the juncture of the small and the large intestines. They are large, prominent, and paired in some species (e.g., in herbivores, most graminivores, and owls) (Fig. 1), whereas in others they may be single, rudimentary, or absent (e.g., in parrots and hawks) (70). Ileocecal valves isolate the ceca from the intestines. Several functions have been attributed to the ceca, but the principal one appears to be that of microbial fermentation of dietary fiber. In view of this finding it is not clear why owls

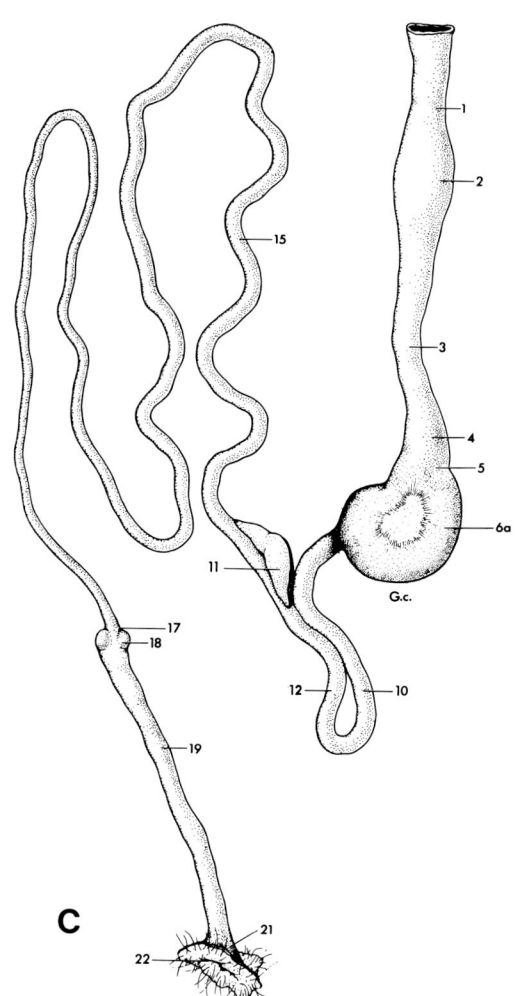

FIG. 1. Digestive tracts of 2.24-kg, 12-wk-old turkey (A); 1.70-kg, adult great horned owl (Bubo virginianus) (B); and 1.22-kg adult red-tailed hawk (Buteo jamaicensis) (C). 1, Precrop esophagus; 2, crop; 3, postcrop esophagus; 4, glandular stomach; 5, isthmus; 6a, muscular stomach; 6, thin craniodorsal muscle; 7, thick cranioventral muscle; 8, thick caudodorsal muscle; 9, thin caudoventral muscle (6–9, muscular stomach of turkey); 10, proximal duodenum; 11, pancreas; 12, distal duodenum; 13, liver; 14, gallbladder; 15, ileum; 16, Meckel's diverticulum; 17, ileocecorectal junction; 18, ceca; 19, rectum; 20, bursa of Fabricius; 21, cloaca; 22, vent; G.C., greater curvature. [From Duke (24).]

have well-developed ceca; it is even more curious that owls have them whereas hawks do not, although these raptors have nearly identical dietary habits. As yet, no function has been ascribed to the ceca of owls.

The rectum extends from the ileocecal junction to the cloaca, and it is relatively short in most species. Histologically it is similar to the small intestine except that it has shorter villi. The cloaca consists of three chambers serving the digestive, urinary, and reproductive tracts. The rectum empties into the coprodeum, the urinary and reproductive tracts terminate at the urodeum, and the proctodeum opens externally through the "vent". The bursa of Fabricius is a dorsal projection of the urodeum. Both the rectum and the cloaca are primarily involved in excretion and in mineral and water balance.

The Remak's nerve serves the rectum and cloaca. It is not clear whether this nerve is of sympathetic or parasympathetic origin (12, 99). There is evidence of noncholinergic excitatory neural activity in the Remak's nerve of the chick (5) that appears to involve a purinergic neurotransmitter (1).

*Liver and Pancreas*

The liver is bilobed (Fig. 1) and relatively large in most birds. It has two ducts, a hepatic and a biliary duct in most species, although not all species (e.g., pigeons) have a gallbladder. The pancreas lies within the duodenal loop and completely fills the loop in turkeys (Fig. 1), which have three lobes with secretions reaching the duodenum via three ducts. The pancreas occupies only one-half of the loop in owls and is even smaller in hawks. As with the ceca, this anatomical difference between hawks and owls poses interesting functional questions. It is clear that turkeys and hawks may have different demands for pancreatic endocrine regulation of carbohydrate metabolism or for exocrine secretions to digest carbohydrate in the diet, because turkeys ingest far more carbohydrate than hawks. Why hawks and owls have different sized pancreata is, however, far less clear and offers another interesting question for future research.

## METHODS OF STUDY OF MOTILITY IN BIRDS

Initial studies of motility involved fluoroscopy, direct observation in laparotomized birds, or measurement of intraluminal pressures (ILP) via inflated balloons inserted into the tract orally, rectally, or through cannulated fistulas. Because the balloons themselves often stimulated motility, sometimes abnormal motility, they were replaced by small open-tipped tubes inserted into the tract and kept filled with saline through constant infusion. Most recently image-intensification radiography with a photomultiplier system has replaced fluoroscopy, and tiny, implantable strain gauge transducers (SGT), which detect contractions, have replaced pressure measurements. Bipolar electrodes also have been employed recently to detect electrical activity associated with muscular depolarization or electrical control potentials. Use of electrodes and SGT allows much greater freedom for the subject than do balloons or tubes, and SGT have even been used telemetrically; this is a significant advantage in working with either wild birds or domestic poultry.

## PREHENSION AND SWALLOWING

The manner in which food is grasped, manipulated, or altered by beak or tongue activity before swallowing varies tremendously among species, depending on feeding habits and on the structure of the beak and tongue (70, 100). It is likely in all species, however, that the presence of food in the mouth stimulates salivation and swallowing.

Swallowing in chickens has been described in detail by White (97) from radiographic studies and by Suzuki and Nomura (91), who used electromyography. The latter authors divide the process into three phases. *1)* Oral phase, during which stimulation of the tongue by food causes rapid and repeated rostrocaudal tongue movements lasting 1–3 s, which move the bolus of food backward along the tongue to the pharynx. *2)* Pharyngeal phase involving the rostrocaudal tongue movements, during which the glottis is closed, the hyoid apparatus is made concave ventrally, the tongue is moved backward, and the esophagus is moved forward. The latter two movements shorten the distance between the oral cavity and the esophagus. *3)* Esophageal phase, during which further tongue movements dislodge the bolus from the tongue into the esophagus, whereupon the glottis, hyoid apparatus, tongue, and esophagus return to their starting positions. Esophageal peristalsis then moves the bolus toward the stomach.

Apparently, similar movements are employed in swallowing either food or fluid, except that fluid is more easily moved to the pharynx by gravity when the head is raised and the beak is pointed upward.

## MOTILITY OF ESOPHAGUS AND CROP

According to early studies of crop motility (see ref. 90), the first bolus of food entering the esophagus of a fasted chicken is likely to move directly to the muscular stomach bypassing the crop, with subsequent boli moving into the crop. More recent radiographic observations have shown that although this may occur, food may also bypass a partially filled crop and pass directly to the muscular stomach or a bolus that has already reached the opening to the glandular stomach may be returned to the crop (G. E. Duke, unpublished observations). The latter reflux was also observed by Vonk and Postma (95). Although further study is needed, it appears that the state of contraction of the muscular stomach at the time when a bolus approaches the opening to the crop determines whether the bolus enters or bypasses the crop. If the muscular stomach is contracting, the bolus enters; if it is relaxed, the bolus bypasses the crop. Pastea et al. (76) found that contractions of the crop and muscular stomach were coordinated and that the stomach may influence crop activity. The fullness of the crop may, in turn, influence gastric activity according to Hill and Strachan (57), who postulate that inhibition of muscular stomach contractions after crop distension may be caused by increased acid secretion by the glandular stomach, which occurs after crop distension (85). In chickens with a full crop, contractions of the crop and of the opposing surface of the esophagus form boli and expel them into the esophagus for passage to the stomach (66).

Crop function appears to be simpler in raptors than in fowl. This could be because raptors eat one or two meals per day, whereas fowl tend to be continuous feeders. Swallowed foods collect in the crop of hawks and are slowly passed to the stomach. In owls, who have no crop, swallowed food items immediately fill the stomach and lower esophagus, but after 20–30 min the entire meal is moved into the muscular stomach (82).

Crop motility, as well as contractions throughout the gastrointestinal tract, may be depressed by excitement or fear (90). During hunger, crop and esophageal contractions are irregular in pigeons and chickens but increase in frequency with increased length of fasting (56).

The esophagus and crop receive parasympathetic excitatory fibers from the vagus and excitatory and inhibitory fibers from the sympathetic system (90). Ohashi (74) found more inhibitory fibers in the esophagus distal to the crop than in the esophagus proximal to it and postulated that this may explain the slower rate of contraction of the distal portion of the esophagus as described by Pintea et al. (78). Stimulation of the peripheral end of the left vagus causes contraction in the left side of the crop (cephalic and dorsal region), and stimulation of the right vagus causes contraction of the right side. Transection of the right vagus alone has little effect on crop motility, but ligation of the left vagus inhibits motility, particularly the ability of the crop to empty itself. The left vagus nerve apparently controls the peristaltic movements of the esophagus, because after ligation of this nerve these movements are abolished. Stimulation of the vagus produces contraction of the circular muscles of the crop, and stimulation of the sympathetic nervous system causes contraction of the longitudinal muscles. These longitudinal muscles are believed to have little influence on normal crop motility [the description of innervation is largely from Sturkie (90)].

MOTILITY OF STOMACH AND DUODENUM

*Motility Patterns: Fowl*

The muscular stomach of fowl consists of two pairs of muscles, the thin and thick muscles (Fig. 1). In each gastrointestinal cycle, these pairs contract alternately, producing a biphasic ILP change or contraction pattern [Fig. 2, tracing D; (27, 48, 68)]. Contrac-

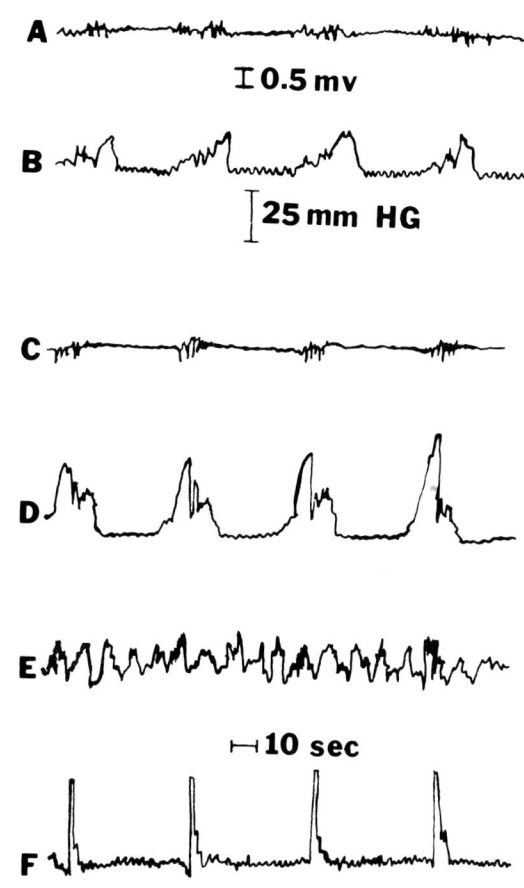

FIG. 2. Tracings of typical records of electrical potential and intraluminal pressure changes from glandular stomach, muscular stomach, and duodenum of turkeys. *Tracings A, C, and E*: electrical potential changes recorded from glandular stomach, thick cranioventral muscle of muscular stomach, and proximal duodenum, respectively. Slow waves with spikes are evident in electrical potential tracings from duodenum (*tracing E*); only electrical spike discharges associated with contractions are evident in glandular stomach (A) and muscular stomach (C) tracings. *Tracings B, D, and F*: intraluminal pressure changes recorded from glandular stomach, muscular stomach, and duodenum, respectively. Muscular stomach contractions cause small intraluminal pressure changes in glandular stomach before each glandular stomach contraction wave. Very small changes in thoracoabdominal pressure due to respiration are recorded between contractions of all 3 organs. Time constant for electrical recording was 1.1 s. [From Duke et al. (43).]

tions of the muscular stomach, glandular stomach, and duodenum are normally fully coordinated in a sequence (Fig. 2) that begins with contraction of the thin muscles followed by the duodenum, thick muscles, and glandular stomach contractions, respectively (Fig. 3). At the end of the contraction of the pair of thin muscles, the pylorus opens, a peristaltic wave begins at the pylorus and sweeps aborad in the duodenum, the thick muscle pair begins to contract, and fluid chyme flows aborad into the duodenum. Within 1–2 s, the pylorus closes, the isthmus opens, and chyme now flows orad into the glandular stomach. Seconds later the glandular stomach begins to contract, forcing flow of chyme back into the muscular stomach. After this flux, the isthmus closes [Fig. 3; (48)].

These gastroduodenal sequences occur at a mean frequency of 3.3 cycles/min in turkeys (Table 1) and at a similar frequency for fowl (90). The highest ILP changes are recorded during contraction of the pair of thick muscles [Table 1; (27)]. The pressures reported by Duke et al. (27) are considerably lower than those reported for chickens and other species by early investigators, i.e., buzzard, 8–26 mmHg; duck, 180 mmHg; hen, 100–150 mmHg; goose, 265–280 mmHg (90). The pressure is much lower in carnivores such as the buzzard, where the muscular stomach is more poorly developed. The higher pressures reported by earlier workers are probably due to the feeding of whole grains (rather than mash diets) that stimulate a greater muscular development of the muscular stomach. The amplitude of contractions is greater in males than in females.

An aspect of normal gastroduodenal motility that is unique to birds is intestinal refluxes (Fig. 4). They may be observed approximately every 15–20 min un-

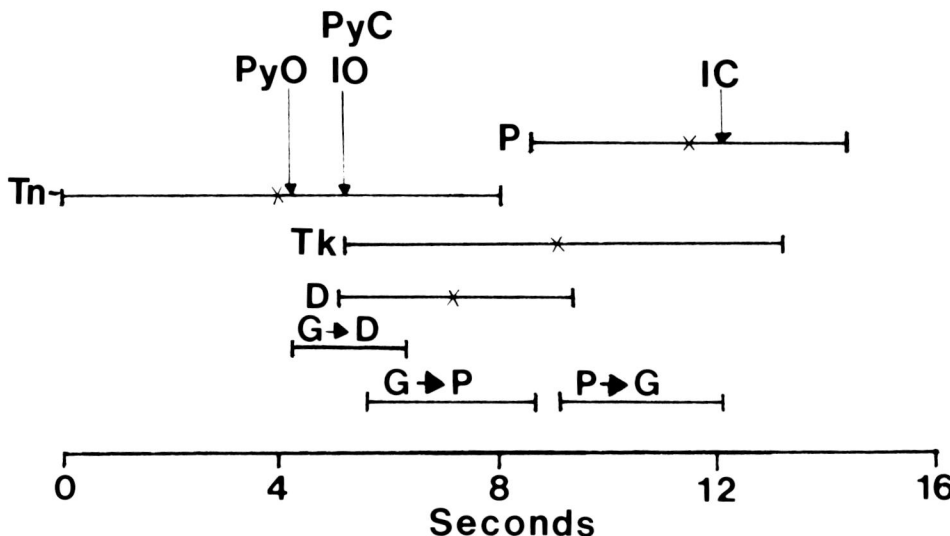

FIG. 3. Relative sequences and duration of events in the gastroduodenal contraction cycle of turkeys. *Horizontal lines*, relative sequence and duration of each event; top 4 lines represent a contractile event, whereas bottom 3 lines represent ingesta flow; end of contraction and beginning of relaxation marked by x in each of top 4 lines. *Vertical arrows*, point in this sequence at which events occur. Tn, thin muscle pair; I, isthmus; Tk, thick muscle pair; Py, pylorus; D, duodenum; O, open; P, glandular stomach; C, closed; G, muscular stomach. [Modified from Dziuk and Duke (48) and Duke (25).]

TABLE 1. *Mean Frequency and Amplitude of Gastroduodenal Intraluminal Pressure Changes, Electrical Action Potentials, and Slow Waves in Turkeys*

| | ILP Changes | | Action Potential | | | Slow Waves | |
|---|---|---|---|---|---|---|---|
| | Frequency, cycles/min | Amplitude, mmHg | Frequency, no./s | No. spikes/burst | Amplitude, mV | Frequency, no./min | Amplitude, mV |
| Glandular stomach | 3.3 ± 0.7 | 34.4 ± 12.9 | 5.3 ± 1.5 | 24.0 ± 9.0 | 0.18 ± 0.1 | | |
| Muscular stomach, thin muscle | 3.3 ± 0.7 | 42.5 ± 42.2 | 4.2 ± 1.4 | 27.2 ± 12.7 | 0.14 ± 0.1 | | |
| Muscular stomach, thick muscle | 3.3 ± 0.7 | 61.6 ± 62.8 | 3.8 ± 1.0 | 22.0 ± 7.3 | 0.42 ± 0.2 | | |
| Duodenum | 9.3 ± 1.2 | 25.0 ± 13.8 | 18.8 ± 3.22 | 11.1 ± 5.7 | 0.44 ± 0.3 | 6.0 ± 0.5 | 0.15 ± 0.1 |

ILP, intraluminal pressure. [From Duke (23).]

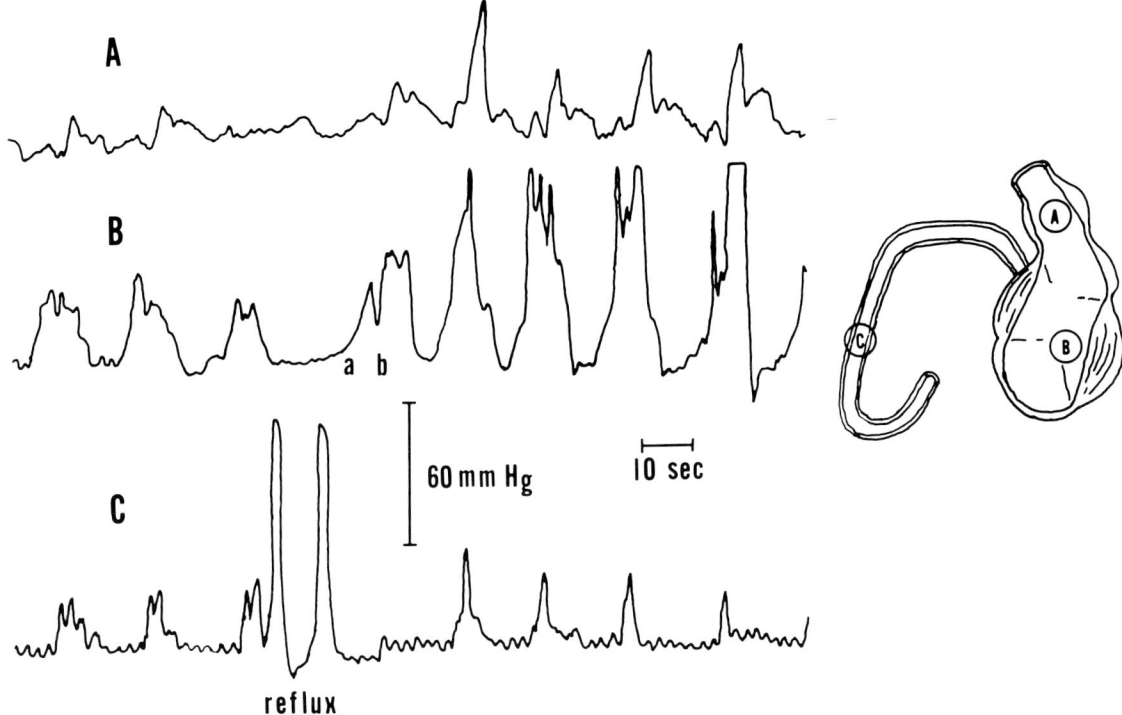

FIG. 4. Tracings of typical records of pressure changes obtained from glandular stomach (*A*), muscular stomach (*B*), and upper proximal duodenum (*C*) of a turkey, showing pressure events during a duodenal reflux. Positions of open-tipped tubes within gastrointestinal tract are indicated by corresponding *circled* letters *A*, *B*, and *C* on the diagram of a sagittal section of stomach. Biphasic pattern of tracing representing contraction of muscular stomach (*B*) is normally quite variable; the 2 phases are identified for 1 cycle: *a*, pressure wave due to contraction of thin muscle pair; *b*, pressure wave due to contraction of thick muscle pair. [From Duke et al. (27).]

der normal circumstances in turkeys (27, 48). The reflux typically involves the entire duodenum and the upper one-third to one-half of the ileum in one or two very powerful antiperistaltic contractions. During the reflux period, apparently because of an intrinsic neural reflex, gastric motility is inhibited.

*Regulation of Motility: Fowl*

A principal regulator of gastrointestinal motility in mammals, the intrinsic, myogenic, electrical slow waves or pacesetter potentials (14, 21, 65) have not been recorded from either the glandular or muscular stomach of turkeys (43). Although they have been recorded from both the small (Fig. 2) and the large intestines and ceca, they apparently have no regulatory function in the duodenum or ceca but may be involved in regulation of ileal and colonic motilities. In the duodenum of turkeys, there are usually 2-3 contractions per duodenal slow wave (Fig. 5); therefore, the slow wave does not set the pace for duodenal motility.

Regulation by slow waves propagated aborad through the stomach and duodenum (as in mammals) may be difficult in most species of birds in view of the complex gastroduodenal contraction sequence in which the most orad part, the glandular stomach, contracts last. Although this sequence is much less complex in birds of prey and is similar to that in the human stomach and duodenum, gastric electrical slow waves have not been recorded in these species either (31, 37).

The gastroduodenal contraction sequence is apparently neurogenically initiated and coordinated via an intrinsic neural network, presumably the myenteric plexus, in both fowl and raptors (43, 71-73).

Gastroduodenal motility in turkeys may be influenced by several factors. A cephalic phase of gastric motility was observed (36) when previously fasted birds were allowed to see food (Fig. 6). In turkeys, great horned owls (*Bubo virginianus*), and red-tailed hawks (*Buteo jamaicensis*) fasted for 24 h, the entry of an attendant into the holding room did not stimulate motility, whereas seeing food (or, in the case of hawks, seeing a package of frozen mice) caused a significant increase in gastric contractile activity (Fig. 6). If after a brief delay the birds were allowed to eat, gastric contractile activity was further increased, indicating the existence of a *gastric phase* of motility.

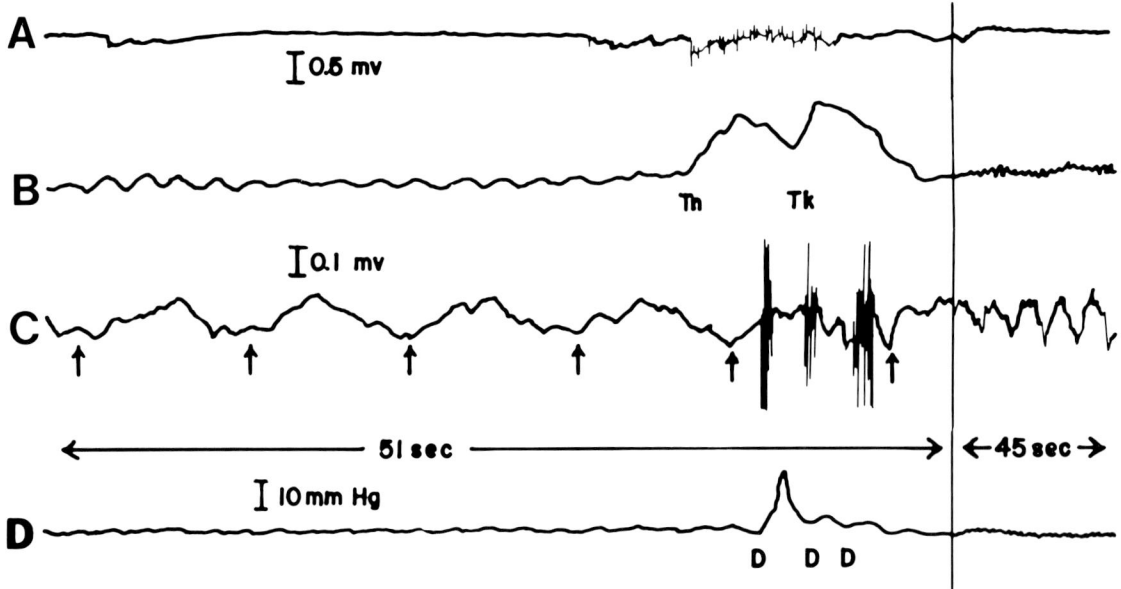

FIG. 5. Tracings of typical records of electrical potential and intraluminal pressure changes from turkey muscular stomach and duodenum. *A* and *C*: tracings of electrical potential changes recorded from thick cranioventral muscle of muscular stomach and from proximal duodenum, respectively. Burst of action potential spikes in *tracing A* is associated with contraction of thick cranioventral muscle. Arrows in *tracing C* indicate beginning of separate slow waves in duodenum and 3 bursts of spike potentials are associated with 3 contractions in *tracing D*. *B* and *D*: tracings of intraluminal pressure changes recorded from muscular stomach and duodenal flexure, respectively. Tn, Tk, and D, beginning of pressure changes associated with contractions of thin muscle pair, thick muscle pair, and 3 contractions in duodenum, respectively. Time constant for electrical recording was 3.2 s. Expanded time scale is in first portion of this record only. [Adapted from Duke et al. (43) and Duke (25).]

An intestinal phase of regulation of gastric motility has also been observed. As in mammals, the chemical nature and volume of duodenal contents may regulate gastric motility, i.e., an enterogastric reflex. Intraduodenal injections of HCl, hypertonic NaCl, amino acid or lipid solutions and distension via balloon inflation all inhibited gastric motility (29, 32). The degree of inhibition was directly related to the concentration and volume introduced into the duodenum. Inhibition was produced within 3–30 s and lasted 2–35 min (depending on dose) for all but lipid solutions, which required 4–6 min to produce inhibition and between 24 and >45 min to recover. The latter inhibitions were believed to be mediated primarily through a humoral mechanism, whereas the former were most likely mainly induced by neural influence.

An interesting aspect of this avian enterogastric reflex was the occurrence of intestinal refluxes during the period of gastroduodenal inhibition. Usually only a single reflux occurred immediately after inhibition began, but during inhibitions caused by hypertonic NaCl or lipid solution refluxes occurred repeatedly. Thus not only did offensive stimuli in the duodenum inhibit further gastric emptying as in mammals but, in birds, the reflux returned the offensive material to the stomach.

Only a few investigations of humoral regulation of gastrointestinal motility have been performed in birds. In fed turkeys, iv injections of the synthetic COOH-terminal octapeptide of cholecystokinin (CCK-8) at 0.5, 5, and 15 µg/kg body wt strongly inhibited gastroduodenal motility but had little or no effect on ileal and cecal motility (87). In fasted turkeys, CCK-8 had much less effect. These injections of CCK-8 caused intestinal refluxes in the duodenum and upper ileum, which lead to speculation as to whether endogenous CCK is involved in the gastroduodenal inhibition and intestinal refluxes of the enterogastric reflex.

Avian pancreatic polypeptide (aPP) also caused depression of gastric and duodenal motilities when injected intravenously (8, 10, 20, and 30 µg/kg body wt). Ileal, cecal, and colonic motility were depressed as well but less than motility of the upper portion of the gastrointestinal tract (42). Intravenous infusions of aPP at levels simulating postprandial plasma concentrations (7.5 and 15 ng of aPP/ml of plasma) also depressed contractile activity (41). The intraluminal presence of HCl, hypertonic NaCl, amino acids, and lipids at the same concentrations that caused an enterogastric reflex in turkeys also caused an increase in the concentration of aPP in the plasma (40). Thus, like CCK, endogenous aPP may also be involved in the enterogastric reflex.

Because both CCK-8 and aPP depress gastroduo-

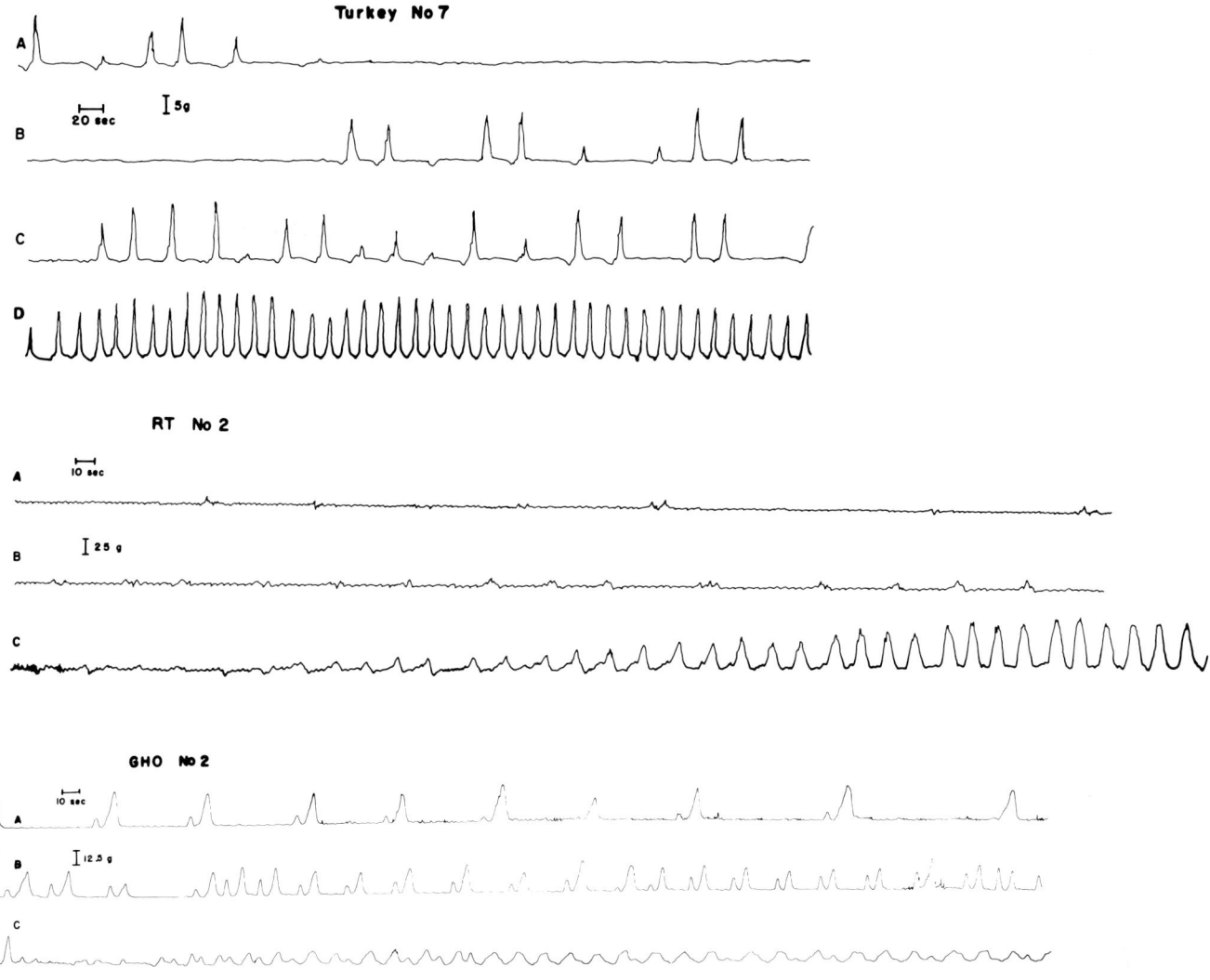

FIG. 6. Tracings of records of contractions occurring after 24-h fasting in muscular stomach of *1*) turkey before entry of an attendant (*A*), after entry (*B*), after seeing food (*C*), and after eating (*D*); *2*) red-tailed hawk (*Buteo jamaicensis*) (RT) and *3*) great horned owl (*Bubo virginianus*) (GHO) in presence of an attendant (*A*), after seeing food (*B*), and after eating (*C*). Lines *A–D* (turkey) or *A–C* (RT and GHO) are 1 continuous recording. Contractions were detected via implanted strain gauge transducers. [From Duke et al. (36).]

denal motility and cause slowing of gastric emptying, both endogenous CCK and aPP may be involved in satiety. Such a role has been proposed for CCK (88).

Diurnal rhythms have also been shown to influence motility of both the muscular stomach of turkeys (30) and ceca of chickens (75). When gastric motility was monitored via implanted SGT for several days before and after a period of 2–3 days of fasting (30), both frequency and amplitude of contractions were increased during daylight and depressed during darkness. The daily increases began slightly before lights were automatically switched on in the holding room, and the decreases were initiated slightly before lights were automatically switched off. The turkeys were, therefore, anticipating changes in illumination, not simply responding to them. During fasting, the diurnal patterns in frequency and amplitude of contractions were less pronounced but they were maintained. This indicates that the diurnal patterns were neither simply caused by food intake during the lighted period nor by lack of food intake in darkness, providing evidence for the existence of some type of intrinsic circadian rhythm.

The diurnal rhythms may be influenced by maturation and ovulation (83). In 26-h-old female chicks there was little depression of gastroduodenal motility during darkness, but as they grew to 30 days old the inhibition of motility during darkness became progressively greater. In the mature laying hen, however, gastroduodenal motility during darkness increased again, i.e., there was less change between light and darkness. This effect was believed to be caused by the increased caloric and calcium requirements during rapid growth as a chick and during egg laying.

*Motility Patterns: Raptors*

In hawks and owls, the motilities of the stomach and duodenum are also coordinated, and the gastroduodenal contraction sequence involves a peristaltic contraction that arises in the glandular stomach and moves through the muscular stomach into the duodenum (62). Radiographically, the peristaltic contraction is most apparent in the muscular stomach as a flattening or an indentation that moves around the greater curvature (62, 82).

When gastric motility was monitored continuously in owls, motility patterns characteristic of ingestion of food (i.e., cephalic and gastric phases of gastric motility, see *Regulation of Motility: Fowl*, p. 1289), digestion, and pellet egestion were discerned. Plotted averages of frequencies of gastric contractions for 10-min periods from food ingestion to pellet egestion indicated phases in the gastric digestion of a meal [Fig. 7; (52)]. The first phase, with relatively rapid and vigorous motility, was called the mechanical digestion phase. The purpose of this phase appeared to be to move the entire meal into the muscular stomach, crush it, and thoroughly mix it with digestive secretions. The second (or chemical digestion) phase (Fig. 7) had low-amplitude and low-frequency contractions that continued to gently mix ingesta with digestive secretions; most digestion was completed during this phase. During the third phase, fluid evacuation from the stomach, pellet formation, and pellet egestion occurred, and the phase was named for the latter two functions (Fig. 7). Several permanently crippled owls were killed at intervals postprandially to help assess the function of each phase. The duration of these phases and of the overall meal-to-pellet interval (MPI) varies directly with the amount eaten by an owl and thus may be used as an estimate of meal size.

When a meal was fed in three portions, e.g., 1 mouse/h for 3h (as would be likely to occur in wild, free-flying owls), a digestive pattern showing the chemical digestion phase interrupted by three mechanical digestion phases was evident [Fig. 7B; (52)].

The single most unique gastrointestinal phenomenon occurring in raptors and in many other avian species (80) is the formation and oral egestion of pellets. Pellets are formed in the stomach and consist of the bones and hair or feathers of ingested prey (55, 62, 81, 82). Egestion involves both gastric activity and esophageal antiperistalsis (37). At ~12-15 min before egestion, muscular stomach contractile amplitude and frequency increase significantly (Fig. 8). Radiographic observations indicated that this contractile activity was both compressing the pellet laterally and pushing it orad into the glandular stomach and eventually into

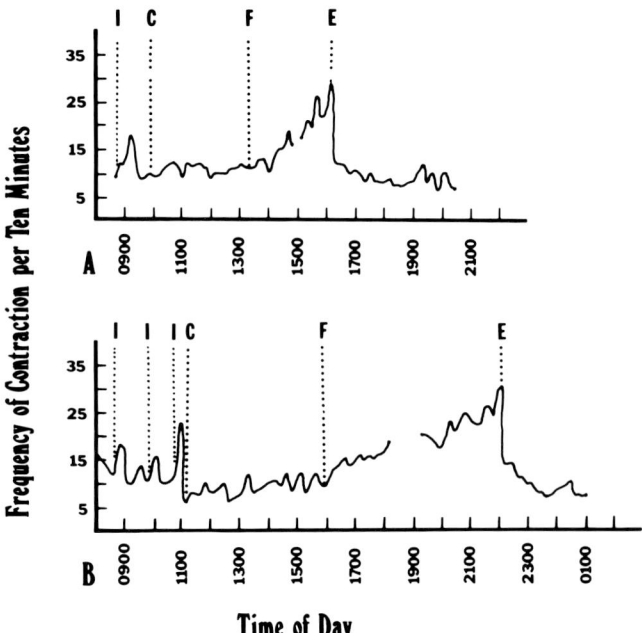

FIG. 7. Frequencies of gastric contractions detected by gastric extraluminal strain gauge transducers in great horned owl (*Bubo virginianus*) plotted by 10-min periods from food ingestion (mice) to pellet egestion for a meal eaten in 1 portion (*A*) or in 3 portions at 1-h intervals (*B*). Interruptions in plot indicate a failure to record data for a brief period, usually because of technical difficulties. I, ingestion; C, start of chemical digestion phase; F, start of pellet formation motility; E, pellet egestion motility. [Modified from Fuller and Duke (52).]

the lower esophagus. At 3-10 s before egestion, gastric motility ceased, and powerful esophageal antiperistalsis moved the pellet orad to the pharynx. As this occurred, owls lowered their heads, opened their mouths, and often shook their heads, apparently to assist passage of the pellet from the upper esophagus and pharynx out of the mouth. Abdominal muscles did not contract during any part of this process (37). Because of this and also because of the prolonged gastric contractile activity before egestion and the occurrence of esophageal antiperistalsis, the mechanism of egestion is considerably different from the mechanisms of either vomiting in mammals with a simple stomach or regurgitation of the cud in ruminants (37), i.e., it is a unique biological process.

*Regulation of Motility: Raptors*

As indicated above, meal size and whether the meal is eaten all at once or in several portions may influence MPI. When MPI was determined in a number of owls under a variety of experimental protocols, several other factors regulating pellet egestion and thus altering the lengths of the three phases and influencing MPI were discerned.

Tests with several species of owls confirmed that MPI is related to meal size in all species (Table 2),

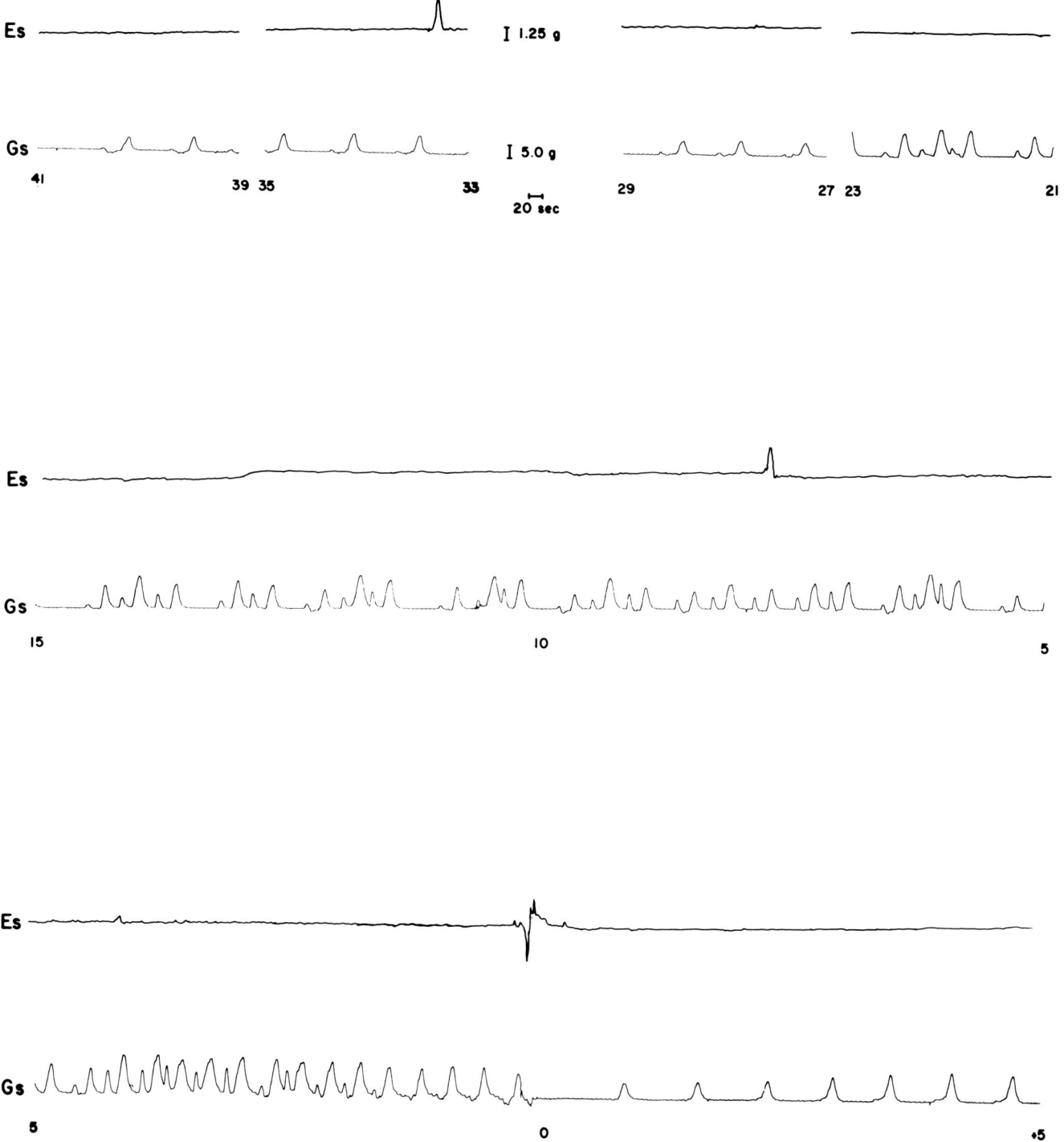

FIG. 8. Tracings of typical records of contractions occurring in esophagus and muscular stomach before, during, and after pellet egestion in great horned owls (*Bubo virginianus*). Es, esophageal contractions obtained with strain gauge implants; Gs, muscular stomach (gastric) contractions. *Numbers below Gs tracings*, times (in min) before or after pellet egestion. [Modified from Duke et al. (37).]

and it was further learned that the MPI tended to be shorter in smaller sized owls (Table 3). These findings indicate that the state of digestion of the meal is very important in regulating pellet egestion (35). To further elucidate the influence of the state of the intragastric environment on pellet egestion, great horned owls were fed 2 mice weighing ~25 g each or 2 mouse skins stuffed with other diets [Table 4; (32)]. The results of

TABLE 2. *Meal-to-Pellet Intervals as Related to Food Consumption in Great Horned Owls, Barred Owls, and Screech Owls Fed Daily at 0900*

| Species | Body Wt, kg | No. of Birds | MPI* at 4 Different Meal Sizes | | | |
|---|---|---|---|---|---|---|
| | | | Meal size† | Average | SD | No. of pellets |
| Great horned owls (*Bubo virginianus*) | 1.77 | 4 | <10 | 11.76 | 0.93 | 4 |
| | | | 10–15 | 12.49 | 1.16 | 11 |
| | | | 15–20 | 13.35 | 1.77 | 12 |
| | | | 20–25 | 14.71 | 1.57 | 9 |
| Barred owls (*Strix varia*) | 0.74 | 2 | <20 | 7.62 | 1.35 | 5 |
| | | | 20–25 | 9.82 | 1.76 | 12 |
| | | | 25–30 | 11.31 | 2.33 | 7 |
| | | | >30 | 11.35 | 0 | 1 |
| Screech owls (*Otus asio*) | 0.15 | 2 | 30–40 | 10.92 | 0.74 | 9 |
| | | | 40–50 | 11.88 | 1.02 | 13 |
| | | | 50–60 | 12.92 | 1.00 | 6 |
| | | | 60–70 | 13.75 | 0 | 1 |

* MPI, meal-to-pellet intervals measured in hours. † Meal size measured in grams of dry matter eaten per kilogram body wt. [Data modified from Duke et al. (35).]

those studies indicated that the presence of any undigested nutrients (e.g., proteins or fats) inhibits egestion until digestion is complete, whereas the absence of nutrients (pellets alone) or possibly the presence of a mass of bones mechanically stimulating the gastric mucosa stimulates egestion. When pellets were fed with mouse skins, MPIs were longer than when pellets were fed alone, presumably because the proteins and fats of the skins had to be digested and passed from the stomach to remove their inhibition of egestion. These findings suggest the possible existence of chemoreceptors in the mucosa of the muscular stomach, which detect the presence or the absence of amino acids or fats and then reflexly inhibit or stimulate pellet egestion, respectively. When mouse skins alone were fed, MPI was as long as with meals of mice and longer than with mouse skins plus pellets or pellets alone. This may indicate that the digested remains of the meal of skins provided so little volume within the stomach that only a weak stimulus for egestion was present. This finding, plus the rapid egestion after a meal of pellets alone, indicated the possible presence of mechanoreceptors within the stomach that are sensitive to volume (or bulk) and that may have a stimulatory function in the reflex regulation of egestion.

Although the intragastric environment seems to be most important in regulation of pellet egestion in owls, other factors may also be involved. Barred owls (*Strix varia*) fed at a submaintenance level until they had lost 10% of their body weight exhibit lengthened MPIs and smaller pellets. Analysis of the pellets disclosed that digestion of the meal is more complete in the hungry owls. Thus the state of hunger may affect MPI (39). Conversely, the constant sight of food shortens MPI in short-eared owls (*Asio flammeus*) (18).

The MPI in owls may also be influenced by environmental stimuli. When great horned owls were fed at either dawn or dusk, it was found that MPIs were directly related to meal size but they were longer for meals eaten at dusk than at dawn, regardless of the size of the meal (38). This is also true for short-eared owls (18). Thus the portion of the daily cycle during which gastric digestion and pellet formation are oc-

TABLE 3. *Meal-to-Pellet Intervals in Six Species of Owls*

| Species | Average Body Wt, kg | No. of Birds | Average MPI, h | SD | No. of Pellets Collected |
|---|---|---|---|---|---|
| Snowy (*Nyctea scandiaca*) | 1.70 | 2 | 12.02 | 4.15 | 33 |
| Great horned (*Bubo virginianus*) | 1.77 | 4 | 13.25 | 1.73 | 36 |
| Barred (*Strix varia*) | 0.741 | 2 | 9.85 | 2.20 | 25 |
| Short-eared (*Asio flammeus*) | 0.432 | 1 | 10.22 | 0.43 | 13 |
| Screech (*Otus asio*) | 0.149 | 2 | 11.86 | 1.20 | 29 |
| Saw-whet (*Aegolius acadicus*) | 0.096 | 1 | 10.04 | 0.63 | 4 |

MPI, meal-to-pellet intervals. [From Duke et al. (35).]

TABLE 4. *Mean Meal-to-Pellet Intervals for Four Great Horned Owls (Bubo virginianus) Fed Various Diets at 1500*

| Diet | Average Meal Wt, g | Average MPI,* h | No. of Pellets Collected |
|---|---|---|---|
| 2 25-g mice | 50 | 15.52 ± 1.76 | 15 |
| 2 mouse skins (with skull) | 15 | 15.26 ± 0.56 | 8 |
| 2 mouse skins + 2 pellets† | 25 | 8.19 ± 0.88 | 11 |
| 2 pellets only‡ | 10 | 2.75 ± 0.65 | 5 |
| 2 mouse skins + 35 g horse meat | 50 | 24.34 ± 3.24 | 10 |
| 2 mouse skins + 9 g suet | 24 | 33.74 ± 7.55 | 11 |

* Meal-to-pellet intervals (MPI) expressed as means ± SD. † Pellets, horse meat, and suet were sewn into mouse skin with silk suture. ‡ Had to be force fed. [Modified from Duke and Rhoades (38).]

curring may affect the MPI. This is an important finding in relation to the influences of daily biorhythms on physiological processes in animals.

Fuller et al. performed an exciting field study in which they attempted to apply the above information and to adapt previously developed techniques for telemetry (M. R. Fuller, K. Daniels, G. E. Duke, and K. E. Zinnel, unpublished observations). In wild, free-flying barred owls, movements were monitored via a tail-mounted locator transmitter, and gastric motility was monitored via telemetry of signals from an implanted SGT to determine *1*) time of ingestion, *2*) time of egestion, *3*) measurement of the lengths of phases in gastric digestion, and thus *4*) estimation of the quantity consumed. It is important to be able to distinguish movements associated with hunting and feeding from other types of movement when trying to understand the behavior of owls, and an estimate of daily food consumption in a free-flying owl is very useful in understanding the energetics of owls.

Although MPI in owls is directly correlated with the quantity eaten, a major stimulus for pellet egestion in hawks is the occurrence of dawn, regardless of the quantity eaten to produce a pellet [Table 5; (4, 35)]. Hawks in a room with dawn at 0700 had MPIs 1–2 h shorter when fed at 1100 than when fed at 0900. In another study involving red-tailed hawks in a room with dawn at 0700, when feeding time was shifted from 0800 to 1600, a delay of 8 h, MPI changed from ~22 h to ~18 h, respectively, a delay of only 4 h. Thus the birds were attempting to egest as early in the day as possible (53). Natural history studies indicate that, although owls may hunt either at night or during the day, hawks require daylight for hunting (53). Thus hawks apparently would benefit by egesting a pellet (i.e., emptying the stomach) early in the day, leaving the rest of the day for capturing and ingesting new prey. Hawks conditioned to eating late in the afternoon in the laboratory or by falconers respond by shifting egestion time to just before the anticipated feeding time (53).

Studies of the gastric and esophageal contractile activity of red-tailed hawks revealed a mechanism of pellet egestion very similar to that of great horned owls (46). When gastric motility was continuously monitored and mean contractile frequency was plotted by 15-min intervals, ingestion motility, phases of chemical digestion and pellet formation, and egestion motility were evident in the plots (Fig. 9). The most striking finding of this study was that gastric motility characteristic of pellet egestion occurred each day approximately at dawn even if the hawks had not eaten the day before or if they had eaten only meat without feathers, fur, or bone! Thus egestion motility is not just the end result of having ingested but is apparently an expression of a circadian rhythm in hawks.

MOTILITY OF ILEUM, CECA, AND RECTUM

Much less is known about avian gastrointestinal motility and its regulation below the level of the duodenum, but descriptions of electrical potential changes and contractile activities are available for the ileum, ceca, and rectum of turkeys.

*Ileum*

Very prominent electric slow waves were recorded from the ileum of turkeys (44), which averaged 0.46 mV in amplitude and had a frequency of 6.1 waves/min (Table 6). Because these waves were very persistent, i.e., they seldom waned in the records (as occurred in records of electrical activity from the duodenum and cecum), and because maximal contraction frequency in the ileum was never >6 contractions/min, it is believed that slow waves may be prominent in regulation of ileal motility. In general ileal contractile and electrical activities are more similar to that of the corresponding portion of the mammalian gut than the activity in any other part of the avian tract.

*Ceca*

Two types of contractions have been recorded from the ceca of turkeys (34), and they are called minor and

TABLE 5. *Meal-to-Pellet Intervals in Seven Species of Hawks*

| | | MPI, h | | | | | |
|---|---|---|---|---|---|---|---|
| Species | No. of Birds | Fed at 0900* | | | Fed at 1100* | | |
| | | $\bar{x}$ | SD | $n$ | $\bar{x}$ | SD | $n$ |
| Bald eagle (*Haliaeetus leucocephalus*) | 3 | 21.7 | 1.3 | 10 | 20.9 | 1.2 | 10 |
| Red-tailed (*Buteo jamaicensis*) | 6 | 22.5 | 0.8 | 72 | 20.4 | 1.1 | 59 |
| Rough-legged (*Buteo lagopus*) | 3 | 21.7 | 0.7 | 79 | | | |
| Broad-winged (*Buteo platypterus*) | 2 | 21.7 | 0.5 | 13 | 20.8 | 0.3 | 5 |
| Goshawk (*Accipiter gentilis*) | 4 | 21.6 | 2.5 | 9 | 20.6 | 1.4 | 65 |
| American kestrel† (*Falco sparverius*) | 1 | 23.6 | 0.2 | 10 | | | |
| Caracara (*Polyborus plancus*) | 1 | | | | 19.6 | 0.3 | 14 |

MPI, meal-to-pellet interval; $\bar{x}$, mean hours; $n$, no. of pellets collected.  *Dawn (lights on in holding room) was at 0700.  †Dawn was at ~0800.  [Data from Duke et al. (35).]

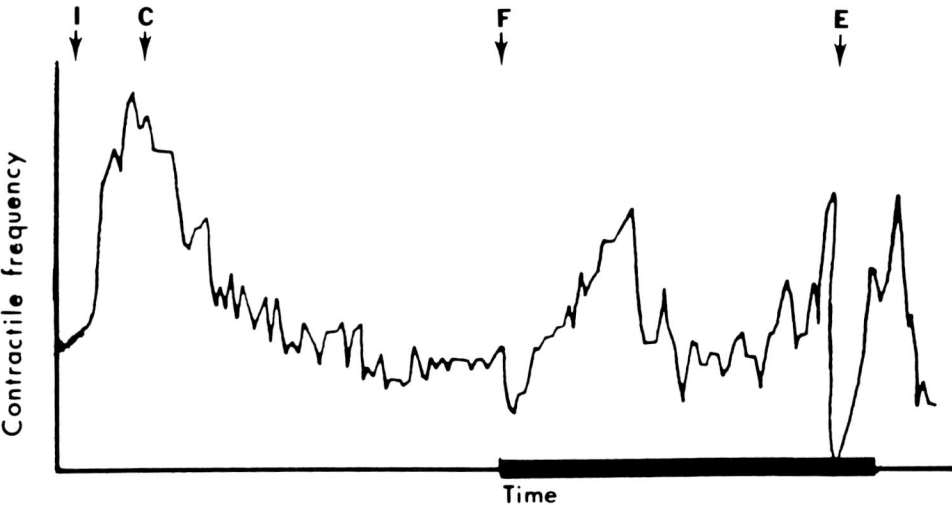

FIG. 9. Graph of mean gastric contractile frequency in red-tailed hawk (*Buteo jamaicensis*) for a 24-h period. I, ingestion; C, start of chemical digestion phase; F, start of pellet formation motility; E, pellet egestion motility. *Thick black bar*, period of lights out. [Modified from Durham (46).]

TABLE 6. *Mean Frequency and Amplitude of Ileal Intraluminal Pressure Changes and Electric Slow Waves in Turkeys*

| ILP Changes | | Slow Waves | | |
|---|---|---|---|---|
| Frequency, cycles/min | Amplitude, mmHg | Frequency, no./min | Amplitude, mV | Persistence,* % |
| 40 ± 2.3 | 16.2 ± 13.0 | 6.7 ± 0.7 | 0.46 ± 0.3 | 97.9 |

ILP, ileal intraluminal pressure. * Persistence of slow waves is proportion of time in which slow waves are evident in recordings of electrical potential changes. [From Duke (23).]

major because of their relatively low and very high amplitudes, respectively (Table 7). Approximately one-half of the time, the minor contractions appear to be coordinated with contractions occurring in the ileum and rectum at the same frequency but slightly out of phase. Interestingly the two ceca are coordinated with each other less than one-half of the time (33). Such coordination can apparently be regulated via extrinsic nerves. Radiographic observations indicate that major contractions are mixing rather than propulsive in nature, whereas major contractions are propulsive and are propagated both orad and aborad (34). Although aborad propagation occurs twice as often as the orad, accumulation of ingesta in the cecal tip is apparently prevented by contractions arising in the distal cecum and moving orad, having a much greater amplitude than those moving aborad. Orad-oriented major contractions appear to be responsible for cecal evacuation (33).

Hodgkiss (59) believed that cecal peristalsis and antiperistalsis are myogenic. Peristalsis can be initiated in isolated cecal segments in response to localized radial distension after treatment with tetrodotoxin or local anesthetics, i.e., intrinsic innervation is not involved. Electric slow waves are rarely recorded in the ceca (Table 7), and are not believed to be involved significantly in regulation of cecal motility (34). The source of myogenic control of peristalsis and antiperistalsis is therefore not clear.

The contents of the ceca are homogeneous, finely textured, and are usually chocolate colored. Cecal contents can be readily distinguished from those from the rectum, and this has been used in determining when the ceca are evacuated. In turkeys fed commercial mash diets, cecal evacuation occurs approximately at dawn (possibly another expression of a diurnal rhythm) and again in late afternoon.

## Rectum

The dominant and most unique aspect of rectal motility is the nearly continuous antiperistalsis. This motility, which can be readily observed radiographically after an enema of $BaSO_4$ solution, is responsible for urinary backflow from the urodeum throughout the rectum and to the ceca (2, 79) for cecal filling.

With a series of implanted SGT and electrodes, two types of electrical slow waves and of contractile activity were recorded in the rectum (63). Low-amplitude, short-duration (sSW) and higher amplitude, long-duration (lSW) slow waves were recorded simultaneously by the two electrodes implanted in the proximal portion of the colon (Fig. 10, tracings A and C), whereas only sSW were recorded by the electrode on the distal colon (tracing E). The sSW were correlated with small contractions (tracings B and D) and the lSW with large contractions (tracing B). Radiographic observations made while recording electrical and contractile activity disclosed that small contractions were correlated with antiperistalsis; however, no movements correlated with large contractions were observed.

A frequency gradient for recorded electric slow waves is a characteristic in the mammalian gut (e.g., 20), and frequency gradients for both the sSW and lSW were observed (Table 8). The frequency of sSW is highest distally, whereas that of the lSW is highest proximally and, in fact, lSW cannot be recorded distally at all (nor could the large contractions) (Fig. 10,

TABLE 7. *Mean Frequency and Amplitude of Cecal Contractile Activity and Electric Slow Waves in Turkeys*

|  | Contractile Activity | | Slow Waves | | |
| --- | --- | --- | --- | --- | --- |
|  | Frequency, cycles/min | Amplitude, g | Frequency, no./min | Amplitude, mV | Persistence,* % |
| Contractions |  |  |  |  |  |
| Major | 1.2 ± 0.3 | 15.7 ± 3.8 |  |  |  |
| Minor | 2.6 ± 0.9 | 2.8 ± 0.3 | 5.1 ± 1.2 | 0.32 ± 0.3 | 6.6 |

* See Table 6 for definition. [From Duke (23).]

TABLE 8. *Mean Frequency and Amplitude of Small and Large Contractions and of Short- and Long-Duration Slow Waves in Rectum of Turkeys*

|  | Contractions | | | | Slow Waves | | | |
| --- | --- | --- | --- | --- | --- | --- | --- | --- |
|  | Small | | Large | | Short | | Long | |
|  | Frequency, cycles/min | Amplitude, g | Frequency, cycles/min | Amplitude, g | Frequency, no./min | Amplitude, mV | Frequency, no./min | Amplitude, mV |
| Proximal* | 14.6 ± 0.85 | 0.45 ± 0.24 | 2.66 ± 0.26 | 0.54 ± 0.20 | 15.4 ± 1.07 | 0.17 ± 0.08 | 2.83 ± 0.26 | 0.21 ± 0.09 |
| Middle |  |  |  |  | 15.8 ± 1.12 | 0.16 ± 0.09 | 2.76 ± 0.24 | 0.12 ± 0.06 |
| Distal | 15.4 ± 0.69 | 0.70 ± 0.33 |  |  | 16.4 ± 2.16 | 0.25 ± 0.12 |  |  |

Values are means ± SD. * *Proximal, middle,* and *distal* refer to electrode implant sites on colon 10 cm, 6 cm, and 1 cm from cloaca, respectively, or to strain gauge transducer implants at 8 cm (proximal) and 3.5 cm (distal) from cloaca. Large contractions were not recorded from distal strain gauge nor were long-duration slow waves recorded from distal electrode. [Adapted from Lai and Duke (63) and Duke (25).]

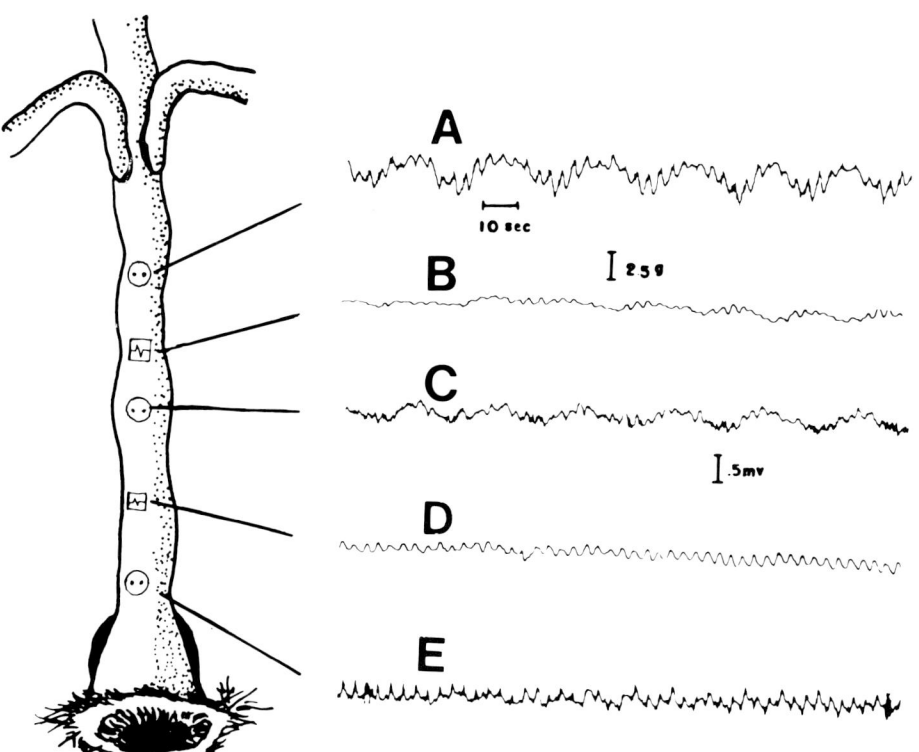

FIG. 10. Electrical potential changes and contractile forces recorded from 3 bipolar electrodes (○) and 2 strain gauges (▣) implanted on rectum of turkey. Electrical potential changes are shown in *tracings A, C,* and *E,* and contractions are shown in *tracings B* and *D.* Both long-duration and short-duration electrical slow waves are evident in *tracings A* and *C*; only short-duration slow waves are evident in *tracing E.* Small contractions are evident in *tracings B* and *D,* but large contractions can be seen only in *tracing B.* [Modified from Lai and Duke (63) and Duke (25).]

tracings *D* and *E*; Table 8). Thus the sSWs are believed to arise in the distal rectum and to be involved in regulation of antiperistalsis, whereas the lSW are believed to arise proximally in the rectum and to be involved in regulation of large contractions. On the basis of the lSW frequency gradient, large contractions appeared to be peristaltic and to be primarily responsible for aboral movement of rectal digesta.

The only interruption in the nearly continuous antiperistalsis so far observed occurs a few seconds before, during, and after defecation (rectal evacuation) (47, 63). At ~10 min before defecation, the amplitude of sSW becomes reduced, and frequency gradient of the lSW is more pronounced. These changes seem to favor depression of antiperistalsis and stimulation of peristalsis. During defecation, a strong contraction begins in the proximal rectum and then appears to be propagated aborally, moving all of the ingesta through the entire length of the rectum and through the cloaca in less than 4 s. These were extremely vigorous contractions (63).

## PASSAGE RATE

The rate of passage of ingesta through the gastrointestinal tract is usually measured by addition of nondigestable, nonabsorbable markers to the diet. A variety of markers may be used, depending primarily on the dietary constituent under study, e.g., iodinated cellulose for determining the transit time of dietary fiber (67), Cr- or Ce-mordanted plant cell walls (94), or radiopaque plastic pellets (15) for determining transit of all solids in the tract. The passage rate of the liquid portion of the digesta can be determined with cobalt-ethylenediaminetetraacetic acid (EDTA) (94) or with phenol red (54); the passage of semisolids may be monitored by the gels of psyllium, guar gum, or polycarbopyil labeled with $^{51}Cr$ (86). Radiography, which allows observation of the rate of passage through specific portions of the tract, may also be used.

In chickens and turkeys, marked excreta first appear within 2–2.5 h, and most of the marker can be recovered within 24 h (22, 93); however, $[^{51}Cr]CrCl_3$ was detected in the cecal excreta of pheasants for up to 72 h after feeding (45). Using radioactive Ba, Imabayashi et al. (60) found that approximately one-half of the label was excreted from chickens within 4–5 h.

Passage rate through healthy birds is largely dependent on the nature of the diet and is affected by consistency, hardness, and water content of the food (90). Fluids pass more rapidly than solids, fiber passes more slowly than other solids, and pelleted diets pass faster than mash (89). Relative content of various nutrients may also be important. Increasing fat levels in a diet progressively decrease passage rate, and the slower passage may improve the digestibility of other nutrients in the diet (64, 69). Higher protein content of the diet also tends to slow passage rate (89). Passage rate is faster in young chicks than in adults (92), and the rate of passage through the adult turkey is similar to that of the adult chicken (58). Factors that affect the overall motility of the tract also influence the rate of food passage. Diseases that depress digestive function slow passage rate (3, 28), and the addition of antibiotics to the feed may also slow it (58). Environmental conditions may affect passage rate as well, e.g., high environmental temperature slows passage in ducks (98). Finally, fasting or overfeeding may slow passage, whereas passage is more rapid in underfed chickens (89).

## REFERENCES

1. AHMAD, A., R. C. P. SINGH, AND B. D. GARG. Evidence of non-cholinergic excitatory nervous transmission in chick ileum. *Life Sci.* 22: 1049–1058, 1978.
2. AKESTER, A. R., R. S. ANDERSON, K. J. HILL, AND G. W. OSBALDISTON. A radiographic study of urine flow in the domestic fowl. *Br. Poult. Sci.* 8: 209–212, 1967.
3. AYLOTT, M. V., O. H. VESTAD, J. F. STEPHENS, AND D. E. TURK. Effect of coccidial infection upon passage rates of digestive tract contents of chicks. *Poult. Sci.* 46: 900–904, 1968.
4. BALGOOYEN, T. G. Pellet regurgitation of captive sparrow hawks. *Condor* 73: 382–385, 1971.
5. BARTLET, A. L., AND T. HASSEN. Contraction of chicken rectum to nerve stimulation after blockade of sympathetic and parasympathetic transmission. *Q. J. Exp. Physiol. Cogn. Med. Sci.* 56: 178–183, 1971.
6. BENNETT, T. The effects of hyoscine and anticholinesterases on cholinergic transmission to the smooth muscle cells of the avian gizzard. *Br. J. Pharmacol.* 37: 585–594, 1969.
7. BENNETT, T. Studies on avian gizzard. Histochemical analysis of extrinsic and intrinsic innervation. *Z. Zellforsch. Mikrosk. Anat.* 98: 188–201, 1969.
8. BENNETT, T. Nerve mediated excitation and inhibition of the smooth muscle cells of avian gizzard. *J. Physiol. Lond.* 204: 669–686, 1969.
9. BENNETT, T. Peripheral and autonomic nervous systems. In: *Avian Biology*, edited by D. S. Farner and J. R. King. London: Academic, 1974, vol. IV, chapt. 1, p. 1–77.
10. BENNETT, T., AND J. L. S. COBB. Studies on avian gizzard morphology and innervation of smooth muscle. *Z. Zellforsch. Mikrosk. Anat.* 96: 173–185, 1969.
11. BENNETT, T., AND J. L. S. COBB. Studies on avian gizzard: Auerbach's plexus. *Z. Zellforsch. Mikrosk. Anat.* 99: 109–120, 1969.
12. BENNETT, T., AND J. MALMFORS. The adrenergic nervous system of domestic fowl (*Gallus domesticus* L.). *Z. Zellforsch. Mikrosk. Anat.* 106: 22–50, 1970.
13. BOLTON, T. B. Physiology of nervous system. In: *Physiology and Biochemistry of Fowl*, edited by D. J. Bell and B. M. Freeman. London: Academic, 1971, vol. 2, chapt. 28, p. 675–705.
14. BORTOFF, A. Digestion: motility. *Annu. Rev. Physiol.* 34:261–290, 1972.
15. BRANCH, J., AND J. H. CUMMINGS. Comparison of radio-opaque pellets and chromium sesquioxide as inert markers in

studies requiring accurate fecal collections. *Gut* 19: 371–376, 1978.
16. BURNSTOCK, C. Evolution of the autonomic innervation of visceral and cardiovascular systems in vertebrates. *Pharmacol. Rev.* 21: 247–324, 1969.
17. CALHOUN, M. *Microscopic Anatomy of the Digestive System.* Ames: Iowa State Univ. Press, 1954, p. 1–127.
18. CHITTY, D. Pellet formation in short-eared owls, *Asio flammeus. Proc. Zool. Soc. Lond.* 108(Series A): 267–287, 1938.
19. CHODNIK, K. S. Cytology of the glands associated with the alimentary tract of the domestic fowl (*Gallus domesticus*). *Q. J. Microsc. Sci.* 89: 75–87, 1948.
20. CHRISTENSEN, J., S. ANURAS, AND R. L. HAUSER. Migrating spike bursts and electrical slow waves in the cat colon. Effect of sectioning. *Gastroenterology* 66: 240–246, 1974.
21. DANIEL, E. E. Digestion: motor function. *Annu. Rev. Physiol.* 31: 203–226, 1969.
22. DANSKY, L. M., AND F. W. HILL. Application of the chromic oxide indicator method to balance studies with growing chickens. *J. Nutr.* 47: 449–459, 1952.
23. DUKE, G. E. Gastrointestinal motility and its regulation. *Poult. Sci.* 61: 1245–1256, 1982.
24. DUKE, G. E. Avian digestion. In: *Duke's Physiology of Domestic Animals* (10th ed.), edited by M. J. Swenson. Ithaca, NY: Cornell Univ. Press, 1983, p. 359–366.
25. DUKE, G. E. Alimentary canal: anatomy, regulation of feeding and motility. In: *Avian Physiology* (4th ed.), edited by P. D. Sturkie. New York: Springer-Verlag, 1986, chapt. 11, p. 269–288.
26. DUKE, G. E. Raptor physiology. In: *Zoo and Wild Animal Medicine* (2nd ed.), edited by M. E. Fowler. Philadelphia, PA: Saunders, 1985, chapt. 27, p. 370–376.
27. DUKE, G. E., H. E. DZIUK, AND O. A. EVANSON. Gastric pressure and smooth muscle electrical potential changes in turkeys. *Am. J. Physiol.* 222: 167–173, 1972.
28. DUKE, G. E., H. E. DZIUK, AND L. HAWKINS. Gastrointestinal transit times in normal and bluecomb turkeys. *Poult. Sci.* 48: 835–842, 1969.
29. DUKE, G. E., AND O. A. EVANSON. Inhibition of gastric motility by duodenal contents in turkeys. *Poult. Sci.* 51: 1625–1636, 1972.
30. DUKE, G. E., AND O. A. EVANSON. Diurnal cycles of gastric motility in normal and fasted turkeys. *Poult. Sci.* 55: 1802–1807, 1976.
31. DUKE, G. E., AND O. A. EVANSON. Gastroduodenal electrical potential changes and contractile activity in birds of prey (Abstract). *Federation Proc.* 35: 303, 1976.
32. DUKE, G. E., O. A. EVANSON, J. G. CIGANEK, J. F. MISKOWIEC, AND T. E. KOSTUCH. Inhibition of gastric motility in turkeys by intraduodenal injections of amino acid solutions. *Poult. Sci.* 51: 1749–1757, 1972.
33. DUKE, G. E., O. A. EVANSON, AND D. R. EPSTEIN. Coordination of cecal motility during cecal evacuation. *Poult. Sci.* 62:545–550, 1983.
34. DUKE, G. E., O. A. EVANSON, AND B. J. HUBERTY. Electrical potential changes and contractile activity of the distal cecum of turkeys. *Poult. Sci.* 59: 1925–1934, 1980.
35. DUKE, G. E., O. A. EVANSON, AND A. A. JAGERS. Meal to pellet intervals in 14 species of captive raptors. *Comp. Biochem. Physiol. A Comp. Physiol.* 53: 1–6, 1976.
36. DUKE, G. E., O. A. EVANSON, AND P. T. REDIG. A cephalic influence on gastric motility upon seeing food in domestic turkeys, Great-horned owls (*Bubo virginianus*) and red-tailed hawks (*Bueto jamaicensis*). *Poult. Sci.* 55: 2155–2165, 1976.
37. DUKE, G. E., O. A. EVANSON, P. T. REDIG, AND D. D. RHOADES. Mechanism of pellet egestion in great-horned owls (*Bubo virginianus*). *Am. J. Physiol.* 231: 1824–1829, 1976.
38. DUKE, G. E., AND D. D. RHOADES. Factors affecting meal to pellet intervals in great-horned owls (*Bubo virginianus*). *Comp. Biochem. Physiol. A Comp. Physiol.* 56: 283–286, 1977.

39. DUKE, G. E., M. R. FULLER, AND B. J. HUBERTY. The influence of hunger on meal to pellet intervals in barred owls. *Comp. Biochem. Physiol. A Comp. Physiol.* 66: 203–207, 1980.
40. DUKE, G. E., J. R. KIMMEL, K. DURHAM, H. G. POLLOCK, R. BERTOY, AND D. RAINS-EPSTEIN. Release of avian pancreatic polypeptide by various intraluminal contents in the stomach, duodenum or ileum of turkeys. *Dig. Dis. Sci.* 27: 782–786, 1982.
41. DUKE, G. E., J. R. KIMMEL, H. P. HUNT, AND H. G. POLLOCK. The influence of avian pancreatic polypeptide on gastric secretion and motility in laying hens. *Poult. Sci.* 64:1231–1235, 1985.
42. DUKE, G. E., J. R. KIMMEL, P. T. REDIG, AND H. G. POLLOCK. Influence of exogenous avian pancreatic polypeptide on gastrointestinal motility of domestic turkeys. *Poult. Sci.* 58: 239–246, 1979.
43. DUKE, G. E., T. E. KOSTUCH, AND O. A. EVANSON. Gastroduodenal electrical activity in turkeys. *Am. J. Dig. Dis.* 20: 1047–1058, 1975.
44. DUKE, G. E., T. E. KOSTUCH, AND O. A. EVANSON. Electrical activity and intraluminal pressure changes in the lower small intestine of turkeys. *Am. J. Dig. Dis.* 20: 1040–1046, 1975.
45. DUKE, G. E., G. A. PETRIDES, AND R. K. RINGER. Chromium-51 in food metabolizability and passage rate studies with the ring-necked pheasant. *Poult. Sci.* 48: 1356–1364, 1968.
46. DURHAM, K. The Mechanism and Regulation of Pellet Egestion in the Red-Tailed Hawk (*Buteo jamaicensis*) and Related Gastrointestinal Contractile Activity. St. Paul: Univ. of Minnesota, 1983. Master's thesis.
47. DZIUK, H. E. Reverse flow of gastrointestinal contents in turkeys (Abstract). *Federation Proc.* 30: 610, 1971.
48. DZIUK, H. E., AND G. E. DUKE. Cineradiographic studies of gastric motility in turkeys. *Am. J. Physiol.* 222: 159–166, 1972.
49. EVERETT, S. D. Pharmacological responses of the isolated innervated intestine of the chick. *Br. J. Pharmacol. Chemother.* 33: 342–348, 1968.
50. FARNER, D. S. Digestion and the digestive system. In: *Biology and Comparative Physiology of Birds*, edited by A. J. Marshall. London: Academic, 1960, vol. I, p. 411–467.
52. FULLER, M. R., AND G. E. DUKE. Regulation of pellet egestion: the effects of multiple feedings on meal to pellet intervals in great-horned owls. *Comp. Biochem. Physiol. A Comp. Physiol.* 62: 439–444, 1978.
53. FULLER, M. R., G. E. DUKE, AND D. L. ESKEDAHL. Regulation of pellet egestion: the influence of feeding time and soundproof conditions on meal to pellet intervals of red-tailed hawks. *Comp. Biochem. Physiol. A Comp. Physiol.* 62: 433–438, 1978.
54. GONALONS, E., R. RIAL, AND J. A. TUR. Phenol red as indicator of digestive tract motility in chickens. *Poult. Sci.* 61: 581–583, 1982.
55. GRIMM, R. J., AND W. M. WHITEHOUSE. Pellet formation in a great-horned owl: a roentgenographic study. *Auk* 80: 301–306, 1963.
56. GROEBBELS, F. *Der Vogel, Erster Band: Atmungswelt und Nahrungswelt.* Berlin: Verlag von Gebruder Borntraeger, 1932.
57. HILL, K. J., AND P. J. STRACHAN. Recent advances in digestive physiology of the fowl. In: *Symp. Zool. Soc. Lond. No. 35,* edited by M. Peaker, London: Academic, 1975, p. 1–12.
58. HILLERMAN, J. P., F. H. KRATZER, AND W. O. WILSON. Food passage through chickens and turkeys and some regulating factors. *Poult. Sci.* 32: 332–335, 1953.
59. HODGKISS, J. P. Peristalsis and antiperistalsis in the chicken caecum are myogenic. *Q. J. Exp. Physiol. Cogn. Med. Sci.* 69: 161–170, 1984.
60. IMABAYASHI, K., M. KAMETAKA, AND T. HATANO. Studies on digestion in the domestic fowl. *Tohoku J. Agric. Res.* 6: 99–11, 1955.
61. JERRETT, S. A., AND W. R. GOODGE. Evidence for amylase in avian salivary glands. *J. Morphol.* 139: 27–46, 1973.
62. KOSTUCH, T. E., AND G. E. DUKE. Gastric motility in great-horned owls. *Comp. Biochem. Physiol. A Comp. Physiol.* 51:

201–205, 1975.
63. LAI, H. C., AND G. E. DUKE. Colonic motility in domestic turkeys. *Am. J. Dig. Dis.* 23: 673–681, 1978.
64. LARBIER, M., N. C. BAPTISTA, AND J. C. BLUM. Effect of diet composition on digestive transit and amino acid intestinal absorption in chickens. *Ann. Biol. Anim. Biochim. Biophys.* 17: 597–603, 1977.
65. LUDWICK, J. R., AND P. BASS. Contractile and electric activity of the extrahepatic biliary tract and duodenum. *Surg. Gynecol. Obstet.* 124: 536–546, 1967.
66. MACOWAN, M. M., AND H. E. MAGEE. Observations on digestion and absorption in fowls. *Q. J. Exp. Physiol. Cogn. Med. Sci.* 21: 275–280, 1932.
67. MALAGELADA, J. R., S. E. CARTER, M. L. BROWN, AND G. L. CARLSON. Radiolabeled fiber, a physiologic marker for gastric emptying and intestinal transit of solids. *Dig. Dis. Sci.* 25: 81–87, 1980.
68. MANGOLD, E. *Die Verdauung bei den Nutztieren.* Berlin: Akademie, 1950, p. 87–93.
69. MATEOS, G. G., J. L. SELL, AND J. A. EASTWOOD. Rate of food passage (transit time) as influenced by level of supplemental fat. *Poult. Sci.* 61: 94–100, 1982.
70. MCLELLAND, J. Digestive system. In: *Form and Function in Birds*, edited by A. S. King and J. McLelland. London: Academic, 1979, p. 69–181.
71. NOLF, P. On the existence in the bird of a system of intrinsic fibers connecting the stomach to the small intestine (Abstract). *J. Physiol. Lond.* 90: 53P–54P, 1937.
72. NOLF, P. L'appareil nerveux de l'automatisme gastrique de l'oiseau. I. Essai d'analyse par la nicotine. *Arch. Int. Physiol. Biochim.* 46: 1–85, 1938.
73. NOLF, P. L'appareil nerveux de l'automatisme gastrique de l'oiseau. II. Etude des effects causés par une ou plusieurs sections de l'anneau nerveaux du gesier. *Arch. Int. Physiol. Biochim.* 46: 441–559, 1938.
74. OHASHI, H. An electrophysiological study of transmission from intramural excitory nerve to smooth muscle cells of the chicken oesophagus. *Jpn. J. Pharmacol.* 21: 585–596, 1971.
75. OSHIMA, S., K. SHIMADA, AND T. TONOUE. Radiotelemetric observations of the diurnal changes in respiration rate, heart rate and intestinal motility of domestic fowl. *Poult. Sci.* 53: 503–507, 1975.
76. PASTEA, E., A. NICOLAU, AND J. ROSCA. Dynamics of the digestive tract in hens and ducks. *Acta Physiol. Hung.* 33: 305–310, 1968.
77. PATTERSON, T. L. Gastric movements in the pigeon with economy of animal material. Comparative studies. V. *J. Lab. Clin. Med.* 12: 1003–1008, 1927.
78. PINTEA, V., V. JARUBESCU, AND M. COTRUT. Contributiuni la studiul esofagului de gaina. *Lucr. Stiint.* 1: 297–310, 1957. [Cited in McLelland (70).]
79. POLIN, D., E. R. WYNOSKY, M. LOUKIDES, AND C. C. PORTER. A possible urinary back flow to ceca revealed by studies on chicks with artificial anus and fed amprolium-$C_{14}$ or thiamine-$C_{14}$. *Poult. Sci.* 46: 89–94, 1967.
80. REA, A. M. Turkey vultures casting pellets. *Auk* 90: 209–210, 1973.
81. REED, C. I., AND B. P. REED. The mechanism of pellet formation in the Great-horned owl (*Bubo virginianus*). *Science* 68: 359–360, 1928.
82. RHOADES, D. D., AND G. E. DUKE. Cineradiographic studies of gastric motility in great-horned owls (*Bubo virginianus*). *Condor* 79: 328–334, 1977.
83. ROCHE, M., AND J. DECERPRIT. Contrôles hormonal et nerveux de la motricité du tractus digestif de la poule. *Ann. Rech. Vet.* 8: 25–40, 1977.
84. ROGERS, F. T. Contribution to the physiology of the stomach. XXXIX. The hunger mechanism of the pigeon and its relation to the central nervous system. *Am. J. Physiol.* 41: 555–570, 1916.
85. ROUFF, H. J., AND K. F. SEWING. Die rolle der kropfs bei der steurung der magensaftsekretion von huhnern. *Naunyn-Schmiedebergs Arch. Exp. Pathol. Pharmakol.* 271: 142–148, 1971.
86. RUSSELL, J., AND P. BASS. Labeling and gastric emptying of gels in dogs (Abstract). *Federation Proc.* 42: 759, 1983.
87. SAVORY, C. J., G. E. DUKE, AND R. W. BERTOY. Influence of intravenous injections of cholecystokinin on gastrointestinal motility in turkeys and domestic fowls. *Comp. Biochem. Physiol. A. Comp. Physiol.* 70: 179–189, 1981.
88. SAVORY, C. J., AND M. J. GENTLE. Intravenous injections of cholecystokinin and caerulin suppress food intake in domestic fowls. *Experientia Basel* 36: 1191–1197, 1980.
89. SIBBALD, I. R. Passage of feed through the adult rooster. *Poult. Sci.* 58: 446–459, 1979.
90. STURKIE, P. D. Alimentary canal: anatomy, prehension, deglutition, feeding, drinking, passage of ingesta and motility. In: *Avian Physiology* (3rd ed.), edited by P. D. Sturkie. New York: Springer-Verlag, 1976, p. 185–195.
91. SUZUKI, M., AND S. NOMURA. Electromyographic studies on the deglutition movement in the fowl. *Jpn. J. Vet. Sci.* 37: 289–293, 1975.
92. THORNTON, P. A., P. J. SCHAIBLE, AND L. F. WOLTERINK. Intestinal transit and skeletal retention of radioactive strontium in the chick. *Poult. Sci.* 35: 1055–1060, 1956.
93. TUCKEY, R., B. E. MARCH, AND J. BIELY. Diet and the rate of food passage in the growing chick. *Poult. Sci.* 37: 786–792, 1958.
94. UDEN, P., P. E. COLUCCI, AND P. J. VAN SOEST. Investigation of chromium, cerium and cobalt as markers in digesta. Rate of passage studies. *J. Sci. Food Agric.* 31: 625–629, 1980.
95. VONK, H. H., AND N. POSTMA. X-ray studies on the movements of the hen's intestine. *Physiol. Comp. Oecol.* 1: 15–23, 1949.
96. WEBB, T. E., AND J. R. COLVIN. The composition, structure and mechanism of formation of the lining of the gizzard of the chicken. *Can. J. Biochem. Physiol.* 42: 59–70, 1964.
97. WHITE, S. S. The Larynx of *Gallus domesticus*. Liverpool: Univ. of Liverpool, 1970. PhD thesis. [Cited in: McLelland (70).]
98. WILSON, E. K., F. W. PIERSON, P. Y. HESTER, R. L. ADAMS, AND W. J. STADELMAN. The effects of high environmental temperature on feed passage time and performance traits of Pekin ducks. *Poult. Sci.* 59: 2322–2330, 1980.
99. YNTEMA, C. L., AND W. S. HAMMOND. Experiments on the origin and development of the sacral autonomic nerves in chick embryo. *J. Exp. Zool.* 129: 375–381, 1952.
100. ZISWILER, V., AND D. S. FARNER. Digestion and digestive system. In: *Avian Biology*, edited by D. S. Farner and J. R. King. London: Academic, 1972, vol. II, chapt. 6, p. 343–430.

# CHAPTER 36

# Histoanatomy and ultrastructure of vasculature of alimentary tract

B. J. GANNON | Department of Anatomy and Histology, School of Medicine, The Flinders University of South Australia, Bedford Park, South Australia, Australia

M. A. PERRY | School of Physiology and Pharmacology, University of New South Wales, Kensington, New South Wales, Australia

## CHAPTER CONTENTS

Vascular Organization of Alimentary Tract
  Vascular supply and drainage of alimentary tract
    Esophagus
    Stomach
    Small bowel—duodenum
    Small bowel—jejunum and ileum
    Large bowel
  Intramural distributive vessels
  Muscle microvessels
  Vasculature of enteric neural plexuses
  Submucosal microvessels
  Mucosal microvessels
    Esophagus
    Stomach
    Small intestine—general
    Small intestine—duodenum
    Colon
Microvascular Ultrastructure and Permeability Characteristics
  Small intestine
    General structure
    Ultrastructure of intestinal capillary wall
    Charge barrier to transcapillary exchange
    Correlation between structure and capillary permeability
  Stomach
    General structure
    Permeability
  Colon
    General structure
    Permeability
Future Directions for Structural Research in Gastrointestinal
       Microvasculature

EACH OF THE VARIOUS TISSUES of the gut subserves its own role in the overall functioning of the alimentary tract, and each has a vascular bed that must be adapted in its spatial organization, density, vessel wall structure, and physiology to serve the particular needs of the tissue it supplies. The diverse range of tissues includes muscle, which is principally visceral smooth muscle but which contains some striated muscle in the upper two-thirds of the esophagus (59); there are extensive layers of connective tissue, adipose tissue, and also nerve plexuses, with about as many neurons as the entire spinal cord (50). The variety of epithelia range from stratified squamous lining the esophagus, through differing columnar epithelia lining the alimentary tract lumen from stomach to colon, to cuboidal epithelia of the intrinsic simple tubular glands (e.g., crypts of Lieberkühn) and branched acinar glands (e.g., Brunner's glands). The extrinsic glands of the alimentary tract—salivary glands, liver plus biliary apparatus, and pancreas are not discussed in this chapter.

Primary roles of the vascular beds supplying each of the tissues of the gut, as elsewhere, are in the delivery of oxygen and nutrients for tissue metabolism and the removal of tissue wastes; however, the specialized roles of the mucosal epithelia and glands of the gut are absorption (131) and secretion (47, 101). The magnitude of this task is readily appreciated when one considers that the gastrointestinal tract receives ~10 liters of fluid each day, comprising 2 liters of ingested water and 8 liters of salivary, gastric, pancreatic, biliary, and intestinal secretions (37, 89). All but 100 ml of this volume load is absorbed. The total flux of fluid (secretion plus absorption) across the gastrointestinal microcirculation is, therefore, ~18 liters every 24 h (alimentary tract lymph volume flows are small compared with absorbed fluid removal via the bloodstream). In addition the capillaries are responsible for the removal of most of the absorbed nutrients, which, in a Western diet, may represent 250–800 g carbohydrate and 70–100 g protein (37, 62). It is not surprising, therefore, that the location, organization, and ultrastructure of the microvessels in this region of the circulation reflect their capacity for fluid and nutrient exchange. A further feature of the circulation of the alimentary tract is the portal arrangement, whereby the venous drainage does not pass directly to the right heart but passes to a second microvascular bed in the liver; the exceptions to this arrangement are the esophagus and the lower rectum

(64, 89). Thus the venous pressures in the branches of the portal venous system draining the gut must necessarily be higher than those of systemic veins; pressures in capillaries of the gut wall are similarly higher than those in other tissues (9, 10).

The vascular beds of the other tissues of the gut (e.g., muscle, connective tissue, nerve plexuses, and fat) serve principally nutritive roles and do not display vascular specializations (e.g., those in the skin for heat regulation and the penis for erection).

In this chapter the vasculature of the alimentary tract is considered from an essentially human viewpoint; consideration of the gut vasculatures of other mammalian species is included in the context of animal models of the human condition or to illustrate interspecies differences that may be relevant in extrapolation of findings from various experimental animal species to humans or to discuss those features examined in most detail to date in mammalian species other than humans. A general comparative approach to alimentary tract vasculature and microvasculature would be a useful contribution in its own right but is not included in this chapter.

We consider first the overall organization of the vascular beds of the alimentary tract, from larger supply/drainage vessels down to the microvessels. The detailed capillary wall ultrastructure and permeability characteristics of the various vascular beds are then considered separately.

## VASCULAR ORGANIZATION OF ALIMENTARY TRACT

The sources of arterial blood supply to, and routes of venous drainage from, the alimentary tract are considered in this section; readers are referred to specific illustrations in a current text (2) for relevant figures. Details of the organization of larger intramural vessels of the wall, the spatial relationships of the microvessels with the surrounding tissues of each of the layers of the gut, and differences in each region of the gut are reviewed.

### Vascular Supply and Drainage of Alimentary Tract

ESOPHAGUS. The esophagus has a sparse vascular bed; surgery to the esophagus is often followed by slow or inadequate healing, and breakdown of surgical anastomosis is not uncommon (156). This organ receives a diverse blood supply by many small branches of vessels supplying other structures. The cervical portion of the esophagus is supplied by branches from the inferior thyroid artery (a branch of the thyrocervical trunk from the subclavian artery), which also supply the lower pharynx (Figs. 1-84 and 1-85 in ref. 2). The thoracic part receives arterial supply from the esophageal arteries, which are direct small branches from the proximal descending aorta and from branches from (principally) the right posterior intercostal and bronchial arteries of the thoracic aorta (Figs. 1-84 and 1-85 in ref. 2). The diverse arterial supply of the abdominal esophagus is derived as two or three branches from the left gastric branch of the celiac artery and from the left inferior phrenic branch of the abdominal aorta; these arteries anastomose through the esophageal opening in the diaphragm with the arterial supply of the thoracic portion of the esophagus (Figs. 1-85 and 2-43 in ref. 2).

The venous drainage of the esophagus is similarly diverse. The cervical part is drained via branches to the inferior thyroid veins. The thoracic part is drained via the azygous, hemiazygous, and accessory hemiazygous veins from an intercommunicating venous plexus on the external surface of the esophagus. The abdominal portion of the esophagus drains into both the azygous vein and the left gastric vein (156). The latter vein is a tributary of the portal vein, whereas all the other drainage routes are via systemic veins. Thus the potential exists for portosystemic redirection of blood from the portal system via the left gastric vein to the lower esophageal venous plexus. This may occur in portal obstruction (e.g., liver cirrhosis) and can result in the development of venous varices in the lower esophagus; these vessels may burst, with resultant hematemesis and possible fatal consequences (156).

STOMACH. The arterial supply of the stomach is from the celiac artery. Blood passes to the stomach along its lesser curvature via a series of arterial branches to its anterior and posterior walls from the anastomotic loop between the left and right gastric arteries (Fig. 2-43 in ref. 2). Along the greater curvature, a similar anastomotic loop between the right gastroepiploic artery (a branch of the gastroduodenal artery) and the left gastroepiploic artery (a branch of the splenic artery) gives off anterior and posterior branches to the stomach wall and inferior branches to the greater omentum. In addition, 4–5 short gastric arteries, derived from the splenic artery, pass to the left end of the greater curve of the stomach through the gastrosplenic ligament, anastomosing with left gastroepiploic, esophageal, and left gastric arteries (2, 156, 165).

Venous drainage of the stomach is via two venous anastomotic loops, the first along the lesser curvature of the stomach joining the right gastric vein (which passes to the pylorus before turning dorsally to join the portal vein) and the left gastric vein (which passes to the portal vein in the left gastropancreatic fold); the left gastric vein also anastomoses with the azygous system via the lower esophageal veins and represents a potential portosystemic venous anastomosis. The second venous drainage loop is along the greater curvature of the stomach between the two layers of the dorsal mesentery of the stomach, and it receives tributaries from anterior and posterior walls of the stomach; this loop is drained at its right end via the right gastroepiploic vein to the superior mesenteric vein and at its left end via the left gastroepiploic vein to the commencement of the splenic vein near the splenic hilum (2, 156, 165).

SMALL BOWEL—DUODENUM. The duodenum arches around the head of the pancreas and shares portions of its blood supply. There are two arterial loops around the head of the pancreas medial to the duodenum (Figs. 2-46–2-48 in ref. 2). These are between superior pancreaticoduodenal arteries (branches of the gastroduodenal branch of the hepatic) and the inferior pancreaticoduodenal arteries (derived from the superior mesenteric artery) anterior and posterior to the head of the pancreas. The wall of the duodenum is supplied by a series of short perforating branches (vasa recta) from each of these two loops (2, 120, 156, 165).

Venous drainage of the duodenum is by pancreaticoduodenal veins that accompany the respective arteries; drainage of the inferior veins is frequently to the right gastroepiploic vein, whereas the upper veins join en route behind the bile duct to directly enter the portal vein (156).

SMALL BOWEL—JEJUNUM AND ILEUM. The arterial supply is from branches from the left side of the superior mesenteric artery (156, 165). These pass between the two layers of the mesentery toward the mesenteric margin of the bowel (Fig. 2-49 in ref. 2). Within the mesentery, each jejunoileal supply artery branches into arcades of vessels; blood reaches the gut wall by straight branches (vasa recta) from these arcades, and the arcades of adjacent vessels anastomose. For the first meter of the jejunum there are one or two tiers of arcades and long (3–5 cm) vasa recta. More distally the number of arcade tiers increases, reaching a maximum of approximately five in the distal ileum (156), with very short vasa recta; however, the vasculature within the mesentery of the distal human small bowel is usually obscured by copious mesenteric fat.

The venous drainage of the jejuno-ileum largely parallels its arterial supply. The main collecting vessel is the superior mesenteric vein, which lies in the mesentery to the right of the superior mesenteric artery. The portal vein is formed by the junction of the superior mesenteric vein with the splanchnic vein. An additional tributary of the superior mesenteric vein is the right gastroepiploic vein (2, 156, 165).

LARGE BOWEL. Arterial supply to the colon is from the superior and inferior mesenteric arteries; the ascending colon and proximal two-thirds of the transverse colon are supplied by ileocolic, right colic, and middle colic arteries arising from the right side of the superior mesenteric artery. There is typically a single anastomotic marginal artery along the mesenteric margin of the large bowel, from which short (2–3 cm) vasa recta pass to the colon wall, with little arcading with adjacent vessels (Figs. 2-50 and 2-52 in ref. 2). The distal one-third of the transverse colon and the descending colon are supplied by the inferior mesenteric artery, which gives a left colic artery at about the midpoint of the descending colon, and two or three sigmoid (or inferior left colic) arteries to the sigmoid colon. These vessels usually anastomose with one another near the colon via a marginal artery (which is continuous with that of the transverse colon) and also show a greater degree of arcading than those to the ascending colon (2, 156, 165).

The upper rectum is supplied from the inferior mesenteric artery by its superior rectal branch (Fig. 2-50 in ref. 2). This artery runs in the sigmoid mesocolon and bifurcates at the third sacral vertebra into left and right branches that run down either side of the rectum, pierce its muscle coat, and continue between muscle and mucosal layers as an anastomotic plexus to the internal anal sphincter. At this level there is anastomosis with arteries not derived from the inferior mesenteric artery; these are the middle rectal (a branch of the internal iliac artery) and the inferior rectal branches (a branch of the internal pudendal) (Fig. 3-42 in ref 2; Figs. 403–407 in ref. 156; ref. 165, p. 665, 670).

Venous drainage of the ascending and traverse colon is to the superior mesenteric vein via the ileocolic, a right colic, and a middle colic vein; straight veins draining the colon wall pass to an anastomosing marginal vein, which connects between these three main vessels and continues distally along the colon. Drainage of the descending and sigmoid colon and upper rectum is to the splenic vein via the inferior mesenteric vein. This latter vessel receives a left colic branch and sigmoid and superior rectal branches. The rectum has two venous plexuses, one between the mucosa and the muscle coat and one external to the muscle coat, which are well interconnected by venous branches that perforate the muscle. The lower region of the external rectal venous plexus drains via the inferior rectal vein to the internal pudendal veins; the middle portion drains via the middle rectal to the internal iliac veins, whereas the upper part of the external plexus together with the internal plexus drains via the superior rectal vein to the inferior mesenteric vein. Thus a free communication exists in the rectal wall between portal and systemic venous systems (2, 156, 165).

The dorsal aspects of the ascending and descending colon are adherent to the posterior abdominal wall, as are the mesenteries that develop embryologically with these sections of the gut. Thus the vessels supplying and draining ascending and descending colons are retroperitoneal rather than lying within mesentery, as is true for vessels of the transverse and sigmoid colons (165).

## Intramural Distributive Vessels

The wall of the gut from lumen outward is typically composed of four layers: *1*) the mucosa, *2*) submucosa, *3*) muscularis, and *4*) serosa (fibrosa in esophagus) (165). The extrinsic vessels of the alimentary tract provide a series of branches that penetrate the outer muscular layer of the gut wall to reach the major distributive arterial and venous plexuses situated in the submucosa. These plexuses are self-anastomotic along the length of the gut and also around the circumference of the small bowel (71, 95, 97), the large bowel (86, 174), and the esophagus, so that anterior and posterior arterial or venous branches from the mesenteric margin of the small bowel continue around the antimesenteric margin. In the stomach, supply/drainage anastomotic loops along the greater and lesser curvatures give a series of subserosal branches to the anterior and posterior walls of the stomach. Penetrating vessels from those vessels reach the submucosal arterial and venous distributive plexuses (120, 122). These plexuses are self-anastomotic, but only relatively small vessels traverse a line midway between greater and lesser curves (129); this is true also for the subserosal vessels (121, 129).

Blood supply/drainage of the greater omentum, an extension of the dorsal mesentery of the stomach, which usually exhibits significant adipose tissue deposition, is principally from inferior branches from the left and right gastroepiploic vessels, which anastomose around the greater curve of the stomach (165). The transverse colon is adherent to the posterior aspect of the omentum (165), and so some cross-communication of small vessels between omentum and the external muscle coat of the transverse colon is expected. Blood supply/drainage of the adipose tissue of the mesentery is from small branches from the arcading jejunal and ileal vessels (48, 57), whereas the vasculature of the appendices epiploicae (fatty protuberances from the colonic wall into the peritoneal cavity) derives from the intramural vessels of the colon.

## Muscle Microvessels

Blood supply to the microvascular bed of the extrinsic muscle coats of the gut is almost exclusively derived from the submucous arterial plexus (3, 10, 107a), the number of orders of branching before capillary supply (10) being a function of the species and of size. Venous drainage is also principally to the submucous venous plexus. However, the arteries that perforate the muscle coat en route to the submucous arterial plexus give small occasional branches, which connect directly into the external muscle vascular bed (107); such connections, although still rare, are more common in the gastric muscularis externa. Similar venous branches from the intramuscular microvascular network to the perforating veins are also found (107) but would apparently account for only a small proportion of total muscle blood flow.

The capillaries of the muscularis externa, where studied, are continuous and nonfenestrated [Fig. 1; (3, 17, 45)]. These microvessels are oriented parallel to the smooth muscle coats in which they lie; there are frequent fine connective tissue strands (collagen fibers) that attach regions of the capillary basal lamina to the basal lamina/endomysium of adjacent visceral smooth muscle cells (13, 14, 29). Such attachments apparently ensure that the capillary network distorts in register with the surrounding muscle as it contracts. Whether capillaries are held open during local muscle contraction by radial tension on their collagen connectives, as has been tentatively suggested (14, 29), awaits definitive proof. The most superficial capillaries of the longitudinal muscle layers of the abdominal portion of the alimentary tract (and also superficial capillaries of the circular muscle layer of the colon between the taeniae coli as well as the capillaries of the mesentery) immediately underlie the simple squamous mesothelium of the serosa; presumably they are important in exchange with peritoneal fluid both normally and during peritoneal dialysis.

In the regions of the gut that are retroperitoneal (duodenum, ascending and descending colons), the capillary bed of the outer visceral smooth muscle layer is in close contact with the fascia of adjacent skeletal muscle, with a high probability of at least microvascular interconnection; a similar situation exists for the rectum. In cases of raised portal pressure, such regions may become significant sites of portosystemic venous anastomosis (165).

The features of the microvascular bed of esophageal striated muscle await investigation but must be presumed to be similar to skeletal muscle beds elsewhere.

## Vasculature of Enteric Neural Plexuses

Between the muscle layers of the gut lie the nodes and internodal connectives of the enteric neural plexus of Auerbach. This plexus is reported to have a separate, sparse, largely planar capillary network (151, 152), as is Meissner's plexus in the submucosa (151). The capillaries of the autonomic plexuses of the gut wall are continuous (76); there is no suggestion that the satellite cells of the ganglia form a component of a blood neuron barrier between the capillaries and the enteric neurons (59, 76).

## Submucosal Microvessels

The submucosa of the gut is only sparsely supplied with microvessels [Fig. 2; (86, 95, 106)], except for the proximal portion of the duodenum, which receives a rich supply to the submucosal acinar glands (of Brunner). There is also a sparse supply to the submucous nerve plexus (of Meissner) (151). The esophageal acinar glands, found in variable numbers in the submucosa of the esophagus in humans but more densely arranged in dogs (165), must also have a well-developed microvessel bed that awaits detailed investigation. The sparse blood supply of the muscularis mu-

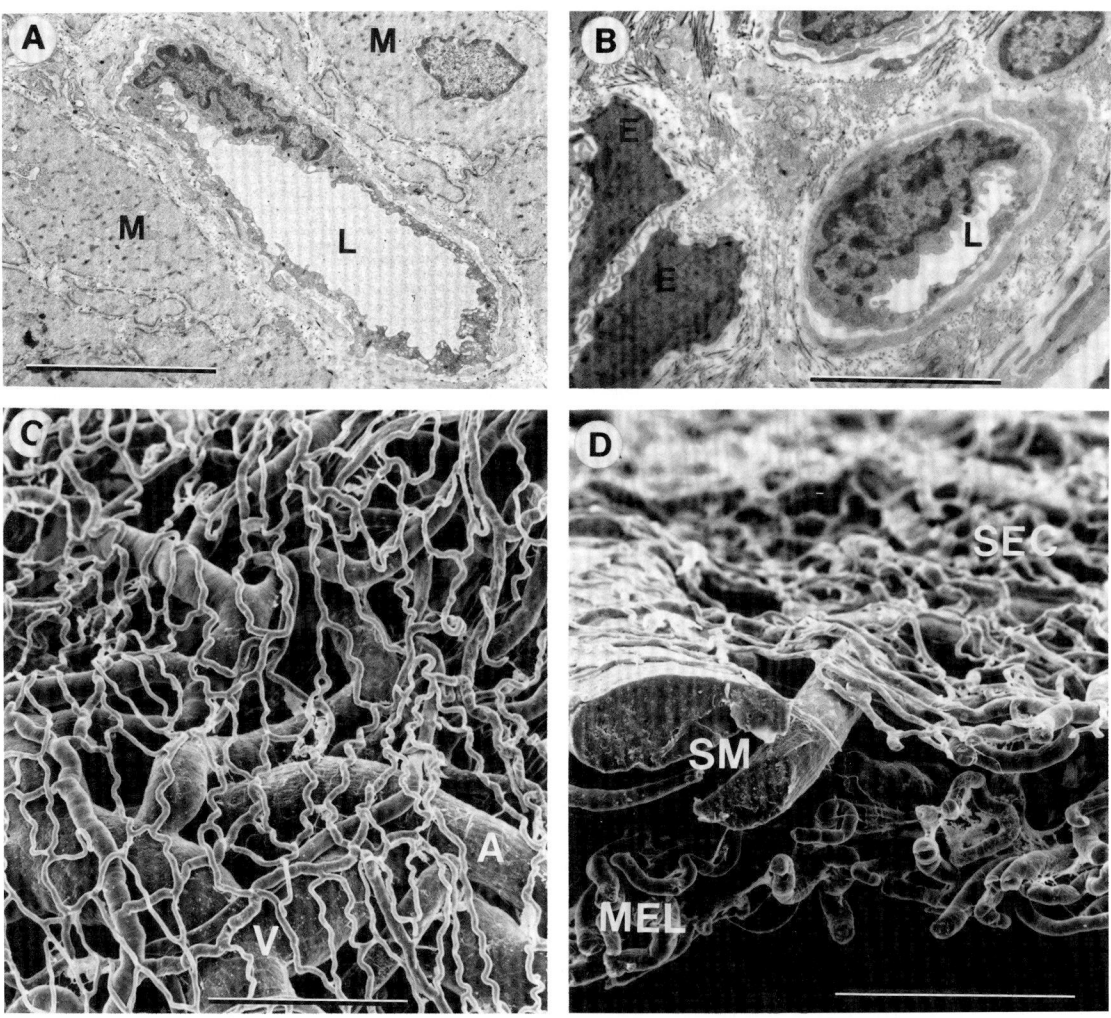

FIG. 1. Electron micrographs of capillaries of rat stomach. A: capillary (L, lumen) from muscularis externa of rat gastric corpus. Endothelium is continuous, with frequent endothelial vesicles, and is largely surrounded by pericyte processes. M, smooth muscle cells. Calibration bar, 5 μm. B: capillary (L, lumen) of subepithelial plexus that underlies basal epithelial cells (E) of forestomach stratified squamous epithelium. Capillary endothelium is continuous with endothelial vesicles and is largely surrounded by pericyte processes. Calibration bar, 5 μm. C: corrosion vascular cast of rat forestomach: view of gastric luminal aspect of cast. Planar array of fine vessels of subepithelial microvascular plexus overlies larger vessels of submucous vascular plexus. A, arteriole; V, venule. Calibration bar, 250 μm. D: corrosion vascular cast of rat forestomach: view of cut edge of cast. Planar array of subepithelial capillaries (SEC) overlies larger submucosal vascular plexus (SM), with capillary network of muscularis externa layer (MEL) below. Calibration bar, 250 μm. [From Browning et al. (17).]

cosa is a continuation of that of the submucosa, and perhaps it is reasonably considered part of that bed.

Also located within the submucosa are the self-anastomosing intramural arterial and venous vascular plexuses (Fig. 2) from which the blood supply/drainage of the muscle, submucosa, and mucosa are derived in parallel with each other (7, 9, 10, 15–17, 52, 53, 85, 86, 104–107a, 125, 126, 160, 174). It is at the level of the submucosa that frequent arteriovenous anastomoses have often been described by earlier workers (5, 6). However, it seems likely that these have been misidentified where arterial and venous vessels cross one another, because of limitations of microscopic resolution in cleared tissue. No convincing arteriovenous anastomoses have been demonstrated; no endothelia similar to the epithelioid segment of the arteriovenous anastomoses in the skin have been reported in histological studies of normal alimentary tract tissues; in vivo microscopy of stomach (17, 52, 53, 66, 67) and small intestinal wall (54, 106) has failed to demonstrate either high-flow or wide-caliber microvessels passing between arterioles and venules within the submucosa. The microsphere evidence (12, 39, 91) of such arteriovenous anastomoses has also been questioned on the grounds of statistical probability that the measured through flow of microspheres is due to

1306    HANDBOOK OF PHYSIOLOGY ~ THE GASTROINTESTINAL SYSTEM I

the presence of a small-diameter microsphere fraction in the injected boluses (96).

*Mucosal Microvessels*

ESOPHAGUS. The microvascular organization of the esophageal mucosa and the other layers of the esophagus remains to be investigated (3, 54). Of interest in the mucosa will be not only the form, density, and diameters of the microvasculature of the stratified squamous epithelium but also that of the intramucosal glands of the esophagus, which are structurally similar to the cardiac glands of the stomach.

In the laboratory rat, the forestomach has a pale lining of stratified squamous epithelia similar to that of the esophagus (17, 58); it has been suggested to represent a dilated lower esophagus (58, 85, 128) and

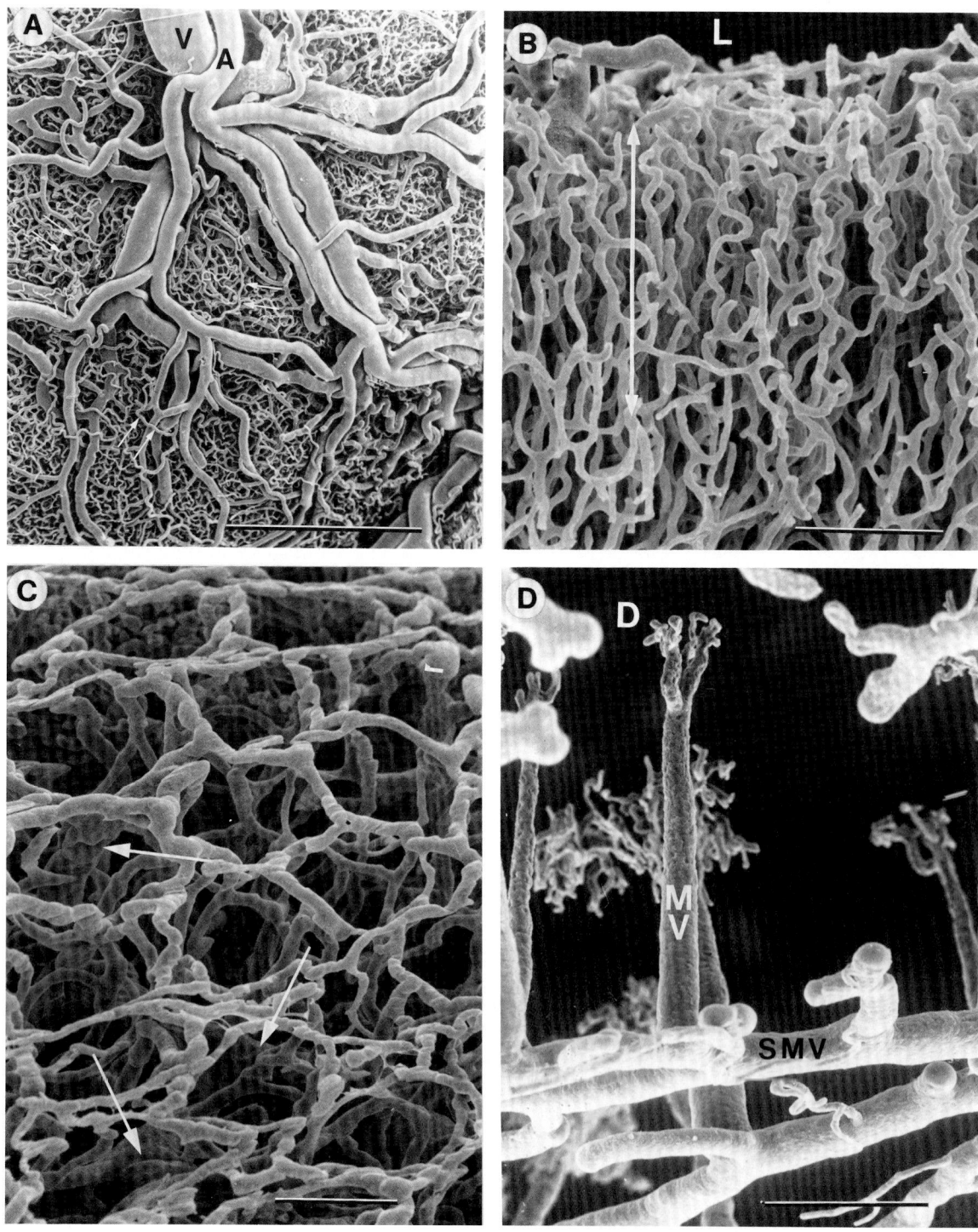

has been used as a model for experimental esophageal ulceration (85). The epithelium of the forestomach is underlaid by a sparse planar array of continuous, nonfenestrated capillaries [see Fig. 1B–D; (17)].

A similar organization might be anticipated in the esophagus, with some gradient in lamina proprial capillary density from pharynx to cardia, because the upper esophagus is reportedly pink at endoscopy, whereas that near the cardia appears gray (see ref. 165, p. 1253).

STOMACH. The microvascular bed of the gastric mucosa is derived from a series of small arterioles, of ~12 $\mu$m luminal diameter, which branch from the submucous arterial plexus (Fig. 2A). These arterioles break up into capillaries at the most abluminal aspect of the mucosa, and the capillaries pass in the lamina propria toward the gastric lumen largely perpendicular to the plane of the gastric surface; there are, however, frequent cross-connections between adjacent capillaries (Fig. 2B). At the most luminal aspect of the lamina propria, the mucosal capillaries form a polygonally arrayed network of capillary rings parallel to the plane of the gastric luminal surface and surrounding the gastric pits (Fig. 2C). Within this polygonal network, subepithelial venules arise that drain to infrequently placed mucosal venules (approximate separation, 300–500 $\mu$m). These mucosal venules pass through the mucosal plane at right angles to reach the submucous venous plexus, receiving no direct capillary tributaries en route (Fig. 2D). This gastric mucosal angioarchitecture, described from both rat gastric corpus and human gastric fundus and body (52, 53), is illustrated in Figure 3.

Transmission electron microscopy has confirmed the close proximity (<0.3 $\mu$m) of the mucosal capillaries to the lamina proprial aspect of the parietal cells [Fig. 4A; (52, 53)] and a preferential spatial association of mucosal capillaries with parietal cells compared with other epithelial cells of the gastric glands (B. J. Gannon and J. Browning, unpublished observations).

Diffusion distances from fenestrated subsurface capillaries to surface mucous cells lining the gastric lumen are typically 0.5–2 $\mu$m. The existence of an intrinsic local portal system for $HCO_3^-$ transport from gastric glands to the surface mucous cells in capillary blood has recently been proposed (Fig. 3, *inset*). The functional significance of this arrangement is presumably to provide additional $HCO_3^-$ to the surface mucous cells; these cells pump $HCO_3^-$ into the mucous layer overlying the gastric luminal surface (1); this mucus-bicarbonate layer produces a barrier to back-diffusing $H^+$ ions (1, 169), thereby protecting the gastric mucosa from acid-induced ulceration (1, 149). The source of this mucosally generated $HCO_3^-$ is the stoichiometrical release of $HCO_3^-$ from the basal (i.e., lamina proprial) surface of parietal cells during $H^+$ secretion (8). This $HCO_3^-$ overflows into venous blood and is observed as the postprandial alkaline tide (37); however, $HCO_3^-$ bypass of the proposed local portal pathway within the mucosa with significant uptake directly into venous blood is unlikely, given that the minimum distance from parietal cells to mucosal venules observed is ~13 $\mu$m and that the mean diffusion distance is much larger because of the infrequency of mucosal venules (52, 53).

This model may explain, at least in part, the observation that the gastric antrum, where the glands lack parietal cells and thus acid-secreting ability, is the most common site of chronic gastric ulcers (107b) rather than the fundus and body of the stomach, which have an oxyntic mucosa, which secretes the acid, and which can therefore be expected to be exposed to the lowest pH levels. Ulceration of oxyntic mucosa is found in conditions where the blood supply is compromised, that is, in aspirin administration, in severely shocked experimental animals, and in shocked patients, where areas of pale oxyntic mucosa indicative of local failure of perfusion are observed (70, 100). The reason for the greater susceptibility of the antral mucosa to chronic ulceration may be related to other factors: leakier tight junctions between epithelial cells and/or a sparser blood supply to this mucosa (108). Quantitative studies of capillary densities of antral compared with oxyntic mucosa are clearly overdue.

Recent studies have indicated the importance of the gastric microvasculature in the prevention of gastric ulceration; there is some evidence that compromise of

FIG. 2. Scanning electron micrographs of microvascular corrosion casts of gastric tissue of rat and human. A: submucosal aspect of cast of rat gastric corpus mucosa plus submucosa; note parallel branching pattern of submucosal arterioles (A) and venules (V). Fine meshwork between is commencement of mucosal capillary network. Note also occasional fine vessels running in plane of submucosa (*arrows*). Calibration bar, 1,000 $\mu$m. B: fractured edge of mucosal cast of rat gastric corpus showing capillaries are oriented principally perpendicular (*arrows*) to plane of gastric luminal surface (L); note, however, frequent cross-connections, which may be important in healing ulcerated gastric mucosa. Calibration bar, 100 $\mu$m. C: luminal aspect of cast of mucosal microvasculature of human gastric body. Note polygonal array of most luminal capillaries, which define openings of gastric pits. Some larger mucosal venule tributaries (*arrows*) are apparent just below most superficial capillaries. Calibration bar, 100 $\mu$m. D: fractured edge of partial vascular cast of rat gastric corpus in which only venules and venous ends of capillaries were filled (by retrograde injection of plastic). Mucosal venule (MV) proceeds from its drainage of subsurface capillaries (D) to submucous venous plexus (SMV) without additional capillary tributaries. Note also infrequency of mucosal venules. Calibration bar, 250 $\mu$m. [A, B, D from Gannon et al. (52); C from Gannon et al. (53).]

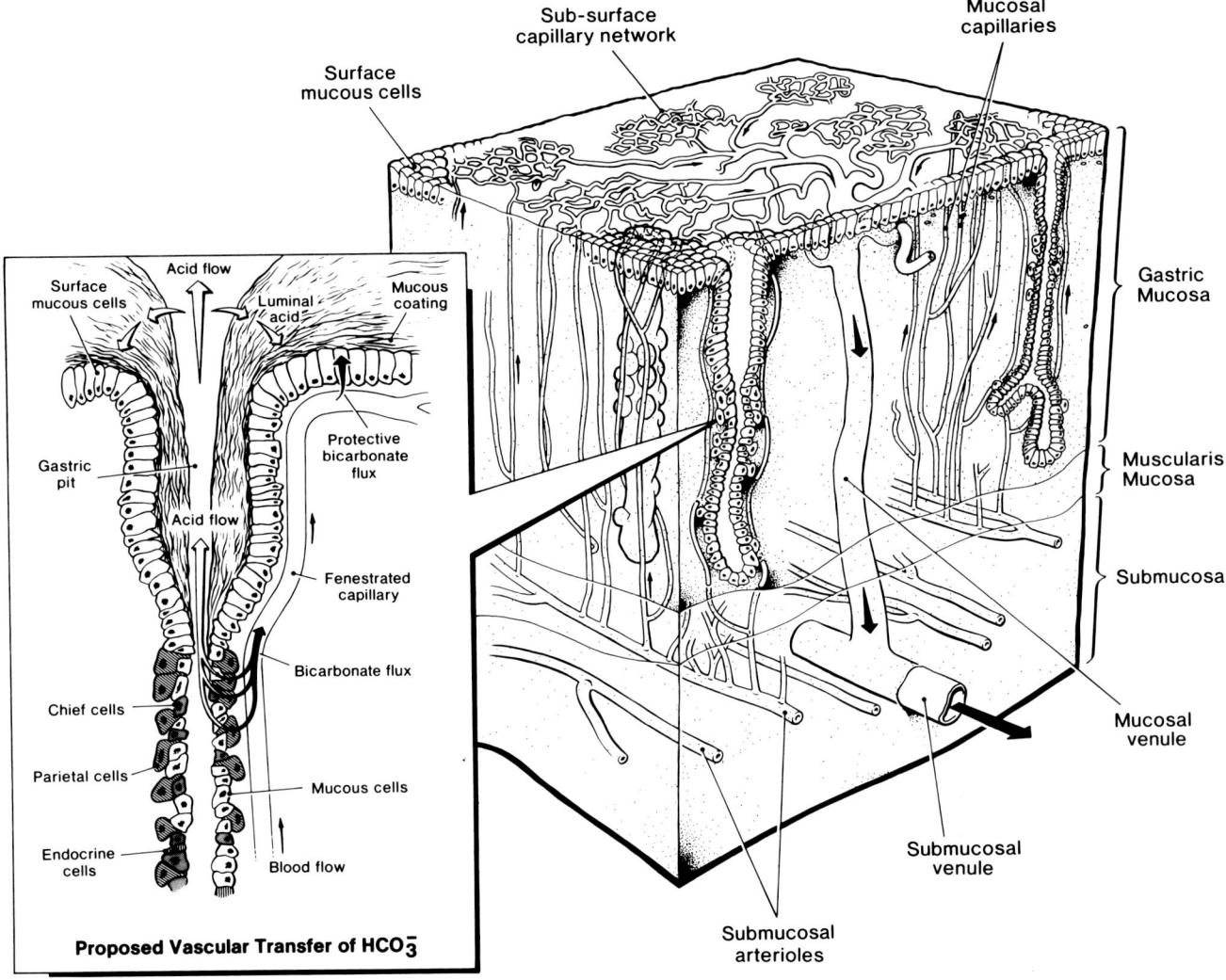

FIG. 3. Microvascular organization of oxyntic mucosa (of stomach) and proposed mechanism for microvascular transport of $HCO_3^-$ produced by parietal cells toward surface mucous cells in a local portal pattern (*inset*). [From Gannon et al. (53).]

gastric mucosal microcirculation may precede breeching of the mucosal surface epithelium (106). The cross-connections between adjacent capillaries within the gastric mucosa may be a vital feature in limiting mucosal injury. In acute ethanol-induced experimental ulceration of rat stomach, the capillaries of the most luminal mucosa are rapidly blocked, but circulation to deeper levels of the mucosa continues [Fig. 4B; (106)]. Given the microvascular organization (Fig. 3), it seems that these capillary cross-connections provide the only pathway for blood perfusing the deeper mucosa to reach adjacent areas of undamaged mucosa where the subsurface vessels remain patent and provide egress to mucosal venules. Healing of mucosal ulcers must presumably be from the remaining microvasculature subjacent to the ulcerated mucosa. Studies of the microvascular architectural changes occurring during the healing phase after establishment of experimental gastric ulcers would be a fruitful area for future investigation.

SMALL INTESTINE—GENERAL. The plane of the intestinal surface epithelium of columnar enterocytes is disturbed topologically by two interspersed frequent distortions: first, the epithelium is formed into the lumen into frequent tongue-shaped projections called villi, which are ~1 mm in length, but which vary in width from ~100–850 μm measured perpendicular to the long axis of the intestine (with significant differences between species), and are ~100 μm in thickness measured along the luminal axis of the intestine. The size and shape of the villi are important, because within each is a core of lamina propria in which are distributed its vasculature and lymphatics; the size of the interface between the lamina propria and the epithelium determines the area available for distribution of the subepithelial capillary network. Between the villi are dispersed the second epithelial distortion—downpocketings of narrow tubular glands into the lamina propria—with a lumen ~20 μm in diameter and ~850 μm deep. Each villus is surrounded by ~8–

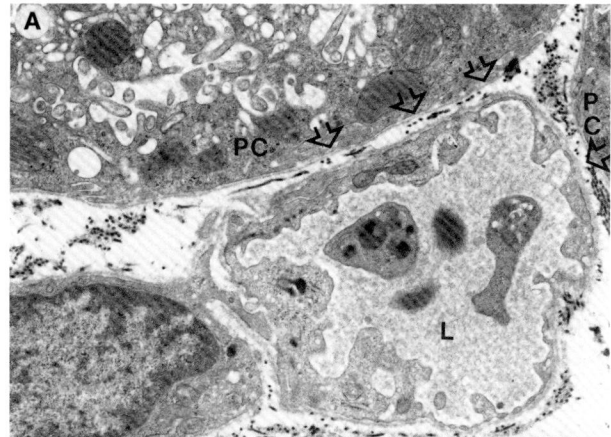
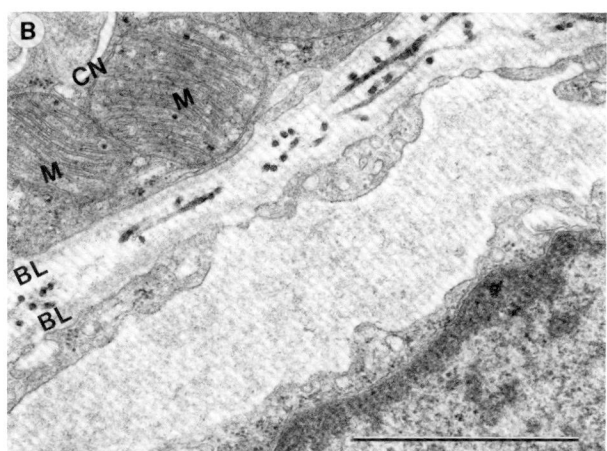
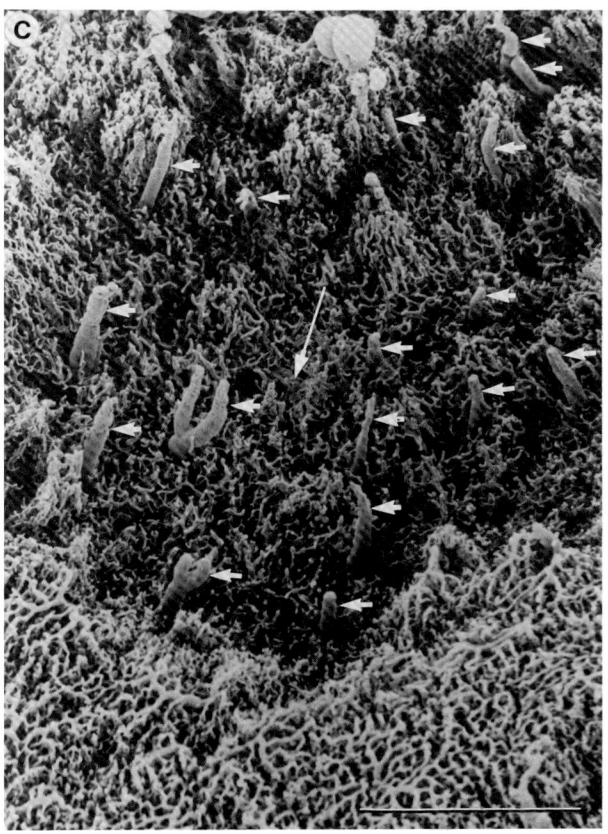

12 of these intestinal glands in human small intestine (Figs. 5 and 6).

The shapes of adjacent villi vary somewhat in human intestine from narrower tongue-shaped villi through to broader leaf-shaped villi [Fig. 6A; (56, 133)]. There is a proximodistal gradient in villus height and width, with larger villi found in the duodenum. The villi of other species have characteristic shapes and are usually more uniform than those found in human intestine. Dog villi are stout cylindrical structures [Fig. 6B; (54, 95)]; cat villi are slender and finger shaped [Fig. 6C; (54, 93, 170)]; those of the pigeon (38) and guinea pig are broad ridges; and rat villi are typically flattened leaf-shaped structures [Fig. 6D; (9, 54, 98, 99, 107, 164)]. An increased frequency of the broader leaf-shaped villi has been reported in samples of human intestine from India compared with those from North America (133); possible reasons suggested for the predominance of these broader villi in India have been dietary differences, racial differences, or differences in rates of alimentary tract infections. In older rats, the lateral margins of adjacent villi are frequently fused together to form broad ridges across the long axis of the gut (98, 99); this lateral fusion of previously distinct villi may be the mode of formation of the broader villus ridges sometimes observed in human intestine (56, 133).

The mucosal microvasculature of the human small intestine is illustrated schematically in Figure 5. An arteriolar supply from the submucous arterial plexus passes directly to the villus tip; at the tip this vessel branches into capillaries in the fountain pattern described by Spanner [Fig. 7; (56, 150)]. A dense plexus of subepithelial capillaries is drained usually by a single venule, which commences high in the villus (at ~80% of villus lamina proprial core height).

The possible existence of arteriovenous anastomoses in the intestine has been debated for a long time. Original reports from injected and cleared tissues (e.g., ref. 150) have now been largely dismissed, as newer techniques with better resolution and less possibility of misidentification have failed to identify such structures (26, 51, 54, 56, 107a).

---

FIG. 4. Electron micrographs of rat gastric microvessels. A: capillary (L, lumen) adjacent to two parietal cells (PC). Note fenestrations in capillary endothelium and close proximity of capillary to parietal cells (open arrowheads). Calibration bar, 2.5 μm. B: higher magnification of capillary close to parietal cells. Note fenestrae with diaphragm and endothelial vesicles in endothelium, separate basal lamina (BL) of capillary and parietal cell, and mitochondria (M) and canaliculi (CN) of parietal cell. Calibration bar, 1.0 μm. C: corrosion microvascular cast of rat gastric corpus after ethanol-induced ulcer formation; view of luminal aspect. Note loss of patency of capillaries throughout much of mucosal thickness almost to submucosa in center of field, so that submucous vascular plexus is just seen (arrow); complete mucosa at bottom. In eroded area, mucosal venules (arrowheads) are cast, presumably by retrograde filling; several ruptures of microvessels are evident at top, permitting extrusion of plastic. Calibration bar, 500 μm. [A, B from Gannon et al. (52); C from O'Brien et al. (106).]

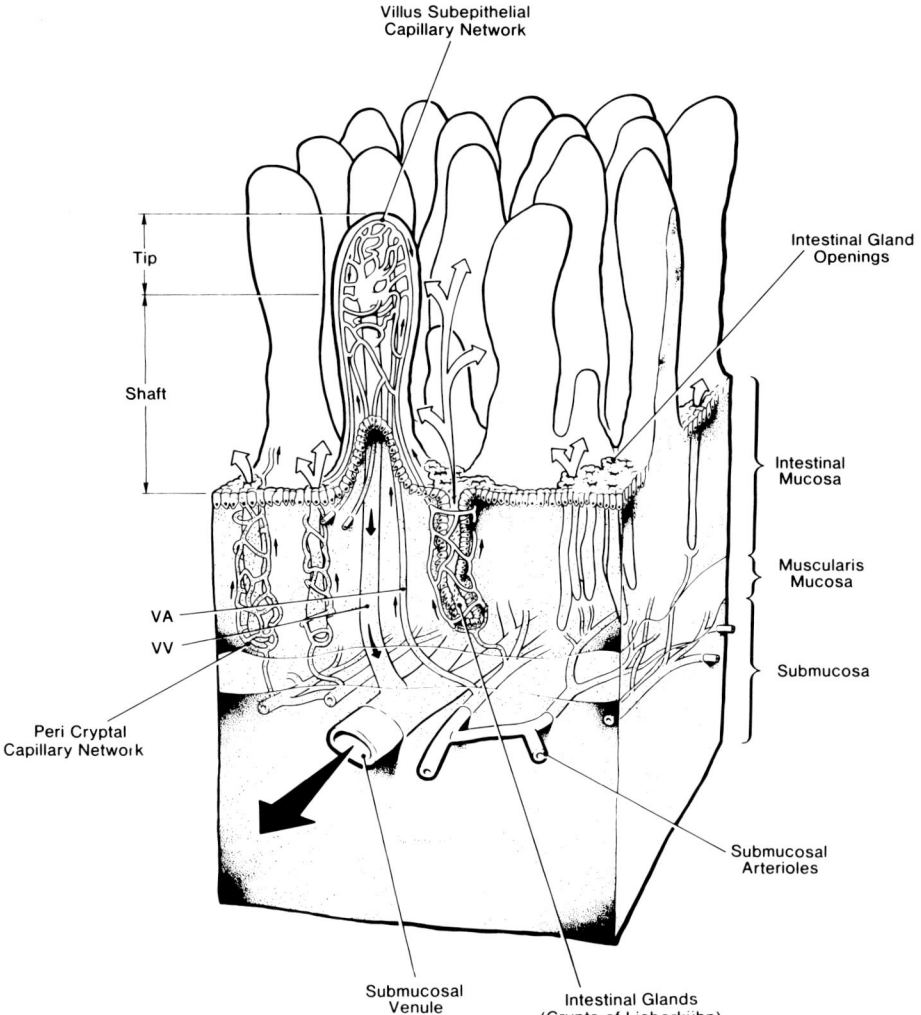

FIG. 5. Mucosal microcirculatory patterns typical of human and rabbit small intestine (except duodenum). VA, villus arteriole; VV, villus venule; *solid arrows* indicate directions of blood flow; *open arrows* indicate intraluminal flux of succus entericus from crypts to villi. [Adapted from Casley-Smith and Gannon (26).]

In the intestine (both large and small) as in the stomach, there have been no reports of tortuous, wide-caliber, arteriolar-to-venular pathways either with or without a specialized endothelial lining reminiscent of the structure of arteriovenous anastomoses of the skin. Recent reports of intestinal arteriovenous anastomoses have not resulted from anatomical findings at all but rather from interpretation of the results of microsphere experiments, wherein a small proportion of microspheres of nominal size, $\leqslant 9$ μm, passed through the gut microvascular bed (12, 39, 91). However, in another recent study of the size distribution in different batches of microspheres that were nominally too large to pass through capillaries, a good correlation was found of the proportion of spheres smaller than the normal size with the number of spheres from those batches that, on injection, traversed the capillary bed. This study showed that the microsphere evidence did not support the presence of intestinal arteriovenous anastomoses (96). The evidence of microvessel diameters as measured from microvascular corrosion casts is perhaps suspect, because most of the investigators using this approach were attempting to determine microvascular connectivity rather than vessel diameters. In those studies the infusion pressures of the plastics were not always appropriately controlled, and so uncritical extrapolation of the dimensions of cast microvessels to the vessel dimensions in vivo is unlikely to be valid. Nevertheless there do appear to be some larger dimension vessels at the tips of villus casts of rabbits and humans (51, 56). In vivo observations in rabbit villi [see Fig. 10A; (51)] suggest the existence of a higher flow channel around the margin of the villus at the tip between arteriole and venule, which might be appropriately termed a preferential channel. This vessel must have a slightly larger diameter than other capillaries of the villus; however, there is no evidence to date that such vessels are capable of opening to become wider-bore vessels capable of carrying very

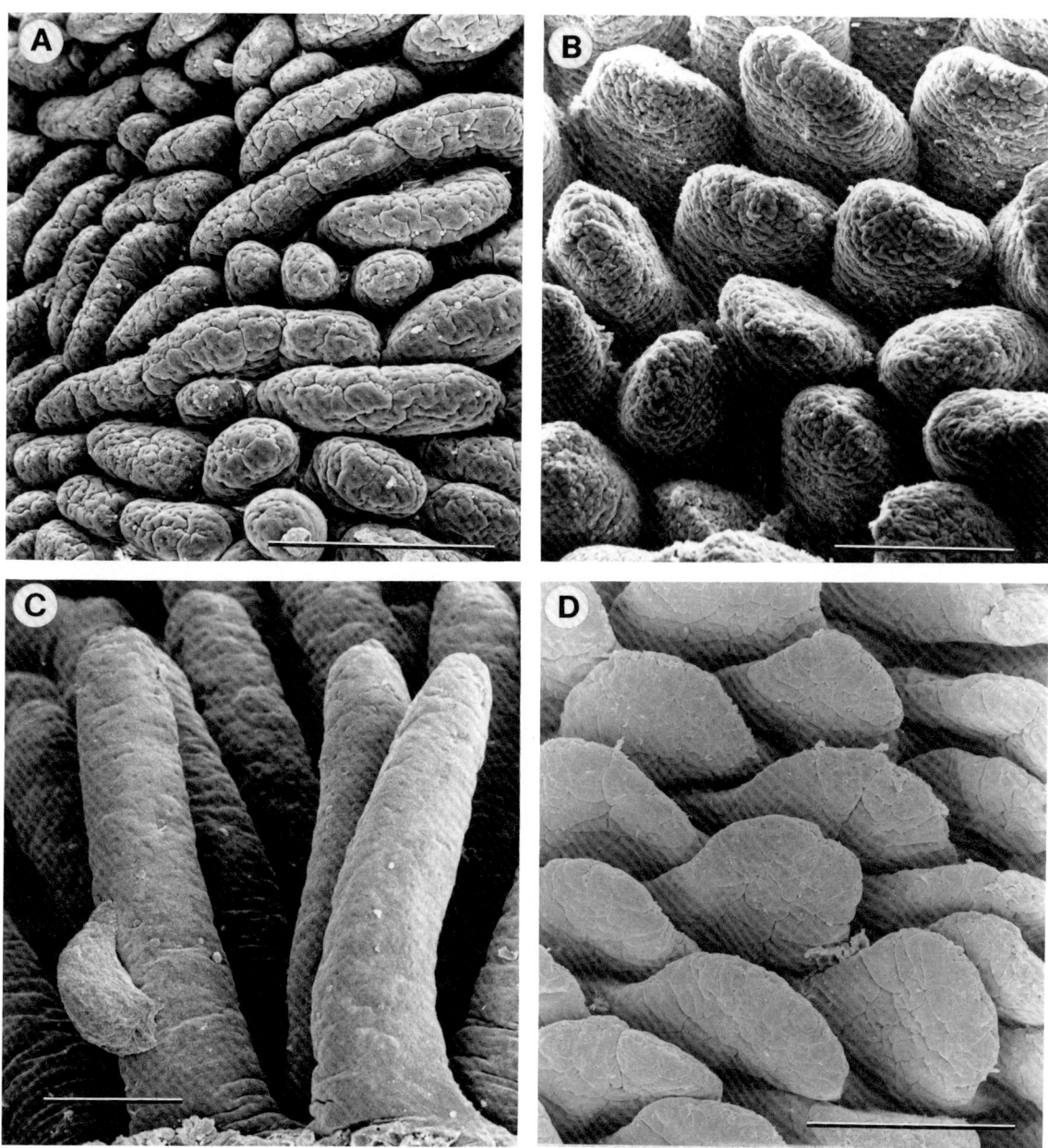

FIG. 6. Scanning electron micrographs of villi of small intestine from several species. *A*: human villi; note variety of villus shapes. *Calibration bar*, 500 μm. *B*: dog villi; note stout cylindrical shape. *Calibration bar*, 250 μm. *C*: cat villi; note slender fingerlike shape. *Calibration bar*, 100 μm. *D*: rat villi; note leaflike flattened shape. *Calibration bar*, 250 μm. [*A* from Gannon et al. (56); *B, C* from Gannon et al. (55).]

high flows and able to permit the passage of large objects (e.g., 15 μm microspheres).

The method by which volume flow of blood through the microvessel bed of each villus is controlled may be somewhat unusual compared with other peripheral tissues, at least in the rat. Knoblach and associates (164) have reported that the central arteriole supplying each rat villus is devoid of a continuous layer of smooth muscle cells from the lower portion of the villus to the tip. They have also observed microfilaments in this arteriolar endothelium and conclude from physiological studies that contractions of these microfilaments are responsible for the regulation of villus blood flow (83, 163). In dog villi (see Fig. 11), however, arteriolar smooth muscle extends all the way up the villus, and so a microfilament control of blood flow is unlikely to occur in dogs. An observation by Uehara and Suyama (159) of an interconnected mesh-

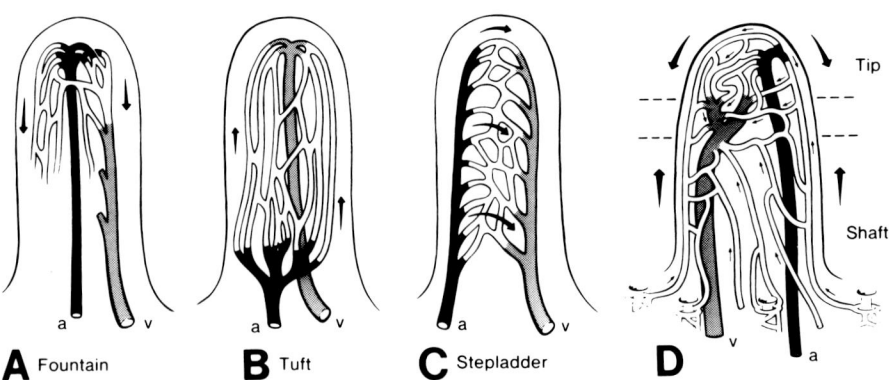

FIG. 7. Models of villus microcirculatory pattern. *A*: fountain pattern of villus blood flow; *B*: tuft pattern; *C*: stepladder pattern; *D*: combined fountain supply to villus tip and tuft supply to villus shaft, as described by Casley-Smith and Gannon (26, 51) for rabbit, rat, and human villi. *Dotted lines* represent watershed region between two blood flow sources to villi (i.e., direct arterial supply to the villus tip and indirect local portal supply via the periglandular capillaries). This watershed level varies in height up the villus with the species. [Adapted from Gannon (51).]

work of myofibroblasts that lies beneath the villus epithelial basal lamina but outside the villus capillary network and completely ensheaths the villus lamina propria (Fig. 8) offers further possibilities of microvessel flow control. Local contraction of the myofilaments in this myofibroblast layer might constrict adjacent capillary lumina, whereas overall contraction of the web would compress the entire villus lamina proprial core and may serve to clear villus interstitial fluid via the villus lacteals.

There is a direct arteriolar supply to the bases of the intestinal glands (107). Each intestinal gland is surrounded by a plexus of capillaries that ends at a capillary ring surrounding the gland opening between the villi (51, 56, 107); adjacent capillary rings are connected by microvessels to each other and to the capillary plexus of the lower portion of the adjacent villi [Figs. 5, 7D, and 8A; (56)]. In rabbit and rat intestine (Fig. 9) it has been shown that blood supply to that portion of the villus capillary plexus below the level of commencement of the villus venule(s) is derived from the pericryptal capillary network [Fig. 10A; (51, 54, 55)]. Given the essentially equivalent microvascular connectivity in human villi to those of rabbits (Fig. 8B) and rats (Fig. 8D), it seems likely that a similar dual blood supply exists to the human villus, with a direct arteriolar supply in fountain pattern to the tip and an indirect tuft pattern of supply to the lower portion of the villus shaft [Fig. 7; (56)].

That the intestinal glands are the sites of intestinal fluid secretion (47) and the villi are the sites of intestinal fluid absorption, long suggested by histologists (130) but dismissed by physiologists (72), has recently been confirmed by physiological experiments (68, 102, 166). Blood flow between the intestinal glands and the lower position of the villi could be thought of as a local portal circulation (Fig. 7D): the blood that passes first through the pericryptal capillary provides on the order of 10–20 liters per day of intestinal secretions (101). Blood effluent from the pericryptal plexus, on reaching the capillaries of the lower portion of the villus, would consequently be at raised colloid osmotic pressure and also at lowered hydrostatic pressure and thus ideally adapted for uptake of fluid from the villus. The direction of this local portal capillary blood flow between pericryptal plexus and the subepithelial capillary plexus of the lower portion of the villus is directly opposite that proposed by Florey (47) and others (e.g., ref. 7) in their scheme of fluid recycling from crypts to villi. The present concept of extraction of fluid (for secretion) from the arteriolar end of a dual capillary network with fluid absorption into the venous end (via the interstitial fluid compartment of the villi from epithelial uptake) seems more probable on hemodynamic grounds. The possible function of the crypt-to-villus fluid flux within the gut lumen (Fig. 5) is to carry digested nutrients by solvent drag to the villus absorptive surface, as suggested by Florey et al. (47) in their fluid-recycling model.

There are substantial interspecies differences in the shape of villi (26, 54, 133), as already noted, and also in their villus microvascular architectures. In particular, the lamina proprial core of cat villi is only ~30 $\mu$m in diameter compared with 30 $\mu$m thick by 100–180 $\mu$m in diameter for human villi. Cat villus microvasculature consists of an arteriole that passes directly from the submucous arterial plexus and breaks up at the tip in a fountain pattern to capillaries that pass parallel to the villus long axis down to the villus base, with occasional cross-connections [Fig. 8C; (26, 93)]. Mucosal venules arise at the level of the villus base and drain both villi and the pericryptal plexus. Cat small intestinal mucosa thus lacks the local portal arrangement between the capillaries of the pericryptal plexus and those of the more basal portion of the villi, as discussed in the rat, rabbit, dog, and human small intestine. Considering the closeness of the incoming arterioles to the outgoing capillary vessels in cat villi and from the results of a series of physiological experiments, Lundgren (93, 94) and Svanvik (153) have

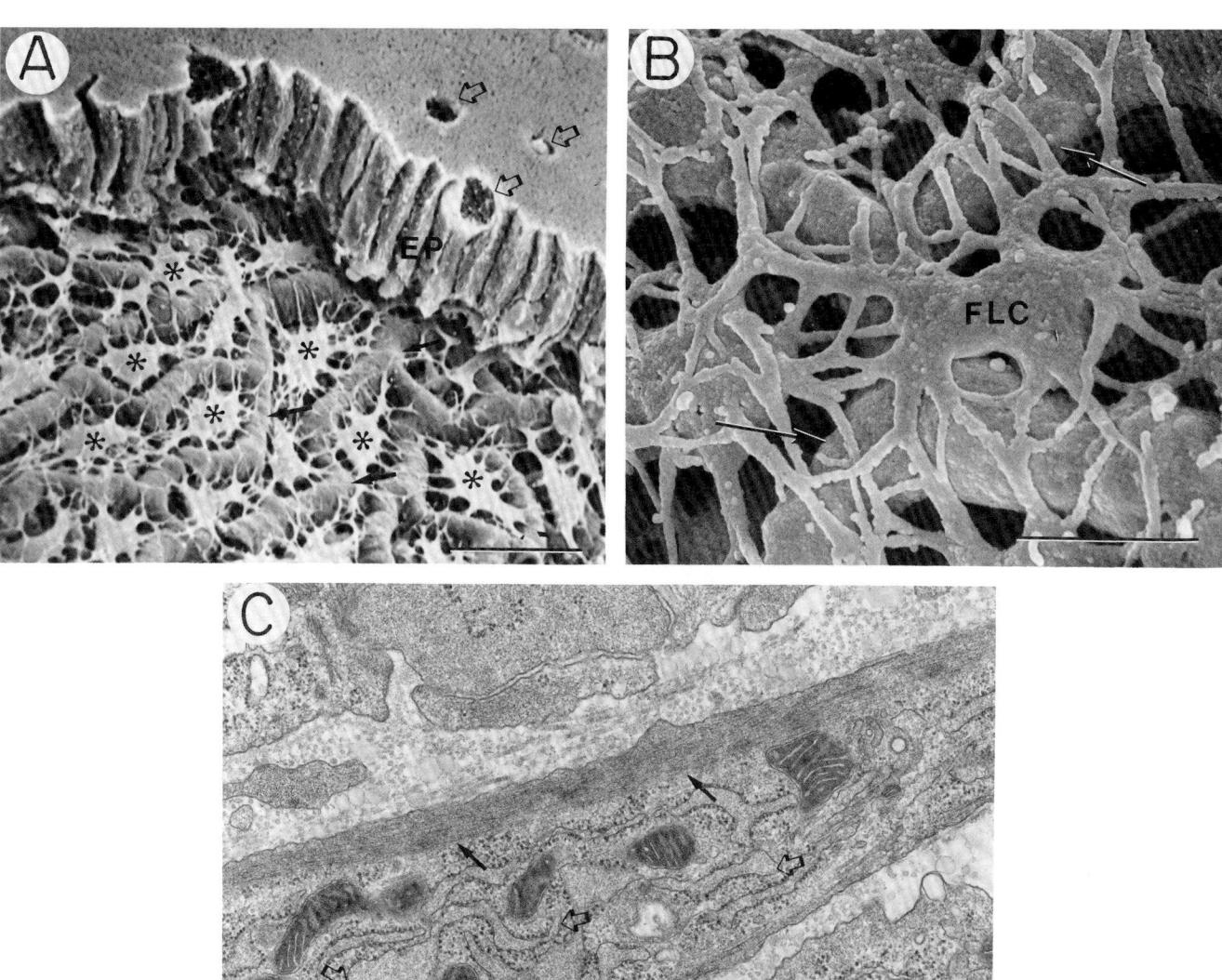

FIG. 8. Scanning and transmission electron micrographs of rat small intestinal villi illustrating myofibroblast-like cells. *A*: low power of rat villus, with epithelial sheet removed in foreground; note cellular network of myofibroblast or fibroblast-like cells (*) that overlie the subepithelial capillary plexus (*solid arrows*). *Open arrows* indicate goblet cell apices. Calibration bar, 20 μm. *B*: higher magnification of fibroblast-like cell (*FLC*) network that overlies villus capillaries (*arrows*). Calibration bar, 5 μm. *C*: Process of fibroblast-like cell; note prominent bundle of 6-nm filaments (*arrows*) and also rough endoplasmic reticulum with distended cisternae (*open arrows*), which is characteristic of these cells. Calibration bar, 1.0 μm. [*A* from Desaki et al. (37a); *B* courtesy of J. Desaki and Y. Euhara; *C* courtesy of J. Desaki.]

proposed the villus vascular countercurrent mechanism; by this mechanism, oxygen delivery to the tips of the villi is thought to be significantly impaired, because it diffuses from incoming arteriole to outgoing capillaries in the basal portion of the villus. Absorbed nutrients and electrolytes, and $CO_2$ generated by villus metabolism, are considered to be inhibited from leaving the villus, diffusing from outgoing capillaries to incoming blood in the arteriole. Further consideration of this countercurrent arrangement is given in the chapter by Jodal and Lundgren in this *Handbook*. The physiological consequences of the anatomical arrangement of the villus microvessels, as discovered in the cat, have been extrapolated from the cat intestine to that of other species, including humans (11, 94). However, there are much larger mean diffusion distances between subepithelial capillaries and the villus arteriole in most other species and also differences in capillary connections and flow directions. Consequently the functional importance of the villus vas-

1314     HANDBOOK OF PHYSIOLOGY ~ THE GASTROINTESTINAL SYSTEM I

cular countercurrent mechanism in species other than the cat has recently been questioned on anatomical (55) and theoretical grounds (84, 170).

The relative roles of the villus capillary blood flow compared with lymphatic drainage in the removal of absorbed fluid from the villus lamina propria, previously calculated from measurements of mucosal venous flow compared with lymph flow and total fluid absorption, has recently been demonstrated in rats (78, 90). In Lee's experiments (90), marked swelling

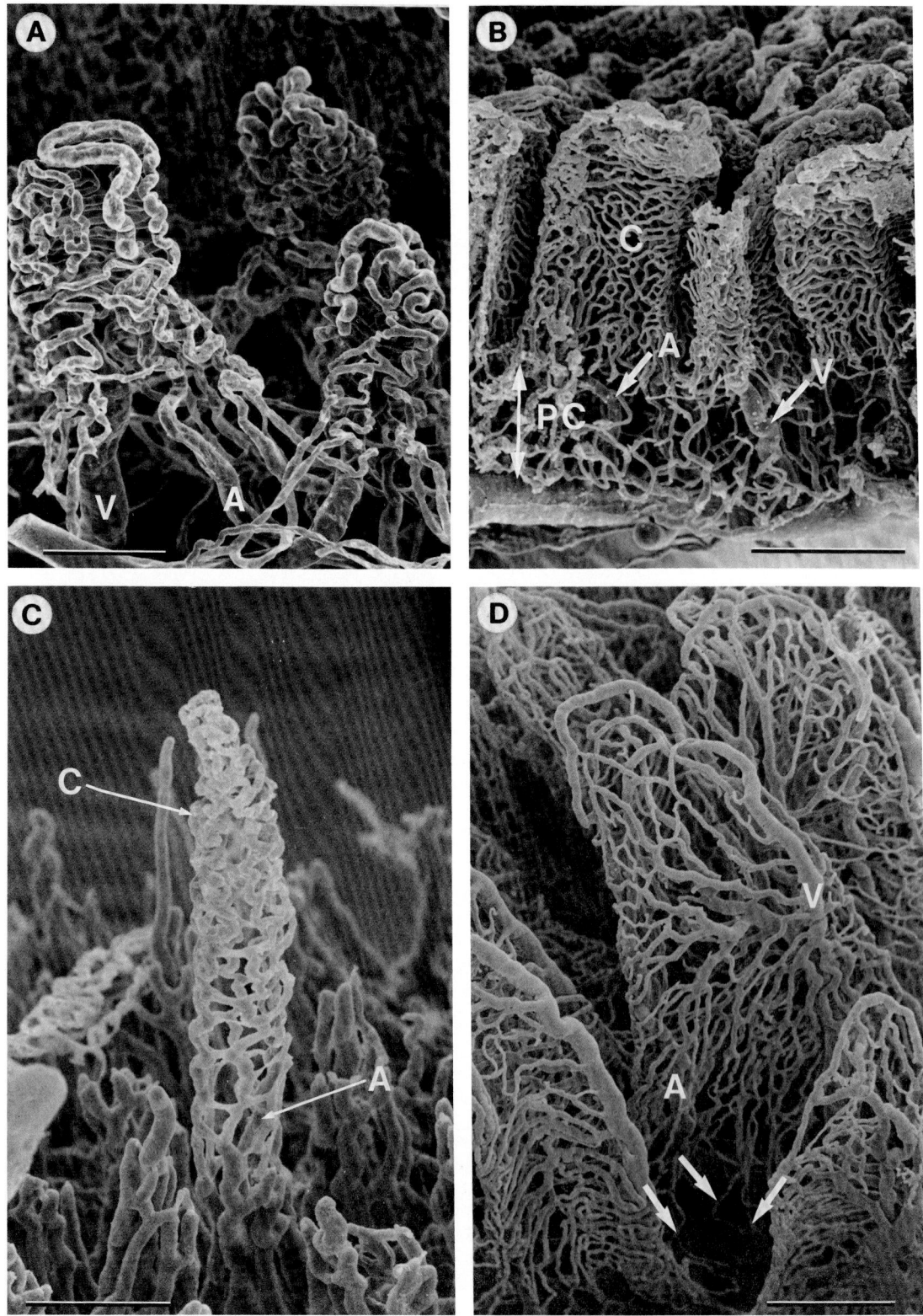

of the villi was observed when villus blood flow was occluded for several minutes, despite the presence of several patent lymphatics in each villus.

SMALL INTESTINE—DUODENUM. In the duodenum, proximal to the site of entry of the common bile duct, are the submucosal duodenal acinar glands of Brunner. The arrangement of Brunner's glands varies from a compact mass, as in the rat (Figs. 10B and 12A), to a diffuse scattering of rosettes, as in the guinea pig (35). The secretion of the proximal duodenal mucosa is rich in both mucus and bicarbonate (73, 74, 113), the latter usually thought to be principally derived from Brunner's glands (69), and is considered to be important in protecting the proximal duodenum from the low pH of the acid gastric chyme passed through the pylorus (82, 171).

The detailed microvascular organization of the Brunner's gland bed has been reported only for rats (15). This study showed that the acini are surrounded by a basketlike plexus (of fenestrated capillaries; see refs. 35, 158), which is interconnected with microvascular plexuses surrounding adjacent acini to form a continuous complex microvascular network, in which no repeating modular organization could be ascertained (Fig. 10B). The arterial supply and venous drainage of Brunner's glands were separate from and parallel to that of the overlying villi [Fig. 12B; (15)]. There were some connections of the Brunner's gland microvascular web with the pericryptal microvascular network. There were also fairly common direct connections from the pericryptal microvascular network to the villus venules en route to the submucosa at the level of the crypts. Thus in the duodenum the capillaries of the lower portion of the villus may not receive a tuft supply of capillary blood from the pericryptal capillary network (Fig. 12B). It is possible that blood from the arteriole supplying the villus tip also supplies the lower portion of the villus via the tip or even that the direction of flow in capillaries of the lower shaft of rat duodenal villi connections between the commencement of the venule and the base of the villi might be reversible under different physiological circumstances.

The parallel arrangement of villi and Brunner's glands vascular beds (Fig. 12B) may be important physiologically, because the secretion of $HCO_3^-$ by Brunner's glands (43) must result, stoichiometrically, in a minor degree of acidification of venous blood effluent from the glands. The supply of acidified blood to the villus enterocytes of the proximal duodenum, which are subjected to a high luminal acid load, would seem an inappropriate arrangement physiologically and is not observed (Fig. 12B); this is in contrast to the vascular connections found in the more distal small intestine between the pericryptal plexus and the lower capillaries of the shaft of the villi [see Fig. 5; (26, 54, 56)].

A further difference in the duodenal vascular bed from the rest of the intestine is that the degree of internal self-anastomosis of the submucosal arterial network is much less than in the more distal small intestine; as a result, the extrinsic arteries to the duodenum can essentially be considered as end arteries from the extramural arcades (121). This paucity of submucous arterial anastomosis, possibly coupled with serosal tension in the duodenum caused by the suspension of an overdistended stomach and heavy omentum in part from the duodenum (which is fixed to the dorsal body wall), thought to be responsible for the susceptibility of the duodenum to ulceration generally and at Mayo's anemic spot of the mucosa in particular (120, 121).

COLON. The topology of the colonic mucosa is similar to that of the stomach. There are frequent tubular downpocketings of the enterocyte layer into the lamina propria—the simple tubular colonic glands.

The organization of the intramural vessels of the colon is also reminiscent of that of the stomach (174). The arterioles from the submucous vascular plexus, which supply the mucosa, break up at the most abluminal level of the mucosa into a capillary network that ramifies in the lamina propria between the colonic glands [Fig. 13; (16)]. The predominant orientation is perpendicular to the plane of the mucosal surface, but there are frequent cross-connections between adjacent capillaries. At the most luminal aspect of the lamina propria, the capillary net of the mucosa is connected with a polygonal plexus of microvessel rings surrounding the necks of the colonic glands (Fig. 13B). This polygonal network is composed of capillaries and perhaps also of some postcapillary venules (depending on the definition of the latter that one adopts), because there is coalescence of flow in parts of the polygonal network as it approaches the origins of the infrequently occurring mucosal venules. These mucosal venules accept small tributaries only imme-

---

FIG. 9. Scanning electron micrographs of microvascular corrosion casts of small intestinal villi of four mammalian species. A: human villi. Note difference in size between adjacent villi and connection of villus capillaries to capillary rings surrounding intestinal gland openings. A, arteriole; V, venule. Calibration bar, 100 μm. B: rat villi, duodenum. Note broad flattened villi arrayed across long axis of gut. C, capillary plexus of villus; PC, pericryptal plexus surrounding intestinal glands; A, arteriole; V, venule. Calibration bar, 250 μm. C: cat villi. Note slender form; plexus consists solely of capillaries (C) and an arteriole (A) in tuft pattern, as seen in partially filled villus at bottom left; there is no villus venule. Mucosal venules commence at level of villus base between adjacent villi. Calibration bar, 100 μm. D: rabbit villi. Note arteriolar breakup near tip and villus capillaries connected to plexus surrounding intestinal gland openings (arrows). A, arteriole; V, venule. Calibration bar, 250 μm. [A from Gannon (51); B from Browning and Gannon (16); C, D from Gannon et al. (55).]

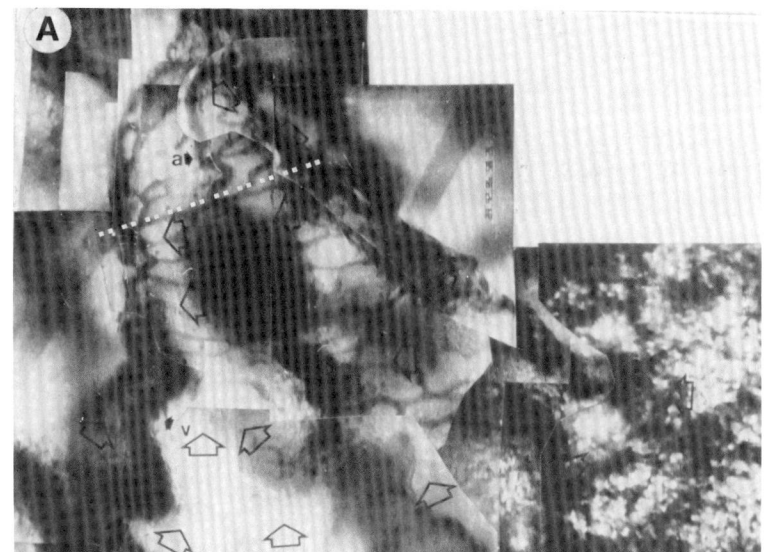

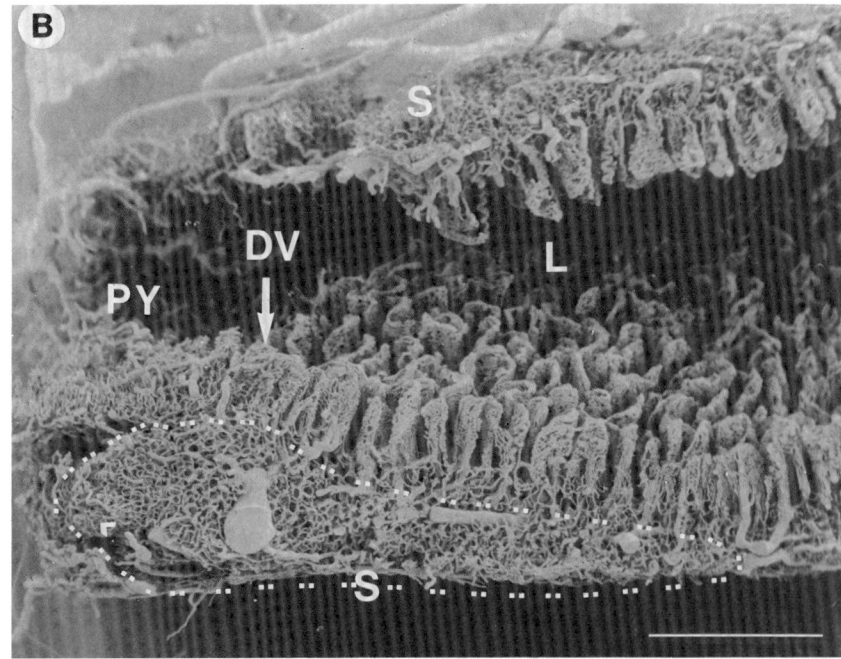

FIG. 10. *A*: montage of in vivo photomicrographs of rabbit intestinal villus (ex video monitor screen). *a*, Arteriole; *v*, venule; *arrows*, principal directions of capillary blood flow; *dotted lines*, division between villus tip and shaft blood flows, as shown in Fig. 5 and Fig. 7D. *Calibration bar*, 250 μm. *B*: vascular corrosion cast of rat pylorus and proximal duodenum, bisected along duodenal long axis. *PY*, pylorus; *DV*, most proximal duodenal villi; *L*, duodenal lumen; *S*, duodenal serosa; *area outlined with dotted line*, compact mass of Brunner's glands. *Calibration bar*, 1,000 μm. [*A* from Gannon (51); *B* from Browning and Gannon (15).]

diately subjacent to the mucosal surfaces and pass perpendicular to the mucosal surface plane to the submucosal venous plexus [Fig. 13C; (16)].

There is no direct arteriolar supply to the luminal portion of the colonic mucosa equivalent to that apparent in the small intestinal villi; indeed the entire circulation of the colonic mucosa appears equivalent to that of the gastric glands of the stomach or of the crypts of Lieberkühn of the small intestine. This colonic microvascular architecture, first determined in rats (16), has now been confirmed in the cottontop marmoset monkey and in humans (J. Browning and B. J. Gannon, unpublished observations). The spatial density of rat colonic mucosal capillaries decreases from the proximal to the distal colon, as does the fenestral frequency per capillary (J. Browning and B. J. Gannon, unpublished observations).

MICROVASCULAR ULTRASTRUCTURE AND PERMEABILITY CHARACTERISTICS

One characteristic of the microcirculation of the gastrointestinal tract is the very large transendothelial exchange of fluid and solutes that occurs during the processes of absorption and secretion. This section reviews the ultrastructure of these exchange vessels and considers the various structures within the capil-

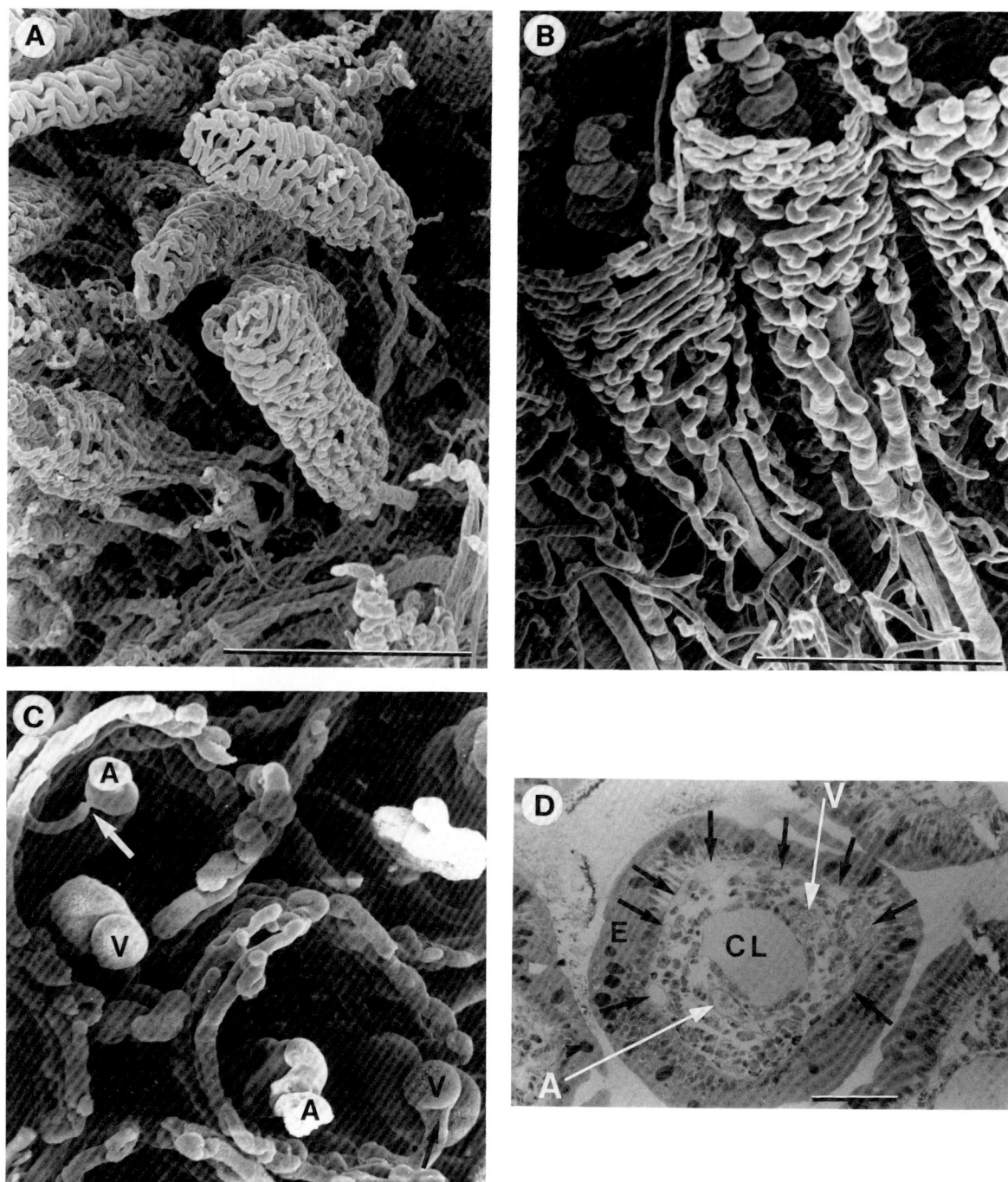

FIG. 11. Micrographs of dog intestinal villi. *A*: cast of dog intestinal villi. Note completely filled villus tip vessels arrayed in fountain pattern. *Calibration bar*, 500 μm. *B*: cast of partially filled dog villi with tips not cast. Capillaries of villus lower shaft connect with capillaries of pericryptal plexus, presumably in tuft pattern. *Calibration bar*, 250 μm. *C*: transverse section of cast of dog villi at middle third of villus; incomplete cast with tip region not filled. Villus arteriole (*A*) serially supplies (*white arrow*) and villus venule (*V*) serially drains (*black arrow*) subepithelial capillary network in stepladder pattern. *Calibration bar*, 100 μm. *D*: transverse section at midshaft of dog villus, 1 μm plastic section, polychrome stain. *A*, arteriole; *V*, venule; *CL*, central lacteal; *black arrows* indicate subepithelial capillaries; *E*, villus epithelium. *Calibration bar*, 100 μm. [From Casley-Smith and Gannon (26).]

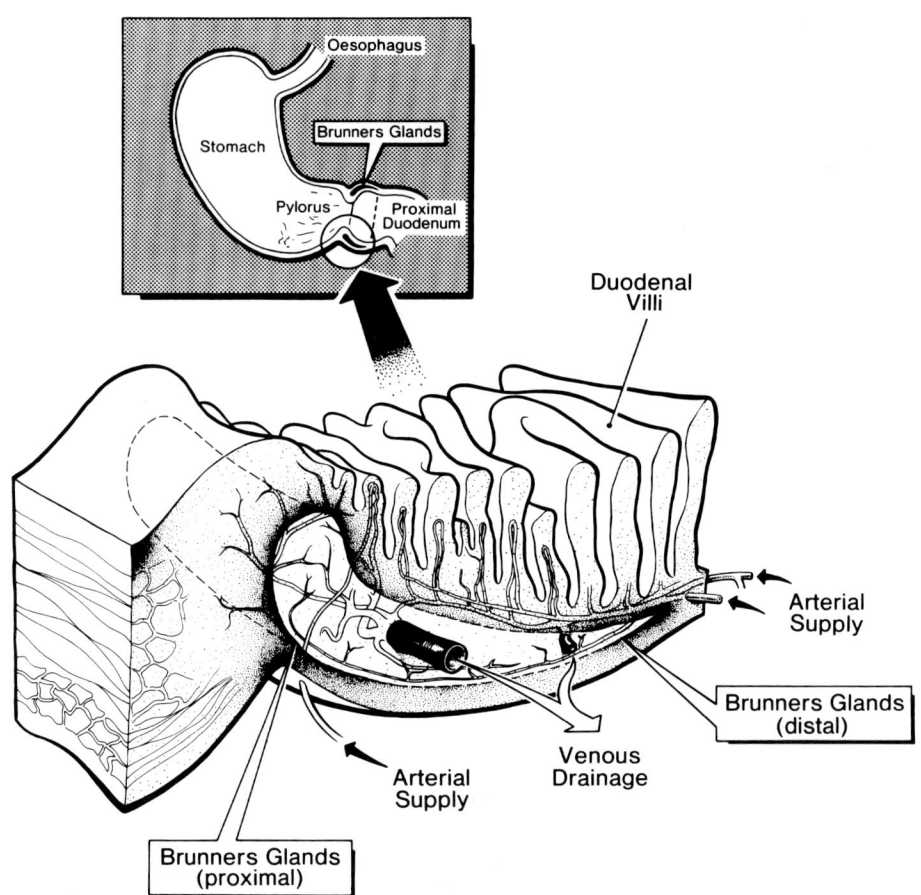

FIG. 12. *A*: major vascular supply and drainage routes of Brunner's gland tissue in rat proximal duodenum. *Inset*, dorsal view of horizontal schematic section of rat stomach, indicating location of Brunner's glands. *B*: parallel nature of separate circulations of Brunner's glands and of villus tip and shaft in duodenum. Note that presumably acidified blood (after $HCO_3^-$ secretion in Brummer's glands) is not supplied to villi, which have to cope with an exogenous $H^+$ load from duodenal lumen (ex gastric juice). [From Browning and Gannon (15).]

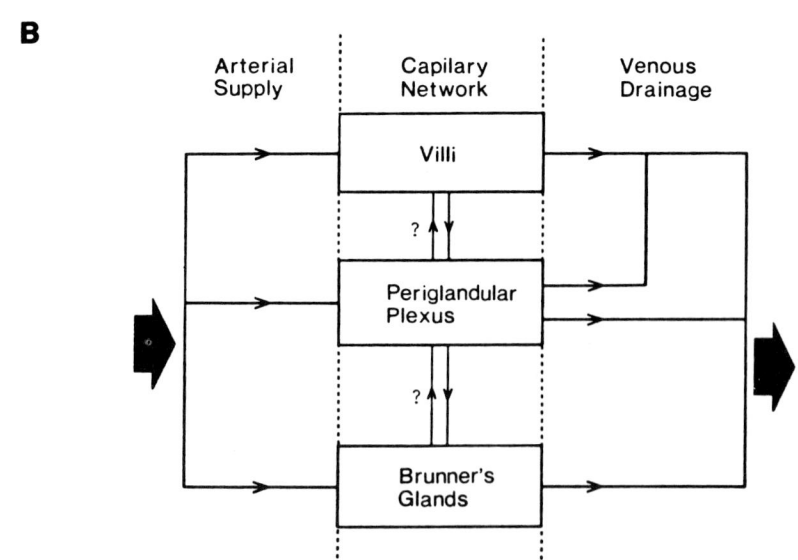

lary wall that may serve as pathways for transendothelial exchange. The ultrastructure of the gastrointestinal circulation has not received as much attention as the microvessels in other vascular beds, such as cardiac muscle and diaphragm. However, recent interest in fenestrated endothelium has led to an increased understanding of the ultrastructure of capillaries in the small intestine, whereas the microcirculation of the stomach and large bowel has not been extensively investigated.

*Small Intestine*

GENERAL STRUCTURE. The small intestine is composed of a number of different layers, including the mucosa (composed of villi, crypts of Lieberkühn, and muscularis mucosae), submucosa, muscularis externa, and the serosa. In the cat the mucosa represents ~25% of the total wall volume and is composed of 16% villi and 9% crypts. The muscularis mucosa, submucosa, and serosa are small structures and collectively represent only 1%–2% of total wall volume. The largest layer is the muscularis externa, which represents 73% of total wall volume (Table 1).

In the mucosa the capillaries are fenestrated, whereas those in the submucosa and muscularis are continuous. In the villi the capillaries are located immediately beneath the mucosal epithelium (Fig. 14) so that the fenestrations are no more than 1–2 $\mu$m from the basal lamina of the epithelial cells (33, 61). The capillaries in this region possess a characteristic asymmetry. The side facing the intestinal epithelium is composed of very thin endothelium <0.1 $\mu$m wide and contains numerous fenestrae, whereas the side facing the center of the villus is thick and contains the nucleus and other organelles (Fig. 15). There are significant differences in the degree of vascularity of the different regions of the intestinal wall. Casley-Smith et al. (28) determined the number of small blood vessels (<25 $\mu$m diam) per square centimeter of thin section and found that the greatest number of vessels was in the tips of the villi and in the crypts, whereas there were fewer vessels in the base of the villi. These observations are consistent with the fountain pattern of the microcirculation in the cat intestine where capillaries originate from a central arteriole at the tip of the villus and coalesce into collecting vessels toward the base (26, 55). The muscularis externa contains relatively fewer capillaries (Table 1). The numbers of vessels together with their diameters have been used to calculate capillary surface area in each region. In the tips of the villi and the crypts the capillary surface area is 5 to 6 times greater than that observed in the villi bases and muscularis externa. The value of 68 $cm^2 \cdot g^{-1}$ calculated for capillary surface area in the muscularis externa is similar to the value recorded in skeletal muscle (111).

ULTRASTRUCTURE OF INTESTINAL CAPILLARY WALL. Interest in the ultrastructure of capillaries arose, in part, from the prediction by physiologists that exchange across the capillary wall could be explained by two separate populations of theoretical pores: small pores of 6 nm radius for the exchange of small solutes and a smaller number of large pores 20–30 nm radius for exchange of macromolecules, including plasma proteins (65, 111, 112). The pore theory assumes that these exchange pathways are uniform structures, either cylindrical pores or slits. Variations in their numbers and dimensions have been used to describe differences in vascular permeability in different tissues (155). However, careful examinations of the capillary wall by electron microscopy have failed to reveal unequivocal ultrastructural counterparts to the theoretical pores predicted from functional studies. The various structures that may act as pathways for transcapillary exchange are shown diagrammatically in Figure 16. In this chapter we consider primarily the ultrastructure and permeability to electron-dense tracers of fenestrated capillaries, because it is the fenestrated capillaries of the mucosa that are associated with the absorptive and secretory sites in the gastrointestinal tract. The continuous capillaries of the submucosal and muscularis layers of the gut appear to be structurally and functionally similar to skeletal muscle capillaries and are likely, therefore, to be far less permeable to fluid and small solutes than fenestrated endothelium (60, 118). Although exchange across the continuous capillaries is likely to be much less than across fenestrated capillaries, the continuous capillaries subjacent to the serosal layer play an important role, which includes the provision of a pathway for exchange between blood and peritoneal fluid. The permeability characteristics of these capillaries are particularly important, therefore, during peritoneal dialysis. Further understanding of their exchange characteristics is likely to come from in vivo microscopy, a technique that has recently been used to investigate the fluid exchange characteristics of single capillaries in intestinal muscle (60). Our present understanding of the role that each of the structures illustrated in Figure 16 plays in the process of transcapillary exchange of fluid and solutes has come from studies of both continuous and fenestrated vascular beds, because many of the pathways are common to both types of endothelium.

*Fenestrae.* In the small intestine the largest surface area of fenestrated capillaries and consequently the greatest number of fenestrae are associated with the tips of the villi and the crypts of Lieberkühn, the sites of absorption and secretion (Table 1). The fenestrae, which are circular openings in the capillary wall ~60 nm diameter, occur in the thin portion of the endothelial cell, where the cytoplasm is <0.1 $\mu$m thick. In general, there are more fenestrae on the venous end of the capillary than on the arterial end (25, 28). However, in the cat there appear to be more fenestrae in the villus tips (28) that represent the arterial end of the microvascular network (56). The fenestrae are often covered by a thin unit membrane or diaphragm, which is a single layer 2–4 nm thick, continuous with the outer leaflet of the plasma membrane. At the center of the diaphragm is a central knob or swelling (33, 41, 92). It appears that not all fenestrae have a diaphragm. In the cat and mouse intestine ~50%–70% of the fenestrae possess a diaphragm (25, 28).

The permeability to water-soluble molecules of the

fenestrae and other structures in the capillary wall has been studied with tracers that can be visualized by electron microscopy. The molecules used range in size from 1-nm radius (hemeoctapeptide) to 15-nm radius (rabbit liver glycogen). The permeability of the capillary wall is assessed by the location and concentration of the tracer at various time intervals after administration.

Of the different pathways available for transcapillary exchange (Fig. 16), it is the fenestrae that appear

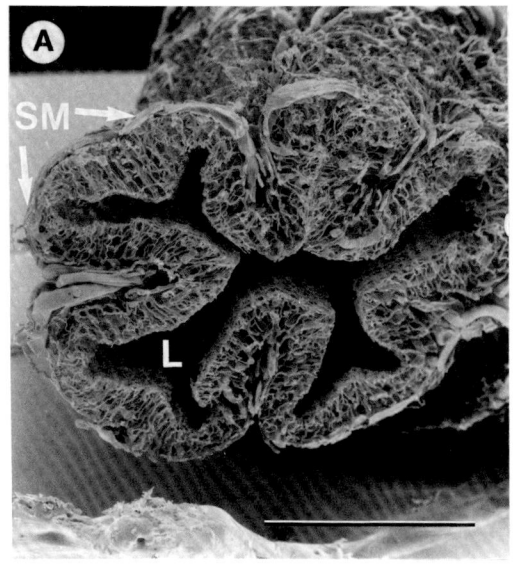
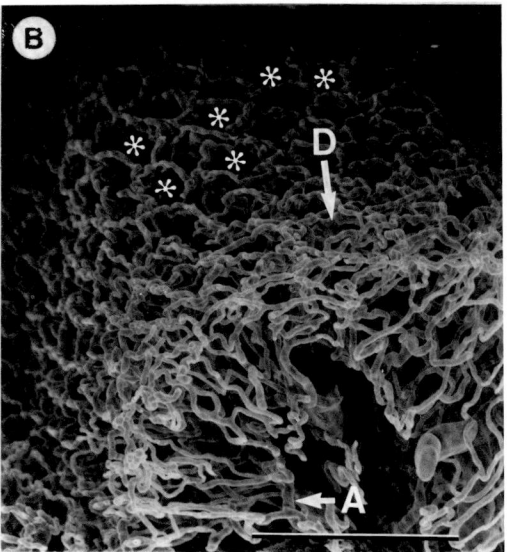
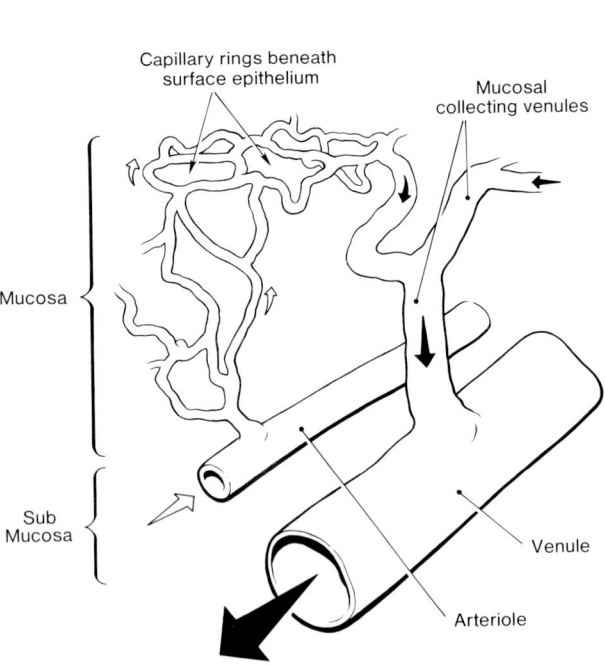
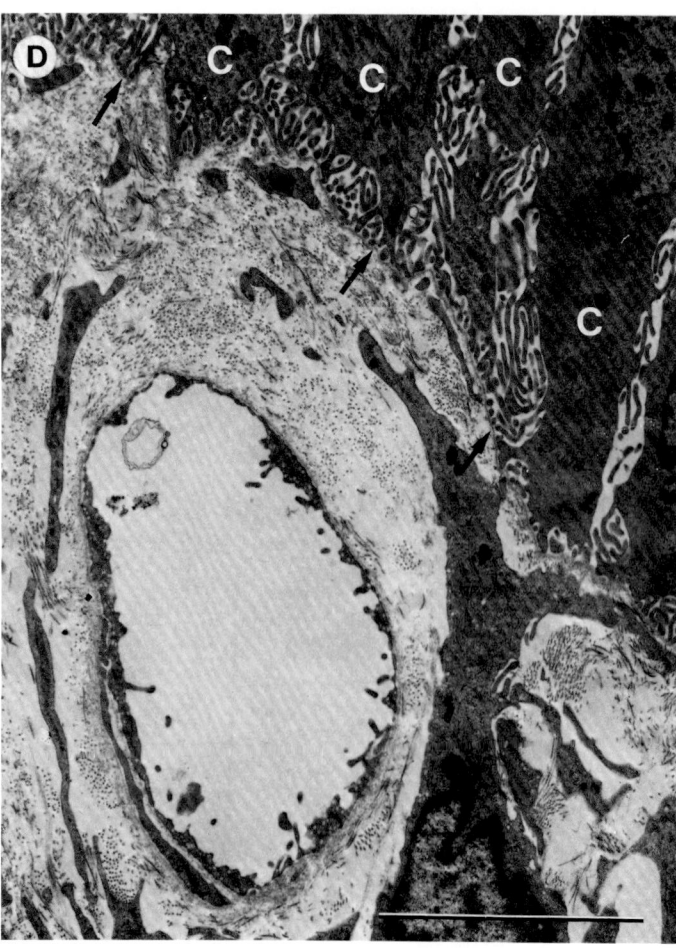

to be the most permeable. Horseradish peroxidase (3 nm radius) rapidly permeates all fenestrae within the intestinal mucosa (33). Within 90 s of injection, horseradish peroxidase was observed in the interstitium opposite the fenestrated portion of the capillary wall. This extravasation of tracer was independent of the presence or absence of a diaphragm across the fenestral opening. However, larger tracers such as ferritin (5.5 nm radius) and glycogen (15 nm radius) leave the circulation at much slower rates (140). It appears that the diaphragms are permeable to tracers <3 nm radius but relatively impermeable to molecules >5.5 nm radius (42, 75, 110). The ability of diaphragmmed fenestrae to restrict molecules >5.5 nm radius means that the concentration of macromolecules within the interstitium is well below the plasma concentration. For example, the interstitial concentration of glycogen (10–15 nm radius) is only 6%–8% of that observed in the capillary lumen (140). Functional studies of the small intestine have found lymph (interstitial fluid)-to-plasma concentration ratios for endogenous plasma proteins that are consistent with the ratio observed with electron-dense tracers (63). Therefore both morphological and functional studies confirm the restrictive nature of the fenestrated endothelium to macromolecules. Fenestrae appear to allow rapid transcapillary passage of tracers <3 nm radius, whereas a substantial proportion of the fenestrae selectively retain larger molecules (>5.5 nm radius) within the circulation.

*Vesicles.* Vesicles are small spherical structures ~70 nm diameter and bounded by a membrane similar in appearance to the plasmalemmal membrane. Approximately 70% of vesicles are attached to either the blood or the interstitial facing membranes of the endothelial cell and the remaining 30% appear free within the endothelial cell cytoplasm (109). The vesicles are connected to the cell surface membrane by short necks that vary from 10 to 40 nm diameter. The openings or stomata may be covered by a thin diaphragm 6–8 nm thick, similar to the diaphragm observed across fenestrae (110).

There are large differences in the number of vesicles encountered *1)* in different regions of the same endothelial cell, *2)* in vessels located in different parts of the microcirculation (e.g., arterioles versus capillaries), and *3)* in different tissues of the body. Vesicles are most numerous in the attenuated periphery of the capillary endothelium. For example, in the continuous capillaries of the rat diaphragm there is a mean of 883 vesicles/$\mu m^3$ in the thin periphery of the endothelial cell compared with 190/$\mu m^3$ in the perikaryon (136). The high density of vesicles observed in the attenuated periphery is characteristic of true capillaries, whereas other microvessels such as arterioles and venules have fewer vesicles. In the mouse diaphragm the number of vesicles is ~200/$\mu m^3$ in the arterioles, 900–1,200/$\mu m^3$ in capillaries, and 300–600/$\mu m^3$ in venules (144). Although the continuous capillaries are rich in vesicles, the highly permeable fenestrated capillaries of the gastrointestinal tract have far fewer. In the mucosa of the rat jejunum the number of vesicles is ~10%–20% of the number observed in the diaphragm and myocardium (136).

The contribution of vesicles to the transport of substances across the capillary wall remains a matter for debate. Vesicles are thought to move in a random fashion by thermal kinetic energy (24, 134). Electron-dense tracers injected into the circulation initially enter vesicles open to the luminal aspect of the endothelial cell and subsequently appear in vesicles that are apparently free within the cytoplasm. The final phase of transport occurs when the vesicles fuse with the membrane of the abluminal aspect of the cell and discharge their contents into the interstitium. Estimates of the time taken for vesicles to cross the endothelial cell range from 0.1 s to 25 s (117, 135, 141). There are differences in the transit time of vesicles across the different regions of the capillary wall. In the parajunctional zone and in the region of the endothelial cell containing organelles there are fewer vesicles, and these vesicles appear to take up tracers more slowly (141).

The entire vesicle population is labeled by and appears to transport smaller molecules (1 nm radius); however, there is a reduction in the proportion of vesicles transporting large tracers, that is, only 90% of vesicles appear to transport molecules with a 1.7 nm radius (142, 144). It is possible that either the presence of a stomatal diaphragm or physical restriction by the neck of some vesicles may limit the entry of larger molecules.

The notion that vesicles are involved in transcapillary transport is not shared by all investigators. Bungaard et al. (21) cut serial, ultrathin sections (15 nm) through the capillary and reconstructed the spatial

---

FIG. 13. Microvasculature of rat colonic mucosa. *A*: corrosion microvascular cast of rat midcolon. Constricted muscle and local absence of fecal pellet produces constricted lumen (*L*). Larger vessels of submucous vascular plexus (*SM*) are evident, but vasculature of muscularis externa is not filled. Calibration bar, 1,000 µm. *B*: fractured cast of rat colonic mucosa; oblique view of luminal aspect. Capillaries nearest lumen are arranged in honeycomb-like plexus surrounding openings of colonic glands (\*). Site where mucosal venule commences drainage (*D*) is also identified. Arterioles (*A*) branch to capillaries only near submucosal aspect. Calibration bar, 250 µm. *C*: microcirculatory pattern of rat colonic mucosa; pattern is analogous to that observed in rat and human stomach (cf. Fig. 3). *D*: fenestrated capillary of rat/human colonic mucosa. Colonocytes (*C*) abut epithelial basal lamina (*arrow*). Calibration bar, 5 µm. [*A, B, C* from Browning and Gannon (16).]

TABLE 1. *Volume and Vascular Dimensions of Different Regions of Cat Jejunum*

|  | Villi Tips | Villi Bases | Crypts | Muscularis Externa |
|---|---|---|---|---|
| Volume, %* | 9.4 ± 0.5 | 7.3 ± 0.3 | 9.9 ± 0.5 | 73.0 ± 1.1 |
| Small vessels/cm² section,† × 10⁴ | 7 ± 1 | 3 ± 0.5 | 11 ± 1 | 2 ± 0.4 |
| Proportion thin endothelium | 0.3 ± 0.04 | 0.02 ± 0.01 | 0.09 ± 0.02 | 0.001 ± 0.001 |
| Fenestrae/capillary cross section | 21 ± 3 | 0.9 ± 0.3 | 5 ± 1 | 0.2 ± 0.1 |
| Proportion fenestrae with diaphragms | 0.6 ± 0.1 |  | 0.5 ± 0.1 |  |
| Calculated fenestra diameter, nm | 53 ± 1 |  | 58 ± 2 |  |
| Fenestra depth, nm | 36 ± 1 |  | 37 ± 1 |  |
| Calculated capillary surface area, cm²·g⁻¹ | 329 ± 54 | 68 ± 11 | 415 ± 48 | 68 ± 15 |

* Calculated with tissue density of 0.956 g/ml.   † Vessels <25 μm diam.   [Data from Casley-Smith et al. (28).]

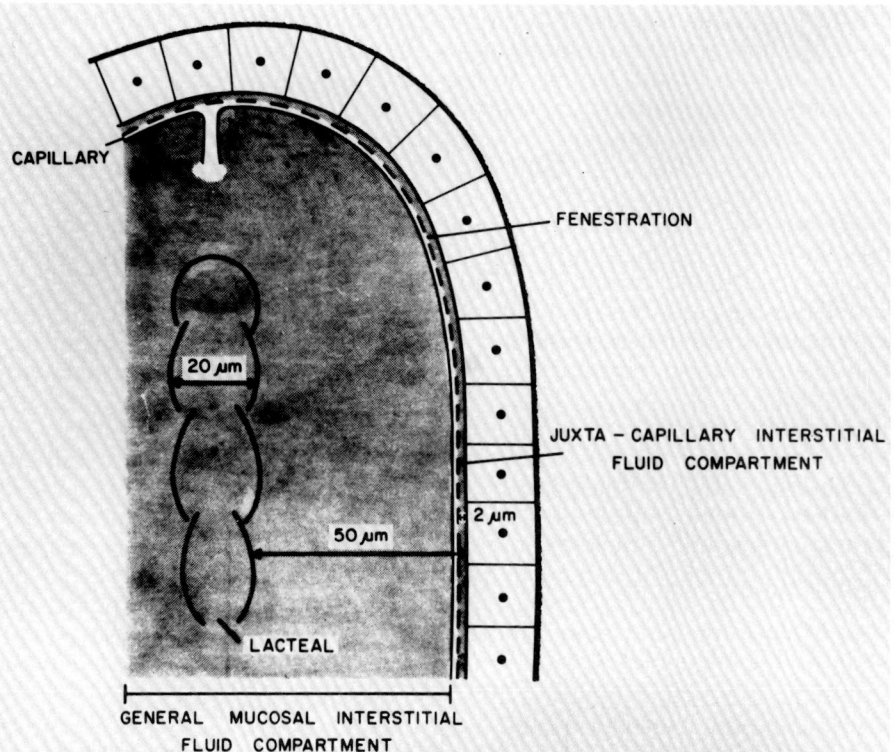

FIG. 14. Blood and lymph microcirculation of intestinal villus, illustrating closeness of fenestrated capillaries to base of mucosal epithelium. [From Granger (61).]

arrangement of vesicles within the wall. Of 921 vesicles examined, they found that none was free in the cytoplasm. All opened either to the capillary lumen or the interstitial space. They concluded that vesicles represent a stationary invagination of the plasmalemmal membrane into the cytoplasm of the endothelial cell and that they do not transport substances across the capillary wall. They did not exclude the possibility that the invaginations from luminal and abluminal sides may coalesce to form a patent vesicle channel across the cell (18, 19, 22, 49).

Although the role that vesicles play in the exchange of substances across the capillary wall remains equivocal, it is apparent that they are unlikely to make a significant contribution to transcapillary exchange in the fenestrated vascular beds of the small intestine. Vesicles are far fewer in number in the fenestrated beds, and the exchange of electron-dense tracers through the fenestrae far exceeds that occurring via the vesicles (140). Simionescu et al. (140) indicate that vesicular transport is at best 6 to 8 times slower than exchange through fenestrae.

*Vesicle channels.* The existence of chains of fused vesicles forming a patent channel across the endothelial cell was first described by Palade and Bruns (109). They occur in both continuous and fenestrated endothelium and are generally located in the attenuated periphery of the endothelial cell where the density of vesicles is greatest. The frequency of transendothelial channels increases toward the venular end of the capillary (144).

The channels are permeable to heme peptides (1 nm radius) and horseradish peroxidase (3 nm radius); however, these tracers do not accumulate in signifi-

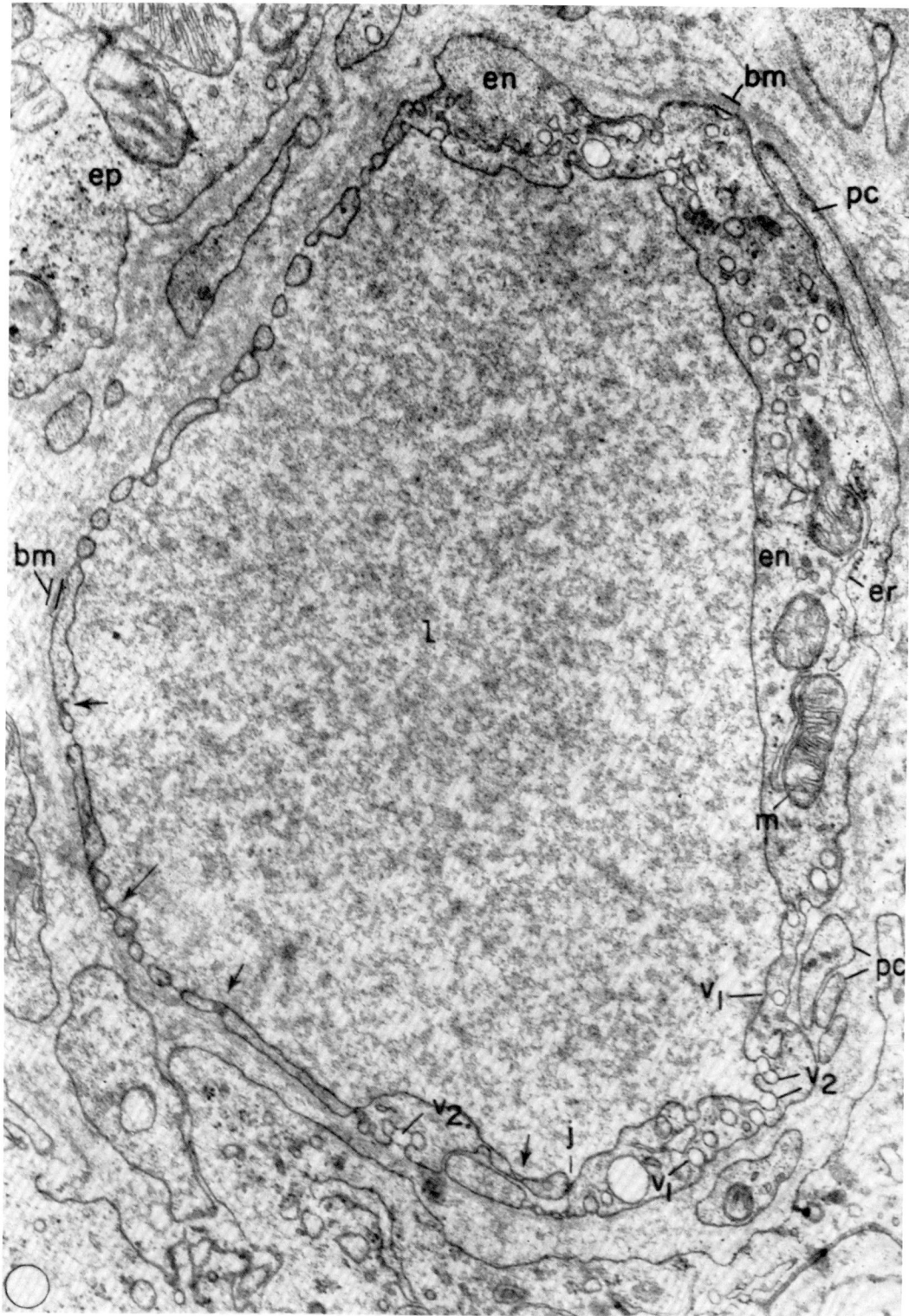

FIG. 15. Cross section of blood capillary in intestinal mucosa of mouse. Endothelial layer (*en*) consists of single cell whose attenuated part faces intestinal epithelium (*ep*). Thicker part (perikaryon) contains cellular organelles and faces center of villus. Attenuated part contains numerous fenestrae with diaphragms; their aggregate area amounts to ~5% of endothelial surface. Thicker part of endothelium is provided with flask-shaped ($v_1$) and apertured ($v_2$) vesicles. *bm*, Continuous basement membrane; *pc*, pericyte pseudopodia. ×29,000. [From Clementi and Palade (33).]

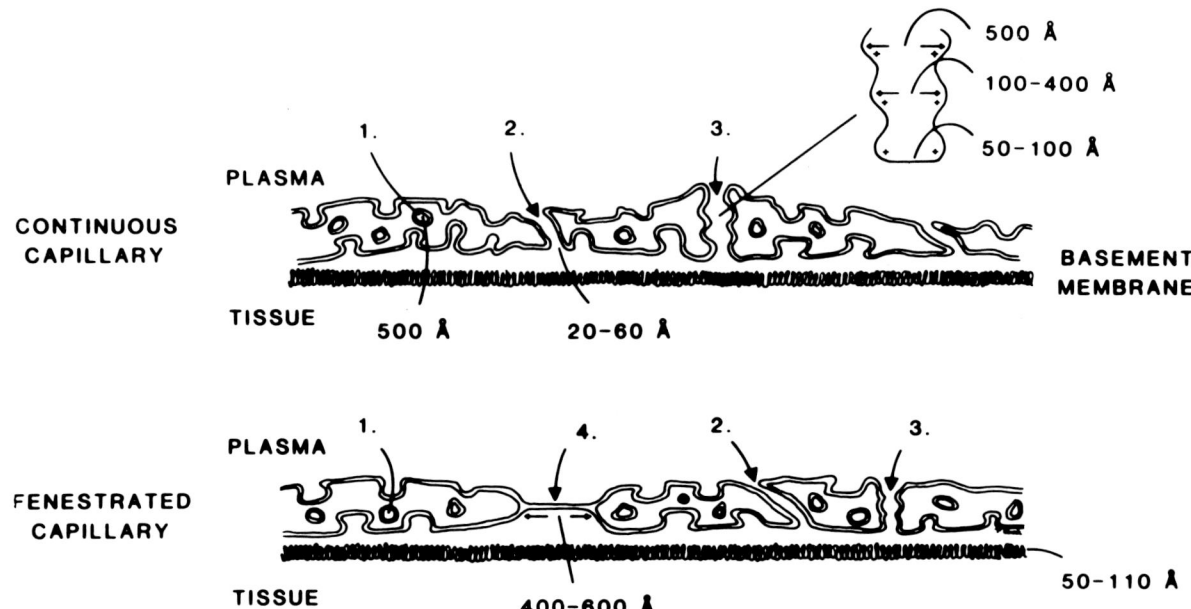

FIG. 16. Continuous and fenestrated capillary walls. *1–4*, Plasmalemmal vesicles, interendothelial junctions, vesicle channels, and fenestrations, respectively. Dimensions of different strictures are indicated in ångströms. Schematic transendothelial channel is shown at *top*, illustrating outer dimensions of channel (500 Å), dimensions of strictures within channel (100–400 Å), and selectivity of diaphragms within channel (50–100 Å). [From Taylor and Granger (154).]

cant quantities within the interstitium adjacent to the channels. This observation has led to the suggestion that the channels may not remain open for long periods of time but act rather as transient hydrophilic pores (142, 144). Larger tracer molecules (>3 nm radius) may be excluded from channels by strictures of ~5 nm radius (located at the fusion sites between the vesicles) or by diaphragms located at the stomata that have similar permeability characteristics to the fenestral diaphragms. Although some investigators suggest that transendothelial channels are relatively common (140, 142, 144), other studies have failed to identify these structures within the capillary wall (18, 172). Because there is no accurate estimate of the frequency or the permeability characteristics of vesicle channels, it is difficult to evaluate their possible contribution to transcapillary exchange. It seems unlikely, however, that they represent a significant pathway for exchange across the fenestrated capillaries of the intestine.

*Junctions.* Another ultrastructural feature of the capillary wall is the narrow cleft or intercellular junction that exists between adjacent endothelial cells. In some junctions there is a resolvable gap between the membranes for the entire length of the junction, forming a patent channel between the capillary lumen and the interstitium. However, in most junctions the outer leaflets of the adjacent plasmalemmas appear either to lie in close apposition or to fuse at one or more points along the junction (Fig. 17). The region of the junction where the membranes appear to touch or fuse probably represents localized points of contact between adjacent endothelial cells, because serial sections through these sites reveal adjacent patent regions where the outer unit membranes are separated (20, 80). Therefore exchange between capillary lumen and interstitium taking place via the junctions would proceed around the points of membrane fusion via adjacent patent regions. Similar interpretation of junctional structure has been made from the appearance of freeze-fracture sections through the junctional complex (172).

In the small intestine, there appear to be fewer junctions than in other vascular beds. There is only one junction per capillary cross section in the small intestine compared with two in muscle (136) and three in lung (114). This means that at any given cross section intestinal capillaries are generally formed by a single endothelial cell, whereas muscle and lung capillaries are formed by two and three cells, respectively. Consequently the area of intercellular junction that is located on the luminal surface of the capillary is only 0.08% of the total luminal surface area in the intestine compared with 0.2% in muscle capillaries (136). The intercellular junctions in the small intestine are also shorter (1.4 µm per µm length of capillary) than those in muscle capillaries (3.2 µm per µm length of capillary), indicating that in the intestine the junc-

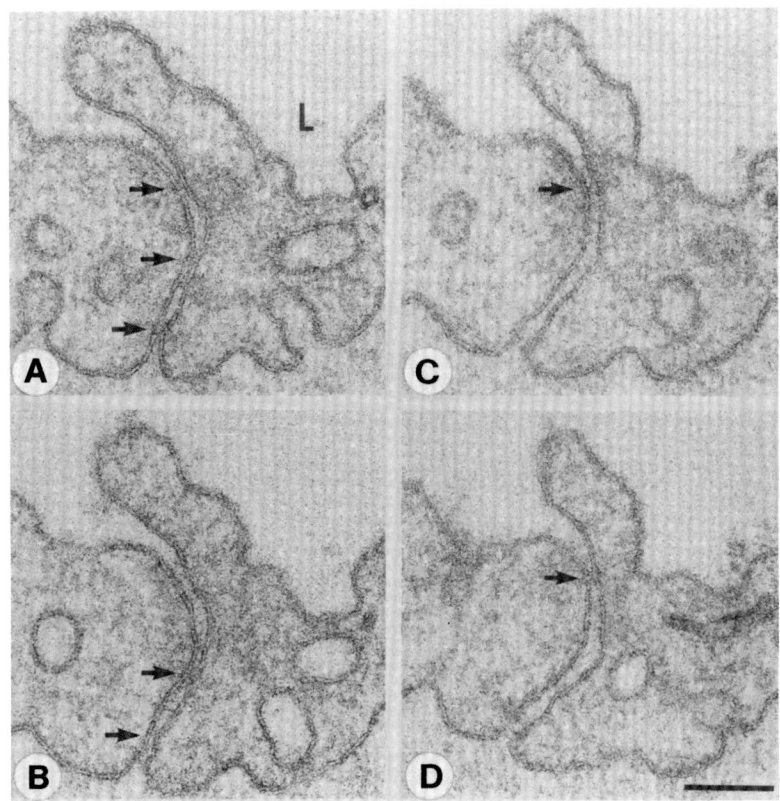

FIG. 17. Four consecutive sections through interendothelial junction in rat heart capillary. *Arrows* mark points of contact between junctional membranes. In serial section, each point of contact appears to open to form a patent pathway through junction around points of membrane apposition. *L*, lumen. [From Bungaard (20).]

tions tend to pass directly from capillary lumen to interstitium, whereas in muscle they follow a more tortuous path (136). In addition, Clementi and Palade (33) have shown that junctions in the small intestine often contain fenestrae that open into the intercellular space, thereby forming a short cut between the capillary lumen and the abluminal aspect of the intercellular junction.

Intercellular junctions are likely to make only a small contribution to total transcapillary exchange in the fenestrated vascular bed of the mucosa; however, they may represent a far more significant pathway for exchange in the continuous vascular bed of the muscular layer of the gut wall, in particular in the serosa and peritoneum where they may constitute a vital pathway for exchange between blood and peritoneal fluid during dialysis. Although studies of the dimensions of the junctions are not available for fenestrated vascular beds, detailed measurements have been made in skeletal muscle (27, 114) and lung (114). In these tissues ~5% of the total junction is narrowed to a width of 5 nm or less, whereas most of the junction (~75%) is between 5 and 15 nm in width (Fig. 18). Calculations based on detailed measurements of junction dimensions indicate that the greatest resistance to filtration as well as the greatest steric restriction to solute exchange occurs in the short, narrow region of the junction, whereas the greatest resistance to diffusional exchange resides in the long length of the junction 5–15 nm in width (27, 114). Although the use of ultrastructural dimensions to predict the functional exchange characteristics of a vascular bed is open to criticism (110), it is nevertheless interesting to note that the values for capillary filtration coefficient and the capillary diffusion coefficients for sodium and inulin calculated from the dimensions of interendothelial junctions are similar to the values recorded in vivo for skeletal muscle and lung capillary beds (27, 114). Such calculations indicate that the junctions in continuous vascular beds represent a feasible pathway for the exchange of fluid and small solute molecules up to the size of inulin (1.3 nm radius).

The permeability of intercellular junctions has been investigated with electron-dense tracers ranging in size from 1 to 15 nm molecular radius. In the intestine the larger tracers (5–15 nm radius) do not penetrate the junctional complex. Horseradish peroxidase (3 nm radius) introduced either into the capillary lumen or the interstitium penetrates the junction as far as the first site of membrane apposition and no farther (33, 143, 172). Smaller tracer molecules such as heme peptides (1 nm radius) have not been used in the intestine, because interpretation of the results is complicated by the fact that the tracers gain rapid access to the interstitium via the fenestrae. Results obtained with small tracers in continuous vascular beds have

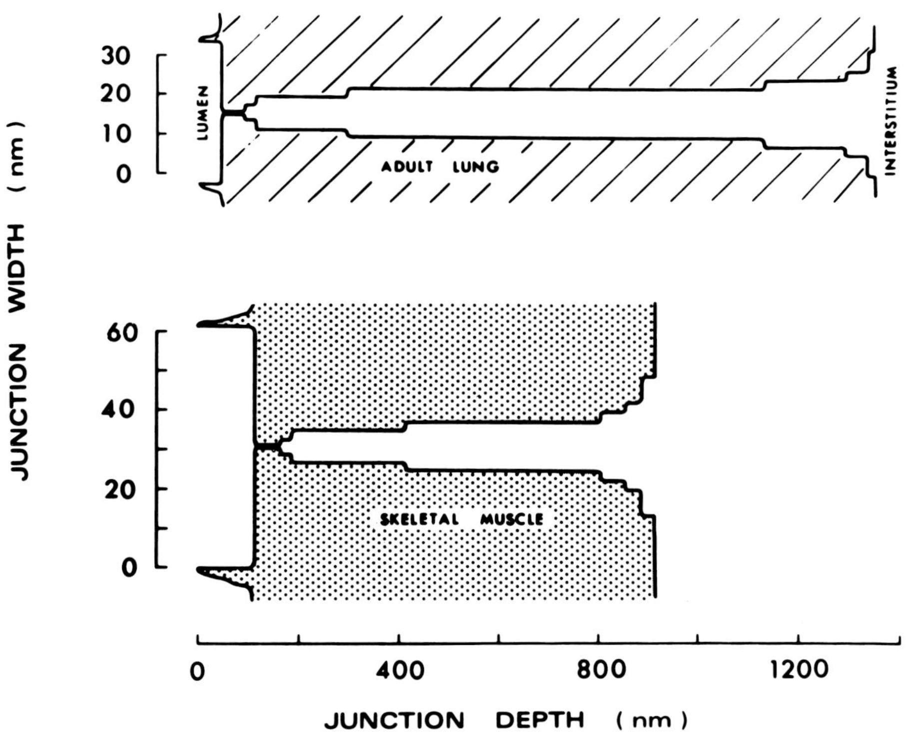

FIG. 18. Mean dimensions of interendothelial junctions in lung (*top*) and skeletal muscle (*bottom*) capillaries in rabbit. To facilitate comparison, widths of junction are shown going from narrowest values (0–5 nm) on luminal side to widest values (>25 nm) on interstitial side, although in reality various widths occur at random along junction. Only a small proportion (5%) of junction is narrowed to width of 0–5 nm, and remainder of junction opens to a width >5 nm. [From Perry (114).]

been conflicting. In rat diaphragm, neither heme peptides nor myoglobin (1.7 nm radius) passed through the intercellular junctions (141, 142), whereas in mouse diaphragm the junctions were found to be permeable to microperoxidase (1 nm radius) (173). These studies suggest that intercellular junctions are impermeable to molecules >1 nm radius, but they may well be permeable to molecules <1 nm radius. In view of the high permeability of the fenestrae to the smaller tracers, it would seem unlikely that the intercellular junctions represent a significant pathway for transcapillary exchange of small solutes in the intestine.

One class of vessel that displays a greater permeability to electron-dense tracers is the pericytic venule that has a diameter of 8–16 μm. Although not investigated in the small intestine, junctions in these vessels in the diaphragm display a range of permeability in which all are permeable to microperoxidase, 50% to horseradish peroxidase, and 5% to hemoglobin. About 30% of the junctions are thought to be open to a width of 3–6 nm. Despite their permeability, pericytic venules are likely to make only a small contribution to normal transvascular exchange because of their relative sparsity (1/10 the number of capillaries) and because the tracer that leaves via these vessels appears to be restricted to the perivenular space and does not extend over long distances into the interstitium of the tissue (145). However, it is possible that these junctions may open into large leaks in response to the mediators of inflammation such as histamine and serotonin, and under these conditions they may contribute significantly to transvascular exchange.

*Basal lamina (basement membrane).* The basal lamina is a continuous layer of fine fibrillar material 50–100 nm thick that surrounds both fenestrated and continuous capillaries. It is composed of three layers: *1*) a dense central layer (lamina densa) surrounded on either side by paler, less dense layers, *2*) the lamina rara interna, and *3*) lamina rara externa. The basal lamina is composed largely of glycoproteins and glycosaminoglycans (31, 79, 81), and its main function remains uncertain. It may act to support and stabilize the capillary wall or it may act as a permeability barrier to the exchange of macromolecules. In the intestine and muscle circulations the basal lamina behaves as a coarse filter that is freely permeable to horseradish peroxidase (3 nm radius) and ferritin (5.5 nm radius) but is less permeable to molecules >10 nm radius (33, 34). The larger tracers may have to diffuse considerable distances before they find a pathway of sufficient size across the basal lamina.

In many organs the basal lamina has associated with it a net negative charge. In the kidney, for example, the basal lamina and foot processes of the glomerular epithelial cells bind positively charged ferritin molecules (124, 132). Loss of this negative charge by infusions of polycations disrupts the integrity of the barrier and results in proteinuria (161). Recent studies (137) indicate that the basal lamina of intestinal capillaries also contains fixed negative charges (see next subsection), although the extent to which they contribute to the permeability characteristics of the intestinal capillary wall has not been established.

CHARGE BARRIER TO TRANSCAPILLARY EXCHANGE. The exchange of molecules across the capillary wall is governed not only by the physical structure of the capillary wall but also by the electrostatic charge associated with each of the exchange pathways. The endothelial cell, like many other cells, carries a net negative charge (36, 148, 167). Because most plasma proteins are also negatively charged at normal body pH, it is likely that electrostatic repulsion plays an important role in retaining plasma proteins within the circulation. The distribution of anionic sites within the endothelial barrier has been studied by injection of positively charged electron-dense tracers. The sites at which the tracer binds is assumed to represent the distribution of anionic sites on the capillary wall. In the mouse jejunum the fenestral diaphragms, coated pits, and coated vesicles were heavily labeled by intravascular cationized ferritin, whereas the plasmalemmal proper was lightly labeled. There was no evidence of labeling of plasmalemmal vesicles, vesicle channels, or their associated diaphragms (146). When injected into the mucosal interstitium, the tracer labeled the lamina rara externa of the basal lamina in discrete clusters that were 100–150 nm apart. After removal of the basal lamina by the enzyme collagenase, the tracer bound to the interstitial aspect of the endothelial plasmalemma, coated pits, and coated vesicles in a similar manner to that described on the luminal aspect. Again the vesicles, channels, and associated diaphragms were unlabeled. The abluminal aspect of the fenestral diaphragm also remained unlabeled, indicating that the anionic sites on this structure are confined to the luminal side (137). These results indicate that the coated pits, coated vesicles, and fenestral diaphragms represent areas of intense negative charge, whereas the plasmalemmal vesicles and vesicle channels are devoid of negative charge. Whether these latter structures are decorated by positive charge remains to be investigated.

To characterize the chemical nature of the anionic sites on the endothelium, Simionescu et al. (138) used enzymes that selectively degrade various components of the endothelial barrier. Protease enzymes of broad specificity removed all of the anonic sites, whereas heparinase removed only those sites associated with the fenestral diaphragm. These results indicate that the anionic sites on the fenestral diaphragm are due to the presence of heparin sulfate or heparin, whereas the remaining sites are of a mixed chemical nature containing acidic glycoproteins and proteoglycans.

Although the functional significance of the pattern of distribution of anionic sites is not completely resolved, it appears that the high density of anionic sites in the fenestral diaphragm would decrease the likelihood of anionic molecules entering this pathway. That is, the negative charge may reduce the otherwise high permeability of the fenestrae to negatively charged macromolecules, including plasma proteins. The conspicuous absence of negative charges associated with vesicles, vesicle channels, and their stomatal diaphragms suggest that these may represent pathways for exchange of anionic molecules. However, the physical dimemsions of the vesicle channels, together with the observation that electron-dense tracers do not accumulate in the interstitium beneath areas of channel formation, indicate that the contribution of this pathway to the total transcapillary exchange of macromolecules may be small. The presence of anionic sites in the basal lamina (31, 32, 138) suggests that this structure also contributes to the charge-selective properties of the capillary wall.

Ultrastructural analysis of the intestinal capillaries and other fenestrated beds such as the pancreas (146) and kidney (162) all reveal fixed negative charges associated with the capillary wall. Functional studies in the kidney support the ultrastructural findings. The combined endothelial and epithelial layers of the glomerular membrane behave as a negatively charged filter that is far less permeable to anionic dextrans (1.8–4.0 nm radius) than neutral dextrans of the same size (30). In the small intestine, however, the capillary wall behaves functionally as a positively charged membrane. For example, the osmotic reflection coefficient for the most positive of the isoenzymes of lactate dehydrogenase was greater (0.95) than that of the most negative isoenzyme (0.71). Similarly, the steady-state, lymph-to-plasma ratio for positively charged dextran was less than that for the neutral dextran of the same size (115). This suggests that elements of the blood-lymph barrier in the intestine are positively charged and reduce the transcapillary exchange of cationic molecules. The electrostatic interaction between charged solute and capillary wall is sufficient to reduce the equivalent pore size in the capillary wall from 55 Å for neutral lactate dehydrogenase to 50 Å for the positively charged isomer (115).

The finding that the intestinal capillary wall behaves as a positively charged filter may have physiological significance. The presence of a positive charge should facilitate the movement of negatively charged plasma proteins into the interstitium of the intestinal mucosa. This would be advantageous for the removal of certain absorbed nutrients, for example, fatty acids that leave the interstitium bound to plasma proteins.

The apparent contradiction between functional studies indicating that the exchange pathways in the intestinal capillary wall are positively charged and ultrastructural studies that have to date only shown anionic sites remains to be resolved. Future studies with anionic electron-dense tracers may reveal the location of cationic sites within the blood-lymph barrier in the intestine.

CORRELATION BETWEEN STRUCTURE AND CAPILLARY PERMEABILITY. The permeability characteristics of intestinal capillaries have been investigated by several physiological techniques. Indicator dilution studies have shown that the intestinal microvascular permeability–surface area products for small molecules such as the trisaccharide raffinose or inulin are 20 times larger than the values recorded in skeletal muscle (Table 2). Allowing for the fact that capillary surface area in the intestine may be 3–4 times greater than in muscle (28, 147), the data indicate that intestinal capillaries are 5 to 7 times more permeable to small molecules than are continuous capillaries. Other fenestrated beds show similar or greater permeability–surface area values. It appears that it is the fenestrae that are responsible for this high permeability because it is through the fenestrae that small electron-dense tracers gain access to the interstitium.

Although the fenestrae are very permeable to small solutes, they are surprisingly impermeable to macromolecules. For example, the osmotic reflection coefficient for total plasma protein in the small intestine is 0.92 (63), higher than the value of 0.90 reported for continuous capillaries (119). The size-limiting structure appears to be the fenestral diaphragm that reduces the permeability of the intestinal capillary wall to plasma protein, while at the same time remaining permeable to small molecules ≦1 nm radius. Analysis of the different molecular weight constituents of lymph and plasma has led to estimates of the pore sizes that would be consistent with the observed degree of blood-lymph exchange. Intestinal capillaries appear to possess two populations of pores of ~4.6 nm and ~20 nm radius (155). It is possible that the fenestrae with diaphragms represent the small pore pathway and open fenestrae represent the large pores, although the total surface area occupied by the fenestrae far exceeds the total area of pores predicted by physiological data. The extent to which junctions, vesicles, vesicle channels, and elements of the basal lamina and interstitium participate in or modify transcapillary exchange remains uncertain.

## Stomach

GENERAL STRUCTURE. The gastric microcirculation possesses both fenestrated and continuous endothelium. In the mucosa the capillaries associated with gastric glands and mucosal epithelial cells are fenestrated, whereas those in the submucosal and muscularis layers of the stomach wall are continuous. The mucosal capillaries are characterized by a thin fenestrated endothelium with numerous endothelial vesicles and a continuous basal lamina. They originate from arterioles deep in the mucosa and pass up beside the gastric glands to form a honeycomb network of vessels immediately beneath the gastric epithelium (see Fig. 3). In both the human (53) and the rat (52), the mucosal capillaries are close to the gastric glands, with a diffusion distance that is often <0.3 µm from parietal cells. The capillaries at the base of the surface epithelial cells are structurally similar to those adjacent to the gastric glands and contain numerous fenestrae and vesicles. The subsurface capillary plexus is close to the mucosal epithelial cells, with diffusion distances of 0.5–1.0 µm in the rat and 3–5 µm in the human. The vascular architecture, together with the fenestrated nature of the capillaries, indicates that the gastric mucosal microcirculation is well suited for the delivery of fluid and nutrients to the secretory cells and for the transport of $HCO_3^-$ from the basal aspect of the parietal cell to the base of the epithelial cells lining the gastric mucosa. The delivery of the alkaline tide to the base of the mucosal epithelium provides the mucosa with optimum protection against the acidic contents of the stomach. Loss of $HCO_3^-$ directly into the venous circulation is prevented by the nature and arrangement of the venules draining the gastric mucosa. The collecting venules originate from capillaries immediately beneath the mucosal surface and pass directly down through the mucosa without receiving further capillary connections. These venules have a continuous endothelium, are few in number, and possess a thick connective tissue sheath. They are separated from the parietal cells by a distance of 10–30 µm and are therefore unlikely to act as an avenue for $HCO_3^-$ removal (52, 53).

PERMEABILITY. There are no quantitative studies of the number, structure, or dimensions of capillaries in the gastric microcirculation, nor has their permeability to electron-dense tracers been investigated. It is not known, for example, how capillary surface area in the stomach compares with other areas of the gastrointestinal tract. The ultrastructural appearance of the gastric microcirculation with its large number of fenestrae suggests a vascular bed that is highly permeable to fluid and small solute molecules. This has been confirmed by functional studies in which the permeability surface area products for small solutes such as raffinose and inulin were found to be 50 times larger in the stomach than in nonfenestrated vascular beds such as skeletal muscle (116) and also larger than values reported for other fenestrated beds such as the small intestine (118) and pancreas (87). Analysis of gastric lymph has been used to assess the permeability

TABLE 2. *Capillary Permeability–Surface Area Products*

|                 | Raffinose | Inulin | Ref. |
|-----------------|-----------|--------|------|
| Small intestine | 42        | 23     | 118  |
| Stomach         | 140       | 70     | 116  |
| Pancreas        |           | 23     | 87   |
| Skeletal muscle | 2.4       | 0.4    | 157  |

Values in $ml \cdot min^{-1} \cdot 100\ g^{-1}$.

of gastric capillaries to macromolecules (116). The data describe the gastric capillaries as possessing two populations of equivalent pores of 4.7 nm and 25 nm radius. The dimensions of the large pores in the stomach are greater than those in other fenestrated beds such as the small intestine (20 nm) and colon (18 nm), suggesting that the stomach is more permeable to macromolecules than are other gastrointestinal organs (see ref. 155). The structural basis for the high permeability of the gastric vasculature to small solutes and macromolecules remains to be investigated.

## Colon

GENERAL STRUCTURE. Like the other organs of the gastrointestinal tract, the large intestine has two ultrastructurally different capillary beds in parallel. The capillaries of the mucosa are fenestrated, whereas those in the muscularis are continuous (44, 88). The mucosal capillaries of the large intestine are similar in appearance to those in the small intestine. They are characterized by thin, fenestrated endothelium, numerous pinocytotic vesicles, and are surrounded by a continuous basal lamina (44). The fenestrae are most abundant in the upper one-third of the mucosa, and they occur on the side of the capillary wall that faces the mucosal epithelium (88). The fenestrae are, in most cases, covered by a thin diaphragm.

A striking feature of the colonic microcirculation is the closeness of the capillaries to the base of the mucosal epithelium. In the dog the distance between the base of the epithelial cells and the fenestrae of the capillaries is 1.0 µm, compared with 2.0 µm in the small bowel (88). Fluid absorbed by the colon enters this small juxtacapillary space and is thought to be removed exclusively by the blood capillaries. This suggestion is supported by the observations that colonic lymphatics are confined to the base of the mucosa, distant from the absorptive epithelium, and that during fluid absorption from the lumen, lymph flow remains unaltered (88).

PERMEABILITY. There has been no systematic analysis of the ultrastructure of colonic capillaries. Early observations by Florey (44) indicated that in the mouse colon the fenestrae were impermeable to ferritin, even after inflammation induced by dilute mustard oil. The permeability of colonic capillaries to endogenous plasma proteins has been assessed by analysis of lymphatic protein flux (127). The osmotic reflection coefficients for plasma proteins were generally less than those reported for the small intestine, indicating that colonic capillaries are slightly more permeable to plasma proteins. The data predict that colonic capillaries possess two populations of equivalent pores of 5.3 and 18 nm radius. Although the dimensions of the pores are similar to those reported for the small intestine, there appears to be a greater proportion of large pores in the colon compared with the small intestine (155).

## FUTURE DIRECTIONS FOR STRUCTURAL RESEARCH IN GASTROINTESTINAL MICROVASCULATURE

Although undoubtedly there are many fruitful areas for future research in gastrointestinal microvascular organization and fine structure, it seems to us that there are some particular aspects of these topics that are currently poorly described and are amenable to investigation with currently available techniques.

As is apparent from comments in this chapter, there is an almost complete lack of documentation of capillary density of the mucosa and of the other layers of the alimentary tract throughout its length. Stereological analyses of capillary density per unit volume of muscle and submucosa and per unit luminal surface area for the epithelia and glands of the esophagus, for the luminal epithelium and glands of the stomach, for the villi and crypts of the small intestine, and for the luminal epithelium and glands of the colon are clearly warranted; specific stereological study of microvessel density in the intramural nerve plexuses is also needed. In such studies, analyses of structural characteristics of capillaries are also important, that is, functional capillary diameters, endothelial cell and basal lamina thicknesses, fenestral frequencies and sizes, endothelial vesicle frequencies and diameters, and interendothelial cell junction lengths and frequencies. Of particular importance may be regional and interspecies differences in such measures and/or the existence of proximodistal gradients. Such data may help to explain particular aspects of gut function: for example, whether the greater susceptibility of the gastric antral compared with oxyntic mucosa to chronic ulceration in humans is due to possible differences in capillary density between these regions of gastric mucosa (108).

Further studies are also required of the microvascular organization of particular tissues of the gut. The microvascular organization of esophageal mucosa, glands, and muscle remains unexplored. Further studies of the microvascular organization of the intramural nerve plexuses throughout the gut, especially of larger species, including humans, are needed, given the current small body of partly conflicting opinion (64, 76).

Virtually nothing is currently known about the effects of diet on enteric microvascular organization and fine structure; once stereological analyses of normal tissue have been documented, this aspect may be fruitfully explored. The effects of changes in dietary volume, including short- to medium-term food deprivation, and also the alimentary tract changes occurring on switching to total parenteral nutrition would also appear appropriate topics for investigation.

Developmental aspects of the microvasculature of

the alimentary tract are also worthy of further investigation. Regarding dietary changes and their effects on the enteric microvasculature, the switch at birth from placental (a naturally occurring form of parenteral nutrition) to enteral nutrition and the change of diet at weaning may be useful natural models of these events. Detailed study of the prenatal development of the capillary beds and especially of the timing and process of development of fenestrae in capillaries would be timely.

Regarding microvascular pathology and experimental pathology, the paucity of knowledge of capillary structure and cell density in normal tissues makes interpretation of structural observations of enteric microvessels in pathological tissues difficult to interpret. Currently there is a good deal of research into the microvascular changes occurring in experimental gastric ulceration (e.g., ref. 106); further studies of this and especially of the microvascular structural changes accompanying the healing of experimental gastric ulcers may aid interpretation of the natural process of ulcer healing. Detailed analyses of the microvascular changes occurring in other diseases of the gut (e.g., celiac disease with attendant disorder of intestinal villi, ulcerative, colitis, diabetes, angiodysplasia of the gut), in experimental gut tumor development, and after substantial ionizing irradiation of the gut (23) seem appropriate starting points to investigate the microvascular correlates of alimentary tract diseases.

REFERENCES

1. ALLEN, A. AND A. GARNER. Mucus and bicarbonate secretion in the stomach and their possible role in mucosal protection. *Gut* 21: 249-262, 1980.
2. ANDERSON, J. E. *Grant's Atlas of Anatomy* (7th ed.). Baltimore, MD: Williams & Wilkins, 1978.
3. BAEZ, S. Skeletal muscle and gastrointestinal microvascular morphology. In: *Microcirculation*, edited by G. Kaley and B. M. Altura. Baltimore, MD: University Park, 1977, vol. 1, p. 69-94.
4. BAKER, S. J., V. I. MATHAN, AND V. CHERIAN. The nature of the villi in the small intestine of the rat. *Lancet* 1: 860, 1963.
5. BARLOW, T. E. Vascular patterns in the alimentary canal. In: *Ciba Symposium Visceral Circulation*, edited by G. E. W. Wotstenholme. London: Churchill, 1952, p. 21-35.
6. BARLOW, T. E., F. H. BENTLEY, AND D. N. WALDER. Arteries, veins and arterio-venous anastomoses in human stomach. *Surg. Gynecol. Obstet.* 93: 657-671, 1951.
7. BELLAMY, J. E. C., W. K. LATSHAW, AND N. O. NIELSEN. The vascular architecture of the porcine small intestine. *Can. J. Comp. Med. Vet. Sci.* 37: 57-62, 1983.
8. BERGLINDH, T., M. HELANDER, AND G. SACHS. Secretion at the parietal cell level—a look at rabbit gastric glands. *Scand. J. Gastroenterol. Suppl.* 14: 7-20, 1979.
9. BOHLEN, H. G., AND R. W. GORE. Preparation of rat intestinal muscle and mucosa for quantitative microcirculatory studies. *Microvasc. Res.* 11: 103-110, 1976.
10. BOHLEN, H. G., H. HEINRICH, R. W. GORE, AND P. C. JOHNSON. Intestinal muscle and mucosal blood flow during direct sympathetic stimulation. *Am. J. Physiol.* 235 (*Heart Circ. Physiol.* 4): H40-H45, 1978.
11. BOND, J. H., D. G. LEVITT, AND M. D. LEVITT. The effect of counter-current exchange on absorption from the small bowel (Abstract). *Gastroenterology* 64: 704, 1973.
12. BOND, J. H., AND M. D. LEVITT. Use of microspheres to measure small intestinal villus blood flow in the dog. *Am. J. Physiol.* 236 (*Endocrinol. Metab. Gastrointest. Physiol.* 5): E577-E583, 1979.
13. BORG, T. K., AND J. B. CAULFIELD. Morphology of connective tissue in skeletal muscle. *Tissue Cell* 12: 197-207, 1980.
14. BORG, T. K., AND J. B. CAULFIELD. The collagen matrix of the heart. *Federation Proc.* 40: 2037-2041, 1981.
15. BROWNING, J., AND B. J. GANNON. The microvascular architecture of rat proximal duodenum, with particular reference to Brunner's glands. *Biomed. Res.* 5: 245-258, 1984.
16. BROWNING, J., AND B. J. GANNON. Mucosal microvascular organization of the rat colon. *Acta Anat.* 126: 73-77, 1986.
17. BROWNING, J., B. J. GANNON, AND P. O'BRIEN. The microvasculature and gastric luminal pH of the forestomach of the rat: a comparison with the glandular stomach. *Int. J. Microcirc. Clin. Exp.* 2: 109-118, 1983.
18. BUNGAARD, M. Transport pathways in capillaries—in search of pores. *Annu. Rev. Physiol.* 42: 325-336, 1980.
19. BUNGAARD, M. Vesicular transport in capillary endothelium: does it occur? *Federation Proc.* 42: 2425-2430, 1983.
20. BUNGAARD, M. The three-dimensional organization of tight junctions in a capillary endothelium revealed by serial section electron microscopy. *J. Ultrastruct. Res.* 88: 1-17, 1984.
21. BUNGAARD, M., J. FRÖKJAER-JENSEN, AND C. CRONE. Endothelial plasmalemmal vesicles as elements in a system of branching invaginations of the cell surface. *Proc. Natl. Acad. Sci. USA* 76: 6439-6442, 1979.
22. BUNGAARD, M., P. HAGMAN, AND C. CRONE. The three-dimensional organisation of plasmalemmal vesicular profiles in the endothelium of rat heart capillaries. *Microvasc. Res.* 25: 358-368, 1983.
23. CARR, N. D., B. R. PULLEN, P. S. HASLETON, AND P. F. SCHOFIELD. Microvascular studies in human radiation bowel disease. *Gut* 25: 448-454, 1984.
24. CASLEY-SMITH, J. R. The Brownian movements of pinocytotic vesicles. *J. R. Microsc. Soc.* 82: 257-261, 1963.
25. CASLEY-SMITH, J. R. Endothelial fenestrae in intestinal villi: differences between arterial and venous ends of the capillaries. *Microvasc. Res.* 3: 49-68, 1971.
26. CASLEY-SMITH, J. R., AND B. J. GANNON. Intestinal microcirculation: spatial organization and fine structure. In: *Physiology of the Intestinal Circulation*, edited by A. P. Shepherd and D. N. Granger. New York: Raven, 1984, p. 9-31.
27. CASLEY-SMITH, J. R., H. S. GREEN, J. L. HARRIS, AND P. J. WADEY. The quantitative morphology of skeletal muscle capillaries in relation to permeability. *Microvasc. Res.* 10: 43-64, 1975.
28. CASLEY-SMITH, J. R., P. J. O'DONOGHUE, AND K. W. J. CROCKER. The quantitative relationships between fenestrae in jejunal capillaries and tissue channels: proof of "tunnel-capillaries." *Microvasc. Res.* 9: 78-100, 1975.
29. CAULFIELD, J. B., AND T. K. BORG. The collagen network of the heart. *Lab. Invest.* 40: 364-372, 1979.
30. CHANG, R. L., W. M. DEEN, C. R. ROBERTSON, AND B. M. BRENNER. Permselectivity of the glomerular capillary wall. III. Restricted transport of polyanions. *Kidney. Int.* 8: 212-218, 1975.
31. CHARONIS, A. S., P. C. TSILIBARY, R. H. KRAMER, AND S. L. WISSIG. Localization of heparan sulfate proteoglycan in the basement membrane of continuous capillaries. *Microvasc. Res.* 26: 108-115, 1983.
32. CHARONIS, A. S., AND S. L. WISSIG. Anionic sites in basement

membranes. Differences in their electrostatic properties in continuous and fenestrated capillaries. *Microvasc. Res.* 25: 265–285, 1982.
33. CLEMENTI, F., AND G. E. PALADE. Intestinal capillaries. I. Permeability to peroxidase and ferritin. *J. Cell Biol.* 41: 33–58, 1969.
34. CLEMENTI, F., AND G. E. PALADE. Intestinal capillaries. II. Structural effects of EDTA and histamine. *J. Cell Biol.* 42: 706–714, 1969.
35. COOKE, A. R. The glands of Brunner. In: *Handbook of Physiology. Alimentary Canal. Secretion*, edited by C. F. Code. Washington, DC: Am. Physiol. Soc., 1967, sect. 6, vol. II, chapt. 61, p. 1087–1095.
36. DANON, D., AND E. SKUTELSKY. Endothelial surface charge and its possible relationship to thrombogenesis. *Ann. NY Acad. Sci.* 275: 47–63, 1976.
37. DAVENPORT, H. *Physiology of the Digestive Tract* (5th ed.). Chicago, IL: Year Book, 1982.
37a. DESAKI J., T. FUJIWARA, AND Y. UEHARA. A cellular reticulum of fibroblast-like cells in the rat intestine: scanning and transmission electron microscopy. *Arch. Histol. Jpn.* 47: 179–186, 1984.
38. DESMETH, M. Developmental variations of the villi along the ileum in newly hatched and adult pigeons. A scanning electron microscopic study. *Z. Mikrosk. Anat. Forsch.* 90: 489–498, 1976.
39. DINDA, P., M. G. BUELL, L. R. DACOSTA, AND L. T. BECK. Simultaneous estimation of arteriolar, capillary, and shunt blood flow of the gut mucosa. *Am. J. Physiol.* 245 (*Gastrointest. Liver Physiol.* 8): G29–G37, 1983.
40. EIDELMAN, S., AND D. LAGUNOFF. The morphology of the normal human rectal biopsy. *Hum. Pathol.* 3: 389–401, 1972.
41. ELFVIN, L. G. The ultrastructure of the capillary fenestrae in the adrenal medulla of the rat. *J. Ultrastruct. Res.* 12: 687–704, 1965.
42. FIELD, J., J. V. HURLEY, AND N. E. W. MCCALLUM. The mechanism of escape of plasma protein from the small blood vessels in the mucosa of the small intestine of the rat. *J. Pathol.* 121: 51–57, 1977.
43. FLEMSTRÖM, G. Stimulation of $HCO_3^-$ transport in isolated proximal bullfrog duodenum by prostaglandins. *Am. J. Physiol.* 239 (*Gastrointest. Liver Physiol.* 2): G198–G203, 1980.
44. FLOREY, H. W. The structure of normal and inflamed small blood vessels of the mouse and rat colon. *Q. J. Exp. Physiol.* 46: 119–122, 1961.
45. FLOREY, H. W. The missing link. The structure of some types of capillary. *Q. J. Exp. Physiol.* 53: 1–5, 1968.
46. FLOREY, H. W., AND H. E. HARDING. Further observations on the secretion of Brunner's glands. *J. Pathol. Bacteriol.* 39: 255–276, 1934.
47. FLOREY, H. W., R. D. WRIGHT, AND M. A. JENNINGS. The secretions of the intestines. *Physiol. Rev.* 21: 36–69, 1941.
48. FRASHER, W. G., JR., AND H. WAYLAND. Repeating modular organization of the microcirculation of cat mesentery. *Microvasc. Res.* 4: 62–76, 1972.
49. FRÖKJAER-JENSEN, J. Three-dimensional organization of plasmalemmal vesicles in endothelial cells. An analysis by serial sectioning of frog mesenteric capillaries. *J. Ultrastruct. Res.* 73: 9–20, 1980.
50. FURNESS, J. B., AND M. COSTA. Types of nerves in the enteric nervous system. *Neuroscience* 5: 1–20, 1980.
51. GANNON, B. J. Co-existence of fountain and tuft patterns of blood supply in intestinal villi of rabbit and man. *Bibl. Anat.* 20: 130–133, 1981.
52. GANNON, B. J., J. BROWNING, AND P. O'BRIEN. The microvascular architecture of the glandular mucosa of rat stomach. *J. Anat.* 135: 667–683, 1982.
53. GANNON, B. J., J. BROWNING, P. O'BRIEN, AND P. ROGERS. Mucosal microvascular architecture of the fundus and body of human stomach. *Gastroenterology* 86: 866–875, 1984.
54. GANNON B. J., J. BROWNING, P. ROGERS, AND B. HARPER. Microvascular organization in the intestine. In: *Microcirculation of the Alimentary Tract—Physiology and Pathology*, edited by A. Koo, S. K. Lam, and L. H. Smaje. Singapore: World Scientific, 1983, p. 39–55. (Proc. Symp. Hong Kong, March 28–30, 1983.)
55. GANNON, B. J., R. W. GORE, AND P. A. W. ROGERS. Is there an anatomical basis for a vascular counter-current mechanism in rabbit and human intestinal villi? *Biomed. Res.* 2, Suppl.: 235–241, 1981.
56. GANNON, B. J., P. A. W. ROGERS, AND P. E. O'BRIEN. Two capillary plexuses in human intestinal villi. *Micron* 11: 447–448, 1980.
57. GANNON, B. J., S. M. ROSENBERGER, T. D. VERSLUIS, AND P. C. JOHNSON. Autoregulatory patterns in the arteriolar network of cat mesentery. *Microvasc. Res.* 26: 1–14, 1983.
58. GARTNER, K., AND J. PFAFF. The forestomach in rats and mice, a food store without bacterial protein digestion. *Zentralbl. Veterinaermed. Reihe A.* 26: 530–541, 1979.
59. GERSHON, M. D., AND S. BURSZTAJN. Properties of the enteric nervous system: limitations of access of intravascular macromolecules to the myenteric plexus and muscularis externa. *J. Comp. Neurol.* 180: 467–487, 1978.
60. GORE, R. W. Fluid exchange across single capillaries in rat intestinal muscle. *Am. J. Physiol.* 242 (*Heart Circ. Physiol.* 11): H268–H287, 1982.
61. GRANGER, D. N. Intestinal microcirculation and transmucosal fluid transport. *Am. J. Physiol.* 240 (*Gastrointest. Liver Physiol.* 3): G343–G349, 1981.
62. GRANGER, D. N., J. A. BARROWMAN, AND P. R. KVIETYS. *Clinical Gastrointestinal Physiology*. Philadelphia, PA: Saunders, 1985.
63. GRANGER, D. N., AND A. E. TAYLOR. Permeability of intestinal capillaries to endogenous macromolecules. *Am. J. Physiol.* 238 (*Heart Circ. Physiol.* 7): H457–H464, 1980.
64. GRANGER, H. J. Digestive system: small and large intestine. In: *Blood Vessels and Lymphatics in Organ Systems*, edited by D. I. Abramson and P. B. Dorbin. Orlando, FL: Academic, 1984, p. 440–446.
65. GROTTE, G. Passage of dextran molecules across the blood-lymph barrier. *Acta Chir. Scand. Suppl.* 211: 1–84, 1956.
66. GUTH, P. H. Vascular factors in ulceration. *Dig. Dis. Sci.* 30: 378, 1985.
67. GUTH, P. H., AND A. ROSENBERG. In vivo microscopy of gastric microcirculation. *Dig. Dis. Sci.* 17: 391–398, 1972.
68. HALLBÄCK, D. A., M. JODAL, A. SJÖQVIST, AND O. LUNDGREN. Evidence for cholera secretion emanating from the crypts. A study of villous tissue osmolality and fluid and electrolyte transport in the small intestine of the cat. *Gastroenterology* 83: 1051–1056, 1982.
69. HARTIALA, K., A. C. IVY, AND M. I. GROSSMAN. Effect of feeding cinchophen on secretion of juice by duodenal glands in dog. *Am. J. Physiol.* 162: 110–114, 1950.
70. HASE, T., AND B. J. MOSS. Microvascular changes of gastric mucosa in the development of stress ulcer in rats. *Gastroenterology* 65: 224–234, 1973.
71. HELLER, A. Über die Blutgerfasse des Dunndarmes. *Ber Sachs Ges Wiss.* 24: 165–171, 1872.
72. HENDRIX T. R., AND T. M. BAYLESS. Digestion: intestinal secretion. *Annu. Rev. Physiol.* 32: 139–164, 1970.
73. HIMAL, H. S., F. MOQTADERI, A. E. KARK, AND J. RUDICK. Hormonal regulation of duodenal secretion: effects of glucagon and secretin. *Curr. Top. Surg. Res.* 3: 453–463, 1971.
74. HIMAL, H. S., AND J. RUDICK. Ionic flux across canine duodenum. Movement of bicarbonate. *Am. J. Gastroenterol.* 67: 574–579, 1977.
75. HURLEY, J. V., AND N. E. W. MCCALLUM. The degree and functional significance of the escape of marker particles from small blood vessels with fenestrated endothelium. *J. Pathol.* 113: 183–196, 1974.
76. JACOBS, J. M. Penetration of systemically injected horseradish

peroxidase into ganglia and nerves of the autonomic nervous system. *J. Neurocytol.* 6: 607–618, 1977.
77. JACOBSON, L. F., AND R. J. NOER. The vascular pattern of the intestinal villi in various laboratory animals and man. *Anat. Rec.* 114: 85–93, 1952.
78. KALIMA, T. The structure and function of intestinal lymphatics and the influence of impaired lymph flow on the ileum of rats. *Scand. J. Gastroenterol.* 16, Suppl. 10: 9–87, 1971.
79. KANWAR, Y. S., AND M. G. FARQUHAR. Isolation of glycosaminoglycans (heparan sulfate) from the glomerular basement membranes. *Proc. Natl. Acad. Sci. USA* 76: 4493–4497, 1979.
80. KARNOVSKY, M. J. The ultrastructural basis of capillary permeability studied with peroxidase as a tracer. *J. Cell Biol.* 35: 213–236, 1967.
81. KATSUYAMA, T., K. C. POON, AND S. S. SPICER. The ultrastructural histochemistry of the basement membranes in the exocrine pancreas. *Anat. Rec.* 188: 371–386, 1977.
82. KING, C. R., AND P. R. SCHLOERB. Gastric juice neutralization in the duodenum. *Surg. Gynecol. Obstet.* 135: 22–28, 1972.
83. KNOBLAUCH, M., C. VOGT, C. HOLLINGER, M. NEFF, AND J. M. METRY. The influence of hormones on the microcirculation of a single jejunal rat villus, with evidence for microfilament mediated vasoconstriction. *Microvasc. Res.* 22: 232, 1981.
84. KOKKO, J. P. Countercurrent exchanger in the small intestine of man: Is there evidence for its existence? (editorial). *Gastroenterology* 74: 791–792, 1978.
85. KOKUE, E., AND Y. KUREBAYASHI. Rat forestomach ulcer induced by drinking glucose solution as an experimental model of gastroesophageal ulcer of swine. *Jpn. J. Vet. Sci.* 42: 395–399, 1980.
86. KUWAMARA, D. Microangiographic study on cancer of the large intestine. *Igaku Kenkyu* 50: 269–296, 1980.
87. KVIETYS, P. R., M. A. PERRY, AND D. N. GRANGER. Permeability of pancreatic capillaries to small molecules. *Am. J. Physiol.* 245 (*Gastrointest. Liver Physiol.* 8): G519–G524, 1983.
88. KVIETYS, P. R., W. H. WILBORN, AND D. N. GRANGER. Effects of rat transmucosal volume flux on lymph flow in the canine colon. *Gastroenterology* 81: 1080–1090, 1981.
89. LANCIAULT, G., AND E. JACOBSON. The gastrointestinal circulation. *Gastroenterology* 71: 851–873, 1976.
90. LEE, J. S. Tissue fluid pressure, lymph pressure, and fluid transport in rat intestinal villi. *Microvasc. Res.* 31: 170–183, 1986.
91. LEVITT, D. G., B. SIRCAR, N. LIFSON, AND E. J. LENDER. Model for mucosal circulation of rabbit small intestine. *Am. J. Physiol.* 237 (*Endocrinol. Metab. Gastrointest. Physiol.* 6): E373–E382, 1979.
92. LUFT, J. H. Fine structure of the diaphragm across capillary pores in mouse intestine. *Anat. Rec.* 148: 307–308, 1964.
93. LUNDGREN, O. Studies on blood flow distribution and countercurrent exchange in the small intestine. *Acta Physiol. Scand. Suppl.* 303: 1–42, 1967.
94. LUNDGREN, O. The alimentary canal. In: *Peripheral Circulation*, edited by P. C. Johnson. New York: Wiley, 1978, p. 225–283.
95. MALL, F. P. Die Blut und Lymphwege in Dunndarm des Hundes. *Abh. Sachs. Ges. Wiss.* 14: 153–189, 1888.
96. MAXWELL, L. C., A. P. SHEPHERD, AND C. A. MCMAHAN. Microsphere passage through intestinal circulation: via shunts or capillaries? *Am. J. Physiol.* 248 (*Heart Circ. Physiol.* 17): H217–H224, 1985.
97. MILLER, B. G., R. I. WOODS, H. G. BOHLEN, AND A. P. EVAN. A new morphological procedure for viewing microvessels. *Anat. Rec.* 203: 493–503, 1982.
98. MILLER, D. S., M. A. RAHMAN, R. TANNER, V. I. MATHAN, AND S. J. BAKER. The vascular architecture of the different forms of small intestinal villi in the rat (*Rattus norvegicus*). *Scand. J. Gastroenterol.* 4: 477–482, 1969.
99. MOHIUDDIN, A. Blood and lymph vessels in the jejunal villi of the white rat. *Anat. Rec.* 156: 83–90, 1965.
100. MOODY, F. G. Role of mucosal blood flow in the pathogenesis of gastric ulcers. In: *International Encyclopedia of Pharmacology and Therapeutics.* Oxford, UK: Pergamon, 1971, sect. 39, p. 339–360.
101. NASSET, E. S. Possible role of succus entericus in amino acid homeostasis in the dog. *Digestion* 16: 108–117, 1977.
102. NASSET, E. S., AND J. S. JU. Micropipet collection of succus entericus at crypt ostia of guinea-pig jejunum. *Digestion* 9: 205–211, 1973.
103. NOPANITAYA, W., J. G. AGHAJANIAN, AND L. D. GRAY. An improved plastic mixture for corrosion casting of the gastrointestinal microvascular system. *Scanning Electron Microsc.* 3: 751–756, 1979.
104. NYLANDER, G., AND S. OLERUD. The vascular pattern of the gastric mucosa of the rat following vagotomy. *Surg. Gynecol. Obstet.* 12: 475–480, 1961.
105. NYLANDER, G., AND S. OLERUD. The vascular pattern of an isolated jejunal loop: a microangiographic study in the rat. *Acta Chir. Scand.* 121: 39–46, 1961.
106. O'BRIEN, P., C. SCHULTZ, B. GANNON, AND J. BROWNING. Prostaglandin E$_2$ protects the microvasculature of the gastric mucosa against ethanol damage. In: *Progress in Lymphology* (10th ed.), edited by J. R. Casley-Smith and N. B. Piller. Adelaide, Australia: Univ. of Adelaide Press, 1985, p. 78–80.
107. OHASHI, Y., S. KITA, AND T. MURAKAMI. Microcirculation of the rat small intestine as studied by the injection replica scanning electron microscope method. *Arch. Histol. Jpn.* 39: 271–282, 1976.
107a. OHTANI, O. Microvasculature as studied by the microvascular casting/scanning electron microscope method. I. Endocrine and digestive system. *Arch. Histol. Jpn.* 46: 1–42, 1983.
107b. OI, M., K. USHIDA, AND S. SUGIMURA. The location of gastric ulcer. *Gastroenterology* 36: 45–56, 1959.
108. OKA, S. Microcirculation of the gastro-intestinal mucosa and the architecture of the blood vessels. *Saishin Igaku Osaka* 25: 1705–1713, 1970.
109. PALADE, G. E., AND R. R. BRUNS. Structural modulations of plasmalemmal vesicles. *J. Cell Biol.* 37: 633–649, 1968.
110. PALADE, G. E., M. SIMIONESCU, AND N. SIMIONESCU. Structural aspects of the permeability of the microvascular endothelium. *Acta Physiol. Scand. Suppl.* 463: 11–32, 1979.
111. PAPPENHEIMER, J. R. Passage of molecules through capillary walls. *Physiol. Rev.* 33: 387–423, 1953.
112. PAPPENHEIMER, J. R., E. M. RENKIN, AND L. M. BORRERO. Filtration, diffusion and molecular sieving through peripheral capillary membranes: a contribution to the pore theory of capillary permeability. *Am. J. Physiol.* 167: 13–46, 1951.
113. PERKINS, W. E., AND T. J. GREEN. Effect of 3,4-toluenediamine on output from in situ rat Brunner's glands pouches. *Proc. Soc. Exp. Biol. Med.* 149: 991–994, 1975.
114. PERRY, M. A. Capillary filtration and permeability coefficients calculated from measurements of interendothelial cell junctions in rabbit lung and skeletal muscle. *Microvasc. Res.* 19: 142–157, 1980.
115. PERRY, M. A., J. N. BENOIT, P. R. KVIETYS, AND D. N. GRANGER. Restricted transport of cationic macromolecules across intestinal capillaries. *Am. J. Physiol.* 245 (*Gastrointest. Liver Physiol.* 8): G568–G572, 1983.
116. PERRY, M. A., W. J. CROOK, AND D. N. GRANGER. Permeability of gastric capillaries to small and large molecules. *Am. J. Physiol.* 241 (*Gastrointest. Liver Physiol.* 4): G478–G486, 1981.
117. PERRY, M., AND D. GARLICK. Transcapillary efflux of gamma globulin in rabbit skeletal muscle. *Microvasc. Res.* 9: 119–126, 1975.
118. PERRY, M. A., AND D. N. GRANGER. Permeability of intestinal capillaries to small molecules. *Am. J. Physiol.* 241 (*Gastrointest. Liver Physiol.* 4): G24–G30, 1981.
119. PERRY, M. A., C. A. NAVIA, D. N. GRANGER, J. C. PARKER, AND A. E. TAYLOR. Calculation of effective pore radii in dog hind-paw capillaries using endogenous lymph and plasma proteins. *Microvasc. Res.* 26: 250–254, 1983.

120. PIASECKI, C. Blood supply to the human gastroduodenal mucosa with special reference to the ulcer-bearing areas. *J. Anat.* 118: 295-335, 1974.
121. PIASECKI, C. Observations on the submucous plexus and mucosal arteries of the dog's stomach and first part of the duodenum. *J. Anat.* 119: 133-148, 1975.
122. PIASECKI, C. Role of ischaemia in the initiation of peptic ulcer. *Ann. R. Coll. Surg. Engl.* 59: 476-478, 1977.
123. POULSEN, S. S., P. KIRKEGAARD, P. OLSEN, AND J. CHRISTIANSEN. Brunner's glands of the rat during cysteamine ulceration. *Scand. J. Gastroenterol.* 16: 459-464, 1981.
124. RENNKE, H. G., R. S. COTRAN, AND M. A. VENKATACHALAM. Role of glomerular charge in glomerular permeability. *J. Cell Biol.* 67: 638-646, 1975.
125. REYNOLDS, D. G., J. BRIM, AND T. W. SHEEHY. The vascular architecture of the small intestine mucosa of the monkey (*Macaca mulatta*). *Anat. Rec.* 159: 211-218, 1967.
126. REYNOLDS, D. G., AND K. G. SWAN. Intestinal microvascular architecture in endotoxic shock. *Gastroenterology* 63: 601-609, 1972.
127. RICHARDSON, P. D. I., D. N. GRANGER, D. MAILMAN, AND P. R. KVIETYS. Permeability characteristics of colonic capillaries. *Am. J. Physiol.* 239 (*Gastrointest. Liver Physiol.* 2): G300-G305, 1980.
128. ROBERTS, A. Proposed terminology for the anatomy of the rat stomach. *Gastroenterology* 60: 344-345, 1971.
129. ROSENBERG, A., AND P. H. GUTH. A method for the in vivo study of the gastric microcirculation. *Microvasc. Res.* 2: 111-112, 1971.
130. SCHAFER, E. A. *Microscopic Anatomy. Quains Elements of Anatomy.* London: Longmans, 1912, vol. 2, p. 539-540.
131. SCHULTZ, S. G. Ion transport by mammalian large intestine. In: *Physiology of the Gastrointestinal Tract*, edited by L. R. Johnson. New York: Raven, 1981, vol. 2, p. 991-1002.
132. SEILER, M. W., H. G. RENNKE, M. A. VENKATACHALAM, AND R. S. COTRAN. Pathogenesis of polycation-induced alterations ("fusion") of glomerular epithelium. *Lab. Invest.* 36: 48-61, 1977.
133. SESSIONS, J. T., JR., S. R. VIEGAS DE ANDRADE, AND E. KOKAS. Intestinal villi: form and motility in relation to function. *Prog. Gastroenterol.* 1: 248-260, 1968.
134. SHEA, S. M., AND M. J. KARNOVSKY. Brownian motion: a theoretical explanation of the movement of vesicles across the endothelium. *Nature Lond.* 212: 353-355, 1966.
135. SHEA, S. M., M. J. KARNOVSKY, AND W. H. BOSSERT. Vesicular transport across endothelium: simulation of a diffusion model. *J. Theor. Biol.* 24: 30-42, 1969.
136. SIMIONESCU, M., N. SIMIONESCU, AND G. E. PALADE. Morphometric data on the endothelium of blood capillaries. *J. Cell Biol.* 60: 128-152, 1974.
137. SIMIONESCU, M., N. SIMIONESCU, AND G. E. PALADE. Preferential distribution of anionic sites on the basement membrane and the abluminal aspect of the endothelium in fenestrated capillaries. *J. Cell Biol.* 95: 425-434, 1982.
138. SIMIONESCU, M., N. SIMIONESCU, J. SILBERT, AND G. E. PALADE. Differentiated microdomains on the luminal surface of the capillary endothelium. II. Partial characterization of their anionic sites. *J. Cell Biol.* 90: 614-621, 1981.
139. SIMIONESCU, N. Cellular aspects of transcapillary exchange. *Physiol. Rev.* 63: 1536-1579, 1983.
140. SIMIONESCU, N., M. SIMIONESCU, AND G. E. PALADE. Permeability of intestinal capillaries. Pathways followed by dextrans and glycogens. *J. Cell Biol.* 53: 365-392, 1972.
141. SIMIONESCU, N., M. SIMIONESCU, AND G. E. PALADE. Permeability of muscle capillaries to exogenous myoglobin. *J. Cell Biol.* 57: 424-452, 1973.
142. SIMIONESCU, N., M. SIMIONESCU, AND G. E. PALADE. Permeability of muscle capillaries to small heme peptides. Evidence of the existence of patent transendothelial channels. *J. Cell Biol.* 64: 586-607, 1975.
143. SIMIONESCU, N., M. SIMIONESCU, AND G. E. PALADE. Structural-functional correlates in the transendothelial exchange of water-soluble macromolecules. *Thromb. Res.* 8, Suppl. 2: 257-269, 1976.
144. SIMIONESCU, N., M. SIMIONESCU AND G. E. PALADE. Structural basis of permeability in sequential segments of the microvasculature of the diaphragm. II. Pathways followed by microperoxidase across the endothelium. *Microvasc. Res.* 15: 17-36, 1978.
145. SIMIONESCU, N., M. SIMIONESCU, AND G. E. PALADE. Open junctions in the endothelium of postcapillary venules of the diaphragm. *J. Cell Biol.* 79: 27-44, 1978.
146. SIMIONESCU, N., M. SIMIONESCU, AND G. E. PALADE. Differentiated microdomains on the luminal surface of the capillary endothelium. I. Preferential distribution of anionic sites. *J. Cell Biol.* 90: 605-613, 1981.
147. SJÖSTRAND, T. On the principles of distribution of blood in the peripheral vascular system. *Skand. Arch. Physiol. Suppl.* 71: 1-150, 1935.
148. SKUTELSKY, E., AND D. DANON. Distribution of surface anionic sites on the luminal front of blood vessel endothelium after interaction with polycationic ligand. *J. Cell Biol.* 71: 232-241, 1976.
149. SMITH, P., P. O'BRIEN, D. FROMM, AND W. SILEN. Secretory state of gastric mucosa and resistance to injury by exogenous acid. *J. Surg.* 133: 81-85, 1977.
150. SPANNER, R. Neue befunde über die Blutwege der Darmwand und ihre functionelle. *Bedeutung Morph. Jahrbuch.* 69: 394-454, 1932.
151. STACH, W. Die Vaskularisation des plexus submucous externus (Schabadasch) und des plexus submucous internus (Meissner) im Dunndarm von Schwein und Katze. *Acta Anat.* 101: 170-178, 1978.
152. STACH, W., N. HUNG, AND S. SCHOOF. Zur Gefaversorsung des plexus myentericus (Auerbach) im Dickdarm der Katze. *Z. Mikrosk. Anat. Forsch. Leipz.* 91: S22-S30, 1977.
153. SVANVIK, J. Mucosal blood circulation and influence on passive absorption in small intestine. *Acta Physiol. Scand. Suppl.* 385: 1-44, 1973.
154. TAYLOR, A. E., AND D. N. GRANGER. Equivalent pore modeling: vesicles and channels. *Federation Proc.* 42: 64-69, 1983.
155. TAYLOR, A. E., AND D. N. GRANGER. Exchange of macromolecules across the microcirculation. In: *Handbook of Physiology. The Cardiovascular System. Microcirculation*, edited by E. M. Renkin and C. C. Michel. Bethesda, MD: Am. Physiol. Soc., 1984, sect. 2, vol. IV, pt. 1, chapt. 11, p. 467-520.
156. THOREK, P. *Anatomy in Surgery* (3rd ed.). New York: Springer-Verlag, 1985.
157. TRAP-JENSEN, J., AND N. A. LASSEN. Capillary permeability for small hydrophilic tracers in exercising skeletal muscle in normal man and in patients with long-term diabetes mellitus. In: *Capillary Permeability*, edited by C. Crone and N. A. Lassen. Copenhagen: Munksgaard, 1970, p. 135. (Alfred Benzon Symp., 2nd, Copenhagen, Denmark, 1969.)
158. TREASURE, T. The ducts of Brunner's glands. *J. Anat.* 127: 299-304, 1978.
159. UEHARA, Y., AND K. SUYAMA. Visualization of the adventitial aspect of the vascular smooth muscle cells under the scanning electron microscope. *J. Electron Microsc.* 27: 157-159, 1978.
160. VAJDA, J., T. RAPOSA, AND Z. HERPAI. Structural bases of blood flow regulation in the small intestine. *Acta Morphol. Acad. Sci. Hung.* 16: 331-340, 1968.
161. VEHASKARI, V. M., E. R. ROOT, F. G. GERMUTH, AND A. M. ROBSON. Glomerular charge and urinary protein excretion: effects of systemic and intrarenal polycation infusion in the rat. *Kidney. Int.* 22: 127-135, 1982.
162. VENKATACHALAM, M. A., AND H. G. RENNKE. The structural and molecular basis of glomerular filtration. *Circ. Res.* 43: 337-347, 1978.
163. VOGT, C., J. P. METRY, C. HOLLINGER, M. ANLIKER, A. VOGEL, AND M. KNOBLAUCH. Evidence for microfilament-mediated vasoconstriction of jejunal villous capillaries. *Bibl.*

*Anat.* 20: 71–74, 1981.
164. VOGT, C., A. VOGEL, C. HOLLIGER, M. RADZYNER, M. ANLIKER, AND M. KNOBLAUCH. The microcirculatory system of the jejunal villus of the rat. Correlation of intravital microscopy, injection casts and electron microscopy. *Bibl. Anat.* 20: 69–70, 1981.
165. WARWICK, R., AND P. L. WILLIAMS. *Gray's Anatomy* (35th ed.). Edinburgh: Longman, 1973.
166. WEISS, L. The cell periphery. *Int. Rev. Cytol.* 26: 63–105, 1970.
167. WELSH, M. J., P. L. SMITH, M. FROMM, AND R. A. FRIZZELL. Crypts are the site of intestinal fluid and electrolyte secretion. *Science Wash. DC* 218: 1219–1221, 1982.
168. WILLIAMS, L. M., AND L. E. BELL. Electron microscopical observations on fetal intestine. *J. Anat.* 132: 301–302, 1981.
169. WILLIAMS, S. E., AND L. A. TURNBERG. Demonstration of a pH gradient across mucus adherent to rabbit gastric mucosa: evidence for a mucus bicarbonate barrier. *Gut* 22: 94–96, 1981.
170. WINNE, D. The influence of villous counter current exchange on intestinal absorption. *J. Theor. Biol.* 53: 145–176, 1975.
171. WINSHIP, D. H., AND J. E. ROBINSON. Acid loss in the human duodenum. Volume changes, osmolal loss, and $CO_2$ production in response to acid loads. *Gastroenterology* 66: 181–188, 1974.
172. WISSIG, S. Identification of the small pore in muscle capillaries. *Acta Physiol. Scand. Suppl.* 463: 33–44, 1979.
173. WISSIG, S. L., AND M. C. WILLIAMS. Permeability of muscle capillaries to microperoxidase. *J. Cell Biol.* 76: 341–359, 1978.
174. WOLFRAM-GABEL, R., C. L. MAILLOT, AND J. G. KORITKE. Systematisation de l'angioarchitectonie de colon chez l'homme adulte. *Acta Anat.* 125: 65–72, 1986.

CHAPTER 37

# Gastrointestinal blood flow–measuring techniques

A. P. SHEPHERD | *Department of Physiology, University of Texas*
J. W. KIEL | *Health Science Center, San Antonio, Texas*

CHAPTER CONTENTS

Microsphere Technique
  Principle of measurement
  Fractionation of intramural blood flow in intestine
    Microsphere size
    Microsphere migration
    Microsphere "shunting"
  Microsphere studies in gastric circulation
Laser-Doppler Velocimetry
  History
  Theory of laser-Doppler blood flowmetry
  Evaluations in gastrointestinal tract
    Linearity
    Spatial selectivity and volume of measurement
    Quantitative use of laser-Doppler velocimetric flowmetry
    Motion noise and other problems
Aminopyrine Clearance and Other pH Trapping Techniques
  Overview of pH trapping methods
  Theoretical background
  Evaluation of aminopyrine clearance
    Initial studies
    Use in nonsecreting stomach
    Comparisons with other methods
    Invalid assumptions
Hydrogen Clearance
  History
  Principle of measurement
  Advantages and disadvantages of hydrogen clearance
  Locally generated hydrogen
Conclusions

TO THE CIRCULATORY PHYSIOLOGIST the gastrointestinal tract offers a particularly intriguing challenge: delineate the mechanisms that regulate blood flow in accordance with gastrointestinal function. However, several significant obstacles stand in the way of that long-sought goal. Adaptations in the complex histology of the stomach and intestine have stratified both structure and function into mucosa for secretion and absorption and into muscularis for propulsion of foodstuffs; a specialized microvascular architecture has adapted each tissue layer and its circulation to its particular function. Thus the relations between blood flow and gastrointestinal function can best be explored by studying local perfusion within the mucosa or muscularis rather than total blood flow to the stomach or intestine.

Methodological limitations now impede our ability to meet this challenge of relating local function to local perfusion and its regulation. Carl Ludwig's famous dictum "Die Methode ist alles" rings especially true for our methods of measuring blood flow within the walls of the gastrointestinal tract, because recent studies have made it increasingly clear that the blood flow–measuring techniques in the armamentarium of the modern circulationist are indeed "all or nothing," depending on whether the results they yield are valid or not. Relations between the circulation and gastrointestinal function, such as that between gastric mucosal blood flow and acid secretion, will have to be carefully reexamined because this long-accepted relationship was founded on invalid measurements with the aminopyrine clearance method for assessing gastric mucosal blood flow. Indeed a vast literature on the gastric mucosal circulation is based on this now-questionable technique and will thus have to be reinterpreted.

Considering these questions about the ability to measure local perfusion within the walls of the stomach and intestine, this review does not exhaustively treat the many methods that have been proposed for assessing the intramural distribution of gastrointestinal blood flow, but instead it focuses on a few of the best evaluated, most often used or misused, or most promising techniques (for comprehensive reviews, see refs. 39, 76). Similarly, because the paramount functions of the gastrointestinal tract are accomplished by the gastrointestinal mucosae (e.g., fluid and foodstuff absorption and acid secretion), the chief emphasis of this review is the measurement of mucosal blood flow in the stomach and intestine.

## MICROSPHERE TECHNIQUE

### Principle of Measurement

The principle of the microsphere technique can best be explained by beginning with a particular application: the fractionation of cardiac output. To measure the distribution of the cardiac output to various organs, a known quantity of radioactively labeled microspheres is injected into the left ventricle to mix the spheres with the blood and allow them to distribute with the cardiac output. The chief assumption of the method is that the probability a given sphere will be deposited in a particular organ is proportional to the fraction of cardiac output that the organ in question receives. It is also assumed that all of the microspheres that reach a particular organ are trapped completely and that none escape to venous blood. It is further assumed that the spheres deposited in the tissue can be recovered when the tissue is sampled and that the relation between the blood flow and sphere delivery is the same at each branch within the arterial tree (104). If these conditions hold, it follows that the fraction of the injected spheres received by a given organ will be in proportion to its share of the cardiac output. If cardiac output is measured by independent means, the organ's blood flow can also be calculated in absolute units rather than simply as a fraction of cardiac output.

Alternatively, the blood flow that a given organ receives could be determined in absolute units if *1*) its share of the cardiac output were determined from the proportion of total radioactivity injected and *2*) the flow to any other organ were determined by independent means. Thus if either cardiac output or the blood flow to any organ is known in absolute units, the radioactive microsphere technique can yield the blood flow in absolute units to any organ in which microspheres can be counted. An ingenious adaptation of this method is the so-called reference organ approach that was suggested by Rudolph and Heymann (108) and subsequently confirmed by Makowski et al. (81) and Domenech et al. (32). In this adaptation of the method, blood is withdrawn into a syringe at a constant known rate by way of a catheter in the arterial tree. Blood withdrawal begins before, continues during the injection of microspheres, and lasts until the injected spheres have passed the sampling site. The syringe thus serves as an organ of known blood flow and one that completely traps the spheres it receives. If one assumes that blood flow is constant during the time in which spheres reach the syringe, the following relationship holds

flow to organ = radioactivity in organ

$$\times \frac{\text{flow to reference organ}}{\text{radioactivity in reference organ}}$$

Because microspheres can be labeled with isotopes of various energy levels, conventional γ-counting equipment can be used to distinguish among microspheres injected at various times during an experiment.

Because the various organs within the systemic circulation are arranged in parallel with one another and because it is relatively easy to ensure (35) that injected spheres are adequately mixed with arterial blood, the microsphere technique has gained great popularity as a method for fractionating cardiac output. In this application the applicable caveats are well known. Moreover, Buckberg et al. (20) have enumerated statistical criteria for acceptable measurements. When spheres are sufficiently large to be completely trapped by the organ in question and when the number injected is not excessive, that is, does not disturb the blood flow level through embolization, the only question that remains is whether a sufficiently large number of spheres is obtained in the tissue sample to reduce inherent statistical variability to acceptable levels for the purposes of the measurement. If the number of microspheres ($N$) is accurately measured in the organ of interest, the coefficient of variation of repeated determinations of $N$ in identical experiments would be the Poisson distribution value of $1/\sqrt{N}$. For $N = 25, 100$, and $400$, the coefficient of variation is 0.20, 0.10, and 0.05, respectively. Thus 400 microspheres is the frequently cited minimum number of microspheres that must be counted to achieve a statistically acceptable level of variability. The same statistical variability applies to values of $N$ both for the reference organ and for the tissue of interest. Finally, it is worth emphasizing that the number of spheres counted, not the total radioactivity, is the important quantity.

*Fractionation of Intramural Blood Flow in Intestine*

Although the fractionation of cardiac output by microspheres is a relatively straightforward procedure, increasing evidence from the renal (9, 26, 37), coronary (69, 142), and intestinal (41, 82, 83, 84) circulations indicates that fractionating blood flow within an organ is fraught with serious problems. Therefore we explore several aspects of the microsphere technique that pertain to fractionating blood flow within an organ.

MICROSPHERE SIZE. In theory the procedure to measure blood flow to a tissue within an organ is simply to count the spheres in the tissue of interest. If the measurement of radioactivity is viewed as a way of counting microspheres, it follows that

$$F_{\text{tissue}} = N_{\text{tissue}} (F/ms)_{\text{reference organ}}$$

where $F$ and $N$ are the blood flow and the number of microspheres in the tissue of interest, respectively, and $F/ms$ is the flow per microsphere in the reference organ (73, 108). As we saw before for determinating blood flow to an organ, errors in the calculated value of $F_{\text{tissue}}$ would occur through errors in the measurement of $N$ or $F/ms$. Here the validity of the calculated blood flow value depends on whether two assumptions hold: *1*) that the sphere composition of the blood reaching the tissue of interest is the same as that upstream in the arterial tree and *2*) that, during the arrival of the injectate, all spheres entering the tissue are trapped and remain there. The effect of microsphere size on the tissue blood flow determination can be explored first by taking two ridiculously extreme examples. A sphere 1 cm in diameter would obviously fail to reach the tissue of interest, because it would be trapped in the aorta or one of its major branches. At the other extreme a 1-μm sphere would pass through the tissues of interest and fail to be trapped at all. In both cases the method would yield a blood flow of zero in the tissue of interest.

Lifson (73) has introduced a simple formalism to facilitate such considerations. The ratio of the calculated tissue blood flow to the true flow is the product of *1*) the fraction (S) of tissue-destined spheres that reach the tissue and *2*) the fraction (T) of those reaching the tissue that are trapped

$$\frac{\text{calculated tissue blood flow}}{\text{actual tissue blood flow}} = \text{ST}$$

The fraction S depends primarily on two frequency distributions. The first is the frequency distribution of sphere diameters in the blood entering the organ. The second is the frequency distribution of the vessels that filter the spheres before they reach the tissues of interest. Thus, as mentioned earlier, S and the calculated values of tissue blood flow should decrease and approach 0 at both ends of the microsphere size spectrum. Additionally S could be either larger or smaller than 1 if processes such as plasma skimming, axial streaming, or right angle branching affect the distribution of microspheres. Needless to say, these effects become more important sources of error as the diameters of the spheres approach the diameters of the vessels in the tissue of interest.

The value of T depends chiefly on the frequency distribution of the diameters of spheres entering the tissue and the frequency distribution of the vessel diameters in the tissue. The value of T should decrease and approach 0 for smaller sphere sizes. Lifson (73) contends that between the two invalid extremes an intermediate sphere size will be found that will give the highest calculated flow values and the most valid measurements. With some skepticism we further explore this possibility, and at this juncture we only point out that even the intermediate-size sphere that gives the highest flow value would still yield a measurement in error to the extent that the product ST is different from unity.

Although microspheres were used as early as 1947 by Prinzmetal et al. (105), it was not until 1958 that Grim and Lindseth (42) attempted to measure the intramural distribution of blood flow in the canine small intestine. Glass microspheres varying in size from 12 to 43 μm were injected intra-arterially into isolated loops of intestine that were subsequently divided into mucosa, submucosa, muscularis, and mesentery. These investigators assumed that microspheres of a particular size measured blood flow in vessels of the same size in the tissue layer in which the spheres were trapped. Microspheres 12 μm in diameter and smaller indicated that blood flow was distributed within the gut wall as follows: mucosa 54%, submucosa 10%, muscularis 19%, and mesentery 17%. However, 28% of the microspheres in this size range appeared in venous blood. For the 12- to 43-μm range, the proportion of spheres in the submucosa was directly related to sphere diameter, whereas the depositions in mucosa and venous blood were inversely related to sphere size. In the muscularis, sphere trapping did not appear to be size dependent. The unstated assumption in this early work was that the mucosa, submucosa, and muscularis constituted three parallel circuits among which the microspheres would be distributed in proportion to the blood flow in each of the three layers.

Despite this early indication that the distribution of microspheres within the gut wall varied with microsphere size, a number of investigators began using the technique to fractionate the intramural distribution of blood flow without paying particular attention to the choice of microsphere size. In 1972 Greenway and Murthy (41) by accident rediscovered the size-dependent distribution of microspheres in the intestine. These investigators had obtained two batches of microspheres both of the same nominal size but with different isotopic markers. Much to their surprise, they found that microspheres with one particular label were distributed primarily to the submucosa, whereas the other batch of microspheres was found predominantly in the mucosa. After sizing the microspheres manually, they found that the microspheres that lodged primarily in the mucosa had a mean diameter of 12 ± 0.15 μm (SE), whereas the microspheres that lodged primarily in the submucosa had a mean diameter of 17 ± 0.16 μm (SE). Greenway and Murthy concluded that, because the largest microspheres were trapped primarily in the submucosa, whereas the smaller spheres were caught in the mucosa, the two layers were arranged in series rather than in parallel. To test this hypothesis, they compared the distribution between mucosa and submucosa and found that, in isolated intestinal loops previously vasoconstricted with vasopressin, a subsequent vasodilation produced by isoproterenol caused microspheres to migrate from submucosa to mucosa. They reasoned, "if the microspheres in the submucosa were impacted in some part of a parallel-coupled vascular bed in the submucosa, it is extremely unlikely that they would move into the mucosa when the vascular bed was subsequently vasodilated. On the other hand, if the submucosal vessels were in series with mucosal vessels, the site of impaction of spheres would depend on the relative sizes of the spheres and vessels as they passed from submucosa to mucosa. This would explain the greater proportion of 12-μm spheres compared with 17-μm spheres in the mucosa and the movement of both types of spheres when the vascular bed was dilated." In this study by Greenway and Murthy, several observations and recommendations were made that have since been verified and studied further by other investigators. These observations were *1*) that larger spheres are trapped primarily in the submucosa, whereas the smaller ones reach the mucosa; *2*) that the size-dependent distribution can be minimized if flow is fractionated into a muscularis compartment and a single combined mucosa-submucosal compartment; and *3*) that microspheres previously lodged in the submucosa can be made to migrate into other tissue layers.

To study the size-dependent distribution of microspheres within the gut wall, Maxwell et al. (84) made intra-arterial injections of microspheres that ranged in size from 7 to 32 μm. After the injection of microspheres, the gut loop was separated into histologically verified tissue layers that were then digested in potassium hydroxide so that the microspheres in each tissue could be reclaimed and sized under a microscope. In addition, venous blood was collected during and for 2 min after the infusion of microspheres. From the diameters of the microspheres thus recovered from tissue and venous blood, frequency histograms were constructed. Typical data are shown in Table 1, which illustrates the distribution of microspheres within the gut wall and venous blood. If blood flow to the different layers occurred independently in parallel circuits with similar filtering capacities, the percentage recovered should be the same for all sizes of microspheres large enough to be trapped. However, these data show that substantial numbers 8- to 11-μm spheres passed through the intestinal vascular bed to venous blood. However, even among the sphere sizes large enough to be trapped completely, the intramural distribution depended markedly on microsphere diameter. Of all the tissue layers, the muscularis showed the least tendency to trap particular microsphere sizes selectively. In the submucosa the percentage of spheres trapped was directly related to sphere size, whereas the number trapped by the mucosa was inversely related to microsphere diameter. This size-dependent distribution is further illustrated in Figure 1, which also shows that there was practically a reciprocal relationship between the mucosal and submucosal fractions.

Both the percentage of spheres trapped and the frequency distribution of spheres showed relatively little size dependence in the muscularis compared with mucosa and submucosa (Table 1 and Fig. 2). Thus it seemed reasonable to assess whether the dependence on size could be eliminated if data from mucosa and submucosa were combined as originally suggested by

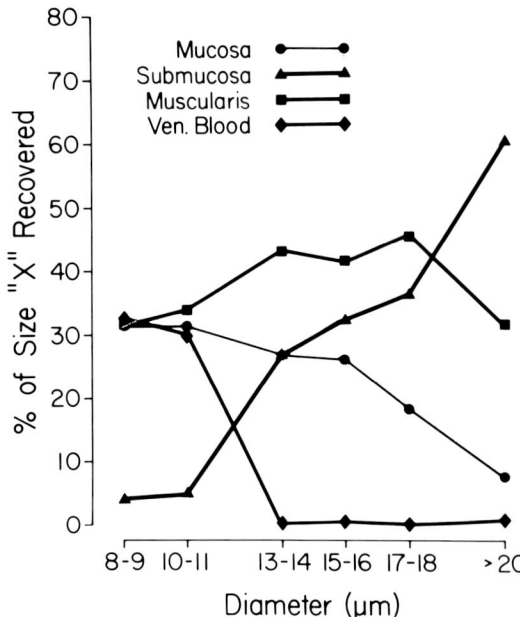

FIG. 1. Size of microspheres determines their distribution within gut wall. Shown are percentages of each microsphere size (X) recovered in canine mucosa, submucosa, muscularis, and venous blood. Note reciprocal relation between mucosal and submucosal trapping of spheres. [From Maxwell et al. (84).]

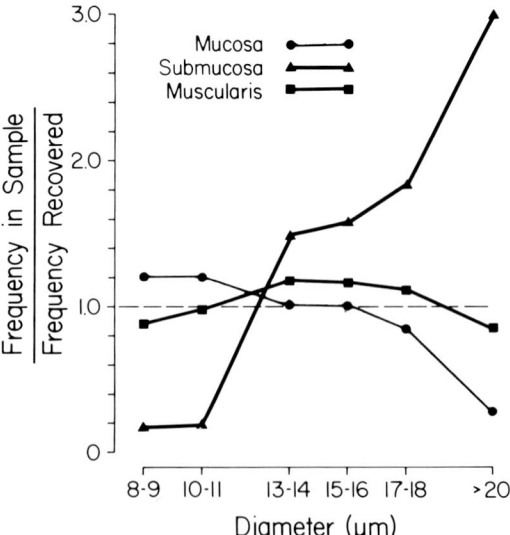

FIG. 2. Size-selective microsphere trapping in intestine. Shown is ratio of frequency of given sphere size in tissue sample to its frequency in injectate or among all spheres recovered. This ratio would be unity if sphere trapping were not size dependent. [From Maxwell et al. (84).]

TABLE 1. *Intramural Distribution of Microspheres*

| Diameter, μm | % Size X Recovered | | | |
|---|---|---|---|---|
| | Mucosa | Submucosa | Muscularis | Venous blood |
| 8–9 | 31.9±7.4 | 4.2±1.6 | 31.3±8.3 | 32.7±8.6 |
| 10–11 | 31.4±6.6 | 4.6±2.1 | 33.8±7.3 | 30.2±8.3 |
| 13–14 | 26.9±5.3 | 29.7±6.5 | 43.4±7.4 | 0±0 |
| 15–16 | 26.3±5.1 | 32.3±5.7 | 41.2±6.6 | 0.2±0.2 |
| 17–18 | 18.0±4.5 | 36.2±7.0 | 45.8±6.4 | 0±0 |
| >20 | 7.6±3.7 | 60.5±6.6 | 31.1±7.1 | 0.8±0.7 |

Values are means ± SE. X, size microsphere. [From Maxwell et al. (84).]

Greenway and Murthy (41). To test for size-dependent distributions, Maxwell et al. (84) established the following criterion: the ratio of the frequency of a particular size sphere in the injectate to the frequency of that size sphere in a given tissue should be 1 if no selective trapping occurred. Although the data for the combined mucosa-submucosa came closer to satisfying their test for size independence than either mucosa or submucosa alone, Maxwell et al. (84) still saw considerable differences from unity for 8- to 14-μm spheres and for spheres >20 μm (Table 2, top). However, when data were limited to the population of spheres between 13 and 18 μm in diameter (i.e., the range found in nominal 15-μm spheres), the ratio of frequencies for combined submucosa and mucosa to the frequencies recovered were not significantly different from 1. This finding thus substantiates the suggestion by Greenway and Murthy that the size-dependent distribution of microspheres in the 15-μm range can be reduced or eliminated by fractionating the intramural distribution of intestinal blood flow into only two compartments (at least under certain conditions).

MICROSPHERE MIGRATION. The common practice in microsphere assessments of blood flow is to infuse microspheres labeled with one nuclide under control conditions and to infuse spheres with a different label during experimental perturbations. Implicit in this approach is the assumption that spheres trapped in the tissue at one time do not subsequently move, because tissue is not sampled until the end of the experiment. In the intestinal vasculature, the series arrangement of large submucosal arterioles that subsequently branch into mucosa and muscularis raises questions about the validity of this assumption. Therefore Maxwell et al. (83) reexamined the problem of sphere migration within the intestinal wall. These investigators used a double loop of perfused canine small bowel to determine whether previously injected spheres could be dislodged by subsequent experimental perturbations. During the control interval, spheres were infused and venous blood was collected. Then the control half of the loop was isolated by ligating the loop itself between the vascular arcades and by tying off the artery and vein that supplied the control half of the perfused loop. Subsequently either isoproterenol was infused or perfusion pressure was elevated. Both venous blood and tissue samples from the two loops were isolated and analyzed separately. As Figure 3 shows, vasodilation significantly elevated the mucosal-to-submucosal ratio of sphere deposition. Thus vasodilation induced both 9-μm and 15-μm spheres to migrate from submucosa to mucosa. Analysis of other data indicated that the spheres lost by the submucosa were gained by both mucosa and muscularis. Elevating perfusion pressure from 90 to 150 mmHg also redistributed microspheres within the intestinal wall. In this case the submucosa lost both 9-μm and 15-μm spheres, the 15-μm spheres apparently going both to the mucosa and muscularis, whereas the 9-μm spheres passed into the venous blood.

The study by Maxwell et al. (83) has serious implications for the use of microspheres to determine the blood flow distribution in the intestinal wall. First, microspheres infused at one time can be induced to migrate by vasodilation or by increased perfusion pressure. Thus if vasodilation or a change in perfusion pressure occurs during an experiment, previously infused spheres no longer represent the conditions under which they were infused. There are undoubtedly other

TABLE 2. *Microsphere Sizes Within Combined Mucosal and Submucosal Tissues*

|  | Diameter, μm | | | | | |
|---|---|---|---|---|---|---|
|  | 8–9 | 10–11 | 13–14 | 15–16 | 17–18 | >20 |
| % Size X | 36.1 ±7.4 | 36.0 ±6.1 | 56.6 ±6.9 | 54.5 ±6.0 | 54.5 ±5.9 | 68.1 ±6.4 |
| Freq X in sample / Freq X in recovered | 0.73 ±0.05 | 0.76 ±0.05 | 1.26 ±0.07 | 1.22 ±0.19 | 1.23 ±0.11 | 1.62 ±0.22 |
|  | 15-μm microspheres | | | | | |
| Freq X in sample / Freq X 13–18 range |  |  | 1.07 ±0.08 | 0.97 ±0.04 | 1.04 ±0.09 |  |

Values are means ± SE. Freq, frequency; X, size microsphere. [From Maxwell et al. (84).]

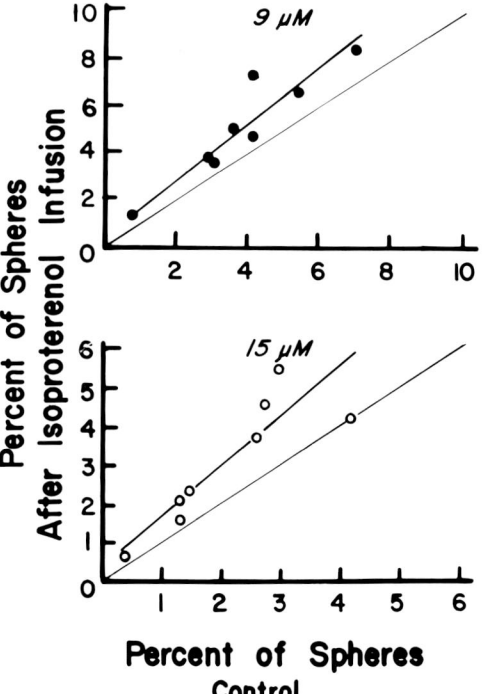

FIG. 3. Microsphere migration induced by vasodilation. Mucosa-to-submucosal ratios of sphere deposition were increased by vasodilation with isoproterenol (no data points fell below line of identity). For both microsphere sizes, control and experimental data were significantly different. [From Maxwell et al. (83).]

experimental perturbations that alter the distribution of previously infused spheres. In such studies a possible redistribution of the previously infused spheres during experimental procedures cannot be excluded. Therefore, if practicable, tissue samples must be taken immediately after each sphere infusion. Second, the practice of combining mucosa and submucosa for analysis was not discredited after vasodilation with isoproterenol. When a redistribution occurs primarily between mucosa and submucosa, combining these two layers into a single compartment facilitates data analysis. However, this procedure should be used with caution because the data from perfusion pressure experiments indicated that a redistribution of spheres was still apparent even when mucosal and submucosal data were combined.

MICROSPHERE "SHUNTING." The intestinal circulation appears to be unique in its ability to allow the arteriovenous passage of microspheres. In contrast to other organs that allow the passage of only a small percentage of the injected microspheres to reach venous blood, the intestinal vasculature allows 20%–33% of the injected 9-$\mu$m spheres to reach venous blood (Table 3). This extent of "shunting" could occur through a population of large-bore vessels or arteriovenous anastomoses. However, modern anatomic studies (38) indicate that large-bore arteriovenous shunts either do not exist in the intestinal circulation or occur very infrequently. The question of how 9-$\mu$m spheres pass through the intestinal circulation is a particularly important one for the microsphere technique, because several methods require using 9-$\mu$m spheres. For example, Dinda et al. (30) claim that simultaneously injected 9-$\mu$m and 15-$\mu$m spheres yield valid measurements of arteriolar, capillary, and shunt blood flow in each of the tissues within the bowel wall. Thus they assume that 9-$\mu$m spheres retained by the tissue provide an estimate of capillary blood flow, and they assume that 9-$\mu$m spheres collected in venous blood estimate shunt blood flow. Similarly, Bond and Levitt (15) and Mickflickier et al. (86) have proposed that 9-$\mu$m spheres be used to measure villus blood flow. As shown in Table 3, how 9-$\mu$m spheres reach venous blood is a quantitatively significant question. If between 20% and 30% of the injected 9-$\mu$m spheres reach venous blood, then this quantity of microspheres either represents shunt blood flow as some investigators believe (30) or it represents a huge error in the measurement—an error that can be corrected only if the tissue route can be identified through which the microspheres pass in reaching venous blood.

Because it appeared unlikely that there were anatomical shunts to explain the shunting of 9-$\mu$m spheres and because spheres of any nominal size actually exhibit a frequency distribution in their diameters, Maxwell et al. (82) sought another explanation. As they noted, the frequency distributions of intestinal capillary diameters and 9-$\mu$m spheres overlap. Hence microspheres could simply pass through capillaries. Therefore they developed simple probabilistic mathematical models to predict both the frequency distribution of microsphere sizes and the percentage of injected spheres that should appear in venous blood. The chief assumptions in their models were that microsphere delivery and sphere diameter are independent and that microspheres pass through capillaries of equal or larger size. The passage of microspheres predicted by the models was consistent with observed values in the canine intestinal circulation and demonstrated that passage through capillaries with a mean diameter of 7.38 ± 1.4 $\mu$m (SD) adequately accounts for the appearance of 9-$\mu$m spheres in venous blood. However, the diameters of nominal 9-$\mu$m spheres were distributed too narrowly to show the sieving effect that one would expect when microspheres are filtered by the intestinal circulation. Therefore Maxwell et al. (82) injected a mixture of microspheres that varied in diameter from 5 to 20 $\mu$m. This mixture demonstrated a marked sieving effect, as shown in Figure 4. The observed distribution of sphere diameters in venous blood agreed reasonably well with the frequency distribution predicted by the mathematical model when it was assumed that the distribution of capillary di-

TABLE 3. *Microsphere Shunting Through Intestinal Circulation*

| Species | Microsphere Diameter, $\mu$m | Passage, % | Radioactive | Reference |
|---|---|---|---|---|
| Dog | 8 | 48 | Yes | Leonard et al. (70) |
| Dog | 7–10 | 28 | Yes | Bond and Levitt (15) |
| Dog | 9 | 20.3 | Yes | Dinda et al. (30) |
| Dog | 9 | 22.2 | Yes | Maxwell et al. (83) |
| Dog (control) | 9 | 24.2±4.1* | Yes | Fan et al. (37) |
| Dog (acidosis) | 9 | 33.3±4.6* | Yes | |
| Dog (control) | 9 | 20.4±2* | Yes | Overbeck (102) |
| Dog (↑PP) | 9 | 28.4±3.7* | Yes | |
| Dog | 9 | 32.7 | No | Maxwell et al. (84) |
| Dog | 12±1.2 | 17–28 | Yes | Grim and Lindseth (42) |
| Rabbit | 7–10 | 16.3 | No | Mickflickier et al. (86) |
| Cat | 12 | <1 | Yes | Greenway and Murthy (41) |

* Values are means ± SE.   PP, perfusion pressure.

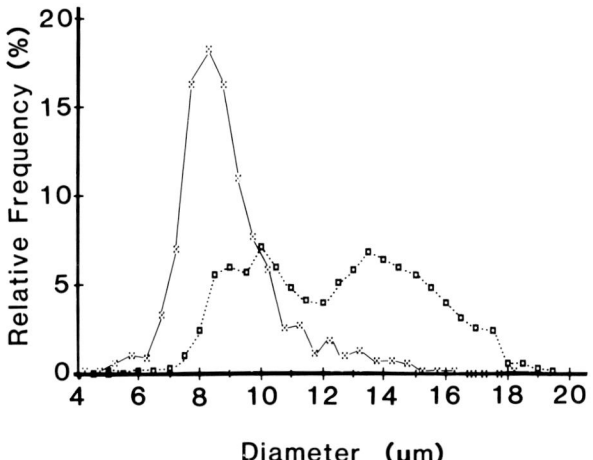

FIG. 4. Microsphere sieving effect. Relative frequency distributions of injected spheres (□) and spheres recovered from venous blood (×). Injectate was mixture of commercial 9-, 10-, 15-, and 20-μm spheres. [From Maxwell et al. (82).]

ameters was Gaussian. Although the sieving effects of a Gaussian capillary bed of mean diameter 7.38 ± 1.4 μm (SD) agreed reasonably with the observed frequency distribution of microsphere diameters in venous blood, the predicted distribution overestimated the relative frequency in the 8- to 9-μm range but underestimated the relative frequency of spheres >10 μm.

To determine whether the discrepancies between predicted values and observed data could be eliminated if the model also included large-bore shunt vessels, Maxwell et al. included in their model a population of vessels that allowed passage of all delivered spheres <20 μm in diameter. When the model had as much as 5% of total blood flow passing through such vessels, the relative frequency of spheres >10 μm in diameter in venous blood was grossly overestimated. Although they did not rigorously evaluate this issue, their calculations suggested that shunt flow through vessels that do not trap 20-μm spheres is not likely to exceed 1%–2% of total blood flow. Because shunts could not adequately account for the frequency distribution of microspheres in venous blood, another approach was used to try to improve the quantitative agreement between the observed and predicted frequency distributions for microspheres in venous blood. When a lognormal rather than a Gaussian distribution of capillary diameters was assumed, the predicted and measured distribution of venous microsphere diameters agreed even more closely (Fig. 5). Compared with the normal distribution, the lognormal distribution includes sufficiently more vessels in the 10- to 14-μm-diameter range so that the estimates of venous spheres >10 μm was elevated to nearly experimental values, and the relative frequency of 8- to 9-μm spheres was reduced to experimental values. The study of Maxwell et al. demonstrated that the passage of spheres through capillaries rather than through shunts adequately accounts for the appearance of spheres in venous blood. Additionally it suggests that the frequency distribution of venous microspheres could provide an in vivo method for estimating the frequency distribution of intestinal capillary diameters. This is a particularly intriguing possibility, because other methods for determining capillary diameters are excruciatingly tedious and time consuming. Other methods are also plagued by significant errors. For example, problems with the vascular casting method include overdistension of blood vessels during the injection of viscous casting medium and shrinkage during its polymerization (10). Problems with in vivo microscopy measurements include uncertainty about depth of focus, inaccuracies with two-dimensional projections of a three-dimensional object, and obscured view of deep vessels by superficial ones (111). Also vascular casts and in vivo microscopy yield estimates of anatomic size distributions, whereas the proposed microsphere method could yield an estimate of vascular size distribution as it relates to microsphere delivery in vivo or physiological blood flow.

Although a number of other investigators (45, 70, 79, 94, 100) had also proposed that microspheres could be used to study the frequency distribution of the diameters of arteriovenous connections, relatively few experimental data are available in the literature. Moreover the mathematical techniques to estimate the frequency distribution of capillary diameters from the frequency distributions of injected and venous microspheres have been relatively primitive. For example, in their modeling Maxwell et al. (82) simply assumed that the frequency distribution of intestinal capillary diameters had some particular mathematical form (i.e., Gaussian or lognormal). By contrast,

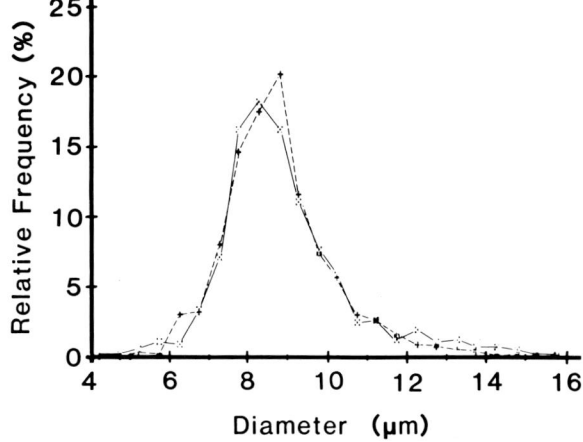

FIG. 5. Predicted (+) and observed (×) relative frequency distributions of spheres recovered from venous blood. Injectate same as in Fig. 4. Assumptions in model were that microsphere delivery to capillaries was $r^4$ function of capillary radius, that mean capillary diameter was 7.38 μm ± SD 1.4, and that frequency distribution was lognormal. [From Maxwell et al. (82).]

McMahan et al. (85) have developed statistical procedures to estimate the frequency distribution of capillary diameters without assuming that these distributions have any particularly mathematical form. Figure 6 shows the estimated probability density obtained by McMahan et al. for intestinal capillaries. The ability of their model to predict the frequency distributions of spheres in venous blood exceeded that shown in Figure 5.

Although the possibility of assessing in vivo capillary sizes from microsphere shunting is a relatively unexplored application of microspheres, several tentative conclusions can be drawn. First, the injectate should include microspheres that range in diameter from those that are completely trapped by the target vascular bed to those that pass through almost completely. Second, the microsphere sizes in both the injectate and venous blood must be determined accurately, and a sufficient number of size bins must be included in the frequency histograms to characterize the distribution accurately. If these precautions are observed and the statistical techniques of McMahan et al. are used, microspheres may be the only practical method for assessing the frequency distribution of capillary diameters in vivo. Clearly such an applications of microspheres appears to be sufficiently promising to warrant additional studies. Combined with modern particle-sizing instrumentation, this method would provide a convenient and rapid method for estimating the frequency distributions of capillary diameters in both normal and pathophysiological conditions.

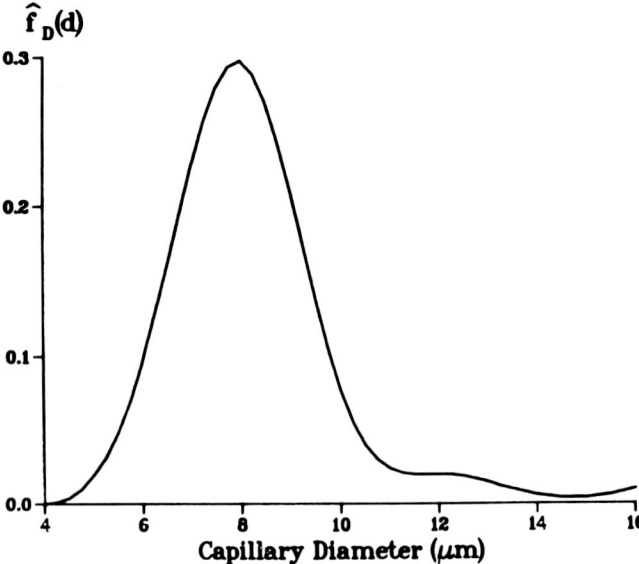

FIG. 6. Relative frequency distribution of intestinal capillary diameters [$\bar{f}_D(d)$]. Frequency distribution calculated from injected and venous microsphere populations without assumptions regarding mathematical form of frequency distribution of intestinal capillary diameters. [From McMahan et al. (85).]

*Microsphere Studies in Gastric Circulation*

The use of microspheres to fractionate the intramural distribution of gastric blood flow was first attempted by Delaney and Grim (28, 29) in 1964. Ten years later, Archibald et al. (2) used the microsphere technique in the gastric chamber preparation developed by Moody and Durbin (93) to examine the effect of isoproterenol on canine gastric mucosal blood flow and acid secretion. Radioactive microspheres (15 ± 5 µm) were used to estimate both total gastric blood flow and its intramural distribution. An unspecified number of spheres was injected into the left ventricle while a simultaneous 80-s reference sample was drawn from the distal aorta. Microsphere measurements of mucosal blood flow were compared with simultaneous assessments by aminopyrine clearance obtained during intravenous infusions of isoproterenol, histamine followed by isoproterenol, and isoproterenol followed by histamine. Although a low but unspecified pH was maintained in the chamber, the aminopyrine clearance measurement of mucosal blood flow was 50% less than the microsphere measurement at rest and 80% less during the isoproterenol infusion. However, both techniques indicated a significant increase in mucosal blood flow during isoproterenol-induced vasodilation.

The following year Archibald et al. (3, 4) applied the microsphere technique to the measurement of gastric mucosal blood flow in a more rigorous fashion. Again the intramural distribution of intraventricularly injected radioactive microspheres (15 ± 5 µm SD) was studied in the canine chambered stomach preparation. Reference samples of 80-s duration were taken from the distal aorta starting 10 s before microsphere injection. Approximately 100,000—500,000 microspheres were used for each injection, and all samples used for calculations contained at least 400 microspheres. In addition, the potential for error due to microsphere shunting was minimal, because fewer than 1% of the injected spheres appeared in venous blood. Furthermore the microsphere injections per se had no apparent effect on systemic blood pressure, cardiac function, gastric $H^+$ secretion, or gastric venous outflow. Microsphere measurements were linearly correlated with independent measurements of total blood flow. The agreement between total blood flow measured by the microspheres and by timed venous collections was particularly good ($r = 0.98$) with no significant difference between the two flow determinations (slope = 0.95). As in their previous study, microsphere measurements of mucosal blood flow were compared with simultaneous measurements by aminopyrine clearance. However, unlike the previous study, mucosal blood flow determinations were obtained during constant acid secretion induced by continuous intravenous infusion of histamine to optimize the aminopyrine clearance measurement. Although the mucosal blood flow measurements with microspheres were linearly correlated ($r = 0.96$) with the aminopyrine clearance measurements, the slope of the regression line (slope = 0.83) indicated that aminopyrine clearance values tended to be consistently less than the microsphere measurements.

As observed previously in the intestine by Grim and Lindseth (42) and by Greenway and Murthy (41), Archibald et al. (4) also found a size-dependent distribution of microspheres in the gastric mucosa and submucosa. Using two sets of differently labeled microspheres (26.5 ± 2.9 μm and 16.1 ± 2.5 μm SD), they noted that the larger spheres tended to be trapped preferentially in the submucosa, whereas the smaller spheres lodged in the mucosa. However, they found that the total radioactivity in the combined mucosa-submucosa was the same regardless of sphere size. Unlike Greenway and Murthy, who postulated a series vascular arrangement to explain the size dependence of the microsphere distribution between the intestinal mucosa and submucosa, Archibald et al. (4) proposed that the preferential trapping of larger spheres in the gastric submucosa was due to axial streaming that increased with increasing sphere size, and they claimed that "the bias of the microsphere technique is to underestimate mucosal flow and overestimate submucosal flow."

Although the use of microspheres for measuring gastric mucosal blood flow became increasingly popular after the work by Archibald et al., lingering doubts concerning the validity and limitations of the method continued to exist. In a recent study, Varhaug et al. (143) addressed the issue of appropriate sphere size by using a mixture of nominal 10-μm (9.5–11.0 μm) and 15-μm (13.0–18.5 μm) spheres in cats. As in previous studies, they found close agreement between sphere estimates of total blood flow and timed venous collections (slope = 0.917, $r = 0.98$ for 15-μm spheres). Similarly, they also observed limited arteriovenous shunting of both sphere sizes: 2% and 0.1% for the 10-μm and 15-μm spheres, respectively. However, unlike previous studies in the stomach, they also sized the spheres microscopically both in the injectate and in tissue sections of the gastric wall. The frequency distributions of the injected and embolized spheres were not significantly different, except for the smallest spheres (<10 μm diam), which presumably failed to lodge in the tissue. They also examined the intramural size distribution of the spheres. In the mucosa the sphere distribution was markedly size dependent; the larger spheres were predominantly located in the lamina propria, whereas the smallest spheres lodged at the glandular bases (Fig. 7). In the submucosa only the largest spheres tended to be trapped. However, unlike previous reports based on γ-counting of dissected tissue, relatively few spheres of any size were found in the submucosa (0.5% and 2.2% of the 10-μm and 15-μm spheres, respectively). Similarly the smaller spheres were also underrepresented in the

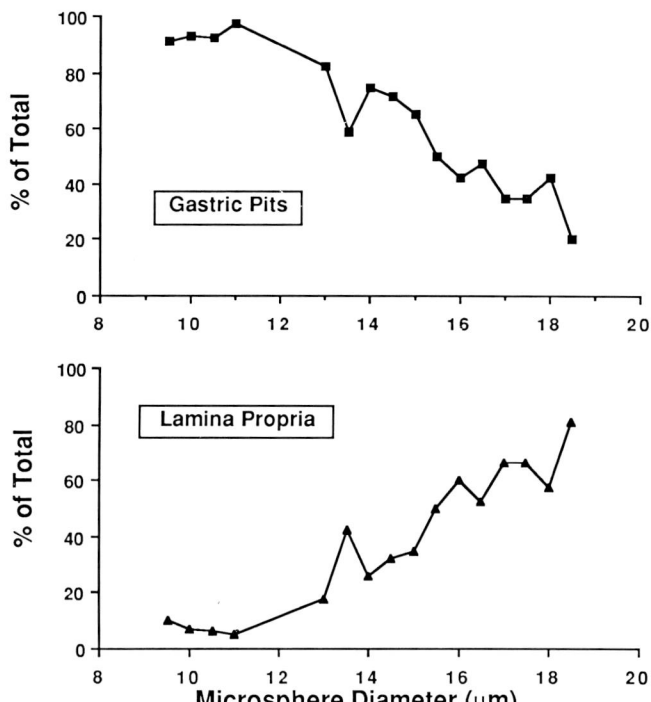

FIG. 7. Spatial distribution of microspheres within stomach wall. Deposition of spheres in gastric pits was inversely related to microsphere size, whereas their accumulation in lamina propria was directly proportional to sphere diameter. [Adapted from Varhaug et al. (143).]

muscularis. Varhaug et al. (143) concluded that "the ideal sphere size for gastric blood flow determination, allowing for representative distribution and minimal arteriovenous shunting or submucosal trapping, seems to be within the range of 10.5–17.0 μm in diameter." Nevertheless the precautions that should be observed to obtain valid microsphere measurements of gastric mucosal blood flow have still not been thoroughly elucidated. Thus application of the microsphere technique in the gastric circulation would greatly benefit from more studies to delineate clearly the pitfalls and the limits of its validity.

## LASER-DOPPLER VELOCIMETRY

### History

Johann Christian Doppler's *On the Colored Light of Double Stars and Some Other Heavenly Bodies* was delivered to the Royal Bohemian Society of Learning in 1842 (145). Since that time the principle that bears his name has been utilized by disciplines of science ranging from astronomy to biochemistry, and the Doppler principle has been used to determine the velocities of objects as large as galaxies and as small as bacteria and macromolecules. In recent years the advent of the laser with its spectral purity has initiated a new era in optical spectroscopy based on the Doppler principle. Of particular interest to the circulatory physiologist are techniques generally known as laser-Doppler velocimetry. These techniques are based on the Doppler principle as it applies to light. The frequency of the radiation scattered by an object moving relative to a radiating source is changed by an amount that depends on the velocity of the object and the scattering geometry. Since the first demonstration (147) of the potential of laser-Doppler velocimetry (LDV) more than 20 years ago, the technique has found numerous applications in industrial settings. Because laser light can traverse a hostile environment with impunity, LDV has been used to study flow velocities in jet exhaust gases and in corrosive fluids—environments in which conventional velocity-measuring instruments would be destroyed. Despite the widespread use of LDV for industrial applications, the history of blood flow measurements with LDV is relatively short.

The use of LDV for blood flow measurements was first introduced in 1972 by Riva et al. (106), who studied red blood cell velocities in the retinal vessels of rabbits. In subsequent studies Tanaka, Riva, and Ben-Sira (141) were eventually able to measure signals that varied with flow velocity in human retinal vessels. In addition to this single-vessel application of laser-Doppler velocimetry, other attempts to measure blood flow have used the Doppler effect. For example, Tanaka and Benedek (140) devised a fiber-optic catheter to measure velocity-dependent Doppler signals in the femoral artery of the rabbit, and other catheter-type LDV systems have also been developed (13, 60, 90). A third example of single-vessel LDV measurements is laser-Doppler microscope systems (18, 36, 66–68, 88) that were used to evaluate flow velocities and velocity profiles in various transparent tissues such as the mesentery of the rabbit and mouse, the toe-web of the frog, and the hamster cheek pouch.

All of the previously mentioned applications of LDV for blood flow measurements are limited to the determination of blood flow velocity in a single vessel. By contrast Stern (131) was the first to suggest that the average blood flow within the microcirculation could be measured from the Doppler broadening of laser light scattered by tissue in which only microscopic blood vessels were present. Subsequently Stern and co-workers (132, 133) demonstrated that blood flow could be measured in several tissues, primarily human skin and the rat renal cortex. After Stern's original studies, reports began to appear that described various designs for LDV blood flowmeters (17, 34, 146), signal processors (17, 98, 144), probe geometries (101, 110), and theories of light scattering by tissue (16, 43). With the availability of commercial instruments in the late 1970s LDV blood flowmetry flourished, and the technique began to be evaluated for numerous clinical and research applications in a wide variety of vascular beds, including the gastrointestinal tract and liver.

*Theory of Laser-Doppler Blood Flowmetry*

Figure 8 illustrates the Doppler effect as it applies to sound waves (80). *Panel A* depicts a stationary source of sound with a particular frequency and a listener some distance from the source. If both listener and source are stationary, the listener receives $Ct/\lambda$ waves in $t$ seconds, where $C$ is the speed of sound and $\lambda$ is the wavelength. *Panel B* illustrates the situation in which the listener moves toward the sound source at velocity $v_L$. Here the listener receives additional

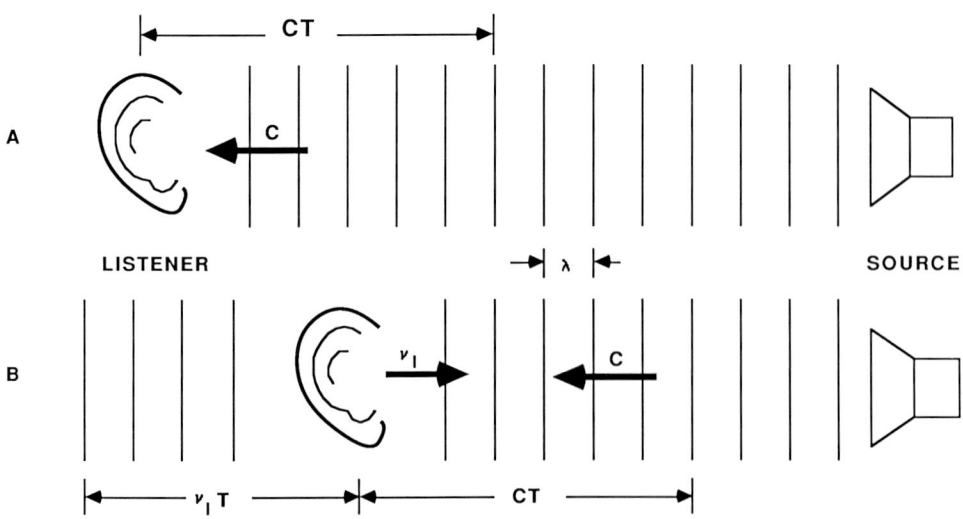

FIG. 8. Doppler effect for sound waves. *A*: if both listener and sound source are stationary, listener hears $Ct/\lambda$ waves in t seconds, where C is speed of sound and $\lambda$ is wavelength. *B*: if listener moves toward source at velocity $v_L$, he will hear additional $v_L t/\lambda$ waves in time $t$. [Adapted from Magnin (80).]

$\nu_L t/\lambda$ waves in time $t$. Because the frequency that the listener experiences ($f_o$) is simply the number of waves per unit time

$$f_o = (Ct/\lambda + \nu_L t/\lambda)/t = (C + \nu_L)/\lambda$$

The frequency at the source that the listener hears when stationary is just $f_s = (C/\lambda)$. The difference between the two perceived frequencies ($f_d$) defines the Doppler frequency shift, which can be expressed as

$$f_d = f_o - f_s = f_s(1 + \nu_L/C) - f_s = \nu_L f_s/C$$

For sound waves the motion of the source has a different Doppler shift frequency from the same motion on the listener's part. In other words, it is not just the relative motion between source and listener that is important but which one is in motion. Additionally, as the velocity of the source approaches the velocity of sound, the Doppler shift frequency becomes infinite. By contrast the situation is fundamentally different for Doppler effects with light. The difference can be explained in terms of Einstein's theory of relativity, which states that the speed of light is a constant in all reference frames. Light needs no material medium for its propagation, and its speed relative to the source or observer is always the same. Therefore it is only the relative motion between the observer and the source that determines the Doppler shift frequency. Thus

$$f_o = [f_s(1 - \nu_{os}/c)/2\sqrt{1 - (\nu_{os}/c)^2}] - f_s$$

where $c$ is the velocity of light and $\lambda_{os}$ is the relative velocity of the source with respect to the observer.

This equation can be applied to light entering tissue, but two other factors must be considered. If light strikes a stationary object and is reflected directly to a receiving detector, the returning light will have the same frequency as the emitted light. However, if the returning light has reflected from an object in motion, such as a red blood cell, the returning light will undergo a Doppler shift that is twice that predicted by the equation. The reason is that the structure reflecting the light acts as both the observer and the source. Because the red blood cell is in motion, the transmitted frequency it receives is Doppler shifted according to the equation, and the reflected light that leaves the red blood cell is shifted again because the red blood cell also acts as a source in motion relative to the stationary receiver. The second factor to consider is that only the component of the velocity vector directed toward or away from the receiver (observer) contributes to the Doppler-shift frequency. Thus, for direct backscattering, one must actually scale the frequency shift by the cosine of the angle between the red blood cell's velocity vector and the line connecting the object to the receiver. Although the Doppler shifts imparted to light by moving red blood cells are quite small compared with the frequency of light, the method is practical because of the spectral purity of laser light.

Having considered the fundamentals of the optical Doppler effect, we now turn our attention to the theory of laser-Doppler blood flowmetry in tissue (16). Figure 9 illustrates the typical optics for measuring blood flow in tissue by LDV. As shown, one optical fiber conducts light to the tissue of interest, and one or more receiving fibers return the scattered light to a photodetector. Figure 10 depicts several scenarios to illustrate the fate of a photon in tissue. When tissue is irradiated with a narrow incident beam, it typically glows with a diffuse backscattered pattern, which in-

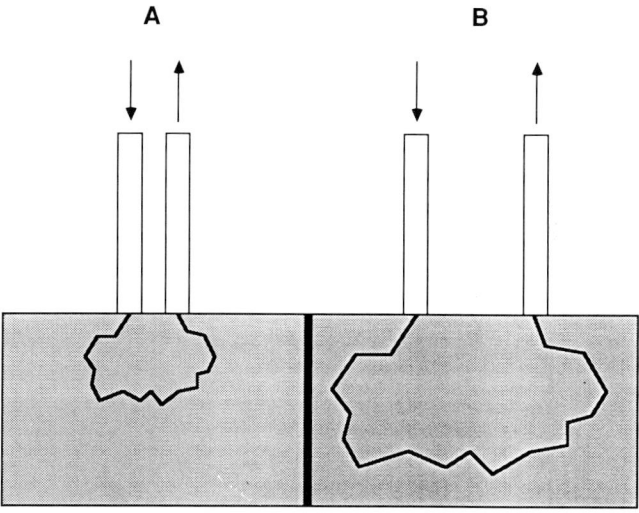

FIG. 9. Typical optics for laser-Doppler velocimetry in tissue. A: coherent light is guided to tissue surface by optical fiber, and one or more receiving fibers return light scattered by tissue to photodetector. B: depth or volume of tissue from which scattered photons are collected increases with greater separation between sending and receiving fibers.

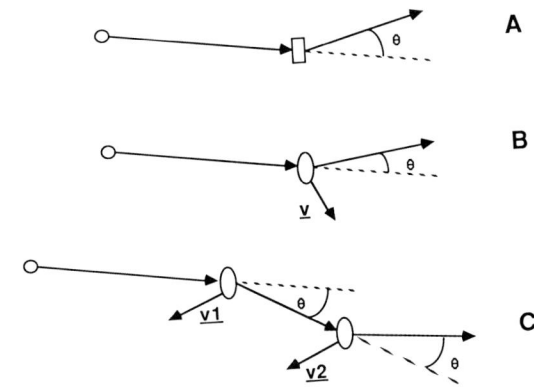

FIG. 10. Interactions between photons and tissue. A: of photons returning to photodetector, most have been scattered by static tissue elements. B: a few photons have experienced a Doppler shift as a result of a single collision with a moving red blood cell. C: other photons experience multiple scattering by moving erythrocytes, but these events are infrequent except in large vessels. [Adapted from Bonner and Nossal (16).]

dicates that photons generally suffer many collisions with stationary somatic cells before interacting with a moving red blood cell. The effect of the collisions between photons and stationary tissue is to randomize the direction of the light that eventually reaches the moving erythrocytes. Because the typical photon–red blood cell interaction results in only a slight deflection of the photon from its original path (mean scattering angle = 5.4°), additional scattering by the stationary tissue matrix is required to return the photon to the detecting fiber at the surface of the tissue. Additionally it is thought that very little (<0.1%) of the returning light consists of photons scattered only by moving red blood cells.

Of the light returning to the photodetector, the photons that have been scattered by moving red blood cells have undergone a Doppler frequency shift, whereas those photons scattered only from stationary tissues have not. When these two kinds of light interfere with each other at the photodetector, they create Doppler beat frequencies. Because red blood cells move at various velocities within perfused tissue, because the photons are scattered at many small angles by the red blood cells, and because the light is diffusely scattered by static tissue, the scattered light exhibits not a single frequency shift but a Doppler broadening over a spectrum of frequencies. The average Doppler shift imparted to a photon by a moving red blood cell is ~0.3 kHz·mm$^{-1}$·s$^{-1}$, and the Doppler frequency spectra thus fall within the audio range (30–20,000 Hz). The first Doppler spectra recorded from the intestinal mucosa are shown in Figure 11.

If the foregoing description of the interactions of coherent light with the static tissue matrix and moving red blood cells is reasonably valid, the following theoretical relationship (16) can be derived as a conceptual framework for measuring tissue perfusion by LDV

$$\bar{\omega} = \frac{(V^2)^{1/2} \beta f(\bar{m})}{(12\xi)a}$$

Here $\bar{\omega}$ is the normalized first moment[1] of the Doppler frequency spectrum, $(V^2)^{1/2}$ is the root-mean-square speed of the moving red blood cells, $a$ is the radius of

---

[1] For readers not familiar with the nomenclature of spectral analysis, the following definitions should be helpful. Imagine the Doppler spectrum as a histogram in which the various frequencies have been sorted into $N$ bins, each with a particular magnitude. To compute the mean frequency of the spectrum, two summations are required. The statistical names of the sums are the zeroth moment and the first moment. The zeroth moment is simply the sum of all $N$ bin magnitudes; the first moment is the sum of all $N$ bin magnitudes multiplied by their corresponding bin number. The mean frequency is the first moment divided by the zeroth moment (49)

$$\text{zeroth moment} = \sum_{\text{bin}=0}^{N} \text{magnitude (bin)}$$

$$\text{first moment} = \sum_{\text{bin}=0}^{N} \text{magnitude (bin)} \times \text{bin}$$

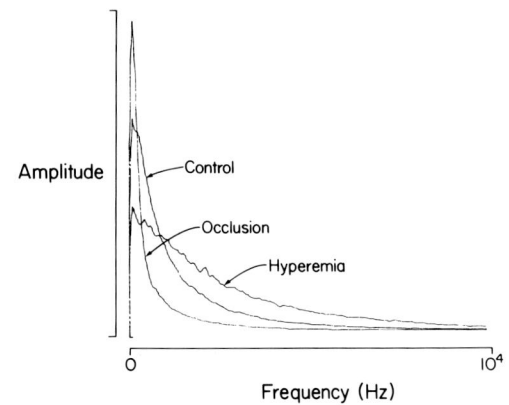

FIG. 11. Doppler frequency spectra recorded from canine intestinal mucosa. In absence of blood flow (artery occluded), instrument noise, imperceptible tissue motion, and unknown factors produce frequency shift in laser light. Average frequency is increased during control blood flow and increased still further during reactive hyperemia (A. P. Shepherd, G. L. Riedel, and J. W. Kiel, unpublished observations).

an equivalent spherical scatterer, $\xi$ is an empirical factor, and $\beta$ is an instrumental factor that depends primarily on the optical coherence of the signal at the detector. The variable $\bar{m}$ is the average number of collisions that a detected photon makes with moving red blood cells. The function $f(\bar{m})$ is linear with low concentrations of red blood cells in the tissue, i.e., when $\bar{m} \ll 1$. When the average number of collisions between detected photons and moving red blood cells is <1, $\bar{\omega}$ increases in an essentially linear fashion with changes in local blood cell concentration. Here the mean frequency $\bar{\omega}$ varies directly with red blood cell flux, i.e., the product of red blood cell concentration and average speed. For higher red blood cell concentrations in the tissue ($\bar{m} \gg 1$), $\bar{\omega}$ is still sensitive to changes in blood flow but varies approximately as $\sqrt{\bar{m}}$. However, $\bar{\omega}$ still varies linearly with $(V^2)^{1/2}$.

According to theory (16), several important microcirculatory variables can be extracted from laser-Doppler frequency spectra and made available in real time as instrumental outputs: *1*) the red blood cell flux or average tissue perfusion, *2*) the concentration of moving erythrocytes in tissue, and *3*) the average red blood cell speed. Additionally, because the measurement is essentially continuous, the pulsatility of blood flow or its oscillations due to vasomotion is also obtained.

Figure 12 is an oversimplified but conceptionally useful illustration of how laser-Doppler signals can be processed into such physiologically meaningful data (47). If only one red blood cell were moving through the tissue at a constant velocity, a photodetector signal with a small alternating current (AC) component and a large direct current (DC) component would result, as shown in Figure 12A. Of all the photons returning to the detector, only a few are Doppler shifted. Thus, as the photons mix on the detector, an average DC

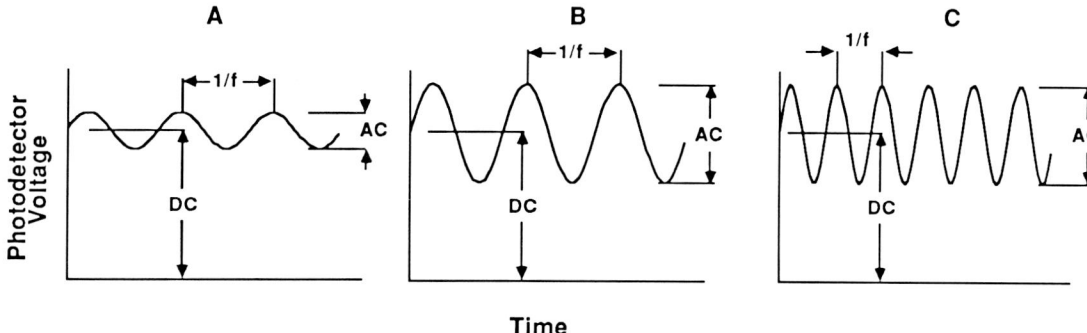

FIG. 12. Idealized scheme of laser-Doppler signal processing. Light returning from tissue consists chiefly of unshifted photons scattered by static tissue and a few Doppler-shifted photons scattered by moving red blood cells. Thus, as the photons mix, a photodetector signal results that has a direct current (DC) offset and a superimposed alternating current (AC) component. *A*: signal for a single red cell moving at constant velocity. *B*: if more red cells were moving at same velocity, magnitude of AC component would increase as more photons are Doppler shifted. *C*: if other factors remained constant and red cell velocity increased, frequency (*f*) of signal would increase. [From Haumschild (47) Reprinted by permission. Copyright © Instrument Society of America 1986. From *Biomedical Sciences Instrumentation*, vol. 22.]

offset voltage is produced upon which an oscillatory (AC) component is superimposed. The AC voltage fluctuation is due to mixing the few Doppler-shifted and the many unshifted photons. As schematically shown in Figure 12*B*, if many more red blood cells were moving through the same volume of tissue, the magnitude of the AC component would increase as more photons are Doppler shifted. If the same number of photons reach the detector, the DC level would be the same. Therefore it is readily apparent that the ratio of AC to DC is proportional to the concentration of moving red blood cells in the tissue. In practice the AC and DC voltages must actually be processed together, because local absorbance changes and other light losses could vary. Figure 12*C* shows how a characteristic Doppler frequency would change if other factors remained constant and only red blood cell velocity increased. In this case the magnitude of neither the AC nor the DC signal would be changed, but the mean frequency of the AC component would increase.

Although this scheme is oversimplified because the complex scattering processes produce many different frequencies rather than one, the process works for each frequency and thus for all. Actually the signal-processing algorithm obtains the mean frequency of the Doppler spectrum to estimate red blood cell speed, and the relative red blood cell concentration is obtained from the AC/DC ratio. The linearized product of red blood cell concentration and red blood cell velocity then yields red blood cell flux or blood flow. Figure 13 is a block diagram of a microprocessor-based LDV blood flowmeter that processes the Doppler signals in such a manner. Table 4 summarizes the various features of commercially available LDV blood flowmeters.

*Evaluations in Gastrointestinal Tract*

LINEARITY. The first studies of LDV flowmetry in the intestinal circulation were reported by Shepherd and Riedel (120), who employed isolated loops of canine small bowel either autoperfused or perfused from a pressurized reservoir of arterial blood. The first aspect of LDV that these investigators examined was its linearity. Because they suspected that local vasoregulatory mechanisms in the gut could possibly cause intramural blood flow to be redistributed unpredictably, they used isoproterenol to vasodilate the preparations. Figure 14 shows the first such evaluation of LDV's linearity. In these experiments total intestinal blood flow was manipulated throughout a wide range by changing the perfusion pressure. The LDV measurements of perfusion in the mucosa were linearly related to total intestinal blood flow that was monitored with an electromagnetic flowmeter.

Figure 15 (*top*) shows a similar demonstration of linearity in the gastric mucosa. Here Kiel et al. (58) used a chambered canine stomach preparation that was also vascularly paralyzed with intra-arterially infused isoproterenol. In both of these studies the LDV flowmeters were "homemade" devices built on the design originally developed at the National Institutes of Health (17). However, most reports with the commercial instruments now indicate that, as in these early studies, laser-Doppler blood flowmeters yield linear measurements of blood flow in a wide variety of vascular beds in which some independent method is available to monitor total perfusion. However, some difficulties have been reported in the gastrointestinal tract. Using a commercially available instrument, Ahn et al. (1) found that the LDV signal apparently saturated when total blood flow increased significantly in

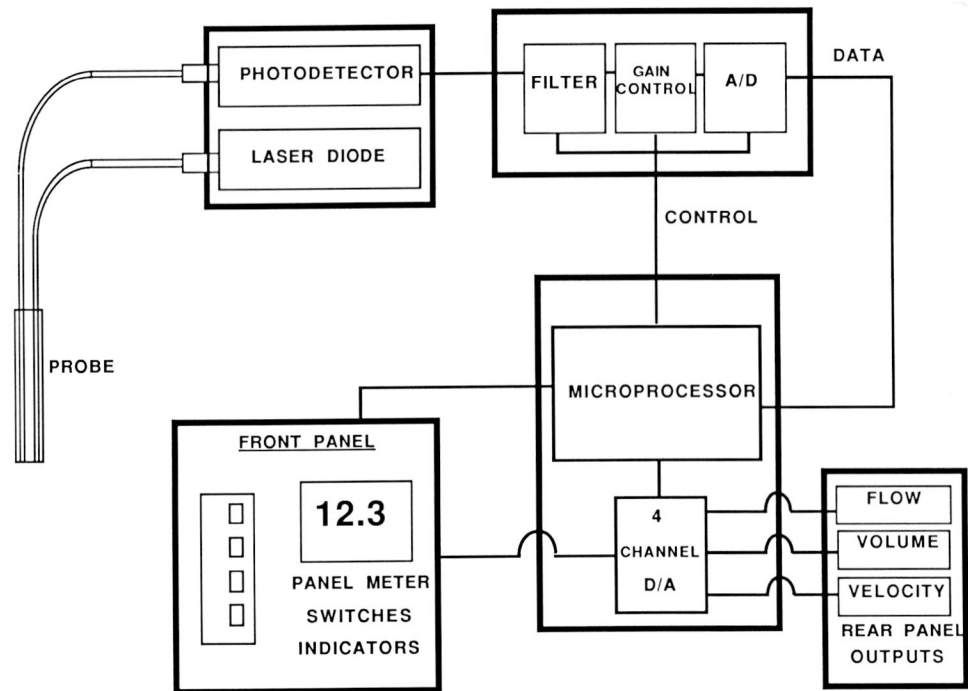

FIG. 13. Block diagram of microprocessor-based laser-Doppler blood flowmeter. Typical signal processing includes setting upper and lower frequency cutoff filters to maximize signal-to-noise ratio and calculations of relative red blood cell flux, local red cell concentration in tissue, and average red cell velocity.

TABLE 4. *Comparison of Laser-Doppler Blood Flowmeters*

| | | | | | | | | | | | Outputs | | |
|---|---|---|---|---|---|---|---|---|---|---|---|---|---|
| Mfg. | Model | Laser | λ, nm | Signal Analysis | Fiber Type | No. Fibers[a] | Diam, μm | Separation,[b] μm | Laser Power, mW | Frequency range[c] | Flow | RBC volume[d] | Velocity |
| MedPacific | LD5000 | He-Ne | 632.8 | Analog | Graded index | 2 | 100 | 500 | 2 | Fixed | + | | |
| Perimed | PF3 | He-Ne | 632.8 | Analog | Step index | 3 | 500 | 750 | 2 | Manual | + | | |
| TSI | BPM 403A | Diode | 780 | Digital | Graded index | 3 | 50 | 500 | 2 | Auto | + | + | + |
| MedPacific | LD6000 | He-Ne | 632.8 | Analog/digital | Graded index | 2 | 100 | 500 | 2 | Fixed | + | + | + |

[a] TSI and Perimed use 1 sending fiber and 2 receiving fibers.   [b] Center-to-center fiber separation.   [c] MedPacific's frequency range is fixed at 100 Hz–20 kHz. Perimed's lower limit is 70 Hz. Upper limit can be set to 4, 12, or 20 kHz. TSI's microprocessor selects frequency range.   [d] Relative red blood cell (RBC) concentration in tissue.   [e] Average RBC speed.

feline gut preparations. The problem apparently arose from the selection of an inappropriately low upper cutoff frequency for the Doppler frequency spectrum. There are other explanations, however, for the apparent lack of a linear relationship between LDV measures of mucosa perfusion and total blood flow. For example, Kiel et al. (59), using LDV flowmetry, have obtained the first evidence that gastric mucosal blood flow is autoregulated, that is, kept relatively constant when perfusion pressure is altered. Their LDV measurements of mucosal blood flow, when plotted versus total blood flow, show a plateau in the LDV values if the preparations are autoregulating mucosal blood flow (Fig. 15, *bottom*). By contrast, maximal vasodilation with isoproterenol greatly increases LDV mucosal blood flow values and "linearizes" their relationship with total gastric perfusion. This finding underscores the need for studies for which LDV measurements of mucosal blood flow are compared, not with total intestinal or gastric blood flow but with another method for selectively measuring mucosal blood flow.

SPATIAL SELECTIVITY AND VOLUME OF MEASUREMENT. A major difficulty in using LDV flowmetry to monitor blood flow in the tissues of the mucosa or muscularis is that the measuring volume is not known precisely in any tissue. Several factors influence the

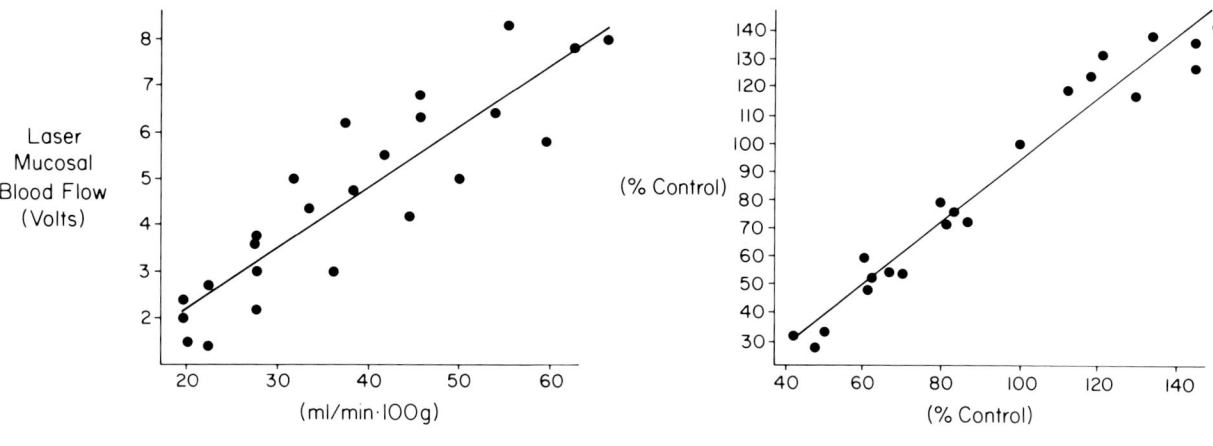

FIG. 14. Linearity of laser-Doppler blood flowmeter in intestine. *Left*: in isolated canine small bowel, raw laser-Doppler velocimetry measurements were linearly related to total blood flow ($r = 0.89$). *Right*: normalizing data to flow values measured at perfusion pressure of 120 mmHg improved correlation (slope, 1.1; $r = 0.97$). Preparations were vasodilated with isoproterenol to eliminate autoregulation and unpredictable redistributions of blood flow. [From Shepherd and Riedel (120).]

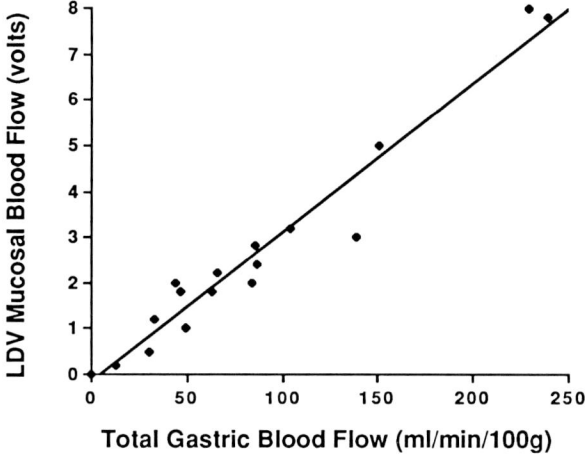

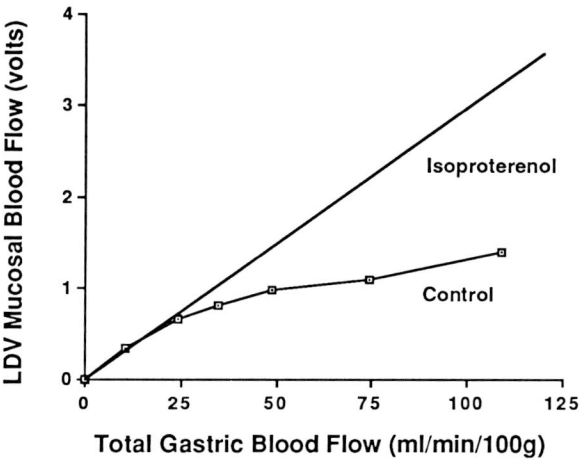

tissue volume or depth in which blood flow is measured with LDV. In all tissues (except those with little ability to scatter coherent light), light becomes isotropically diffuse after passing through 300–600 μm of tissue. This mean path for light diffusion and the spatial separation of the light-conducting fibers are primary determinants of the tissue volume sampled by LDV. Figure 9 illustrates that increasing the distance between sending and receiving fibers increases the depth or volume from which scattered photons are collected by the receiving fiber. For a 500- to 600-μm fiber separation and a typical tissue, the depth of the sampled tissue is estimated to be 0.6–1.2 mm. Except for skin and blood, the optical properties of living, perfused tissue are poorly understood. Thus the optical theory described in this section is little help in answering definitively the question of LDV's precise volume of measurement. Therefore a physiological approach is required.

Several physiological observations in the intestinal circulation indicate that, indeed, LDV yields a selective, superficial measure of blood flow just beneath the surface of the tissue to which the fiber-optic probe is applied. First, when selective vasodilators are infused intra-arterially, the mucosal and muscularis blood flow signals often change in opposite directions

FIG. 15. Linearity of laser-Doppler velocimetric (LDV) measurements of gastric mucosal blood flow. *Top*: in chambered canine stomach flaps vasodilated with isoproterenol, LDV-measured blood flow was linearly related to total gastric perfusion ($r = 0.98$). Flow was changed by altering perfusion pressure. *Bottom*: in preparations not vasodilated with isoproterenol, curve deviated from apparent linearity because gastric mucosal blood flow was autoregulated, as indicated by analysis of pressure versus flow relationship (not shown). For comparison, regression line from isoproterenol data is also shown. [From Kiel et al. (58).]

(125). Isoproterenol increases mucosal blood flow but simultaneously depresses muscularis perfusion. The opposite pattern is observed with adenosine, which selectively increases perfusion of the muscularis at the expense of the mucosa (125). Microsphere measurements confirm these directionally opposite changes with these two selective vasodilators (40, 124). Clearly, directionally opposite changes in the two circulations could not possibly be registered if LDV flowmeters simply respond to blood flow throughout the gut wall. Second, LDV blood flowmeters register a reactive hyperemia in the mucosa at the same time that no reactive hyperemia is seen in the muscularis (118). Third, if nonperfused small bowel tissue is placed between the optical probe and the perfused feline intestine, the LDV signal drops to the same level observed during occlusion of the supply artery. Furthermore with such nonperfused tissue between the probe and the perfused gut, the LDV signal records very little of the mucosal reactive hyperemia that is registered with another probe directly on the perfused mucosa (64). Similar observations have also been made in the gastric mucosa (59). Fourth, and more physiologically, several studies with microspheres have shown that nonlipid, nonprotein test meals such as glucose induce a functional hyperemia that is confined to the intestinal mucosa (23, 103, 149). The same results are obtained with LDV blood flowmetry (117). Fifth, other techniques commonly used to measure mucosal blood flow, such as hydrogen clearance (64) and microspheres (64), yield significant linear correlations with laser-Doppler estimates of mucosal perfusion.

QUANTITATIVE USE OF LASER-DOPPLER VELOCIMETRIC FLOWMETRY. Laser-Doppler velocimetric blood flowmetry affords the considerable advantages of continuous, linear measurements with a high degree of spatial resolution. However, at the present state in its evolution, several problems impair the quantitative use of LDV flowmetry: reproducibility, its nonzero signal at zero blood flow, and the lack of calibration in conventional flow units, for example, milliliters per minute or milliliters per minute per gram.

In all of the tissues studied, appropriately used LDV flowmetry exhibited significant linear relationships with measurements of total blood flow. For example, Figure 16 shows that in an isolated rat liver preparation LDV values and total blood flow values were significantly correlated. However, repetition of the protocol, in which perfusion pressure was altered to change blood flow, did not yield identical results. In fact the relationships between LDV and total blood flow values, although still linear, had markedly different slopes. There are several possible explanations for this alarming lack of reproducibility that has been noted in many other organs (55, 125, 128): instability in the instrument itself, the lack of reproducible

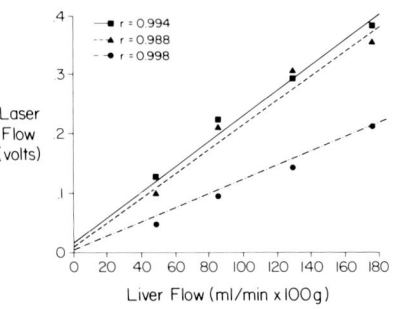

FIG. 16. Lack of reproducibility with laser-Doppler blood flowmetry. Manipulating portal venous perfusion pressure to alter blood flow to isolated rat liver preparation resulted in highly linear relation between total hepatic perfusion and laser-Doppler velocimetry-measured blood on liver surface, but slopes of lines were not consistently reproducible. [From Shepherd et al. (125).]

changes in local perfusion beneath the LDV probe, and site-to-site variability in capillary density or the number of red blood cells in motion. Tests with mechanical models (98, 99, 117) show that the instruments themselves are quite stable and that they yield very reproducible results. Thus the most plausible explanation for the lack of reproducibility in the data from perfused tissue is that local blood flow in the small volume of tissue sampled by the LDV flow probe does not always accurately reflect total blood flow in the whole organ.

The same conclusion was reached by Johnson et al. (55), who found great variability in the slopes of the relationships between LDV and plethysmographic measurements of blood flow in the skin of the human forearm. They speculated that one explanation for this variability was differences in capillarity from one site to another, and they showed that LDV readings of resting cutaneous blood flow varied sufficiently from one site to another on a given subject's forearm to explain the variability among subjects. Thus the high degree of spatial resolution that LDV blood flowmetry affords is both an advantage and a disadvantage. The ability of LDV flowmeters to monitor blood flow in a small volume of tissue estimated to be in the 1–2 mm$^3$ range is advantageous if an investigator wishes to record blood flow in the healing edge of an ulcer or other lesion, but such high selectivity risks sampling blood flow in a minute volume that may not be representative of the target tissue.

Two solutions to this dilemma have been suggested. One is to move the LDV flow probe to various sites, make multiple measurements, and average the results. This can be accomplished with a single LDV flowmeter, but it is tedious and time consuming. The second approach suggested by Salerud (110) is a new design for the flow probe. His design is a probe that contains seven optical fibers, collecting scattered light from seven relatively widely spaced sites. At six different adjacent sites on the human forearm, he measured resting cutaneous blood flow with conventional, single-return-fiber probes and the seven-return-fiber probes. As predicted by statistical theory, the site-to-site variability with the multiple-fiber probe was reduced approximately by the factor of $\sqrt{7}$.

The lack of a calibration constant to convert the voltage of LDV flowmeters into conventional flow units does not preclude use of the method for many significant purposes in studies of gastrointestinal blood flow. In fact the method has made it possible to observe phenomena that were previously impossible or impractical to study with conventional methods and to confirm results reported with more cumbersome, discontinuous techniques. Examples of previously unreported findings made possible by LDV are *1)* the different propensities of the intestinal mucosa and muscularis to display reactive hyperemia (122), *2)* the demonstration of a "vascular steal" mechanism through which selective vasodilators can induce the mucosa or muscularis to rob one another of blood flow (124), and *3)* the demonstration of reactive hyperemia and autoregulation in the gastric mucosal circulation (58, 59). Examples of LDV findings that confirm previous results from measurements of total (116, 121) and regional perfusion are *1)* the glucose-induced intestinal hyperemia that is confined to the mucosa (123) and *2)* the increase in gastric mucosal blood flow that accompanies acid secretion (A. P. Shepherd and J. W. Kiel, unpublished observations).

Despite these advances made possible by the present state of laser-Doppler blood flowmetry, calibration in absolute flow units would be highly desirable, and it would greatly facilitate comparisons among laboratories, among tissues, and from one location to another on a given preparation. Unfortunately at this writing a universally applicable calibration constant has not been attained. For example, even within skeletal muscle, the slopes of the relation between LDV and microsphere estimates of blood flow are different for gracilis and cremaster muscles (128). Thus because of local variations possibly in the optical properties of tissue, local red blood cell concentrations, vascular density or geometry, or other factors, it has not been possible to apply in one tissue a calibration factor obtained in another, although claims to the contrary have been made (33).

MOTION NOISE AND OTHER PROBLEMS. Laser-Doppler velocimetric blood flowmeters are exquisitely sensitive motion detectors. Unfortunately many extraneous sources of noise cause mechanical vibrations in the same frequency range as Doppler shifts produced by red blood cells perfusing tissue. Examples are recorder chart motors, perfusion pumps, skeletal muscle fasciculations, and the diffusion of macromolecules. In fact when the vascular supply to a perfused preparation is occluded, the LDV signal usually drops to a low, small-positive value. In this instance imperceptible tissue motion relative to the probe, internal tissue motion, macromolecular diffusion, vasomotion, red blood cell setting, and other factors could contribute to the signal that was not zero in the absence of net blood flow. Additionally the relations between LDV and independent measurements of total blood flow, when extrapolated to zero blood flow, yield a positive intercept on the LDV axis (55, 132). Because most physiologists trust an "occlusive zero" value, this problem can easily be overcome in isolated perfused preparations, but it cannot be eliminated at a tissue locus that precludes vascular occlusion to obtain a zero.

In the gastrointestinal tract, motion artifacts can be a major problem because of the inherent motility of the stomach and intestine. As Figure 17 shows, spikes in the LDV signal occurred during arterial occlusion. These artifacts can only be due to motility. Also a more complicated issue is the rhythmic oscillations that frequently occur in the LDV signals regardless of whether the signal is obtained from the mucosa or muscularis (Fig. 18). These oscillations could be due entirely to motion artifacts or to motility-related oscillations in gastric mucosal blood flow. At this writing it is not clear which explanation is correct; however, it is worth noting that other techniques such as thermal probes and in vivo microscopy also indicate that gastric mucosal blood flow oscillates at approximately the same frequency as gastric motility. In addition to creating artifacts in the LDV signal or causing true oscillations in mucosal blood flow, gastrointestinal motility can cause another complication, the loss of optical coupling between the probe and the tissue of interest. The loss of optical coupling and motility artifacts are significant obstacles that will have to be overcome before laser-Doppler blood flowmetry can be used in combination with endoscopy. Regarding optical coupling, laser-Doppler blood flowmeters vary in their performance depending on their optical design. Some can operate only if the optical probe is brought into light contact with tissue, whereas others provide a useful signal even if the probe tip is 1–2 mm away from the tissue of interest. Additionally the loss of optical coupling can readily be recognized in those instruments that provide a readout of the DC intensity level.

## AMINOPYRINE CLEARANCE AND OTHER pH TRAPPING TECHNIQUES

### Overview of pH Trapping Methods

The pH trapping techniques, particularly aminopyrine clearance, played a unique and pivotal role in the evolution of our current techniques for measuring mucosal blood flow. When the aminopyrine clearance technique was first proposed by Jacobson et al. (53) in 1966, it appeared to be the ideal method for meas-

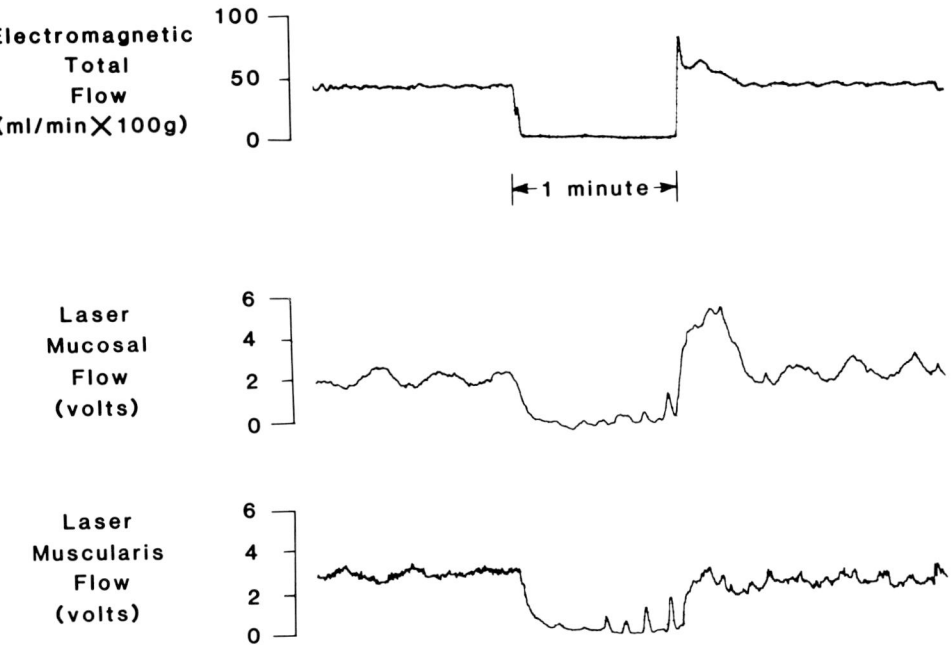

FIG. 17. Reactive hyperemia and motility artifacts in laser-Doppler blood flow tracings. In isolated loop of canine small bowel, spikes in laser-Doppler velocimetry tracings during arterial occlusion are motility artifacts. Both mucosal and muscularis perfusion seem to undergo motility-related oscillations (also see Fig. 18). Note that following arterial occlusion both total and mucosal blood flow tracings displayed characteristic reactive hyperemia, but reactive hyperemia was absent in muscularis. [From Shepherd and Riedel (122).]

uring gastric mucosal blood flow and the fulfillment of a quest that began with Beaumont's observations of the mucosal color variations in St. Martin's stomach. As a research tool, aminopyrine clearance not only allowed for repeated measurements in the same stomach in a conscious animal, but most significantly it also provided a quantitative measurement in milliliters per minute. Partly because of the apparent simplicity of its underlying principles and largely because its results concurred with longstanding speculations on the relationship between mucosal function and blood flow, aminopyrine clearance rapidly became the gold standard for measuring gastric mucosal blood flow.

Although limitations and peculiar results were noted almost immediately after the method was introduced, the lack of an accepted, alternative technique precluded a completely objective assessment of aminopyrine clearance. Furthermore the availability of any technique with the potential capability of measuring gastric mucosal blood flow led to the acceptance of its underlying assumptions largely on circumstantial evidence. However, with the advent of alternative techniques, a growing number of experimental situations were identified in which the results obtained with aminopyrine clearance conflicted with those yielded by other methods for assessing gastric mucosal blood flow. Then in the late 1970s it was found that aminopyrine accumulated not only in the gastric lumen but also in isolated gastric glands and parietal cells. Furthermore the accumulation of aminopyrine depended on parietal cell function. Finally in the early 1980s it was shown that aminopyrine clearance measurements reflected not only mucosal blood flow but parietal cell function as well.

It is now clear that the passage of aminopyrine from the blood to the gastric lumen is not the simple blood flow–limited process portrayed by the pH partition hypothesis (see *Theoretical Background*, below) and that the clearance of aminopyrine depends on other factors in addition to mucosal blood flow. Consequently it must be concluded that aminopyrine clearance is not a valid technique for measuring mucosal blood flow. Although the other pH trapping techniques (i.e., aniline clearance, neutral red clearance, and barbital clearance) have not been critically investigated to the same extent as aminopyrine clearance, they are based on the same basic principles, they yield similar results, and they should also be viewed with caution.

*Theoretical Background*

Aminopyrine clearance and other pH trapping techniques for measuring gastric mucosal blood flow are based on the pH partition hypothesis developed by Shore et al. in 1956 (127). To explain the accumulation

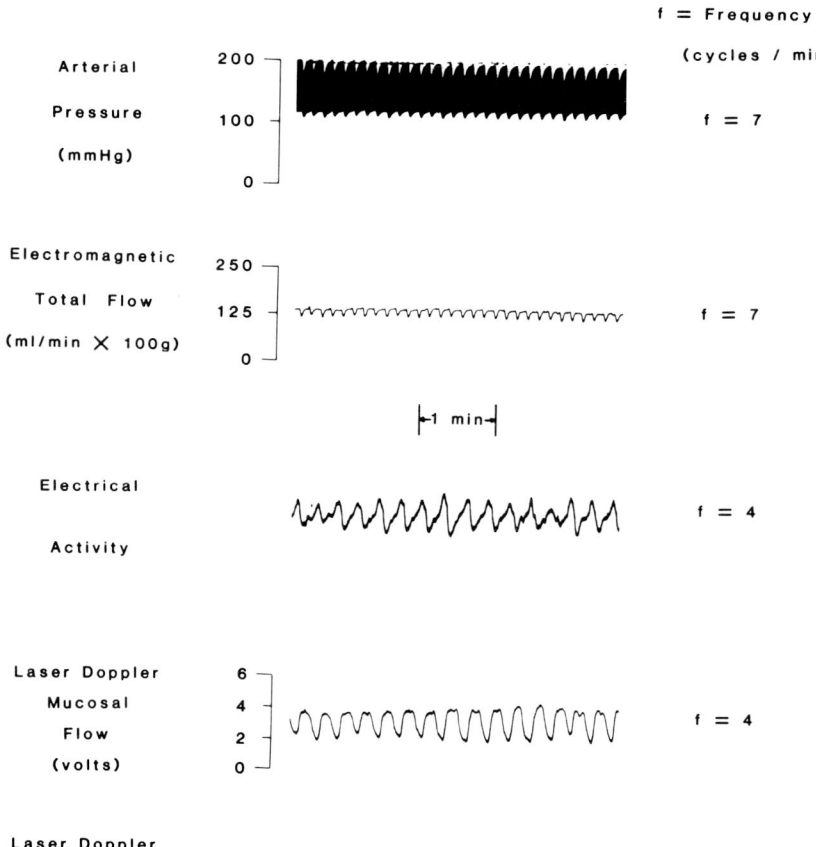

FIG. 18. Motility artifacts or motility-related oscillations in gastric blood flow? In chambered canine stomach flaps, laser-Doppler blood flow tracings oscillate at same frequency as electrical activity in muscularis. [From Kiel et al. (58).]

of parenterally administered weak bases in gastric juice, these investigators proposed that the gastric mucosa be viewed as a simple two-compartment model: one compartment represents the blood plasma and the other the gastric juice. A lipid barrier selectively permeable to undissociated compounds separates the two compartments (Fig. 19). In the presence of a substantial pH gradient, undissociated weak bases in the plasma compartment readily diffuse across the barrier and dissociate at the low pH of the gastric juice. Because the lipid barrier is impermeable to the ionized form of the base, the base is trapped and thus accumulates in the gastric lumen.

According to the Henderson-Hasselbalch equation for weak bases

$$\text{pH} - pK_a = \log([U]/[D]) \qquad (1)$$

where [U] and [D] are the concentrations of undissociated and dissociated weak base, respectively. Equation 1 can be simplified to

$$[D] = [U] \cdot 10^{(pK_a - \text{pH})} \qquad (2)$$

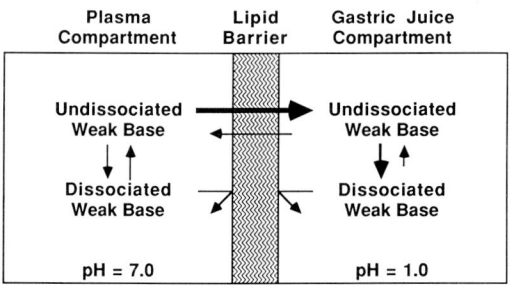

FIG. 19. Two-compartment model of the pH partition hypothesis. Gastric mucosa is represented as a plasma compartment and a gastric juice compartment separated by a lipoidal barrier selectively permeable to undissociated weak base. At plasma pH, weak base is predominantly undissociated, readily diffuses across barrier, and is "trapped" when dissociated in the low pH of gastric juice.

If R equals the concentration ratio of weak base in the gastric (g) and plasma (p) compartments, it follows that

$$R = \frac{[U]_g + [D]_g}{[U]_p + [D]_p} \qquad (3)$$

Substituting Equation 2 into Equation 3 gives

$$R = \frac{[U]_g + [U]_g \cdot 10^{(pK_a-pH)_g}}{[U]_p + [U]_p \cdot 10^{(pK_a-pH)_p}} \quad (4)$$

At equilibrium, $[U]_g = [U]_p$, and therefore Equation 4 simplifies to

$$R = \frac{1 + 10^{(pK_a-pH)_g}}{1 + 10^{(pK_a-pH)_p}} \quad (5)$$

For a weak base with $pK_a = 5$ and when plasma pH = 7.0 and gastric juice pH = 1.0

$$R = \frac{1 + 10^{(5-1)}}{1 + 10^{(5-7)}} \approx 1 \times 10^4 \quad (6)$$

In canine Heidenhain pouches maximally stimulated with histamine, Shore et al. (127) found that, for weak bases, the concentration ratio (R) between gastric juice and plasma increased as the negative log of the dissociation constant ($pK_a$) of the base increased. However, for weak bases with $pK_a$ values $\geq 5$, R did not increase with increasing $pK_a$ but remained relatively constant. According to the mucosal two-compartment model and calculations based on the Henderson-Hasselbalch equation, the predicted R for a weak base (e.g., aminopyrine) with $pK_a = 5$ should be $\sim 1 \times 10^4$ at a plasma pH of 7 and a gastric juice pH of 1. However, the ratio obtained experimentally was 40. The two-compartment model assumes that, at equilibrium, R depends solely on the $pK_a$ of the base, the pH gradient, and the permeability characteristics of the lipid barrier. An additional implicit assumption is that the delivery of the base into the system is infinite and that equilibrium is established independently of blood flow. However, because gastric mucosal blood flow is not infinite and because of the large discrepancy between the predicted and observed R, Shore et al. (127) concluded that the gastric luminal appearance of weak bases with $pK_a \geq 5$ was in fact blood flow dependent. Furthermore measurements of the arteriovenous concentration difference for aniline ($pK_a = 5$) showed that roughly two-thirds of the aniline in gastric blood was removed during passage through the stomach. This extraction ratio (64%) seemed to approximate the fraction of total blood flow passing through the mucosa. Therefore Shore et al. also concluded that the stronger bases ($pK_a \geq 5$) were completely cleared from mucosal blood and that their clearance by the stomach could possibly be used to measure mucosal blood flow. The fact that a wide variety of compounds, dissimilar except for their $pK_a$ values, were cleared by the stomach was taken as evidence that the process did not involve an active transport mechanism.

Clearance by definition is the volume of plasma from which a substance has been completely removed in a given period of time. The clearance technique was originally developed for the determination of renal glomerular filtration and subsequently was adapted for measuring renal plasma flow. For use in the kidney, clearance is formulated as

$$C_p = U_x \cdot V/P_x$$

where $C_p$ is the plasma clearance in milliliters per minute, $U_x$ and $P_x$ are the concentrations of the clearance marker (x) in urine and plasma, respectively, and V is the urine flow. To measure blood flow accurately with a clearance technique, the clearance marker must meet certain basic requirements. Because clearance is an application of the Fick principle and the law of conservation of mass, it is essential that the disposition of the marker be accounted for in a quantitative fashion (51). In practical terms this means that *1*) the concentrations of the marker in the appropriate fluids and the volume flow rate must be accurately determined; *2*) the marker must not be synthesized, degraded, or retransported (either excreted or reabsorbed) during or after the clearance process; *3*) the marker must not be modified or cleared by other organ systems; *4*) the marker must be physiologically inert; and (5) the marker must be either completely cleared or extracted at a known and constant rate from the circulation of interest. The validity of any clearance measurement ultimately depends on the satisfactory fulfillment of these conditions by the clearance marker.

*Evaluation of Aminopyrine Clearance*

INITIAL STUDIES. Aminopyrine ($pK_a = 5$) was one of the weak bases investigated by Shore et al. (127) that appeared to be cleared by the stomach in a flow-dependent fashion. In 1966 Jacobson et al. (53) evaluated aminopyrine clearance as a technique for measuring mucosal blood flow in canine Heidenhain pouch preparations. Although aminopyrine accumulation was significantly greater during stimulated acid secretion than when exogenous acid was placed in the lumen, they confirmed that the accumulation of aminopyrine depended on a low luminal pH. They also noted that, during stimulated acid secretion, R was relatively constant over time (R ≈ 40) and that R was relatively unaffected by changes in blood aminopyrine concentration. Because R was independent of the blood aminopyrine concentration, they concluded that the blood concentrations of aminopyrine in their animals were below the transport maximum for the mucosal barrier and that aminopyrine was completely cleared from the mucosal blood.

To test whether the process by which aminopyrine was removed from the blood fulfilled the requirements of the Fick principle, Jacobson et al. (53) demonstrated that aminopyrine was not removed from the blood by organs other than the stomach, that 58% of the aminopyrine in gastric blood was removed during passage through the stomach, that all the aminopyrine removed from the gastric blood was fully recoverable from the gastric juice, and that acidified aminopyrine in the gastric lumen was not reabsorbed. They also noted that large doses of aminopyrine did not alter the volume rate of secretion or the acid concentration in the gastric juice during stimulated acid secretion. Because there was no unaccountable loss of aminopyrine and because aminopyrine appeared to be completely cleared from mucosal blood, they concluded that the accumulation of aminopyrine by the stomach met the requirements of the Fick principle and that the clearance of aminopyrine could be used to measure mucosal blood flow. For the stomach

$$C_p = [AP]_g \cdot V/[AP]_p$$

where $C_p$ is the plasma clearance of aminopyrine in milliliters per minute, $[AP]_g$ and $[AP]_p$ are the aminopyrine concentrations in gastric juice and plasma, respectively, and V is the volume rate of gastric secretion. They also pointed out that, if the clearance relationship were valid and $R = [AP]_g/[AP]_p$, then $R = C_p/V$ as well. In other words, R would also reflect the ratio of mucosal blood flow to secretory rate. For example, if $R = 40$, then 40 ml of blood were required for each milliliter of gastric juice secreted.

In establishing their technique for measuring gastric mucosal blood flow, Jacobson et al. (53) also investigated the relationship between acid secretion and aminopyrine clearance. In response to graded infusions of either histamine or gastrin, gastric acid and volume secretion increased in parallel so that the concentration of HCl remained relatively constant except at the lowest secretory rates. As secretion increased in response to both secretagogues, R rapidly declined from initially high values at low secretory rates to a consistent plateau value of 30–40 when secretion was near maximal. Over the entire secretory range, there was a strong linear correlation between plasma aminopyrine clearance and the volume rate of gastric juice secretion.

They also investigated the effect of several secretory inhibitors during stimulated acid secretion and again found a linear correlation between plasma aminopyrine clearance and gastric secretion (i.e., when secretion was inhibited, aminopyrine clearance also fell). However, the response to two levels of isoproterenol infusion during histamine-stimulated acid secretion was particularly noteworthy, as shown in Figure 20. At the low dosage of isoproterenol, gastric volume secretion was relatively unaffected, but there was a significant increase in R. Consequently, plasma aminopyrine clearance was also increased. At the higher dosage of isoproterenol, there was a further increase in R, but gastric volume secretion fell to a greater extent so that plasma aminopyrine clearance also decreased. Based on the observation that low doses of isoproterenol caused an increase in plasma aminopyrine clearance without the corresponding change in gastric secretion seen in their other experiments, Jacobson et al. (53) concluded that "secretory changes induce corresponding circulatory alterations, but the reverse relationship, that is, alteration of secretion by a change in blood flow, is seen only when blood flow is reduced to a limiting value." Furthermore, the fact that secretion and aminopyrine clearance could be dissociated was taken as evidence that the two pro-

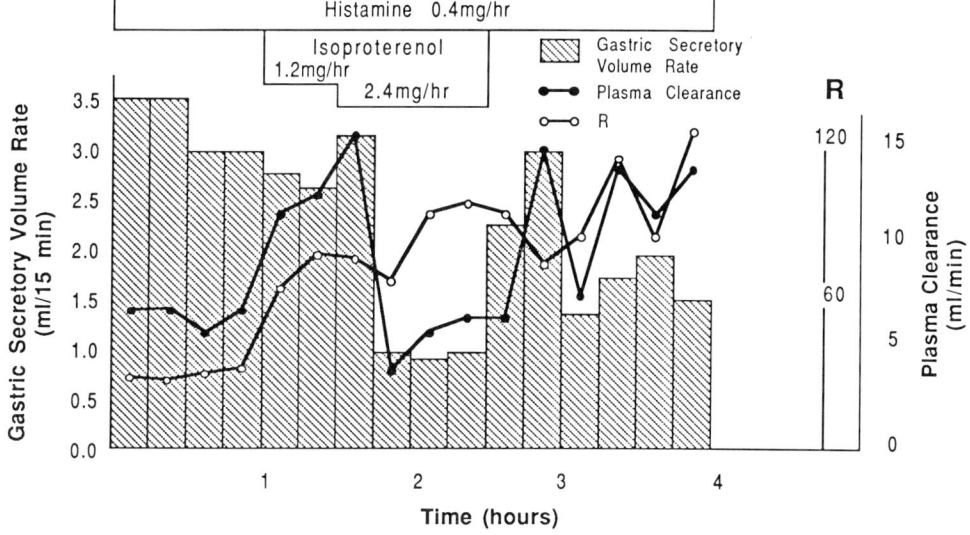

FIG. 20. Dissociation of gastric secretion and aminopyrine clearance. In a histamine-stimulated Heidenhain pouch, a low dose of isoproterenol greatly increased aminopyrine clearance but did not change gastric volume secretion. However, the higher dose depressed both aminopyrine clearance and gastric secretion. R, concentration ratio. [Adapted from Jacobson et al. (53).]

cesses were not inextricably linked and that aminopyrine was not actively secreted by the gastric mucosa.

Although the initial experiments with aminopyrine clearance provided circumstantial evidence of its validity, the other techniques then available for measuring gastric mucosal blood flow (e.g., thermal conductivity or $^{42}$K distribution) were not generally accepted. Consequently a rigorous comparison of gastric mucosal blood flow measurements by aminopyrine clearance and another technique was not performed. However, in subsequent studies Jacobson et al. (52) and Swan and Jacobson (137) made simultaneous measurements of gastric volume secretion, aminopyrine clearance, and total blood flow in canine Heidenhain pouches stimulated with histamine and gastrin. As previously observed by Jacobson et al. (53), the increase in gastric secretion was paralleled closely by increases in aminopyrine clearance during graded infusions of both secretagogues. However, total blood flow was not significantly increased by graded infusions of either secretagogue. Even though total blood flow did not increase, aminopyrine clearance increased by roughly 300% and 200% during the graded infusions of histamine and gastrin, respectively. At the lowest infusion rate for both secretagogues, mucosal blood flow measured by aminopyrine clearance represented ~20% of the total blood flow, but during maximal secretion this fraction increased to ~50% (Fig. 21).

Simultaneous measurements of aminopyrine clearance and total blood flow were also made in canine chambered-stomach preparations by Moody (91, 92). As in the previous studies, Moody (91) found that aminopyrine clearance was directly related to acid secretion ($r = 0.89$), but unlike the previous studies, he found that aminopyrine clearance was a constant

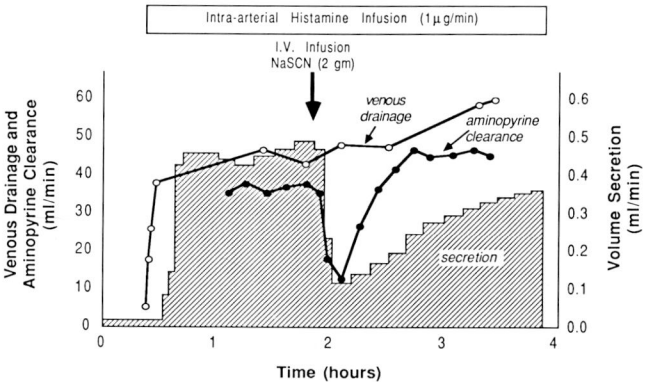

FIG. 22. Dissociation of total gastric blood flow and aminopyrine clearance during inhibition of acid secretion. In chambered canine stomach flap stimulated with histamine, thiocyanate poisoning greatly depressed aminopyrine clearance and secretion of gastric juice but did not alter total blood flow. [Adapted from Moody (91).]

fraction of total gastric blood flow (i.e., 59%) and that aminopyrine clearance was linearly correlated with total blood flow, which increased dramatically during graded infusions of histamine. In addition, Moody also investigated the vascular and secretory responses during thiocyanate inhibition of histamine-stimulated acid secretion, as shown in Figures 22 and 23. Figure 22 shows that, after administration of thiocyanate, the decrease in gastric secretion was paralleled by a fall in aminopyrine clearance, although total blood flow was unchanged. Similarly in Figure 23 gastric acid secretion and aminopyrine clearance were both severely attenuated by thiocyanate, but total blood flow and oxygen consumption were unaffected. Furthermore, the distribution of $^{42}$K between the gastric layers was also unaffected by thiocyanate, indicating that no redistribution of total blood flow had occurred (92).

The fall in aminopyrine clearance with acid secretion, despite the fact that the pH of the mucosal bathing solution was sufficient to support "a large movement of aminopyrine" and the lack of change in total blood flow, oxygen consumption, or blood flow distribution led Moody to conclude that "aminopyrine is not a true measure of mucosal perfusion during thiocyanate administration" and that the luminal pH might not "reflect the true pH at the sites where aminopyrine passes from the blood to the gastric lumen" (92). He further speculated that "the aminopyrine technique was measuring only a fraction of mucosal blood flow" and that "it is quite possible that aminopyrine is cleared from that portion of the capillary bed that perfuses the region of the acid-secreting cells" (91). These speculations were supported by the consistent linear correlation between aminopyrine clearance and acid secretion.

USE IN NONSECRETING STOMACH. Although Jacobson et al. (53) had shown that aminopyrine accumulation was significantly greater during stimulated acid secre-

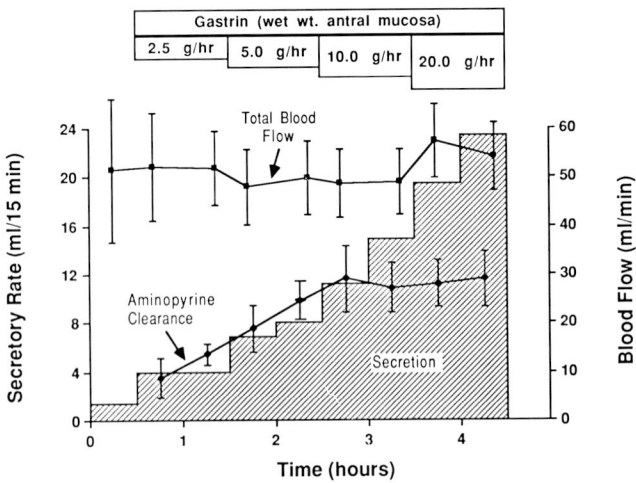

FIG. 21. Dissociation of total gastric blood flow and aminopyrine clearance during stimulated acid secretion. In Heidenhain pouch, graded gastrin infusion greatly increased aminopyrine clearance without changing total blood flow. [Adapted from Swan and Jacobson (137).]

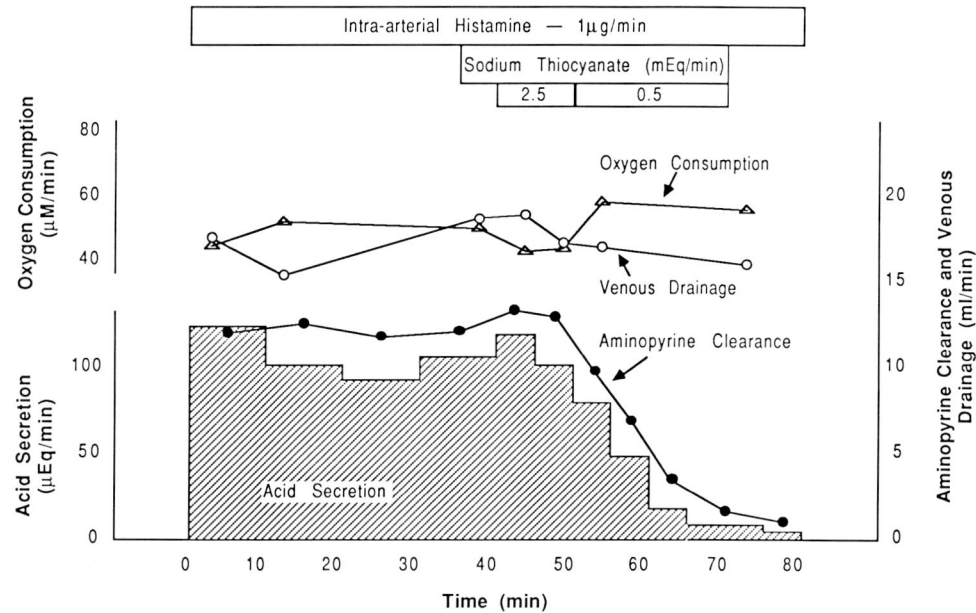

FIG. 23. Dissociation of gastric oxygen consumption and aminopyrine clearance during inhibition of acid secretion. In chambered canine stomach flap stimulated with histamine, thiocyanate poisoning depressed aminopyrine clearance nearly to zero without altering either total blood flow or gastric oxygen uptake. [Adapted from Moody (92).]

tion than in the resting stomach at a comparable luminal pH and although Moody (91, 92) had demonstrated that aminopyrine clearance was invalid during the inhibition of acid secretion despite the presence of luminal acid, the pH partition hypothesis implies that resting mucosal blood flow measurements can be made providing the pH gradient is maintained. Therefore a number of investigators attempted to measure resting mucosal blood flow by aminopyrine clearance with exogenous hydrochloric acid instilled into the gastric lumen. In 1968 Harper et al. (46) compared aminopyrine clearance and total blood flow in isolated feline stomachs under resting and stimulated conditions. In response to histamine or gastrin, aminopyrine clearance and total blood flow were linearly correlated with acid secretion. Previous studies with these two secretagogues showed that aminopyrine clearance increased, whereas total blood flow was unchanged (52, 137) or that aminopyrine clearance was a constant fraction of total blood flow (91). However, Harper et al. (46) found that "the increase in total flow was due to the increase in mucosal flow, nonmucosal flow remaining almost unchanged over the whole secretory range." This conclusion was based on the observation that when total blood flow was held constant at three different flow rates, aminopyrine clearance was still linearly correlated with acid secretion. Furthermore, they also noted that the aminopyrine clearance values obtained in resting stomachs instilled with exogenous acid were identical to the clearance values calculated from the linear regression line at zero secretion. Therefore they also concluded that "the aminopyrine technique of measuring mucosal blood flow is no less valid when acid is instilled into the resting stomach than during secretion." Similar findings and conclusions were subsequently made by Rudick et al. (107) with canine fundic pouches. Rudick et al. also used aminopyrine clearance in antral pouches containing exogenous acid and found appropriate directional changes in mucosal flow in response to various vasodilators.

To study the gastric circulatory responses to secretory inhibitors, Cowley and Code (27) employed aminopyrine clearance in resting canine stomachs instilled with 0.1 N HCl. Based on the aminopyrine concentration difference between jugular and gastroepiploic venous blood, they calculated that the mean aminopyrine extraction ratio in the unstimulated stomach was 25% as opposed to the 64% (analine) and 58% in histamine-stimulated stomachs noted by Shore et al. (127) and Jacobson et al. (53), respectively. Consequently they concluded that the clearance of aminopyrine was probably incomplete in the resting stomach despite the presence of exogenous acid in the lumen. However, the clearance values were sufficiently consistent that they also concluded that the extraction ratio was relatively fixed and that aminopyrine clearance could be used to determine qualitative changes in mucosal blood flow in nonsecreting, passively acidified stomachs. In response to vasopressin, norepinephrine, and a single bolus of gastrin, aminopyrine clearance in resting canine Heidenhain pouches decreased significantly, indicating a fall in mucosal blood flow, whereas in response to epinephrine, mucosal blood flow increased.

COMPARISONS WITH OTHER METHODS. The initial appeal and rapid acceptance of the aminopyrine clearance technique as the de facto standard for measuring gastric mucosal blood flow was due in part to the plausibility of the pH partition hypothesis, the general agreement of the aminopyrine clearance data with the pH partition hypothesis, and the desire for an accurate, quantitative technique for measuring mucosal blood flow. It should also be noted though that the almost universal acceptance of the aminopyrine clearance technique was largely due to the fact that the other techniques available for measuring gastric mucosal blood flow were seriously questioned. Consequently no comparative studies were performed to validate the method. However, when Archibald et al. (2) introduced the microsphere technique for measuring gastric mucosal blood flow in 1974 (see MICROSPHERE TECHNIQUE, p. 1335), a number of investigators began challenging the accuracy and validity of aminopyrine clearance.

In their initial study, Archibald et al. (2) compared measurements of mucosal blood flow determined by aminopyrine clearance and microspheres [15 ± 5 (SD) μm diam] in resting canine chambered-stomach preparations. Despite the presence of exogenous acid, aminopyrine clearance estimates of mucosal blood flow were significantly less than microsphere estimates during control (2.4 vs. 5.5 ml/min) and following isoproterenol (4.5 vs. 20.3 ml/min). Although both techniques showed an increase in mucosal blood flow with isoproterenol, microspheres indicated a 270% increase, whereas aminopyrine clearance indicated only an 80% increase. Consequently they concluded that "aminopyrine clearance does not correlate with microsphere measured mucosal flow during isoproterenol infusion, despite the presence of exogenous acid on the mucosal surface."

In a subsequent study Archibald et al. (3) compared the two techniques in a more rigorous fashion during infusions of histamine or isoproterenol. As shown in Figure 24, over a wide range of flow, aminopyrine clearance was linearly correlated with mucosal blood flow measured by the microsphere technique during administration of histamine ($r = 0.96$) and isoproterenol ($r = 0.78$). However, in both cases, aminopyrine clearance significantly underestimated the microsphere-determined mucosal blood flow. Analysis of the slopes of the two regression lines showed that the discrepency between the two techniques was relatively minor during histamine administration but very pronounced during isoproterenol administration. During histamine administration, aminopyrine clearance was 83% of the microsphere measurement, but during isoproterenol administration, aminopyrine clearance

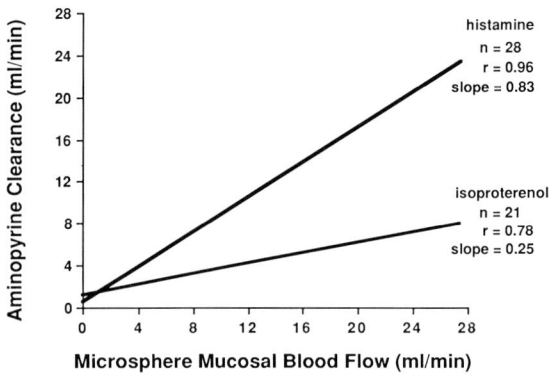

FIG. 24. Comparison of gastric mucosal blood flow measurements by aminopyrine clearance and microspheres. During infusions of histamine or isoproterenol, aminopyrine clearance values showed significant linear correlation with microsphere determinations in chambered canine stomach flaps. However, slopes of regression lines show that aminopyrine clearance consistently underestimated blood flow measured by microspheres. Furthermore discrepancy between the two methods was even greater in the absence of acid secretion (isoproterenol). Linear regression lines are shown; data points omitted for clarity. [Adapted from Archibald et al. (3).]

reflected only 25% of microsphere-determined mucosal blood flow.

Additionally Archibald et al. (3) verified that mucosal blood flow measured by either aminopyrine clearance or microspheres was linearly related to the rate of histamine-stimulated acid secretion. Interestingly the ratio of microsphere-determined mucosal blood flow to aminopyrine clearance was relatively constant at 1.25 over most of the secretory range; however, at lower secretory rates the ratio increased dramatically (Fig. 25). This increase in the ratio of microsphere-to-aminopyrine clearance was taken as evidence that the fraction of mucosal blood flow measured by aminopyrine clearance varied depending on the secretory state of the mucosa. Furthermore, the aminopyrine-to-microsphere clearance ratio or "clearance fraction" was also shown to decline with increasing blood flow in resting and isoproterenol-treated segments. Archibald et al. (3) concluded that "since the clearance fraction can vary, caution seems advisable in comparing clearances obtained under different experimental conditions unless it can be demonstrated that the clearance fraction has not been altered." Marked discrepancies between mucosal blood flow determinations by microspheres and aminopyrine clearance were subsequently noted by Cheung et al. (21) after mucosal injury with aspirin, bile salt, and ethanol. Later Miller et al. (87) also concluded that aminopyrine clearance was inaccurate in aspirin-damaged gastric mucosa.

From a practical standpoint, there were a number of technical problems associated with the use of the original aminopyrine clearance technique, most notably the complicated and time-consuming photometric assay procedure (19) and the toxicity of aminopyrine

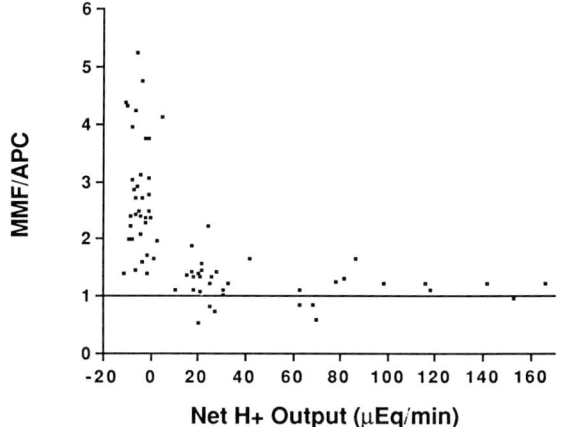

FIG. 25. Effect of acid secretion rate on ratio of microsphere-measured mucosal blood flow to aminopyrine clearance (MMF/APC). If two techniques measured same quantity, ratio would equal one. Most data points lie above *solid line* showing aminopyrine clearance underestimated microsphere determinations. Note disparity increased markedly at low rates of acid secretion. [Adapted from Archibald et al. (3).]

to both humans and animals at the plasma concentrations necessary to achieve measurable concentrations (51). In 1976 Tague and Jacobson (138) proposed the use of [$^{14}$C]aminopyrine as a clearance marker in place of unlabeled aminopyrine. In autoperfused, chambered canine gastric segments under control conditions or after administration of histamine or histamine plus vasopressin, they found no significant difference between the clearances of simultaneously administered [$^{14}$C]aminopyrine and unlabeled aminopyrine. Similarly, when [$^{14}$C]aminopyrine alone was used, the clearance values were not significantly different from the clearance values obtained when both [$^{14}$C]aminopyrine and unlabeled aminopyrine were used. However, even though regression analysis of the clearance measurements with the two markers showed a strong linear correlation ($r = 0.87$), the slope of the regression line was significantly less than 1.0, indicating that the [$^{14}$C]aminopyrine clearance was consistently less than the unlabeled aminopyrine clearance (Fig. 26). This discrepancy between measurements by the two markers was not due to competitive inhibition of an active transport mechanism, because they also found that [$^{14}$C]aminopyrine clearance during histamine infusion was unaffected by a large bolus of unlabeled aminopyrine.

Because [$^{14}$C]aminopyrine could be detected at much smaller and less toxic concentrations than unlabeled aminopyrine, Guth et al. (44) evaluated [$^{14}$C]-aminopyrine for clearance measurements of gastric mucosal blood flow in humans during graded infusions of pentagastrin. As previously apparent in animal studies with unlabeled aminopyrine, they found that R was inversely related to acid secretion and that there was a strong linear relationship between acid secretion and [$^{14}$C]aminopyrine clearance. No toxic effects of aminopyrine were noted in any of the subjects at the dosage levels administered. Because of the similarity between the results with humans and animals and because of the lack of toxicity, Guth et al. (44) concluded that "the [$^{14}$C]aminopyrine clearance procedure appears to be a satisfactory and potentially useful technique for studying gastric mucosal blood flow in man."

Despite the simplification of the clearance technique by Tague and Jacobson (138) and the optimism of Guth et al. (44), new techniques for measuring gastric mucosal blood flow continued to yield measurements in sharp disagreement with aminopyrine clearance measurements. In 1982 Murakami et al. (96) developed the contact electrode hydrogen gas clearance technique (see HYDROGEN CLEARANCE, p. 1361) for measuring mucosal blood flow. Simultaneous measurements of mucosal blood flow by aminopyrine clearance and hydrogen gas clearance were made in rats during graded infusions of pentagastrin and isoproterenol. Aminopyrine clearance was linearly related to hydrogen gas clearance during administration of both pentagastrin ($r = 0.935$) and isoproterenol ($r = 0.777$); however, as seen previously with the microsphere technique, aminopyrine clearance significantly underestimated mucosal blood flow as measured by hydrogen gas clearance during isoproterenol infusion. Of greater importance was the observation that at the highest dosage of pentagastrin, the relative increase in mucosal blood flow measured by aminopyrine clearance was significantly greater than by hydrogen gas clearance. This overestimation of mucosal blood flow by aminopyrine clearance during pen-

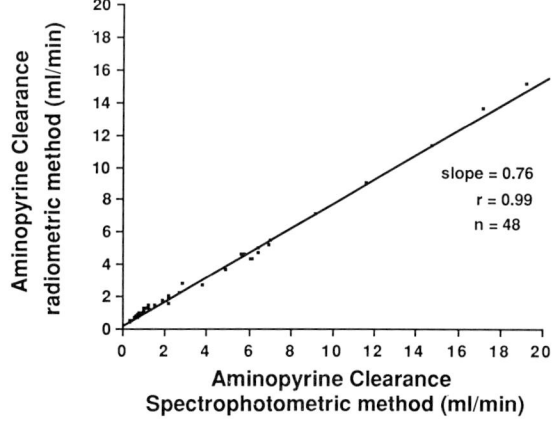

FIG. 26. Comparison of aminopyrine clearances determined spectrophotometrically and with $^{14}$C-labeled aminopyrine. Although measurements were highly correlated, slope of regression line, which is significantly different from 1.0, indicates that spectrophotometric method overestimated [$^{14}$C]aminopyrine clearance. Spectrophotometric method requires much higher plasma concentrations of aminopyrine than isotope method. [Data from Tague and Jacobson (138).]

tagastrin-stimulated acid secretion was subsequently confirmed by Leung et al. (71) with hydrogen gas clearance in rabbits. In response to pentagastrin infusion, aminopyrine clearance increased 216%, whereas hydrogen gas clearance and left gastric artery electromagnetic blood flow increased only 22% and 17%, respectively (Fig. 27). Similarly, Holm-Rutili and Berglindh (48) also found that aminopyrine clearance overestimated mucosal blood flow in rats during pentagastrin stimulation when compared with laser-Doppler velocimetry and single-vessel blood flows calculated from velocity measurements made during in vivo microscopy.

INVALID ASSUMPTIONS. The preceding evidence indicates that aminopyrine clearance does not accurately reflect gastric mucosal blood flow as measured by various other techniques in a number of experimental situations. These findings do not necessarily invalidate the aminopyrine clearance technique, but they do impose severe limitations on when and how the technique can be used. For a measuring technique to be considered invalid, particularly a technique that has achieved the status of aminopyrine clearance, it must be demonstrated that the technique does not obey or fulfill the fundamental principles and assumptions on which the technique is based.

As discussed, aminopyrine clearance is based on the pH partition hypothesis. In the pH partition hypothesis the gastric mucosa is divided into two fluid compartments, the plasma and the gastric juice, separated by a simple lipoidal barrier. When a substantial pH gradient is established between the two compartments, weak bases such as aminopyrine are un-ionized at plasma pH and are able to diffuse across the lipid barrier where they become trapped as they are ionized by the low pH of the gastric juice. In the original two-compartment model, Shore et al. (127) assumed that at equilibrium the net flux of a weak base is zero and, given a plasma pH of 7 and a gastric juice pH of 1, the predicted concentration ratio between gastric juice and plasma should be $1 \times 10^4$ for a weak base with a $pK_a$ of 5 (see Fig. 19). However, the experimentally determined R value was 40 rather than $1 \times 10^4$. Therefore the net flux could not be equal to 0. Consequently, according to the model, the movement of aminopyrine from the plasma compartment to gastric juice compartment must be limited either by the diffusion characteristics of aminopyrine in the barrier (diffusion limited), or by the convective delivery of aminopyrine to the barrier (blood flow limited), or by a combination of both.

The two-compartment model is a gross oversimplification of the gastric mucosa. Although it provides an explanation for the accumulation of weak bases in the gastric lumen, it is a static model, it does not address temporal aspects of the accumulation process, it ignores the dynamic range of gastric function, and it obviously oversimplifies the epithelial and micro-

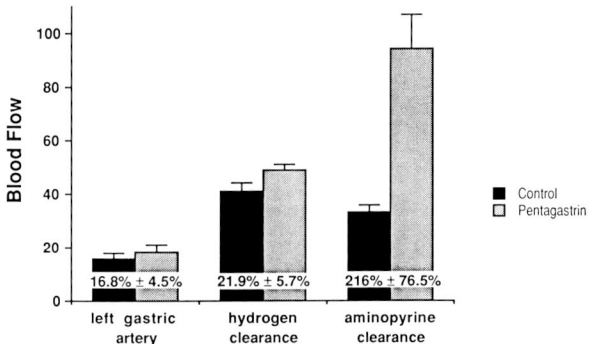

FIG. 27. Aminopyrine clearance overestimates gastric mucosal blood flow during stimulated acid secretion. In rabbits, pentagastrin increased blood flow measured by all 3 techniques. Measurements by electromagnetic flow probe and hydrogen clearance showed similar increases in blood flow (17% and 22%, respectively), but an inordinate increase in aminopyrine clearance (216%) occurred that was quantitatively inconsistent with the other two measurements. Flow units are left gastric artery, ml/min; aminopyrine and hydrogen clearance, $ml \cdot min^{-1} \cdot 100\ g^{-1}$. [Data from Leung et al. (71).]

vascular components of the gastric mucosal barrier. Based on circumstantial evidence, Shore et al. (127) concluded that weak bases were probably completely cleared from mucosal blood and that the process was therefore blood flow limited. However, as pointed out earlier, the validity of the clearance technique as an accurate measure of blood flow depends ultimately on the complete or fixed extraction of the clearance marker. For the gastric mucosal clearance of aminopyrine, the true extraction of aminopyrine cannot be determined because it is not possible to obtain pure mucosal venous blood.

In their initial feasibility study, Jacobson et al. (53) also concluded that aminopyrine was completely cleared from gastric mucosal blood. This conclusion was based on the fact that, during stimulated secretion, the measured R values were relatively constant over a range of plasma aminopyrine concentrations; if clearance were less than complete, the R value should have decreased with increasing plasma aminopyrine concentration. They further reasoned that, if mucosal extraction were significantly less than 100%, nonmucosal blood flow would have to approach zero to account for the observed total aminopyrine extraction (≈60%). Because of the various dissimilar compounds that were cleared by the stomach, they also concluded that an active transport mechanism was not involved in the clearance process. However, as later noted by Jacobson (51), "these arguments do not, of themselves, prove that the gastric mucosa completely clears aminopyrine from its circulation. This evidence merely makes that assumption a likely one."

In 1976 Berglindh et al. (11, 12) developed a technique for isolating rabbit gastric glands and proposed using aminopyrine accumulation as an index of acid production and parietal cell activity. Significant accumulation of aminopyrine occurred in both resting and stimulated gastric glands. Although it was not surprising that aminopyrine accumulated in the stimulated glands because, as they pointed out, "in a stimulated, secreting gland the HCl is formed inside the parietal cells, probably in the intracellular canaliculi, where the aminopyrine would accumulate," it was somewhat surprising that aminopyrine accumulated in the resting glands. To explain the resting accumulation, they speculated that "the only conceivable structure fit to contain preformed acid in a resting parietal cell would be the cytoplasmic tubulo-vesicles." As shown in Figure 28, accumulations of aminopyrine were also observed by Sonnenberg et al. (129, 130) in isolated parietal cells under both resting and stimulated conditions.

Because aminopyrine was accumulated in both resting and stimulated parietal cells, Sonnenberg and Blum (129) investigated aminopyrine clearance in healthy human subjects and in subjects with pernicious anemia. In healthy subjects, bolus injections followed by continuous infusions of [$^{14}$C]aminopyrine caused an initial rapid rise and subsequent exponential decline in both the R and clearance values, despite a relatively constant acid secretion. Similarly infusions of pentagastrin also caused transient spikes in both the R and clearance values, although acid secretion remained elevated. However, in patients with pernicious anemia without a significant parietal cell population, they observed no initial increase and a subsequent fall in the R or clearance values after bolus injections of [$^{14}$C]aminopyrine, nor were there any spikes following pentagastrin infusion. If the gastric mucosa behaved as a two-compartment model and aminopyrine clearance were limited only by blood flow, the transient changes in the R and clearance values should not have occurred after either the bolus infusions of aminopyrine or the pentagastrin infusions, because the acid secretory state was stable. The fact that these transients did not occur in patients with pernicious anemia and the fact that aminopyrine is sequestered by isolated parietal cells led Sonnenberg and Blum (129) to conclude that the mucosa behaves as a three-compartment model with the parietal cells serving as a storage compartment. The transient changes could thus be attributed to storage of aminopyrine after the initial bolus and a volume washout during stimulated acid secretion.

The results of Sonnenberg and Blum (129) were subsequently confirmed by Müller-Lissner et al. (95) in both humans and dogs. Müller-Lissner et al. also concluded that the observed peaks could be explained by volume washout of aminopyrine previously stored in parietal cells and that "the peaks might reflect parietal cell function and the steady state levels might reflect both parietal cell function and gastric mucosal blood flow." They further stated that because "in many instances there is a parallel change of gastric mucosal blood flow and of parietal cell function, changes in aminopyrine clearance has [sic] the following limitations: (1) it is only a relative measure of gastric mucosal blood flow; (2) steady state conditions in plasma and gastric juice are required (up to 2 hrs after the initial bolus); and (3) the acid secretion rate should remain constant during the experiment."

When taken in conjunction with the previously cited situations in which discrepancies were noted between aminopyrine clearance and other measurements of gastric mucosal blood flow, the limitations imposed on the technique by Müller-Lissner et al. (95) render aminopyrine clearance practically useless for experimental studies of gastric mucosal blood flow (109). However, the real significance of the variable storage and release of aminopyrine by parietal cells is that it invalidates the assumption that aminopyrine is completely cleared from mucosal blood, and it underscores the fact that the gastric mucosa is considerably more complicated than the simple, two-compartment model portrayed by the pH partition hypothesis. The facts that aminopyrine is stored in parietal cells and that the movement of aminopyrine into the gastric lumen varies with the level of parietal cell activity indicate that aminopyrine cannot be completely cleared from the mucosa and that the clearance fraction varies with parietal cell activity. These findings also show that processes other than diffusion and blood flow participate in the net transport of aminopyrine from blood to lumen. Because the accuracy of the clearance technique is crucially dependent on a constant extraction of the marker and because the extraction of aminopyrine is not only less than complete but also variable, the clearance of aminopyrine cannot be considered a valid technique for measuring gastric mucosal blood flow.

## HYDROGEN CLEARANCE

### History

Hydrogen clearance is rapidly gaining popularity as a technique for measuring gastric mucosal blood flow, but the method has not been used extensively in the

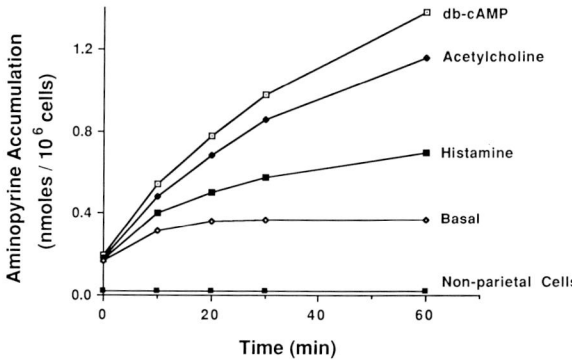

FIG. 28. Sequestration of aminopyrine by isolated parietal cells. Parietal cells accumulate significant quantities of aminopyrine; this sequestration is enhanced by agents listed. [Adapted from Sonnenberg et al. (130).]

gastrointestinal tract. The hydrogen clearance method, however, has a long history in other vascular beds, particularly in the cerebral circulation. For that use of hydrogen clearance as well as the general principles of polarography, Young (148) has provided an extensive review.

The use of inert gases as blood flow markers had its major beginnings in 1945 with the description by Kety and Schmidt (57) of the nitrous oxide method for determining cerebral blood flow. In his classic 1951 review of blood flow tracers, Kety (56) named hydrogen gas as a potential blood flow marker, and he noted that it was both metabolically inert and not normally present in the body. The other important properties of hydrogen are its solubility in lipids, its diffusibility in tissues, its low water-gas partition coefficient (0.018), and its rapid elimination by the pulmonary circulation. Although these properties qualified hydrogen gas as a potential blood flow tracer, methods for measuring dissolved hydrogen in tissue were not available until 1956 when Misrahy and Clark (89) recorded hydrogen potentials in the cerebral cortex of animals ventilated with hydrogen gas. Perturbations known to influence cerebral blood flow, such as $CO_2$ inhalation, indicated that the hydrogen potential did indeed reflect alterations in cerebral perfusion. In 1959 Clark and Bargeron (24, 25) used hydrogen electrodes placed intravascularly to detect cardiac shunts. In both of these early uses of hydrogen electrodes, blood flow assessments were only qualitative because the potentiometric method was neither linear nor selective for changes in hydrogen concentration.

Hydrogen polarography is based on the principle that the oxidation of hydrogen generates electrons: $H_2 \rightarrow 2H^+ + 2e^-$. Thus the reaction donates electrons to the electrode and causes current flow. Instead of recording potentials generated by the spontaneous oxidation of hydrogen, Hyman (50) in 1961 introduced the innovation of monitoring the current generated by a platinum electrode that catalyzed the reaction. The next advance in the $H_2$-electrode art was the realization that a positive voltage facilitated the electrode's acceptance of electrons liberated by the oxidation of hydrogen. In 1964 Aukland et al. (8) modified Hyman's polarographic method by biasing the electrode at +250 mV, and they showed that the electrode gave linear measurements of hydrogen concentration and that interference by other substances such as oxygen, hydrogen ion, and ascorbate was acceptably small. Aukland et al. (8) used an electrode inserted into tissue to demonstrate that hydrogen clearance correlated well with venous outflow in the canine myocardium and renal cortex. They employed both inspired hydrogen and close intra-arterial injections of hydrogen-saturated saline. The work of Aukland et al. (7, 8) thus founded hydrogen clearance as a flow-measuring technique; its applicability in the cerebral circulation was quickly established and it flourished.

By contrast, the application of hydrogen clearance in the gastrointestinal circulations has evolved very slowly. Until recently relatively few gastrointestinal studies have used hydrogen clearance. Mackie and Turner (77, 78) were the first to measure blood flow in the gastrointestinal tract with hydrogen clearance. In 1971, using two indicating electrodes, Mackie and Turner made simultaneous measurements of blood flow within the cardiac and pyloric regions of the rat stomach. Their electrodes were chronically implanted in the submucosa, they could not be used to measure mucosal blood flow, and they gave multiexponential washout curves. However, the method could be used in conscious animals, and it showed that gastric blood flow was reduced after vagotomy and hypoxia. Subsequently Semb (112) in 1979 inserted electrodes into the mucosa and submucosa of the dog stomach and found, using either hydrogen-saturated saline or inhaled hydrogen, that blood flow could be determined both in the antrum and the corpus. In subsequent studies with cats, Semb (113, 114, 115) used hydrogen clearance to study gastric mucosal blood flow changes in response to histamine, pentagastrin, isoproterenol, epinephrine, and test meals.

The current interest in hydrogen clearance as a method for measuring gastric mucosal blood flow began with the report of Murakami et al. (96), whose innovation was a surface electrode that consisted of an insulated platinum wire in the form of a coil spring. The surface electrode not only avoided the problem of tissue trauma that penetrating electrodes inflict but also had the advantage of generally yielding monoexponential washout curves in contrast to the multiexponential curves that Semb (112) and Mackie and Turner (77, 78) had obtained with penetrating electrodes. To test their method, Murakami et al. (96) compared hydrogen clearance curves obtained in rats with surface and penetrating electrodes, examined the extent of hydrogen loss into the gastric lumen, and compared hydrogen and aminopyrine clearances during infusions of isoproterenol or pentagastrin. Results obtained with contact electrodes were significantly correlated with aminopyrine clearance during the vasodilation induced by isoproterenol and pentagastrin. In a subsequent study Murakami et al. (97) showed that hydrogen clearance measurements of gastric mucosal blood flow were also significantly correlated with those obtained by LDV.

After the report by Murakami et al. (96) other investigators rapidly began to evaluate the hydrogen clearance method for measuring gastric mucosal blood flow with surface electrodes. Chueng and Sonnenschein (22) showed that hydrogen clearance measurements of gastric mucosal perfusion were significantly correlated with total venous outflow. The slope of the relationship was 1.21. This slope indicates that the ratio of hydrogen gas clearance to total gastric blood flow was ~82%, a value that agrees roughly with the finding of Archibald et al. (4), who used radioactive microspheres and reported that the ratio of mucosal to total gastric blood flow in dogs was 68% in the resting stomach and 87% during histamine stimulation.

Subsequent refinements were made by Ashley and Cheung (5), who used 3% hydrogen to eliminate the flammability and the hypoxia-producing effect of 100% hydrogen. With a slightly modified and more sensitive hydrogen electrode, they also showed that hydrogen gas clearance measurements were significantly correlated with microsphere estimates of gastric mucosal blood flow and that the slope of this relationship was 0.65 (Fig. 29). The slope of 0.65 suggested that mucosal blood flow as measured by hydrogen clearance was somewhat less than that of microsphere-determined blood flow. In a subsequent study, Leung et al. (71) further evaluated the use of 3% hydrogen. Saturation of tissues with the indicator is a basic requirement of all inert gas washout techniques for blood flow measurements. However, such equilibrium conditions cannot be achieved with pure hydrogen because it produces severe hypoxia. Leung et al. showed that with 3% hydrogen, an average of 15 min was required to reach a plateau in the rat gastric mucosa. With shorter periods of hydrogen administration, blood flow was overestimated, presumably because diffusion from hydrogen-saturated to hydrogen-poor regions contributes to the local clearance of hydrogen. A modification of the method has been used in combination with endoscopy to measure gastric mucosal blood flow in conscious dogs (6, 72).

*Principle of Measurement*

The Kety-Schmidt method (57) for accessing blood flow by the accumulation or washout of inert gases has been reviewed extensively elsewhere (56, 65). Fig-

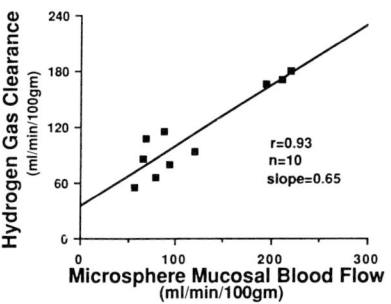

FIG. 29. Hydrogen gas clearance values significantly correlated with microsphere-measured gastric mucosal blood flow. In anterior corpus of canine stomach at gastrotomy, hydrogen underestimated microsphere-measured gastric mucosal perfusion as indicated by slope of regression line. [From Ashley and Cheung (5).]

ure 30 illustrates the principle of the inert gas method. As originally proposed by Kety and Schmidt, blood flow was assessed during the saturation of tissue by an inhaled inert gas. If an inert gas is inhaled or delivered in arterial blood until an equilibrium is obtained between blood and tissue, then at equilibrium the concentration in tissue is given by

$$100\, C_{tissue} = F \int_0^\infty C_{in(t)}\, dt - F \int_0^\infty C_{out(t)}\, dt$$

or

$$\text{tissue residue} = \text{entering} - \text{leaving}$$

where F is defined as blood flow per 100 g tissue and $C_{in}$ and $C_{out}$ are the indicator's concentrations in arterial and venous blood, respectively. At infinite time the tissue concentration is related to that of the blood by the partition coefficient $\lambda = C_{tissue}/C_{blood}$. Hence

$$100\, C_{tissue} = 100\, \lambda\, C(\infty)$$

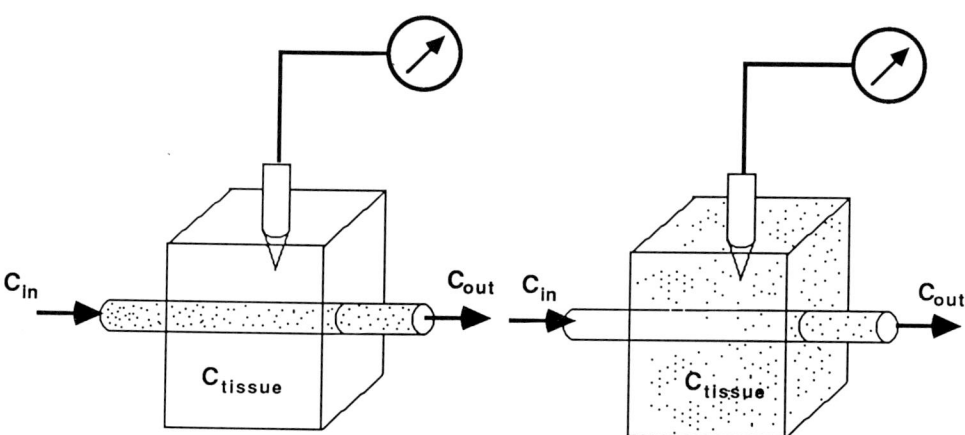

FIG. 30. Principle of hydrogen clearance technique for measuring blood flow. If instantaneous arterial ($C_{in}$) and venous ($C_{out}$) concentrations of indicator gas were known, blood flow could be determined from either tissue uptake or washout of hydrogen, but in practice only relative tissue hydrogen concentration is recorded. Also see Figs. 31 and 32.

Therefore, from these two equations it follows that

$$F = 100 \, \lambda \, \frac{C(\infty)}{\int_0^\infty C_{in(t)} - C_{out(t)} dt} = 100 \, \lambda \, \frac{\text{height}}{\text{area}}$$

Thus blood flow could be obtained from the tissue uptake or saturation curves, as shown in Figure 31, if the area between the arterial and venous saturation curves were known from time zero and if equilibrium were reached when $C_{in} = C_{out}$. However, this time may not be reached in saturation experiments with hydrogen and it cannot be determined with certainty, because only the tissue concentration of the indicator is usually monitored. Therefore one must also assume that equilibrium has been reached. If an approximate equilibrium value for $C(\infty)$ is used, the true flow will be overestimated.

In the desaturation experiment, typical of hydrogen clearance measurements, one assumes that an equilibrium has been reached after which the washout or desaturation is registered, as shown in Figure 32. It is also assumed that the arterial hydrogen concentration instantly falls to zero on the cessation of hydrogen administration. Here flow is also given by

$$F = 100 \, \lambda \cdot (\text{height/area})$$

but the area of interest is that below the washout curve, as shown in Figure 32.

If it is further assumed that the indicator (hydrogen) is being removed from a single well-mixed compartment, a monoexponential curve should result from which the half time ($t_{1/2}$) can be obtained. Thus

$$F = \ln(2)/t_{1/2} = 0.693/t_{1/2}$$

The advantage of the height-over-area algorithm is that it does not require the assumption of a monoexponential washout. The disadvantage is that the area under the entire washout curve must be integrated, whereas the monoexponential method is applied to a portion of the washout curve that is extrapolated to infinite time. In both cases the object is essentially the same, i.e., to obtain the indicator's mean transit time, because $t_{1/2}$ = area/height.

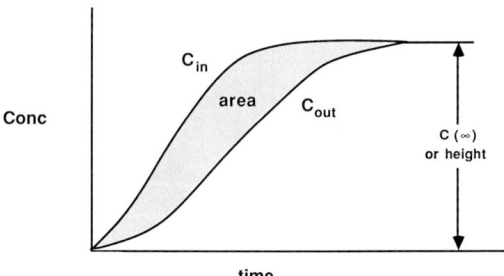

FIG. 31. Blood flow determined from tissue saturation or uptake of indicator. Blood flow could be determined from tissue uptake of hydrogen if instantaneous arterial ($C_{in}$) and venous ($C_{out}$) concentrations of hydrogen were known.

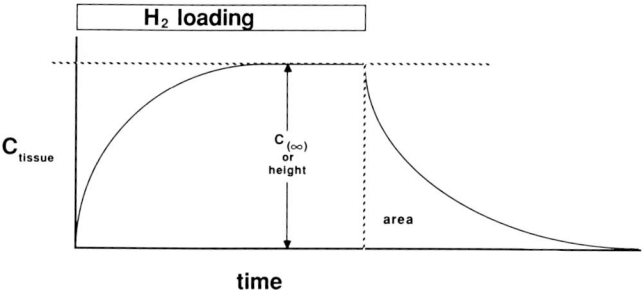

FIG. 32. Blood flow determined from washout of hydrogen. If it can be assumed that hydrogen reaches equilibrium with tissue ($C_\infty$), blood flow can be determined by monitoring only instantaneous tissue hydrogen concentration and integrating area under washout curve.

In the theory of inert gas clearance, four troubling assumptions are made: *1*) hydrogen achieves rapid equilibrium between blood and tissue; *2*) arterial delivery of hydrogen is zero during the washout curve; *3*) hydrogen is removed from the measuring site only by blood flow; *4*) the electrode measures only hydrogen.

*Advantages and Disadvantages of Hydrogen Clearance*

Hydrogen clearance possesses four distinct advantages over other blood flow–measuring techniques. *1*) In contrast to the microsphere method, which is limited by the number of isotopes that can be distinguished by their energy levels (usually 4 or 5), numerous hydrogen clearance assessments can be made repetitively in a given experiment. *2*) Provided the electrode response is linear and has constant sensitivity during the washout period, blood flow can be assessed independently of the absolute amplitudes of the hydrogen potential. *3*) Unlike microsphere and aminopyrine clearance, hydrogen clearance provides an assessment of blood flow in a relatively small, discrete volume of tissue. *4*) The hydrogen clearance method is relatively easy to implement in that the gas and the electronic circuitry are inexpensive and readily available.

Of course the method has disadvantages as well. *1*) For penetrating electrodes the tissue damaged and made edematous by the electrode can serve as a barrier to the diffusion of hydrogen as well a have an abnormal blood flow. *2*) Hydrogen clearance curves (even those obtained on the gastric mucosa with surface electrodes) are often multiexponential and thus should be analyzed by the height-over-area algorithm rather than by the monoexponential method. This requires more extensive recording and analysis of the data. *3*) Investigators have questioned the assumption that the arterial concentration of hydrogen falls instantly to zero upon the cessation of hydrogen breathing (134). *4*) Platinum electrodes are sensitive to oxygen as well as hydrogen.

The presence of a countercurrent mechanism (14,

54, 75) in the intestinal villus may also preclude the use of hydrogen clearance for assessing intestinal mucosal blood flow, particularly in low-flow states when the efficiency of countercurrent shunting would be greatest. However, in a preliminary study with cats, Kvietys et al. (64) found that hydrogen clearance assessments of intestinal mucosal blood flow were significantly correlated both with microsphere and laser-Doppler measurements of mucosal perfusion. Predictably, the countercurrent shunting of hydrogen between arteriole and venule at the base of the villus should lead to an underestimation of mucosal blood flow by hydrogen clearance. However, in the study of Kvietys et al. (64), hydrogen clearance appeared to yield adequate assessments of intestinal mucosal blood flow in the range of 25 to 75 ml·min$^{-1}$·100 g$^{-1}$ of total blood flow.

As shown in *History*, p. 1343, various modifications of the technique have been developed to overcome these disadvantages. Tissue injury has been reduced or eliminated by using smaller penetrating electrodes or by placing the electrode on the surface of the tissue. Approaches to multiexponential washout curves include curve-stripping methods to separate flow into two or more apparent "compartments."

Because polarographic electrodes monitor local hydrogen concentrations, many investigators claim that hydrogen clearance measures blood flow in a small volume of tissue immediately adjacent to the electrode. The volume of measurement is a function of electrode geometry and has been claimed to be on the order of 1 mm$^3$ (61). However, some evidence from the cerebral circulation indicates that this is not true. Hydrogen generated 2–5 mm from the recording electrode contributes significantly to the recorded signal within the time course of a 10- to 20-min clearance curve (74). Similar arguments (148) against the purported spatial resolution of 1 mm$^3$ have been based on observations in thin and thick layers of gray matter that should be well perfused in comparison to adjacent white matter.

*Locally Generated Hydrogen*

In 1970 Stosseck and Lübbers (135) introduced a new approach to measuring blood flow by hydrogen clearance. Their method employs a second electrode to generate hydrogen electrochemically within the vicinity of the measuring electrode, as shown in Figure 33. Stosseck and Lübbers originally hoped to generate a brief spike of hydrogen in the tissue and thus to be able to make rapid repetitive determinations of blood flow in a relatively small volume of tissue. However, their technique was based on questionable assumptions regarding the homogeneity and constancy of blood flow during the local clearance measurement. Moreover, values estimated with locally generated hydrogen differed markedly from those obtained by the standard hydrogen inhalation measurement.

More recently the locally generated hydrogen

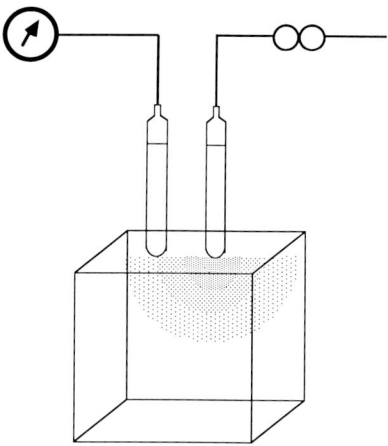

FIG. 33. Proposed method for measuring blood flow by local generation of hydrogen. One electrode measures local H$_2$ concentration while a second electrode connected to a constant current source generates hydrogen electrochemically. Tissue is first saturated with hydrogen, then H$_2$-generating current is shut off, and washout curve is recorded.

method has been further evaluated by Koshu et al. (62), who used the method in the cerebral circulation of dogs. As further developed by Koshu et al. (63), electrochemically generated hydrogen yielded values that were well correlated with conventional measurements with inhaled hydrogen. Their refinements of the technique included using greater electrical currents to generate more hydrogen within the vicinity of the recording electrode and generating hydrogen for longer periods of time than Stosseck et al. (136). Thus the spuriously high hydrogen clearance values reported by Stosseck et al. appear to have been due to the diffusive loss of hydrogen from the generating site to adjacent tissue regions containing little or no hydrogen. Shima et al. (126) have studied blood flow in the bone marrow of rabbits and showed that values obtained with the electrochemically generated hydrogen method correlated well with those obtained by conventionally inhaled hydrogen. Finally, preliminary experiments have been conducted in the gastric mucosa by Shepherd and co-workers (117), who showed that locally generated hydrogen clearance measurements were significantly correlated with gastric mucosal blood flow values obtained by LDV.

CONCLUSIONS

Many methods have been promoted for fractionating blood flow within the walls of the gastrointestinal tract, particularly for assessing mucosal perfusion. Some have been used in only one or two reports, whereas others have never been used outside the laboratory in which they were first developed. Thus this anthology reflects the authors' biased choice of those most extensively evaluated and those that hold the greatest promise of producing the sound results that will be required to establish firmly the relationships between the behavior of the regional circulations of the gastrointestinal tract and their physiological functions.

Of the methods reviewed here, aminopyrine clearance has clearly been used most extensively for gastrointestinal blood flow studies. Nevertheless, as we saw, it has reached the end of its useful life. There are too many situations in which clear and convincing data show that aminopyrine clearance yields invalid results. In spite of this a historical momentum perpetuates its use; reports still appear regularly in which aminopyrine clearance is used as the standard method of measuring gastric mucosal blood flow (139). However, to pay aminopyrine clearance its due, it is fair to say that before the advent of aminopyrine clearance, gastric mucosal blood flow was seldom studied. Nothing has done as much to stimulate the study of the gastric mucosal circulation since Beaumont's original observations on the color changes in St. Martin's gastric mucosa. Nevertheless it is time to abandon the use of aminopyrine clearance and to place it on the museum shelf with the Stromuhr and other honored but antiquated techniques.

Next in terms of extent of use in the gastrointestinal tract is the radioactive microsphere technique. Many of the problems associated with this technique have now been identified (118, 119), but the limits of its validity in some situations have still not been thoroughly explored. However, when used conservatively it is usually capable of fractionating intestinal blood flow into the two chief compartments of interest: the muscularis-serosa and the mucosa-submucosa compartments. In gastric applications more work needs to be done to identify the limitations of the microsphere method that have already been delineated in the gut.

The hydrogen clearance method has a long history of use in other organs, but with the exception of a few early reports, its application in the gastrointestinal tract is relatively new. The advent of the surface electrode and the wealth of experience and literature from other vascular beds should greatly facilitate its further use and development as a technique for measuring blood flow in the gastrointestinal tract. In addition the technique of generating hydrogen electrochemically with a second electrode could greatly increase the convenience of the method by eliminating the need for tanks of hydrogen and by making faster, more numerous measurements possible than with inhaled hydrogen. However, the locally generated hydrogen technique suffers from motion artifacts because gastrointestinal motility can move the hydrogen-recording electrode in and out of the hydrogen-rich area created by the generating electrode. Finally the locally generated hydrogen technique could possibly be converted to a continuous measurement. In one scheme (31) the hydrogen concentration signal would be fed back to regulate the rate of hydrogen generation and to maintain a constant tissue hydrogen level. In such a paradigm the regulated hydrogen generation rate would provide a continuous measure of the blood flow responsible for $H_2$ removal.

Despite the availability of commercially made LDV blood flowmeters, LDV is still in its infancy, but it holds great promise. None of the other methods reviewed here is capable of the frequency response and the continuous measurements of local perfusion that LDV blood flowmetry provides. Only hydrogen clearance approaches the spatial resolution of LDV's fiber-optic probes. Uncertainty about the measuring volume, technical difficulties such as motion artifacts and the maintenance of optical coupling between flow probe and tissue, inadequate data on the optical properties of gastrointestinal tissues, and the lack of a calibration in conventional flow units now hamper its use. If these problems can be overcome, LDV could significantly advance blood flowmetry in the gastrointestinal tract. If LDV flowmetry were combined with multiple wavelength spectroscopy and if both of these technologies were combined with the endoscope, a wealth of information about mucosal physiology would be available to the gastroenterologist: the redox state of the tissue, the oxyhemoglobin saturation of capillary blood, and a quantitative measure of mucosal blood flow. If the fiber-optic LDV flowmeter can be combined with the endoscope, the potential clinical applications include delineating small ischemic foci that are undetectable with other methods, monitoring the efficacy of vasopressin therapy to staunch gastrointestinal bleeding, determining the role of mucosal blood flow changes during the progression of disease such as nonocclusive mesenteric ischemia and inflammatory bowel disease, defining the regions of compromised perfusion during bowel resection, and determining the role of mucosal blood flow changes in ulcerogenesis and ulcer healing. If further research and development achieve even a few of these goals, the laser will have ushered in a new era of gastrointestinal blood flow measurements.

The fine line between the proper and improper use of a blood flow–measuring technique is easily crossed; trespassing beyond the bounds of a method's validity yields results that are useless. Moreover the boundaries that circumscribe the valid and proper use of the techniques for measuring blood flow within the walls of the gastrointestinal tract in many cases are only faintly blazed. Therefore investigators who employ these methods should also scout the boundaries and thus mark the limits of the validity of these flow-measuring techniques. For only then can we obtain a meaningful measure of gastrointestinal blood flow and only then can we harness "the Pythagorean power by which number holds sway above the flux."

The authors express their gratitude to K. Morren for secretarial assistance and to G. Riedel for preparation of the figures.

The authors' original investigations were supported by National Institutes of Health research grants AM-33024 and HL-36080.

# REFERENCES

1. AHN, H., J. LINDHAGEN, G. E. NILSSON, E. G. SALERUD, M. JODAL, AND O. LUNDGREN. Evaluation of laser-Doppler flowmetry in the assessment of intestinal blood flow in cat. *Gastroenterology* 88: 951–957, 1985.
2. ARCHIBALD, L. H., F. G. MOODY, AND M. SIMONS. Effect of isoproterenol on canine gastric acid secretion and blood flow. *Surg. Forum.* 25: 409–411, 1974.
3. ARCHIBALD, L. H., F. G. MOODY, AND M. A. SIMONS. Comparison of gastric mucosal blood flow as determined by aminopyrine clearance and gamma-labeled microspheres. *Gastroenterology* 69: 630–635, 1975.
4. ARCHIBALD, L. H., F. G. MOODY, AND M. SIMONS. Measurement of gastric blood flow with radioactive microspheres. *J. Appl. Physiol.* 38: 1051–1056, 1975.
5. ASHLEY, S. W., AND L. Y. CHEUNG. Measurement of gastric mucosal blood flow by hydrogen gas clearance. *Am. J. Physiol.* 247 (*Gastrointest. Liver Physiol.* 10): G339–G345, 1984.
6. ASHLEY, S. W., Z. Y. YAN, D. I. SOYBEL, AND L. Y. CHEUNG. Endoscopic measurements of gastric mucosal blood flow in dogs. *J. Surg. Res.* 38: 416–423, 1985.
7. AUKLAND, K. Hydrogen polarography in measurement of local blood flow, theoretical and empirical basis. *Acta Neurol. Scand.* 41, Suppl. 14: 42–45, 1965.
8. AUKLAND, K., B. F. BOWER, AND R. W. BERLINER. Measurement of local blood flow with hydrogen gas. *Circ. Res.* 14: 164–187, 1964.
9. BANKIR, L. M., T. T. TAN, AND J. GRUNFELD. Measurement of glomerular blood flow in rabbits and rats: erroneous findings with 15-μm microspheres. *Kidney Int.* 15: 126–133, 1979.
10. BASSINGTHWAIGHTE, J. B., T. YIPINTSOI, AND R. B. HARVEY. Microvasculature of the dog left ventricular myocardium. *Microvasc. Res.* 7: 229–249, 1974.
11. BERGLINDH, T., H. F. HELANDER, AND K. J. ÖBRINK. Effects of secretagogues on oxygen consumption, aminopyrine accumulation and morphology in isolated gastric glands. *Acta Physiol. Scand.* 97: 401–414, 1976.
12. BERGLINDH, T., AND K. J. ÖBRINK. A method for preparing isolated glands from the rabbit gastric mucosa. *Acta Physiol. Scand.* 96: 150–159, 1976.
13. BHARADVAJ, B. K., R. F. MABON, AND D. P. GIDDENS. Steady flow in a model of the human carotid bifurcation. Part II—laser-Doppler anemometer measurements. *J. Biochem.* 15: 363–378, 1982.
14. BIBER, B., O. LUNDGREN, AND J. SVANVIK. The influence of blood flow on the rate of absorption of $^{85}$Kr from the small intestine of the cat. *Acta Physiol. Scand.* 89: 227–238, 1973.
15. BOND, J. H., AND M. D. LEVITT. Use of microspheres to measure small intestinal villus blood flow in the dog. *Am. J. Physiol.* 236 (*Endocrinol. Metab. Gastrointest. Physiol.* 5): E577–E583, 1979.
16. BONNER, R. F., AND R. NOSSAL. A model for laser Doppler measurements of blood flow in tissue. *Appl. Opt.* 20: 2097–2107, 1981.
17. BONNER, R. F., T. R. CLEM, P. D. BOWEN, AND R. L. BOWMAN. Laser-Doppler continuous real-time monitor of pulsatile and mean blood flow in tissue microcirculation. In: *Scattering Techniques Applied to Supramolecular and Non-Equilibrium Systems*, edited by S. H. Chen, B. Chu, and R. Nossal. New York: Plenum, 1981, p. 685–702.
18. BORN, G. V. R., A. MELLING, AND J. H. WHITELAW. Laser Doppler microscope for blood velocity measurements. *Biorheology* 15: 163–172, 1978.
19. BRODIE, B. B., AND J. AXELROD. The fate of aminopyrine (pyramidon) in man and methods for the estimation of aminopyrine and its metabolites in biological material. *J. Pharmacol. Exp. Ther.* 99: 171–184, 1950.
20. BUCKBERG, G. D., J. C. LUCK, D. B. PAYNE, J. I. E. HOFFMAN, J. P. ARCHIE, AND D. E. FIXLER. Some sources of error in measuring regional blood flow with radioactive microspheres. *J. Appl. Physiol.* 31: 598–604, 1971.
21. CHEUNG, L. Y., F. G. MOODY, AND R. S. REESE. Effect of aspirin, bile salt, and ethanol on canine gastric mucosal blood flow. *Surgery St. Louis* 77: 786–792, 1975.
22. CHEUNG, L. Y., AND L. A. SONNENSCHEIN. Measurement of regional gastric mucosal blood flow by hydrogen gas clearance. *Am. J. Surg.* 147: 32–37, 1984.
23. CHOU, C. C., C. P. HSIEH, Y. M. YU, P. KVIETYS, L. C. YU, R. PITTMAN, AND J. M. DABNEY. Localization of mesenteric hyperemia during digestion in dogs. *Am. J. Physiol.* 230: 583–589, 1976.
24. CLARK, L. C., JR., AND L. M. BARGERON. Left to right shunt detection by an intravascular electrode with hydrogen as an indicator. *Science Wash. DC* 130: 709–710, 1959.
25. CLARK, L. C., JR., AND L. M. BARGERON. Detection and direct recording of right to left shunts with a hydrogen electrode catheter. *Surgery St. Louis* 46: 797–804, 1959.
26. CLAUSEN, G., A. KIRKEBO, I. TYSSEBOTN, E. S. OFJORD, AND K. AUKLAND. Erroneous estimates of intrarenal blood flow distribution in the dog with radiolabelled microspheres. *Acta Physiol. Scand.* 107: 385–387, 1979.
27. COWLEY, D. J., AND C. F. CODE. Effects of secretory inhibitors on mucosal blood flow in nonsecreting stomach of conscious dogs. *Am. J. Physiol.* 218: 270–274, 1970.
28. DELANEY, J. P., AND E. GRIM. Canine gastric blood flow and its distribution. *Am. J. Physiol.* 207: 1195–1202, 1964.
29. DELANEY, J. P., AND E. GRIM. Experimentally induced variations in canine gastric blood flow and its distribution. *Am. J. Physiol.* 208: 353–358, 1965.
30. DINDA, P. K., M. G. BUELL, L. R. DACOSTA, AND I. T. BECK. Simultaneous estimation of arteriolar, capillary, and shunt blood flow of the gut mucosa. *Am. J. Physiol.* 245 (*Gastrointest. Liver Physiol.* 8): G29–G37, 1983.
31. DIRESTA, G. R. The Measurement of Tissue Perfusion Using a $H_2$-Clamp Technique. Brooklyn, NY: Polytechnic Inst. of New York, 1982. Dissertation. (Dissertation Abstracts Order #DA8217322.)
32. DOMENECH, R. J., J. I. E. HOFFMAN, M. I. M. NOBLE, K. B. SAUNDERS, J. R. HENSON, AND S. SUBIJANTO. Total and regional coronary blood flow measured by radioactive microspheres in conscious and anesthetized dogs. *Circ. Res.* 25: 581–596, 1969.
33. DRUCE, H. M., R. F. BONNER, C. PATOW, P. CHOO, R. J. SUMMERS, AND M. A. KALINER. Response of nasal blood flow to neurohormones as measured by laser-Doppler velocimetry. *J. Appl. Physiol.* 57: 1276–1283, 1984.
34. DUTEIL, L., J. C. BERNENGO, AND W. SCHALLA. A double wavelength laser-Doppler system to investigate skin microcirculation. *IEEE Trans. Biomed. Eng.* 32: 439–447, 1985.
35. EDLICH, R. F., I. GROTENHUIS, AND R. J. BUCHIN. Radioactive microspheres. Effect of their physical properties on vascular distribution. *Proc. Soc. Exp. Biol. Med.* 128: 909–913, 1968.
36. EINAV, S., H. J. BERMAN, R. L. FUHRO, P. R. DIGIOVANNI, J. D. FRIDMAN, AND S. FINE. Measurement of blood flow in vivo by laser Doppler anemometry through a microscope. *Biorheology* 12: 203–205, 1975.
37. FAN, F., G. B. SCHUESSLER, R. Y. Z. CHEN, AND S. CHIEN. Determinations of blood flow and shunting of 9- and 15-μm spheres in regional beds. *Am. J. Physiol.* 237 (*Heart Circ. Physiol.* 6): H25–H33, 1979.
38. GANNON, B. J., R. W. GORE, AND P. A. W. ROGERS. Is there an anatomical basis for a vascular counter-current mechanism in rabbit and human intestinal villi? *Biomed. Res.* 2: 235–241, 1981.
39. GRANGER, D. N., AND G. B. BULKLEY. *Measurement of Blood Flow. Applications to the Splanchnic Circulation.* Baltimore, MD: Williams & Wilkins, 1981.
40. GRANGER, D. N., J. D. VALLEAU, R. E. PARKER, R. S. LANE, AND A. E. TAYLOR. Effects of adenosine on intestinal hemodynamics, oxygen delivery, and capillary fluid exchange. *Am. J. Physiol.* 235 (*Heart Circ. Physiol.* 4): H707–H719, 1978.

41. GREENWAY, C. V., AND V. S. MURTHY. Effects of vasopressin and isoprenaline infusions on the distribution of blood flow in the intestine; criteria for the validity of microsphere studies. *Br. J. Pharmacol.* 46: 177–188, 1972.
42. GRIM, E., AND E. O. LINDSETH. Distribution of blood flow to the tissues of the small intestine of the dog. *Med. Bull. Univ. Minn.* 30: 138–145, 1958.
43. GUSH, R. J., T. A. KING, AND M. I. V. JAYSON. Aspects of laser light scattering from skin tissue with application to laser Doppler blood flow measurement. *Phys. Med. Biol.* 29: 1463–1476, 1984.
44. GUTH, P. H., H. BAUMANN, M. I. GROSSMAN, D. AURES, AND J. ELASHOFF. Measurement of gastric mucosal blood flow in man. *Gastroenterology* 74: 831–834, 1978.
45. HALES, J. R. S., A. A. FAWCETT, AND J. W. BENNET. Differential influences of CNS and superficial body temperatures on the partition of cutaneous blood flow between capillaries and arteriovenous anastomoses (AVA's). *Pfluegers Arch.* 361: 105–106, 1975.
46. HARPER, A. A., J. D. REED, AND J. R. SMY. Gastric blood flow in anaesthetized cats. *J. Physiol. Lond.* 194: 795–807, 1968.
47. HAUMSCHILD, D. J. An overview of laser Doppler flowmetry. In: *Biomedical Sciences Instrumentation, Proc. 23rd Annual Rocky Mountain Bioengineering Symp. and 23rd Int. ISA Biomedical Sciences Instrumentation Symp.*, edited by A. W. Hahn. Columbia, MO: Univ. of Missouri, 1986, vol. 22, p. 35–40.
48. HOLM-RUTILI, L., AND T. BERGLINDH. Pentagastrin and gastric mucosal blood flow. *Am. J. Physiol.* 250 (*Gastrointest. Liver Physiol.* 13): G575–G580, 1986.
49. HUNT, B. F., S. C. LEAVITT, AND D. C. HEMPSTEAD. Digital processing chain for a Doppler ultrasound subsystem. *Hewlett-Packard J.* 37: 45–48, 1986.
50. HYMAN, E. S. Linear system for quantitating hydrogen at a platinum electrode. *Circ. Res.* 9: 1093–1097, 1961.
51. JACOBSON, E. D. Clearances of the gastric mucosa. *Gastroenterology* 54: 434–448, 1968.
52. JACOBSON, E. D., M. M. EISENBERG, AND K. G. SWAN. Effects of histamine on gastric blood flow in conscious dogs. *Gastroenterology* 51: 466–472, 1966.
53. JACOBSON, E. D., R. H. LINFORD, AND M. I. GROSSMAN. Gastric secretion in relation to mucosal blood flow studied by a clearance technic. *J. Clin. Invest.* 45: 1–13, 1966.
54. JODAL, M., U. HAGLUNG, AND O. LUNDGREN. Countercurrent exchange mechanisms in the small intestine. In: *Physiology of the Intestinal Circulation*, edited by A. P. Shepherd and D. N. Granger. New York: Raven, 1984, p. 83–98.
55. JOHNSON, J. M., W. F. TAYLOR, A. P. SHEPHERD, AND M. K. PARK. Laser-Doppler measurement of skin blood flow: comparison with plethysmography. *J. Appl. Physiol.* 56: 798–803, 1984.
56. KETY, S. S. The theory and application of the exchange of inert gas at the lungs and tissues. *Pharmacol. Rev.* 3: 1–41, 1951.
57. KETY, S. S., AND C. F. SCHMIDT. The determination of cerebral blood flow in man by the use of nitrous oxide in low concentrations. *Am. J. Physiol.* 143: 53–66, 1945.
58. KIEL, J. W., G. L. RIEDEL, G. R. DIRESTA, AND A. P. SHEPHERD. Gastric mucosal blood flow measured by laser-Doppler velocimetry. *Am. J. Physiol.* 249 (*Gastrointest. Liver Physiol.* 12): G539–G545, 1985.
59. KIEL, J. W., G. L. RIEDEL, AND A. P. SHEPHERD. Autoregulation of gastric mucosal blood flow (Abstract). *Proc. Int. Congr. Physiol. Sci. 30th, Vancouver, Canada*, 1986, vol. 16, p. 123.
60. KILPATRICK, D., J. V. TYBERG, AND W. W. PARMLEY. Blood velocity measurement by fiber optic laser Doppler anemometry. *IEEE Trans. Biom. Eng.* 29: 142–145, 1982.
61. KOBRINE, A. I., T. F. DOYLE, AND A. N. MARTINS. Spinal cord blood flow in the rhesus monkey by the hydrogen clearance method. *Surg. Neurol.* 2: 197–200, 1974.
62. KOSHU, K., K. KAMIYAMA, N. OKA, S. ENDO, A. TAKAKU, AND T. SAITO. Measurement of regional blood flow using hydrogen gas generated by electrolysis. *Stroke* 13: 483–487, 1982.
63. KOSHU, K., J. NAKADA, Y. HIRASHIMA, S. ENDO, A. TAKAKU, AND T. SAITO. Measurement of regional cerebral blood flow by an electrolytic method using a monopolar electrode. *J. Cereb. Blood Flow Metab.* 3: S111–S112, 1983.
64. KVIETYS, P. R., A. P. SHEPHERD, AND D. N. GRANGER. Laser-Doppler, $H_2$ clearance, and microsphere estimates of mucosal blood flow. *Am. J. Physiol.* 249 (*Gastrointest. Liver Physiol.* 12): G221–G227, 1985.
65. LASSEN, N. A., AND W. PERL. *Tracer Kinetic Methods in Medical Physiology*. New York: Raven, 1979.
66. LE-CONG, P. *Development of a Laser Doppler Velocimeter and Its Applications to Microcirculation Studies*. Univ. of California, San Diego, 1976. Dissertation. University Microfilm Order No. 77-522.
67. LE-CONG, P., AND R. H. LOVEBERG. Analysis of dual beam laser velocimeter applied to microcirculation studies. *Rev. Sci. Instrum.* 51: 565–574, 1980.
68. LE-CONG, P., AND B. W. ZWEIFACH. In vivo and in vitro velocity measurements in microvasculature with a laser. *Microvasc. Res.* 17: 131–141, 1979.
69. LEKVEN, J., AND K. S. ANDERSON. Migration of 15 micron microspheres from infarcted myocardium. *Cardiovasc. Res.* 14: 280–287, 1980.
70. LEONARD, J. J., R. W. EMERY, S. EINZIG, D. M. NICOLOFF, AND I. J. FOX. Evidence for arteriovenous communications in the gastrointestinal tract. *Surg. Forum* 28: 419–421, 1977.
71. LEUNG, F. W., P. H. GUTH, O. U. SCREMIN, E. M. GOLANSKA, AND G. L. KAUFFMAN, JR. Regional gastric mucosal blood flow measurements by hydrogen gas clearance in the anesthetized rat and rabbit. *Gastroenterology* 87: 28–36, 1984.
72. LEUNG, F. W., J. WASHINGTON, G. L. KAUFFMAN, JR., AND P. H. GUTH. Endoscopic measurement of gastric corpus mucosal blood flow in conscious dogs. *Dig. Dis. Sci.* 31: 625–630, 1986.
73. LIFSON, N. Use of microspheres to measure intraorgan distribution of blood flow in the splanchnic circulation. In: *Measurement of Blood Flow. Applications to the Splanchnic Circulation*, edited by D. N. Granger and G. B. Bulkley. Baltimore, MD: Williams & Wilkins, 1981, p. 177–194.
74. LÜBBERS, D. W., R. WODICK, K. STOSSECK, AND H. ACKER. Problems concerning the $H_2$ inhalation technique to determine the cerebral blood flow by means of palladinized Pt electrodes. In: *Cerebral Blood Flow: Clinical and Experimental Results*, edited by M. Brock, C. Fieschi, D. H. Ingvar, N. A. Lassen, and K. Schürmann. Berlin: Springer-Verlag, 1969, p. 39–41.
75. LUNDGREN, O. Studies on blood flow distribution and countercurrent exchange in the small intestine. *Acta Physiol. Scand.* 303: 5–42, 1967.
76. LUNDGREN, O. Microcirculation of the gastrointestinal tract and pancreas. In: *Handbook of Physiology. The Cardiovascular System. Microcirculation*, edited by E. M. Renkin and C. C. Michel. Bethesda, MD: Am. Physiol. Soc., 1984, sect. 2, vol. IV, pt. 2, chapt. 17, p. 799–863.
77. MACKIE, D. B., AND M. D. TURNER. Long-term blood flow studies in the gastric submucosa of unanesthetized rats. *Arch. Surg.* 103: 500–503, 1971.
78. MACKIE, D. B., AND M. D. TURNER. Vagotomy and submucosal blood flow. *Arch. Surg.* 102: 626–629, 1971.
79. MADDEN, R. E., A. PAPARO, AND M. SCHWARTZ. Limiting vascular diameters in various organs. *Arch. Surg.* 96: 130–137, 1968.
80. MAGNIN, P. A. Doppler effect: history and theory. *Hewlett-Packard J.* 37: 26–31, 1986.
81. MAKOWSKI, E. L., G. MESCHIA, W. DROEGEMUELLER, AND F. C. BATTAGLIA. Measurement of umbilical arterial blood flow

to the sheep placenta and fetus in utero. *Circ. Res.* 23: 623–631, 1968.
82. MAXWELL, L. C., A. P. SHEPHERD, AND C. A. MCMAHAN. Microsphere passage through intestinal circulation: via shunts or capillaries? *Am. J. Physiol.* 248 (*Heart Circ. Physiol.* 17): H217–H224, 1985.
83. MAXWELL, L. C., A. P. SHEPHERD, AND G. L. RIEDEL. Vasodilation or altered perfusion pressure moves 15-$\mu$m spheres trapped in the gut wall. *Am. J. Physiol.* 243 (*Heart Circ. Physiol.* 12): H123–H127, 1982.
84. MAXWELL, L. C., A. P. SHEPHERD, G. L. RIEDEL, AND M. D. MORRIS. Effect of microsphere size on apparent intramural distribution of intestinal blood flow. *Am. J. Physiol.* 241 (*Heart Circ. Physiol.* 10): H408–H414, 1981.
85. MCMAHAN, C. A., L. C. MAXWELL, AND A. P. SHEPHERD. Estimation of the distribution of blood vessel diameters from the arteriovenous passage of microspheres. *Biometrics* 42: 371–380, 1986.
86. MICKFLICKIER, A. B., J. H. BOND, B. SIRCAR, AND M. D. LEVITT. Intestinal villus blood flow measured with carbon monoxide and microspheres. *Am. J. Physiol.* 230: 916–919, 1976.
87. MILLER, T. A., J. M. HENAGAN, AND T. M. LOY. Impairment of aminopyrine clearance in aspirin-damaged canine gastric mucosa. *Gastroenterology* 85: 643–649, 1983.
88. MISHINA, H., T. KOYAMA, AND T. ASAKURA. Velocity measurements of blood flow in the capillary and vein using a laser-Doppler microscope. *Appl. Opt.* 14: 2326–2327, 1975.
89. MISRAHY, G. A., AND L. C. CLARK. Use of the platinum black cathode for local blood flow measurements in vivo (Abstract). *Proc. Int. Cong. Physiol. Sci., 22nd, Brussels*, vol. 1, 1956, p. 650.
90. MITO, K. Measurement of arterial blood flow profile by an optical fiber laser Doppler flowmeter. *Jpn. J. Med. Electron. Biol. Eng.* 19: 383–389, 1981.
91. MOODY, F. G. Gastric blood flow and acid secretion during direct intraarterial histamine administration. *Gastroenterology* 52: 216–224, 1967.
92. MOODY, F. G. Oxygen consumption during thiocyanate inhibition of gastric acid secretion in dogs. *Am. J. Physiol.* 215: 127–131, 1968.
93. MOODY, F. G., AND R. P. DURBIN. Effects of glycine and other instillates on concentration of gastric acid. *Am. J. Physiol.* 209: 122–126, 1965.
94. MØRKRID, L., J. OFSTAD, AND Y. WILLASSEN. Diameter of afferent arterioles during autoregulation estimated from microsphere data in the dog kidney. *Circ. Res.* 42: 181–191, 1978.
95. MÜLLER-LISSNER, S. A., A. SONNENBERG, AND A. L. BLUM. Does gastric aminopyrine reflect gastric mucosal blood flow or parietal cell function. *Gut* 23: 997–1002, 1981.
96. MURAKAMI, M., M. MORIGA, T. MIYAKE, AND H. UCHINO. Contact electrode method in hydrogen gas clearance technique: a new method for determination of regional gastric mucosal blood flow in animals and humans. *Gastroenterology* 82: 457–467, 1982.
97. MURAKAMI, M., H. SAIDA, M. SEKI, AND T. MIYAKE. Measurement of gastric mucosal blood flow by laser-Doppler velocimetry. *Nippon Shokakibyo Gakkai Zasshi* 80: 2275–2276, 1983.
98. NILSSON, G. E. Signal processor for laser Doppler tissue flowmeters. *Med. Biol. Eng. Comput.* 22: 343–348, 1984.
99. NILSSON, G. E., T. TENLAND, AND P. A. ÖBERG. Evaluation of a laser Doppler flowmeter for measurement of tissue blood flow. *IEEE Trans. Biomed. Eng.* 27: 597–604, 1980.
100. OFSTAD, J., L. MÖRKRID, AND Y. WILLASSEN. Diameter of afferent arteriole in the dog kidney estimated by the microsphere method. *Scand. J. Clin. Lab. Invest.* 35: 767–774, 1975.
101. OLLKKONEN, H., P. SIMONEN, T. IMMONEN, T. JAASKELAINEN, AND J. FRAKI. Dual diode transducer for laser-Doppler skin blood velocimeter. *J. Biomed. Eng.* 6: 75–77, 1984.
102. OVERBECK, H. W. Intestinal circulation during arterial hypertension. In: *Physiology of the Intestinal Circulation*, edited by A. P. Shepherd and D. N. Granger. New York: Raven, 1984, p. 349–360.
103. PAWLIK, W. W., J. D. FONDACARO, AND E. D. JACOBSON. Metabolic hyperemia in canine gut. *Am. J. Physiol.* 239 (*Gastrointest. Liver Physiol.* 2): G12–G17, 1980.
104. PHIBBS, R. H., AND L. DONG. Nonuniform distribution of microspheres in blood flowing through a medium sized artery. *Can. J. Physiol. Pharmacol.* 48: 415–421, 1970.
105. PRINZMETAL, M., B. SIMKIN, H. C. BERGMAN, AND H. E. KRUGER. Studies on the coronary circulation. II. The collateral circulation of the normal human heart by coronary perfusion with radioactive erythrocytes and glass spheres. *Am. Heart J.* 33: 420–442, 1947.
106. RIVA, C. E., B. ROSS, AND G. B. BENEDEK. Laser-Doppler measurements of blood flow in capillary tubes and retinal arteries. *Invest. Ophthalmol.* 11: 936–944, 1972.
107. RUDICK, J., J. L. WERTHER, M. L. CHAPMAN, D. A. DREILING, AND H. D. JANOWITZ. Mucosal blood flow in canine antral and fundic pouches. *Gastroenterology* 60: 263–271, 1971.
108. RUDOLPH, A. M., AND R. A. HEYMANN. The circulation of the fetus in utero. *Circ. Res.* 21: 163–184, 1967.
109. RUPPIN, R., AND L. DEMLING. Gastric aminopyrine clearance—an obsolete technique? *Hepato-Gastroenterology* 31: 155–157, 1984.
110. SALERUD, G. Laser-Doppler Tissue Flowmetry. Fiberoptic Methods in Microvascular Research. Linkoping, Sweden: Linkoping Univ., 1986. Dissertation. (Linkoping Studies in Science and Technology Dissertations, No. 137, Linkoping University Medical Dissertations, No. 216.)
111. SARELIUS, I. H., L. C. MAXWELL, S. D. GRAY, AND B. R. DULING. Capillarity and fiber types in the cremaster muscle of rat and hamster. *Am. J. Physiol.* 245 (*Heart Circ. Physiol.* 14): H368–H374, 1983.
112. SEMB, B. K. H. Gastric flow measured with hydrogen clearance technique. *Scand. J. Gastroenterol.* 14: 641–646, 1979.
113. SEMB, B. K. H. Changes of regional gastric flow measured by hydrogen clearance technique after histamine stimulation in conscious animals. *Scand. J. Gastroenterol.* 16: 795–800, 1981.
114. SEMB, B. K. H. The effect of catecholamines on gastric mucosal flow. *Scand. J. Gastroenterol.* 17: 663–670, 1982.
115. SEMB, B. K. H. Regional gastric flow changes after meal stimulation measured by the hydrogen clearance technique in conscious cats. *Scand. J. Gastroenterol.* 17: 839–842, 1982.
116. SHEPHERD, A. P. Intestinal blood flow autoregulation during foodstuff absorption. *Am. J. Physiol.* 239 (*Heart Circ. Physiol.* 8): H156–H162, 1980.
117. SHEPHERD, A. P., G. R. DIRESTA, J. W. KIEL, AND G. L. RIEDEL. Hybrid blood flow-probe for simultaneous $H_2$ clearance and laser-Doppler velocimetry (Abstract). *Proc. Int. Congr. Physiol. Sci. 30th, Vancouver, Canada*, 1986, vol. 16, p. 123.
118. SHEPHERD, A. P., L. C. MAXWELL, AND E. D. JACOBSON. Limitations of the microsphere technique to fractionate intestinal blood flow. In: *Measurement of Blood Flow. Applications to the Splanchnic Circulation*, by D. N. Granger and G. B. Bulkley. Baltimore, MD: Williams & Wilkins, 1981, p. 195–200.
119. SHEPHERD, A. P., L. C. MAXWELL, AND G. L. RIEDEL. Microsphere fractionation of intestinal blood flow. *Am. J. Physiol.* 246 (*Gastrointest. Liver Physiol.* 9): G644–G645, 1984.
120. SHEPHERD, A. P., AND G. L. RIEDEL. Continuous measurement of intestinal mucosal blood flow by laser-Doppler velocimetry. *Am. J. Physiol.* 242 (*Gastrointest. Liver Physiol.* 5): G668–G672, 1982.
121. SHEPHERD, A. P., AND G. L. RIEDEL. Effect of pulsatile pressure and metabolic rate on intestinal autoregulation. *Am. J. Physiol.* 242 (*Heart Circ. Physiol.* 11): H769–H775, 1982.
122. SHEPHERD, A. P., AND G. L. RIEDEL. Differences in reactive

hyperemia between the intestinal mucosa and muscularis. *Am. J. Physiol.* 247 (*Gastrointest. Liver Physiol.* 10): G617–G622, 1984.
123. SHEPHERD, A. P., AND G. L. RIEDEL. Laser-Doppler blood flowmetry of intestinal mucosal hyperemia induced by glucose and bile. *Am. J. Physiol.* 248 (*Gastrointest. Liver Physiol.* 11): G393–G397, 1985.
124. SHEPHERD, A. P., G. L. RIEDEL, L. C. MAXWELL, AND J. W. KIEL. Selective vasodilators redistribute intestinal blood flow and depress oxygen uptake. *Am. J. Physiol.* 247 (*Gastrointest. Liver Physiol.* 10): G377–G384, 1984.
125. SHEPHERD, A. P., G. L. RIEDEL, AND W. F. WARD. Laser-Doppler measurements of blood flow within the intestinal wall and on the surface of the liver. In: *Microcirculation of the Alimentary Tract-Physiology and Pathology*, edited by A. Koo, S. K. Lam, and L. H. Smaje. Singapore: World Scientific, 1983, p. 115–129.
126. SHIMA, I., S. YAMAUCHI, T. MATSUMOTO, M. KUNISHITA, K. SHINODA, N. YOSHIMIZU, S. NOMURA, AND M. YOSHIMURA. A new method for monitoring circulation of grafted bone by use of electrochemically generated hydrogen. *Clin. Orthop. Relat. Res.* 198: 244–249, 1985.
127. SHORE, P. A., B. B. BRODIE, AND C. A. M. HOGBEN. The gastric secretion of drugs: a pH partition hypothesis. *J. Pharmacol. Exp. Ther.* 119: 361–369, 1957.
128. SMITS, G. J., R. J. ROMAN, AND J. H. LOMBARD. Evaluation of laser-Doppler flowmetry as a measure of tissue blood flow. *J. Appl. Physiol.* 61: 666–672, 1986.
129. SONNENBERG, A., AND A. L. BLUM. Limitations to measurement of gastric mucosal blood flow by [$^{14}$C]aminopyrine clearance. In: *Gastrointestinal Mucosal Blood Flow*, edited by L. P. Fielding. New York: Churchill Livingstone, 1980, p. 43–58.
130. SONNENBERG, A., T. BERGLINDH, M. J. M. LEWIN, J. A. FISCHER, G. SACHS, AND A. L. BLUM. Stimulation of acid secretion in isolated gastric cells. In: *Hormone Receptors in Digestion and Nutrition*, edited by G. Rosselin, P. Fromageot, and S. Bonfils. Amsterdam: Elsevier/North-Holland, 1979, p. 337–348.
131. STERN, M. D. In vivo evaluation of microcirculation by coherent light scattering. *Nature Lond.* 254: 56–58, 1975.
132. STERN, M. D., P. D. BOWEN, R. PARMA, R. W. OSGOOD, R. L. BOWMAN, AND J. H. STEIN. Measurement of renal cortical and medullary blood flow by laser-Doppler spectroscopy in the rat. *Am. J. Physiol.* 236 (*Renal Fluid Electrolyte Physiol.* 5): F80–F87, 1979.
133. STERN, M. D., D. L. LAPPE, P. D. BOWEN, J. E. CHIMOSKY, G. A. HOLLOWAY, JR., H. R. KEISER, AND R. L. BOWMAN. Continuous measurement of tissue blood flow by laser-Doppler spectroscopy. *Am. J. Physiol.* 232 (*Heart Circ. Physiol.* 1): H441–H448, 1977.
134. STOSSECK, K. Hydrogen exchange through the pial vessel wall and its meaning for the determination of local cerebral blood flow. *Pfluegers Arch.* 320: 111–119, 1970.
135. STOSSECK, K., AND D. W. LÜBBERS. Determination of microflow of the cerebral cortex by means of electrochemically generated hydrogen. In: *Brain and Blood Flow*, edited by R. W. R. Russell. London: Pitman, 1970, p. 80–84.
136. STOSSECK, K., D. W. LÜBBERS, AND N. COTTIN. Determination of local blood flow (microflow) by electrochemically generated hydrogen: Construction and application of the measuring probe. *Pfluegers Arch.* 348: 225–238, 1974.
137. SWAN, K. G., AND E. D. JACOBSON. Gastric blood flow and secretion in conscious dogs. *Am. J. Physiol.* 212: 891–896, 1967.
138. TAGUE, L. L., AND E. D. JACOBSON. Evaluation of [$^{14}$C]-aminopyrine clearance for determination of gastric mucosal blood flow. *Proc. Soc. Exp. Biol. Med.* 151: 707–710, 1976.
139. TAKESHITA, H., Y. KOTANI, AND S. OKABE. Comparative study of hydrogen and aminopyrine clearance methods for determination of gastric mucosal blood flow in dogs. *Dig. Dis. Sci.* 29: 841–847, 1984.
140. TANAKA, T., AND G. B. BENEDEK. Measurement of velocity of blood flow (in vivo) using a fiber optic catheter and optical mixing spectroscopy. *Appl. Opt.* 14: 189–200, 1975.
141. TANAKA, T., C. RIVA, AND I. BEN-SIRA. Blood velocity measurements in human retinal vessels. *Science Wash. DC* 186: 830–831, 1974.
142. UTLEY, J., E. L. CARLSON, J. I. E. HOFFMAN, H. M. MARTINEZ, AND G. D. BUCKBERG. Total and regional myocardial blood flow measurements with $25\mu$, $15\mu$, $9\mu$, and filtered 1-10$\mu$ diameter microspheres and antipyrine in dogs and sheep. *Circ. Res.* 34: 391–405, 1974.
143. VARHAUG, J.-E., K. SVANES, C. SVANES, AND J. LEKVEN. Gastric blood flow determination: intramural distribution and arteriovenous shunting of microspheres. *Am. J. Physiol.* 247 (*Gastrointest. Liver Physiol.* 10): G468–G479, 1984.
144. WATKINS, D. W., AND G. A. HOLLOWAY. An instrument to measure cutaneous blood flow using the Doppler shift of laser light. *IEEE Trans. Biomed. Eng.* 25: 28–33, 1978.
145. WHITE, D. N. Johann Christian Doppler and his effect—a brief history. *Ultrasound Med. Biol.* 8: 583–591, 1982.
146. WUNDERLICH, R. W., R. L. FOLGER, D. B. GIDDON, AND B. R. WARE. Laser-Doppler blood flow meter and optical plethysmograph. *Rev. Sci. Instrum.* 51: 1258–1262, 1980.
147. YEH, Y., AND H. Z. CUMMINGS. Localized fluid flow measurements with an He-Ne laser spectrometer. *Appl. Phys. Lett.* 4: 176–178, 1964.
148. YOUNG, W. $H_2$ clearance measurement of blood flow: a review of technique and polarographic principles. *Stroke* 11: 552–564, 1980.
149. YU, Y. M., L. C. YU, AND C. C. CHOU. Distribution of blood flow in the intestine with hypertonic glucose in the lumen. *Surgery St. Louis* 78: 520–525, 1975.

CHAPTER 38

# Physiology of gastric circulation

PAUL H. GUTH — *Veterans Administration Medical Center and Center for Ulcer Research and Education (CURE), West Los Angeles, and University of California, Los Angeles, California*

FELIX W. LEUNG — *Division of Gastroenterology, Sepulveda Veterans Administration Medical Center, University of California, Los Angeles, and CURE, West Los Angeles, California*

GORDON L. KAUFFMAN, JR. — *Division of General Surgery, Milton S. Hershey Medical Center, Pennsylvania State University, University Park, Pennsylvania, and CURE, West Los Angeles, California*

## CHAPTER CONTENTS

Anatomy
  Supplying vessels
  Microvessels
    Muscularis externa
    Submucosa
    Arteriovenous anastomoses
    Mucosa
  Modification of stomach wall blood flow
  Gastric lymphatic system
Techniques for Measuring Gastric Blood Flow
  Gross flow
  Mucosal blood flow
    Clearance techniques based on $pK_a$
    Indicator-dilution (fractional extraction) techniques
    Inert-gas clearance techniques
    Other techniques
  Techniques for studying gastric microvasculature
    In vivo microscopy
    Injection and fixation
    In vitro arterial strips
Control of Gastric Blood Flow
  Neural
    Central nervous system
    Autonomic nervous system
  Biogenic amines
    Catecholamines
    Histamine
  Gastrointestinal hormones
    Gastrin
    Vasoactive intestinal peptide
    Vasopressin
    Glucagon
    Somatostatin
    Secretin
    Neurotensin
    Met-enkephalin and morphine
    Norleucine motilin
  Prostaglandins
    Prostaglandins and resting gastric mucosal blood flow
    Prostaglandins, gastric acid secretion, and blood flow
    Prostaglandin-induced mucosal protection and gastric blood flow
  Leukotrienes
Gastric Mucosal Blood Flow in Gastric Physiology
  Acid secretion
    Stimulation of acid secretion
    Inhibition of acid secretion
  Autoregulation
  Eating
  Changes in gastric blood flow with age
  Gastric motility
  Pulse pressure
Gastric Mucosal Blood Flow in Gastric Pathophysiology
  Effect of disruption of gastric mucosal barrier to acid backdiffusion
  Prevention of mucosal injury
  Role of oxygen-derived free radicals in ischemic gastric injury
  Effect of local and systematic hypothermia
  Effect of portal hypertension
  Effect of nicotine and cigarette smoke
  Measurement of gastric hemodynamics in humans

---

OUR UNDERSTANDING of the gastric circulation and its role in gastric physiology and pathophysiology has increased significantly in recent years. Improved techniques to study the anatomical organization of the gastric microvasculature and its regulation and to measure gastric mucosal blood flow under various conditions have played a major role in this advance. This chapter begins with a description of the anatomic organization of both the gross and microscopic vascular supply of the stomach, including a delineation of areas of controversy and areas of deficient knowledge. Next the major techniques used to study the gastric circulation, the principles underlying each, and their advantages and disadvantages are described. Such information is essential for evaluating studies reviewed in the subsequent sections. In some studies contradictory data are reported, and differences in the techniques used may, in part, explain the differing results. Factors controlling gastric blood flow—e.g., nerves, biogenic amines, hormones, and prostanoids—are presented. Next the role of blood flow in gastric physiology is reviewed, including studies that challenge previously held concepts of the relationship between acid secretion and blood flow. Finally the role of blood flow in gastric pathophysiology, including mucosal injury in experimental animals as well as in humans, is discussed.

## ANATOMY

### Supplying Vessels

The celiac artery (axis), which arises from the front of the aorta between the 12th thoracic and 1st lumbar vertebrae, provides the principal arterial supply to the stomach. This short major vessel gives rise to the left gastric, hepatic, and splenic arteries. Classic descriptions, such as those of Michels (170), and the more recent angiographic studies (188) indicate that these vessels or branches from them comprise the six main arteries supplying the stomach, that is, the left and right gastric, the left and right gastroepiploic, the short gastric branches of the splenic, and the small branches from the gastroduodenal arteries. Six other secondary arteries have also been described as frequently sending branches to the stomach. These are the superior pancreaticoduodenal artery of Wilkie (which supplies the pylorus and duodenum), the retroduodenal (which frequently gives off one or more pyloric branches), the transverse pancreatic, the dorsal pancreatic, and the left inferior phrenic arteries. All the supplying vessels anastomose extensively among themselves and with vessels arising from the superior mesenteric artery. Atypical vascular patterns often occur. Some of these have been described in detail by Michels (170) in human cadaver studies and by others (187) in angiographic studies.

The typical pattern of arterial supply to the stomach is diagramed in Figure 1. The left gastric artery reaches the lesser curvature at the level of the cardia, where it turns downward and branches into vessels that supply the anterior and posterior surfaces of the body and fundus of the stomach. The branch to the lesser curvature descends to the right toward the pylorus and anastomoses with the right gastric artery. The right gastric artery is smaller than the left. It is a branch of the hepatic artery and courses along the lesser curvature from the pylorus toward the left. The right and left gastric arteries, as they traverse the lesser curvature, send branches at intervals to the anterior and posterior walls of the antrum. The right

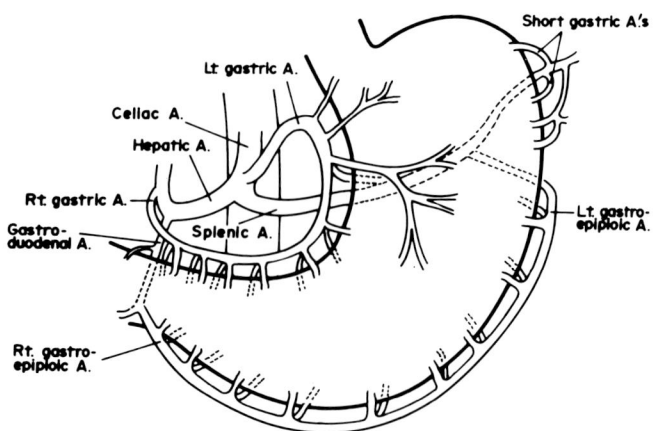

FIG. 1. Arterial supply of the stomach. [From Guth and Ballard (79a). In: *Physiology of the Gastrointestinal Tract*, © 1981, Raven Press, New York.]

gastroepiploic (a branch from the gastroduodenal artery) and left gastroepiploic (a branch from the splenic artery) arteries traverse the greater curvature and send branches at intervals to the anterior and posterior walls of the antrum and corpus. The short gastric arteries arise from the splenic artery as it passes behind the greater curvature of the fundus, and they also supply branches to the anterior and posterior walls of the stomach in this region.

### Microvessels

MUSCULARIS EXTERNA. There is no definitive description of the vascular supply of the muscle layer of the stomach. Our current knowledge is based on in vivo studies of the rat gastric microcirculation (83) and vascular injection studies of human postmortem material (208).

In vivo microscopic studies of the rat gastric microcirculation revealed that as the branches from the supplying arteries pierce the muscle coat, they send branches to the muscle (83). These in turn branch and ultimately divide into capillaries, which course in the superficial and deep muscle layers. There is free communication between the capillaries in the same plane, as well as between capillaries in different planes. Although the terminal arteriole usually divides into capillaries, thoroughfare channels are seen in rare instances. This type of communication differs from the short arteriovenous anastomosis. The thoroughfare channel is formed by an arteriole that has reached near capillary size (metarteriole) but continues for some distance to terminate in a venule, thereby short-circuiting the capillary bed. The capillary network drains into venules accompanying the arterioles. These in turn drain into veins emerging from the submucosal plexus. In a scanning electron-microscopic study of vascular casts of the rat stomach, Browning et al. (28) described the capillaries as showing two orientations that are at right angles to each other and related to the axial orientations of the muscle cells of the external muscle layers. In vascular injection studies of human stomach, Piasecki (208) described the presence of a subserosal and a deep muscle vascular plexus.

SUBMUCOSA. After piercing the muscle coat, the supplying arteries pass to the outer portion of the submucosa and form primary arterial arcades by anastomosing among themselves (15, 83). These provide smaller anastomosing branches, which finally supply anastomosing branches that course in the muscularis mucosae or in the base of the mucosa just above the muscularis mucosae (79). The latter are clearly seen in india ink injection studies (Fig. 2A). These in turn send short branches (mucosal arterioles) into the deep mucosa that supply capillaries at the base of the mucosa. In addition, in vivo microscopic studies have revealed that in some areas arteriolar branches from the submucosal arteriolar plexus go back up to the muscle layer to also supply that microvascular bed.

The lesser curvature in the rat appears to have a much less extensive arterial anastomotic network than the other gastric regions. The mucosal arterioles arise from the primary arcade. Barlow et al. (15) and Piasecki (208) described end arteries in the lesser curvature of the human stomach, that is, some mucosal arterioles come directly from the branches of the right and left gastric arteries.

The submucosal veins follow the pattern of the arteries. Collecting veins, which pass perpendicularly through the mucosa, carry blood from the mucosa to venules coursing in or just above the muscularis mucosae (Fig. 2B), which, in turn, enter venules that form the submucosal venular plexus (Fig. 3). The submucosal venules and arterioles generally run in pairs, with the venules exhibiting a larger diameter and a much slower red cell velocity than the corresponding arterioles (64). In turn, the plexus drains into veins that follow the same course as the primary arterial branches to the stomach. Just before the veins leave the muscle, they receive branches from veins draining the muscle layer.

In addition there are a few submucosal capillaries. These branch from submucosal arterioles and run for long distances as single vessels in the plane of the submucosa, external to the submucosal vascular plexus of larger vessels, and drain into submucosal venules (64). They usually exhibit rapid flow.

ARTERIOVENOUS ANASTOMOSES. Based on intravascular dye injection studies of human stomachs, Barlow et al. (15) described the presence of arteriovenous anastomoses or shunts in the submucosa. This structural arrangement offered a possible mechanism for the control of blood flow to the mucosa. On the basis of glass microsphere studies in the dog, Walder (264) concluded that mucosal blood flow is a function of

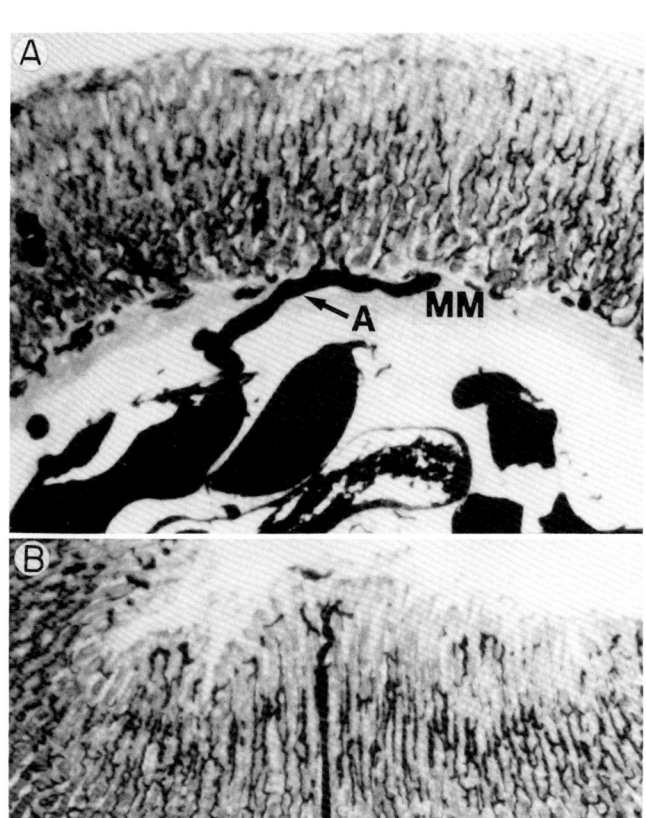

FIG. 2. Photomicrograph of histological section taken after intravascular injection of india ink. A: terminal arcade (A) of submucosal arteriolar plexus actually courses in the base of the mucosa, in or just above muscularis mucosae (MM). Short mucosal arterioles arise from arcade to supply capillaries at base of mucosa. B: collecting venule (CV) also actually lies in the base of mucosa in or just above muscularis mucosae (MM). [From Guth (79).]

mucosal arteriolar resistance and shunt resistance. In studies of the gastric circulation, the role of submucosal arteriovenous anastomoses has frequently been used to explain experimental results. More recently, however, considerable physiological and anatomical data that question the existence of shunts have been published.

In vivo microscopic studies in the rat (64, 83, 102) and cat (89) have failed to reveal evidence of shunts. Utilizing a fluorescent in vivo microscopy technique in the rat, Guth and Moler (81) were able to follow the flow of fluorescein-labeled albumen through the submucosal arterioles to mucosal capillaries and did not see any flow directly from submucosal arterioles to submucosal venules. Finally, Piasecki (208), in an

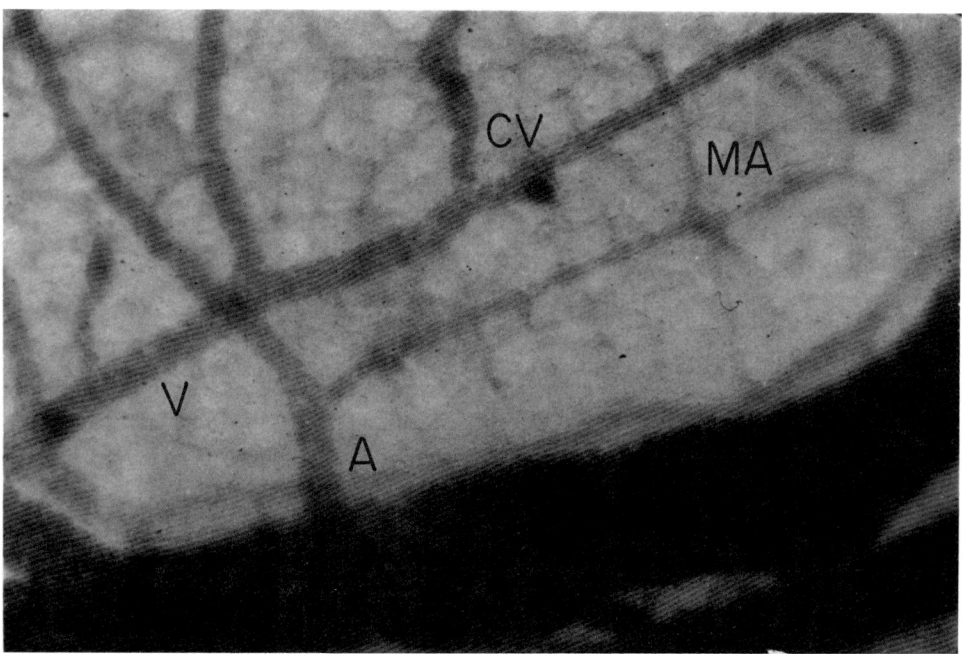

FIG. 3. In vivo photomicrograph of rat gastric submucosal vascular bed. Characteristic submucosal arterial (A) and venous (V) plexi are seen. Venous network can be distinguished by larger diameter of its vessels and presence of collecting veins (CV), seen in cross-section, which drain into venous anastomotic network. Arterial arcade gives rise to mucosal arteriole (MA), which divides and enters the capillary network. This mucosal arteriole appears to be entering a vein; in actuality, it goes beneath the vein to enter the mucosa. Honeycomb-like appearance of mucosal capillary bed is barely visible. × 80. [From Guth and Smith (86), © by Williams & Wilkins, 1975.]

injection study similar to that of Barlow et al. (15), and Gannon et al. (65), in a vascular casting scanning electron-microscopic study, were unable to confirm the presence of submucosal arteriovenous anastomoses in the human stomach.

The anatomic description of the arteriovenous anastomoses by Barlow et al. (15) was based on injection studies. There are several factors that may lead to misinterpretation of these specimens. Staubesand and Hammersen (247) demonstrated that, with two-dimensional viewing, overlapping vessels may appear to be anastomosing. An apparent arteriovenous anastomosis must be viewed from various angles (three-dimensionally) to avoid this error. In addition, pressure-flow relationships and anatomy are distorted by injection techniques, as a result of either the injection pressure or the injection material occluding vessels.

Similarly, the conclusions drawn from microsphere studies, such as those of Walder (264), have been questioned by more recent investigations with improved, accurately sized microspheres with radioactive labels. These permit quantitative estimates of shunt flow. In studies in the baboon, dog, and rat (3, 30, 234, 280), shunt flow was reported as 0%–5.2% of total flow. Thus if shunt flow does exist, it is relatively insignificant, accounting for no more than 5% of total flow.

In conclusion, although there are some recent studies using injection (96) or dye dilution (18) techniques that suggest the presence of shunts, the predominance of current evidence is against their presence.

MUCOSA. The mucosal arterioles divide into several branches, each of which in turn divides into several capillaries in the base of the mucosa (Fig. 2A). The mucosal arterioles are interconnected by slender anastomosing channels, but there are no direct anastomoses with mucosal veins. Most gastric glands are supplied by two to three capillaries, which run between, parallel to, and in close approximation to them. The capillaries thus pass perpendicular to the mucosal surface but do interconnect by short channels at right angles to the axis of the gland tubules (15, 64). Some investigators (193) claimed that the arterioles also course through the mucosa parallel to the glands. More recent work by others (64, 83), however, clearly demonstrated that the arterioles do not extend beyond the base of the mucosa. The capillaries at the mucosal surface branch into loops around the gland openings [Fig. 4; (15, 83, 87)]. Blood from the capillary bed drains into collecting veins distributed throughout the mucosa. The capillaries enter collecting veins only immediately below the mucosal surface. There are no capillary connections to collecting veins deeper in the mucosa [Fig. 5; (64, 65)]. The collecting veins course perpendicularly from the superficial mucosa to the muscularis mucosae, where they enter the submucosal venous plexus.

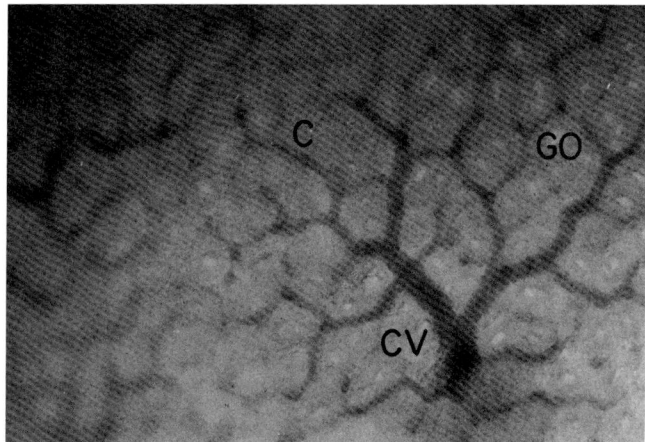

FIG. 4. In vivo photomicrograph of surface of rat gastric mucosa. Honeycomb-like appearance of capillaries (C) surrounding glands and ultimately draining into collecting veins (CV) is clearly seen. Orifices (GO) of glands in center of surrounding capillaries can be seen in some areas. × 75. [From Guth and Smith (86), © by Williams & Wilkins, 1975.]

The direction of blood flow in mucosal capillaries is from the base of the mucosa to the surface. Therefore, blood passing the oxyntic cells in the middle of the mucosa may receive $HCO_3^-$ from these cells during acid secretion (alkaline tide) and carry it to the mucosal surface cells. Gannon et al. (64) have proposed such an intramucosal transfer of $HCO_3^-$ and have postulated that this might assist in protecting the gastric surface epithelium against backdiffusing $H^+$.

*Modification of Stomach Wall Blood Flow*

As can be seen from the preceding description and from Figure 6, the submucosal and mucosal microvessels are connected in series. The main supplying artery sends a branch to the muscle layer and then continues to the submucosa to form the submucosal arteriolar plexus; thus the muscle vascular bed is in parallel with the submucosal-mucosal vascular bed. This latter arrangement provides an anatomical explanation for the changes in distribution of flow between muscle and submucosa-mucosa under certain experimental conditions. For example, Delaney and Grim (49), using the $^{42}K$ indicator-dilution technique, found that in the corpus of the canine stomach the mucosa received >70% of the blood flow, the remainder being divided about equally between the submucosa and the muscularis. With norepinephrine infusion, gastric perfusion decreased from 0.54 to 0.40 $ml \cdot min^{-1} \cdot g^{-1}$ and there was redistribution of flow from mucosa (from 72% to 64%) to the muscularis (from 15% to 22%).

The overall anatomical arrangement of the submucosal arteriolar network explains the importance of this network in controlling blood flow to the mucosa. Mucosal flow is decreased by constriction of these vessels and is increased by dilatation of these vessels. In vivo microscopic observations (86) revealed that stimulation of the splanchnic nerve caused constriction of the submucosal arterioles followed by dilatation of the arterioles toward control diameters, despite continued splanchnic nerve stimulation (escape from

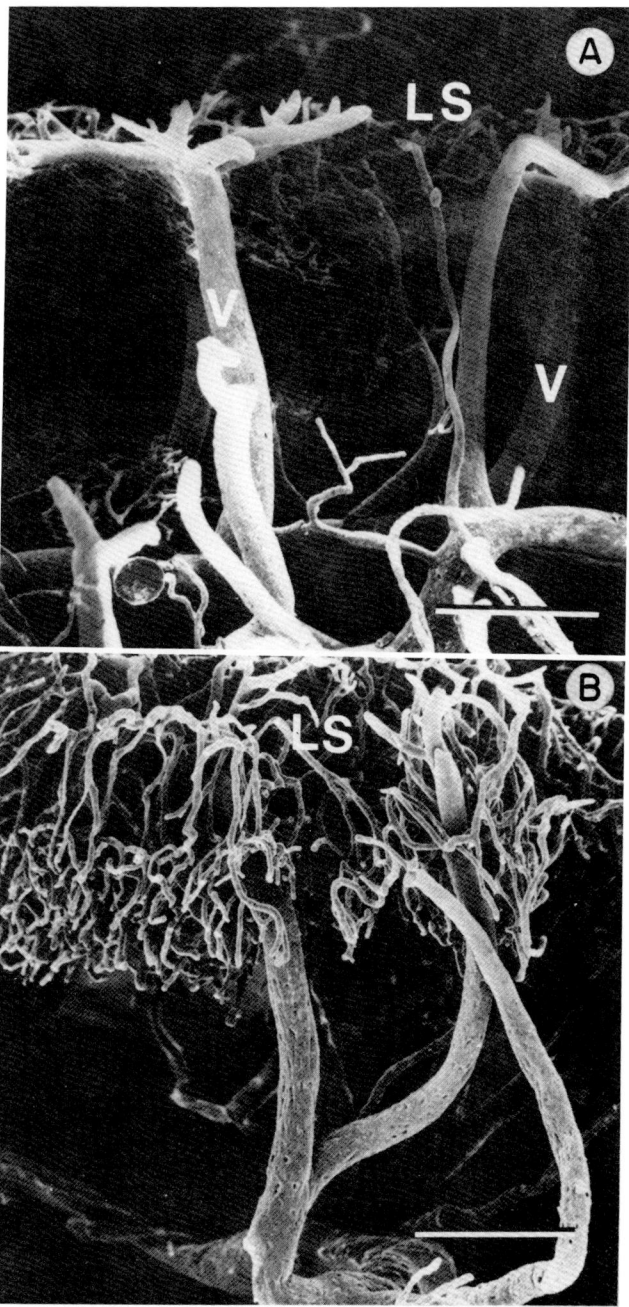

FIG. 5. Gastric mucosal venous vasculature. Scanning electron micrographs of (retrograde) venous partial casts; i.e., only venous vessels and venous portions of capillary network are filled with casting medium. A: mucosal venules (V) receive capillary tributaries at luminal surface (LS) but then penetrate mucosal region without further capillary connections. Bar, 0.3 mm. B: as seen in Fig. 3A, with greater filling of venous end of capillary network adjacent to luminal surface (LS). Venules converge within mucosal region but again are without further direct capillary tributaries en route to submucosa. Bar, 0.25 mm. [From Gannon et al. (64).]

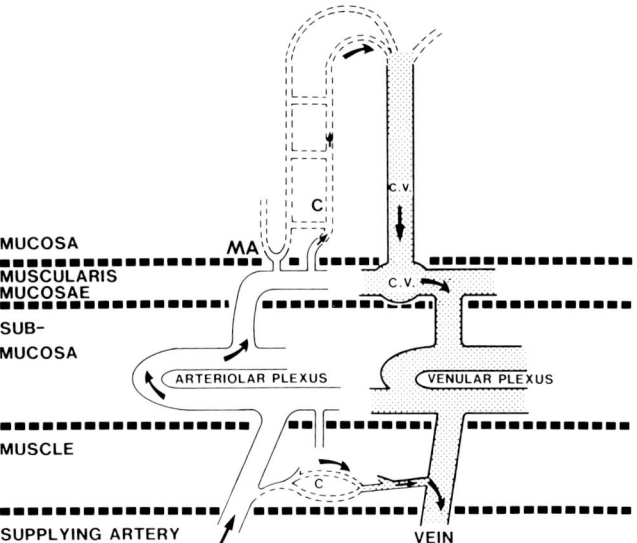

FIG. 6. Gastric microcirculation. MA, mucosal arteriole; C, capillary; CV, collecting vein. Microvasculature of muscle layer is in parallel with that of mucosa, while microvasculature of submucosa is in series with that of mucosa. There are no arteriovenous anastomoses. [From Guth and Leung (80a). In: *Physiology of the Gastrointestinal Tract*, © 1987, Raven Press, New York.]

adrenergic vasoconstriction). Observation of flow in capillaries in the superficial mucosa during splanchnic nerve stimulation revealed cessation of flow followed by partial resumption of flow. The time course of events in the submucosa and mucosa was consistent with the concept that constriction of the submucosal arterioles decreased mucosal blood flow, and dilatation of the submucosal arterioles increased blood flow.

## Gastric Lymphatic System

There has been a dearth of studies in recent years concerning the gastric lymphatic system. Nagata and Guth (184) studied the anatomy of the lymphatic system in the rat stomach by means of fluorescent in vivo microscopy. A fluorescein-albumin conjugate was injected via a micropipette into the mucosa, submucosa, or muscularis externa. The conjugate movement was visualized with a closed-circuit television system. When injected into the base of the mucosa, the conjugate flowed from the deposited pool. These fluorescent streams, 21–53 $\mu$m diam, formed a network in the base of the mucosa and superficial submucosa. They were in close approximation to, but separate from, the arterioles and venules. These fluorescent channels probably represent lymphatic microvessels, as they were connected to larger lymphatic microvessels running parallel to the large arterioles and venules in the deep submucosa. These larger lymphatic vessels passed through the muscularis externa and drained into extragastric lymphatic vessels on the lesser or greater curvature. There was no network of lymphatic microvessels in the deep submucosa or muscularis externa. The extragastric lymphatic vessels, 50–340 $\mu$m diam, had valves and displayed spontaneous contractions, moving the conjugate toward the lymph nodes.

## TECHNIQUES FOR MEASURING GASTRIC BLOOD FLOW

### Gross Flow

The oldest method for measuring blood flow in an organ is by collection of venous effluent. This technique assumes that venous drainage reflects arterial inflow; it necessitates the surgical isolation of a vein, for example, the gastrosplenic, in which case complete splenectomy often is performed. In some instances the omentum also is removed. Scrupulous attention must be paid to the ligation of all drainage channels other than the one from which effluent is to be collected. It is especially difficult to isolate gastric blood flow from that of the pancreas and duodenum. In many studies an isolated flap of stomach supplied by one artery and one vein is used.

The use of the electromagnetic flowmeter, developed by Kolin (133), is a less traumatic technique. When a conducting fluid, that is, one with ions, such as blood, moves through a magnetic field, an electromagnetic force proportional to the flow rate is created. In practice, a cuff transducer is placed around the vessel to pick up the electrical signal for amplification and recording. A distinct advantage for this method is that the electromagnetic flowmeter is virtually insensitive to the velocity profile in the vessel.

Although there is surgical trauma during placement of the cuff, the incision can be closed and the animal allowed to recover (112). In earlier models of electromagnetic flowmeters, the vessels had to be repeatedly occluded to determine base-line or zero flow; this is achieved electronically, without occlusion, in newer models.

### Mucosal Blood Flow

CLEARANCE TECHNIQUES BASED ON $pK_a$. Gastric clearance techniques, based on principles described by Shore et al. (236) and developed by Jacobson et al. (113), were widely used until recently. They can be used in either anesthetized or unanesthetized animals. Gastric secretion and blood flow can both be measured simultaneously. The method is based on the principle that diffusion of weak organic compounds, such as weak bases, through lipid membranes depends on the degree of ionization of the compound. Lipid membranes are selectively permeable to the undissociated form of the molecule. The cell membrane, which separates plasma and gastric juice, is a lipid barrier; at the pH of blood, the un-ionized base diffuses freely through the membrane. When it comes in contact with the markedly lower pH of the gastric juice, the base dissociates; because it is no longer so lipid soluble, it cannot diffuse back into the blood. This marked difference in pH accounts for the difference in concentration of the ionized molecule in the gastric juice and plasma phases; the extent of this difference depends on the $pK_a$ of the compound. Drugs with a $pK_a$ of 5–10 will diffuse from the plasma and accumulate in the gastric juice, provided the pH is below the $pK_a$.

Aminopyrine clearance is the most widely used technique based on this principle (113). A loading dose of aminopyrine is followed by a continuous intravenous infusion of a maintenance dose throughout the experiment to stabilize plasma aminopyrine concentration. Gastric juice samples are collected at intervals and the volume, $H^+$ concentration, and aminopyrine concentration are determined. Venous blood samples also are taken at intervals and analyzed for aminopyrine concentration. The clearance, which represents pouch mucosal plasma flow, is calculated from the equation $C = GV/P$, where C is the clearance (ml/min), G is gastric juice concentration, P is plasma aminopyrine concentration (mg/ml), and V is the gastric secretory rate (ml/min). The ratio of G/P, designated as R, tells us how much plasma flow in the mucosa occurred per unit of secretory volume (substituting R for G/P in the clearance equation yields $C = RV$ or $R = C/V$). Cowley et al. (43) demonstrated that, by the intragastric instillation of exogenous acid, aminopyrine clearance could be used to measure gastric mucosal blood flow in the nonsecreting state.

Other compounds utilizing this same principle that have been used to measure gastric clearance include [$^{14}C$]aminopyrine (80, 252), $^{14}C$-labeled aniline (32, 45, 236), technetium-99 (254), and neutral red (128–131).

*Critique of aminopyrine clearance.* Recent studies have raised serious questions about the validity of the amionpyrine-clearance technique as a measure of just mucosal blood flow. Because aminopyrine diffuses down a hydrogen ion gradient [accumulation of aminopyrine is used as a measure of acid secretion in isolated parietal cell studies (241)], it has been suggested that aminopyrine clearance reflects parietal cell function as well as mucosal blood flow. In human studies, Sonnenberg and Blum (242) observed a rapid rise and subsequent fall in clearance after aminopyrine administration, and a rapid, transient rise in clearance during pentagastrin infusion, although acid secretion remained at a constant high level. In patients with pernicious anemia, these two phenomena were not observed, and the maximal aminopyrine clearance was half as high as the minimal aminopyrine clearance of the nonstimulated stomach of healthy controls. Sonnenberg and Blum believe three phenomena are taking place within the gastric mucosa and may be responsible: *1*) a diffusion limit between the blood compartment and the gastric lumen, *2*) facilitated excretion of aminopyrine by bulk flow, and *3*) storage within the mucosa. Sonnenberg and Blum concluded that a diffusion barrier alone could not account for their data. Instead they felt the only reasonable explanation was a combination of aminopyrine storage and consecutive washout by basal and stimulated volume flow. Based on an extensive mathematical analysis, both theoretical and of Jacobson's data (110), Dugas and Wechsler (53) concluded that the rate-limiting step for aminopyrine to gastric juice is the resultant of, at least, blood flow and diffusion limitations. In a study designed to compare this technique with two others (146), gastric mucosal blood flow changes were measured by hydrogen gas clearance and aminopyrine clearance. These changes were then compared with left gastric artery flow changes measured by an electromagnetic flow probe. During pentagastrin stimulation, blood flow measurements by hydrogen gas clearance and the electromagnetic flow probe increased by 22% ± 6% and 17% ± 5%, respectively, whereas by aminopyrine clearance it increased by 216% ± 77%. The close agreement between the hydrogen gas clearance and left gastric artery flow changes is in agreement with radiopotassium (49) and microsphere (33) studies that showed that changes in mucosal blood flow are proportional to alterations in total blood flow. The extremely high aminopyrine clearance suggests that it reflects acid secretion as well as mucosal blood flow.

INDICATOR-DILUTION (FRACTIONAL EXTRACTION) TECHNIQUES. *Potassium-42 and rubidium-86.* The indicator-dilution technique, using $^{42}K$ and $^{86}Rb$, has been used to determine gastric blood flow and its distribution under basal and experimental conditions (48, 49, 78, 225, 232, 274). This technique is based on the assumption that the fraction of the injected isotope in an organ 30–60 s after injection of a small bolus of the isotope is equal to the fraction of the cardiac output perfusing that organ. Theoretically all the $^{42}K$ or $^{86}Rb$ in the blood flowing through an organ exchanges with intracellular K in a single passage through the organ. The blood flow of an organ is obtained by multiplying cardiac output by the fraction of injected isotope in that organ.

*Radioactive-labeled microspheres.* One form of the indicator-dilution method is the radioactive-labeled microsphere technique. Microspheres of a uniform size are injected into the left ventricle. The spheres are distributed to the different organs according to the fraction of the cardiac output going to the respective organs. The microspheres are trapped in vessels smaller than the diameter of the spheres. From the radioactivity of the tissue in which the investigator is interested, the total amount of radioactivity injected, and the cardiac output, the flow in milliliters per minute to that tissue can be calculated. The critical assumption of the microsphere is different from that of the $^{42}K$ and $^{86}Rb$ methods. The question regarding the microspheres is whether they distribute at arterial bifurcations in proportion to blood flow. The questionable assumption in the $^{42}K$ or $^{86}Rb$ technique is that all tissues have the same extraction ratio for the isotope. For the microspheres, all vessels less than the diameter of the spheres should extract 100% of those entering; in the absence of significant arteriovenous shunt flow, all tissues would have equal extractions for the spheres. Delaney and Grim (48) found close agreement between the mean distribution in the mucosa, submucosa, and muscularis of the dog stomach of 16- or 10-μm-diam microspheres and $^{42}$K.

Comparison with aminopyrine clearance. Archibald et al. (3) studied radioactive-labeled microsphere and aminopyrine-clearance measurements simultaneously in anesthetized dogs. Although there was a reasonably close relationship between the two methods in estimating mucosal perfusion during histamine stimulation (clearance averaged 90% of the microsphere value), during isoproterenol infusion and in the resting state, aminopyrine clearance averaged only 38% and 46%, respectively, of the microsphere value. Archibald et al. conclude that aminopyrine clearance reflects only a small fraction of mucosal blood flow in the nonsecreting stomach, even in the presence of exogenous acid. They speculate that externally applied acid in the resting stomach may not provide as effective a pH gradient for cells lining the glands as when they are continuously exposed to a fresh supply of acid in the secreting stomach.

Advantages and disadvantages. An advantage of the microsphere technique over the isotope technique is that microspheres with different labels, for example, $^{85}$Sr, $^{141}$Ce, and $^{51}$Cr, can be injected at different times during an experiment (with cardiac output determined each time by obtaining an integrated blood sample from the aorta using a withdrawal pump at a constant rate for a short period of time). When the animal is killed at the end of the experiment, the organ blood flow at the different times during the course of the study is obtained from the organ concentration of the different labels and the cardiac output for the time the label was injected.

Serious questions have been raised by Greenway and Murthy (77) about the validity of the microsphere technique in assessing distribution of blood flow when the blood vessels of the area studied are in series rather than in parallel. In a study of the distribution of blood flow in the intestine, Greenway and Murthy found that the distribution of microspheres between the mucosa and submucosa depended on the size of the microspheres. The smaller the spheres, the more were found in the mucosa, for example, 47.4% of 12-μm spheres as compared with 26.3% of 17-μm spheres. The distribution also depended on the state of the vascular bed. When given during an infusion of vasopressin, the mucosa-submucosa distribution of 17-μm spheres was 20.9% to 79.1%. A subsequent infusion of isoprenaline resulted in movement of some of the spheres from the submucosa into the mucosa, the distribution becoming 44.4% to 55.6%. The data of Greenway and Murthy suggest that the intestine consists of two parallel-coupled circuits, one to the muscle and the other through the submucosa to the mucosa. The vessels in the submucosa are in series with those in the mucosa, and submucosal shunts do not exist. On the basis of in vivo microscopic studies, the same is true of the microvascular bed of the stomach (Fig. 6). Maxwell et al. (163) reported similar findings in the canine intestine, even when vessels were not initially constricted. Vasodilatation with isoproterenol or increasing perfusion pressure caused migration of microspheres infused earlier. The combined mucosal-plus-submucosal compartments, however, were relatively constant even after vasodilatation with isoproterenol. Maxwell et al. conclude that when redistribution occurs primarily between mucosa and submucosa, combining these two layers into a single compartment may facilitate data analysis.

INERT-GAS CLEARANCE TECHNIQUES. *Hydrogen gas clearance.* The recently validated hydrogen gas-clearance technique (6, 39, 146, 181) using platinum contact electrodes permits regional gastric mucosal blood flow measurements to be obtained in conscious and anesthetized animals as well as in humans. This technique is based on the dissociation of molecular hydrogen at the surface of platinum into hydrogen ions and electrons. A platinum electrode positioned against the gastric mucosa and a calomel or a Ag-AgCl reference electrode placed in the abdominal cavity or on the skin are connected to a polarographic unit and chart recorder. As hydrogen gas is inhaled, it accumulates in the gastric mucosa, and the circuitry permits the current resulting from the hydrogen dissociation ($H_2 \xrightarrow{Pt} 2H^+ + 2e^-$, where $e$ is electron) to be recorded. In in vitro systems these current measurements are unaffected by pH changes in the vicinity of the electrode (10, 146, 181). When the external hydrogen gas is discontinued, the current gradually falls. Because the hydrogen gas can be removed from the tissue only by blood flow, the fall in current is proportional to blood flow. Points along the desaturation current tracing are plotted on semilogarithmic paper. The half time, $t_{1/2}$ (min), is determined from this plot. Flow in ml·min$^{-1}$·100 g$^{-1}$ is given by the following equation: flow = $0.693/t_{1/2} \times 100$.

Despite variations in the technique used by different investigators, the following results are consistently demonstrated. Mucosal blood flow is higher in the antrum than in the corpus in the resting state (39, 146, 181). Secretagogue stimulation increases corpus but not antral mucosal blood flow (39, 146, 181). Vasopressin infusion decreases both antral and corpus mucosal blood flow (39, 146).

When hydrogen gas clearance, venous outflow, and microsphere measurements are compared, good correlation is revealed (6, 39). Aminopyrine clearance and hydrogen gas clearance give similar directional changes with pentagastrin (146, 181) or vasopressin (146) stimulation, with much greater percent changes demonstrated by aminopyrine clearance (146). Under pentagastrin stimulation, simultaneous aminopyrine-clearance and hydrogen gas–clearance measurements and electromagnetic-flow-probe measurement of left gastric artery flow provide additional data to resolve the discrepancy (146). The increases measured by hydrogen gas clearance and electromagnetic flow probe are of the same order of magnitude (22% ± 6% and 17% ± 5%, respectively), whereas that measured by aminopyrine clearance is of much higher order of magnitude (216% ± 77%). These data, together with earlier reports that aminopyrine clearance reflects not just mucosal flow but also parietal cell function (179, 242), call into question the validity of aminopyrine clearance for the measurement of gastric mucosal blood flow.

Limitations of hydrogen gas clearance. Saturation of all tissues with the gas is a basic requirement of all inert-gas washout techniques for blood-flow measurements (124). This is not possible with the inhalation of pure hydrogen, as was initially used by Murakami et al. (181) and Cheung and Sonnenschein (39). Inhalation of 100% hydrogen gas, even briefly, results in hypoxia. Leung et al. (146) reported the use of 3% hydrogen in air to avoid the explosive hazard of >4% hydrogen in air mixtures, and hypoxia. Full tissue saturation can be achieved, and an average of 10–15 min is required for the current tracing to reach plateau. With shorter periods of hydrogen gas administration, hydrogen partial pressure is not equalized in all tissue compartments. Under these conditions, hydrogen gas–clearance curves reflect not only tissue blood flow but also diffusion of hydrogen from tissue compartments of high concentration to those of low concentration (92) and yield artifactually high flow values (146). Discrepancies in the absolute values of mucosal blood flow among different laboratories (39, 146, 181) are most likely explainable by this theoretical consideration. Takeshita et al. (253) have reported that hydrogen gas clearance is unable to detect increases in flow induced by pentagastrin.

Advantages of hydrogen gas clearance. The technique of hydrogen gas clearance permits repeated measurement of gastric mucosal blood flow in focal areas. The contact electrode method has been applied not only in anesthetized rats (146, 181), rabbits (146), and dogs (39) but also in conscious humans (181). The potential applicability in conscious human studies is a distinct advantage over other techniques. Pure hydrogen, already reported for use in human studies by Murakami et al. (181), is unlikely to gain widespread acceptance because of the explosive and hypoxic hazard. The applicability of 3% hydrogen in air in human studies remains to be confirmed.

Radiolabeled inert-gas washout. Washout of radiolabeled inert gases, for example, $^{85}$Kr or $^{133}$Xe, has also been used to estimate blood flow (19, 152). These gases are lipid soluble and pass rapidly across the blood-tissue interface, being limited only by blood flow. They are almost completely eliminated by the lungs in one passage, so that practically no recirculation occurs. A bolus of known concentration of indicator is either injected intra-arterially or is placed in the gastric lumen and the disappearance of the isotope with time recorded. The radioactive decay rate versus time is plotted on semilog paper. For a single-compartment vascular bed, the curve is monoexponential. Most organs, however, are heterogeneous, and more than one flow rate to different compartments occurs. The resulting multiexponential curve must be analyzed by a curve peeling procedure, which makes the assumption that the components of the curve each have exponential washout curves that can be added for the total curve. Ivarsson et al. (107) recently described a modification of the $^{85}$Kr-elimination method that permitted the determination of total gastric blood flow and muscle blood flow, and, by subtraction, submucosa-mucosa blood flow. Krypton-85 was injected intra-arterially and a scintillation detector was used to record the disappearance of $\alpha$-activity from the entire gastric wall, and a Geiger-Müller tube was used to record the disappearance of $\beta$-activity from the muscle layer.

OTHER TECHNIQUES. *Reflectance spectrophotometry.* The technique of reflectance spectrophotometry has been used by Sato et al. (226) to determine the hemoglobin concentration of the rat gastric mucosa. Two fiberoptic coaxial light guides couple the mucosal surface to a spectrophotometer. The coaxial light guide is gently applied to the mucosa. Incident light from a monochromator is carried by the outer light guide to the mucosa. Reflected light from the mucosa is carried back by the central guide to the spectrophotometer. The difference in absorption between 560 nm (the isobestic point of oxy- and deoxyhemoglobin) and 650 nm (beyond the hemoglobin absorption spectrum) showed a linear correlation with hemoglobin concentration up to 150 nmol hemoglobin/g mucosa. The intensity of the spectrum was greater in the corpus than the antral mucosa. Both fell with hemorrhagic shock. By appropriate spectral analysis, the oxygen saturation of mucosal hemoglobin can also be determined. The spectrophotometer is connected to a computer and both total hemoglobin concentration and oxygen saturation determinations are rapidly obtained. Multiple readings at different points in the gastric mucosa can be made quickly and easily.

Reflectance spectrophotometry also can be used in humans by passing the coaxial light guide through the biopsy channel of an endoscope. In a study of 27 patients with thermal or head injury, Kamada et al. (120) reported that when gastric mucosal blood volume (hemoglobin concentration) was ~36% of age-matched controls, acute gastric mucosal lesions developed a few days later. Mucosal lesions did not develop in those patients whose mucosal blood volume on admission was normal or only slightly decreased on admission. In a study of patients with gastric ulcer, mucosal blood volume in the ulcer margin rose ~33% above that in the intact surrounding mucosa during healing. This rise did not occur in those ulcers that failed to heal after 3 mo therapy.

*Laser-Doppler velocimetry.* Laser-Doppler velocimetry (LDV) is based on the principle that light scattered by moving red blood cells experiences a shift in its frequency, and the mean Doppler frequency therefore provides an estimate of blood flow (25). A fiberoptic guide conducts laser light to the tissue and carries backscattered light to a photodetector. The advantages are that it provides a continuous measurement of flow in a limited region and it can be used endoscopically to measure mucosal flow. The LDV technique has limitations: maintaining constant optical coupling between the probe and tissue is difficult (due to peristalsis), and excessive pressure can cause ischemia (72). Although there are several studies of the use of LDV to measure intestinal blood flow in experimental animals (59, 233), there is only a preliminary report concerning its use to measure gastric mucosal blood flow. Simultaneously, Saita et al. (222) estimated gastric corpus mucosal blood flow in the rat by LDV and hydrogen gas clearance. The laser-Doppler flow signal is in electrical units (voltage) and not absolute blood-flow units. Saita et al. observed a good correlation ($r = 0.8$) between the LDV signal and hydrogen gas clearance (which measures blood flow in $ml \cdot min^{-1} \cdot 100\ g^{-1}$) as mucosal flow was decreased by vasopressin or bleeding or increased by pentagastrin administration.

*Iodoantipyrine clearance.* In 1945, Kety (124) established the theoretical basis for the estimation of tissue blood flow making use of inert tracers. In 1982, Dugas and Wechsler (54) validated the use of radiolabeled iodoantipyrine clearance for measuring gastrointestinal tissue blood flow using tissue sampling. Most recently iodo-$^{14}$C-labeled antipyrine autoradiography has been used to measure regional blood flow in the stomach and duodenum by Hudson et al. (101a). These iodoantipyrine-clearance techniques are based on the Fick principle, which states that the time rate of change of tissue concentration of a biologically inert, diffusible tracer is equal to the difference between the rates at which the tracer is brought to the tissue in arterial blood and removed from it by the venous blood. Kety (124) has shown that when extraction is complete, the relationship can be expressed mathematically as

$$Ci_{(T)} = \lambda k \int_0^T Ca_{(t)} e^{-k(T-t)} dt$$

where $Ci_{(T)}$ is the concentration of the tracer in the tissue at time $T$ when the circulation is stopped, $\lambda$ is the tissue-blood partition coefficient specific for the tracer and tissue under consideration, $k$ is the rate of blood flow per unit weight of tissue multiplied by the reciprocal for that tissue, Ca is the concentration of tracer in the arterial blood at each time interval ($t$) during the tracer infusion, and $e$ is the base for natural logarithms.

Because this equation cannot be solved for flow, a table listing $Ci_{(T)}$ values for a wide range of blood flows can be generated using the arterial concentration values from a given experiment. This can be accomplished by use of an iterative program and a microcomputer. After $Ci_{(T)}$ values are obtained from tissue samples or autoradiographs of that experiment, the corresponding flow values can be read from the table.

In practice, the labeled iodoantipyrine is infused intravenously over 30–60 s; during this period arterial blood samples are obtained every 3–5 s. Immediately prior to completion of the infusion, cardiac arrest is induced by the rapid intravenous injection of KCl. Tissue samples are quickly obtained and rapidly frozen (in isopentane cooled to dry ice temperature, for example). Subsequently the blood radioactivity is determined and either tissue radioactivity is determined (tissue-sampling technique) or frozen sections are cut and autoradiographs are prepared (autoradiography technique).

Dugas and Wechsler (54) used the tissue-sampling technique to obtain blood-flow values for different segments of the gastrointestinal tract that were within the range obtained with standard, accepted techniques. The autoradiography technique permits evaluation of distribution of blood flow among tissue layers, but also within a single layer such as the mucosa (101a).

*Heat clearance.* Mucosal blood flow has been measured in unanesthetized animals by a heat-clearance technique (20) and with a thermocouple (70, 74, 132, 248). These methods are based on the assumption that change in blood flow in a tissue will result in altered thermal conductivity of the tissue. In the heat-clearance technique, a small heater coil is affixed to the mucosal wall and maintained there by continuous suction of ~ 5 mmHg. The coil contains a thermistor to measure temperature within the coil. Energy is applied to the heater at constant rate, and changes in blood flow result in altered thermal conductivity. A second, remote thermistor picks up the ambient tissue temperature. Thermal conductivity (flow) is given by

$$\lambda = KI^2/\phi$$

where $\lambda$ is thermal conductivity (flow), $K$ is the instrument constant, $\phi$ is the temperature difference between the two thermistors, and $I^2$ is current supplying the heater coil. Because $I^2$ is constant, for any particular instrument, flow ($\lambda$) = $1/\phi$. Although this technique can be used in conscious animals with appropriate chronic gastric pouches, it has several disadvantages. One is that measurements are only qualitative; that is, results are expressed in units such as millivolts and not milliliters per minute. Another disadvantage is that the suction required to attach the device to the mucosa may interfere with the record and cause electrical interference.

*Constant flow and variable pressure.* Change in vascular tone within an organ can be measured by perfusing the organ through the arterial system at a constant rate while measuring perfusion pressure (112, 134). The artery that is perfused must be the sole artery supplying that organ. Venous drainage is usually returned to the perfusion system. The perfusate is an oxygenated nutrient solution at 37°C or heparinized blood.

A pressure transducer placed in the circuit between the pump and the organ will monitor perfusion pressure. Under conditions of increased vascular tone, perfusion pressure will increase and vice versa. This technique does not provide information required to distinguish between arteriolar and venous effects.

With this technique, pharmacological effects of vasoactive compounds can be studied in an organ in situ. The effect of neural stimulation on vascular tone can also be studied. Physiological studies requiring an unanesthetized animal cannot make use of this technique.

*Techniques for Studying Gastric Microvasculature*

IN VIVO MICROSCOPY. Recent advances in in vivo study of microcirculation have led to methods for observing the gastric circulation in the living animal (83, 102, 220). A fasted rat is anesthetized, the abdomen opened, and the stomach exteriorized. An incision is made in the duodenum just distal to the pylorus, and a clad fiberglass rod is passed retrograde to the stomach.

Transillumination of the gastric wall is achieved by passing light from a high-intensity light source through the rod. Removal of the muscle and serosal layers from a small area on the anterior wall permits visualization of blood flow through the submucosal arterial network, down to the deep layer of mucosa, and back through mucosal venules to the submucosal venous network (see Fig. 3). The area under study is kept moist and warm by bathing it continuously with Krebs solution. The superficial mucosa can be visualized with a different preparation. A long incision is made in the anterior wall of the forestomach just proximal to the "ruminal ridge." Part of the adjacent posterior wall of the glandular stomach is then everted through the incision, thus exposing the mucosa to direct visualization. The fiberglass rod is placed beneath the serosa of the everted portion of the stomach. The flow of red blood cells through the capillaries around the mouth of the gastric glands and into the collecting veins can be seen clearly in this preparation (see Fig. 4).

In vivo fluorescence microscopy has been developed for the study of vascular permeability—the movement of large molecules across microvessels (185, 268). A microscope with a vertical illuminator and appropriate filters is used. Fluorescein isothiocyanate conjugated to serum albumin is injected intravenously. A closed-circuit television system using a video camera with an extremely light-sensitive silicon intensifier target permits video monitoring and videotaping of the flow of the fluorescent conjugate through the microvessels and, under appropriate experimental conditions, diffusion out of the vessels into the interstitium. This technique has recently been adapted for the study of gastric microcirculation (82, 182, 183).

INJECTION AND FIXATION. Injection and fixation of the vascular bed has been attempted since before the discovery of circulation by Harvey (95). Barlow (14) injected radiopaque substances at 150 mmHg pressure into one of the gastric gastroepiploic arteries of stomachs excised at surgery or removed from cadavers. Bismuth oxychloride was used to fill the larger vessels, and silver iodide the smaller vessels. Piasecki (208, 209) injected india ink in 2% gelatin or a barium sulfate suspension in his studies of canine and human gastric vasculature. The tissues were fixed in formalin and sectioned or were cleared (Spalteholz technique) and examined under a dissecting microscope.

To preserve the living vascular geometry, silicone elastomer microvascular filling techniques have been used (31, 96, 240). These room temperature, vulcanizing silicone rubbers are infused at normal systemic pressure. Special care is taken to maintain pressure relationships until the cast is hardened. The specimen is then cleared in glycerol, or the parenchymal tissue is dissolved with caustic (for example, KOH) and embedded in plastic.

It is difficult to completely fill the capillary bed with injected material. The viscosity, surface tension, and size of particles of the filling agent must be considered. Injection at nonphysiological pressures can distort the true geometry of the vessels.

Most recently, Gannon and his colleagues (64, 65) have applied the corrosion vascular casting–scanning electron-microscopy technique to the study of the gastric microvasculature. Blood is washed out with a colloid containing saline via a thoracic aorta cannula (the thoracic posterior vena cava is cut to permit outflow), then an acrylic casting medium is infused. The casts are then hardened and the tissue digested and prepared for scanning electron microscopy and stereophotomicrography. The resultant elegant casts and photography have enabled Gannon's group to make detailed descriptions of the gastric microvasculature.

IN VITRO ARTERIAL STRIPS. In vitro preparations of arteries and veins for studies of vascular reactivity to various stimuli have been used widely. The vessels can be cut into ring segments 2–5 mm in length or into helical strips, or they can be incised in intact, unbranched lengths of several centimeters (260). The ring segments and helical strips can be suspended and coupled to a force transducer for measurements of tension development. Longer unbranched segments of large- and medium-sized vessels are suitable for in vitro perfusion. When perfused at constant flow, contraction or relaxation of the vessel will be reflected in changes in perfusion pressure.

## CONTROL OF GASTRIC BLOOD FLOW

### Neural

CENTRAL NERVOUS SYSTEM. The following description by Beaumont (16), based on observations of the exposed gastric mucosa of his patient St. Martin in the early nineteenth century, is probably the first evidence that the central nervous system plays a role in gastric function, including blood flow. Observations of this nature were extended by Wolf (273) in the study of the gastrostomy of his patient, Tom.

> In... predisposition, from whatever cause... fear, anger, or whatever depresses or disturbs the nervous system—the villous coat (of the stomach) becomes sometimes red and dry, at other times pale and moist, and loses its smooth and healthy appearance.

Beaumont describes two opposing patterns of gastric reaction to emotional conflicts. One, an arousal pattern, was characterized by vascular engorgement of the mucosa, increased secretion of HCl, and increased motor activity. The other, marked by a general attitude of withdrawal, was characterized by pallor of the mucosa and a decrease in acid secretion and motor activity.

Using a stereotactic method to implant electrodes in dogs, Leonard and his colleagues (144) studied the effect of anterior and posterior hypothalamic stimulation on left gastric artery blood flow (via an electromagnetic flowmeter probe) and acid secretion. Low-frequency stimulation (25 cycles/s) of the anterior hypothalamus resulted in a parasympathetic vascular and secretory pattern, that is, increased blood flow and acid secretion. Vagotomy abolished this effect, and stimulation of the distal end of the cut vagus nerve increased blood flow. Stimulation of the posterior hypothalamus resulted in a sympathetic vascular and secretory pattern, that is, a marked decrease in gastric blood flow, and inhibition of histamine-stimulated acid secretion. Celiac ganglionectomy abolished the gastric blood flow change.

Osumi et al. (196) studied changes in gastric mucosal blood flow, using the aminopyrine-clearance technique, and acid secretion following electrical stimulation of the lateral hypothalamic area in the rat. Repetitive stimulation at 10 cycles/s for 10 min elicited a significant, reproducible increase in both gastric mucosal blood flow and acid output. Because the injection of norepinephrine into the lateral ventricle blocked these increases, the authors also speculated that a central noradrenergic inhibitor mechanism is involved in the regulation of gastric mucosal blood flow and acid secretion.

Ishikawa et al. (103) showed that electrical stimulation of the caudal portion of the ventromedial hypothalamus (VMH) produced a significant increase in gastric acid output and mucosal blood flow. When gastric acid output was stimulated by 2-deoxy-D-glucose, electrical stimulation of the VMH significantly reduced the level of these parameters. These findings suggest that the VMH is not a homogeneous neuron group but consists of both excitatory and inhibitory neurons.

Osumi et al. (197) demonstrated that in the anesthetized rat, unilateral electrical stimulation of the locus coeruleus and microinjection of norepinephrine into the ala cinerea decreased basal gastric acid output and mucosal blood flow. They speculated that central noradrenergic inhibitory mechanisms originating from the locus coeruleus might be involved in the regulation of gastric functions, probably at the level of the brain stem ala cinerea.

Ishikawa et al. (104) showed that the parallel increase in gastric acid output and mucosal blood flow produced by microinjection of nicotine into the caudal portion of the VMH and ala cinerea could be blocked by concomitant administration of hexamethonium. The increase induced by intraventricular nicotine could be blocked by bilateral destruction of the VMH. Ishikawa and his colleagues speculated that cholinergic nicotine receptors in the VMH were involved in regulation of gastric functions.

The results of the preceding studies can be accepted only with reservation, pending confirmation by other investigators. There have been many more studies on the effect of central nervous stimulation on gastric acid secretion than on blood flow; the results are highly discrepant. Thus Sen and Anand (231), like Porter et al. (211), reported that anterior hypothalamic stimulation increased acid secretion but posterior stimulation did not; Feldman et al. (60) reported that posterior stimulation increased gastric acid secretion but anterior stimulation did not; Porter et al. (211) observed an increase in acid secretion with both anterior and posterior stimulation, although the posterior response was a delayed one; and finally, both Smith and McHugh (239) and Zukoski et al. (281) reported no change in acid secretion on either anterior or posterior hypothalamic stimulation.

AUTONOMIC NERVOUS SYSTEM. *Sympathetic.* The sympathetic nerve supply to the stomach is derived from the 6th to the 10th spinal nerves and terminates in the celiac ganglia. From here, postganglionic fibers reach the stomach as discrete nerves, as nerves mixed with vagal fibers, or as nerves accompanying the arteries. Using a fluorescent histochemical method, Furness (63) found that the arteries to the stomach were richly supplied by adrenergic nerves, as were those penetrating the musculature. There was a profusion of heavily innervated arteries in the submucosa.

On histological section, the adrenergic nerves were seen at the outer edge of the media of the arteries. The smaller branches (mucosal arteries), which crossed the muscularis mucosae to supply the mucosal capillaries, also were accompanied by adrenergic axons. The capillaries were almost exclusively without adrenergic innervation. The veins within the stomach wall were sparsely innervated. In the submucosa, a few of the larger veins (100–200 µm) had adrenergic fibers with them, but veins of <100 µm were generally not innervated. The smaller veins carrying blood away from the stomach were all innervated but less densely than the accompanying arteries. As the veins became larger, their density of innervation became greater but still less so than the adjacent artery. These studies by Furness (63) were performed in the guinea pig, rat, cat, and rabbit. Similar findings were reported by Jacobowitz (108), in that blood vessels in the submucosa and basal parts of the mucosa were fairly densely innervated, while those in the superficial parts of the mucosa were almost devoid of adrenergic fluorescence. Nakamura et al. (186), however, did identify adrenergic nerves in the basal and middle zones of the mucosa of the rat. They appeared to innervate the capillary endothelium. In rats pretreated with 6-hydroxydopamine, there was a widening of the gap between the nerve ending and the capillary endothelial cells, suggesting that adrenergic hypofunction resulted in increased capillary permeability.

Electrical stimulation of the sympathetic fibers to the stomach resulted in decreased total blood flow (venous outflow measurement) (116), celiac (89) and gastroepiploic (206) artery flow (electromagnetic flow probe), and gastric mucosal blood flow (aminopyrine-clearance technique) (22, 214). Using a study of histological sections of stomachs following intravascular injection of colored dyes or india ink, Schnitzlein (227) observed that stimulation of the celiac ganglion caused contraction of the arterioles and relative ischemia of the gastric mucosa. Arabehety et al. (2) observed that splanchnic section resulted in a marked increase in filling of gastric mucosal capillaries with india ink. Thus several independent investigators, using different techniques, came to the same conclusion: stimulation of the sympathetic fibers to the stomach decreases both total and mucosal blood flow to the stomach.

Jansson et al. (116) observed that when stimulation of sympathetic fibers was prolonged, blood flow, following the initial fall, increased and reached a new steady-state flow level within 3–4 min. This phenomenon has been termed autoregulatory escape from adrenergic vasoconstrictor influence. Ross (221) suggested this term to avoid confusion with autoregulation (maintenance of blood flow to a tissue despite alterations in perfusion pressure) and because the escape phenomenon occurs with adrenergic agents but not with vasopressin. Originally the escape was attributed to a flow redistribution in the stomach wall due to the opening of submucosal arteriovenous anastomoses during sympathetic stimulation (61). Both in vitro arterial segment studies (58) and in vivo microscopic observations (84, 87), however, indicate that escape is due to relaxation of initially constricted vessels and not to the opening of shunts.

The in vivo microscopic studies also demonstrated the important role of constriction and dilatation of submucosal arterioles in regulating gastric mucosal blood flow in the rat (86) and cat (89). Stimulation of the left splanchnic nerve for 3 min caused an initial constriction of submucosal arterioles followed by partial escape. No arteriovenous anastomoses were seen either in the resting state or during nerve stimulation. In vivo microscopic observations of the superficial mucosal blood flow during splanchnic nerve stimulation revealed a slowing of flow with progressively fewer red blood cells present in the capillaries and in the collecting veins into which they feed. Finally, there was a complete cessation of flow with no red blood cells seen in the majority of capillaries, and the mucosa appeared blanched. After a while, even though splanchnic stimulation was continuing, escape occurred with a partial return of flow. There was no statistically significant difference between the mean time to maximum constriction of submucosal arterioles and to maximum blanching of the mucosa, or between time to escape in the two areas. Thus the submucosal arterioles appear to be the vascular segment controlling gastric mucosal blood flow; constriction of these arterioles decreases and dilatation increases mucosal blood flow.

Yokotani et al. (276) showed that greater splanchnic nerve stimulation reduced significantly both gastric acid secretion and mucosal blood flow. Stimulation of the splanchnic postganglionic nerve reduced acid secretion to a greater extent than blood flow. Stimulation of the adrenal branch reduced both the acid secretion and blood flow. Infusion of epinephrine reduced mucosal blood flow to a greater extent than acid secretion. Phentolamine antagonized the inhibitory effect of these manipulations. Yokotani et al. speculated that catecholamines released from the splanchnic postganglionic nerve terminals inhibit gastric acid secretion through $\alpha$-adrenergic receptors in the stomach, independent of mucosal blood flow, and that circulating catecholamines released from the adrenal medulla inhibit both acid secretion and mucosal blood flow through $\alpha$-adrenergic receptors in the stomach. Yano et al. (275), however, did demonstrate a direct vasoconstrictor effect of sympathetic stimulation. They measured gastric blood flow in rats by the cross-thermocouple method. Stimulation of the periarterial nerve bundle along the left gastric artery produced a decrease in gastric blood flow, which was antagonized by phenoxybenzamine.

*Parasympathetic.* Effect of vagus nerve stimulation.

The parasympathetic supply to the stomach is via the vagus nerves. Martinson (162) and Jansson (115) demonstrated that in the cat the vagus nerves may be divided into low- and high-threshold groups of fibers (duration of electrical stimulus, less than or greater than 0.5 ms). Stimulation of the high-threshold set induced an atropine-resistant, nonadrenergic relaxation of the stomach. Martinson (161) showed that stimulation of the vagal relaxatory fibers caused a concomitant augmentation of gastric blood flow (venous outflow measurement) and secretion. Atropine reduced the blood flow increase and completely abolished the secretory response.

These observations led Jansson et al. (117) to conclude that the blood flow increase to the stomach during vagal stimulation is largely secondary to an augmented secretion. Careful scrutiny of graphs published by Martinson (161), however, shows an increase in blood flow within 1 min of the onset of vagal stimulation. This suggests a direct dilator effect of vagal stimulation preceding acid secretion (which takes several minutes), as well as the increase in blood flow initiated by the increase in acid secretion.

Zinner et al. (278) used the microsphere technique in cats to demonstrate that with vagus nerve stimulation at the thoracic level, there was a selective increase in gastric blood flow not accompanied by a flow increase to other viscera or change in central hemodynamics.

Yano et al. (275) used the cross-thermocouple method for measuring gastric blood flow in rats. Vagus nerve stimulation produced an increase in gastric blood flow within 20 s. The increase was not affected by atropine or pretreatment with phentolamine, propranolol, indomethacin, or aprotinin but was blocked by hexamethonium. A noncholinergic primary dilator effect of vagus nerve stimulation on the gastric blood vessel was postulated.

Bell and Battersby (19) used an $^{85}$Kr-clearance technique to measure gastric mucosal blood flow in the dog. Vagotomy caused a statistically significant reduction in gastric mucosal blood flow, which occurred within 5 min of nerve section (the earliest measurement made), suggesting a direct vagal effect on the vasculature.

An in vivo microscopy technique in the rat was used by Guth and Smith (86) to study the possible direct vascular effect of vagal nerve stimulation. Gastric submucosal arteriolar diameter was measured immediately before and after vagal nerve stimulation (8 V, 2 ms duration, 6 impulses/s). In 45 or 51 stimulation episodes in 11 rats, the arterioles dilated within 10 s of beginning stimulation and constricted within 10 s of cessation of stimulation. These changes were significant at $P < 0.001$. Similar results were obtained in the cat (89). The findings of immediate submucosal arteriolar dilatation with vagal stimulation and constriction on cessation of stimulation are compatible with a direct dilator effect of vagal stimulation on the vascular smooth muscle of these vessels. This does not deny the important role of other factors secondary to augmented acid secretion in enhancing blood flow to the stomach. The immediate "on-off" response observed in the in vivo microscopic study, however, is too rapid to be explained by factors secondary to acid secretion. In a preliminary report, Morishita and Guth (178) observed that the prompt dilatation of submucosal arterioles was not inhibited by atropine. This supports the postulate of Yano et al. (275) that the direct gastric vasodilator effect of vagal nerve stimulation is not mediated by cholinergic fibers.

These data indicate that vagus nerve stimulation does have a direct vasodilatory effect on the gastric vasculature. Blockade of acid secretion (other than by an anticholinergic agent) during vagus nerve stimulation is an important area for further research. It may provide an answer to the question whether the sustained increase in gastric blood flow during vagus nerve stimulation is due to the augmented acid secretion or is a persistent vasodilatory effect of stimulating the vagus nerve.

Effect of vagotomy. Nakamura et al. (185) used the aminopyrine-clearance technique to study gastric mucosal blood flow and the venous outflow procedure to measure total blood flow in the dog before and after vagotomy. They found a decrease in both total and gastric mucosal blood flow during the immediate postvagotomy period. This reduction was maintained in dogs studied 3 mo after vagotomy. These observations were confirmed by Mackie and Turner (156), who used the hydrogen gas–clearance technique to measure gastric submucosal blood flow in conscious dogs. After bilateral truncal vagotomy, there was an immediate and significant reduction in flow that was maintained for at least 5 wk. Although there is a consensus concerning the early effects of vagotomy on gastric mucosal blood flow, there is controversy concerning the long-term effects. Bell and Shelley (20) reported that no long-term effect of vagotomy was found on mucosal blood flow as measured by the heat-clearance technique. Similarly, Delaney (47), using the radiorubidium indicator-dilution technique, found no significant change in corpus blood flow 4–6 wk after truncal vagotomy; gastric antral flow, however, was increased. These investigators speculate that either the decrease in antral muscle tonus following denervation or reflux of duodenal content through the pyloroplasty might account for the increase in antral blood flow. Analogous findings in in vivo microscopic studies in the rat were described by Hunter et al. (102), in which there was decreased submucosal blood flow in the corpus but increased flow in the antral submucosal microvessels for up to 1 h after vagotomy. Levine et al. (149) measured gastric mucosal blood flow in conscious miniature swine with microspheres 4 wk after either truncal or selective vagotomy and reported that vagotomy did not alter normotensive flow or flow after 5 or 90 min of shock.

The reduction in gastric blood flow immediately after vagotomy suggests that vagal vasodilatory stimuli play a role in establishing basal vessel tone. The lack of long-term effect of vagotomy suggests that an undefined compensatory mechanism restores the basal vasodilatory tone present prior to vagotomy.

*Parasympathetic-sympathetic interaction.* Evidence for cholinergic inhibition of adrenergic neurotransmission in the canine gastric artery has been presented by Van Hee and Vanhoutte (260). In studies on dog gastric artery strips, they found that tetrodotoxin and phenoxybenzamine abolished the contractile response to electrical stimulation, indicating that the contractions were induced by release of endogenous norepinephrine from adrenergic nerve endings. Acetylcholine, which by itself had no effect on basal tension, inhibited the response to electrical stimulation. This suggests that there are muscarinic receptors on the sympathetic nerve endings, the activation of which mediates inhibition of adrenergic neurotransmission.

Left gastric artery perfusion studies were performed in the intact dog (260). Vagal stimulation depressed the vasoconstrictor response to sympathetic (celiac plexus) nerve stimulation significantly more than those induced by exogenous norepinephrine. According to these data, in the blood vessels of the stomach, endogenously released acetylcholine exerts an inhibitory influence on adrenergic neurotransmission. In the resting state, vagal stimulation caused a prompt decrease in perfusion pressure, consistent with the data presented in the previous section of a direct vascular dilatatory effect of vagal stimulation.

*Biogenic Amines*

CATECHOLAMINES. The literature concerning the effect of catecholamines on gastric blood flow presents markedly discrepant findings. Using bubble flowmeters, Cumming et al. (44) found epinephrine to be a dilator and norepinephrine a constrictor of the canine gastric circulation when infused intravenously, whereas, in the cat, Thompson and Vane (257) observed constrictor responses when epinephrine was infused at a high dose. Using the $^{42}$K indicator-dilution technique in the dog, Delaney and Grim (49) found that epinephrine increased and norepinephrine decreased gastric perfusion. Nicoloff et al. (190) measured left gastric and splenic arterial blood flows electromagnetically and observed vasoconstriction in response to the intravenous infusion of norepinephrine, but they observed dilatation in some dogs and constriction in others with the same dose of epinephrine. Using the aminopyrine-clearance technique, Jacobson et al. (113) showed a reduction in gastric mucosal blood flow by intravenous epinephrine during gastrin stimulation and Cowley and Code (42) found an increase in the nonsecreting canine pouch.

Variations in the method of measuring blood flow; dose, route, and duration of drug administration; type of anesthesia; species; and animal preparation may be responsible for these different observations with the intravenous administration of vasoactive agents. In addition, the direct effect of these agents on the gastric circulation is confounded by their effects on cardiac output and other vascular beds. In vitro studies of the effect of agents on arterial strips, in vivo microscopic study of the topical application of agents, and the close intra-arterial infusion of agents permit study of the direct gastric vascular effects of the agents.

Van Hee and Vanhoutte (260) performed in vitro studies on isolated helical strips of canine gastric arteries. Contractile responses were obtained to increasing concentrations of both epinephrine and norepinephrine. Epinephrine produced a greater maximal tension, but there was no significant difference between the dose-response curves for the two catecholamines when the results were expressed as percentage of the maximal response obtained with each catecholamine. The adrenergic blocking agent phenoxybenzamine caused dose-dependent inhibition of the response to both epinephrine and norepinephrine. The $\beta$-agonist isoproterenol neither caused a significant change in tension nor significantly affected the contractile response to epinephrine. The direct constricting effect of both catecholamines was also demonstrated in the intact animal in in vivo microscopic studies in the rat (81, 85). Application of epinephrine (85) and norepinephrine (81) to the intact, exposed gastric submucosal vascular bed produced prompt constriction of the arterioles.

Zinner et al. (279) studied the effects of the close intra-arterial injection of adrenergic agents on the gastric circulation in anesthetized dogs, measuring blood flow through the right and left gastric arteries electromagnetically. Intra-arterial epinephrine and norepinephrine caused constriction, followed by dilatation (escape from adrenergic constriction) in both circulations. The constrictor components were attenuated or abolished by $\alpha$-blockade with phenoxybenzamine, and the dilator components by $\beta$-adrenergic blockade with propranolol. The $\beta$-agonist isoproterenol produced vasodilatation of both right and left gastric circulations; this effect was attenuated by $\beta$-adrenergic blockade. The constrictor response was similar in both circulations, but the dilator response was greater in the left gastric circulation. With epinephrine, the dilator response after the initial constriction in the left gastric artery resulted in a blood flow after 3 min that was significantly greater than the control flow. This may explain the dilator effect of epinephrine infusions reported by several investigators.

Zinner et al. (280) also studied the effect of close

intra-arterial injection of epinephrine in the baboon, measuring total gastric blood flow electromagnetically and using radioactive microspheres to determine regional distribution. Control flow was 55 ml·min$^{-1}$, with 77% of flow going to the gastric mucosa and 2% of injected spheres appearing in the liver. In contrast to the studies on dogs, epinephrine infusion resulted in a sustained vasoconstriction, with no escape from adrenergic constriction. There was neither redistribution of flow (change in percent of flow to the gastric mucosa) nor change in arteriovenous shunting (percent of spheres appearing in the liver). Levine et al. (150) showed that after celiac ganglionectomy, gastric mucosal blood flow was preserved during shock, and gastric mucosal lesion formation was reduced.

These in vitro and in vivo microscopic close arterial injection studies indicate that both norepinephrine and epinephrine initially constrict gastric arteries and decrease gastric blood flow. Escape from adrenergic vasoconstriction occurs (increase in blood flow despite the continued presence of the catecholamine) in dogs but not in baboons. Vasoconstriction in the gastric vascular bed is mediated by $\alpha$-receptor stimulation, and vasodilatation, including the escape phenomenon in dogs, by $\beta$-receptor stimulation.

HISTAMINE. The importance of considering the route of administration and dosage in studying the effects of agents on the gastric circulation is clearly demonstrated in studies in which histamine is given. Over 20 years ago, Peter et al. (207) and Jacobson (109) found that histamine dilates the gastric circulation and increases gastric blood flow when infused locally, under circumstances in which it has no effect on systemic arterial pressure, or when infused systemically in small doses. Conversely, Menguy (167) observed that the administration of large amounts of histamine by a systemic route can cause abrupt hypotension and, presumably, a sympathetic discharge resulting in constriction and a decreased blood flow to the stomach.

Histamine acts via two types of receptors: *1*) those blocked by the older antihistamine agents, such as mepyramine (e.g., the receptors mediating bronchial constriction), termed $H_1$ (5); and *2*) those not blocked by mepyramine (e.g., the receptors mediating gastric acid secretion), termed $H_2$ (21). The recently developed $H_2$ antagonists (21) block the latter receptors.

Main and Whittle (160) studied the types of histamine receptors in the gastric mucosa using the $^{14}$C-aniline–clearance technique to measure gastric mucosal blood flow. They found that when acid secretion was inhibited by either of the histamine $H_2$-receptor antagonists, burimamide or metiamide, histamine still produced an increase in gastric mucosal blood flow. The selective histamine $H_1$-receptor agonist, 2-pyridylethylamine, had no effect on acid output but increased resting mucosal blood flow. These results suggested that histamine $H_2$ receptors, primarily concerned with acid secretion, and $H_1$ receptors, concerned with vasodilatation, are both present in the gastric mucosa.

Guth and Smith (90) studied the types and functions of histamine receptors in the submucosal arterioles of the corpus and antrum of rat and cat stomachs using an in vivo microscopy technique. Change in arteriolar diameter in response to superfusion of the exposed submucosal vascular bed with histamine (with and without the $H_1$ antagonist mepyramine and the $H_2$ antagonist metiamide) was measured by an image-splitting technique. Histamine $H_1$ and $H_2$ receptors subserving vasodilatation were demonstrated in both areas in both species. In a subsequent study Guth et al. (91) demonstrated similar vasodilatation of gastric submucosal arterioles in response to superfusion with the $H_1$ agonists 2-pyridylethylamine and 2-thiazole-ethylamine and the $H_2$ agonist dimaprit. These studies indicate that histamine increases gastric blood flow by stimulating both $H_1$ and $H_2$ histamine receptors on the gastric submucosal arterioles.

In contrast to the findings of Main and Whittle (160) in the rat, Konturek et al. (141) observed in dogs that with metiamide, inhibition of histamine-stimulated acid secretion was always associated with a marked reduction in mucosal blood flow. One possible explanation for these different findings, besides species difference, is a difference in experimental design. Main and Whittle (160) infused metiamide first to study its effect on resting flow (no effect) and then added the histamine infusion and obtained an increase in mucosal flow but not acid secretion. Konturek et al. (141) first infused histamine to obtain a marked rise in acid secretion and mucosal blood flow and then added metiamide, with a resultant decrease in both parameters. Because resting blood flow and acid secretion were not measured, they could not be compared with the histamine plus metiamide measurements.

A species difference has been shown between the rabbit and the rat. Using an isolated vascular perfused stomach preparation, Salvati and Whittle (224) demonstrated that in the rabbit, the $H_1$ agonist (2-pyridylethylamine) constricted, whereas the $H_2$ agonist (dimaprit) dilated the gastric vasculature. In the rat, both agents dilated the gastric vasculature. Curwain and Turner (46) also demonstrated in the rabbit that an $H_2$ agonist caused an increase in gastric mucosal blood flow and acid secretion while an $H_1$ agonist inhibited this blood flow increase.

The $H_2$-receptor antagonists have no effect on resting mucosal blood flow in either the anesthetized rat (160) and cat (94) with metiamide, using the $^{14}$C-aniline– or aminopyrine-clearance technique, or in the rat (200) and dog (50) with cimetidine, using a radiolabeled-microsphere technique.

The effect of $H_2$-receptor antagonists on gastric mucosal blood flow in animals that are subjected to ulcerogenic procedures is controversial. Treatment with cimetidine reduced gastric ischemia in hemorrhagic shock in miniature pigs (151) but not in rats (200), and metiamide reduced gastric ischemia in rats subjected to restraint stress (228). The reason for these discrepant findings is not clear.

An interaction between histamine and sympathetic nerve stimulation has been described. McGrath and Shepherd (164) found that histamine inhibited both norepinephrine release and vasoconstriction caused by sympathetic nerve stimulation in isolated blood vessels. The effect was blocked by metiamide and mimicked by an $H_2$-receptor agonist. In the isolated, perfused gracilis muscle, Powell (212) observed that histamine reduced vasoconstriction caused by sympathetic nerve stimulation, but not norepinephrine infusion. This effect was prevented by treatment with metiamide and mimicked by dimaprit, an $H_2$ agonist. These results indicate that, in some vascular beds, histamine can modulate sympathetic vasoconstriction by a prejunctional mechanism through an interaction with $H_2$ receptors. This could be of pathophysiological significance because of the high quantities of histamine contained in sympathetic nerves and vascular tissue. Analogous studies have not been performed in the gastric vasculature.

Tepperman et al. (256) have challenged the concept of the specificity of the gastric histamine receptors. The intra-arterial injection of tripelennamine, an $H_1$-receptor antagonist, inhibited the stimulation of acid secretion by histamine, and the $H_2$ antagonist metiamide inhibited the vasodilatory response to the $H_1$-receptor agonist, 2-methylhistamine. These findings have been questioned, however, because of the large dose of tripelennamine required to inhibit histamine-stimulated acid secretion, and 2-methylhistamine is not a pure $H_1$ agonist (199).

Nagata and Guth (182) have applied the fluorescent in vivo microscopy technique to the study of the effect of histamine on microvascular permeability in the rat stomach. Both histamine and an $H_1$ (but not an $H_2$) agonist caused dose-dependent leak of the fluorescein-albumin conjugate from venules in the muscularis externa when applied topically to the serosal surface of the stomach. An $H_1$ (but not an $H_2$) antagonist decreased the histamine-induced leak. In the submucosa, histamine caused dose-dependent dilatation of arterioles but no leak of conjugate (182). Perfusion of the gastric lumen with histamine increased acid output to the same maximum values attained by intravenous or subcutaneous histamine. However, only in rats pretreated with a $\beta$-adrenergic antagonist did histamine cause leak of the conjugate from mucosal collecting venules (not capillaries). An $H_1$-receptor antagonist, but not an $H_2$-receptor antagonist, significantly reduced the histamine-induced leaks. Thus, via $H_1$ receptors, histamine increases venular permeability to macromolecules in both the muscularis externa and the mucosa. This effect in the mucosa is manifest only when $\beta$-adrenergic receptors are blocked and initiation of the permeability change requires a larger dose of histamine than for initiating the acid secretory response.

In summary, histamine increases gastric mucosal blood flow in the rat via stimulation of $H_1$, and probably $H_2$, receptors and increases venular permeability via $H_1$ receptors. In contrast, in the rabbit, $H_1$-receptor stimulation causes gastric vascular constriction.

*Gastrointestinal Hormones*

GASTRIN. It has been clearly demonstrated in a number of investigations that both gastrin and pentagastrin are potent stimulants of gastric acid secretion. Associated with the increase in acid secretion, there is an increase in gastric mucosal blood flow. This has been found in dogs (113), cats (93), rats (158), and humans (80, 107, 128). Evidence that the increase in blood flow is secondary to the increase in acid secretion is based on the finding that the ratio of gastric mucosal blood flow to acid secretion remains constant as both increase in response to increasing doses of pentagastrin. Jacobson and Chang (111) compared histamine and gastrin effects (using aminopyrine clearance) and found the ratio to be greater for histamine. This suggested that the increased mucosal flow due to histamine, in contrast to that due to gastrin, represented both a direct dilating property and an indirect metabolic effect secondary to secretion. This was confirmed by in vivo microscopic observations in the cat by Guth and Smith (88). The close intra-arterial infusion of histamine, but not pentagastrin, in doses approximating 3% of the intravenous $D_{50}$ dose for stimulation of acid secretion, caused prompt dilatation of gastric submucosal arterioles.

VASOACTIVE INTESTINAL PEPTIDE. Using the aminopyrine-clearance technique in the dog, Konturek et al. (135) found that vasoactive intestinal peptide (VIP) decreased pentagastrin-stimulated acid secretion, accompanied by a fall in gastric mucosal blood flow. The ratio of blood flow to acid secretion remained unchanged, suggesting that the fall in blood flow was secondary to the inhibition of acid secretion.

The inhibitory effect of VIP on acid and pepsin secretions in dogs was not found in cats by Vagne et al. (258), who showed that VIP induced an increase in pentagastrin-stimulated gastric acid and pepsin secretions and mucosal blood flow measured by aminopyrine clearance in the cat.

VASOPRESSIN. Vasopressin decreased gastric blood flow in baboons (electromagnetic blood-flow measurement) (280), dogs (aminopyrine clearance) (113), cats (radiolabeled microspheres) (237), and rats (hydrogen gas clearance) (146). Angiographic studies in humans (8) revealed marked constriction of the gastric arteries in response to the close intra-arterial infusion of vasopressin. Evidence for escape from vasopressin vasoconstriction has not been demonstrated in the studies in baboons and humans.

GLUCAGON. Results of studies on the effect of glucagon on gastric blood flow are discrepant. Glucagon decreased pentagastrin- and histamine-stimulated acid secretion and mucosal blood flow in the dog (154). The ratio of blood flow to acid secretion remained unchanged. On the other hand, Bond and Levitt (23) used the microsphere technique to show that glucagon increased gastric blood flow under normal conditions and during hypovolemic shock. In prolonged shock, glucagon caused cardiovascular collapse unless the lost blood was replenished. Lockenvitz et al. (155) showed that glucagon did not have any effect on gastric mucosal blood flow in nonstressed rats. In rats under immobilization stress, mucosal blood flow was increased by glucagon. In in vivo microscopic studies of the anesthetized cat and rat (88), the close intra-arterial infusion of glucagon had no effect on the diameter of the gastric submucosal arterioles. This suggests that glucagon does not have a direct effect on the gastric microcirculation. The discrepant findings of the various studies of the effect of glucagon on gastric blood flow might be due to the effect of glucagon on systemic blood pressure.

SOMATOSTATIN. In dogs with gastric fistulas and Heidenhain pouches, somatostatin inhibited acid and pepsin responses to pentagastrin, urecholine, and a peptone meal (140) that was associated with a marked reduction in aminopyrine clearance. The ratio of aminopyrine concentration in gastric juice and blood plasma was not significantly changed, suggesting that the change in mucosal blood flow was secondary to an inhibition of gastric secretion. A similar inhibition of gastric secretion and blood flow was obtained in cats with chronically implanted gastric fistulas (1). Lin et al. (153), using aminopyrine clearance, confirmed that somatostatin decreased tetragastrin-stimulated gastric mucosal blood flow. Using the hydrogen gas-clearance technique, Leung and Guth (145) demonstrated an inhibition of pentagastrin-stimulated gastric acid secretion associated with an enhancement of gastric corpus mucosal blood flow in anesthetized rats given somatostatin. Doertenbach et al. (52) and Price et al. (213) showed that somatostatin significantly reduced basal gastric corpus mucosal blood flow measured by microspheres in anesthetized and conscious dogs, respectively. On the other hand, Leung and Guth (145) reported that antisecretory doses of somatostatin had no significant effect on basal antral or corpus mucosal blood flow measured by hydrogen gas clearance in anesthetized rats. Sonnenberg and West (244) used neutral red clearance to measure gastric mucosal blood flow in humans. Somatostatin produced a greater reduction in pentagastrin-stimulated mucosal blood flow than acid secretion when given to normal subjects. In patients with cirrhosis, pentagastrin had a lesser effect on acid secretion, while somatostatin did not affect pentagastrin-stimulated mucosal blood flow, although acid secretion was slightly decreased. Sonnenberg and West concluded that somatostatin can affect gastric mucosal blood flow independently of acid secretion. Therefore, although somatostatin is a potent gastric acid secretory inhibitor, the effect of this peptide on gastric mucosal blood flow varies with the technique used to assess blood flow.

SECRETIN. The immediate effect of close intra-arterial infusion of secretin on cat gastric submucosal arteriolar diameter was studied by Guth and Smith (88) using an in vivo microscopic technique. Natural, but not synthetic, secretin caused arteriolar dilatation, suggesting the presence of a contaminating vasoactive agent in the former. Using the aminopyrine-clearance technique in the dog, Konturek et al. (135) found that secretin decreased both pentagastrin-stimulated acid secretion and gastric mucosal blood flow. The ratio of blood flow to acid secretion remained unchanged, suggesting that the fall in blood flow was secondary to the inhibition of acid secretion. These findings indicate that secretin does not have a direct vasoactive effect on gastric blood flow.

NEUROTENSIN. Osumi et al. (198) found a reduction in both basal gastric acid output and mucosal blood flow measured by aminopyrine clearance when neurotensin was injected into the lateral ventricle in anesthetized rats. The reduction was blocked by pretreatment with reserpine or 6-hydroxydopamine intraventricularly.

Nemeroff et al. (189) showed that centrally administered neurotensin, which had been shown to inhibit both gastric acid secretion and mucosal blood flow, significantly inhibited the development of gastric ulcers induced by cold-restraint stress in the rat.

MET-ENKEPHALIN AND MORPHINE. Walu et al. (265) reported that when Met-enkephalin or morphine was infused intra-arterially, there was a potentiation of histamine-induced acid and pepsin secretion and mucosal and total gastric blood flow, which were significantly blocked by naloxone and nalorphine. Both opiates induced no secretory changes in the resting stomach but did increase mucosal and total blood flow.

Konturek et al. (139) showed that systemic or portal infusion of Met-enkephalin, enkephalin analogue, or morphine caused a dose-dependent increase in acid secretion and blood flow under basal conditions as well as under pentagastrin or histamine stimulation.

NORLEUCINE MOTILIN. Norleucine motilin decreased both pentagastrin-stimulated acid secretion and gastric mucosal blood flow in the dog (aminopyrine-clearance technique) (134). The ratio of blood flow to acid secretion remained unchanged, suggesting that the fall in blood flow was secondary to the inhibition of acid secretion.

*Prostaglandins*

Prostaglandins (PG) are natural compounds that act locally (4). They produce effects close to their cell origin and usually are metabolized before they reach the arterial circulation (259). Prostaglandins synthesized intramurally in blood vessels can act by directly modifying vascular smooth muscle tension (76), by altering vessel responsiveness to other vasoactive substances (99, 269), or by changing amounts of adrenergic neurotransmitter released from sympathetic nerve endings (98).

Prostaglandins are products of arachidonic acid metabolism [see Fig. 5; (175)]. Arachidonic acid is released from cell membranes by the action of the enzyme phospholipase $A_2$. A cyclooxygenase then generates cyclic endoperoxides, $PGG_2$ and $PGH_2$, from this precursor. The endoperoxides are enzymatically (prostaglandin synthetase) converted to a variety of products: by an isomerase and by a reductase to $PGE_2$, $PGD_2$, and $PGF_{2\alpha}$; by thromboxane synthetase to thromboxane $A_2$, which causes blood vessels to contract and platelets to aggregate; or by 6,9-oxycyclase into prostacyclin ($PGI_2$), which relaxes most blood vessels and inhibits platelet aggregation. Whereas thromboxane $A_2$ is the major metabolite of arachidonic acid in platelets, $PGI_2$ is the major metabolite in endothelium. Formation of $PGI_2$, followed by spontaneous breakdown to 6-oxo-$PGF_{1\alpha}$, is also the major route of endoperoxide metabolism in the rat stomach. Drugs (such as aspirin) and indomethacin inhibit the cyclooxygenase enzyme and thus inhibit the production of endoperoxides and all their derivatives.

It has been demonstrated that $PGI_2$ is formed not only by vascular tissue (173) but is avidly generated by the gastric mucosa of all species tested (174): rat, rabbit, cat, dog, guinea pig, and mouse. Prostaglandin-metabolizing enzymes have been demonstrated in human biopsy specimens of the esophagus, gastric fundus, gastric corpus, gastric antrum, and duodenum (205). Prostaglandin-forming cyclooxygenase was demonstrated, by an immunohistofluorescence procedure, in the lamina propria of the mucosa and in blood vessels of the submucosa, muscularis externa, and serosa of the porcine stomach (17). Other than capillary endothelium, the cells responsible for the generation of prostaglandins in the gastric mucosa are unknown.

PROSTAGLANDINS AND RESTING GASTRIC MUCOSAL BLOOD FLOW. Using a $^{14}C$-aniline–clearance technique to measure gastric mucosal blood flow in the rat, Main and Whittle (159) observed that indomethacin, in doses sufficient to inhibit prostaglandin formation, significantly reduced resting gastric mucosal blood flow. Similarly, Kauffman et al. (121) found that indomethacin decreased basal gastric mucosal blood flow in the conscious dog. In in vivo microscopic studies in the rat, indomethacin decreased the diameter of gastric submucosal arterioles, the vessels controlling blood flow to the mucosa (81). Skarstein (238) showed that indomethacin (3 mg·$kg^{-1}$ iv) reduced basal gastric mucosal blood flow measured by microspheres in the anesthetized cats by ~50%.

Konturek et al. (136) showed that basal gastric mucosal blood flow was significantly reduced in healthy volunteers after treatment with indomethacin. These findings indicate that endogenous prostaglandins may be one factor in the maintenance of basal gastric mucosal blood flow in animals and humans.

In rats, $PGI_2$ (271) and prostaglandins of the E and A series (158) increased resting mucosal blood flow. In in vivo microscopic studies, Guth and Moler (81) observed that superfusion of the exposed submucosal vascular bed with $PGE_2$ resulted in a dose-related dilatation of the submucosal arterioles. Holm-Rutili and Obrink (100a), using an in vivo microscopy technique in the anesthetized rat, calculated gastric mucosal blood flow from measurements of red blood cell velocity and vessel diameter. Luminal $PGE_1$ but not intravenous $PGE_1$ increased flow. Intravenous $PGE_1$ but not luminal $PGE_1$ inhibited basal gastric acid secretion. Konturek et al. (137) reported that, in the dog, $PGI_2$ but not $PGE_2$ increased resting gastric mucosal blood flow. In the totally isolated ex vivo canine stomach, Kowalewski and Kolodej (142) found that $PGE_2$ had a potent vasodilator action on the gastric circulation, reducing gastric peripheral resistance and the gastric arterial perfusion pressure. Cheung (33) found that in the nonstimulated stomach topical 16,16-dimethyl $PGE_2$ caused an increase in total gastric blood flow. Exogenous $PGE_2$ and $PGI_2$ administration appear to produce significant mucosal blood flow increases primarily by reducing gastric vascular resistance (increasing arteriolar diameter).

Kauffman and Whittle (122) showed that the vasoactive response to arachidonic acid by the gastric vasculature depends on the experimental conditions. Administration of arachidonic acid by close intra-arterial injection, so that it reached the gastric vasculature within 3 s, produced vasodilation, evidenced by a drop in the perfusion pressure. In contrast, when given in the same dose from a more distant site and incubating with blood components for 30 s before reaching the gastric vasculature, a significant vasoconstrictive response, evidenced by a rise in perfusion pressure, was observed. These findings suggest that arachidonic acid, given by close intra-arterial injection, is converted in the gastric vascular endothelium mainly to vasodilator substances, presumably $PGI_2$ or $PGE_2$; whereas when allowed to mix with blood platelets for 30 s, it is converted mainly to a vasoconstrictor substance, presumably thromboxane $A_2$.

PROSTAGLANDINS, GASTRIC ACID SECRETION, AND BLOOD FLOW. Prostaglandins are potent inhibitors of gastric acid secretion. The effect of exogenously administered prostaglandin on secretagogue-stimulated gastric blood flow is dependent on the technique used for measuring blood flow and the route of administration. The aminopyrine- (137, 139, 172) and aniline-clearance (158) techniques consistently demonstrate a parallel reduction in mucosal blood flow and inhibition of acid secretion. A dissociation of the effects of close intra-arterial administration of prostaglandins on stimulated gastric acid secretion, which is inhibited, and total gastric blood flow and gastric mucosal blood flow, which increases, has been demonstrated by the electromagnetic flow probe (67, 68), the venous-outflow technique (35), and the radiolabeled microspheres (35, 67). Luminal prostaglandin administration, in contrast, was shown to result in a reduction in histamine-stimulated gastric acid secretion and a decrease in total and mucosal blood flow measured by venous outflow and microspheres, respectively (33).

Gerkins et al. (69) obtained data suggesting an important role for locally synthesized prostaglandins as modulators of gastric secretory function. In the anesthetized dog, both aspirin and indomethacin potentiated pentagastrin-stimulated acid output while decreasing gastric blood flow. The implication is that pentagastrin increases the output of vasodilatory and acid-inhibiting prostaglandins. Kauffman et al. (123) measured plasma concentrations of 6-oxo-$PGF_{1\alpha}$, $PGE_2$, and thromboxane $B_2$ in an attempt to identify an increase in portal venous prostaglandin levels during stimulated gastric acid secretion. Under nonstimulated conditions, gastric venous plasma contained significantly higher levels of these prostanoids than gastric arterial plasma. No increase in gastric venous prostanoid concentrations was identified during near-maximum pentagastrin- or histamine-stimulated acid secretion. In contrast to the findings of Gerkins et al. (69), these data questioned the role of endogenous prostaglandins in modulating stimulated gastric acid secretion.

PROSTAGLANDIN-INDUCED MUCOSAL PROTECTION AND GASTRIC BLOOD FLOW. Because exogenous prostaglandins are protective against a variety of noxious agents and stimulate gastric mucosal blood flow, a number of investigators have attempted to define the role of mucosal blood flow under conditions of prostaglandin-induced protection. Reports that prostaglandins in antisecretory doses would increase basal gastric mucosal blood flow (27, 33, 137, 142, 158, 271) prompted the speculation that prostaglandin cytoprotection might be mediated by an increase in gastric mucosal blood flow (69, 138). Leung et al. (148) tested that hypothesis by determining the effect of a cytoprotective (nonantisecretory) dose of 16,16-dimethyl $PGE_2$ on basal gastric mucosal blood flow. This dose of prostaglandin did not produce an increase in gastric mucosal blood flow at a time when the cytoprotective effect of the prostaglandin was expected to be present. Despite this, although blood flow was completely absent in the mucosal lesions induced by absolute ethanol, in prostaglandin-pretreated stomachs blood flow was maintained and no lesions developed. These observations suggest that maintenance of mucosal blood flow by prostaglandins may be an important element of prostaglandin-induced gastric mucosal protection against ethanol-induced injury.

Szabo et al. (251) observed extravasation of intravenously injected Evans blue into the gastric wall, an indication of increased vascular permeability, 1–3 min after the intragastric administration of 75% and 100% ethanol in rats, while monastral blue labeling of injured gastric mucosal vessels was seen within 1 min. Pretreatment with $PGF_{2\beta}$ reduced these changes. In a preliminary report utilizing in vivo microscopy, Ohya and Guth (195) observed a similar rapid onset of leak of albumin from mucosal microvessels within 1 min of the topical application of 100% ethanol and an equally rapid stasis of mucosal blood flow. It would appear then that prostaglandins reduce various forms of vascular permeability and/or injury, which may be another element of importance in prostaglandin-induced protection.

### Leukotrienes

The leukotrienes are a more recently described family of $C_{20}$-carboxylic acids biosynthesized from arachidonic acid by the enzyme lipoxygenase [Fig. 7; (75)]. Leukotriene (LT) $C_4$ and $D_4$ increase microvascular permeability and constrict bronchi. It has been suggested that they act as mediators of the bronchospasm of bronchial asthma and other immediate hypersensitivity reactions. Leukotrienes $B_4$, $C_4$, $D_4$, and $E_4$ induce contractions in a number of guinea pig smooth muscle preparations.

Whittle et al. (272) studied the effect of leukotrienes $B_4$, $C_4$, and $D_4$ in vivo in the submucosal microcirculation of the anesthetized rat using direct microscopy techniques. The topical application to the exposed mucosa of $LTB_4$ and $LTD_4$ did not have any significant vasoactive effect. In contrast, $LTC_4$ induced vasoconstriction in the venules that was more pronounced than in the arterioles, reaching peak responses within 1–1.5 min, and that was unaffected by indomethacin administration. Intense focal vasoconstriction in the venules was clearly demonstrated, leading to sluggish blood flow and stasis within the vessel. A similar intense, focal venoconstriction was seen also with the topical application of the epoxymethano endoperoxide analogue (U-46618), a thromboxane mimetic compound. These potent venular vasoconstrictor actions of $LTC_4$ and the thromboxane mimetic compound in the gastric submucosal microcirculation identify this leukotriene and naturally occurring thromboxane $A_2$ as potential endogenous ulcerogenic agents. This suggests that these cyclooxygenase and lipoxygenase arachidonate products could play a role in microcirculatory events accompanying gastric ulcer formation.

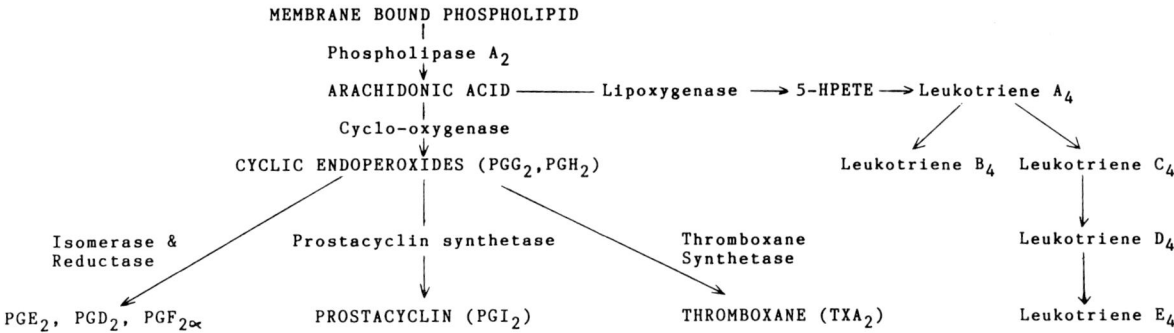

FIG. 7. Pathways of arachidonic acid metabolism. [From Guth and Leung (80a). In: *Physiology of the Gastrointestinal Tract*, © 1987, Raven Press, New York.]

## GASTRIC MUCOSAL BLOOD FLOW IN GASTRIC PHYSIOLOGY

### Acid Secretion

STIMULATION OF ACID SECRETION. During stimulated gastric acid secretion, there is a parallel increase in gastric acid secretion and mucosal blood flow as measured by aminopyrine clearance (110, 113). The lack of increase in total gastric blood flow, as measured by an electromagnetic flow probe in the presence of significant increases in mucosal blood flow, was explained by a redistribution of the circulation from nonmucosal tissues to the mucosa. This hypothesis has been brought into serious question by several lines of evidence. It has been shown, using the radiolabeled-microsphere technique, that mucosal blood flow is a relatively constant fraction (~70%–80%) of total gastric blood flow under basal conditions and during secretagogue stimulation (33, 49). Careful analysis of the original data of Jacobson et al. (112, 113) reveals that redistribution alone could not account for the increase in mucosal flow in the absence of an increase in total gastric blood flow.

Recent observations suggest that aminopyrine clearance reflects acid secretion as well as blood flow (see discussion of aminopyrine clearance in *Mucosal Blood Flow*, p. 1376). This casts serious doubt on the validity of the conclusions concerning relationships between acid secretion and blood flow when aminopyrine clearance is used to measure blood flow. Several studies have shown that, when the gastric vasculature is adequately perfused, secretagogue-stimulated gastric acid secretion can vary independently of gastric blood flow (203, 210). In an isolated, blood-perfused canine stomach preparation, Perry et al. (203) studied the relationship between gastric oxygen consumption, acid secretion, and gastric blood flow during intraarterial infusion of pentagastrin. When blood flow was increased above 38 ml·min$^{-1}$·100 g$^{-1}$ by pump perfusion, gastric oxygen consumption and acid secretion remained constant. When blood flow was reduced below this value by arterial occlusion, there was a linear correlation between gastric oxygen consumption, acid secretion, and gastric blood flow. Based on these experimental observations, a model was proposed by Perry et al. in which, at low flow rates, the delivery of oxygen is inadequate and therefore limits the stomach's ability to produce acid, leading to an apparent dependency of acid secretion on blood flow. When flow values exceed 38 ml·min$^{-1}$·100 g$^{-1}$, or when all the gastric tissue is fully perfused, gastric acid secretion can vary independently of blood flow. Blood flow may increase or decrease without affecting acid secretion, or acid production may be increased without altering blood flow. These findings in the isolated, blood-perfused canine gastric preparation are supported by two studies in the intact animal. Using the radiolabeled-microsphere technique in the dog, Polansky et al. (210) were unable to demonstrate any rise in submucosal-mucosal flow when gastric acid secretion was stimulated by histamine or peptone. Basal blood flow was extremely high, ~100 ml·min$^{-1}$·100 g$^{-1}$, however, in that study. Using in vivo microscopy and LDV in the rat, Holm-Rutili and Berglindh (100) observed an increase in gastric mucosal blood flow of ~40%, regardless of the degree of pentagastrin-stimulated acid secretion. The controversial nature of the data regarding the relationship between stimulated gastric acid secretion and gastric mucosal blood flow will continue to capture the interest of investigators.

INHIBITION OF ACID SECRETION. Table 1 summarizes the observations on the change in gastric mucosal blood flow during inhibition of secretagogue-stimulated gastric acid secretion by a variety of agents and manipulations. The aminopyrine-clearance technique consistently shows a parallel reduction as gastric acid secretion is inhibited. Dissociated effects on mucosal blood flow and acid secretion are demonstrated by venous outflow, microspheres, and hydrogen gas clearance. The parietal cells undergo predictable structural changes (electron-microscopy studies) when stimulated by secretagogues, with the formation of the needed structural secretory apparatus. With discontinuation of secretagogue stimulation, the structure of the parietal cell returns to the resting state.

TABLE 1. *Secretory Inhibition: Change in Mucosal Blood Flow*

| Stimulant | Inhibitor | Gastric Blood Flow Technique | MBF Change | Ref. |
|---|---|---|---|---|
| | Thiocyanate | APC | Decrease | 176 |
| | | Venous outflow | No change | 176 |
| | Gastrin | APC | Decrease | 42 |
| Histamine | Gastrone | | | |
| | Intra-arterial $PGE_1$ | Microsphere | Increase | 35 |
| | Topical $dmPGE_2$ | Microsphere | Decrease | 33 |
| | Intra-arterial $PGE_2$ | EMFP | Increase | 67 |
| | Intra-arterial $PGI_2$ | Microsphere | Increase | 67 |
| | Arachidonic acid | Microsphere | Increase | 67 |
| | Cimetidine | Microsphere | Decrease | 38 |
| Pentagastrin | Somatostatin | APC | Decrease | 140 |
| | | HGC | Increase | 145 |
| | Gastric devascularization | Microsphere | Decrease | 262 |
| | Hypovolemia | Microsphere | Decrease | 11, 250 |
| | | Regulated flow | Decrease | 203 |
| | Vasopressin | $^{99m}$Tc-4-methylaminophenozone | Decrease | 51 |
| | Omeprazole | Microsphere | No change | 143 |
| Tetragastrin | Somatostatin | APC | Decrease | 153 |

MBF, mucosal blood flow; APC, aminopyrine clearance; EMFP, electromagnetic flow probe; HGC, hydrogen gas clearance. [Data from Guth and Leung (80a).]

Inhibition of gastric acid secretion by $PGE_2$ (105) and thiocyanate (277) is accompanied by a return to resting parietal cell structure in the former but not in the latter situation. Cheung and Lowry (35) showed that 16,16-dimethyl $PGE_2$–induced inhibition of acid secretion produced a reduction of oxygen consumption to resting levels, but oxygen consumption did not decrease appreciably during thiocyanate-induced inhibition of acid secretion. Moody (176) used the microsphere technique to show that thiocyanate inhibition of histamine-stimulated gastric acid secretion was not accompanied by a reduction in total gastric blood flow in an exteriorized gastric flap preparation. To sustain the structural changes in the parietal cells when acid secretion is inhibited by thiocyanate, it appears that gastric blood flow must be maintained at the stimulated level. Preliminary data with substituted benzimidazoles, which are potent antisecretory agents, support this hypothesis. Picaprazole, a specific $H^+$-$K^+$-ATPase inhibitor, inhibits the production of acid but further increases the secretory surface of the parietal cell (249). Omeprazole, also a specific $H^+$-$K^+$-ATPase inhibitor, does not reduce stimulated gastric blood flow measured by microspheres (143). Thus the study of gastric mucosal blood flow and the structural changes in the parietal cell during inhibition of stimulated gastric acid secretion may provide insight into the source of the signal for, and the precise supportive role of, increased mucosal blood flow during stimulated gastric acid secretion.

*Autoregulation*

The term *autoregulation* is used to describe the intrinsic ability of an organ to maintain a relatively constant blood flow in the face of a fluctuating arterial pressure (118). Study of the resistance-flow relationship in the innervated gastric vascular bed indicated that autoregulation did not occur to any appreciable degree in the stomach (114). In the isolated pump-perfused canine stomach, Holm-Rutili et al. (101) showed that the ability of the stomach to regulate blood flow and oxygen uptake was significantly improved after sympathetic denervation. Under these circumstances, when arterial pressure was reduced, vascular resistance decreased and oxygen uptake remained relatively constant. In the same preparation, Perry et al. (204) showed that histamine enhanced the ability of the stomach to autoregulate its blood flow. The mechanism underlying the enhanced autoregulation after sympathetic denervation has not been determined.

*Eating*

In general, gastric blood flow increases with eating. The change appears to vary with time after meal ingestion and with the type of meal. Bond et al. (24) used a radiolabeled-microsphere technique to study the effect of feeding on blood flow to the different tissue layers of the stomach of conscious dogs. Flow measurements were obtained 45 min after ingestion of a high-protein meal, at which time the bulk of the meal was in the stomach and jejunum. After feeding, blood flow to the whole stomach wall increased significantly, which was entirely due to increased flow to the mucosa; the submucosa and muscularis flow remained unchanged. Taylor et al. (255), using the $^{86}$RbCl indicator-dilution technique in the rat, determined that having food in the stomach markedly increased antral as well as corpus blood flow. With progressive starvation, the antral-corpus flow ratio decreased.

Semb (230), using the hydrogen gas–clearance technique, reported that 30 min after feeding concentrated fish broth to conscious cats there was a significant increase in corpus mucosal-submucosal blood flow but a decrease in antral mucosal-submucosal blood flow. Two hours after the feeding, the changes in corpus and antral mucosal blood flow were reversed. Nowicki et al. (192) used microspheres to measure gastric mucosal-submucosal blood flow in conscious newborn piglets, and no change after feeding was observed. The mechanism underlying the postprandial increase in gastric mucosal blood flow may be due to gastric distension, the accompanying rise in gastric acid secretion, or direct stimulation by nutrients. The exact contribution of each remains to be determined.

### Changes in Gastric Blood Flow With Age

Varga and Csaky (261) studied changes in blood supply to various parts of the rat gastrointestinal tract with age using the $^{86}$Rb indicator-dilution technique. Cardiac output, in relative values, decreased with age. The total weight of the alimentary tract as a percent of body weight declined with age from 6.6% in 25- to 28-day-old rats to 1.9% in 240-day-old rats. The proportional weight of the various parts of the gastrointestinal tract was the same in all age groups, with the exception of the cecum, which increased. Blood flow to the glandular stomach rose from 0.228 ml·min$^{-1}$·g$^{-1}$ in 25- to 28-day-old rats to 0.424 ml·min$^{-1}$·g$^{-1}$ in 29- to 34-day-old rats and then progressively fell to 0.177 and 0.114 ml·min$^{-1}$·g$^{-1}$ in 45- to 66- and 240-day-old rats. Ballard et al. (12) found that sensitivity of gastric submucosal arterioles to norepinephrine constriction did not change with age until 25 mo of age, when sensitivity increased. It remains to be determined whether the decline in blood flow and the increased vascular sensitivity to norepinephrine (vasoconstriction) with aging affect the susceptibility of the gastric mucosa to injury.

### Gastric Motility

Chou and Grassmick (41) investigated the effect of increasing motility and intraluminal pressure on blood-flow distribution within the wall of the dog stomach using radiolabeled microspheres. The infusion of physostigmine markedly elevated luminal pressure of the small intestine, indicating that the motility response to this agent was a tonic contraction. Total flow to the gastric body decreased, solely because of a significant decrease in blood flow to the mucosa and submucosa. The muscularis and serosa escaped the mechanical compression of increased wall tension with no observed reduction in blood flow. This may be attributable to an activity-related hyperemia, as has been shown for skeletal muscle (13).

### Pulse Pressure

With the increasing use of cardiopulmonary bypass, the importance of an arterial pulse pressure in the regulation of organ blood flow and cardiac output distribution has come under investigation. There have been contradictory results. An increase in peripheral vascular resistance with nonpulsatile cardiopulmonary bypass has been demonstrated by some investigators (55) and a decrease by others (26). Shoor et al. (235) studied the effect of nonpulsatile arterial perfusion on gastric blood flow and intraorgan flow distribution in anesthetized dogs using radiolabeled microspheres. Total gastric blood flow, as well as the partitioning of that flow between antrum and corpus and mucosa and muscle layers, was not significantly altered by nonpulsatile arterial perfusion.

## GASTRIC MUCOSAL BLOOD FLOW IN GASTRIC PATHOPHYSIOLOGY

### Effect of Disruption of Gastric Mucosal Barrier to Acid Backdiffusion

There are conflicting reports concerning the effect of disruption of the gastric mucosal barrier on blood flow (9, 194, 217, 270). Bruggeman et al. (29) studied this problem using a perfused isolated segment of dog stomach in which it was observed that bathing the mucosal surface with salicylic acid in 160 mM HCl resulted in a prompt fall in vascular resistance (increase in flow). Salicylic acid in neutral solution had no effect, but subsequent replacement of the bathing solution with 160 mM HCl caused an immediate fall in resistance. Therefore backdiffusion of acid was thought to be the proximate cause of vasodilatation. Pretreatment with pyrilamine, a histamine $H_1$-receptor antagonist plus cimetidine, an $H_2$-receptor antagonist, largely blocked the fall in resistance, suggesting that mucosal histamine liberated during acid backdiffusion mediated the vasodilatation. Because the block was not complete, backdiffusing acid acting directly on resistance vessels also might play a role. Starlinger et al. (246) confirmed this concept in a study in the anesthetized rabbit in which they demonstrated a direct linear correlation between gastric luminal H$^+$ concentration and gastric mucosal blood flow measured by microspheres.

Cheung et al. (36) studied the relationship between blood flow and gastric mucosal barrier disruption using both aminopyrine clearance and radiolabeled microspheres to measure mucosal flow and using venous outflow to measure total flow in a canine gastric chamber preparation. Topical aspirin, sodium taurocholate, and ethanol, all barrier "breakers," caused a significant increase in both total venous flow and microsphere-measured mucosal blood flow. Aminopyrine clearance increased to a much smaller degree with aspirin and taurocholate but did not increase with ethanol. These results suggest that aminopyrine clearance may be unreliable in quantitating mucosal blood flow changes in the presence of mucosal injury. This was confirmed by Miller et al. (171), who demonstrated "trapping" of aminopyrine in the injured epithelium. Cheung et al. (36) also noted that aspirin-induced erosions occur at discrete sites and are usually preceded by focal pallor, suggesting focal ischemia. They postulate that the increase in overall gastric mucosal blood flow may be a secondary defensive response to damage. McGreavy and Moody (166), however, measured gastric mucosal blood flow with microspheres in dogs exposed to luminal aspirin. Twenty minutes after aspirin exposure, mucosal blood flow to areas that eventually become injured was greater than the blood flow to areas that remained visibly normal. These authors argued against the hypothesis that reduced blood flow plays a role in the pathogenesis of aspirin-induced mucosal lesion. Ashley et al. (7) demonstrated that in the gastric mucosa of isolated stomach segments exposed to aspirin, despite an increase in blood flow measured by venous outflow and a rise in mucosal blood flow measured by hydrogen gas clearance in the nonulcerated area, a fall in mucosal blood flow was recorded in the aspirin-induced lesion area by hydrogen gas clearance. There appears to be no clear consensus as to the role of local blood flow in areas that ulcerate when exposed to luminal aspirin.

*Prevention of Mucosal Injury*

Experimental evidence has accumulated in recent years that increasing mucosal blood flow confers a significant degree of protection on the gastric mucosa. Two lines of evidence have been developed in support of this concept.

First, a reduction in mucosal blood flow predisposes the gastric mucosa to injury. Mersereau and Hinchey (169) observed that while 150 mM HCl caused no gastric damage in the normotensive rat, the gastric mucosa in the hypotensive rat was ischemic, and as little as 50 mM HCl produced erosions. In both the dog (217) and rat (270), bile salt–induced gastric lesions were significantly increased by reducing gastric mucosal blood flow with either vasopressin or indomethacin. Cheung and Chang (34) observed that luminal $p$-chloromercuribenzene sulfonate did not cause gross damage unless mucosal ischemia, produced by hemorrhagic shock, was present. Apparently there was a critical relationship between the level of mucosal perfusion and the rate of $H^+$ backdiffusion, lesions occurring only when there was a marked reduction in the ratio of mucosal blood flow to $H^+$ loss.

Using the hemorrhagic shock model, Leung et al. (147) demonstrated a one-to-one linear correlation between reduction in gastric mucosal blood flow and reduction in mean blood pressure. Mean blood pressure and hence, by inference, mucosal blood flow had to be reduced to well below 40% of base-line values for significant increase of acid-induced gastric mucosal lesions. A threshold appears to exist for the formation of acid-induced mucosal lesion as mucosal blood flow is reduced.

Second, increasing mucosal blood flow protects against gastric mucosal injury. Intra-arterial infusion of isoproterenol significantly decreased gastric damage produced by either topical bile salts plus hemorrhagic shock (218) or topical aspirin (165). Whittle (270) observed that the administration of a prostaglandin analogue increased mucosal blood flow and protected rats against lesions produced by the combination of bile salts, acid, and indomethacin. This suggests that one means by which prostaglandin may exert its protective effect is by increasing gastric mucosal blood flow. In support of this concept of protection by increased blood flow, Levine et al. (150) showed that after celiac ganglionectomy, gastric mucosal blood flow was preserved during shock and gastric mucosal lesion formation was reduced. Esplugues et al. (57) showed that the $\beta$-adrenoreceptor agonist salbutanol produced a dose-related increase in mucosal blood flow and accelerated the healing of experimental chronic gastric ulcer.

In contrast to reports using the endotoxin model, which have shown that gastric mucosal blood flow is decreased during sepsis (37), when bacteremia was produced by live *Escherichia coli*, gastric mucosal blood flow was shown to either remain unchanged (215) or actually increase (66, 191). Because indomethacin blocked this increase, Nilsson et al. (191) speculated that the increase might be mediated by prostaglandin.

In a canine model of *E. coli* sepsis, Payne and Bowen (202) found that despite the absence of a significant change in total gastric blood flow, there were significant and persistent reductions in epithelial oxygen tension and potential difference in the gastric mucosa. Treatment with methylprednisolone 30 min after the start of sepsis ameliorated mucosal hypoxia, restored potential difference to normal, and prevented the focal superficial epithelial histopathological changes. Although only total gastric blood flow was measured by an electromagnetic flow probe, Payne and Bowen postulated the methylprednisolone-enhanced nutrient microcirculatory blood flow to the apical gastric epithelium. Rees et al. (216) further demonstrated that treatment of the septic dogs with naloxone reversed the cellular hypoxia and change in potential difference induced by infusion of live *E. coli*, although naloxone did not alter gastric blood flow in either the control or the septic preparations.

Menguy and Masters (168) demonstrated that the gastric mucosa is extremely sensitive to a deficit in energy metabolism. In rats subjected to hemorrhagic shock, a greater reduction in energy substrates developed in the gastric mucosa than in other organs, which could result in cell death with formation of mucosal lesions. These findings suggest that by maintaining adequate tissue oxygenation, mucosal blood flow plays an important role in preventing mucosal injury.

Maintenance of mucosal acid-base balance has been proposed by Kivilaakso et al. (127) and Moody et al. (177) as an alternative role for blood flow in protecting against mucosal injury. Using an intramucosal pH probe, Kivilaakso et al. (127) demonstrated a profound drop in intramucosal pH following hemorrhagic shock in the rabbit. They suggested that the critical determinant of ulceration during shock is not tissue anoxia but an impaired capacity of the mucosa to remove or buffer the influx of acid. Moody et al. (177) postulated that increasing blood flow protects against mucosal damage by topical noxious agents by disposing of $H^+$ "by buffer, dilution, or other processes that allow the surface cells to withstand increased permeation of $H^+$ ion."

Others have confirmed the importance of the acid-base status of the gastric mucosa in mucosal defense and injury. Cheung et al. (40) infused HCl intra-arterially to reduce gastric mucosal pH and observed that, although gastric mucosal blood flow remained unchanged, acidified sodium taurocholate–induced mucosal injury was significantly increased. Bicarbonate delivery to the gastric mucosa plays an important role in preventing the formation of acid-induced gastric mucosal ulceration during shock, as demonstrated by Starlinger et al. (246). In the anesthetized rat, despite an improvement in gastric blood flow produced by prostacyclin, acid-induced ulcerations still occurred in experimental stomachs during shock. Intra-arterially infused $HCO_3^-$, which corrected mucosal acidosis, completely prevented the formation of such acid-induced ulceration, while blocking carbonic anhydrase, and the production of bicarbonate with acetazolamide completely abolished this protective effect.

Thus the role of mucosal blood flow in protecting the gastric mucosa against injury involves maintenance of oxygenation and acid-base balance in the mucosa.

*Role of Oxygen-Derived Free Radicals in Ischemic Gastric Injury*

Granger et al. (73) have provided strong evidence for oxygen-derived free radicals playing a role in ischemia-induced intestinal injury. This has been termed *ischemia-reperfusion* injury. During the ischemic period the stage is set for oxyradical formation: mucosal ATP is catabolized ultimately to hypoxanthine, and mucosal xanthine dehydrogenase is converted to the xanthine oxidase (XOD) form. With reperfusion, oxygen is available and there is a burst of oxyradical formation: hypoxanthine + $O_2 \xrightarrow{XOD} O_2^-$ + xanthine. The superoxide radical ($O_2^-$) undergoes further conversion to $H_2O_2$ and $HO\cdot$. Lipid peroxidation by these highly reactive oxyradicals may cause significant tissue damage. Using the rat hemorrhagic shock model of gastric mucosal injury, Itoh and Guth (106) demonstrated that a similar mechanism may be involved in gastric ischemic injury. In the presence of 0.1 N HCl in the stomach, the gross erosions produced by 20 min of hemorrhagic hypotension followed by reperfusion of shed blood were significantly reduced by allopurinol, an inhibitor of XOD, and superoxide dismutase, a scavenger of $O_2^-$. However, the lack of a protective effect with dimethyl sulfoxide, an $HO\cdot$ scavenger, at the concentrations used, remains to be explained. It has to be demonstrated that directly generated oxygen-derived free radicals will produce an injurious effect on the gastric mucosa to provide firm support for this hypothesis.

*Effect of Local and Systemic Hypothermia*

Iced water or iced saline gastric lavage is widely used to arrest bleeding from acute erosive gastritis. Although controlled clinical studies to evaluate the effectiveness of this procedure have not been performed, several animal experimental studies have, with differing results on the effect of irrigation on blood flow. In the normal canine stomach, gastric iced water lavage, but not lavage with water at body temperature, reduced gastric blood flow by ~65%, as measured by venous outflow (223, 266) or the electromagnetic flowmeter techniques (267). In contrast, in cats in which acute gastritis had been induced by the gastric instillation of 10% acetic acid, neither iced water nor warm water gastric lavage significantly affected blood flow to the mucosa or muscle layer, as measured by the radiolabeled-microsphere technique (245). The latter study suggests that local hypothermia may not affect the gastric circulation in stomachs with acute gastritis. Furthermore, in anesthetized cats, Semb (229) found no reduction in gastric mucosal or submucosal blood flow using the hydrogen gas–clearance technique with reduction of gastric mucosal temperature to 15°C.

Total-body hypothermia has also been used to control massive upper gastrointestinal hemorrhage in humans (71). The effect of lowering body temperature to 31°C on gastric blood flow was studied in normal dogs using the radiorubidium-clearance technique (56). There was a significant 60% reduction in blood flow to all layers of the corpus but not to the antrum. A similar result was obtained by Murakami et al. (180). Hypothermia was associated with an increase in blood viscosity, a decrease in gastric mucosal blood flow measured by hydrogen clearance, and an increase in gastric mucosal lesions. In contrast, in the anesthetized rat, reduction of core temperature from 37°C to 24°C by cold water immersion for up to 3 h did not produce any significant change in gastric mucosal blood flow measured by aminopyrine clearance (125). Garrick et al. (65a) also found no decrease in gastric mucosal blood flow after 1, 2, and 3 h of cold water immersion, which reduced core temperature from 35°C to 25°C in anesthetized rats. There is no consensus regarding the effect of local gastric or systemic hypothermia on gastric mucosal blood flow.

## Effect of Portal Hypertension

Two hypotheses regarding splanchnic hemodynamics in patients with portal hypertension have been advanced, that of backward flow and that of forward flow. Vorobioff et al. (263), in a portal vein–stenotic rat model, showed that portal venous blood flow was increased with a corresponding decrease in splanchnic arteriolar resistance, thus providing data to support the forward-flow theory. In particular, the gastric blood flow in the portal vein–stenotic rats was twice that in the controls. The reason for the increase in portal venous flow is not known, but postulates include altered gastric vascular sensitivity to norepinephrine (126) and the formation of gastric arteriovenous shunts (97).

## Effect of Nicotine and Cigarette Smoke

Pawlik et al. (201) examined the acute effect of a 10-min infusion of nicotine on total gastric blood flow measured by an electromagnetic flow probe in anesthetized dogs. Control flow value was $65.4 \pm 8$ ml·min$^{-1}$·100 g$^{-1}$ tissue. Intra-arterial infusion of 25 and 50 $\mu$g·min$^{-1}$·kg$^{-1}$ body wt produced significant sustained increases of $8.7\% \pm 2\%$ and $14.3\% \pm 2\%$, respectively. Intravenous administration of 5 and 20 $\mu$g·min$^{-1}$·kg$^{-1}$ body wt transiently but significantly increased flow by 10% and $46\% \pm 2\%$, respectively.

Sonnenberg and Husmert (243) examined the effect of intravenous nicotine on pentagastrin-stimulated gastric acid output and neutral red clearance in humans. They observed that volume secretion was inhibited more than neutral red clearance and concluded that nicotine increased blood flow to the gastric mucosa relative to reduced gastric secretion.

Robert et al. (219) found that a 30-min inhalation of tobacco or nicotine-free cigarette smoke or a 1-h infusion of intravenous nicotine had no effect on either antral or corpus mucosal blood flow measured by hydrogen gas–clearance in the anesthetized rat. When administered after gastric acid secretion was stimulated by pentagastrin for 1 h, the high dose significantly reduced stimulated gastric acid secretion and corpus mucosal blood flow to $55\% \pm 9\%$ and $84\% \pm 4\%$ of stimulated value, respectively.

Differences in the time of observation, route of drug administration, and technique for measuring blood flow may account for the discrepancy in these observations.

## Measurement of Gastric Hemodynamics in Humans

In recent years, a number of techniques have been developed for measuring gastric mucosal hemodynamics in humans. Prior to the application of these techniques in human studies, much of what we know concerning the role of blood flow in gastric physiology and pathophysiology has been derived from animal studies. The development of these techniques offers the exciting possibility of testing hypotheses concerning the role of blood flow in human gastric physiology and disease.

The [$^{14}$C]aminopyrine- and neutral red–clearance techniques were used to examine the relationship between gastric acid secretion and mucosal blood flow. Parallel changes in gastric acid secretion and mucosal blood flow were documented during secretagogue stimulation and inhibition of acid secretion (80, 128–131). Sonnenberg and Husmert (243) used the neutral red–clearance technique to measure gastric mucosal blood flow in healthy nonsmokers. Nicotine reduced pentagastrin-stimulated acid secretion and neutral red–clearance in a dose-dependent manner. In five healthy smokers, smoking five cigarettes over 2 h induced similar changes to the intravenous infusion of nicotine. Because volume secretion was inhibited more than neutral red clearance, Sonnenberg and Husmert speculated that nicotine increases blood supply to the gastric mucosa relative to the reduced gastric secretion. Sonnenberg and West (244) used the same technique and found that patients with cirrhosis were less sensitive to pentagastrin stimulation, and somatostatin had no effect on either acid secretion or mucosal blood flow during pentagastrin stimulation. Conversely in normal subjects somatostatin decreased both gastric acid secretion and mucosal blood flow (4 $\mu$g·kg$^{-1}$·h$^{-1}$ somatostatin inhibited mucosal blood flow more than acid secretion). Because neutral red clearance is based on the same principle as aminopyrine clearance, the conclusions from these studies are difficult to interpret. Meaningful interpretation of these human studies will have to await further validation of the technique to determine if true blood flow is being measured.

Ivarsson et al. (107) used the $^{85}$Kr-elimination method to measure antral and corpus mucosal blood flow in anesthetized human subjects undergoing abdominal surgery and found that during pentagastrin stimulation there was a 5- and a 12-fold increase in corpus mucosal blood flow in control subjects and in duodenal ulcer patients, respectively, and a significant reduction of flow distribution to the muscle layer. There was a linear relationship between the increased rates of acid secretion and mucosal blood flow. Pentagastrin produced no change in antral mucosal blood flow. Confirmation of these observations by techniques other than the [$^{14}$C]aminopyrine (80) or neutral red clearance (128, 130) has not been reported.

Kamada et al. (119, 120) used the reflectance-spectrophotometry technique to measure an index of mucosal hemoglobin concentration in patients. In patients with active gastric ulcer (119), the index of mucosal hemoglobin concentration decreased significantly in most regions of the stomach compared with control patients. During the healing stage, there was a 33% rise in the index of mucosal hemoglobin concentration at the edge of the ulcer in those ulcers that healed in 3 mo. In those ulcers that failed to heal, the rise was only 2%. This finding implies that an impaired blood supply to the ulcer bed may be a factor in ulcer persistence. In patients admitted to the hospital with thermal or head injury (120), when the index of mucosal hemoglobin concentration was 27% of the level of young healthy controls or 36% of age-matched controls, gastric mucosal lesions developed within a few days after admission. This finding implies that a marked reduction in mucosal blood flow may be a pathogenetic factor in the development of stress-induced gastric mucosal lesions.

Murakami et al. (181) measured gastric mucosal blood flow in nine human subjects by hydrogen gas clearance. Reproducible results of consecutive measurements were obtained. In one patient with gastric ulcer, a progressive increase in mucosal blood flow around the ulcer was observed as the ulcer healed.

Fukutomi et al. (62) used hydrogen gas clearance and inserted a platinum electrode to measure gastric mucosal blood flow in humans. There was no significant difference between patients with gastric ulcer and control patients. A progressive increase in gastric mucosal blood flow at the edge of the ulcer as the ulcer was healing was documented. In patients with non-healing ulcers, blood flow at the margin of the ulcer was markedly lower than in the healing group.

Both the hydrogen gas–clearance technique and reflectance-spectrophotometry technique suggest a reduced flow or index of mucosal hemoglobin concentration in the tissue adjacent to gastric ulceration, and recovery toward normal is associated with healing. Confirmation of these observations is important. Whether the reduced flow or index of mucosal hemoglobin concentration precedes the formation of the ulceration or is secondary to the presence of the ulceration will have to be studied next. It is important to test the hypothesis that measures to increase blood flow around an active ulcer may hasten ulcer healing, particularly ulcers that are resistant to conventional therapy.

We are indebted to J. Hartman and D. Claus for invaluable secretarial assistance.

This work was supported by National Institute of Arthritis, Diabetes, and Digestive and Kidney Diseases Grants AM-25891, AM-27465, and AM-34840; American Society for Gastrointestinal Endoscopy Grant H850208; and Veterans Administration Research Funds.

## REFERENCES

1. Albinus, M., E. L. Blair, R. M. Case, D. H. Coy, A. Gomez-Pan, B. H. Hirst, J. D. Reed, A. V. Schally, B. Shaw, P. A. Smith, and J. R. Smy. Comparison of the effect of somatostatin on gastrointestinal function in the conscious and anaesthetized cat and on the isolated cat pancreas. *J. Physiol. Lond.* 269: 77–91, 1977.
2. Arabehety, J. T., H. A. Dolcini, and S. J. Gray. Sympathetic influences on circulation of the gastric mucosa of the rat. *Am. J. Physiol.* 197: 915–922, 1959.
3. Archibald, L. H., F. G. Moody, and M. Simons. Measurement of gastric blood flow with radioactive microspheres. *J. Appl. Physiol.* 38: 1051–1056, 1975.
4. Armstrong, J. M., G. J. Dusting, S. Moncada, and J. R. Vane. Cardiovascular actions of prostacyclin ($PGI_2$), a metabolite of arachidonic acid which is synthesized by blood vessels. *Circ. Res.* 43, Suppl. 1: 112–119, 1978.
5. Ash, A. S. F., and H. O. Schild. Receptors mediating some actions of histamine. *Br. J. Pharmacol.* 27: 427–439, 1966.
6. Ashley, S. W., and L. Y. Cheung. Measurement of gastric mucosal blood flow by hydrogen gas clearance. *Am. J. Physiol.* 247 (*Gastrointest. Liver Physiol.* 10): G339–G345, 1984.
7. Ashley, S. W., L. A. Sonnenschein, and L. Y. Cheung. Focal gastric mucosal blood flow at the site of aspirin-induced ulceration. *Am. J. Surg.* 149: 53–59, 1985.
8. Athanasoulis, C. A., S. Baum, A. C. Waltman, E. J. Ring, A. Imbembo, and T. J. VanderSalm. Control of acute gastric mucosal hemorrhage. Intra-arterial infusion of posterior pituitary extract. *N. Engl. J. Med.* 290: 603–610, 1974.
9. Augur, N. A. Gastric mucosal blood flow following damage by ethanol, acetic acid or aspirin. *Gastroenterology* 58: 311–320, 1970.
10. Aukland, K., B. F. Bower, and R. W. Berliner. Measurement of local blood flow with hydrogen gas. *Circ. Res.* 14: 164–187, 1964.
11. Bakke, A., P. Holme, and K. Svanes. The significance of gastric mucosal blood flow and acid secretion in erosive gastritis following hemorrhagic shock in cats. *Acta Chir. Scand.* 148: 113–119, 1982.
12. Ballard, K. W., G. Paulsen, N. Oren-Wolman, and P. H. Guth. Age-related changes in the gastric submucosal arterioles and gastric acid secretion. *Microvasc. Res.* 25: 176–185, 1983.
13. Barcroft, H. Circulation in skeletal muscle. In: *Handbook of Physiology. Circulation*, edited by W. F. Hamilton. Washington, DC: Am. Physiol. Soc., 1963, sect. 2, vol. II, p. 1353–1385.
14. Barlow, T. E. Vascular patterns in the alimentary canal. In: *Visceral Circulation*, edited by G. E. W. Wolstenholme. London: Churchill, 1952, p. 21–35. (Ciba Symp.)
15. Barlow, T. E., F. H. Bentley, and D. N. Walder. Arteries, veins and arteriovenous anastomoses in the human stomach. *Surg. Gynecol. Obstet.* 93: 657–671, 1951.
16. Beaumont, W. *Experiments and Observations on the Gastric Juice and the Physiology of Digestion.* New York: Dover, 1833.
17. Bebiak, D. M., E. R. Miller, R. L. Huslig, and W. L. Smith. Distribution of prostaglandin-forming cyclooxygenase in the porcupine stomach (Abstract). *Federation Proc.* 38: 884, 1979.
18. Bell, P. R. F. Gastric arterio-venous shunts. An investigation using a dye solution technique. *Scand. J. Gastroenterol.* 2: 59–67, 1967.
19. Bell, P. R. F., and C. Battersby. Effect of vagotomy on gastric mucosal blood flow. *Gastroenterology* 54: 1032–1037, 1968.
20. Bell, P. R. F., and T. Shelley. Gastric mucosal blood flow and acid secretion in conscious animals measured by heat clearance. *Am. J. Dig. Dis.* 13: 685–696, 1968.
21. Black, J. W., W. A. M. Duncan, C. J. Durant, C. R. Ganellin, and M. E. Parsons. Definition and antagonism of histamine $H_2$-receptors. *Nature Lond.* 236: 385–390, 1972.
22. Blair, E. L., E. R. Grund, J. D. Reed, D. J. Sanders, G. Sanger, and B. Shaw. The effect of sympathetic nerve stimulation on serum gastrin, gastric acid secretion and mucosal blood flow responses to meat extract stimulation in anaesthetized cats. *J. Physiol. Lond.* 253: 493–504, 1975.
23. Bond, J. H., and M. D. Levitt. Effect of glucagon on gastrointestinal blood flow of dogs in hypovolemic shock. *Am. J. Physiol.* 238 (*Gastrointest. Liver Physiol.* 1): G434–G439, 1980.
24. Bond, J. H., R. A. Prentiss, and M. D. Levitt. The effects

of feeding on blood flow to the stomach, small bowel, and colon of the conscious dog. *J. Lab. Clin. Med.* 93: 594–599, 1979.

25. BONNER, R., AND R. NOSSAL. A model for laser Doppler measurements of blood flow in tissue. *Appl. Opt.* 20: 2097–2107, 1981.
26. BOUCHER, J. K., L. W. RUDY, JR., AND H. EDMUNDS, JR. Organ blood flow during pulsatile cardiopulmonary bypass. *J. Appl. Physiol.* 36: 86–90, 1974.
27. BOUGHTON-SMITH, N. K., J. R. VANE, AND B. J. R. WHITTLE. Effects of prostacyclin ($PGI_2$), $PGI_1$ and 6-oxo-$PGF_{1\alpha}$ on the rat gastric mucosa. *Br. J. Pharmacol.* 62: 413P, 1978.
28. BROWNING, J., B. J. GANNON, AND P. O'BRIEN. The microvasculature and gastric luminal pH of the forestomach of the rat: a comparison with the glandular stomach. *Int. J. Microcirc. Clin. Exp.* 2: 109–118, 1983.
29. BRUGGEMAN, T. M., J. G. WOOD, AND H. W. DAVENPORT. Local control of blood flow in the dog's stomach: vasodilatation caused by acid back-diffusion following topical application of salicylic acid. *Gastroenterology* 77: 736–744, 1979.
30. BUCHIN, R. F., AND R. F. EDLICH. Quantitation of gastric arteriovenous blood flow by the microsphere clearance technique. *Arch. Surg.* 99: 579–581, 1969.
31. BULKLEY, G., H. GOLDMAN, L. TRENCIS, AND W. SILEN. Gastric microcirculatory changes in hemorrhagic shock. *Surg. Forum* 21: 27–30, 1970.
32. CHAHAL, P., P. HOLTON, AND J. A. KING. Comparison of neutral red and other markers used for the estimation of gastric mucosal blood flow. *J. Physiol Lond.* 256: 29P, 1976.
33. CHEUNG, L. Y. Topical effects of 16,16-dimethyl prostaglandin $E_2$ on gastric blood flow in dogs. *Am. J. Physiol.* 238 (*Gastrointest. Liver Physiol.* 1): G514–G519, 1980.
34. CHEUNG. L. Y., AND N. CHANG. The role of gastric mucosal blood flow and $H^+$ back-diffusion in the pathogenesis of acute gastric erosions. *J. Surg. Res.* 22: 357–361, 1977.
35. CHEUNG, L. Y., AND S. F. LOWRY. Effects of intra-arterial infusion of prostaglandin $E_1$ on gastric secretion and blood flow. *Surgery St. Louis* 83: 699–704, 1978.
36. CHEUNG, L. Y., F. G. MOODY, AND R. S. REESE. Effect of aspirin, bile salt, and ethanol on canine gastric mucosal blood flow. *Surgery St. Louis* 77: 786–792, 1975.
37. CHEUNG, L. Y., R. S. REESE, AND F. G. MOODY. Direct effect of endotoxin on the gastric mucosal microcirculation and electrical gradient. *Surgery St. Louis* 79: 564–568, 1976.
38. CHEUNG, L. Y., AND L. A. SONNENSCHEIN. Effect of cimetidine on canine gastric mucosal pH and blood flow. *Am. J. Surg.* 145: 24–28, 1983.
39. CHEUNG, L. Y., AND L. A. SONNENSCHEIN. Measurements of regional gastric mucosal blood flow by hydrogen gas clearance. *Am. J. Surg.* 147: 32–37, 1984.
40. CHEUNG, L. Y., A. A. TOENJES, AND L. A. SONNENSCHEIN. Acidification of arterial blood enhances gastric mucosal injury induced by bile salts in dogs. *Am. J. Surg.* 143: 74–79, 1982.
41. CHOU, C. C., AND B. GRASSMICK. Motility and blood flow distribution within the wall of the gastrointestinal tract. *Am. J. Physiol.* 235 (*Heart Circ. Physiol.* 4): H34–H39, 1978.
42. COWLEY, D. J., AND C. F. CODE. Effects of secretory inhibitors on mucosal blood flow in nonsecreting stomach of conscious dogs. *Am. J. Physiol.* 218: 270–274, 1970.
43. COWLEY, D. J., C. F. CODE, AND R. FIASSE. Gastric mucosal blood flow during secretory inhibition by gastrin pentapeptide and gastrone. *Gastroenterology* 56: 659–665, 1969.
44. CUMMING, J. D., A. L. HAIGH, E. H. L. HARRIES, AND M. E. NUTT. A study of gastric secretion and blood flow in the anaesthetized dog. *J. Physiol. Lond.* 168: 219–233, 1963.
45. CURWAIN, B. P., AND P. HOLTON. The measurement of dog gastric mucosal blood flow by radioactive aniline clearance compared with aminopyrine clearance. *J. Physiol. Lond.* 229: 115–131, 1973.
46. CURWAIN, B. P., AND N. C. TURNER. Comparison of the agonist activity of impromidine (SK & F 92676) in anaesthetized rabbits and on the rabbit isolated fundic mucosa. *Br. J. Pharmacol.* 73: 917–919, 1981.
47. DELANEY, J. P. Chronic alterations in gastrointestinal blood flow induced by vagotomy. *Surgery St. Louis* 62: 155–158, 1967.
48. DELANEY, J. P., AND E. GRIM. Canine gastric blood flow and its distribution. *Am. J. Physiol.* 207: 1195–1202, 1964.
49. DELANEY, J. P., AND E. GRIM. Experimentally induced variations in canine gastric blood flow and its distribution. *Am. J. Physiol.* 208: 353–358, 1965.
50. DELANEY, J. P., H. M. MICHEL, AND J. BOND. Cimetidine and gastric blood flow. *Surgery St. Louis* 84: 190–193, 1978.
51. DOBRONTE, Z., J. LANG, I. SAGI, AND V. VARRS. Measurement of gastric mucosal blood flow in dogs by the $^{99m}$Tc-4-methylaminophenazone clearance technique. *Gastroenterology* 83: 279–284, 1982.
52. DOERTENBACH, J. G., C. HOTTENROTT, U. SCHWEDES, K. H. USADEL, AND A. ENCKE. Haemodynamic effects of somatostatin in acute gastrointestinal hemorrhage in dogs. *Resuscitation* 10: 57–61, 1982.
53. DUGAS, M. C., AND R. L. WECHSLER. Analysis of aminopyrine clearance to measure gastric mucosal blood flow: insight derived from mathematical models. In: *Gastrointestinal Mucosal Blood Flow*, edited by L. P. Fielding. Edinburgh: Churchill Livingstone, 1980, p. 35–42.
54. DUGAS, M. C., AND R. L. WECHSLER. Validity of iodoantipyrine clearance for measuring gastrointestinal tissue blood flow. *Am. J. Physiol.* 243 (*Gastrointest. Liver Physiol.* 6): G155–G171, 1982.
55. DUNN, J., M. KIRSH, J. HARNESS, M. CARROLL, J. STRAKER, AND H. SLOAN. Hemodynamic, metabolic, and hematologic effects of pulsatile cardiopulmonary bypass. *J. Thorac. Cardiovasc. Surg.* 68: 138–147, 1974.
56. EDLICH, R. F., J. W. BORNER, AND O. H. WANGENSTEEN. Gastric blood flow: its distribution during systemic hypothermia. *Am. J. Surg.* 120: 38–40, 1970.
57. ESPLUGUES, J., J. M. LLORIS, E. MARTÍ-BONMATÍ, AND E. J. MORCILLO. Effects of beta-adrenoceptor drug stimulation on various models of gastric ulcer in rats. *Br. J. Pharmacol.* 76: 587–594, 1982.
58. FARA, J. W., AND G. ROSS. Escape from drug-induced constriction of isolated arterial segments from various vascular beds. *Angiologica* 9: 27–33, 1972.
59. FELD, A. D., J. D. FONDACARO, G. HOLLOWAY, AND E. D. JACOBSON. Laser Doppler velocimetry: a new technique for the measurement of intestinal mucosal blood flow. *Gastrointest. Endosc.* 30: 225–230, 1984.
60. FELDMAN, S., D. BIRNBAUM, AND A. J. BEHAR. Gastric secretion and acute gastroduodenal lesions following hypothalamic and preoptic stimulation. *J. Neurosurg.* 18: 661–670, 1961.
61. FOLKOW, B., D. H. LEWIS, O. LUNDGREN, S. MELLANDER, AND I. G. WALLENTIN. The effect of graded vasoconstrictor fiber stimulation on the intestinal resistance and capacitance vessels. *Acta Physiol. Scand.* 61: 445–457, 1964.
62. FUKUTOMI, H., J. MIYOMOTO, AND T. SAKITA. Endoscopical measurement of gastric blood flow of patients suffering from gastric ulcer. In: *Basic Aspects of Microcirculation. Proc. Int. Symp. Microcirc. Tokyo, July 26, 1981*, edited by M. Tsuchya, M. Asano, and M. Oda. Amsterdam: Excerpta Med., 1982, p. 251–258.
63. FURNESS, J. B. The adrenergic innervation of the vessels supplying and draining the gastrointestinal tract. *Z. Zellforsch. Mikrosk. Anat.* 113: 67–82, 1971.
64. GANNON, B., J. BROWNING, AND P. O'BRIEN. The microvascular architecture of the glandular mucosa of rat stomach. *J. Anat.* 135: 667–683, 1982.
65. GANNON, B., J. BROWNING, P. O'BRIEN, AND P. ROGERS. Mucosal microvascular architecture of the fundus and body of human stomach. *Gastroenterology* 86: 866–875, 1984.
65a. GARRICK, T., F. W. LEUNG, S. BUACK, K. HIRABAYASHI, AND P. H. GUTH. Gastric motility is stimulated but flow is unaffected during cold restraint-induced lesion formation in the rat. *Gastroenterology* 91: 141–148, 1986.

66. GENTER, B., A. M. STONE, T. A. STEIN, AND L. WISE. Gastric mucosal blood flow and *Escherichia coli* bacteremia. *Am. J. Surg.* 145: 364–368, 1983.
67. GERBER, J. G., AND A. S. NIES. Canine gastric mucosal vasodilation with prostaglandins and histamine analogs. *Dig. Dis. Sci.* 27: 870–874, 1982.
68. GERKINS, J. F., J. G. GERBER, D. G. SHAND, AND R. A. BRANCH. Effect of $PGI_2$, $PGE_2$ and 6-keto-$PGF_1$ on canine gastric blood flow and acid secretion. *Prostaglandins* 16: 815–823, 1978.
69. GERKINS, J. F., D. G. SHAND, C. FLEXNER, A. S. NIES, J. A. OATES, AND J. L. DATA. Effect of indomethacin and aspirin on gastric blood flow and acid secretion. *J. Pharmacol. Exp. Ther.* 203: 646–652, 1977.
70. GIBBS, F. A. A thermoelectric blood flow recorder in the form of a needle. *Proc. Soc. Exp. Biol. Med.* 31: 141–146, 1933.
71. GOWEN, G. F., AND W. W. LINDEMUTH. General hypothermia for managing gastrointestinal hemmorrhage. A report of 3 cases in which total body hypothermia was used to control massive gastrointestinal hemmorrhage. *J. Am. Med. Assoc.* 175: 29–33, 1961.
72. GRANGER, D. N., AND D. N. KVIETYS. Recent advances in measurement of gastrointestinal blood flow. *Gastroenterology* 88: 1073–1076, 1985.
73. GRANGER, D. N., G. RUTILI, AND J. M. MCCORD. Superoxide radicals in feline intestinal ischemia. *Gastroenterology* 81: 22–29, 1981.
74. GRAYSON, J. Internal calorimetry in the measurement of blood flow. *J. Physiol. Lond.* 118: 54–72, 1952.
75. GREEN, R. H., AND P. F. LAMBETH. Leukotrienes. *Tetrahedron* 39: 1687–1721, 1983.
76. GREENBERG, R. A., AND H. V. SPARKS. Prostaglandins and consecutive vascular segments of the canine hindlimb. *Am. J. Physiol.* 216: 567–571, 1969.
77. GREENWAY, C. V., AND V. S. MURTHY. Effects of vasopressin and isoprenaline infusions on the distribution of blood flow in the intestine: criteria for the validity of microsphere studies. *Br. J. Pharmacol.* 46: 177–188, 1972.
78. GUTH, P. H. Gastric blood flow in restraint stress. *Am. J. Dig. Dis.* 17: 807–813, 1972.
79. GUTH, P. H. Microvascular organization in the stomach. In: *Microcirculation of the Alimentary Tract*, edited by A. Koo, S. K. Lam, and L. H. Smaje. Singapore: World Sci., 1983, p. 17–27.
79a. GUTH, P. H., AND K. W. BALLARD. Physiology of the gastric circulation. In: *Physiology of the Gastrointestinal Tract* (1st ed.), edited by L. R. Johnson. New York: Raven, 1981, p. 709–731.
80. GUTH, P. H., H. BAUMANN, M. I. GROSSMAN, D. AURES, AND J. ELASHOFF. Measurement of gastric mucosal blood flow in man. *Gastroenterology* 74: 831–834, 1978.
80a. GUTH, P. H., AND F. L. LEUNG. Physiology of the gastric circulation. In: *Physiology of the Gastrointestinal Tract* (2nd ed.), edited by L. R. Johnson. New York: Raven, 1987, vol. 2, p. 1031–1053.
81. GUTH, P. H., AND T. L. MOLER. Endogenous prostaglandins in the regulation of the rat gastric microcirculation (Abstract). *Microvasc. Res.* 17: S15, 1979.
82. GUTH, P. H., AND T. L. MOLER. In vivo fluorescence microscopy of the gastric microcirculation (Abstract). *Gastroenterology* 76: 1147, 1979.
83. GUTH, P. H., AND A. ROSENBERG. In vivo microscopy of the gastric microcirculation. *Am. J. Dig. Dis.* 17: 391–398, 1972.
84. GUTH, P. H., G. ROSS, AND E. SMITH. Changes in intestinal vascular diameter during norepinephrine vasoconstrictor escape. *Am. J. Physiol.* 230: 1466–1468, 1976.
85. GUTH, P. H., AND E. SMITH. Vasoactive agents and the gastric microcirculation. *Microvasc. Res.* 8: 125–131, 1974.
86. GUTH, P. H., AND E. SMITH. Neural control of gastric mucosal blood flow in the rat. *Gastroenterology* 69: 935–940, 1975.
87. GUTH, P. H., AND E. SMITH. Escape from vasoconstriction in the gastric microcirculation. *Am. J. Physiol.* 228: 1893–1895, 1975.
88. GUTH, P. H., AND E. SMITH. The effect of gastrointestinal hormones on the gastric microcirculation. *Gastroenterology* 71: 435–438, 1976.
89. GUTH, P. H., AND E. SMITH. Nervous regulation of the gastric microcirculation. In: *Nerves and the Gut*, edited by F. P. Brooks and P. W. Evers. New York: Slack, 1977, p. 365–373.
90. GUTH, P. H., AND E. SMITH. Histamine receptors in the gastric microcirculation. *Gut* 19: 1059–1063, 1978.
91. GUTH, P. H., E. SMITH, AND T. MOLER. $H_1$ and $H_2$ receptors in rat gastric submucosal arterioles. *Microvasc. Res.* 19: 320–328, 1980.
92. HALSEY, J. H., N. F. CAPRA, AND R. S. MCFARLAND. Use of hydrogen for measurement of regional cerebral blood flow: problem of intercompartmental diffusion. *Stroke* 8: 351–357, 1977.
93. HARPER, A. A., J. D. REED, AND J. R. SMY. Gastric blood flow in anaesthetized cats. *J. Physiol. Lond.* 194: 795–807, 1968.
94. HARRIS, D. W., J. R. SMY, J. D. REED, AND C. W. VENABLES. The effects of burimamide and metiamide on basal gastric function in the cat. *Br. J. Pharmacol.* 53: 293–297, 1975.
95. HARVEY, W. *Movement of the Heart and Blood in Animals. An Anatomical Essay* [1628], translated by K. J. Franklin. Oxford, UK: Blackwell, 1957.
96. HASE, T., AND B. J. MOSS. Microvascular changes in the development of stress ulcer in rats. *Gastroenterology* 65: 224–234, 1973.
97. HASHIZUME, M., K. TANAKA, AND K. INOKUCHI. Morphology of gastric microcirculation in cirrhosis. *Hepatology Baltimore* 3: 1008–1012, 1983.
98. HEDQUIST, P. Autonomic neurotransmission. In: *The Prostaglandins*, edited by P. W. Ramwell. New York: Plenum, 1973, p. 101–131.
99. HOLMES, S. W., E. W. HORTON, AND I. H. M. MAIN. The effect of prostaglandin $E_1$ on responses of smooth muscle to catecholamines, angiotensin and vasopressin. *Br. J. Pharmacol.* 21: 538–543, 1963.
100. HOLM-RUTILI, L., AND T. BERGLINDH. Pentagastrin and gastric mucosal blood flow. *Am. J. Physiol.* 250 (*Gastrointest. Liver Physiol.* 13): G575–G580, 1986.
100a. HOLM-RUTILI, L., AND K. J. OBRINK. Effects of prostaglandin $E_1$ and gastric mucosal microcirculation and spontaneous acid secretion in the rat. In: *Mechanisms of Mucosal Protection in the Upper Gastrointestinal Tract*, edited by A. Allen, G. Flemström, A. Garner, W. Silen, and L. A. Turnberg. New York: Raven, 1984, p. 279–283.
101. HOLM-RUTILI, L., M. A. PERRY, AND D. N. GRANGER. Autoregulation of gastric blood flow and oxygen uptake. *Am. J. Physiol.* 241 (*Gastrointest. Liver Physiol.* 4): G143–G149, 1981.
101a. HUDSON, D., O. U. SCREMIN, AND P. H. GUTH. Measurement of regional gastroduodenal blood flow with iodo [$^{14}$C]antipyrine autoradiography. *Am. J. Physiol.* 248 (*Gastrointest. Liver Physiol.* 11): G539–G544, 1985.
102. HUNTER, G. C., J. GOLDSTONE, R. VILLA, AND L. W. WAY. Effect of vagotomy upon intragastric redistribution of microvascular flow. *J. Surg. Res.* 26: 314–319, 1979.
103. ISHIKAWA, T., M. NAGATA, AND Y. OSUMI. Dual effects of electrical stimulation of ventromedial hypothalamic neurons on gastric acid secretion in rats. *Am. J. Physiol.* 245 (*Gastrointest. Liver Physiol.* 8): G265–G269, 1983.
104. ISHIKAWA, T., Y. OSUMI, M. FUJIWARA, AND M. NAGATA. Possible roles of central cholinergic nicotine mechanisms in regulation of gastric functions. *Eur. J. Pharmacol.* 80: 331–336, 1982.
105. ITO, S., AND G. C. SCHOFIELD. Studies on the depletion and accumulation of microvilli and changes in the tubulovesicular compartment of mouse parietal cells in relation to gastric acid secretion. *J. Cell Biol.* 63: 364–382, 1974.
106. ITOH, M., AND P. H. GUTH. Role of oxygen-derived free radicals in hemorrhagic shock-induced gastric lesions in the rat. *Gastroenterology* 88: 1162–1167, 1985.
107. IVARSSON, L. E., N. DARLE, L. HULTÉN, J. LINDHAGEN, AND

107. O. LUNDGREN. Gastric blood flow and distribution: the effect of pentagastrin in anesthetized cat and man as studied by an inert gas elimination method. *Scand. J. Gastroenterol.* 17: 1037–1048, 1982.
108. JACOBOWITZ, D. Histochemical studies on the autonomic innervation of the gut. *J. Pharmacol. Exp. Ther.* 149: 358–364, 1965.
109. JACOBSON, E. D. Effects of histamine, acetylcholine, and norepinephrine on gastric vascular resistance. *Am. J. Physiol.* 204: 1013–1017, 1963.
110. JACOBSON, E. D. Clearance of the gastric mucosa. *Gastroenterology* 54: 434–448, 1968.
111. JACOBSON, E. D., AND A. C. K. CHANG. Comparison of gastrin and histamine on gastric mucosal blood flow. *Proc. Soc. Exp. Biol. Med.* 130: 484–486, 1969.
112. JACOBSON, E. D., M. M. EISENBERG, AND K. G. SWAN. Effects of histamine on gastric blood flow in conscious dogs. *Gastroenterology* 51: 466–472, 1966.
113. JACOBSON, E. D., R. H. LINFORD, AND M. I. GROSSMAN. Gastric secretion in relation to mucosal blood flow studied by a clearance technique. *J. Clin. Invest.* 45: 1–13, 1966.
114. JACOBSON, E. D., J. B. SCOTT, AND E. D. FROHLICH. Hemodynamics of the stomach. I. Resistance-flow relationship in the gastric vascular bed. *Am. J. Dig. Dis.* 7: 779–785, 1962.
115. JANSSON, G. Extrinsic nervous control of gastric motility. *Acta Physiol. Scand. Suppl.* 326: 1–42, 1969.
116. JANSSON, G., M. KAMPP, O. LUNDGREN, AND J. MARTINSON. Studies on the circulation of the stomach (Abstract). *Acta Physiol. Scand. Suppl.* 277: 91, 1966.
117. JANSSON, G., O. LUNDGREN, AND J. MARTINSON. Neurohormonal control of gastric blood flow. *Gastroenterology* 58: 425–429, 1970.
118. JOHNSON, P. C. Origin, localization, and homeostatic significance of autoregulation in the intestine. *Circ. Res.* 15, Suppl. 1: 225–233, 1964.
119. KAMADA, T., S. KAWANO, N. SATO, M. FUKUDA, H. FUSAMOTO, AND H. ABE. Gastric mucosal blood distribution and its changes in the healing process of gastric ulcer. *Gastroenterology* 84: 1541–1546, 1983.
120. KAMADA, T., N. SATO, S. KAWANO, H. FUSAMOTO, AND H. ABE. Gastric mucosal hemodynamics after thermal or head injury. *Gastroenterology* 83: 535–540, 1982.
121. KAUFFMAN, G. L., JR., D. AURES, AND M. I. GROSSMAN. Indomethacin decreases basal gastric mucosal blood flow (Abstract). *Gastroenterology* 76: 1165, 1979.
122. KAUFFMAN, G. L., JR., AND B. J. R. WHITTLE. Gastric vascular actions of prostanoids and the dual effect of arachidonic acid. *Am. J. Physiol.* 242 (*Gastrointest. Liver Physiol.* 5): G582–G587, 1982.
123. KAUFFMAN, G. L., JR., B. J. R. WHITTLE, AND J. A. SALMON. Gastric venous prostaglandin concentrations during basal and stimulated acid secretion in dog. *Proc. Soc. Exp. Biol. Med.* 169: 233–238, 1982.
124. KETY, S. S. Theory of blood-tissue exchange—its application to measurement of blood flow. In: *Methods in Medical Research VIII*, edited by H. D. Bruner. Chicago, IL: Year Book, 1960, p. 223–227.
125. KITAGAWA, H., M. FUJIWARA, AND Y. OSUMI. Effects of water-immersion stress on gastric secretion and mucosal blood flow in rats. *Gastroenterology* 77: 298–302, 1979.
126. KITANO, S., K. INOKUCHI, K. SUGIMACHI, AND N. KOYANAGI. Hemodynamic and morphological changes in the stomach of portal hypertensive rats. *Eur. Surg. Res.* 13: 227–235, 1981.
127. KIVILAAKSO, E., D. FROMM, AND W. SILEN. Relationship between ulceration and intramural pH of gastric mucosa during hemorrhagic shock. *Surgery St. Louis* 84: 70–78, 1978.
128. KNIGHT, S. E., AND R. L. McISAAC. Neutral red clearance as an estimate of gastric mucosal blood flow in man. *J. Physiol. Lond.* 272: 62P–63P, 1977.
129. KNIGHT, S. E., R. L. McISAAC, AND L. P. FIELDING. The effect of the histamine-$H_2$-antagonist cimetidine on gastric mucosal blood flow (Abstract). *Gut* 18: A948, 1977.
130. KNIGHT, S. E., R. L. McISAAC, AND L. P. FIELDING. Comparison of gastric mucosal blood flow (GMBF) in normal subjects and patients with duodenal ulcer (Abstract). *Br. J. Surg.* 64: 824, 1977.
131. KNIGHT, S. E., R. L. McISAAC, AND L. P. FIELDING. The effect of highly selective vagotomy on the relationship between gastric mucosal blood flow and acid secretion in man. *Br. J. Surg.* 65: 721–723, 1978.
132. KOCH, H., AND L. DEMLING. The value of the thermocouple in the measurement of the gastric mucosal blood flow. *Res. Exp. Med.* 167: 784, 1976.
133. KOLIN, A. Blood flow determination by electromagnetic method. *Med. Phys.* 3: 141–155, 1960.
134. KONTUREK, S. J., A. DEMBINSKI, R. KROL, AND E. WUNSCH. Effect of 13-NLE-motilin on gastric secretion, serum gastrin level and mucosal blood flow in dogs. *J. Physiol. Lond.* 264: 665–672, 1977.
135. KONTUREK, S. J., A. DEMBINSKI, P. THOR, AND R. KROL. Comparison of vasoactive intestinal peptide (VIP) and secretin in gastric secretion and mucosal blood flow. *Pfluegers Arch.* 361: 175–181, 1976.
136. KONTUREK, S. J., N. KWIECIEN, W. OBTULOWICZ, A. KIEC-DEMBINSKA, M. POLANSKI, B. KOPP, E. SITO, AND J. OLEKSY. Effect of carprofen and indomethacin on gastric function, mucosal integrity and generation of prostaglandins in man. *Hepato-Gastroenterology* 29: 267–270, 1982.
137. KONTUREK, S. J., C. LANCASTER, A. J. HANACHAR, J. E. NEZAMIS, AND A. ROBERT. The influence of prostacyclin on gastric mucosal blood flow resting and stimulated canine stomach (Abstract). *Gastroenterology* 76: 1173, 1979.
138. KONTUREK, S. J., AND A. ROBERT. Cytoprotection of canine gastric mucosa by prostacyclin: possible mediation by increased mucosal blood flow. *Digestion* 25: 155–163, 1982.
139. KONTUREK, S. J., A. ROBERT, A. J. HANCHAR, AND J. E. NEZAMIS. Comparison of prostacycline and prostaglandin $E_2$ on gastric secretion, gastrin release, and mucosal blood flow in dogs. *Dig. Dis. Sci.* 25: 673–679, 1980.
140. KONTUREK, S. J., J. TASLER, M. CIESKOWSKI, D. H. COY, AND A. V. SCHALLY. Effect of growth hormone release-inhibiting hormone on gastric secretion, mucosal blood flow, and serum gastrin. *Gastroenterology* 70: 737–741, 1976.
141. KONTUREK, S. J., J. TASLER, W. OBTULOWICZ, AND J. F. REHFELD. Effect of metiamide, a histamine $H_2$-receptor antagonist on mucosal blood flow and serum gastrin level. *Gastroenterology* 66: 982–986, 1974.
142. KOWALEWSKI, K., AND A. KOLODEJ. Effect of prostaglandin-$E_2$ on gastric secretion and on gastric circulation of totally isolated ex vivo canine stomach. *Pharmacology* 11: 85–94, 1974.
143. LARSEN, K. R., V. A. MAAS, AND E. CARLSSON. The effects of omeprazole, a proton pump inhibitor, on pentagastrin-stimulated blood flow and oxygen consumption in the ex-vivo canine gastric chamber (Abstract). *Gastroenterology* 86: 1153, 1984.
144. LEONARD, A. S., D. LONG, L. A. FRENCH, E. T. PETER, AND O. H. WANGENSTEEN. Pendular pattern in gastric secretion and blood flow following hypothalamic stimulation—origin of stress ulcer? *Surgery St. Louis* 56: 109–120, 1964.
145. LEUNG, F. W., AND P. H. GUTH. Dissociated effects of somatostatin on gastric acid secretion and mucosal blood flow. *Am. J. Physiol.* 248 (*Gastrointest. Liver Physiol.* 11): G337–G341, 1985.
146. LEUNG, F. W., P. H. GUTH, O. U. SCREMIN, E. M. GOLANSKA, AND G. L. KAUFFMAN, JR. Regional gastric mucosal blood flow measurements by hydrogen gas clearance in the anesthetized rat and rabbit. *Gastroenterology* 87: 28–36, 1984.
147. LEUNG, F. W., M. ITOH, K. HIRABAYASHI, AND P. H. GUTH. Role of blood flow in gastric and duodenal mucosal injury in the rat. *Gastroenterology* 88: 281–289, 1985.

148. LEUNG, F. W., A. ROBERT, AND P. H. GUTH. Gastric mucosal blood flow in rats after 16,16-dimethyl prostaglandin E$_2$ given at a cytoprotective dose. *Gastroenterology* 88: 1948–1953, 1985.
149. LEVINE, B. A., V. H. GASKILL III, AND K. R. SIRINEK. Lack of sustained vagal control of gastric mucosal blood flow. Why vagotomy is not effective in preventing recurrent hemorrhage from stress ulcers. *Surgery St. Louis* 90: 631–636, 1981.
150. LEVINE, B. A., H. V. GASKILL III, AND K. R. SIRINEK. Gastric mucosal cytoprotection by splanchnicectomy is based on protection of gastric mucosal blood flow. *J. Trauma* 23: 278–284, 1983.
151. LEVINE, B. A., W. H. SCHWESINGER, K. R. SIRINEK, D. JONES, AND B. A. PRUITT. Cimetidine prevents reduction in gastric mucosal blood flow during shock. *Surgery St. Louis* 84: 113–119, 1978.
152. LEVITT, M. D., AND D. G. LEVITT. Use of inert gases to study the interaction of blood flow and diffusion during passive absorption from the gastrointestinal tract of the rat. *J. Clin. Invest.* 52: 1852–1862, 1973.
153. LIN, T.-M., D. C. EVANS, C. J. SHAAR, AND M. A. ROOT. Action of somatostatin on stomach, pancreas, gastric mucosal blood flow, and hormones. *Am. J. Physiol.* 244 (*Gastrointest. Liver Physiol.* 7): G40–G45, 1983.
154. LIN, T. M., AND M. W. WARRICK. Effect of glucagon on pentagastrin-induced gastric acid secretion and mucosal blood flow in the dog. *Gastroenterology* 61: 328–331, 1971.
155. LOCKENVITZ, E., P. O. SCHWILL, E. HANISCH, AND W. ENGELHARDT. Influence of exogenous glucagon on gastric acid secretion, mucosal blood flow, and stress ulcers in the rat: dose-response results under non-stress conditions and immobilization stress. *Stress Res. Exp. Med.* 182: 245–253, 1983.
156. MACKIE, D. B., AND M. D. TURNER. Vagotomy and submucosal blood flow. *Arch. Surg.* 102: 626–629, 1971.
157. MAIN, I. H. M., AND B. J. R. WHITTLE. The effects of E and A prostaglandins on gastric mucosal blood flow and acid secretion in the rat. *Br. J. Pharmacol.* 49: 428–436, 1973.
158. MAIN, I. H. M., AND B. J. R. WHITTLE. Gastric mucosal blood flow during pentagastrin- and histamine-stimulated acid secretion in the rat. *Br. J. Pharmacol.* 49: 534–542, 1973.
159. MAIN, I. H. M., AND B. J. R. WHITTLE. Investigation of the vasodilator and antisecretory role of prostaglandins in the rat gastric mucosa by use of non-steroidal anti-inflammatory drugs. *Br. J. Pharmacol.* 53: 217–224, 1975.
160. MAIN, I. H. M., AND B. J. R. WHITTLE. A study of the vascular and acid-secretory responses of the rat gastric mucosa to histamine. *J. Physiol. Lond.* 257: 407–418, 1976.
161. MARTINSON, J. The effect of graded vagal stimulation on gastric motility, secretion and blood flow in the cat. *Acta Physiol. Scand.* 65: 300–309, 1965.
162. MARTINSON, J. Studies on the efferent vagal control of the stomach. *Acta Physiol. Scand. Suppl.* 255: 1–24, 1965.
163. MAXWELL, L. C., A. P. SHEPHERD, AND G. L. RIEDEL. Vasodilatation or altered perfusion pressure moves 15-$\mu$m spheres trapped in the gut wall. *Am. J. Physiol.* 243 (*Heart Circ. Physiol.* 12): H123–H127, 1982.
164. MCGRATH, M. A., AND J. T. SHEPHERD. Inhibition of adrenergic neurotransmission in canine vascular smooth muscle by histamine. *Circ. Res.* 39: 566–573, 1976.
165. MCGREAVY, J. M., AND F. G. MOODY. Protection of gastric mucosa against aspirin-induced erosions by enhanced blood flow. *Surg. Forum* 28: 357–359, 1977.
166. MCGREAVY, J. M., AND F. G. MOODY. Focal microcirculatory changes during the production of aspirin-induced gastric mucosal erosions. *Surgery St. Louis* 89: 337–341, 1981.
167. MENGUY, R. Effects of histamine on gastric blood flow. *Am. J. Dig. Dis.* 7: 383–393, 1962.
168. MENGUY, R., AND Y. F. MASTERS. Gastric mucosal energy metabolism and "stress ulceration." *Ann. Surg.* 180: 538–548, 1974.
169. MERSEREAU, W. A., AND E. J. HINCHEY. Effect of gastric acidity on gastric ulceration induced by hemorrhage in the rat, utilizing a gastric chamber technique. *Gastroenterology* 64: 1130–1135, 1973.
170. MICHELS, N. A. *Blood Supply and Anatomy of the Upper Abdominal Organs.* Philadelphia, PA: Lippincott, 1955.
171. MILLER, T. A., J. M. HENAGAN, AND T. M. LOG. Impairment of aminopyrine clearance in aspirin-damaged canine gastric mucosa. *Gastroenterology* 85: 643–649, 1983.
172. MILLER, T. A., J. M. HENAGAN, AND A. ROBERT. Effect of 16,16-dimethyl PGE$_2$ on resting and histamine- stimulated gastric mucosal blood flow. *Dig. Dis. Sci.* 25: 561–567, 1980.
173. MONCADA, S., R. GRYGLEWSKI, S. BUNTING, AND J. R. VANE. An enzyme isolated from arteries transforms prostaglandin endoperoxides to an unstable substance that inhibits platelet aggregation. *Nature Lond.* 663–665, 1976.
174. MONCADA, S., J. A. SALMON, J. R. VANE, AND B. J. R. WHITTLE. Formation of prostacyclin (PGI$_2$) and its product, 6-oxo-PGF$_{1\alpha}$ by the gastric mucosa of several species. *J. Physiol. Lond.* 275: 4P–5P, 1978.
175. MONCADA, S., AND J. R. VANE. The role of prostacyclin in vascular tissue. *Federation Proc.* 38: 66–71, 1979.
176. MOODY, F. G. Oxygen consumption during thiocyanate inhibition of gastric acid secretion in dogs. *Am. J. Physiol.* 215: 127–131, 1968.
177. MOODY, F. G., J. MCGREAVY, C. ZALEWSKY, L. Y. CHEUNG, AND M. SIMONS. The cytoprotective effect of mucosal blood flow in experimental erosive gastritis. *Acta Physiol. Scand. Special Suppl. 1978*, p. 35–43.
178. MORISHITA, T., AND P. H. GUTH. Vagal nerve stimulation causes noncholinergic dilatation of gastric arterioles. *Am. J. Physiol.* 250 (*Gastrointest. Liver Physiol.* 13): G660–G664, 1986.
179. MULLER-LISSNER, S. A., A. SONNENBERG, AND A. BLUM. Does gastric aminopyrine clearance reflect gastric mucosal blood flow or parietal cell function? *Gut* 23: 997–1002, 1981.
180. MURAKAMI, M., S. K. LAM, M. INADA, AND T. MIYAKE. Pathophysiology and pathogenesis of acute gastric mucosal lesions after hypothermic restraint stress in rats. *Gastroenterology* 88: 660–665, 1985.
181. MURAKAMI, M., M. MORIGA, T. MIYAKE, AND H. UCHINO. Contact electrode method in hydrogen gas clearance technique: a new method for determination of regional gastric mucosal blood flow in animals and humans. *Gastroenterology* 82: 457–467, 1982.
182. NAGATA, H., AND P. H. GUTH. Effect of histamine on microvascular permeability in the rat stomach. *Am. J. Physiol.* 245 (*Gastrointest. Liver Physiol.* 8): G201–G207, 1983.
183. NAGATA, H., AND P. H. GUTH. Effect of topical histamine on mucosal microvascular permeability and acid secretion in the rat stomach. *Am. J. Physiol.* 246 (*Gastrointest. Liver Physiol.* 9): G654–G659, 1984.
184. NAGATA, H., AND P. H. GUTH. In vivo observation of the lymphatic system in the rat stomach. *Gastroenterology* 86: 1443–1450, 1984.
185. NAKAMURA, K., K. ISHI, M. KUSANO, AND S. HAYASHI. Acute and long-term effects of vagotomy on gastric mucosal blood flow. In: *Vagotomy. Latest Advances with Special Reference to Gastric and Duodenal Ulcer,* edited by F. Halle and S. Andersson. New York: Springer-Verlag, 1974, p. 109–111.
186. NAKAMURA, M., N. WATANABE, N. TSUKUDA, M. ODA, AND M. TSUCHIYA. Demonstration of the adrenergic nerves in the rat gastric mucosa. A histofluorescence and electron microscopic study in comparison with the distribution of the cholinergic nerves. *Okajimas Folia Anat. Jpn.* 59: 65–86, 1982.
187. NAKAMURA, Y., AND H. WAYLAND. Macromolecular transport in the cat mesentery. *Microvasc. Res.* 9: 1–21, 1975.
188. NEBESAR, R. A., P. L. KORNBLITH, J. J. POLLARD, AND N. A. MICHELS. *Celiac and Superior Mesenteric Arteries. A Correlation of Angiograms and Dissections.* Boston, MA: Little, Brown, 1969.

189. NEMEROFF, C. B., D. E. HERNANDEZ, R. C. ORLANDO, AND A. J. PRANGE, JR. Cytoprotective effect of centrally administered neurotensin on stress-induced gastric ulcers. *Am. J. Physiol.* 242 (*Gastrointest. Liver Physiol.* 5): G342–G346, 1982.
190. NICOLOFF, D. M., E. T. PETER, N. H. STONE, AND O. H. WANGENSTEEN. Effects of catecholamines on gastric secretion and blood flow. *Ann. Surg.* 159: 32–36, 1964.
191. NILSSON, L. O., A. M. STONE, T. A. STEIR, AND L. WISE. Indomethacin and the gastric mucosal blood flow changes of sepsis. *Ann. Surg.* 198: 592–595, 1983.
192. NOWICKI, P. T., B. S. STONESTREET, N. B. HANSEN, A. C. YAO, AND W. OH. Gastrointestinal blood flow and oxygen consumption in awake newborn piglets: effect of feeding. *Am. J. Physiol.* 245 (*Gastrointest. Liver Physiol.* 8): G697–G702, 1983.
193. NYLANDER, G., AND S. OLERUD. The vascular pattern of the gastric mucosa of the rat following vagotomy. *Surg. Gynecol. Obst.* 112: 475–480, 1961.
194. O'BRIEN, P., AND W. SILEN. Effects of bile salts and aspirin on the gastric mucosal blood flow. *Gastroenterology* 64: 246–253, 1973.
195. OHYA, Y., AND P. H. GUTH. Effect of topical ethanol on rat gastric mucosal microcirculation (Abstract). *Clin. Res.* 33: 37A, 1985.
196. OSUMI, Y., S. AIBARA, K. SAKAE, AND M. FUJIWARA. Central noradrenergic inhibition of gastric mucosal blood flow and acid secretion in rats. *Life Sci.* 20: 1407–1416, 1977.
197. OSUMI, Y., T. ISHIKAWA, Y. OKUMA, Y. NAGASAKA, AND M. FUJIWARA. Inhibition of gastric function by stimulation of rat locus coeruleus. *Eur. J. Pharmacol.* 75: 27–35, 1981.
198. OSUMI, Y., Y. NAGASAKA, L. H. FU, AND M. FUJIWARA. Inhibition of gastric acid secretion and mucosa blood flow induced by intraventricularly applied neurotensin in rats. *Life Sci.* 23: 2275–2280, 1978.
199. OWEN, D. A. A. The effects of histamine and some histamine-like agonists on blood pressure in the cat. *Br. J. Pharmacol.* 55: 173–179, 1975.
200. OWEN, D. A. A. Reduction by cimetidine of acute gastric hemorrhage caused by reinfusion of blood after exposure to exogenous acid during gastric ischemia in rats. *Gastroenterology* 77: 979–985, 1979.
201. PAWLIK, W. W., R. O. BANKS, AND E. D. JACOBSEN. Hemodynamic actions of nicotine on the canine stomach. *Proc. Soc. Exp. Biol. Med.* 177: 447–454, 1984.
202. PAYNE, J. G., AND J. C. BOWEN. Hypoxia of canine gastric mucosa caused by *Escherichia coli* sepsis and prevented with methylprednisolone therapy. *Gastroenterology* 80: 84–93, 1981.
203. PERRY, M. A., G. J. HAEDICKE, G. B. BULKLEY, P. R. KVIETYS, AND D. N. GRANGER. Relationship between acid secretion and blood flow in the canine stomach: role of oxygen consumption. *Gastroenterology* 85: 529–534, 1983.
204. PERRY, M. A., D. MURPHREE, AND D. N. GRANGER. Oxygen uptake as a determinant of gastric blood flow autoregulation. *Dig. Dis. Sci.* 27: 675–679, 1982.
205. PESKAR, B. M. Regional distribution of prostaglandin-metabolizing enzymes in the mucosa of the human upper gastrointestinal tract. *Acta Hepato-Gastroenterology* 25: 49–51, 1978.
206. PETER, E. T., D. M. NICOLOFF, A. S. LEONARD, A. I. WALDER, AND O. H. WANGENSTEEN. Effect of vagal and sympathetic stimulation and ablation on gastric blood flow. *J. Am. Med. Assoc.* 183: 1003–1005, 1963.
207. PETER, E. T., D. M. NICOLOFF, H. SOSIN, A. I. WALDER, AND O. H. WANGENSTEEN. Relationship between gastric blood flow and secretion (Abstract). *Federation Proc.* 21: 264, 1962.
208. PIASECKI, C. Blood supply to the human gastroduodenal mucosa with special reference to the ulcer-bearing areas. *J. Anat.* 118: 295–335, 1974.
209. PIASECKI, C. Observations on the submucous plexus and mucosal arteries of the dog's stomach and first part of the duodenum. *J. Anat.* 119: 133–148, 1975.
210. POLANSKY, D. B., S. S. SHIRAZI, AND D. COON. Lack of correlation of gastric acid secretion and blood flow. *J. Surg. Res.* 26: 320–325, 1979.
211. PORTER, R. W., H. J. MOVIUS, AND J. D. FRENCH. Hypothalamic influences on hydrochloric acid secretion of the stomach. *Surgery St. Louis* 33: 875–880, 1953.
212. POWELL, J. R. Effects of histamine on vascular sympathetic neuroeffector transmission. *J. Pharmacol. Exp. Ther.* 208: 360–365, 1979.
213. PRICE, B. A., B. M. JAFFE, AND M. J. ZINNER. Effect of exogenous somatostatin infusion on gastrointestinal blood flow and hormones in the conscious dog. *Gastroenterology* 88: 80–85, 1985.
214. REED, J. D., D. J. SANDERS, AND V. THORPE. The effect of splanchnic nerve stimulation on gastric acid secretion and mucosal blood flow in the anaesthetized cat. *J. Physiol. Lond.* 214: 1–13, 1971.
215. REES, M., AND J. C. BOWEN. Stress ulcers during live *Escherichia coli* sepsis. The role of acid and bile. *Ann. Surg.* 195: 646–652, 1982.
216. REES, M., J. G. PAYNE, AND J. C. BOWEN. Naloxone reverses tissue effects of live *Escherichia coli* sepsis. *Surgery St. Louis* 91: 81–86, 1982.
217. RITCHIE, W. P., JR. Acute gastric mucosal damage induced by bile salts, acid, and ischemia. *Gastroenterology* 68: 699–707, 1975.
218. RITCHIE, W. P., JR., AND E. W. SHEARBURN III. Influence of isoproterenol and cholestyramine on acute gastric mucosal ulcerogenesis. *Gastroenterology* 73: 62–65, 1977.
219. ROBERT, A., F. W. LEUNG, K. HIRABAYASHI, AND P. H. GUTH. Effect of nicotine and cigarette smoke on gastric mucosal blood flow in rats (Abstract). *Gastroenterology* 88: 1717, 1985.
220. ROSENBERG, A., AND P. H. GUTH. A method for the in vivo study of the gastric microcirculation. *Microvasc. Res.* 2: 111–112, 1970.
221. ROSS, G. Escape of mesenteric vessels from adrenergic and nonadrenergic vasoconstriction. *Am. J. Physiol.* 221: 1217–1222, 1971.
222. SAITA, H., M. MURAKAMI, M. SEKI, AND T. MIYAKE. Evaluation of the measurement of gastric mucosal blood flow by laser Doppler velocimetry in rats (Abstract). *Gastroenterology* 86: 1228, 1984.
223. SALMON, P. A., W. O. GRIFFIN, AND O. H. WANGENSTEEN. Effect of intragastric temperature changes upon gastric blood flow. *Proc. Soc. Exp. Biol. Med.* 101: 442–444, 1959.
224. SALVATI, P., AND B. J. WHITTLE. Vascular responses of the isolated perfused stomach of rabbit and rat to histamine. *Eur. J. Pharmacol.* 89: 63–68, 1983.
225. SAPIRSTEIN, L. A. The indicator fractionation technique for the study of regional blood flow. *Gastroenterology* 52: 365–371, 1967.
226. SATO, N., T. KAMADA, M. SCHICHIRI, S. KAWANO, H. ABE, AND B. HAGIHARA. Measurement of hemoperfusion and oxygen sufficiency in gastric mucosa in vivo. *Gastroenterology* 76: 814–819, 1979.
227. SCHNITZLEIN, H. N. Regulation of blood flow through the stomach of the rat. *Anat. Rec.* 127: 735–754, 1957.
228. SCHWILLE, P. O., G. LANG, AND P. HOFMANN. Rat gastric secretion and mucosal blood flow during restraint stress-effect of a low dose metiamide. *Res. Exp. Med.* 171: 205–210, 1977.
229. SEMB, B. K. H. Regional gastric flow determined by a hydrogen clearance technique in anesthetized and conscious animals. *Scand. J. Gastroenterol.* 15: 569–576, 1980.
230. SEMB, B. K. H. Regional gastric flow changes after meal stimulation measured by the hydrogen gas clearance technique in conscious cats. *Scand. J. Gastroenterol.* 17: 839–842, 1982.
231. SEN, R. N., AND B. K. ANAND. Effect of electrical stimulation of the hypothalamus on gastric secretory activity and ulceration. *Indian J. Med. Res.* 45: 507–513, 1957.
232. SETCHELL, B. P., AND J. L. LINZELL. Soluble indicator tech-

niques for tissue blood flow measurement using $^{86}$RbCl, urea, antipyrine (phenazone) derivatives of $^3$H-water. *Clin. Exp. Pharmacol. Physiol.* 1, Suppl.: 15–29, 1974.
233. SHEPHERD, A. P., AND G. L. RIEDEL. Continuous measurement of intestinal mucosal blood flow by laser-Doppler velocimetry. *Am. J. Physiol.* 242 (*Gastrointest. Liver Physiol.* 5): G668–G672, 1982.
234. SHOEMAKER, C. P., JR., AND S. R. POWERS, JR. The absence of large functional arteriovenous shunts in the stomach of the anesthetized dog. *Surgery St. Louis* 60: 118–126, 1966.
235. SHOOR, P. M., L. D. GRIFFITH, R. B. DILLEY, AND E. F. BERNSTEIN. Effect of pulseless perfusion on gastrointestinal blood flow and its distribution. *Am. J. Physiol.* 236 (*Endocrinol. Metab.* 1): E28–E32, 1979.
236. SHORE, P. A., B. B. BRODIE, AND C. A. M. HOGBEN. The gastric secretion of drugs: a pH partition hypothesis. *J. Pharmacol. Exp. Ther.* 119: 361–369, 1957.
237. SKARSTEIN, A. Effect of vasopressin on blood flow distribution in the stomach of cats with gastric ulcer. *Scand. J. Gastroenterol.* 13: 783–788, 1978.
238. SKARSTEIN, A. Effect of indomethacin on blood flow distribution in the stomach of cats with acute gastric ulcer. *Scand. J. Gastroenterol.* 14: 905–911, 1979.
239. SMITH, G. P., AND P. R. MCHUGH. Gastric secretory response to amygdaloid or hypothalamic stimulation in monkeys. *Am. J. Physiol.* 213: 640–644, 1967.
240. SOBIN, S. S. Vascular injection methods. In: *Methods in Medical Research*, edited by C. A. Weiderhielm. Chicago, IL: Year Book, 1966, p. 233–238.
241. SOLL, A. H. Prostaglandin inhibition of histamine-stimulated aminopyrine uptake and cyclic AMP generation by isolated canine parietal cells (Abstract). *Gastroenterology* 74: 1146, 1978.
242. SONNENBERG, A., AND A. L. BLUM. Limitations to measurement of gastric mucosal blood flow by $^{14}$C-aminopyrine clearance. In: *Gastrointestinal Mucosal Blood Flow*, edited by L. P. Fielding. Edinburgh: Churchill Livingstone, 1980, p. 43–58.
243. SONNENBERG, A., AND N. HUSMERT. Effect of nicotine on gastric mucosal blood flow and acid secretion. *Gut* 23: 532–535, 1982.
244. SONNENBERG, A., AND C. WEST. Somatostatin reduces gastric mucosal blood flow in normal subjects but not in patients with cirrhosis of the liver. *Gut* 24: 148–153, 1983.
245. SØREIDE, O., T. SVANES, J. E. VARHAUG, AND K. SVANES. Acute gastritis in cats. Effect of water lavage and local hypothermia on gastric blood flow. *Digestion* 18: 248–260, 1978.
246. STARLINGER, M., R. JAKESZ, J. B. MATTHEWS, C. YOON, AND R. SCHIESSEL. The relative importance of $HCO_3^-$ and blood flow in the protection of rat gastric mucosa during shock. *Gastroenterology* 81: 732–735, 1981.
247. STAUBESAND, J., AND F. HAMMERSEN. Zur Problematik des Nachweises arterio-venoser Anastomosen im Injektionspraparat. Beobachtungen an Menschlichen Nierenbenken. *Z. Anat. Entwicklungsgech.* 119: 365–370, 1956.
248. STOW, R. W. Thermal measurement of tissue blood flow. *Trans. NY. Acad. Sci.* 27: 748–758, 1965.
249. SUNDELL, G., AND H. F. HELANDER. Parietal cell ultrastructure during inhibition of acid secretion. *Acta Physiol. Scand. Suppl.* 508: 65, 1982.
250. SVANES, K., J. E. VARHAUG, P. HOLM, A. BAKKE, AND I. ROMSLO. Effects of hemorrhagic shock on gastric blood flow and acid secretion in cats. *Acta Chir. Scand.* 147: 81–88, 1981.
251. SZABO, S., J. S. TRIER, A. BROWN, AND J. SCHNOOR. Early vascular injury and increased vascular permeability in gastric mucosal injury caused by ethanol in the rat. *Gastroenterology* 88: 228–236, 1985.
252. TAGUE, L. L., AND E. D. JACOBSON. Evaluation of $^{14}$C-aminopyrine clearance of determination of gastric mucosal blood flow. *Proc. Soc. Exp. Biol. Med.* 151: 707–710, 1967.
253. TAKESHITA, H., Y. KOTANI, AND S. OKABE. Comparative study of hydrogen and aminopyrine clearance methods for determination of gastric mucosal blood flow in dogs. *Dig. Dis. Sci.* 29: 841–847, 1980.
254. TAYLOR, T. V., B. R. PULLAN, J. B. EDLER, AND B. TORRANCE. Observations of gastric mucosal blood flow using $^{99}$Tcm in rat and man. *Br. J. Surg.* 62: 788–791, 1975.
255. TAYLOR, T. V., B. R. PULLAN, AND B. TORRANCE. Effect of fasting on mucosal blood flow in antrum and corpus of the stomach. *Eur. Surg. Res.* 8: 227–235, 1976.
256. TEPPERMAN, B. L., L. I. TAGUE, AND E. D. JACOBSON. Inhibition of canine gastric acid secretion by an $H_1$ receptor antagonist to histamine. *Dig. Dis. Sci.* 23: 801–808, 1978.
257. THOMPSON, J. E., AND J. R. VANE. Gastric secretion induced by histamine and its relationship to the rate of blood flow. *J. Physiol. Lond.* 121: 433–444, 1953.
258. VAGNE, M., S. J. KONTUREK, AND J. A. CHAYVIALLE. Effect of vasoactive intestinal peptide on gastric secretion in the cat. *Gastroenterology* 83: 250–255, 1982.
259. VANE, R. The release and fate of vasoactive hormones in the circulation. *Br. J. Pharmacol.* 35: 209–242, 1969.
260. VAN HEE, R. H., AND P. M. VANHOUTTE. Cholinergic inhibition of adrenergic neurotransmission in the canine gastric artery. *Gastroenterology* 74: 1266–1270, 1978.
261. VARGA, F., AND T. Z. CSAKY. Changes in the blood supply of the gastrointestinal tract in rats with age. *Pfluegers Arch.* 364: 129–133, 1976.
262. VARHAUG, J. E., AND K. SVANES. Gastric ulceration and changes in acid secretion and mucosal blood flow after partial gastric devascularization in cats. *Acta Chir. Scand.* 145: 313–319, 1979.
263. VOROBIOFF, J., J. E. BREDFELDT, AND R. J. GROSZMANN. Hyperdynamic circulation in portal-hypertensive rat model: a primary factor for maintenance of chronic portal hypertension. *Am. J. Physiol.* 244 (*Gastrointest. Liver Physiol.* 7): G52–G57, 1983.
264. WALDER, D. N. Arteriovenous anastomoses of the human stomach. *Clin. Sci. Lond.* 11: 59–71, 1952.
265. WALU, K. M., W. PAWLIK, S. J. KONTUREK, AND A. V. SCHALLY. Effect of met-enkephalin and morphine on gastric secretion and blood flow. *Acta Physiol. Pol.* 32: 383–392, 1981.
266. WANGENSTEEN, O. H., P. A. SALMON, W. O. GRIFFEN, JR. S. PATERSON, AND F. FATTAH. Studies of local gastric cooling as related to peptic ulcer. *Ann. Surg.* 150: 346–358, 1959.
267. WATERMAN, N. G., AND J. L. WALKER. Effect of a topical adrenergic agent on gastric blood flow. *Am. J. Surg.* 127: 241–243, 1974.
268. WAYLAND, H., J. R. FOX, AND M. D. ELMORE. Quantitative fluorescent tracer studies in vivo. *Bibl. Anat.* 13: 61–64, 1975.
269. WEINER, R., AND G. KALEY. Influence of prostaglandin $E_1$ on the terminal vascular bed. *Am. J. Physiol.* 217: 563–566, 1969.
270. WHITTLE, B. J. R. Mechanisms underlying gastric mucosal damage induced by indomethacin and bile salts, and the actions of prostaglandins. *Br. J. Pharmacol.* 60: 455–460, 1977.
271. WHITTLE, B. J. R., N. K. BOUGHTON-SMITH, S. MONCADA, AND J. R. VANE. Actions of prostacyclin ($PGI_2$) and its product 6-oxo-$PGF_1$ on the rat gastric mucosa in vivo and vitro. *Prostaglandins* 15: 955–968, 1978.
272. WHITTLE, B. J. R., N. OREN-WOLMAN, AND P. H. GUTH. Gastric vasoconstrictor actions of leukotriene $C_4$, $PGF_{2\alpha}$, and a thromboxane mimetic U-46619 on the rat submucosal microcirculation in vivo. *Am. J. Physiol.* 248 (*Gastrointest. Liver Physiol.* 11): G580–G586, 1985.
273. WOLF, S. Gastric function throughout one eventful year. In: *The Stomach.* New York: Oxford Univ. Press, 1965, p. 179–193.
274. WOOD, E. H. Symposium on use of indicator-dilution techniques in the study of the circulation. *Circ. Res.* 10: 377–581, 1962.
275. YANO, S., A. FUJIWARA, Y. OZAKI, AND M. HARADA. Gastric blood flow responses to autonomic nerve stimulation and

related pharmacological studies in rats. *J. Pharm. Pharmacol.* 35: 641–646, 1983.
276. YOKOTANI, K., I. MURAMATSU, AND M. FUJIWARA. Effects of the sympathetic nervous system on bethanechol-induced elevation of gastric acid secretion and mucosal blood flow in rats. *J. Pharmacol. Exp. Ther.* 227: 478–483, 1983.
277. ZALEWSKY, C. A., AND F. G. MOODY. Stereological analysis of the parietal cell during acid secretion and inhibition. *Gastroenterology* 73: 66–74, 1977.
278. ZINNER, M. J., B. M. JAFFE, L. DEMAGISTRIS, A. DAHLSTROM, AND H. AHLMAN. Effect of cervical and thoracic vagal stimulation on luminal serotonin release and regional blood flow in cats. *Gastroenterology* 82: 1403–1408, 1982.
279. ZINNER, M. J., J. C. KERR, AND D. G. REYNOLDS. Adrenergic mechanisms in canine gastric circulation. *Am. J. Physiol.* 229: 977–982, 1975.
280. ZINNER, M. J., J. C. KERR, AND D. G. REYNOLDS. Distribution and arteriovenous shunting of gastric blood flow in the baboon: effect of epinephrine and vasopressin infusions. *Gastroenterology* 71: 299–302, 1976.
281. ZUKOSKI, C. F., H. M. LEE, AND D. M. HUME. Effect of hypothalamic stimulation on gastric secretion and adrenal function in the dog. *J. Surg. Res.* 3: 301–306, 1963.

CHAPTER 39

# Microcirculation of the intestinal mucosa

D. NEIL GRANGER
PETER R. KVIETYS
RONALD J. KORTHUIS

*Department of Physiology, Louisiana State University Medical Center, Shreveport, Louisiana*

ANDRE J. PREMEN

*Department of Physiology, Uniformed Services University of the Health Sciences, F. Edward Hebert School of Medicine, Bethesda, Maryland*

CHAPTER CONTENTS

Intrinsic Regulation of Blood Flow and Oxygenation
  Basic concepts
  Vascular response to arterial pressure alterations
  Vascular response to venous pressure elevation
  Reactive hyperemia
  Vascular response to alterations in arterial blood gases and hematocrit
  Postprandial intestinal hyperemia
    Anticipatory/ingestion phase
    Digestion/absorption phase
    Localization of postprandial hyperemia
    Luminal stimuli responsible for intestinal hyperemia
    Mechanisms of postprandial intestinal hyperemia
Influence of Blood Flow on Intestinal Transport
  Washout of flow-limited solutes
  Effects of oxygen delivery on absorption
Countercurrent Exchange
  Anatomical basis
  Theoretical considerations
  Experimental evidence
    Countercurrent exchanger
    Countercurrent multiplier
Vascular Capacitance
Vasoactive Agents and Intestinal Oxygen Uptake
  Relation between blood flow and oxygen uptake
  Oxidative metabolism
  Effective capillary density
  Intramural blood flow distribution
Angiotensin II and Vasopressin
Effects of Experimental Conditions on the Intestinal Circulation
  Anesthesia and adjuvants
  Respiration and blood gases
  Laparotomy and visceral manipulation
  Temperature
Transcapillary Fluid and Solute Exchange
  Starling hypothesis
  Rate of transcapillary fluid movement (lymph flow)
  Capillary filtration coefficient
  Capillary hydrostatic pressure
  Interstitial hydrostatic pressure
  Osmotic reflection coefficient
  Transcapillary oncotic pressure gradient
  Interaction of capillary and interstitial forces
    Edema safety factors
    Venous pressure elevation
    Arterial pressure reduction
    Sympathetic stimulation
    Net fluid absorption
    Net fluid secretion
Small-Solute and Macromolecule Exchange
  Small solutes
  Macromolecules
  Factors influencing permeability
  Pathways for macromolecule exchange
Conclusions

---

THE INTESTINE CAN BE DISTINGUISHED from other vascular beds by its relatively high rates of blood flow, $O_2$ utilization, and transcapillary exchange of fluid and solutes. These processes are presumed to proceed at accelerated rates as a result of the demands imposed on the microvasculature by the epithelial cells of the mucosal layer. It is well recognized that ~80% of total intestinal blood flow is supplied to the metabolically active mucosal layer under resting conditions. This fact, coupled to other known characteristics of the mucosal circulation, has lead most investigators to assume that measurements of total intestinal blood flow, $O_2$ utilization, and transcapillary fluid and solute exchange provide reasonable estimates of these parameters in the mucosal layer. Although examples are provided, both here and in the chapters by Shepherd and Kiel in this *Handbook*, that refute this general assumption, the overwhelming majority of information lends support to it. The objective of this chapter is to summarize the available literature and current concepts regarding the regulation of blood flow, $O_2$ delivery, and transcapillary exchange in the intestinal mucosa. Because of the constraints imposed by the dearth of information on the mucosal microcirculation per se, this summary is largely derived from whole-organ studies of the intestinal circulation.

## INTRINSIC REGULATION OF BLOOD FLOW AND OXYGENATION

### Basic Concepts

It is well recognized that the intestine is endowed with the capacity to regulate its blood flow and degree of oxygenation when nervous and hormonal influences are eliminated. This intrinsic ability to control tissue perfusion and blood-tissue exchange has been ascribed to specific segments of the microvasculature. Because intravascular pressure measurements demonstrate that a major fraction of total pressure dissipation occurs at the arterioles (144), this vascular segment is designated as the resistance vessel that controls blood flow. In the mucosa of the rat small intestine, the greatest dissipation of pressure occurs between the distributing arteriole (also called the marginal vessel) and villus capillaries (144), indicating that these are the major resistance vessels for villus perfusion. The major resistance vessel for perfusion of the crypts remains undefined; however, it is likely that the arterial connections from the submucous vascular network are important in this regard (60, 326). Although there are little data regarding differential control of villus and crypt blood flows, it is clear that the microvascular architecture favors this possibility. Thus at any given moment local and extrinsic stimuli exert control over the caliber of the resistance vessels. In doing so, these signals modulate blood flow in the villous and crypt regions of the intestinal mucosa.

The capillaries are the major exchange vessels in the intestinal mucosa; across the surface of these microvessels diffuse all the nutrients required to sustain the parenchymal cells. Evidence indicates that only a fraction of the intestinal capillaries are perfused under normal conditions (397, 399, 428). The term *precapillary sphincter* has been used to describe the microvascular element that exerts control over the number of perfused capillaries. Although this term is widely used as a functional descriptor of exchange-vessel regulation, it remains unclear whether there is an anatomical equivalent to the precapillary sphincter in the small intestine (269). Bohlen et al. (33) have noted precapillary sphincters in the rat small intestine by using intravital microscopy. The sphincter was described as a single vascular smooth muscle cell encircling the initial segment of each villous capillary. This spontaneously contractile cell has the physiological and anatomical characteristics of a precapillary sphincter (33, 144). Other investigators contend that arterioles in the villi have smooth muscle in their initial segment, to the level of the tops of the crypts, but they lack smooth muscle within the villus proper (60). They therefore contend that microfilaments in the pericytes surrounding villous capillaries (rather than muscular sphincters) modulate the number of perfused capillaries. Irrespective of the anatomical nature of the putative precapillary sphincter, there is an overwhelming body of physiological data that clearly indicates that perfused capillary density can change independently of total vascular resistance, suggesting that the arterioles do not represent the sphincters.

Both resistance and exchange vessels play a role in the regulation of tissue oxygenation (190, 194, 429). Oxygen is carried, by convection, in the stream of blood that courses through the microcirculation. Consequently the rate of $O_2$ delivery to a tissue depends on blood flow and the $O_2$ concentration in arterial blood. Physiological control of $O_2$ convection is thus achieved by modulation of blood flow through appropriate alterations in arteriolar tone. This blood flow control system serves to stabilize capillary partial pressure of $O_2$ ($P_{O_2}$), which drives $O_2$ from blood to tissue. Inasmuch as capillary surface area and capillary-to-cell diffusion distance are major determinants of the diffusive flux of $O_2$ across capillaries, modulation of perfused-capillary density by precapillary sphincters also plays a role in the regulation of tissue oxygenation. Filtration coefficient (161, 285, 397) and permeability–surface area product (PS) (427) measurements in the intestine indicate that only 20%–30% of the exchange vessels are perfused under normal conditions. Capillary recruitment during stress enhances blood-to-tissue diffusion of $O_2$, thereby preventing large reductions in tissue $P_{O_2}$. Thus the tone of both arterioles and precapillary sphincters has been considered in studies of intestinal oxygenation.

Although many factors have been implicated in intestinal vasoregulation, two mechanisms have been repeatedly invoked to explain the intrinsic vascular responses to the aforementioned stresses, i.e., metabolic and myogenic mechanisms (171, 176, 246). The metabolic hypothesis states that tissue metabolism and arteriolar smooth muscle constitute a local control system that provides the necessary coupling between blood flow and tissue nutritional requirements. Any condition causing an imbalance between tissue $O_2$ supply and demand will produce an outpouring of metabolites into the interstitial fluid. The metabolites then diffuse to the arterioles and precapillary sphincters to cause vasodilation and capillary recruitment. The increased blood flow and/or $O_2$ extraction restores the $O_2$ supply to a level compatible with tissue $O_2$ demand. Thus the metabolic model of intestinal blood flow regulation predicts that the $O_2$ delivery to tissues, not blood flow per se, is the controlled variable [Fig. 1; (430)]. Many agents have been proposed as candidates for the vasodilator metabolite, and it is quite possible that more than one substance may function as the mediator of local blood flow regulation (204). Metabolites that exhibit demonstrable vasodilator effects on the mesenteric circulation include $K^+$ (66, 83, 462), $H^+$ (343, 363, 401, 457), adenosine (187, 193), the adenine nucleotides (110, 202, 325), and the level of osmolality (68, 304). A clear role played by any of these "metabolites" in intestinal vasoregulation has

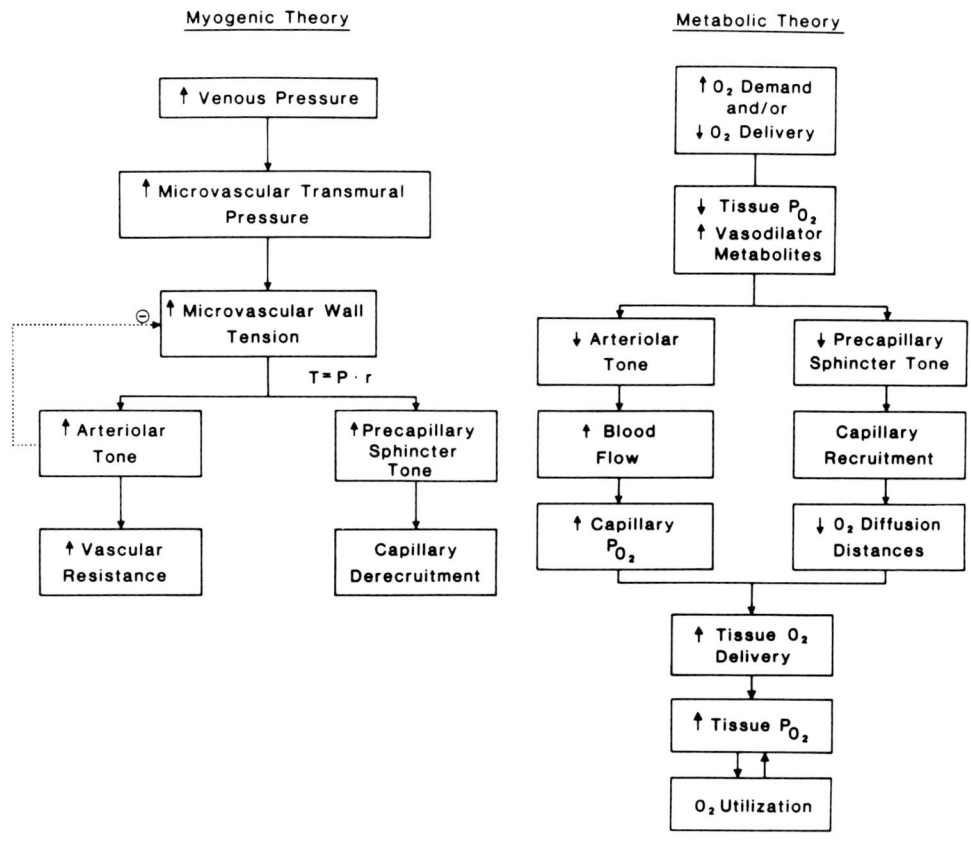

FIG. 1. Metabolic and myogenic theories of intestinal blood flow regulation.

not been firmly established; of the aforementioned factors, adenosine has received the greatest attention. A correlation between venous blood adenosine concentration and the reactive hyperemic response to arterial occlusions of varying duration has been demonstrated (347). The role of adenosine in local intestinal vasoregulation has been assessed with theophylline, a competitive inhibitor of adenosine action, and dipyridamole, an inhibitor of parenchymal reuptake of adenosine (193). The results obtained from these studies indicate that, in the fasted state, adenosine does not contribute to prevailing vascular tone and does not participate in the vascular responses to mild stresses such as reductions of perfusion pressure or moderate increases in $O_2$ demand. By contrast, adenosine appears to play an important role in intestinal vasoregulation under conditions of severe stress, i.e., reactive hyperemia, and pressure-flow autoregulation in hypermetabolic states (193). There is also evidence undermining the role of adenosine in regulating intestinal blood flow. Close intra-arterial infusions of adenosine in the intestine decrease capillary exchange capacity and $O_2$ consumption (187, 436). Furthermore adenosine infusions appear to redistribute intestinal blood flow from the mucosa-submucosa layer to the muscularis layer (436). This apparent vasoconstriction of the mucosal vasculature by adenosine is inconsistent with the documented responses of mucosal blood flow to various stress states.

Another version of the metabolic hypothesis suggests that interstitial $P_{O_2}$ is the important link between parenchymal metabolism and microvascular tone. The oxidative requirements of intestinal vascular smooth muscle are high, thereby enhancing the susceptibility of intestinal blood vessels to changes in interstitial $P_{O_2}$ (149). Indirect support for the role played by tissue $P_{O_2}$ is provided by the intestinal hyperemia and capillary recruitment produced by hypoxemia (422, 457) and by the fact that conditions that reduce tissue $P_{O_2}$ also cause vasodilation (28). Direct measurements of tissue $P_{O_2}$ and blood flow in the rat intestine reveal an inverse correlation between these parameters (29). Furthermore Bohlen (29) has determined that more than one-fourth of the hyperemia induced by glucose absorption in the rat small bowel can be attributed to a reduction in tissue $P_{O_2}$. Although the specific features of the metabolite and $P_{O_2}$ theories differ, their ultimate functions are identical: to maintain intracellular $P_{O_2}$ above the critical level at which $O_2$ availability limits oxidative metabolism. Despite the wealth of data that supports the involvement of a metabolic mechanism in intestinal vasoregulation, the relative roles of tissue $P_{O_2}$ and metabolites remain poorly understood.

The myogenic theory of local blood flow control is based on the assumption that vascular resistance is directly proportional to transmural pressure at the arteriolar level (109, 240, 245) because of the effect of stretch on vascular smooth muscle activity (Fig. 1). In essence, this theory proposes the existence of arteriolar tension receptors that, in denervated preparations, modulate vascular smooth muscle tone in response to changes in transmural pressure. Because vascular wall tension is determined by the product of transmural pressure and vessel diameter, one would predict that, based on a myogenic mechanism, an increase in vascular transmural pressure results in arteriolar vasoconstriction and an increased vascular resistance. In many respects the predicted effects of a myogenic mechanism are very similar to those of a metabolic mechanism. Both theories predict a reduced vascular resistance in response to a fall in arterial pressure ($P_a$), the myogenic theory because of a fall in vascular transmural pressure and metabolic theory because of a reduction in tissue $P_{O_2}$ and/or accumulation of vasodilator metabolites. One experimental perturbation that allows clear differentiation between the two mechanisms is acute venous pressure ($P_v$) elevation. The myogenic theory predicts an increased vascular resistance in response to the increased transmural pressure, whereas the metabolic theory predicts a fall in vascular resistance in response to the reductions in blood flow and $O_2$ supply to the tissue.

An additional component of the myogenic control system in the intestine is the dependence of precapillary sphincter tone on transmural pressure. There is evidence that the number of perfused capillaries is inversely related to microvascular pressure (167, 178, 249, 348, 421). This relationship is generally used to support the contention that there are also tension receptors in precapillary sphincter smooth muscle that respond to alterations in vascular transmural pressure. From a homeostatic viewpoint the myogenic mechanism appears to be directed more to keeping intestinal capillary hydrostatic pressure ($P_c$) and transcapillary fluid exchange constant (243), whereas the metabolic mechanism is directed toward maintaining adequate blood flow and $O_2$ delivery.

A variety of experimental perturbations have been used to assess the relative contributions of metabolic and myogenic factors in intrinsic regulation of intestinal blood flow and oxygenation. The most commonly used perturbations are alterations in $P_a$, $P_v$, arterial $O_2$ concentration, and parenchymal oxidative metabolism. The responses of the intestinal circulation to these and other perturbations are described next, and their significance in regard to intrinsic vasoregulation is discussed.

*Vascular Response to Arterial Pressure Alterations*

The term *autoregulation* is commonly used to describe the intrinsic ability of an organ to maintain a constant blood flow in the presence of a fluctuating $P_a$ (243). The relationship between blood flow and $P_a$ has been defined in the small intestine of the dog (211, 213, 221, 241, 247, 351, 417, 463), cat (167), and rat (5) as well as in the dog colon (158, 214, 275, 276, 283). These studies indicate that autoregulation in the intestine is not the intense phenomenon seen in other organs (e.g., brain, kidney) because a reduction in perfusion pressure is usually accompanied by a reduction in blood flow while total vascular resistance falls by a modest extent. Several investigators have recently employed feedback gain estimates to quantitate the degree of pressure-flow autoregulation (167, 192, 193, 275, 351, 360, 399, 423, 433). The most frequently used equation for calculation of closed loop gain ($G_c$) is

$$G_c = 1 - [(\Delta F/F)/(\Delta P/P)] \qquad (1)$$

where $(\Delta F/F)/(\Delta P/P)$ is the slope of the normalized pressure-flow curve at a given point. If $G_c = 1.0$, the flow is independent of perfusion pressure, i.e., there is perfect flow autoregulation. In a purely passive (nonautoregulating) vascular bed, flow varies proportionally with pressure, and $G_c = 0$. If the flow regulator compensates for 50% of the applied disturbance, then $G_c = 0.5$. Closed loop gain values for the resting small bowel range between −0.10 and +0.70 (192, 351, 360, 423, 433). In the resting colon $G_c$ is generally negative, indicating that passive distension or elastic recoil of blood vessels occurs during the pressure alterations (275). The degree of flow autoregulation ($G_c$) diminishes with decreasing perfusion pressure [Fig. 2; (192, 351, 360)]. The lower limit for intestinal autoregulation generally lies between 40 and 60 mmHg.

Autoregulation in the intestine is a labile phenomenon and is infrequently present in preparations in which pumps and external perfusion circuits are employed (243). The site of autoregulation in the intes-

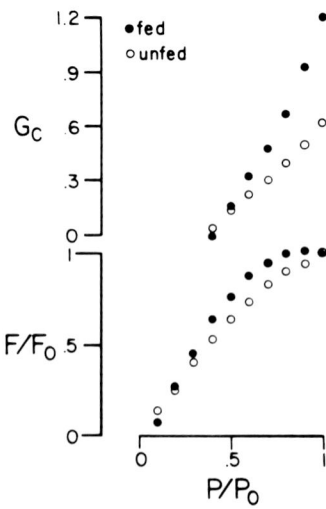

FIG. 2. Dependence of superior mesenteric blood flow ($F/F_0$, blood flow normalized to control) and autoregulatory closed-loop gain ($G_c$) on perfusion pressure ($P/P_0$, arterial pressure normalized to control) in fed and fasted animals. [From Norris et al. (351).]

tine has been localized to the precapillary resistance vessels (arterioles) (213). An increase in the resistance to blood flow in the venous portion of the circulation is observed when intestinal perfusion pressure is decreased. Thus the precapillary-to-postcapillary resistance ratio ($R_a/R_v$) falls as $P_a$ is reduced (167, 247). Evidence obtained with nerve blocking agents and chronically denervated segments of intestine indicates that the adjustments of pre- and postcapillary resistances ($R_a$ and $R_v$, respectively) to alterations in perfusion pressure may be mediated by a local arteriovenous reflex (213).

Studies of the small (313) and large (158) bowel indicate that mucosal blood flow is autoregulated to a greater extent than total blood flow. Using an indicator dilution technique in the cat small intestine, Lundgren and Svanvik (313) demonstrated that villous plasma flow was virtually unchanged when perfusion pressure was reduced from 100 mmHg to 25 mmHg while total blood flow fell by ~43% (Fig. 3). Comparable results have been reported for the dog colon (158) in which absorptive-site blood flow, measured with a [$^3$H]H$_2$O clearance technique, is almost perfectly autoregulated over a $P_a$ range of 140 mmHg to 30 mmHg, while total flow falls in proportion to $P_a$. The observation that mucosal blood flow autoregulation is more intense than total flow autoregulation is generally attributed to the high metabolic activity of the enterocytes (176).

The influence of a specific agent and/or an experimental perturbation on the ability of the intestine to autoregulate blood flow was examined in several studies. The autoregulatory ability of the small intestine is unaffected by acute (360) or chronic (213) sympathetic denervation, sympatholytic agents (213), and alterations in pulse pressure (433). Blood flow autoregulation is depressed or abolished by intraenteric distension (212), intra-arterial cyanide (243), and isoflurane anesthesia (360). A significant improvement in intestinal blood flow autoregulation after feeding or intraenteric placement of nutrients in isolated segments was demonstrated in recent studies (192, 275, 351, 426, 433). Norris and co-workers (351) first noted that the intensity of blood flow autoregulation in the superior mesenteric artery is much greater in fed ($G_c$ = 1.2) than in fasted ($G_c$ = 0.60) dogs (Fig. 2). They subsequently proposed that the influence of feeding on blood flow autoregulation resulted from the increased O$_2$ demand imposed by nutrient absorption (192). The fact that metabolic factors play a role in the enhanced autoregulation induced by feeding is supported by the observation that dinitrophenol-induced increases in intestinal O$_2$ uptake are also associated with improved autoregulation (192). The observation that blood flow autoregulation in the small intestine of fasted rats is very intense in comparison with the results obtained in dogs and cats has also been attributed to the high basal O$_2$ consumption of the rat intestine (5). The contention that a metabolic control system, rather than a myogenic one, is involved in intestinal blood flow autoregulation is supported by the observation that hypermetabolic states exert a greater influence on autoregulation intensity than do alterations in pulse pressure (433). The nature of the metabolic mediator of intestinal blood flow autoregulation remains unclear, although adenosine has been recently implicated. Granger and Norris (193) have demonstrated that theophylline reduces whereas dipyridamole enhances intestinal blood flow autoregulation in fed, but not in fasted, dogs.

Based on the observations regarding the influence of metabolic rate on blood flow autoregulation one would expect a greater intensity of autoregulation in the intestine of neonatal rather than adult animals, because basal O$_2$ uptake is much higher in the former. Buckley et al. (50) have observed that the intestine behaves as a passive vascular bed ($G_c$ = 0) when $P_a$ is reduced in the 1- to 14-day-old pig. By 1 mo of age autoregulation maintains intestinal blood flow within 95% of control values until $P_a$ is reduced to <65 mmHg. Thus despite the higher metabolic demands of the neonate, intestinal autoregulation is negligible at birth, yet it is fully developed after postnatal wk 2. The contention that intrinsic vasoregulation is weak or absent at birth is supported by the observation that autoregulatory escape to sympathetic stimulation is absent in the 2-day-old pig yet intense after postnatal wk 2 (51).

Intestinal blood flow autoregulation is significantly altered in animals with chronic arterial hypertension, and it contributes to the overall disturbance in blood pressure control in some forms of hypertension (155, 340). Studies comparing autoregulatory ability in the intestines of normotensive Wistar-Kyoto (WKY) and spontaneously hypertensive (SHR) rats indicate that autoregulation is demonstrable in WKY yet absent in SHR (155). The absence of autoregulation in SHR has been attributed to the vascular hypertrophy associated with chronic arterial hypertension inasmuch as an increased vascular wall thickness would reduce the internal diameter even during complete smooth muscle relaxation, thereby limiting autoregulatory capacity. The limited autoregulatory ability of the intestine in SHR may also be related to the higher control blood flow. According to the metabolic theory, auto-

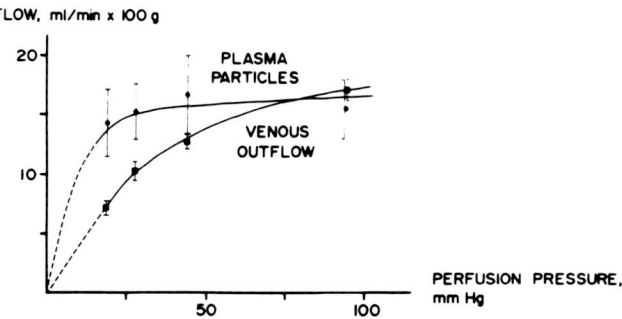

FIG. 3. Effects of varying perfusion pressure on total intestinal blood flow (venous outflow) and villous plasma flow (plasma particles). [From Lundgren (311).]

regulation should be diminished when control blood flow is high.

Data derived from rats with renovascular hypertension indicate that a large portion of the increased vascular resistance results from a compensatory autoregulatory response to the increased systemic $P_a$ (340). It appears that as much as 74% of the increase in intestinal resistance in fed hypertensive rats and 64% of the increase in fasted hypertensive rats may be attributable to a local pressure or flow-dependent autoregulatory mechanism. The intestinal vasoconstriction associated with renovascular hypertension is significantly blunted if the superior mesenteric artery is protected against the hypertension by a servocontrolled cuff placed around the vessel.

Alterations in $P_a$ influence the degree of perfusion of both resistance and exchange vessels. When $P_a$ and blood flow are reduced in a stepwise fashion, intestinal capillary exchange capacity progressively increases (161). The changes in capillary exchange capacity are accompanied by corresponding changes in $O_2$ extraction, suggesting a direct functional link between these parameters. The role of $O_2$ in mediating the exchange vessel response to perfusion pressure alterations is demonstrated by the observation that capillary exchange capacity is well correlated with both $O_2$ extraction and $O_2$ delivery-to-demand ratio, irrespective of whether $O_2$ delivery or demand is varied (285). Figure 4 presents the relationships between capillary filtration coefficient ($K_{f,c}$), arteriovenous $O_2$ difference [(a-v)$O_2$], and $O_2$ delivery-to-demand ratio in the canine ileum.

In contrast to blood flow, $O_2$ uptake is maintained at a normal level even when $P_a$ is reduced to <40 mmHg in the small intestine (192) and <60 mmHg in the colon (283). This apparent autoregulation of $O_2$ uptake occurs with equal intensity in both fasted and fed preparations (Fig. 5). Two factors play a role in maintaining a constant $O_2$ uptake when perfusion pressure is reduced: blood flow autoregulation and increased $O_2$ extraction. In the fasting state, intestinal venous $O_2$ content is high and increased $O_2$ extraction is the major mechanism that maintains $O_2$ uptake inasmuch as blood flow autoregulation is weak or absent. However, blood flow autoregulation is more important in maintaining intestinal $O_2$ uptake in fed animals in which the venous $O_2$ content is initially low because of the increased metabolic demand. As the degree of autoregulation falls at low perfusion pressures, the contribution of increased $O_2$ extraction rises. Thus despite the different sensitivities of resistance vessels to pressure reductions in fasted and fed dogs, the concerted operation of local flow control and modulation of $O_2$ extraction maintains adequate in-

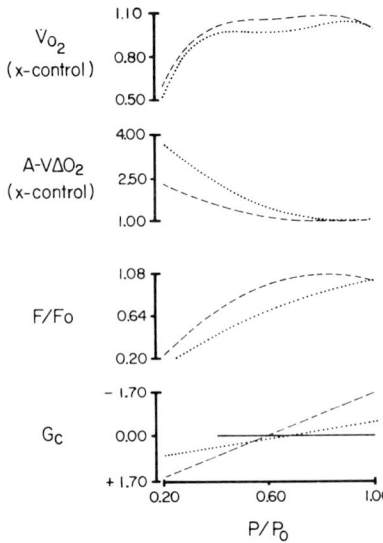

FIG. 5. Dependence of intestinal $O_2$ uptake ($\dot{V}_{O_2}$), arteriovenous $O_2$ difference (A-V$\Delta O_2$), normalized blood flow (F/$F_0$), and autoregulatory closed-loop gain ($G_c$) on arterial pressure (P/$P_0$) in fed (*dashed lines*) and fasted (*dotted lines*) dogs. [From Granger and Norris (192).]

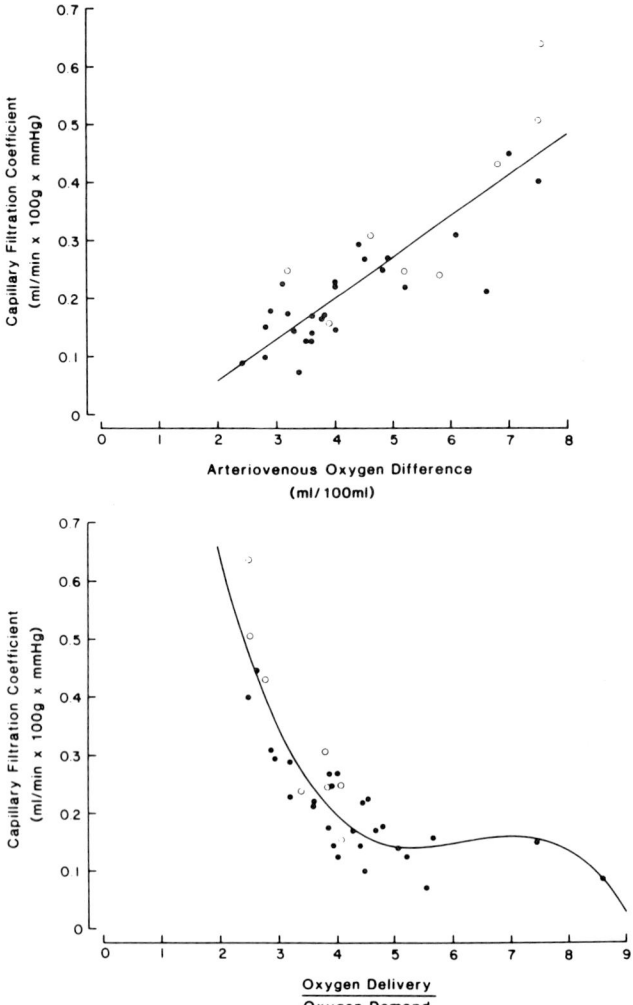

FIG. 4. Relationships between capillary filtration coefficient, arteriovenous $O_2$ difference, and $O_2$ delivery-to-demand ratio in the canine ileum. [From Kvietys et al. (285).]

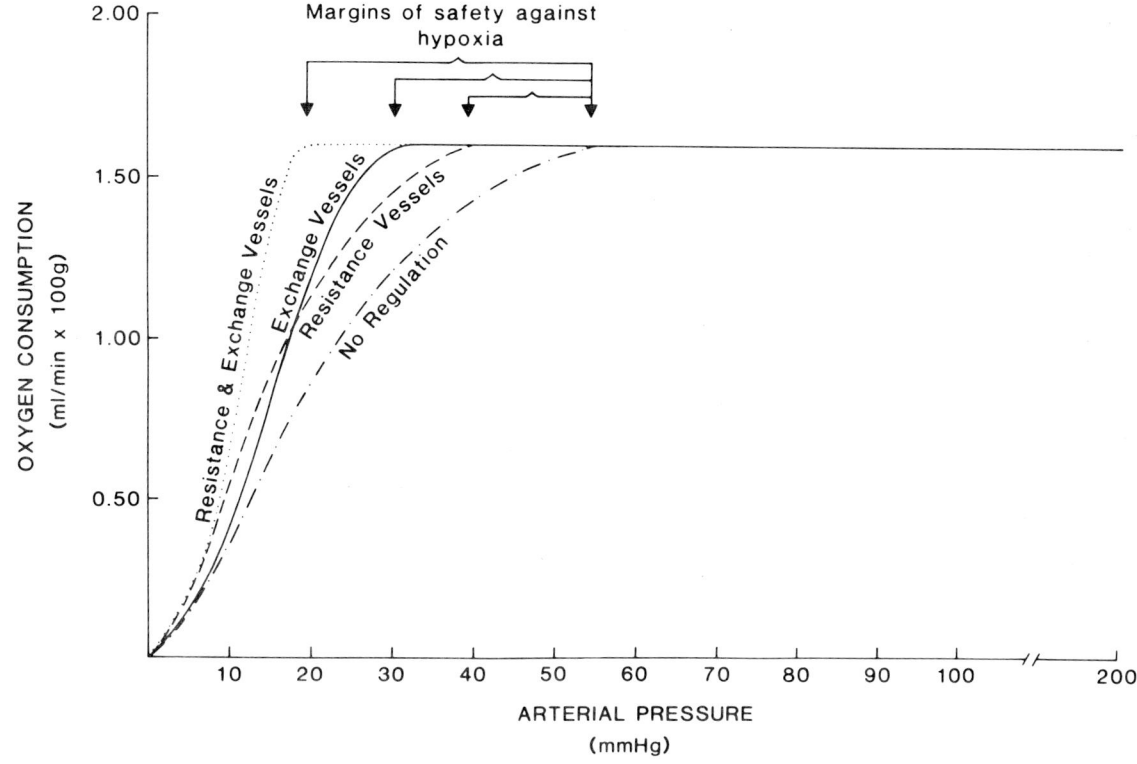

FIG. 6. Steady-state relation between intestinal $O_2$ consumption and arterial pressure predicted by mathematical model for a passive system (no regulation of exchange or resistance vessels), resistance vessel regulation only, exchange vessel regulation only, and regulation of both resistance and exchange vessels. Difference to inflection points of $O_2$ consumption–arterial pressure curves provides a measure of margin of safety against hypoxia afforded by resistance and/or exchange vessel regulation. [From Granger and Granger (152).]

testinal oxygenation in both groups over a wide range of perfusion pressures (192, 275, 426).

The ability of the intestine to maintain adequate oxygenation for normal oxidative metabolism in the presence of fluctuations in $P_a$ has been attributed to intrinsic alterations of arteriolar and precapillary sphincter tone, i.e., to blood flow autoregulation and capillary recruitment (161, 194, 428). The quantitative significance of autoregulation and capillary recruitment in maintaining intestinal oxygenation has been recently assessed with a mathematical model based on data relating intestinal vascular resistance and perfused capillary density to the $O_2$ delivery-to-demand ratio (152). The model predicts that recruitment of capillaries is of greater quantitative significance than blood flow autoregulation (Fig. 6). This prediction is not entirely surprising in light of the modest tendency of the intestinal vasculature to autoregulate blood flow and the responsiveness of intestinal capillary exchange capacity to alterations in $O_2$ availability-to-demand ratio. It appears that there is a larger margin of safety against hypoxia when blood flow autoregulation and capillary recruitment work in unison. For a purely passive system (absence of autoregulation and recruitment), the model predicts that tissue hypoxia results when $P_a$ is reduced to <55 mmHg. With regulation of both resistance and exchange vessels, $P_a$ must be reduced to <20 mmHg before the tissue becomes hypoxic. This prediction agrees with experimental observations (313). Thus the responses of the model to alterations in perfusion pressure indicate that the intensity of blood flow autoregulation and capillary recruitment reported for the small intestine is quantitatively significant in preventing cellular hypoxia.

*Vascular Response to Venous Pressure Elevation*

The effect of $P_v$ elevation is an important criterion for determining whether metabolic or myogenic mechanisms are involved in local vasoregulation. The metabolic hypothesis predicts that elevation of $P_v$ causes vasodilation and an increased capillary density as a result of the reduced blood flow and vasodilator accumulation. According to the myogenic hypothesis, vascular resistance increases and capillary density decreases during $P_v$ elevation because of a rise in intravascular (transmural) pressure at the arteriolar and precapillary sphincter levels. In the small intestine of the dog (240, 246, 249, 421, 433) and cat (178, 346, 348) as well as in the dog colon (158, 214, 215, 275, 276, 283), $P_v$ elevation results in an increased vascular resistance, which is consistent with a myogenic mechanism. Vascular resistance is virtually unaltered by $P_v$ elevation in the rat small intestine (155). The increased vascular resistance frequently observed during $P_v$ elevations results from intense precapillary constriction (245). Active responses of the intestinal vasculature must be involved, because the increased vascular resistance caused by $P_v$ elevation is abolished by cyanide (240).

The rise in vascular resistance produced by $P_v$ elevation in the dog and cat small intestine is generally associated with a reduction in the $K_{f,c}$ or PS for rubidium (178, 246, 249, 348, 421), indicating that the precapillary sphincters are also under myogenic control. The $K_{f,c}$ in the cat intestine is inversely related to $P_c$, irrespective of whether $P_c$ is changed by alterations in $P_v$ or $P_a$ (Fig. 7). However, there is a direct linear correlation between $K_{f,c}$ and $P_c$ in the rat small intestine; this tendency for $K_{f,c}$ to rise when $P_v$ is elevated has been attributed to the high metabolic rate in the rat intestine (5, 147). In the dog colon, $P_v$ elevation causes a concomitant increase in total vascular resistance and $K_{f,c}$, indicating that metabolic factors are more important in regulating precapillary sphincter tone, whereas myogenic factors exert predominant control over resistance vessels.

When $P_v$ is elevated intestinal blood flow falls, and consequently $O_2$ extraction rises. In the feline ileum the increase in $O_2$ extraction is proportionally greater than the reduction in blood flow, thus $O_2$ consumption is significantly elevated (346). The elevated intestinal $O_2$ utilization during acute venous hypertension has been attributed to increased motility. This assertion is supported by the observation that atropine inhibits both the enhanced motility and elevated $O_2$ utilization induced by venous hypertension in the feline ileum (344). An increased $O_2$ consumption induced by $P_v$ elevation is noted in the dog small intestine only when blood flow is low (421); at a normal blood flow, $O_2$ extraction rises only enough to maintain a constant rate of $O_2$ utilization. The rise in $O_2$ extraction is not sufficient to maintain normal oxidative metabolism when $P_v$ is elevated in the dog colon (50).

The intensity and direction of the intestinal vascular response to $P_v$ elevation is influenced by oxidative requirements, blood flow, and extravascular pressure. There are conflicting reports regarding the influence of enhanced oxidative metabolism on the response of the intestinal vasculature to $P_v$ elevation. Some investigators (192, 275) have demonstrated that an increased $O_2$ demand, resulting from stimulation of nutrient absorption or dinitrophenol administration, significantly reduces or abolishes the rise in vascular resistance produced by acute venous hypertension; these findings are consistent with the metabolic hypothesis. Other researchers (426) have noted an exaggerated resistance response to venous hypertension during a hypermetabolic state. However, the contention that the myogenic mechanism plays a minor role in local control of intestinal blood flow when the parenchymal $O_2$ availability-to-demand ratio is lower than normal is supported by the observation that intestinal preparations perfused at normal blood flows exhibit marked arteriolar and precapillary sphincter constriction in response to $P_v$ elevation, whereas in underperfused preparations vascular resistance decreases and capillary density increases (421). Furthermore arterial hypoxemia abolishes the increased vascular resistance induced by acute venous hypertension (457).

The increment of intestinal vascular resistance produced by $P_v$ elevation also depends on extravascular pressure (159, 464). If intraenteric pressure is elevated (spontaneously, pharmacologically, or mechanically), the myogenic vasoconstriction induced by acute venous hypertension is either reduced or abolished. The effects of extravascular pressure on intestinal blood flow are consistent with the "vascular waterfall" phenomenon. Generally, the driving pressure for blood flow through the intestinal vasculature is the difference between $P_a$ and $P_v$. However, when interstitial hydrostatic pressure ($P_t$) increases (because of luminal pressure elevation) to exceed $P_v$, a constriction develops at the venular level. The pressure at the collapse point (upstream) equals $P_t$, because the veins do not resist collapse. Under these conditions outflow $P_v$ no longer influences blood flow, and the driving pressure becomes $P_a$ minus $P_t$. Thus when lumen pressure is maintained at atmospheric pressure, $P_v$ elevation results in a progressive decrease in blood flow, but when lumen pressure is held constant at an elevated level, no significant effect on blood flow is exerted by $P_v$ elevation until $P_v$ exceeds lumen pressure (159). These observations are consistent with the hypothesis that

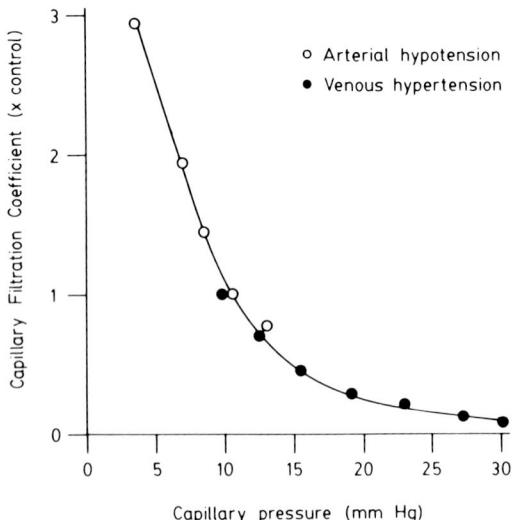

FIG. 7. Relationship between capillary filtration coefficient and capillary pressure in the cat small intestine. Capillary pressure was altered by venous pressure elevation or arterial pressure reduction. The inverse correlation is believed to result from myogenic control of perfused capillary density. [From Granger and Barrowman (147).]

luminal pressure (when it is >$P_v$) exerts a waterfall effect on the intestinal vasculature.

There is evidence that acute venous hypertension alters the distribution of blood flow within the bowel wall. Blood flow to the mucosa-submucosa layer, which normally accounts for ~80% of total flow in the small intestine, progressively decreases as $P_v$ is elevated from 0 mmHg to 20 mmHg, while muscularis flow increases over the same pressure range [Fig. 8; (178)]. Blood flow is distributed approximately equally between the mucosa-submucosa and muscularis layers at $P_v \geqq 20$ mmHg. Studies of $K_{f,c}$ indicate that a reduction in capillary density also occurs predominantly between $P_v$ of 0 mmHg and 20 mmHg (178, 249, 348). These studies indicate that the constriction of arteriolar and precapillary sphincter smooth muscles during $P_v$ elevation may be predominantly in the mucosa-submucosal layer of the intestine. In addition the blood flow distribution studies suggest that the vasculature of the muscularis dilates in response to $P_v$ elevation. These findings and interpretations are supported by intravital microscopic studies in the rat intestine that demonstrate constriction of submucosal arterioles and dilation of arterioles in the muscularis layer when $P_v$ is elevated (84). In the colon, $P_v$ elevation reduces total blood flow and increases vascular resistance, yet it has no effect on absorptive-site blood flow (158).

The responses of the intestinal vasculature to $P_v$ elevation are different in normotensive WKY and in SHR rats (155). Increments in $P_v$ do not alter vascular resistance in WKY yet significantly increase total vascular resistance in SHR. The latter effect is caused entirely by a rise in $R_a$. These findings indicate that, unlike in the normotensive rat, there is a pronounced myogenic response of the intestinal vasculature in SHR to acute venous hypertension. The intense vasoconstriction in response to $P_v$ elevation is consistent with the concept of an enhanced vascular sensitivity to vasoconstrictor stimuli resulting from vascular smooth muscle hypertrophy. According to this concept a given degree of smooth muscle contraction in a hypertrophied resistance vessel will lead to a greater reduction in lumen diameter and therefore a greater increase in resistance than in a thin-walled vessel (111). It is conceivable, therefore, that a weak myogenic response, which is not expressed in the WKY, is fully expressed in the SHR as a result of the structural adaptations of the vasculature. The enhanced myogenic responsiveness of the vasculature in SHR may play an important role in the maintenance of arterial hypertension.

In contrast to the increased vascular resistance and reduced blood flow produced by acute $P_v$ elevation, chronic portal hypertension is associated with intense vasodilation in the small intestine (18, 27, 479). Cross-perfusion studies indicate that arterial blood from portal hypertensive rats contains a humoral factor that increases intestinal blood flow in control animals. It is suggested that an elevated circulating glucagon level may account for ~40% of the portal hypertension-induced intestinal hyperemia (18). A reduced sensitivity of the intestinal vasculature to norepinephrine has also been observed in chronic portal hypertensive animals (263). Chronic portal hypertension does not alter intestinal $O_2$ consumption (18) or intramural blood flow distribution (19).

*Reactive Hyperemia*

The small and large intestines exhibit a characteristic hyperemia after brief periods of arterial occlusion (283, 346, 367, 418, 435). The magnitude and duration of the reactive hyperemic response are related to the duration of occlusion. After a 60-s arterial occlusion, blood flow increases to approximately twice control values. Intestinal motility increases during the ischemic period, with a rise in intraluminal pressure that becomes more prominent with greater durations of occlusion (15, 367, 417, 418). In the small bowel the magnitude of the reactive hyperemic response to arterial occlusion alone is greater than that observed with simultaneous arterial and venous occlusion and venous occlusion alone (346, 418). The latter obser-

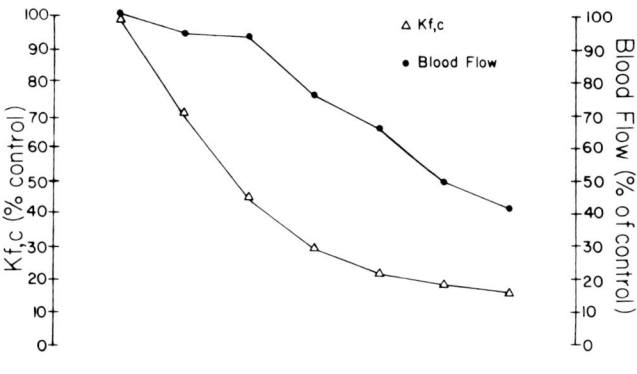

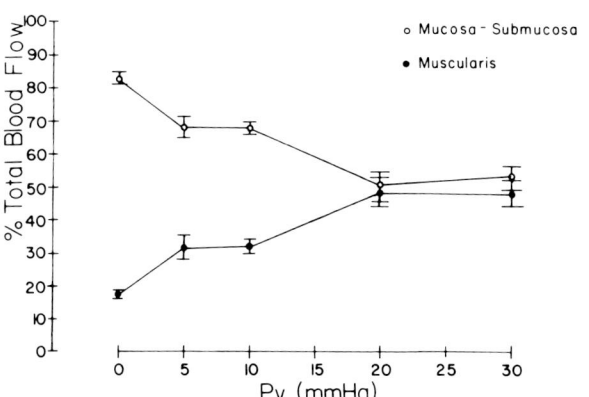

FIG. 8. Percentage of total intestinal blood flow in mucosa-submucosa and muscularis at various venous pressures ($P_v$); $K_{f,c}$, capillary filtration coefficient. [From Granger et al. (178).]

vation can be explained by *1*) erythrocyte drainage from the tissue during the arterial occlusion (thereby decreasing $O_2$ reserve for utilization during the ischemic period) or *2*) prevention of a dramatic decrease in vascular transmural pressure during venous occlusion (thereby minimizing myogenic vasodilation on release of the occlusion). In the colon, the postocclusion period is characterized by a hypoemia rather than a hyperemia (283). The hypoemic response has the general appearance of a reactive hyperemia but is displaced below the preocclusion blood flow.

Both the metabolic and myogenic hypotheses predict active dilation during arterial occlusion. The metabolic model predicts vasodilation secondary to tissue $P_{O_2}$ reduction and/or accumulation of vasodilator metabolites during arterial and/or venous stasis. The effect of duration of occlusion on peak hyperemic flow and on duration of hyperemia suggests that the vascular response is caused by metabolite accumulation and/or $O_2$ deficiency. Tissue $P_{O_2}$ reduction and purine metabolite accumulation have both been observed during arterial occlusion in the small intestine (28, 229, 347). Although adenosine concentration in venous blood increases fourfold at peak hyperemia (347), competitive inhibitors of adenosine reduce the peak hyperemic response to arterial occlusion by 15% (187) and shorten the duration of the hyperemia by 50% (193).

Although the myogenic model also predicts vasodilation after the release of arterial occlusion (due to marked reduction in vascular transmural pressure during the occlusion period), vascular resistance should increase during venous occlusion because of elevation of intravascular pressure at the microvessel level. The fact that the hyperemic response to arterial occlusion is greater than that observed after venous occlusion in the small intestine lends support to myogenic involvement in the hyperemic response (346). The reactive hypoemic response observed in the colon is also consistent with myogenic control, inasmuch as the return of blood flow to the preocclusion level corresponds with the gradual decline in vascular transmural pressure after the release of the venous occlusion (283).

The ability of the small intestine to repay the $O_2$ debt incurred during vascular occlusions largely depends on which vessel is occluded, i.e., artery or vein (346). With arterial occlusions there is inadequate repayment of the $O_2$ debt, inasmuch as $O_2$ extraction is depressed during the postocclusion hyperemia. The magnitude of the $O_2$ deficit is proportional to the duration of arterial occlusion. In contrast, venous occlusions are associated with an overpayment of $O_2$ in the postocclusion period, the magnitude of which is related to the duration of occlusion. It is suggested that arterial occlusions depress, whereas venous occlusions enhance, oxidative metabolism in the small intestine (346). The latter effect may result from the intense motility associated with venous occlusion.

An assumption inherent in most studies is that the hyperemic response to arterial occlusion occurs uniformly throughout the wall of the small intestine. Microsphere analysis of blood flow distribution within the wall of the small intestine suggests that relatively uniform increases in intestinal wall blood flow occur only for an occlusion period of 60 s (367). Increasing the duration of arterial occlusion results in a predominant hyperemia in the muscularis layer. The greater hyperemic response in the muscularis at longer occlusion periods (>60 s) has been attributed to the enhanced motility observed with longer lasting occlusion (367). The results obtained with the microsphere technique have not been confirmed with the newly developed laser Doppler velocimeter (435). The laser Doppler studies indicate that mucosal and total blood flow consistently show reactive hyperemia in response to a 60-s arterial occlusion but the muscularis does not. The blood flow payback-to-debt ratio was ~0.2 for both total and mucosal blood flows (Fig. 9). Increasing basal intestinal $O_2$ consumption by intraenteric placement of nutrients prolonged the reactive hyperemic response and increased the payback-to-debt ratio to 0.4 (435).

*Vascular Response to Alterations in Arterial Blood Gases and Hematocrit*

Because the metabolic theory predicts that any reduction in the $O_2$ availability-to-demand ratio should elicit vasodilation and capillary recruitment, arterial hypoxia has been used to study the ability of the intestine to maintain tissue oxygenation. The effects of hypoxemia on intestinal resistance and exchange vessels have been examined in two studies (422, 457). Svanvik et al. (457) studied feline intestine perfused at constant $P_a$ and found that blood flow increased 48% when the inspired $P_{O_2}$ was reduced to 55 mmHg.

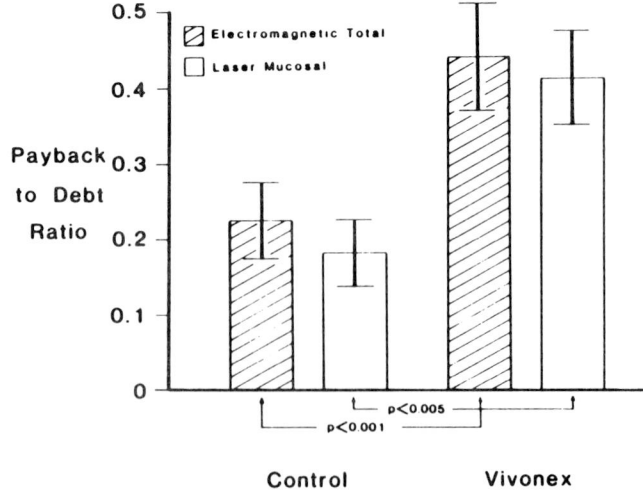

FIG. 9. Effect of metabolic rate on total and mucosal blood flow payback-to-debt ratio after a 60-s arterial occlusion in the canine intestine. [From Shepherd and Riedel (435).]

Capillary exchange capacity, estimated by $K_{f,c}$ measurements, increased by 60%. These findings have been confirmed in canine intestinal preparations perfused at constant pressure in which blood flow increased by 46% when arterial $P_{O_2}$ was reduced to 50 mmHg (422). The same level of arterial hypoxia increased the capillary exchange capacity (PS for $^{86}$Rb) 60% above control value during constant flow perfusion (Fig. 10). Thus both studies indicate that resistance and exchange vessels respond to arterial hypoxia as predicted by a metabolic mechanism. Both the vasodilation and the capillary recruitment should tend to maintain tissue oxygenation despite the reduced $O_2$ supply. When blood flow is held constant, the intestine maintains $O_2$ uptake within 48% of control value during arterial hypoxia. However, when both blood flow and capillary density are free to increase, $O_2$ uptake remains within 26% of control value despite the hypoxia (422). Skeletal muscle apparently maintains its $O_2$ consumption within 15% of control value at comparable hypoxic levels (191). Thus the intestine appears to be slightly less effective than skeletal muscle in regulating its oxygenation during arterial hypoxia. The nearly fivefold greater $O_2$ demands of the intestine may partly explain this difference.

Studies in awake dogs indicate that hypoxemia produced by breathing an 8% $O_2$-$N_2$ mixture leads to a 20% increase in intestinal blood flow, whereas colonic blood flow is unaltered (89). The intestinal vascular response to hypoxemia in conscious animals is influenced by the arterial $CO_2$ content (265). This $CO_2$-hypoxic interaction was found to depend on sinoaortic reflexes. The denervated intestinal vascular bed responds differently to hypercapnia [partial pressure of $CO_2$ ($P_{CO_2}$) = 80 mmHg] (457). As during hypoxia, there is marked relaxation of resistance vessels during hypercapnia. Unlike hypoxia, however, the precapillary sphincters constrict, and capillary density decreases during hypercapnia. In addition the myogenic reactivity of the resistance vessels to $P_v$ elevation is preserved during hypercapnia. The ability of the small bowel to maintain adequate $O_2$ delivery during hypercapnia has not been studied.

The intestinal vascular responses to arterial hypoxia have been studied in both fetal and neonatal lambs. Fetal hypoxemia, induced by administration to the mother of a gas mixture low in $O_2$, generally does not affect intestinal blood flow until the degree of hypoxemia is severe, at which point vascular resistance rises and blood flow falls [Fig. 11; (96, 332, 372)]. The $O_2$ extraction increases sufficiently to maintain a normal intestinal $O_2$ consumption during moderate hypoxemia. However, when the hypoxemia is severe ($O_2$ supply reduced by >45%), $O_2$ consumption falls. In the neonatal intestines, hypoxemia evokes vascular responses that are qualitatively similar to those seen in the fetal intestines [Fig. 11; (98)]. A major difference between the fetal and neonatal intestines is the relationship between $O_2$ consumption and blood flow (97). In the fetal intestine, $O_2$ consumption is linearly related to blood flow, indicating that $O_2$ uptake is blood flow limited even when blood flow is 50% above normal. In contrast, blood flow can be varied over a wide range without affecting $O_2$ consumption in the neonate; comparable results were obtained in adult animals (50, 51).

Alterations of arterial hematocrit have also been used as a model for studying the influence of $O_2$ delivery on intestinal hemodynamics and oxygenation (97, 125, 224, 434). Studies in adult dogs indicate that there is an inverse, linear correlation between intestinal blood flow and hematocrit and a direct linear correlation between the (a–v)$O_2$ difference and hematocrit (Fig. 12). The relationship between intestinal $O_2$ uptake and hematocrit is parabolic, showing a

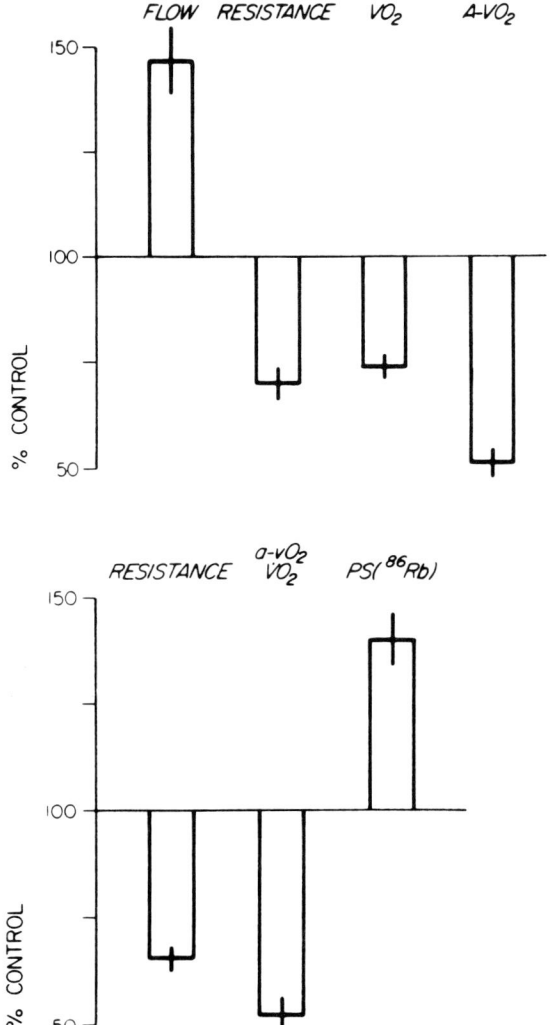

FIG. 10. Effects of arterial hypoxia [partial pressure of $O_2$ ($P_{O_2}$) ≤50 mmHg] on hemodynamics and oxygenation in canine intestinal segments perfused either under constant pressure (*upper panel*) or constant flow (*lower panel*) conditions. $O_2$ consumption ($V_{O_2}$); (a–v)$O_2$, arteriovenous $O_2$ difference (A-V$O_2$); PS, permeability–surface area product. [From Shepherd (422).]

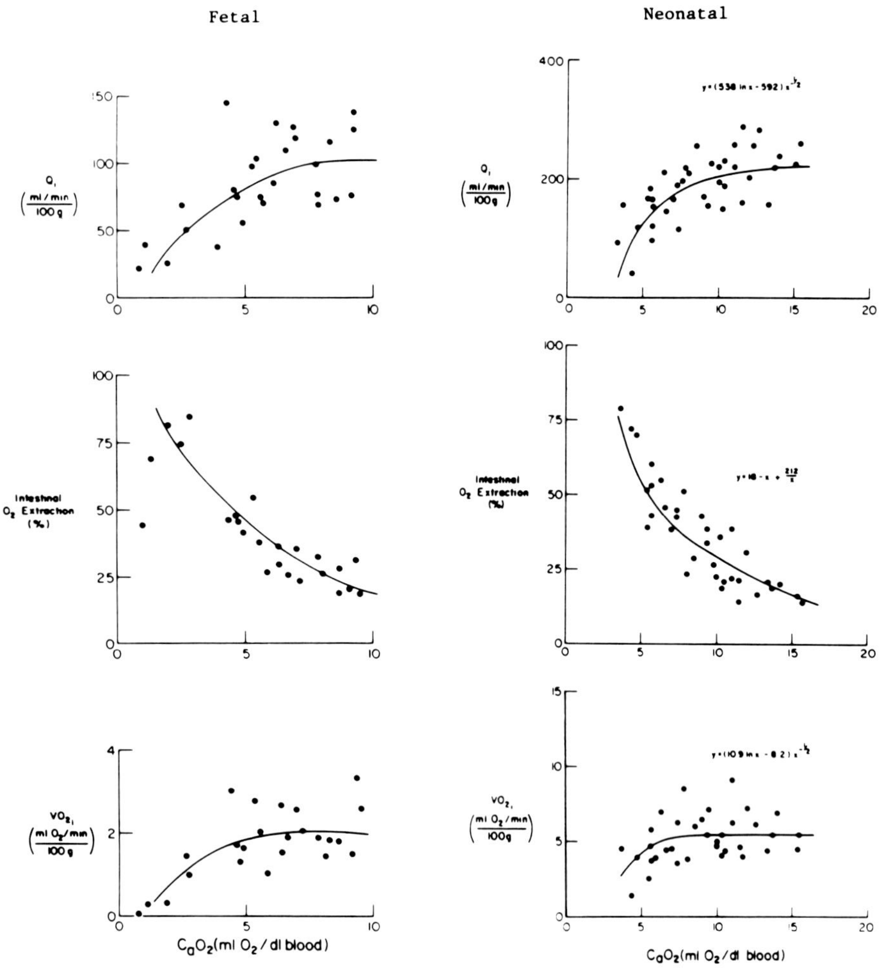

FIG. 11. Effects of alterations in arterial blood $O_2$ content ($C_aO_2$) on intestinal blood flow ($Q_i$), $O_2$ extraction and $O_2$ consumption ($V_{O_{2i}}$) in fetal and neonatal lambs. [From Edelstone and Holzman (97).]

maximal $O_2$ uptake at an hematocrit of 48.7% (optimal hematocrit). Raising perfusion pressure from 120 to 180 mmHg does not alter the optimal hematocrit for intestinal $O_2$ uptake. However, intraenteric placement of nutrients increases the optimal hematocrit to 57.1%. The finding that the optimal hematocrit in the resting bowel (48.7%) is somewhat above the normal range was explained by the plasma skimming known to occur in the intestinal mucosa (434).

The optimal hematocrit for intestinal oxygenation in fetal lambs is 33% (125). The normal hematocrit for the fetal lamb in utero is 32%. Intestinal blood flow varies little over a range of hematocrit from 12% to 40% yet decreases significantly at hematocrits >45%. In neonatal lambs, intestinal blood flow is unaltered by hematocrit alterations over a range from 10% to 54% (224). Intestinal $O_2$ consumption also remains constant over this range of hematocrits. Thus increases in $O_2$ extraction play a major role in maintaining a normal rate of $O_2$ utilization when intestinal $O_2$ delivery is reduced by lowering the hematocrit.

*Postprandial Intestinal Hyperemia*

It is well established that after ingestion of a meal a functional (postprandial) hyperemia occurs within the splanchnic circulation (10, 67, 74, 103, 130, 156, 160, 176, 314). Essex et al. (101) and Herrick et al. (220) demonstrated in their pioneering work that after ingestion of a test meal blood flow is elevated to the carotid, coronary, femoral, and superior mesenteric arteries in conscious dogs. These authors were first to indicate that the increased blood flow to the splanchnic vasculature is not obtained at the expense of blood flow to somatic tissues (220).

In the past two decades investigations have indicated that the ingestion of foodstuffs results in a dual hemodynamic response within the splanchnic circulation: *1*) an initial response during the anticipation

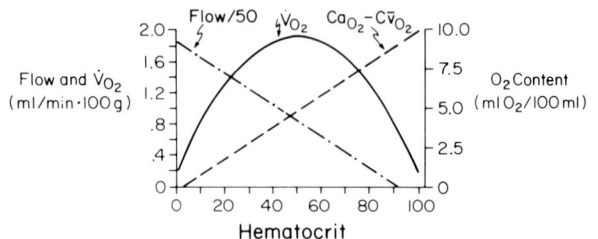

FIG. 12. Effects of hematocrit on canine intestinal blood flow, $O_2$ consumption ($\dot{V}_{O_2}$), arterial $O_2$ content, and arteriovenous $O_2$ difference ($C_aO_2 - C\bar{v}_{O_2}$). [From Shepherd and Riedel (434).]

and ingestion of food and 2) a subsequent response during the digestion and absorption of chyme from the intestinal lumen.

ANTICIPATORY/INGESTION PHASE. The anticipatory/ingestion phase of digestion is characterized by transient increases in heart rate, cardiac output, aortic pressure, and renal vascular resistance (123, 124, 475–477). Concurrently coronary vascular resistance decreases (476, 477), while splanchnic resistance either increases (475–477) or is not altered (123, 124). Vascular resistance in the limbs and skeletal muscle has been reported to either decrease (124, 476, 477) or increase (124) during this time. These transient hemodynamic responses appear to be mediated by a generalized arousal of the sympathetic nervous system because they can be attenuated by adrenergic blocking agents (475).

DIGESTION/ABSORPTION PHASE. The cardiovascular responses to digestion appear to be confined to the gastrointestinal organs. Within 5–30 min after meal ingestion, the cardiac output, heart rate, aortic pressure, and flows to both coronary and renal vascular beds return to preprandial (base line) values. Simultaneously blood flow to the intestine and pancreas starts to increase with peak hyperemias achieved 30–90 min postprandially (39, 54, 123, 124, 131, 475–477).

The augmented intestinal blood flow is not uniformly distributed throughout the gastrointestinal tract. In conscious dogs, blood flow to the stomach, duodenum, jejunum, and pancreas increases within 30–90 min postprandially (38, 131). The decreased splanchnic vascular resistance represents, on the average, an increase in superior mesenteric artery (SMA) blood flow between 28% and 132% (123, 124, 473, 475). Blood flow to the terminal ileum does not increase until 45–90 min postprandially, whereas colonic blood flow does not change after meal ingestion (39, 131). Transient decreases in distal colon blood flow have been observed 30 min postprandially, apparently caused by tonic colonic contractions produced by the gastrocolic reflex (131, 453). Recent data indicate that the discrepancy between the magnitudes of the splanchnic hyperemia in isolated intestinal preparations and in conscious animals may be due to the state of anesthesia, inasmuch as postprandial intestinal hyperemia is much higher in conscious than in anesthetized animals (219). The splanchnic vasodilation may last for 4–7 h, depending on the nature and quantity of the meal (67, 103).

During digestion, blood flow to the limbs and skeletal muscle is either decreased (124, 476, 477) or unaltered (131), apparently depending on the level of exercise. At rest, blood flow is decreased, but if the animal changes position, the decrement in flow can be abolished or even reversed (131, 476, 477). Exercise enhances blood flow to the periphery during the postprandial state; however, flow through the SMA remains elevated (54, 123, 473, 475), suggesting that the augmented limb flow is due to an elevation in cardiac output. Blood flows to the adrenal glands and various regions of the brain including cerebellum, cortex, hypothalamus, medulla, and pituitary do not change postprandially, whereas adipose tissue blood flow has been shown to decrease (131).

The renal vascular response to feeding is somewhat complex. Different dietary components appear to elicit different hemodynamic responses in the kidneys. Mixed meals or meals rich in fat or carbohydrate (123, 356, 377, 383, 420, 476) do not elicit significant postprandial increases in renal hemodynamics. However, ingestion of protein-rich meat meals markedly increases renal blood flow and glomerular filtration rate by 40%–100% in humans and dogs (43, 250, 300, 356, 378, 383, 391, 393, 420). These hemodynamic responses occur within 30–60 min postprandially and attain peak responses 60–120 min after meat ingestion. The renal postprandial hyperemia may last for several hours, similar to the hyperemia seen within the splanchnic vascular bed (300, 356, 383, 393).

Protein alone appears to mediate substantial increases in renal hemodynamics, and the elevation in renal blood flow is similar in magnitude and duration to the splanchnic hemodynamic responses obtained after ingestion of a mixed meal. The blood-borne mediator(s) of the renal postprandial hyperemia has yet to be identified and characterized. Pancreatic glucagon, once thought to be a prime hormonal candidate in mediating the renal hemodynamic responses to protein-rich meals, appears to have relatively little importance in directly mediating the renal vascular response to protein meals (21, 381, 383).

In summary, although the cardiovascular response during the anticipatory/ingestion phase of digestion can be attributed to a generalized sympathetic discharge, the responses elicited during the digestion/absorption phase appear to be confined to the gastrointestinal organs, except after high protein intake, where meat appears to significantly elevate renal hemodynamics and to increase splanchnic blood flow.

LOCALIZATION OF POSTPRANDIAL HYPEREMIA. The specificity of the postprandial hyperemic response is still controversial. The upper small intestine (duodenum and jejunum) vasodilates after feeding or as a result of intraduodenal placement of corn oil, but the vascular responses of the ileum and colon vary to this stimulus (39, 105, 131). Some workers have shown that the hyperemia in the upper small intestine is restricted to the segment exposed to food, whereas others regard it as a more diffuse phenomenon. Feeding or placement of corn oil into the cat duodenum produces a diffuse intestinal hyperemia involving segments of the intestine that do not contain the food or oil (39, 105). Feeding, perfusion of the duodenum, or placement of low-fat food into one of two isolated jejunal segments produce a localized hyperemia confined to the segment exposed to food (73, 131, 286). In addition placement of glucose, amino acids, and/or fatty acids into one of two isolated jejunal segments increases blood flow to the segment containing the nutrients while not affecting blood flow to the adjacent segment (68, 76, 469, 498). In conscious rats, however, a hyperemia in response to a mixed meal is not only detected in bowel segments exposed to chyme, but also observed in distal (unexposed) segments (219).

Some investigators have shown (by injecting 7–10 $\mu$m radioactive microspheres) that the intestinal hyperemia is apparent in all layers (mucosa-submucosa and muscularis-serosa) of the intestinal wall (39), whereas others (using 13–15 $\mu$m microspheres) have shown that the hyperemia is limited to only the mucosal layer (73, 131, 368, 498). Direct observation (in vivo microscopy) of the rat intestinal microvasculature during glucose absorption reveals that intestinal blood flow doubles concomitant with arteriolar vasodilation occurring throughout the intestinal wall, suggesting that the absorptive hyperemia is not limited to the mucosal circulation of the rat (28). Yet, after luminal placement of a mixture of 5% bile and glucose in isolated, vascularly perfused dog ileal loops, laser Doppler velocimetry reveals that superficial mucosal blood flow increases 42%, whereas muscularis-serosal flow falls 10% concomitantly with a 21% increase in total segmental blood flow (436). These divergent compartmental hemodynamic responses in rats and dogs during glucose-mediated absorptive hyperemia may be related to the relative thickness of the intestinal wall and/or to the techniques used to measure blood flow (436).

LUMINAL STIMULI RESPONSIBLE FOR INTESTINAL HYPEREMIA. Chyme in the intestinal lumen could affect intestinal blood flow through mechanical stimulation of the mucosa. Sliding a plastic or vinyl tube back and forth intraluminally in an isolated jejunal segment results in increases in local blood flow and venous plasma vasoactive intestinal polypeptide (VIP) concentration (22, 99, 102). However, chyme per se does not appear to produce the degree of mechanical stimulation necessary to elicit an increase in intestinal blood flow. Luminal placement of digested food significantly increases jejunal blood flow, but undigested food has no vascular effect (76). It has been hypothesized that the mesenteric vasodilation ascribed to mechanical mucosal stimulation may be due to the activation of a local neural reflex releasing serotonin from enterochromaffin cells and ultimately releasing VIP from intramural neurons (22, 99, 102) (see MECHANISMS OF POSTPRANDIAL INTESTINAL HYPEREMIA, p. 1420).

Changes in luminal pH during the postprandial state may also affect intestinal blood flow. Intraduodenal placement of hydrochloric acid (pH ~0.9) increases SMA blood flow (105). Perfusion of the duodenal lumen with an electrolyte solution (pH between 1.5 and 2.0) increases local blood flow, whereas perfusion with solutions of higher pH (between 2.5 and 11) fails to alter blood flow (71, 227). During the postprandial state, however, intraduodenal pH normally fluctuates between 3.5 and 7.4 (41, 118). Thus it is apparent that changes in intraluminal pH are unlikely to contribute significantly to the postprandial intestinal hyperemia.

After ingestion of food or intestinal placement of hypertonic solutions, an intestinal hyperemia could be produced subsequent to an elevation in luminal osmolality. Placement of hypertonic glucose or mannitol solutions in the intestinal lumen produces a greater hyperemia than that elicited by corresponding isotonic solutions (68, 368). Intrajejunal placement of a solution of polyethylene glycol (PEG), which has an osmolality of 3,000 mosmol/kg, increases local intestinal blood flow. However, placement of PEG solutions with osmolalities <1,500 mosmol/kg fails to alter blood flow. Likewise, correlations between changes in intestinal blood flow and osmolality (100–1,000 mosmol/kg) after various test meals is poor (68, 286). Normally the osmolality of the intestinal chyme fluctuates between 220 and 320 mosmol/kg (118). Therefore, although the intestinal vasculature has been reported to be more sensitive to changes in plasma osmolality than other organs (304), it is doubtful that changes in luminal osmolality per se are big enough postprandially to elicit significant increases in intestinal blood flow. The importance of tissue hyperosmolality is discussed in MECHANISMS OF POSTPRANDIAL INTESTINAL HYPEREMIA, p. 1420.

The importance of vasoactive cations as mediators of the intestinal hyperemia has been assessed. Placement of isosmotic solutions of $NaCl$, $MgCl_2$, or $CaCl_2$ in the ileal lumen decreases blood flow ~5%, whereas isosmotic KCl produces variable effects (65). Intraluminal placement of either isosmotic Tyrode's solution or NaCl also produces variable effects on intestinal blood flow (73, 286, 468, 472). In conscious rats, Tyrode's solution markedly increases small intestinal blood flow (219). Although the physiological importance of vasoactive cations as direct mediators of the intestinal postprandial hyperemia appears unimportant (74), changes in electrolyte concentration may indirectly influence splanchnic blood flow through their active cotransport ($Na^+$) with glucose and amino acids.

The major constituents of chyme are digested and undigested foodstuffs, pancreatic enzymes, and bile. Food, digested in vitro by a pancreatic enzyme preparation, significantly increases local blood flow when placed in the canine jejunum (73, 76, 286). However, after luminal placement of either undigested food or the enzyme preparation alone, intestinal blood flow does not change (76, 286). When the digested food was centrifuged and separated into liquid and solid phases, it was found that the vasoactive properties of digested food are solely attributable to factors contained within the liquid phase (76). These findings indicate that the substances responsible for the intestinal hyperemia during the postprandial state are most likely the hydrolytic products of food digestion.

Studies have been conducted to ascertain the importance of bile during food-induced intestinal hyperemia (76, 273). After luminal placement of physiological concentrations of either glucose, amino acids, oleic acid, or monolein alone in the jejunum (major end products of food digestion), only physiological concentrations of glucose (150 mM) increased blood flow (5%). Although the long-chain fatty acid, oleic acid, and the monoglyceride monolein are unable to alter intestinal blood flow when placed within the small bowel in aqueous solution, solubilization of these constituents of chyme results in a significant intestinal hyperemia (75, 76, 273). The increase of the pH of the solution to 9 (75), addition of gallbladder bile (273), or addition of sodium taurocholate (76) to these lipids result in an increase in intestinal blood flow between 20% and 40%.

During the early phase of digestion, bile in the intestinal lumen is ~33% of the concentration found in the gallbladder. As time passes, the concentration of bile decreases to a steady-state value of 10% of that in the gallbladder (273). When placed within the jejunum lumen at these concentrations, bile fails to increase intestinal blood flow; however, it does appear to render most of the constituents of chyme vasoactive. At a concentration of 10% of that within the gallbladder, bile not only renders long-chain fatty acids (oleic acid) vasoactive but also enhances the hyperemic effect of luminally placed glucose (273). Moreover the increase in the bile concentration to 33% of that in the gallbladder renders both short-chain fatty acids (caproic acid) and amino acids (a physiological mixture) vasoactive, while further enhancing glucose-induced intestinal hyperemia. This concentration of bile, however, does not further enhance oleic acid–induced hyperemia (273). These findings regarding bile indicate that physiological concentrations of the substance fail to directly increase jejunal blood flow when placed within the intestinal lumen alone (76, 273). However, endogenous bile does appear to play a major indirect role in initiating jejunal hyperemia inasmuch as bile, at physiological concentrations, renders most of the constituents of chyme vasoactive within the jejunal lumen. Thus, in effect, bile acts as a modulator of food-induced intestinal hyperemia.

The bile contained in intestinal chyme appears to be more important in directly initiating postprandial intestinal hyperemia in the lower small bowel (ileum). Although it lacks a direct vasoactive effect in the jejunum (76, 273), intraluminal placement of either endogenously or synthetically derived bile alone increases ileal blood flow by ~100% (76, 282). Furthermore, of the major constituents of bile (bile salts, bilirubin, cholesterol, and lecithin), bile salts appear largely responsible for the bile-induced ileal hyperemia since intraluminal placement of a bile salt solution readily reproduces the ileal hyperemia produced by either endogenously or synthetically derived bile. Moreover cholestyramine, a bile salt sequestering resin, negates the vasodilatory effects of endogenous bile on ileal blood flow (282).

The importance of protein and metabolites of protein digestion as contributors to the intestinal hyperemia coincident with the digestive process was initially brought up by Brodie and co-workers in 1910 (48). In an isolated jejunal segment, they noted that local blood flow increased significantly after intraluminal placement of a peptide solution. Later studies have corroborated the importance of protein inasmuch as ingestion of protein-rich meals in humans (46) or gastric placement of protein in conscious rats (219) produces marked increases in splanchnic blood flow. Similarly, in exteriorized canine jejunal loops a protein-rich test diet was shown to increase intestinal blood flow to approximately the same degree as a carbohydrate-rich test diet (64% and 68%, respectively) (445).

The major hydrolytic products of protein digestion include small peptides (di- and tripeptides) and individual amino acids (196, 350). Intraluminal placement of glutamic acid (28 mM), aspartic acid (20 mM), phenylalanine (127 mM), or glycine (300 mM) increases intestinal blood flow (76, 105, 472). However, these luminal concentrations of amino acids far exceed those found in the lumen after meal ingestion (1, 350, 358), suggesting that the vasodilatory effect of individual amino acids is pharmacological in nature; when postprandial concentrations of 16 different amino acids and 3 different peptides are individually placed in the jejunal lumen, blood flow fails to increase. Furthermore even when the 16 amino acids are instilled simultaneously, they do not increase intestinal blood flow (76). Perfusion of the distal jejunum with alanine (6 mM), however, slightly increases (7%) SMA blood flow (368). Intraluminal placement of three dipeptides, Gly-Gly, Pro-Leu, and Gly-Asp, at a concentration of 37.5 mM also fails to increase jejunal blood flow (273).

Although it does not appear that the major hydrolytic products of protein digestion (individual amino acids and dipeptides) are important contributors to food-induced intestinal hyperemia, a recent review by Gallavan and Chou (130) suggests that certain by-products of protein digestion may be potent vasodilators in the intestinal circulation. Based on previous observations during protein administration (46, 48), these authors suggest that fragments cleaved off the parent protein molecule may possess amino acid sequences similar to those found in known vasoactive regulatory peptides of the intestine. The nature and vasoactivity of these protein-derived fragments remain to be clarified and further examined.

The major end product of carbohydrate metabolism

is the 6-carbon hexose, glucose. Postprandially the luminal concentration of glucose fluctuates between 28 and 222 mM, rarely exceeding 300 mM (41). Although glucose has been repeatedly shown to increase intestinal blood flow (68, 76, 468), perfusion of either the duodenum or jejunum with isotonic glucose solutions does not alter local blood flow (354, 459). However, a slight hyperemia (between 5%–10% above control values) is observed with 20–278 mM glucose if the hexose is placed in the lumen of isolated jejunal or ileal segments and local venous outflow measured (68, 76, 468, 472). Furthermore, when blood flow is calculated using red blood cell velocity and vessel diameter measurements (in vivo microscopy), total intestinal blood flow (whole-wall) increases to 200%–210% of control values with a concomitant 20–25% dilation of submucosal vessels when the mucosa is exposed to glucose concentrations between 1.39 and 27.8 mM (28). These unusually large increases in intestinal blood flow are not in accord with previous observations using other techniques in whole-organ studies. However, a recent study, which also utilized measurements of red blood cell velocity and arteriolar diameter, has shown that at glucose concentrations between 13.9 and 55.5 mM intestinal blood flow increases by only 18%–45%. Also, solution osmolality has no effect on either the time course or the magnitude of the hyperemia at a given glucose concentration (388). These new findings are in contrast to the previously reported results obtained with the same technology (28), and the divergence appears to be related to the methods employed to calculate arteriolar blood flow (388). The 18%–21% increase in blood flow observed at a glucose concentration of 13.9 mM (388) concurs with previous data obtained by measuring whole-organ blood flow during glucose-induced absorptive hyperemia (68, 219, 354, 425, 446, 449, 468). In summary, although intraluminal glucose can increase intestinal blood significantly, present data suggest that it probably only plays a small role in the postprandial intestinal hyperemia.

The major end products of lipid digestion are 2-monoglycerides and free fatty acids. When long-chain lipolytic products of fat digestion, monolein, and oleic acid are instilled in the intestinal lumen alone at physiological concentrations (20 mM) (223), they fail to elevate intestinal blood flow (76, 273). However, if solubilized by increasing solution pH to 9 or by adding a bile salt solution or 10% gallbladder bile, these lipids elicit a 20%–40% increase in intestinal blood flow (76, 273, 287). Thus it appears that micellar lipids are very potent vasodilators of the intestinal vasculature. When the short-chain fatty acid (20-mM caproic acid) is placed in the intestinal lumen alone, in a bile salt solution, or in 10% gallbladder bile it does not affect intestinal blood flow. However, when solubilized in 33% gallbladder bile, caproic acid increases intestinal blood flow by 13% (76, 273). Because a luminal bile concentration of 10% of that in the gallbladder appears to be a more physiological concentration, the observations noted above suggest that long-chain, but not short-chain, lipolytic products of fat digestion contribute significantly to the intestinal postprandial hyperemia observed after meal ingestion.

Recent observations in anesthetized dogs indicate that of the three major dietary components (fat, protein, and carbohydrate), fat (on a weight basis) produces the greatest jejunal hyperemia (30%), followed by protein (24%) and carbohydrate (18%). However, it was concluded that the hyperemia ascribed to protein and carbohydrate was not insignificant and that the postprandial intestinal hyperemia results from a synergistic effect of all three dietary components (445). A recent study in conscious rats corroborates the importance of all three dietary components as contributors to the intestinal postprandial hyperemia (219).

Finally, although the majority of the constituents of chyme are absorbed proximally to the large bowel, a significant amount of carbohydrates reach the colon and are subsequently converted to volatile fatty acids (acetic, propionic, and butyric acids) (7, 35, 38, 41, 456). In a canine colon preparation, luminal placement of a cocktail containing acetic (75 mM), propionic (30 mM), and butyric (30 mM) acids significantly increases colonic blood flow (23.5%) and $O_2$ uptake (18.4%). Moreover, of the three fatty acids only acetic acid could mimic the effects of the entire mixture on colonic hemodynamics and $O_2$ uptake, suggesting that physiological concentrations of volatile fatty acids (especially acetic acid) significantly alter colonic blood flow (274).

Figure 13 illustrates the intestinal vascular response to various constituents of chyme. Note the importance of bile in the jejunal vascular response to a meal and the importance of bile salts during postprandial ileal hyperemia.

MECHANISMS OF POSTPRANDIAL INTESTINAL HYPEREMIA. Although the existence of a postprandial intestinal hyperemia has been established and well documented, the precise mechanisms governing chyme-induced increases in intestinal blood flow are not as yet clearly defined. Several different mechanisms have been implicated in the absorptive hyperemia associated with ingestion of a meal. These mechanisms include: *1*) direct effect of constituents of chyme on the intestinal vasculature; *2*) activation of intrinsic nerves; *3*) tissue hyperosmolality; *4*) metabolic factors; *5*) release of blood-borne vasoactive gastrointestinal hormones; and *6*) release of vasoactive autacoids. The importance of various constituents of chyme in the initiation of postprandial intestinal hyperemia and their various possible mechanisms of action are discussed in a number of reviews (10, 74, 103, 130, 160, 176).

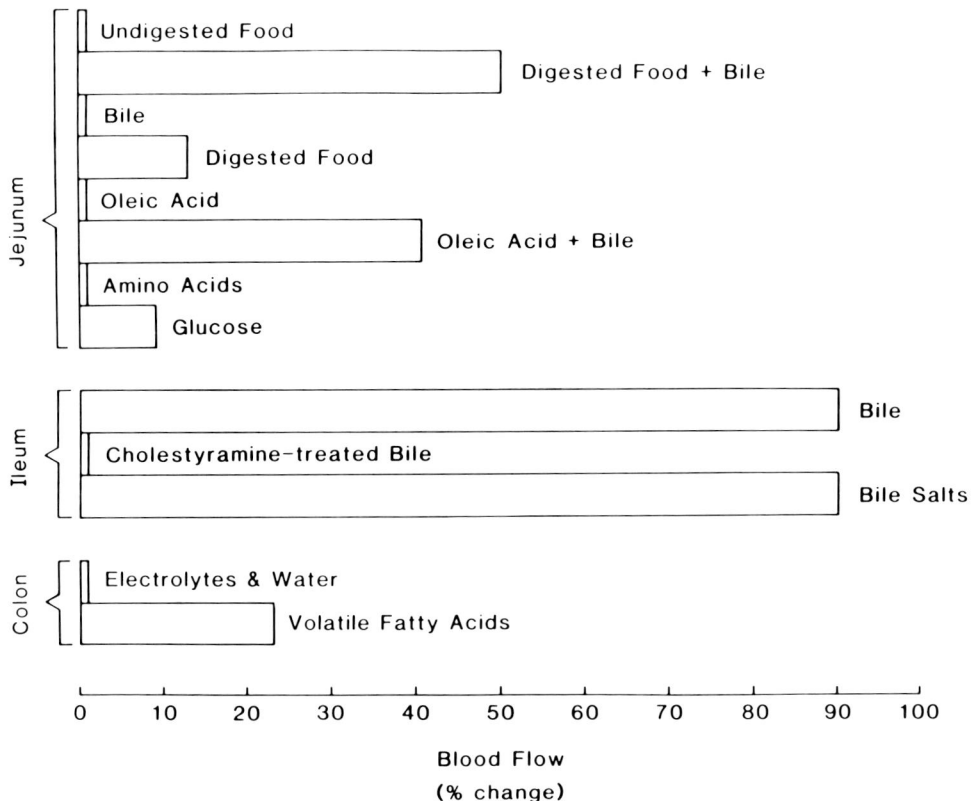

FIG. 13. Effects of intraluminal placement of various constituents of chyme on intestinal blood flow. [Modified from Granger et al. (160).]

*Direct vasoactive action by constituents of chyme.* It appears that at least two constituents of chyme directly affect the intestinal vasculature. At a blood concentration of 60 $\mu$M, oleic acid produces a significant vasodilation of the jejunal vasculature in the dog (448). Also, intra-arterial infusion of bile salts (taurocholate, taurodeoxycholate, and taurochenodeoxycholate), attaining blood concentrations between 0.6 and 0.8 mM, elicits dose-dependent and highly correlated increases in ileal blood flow of 80%–120% (282). Although these studies support the notion that selected constituents of chyme do exert a direct vasoactive effect on the intestinal vasculature, they do not preclude the existence or importance of local regulatory mechanisms activated by oleic acid and/or bile salts.

*Intrinsic nerves.* The intestinal hyperemia observed during digestion may involve the activation of local nerves and/or local neural reflexes. Early work suggested that the mesenteric vasodilation ascribed to mechanical mucosal stimulation by vinyl tubes (mimicking movement of chyme) is due to an activation of a local neural reflex involving interactions between serotonin and VIP (22, 23, 99, 102). However, as described in LUMINAL STIMULI RESPONSIBLE FOR INTESTINAL HYPEREMIA, p. 1418, chyme per se does not appear to produce enough mechanical stimulation to elicit an impressive rise in local blood flow.

Evidence indicates that local nerves contribute importantly during food-induced intestinal hyperemia. Prior treatment of the intestinal mucosa with a local anesthetic dibucaine attenuates or actually abolishes the local hyperemic response to intrajejunal placement of glucose or digested food solutions (68, 380, 498). The fall in SMA resistance during digestion can be attenuated or abolished by atropine, but not by phenoxybenzamine ($\alpha$-adrenergic antagonist), propranolol ($\beta$-adrenergic antagonist), or by acute bilateral splanchnicectomy (105, 475–477). These observations suggest that cholinergic, but not adrenergic, mechanisms may be involved during the postprandial intestinal hyperemic response.

However, recent data indicate that the importance of local nerves and/or cholinergic mechanisms is not as great as previously thought. In jejunal segments of anesthetized dogs, nutrient-induced intestinal hyperemia (by either intraluminal glucose or oleic acid) is not attenuated or abolished by infusion of methysergide (serotonergic antagonist), hexamethonium (ganglionic blocking agent), or tetrodotoxin (specific blocker of $Na^+$ channels in membranes of excitable cells) or by extrinsically denervating the jejunal segment (354). Although prior exposure of the mucosa to dibucaine does attenuate or even block glucose- or oleic acid–mediated elevations in intestinal blood flow and $O_2$ uptake, the effect does not appear to be primarily due to an alteration in vascular sensitivity to vasoactive agents inasmuch as dibucaine does not alter the intestinal vascular response to norepinephrine or isoproterenol. The blocking action of dibucaine during nutrient-induced intestinal hyperemia appears to be attributable instead to its inhibitory effect on glucose transport and $O_2$ consumption, because the anesthetic markedly inhibits active but enhances passive transport of glucose across rat intestinal sacs in vitro and also inhibits jejunal mucosal $O_2$ uptake in the dog (354). These findings suggest that local metabolic (rather than neural) mechanisms are more important during food-induced intestinal hyperemia.

Also, recent evidence indicates that cholinergic mechanisms may be unimportant during postprandial intestinal hyperemia. In an autoperfused canine jejunal segment, cholinergic blockade with atropine fails to alter increases induced by bile oleic acid in jejunal blood flow (40%) and $O_2$ uptake (15%). In fact, during the first 4–5 min the hyperemia elicited by the micellar fat solution is actually greater after cholinergic blockade (287). Similar findings were reported regarding the apparent enhancement of food-induced intestinal hyperemia after atropine pretreatment (353). Thus, if a cholinergic mechanism is involved during postprandial intestinal hyperemia, its role is, most likely, small. There is, however, the possibility that activation of noncholinergic, nonadrenergic vagal fibers may participate in the intestinal vascular response to a meal. In conscious rats, truncal vagotomy abolishes the duodenal and significantly attenuates the jejunal hyperemia associated with gastric instillation of a mixed meal (219). Furthermore, because the proximal small intestinal hyperemia is not affected by atropine pretreatment (219), vagotomy-induced decreases in intestinal blood flow suggest that if a neural component contributes during postprandial intestinal hyperemia, one would have to postulate the existence of an important noncholinergic, nonadrenergic mechanism.

*Tissue hyperosmolality.* As a result of active cotransport of electrolytes with nutrients, the osmolality of the mucosal interstitium increases after the ingestion of a meal (30). The intestinal vasculature appears to be extremely sensitive to alterations in plasma (and, presumably, interstitial) osmolality inasmuch as each 1% increment in plasma osmolality produces a 3% decrease in vascular resistance (304). These observations suggest that changes in tissue osmolality may contribute to the intestinal vascular response to a meal.

However, the importance of tissue hyperosmolality in the complex mechanisms of postprandial intestinal hyperemia remains a debatable issue. Evidence indicates that intestinal villus hyperosmolality, subsequent to coupled active transport of $Na^+$ with glucose, increases submucosal osmolality and initiates significant dilation of submucosal vessel in the rat. The time courses of increased tissue osmolality and submucosal vasodilation are essentially identical. Thus a naturally occurring osmotic vasodilatory component during absorptive hyperemia may exist (30). A more recent study demonstrated, however, that suffusion of the rat jejunal mucosa with either hypertonic or isotonic glucose solutions causes a similar increase in submucosal blood flow; that hypertonic solutions fail to maintain an intestinal hyperemia; and that there is no effect of solution osmolality on either the time course or magnitude of the hyperemia at a given glucose concentration (388). The role of tissue hyperosmolality in the glucose-induced absorptive hyperemia was not confirmed by these findings. It remains uncertain, however, whether the alterations in luminal osmolality lead to predictable changes in the osmolality of interstitial fluid surrounding the submucosal arterioles.

*Metabolic factors.* Intestinal absorption, secretion, and motility are $O_2$-consuming processes. During the postprandial state, all of these functions are greatly stimulated. It is well established that intestinal $O_2$ consumption rises markedly in response to the presence of food in the lumen (46, 48, 128, 273, 286, 368, 425, 447, 468, 472). According to the metabolic theory of local blood flow regulation, arteriolar and precapillary sphincter tone are closely linked to the metabolic status of the tissue. Therefore one can predict that increases in oxidative metabolism are associated with vasodilation and capillary recruitment.

There is relatively little information regarding the quantitative relationship between the rate of nutrient absorption and the intensity of the absorptive hyperemia. There is some evidence that the increment in intestinal blood flow produced by intraluminal placement of glucose solutions is correlated with the rate of glucose-coupled $H_2O$ absorption (Fig. 14). Whether such a correlation exists for other actively transported nutrients remains to be determined. The magnitude of the absorptive hyperemia need not always be correlated with blood flow, because $O_2$ extraction may increase sufficiently to meet the increased $O_2$ demand, thereby obviating the hyperemic response (163, 368, 425). This possibility is supported by the observation that intestinal $O_2$ uptake (the product of blood flow and $O_2$ extraction) is usually more closely correlated with intestinal function than is blood flow (Fig. 14). Highly significant correlations between $O_2$ uptake and absorption rate have been reported for both the small (468) and the large bowel (275).

The degree of correlation between changes in intestinal $O_2$ uptake and blood flow during the postprandial state appears to be related to the nature of the luminal contents. The increased $O_2$ demand produced by luminal placement of Tyrode's solution or of Tyrode's solution plus glucose is met by an increase in blood flow. After luminal placement of Tyrode's solution plus taurocholate, the enhanced metabolic demand is

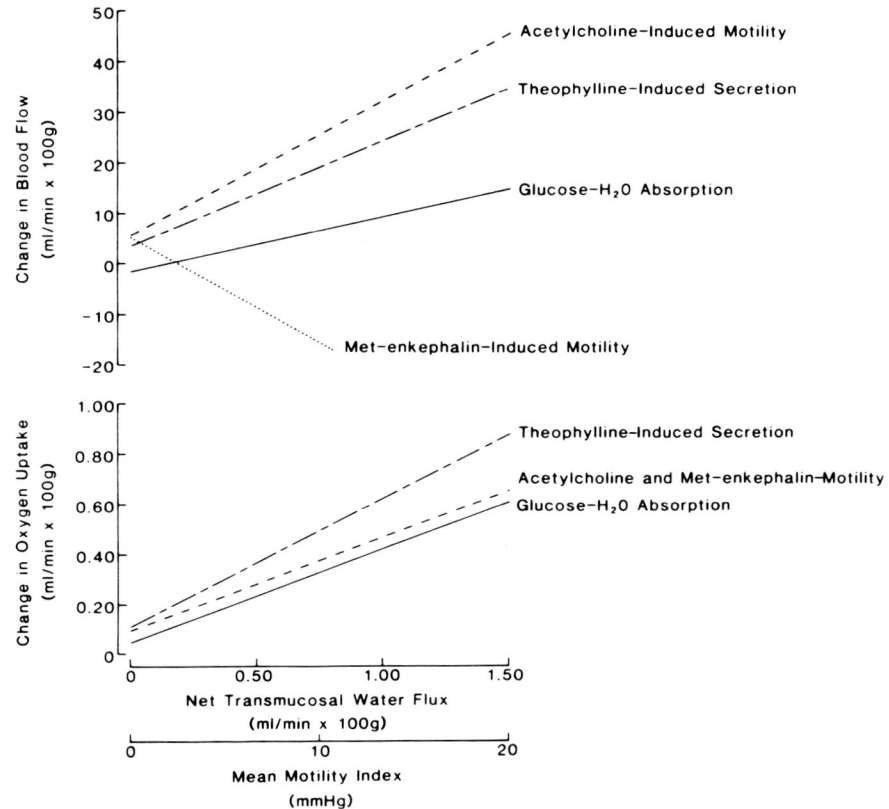

FIG. 14. Relationship between intestinal blood flow (*upper panel*), $O_2$ uptake (*lower panel*), and various functional activities (absorption, secretion, motility). [From Granger et al. (160).]

met by an increase in $O_2$ extraction (468). However, a significant correlation is found between $O_2$ uptake and intestinal blood flow after luminal placement of digested food and bile (129, 328). The precise relationship between $O_2$ uptake and blood flow may depend on the initial value of $(a-v)O_2$ in the intestine (192). The greater the initial $(a-v)O_2$, the greater the intestinal hyperemia at a given $O_2$ uptake. Figure 15 demonstrates that for the identical $O_2$ uptake the corresponding increase in superior mesenteric blood flow is greater when the $(a-v)O_2$ is >6 vol% than when it is <6 vol%. These findings suggest that the food-mediated increase in intestinal blood flow depends on the resting $(a-v)O_2$ in the gut.

Studies with glucose and glucose analogues support the contention that intraluminal placement of nutrients elicits an intestinal hyperemia caused by stimulation of absorptive processes and tissue metabolism. Glucose-mediated absorptive hyperemia is characterized by small increases in blood flow (7%–9%) coupled with larger increases in $O_2$ uptake (12%–25%) and increases in the capillary PS (18%–36%) (75, 368, 425, 446, 472). Moreover both glucose and 3-$O$-methylglucose (which is actively transported but not metabolized) elicit an intestinal hyperemia when placed in the jejunal lumen; yet, 2-deoxyglucose (which is neither actively transported nor metabolized) does not.

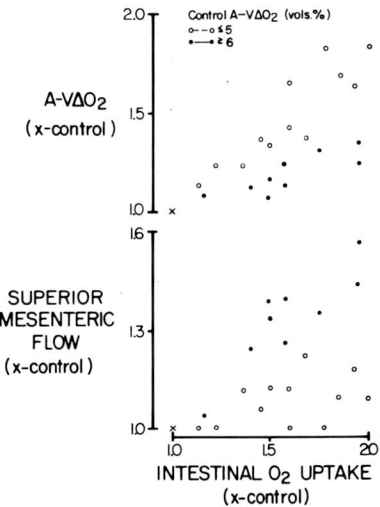

FIG. 15. Changes in intestinal blood flow and $O_2$ extraction produced by intraluminal placement of food in the small bowel. *Solid circles*, data obtained at a control arteriovenous $O_2$ difference $(a-v)O_2 \geq 6$ vol%; *open circles*, data obtained at a control $(a-v)O_2 \leq 5$ vol%; ×, control values for blood flow and $O_2$ extraction. [From Granger and Norris (192).]

Glucose increases, but 3-$O$-methylglucose does not alter $O_2$ uptake, and the hyperemia elicited by glucose (19%) is greater than that produced by the actively transported analogue (7%) (449). These findings suggest that about two-thirds of the hyperemic effect of luminally placed glucose is strongly associated with both absorptive processes and an enhancement of oxidative metabolism.

Estimates of functional capillary exchange capacity (perfused capillary density) have been derived in the absorbing small bowel. Based on rubidium clearance time and $K_{f,c}$ determinations, capillary exchange capacity is predicted to increase by 15%–50% during glucose absorption (285, 368, 425). This is generally considered to reflect capillary recruitment caused by relaxation of precapillary sphincter smooth muscle. The capillary recruitment induced by glucose absorption is presumed to occur exclusively in the mucosal layer thereby providing a greater surface area for delivery of $O_2$ to the absorptive epithelia. The observation that capillary recruitment is generally associated with a rise in tissue $O_2$ extraction supports the latter contention (285). If the increased $O_2$ demand imposed by glucose absorption is met primarily by an increase in blood flow (rather than $O_2$ extraction), minimal alterations in capillary exchange capacity are observed.

A mathematical model has been used to determine the relative contribution of increases in blood flow and $O_2$ extraction and of capillary recruitment in ensuring adequate intestinal oxygenation in the hypermetabolic state associated with feeding (152). An interesting prediction by the model is that $O_2$ extraction is quantitatively more important than blood flow in providing additional $O_2$ to the cells when metabolic demand is increased, irrespective of which control system (resistance or exchange vessel) is operating (Fig. 16). In the uncontrolled system (no regulation) $O_2$ extraction rises in proportion to the increment in $O_2$ consumption, because the capillary-to-cell $P_{O_2}$ gradient increases sufficiently to provide a greater than normal transcapillary $O_2$ flux. This can occur because the intestinal cell $P_{O_2}$ is operating well above the critical level required to maintain normal oxidative metabolism. Simulation results obtained assuming only exchange vessel regulation were similar to those obtained assuming an uncontrolled system, i.e., an increased $O_2$ extraction accounted for essentially all of the increment in $O_2$ uptake. Recruitment, however, was advantageous in that it minimized the fall in tissue $P_{O_2}$ produced by an increased metabolic rate. With arteriolar (resistance vessel) feedback (either alone or coupled to exchange vessel regulation) blood flow plays a significant role in providing the additional $O_2$ required during hypermetabolic states. The increments in blood flow produced by arteriolar dilation enhance $O_2$ delivery by stabilizing capillary $O_2$ tension, thereby leading to a smaller rise in $O_2$ extraction than observed in the absence of resistance vessel regulation. However, for increments in $O_2$ consumption observed experimentally (20%–30%), the model predicted that

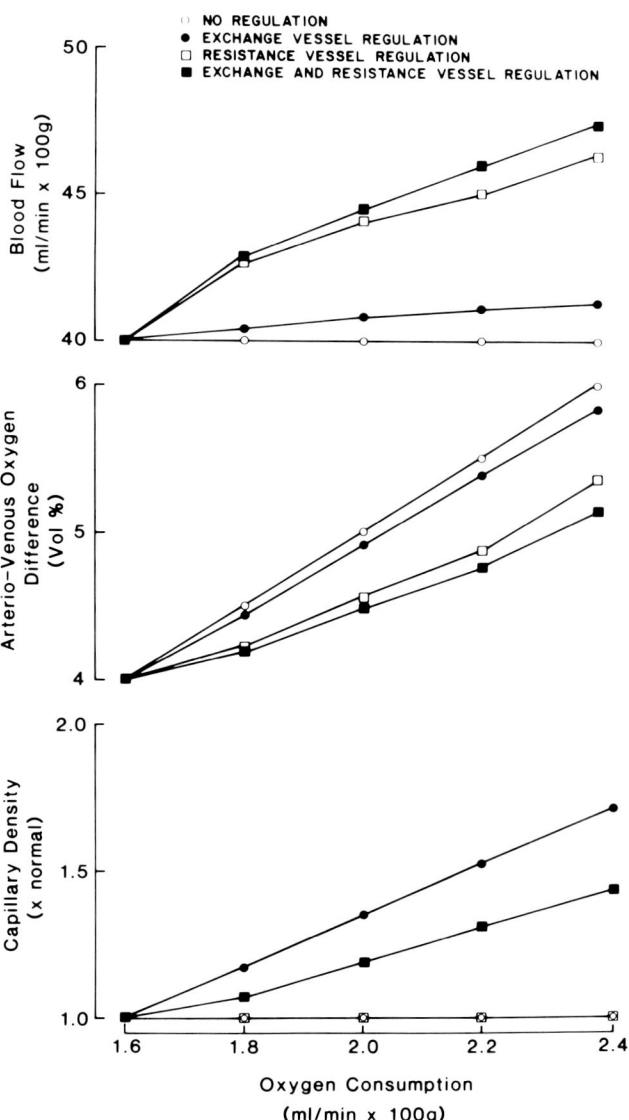

FIG. 16. Role of arteriolar feedback, precapillary sphincter feedback, and passive factors in augmenting transcapillary $O_2$ flux after graded elevations in intestinal $O_2$ demand. [From Granger and Granger (152).]

the metabolic hyperemia is proportionally smaller than the increment in $O_2$ extraction.

Alterations in tissue $P_{O_2}$ have been suggested to explain the metabolically mediated intestinal hyperemia produced by glucose. In the rat small intestine, glucose-induced absorptive hyperemia appears to be strongly related to a precipitous fall (53%) in tissue $P_{O_2}$ (28). Moreover the hyperemic response to glucose is quantitatively and temporally related to the fall in mucosal $P_{O_2}$ (29). These data (28, 29) indicate that at least one-third of the glucose-induced intestinal hyperemia can be ascribed to a marked fall in tissue $P_{O_2}$. The observation that the degree of capillary recruitment produced by absorption is inversely correlated to the $O_2$ availability-to-demand ratio (an index of tissue oxygenation) further explains the role of metabolic factors (285).

The role of adenosine in the postprandial hyperemia is demonstrated by the observation that intra-arterial infusion of the nucleoside elicits a dose-dependent increase in ileal blood flow and $O_2$ uptake (482). Moreover direct application of either adenosine deaminase or theophylline to the extracellular space of the rat jejunal muscularis significantly reduces the absorptive hyperemia induced by a mucosal suffusate containing glucose (56 mM) and oleic acid (20 mM) (390). Although these observations demonstrate that adenosine is an important metabolic mediator, the latter study (390) also demonstrates that while suffusion of the muscularis with adenosine produces a dose-dependent increase in blood flow, mucosal suffusion with adenosine fails to alter blood flow. These divergent compartmental hemodynamic responses to adenosine are problematic because many investigators have shown that nutrient-induced intestinal hyperemia is either confined to the mucosa (73, 131, 368, 436, 498) or apparent in all layers (28, 39) of the intestine.

Other investigators have questioned the importance of adenosine as a metabolic mediator of intestinal hyperemia. Luminal placement of a predigested low-fat, low-protein food mixture increases SMA blood flow by 15%, a response that is not modified by pretreatment with either theophylline or dypyridamole (193). Furthermore exogenous administration of adenosine has been shown to decrease ileal $O_2$ uptake, cause capillary derecruitment, constrict the mucosal vasculature, and redistribute blood flow away from the mucosa to the muscularis (187, 437). It has also been suggested that adenosine redistributes wall blood flow through a "vascular steal" mechanism because adenosine appears to be a more potent vasodilator in the muscularis than in the mucosa (437). Inasmuch as these aforementioned responses to adenosine (187, 437) are opposite to those observed during absorptive hyperemia, the physiological importance of adenosine as a metabolic contributor to the postprandial intestinal hyperemia remains questionable.

Further study is required to unravel the divergent intestinal hemodynamic responses to adenosine. Determination of intestinal tissue concentrations of adenosine, along with nucleoside secretory rates, during the postprandial state will help clarify the importance of adenosine as a metabolic mediator of postprandial intestinal hyperemia.

*Gastrointestinal hormones and peptides.* A physiological role of a humoral component during postprandial intestinal hyperemia was suggested by Burns and Schenk (53) in 1967 when they reported that intravenous infusions of gastrin and secretin significantly increase SMA blood flow. The involvement of humoral substances (e.g., endogenous gastrointestinal hormones) during the intestinal vascular response to a meal is suggested by bioassay and cross-perfusion experiments.

Intraduodenal infusion of food or acid increases local blood flow and decreases the vascular resistance in an isolated jejunal segment perfused by the duodenal venous outflow (226). Moreover intraduodenal instillation of corn oil, acid, or phenylalanine in cats produces a selective increase in mesenteric blood flow, associated with increases in gallbladder and duodenal motility, and an elevation in pancreatic secretion, responses that can be reproduced by intravenous infusions of low doses of secretin and cholecystokinin (CCK). Cross-perfusion studies indicate that intraduodenal instillation of corn oil increases intestinal blood flow in both the test animal and in a cross-perfused recipient animal (105). These findings suggest that contact of chyme with the intestinal mucosa can cause the release of vasoactive agents (including gastrointestinal hormones) into the general circulation.

The humoral candidates have included the three well established gastrointestinal hormones: gastrin, secretin, and CCK. These hormones are released into the systemic circulation after a meal and are known to mediate changes in intestinal secretory and motility patterns coincident with the digestive process. Studies have been conducted that explored the vasodilatory actions (and possible physiological significance) of these three hormones and a host of others (glucagon, neurotensin, substance P, glucose-dependent insulinotropic peptide (GIP), and VIP). The vasoactivity of these and other hormones in the splanchnic vascular bed is examined in several reviews (74, 77, 103, 176) and is not discussed here. To implicate gastrointestinal peptides in the postprandial hyperemia, it must be shown that they have vasodilatory effects at postprandial blood concentrations. It appears that the vasodilatory effect ascribed to a majority of gastrointestinal peptides in the intestine is pharmacological, because blood levels of the hormones far exceed postprandial concentrations needed to dilate the intestinal vasculature (77). However, it has been suggested that CCK in the duodenum and jejunum and neurotensin in the ileum may function as important blood-borne mediators of postprandial intestinal hyperemia (77, 103).

Chou et al. (72) conducted the first systematic study in the dog, exploring the cardiovascular effects of physiological blood levels of gastrin, secretin, and CCK on a variety of vascular beds, including the small intestine. Their studies suggest that CCK could contribute, as a blood-borne hormone, to postprandial intestinal hyperemia because at blood levels comparable to those reported as "postprandial" CCK selectively dilates the duodenum and jejunum. Other nondigestive organs (heart, kidney, forelimb, spleen, skin, and muscle), which are known not to be hemodynamically altered postprandially, are unaffected by

CCK. Gastrin, although selectively dilating only the duodenum and jejunum, does so at a blood level ~400–900 times greater than reported postprandial concentrations. Secretin appears to be a nonselective vasodilator decreasing vascular resistance in both digestive and nondigestive organs. Moreover the blood concentration of secretin necessary to induce intestinal vasodilation is considerably higher than reported postprandial blood levels. Based on these and other pertinent data (77, 103), including the observation that local intra-arterial infusion of CCK redistributes blood flow within the intestinal wall with a preferential increase in mucosal flow (104), CCK has emerged as a viable hormonal mediator of the postprandial intestinal hyperemia.

Although recent studies, performed with pure synthetically derived hormones, have corroborated the pharmacological nature of the intestinal dilation produced by several gastrointestinal hormones, these studies have also shown that synthetically derived CCK acts in the intestine as a pharmacological agent, rather than a blood-borne physiological hormone (175a, 384, 385). In a constant-flow canine ileum preparation, intra-arterial infusion of physiological concentrations of gastrin, secretin, GIP, or cholecystokinin COOH-terminal octapeptide (CCK-8) failed to alter ileal perfusion pressure. However, at a blood concentration ~100 times greater than levels measured postprandially, secretin decreased ileal perfusion pressure by ~12%. A similar decrease in perfusion pressure was produced by GIP at an arterial blood level ~10 times greater than reported postprandial levels (385).

The observation of the hemodynamic action of CCK-8 is interesting because previous studies have demonstrated its role as a physiological blood-borne intestinal vasodilator (72, 77, 103). Although a case could be made in regard to the area of testing in the intestine (duodenum and jejunum vs. ileum), the purity of the used hormone preparation appears to be more crucial. In most of the previous studies demonstrating marked increases in intestinal blood flow with CCK at physiological blood levels, the hormone was derived from natural sources (extracted, partially purified forms). These CCK preparations may have been contaminated with other vasoactive agents. This is particularly apparent in the classic study by Chou and co-workers (72) who used a 17%-pure extract (pure, synthetically derived CCK-8 was unavailable at that time). Thus a vasodilatory action by contaminants cannot be ruled out in the studies with extracted, partially purified CCK (72, 77, 103).

The influence of postprandial blood levels of CCK on intestinal hemodynamics has been reassessed recently, based on reported levels of the peptide (329, 330, 384). Using this new information, Premen et al. (384) have found that in the autoperfused canine jejunum postprandial blood levels of CCK-8 fail to elevate intestinal blood flow. Likewise, blood flow is not affected by postprandial blood levels of secretin or neurotensin. Moreover, when infused simultaneously (to determine the possibility of a mutually potentiating action on intestinal blood flow), the combination of secretin, neurotensin, and CCK-8 also fails to elevate jejunal blood flow. However, when infused at rates that produce arterial blood levels ~100 times greater than postprandial, each hormone alone—as well as in combination—elicits marked increases in blood flow (384).

These new hemodynamic data obtained with pure, synthetically derived gastrointestinal hormones (384, 385) indicate that gastrin, secretin, neurotensin, GIP, and CCK-8 are not of quantitative importance in regulating intestinal blood flow during the postprandial state. However, higher (presumably pharmacological) blood levels of these hormones do elevate intestinal blood flow, a finding that corroborates previous studies (74, 77, 103, 176). Furthermore recent data indicate that after micellar fat placement in the jejunal lumen, the release of CCK, glucagon (127), and neurotensin (134) is transient and generally too low to account for the lipid-induced elevations in jejunal blood flow. Data do exist, however, suggesting that neurotensin (218, 267) and substance P (382) may be of physiological importance in modulating ileal blood flow during the postprandial state.

Neurotensin has recently been proposed as an important blood-borne hormone regulating ileal hemodynamics (218, 267) because, at arterial blood levels calculated to be intermediate among published postprandial values, the hormone increases ileal blood flow in the cat by 28% (218). Because neurotensin is found in greatest concentrations in the ileum and is released from mucosal endocrine cells by the presence of bile in the intestinal lumen (120, 267, 379), the hormone could mediate bile-induced increases in ileal hemodynamics (282). However, one study has shown that at postprandial blood levels neurotensin only increases canine ileal muscularis blood flow. Mucosal flow is not altered, not even at higher blood concentrations that increase duodenal and jejunal muscularis blood flow (9). Although neurotensin does not appear to contribute significantly to postprandial jejunal hyperemia (134, 384), it may contribute to the postprandial ileal hyperemia. Further studies are required to characterize the distribution of intestinal blood flow in the wall of the ileum during neurotensin infusion.

The intestinal hemodynamic actions of substance P have recently been reviewed (77, 373). It is generally agreed that substance P is one of the most potent vasodilating compounds known (373). In fact, on a molar basis, substance P appears to be the most powerful intestinal vasodilator tested thus far (415). It has been suggested, however, that the vasodilatory action ascribed to substance P represents a pharmacological effect, because the intestinal vasodilation elicited by the peptide is produced at substance P blood levels higher than those present in the circulation postprandially (77). This contention has recently been challenged: reported postprandial blood levels of substance P were measured from peripheral venous blood and not from within the intestinal circulation where blood levels of substance P may be considerably higher (382).

In a canine ileum preparation, substance P significantly dilates the ileal vasculature at a calculated arterial blood concentration of 47 pM (382). Although this blood level of the peptide is higher than the reported postprandial blood concentration of 27.5 pM (3), the latter measurement was taken from peripheral blood. Thus it may represent an underestimate of the true splanchnic (i.e., portal) postprandial blood concentration. These observations suggest that the vasodilatory action of substance P at 47 pM might prove to be physiologically important. Once the postprandial blood concentration of substance P is accurately determined within the splanchnic vascular bed, further clarification of the physiological importance of blood-borne substance P on intestinal blood flow can be ascertained.

Although recent data (384, 385) indicate that gastrointestinal hormones are not quantitatively important contributors (as blood-borne agents) to the postprandial intestinal hyperemia, one cannot exclude the possibility that these hormones may exert a local physiological effect (i.e., function as paracrine agents) in the intestinal vascular response to food. After their release from mucosal endocrine cells, the hormones could achieve tissue concentrations far greater than those reported in the circulation during the postprandial state. Likewise, it is not absolutely certain whether postprandial blood levels of these hormones accurately reflect their respective physiologically effective concentrations at target sites. Previous studies with gastrointestinal hormones did not measure interstitial tissue concentrations of the hormones or hormone secretory rates after food absorption. Because of the marked increases in intestinal blood flow reported at pharmacological blood levels (e.g., 10–100 times postprandial) it is reasonable to suggest that gastrointestinal hormones could play a role as paracrine rather than endocrine agents in the postprandial regulation of intestinal blood flow.

Gallavan et al. (127) have recently provided strong evidence in support of a paracrine role for VIP in significantly contributing to micellar fat-mediated increases in jejunal blood flow. Micellar fat, in the form of a bile–oleic acid mixture, significantly increases both intestinal blood flow (21%) and VIP release (118%) measured as the product of the arteriovenous peptide concentration gradient and blood flow. However, no significant changes in either glucagon or CCK release are observed during the micellar fat-induced hyperemia. Moreover there is a close temporal relationship between VIP release and the jejunal hyperemia induced by bile and oleic acid mixture. Subsequent studies with local intra-arterial infusions of VIP provided evidence that although the peptide does not reproduce the micellar fat–induced intestinal hyperemia at postprandial blood levels, higher doses of VIP (10–100 times greater than that released in response to the bile–oleic acid mixture) do so. Taking into account that the intestinal vasculature is richly innervated with VIPergic nerves (467) and that VIP is found only in neuronal tissue (290), these investigators (127) reasoned that micellar fat–induced release of VIP may produce a relatively high concentration of the peptide in synaptic clefts before slowly diffusing into the interstitial spaces. Thus it would be necessary to infuse VIP at concentrations considerably higher than those released endogenously in response to micellar fat to achieve similar tissue concentrations of the peptide in the vicinity of arterial receptors for VIP. This notion of the paracrine role played by gastrointestinal hormones/peptides in the regulation of intestinal blood flow was first suggested in the late 1970s by Eklund et al. (100) and Fahrenkrug et al. (102). Their combined data indicated that intra-arterial infusion of VIP can reproduce the physiological effects observed after activation of noncholinergic, nonadrenergic nerves (i.e., VIPergic nerves) in the intestine but only at arterial blood levels far greater than those measured after its release from intrinsic nerves. Neurally induced release of VIP into the circulation is only ~1/10,000 of the arterial blood concentration of the peptide necessary to produce similar physiological effects (i.e., elevations in blood flow) after intra-arterial infusion of VIP.

It is likely that postprandial blood levels of VIP grossly underestimate the true postprandial concentration of the peptide at target sites. After neural release, VIP appears to act locally as a neurocrine agent and then is apparently inactivated before attaining vasoactive levels in the circulation. Consequently one would expect that arterial blood concentrations of VIP would have to be markedly elevated to mimic the neurogenically mediated responses (elevations in blood flow), because mechanisms for reuptake by presynaptic nerves and/or local metabolizing enzymes are quite likely to exist (as they do for other neurotransmitters) at the synaptic clefts. Therefore it appears that VIP may contribute to postprandial intestinal hyperemia by acting as a local modulator (i.e., a neurocrine agent) on the intestinal vasculature.

*Endogenous autacoids.* A variety of endogenous autacoids have been implicated as local paracrine mediators in the regulation of intestinal blood flow. These substances are diversified in regard to structure and overall biological activity but appear to have at least one function in common, i.e., vasodilation of the intestinal vasculature. Members of this diversified group include two amines: histamine and serotonin (also known as 5-hydroxytryptamine, 5HT, and enteramine); one polypeptide bradykinin; and the arachidonic acid derivatives—the prostaglandins. Available data suggest that these naturally occurring autacoids may play a role in the regulation of postprandial intestinal hyperemia.

Serotonin is chiefly concentrated in mucosal enterochromaffin cells with a smaller distribution in neurons of the myenteric plexus. The biological actions of this amine in the gastrointestinal tract have recently been reviewed (359). Feeding, intraduodenal instillation of hypertonic glucose solutions, and acid perfusion of the duodenum all produce an elevation of serotonin levels in portal venous blood (26, 260, 261, 316). Vagal nerve stimulation elevates portal venous serotonin concentration and releases the amine into the intestinal lumen (2, 440). Serotonin appears to have variable effects on intestinal blood flow depending on the dose employed, species used, experimental preparation, and the intestinal motor activity (69, 359, 461). Because serotonin is an intestinal vasodilator at low doses in sympathetically innervated preparations (176), the amine could be involved in the postprandial intestinal hyperemia. It appears that the vasodilatory effect of CCK may be mediated through serotonin, because CCK-mediated vasodilation can be abolished by the serotonergic antagonist dihydroergotamine or by making the intestinal vasculature tachyphylactic to serotonin (22, 176). These data imply that if CCK plays a role in the intestinal vascular response to food (as a paracrine agent?), its actions could involve a serotonergic component. Serotonin has also been implicated in the mesenteric vasodilation ascribed to mechanical mucosal stimulation (see LUMINAL STIMULI RESPONSIBLE FOR INTESTINAL HYPEREMIA, p. 1418). The physiological importance of serotonin as a mediator of the postprandial intestinal hyperemia remains to be clearly defined.

Bradykinin has been implicated in the functional intestinal hyperemia associated with food ingestion. Infusion of the polypeptide produces intestinal vasodilation in many species (107, 177, 202, 413). Local intra-arterial infusion of bradykinin significantly dilates the canine intestinal vascular bed (413). Furthermore bradykinin is elevated in the portal venous blood of conscious dogs after intraduodenal instillation of hypertonic glucose solutions (316). Inasmuch as bradykinin has been implicated in the functional hyperemia in both salivary glands and pancreas [(452); see also the chapter by Kvietys, Harper, and Granger in this *Handbook*] the polypeptide could also contribute to postprandial intestinal hyperemia. Further studies are required to delineate the physiological importance of bradykinin in intestinal vasoregulation.

Histamine is an endogenous biologically active amine with an ubiquitous distribution. Histamine is found in large concentrations in the vascular endothelium (225) and in mast cells. It is well documented that the intestinal vasculature dilates in the presence of histamine and that both histamine $H_1$ and $H_2$ receptors are present in the intestinal circulation (63, 108, 199, 345, 371). Studies have implicated histamine in the regulation of postprandial motor activity and alkaline secretion (122, 268). Furthermore, histamine is released from its intestinal storage sites after a meal (412, 495), which suggests that this vasoactive amine may also contribute to postprandial intestinal hyperemia. A recent investigation by Chou and Siregar (78), conducted in exteriorized canine jejunal loops, demonstrated that endogenous histamine may play a role in the functional hyperemia. These researchers found that intrajejunal placement of a mixed meal increases intestinal blood flow by 30%, a response that was attenuated to 15% after pretreatment with the $H_1$-receptor antagonist tripelennamine. This antagonist also blocks the food-induced increase in intestinal $O_2$ uptake. Pretreatment with the $H_2$-receptor antagonist metiamide fails to alter food-mediated increases in blood flow and $O_2$ uptake. Pretreatment with both $H_1$ and $H_2$ blockers produces a response similar to that observed with $H_1$ receptor blockade alone (78). These findings suggest that endogenous histamine acting on $H_1$ receptors may modulate the postprandial intestinal hyperemia. Endogenous histamine may directly dilate the vasculature or work indirectly by stimulating parenchymal cell metabolism. The actual mechanism(s) mediating histamine-induced elevations in blood flow and $O_2$ uptake remain to be delineated.

Prostaglandins are endogenous substances (20-carbon fatty acids) derived from arachidonic acid. These substances have been found in almost every tissue studied, including the splanchnic organs. Prostaglandins encompass a diversified group of compounds with different vasoactivity on the intestinal vasculature. Prostaglandins of the A, B, E, and I type are intestinal vasodilators, whereas those of the F type are vasoconstrictors (461). Prostaglandins of the D type appear to demonstrate both vasodilatory and vasoconstrictor activities (116, 133). Experiments have shown that prostaglandins are synthesized within the splanchnic viscera (17, 106, 264, 410) and that they may regulate gastrointestinal blood flow under steady-state resting conditions (25, 126, 258, 352, 410). Furthermore a recent study in pigs has demonstrated a postprandial rise in intestinal prostaglandin concentration after ingestion of a liquid nutrient meal (93). These findings support the possibility that prostaglandins may contribute to the postprandial intestinal hyperemia.

Investigations conducted in dog and rat jejunal preparations (129, 328, 389) have provided evidence that endogenous prostaglandins may regulate intestinal blood flow during the postprandial state. Intra-arterial or intravenous infusion of the cyclooxygenase inhibitors indomethacin and mefenamic acid reduces resting blood flow and greatly enhances food-mediated increases in jejunal blood flow and $O_2$ uptake (129). Conversely, intravenous or intra-arterial infusion or intraluminal placement of arachidonic acid markedly attenuates food-induced elevations in jejunal blood flow. Luminal arachidonic acid also attenuates food-mediated increases in jejunal $O_2$ uptake (328). The results from these studies suggest that endogenous intestinal prostaglandins may regulate postprandial intestinal hyperemia by limiting food-induced increases in intestinal blood flow and $O_2$ uptake. Although the identity of the specific prostaglandins involved and their mechanism(s) of action are not known, some putative mechanisms have been reported recently: *1*) an antagonistic effect by prostaglandins on endogenous histamine, and *2*) prostaglandin-mediated inhibition of nutrient absorption (10, 130). However, the results of one study suggest that prostacyclin ($PGI_2$) is not an important mediator of the postprandial intestinal hyperemia, because the intestinal vascular and metabolic responses to $PGI_2$ infusion are inconsistent with the responses during an absorptive hyperemia stimulated by active cotransport of glucose with $Na^+$ (115).

INFLUENCE OF BLOOD FLOW
ON INTESTINAL TRANSPORT

*Washout of Flow-Limited Solutes*

Passive absorption of substances from the gut lumen to the circulation involves two major steps. *1*) Diffusion of the solute across the mucosal barrier (unstirred $H_2O$ layer and enterocyte) into the interstitium; this process is governed by the luminal and interstitial concentrations of the absorbed substance, the surface area available for exchange, and the permeability characteristics of the membrane. *2*) Entrance of the absorbed substance into the blood; this stage is determined by the concentration gradient of the absorbed substance between the interstitium and blood, as well as the PS of the capillaries for the solute.

If villous capillary blood flow is zero, the concentration of the absorbed substance will reach diffusion equilibrium between the lumen, interstitium, and blood compartments. Under this condition the concentration gradients driving the passive absorptive process are dissipated and the net solute absorption ceases. The blood flowing through the villous capillaries can sustain passive solute absorption by continuously removing the absorbed substance and thereby maintaining a steep lumen-to-interstitium concentration gradient. The quantitative importance of blood flow in passive solute absorption is determined by the diffusibility of the absorbed substance and the rate of blood flow. For highly diffusible substances, the interstitial solute concentration tends to approximate that in the lumen. In this instance, the rate of blood flow determines the rate of solute absorption, and the absorptive process is flow limited. Similarly, if the absorbed substance is poorly diffusible, the solute concentration in the interstitium is virtually uninfluenced by blood flow. Under these conditions, the rate of diffusion of the solute across the mucosal membrane determines the rate of absorption, i.e., absorption is diffusion limited (320, 321, 490, 491).

There are several reports (317–319, 322–324, 483–489, 492) that describe significant positive correlations between the rate of absorption of highly diffusible substances (e.g., tritiated $H_2O$) and blood flow in the small bowel (Fig. 17). The same researchers also demonstrated that the absorption of less diffusible substances is poorly correlated with blood flow. For example, ethanol absorption was only partially dependent on blood flow, whereas ribitol absorption was completely independent of blood blow. The absorption of highly diffusible (blood flow–limited) substances has been used by several investigators to measure absorptive-site blood flow and total intestinal blood flow (323). The validity of these absorptive-site flow measurements have been questioned on the grounds that highly diffusible solutes are absorbed at a slower rate than predicted because of the countercurrent exchange in the villi. Proponents of the countercurrent theory contend that a significant proportion of some passively absorbed substances diffuse from the venules to arterioles at the villous base. This exchange process should reduce the interstitium-to-blood concentration gradient of the absorbed substance at the villus tip and thereby reduce the absorption rate. Thus a physiological implication of the countercurrent exchange mechanism is that the rate of absorption of highly diffusible solutes is reduced, particularly at low blood flows (310a, 490, 491).

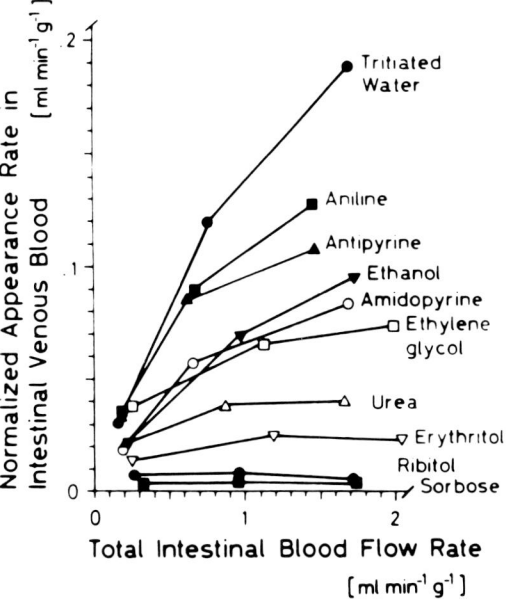

FIG. 17. Dependence of passive solute absorption rate on jejunal blood flow in the rat. [Modified from Winne (491).]

## Effects of Oxygen Delivery on Absorption

Reductions in blood flow not only decrease the rate of removal of flow-limited solutes from the absorptive site, but they may also affect absorption by limiting $O_2$ availability. In the normal small intestine, increasing blood flow above the control value does not alter $O_2$ uptake or glucose absorption rate, which indicates that blood flow is not a limiting factor in $O_2$ delivery or glucose transport. However, if blood flow is reduced, either mechanically or with vasoconstrictors, $O_2$ uptake becomes blood flow dependent (278). Varro et al. (471) have demonstrated that a 50% reduction in canine intestinal blood flow has negligible effects on $O_2$ uptake and glucose absorption rate. When blood flow was reduced by >50%, both absorption rate and $O_2$ uptake declined in a linear fashion, indicating that $O_2$ availability becomes a limiting factor in glucose transport at low blood flows. The effects of reductions in blood flow and $O_2$ delivery on fluid and electrolyte secretion have not been assessed.

## COUNTERCURRENT EXCHANGE

The concept that solutes are exchanged between the venous and arterial limbs of the villous vasculature because of diffusion was first proposed by Butterworth (55, 56, cf. 311) in 1962. However, Lundgren and his co-workers (252–255, 308) have obtained considerable experimental evidence that supports the concept of countercurrent exchange, and they have become the major proponents of the concept. We briefly review in this chapter the anatomical and theoretical bases for the intestinal countercurrent exchanger and the experimental support for its existence. For detailed reviews the reader is referred to several excellent treatises (234, 311, 312, 486).

## Anatomical Basis

The minimal anatomical requirement for a countercurrent exchanger is the presence of parallel blood vessels (artery and vein or artery and capillaries) in which blood is flowing in opposite directions. In some species, i.e., cats, the vascular arrangement in villi of the small intestine meets this minimal requirement because there is an arteriole located centrally in the villous core that gives rise to a plexus of subepithelial capillaries that extend from villous tip to base (60, 136). This hairpin arrangement in which the main directions of blood flow in the two limbs are opposite over a long distance (750 $\mu$m) may not be applicable to other species, such as rabbits and humans. Using scanning electron microscopy of microvascular casts as well as intravital microscopy Gannon et al. (135, 137) demonstrated that villus venules in rabbits and humans drain into a subepithelial capillary plexus only a short distance below the villous tip (~30% of villus height). From this level the subepithelial capillaries receive blood from the villous base and crypts. Thus, in over 60% of the height of the villus, capillary blood flows concurrently to flow in the central arteriole.

Another important anatomical requisite for countercurrent exchange is that all (or most) of the subepithelial capillaries must be situated in close distance from the central villous arteriole. In the cat intestine, this criterion is clearly met inasmuch as the central arteriole and subepithelial capillaries are separated by only 15–20 $\mu$m (308, 486). However, in other species, such as rabbits and humans, the distance from the villous arteriole to subepithelial capillaries ranges between 20 and 250 $\mu$m, with most capillaries situated >75 $\mu$m from the arteriole (137). Thus in human and rabbit villi a countercurrent mechanism is highly unlikely because most of the capillaries are too far from the arteriole and because blood flows in the arteriole and subepithelial capillaries are probably concurrent for most of the villous height.

The efficiency of a villous countercurrent exchanger depends on the permeability characteristics of the central villous arteriole and the subepithelial capillaries. The permeability characteristics of villous capillaries resemble those of other organs, i.e., the capillaries are highly permeable to lipid-soluble compounds (e.g., gases) and small water soluble solutes (e.g., NaCl) yet relatively impermeable to macromolecules (e.g., plasma proteins). The villous capillary plexus can be distinguished from other vascular beds by the large surface area that it provides for the exchange of solutes. In the cat jejunum, the capillary surface area in villi is estimated to be 0.34 $m^2$/100 g of intestine (60). The surface area and solute permeabilities of the central arteriole are likely to be much lower than those of the subepithelial capillary plexus. Thus it is likely that the rate of exchange of compounds between the two limbs of the hairpin loop is limited by the low permeability and surface area of the central arteriole. Whether this factor significantly impairs the efficiency of the intestinal countercurrent exchanger remains uncertain.

## Theoretical Considerations

If countercurrent exchange takes place in intestinal villi then blood-borne solutes may diffuse from the central arteriole to the subepithelial capillary network (Fig. 18A), provided there is a concentration gradient between the two vascular segments and the solute can readily diffuse within the interstitial compartment separating the vessels. This process tends to impair the net transport of the solute to the villous tips via the blood. Conversely, net blood absorption of a highly diffusible solute placed in the gut lumen may be delayed because of the diffusion from the subepithelial capillary network to the central arteriole (Fig. 18B). In this situation the absorbed solute is returned to the villous tip via the central arteriole where it is trapped, and its appearance in the venous drainage from the mucosa is delayed.

An essential requirement for efficient countercurrent exchange within intestinal villi is that the time required for solute diffusion between the central arteriole and subepithelial capillaries must be a minor fraction of the mean transit time for plasma in the villous vasculature. Lundgren and co-workers (24, 314) have estimated the mean transit time in cat villi with an indicator-dilution technique, using $^{198}$Au-labeled colloid particles. This mean transit time is ~5 s at a resting blood flow and it is increased to 20–25 s

at very low blood flows and decreased to 1 s during intense vasodilation (Fig. 19B). The time required for diffusion equilibrium of a solute with a diffusion constant of $10^{-5}$ cm/s (~2 times that of Xe) within the center of a cylinder of various radii has been calculated [Fig. 19A; (238)]. The predicted diffusion time for the hypothetical solute in a cylinder with a radius of 20 $\mu$m (which mimics the situation in cat villi) is only a minor fraction of the villous mean transit time even during maximal vasodilation. However, increasing the radius of the cylinder to 75 $\mu$m (which mimics the situation in rabbits and humans) dramatically prolongs the time for diffusion equilibrium, such that the diffusion time may become a major fraction of the villous mean transit time. Thus one can assume that highly diffusible solutes can rapidly diffuse between vascular limbs of the hairpin loop in cat villi and are therefore easily trapped in the exchanger; however, the efficiency of trapping of the same solute in rabbit and human villi may be relatively impaired because of the long distances involved.

It has also been suggested that the villous microvasculature may function as a countercurrent multiplier (207, 232, 233, 235). This hypothesis implies that the concentration gradient between the subepithelial capillary plexus and central arteriole, created by active-solute transport across the enterocytes, is amplified (or multiplied) because of the relatively slow flow of blood through the hairpin vessels. It is assumed that the $Na^+$-$K^+$ pump (and other transport processes) increases the osmolality in the subepithelial capillaries in the villous tips, and this increase in osmolality is multiplied along the length of the villus because of the

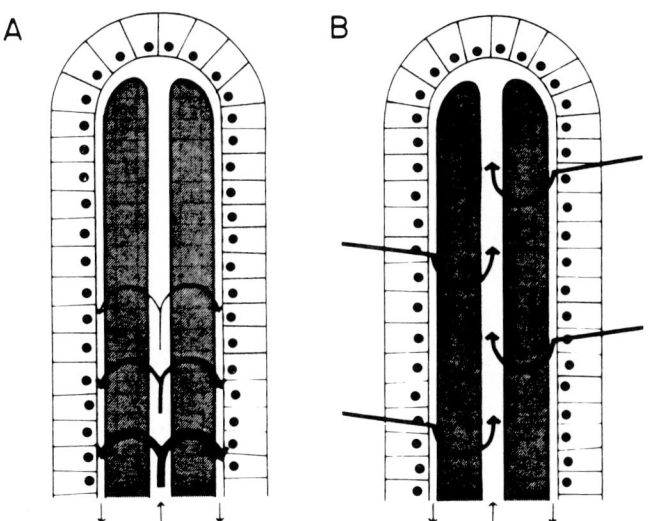

FIG. 18. Patterns of countercurrent exchange of blood-borne (A) and luminally derived (B) solutes. [Modified from Lundgren (311).]

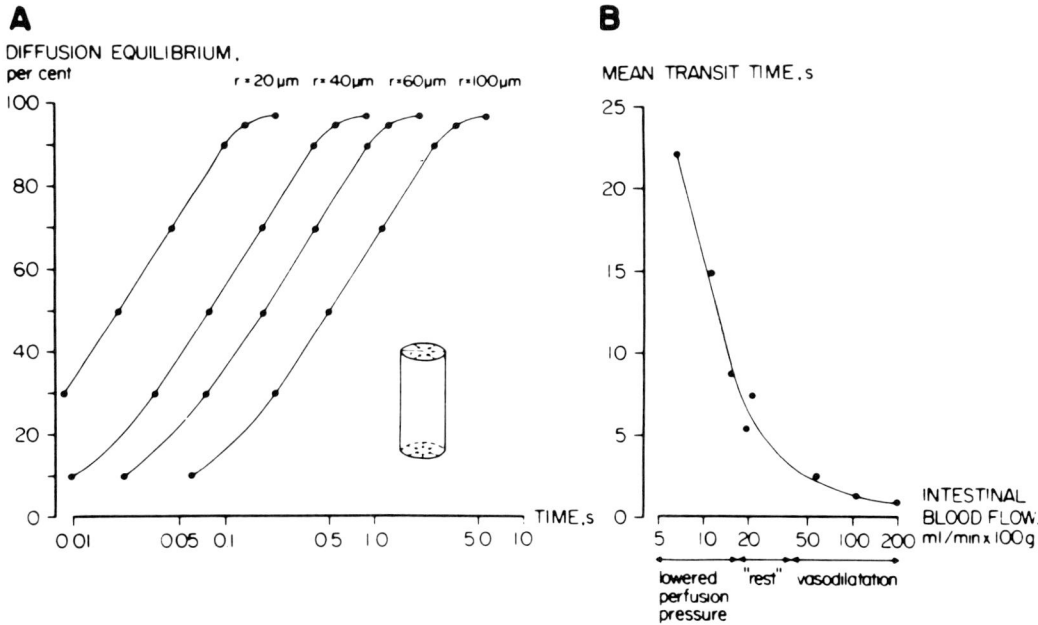

FIG. 19. A, time estimated for attainment of diffusion equilibrium between outer surface and center of cylinders of various radii (r); B, mean transit time of plasma in villous vascular loops of the cat versus total intestinal blood flow. [From Lundgren (311).]

exchange of solutes or water (by osmosis) between the two limbs of the hairpin loop. A number of factors can influence the efficiency of such a countercurrent multiplier: *1*) the solute transport capacity of the enterocytes; *2*) the hydraulic conductivities of the epithelium, subepithelial capillaries, and central arteriole; *3*) the permeability coefficients and osmotic reflection coefficient ($\sigma_d$) for the solute in both limbs of the hairpin loop; and *4*) the rate of villous blood flow. Although the putative villous countercurrent multiplier is often compared with that of the renal medulla, there are significant structural and functional differences between these systems (266). In the kidney, NaCl absorption by the thick segment of the loop of Henle functions as the multiplier, inasmuch as solutes pumped out by the ascending limb continuously reenter into the descending limb. For such a multiplication effect to occur in the intestine, the vascular limbs of the hairpin loop must act as an amplifier. However, this would require active transport of the solute by the capillary endothelium as well as low solute and water permeabilities of villous microvessels. Even the exchange of NaCl or $H_2O$ (driven by osmosis) between the two limbs of the hairpin loop is difficult to envision in light of the high permeability and low $\sigma_d$ value of villous capillaries. Nonetheless there is experimental evidence, albeit indirect, consistent with countercurrent exchange and multiplication of NaCl.

*Experimental Evidence*

COUNTERCURRENT EXCHANGER. The absorption of $H_2$, He, $CH_4$, $^{131}Xe$ from the lumen of the small bowel has been assessed in dogs and compared with their predicted theoretical absorption rates based on the existing villous blood flow and the blood solubility of the gases (36). The measured rates of absorption for these inert gases were substantially lower than predicted. It was concluded that ~85% of $H_2$, He, and $CH_4$ and 56% of $^{131}Xe$ initially taken up by the blood at the villous tip was trapped or shunted during passage down the villus. In cats $^{85}Kr$ absorption was also found to be significantly less than expected for this highly diffusible gas (251). In contrast with the results obtained in the dog and cat, the absorption rate of various inert gases from the rat (306) and rabbit (37) small intestine was in close agreement to predicted rates, i.e., there was no evidence of countercurrent exchange of inert gases. Two possible explanations for the discrepancies can be proposed: *1*) the anatomical basis for a countercurrent exchange system may not be present in the rat or rabbit [this appears to be true for the rabbit (137)] and/or *2*) the relatively widely spaced villi in the rat and rabbit allow the gases to be absorbed at the villous base, thereby bypassing any exchange process that may exist along the villus (234).

During the absorption of radiolabeled long- and short-chain fatty acids a concentration gradient along the villus has been demonstrated autoradiographically in the cat (236, 237). The concentration of absorbed lipids was highest at the tip and lowest at the base. The concentration gradient was steeper during the absorption of the long-chain fatty acid. The gradient for both long- and short-chain fatty acids can be substantially reduced by vasodilation or ischemia. These observations have been offered in support of countercurrent exchange of lipophilic substances within the villi; with the less lipid soluble, short-chain fatty acids are less effected by the exchanger. However, it seems highly unlikely that fatty acid molecules bound to albumin in the vasculature can easily traverse the 25 μm of interstitium separating the two limbs of the exchanger.

A concentration gradient along the villus has also been demonstrated for $[^3H]H_2O$ during absorption from the lumen of the canine intestine (408). The concentration of $[^3H]H_2O$ was twice as great at the tips as at the base of the villi. The concentration gradient for $[^3H]H_2O$ extended all the way down to muscle layer of the small bowel, i.e., the concentration of $[^3H]H_2O$ in the muscle was one-eighth that at the villous tip. These observations suggest that there must be an alternative explanation for the development of a concentration gradient for highly diffusible and permeable substances during their absorption.

Lipophilic solutes should also undergo countercurrent exchange when they arrive at the villi from the blood side. Intra-arterial administration of [*N*-methyl-$^{14}C$]antipyrine resulted in the establishment of a concentration gradient within cat villi (255). Autoradiographic analysis indicated that the labeled antipyrine was localized almost entirely at the base of the villus, as would be expected if there was significant exchange of antipyrine entering the villus. This concentration gradient was abolished by vasodilation.

Oxygen is a highly diffusible gas that has been reported to be shunted at the base of the villus. Because of the physiological implications of this phenomenon, a great deal of attention has been focused on the countercurrent exchange of $O_2$. The shunting of $O_2$ in the villous exchanger has been inferred from the following observations. Oxygen appears 1–2 s earlier than red blood cells in the venous blood after intra-arterial administration (253). A concentration gradient for $O_2$ has been demonstrated in the rat villus with a mean $P_{O_2}$ of 13 mmHg at the tip and 25 mmHg at the base (28). An alternative explanation for the $P_{O_2}$ gradient from the villous base to the tip is that the greater metabolic activity of the enterocytes at the villous tip results in a greater $O_2$ consumption in this region. Levitt et al. (305) in their analysis of countercurrent exchange of $O_2$ suggest that the lower $P_{O_2}$ at the villous tip due to countercurrent exchange is negligible compared with the influence of metabolic activity.

The development of a concentration gradient for $[^3H]H_2O$ from the base to the tip of the villus has been observed during intra-arterial administration of the labeled molecule (408). However, the gradient for [³H]H₂O extended across the entire gut wall with the muscle concentration of [³H]H₂O being roughly 2–3 times that at the villous tip. The establishment of a concentration gradient along regions of the small bowel where no exchanger exists suggests that there must be an alternative explanation for these findings.

COUNTERCURRENT MULTIPLIER. Evidence in favor of the existence of a countercurrent multiplier is based on the demonstration of ionic gradients along the villus. The concentration of Na⁺ has been shown to be higher at the villus tip than at the base during absorption of glucose and electrolytes (30, 207). This gradient is considerably reduced by vasodilation, ischemia, and ouabain (207). Cryoscopic methods have allowed for measurements of tissue osmolalities within different regions of the villi. An osmolality gradient from the villous tip to the base has been described for the cat small intestine (209, 210, 235). The gradient can be reduced by vasodilation and ischemia (235). An osmolality gradient along the villus has also been described in humans (206) and rabbits (311). The latter observations are rather surprising, because the anatomical arrangement of the intervillous circulation as well as the concurrent flow of blood along most of the villus height in humans and rabbits argue against the existence of a countercurrent exchanger, let alone a multiplier, in these two species. An alternative explanation for the tip-to-base osmolality gradient is a corresponding gradient of active NaCl transport along the length of the villus (266).

VASCULAR CAPACITANCE

*Vascular capacitance* is a term applied to the relationship between the total volume contained in the vasculature and the existing transmural pressure (205, 402). The overall capacitance of the intestinal vascular bed is the sum of the capacitance of the arterial, capillary, and venular segments of the vasculature. Inasmuch as 75% (or more) of the total intestinal blood volume is contained within the veins, these vessels are generally referred to as the primary capacitance vessels. Pressure-volume relationships can be obtained in individual mesenteric veins or whole-organ preparations of the intestine (Fig. 20). In general the pressure-volume curves in isolated vessels are curvilinear, (444) whereas those in intestinal segments are linear (248, 404). When the pressure-volume curve is linear, the slope of the relationship (Δvolume/Δpressure) is equal to compliance. Estimates of intestinal vascular compliance range from 0.22 to 0.34 ml·100 g⁻¹·mmHg⁻¹ (248, 404, 405), with a value of 0.25 ml·100 g⁻¹·mmHg⁻¹ taken as the mean (402, 403).

Studies on isolated intestinal veins in vivo or in vitro are limited to large veins and do not include the contribution of the numerous small venules to the

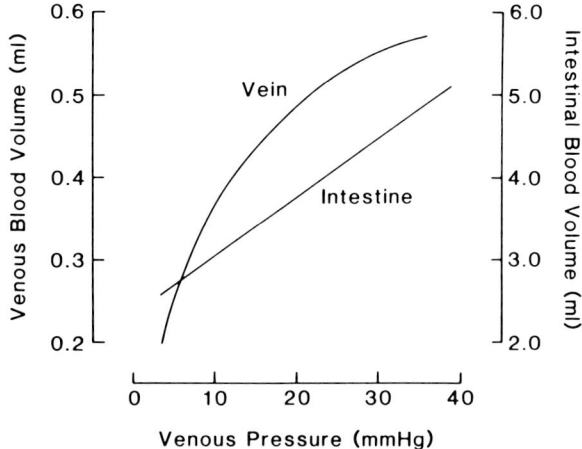

FIG. 20. Relationship between venous pressure and blood volume in an isolated intestinal vein [data from Simon et al. (444)] and in an entire intestinal loop [data from Rothe et al. (404)].

capacitance response. As shown in Figure 20, the blood volume at a normal $P_v$ in an isolated intestinal vein is ~1/10 the blood volume of the segment it drains. Whole-organ approaches, while incorporating the entire venular tree in the capacitance response, suffer from the difficulty in obtaining complete pressure-volume curves. The large increments in $P_v$ (>10 mmHg) necessary to obtain pressure-volume curves also produce large increments in interstitial volume (because of capillary filtration) thereby overestimating the change in blood volume.

The blood volume of the intestine has been estimated to be between 8 and 15 ml/100 g tissue (90, 114, 403) under resting conditions, i.e., normal vascular pressures and blood flows. The blood content of the intestine can be altered by passive and/or active mechanisms. Passive changes in volume are due to elastic recoil or distension of the veins in response to alterations in blood flow or venous (transmural) pressure (403). A doubling of blood flow or $P_v$ will cause an increase in vascular volume of ~20%–30% (405). If blood flow is reduced to zero, while maintaining a normal $P_v$ (~10 mmHg), intestinal volume is reduced by 40%. If $P_v$ is allowed to drop to zero during the no-flow state, the reduction in blood volume is ~65%. Thus the maximum amount of blood that can be expelled from the intestine by passive elastic recoil of the veins is 65% of the resting volume. The intravascular volume remaining in the small intestine when $P_v$ and blood flow are zero is referred to as the unstressed volume (403).

Active changes in intestinal volume are a result of relaxation or contraction of venular smooth muscle. Constriction of the veins increases vessel wall tension and/or decreases the intravascular volume (Fig. 21). Curve A in Figure 21 depicts the effects of venular constriction that results in a decreased compliance with no change in unstressed volume. Curve B is an example of venular constriction that decreases un-

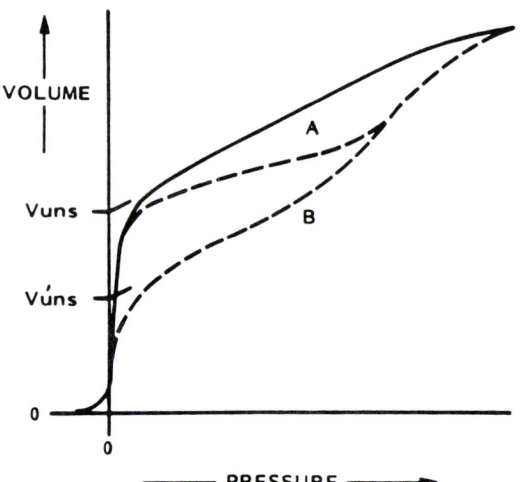

FIG. 21. Effects of venoconstriction on the intestinal pressure-volume relationship. $V_{uns}$, unstressed volume obtained by linear extrapolation of the pressure-volume curve to the volume at zero pressure; curve A, relationship produced by venoconstriction that causes a reduced compliance (slope of curve) without a change in unstressed volume; curve B, relationship produced by venoconstriction that causes a reduced unstressed volume ($V'_{uns}$) without a change in compliance. [From Rothe (403).]

stressed volume yet does not affect compliance. Usually venoconstriction involves decreases in both compliance and unstressed volume. However, Rothe (403) suggests that decreases in unstressed volume play a more important role than decreases in compliance in the intestinal capacitance response to vasoconstrictor stimuli.

Responses of capacitance vessels to various physiological and pathological perturbations are expressed as displacements of the pressure-volume curves (see Fig. 21). Sympathetic nerve stimulation expels 40%–60% of the intestinal blood volume (90, 402). Almost half of the blood volume is mobilized because of passive responses of the vasculature, i.e., elastic recoil due to decreased blood flow (90). Administration of norepinephrine decreases intestinal blood volume, an effect attributed to a decrease in both compliance and unstressed volume (239). Vasodilation with either isoproterenol (405) or papaverine (239) increases unstressed volume with little change in compliance. Arterial hypertension is associated with a decrease in intestinal vascular compliance (444).

Although it is generally agreed that the major site of vascular capacitance lies somewhere distal to the capillaries, the exact site along the venous system is still unresolved. The finding that villous plasma volume is unaffected by elevation in $P_v$ while mucosal blood volume increases suggests that the blood vessels of the villi contribute little to the total vascular capacitance of the intestine (313). However, the observation that the venous occlusion technique and the stop-flow isogravimetric method yield the same values for $P_c$ (174) indicates that the major sites of vascular capacitance and capillary filtration are located in the same segment of the circulation, i.e., at or near the capillaries. More systematic studies to determine the precise location of the major capacitance vessels are warranted.

VASOACTIVE AGENTS AND INTESTINAL OXYGEN UPTAKE

In recent years considerable attention has been devoted to the effects of vasoactive agents on intestinal $O_2$ uptake. The underlying theme of most of these studies is the relation between $O_2$ uptake and blood flow under various physiological and pathological conditions. The effects of vasoactive agents on $O_2$ uptake have been used to assess the relationship between intestinal functional activity and oxygenation (156, 163, 187, 193, 272, 274, 282). Vasoactive agents have not only been used to simulate various circulatory disorders (52, 117, 369, 416) but have also been assessed for their potential usefulness as therapeutic agents in these disorders (45, 52, 117, 416). In this section, the effects of vasodilators and vasoconstrictors on intestinal $O_2$ uptake are discussed in terms of their effects on total (and intramural) blood flow, oxidative metabolism, and perfused capillary density.

*Relation Between Blood Flow and Oxygen Uptake*

Figure 22 illustrates the relations between intestinal blood flow and $O_2$ uptake observed when blood flow is altered with a pump or through graded reductions in perfusion pressure, i.e., in the absence of vasoactive agents. The most frequently observed relationship is one where $O_2$ uptake remains virtually constant over a wide range of blood flows, i.e., $O_2$ uptake is blood flow independent (Fig. 22, curve A). Oxygen uptake is compromised only when blood flow reaches a critically low level. Below this critical blood flow, $O_2$ uptake is considered to be blood flow dependent. Resting intes-

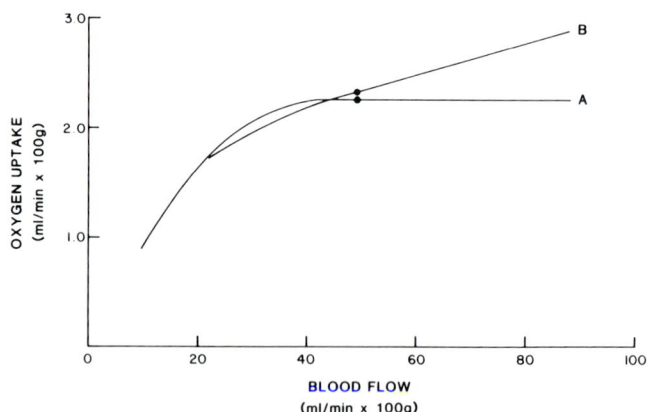

FIG. 22. Examples of blood flow–independent (A) and blood flow–dependent (B) $O_2$ uptake curves for the small intestine. Control value indicated by *closed circle*. [Adapted from Kvietys et al. (285; *curve A*) and from Shepherd (426; *curve B*).]

tinal blood flow is usually greater than the critical blood flow at which $O_2$ uptake is blood flow dependent.

The reduction in $O_2$ uptake below a critical blood flow may be explained in terms of the normal relation between $O_2$ uptake and cell $P_{O_2}$. The relation between $O_2$ uptake and cell $P_{O_2}$ is qualitatively similar to the relation between $O_2$ uptake and blood flow, i.e., $O_2$ uptake remains constant over a wide range of cell $P_{O_2}$ and becomes compromised only at a very low $P_{O_2}$ (the critical $P_{O_2}$) (194, 231). It is generally believed that the normal resting cell $P_{O_2}$ is well above this critical level (194). There is experimental evidence indicating that graded reductions in blood flow produce concomitant reductions in cell $P_{O_2}$ without altering $O_2$ uptake (44). However, at very low blood flows the rate of $O_2$ diffusion to the cells is so low that the intracellular $P_{O_2}$ falls below the critical level required to maintain normal intracellular metabolism. Thus the reduction in $O_2$ uptake observed at low blood flows may simply reflect a depression in oxidative metabolism due to a limited availability of $O_2$.

A less frequently observed relationship between intestinal blood flow and $O_2$ uptake is one where $O_2$ uptake is dependent on blood flow over the entire range of blood flows studied (Fig. 22, curve B). Such relationships between blood flow and $O_2$ uptake have been observed under various experimental conditions. One condition that markedly affects the ability of the intestine to maintain its $O_2$ uptake over a wide range of blood flows is luminal distension. In a preparation of the cat small intestine, $O_2$ uptake is blood flow independent under resting conditions, whereas $O_2$ uptake is blood flow dependent after distension of the bowel to 20 mmHg (357). Another factor that can alter the relation between intestinal blood flow and $O_2$ uptake is the $O_2$-carrying capacity of the blood. Alterations in the hematocrit of arterial blood from normal values impair the ability of the intestine to maintain its $O_2$ uptake during mechanical alterations in blood flow (432). Finally, underperfusion of an organ could result in a situation in which $O_2$ uptake appears to be blood flow dependent. Oxygen uptake is blood flow independent in isolated colon preparations perfused via the caudal mesenteric and middle colic arteries (total perfusion) (52), whereas $O_2$ uptake is blood flow dependent in colons partially perfused via only the caudal mesenteric artery (275, 283). The blood flow dependency of $O_2$ uptake induced by luminal distension, altered hematocrit, or partial perfusion may reflect a significant reduction in $P_{O_2}$ below the critical level in some cells.

The possibility that some of the parenchymal cells may have a $P_{O_2}$ below the critical level even under normal conditions has been addressed (230). It was proposed that the intestine is composed of two regions: one region in which $O_2$ uptake is blood flow independent (well perfused and normoxic) and a second region in which $O_2$ uptake is blood flow dependent (underperfused and hypoxic). According to this conceptual model of the intestinal circulation an increase in blood flow does not alter total intestinal $O_2$ uptake if the increment in flow is directed solely to the normoxic region. An increase in intestinal $O_2$ uptake would occur only if all, or a portion, of the hyperemia is directed to the hypoxic region. A quantitative assessment of this two-component model has been undertaken to predict the various boundary conditions (i.e., assumptions) that must be imposed on the model in order for it to simulate experimental observations (284). The mathematical model used in the analysis was based on current concepts and available data regarding intestinal hemodynamics and $O_2$ exchange. The simulations predict that 30%–70% of the intestine must be hypoxic (regions where $O_2$ uptake is blood flow dependent) in order for the two-component model to adequately explain published observations (132). The existence of such an extensive hypoxic region seems unlikely for the normal intestine. Thus, of the two types of relationships depicted in Figure 22, the one that is most consistent with current concepts regarding intestinal $O_2$ supply and demand (156, 194, 427) is one where $O_2$ uptake is independent of blood flow (curve A).

*Oxidative Metabolism*

The portion of curve A in Figure 22 where $O_2$ uptake is blood flow independent presumably reflects the basal oxidative requirements of the intestine. With this concept in mind one can predict that stimulation or inhibition of oxidative metabolism will shift the plateau of the blood flow–$O_2$-uptake curve upward and downward, respectively. Stimulation of motor (272) or transport (285, 433) activities raises the plateau of the blood flow–$O_2$-uptake curve. Conversely, decreasing intestinal temperature and thereby metabolic rate lowers the plateau [Fig. 23; (285)].

The effects of various vasodilator agents on intestinal $O_2$ uptake can be explained in terms of the relation between blood flow and $O_2$ uptake. Vasodilators that increase oxidative metabolism are expected to shift the plateau of the blood flow–$O_2$-uptake curve upward as shown by pathway A in Figure 24. Drugs that do not affect oxidative metabolism follow the normal curve, as indicated by pathway B. Vasodilators that depress oxidative metabolism shift the plateau downward, as indicated by pathway D. In intestinal preparations that have been shown to exhibit a blood flow–independent $O_2$-uptake curve, the effects of vasodilators on $O_2$ uptake are consistent with the theoretical predictions shown in Figure 24. Dinitrophenol, which increases $O_2$ demand in vitro (262, 302), increases $O_2$ uptake in vivo in a manner consistent with pathway A in Figure 24 (277). Isoproterenol, a drug that does not affect $O_2$ demand in vitro, does not alter $O_2$ uptake in vivo as predicted by pathway B (277). Adenosine, an agent reported to decrease $O_2$ consumption in vitro, decreases $O_2$ uptake in accord with

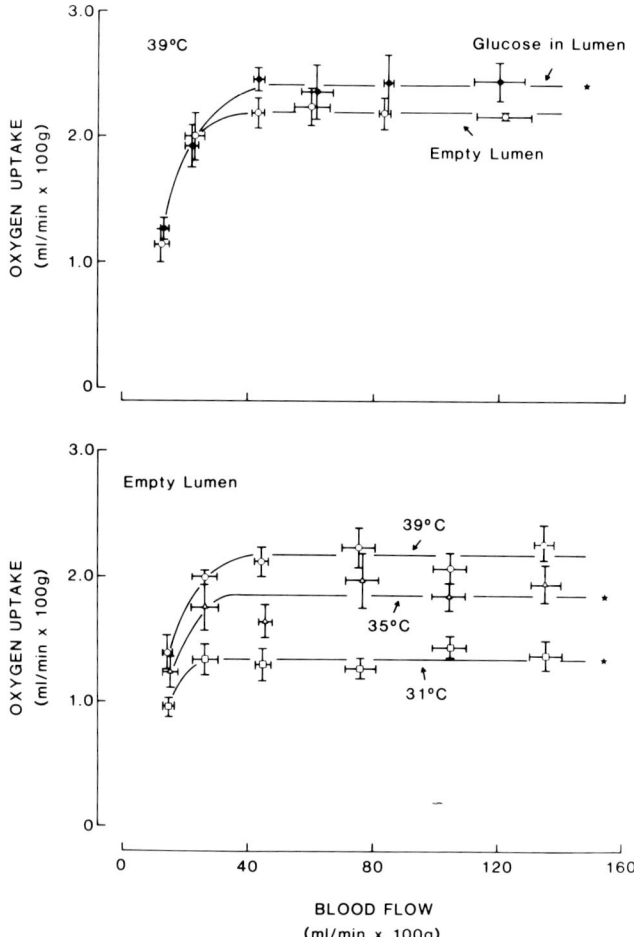

FIG. 23. Effects of intraluminal placement of glucose (*upper panel*) and reductions in luminal temperature (*lower panel*) on relation between ileal $O_2$ demand and blood flow. Relations were obtained by altering blood flow with a pump. *Asterisks* indicate significant ($P < 0.05$) differences in plateau portion of curves from control values (empty lumen at 39°C). [From Kvietys et al. (285).]

pathway D (187, 193, 277). These results suggest that vasodilators will not alter intestinal $O_2$ uptake in autoperfused preparations in which $O_2$ uptake is independent of blood flow, unless they exert an effect (either direct or indirect) on oxidative metabolism.

The available data indicate that vasodilators tend to increase intestinal $O_2$ uptake irrespective of their effects on oxidative metabolism (74, 278). These observations have been attributed (278) to the use of intestinal preparations in which $O_2$ uptake is dependent on blood flow (Fig. 22, curve A). If vasodilators are infused in these preparations, they are expected to increase $O_2$ uptake in accordance with the rise in blood flow. This assumption underscores the importance of establishing the relationship between blood flow and $O_2$ uptake in the same autoperfused preparation in which the effects of vasodilators on $O_2$ uptake are to be assessed.

The effects of vasoconstrictors on $O_2$ uptake can also be predicted from the relation between blood flow and $O_2$ uptake. A vasoconstrictor that decreases oxidative metabolism is expected to shift the blood flow–$O_2$-uptake curve downward, as shown by pathway E in Figure 24. Agents that do not affect oxidative metabolism are expected to decrease $O_2$ uptake by simply following the normal curve, as indicated by pathway G. A vasoconstrictor that increases oxidative metabolism is predicted to either increase, not affect, or decrease $O_2$ uptake (depending on the magnitude of the reduction in blood flow) as indicated by pathway I.

The available data (74, 278) indicate that vasoconstrictors generally decrease intestinal $O_2$ uptake in preparations exhibiting either a normal or an abnormal relation between blood flow and $O_2$ uptake. Agents that depress $O_2$ uptake in vitro [e.g., vasopressin (183) and ouabain (121)] decrease $O_2$ uptake in a manner predicted by pathway E in Figure 24. Angiotensin II, prostaglandin $F_{2\alpha}$ ($PGF_{2\alpha}$), and epinephrine are the only vasoconstrictors that do not consistently decrease intestinal $O_2$ uptake in vivo (74, 278). One possible explanation for the inconsistent effects of angiotensin II and $PGF_{2\alpha}$ on $O_2$ uptake is that when these agents stimulate motility they either do not change or they increase or decrease (370) intestinal $O_2$ uptake (481). Because increases in motility would increase oxidative metabolism (272), the responses to angiotensin II and $PGF_{2\alpha}$ could represent the theoretically predicted effects of vasoconstrictors that increase oxidative metabolism (pathway I in Fig. 24). The ability of epinephrine to decrease intestinal blood

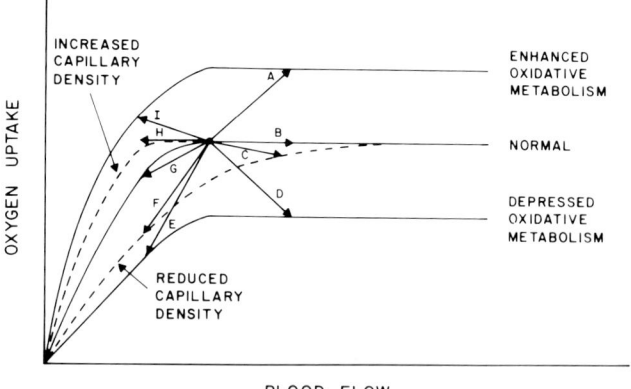

FIG. 24. Relation between blood flow and $O_2$ uptake and factors that alter this relationship. Note that alterations in tissue oxidative metabolism shift curves vertically, whereas alterations in capillary density shift curves horizontally. *Dot* represents control blood flow under normal conditions. *Pathway A*, vasodilator that increases oxidative metabolism; *pathway B*, vasodilator that either does not affect metabolism or increases capillary density; *pathway C*, vasodilator that decreases capillary density; *pathway D*, vasodilator that decreases metabolism; *pathway E*, is taken by vasoconstrictor that decreases metabolism; *pathway F*, vasoconstrictor that decreases capillary density; *pathway G*, vasoconstrictor that does not affect metabolism or capillary density; *pathway H*, vasoconstrictor that increases capillary density; *pathway I*, vasoconstrictor that increases metabolism. [From Kvietys and Granger (278).]

perature is consistent with a $Q_{10}$ for $O_2$ consumption of 2.7 (281). These observations indicate that variations in ambient temperature may explain the wide range of reported intestinal $O_2$ uptake values.

TRANSCAPILLARY FLUID AND SOLUTE EXCHANGE

*Starling Hypothesis*

It has long been recognized that large amounts of water and solutes escape the circulation to enter the interstitium of the intestine. Because the exchange of fluid between the blood and the interstitium is governed by the hydrostatic and colloid osmotic pressure gradients exerted across the microvascular wall and by the permeability and hydraulic conductance characteristics of the capillary barrier, transcapillary fluid exchange is discussed in regard to the Starling relation (455)

$$J_{v,c} = K_{f,c}[(P_c - P_t) - \sigma_d(\pi_c - \pi_t)] \quad (2)$$

where $J_{v,c}$ is the rate of transcapillary fluid movement (filtration occurs when $J_{v,c}$ is positive, and absorption occurs when $J_{v,c}$ is negative), $\pi_c$ is the plasma oncotic pressure, and $\pi_t$ is the interstitial oncotic pressure.

Because the magnitude and direction of water and solute movement between the vascular and interstitial compartments vary with the functional state of the bowel, adjustments in these forces and membrane parameters allow the microcirculation to provide the fluid for epithelial transport during secretion and to remove fluid from the interstitium during absorption without overhydration of the interstitial spaces. However, alterations in the permeability and/or hydraulic conductance characteristics of the microvasculature can lead to an engorgement of the interstitium with capillary filtrate. Interstitial edema is a common feature of diseases of the intestine.

*Rate of Transcapillary Fluid Movement (Lymph Flow)*

It is generally assumed that the rate of lymph flow from a tissue reflects the $J_{v,c}$ value under isogravimetric or isovolumetric conditions (i.e., when the tissue is neither gaining nor losing weight or volume). Steady-state, resting lymph flow values for the small intestine range between 0.02 and 0.08 ml·min$^{-1}$·100 g$^{-1}$ in cats (148, 165, 175, 182, 348) and between 0.13 and 0.38 ml·min$^{-1}$·100 g$^{-1}$ in rats (5, 12). Colonic lymph flow averages approximately one-third the rate measured in the small intestine (170). Some of these differences may not truly reflect differences in the rate of transcapillary fluid movement if significant transepithelial fluid secretion or absorption occurred during the period of lymph flow measurement; i.e., during secretion the rate of transcapillary fluid movement may be significantly underestimated when using lymph flow measurements because a part of the capillary filtrate is removed from the interstitium by the transporting epithelium rather than by the lymphatics. During net transepithelial fluid absorption, lymph flow does not reflect the rate of transcapillary fluid movement, because the absorbed fluid rather than capillary filtrate is removed from the interstitium via the mucosal lymphatics. However, the lymph flow data presented above probably represent reasonable estimates of the rate of transcapillary fluid movement, because these values were usually obtained under conditions favoring minimal transepithelial fluid transport.

The rate of intestinal lymph flow is altered by a variety of conditions that influence transvascular fluid exchange. For example, acute elevation of $P_v$ increases lymph flow in the small intestine and colon (5, 270, 348, 398). Acute elevation of $P_v$ to 30 mmHg can increase lymph flow by as much as 30-fold in the small intestine. Theoretically a 10-mmHg reduction in $\pi_c$ should produce a similar increase in lymph flow as a 10-mmHg increment in $P_v$. However, plasma dilution causes a larger increase in intestinal lymph flow than does venous hypertension (170). Several different hypotheses may explain this observation. *1*) Elevation of $P_v$ may invoke a myogenic constriction of the arterioles thereby minimizing the increase in microvascular pressure, which might otherwise occur with venous hypertension (348). *2*) Although the increase in microvascular hydrostatic pressure is greatest in the venules and least in the arterial capillaries, all microvessels are exposed to the same hypooncotic stress when plasma protein concentration is reduced. *3*) The increased venular diameter associated with venous hypertension may mechanically compress the interstitium and raise interstitial fluid pressure which, in turn, would partially oppose the effect of increased microvascular pressure. Finally *4*), hemodilution may result in vasodilation and thereby increase $P_c$ concomitant with the reduction in $\pi_c$. Further investigation is required to explain the apparent discrepancy between venous hypertension and hypoproteinemia in relation to their effects on fluid exchange.

In addition to venous hypertension and hypoproteinemia, several vasodilator agents and hormones increase intestinal lymph flow, including histamine (345), bradykinin (13), isoproterenol (177), glucagon (164), CCK (173, 466), secretin (173, 291), prostaglandin $E_1$ (PGE$_1$) (181), and diuretics (458). Lymph flow from the small intestine also increases during net fluid absorption (11, 173). However, lymph flow falls during net fluid secretion (151, 168), arterial hypotension (180), and local intra-arterial infusion of hypertonic glucose (304), vasopressin (392), theophylline, and VIP (169).

According to the classic view of lymph formation and flow, the interstitial-to-lymphatic hydrostatic pressure gradient provides the major driving force for lymphatic filling and thus is the primary determinant of lymph flow (349). Although there is direct evidence to support this concept in studies in collecting lymph vessels of rat and guinea pig mesentery (188, 217), no direct evidence exists for whole organs. Nevertheless there is convincing evidence that small intestinal lymph flow is related to steady-state interstitial hydrostatic pressures (348).

*Capillary Filtration Coefficient*

The $K_{f,c}$ provides a direct measure of transcapillary hydraulic conductance which, in turn, represents a product of the microvascular surface area available for exchange and permeability to filtered fluid (366, 397, 399). As such, $K_{f,c}$ is influenced by the size and number of pores in each capillary as well as by the number of perfused capillaries. Thus $K_{f,c}$ relates net fluid filtration (or absorption) to a pressure gradient across the microvascular barrier. In principle the surface area available for exchange may be influenced by at least two factors: the degree of distension of individual capillaries and the number of open capillaries. Although tension in the wall of capillaries is low because of their small radius of curvature, they are not very distensible, and changes in transmural pressure appear to have very little effect on capillary diameter. Consequently the most important influence on surface area is the number of open capillaries.

Most estimates of the $K_{f,c}$ in the intestine have been obtained using gravimetric (volumetric) techniques. These methods involve a sudden elevation of $P_v$. The ensuing volume or weight change consists of two phases: an initial, rapid increase in weight, which is generally attributable to vascular volume changes, and a slower, more prolonged increase caused by transcapillary filtration. The $K_{f,c}$ is then calculated by dividing the slope of the slow (filtration rate) component by the imposed change in $P_c$. The gravimetric (volumetric) techniques suffer from two major potential problems (366, 399). *1*) It is difficult to determine the end point of the vascular distension phase and the beginning of the filtration component, i.e., the magnitude of the elevated filtration rate induced by venous hypertension may be obscured by intravascular volume changes associated with stress relaxation (viscoelastic creep or delayed compliance) of the veins. *2*) The rate of fluid filtration induced by venous hypertension is not constant with time because of readjustments of interstitial forces; as fluid filters out of the blood into the tissues, the $\pi_t$ is reduced and tissue fluid pressure increases. These changes tend to oppose the increase in $P_c$ and thereby limit the accumulation of fluid in the tissues. However, the zero-flow equilibration modification of the standard gravimetric technique minimizes these difficulties (178). In addition, a new method for estimating intestinal $K_{f,c}$ has been described that eliminates the need for weighing an organ or placing it in a plethysmograph (64). The technique, although not in widespread use, should minimize several potential problems associated with traditional techniques, including denervation, tissue manipulation, and problems associated with exteriorization.

A wide variety of pharmacological agents alter $K_{f,c}$ in the intestines (Table 1). In general vasodilators increase whereas vasoconstrictors reduce the $K_{f,c}$ (399). For example, isoproterenol produces a dose-dependent increase in $K_{f,c}$ (114). This direct correlation results from simultaneous relaxation of vascular smooth muscle in resistance vessels and precapillary sphincters. Neither metabolic nor myogenic mechanisms can explain the direct correlation between $K_{f,c}$ and blood flow produced by most vasodilators and vasoconstrictors. Rather, the responses produced by these pharmacological agents indicate that vascular elements controlling perfused capillary density (precapillary sphincters) possess specific receptors for a wide variety of humoral substances and drugs. Although the notion that vasodilators increase $K_{f,c}$ and vasoconstrictors decrease $K_{f,c}$ is generally true, there are some notable exceptions. For example, adenosine produces vasodilation of the small intestine but reduces $K_{f,c}$ (187). This observation may be explained by the fact that adenosine infusion is associated with a redistribution of blood flow away from the mucosa-submucosa to the muscularis (187, 437).

Although most of the $K_{f,c}$ changes listed in Table 1 have been attributed to increased microvascular surface area, some of the physiological, pharmacological, and pathological interventions may produce an increased $K_{f,c}$ as a result of increased vascular permeability. These include hemorrhagic shock (179), bradykinin (177), histamine (345), glucagon (164), and arterial hypoxemia (376). Attempts to attribute changes in $K_{f,c}$ to changes in surface area or permea-

TABLE 1. *Effects of Physiological, Pathological, and Pharmacological Conditions on Capillary Filtration Coefficient in Small Intestine*

| Conditions or Agents That Increase $K_{fc}$ | |
|---|---|
| Glucose absorption | Histamine |
| Arterial hypotension | Secretin |
| Hyperthermia | Aminophylline |
| Denervation | Glucagon |
| Hemorrhagic shock | Acetylcholine |
| Nitroglycerin | Serotonin |
| Isoproterenol | Cholecystokinin |
| Phentolamine | Prostaglandin $E_1$ |
| Neostigmine | Propranolol |
| Bradykinin | Epinephrine |
| Sodium nitroprusside | Cholera toxin |
| Sodium nitrite | Hypoxia |
| Conditions or Agents That Decrease $K_{fc}$ | |
| Sympathetic nerve stimulation | Pentagastrin |
| Luminal distension | Adenosine |
| Portal hypertension | Norepinephrine |
| Acute arterial hypertension | Phenylephrine |
| Hypothermia | Angiotensin II |
| Serotonin | Ergotamine |

$K_{f,c}$, capillary filtration coefficient. [From Granger et al. (162).]

bility are often complicated by the fact that some interventions may produce opposing influences on surface area and permeability. For example, luminal distension is associated with a reduction in the $K_{f,c}$ but may increase vascular permeability (159). Although small changes in capillary pore size should markedly increase $K_{f,c}$ (because flow through cylindrical channels varies by the fourth power of the radius), intestinal $K_{f,c}$ rarely changes by 100% even in conditions (e.g., absorption, ischemia) or with agents (e.g., histamine, $O_2$ radicals) that dramatically alter the permeability of intestinal capillaries to macromolecules. This apparent discrepancy may be explained by the fact that most of the hydraulic conductance across intestinal capillaries occurs through the relatively abundant small pores (47-Å radius), whereas most agents that increase capillary permeability to macromolecules do so by affecting the relatively few large pores (250-Å radius) (460).

The hydraulic conductivity ($L_p$) of single capillaries in intestinal muscle has been measured with microocclusion techniques (143, 145). These data suggest that a high axial gradient in $L_p$ occurs along the length of the capillaries. The $L_p$ may vary by as much as sevenfold between the arterial and the venous ends of the capillary. This technique has not yet been applied to the mucosal capillaries of the small intestine or the colon.

*Capillary Hydrostatic Pressure*

If blood flow and volume of blood in the capillaries are in a steady state, mean $P_c$ can be defined as follows

$$P_c = \dot{Q}_c R_v + P_v \qquad (3)$$

where $\dot{Q}_c$ is capillary blood flow. We can substitute for $\dot{Q}_c$ in terms of pressure and resistance so that

$$P_c = \frac{P_a + P_v(R_a/R_v)}{1 + R_a/R_v} \qquad (4)$$

By this formulation, $P_c$ is localized to a finite point along the length of the capillary, with all the resistance to blood flow located either upstream ($R_a$) or downstream ($R_v$) from this point. However, there is no single anatomical site that corresponds with the location of mean $P_c$ under all conditions. In fact, mean $P_c$ in one capillary may favor filtration, whereas in an adjacent capillary, $P_c$ may be somewhat lower and favor absorption. Although Equations 3 and 4 represent a simplified view of the microcirculation, they can be used as a framework for discussing the factors that determine $P_c$ at any given time.

Capillary pressure has been estimated by gravimetric and venous occlusion methods in the small intestine of dogs, rats, and cats (5, 174, 247). The resting value of $P_c$ in these species at normal portal pressure is 15.5–17.0 mmHg. This value is lower than that measured in skeletal muscle (20 mmHg), which presumably reflects the higher $R_a/R_v$ ratio in the intestine (15:1) than in the skeletal muscle (5:1). The low $P_c$ in the small intestine (compared to skeletal muscle) may be of homeostatic significance, because it prevents excessive capillary filtration in a tissue with a high capillary exchange capacity. The $P_c$ in the colon has not been measured.

It is evident from Equation 4 that intestinal $P_c$ is largely influenced by the $P_a$ and $P_v$ levels. When $P_a$ is increased, only 5%–10% of the incremental change is transmitted to intestinal capillaries. However, an elevation in $P_v$ has a much more profound effect, with 60%–70% of the incremental change transmitted to the capillaries in the cat (247, 348). Venous pressure elevation over a range of 0–30 mmHg is associated with a progressive rise in $R_a$ and a fall in $R_v$ (247). The progressive increase in $R_a/R_v$ ratio caused by venous hypertension reduces the potential change in $P_c$ (assuming $R_a/R_v$ ratio remains at a control level during $P_v$ elevation) by 6.5 mmHg (348). In contrast to the results from the cat small intestine, ~85%–97% of the increment in $P_v$ is transmitted to rat intestinal capillaries (5).

The distribution of pressures across the microcirculation has been measured in the rat (Fig. 26). The results of micropuncture studies clearly indicate that the $P_c$ in the mucosal villi is significantly lower than the $P_c$ in the muscle layers (31). The lower mucosal $P_c$ is primarily determined by the very low resistance of the mucosal venules. A weighted average $P_c$ of 16.8 mmHg for the whole small intestine has been calculated using capillary pressures and relative flows in the various layers (144). This value is in excellent agreement with $P_c$ obtained with the venous occlusion technique (16.6 mmHg) and also compares favorably with $P_c$ estimates derived from volumetric techniques in the cat (15.5 mmHg; ref. 348) and dog (16.4 mmHg; ref. 247).

A variety of humoral and pharmacological agents

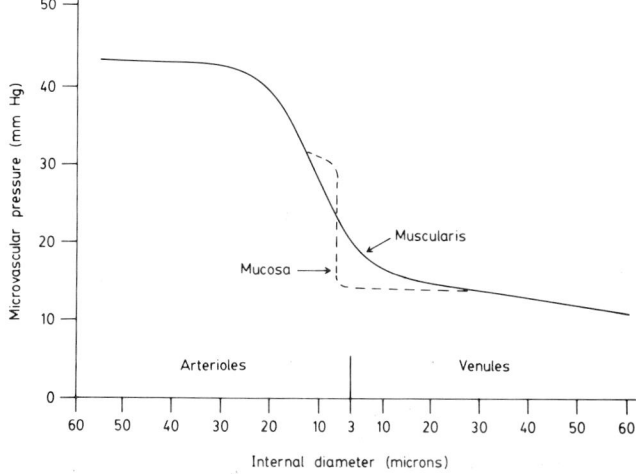

FIG. 26. Distribution of pressures in the microcirculation of the rat small intestine. [From Bohlen and Gore (31).]

alter $P_c$ in the small intestine. In general vasodilators such as glucagon (164), adenosine (187), bradykinin (13), and nitroglycerine (64) increase $P_c$, whereas vasoconstrictors such as vasopressin (392) decrease $P_c$. However, an important factor in considering the net effect of pharmacological agents on $P_c$ is the route of administration. For example, local intra-arterial administration of a vasodilator may cause a decrease in arterial resistance with no change in systemic $P_a$ and thus result in an increase in blood flow and $P_c$. The same drug administered systemically may cause a decrease in arterial resistance as well as a reduction in $P_a$, therefore, blood flow and $P_c$ either remain unaltered or decrease.

### Interstitial Hydrostatic Pressure

Estimates of $P_t$ have been obtained for the small intestine (166) with Guyton's capsule method. Values for $P_t$ have also been determined with micropuncture techniques (295). A final indirect method involves calculation of $P_t$ when the other factors in the Starling relation are known (348); i.e., $P_t = P_c - \sigma_d(\pi_p - \pi_t) - J_L/K_{f,c}$, where $J_L$ is steady-state lymph flow. Although a potential limitation of the capsule technique is that the size of the fluid-pressure measuring device precludes measurements of $P_t$ within a single layer of the small intestine, the $P_t$ values obtained with this method compare favorably with calculated values (166). In general $P_t$ ranges between $-2$ and 2.4 mmHg when $P_a$ is normal and portal pressure is 0–5 mmHg (13, 175, 348). When portal pressure exceeds 5 mmHg, $P_t$ is consistently positive. Micropuncture techniques yield a value of 0.5–1.0 mmHg in the mucosa of the rat small intestine (295).

The value of $P_t$ is determined primarily by the interstitial fluid volume. The relation between interstitial fluid volume and pressure is depicted in Figure 27. The interstitial compliance curve indicates that at normal tissue hydration small changes in interstitial volume cause large changes in interstitial pressure, yet when the tissue becomes edematous, a considerable volume of interstitial fluid can accumulate without altering $P_t$. Thus there are two distinct components to this curve: a low compliance region (0.4 ml·mmHg$^{-1}$·100 g$^{-1}$) at interstitial pressures between $-2$ and 3 mmHg (portal pressure <15 mmHg) and a high compliance region (4.0 ml·mmHg$^{-1}$·100 g$^{-1}$) at $P_t > 3$ mmHg ($P_v > 15$ mmHg) (348). Interstitial fluid pressure has been shown to increase in the intestine during intra-arterial infusion of glucagon (164) or bradykinin (13) and during intestinal absorption (175). Cholera toxin–induced intestinal secretion (297), local arterial hypotension (180), and sympathetic stimulation (148) are associated with a reduction of $P_t$.

### Osmotic Reflection Coefficient

The value of $\sigma_d$ describes the degree of macromolecule restriction by the microvascular wall and as such is the most significant measurement of macromolecule restriction in relation to transcapillary fluid exchange. Because intestinal capillaries are permeable to plasma proteins, only part of the oncotic pressure generated by plasma proteins is exerted across the capillary wall. Thus the $\sigma_d$ describes the fraction of total osmotic pressure generated across a capillary membrane (impermeant proteins generate 100% of their maximum osmotic pressure and $\sigma_d = 1$, whereas freely permeable proteins do not generate an effective oncotic pressure and $\sigma_d = 0$). Estimates of $\sigma_d$ for total protein and various plasma protein fractions have been recently obtained with lymph data (184); a $\sigma_d$ value of $\sim$0.92 has been obtained for cat (184), rat (297), and dog (289, 355). Accordingly, 92% of the oncotic pressure gradient is transmitted across the wall of intestinal capillaries under resting conditions.

### Transcapillary Oncotic Pressure Gradient

If one assumes that lymph provides a valid reflection of interstitial fluid, the transcapillary oncotic pressure can be estimated from lymph and plasma either with an oncometer or from equations that relate protein concentration to oncotic pressure. A recent report demonstrates that lymph in the mesenteric duct of rats has a protein concentration comparable to that of lacteal lymph, which indicates that the collecting duct lymph provides a valid reflection of mucosal interstitial fluid (499). The transcapillary oncotic pressure gradient in the normal resting intestine is $\sim$10 mmHg. Because $\sigma_d > 0$ in intestinal capillaries, a change in capillary filtration rate should alter the transcapillary oncotic pressure gradient, the magnitude of the change being dependent on capillary surface area, $\sigma_d$, lymph flow, interstitial compliance, and the degree of solute exclusion by the interstitial matrix. The transcapillary oncotic pressure gradient increases in response to an increase in $P_c$ if capillary permeability is unaltered. This is primarily a result of

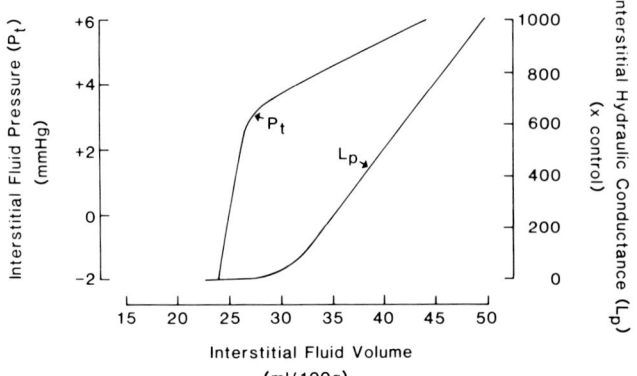

FIG. 27. Steady-state relationship among intestinal interstitial fluid volume, interstitial fluid pressure, and interstitial hydraulic conductance. [From Granger et al. (162).]

dilution of interstitial proteins by an expanded interstitial volume (162).

*Interaction of Capillary and Interstitial Forces*

In the nonabsorbing intestine, the balance of the hydrostatic and oncotic forces governing transcapillary fluid exchange favors net filtration of fluid from the vascular to extravascular compartments (Fig. 28). To maintain a constant interstitial volume, the rate of transcapillary fluid filtration is balanced by an equal outflow of fluid by the lymphatics. However, when excessive fluid enters the interstitium via the blood or lumen, the interstitial forces readjust to prevent dramatic increases in interstitial volume. The interaction between the interstitial forces and lymph flow during $P_v$ elevation, $P_a$ reduction, sympathetic stimulation, net fluid absorption, and net fluid secretion is discussed next.

EDEMA SAFETY FACTORS. Under normal conditions, almost all the fluid present in the interstitium of the intestine is immobilized within the tissue gel. However, alterations in the balance of forces and in the membrane parameters governing capillary fluid exchange may lead to excessive accumulation of free fluid in the interstitial spaces, i.e., to interstitial edema. For example, increased filtration may result from an increase in $P_c$ or $\pi_t$ or from a reduction in $\pi_c$ or lymph flow. If such increases in filtration forces are of sufficient magnitude, edema ensues. However, the intestine, like most other tissues, has the ability to oppose excessive fluid accumulation. This ability has been described as the margin of safety or the safety factor against edema (201). The edema safety factor is quantifiable in terms of mmHg. For example, the safety factor against edema in the small intestine is ~15 mmHg. This implies that the intestine can withstand a 15 mmHg increase in $P_c$ or a 15 mmHg reduction in $\pi_c$ without an excess accumulation of interstitial fluid. However, a rise in $P_c$ in excess of 15 mmHg does produce edema.

Several factors account for the ability of the intestine to resist edema formation. For example, when $P_c$ is increased, fluid is filtered into the interstitium at an increased rate. However, interstitial volume does not increase significantly because of the compliance characteristics of the intestinal interstitium (Fig. 27); i.e., because the interstitium is very noncompliant when $P_t$ is negative, a very small increase in interstitial volume produces a relatively large increase in $P_t$. The rise in $P_t$ effectively opposes the rise in $P_c$. Thus the normal negativity of $P_t$ in the intestine provides one important component of the edema safety factor. However, when $P_t$ exceeds 3 mmHg, interstitial compliance increases dramatically. In this situation, $P_t$ increases only by a small amount when interstitial volume is increased further, and the interstitial pressure component of the margin of safety is no longer effective in attenuating the increase in tissue volume.

A second important component of the edema safety factor is the ability of intestinal lymphatics to remove large quantities of fluid from the tissue spaces when

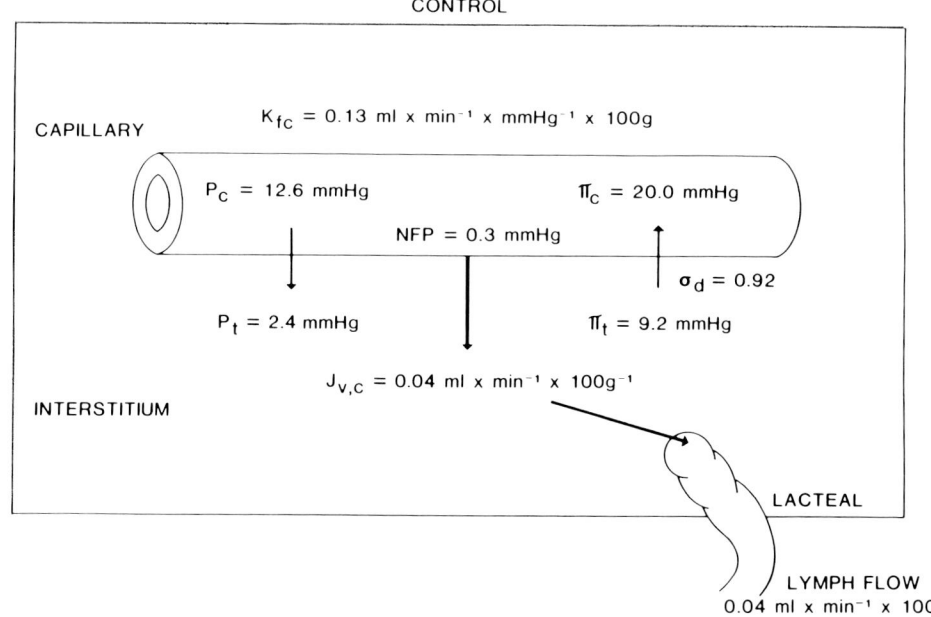

FIG. 28. Starling forces and capillary membrane parameters in the small intestine under control (nontransporting) conditions. $J_{v,c}$, rate of transcapillary fluid movement; $K_{f,c}$, capillary filtration coefficient; $P_c$, capillary hydrostatic pressure; $P_t$, interstitial hydrostatic pressure; $\sigma_d$, osmotic reflection coefficient; $\pi_c$, plasma oncotic pressure; $\pi_t$, interstitial oncotic pressure; NFP, net capillary filtration pressure. [From Granger et al. (162).]

$P_t$ rises. From Figure 27 it is apparent that any perturbation that enhances fluid filtration can cause $P_t$ to rise from its normal value (−2 mmHg) to approximately +3 mmHg. This increase in $P_t$ is associated with a 2- to 3-fold increase in lymph flow. However, when enough fluid has filtered to increase $P_t$ above +3 mmHg, lymph flow increases 10–30-fold. Apparently this biphasic response of lymph flow is the result of alterations in the interstitial resistance to fluid flow. When $P_t$ is less than +3 mmHg, the solid tissue elements (including the mucopolysaccharide gel reticulum) are compacted upon themselves and the tissue fluids are almost entirely entrapped in the gel phase (200, 201). Thus the resistance to fluid flow from the interstitium to initial lymphatics is extremely high. On the other hand, when enough fluid accumulates in the interstitium to raise $P_t$ above a critical level (+3 mmHg), interstitial volume suddenly and rapidly increases (200, 201). This phenomenon is apparently related to the fact that when tissue hydration exceeds a critical level, the tissue elements are no longer compacted, and the elastic rigidity of the interstitium is lost. Consequently much of the tissue fluid becomes free fluid, and the resistance to movement of free fluid in the interstitium decreases dramatically. Thus a high $P_t$ coupled to a low interstitial hydraulic resistance may account for the sudden and dramatic increase in intestinal lymph flow.

The reduction in $\pi_t$ associated with interstitial fluid accumulation also contributes to the edema safety factor. The increased lymph flow that occurs before the development of interstitial edema carries large quantities of relatively protein-rich fluid out of the interstitial spaces. This fluid is replaced by protein-poor capillary filtrate, thereby decreasing the $\pi_t$. The reduction in $\pi_t$ tends to limit further accumulation of edema fluid by opposing capillary filtration. The reduction in $\pi_t$ at high capillary filtration rates involves both the washout and the dilution of interstitial proteins.

VENOUS PRESSURE ELEVATION. The most frequently employed perturbation for study of the interaction of capillary and interstitial forces in the small intestine is acute $P_v$ elevation (244, 247, 348, 480). Wallentin (480) and Johnson (244) were the first to propose that the accumulation of interstitial fluid caused by elevation of intestinal $P_v$ produces compensatory adjustments in the interstitial forces that allow the intestine to regain an isogravimetric state. Wallentin (480) proposed that changes in $P_t$ constitute the major force adjustment caused by elevated $P_c$. However, Johnson (244) and later Yablonski and Lifson (496) suggested that a reduction in $\pi_t$ is the major factor counteracting excessive capillary filtration after $P_v$ elevation.

Mortillaro and Taylor (348) were first to systematically analyze the interactions of capillary and interstitial forces and lymph flow in response to $P_v$ elevation. In their study, estimates of $P_c$, $P_t$, $K_{f,c}$, transcapillary oncotic pressure gradient, and $J_{v,c}$ (lymph flow) were obtained over a range of $P_v$ (0–30 mmHg) in the cat small intestine. These results indicate that $P_v$ elevations induce an increase in both transvascular filtration rate and lymph flow. Accompanying these changes was a progressive reduction in the $K_{f,c}$ and increases in $P_t$ and the transcapillary oncotic pressure gradient (348). These changes tended to limit the accumulation of interstitial fluid in response to increased $P_v$. Thus interstitial fluid volume increased only slightly for $P_v$ elevations of <20 mmHg. However, when portal pressure exceeded 20–30 mmHg, a rapid accumulation of interstitial fluid was observed (348).

Figure 29 compares the safety factors against edema in cat small intestine (348) and in dog colon (398) for an increment in $P_c$ of 12–13 mmHg. The data indicate that the relative contribution of each safety factor to the prevention of edema differs between these organs. In both tissues, the increased oncotic pressure gradient and the increased $P_t$ are the major safety factors, whereas lymph flow plays a less important role, particularly in the colon.

ARTERIAL PRESSURE REDUCTION. The intestinal vascular bed exhibits an intrinsic ability to maintain a relatively constant blood flow over a range of arterial perfusion pressures. Inasmuch as the reduction in total vascular resistance produced by reductions in $P_a$ is generally attributed to a fall in $R_a$, it has been proposed that intestinal $P_c$ and transvascular filtration rate are also autoregulated variables (243, 247). This concept of $P_c$ autoregulation is homeostatically appealing, because with its high $K_{f,c}$ it protects the intestine against drastic loss or accumulation of interstitial fluid in the event of an accidental reduction or elevation in $P_a$. Furthermore, one would expect autoregulation of $P_c$ to be more important in the mucosal layer, because this region of the small bowel exhibits a much higher exchange capacity than other regions of the intestinal wall (243).

Johnson and Hanson (247) were first to propose that $P_c$ is autoregulated in the small intestine. In their

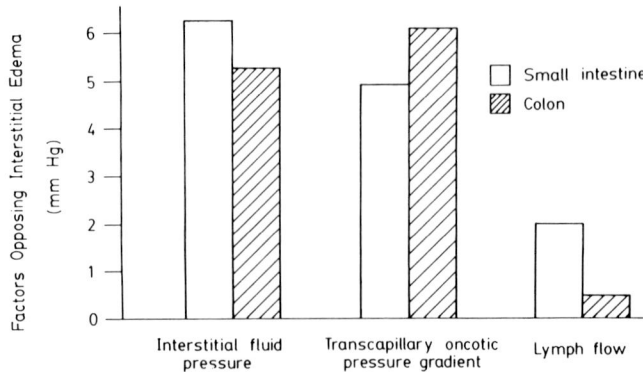

FIG. 29. Safety factors against interstitial edema in the small intestine and the colon for an increment in capillary pressure of 12–13.2 mmHg. [From Granger and Barrowman (147).]

study the zero-flow extrapolation method (366) of estimating $P_c$ was used to examine the effects of changes in $P_a$ on arterial and venous resistances in the isolated dog intestine. With this method it is usually necessary to elevate $P_v$ when $P_a$ is reduced in order to maintain an isogravimetric state and hold $P_c$ constant. In some instances, however, the researchers (247) observed that it was not necessary to increase $P_v$ to maintain an isogravimetric state after $P_a$ reduction. They concluded from this observation that $P_c$ in the intestine is maintained over a wide range of $P_a$ by adjustments in the $R_a/R_v$ ratio (247). Furthermore Johnson and Hanson deduced that an increased $R_v$ is primarily responsible for maintaining $P_c$ when $P_a$ is reduced (247).

Although the hypothesis of Johnson and Hanson is widely accepted, there is some recent evidence that opposes the concept of $P_c$ autoregulation in the small intestine. Bohlen and Gore (31) obtained direct measurements of $P_c$ in rat intestinal muscle at varying $P_a$ values and found that $P_c$ changes in direct linear proportion to systemic $P_a$. The concept of $P_c$ autoregulation has also been reevaluated with a whole-organ approach (167) similar to that used by Johnson and Hanson with one important difference; rather than employing the zero-flow extrapolation method (366), the stop-flow isovolumetric technique was used to measure $P_c$ (244). The latter technique allows the measurement of the $P_c$ at each $P_a$ level. Lymph flow, $K_{f,c}$, and the plasma-lymph oncotic pressure gradient were also monitored to assess the influence of $P_a$ reduction in intestinal transcapillary fluid balance.

A basic premise of this analysis was that autoregulation of $P_c$ should serve to maintain the $J_{v,c}$ (and lymph flow) relatively constant during decreases in $P_a$. However, as $P_a$ was reduced, the lymph flow, the $P_c$, and the transcapillary oncotic pressure gradient decreased while the $K_{f,c}$ increased (167). Although the changes in $R_a$ and $R_v$ during $P_a$ reduction in this study were qualitatively similar to those reported by John-

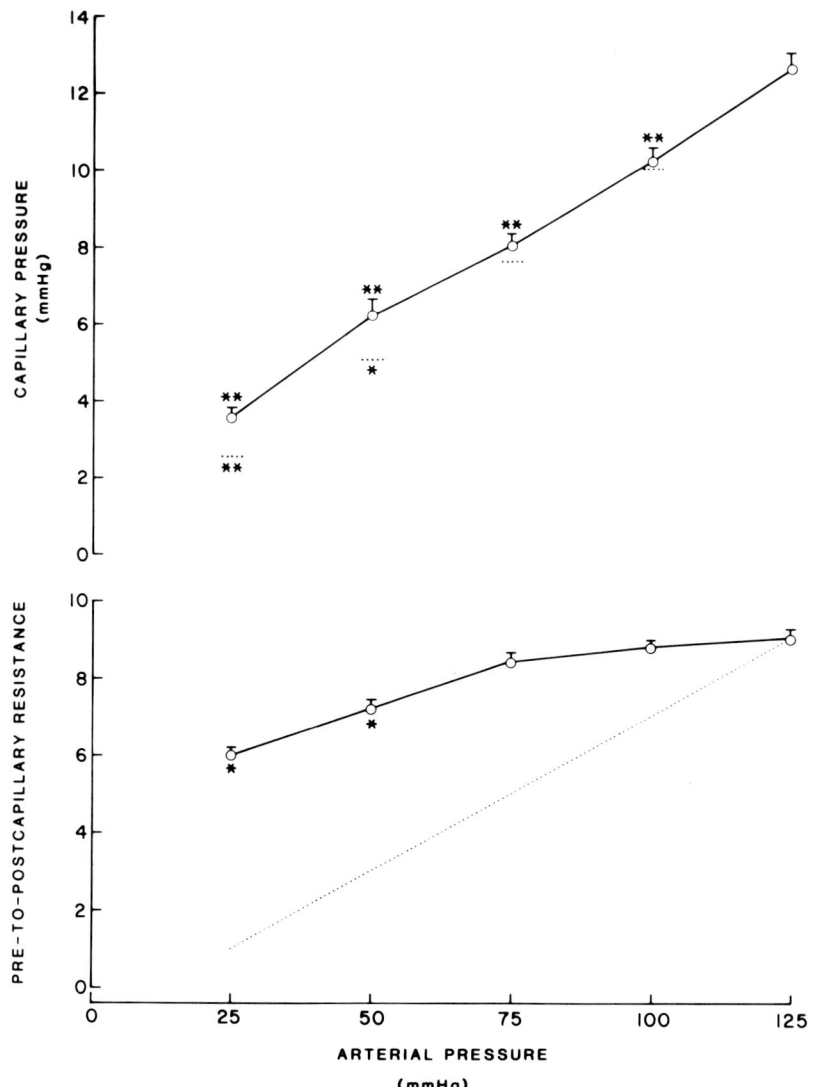

FIG. 30. Relations among intestinal capillary pressure, precapillary-to-postcapillary resistance ratio ($R_a/R_v$), and arterial pressure. *Dotted lines* in *upper panel* represent predicted mean values for capillary pressure, assuming $R_a/R_v$ remained at value obtained at 125 mmHg arterial pressure. *Dotted line* in *lower panel*, $R_a/R_v$ required for perfect autoregulation of capillary pressure. *Asterisks*, statistical significance at $P < 0.05$ (*) and $P < 0.01$ (**) levels as compared with values at 125 mmHg arterial pressure. [From Granger et al. (167).]

son and Hanson (247), the magnitude of the changes in the $R_a/R_v$ ratio were clearly insufficient to keep $P_c$ from falling as $P_a$ was reduced [Fig. 30; (167)]. Over the $P_a$ range of 75–125 mmHg, $P_c$ decreased in a fashion expected from a rigid system. At $P_a$ values of 25–50 mmHg, $R_a/R_v$ ratios fell significantly and the $P_c$ decreased less than predicted for a passive system (167).

The significant reduction in intestinal lymph flow produced by $P_a$ reduction supports the contention that $P_c$ is poorly autoregulated (167). If $P_c$ were well autoregulated, one would expect $J_{v,c}$ (lymph flow) to be relatively unaffected by $P_a$ reduction. However, the decrease in lymph flow is proportionally greater than the decrease in $P_c$ when $P_a$ is reduced. With a reduction in $P_c$, the $P_t$ should decrease while $\pi_t$ should rise. Such changes in interstitial forces would then serve to minimize the decrease in capillary filtration rate produced by a given decrement of $P_c$ (Fig. 31). Calculation of $P_t$ from the mean values of the other factors in Equation 1 indicate a progressive reduction in $P_t$ as $P_a$ is reduced. Because $P_t$ is considered to be the major driving force for lymphatic filling, it is likely that the proportionally large reductions in lymph flow are due to the dramatic decline in $P_t$ as $P_a$ is reduced (167). Thus readjustments in interstitial hydrostatic and oncotic forces and a reduction in lymph flow help to prevent excess dehydration of the intestinal interstitium when $P_a$ is reduced (Fig. 31).

SYMPATHETIC STIMULATION. Stimulation of sympathetic nerve fibers to the small intestine produces several physiological effects. These include vasoconstriction, reductions in capillary exchange capacity ($K_{f,c}$ and PS) and in $O_2$ uptake, and stimulation of $H_2O$ absorption (49, 112–114, 307, 309, 424). The vascular effect of sympathetic stimulation is characterized by an initial marked reduction in blood flow followed by a gradual return of blood flow toward normal values (autoregulatory escape) (112). It has been proposed (310) that mean intestinal $P_c$ and $J_{v,c}$ remain largely unchanged from control values during the steady-state phase of sympathetic vasoconstriction, i.e., after autoregulatory escape.

The concept of $P_c$ autoregulation is based entirely on the observation that intestinal weight remains fairly constant during the steady-state phase of sympathetic vasoconstriction (112, 307). However, direct micropuncture measurements of microvascular pressures in the intestinal muscle layer indicate that $P_c$ is significantly reduced during sympathetic activation, suggesting that $P_c$ is not autoregulated (32). This phenomenon has recently been reevaluated in cat small intestine; whole-organ estimates of $P_c$, $P_t$, $K_{f,c}$, transcapillary oncotic pressure gradient, and $J_{v,c}$ (lymph flow) were obtained prior to and during postganglionic sympathetic nerve stimulation (148). The results of this study indicate that sympathetic activation significantly reduces both $P_c$ and $J_{v,c}$ in the cat

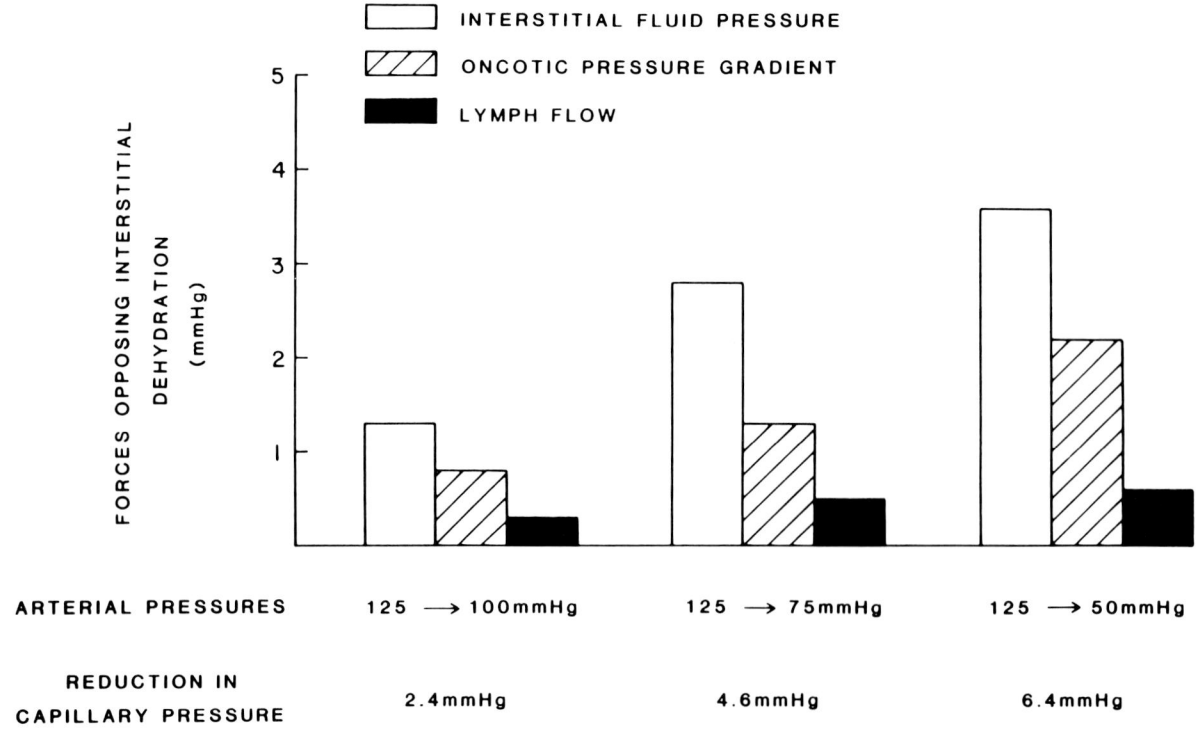

FIG. 31. Effects of changes in lymph flow, interstitial fluid pressure, and interstitial oncotic pressure on preventing interstitial dehydration in intestine during reductions in arterial and capillary pressures. [From Granger et al. (167).]

small intestine (148). The reduction in $P_c$ induced by sympathetic stimulation resulted primarily from an increased $R_a$ while $R_v$ was largely unaltered (148). It was also noted that $P_t$ and the transcapillary oncotic pressure gradient were reduced by sympathetic stimulation (Fig. 32), which is similar to the response to interstitial dehydration (148). These readjustments in tissue forces (decreased $P_t$, increased $\pi_t$) are qualitatively similar to those produced by lowering $P_a$ to the gut and serve to oppose excess dehydration of the interstitial spaces.

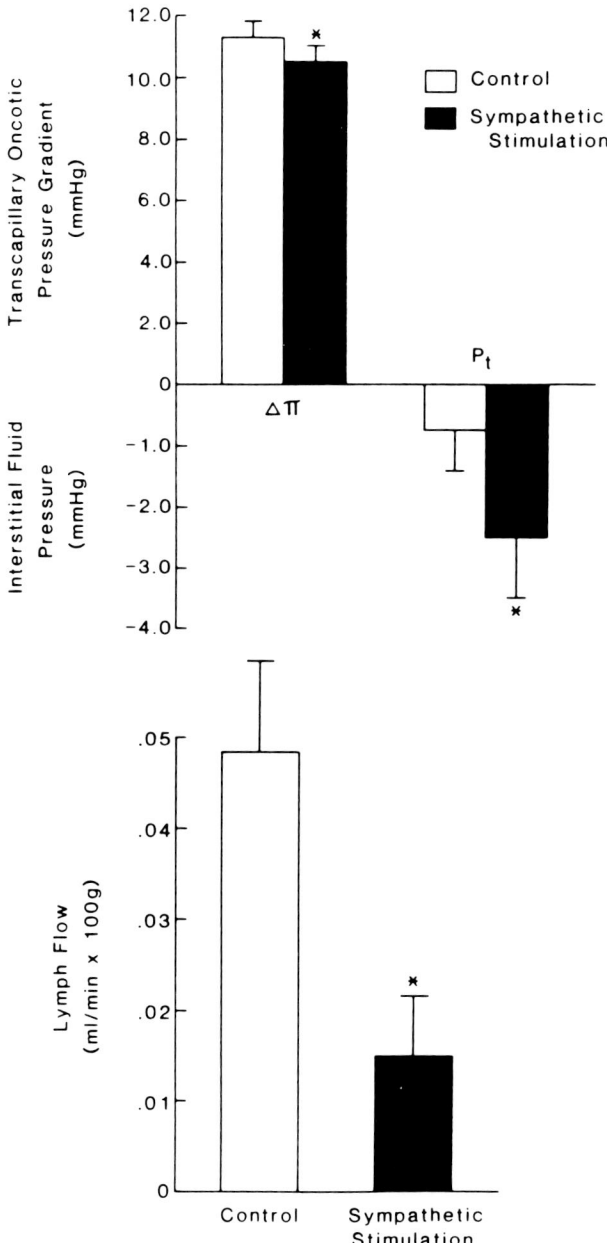

FIG. 32. Effects of sympathetic stimulation on intestinal transcapillary fluid exchange. $P_t$, interstitial fluid pressure; $\Delta\pi$, transcapillary oncotic pressure difference; *, $P < 0.05$. [From Granger et al. (148).]

In addition to the aforementioned changes in the Starling forces, sympathetic stimulation is also associated with a persistent reduction in the $K_{f,c}$ (148). This observation is consistent with the results of several published reports that indicate that there is a sustained increase in precapillary sphincter tone in the intestine during sympathetic activation (113, 424). The dramatic capillary derecruitment produced by sympathetic stimulation significantly reduces the transport capacity of the intestinal microvasculature and thereby limits the amount of fluid filtered for a given net filtration pressure. The relative magnitudes of the decrements of $K_{f,c}$ and lymph flow are comparable, which indicates that net capillary filtration pressure is only slightly reduced (because of the readjustment of tissue forces) and that the reduction in $K_{f,c}$ is the primary factor accounting for the decreased $J_{v,c}$ (lymph flow) during sympathetic stimulation (148).

NET FLUID ABSORPTION. *Role of the interstitium.* The first compartment exposed to absorbed $H_2O$ in the intestine is the interstitium. Accumulation of absorbed $H_2O$ in the interstitial spaces of the lamina propria initiates a series of physical changes in the interstitial matrix that ultimately facilitate the removal of absorbed fluid via blood and lymph capillaries.

Whole-organ studies using different extracellular markers (e.g., sucrose) indicate that interstitial volume in the nonabsorbing small bowel is 18–27 ml/100 g tissue (162, 165, 257). In vitro estimates of the extracellular space in the mucosal and serosal layers of everted rat jejunum indicate that the mucosal extracellular space is four times smaller than that of the serosa (162). The effect of net $H_2O$ absorption on total wall interstitial volume has been examined in autoperfused segments of cat ileum (165). As illustrated in Figure 33 there is a positive linear correlation between interstitial volume and net fluid absorption rate. On the basis of this relationship, a doubling of interstitial volume is predicted at absorption rates >1.80 ml·min$^{-1}$·100 g$^{-1}$. If one assumes that the increment in interstitial volume occurs exclusively in the mucosal layer of the bowel wall and that this compartment comprises one-fourth to one-fifth the total organ interstitial volume (162), substantially larger increments in interstitial volume may occur in the mucosa during absorption (186).

There are several physiological consequences of the interstitial volume expansion that are observed during net fluid absorption in the intestine. These include *1*) an increased hydraulic conductivity of the interstitial matrix, *2*) a reduction in the ability of the interstitium to retard the diffusive and convective migration of solutes, *3*) an increase in $P_t$, and *4*) a reduction in $\pi_t$.

*Interstitial hydraulic conductance.* Because mucopolysaccharides tend to immobilize interstitial fluid, the hydraulic conductivity of the normally hydrated

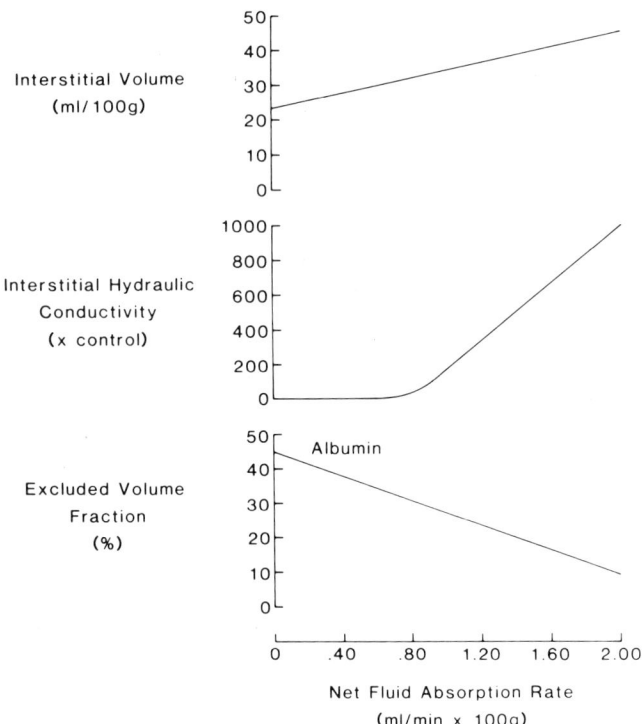

FIG. 33. Effects of net fluid absorption rate on intestinal interstitial volume, interstitial hydraulic conductivity, and the excluded volume fraction of albumin. [From Granger et al. (162).]

interstitium is quite low (165, 188, 189, 195). In vitro and in vivo studies have clearly demonstrated that interstitial hydraulic conductivity increases greatly as matrix hydration increases. Figure 33 illustrates the effects of interstitial volume expansion caused by net fluid absorption on tissue hydraulic conductivity predicted from the aforementioned studies. This relationship indicates that interstitial hydraulic conductivity increases to ~200 times the nonabsorptive value at an absorption rate of 1.0 ml·min$^{-1}$·100 g$^{-1}$ and increases 1,000-fold at a rate of 2.0 ml·min$^{-1}$·100 g$^{-1}$. Such profound changes in hydraulic conductivity should allow small hydrostatic pressure gradients within the mucosal interstitium to move large amounts of fluid between the epithelia and microvessels (blood and lymph).

Solute mobility. The effects of the interstitial matrix on solute diffusion are nearly as dramatic as its impact on the hydraulic flow of $H_2O$ (189, 195). The restricted diffusion of solutes (e.g., albumin) through the normally hydrated interstitium results from the exclusion phenomenon and the frictional interaction of solutes with the matrix. The exclusion phenomenon describes the ability of a gel (e.g., the interstitium) to exclude solutes from a portion of the available intragel $H_2O$. Albumin is normally distributed in only 40% of the total matrix $H_2O$ volume, because it cannot fit into certain parts of the meshwork with a high matrix density. The interstitial volume expansion associated with fluid absorption leads to a reduction in the extent of albumin exclusion within the intestinal interstitium (Fig. 33). On the basis of albumin exclusion estimates in the nonabsorptive state, one can predict that the rate of diffusion of albumin in the interstitium is reduced by at least one-third its velocity in $H_2O$, because the volume or effective surface area for diffusion is limited by the exclusion effect. A further reduction of albumin movement (both diffusive and convective) through the interstitium occurs as a result of steric interaction between the solute and that portion of the matrix that it can penetrate. A dramatic rise in the diffusive and convective movement of albumin in the matrix occurs during absorption. The degree of albumin exclusion falls to <10% at high absorption rates. Therefore the area available for diffusive exchange increases significantly. A more substantial increment in interstitial solute mobility results from the diminished steric interaction between the solute and matrix associated with interstitial volume expansion. In fact, the equivalent pore radius of the matrix rises from ~200 Å in the nonabsorptive state to >1,000 Å in the absorptive state (165, 186).

Hydrostatic and oncotic forces. The most important physiological consequence of the interstitial volume expansion associated with intestinal fluid absorption is the alteration of interstitial hydrostatic and oncotic pressures. Mathematical analyses (429) and results from capillary filtration studies in the intestine (348) suggest that the magnitude of the increment in interstitial volume during fluid absorption significantly alters the interstitial forces, i.e., increases $P_t$ and decreases $\pi_t$. These changes enhance the removal of absorbed fluid from the lamina propria by 1) opposing further capillary filtration and converting filtering capillaries to absorbing capillaries and 2) providing an increased hydrostatic pressure gradient for lymphatic filling (186).

There are relatively few estimates of $P_t$ during absorption (175). Two indirect approaches have been used to obtain them: micropuncture measurements of central lacteal pressure (295) and calculation of interstitial pressure from Starling force measurements (175). Because of the highly permeable nature of the lymphatic wall, it can be assumed that central lacteal pressure should approximate $P_t$ under steady-state conditions. The relation between $P_t$ (lacteal) and net fluid absorption rate is presented in Figure 34. Although lacteal pressure was measured over a narrow range of absorption rates, it appears that $P_t$ increases significantly as absorption rate increases, presumably because of progressive interstitial volume expansion. Interstitial hydrostatic pressure calculated from Starling force measurements in the absorptive state indicates that $P_t$ approaches a maximal value at absorption rates >0.50 ml·min$^{-1}$·100 g$^{-1}$. On the basis of these data and the reported changes in interstitial volume during fluid absorption (Fig. 33), an interstitial compliance of 3.5 ml/mmHg is predicted. This value agrees favorably with the interstitial compliance (4.0

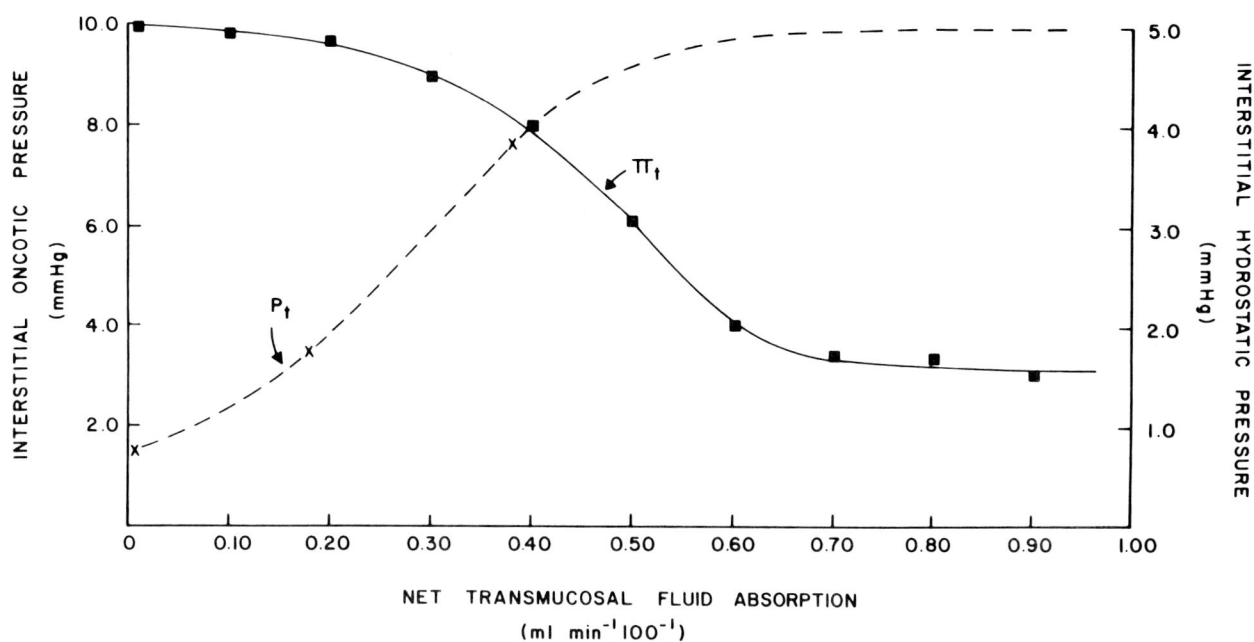

FIG. 34. Steady-state relations between interstitial hydrostatic ($P_t$) and oncotic ($\pi_t$) pressures and net fluid absorption rate. [From Granger (146).]

ml/mmHg/100 g) reported for the same preparation during periods of enhanced capillary filtration (348).

Direct measurements of $\pi_t$ changes induced by net fluid absorption have not been performed to date because of the limited size of the interstitial spaces. However, the indirect approach of using lymph oncotic pressure as an estimate of interstitial fluid oncotic pressure has been extensively applied to the small bowel (147). There are several studies that describe the influence of net fluid absorption on intestinal lymph protein concentration or lymph oncotic pressure (11, 14, 20, 49, 182, 296, 299, 466). The results obtained from these studies indicate that $\pi_t$ is reduced by 2–7 mmHg (from a normal value of 10 mmHg) during fluid absorption. Furthermore the results indicate that the magnitude of the reduction in $\pi_t$ is dependent on net fluid absorption rate (Fig. 34). At absorption rates <0.30 ml·min$^{-1}$·100 g$^{-1}$ the $\pi_t$ is minimally reduced (when $P_t$ is increasing). However, at higher rates of fluid absorption, $\pi_t$ decreases by as much as 6–7 mmHg.

The dependence of the interstitial (hydrostatic and oncotic) pressures on net fluid absorption rate has been attributed to differences in interstitial compliance at normal and increased interstitial volumes. Mortillaro and Taylor (348) have demonstrated a significant increase (0.40–4.00 ml/mmHg) in interstitial compliance when interstitial volume is increased by >3.0 ml/100 g intestine because of enhanced capillary filtration. Increments in interstitial volume <3.0 ml/100 g produce a dramatic increase in $P_t$, yet $\pi_t$ is minimally altered. This contrasts with the large reductions in $\pi_t$ and the slight changes in $P_t$ observed when interstitial volume increases by >3.0 ml/100 g.

During net fluid absorption, interstitial volume does not increase by 3.0 ml/100 g until the absorption rate exceeds 0.30 ml·min$^{-1}$·100 g$^{-1}$, the point at which $\pi_t$ is significantly influenced by absorption rate. Therefore the interstitial hydrostatic and oncotic pressure changes induced by varying absorption rates are consistent with the capillary filtration studies of Mortillaro and Taylor (348) and the hypothesis that the compliance of the interstitium increases when it is sufficiently expanded.

*Role of the lymphatics.* The rise in $P_t$ produced by net fluid absorption should lead to an increased rate of intestinal lymph formation. There are numerous reports describing an increased intestinal or thoracic duct lymph flow after a meal or fluid ingestion (11, 14, 20, 42, 49, 292, 293, 298). Intestinal lymph flow in the cat in the nonabsorptive state generally ranges between 0.02 and 0.08 ml·min$^{-1}$·100 g$^{-1}$. During net fluid absorption, lymph flow can increase to values as high as 0.45 ml·min$^{-1}$·100 g$^{-1}$ (165). The magnitude of the increase in lymph flow during fluid absorption appears to be quite variable. This variability has been attributed to factors such as tonicity of fluid placed in the lumen, portal vein pressure, intraenteric pressure, motility, and the use of lymph contaminated by contributions from other tissues (e.g., liver). If these factors are held constant or eliminated, the rate of fluid absorption becomes a major determinant of intestinal lymph flow. The dependence of lymph flow on fluid absorption rate presumably results from the fact that interstitial volume and hydrostatic pressure are directly related to absorption rate.

The relative fraction of absorbed fluid that is removed from the mucosal interstitium by the lymphatics and capillaries has been studied by numerous investigators (11, 14, 20, 42, 49, 298). In 1684 Leeuwenhoek (cf. 162) concluded, based on microscopic observations of the blood and lymph circulations of intestinal villi, that capillaries are the primary conduits for removal of absorbed nutrients and $H_2O$. Although twentieth century estimates of the fraction of $H_2O$ leaving the intestine via lymph vessels range between 1% and 85% (146), most of the recent studies support Leeuwenhoek's assertion. Only at low absorption rates does the lymphatic contribution exceed 50% (Fig. 35). At absorption rates >0.20 $ml \cdot min^{-1} \cdot 100\ g^{-1}$, the capillaries are the major route for removal of absorbed fluid from the interstitium, accounting for ≦85% of the total volume removed.

The differential role of capillaries and lymphatics in removing absorbed fluid when absorption rate is altered is consistent with the concept of a change in interstitial compliance at a low absorption rate. At low absorption rates, $P_t$ increases but $\pi_t$ is virtually unaltered (Fig. 34). The increased hydrostatic pressure should preferentially drive fluid into the lymphatics, because the hydraulic conductance of these vessels is greater than that of the capillaries. As fluid absorption rate is increased, $\pi_t$ falls, and the driving force for lymphatic filling increases by only a small amount (because both interstitial forces act across the capillary wall, but only the hydrostatic pressure is involved in lymphatic filling). Thus absorbed fluid is preferentially removed through the capillaries at high absorption rates (186).

*Role of the capillaries.* Although the available evidence indicates that the change in interstitial forces induced by interstitial volume expansion is the primary event leading to vascular removal of absorbed fluid, alterations in capillary forces, surface area, and permeability appear to modify this response.

Capillary pressure. The $P_c$ may increase during net fluid absorption because of the well-documented intestinal hyperemia associated with food ingestion or placement of nutrients in the bowel lumen (160). The postprandial intestinal hyperemia usually involves an increase in blood flow between 10% and 60%, and the magnitude of the increase depends on the nutrients placed in the lumen (see *Postprandial Intestinal Hyperemia*, p. 1416). If the reduction in vascular resistance during absorption occurs exclusively in the mucosal layer and it is limited to the precapillary (arteriolar) segment of the vasculature, one might expect an increment in $P_c$ ranging between 0.5 and 3.0 mmHg. The only available estimate of $P_c$ during absorption was derived from whole-organ gravimetric procedures and involved luminal perfusion with a glucose-electrolyte solution (175). The 16% increase in blood flow induced by glucose absorption produced a 1.1-mmHg increase in intestinal $P_c$. Although this increment in $P_c$ appears small and inconsequential, the fact that it is ~½ the net capillary absorptive force indicates that it significantly reduces the driving force for movement of absorbed fluid from the interstitium into the capillaries. The physiological advantage of the "braking effect" of $P_c$ on capillary fluid exchange during absorption remains uncertain. However, there is evidence that large increases in $P_c$ induced by local intraarterial infusion of a selective mucosal vasodilator do not alter the absolute or relative amounts of absorbed fluid removed by intestinal capillaries (49).

Plasma oncotic pressure. Another important intracapillary force that may influence the rate of entry of absorbed fluid into the capillary is $\pi_c$. One might

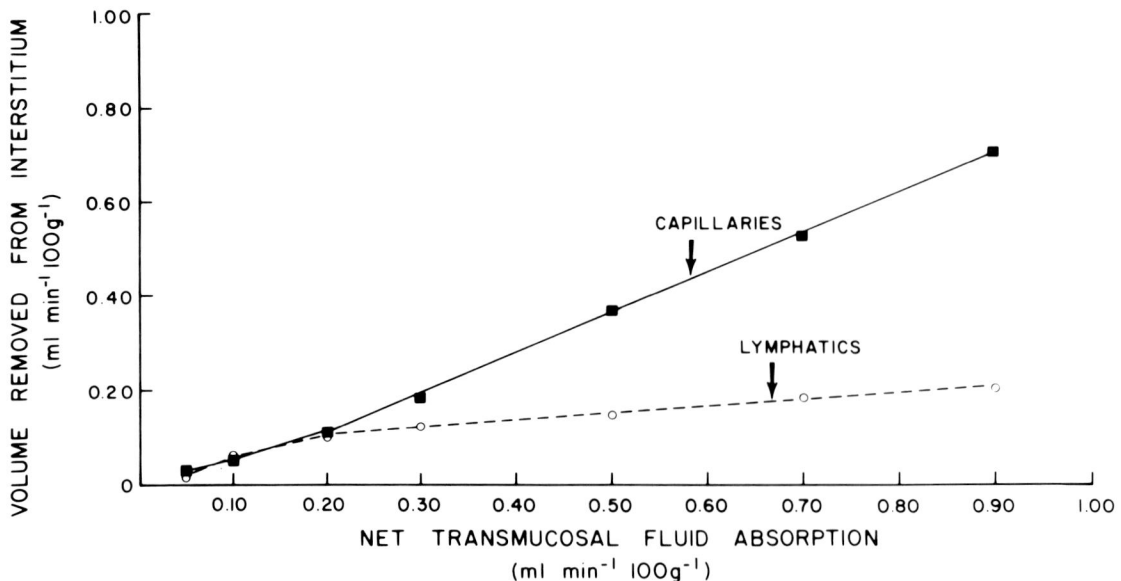

FIG. 35. Steady-state relations between rate of removal of absorbed fluid by intestinal capillaries and lymphatics and net fluid absorption rate. [From Granger (146).]

expect capillary oncotic pressure to be reduced if absorbed fluid enters the capillary at a rate sufficient to dilute plasma proteins, as occurs in the peritubular capillaries of the kidney. Because net fluid absorption rate is usually <5% of total intestinal plasma flow, it is not surprising that arteriovenous oncotic pressure differences cannot be detected in whole-organ preparations. However, if estimates of villus or absorptive-site blood flow are considered, then the extent of plasma dilution in those subepithelial capillaries involved in the absorptive process may be large. Estimates of absorptive-site blood flow, based on inert-gas clearance, indicator dilution, or microsphere techniques, generally range between 5 and 8 ml·min$^{-1}$·100 g$^{-1}$ intestine (323). On the basis of a net H$_2$O absorption rate of 1.0 ml·min$^{-1}$·100 g$^{-1}$, $\pi_c$ is predicted to fall by 3–4 mmHg because of dilution of blood at the absorptive site. If capillary oncotic pressure is indeed reduced by this amount, the net driving force for movement of absorbed fluid from interstitium to blood will be greatly diminished along the length of the capillaries.

*Capillary filtration coefficient.* There are several studies that demonstrate an effect of glucose-electrolyte absorption on the intestinal $K_{f,c}$ (175, 285, 425). The $K_{f,c}$ increases by 43%–300% during glucose absorption, an effect attributed to capillary recruitment. The contention that capillary recruitment is responsible for the rise in $K_{f,c}$ associated with absorption is supported by reports that PS for rubidium is also increased during absorption (425). Regardless of whether the absorption-induced increase in $K_{f,c}$ is entirely due to capillary recruitment or is a combination of increased vascular permeability and recruitment, the fact that capillary hydraulic conductance increases during absorption is of great physiological importance, because $K_{f,c}$ determines the imbalance in transcapillary forces that is required to move a given volume of absorbed fluid from the interstitium to blood. For example, a net absorptive force of only 2.0 mmHg is required to move 0.60 ml·min$^{-1}$·100 g$^{-1}$ of fluid into the capillaries when $K_{f,c}$ is 0.30 ml·min$^{-1}$·mmHg$^{-1}$·100 g$^{-1}$ (double normal), whereas a force of 4.0 mmHg is required if $K_{f,c}$ is unchanged from control (186).

*Osmotic reflection coefficient.* Although intestinal vascular permeability is not altered during the absorption of glucose or electrolytes, fat absorption is associated with a pronounced reduction in the $\sigma_d$ from 0.92 to 0.70 (174). It is clear that such a dramatic reduction should modify the rate of removal of absorbed fluid via the capillaries. A reduction in the $\sigma_d$ from 0.92 to 0.70 could decrease the effective absorptive force, due to the transcapillary oncotic pressure gradient, by as much as 3.0 mmHg. A decrement in the net absorptive force of this magnitude would dramatically reduce the effectiveness of capillaries in removing absorbed fluid, provided $K_{f,c}$ remains unchanged. Because an increased vascular permeability should lead to a rise in $K_{f,c}$, it is possible that the resulting small absorptive force is still sufficient to drive fluid into the capillaries.

*Interplay of interstitium, lymphatics, and capillaries during absorption.* Our knowledge of the reactions initiated within the interstitial spaces, capillaries, and lymphatics during absorption is now sufficient to quantitatively describe the process by which absorbed fluid is removed from the intestinal interstitium (186). Figure 36 summarizes the changes in capillary filtration forces produced by glucose-coupled fluid absorption in the cat ileum (175). For the nonabsorptive state (see Fig. 28), there is a small (0.30 mmHg) imbalance of forces across the capillary wall that favors net fluid filtration into the interstitium. To maintain the normal interstitial volume, the rate of capillary filtration is balanced by an equal outflow of fluid via the lymphatics.

Perfusion of the intestinal lumen with a glucose-electrolyte solution leads to net transmucosal fluid absorption (at a rate of 0.74 ml·min$^{-1}$·100 g$^{-1}$) and a rise in interstitial volume (31%). Interstitial volume expansion produces an increase in $P_t$ (2.0 mmHg) and a reduction in $\pi_t$ (1.8 mmHg). Associated with the changes in interstitial forces are an increase in $P_c$ (1.1 mmHg) and a doubling of capillary hydraulic conductance. Because vascular permeability is not altered by glucose absorption, the $\sigma_d$ remains the same. The absorption-induced changes in capillary and interstitial forces modify the balance of pressures across intestinal capillaries to produce a net absorptive force of 2.3 mmHg. This force, coupled to the elevated capillary hydraulic conductance, drives 82% of the absorbed fluid into the capillaries. Intestinal lymph flow also increases during absorption because of the increased lymphatic filling caused by the rise in $P_t$. The enhanced lymph flow removes the remaining 18% of absorbed fluid from the mucosal interstitium.

Stimulation of fluid absorption does not affect colonic lymph flow. This observation indicates that the absorbed volume is removed from the colonic interstitium exclusively via the capillaries. In the colon the fenestrated capillaries are much closer to the epithelium than their counterparts in the small intestine, which seems to be advantageous for the removal of absorbed fluid. Although no information is available on the mechanisms by which filtering capillaries are converted to absorbing capillaries, it is likely that the mechanisms are similar to those described for the small intestine. Because the juxtacapillary space in the colonic mucosa is much smaller than that in the mucosa of the small intestine, the interstitial forces may change to a greater extent at a given net fluid absorption rate in the colon than in the small intestine (288).

NET FLUID SECRETION. *Filtration secretion.* In the small intestine, increments in intestinal $P_c$ in excess

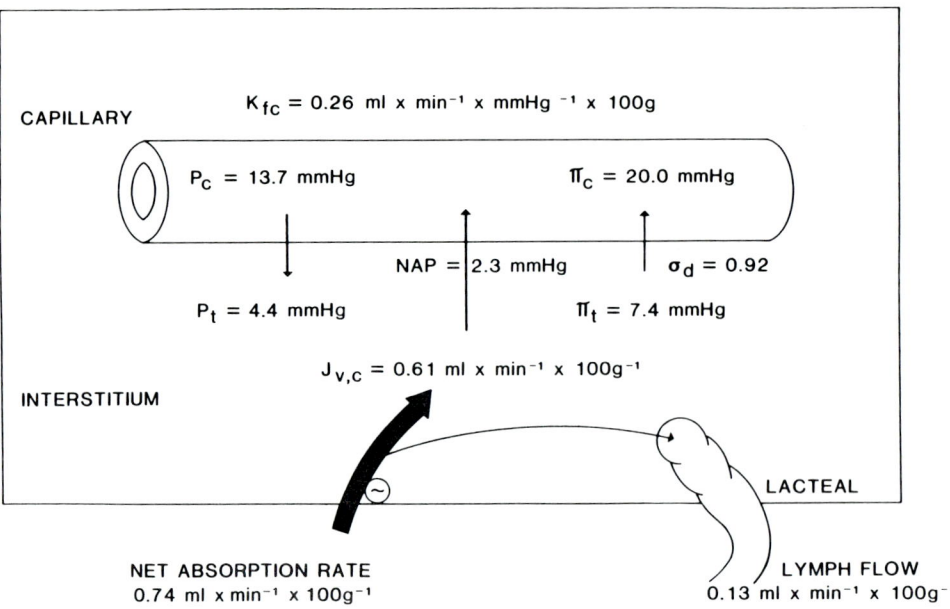

FIG. 36. Effects of net fluid absorption on Starling forces and capillary membrane parameters in the small intestine. $J_{v,c}$, rate of transcapillary fluid movement; $K_{f,c}$, capillary filtration coefficient; $P_c$, capillary hydrostatic pressure; $P_t$, interstitial hydrostatic pressure; $\sigma_d$, osmotic reflection coefficient; $\pi_c$, plasma oncotic pressure; $\pi_t$, interstitial oncotic pressure; NAP, net capillary absorptive pressure. [From Granger et al. (162).]

of 15 mmHg lead to unrestrained interstitial edema and ultimately to an exudation of interstitial fluid into the lumen. The terms *filtration secretion* and *secretory filtration* are used to describe the latter process. An imbalance in forces across the capillary wall in excess of 12–15 mmHg can be induced by acute portal hypertension, increased intraenteric pressure, plasma dilution, lymphatic obstruction, and by substances that increase capillary permeability or pressure, or both (147). Filtration secretion does not occur with imbalances in the capillary forces <12 mmHg (threshold value) because of two factors: a low mucosal hydraulic conductance and a low mucosal $P_t$ (496). When the net capillary filtration pressure exceeds the threshold value, sustained net capillary filtration occurs. The increased capillary filtration causes mucosal interstitial volume to increase, which in turn causes an increased mucosal fluid pressure (348, 496). When mucosal fluid pressure increases by >5 mmHg, large channels are opened in the mucosal membrane at the villus tips (150, 206). The width of the intercellular channels between mucosal epithelium, which is ~8–10 Å under normal conditions (119), increases sufficiently to allow solutes >37 Å in radius (e.g., albumin) to enter the lumen (Table 2), and the hydraulic conductance of the mucosal membrane increases (496). Ultrastructurally, the changes in the mucosal membrane vary from a widening of the mucosal intercellular space during plasma volume expansion (92) to villus tip erosion with prostaglandin $E_1$ ($PGE_1$) (181) and glucagon (164) infusions, and bile–oleic acid in-

TABLE 2. *Effects of Various Secretagogues on Intestinal Lymph Flow and Protein Concentration of Secreted Fluid*

| Secretagogue | Lymph Flow, × control | Protein Concentration, mg/100 ml |
|---|---|---|
| Venous pressure elevation | 22.8±3.2 | 650±48 |
| Plasma dilution | 42.1±10 | |
| Cholera toxin | 0.03±0.02 | Not detectable |
| Prostaglandin $E_1$ | 8.9±1.1 | 770±85 |
| Glucagon | 5.6±0.82 | 831±150 |
| Histamine | 20.0±1.44 | 1,660±110 |
| Ricinoleic acid | 5.3±1.2 | 566±91 |
| Vasoactive intestinal polypeptide | 0.39±0.05 | Not detectable |
| Theophylline | 0.081±0.04 | Not detectable |
| Carcinoid serum | 0.043±0.027 | |

From Granger et al. (151).

stillation in the lumen (287). The increased mucosal conductance allows for filtration secretion rates of ~1.0 ml·min⁻¹·100 g⁻¹ at a portal pressure of 30 mmHg (168). If the mucosal fluid pressure remains at 5 mmHg, the mucosal hydraulic conductance is ~0.20 ml·min⁻¹·mmHg⁻¹·100 g⁻¹, a value 2,000 times greater than that reported for normal mucosa (119). Because of the structural changes in the mucosal membrane the composition of the secreted fluid closely resembles lymph (151, 496), suggesting that the process represents an exudation of interstitial fluid into the lumen from the mucosa. Figure 37 illustrates the changes in capillary and interstitial forces that

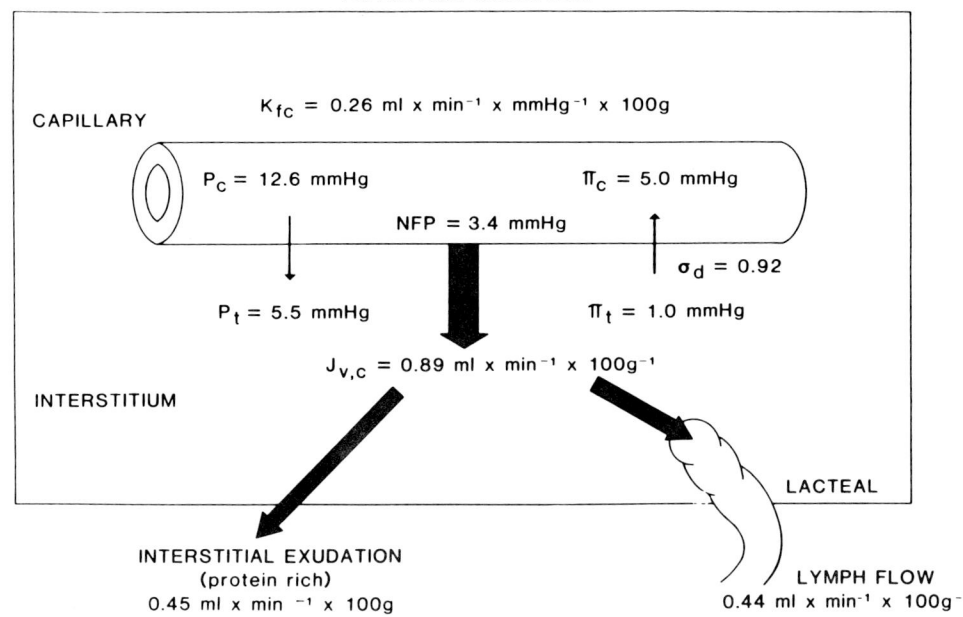

FIG. 37. Changes in Starling forces and capillary membrane parameters that lead to filtration secretion. $J_{v,c}$, rate of transcapillary fluid movement; $K_{f,c}$, capillary filtration coefficient; $P_c$, capillary hydrostatic pressure; $P_t$, interstitial hydrostatic pressure; $\sigma_d$, osmotic reflection coefficient; $\pi_c$, plasma oncotic pressure; $\pi_t$, interstitial oncotic pressure; NFP, net capillary filtration pressure. [From Granger et al. (162).]

occur when filtration secretion is induced by lowering $\pi_c$ to 5 mmHg.

Transient analysis of the relationship between intestinal lymph flow and filtration secretion rate indicates that lymph flow increases rapidly to 20 times control values after elevating portal pressure to 30 mmHg, after which time lymph flow progressively decreases. Concomitant to the rapid decrease in lymph flow is a rapid increase in intestinal fluid secretion rate. A correlation between the onset of intestinal secretion and a decline in intestinal lymph flow is also observed during plasma dilution–induced, $PGE_1$-induced, and histamine-induced secretions (151, 168, 181). The reduction in lymph flow, once filtration secretion is observed, suggests that the changes resulting in the increased mucosal conductance may also be responsible for the decrease in lymph flow. A likely explanation is that the mucosal interstitial compliance is dramatically altered immediately after rupture of mucosal membrane; venting of fluid by epithelia allows for decompression of the interstitium, a reduction in mucosal fluid pressure, and thus a smaller gradient for lymphatic filling.

*Active secretion.* Although it is recognized that the small bowel can act as a net $H_2O$ secreting organ under certain conditions (e.g., cholera), very little attention has been given to the role of the interstitium, capillaries, and lymphatics in providing fluid for the active secretory process. We summarize here the available data regarding the role of the microcirculation in active fluid secretion and develop a working hypothesis on the capillary, interstitial, and lymphatic alterations that are produced by net fluid secretion.

Stimulation of active transport processes in the mucosal epithelium can cause net fluid and solute movement into the lumen of the small bowel (e.g., choleragenic secretion). The active secretory process is characterized by an intact mucosal membrane with active $Cl^-$ (or NaCl) secretion acting as the driving force. Unlike filtration secretion, which is characterized by a secreted fluid rich in plasma proteins, the secretions of cholera are devoid of plasma proteins (Table 2), hence supporting the concept that the mucosal membrane remains intact. Simulations from mathematical models of intestinal capillary fluid exchange indicate that choleragenic secretions should significantly alter interstitial, capillary, and lymphatic flows and forces in the small bowel (429). As the protein-free fluid is secreted into the lumen, mucosal interstitial fluid volume decreases causing $\pi_t$ to increase and tissue fluid pressure to decrease. The reduction of $P_t$ causes a concomitant decrease in lymph flow. The changes in interstitial forces tend to enhance capillary filtration, which in turn serves to provide the fluid ($H_2O$) necessary for the active pump. Experimental support for the model predictions is provided by the fact that villus lymph (lacteal) pressure (297) and total intestinal lymph flow (151, 168) decrease or cease after the administration of cholera enterotoxin, VIP, and theophylline (Table 2). The reduction of lymph flow produced by active secretagogues is consistent with the concept that active secretion decreases interstitial fluid volume and pressure.

Most active secretagogues are potent vasodilators and therefore increase both $P_c$ and $K_{f,c}$ in the small intestine. Cedgard et al. (62) have reported that cholera enterotoxin produces a significant increase in intestinal $K_{f,c}$ and in $P_c$. The enhanced net filtration pressure coupled to the elevated $K_{f,c}$ should greatly increase intestinal $J_{v,c}$. Thus the enhanced fluid requirements of the secretory pump are met because of the alterations in capillary and interstitial forces and perfused capillary surface area.

Figure 38 describes the changes in Starling forces and capillary membrane parameters, predicted to occur during periods of active fluid secretion in the small bowel. As protein-free fluid is transported out of the interstitium by the epithelial cells, interstitial fluid volume decreases, thereby causing $\pi_t$ to increase and $P_t$ to fall. Assuming a normal (low) interstitial compliance, a 5% reduction in interstitial volume caused by active secretion would produce a 2.25-mmHg reduction in $P_t$ and a 0.75-mmHg increase in $\pi_t$. These changes in interstitial forces coupled to a 1-mmHg rise in $P_c$ (produced by vasodilation) should increase the net filtration pressure from 0.30 mmHg to 4.20 mmHg. The increased net capillary filtration pressure, in association with a 30% increase in $K_{f,c}$, will lead to a $J_{v,c}$ of 0.71 ml·min$^{-1}$·100 g$^{-1}$. Inasmuch as lymph flow ceases because of the fall in $P_t$, all of the capillary filtrate is available for the secretory epithelium. Although currently available data are generally consistent with the hypothesis presented, the reader should bear in mind that a complete steady-state analysis of capillary fluid dynamics during fluid secretion has not been reported.

SMALL-SOLUTE AND MACROMOLECULE EXCHANGE

A variety of different techniques have been used to study intestinal vascular permeability. Small-solute permeability has been studied with the multiple indicator–dilution and osmotic transient techniques, whereas macromolecule permeability has been investigated by steady-state analysis of lymph protein composition. We present here a brief description of the information provided by these techniques.

Small Solutes

The permeability characteristics of capillaries in the cat small intestine have been investigated using the multiple indicator–dilution technique (375). The diffusible tracers used were raffinose (5.7-Å radius), inulin (15-Å radius), and β-lactoglobulin A (28-Å radius). Blood flow to the intestine was increased from ~15 to 50 ml·min$^{-1}$·100 g$^{-1}$ by gradually increasing the rate of local intra-arterial infusion of isoproterenol (a selective mucosal vasodilator). Under resting conditions ~80% of the blood flow is distributed to the mucosa-submucosa of the cat small intestine and 20% to the muscularis-serosa (178, 308). Isoproterenol al-

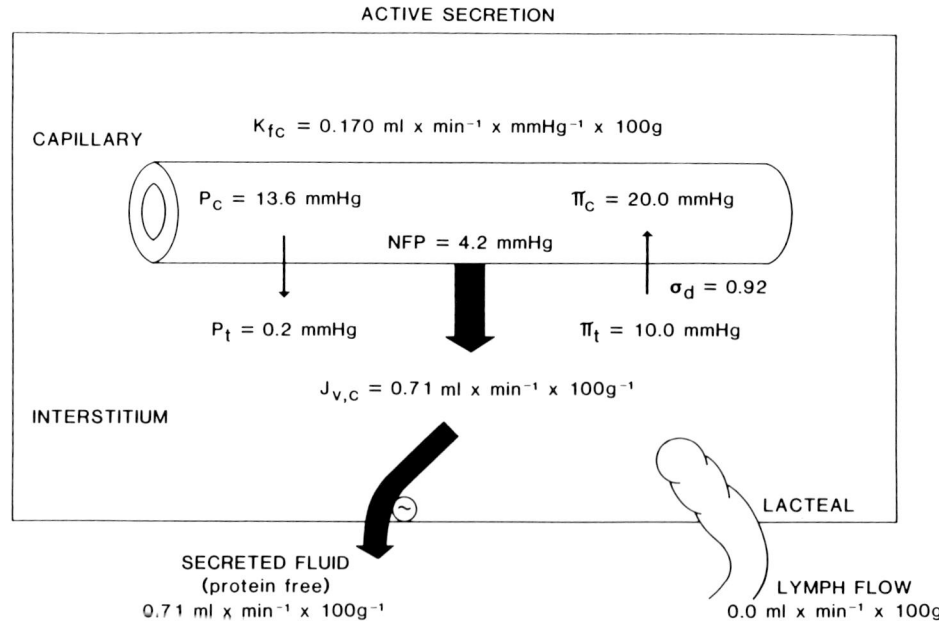

FIG. 38. Effects of active (solute-coupled) fluid secretion on Starling forces and capillary membrane parameters in the small intestine. $J_{v,c}$, rate of transcapillary fluid movement; $K_{f,c}$, capillary filtration coefficient; $P_c$, capillary hydrostatic pressure; $P_t$, interstitial hydrostatic pressure; $\sigma_d$, osmotic reflection coefficient; $\pi_c$, plasma oncotic pressure; $\pi_t$, interstitial oncotic pressure; NFP, net capillary filtration pressure. [From Granger et al. (162).]

ters this distribution in favor of the mucosa-submucosa, therefore PS values obtained during isoproterenol infusion reflect predominantly the permeability characteristics of the fenestrated capillaries of the mucosal-submucosal regions of the small intestine. The PS values for all three tracers increased with increasing plasma flow rate. At the highest plasma flow rate studied (50 ml·min$^{-1}$·100 g$^{-1}$) the PS values for raffinose, inulin, and $\beta$-lactoglobulin A were 42, 23, and 3.5 ml·min$^{-1}$·100 g$^{-1}$, respectively. The increase in PS with increasing plasma flow rate presumably resulted from capillary recruitment induced by isoproterenol. Raffinose appeared to be flow limited over the entire range of flow rates studied, i.e., the PS value for raffinose was governed by plasma flow rate and not by the restrictive properties of the capillary wall. There was, however, restricted diffusion of $\beta$-lactoglobulin A compared to inulin. This restriction reduced PS$_\text{lactoglobulin}$ and consequently the ratio PS$_\text{inulin}$/PS$_\text{lactoglobulin}$ (7.6) was greater than the ratio of their respective free-diffusion coefficients (1.73). These data are consistent with an equivalent pore radius of 59 Å for the capillaries in the mucosa-submucosa of the small intestine. The PS values reported for the small intestine are 20 times larger than those observed for raffinose and inulin in skeletal muscle (139). The proportion of this difference, which is caused by the greater capillary surface area in the intestine, remains uncertain. Even if the capillary surface area in the small intestine was as much as three- to fourfold greater than in skeletal muscle, this would mean that the fenestrated capillaries of the intestine were still 5–7 times more permeable to small solutes than the continuous capillaries of skeletal muscle.

Adenosine is known to selectively dilate the muscularis layer of the small intestine (187) and has recently been used in indicator dilution studies to investigate the permeability characteristics of capillaries in intestinal smooth muscle (375). The transit time of tracers through the muscularis vessels is less than that through the tortuous vessels of the mucosa-submucosa. Therefore during adenosine infusion the initial samples on the indicator dilution curve predominantly represent blood from the muscularis region of the small bowel (375), whereas later samples mainly represent blood from the mucosal-submucosal region. The PS values for raffinose and inulin obtained in the cat small intestine during adenosine infusion differed from those measured during isoproterenol infusion. Although this approach does not allow complete separation of blood perfusing the muscularis from the blood perfusing the mucosal region of the small intestine, the results indicate that the equivalent pore dimensions of capillaries in the muscularis are close to the 40–45-Å radius observed in skeletal muscle capillaries and smaller than the 59-Å radius observed in mucosal capillaries.

Results from osmotic transient studies indicate that the $\sigma_\text{d}$ values of intestinal capillaries for NaCl, urea, glucose, and maltose range between 0.0006 and 0.0017, with no correlation between $\sigma_\text{d}$ and solute size (153). These values are $\frac{1}{10}$–$\frac{1}{100}$ the values obtained for organs perfused primarily by continuous capillaries, i.e., skeletal muscle (87), heart (470), and mesentery (341). The equivalent radius of capillary pores predicted with this technique in the small bowel ranges between 200 and 350 Å (153), which contrasts with the 35–45-Å radius pores predicted for skeletal muscle and heart capillaries. Although the results obtained with the osmotic transient method tend to agree with ultrastructural estimates of pore dimensions in the fenestrated capillaries of the intestine, several difficulties with the technique in general and in its application to small intestine (not the least of which is that the osmotic bolus increases capillary permeability) tend to limit the reliability of the results (153).

*Macromolecules*

It is well recognized that the intestine accounts for a large proportion of the total transcapillary escape rate of proteins in humans and in cats, dogs, and rats (407, 497). The rate of protein leakage across colonic capillaries is ~0.50 mg·min$^{-1}$·100 g$^{-1}$ (398). In the nonabsorbing small intestine, protein leaks across capillaries at a rate of approximately 1.5 mg·min$^{-1}$·100 g$^{-1}$ (172), a value ~10 times greater than that reported for skeletal muscle (459). The relatively high rate of capillary protein leak in the intestine is generally attributed to a large capillary surface area and a high permeability to macromolecules. Because the $\sigma_\text{d}$ value of intestinal capillaries to plasma proteins generally exceeds the values reported for other organs, capillary surface area may be the more important factor accounting for the high rates of protein leak.

The results of several studies (8, 138, 185, 331, 398, 478) clearly establish that intestinal capillaries selectively restrict blood-to-interstitium movement of macromolecules in accordance with the solute size. At normal capillary filtration rates, the data show a steep fall in the permeation of solutes with a radius <60 Å. Above 60 Å there is an extension of residual permeability with no decrement in permeability for molecules as large as 135-Å radius. The steep fall in permeability with solute radius below 60 Å suggests that there are restrictive porosities approximating this dimension. The constant residual permeability between 60 and 135-Å radius has been attributed to either large pores (>135-Å radius) or vesicular transport (138).

A technique was recently developed to quantitatively assess vascular permeability to macromolecules in the intestine (184). This method is based on the relationship between lymph-to-plasma solute concentration ratio (L/P) and lymph flow (Fig. 39). When lymph flow is increased by graded increases in P$_\text{v}$, the

L/P ratio for any given macromolecule decreases. This is called the filtration rate–dependent portion of the relationship. At high lymph flows (>10 times control values) the L/P ratio becomes constant despite further increases in lymph flow (filtration rate–independent values). At a normal portal pressure, the exchange of macromolecules across the intestinal capillary wall occurs by both diffusion and convection. Elevation of $P_v$ increases the convective movement of macromolecules across the capillary wall, while the diffusive contribution to total exchange is reduced to a negligible level. Only when the L/P ratio is filtration rate independent can the true sieving characteristics of the capillary wall be assessed, at which time $1 - L/P$ (filtration rate independent) is equal to $\sigma_d$. There is both theoretical and experimental evidence to support the contention that $\sigma_d = 1 - L/P$ at high capillary filtration rates (47, 184, 460).

The relationship between total protein L/P ratio and lymph flow rate obtained experimentally in the small intestine of cat and rat is shown in Figure 40. The $\sigma_d$ for total protein (calculated assuming $\sigma_d = 1 - L/P$ when L/P is filtration rate independent) is 0.92. Analysis of the different molecular weight con-

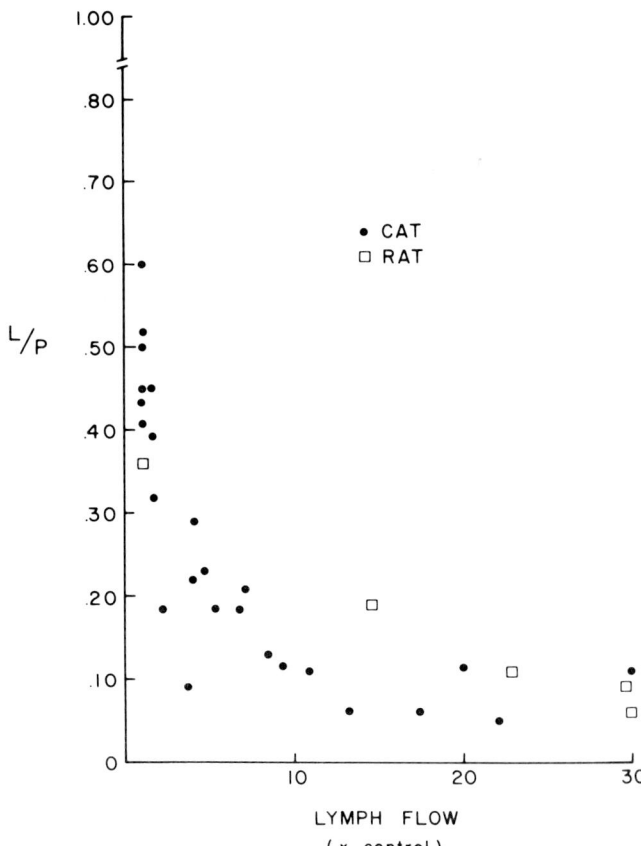

FIG. 40. Experimental data from cat and rat small intestine showing relationship between lymph flow and lymph-to-plasma protein concentration ratio (L/P). [From Taylor and Granger (460).]

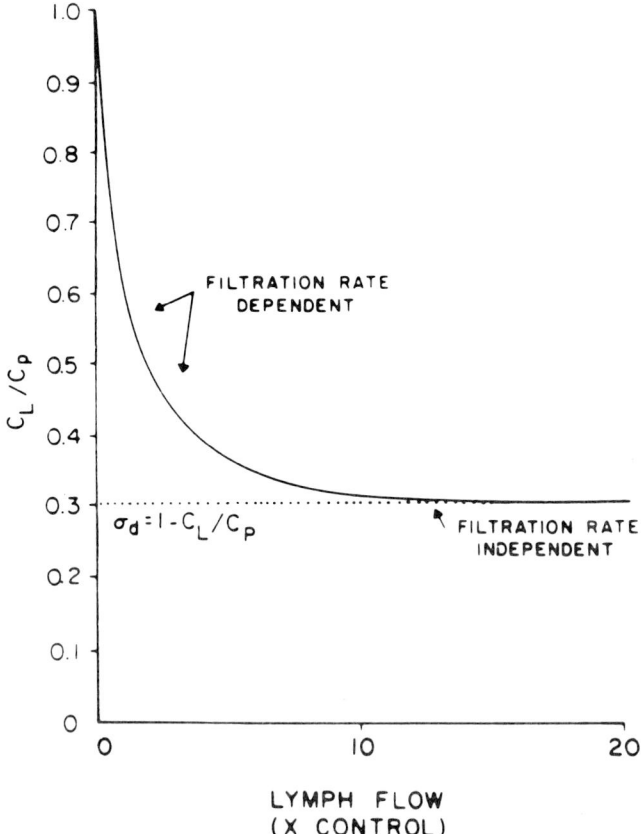

FIG. 39. Theoretical relationship between lymph-to-plasma protein concentration ratio ($C_L/C_P$) and lymph flow. The osmotic reflection coefficient ($\sigma_d$) can be estimated from relation $\sigma_d = 1 - C_L/C_P$ when $C_L/C_P$ is filtration rate independent. [From Granger and Taylor (184).]

stituents of lymph and plasma samples has provided estimates of the $\sigma_d$ values for a variety of proteins of different sizes in the small and large intestine (Table 3).

The $\sigma_d$ values of molecules of different sizes may be used to describe the permeability characteristics of the vascular bed in terms of equivalent pore theory (396). An example of such an analysis is shown in Figure 41, where $1 - \sigma_d$ is plotted as a function of solute radius. The plot shown in Figure 41 can be described by fitting the data with two sets of equivalent pores. This is done by first fitting a theoretical large pore line to the points representing the large solutes. Then by a curve-peeling process the resulting values of $1 - \sigma_d$ for small solutes are fitted with a smaller theoretical pore curve. The ordinate intercept predicts the percentage of the total hydraulic conductance occurring through each set of pores. With this approach, the permeability of intestinal capillaries to macromolecules under control conditions can be described by two populations of equivalent pores of 46-Å and 200-Å radius (Fig. 41). There are 6,400 small pores for every large pore, and 95% of the total hydraulic conductance across the intestinal capillary occurs through small pores whereas only 5% occurs through large pores.

TABLE 3. *Capillary Reflection Coefficients Calculated With L/P Data Obtained at High Capillary Filtration Rates in Small and Large Intestine*

| Solute Radius, Å | Small Intestine | Large Intestine |
|---|---|---|
| Total protein | 0.92 | 0.85 |
| 37 | 0.90 | 0.75 |
| 38 | 0.92 | |
| 39 | 0.94 | |
| 40 | | 0.82 |
| 42 | 0.96 | |
| 44 | | 0.87 |
| 48 | | 0.88 |
| 96 | 0.98 | |
| 100 | | 0.95 |
| 120 | 0.99 | 0.98 |

L/P, lymph-to-plasma solute concentration ratio. [From Granger et al. (162).]

Until recently little was known about the charge-selective properties of the intestinal capillary wall. Studies of endogenous lactate dehydrogenase (LDH) isoenzymes in plasma and intestinal lymph (374) indicate that the degree of restriction to blood-lymph exchange increases with increasing positive charge of the molecule. Furthermore, the $\sigma_d$ for LDH isoenzymes decrease from 0.95 for the most positive isoenzyme [isoelectric point (pI) = 8.3] to 0.71 for the most negative isoenyzmes (pI = 5.2). That is, the blood-lymph barrier in the intestine behaves as if it were positively charged. Studies with charged dextran molecules ($M_r$ = 24,000) support this finding (374). The steady-state L/P ratio of neutral dextran is twice that of a positive dextran of the same molecular weight, indicating selective restriction of the positive molecule compared to neutral dextran by the intestinal blood-lymph barrier. Ultrastructural studies (443) indicate that plasmalemmal vesicles and/or transendothelial channels may represent the positively charged pathways across intestinal capillaries, because cationic ferritin labeled all but these two structures in the endothelial cell wall. The findings in the intestine contrast with those in the kidney, where the existence of a negatively charged barrier is well established. The physiological significance of a positive-charge barrier associated with intestinal capillaries may be to facilitate the movement of negatively charged proteins, e.g., albumin, into the interstitium of the intestinal mucosa. This would be advantageous for certain absorbed nutrients, e.g., fatty acids, which leave the interstitium, in part, bound to proteins. The effects of solute configuration on transcapillary exchange have not been systematically analyzed in the intestine. Ultrastructural studies have demonstrated, however, that large dextrans (linear polymers) appear to unravel and move end on through the fenestral diaphragm of intestinal capillaries (441).

The mechanisms that account for the transfer of macromolecules across capillaries in the intestine are poorly understood. Convection, duffusion, and vesicular exchange are considered to be the principal mechanisms by which macromolecules cross the capillary wall. The relative contributions of diffusion and convection to macromolecule transport across intestinal capillaries has been estimated from lymphatic protein flux data in humans (493) and cats (172). From the relationship between lymphatic protein clearance and lymph flow in the intestine of cirrhotic patients, Witte et al. (493) have deduced that diffusion is the dominant process responsible for transcapillary protein exchange in the intestine. Lymphatic protein flux data from the cat intestine, which was analyzed using phenomenological transport equations, indicate, however, that convection accounts for 80%–90% of total transcapillary protein movement at normal and increased capillary filtration rates.

*Factors Influencing Permeability*

A variety of physiological, pharmacological, and pathological interventions are known to enhance capillary protein leakage in the intestine. Whether the increased transcapillary protein flux is a result of an increase in the perfused capillary surface area or is due to an increase in vascular permeability is unknown in many instances. Many agents (Table 4) increase vascular permeability (by reducing $\sigma_d$ for total plasma proteins), however, it is uncertain whether they also increase capillary surface area. Other substances such as isoproterenol and secretin increase capillary protein

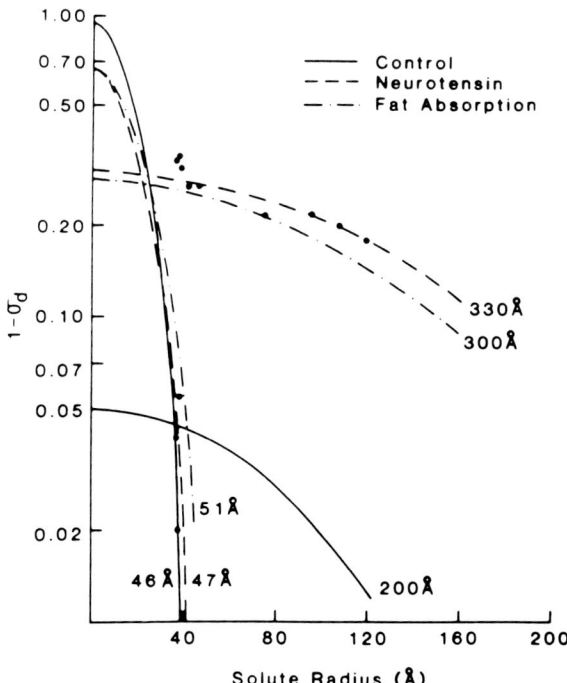

FIG. 41. Application of pore-stripping analysis to osmotic reflection coefficient ($\sigma_d$); *dashed lines*, data acquired during neurotensin infusion; *solid lines*, data acquired in control animals; *dot/dashed lines*, data acquired during fat absorption. [From Harper et al. (218).]

TABLE 4. *Effects of Various Physiological and Pharmacological Interventions on Osmotic Reflection Coefficient for Total Plasma Proteins in Intestinal Circulation*

| Experimental Condition | Osmotic Reflection Coefficient |
|---|---|
| Physiological | |
|   Control | 0.92 |
|   Fat absorption | 0.70 |
|   Glucose absorption | 0.92 |
| Drugs and hormones | |
|   Isoproterenol | 0.92 |
|   Bradykinin | 0.65 |
|   Secretin | 0.91 |
|   Cholecystokinin | 0.89 |
|   Glucagon | 0.81 |
|   Histamine | 0.56 |
|   Cimetidine and histamine | 0.90 |
|   Benadryl and histamine | 0.56 |
|   Compound 48/80 | 0.76 |
|   Angiotensin II | 0.93* |
|   Neurotensin | 0.73 |
| Pathological | |
|   Ischemia | 0.59 |
|   Ischemia and superoxide dismutase | 0.86 |
|   *Escherichia coli* endotoxin | 0.78 |
|   Goldblatt hypertension | 0.55* |
|   Arterial hyperglycemia (20 mM) | 0.64 |
|   Ethanol | 0.88* |

* Values derived from dog; all other values from cat. [From Granger et al. (162).]

(11, 42, 173, 466, 494). This increased protein flux may be the result of an increase in perfused capillary surface area or it may be due to an increase in capillary permeability. The $K_{f,c}$ and the PS for rubidium, two common indices of capillary exchange capacity, also increase during absorption (175, 425). However, neither of these measurements can discriminate between a change in capillary surface area and a change in permeability. Recent studies of capillary permeability during intestinal absorption indicate that either cream or a mixture of bile and oleic acid produced a four- to sevenfold increase in lymphatic protein flux and an increase in vascular permeability (173). The index of capillary permeability used in this study was the $\sigma_d$, which decreased from a normal value of 0.92 to 0.68 after luminal instillation of bile and oleic acid and to 0.71 after cream feeding (Fig. 42).

The $\sigma_d$ for protein molecules of different sizes has been used to calculate equivalent pore sizes in the intestinal capillary wall during fat absorption. There was no change in the size of the small pores during fat absorption (51 Å) compared with control values (46 Å); however, the large pores increased from 200-Å to 300-Å radius (Fig. 41). Pretreatment of the animal with $H_1$- and $H_2$-receptor antagonists or indomethacin

leakage without altering vascular permeability, suggesting that capillary recruitment occurs. Certain conditions that increase vascular permeability do so by preferentially increasing the dimensions of the large pores. After 1 h of intestinal ischemia there is a reduction in the $\sigma_d$ values for endogenous proteins, consistent with an increase in the size of the large pores from 200-Å to 330-Å radius, whereas the small-pore dimensions remain relatively constant at 46–50 Å. The mechanism by which certain conditions selectively influence the large-pore system is not readily apparent. In vivo microscopic studies in tissues such as mesentery indicate that various pharmacological agents reversibly increase vascular leakage of tracers by forming large interendothelial gaps (large pores) in venous capillaries (6). The gaps are believed to be formed as a result of receptor-mediated contraction and subsequent separation of endothelial cells.

The only condition that appears to selectively influence the small-pore population is arterial hypoxemia (376). Reduction in the arterial $P_{O_2}$ from 118 mmHg to 35 mmHg for a period of 10 min increases the small-pore radius by 8 Å (as measured by the multiple indicator–dilution technique) while lymph protein clearance remains unchanged. These observations suggest that physiological conditions that produce a dramatic fall in tissue $P_{O_2}$ may selectively increase the size of the small pores in intestinal capillaries.

It has long been known that absorption, particularly of fats, produces an increase in lymphatic protein flux

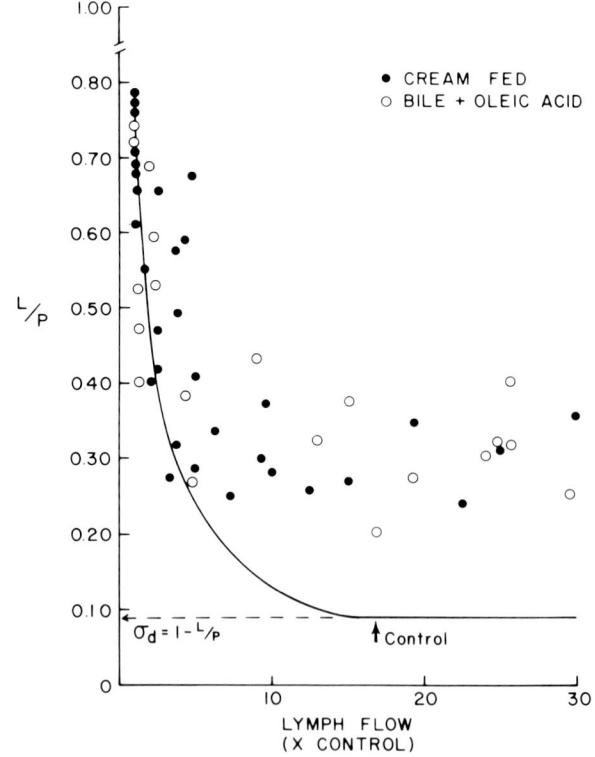

FIG. 42. Steady-state relation between intestinal lymph-to-plasma total protein concentration ratio (L/P) and lymph flow after cream feeding and intraluminal placement of bile–oleic acid. *Solid line* represents control relationship established in fasted animals. Osmotic reflection coefficient ($\sigma_d$) was estimated from relation $\sigma_d = 1 - L/P$ when L/P is filtration rate independent. [From Granger et al. (173).]

did not prevent the increase in permeability during fat absorption, whereas infusions of CCK and secretin had no effect on vascular permeability in control preparations, suggesting that none of these agents is responsible for the change observed during fat absorption. However, the intestinal polypeptide neurotensin has been shown to decrease the $\sigma_d$ in a manner similar to that observed during fat absorption [Table 4; (218)]. Furthermore neurotensin selectively increased the size of the large pores (Fig. 41) to 330-Å radius, which is similar to that observed during fat absorption. These findings suggest that neurotensin may mediate the vascular permeability changes produced by fat absorption.

In contrast to the results obtained during fat absorption, intestinal vascular permeability is not affected by the absorption of glucose or electrolytes (162). Despite the absence of a vascular permeability change, there is a six- to sevenfold increase in intestinal lymph protein flux during glucose absorption (182). This may be explained by the recent observation that $K_{f,c}$ can increase by three times during glucose absorption (175). A threefold increase in capillary surface area, coupled to a doubling of the diffusional gradient caused by dilution of interstitial proteins with absorbed fluid, could produce the large increments in capillary and lymph protein fluxes.

A major influence of the increased vascular permeability during fat absorption is the dramatic increase in plasma protein flux across the capillary wall. The true magnitude of this change is apparent only when the convective, diffusive, and net movements of plasma proteins across the capillary wall are compared in absorbing and nonabsorbing intestines (Fig. 43). In the nonabsorbing small intestine, small quantities of fluid are filtered across the capillary wall (172). Therefore plasma proteins move by both convection and diffusion from the capillary lumen to interstitium in the nonabsorptive state. In contrast, the movement of fluid in the absorbing intestine is from interstitium to blood. Under this condition, diffusion and convection are moving proteins in opposite directions across the capillary wall, and lymphatic protein flux is now the net result of two much larger and opposing fluxes. Therefore during absorption large quantities of plasma proteins enter the mucosal interstitium. Most of this protein returns to the circulation directly (by convection) across the walls of absorbing capillaries, whereas the remainder returns through the lymphatics. The reason for this large interstitial turnover of

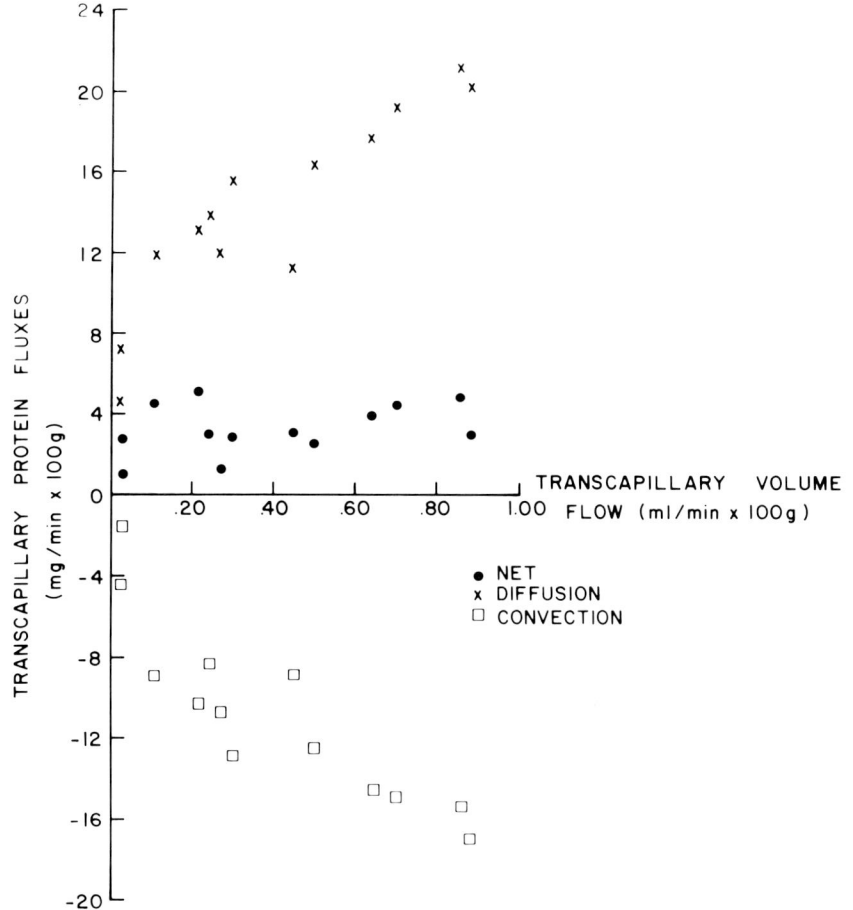

FIG. 43. Relation between intestinal transcapillary protein fluxes (net, diffusive, and convective) and transcapillary volume flow when capillaries are in an absorbing state. Positive values denote blood-to-interstitium movement, whereas negative values indicate interstitium-to-blood movement. [From Granger et al. (172).]

plasma protein remains uncertain; however, it may provide a mechanism whereby absorbed nutrients are removed from the interstitium bound to plasma protein. That is, unbound protein diffuses out of the circulation, binds to the absorbed nutrient, and is carried back into the circulation by the convective movement of absorbed fluid. This may be an important mechanism for the absorption of many substances including those medium- and long-chain fatty acids that are not incorporated into chylomicrons but enter the circulation in significant quantities bound to albumin (11, 333).

*Pathways for Macromolecule Exchange*

The structural equivalents to the small- and large-pore populations predicted for intestinal capillaries have not been firmly established (292, 361, 362, 394, 395, 400, 409, 441, 442, 454). It is likely, however, that the structural equivalent of the large pores is the open fenestrae (200–400-Å radius). The internal radius of the cytoplasmic vesicles (~250 Å) is also in agreement with the physiological large-pore estimates. It is also possible that differential porosities within the fibrillar structure of the basement membrane account for a component of the large-pore equivalency. Although the permeability of the fenestral diaphragm is unknown, it is generally considered that the porosity of this structure is the morphological equivalent to the small-pore system (57–59, 79–82, 256, 362, 442). The concept that the presence or the absence of size-limiting structures within the fenestral diaphragms differentiates subpopulations that correspond to small- and large-pore systems seems tenable, yet the relative frequency of open and diaphragmed fenestrae (61) appears to be much higher than the relative frequency of small and large pores predicted by the physiological data.

CONCLUSIONS

Based on the information presented in this chapter several conclusions can be drawn regarding the physiology of the intestinal circulation. *1*) Intrinsic regulation of blood flow is mediated by both metabolic and myogenic factors. Myogenic factors appear to play a more important role under resting conditions, whereas metabolic factors dominate when the ratio of $O_2$ availability-to-$O_2$ demand is reduced. *2*) Adjustments of blood flow and/or $O_2$ extraction account for the ability of the intestine to maintain an adequate $O_2$ supply when either $O_2$ delivery or $O_2$ demand is altered. Capillary recruitment plays an important role in preventing cell hypoxia when blood flow is reduced or $O_2$ demand is increased. *3*) The postprandial hyperemia is elicited by the presence of specific constituents (e.g., long-chain fatty acids) of chyme in the bowel lumen. The mechanism(s) responsible for the hyperemia remain undefined. *4*) Blood-borne gastrointestinal hormones and peptides appear to play a minimal role in regulating intestinal blood flow. Paracrine control of the circulation is a viable yet untested possibility. *5*) Highly diffusible gases undergo countercurrent exchange within the villous circulation. However, the extent and importance of exchange of physiological gases (e.g., $O_2$) and solutes (NaCl) between the arterial and venous limbs of the villous hairpin loop remain unclear. *6*) The available data regarding the influence of vasoactive agents on $O_2$ utilization can be largely explained in terms of the normal relationship between intestinal $O_2$ uptake and blood flow. Vasoactive agents may also alter $O_2$ uptake through changes in intramural blood flow distribution, perfused capillary density, and oxidative metabolism. *7*) Angiotensin II and vasopressin are important physiological vasoconstrictors in the intestine. The vasopressin and the angiotensin systems are overlapping mechanisms governing vascular resistance, i.e., when one system is inhibited, the other compensates to maintain resting vascular tone. *8*) A variety of conditions or perturbations are imposed during the course of an experiment that may alter resting intestinal blood flow and oxygenation and modify the responsiveness of the vasculature to pharmacological and physiological stimuli. These factors include anesthesia, adjuvants to anesthesia, artificial ventilation, surgery, visceral manipulation, and thermoregulation. *9*) The rate and direction of fluid movement across intestinal capillaries vary in relation to intestinal function. Net capillary fluid movement is modulated by the balance of hydrostatic and oncotic pressures exerted across the capillary wall. Adjustments of these forces and of perfused capillary surface area allow the microcirculation to provide the fluid for epithelial transport during periods of net fluid secretion and to remove fluid from the interstitium during periods of net fluid absorption. *10*) Intestinal capillaries are highly permeable to small solutes (e.g., glucose) yet relatively impermeable to macromolecules (e.g., albumin). Vascular permeability is also influenced by the electrical charge and configuration of the solute. Transient structural alterations in the capillary wall enhance the movement of fluid and proteins between the vascular and extravascular compartments during fat absorption, an effect that may be mediated by neurotensin.

There are several unexplored areas of research on the intestinal circulation that warrant attention. Particular emphasis should be placed on defining the characteristics of the circulation in the individual layers of the bowel wall. New techniques and approaches for measuring blood flow and microvascular exchange of $O_2$, $H_2O$, and $H_2O$-soluble solutes within discrete tissue regions are necessary to meet this objective. There is a limited number of published reports that support the feasibility of such technological advances in the near future. This new technology, coupled to investigative innovation, should greatly improve our understanding of the mucosal microcirculation.

The authors thank Sandy Worley and Ursula Romano for typing the manuscript and Penny Cook for preparing the illustrations. We also thank Dr. Aubrey Taylor for his support and encouragement.

REFERENCES

1. ADIBI, S. A., AND D. W. MERCER. Protein digestion in human intestine as reflected in luminal, mucosal, and plasma amino acid concentrations after meals. *J. Clin. Invest.* 52: 1586–1594, 1973.
2. AHLMAN, H., L. DEMAGISTRIS, M. ZINNER, AND B. M. JAFFE. Release of immunoreactive serotonin into the lumen of the feline gut in response to vagal nerve stimulation. *Science Wash. DC* 213: 1254–1255, 1981.
3. AKANDE, B., P. REILLY, I. M. MODLIN, AND B. M. JAFFE. Radioimmunoassay measurement of substance P release following a meat meal. *Surgery St. Louis* 89: 378–383, 1981.
4. AMORY, D. W., J. L. STEFFENSON, AND R. P. FORSYTH. Systemic and regional blood flow changes during halothane anesthesia in the rhesus monkey. *Anesthesiology* 35: 81–90, 1971.
5. ANZUETO, L., J. N. BENOIT, AND D. N. GRANGER. A rat model for studying the intestinal circulation. *Am. J. Physiol.* 246 (*Gastrointest. Liver Physiol.* 9): G56–G61, 1984.
6. ARFORS, K. E., G. RUTILI, AND E. SVENSJO. Microvascular transport of macromolecules in normal and inflammatory conditions. *Acta Physiol. Scand.* 463: 93–103, 1979.
7. ARGENZIO, R. A., M. SOUTHWORTH, AND C. E. STEVENS. Sites of organic acid production and absorption in the equine gastrointestinal tract. *Am. J. Physiol.* 226: 1043–1050, 1974.
8. ARTURSON, G., AND K. GRANATH. Dextrans as test molecules in studies of the functional ultrastructure of biological membranes. *Clin. Chim. Acta* 37: 309–322, 1972.
9. BACA, I., U. MITTMANN, G. E. FEURLE, M. HAAS, AND T. MULLER. Effect of neurotensin on regional intestinal blood flow in the dog. *Res. Exp. Med.* 179: 53–58, 1981.
10. BANKS, R. O., R. H. GALLAVAN, JR., M. J. ZINNER, G. B. BULKLEY, S. L. HARPER, D. N. GRANGER, AND E. D. JACOBSON. Vasoactive agents in control of the mesenteric circulation. *Federation Proc.* 44: 2743–2749, 1985.
11. BARROWMAN, J. A. *Physiology of the Gastrointestinal Lymphatic System.* Cambridge, UK: Cambridge Univ. Press, 1978.
12. BARROWMAN, J. A., AND D. N. GRANGER. Effects of experimental cirrhosis on splanchnic microvascular fluid and solute exchange in the rat. *Gastroenterology* 87: 165–172, 1984.
13. BARROWMAN, J. A., M. A. PERRY, P. R. KVIETYS, M. ULRICH, AND D. N. GRANGER. Effects of bradykinin on intestinal transcapillary fluid exchange. *Can. J. Physiol. Pharmacol.* 59: 786–789, 1981.
14. BARROWMAN, J. A., AND K. B. ROBERTS. The role of the lymphatic system in the absorption of water from the intestine of the rat. *Q. J. Exp. Physiol. Cogn. Med. Sci.* 52: 19–30, 1967.
15. BEAN, J. W., AND M. M. SIDKY. Effects of low $O_2$ on intestinal blood flow, tonus, and motility. *Am. J. Physiol.* 189: 541–547, 1957.
16. BECKER, H., A. MANGANARO, H. LAZER, D. G. MULDER, G. D. BUCKBERG. Limitations of studying splanchnic blood flow during anesthesia. *Surg. Forum* 30: 347–349, 1979.
17. BENNET, A., I. F. STANFORD, AND H. L. STOCKLEY. Estimation and characterization of prostaglandins in the human gastrointestinal tract. *Br. J. Pharmacol.* 61: 579–586, 1977.
18. BENOIT, J. N., J. A. BARROWMAN, S. L. HARPER, P. R. KVIETYS, AND D. N. GRANGER. Role of humoral factors in the intestinal hyperemia associated with chronic portal hypertension. *Am. J. Physiol.* 247 (*Gastrointest. Liver Physiol.* 10): G486–G493, 1984.
19. BENOIT, J. N., W. A. WOMACK, R. J. KORTHUIS, W. A. WILBORN, AND D. N. GRANGER. Chronic portal hypertension: effects on gastrointestinal blood flow distribution. *Am. J. Physiol.* 250 (*Gastrointest. Liver Physiol.* 13): G535–G539, 1986.
20. BENSON, J. A., P. R. LEE, J. F. SCHOLER, K. S. KIM, AND J. L. BOLLMAN. Water absorption from the intestine via portal and lymphatic pathways. *Am. J. Physiol.* 184: 441–444, 1956.
21. BERGSTROM, J., M. AHLBERG, AND A. ALVESTRAND. Influence of protein intake on renal hemodynamics and plasma hormone concentrations in normal subjects. *Acta Med. Scand.* 217: 189–196, 1985.
22. BIBER, B., J. FARA, AND O. LUNDGREN. A pharmacological study of intestinal vasodilator mechanisms in the cat. *Acta Physiol. Scand.* 90: 673–683, 1974.
23. BIBER, B., O. LUNDGREN, AND J. SVANVIK. Studies on the intestinal vasodilation observed after mechanical stimulation of the mucosa of the gut. *Acta Physiol. Scand.* 82: 177–190, 1971.
24. BIBER, B., O. LUNDGREN, AND J. SVANVIK. Intramural blood flow and blood volume in the small intestine of the cat as analyzed by an indicator-dilution technique. *Acta Physiol. Scand.* 87: 391–403, 1973.
25. BILL, A. Effects of indomethacin on regional blood flow in conscious rabbits: a microsphere study. *Acta Physiol. Scand.* 105: 437–442, 1979.
26. BLACK, J. W., E. W. FISHER, AND A. N. SMITH. The effects of precursors of 5-hydroxytryptamine on gastric secretion in anesthetized dogs. *J. Physiol. Lond.* 146: 10–17, 1959.
27. BLANCHET, L., AND D. LEBREC. Changes in splanchnic blood flow in portal hypertensive rats. *Eur. J. Clin. Invest.* 12: 327–330, 1982.
28. BOHLEN, H. G. Intestinal tissue $P_{O_2}$ and microvascular responses during glucose exposure. *Am. J. Physiol.* 238 (*Heart Circ. Physiol.* 7): H164–H171, 1980.
29. BOHLEN, H. G. Intestinal mucosal oxygenation influences absorptive hyperemia. *Am. J. Physiol.* 239 (*Heart Circ. Physiol.* 8): H489–H493, 1980.
30. BOHLEN, H. G. $Na^+$-induced intestinal interstitial hyperosmolality and vascular responses during absorptive hyperemia. *Am. J. Physiol.* 242 (*Heart Circ. Physiol.* 11): H785–H789, 1982.
31. BOHLEN, H. G., AND R. W. GORE. Comparison of microvascular pressures and diameters in the innervated and denervated rat intestine. *Microvasc. Res.* 14: 251–264, 1977.
32. BOHLEN, H. G., AND R. W. GORE. Microvascular pressure in rat intestinal muscle during direct nerve stimulation. *Microvasc. Res.* 17: 27–37, 1979.
33. BOHLEN, H. G., P. M. HUTCHINS, C. E. RAPELA, AND H. D. GREEN. Microvascular control in intestinal mucosa of normal and hemorrhaged rats. *Am. J. Physiol.* 229: 1159–1164, 1975.
34. BOLEY, S. J., G. P. AGARWAL, A. R. WAREEN, F. J. VEITH, B. S. LEVOWITZ, W. TRIEBER, J. DOUGHERTY, S. S. SCHWARTZ, AND M. L. GLEIDMAN. Pathophysiologic effects of bowel distension on intestinal blood flow. *Am. J. Surg.* 117: 228–234, 1969.
35. BOND, J. H., B. E. CURRIER, AND H. BUCHWALD. Colonic conservation of malabsorbed carbohydrate. *Gastroenterology* 78: 444–447, 1980.
36. BOND, J. H., D. G. LEVITT, AND M. D. LEVITT. Quantitation

of countercurrent exchange during passive absorption from the dog small intestine. *J. Clin. Invest.* 59: 308–318, 1977.
37. BOND, J. H., D. G. LEVITT, AND M. D. LEVITT. Use of inert gases and carbon monoxide to study the possible influence of countercurrent exchange on passive absorption from the small bowel. *J. Clin. Invest.* 54: 1259–1265, 1978.
38. BOND, J. H., AND M. D. LEVITT. Fate of soluble carbohydrate in the colon of rats and man. *J. Clin. Invest.* 57: 1158–1164, 1976.
39. BOND, J. H., R. A. PRENTISS, AND M. D. LEVITT. The effects of feeding on blood flow to the stomach, small bowel, and colon of the conscious dog. *J. Lab. Clin. Med.* 93: 594–599, 1979.
40. BOND, J. H., R. A. PRENTISS, AND M. D. LEVITT. The effect of anesthesia and laparotomy on blood flow to the stomach, small bowel, and colon of dog. *Surgery St. Louis* 87: 313–318, 1980.
41. BORGSTROM, B., A. DAHLQUIST, G. LUNDH, AND J. SJOVALL. Studies of intestinal digestion and absorption in the human. *J. Clin. Invest.* 36: 1521–1536, 1958.
42. BORGSTROM, B., AND C. B. LAURELL. Studies on lymph and lymph-proteins during absorption of fat and saline by rats. *Acta Physiol. Scand.* 29: 264–280, 1953.
43. BOSCH, J. P., A. SACCAGI, A. LAUER, M. BELLEDONNE, AND S. GLABMAN. Effect of diet on glomerular filtration rate (GFR): functional reserve (FR) of the normal kidney (Abstract). *Kidney Int.* 23: 118, 1983.
44. BOWEN, J. C., D. K. GARG, P. D. SALVATO, AND E. D. JACOBSON. Differential oxygen utilization in the stomach during vasopressin and tourniquet ischemia. *J. Surg. Res.* 25: 15–20, 1978.
45. BOWEN, J. C., W. PAWLIK, W. F. FANG, AND E. D. JACOBSON. Pharmacologic effects of gastrointestinal hormones on intestinal oxygen consumption and blood flow. *Surgery St. Louis* 78: 515–519, 1975.
46. BRANDT, J., L. CASTLEMAN, H. RUSKIN, J. GREENWALD, AND J. KELLEY. The oral protein and glucose feeding on splanchnic blood flow and oxygen utilization in normal and cirrhotic subjects. *J. Clin. Invest.* 34: 1017–1025, 1955.
47. BRESLER, E. H., AND L. J. GROOME. On equations for combined convective and diffusive transport of neutral solute across porous membranes. *Am. J. Physiol.* 241 (*Renal Fluid Electrolyte Physiol.* 10): F469–F476, 1981.
48. BRODIE, T. G., W. CULLIS, AND W. HALLIBURTON. The gaseous metabolism of the small intestine. II. The gaseous exchanges during the absorption of Witte's peptone. *J. Physiol. Lond.* 40: 173–189, 1910.
49. BRUNSSON, I., S. EKLUND, M. JODAL, O. LUNDGREN, AND H. SJOVALL. The effect of vasodilation and sympathetic nerve activation on net water absorption in the cat's small intestine. *Acta. Physiol. Scand.* 106: 61–68, 1979.
50. BUCKLEY, N. M., P. BRAZEAU, AND I. D. FRASIER. Postnatal development of autoregulation of blood flow to the small intestine (Abstract). *Federation Proc.* 43: 1011, 1984.
51. BUCKLEY, N. M., M. JARENWATTANANON, P. M. GOOTMAN, AND I. D. FRASIER. Autoregulatory escape from neural control of intestinal circulation in developing swine. *Physiologist* 28: 289, 1985.
52. BULKLEY, G. B., P. R. KVIETYS, M. A. PERRY, AND D. N. GRANGER. Effects of cardiac tamponade on colonic hemodynamics and oxygen uptake. *Am. J. Physiol.* 244 (*Gastrointest. Liver Physiol.* 7): G604–G612, 1983.
53. BURNS, G. P., AND W. G. SCHENK. Intestinal blood flow in the conscious dog. *Surg. Forum* 18: 313–315, 1967.
54. BURNS, G. P., AND W. G. SCHENK. Effect of digestion and exercise on intestinal blood flow and cardiac output. *Arch. Surg.* 98: 790–794, 1969.
55. BUTTERWORTH, C. E., JR. General discussion. In: *Intestinal Biopsy*, edited by G. E. W. Wolstenholme and M. P. Cameron. Boston, MA: Little, Brown, 1962, p. 109–112.
56. BUTTERWORTH, C. E., JR. The bayonet tube and the intestinal villus. In: *Malabsorption Syndromes*. Basel: Karger, 1963, p. 80–83. Symp. 2nd World Congr. Gastroenterol., Munich, 1962.
57. CASLEY-SMITH, J. R. The identification of chylomicra and lipoproteins in tissue sections and their passage into jejunal lacteals. *J. Cell Biol.* 15: 259–277, 1962.
58. CASLEY-SMITH, J. R. Endothelial fenestrae in intestinal villi: differences between the arterial and venous ends of the capillary. *Microvasc. Res.* 3: 49–68, 1971.
59. CASLEY-SMITH, J. R. The functioning and interrelationships of blood capillaries and lymphatics. *Experientia* 32: 1–12, 1976.
60. CASLEY-SMITH, J. R., AND B. J. GANNON. Intestinal microcirculation: spatial organization and fine structure. In: *Physiology of the Intestinal Circulation*, edited by A. P. Shepherd and D. N. Granger. New York: Raven, 1984, p. 9–33.
61. CASLEY-SMITH, J. R., P. J. O'DONOGHUE, AND K. W. J. CROCKER. The quantitative relationship between fenestrae in jejunal capillaries and connective tissue channels: proof of "tunnel capillaries." *Microvasc. Res.* 9: 78–100, 1975.
62. CEDGARD, S., D. A. HALLBACK, M. JODAL, O. LUNDGREN, AND S. REDFORS. The effects of cholera toxin on intramural blood flow distribution and capillary hydraulic conductivity in the cat small intestine. *Acta Physiol. Scand.* 102: 148–158, 1978.
63. CHARBON, G. A., H. A. A. BROUWERS, AND A. SALA. Histamine $H_1$- and $H_2$-receptors in the gastrointestinal circulation. *Naunyn-Schmiedebergs Arch. Pharmacol.* 312: 123–129, 1980.
64. CHEN, H. I., F. C. YEH, AND W. HO. Direct effects of nitroglycerin on the resistance, exchange and capacitance functions of canine intestinal vasculature. *J. Pharmacol. Exp. Ther.* 218: 497–503, 1981.
65. CHEN, W. T. *Blood Flow in the Canine Ileum as Affected by Luminal Isosmotic and Hypertonic Solutions*. East Lansing: Michigan State Univ., 1970. Master's thesis.
66. CHOU, C. C. Effect of potassium chloride on intestinal blood flow. *J. Lab. Clin. Med.* 75: 729–741, 1970.
67. CHOU, C. C. Splanchnic and overall cardiovascular hemodynamics during eating and digestion. *Federation Proc.* 42: 1548–1551, 1983.
68. CHOU, C. C., T. D. BURNS, C. P. HSIEH, AND J. M. DABNEY. Mechanism of local vasodilation with hypertonic glucose in the jejunum. *Surgery St. Louis* 71: 380–387, 1972.
69. CHOU, C. C., AND J. M. DABNEY. Interrelation of ileal wall compliance and vascular resistance. *Am. J. Dig. Dis.* 12: 1198–1208, 1967.
70. CHOU, C. C., AND B. GRASSMICK. Motility and blood flow distribution within the wall of the gastrointestinal tract. *Am. J. Physiol.* 235 (*Heart Circ. Physiol.* 4): H34–H39, 1978.
71. CHOU, C. C., C. P. HSIEH, T. D. BURNS, AND J. M. DABNEY. Effects of lumen pH and osmolarity on duodenal blood flow and motility (Abstract). *Gastroenterology* 60: 648, 1971.
72. CHOU, C. C., C. P. HSIEH, AND J. M. DABNEY. Comparison of vascular effects of gastrointestinal hormones on various organs. *Am. J. Physiol.* 232 (*Heart Circ. Physiol.* 1): H103–H109, 1977.
73. CHOU, C. C., C. P. HSIEH, Y. M. YU, P. KVIETYS, L. C. YU, R. PITTMAN, AND J. M. DABNEY. Localization of mesenteric hyperemia during digestion in dogs. *Am. J. Physiol.* 230: 583–589, 1976.
74. CHOU, C. C., AND P. R. KVIETYS. Physiological and pharmacological alterations in gastrointestinal blood flow. In: *The Measurement of Splanchnic Blood Flow*, edited by D. N. Granger and G. B. Bulkley. Baltimore, MD: Williams & Wilkins, 1981, p. 475–509.
75. CHOU, C. C., P. KVIETYS, R. GALLAVAN, AND R. NYHOF. Blood flow, oxygen consumption and absorption of glucose and oleic acid in the canine jejunum (Abstract). *Gastroenterology* 76: 1114, 1979.
76. CHOU, C. C., P. KVIETYS, J. POST, AND S. P. SIT. Constituents of chyme responsible for postprandial intestinal hyperemia. *Am. J. Physiol.* 235 (*Heart Circ. Physiol.* 4): H677–H682, 1978.
77. CHOU, C. C., M. J. MANGINO, AND D. R. SAWMILLER. Gas-

trointestinal hormones and intestinal blood flow. In: *Physiology of the Intestinal Circulation*, edited by A. P. Shepherd and D. N. Granger. New York: Raven, 1984, p. 121-130.
78. CHOU, C. C., AND H. SIREGAR. Role of histamine $H_1$- and $H_2$-receptors in postprandial intestinal hyperemia. *Am. J. Physiol.* 243 (*Gastrointest. Liver Physiol.* 6): G248-G252, 1982.
79. CLEMENTI, F., AND G. E. PALADE. Intestinal capillaries. I. Permeability to peroxidase and ferritin. *J. Cell Biol.* 41: 33-58, 1969.
80. CLEMENTI, F., AND G. E. PALADE. Intestinal capillaries. II. Structural effects of EDTA and histamine. *J. Cell Biol.* 42: 706-724, 1969.
81. COLLAN, Y., AND T. V. KALIMA. Topographic relations of lymphatic endothelial cells in the initial lymphatic of the intestinal villus. *Lymphology* 7: 175-184, 1974.
82. COOPERMAN, L. H. Effects of anaesthetics on the splanchnic circulation. *Br. J. Anaesth.* 44: 967-970, 1972.
83. DABNEY, J. M., J. B. SCOTT, AND C. C. CHOU. Effects of cations on ileal wall compliance and blood flow. *Am. J. Physiol.* 212: 835-839, 1967.
84. DAVIS, M. J., AND R. W. GORE. Capillary pressures in rat intestinal muscle and mucosal villi during venous pressure elevation. *Am. J. Physiol.* 249 (*Heart Circ. Physiol.* 18): H174-H187, 1985.
85. DHASMANA, K. M., O. PRAKASH, AND P. R. SAXEMA. Effects of fentanyl, and the antagonism by naloxane, on regional blood flow and biochemical variables in conscious rabbits. *Arch. Int. Pharmacodyn. Ther.* 260: 115-129, 1982.
86. DHASMANA, K. M., P. R. SAXENA, O. PRAKASH, AND H. T. VAN DER ZEE. A study on the influence of ketamine on systemic and regional hemodynamics in conscious rabbits. *Arch. Int. Pharmacodyn. Ther.* 269: 323-334, 1984.
87. DIANA, J. N., S. C. LONG, AND H. YAO. Effect of histamine on equivalent pore radius in capillaries of isolated dog hindlimb. *Microvasc. Res.* 4: 413-437, 1972.
88. DOBBINS, W. O., AND E. L. ROLLINS. Intestinal mucosal lymphatic permeability: an electron microscopic study of endothelial vesicles and cell junctions. *J. Ultrastruct. Res.* 33: 29-59, 1970.
89. DOHERTY, J. U., AND C. S. LIANG. Arterial hypoxemia in awake dogs. *J. Lab. Clin. Med.* 104: 665-677, 1984.
90. DONALD, D. E., AND L. L. AARHUS. Active and passive release of blood from canine spleen and small intestine. *Am. J. Physiol.* 227: 1166-1172, 1974.
91. DRAGSTEDT, C. A., V. F. LANG, AND R. F. MILLET. The relative effects of distension on different portions of the intestine. *Arch. Surg.* 18: 2257-2286, 1929.
92. DUFFY, P. A., D. N. GRANGER, AND A. E. TAYLOR. Intestinal secretion induced by volume expansion in the dogs. *Gastroenterology* 75: 413-418, 1978.
93. DUPONT, J., S. MEYDANI, G. L. CASE, R. V. PHILLIPS, AND L. D. LEWIS. Prostaglandins and their metabolites in the gastrointestinal tract of Yucatan miniature swine. *Am. J. Clin. Nutr.* 34: 2048-2053, 1981.
94. DURBIN, T. J., N. A. MORTILLARO, AND W. H. WILBORN. Effects of endogenous histamine on capillary permeability in the feline ileum (Abstract). *Federation Proc.* 41: 1742, 1982.
95. EADE, M. N., AND R. W. GINN. The distribution of blood flow along the small intestine of the dog. *Proc. Soc. Exp. Biol. Med.* 157: 390-392, 1978.
96. EDELSTONE, D. I., AND I. R. HOLZMAN. Fetal intestinal oxygen consumption at various levels of oxygenation. *Am. J. Physiol.* 242 (*Heart Circ. Physiol.* 11): H50-H54, 1982.
97. EDELSTONE, D. I., AND I. R. HOLZMAN. Fetal and neonatal circulations. In: *Physiology of the Intestinal Circulation*, edited by A. P. Shepherd and D. N. Granger. New York: Raven, 1984, p. 179-190.
98. EDELSTONE, D. I., D. R. LATTANZI, M. E. PAULONE, AND I. R. HOLZMAN. Neonatal intestinal oxygen consumption during arterial hypoxemia. *Am. J. Physiol.* 244 (*Gastrointest. Liver Physiol.* 7): G278-G283, 1983.
99. EKLUND, S., J. FAHRENKRUG, M. JODAL, O. LUNDGREN, O. B. SCHAFFALITZKY DE MUCKADELL, AND A. SJOQUIST. Vasoactive intestinal polypeptide, 5-hydroxytryptamine, and reflex hyperemia in the small intestine of the cat. *J. Physiol. Lond.* 302: 549-557, 1980.
100. EKLUND, S., M. JODAL, O. LUNDGREN, AND A. SJOQUIST. Effects of vasoactive intestinal polypeptide on blood flow, motility, and fluid transport in the gastrointestinal tract of the cat. *Acta Physiol. Scand.* 105: 461-468, 1979.
101. ESSEX, H. E., J. R. HERRICK, E. J. BALDES, AND E. J. MANN. Blood flow on the circumflex branch of the left coronary artery of the intact dog. *Am. J. Physiol.* 117: 271-279, 1936.
102. FAHRENKRUG, J., U. HAGLUND, M. JODAL, O. LUNDGREN, L. OLBE, AND O. B. SCHAFFALITZKY DE MUCKADELL. Nervous release of vasoactive intestinal polypeptide in the gastrointestinal tract of cats: possible physiological implications. *J. Physiol. Lond.* 284: 291-305, 1978.
103. FARA, J. W. Postprandial mesenteric hyperemia. In: *Physiology of the Intestinal Circulation*, edited by A. P. Shepherd and D. N. Granger. New York: Raven, 1984, p. 99-106.
104. FARA, J. W., AND K. S. MADDEN. Effect of secretin and cholecystokinin on small intestinal blood flow distribution. *Am. J. Physiol.* 229: 1365-1370, 1975.
105. FARA, J. W., E. H. RUBINSTEIN, AND R. R. SONNENSCHEIN. Intestinal hormones in mesenteric vasodilation after introduodenal agents. *Am. J. Physiol.* 223: 1058-1067, 1972.
106. FERREIRA, S. H., A. G. HERMAN, AND J. R. VANE. Prostaglandin production by rabbit isolated jejunum and its relationship to the inherent tone of the preparation. *Br. J. Pharmacol.* 56: 469-477, 1976.
107. FERUGLIO, F. S., F. GRECO, AND L. CESANO. Effect of drug infusion on the systemic and splanchnic circulation. I. Bradykinin infusion in normal subjects. *Clin. Sci.* 26: 487-491, 1964.
108. FLYNN, S. B., AND D. A. OWENS. Histamine receptors in peripheral vascular beds in the cat. *Br. J. Pharmacol.* 55: 181-188, 1975.
109. FOLKOW, B. Intravascular pressure as a factor regulating the tone of small vessels. *Acta Physiol. Scand.* 17: 289-310, 1949.
110. FOLKOW, B. The vasodilator action of adenosine triphosphate. *Acta Physiol. Scand.* 17: 311-317, 1949.
111. FOLKOW, B., AND M. I. L. HALLBACK. Physiopathology of spontaneous hypertension in rats. In: *Hypertension: Physiopathology and Treatment*, edited by J. Genest, E. Koiw, and O. Kuchel. New York: McGraw-Hill, 1977, p. 507-529.
112. FOLKOW, B., D. H. LEWIS, O. LUNDGREN, S. MELLANDER, AND I. WALLENTIN. The effect of graded vasoconstrictor fiber stimulation on intestinal resistance and capacitance vessels. *Acta Physiol. Scand.* 61: 445-457, 1964.
113. FOLKOW, B., D. H. LEWIS, O. LUNDGREN, S. MELLANDER, AND I. WALLENTIN. The effect of sympathetic vasoconstrictor fibers on the distribution of capillary flow in the intestine. *Acta Physiol. Scand.* 61: 458-466, 1964.
114. FOLKOW, B., O. LUNDGREN, AND I. WALLENTIN. Studies on the relationship between flow resistance, capillary filtration coefficient and regional blood volume in the intestine of the cat. *Acta Physiol. Scand.* 57: 270-283, 1963.
115. FONDACARO, J. D., AND E. D. JACOBSON. The role of prostacyclin ($PGI_2$) in metabolic hyperemia. *Prostaglandins* 21, Suppl. V: 25-32, 1981.
116. FONDACARO, J. D., M. M. SCHWAIGER, AND E. D. JACOBSON. Effects of prostacyclin ($PGI_2$) and prostaglandin $D_2$ ($PGD_2$) on the ischemic canine mesenteric circulation (Abstract). *Gastroenterology* 76: 1134, 1979.
117. FONDACARO, J. D., K. M. WALUS, M. SCHWAIGER, AND E. D. JACOBSON. Vasodilation of the normal and ischemic canine mesenteric circulation. *Gastroenterology* 80: 1542-1549, 1981.
118. FORDTRAN, J. S., AND T. W. LOCKLEAR. Ionic constituents and osmolality of gastric and small-intestinal fluids after eating. *Am. J. Dig. Dis.* 11: 503-521, 1966.
119. FORDTRAN, J. S., F. C. RECTOR, M. F. EWTON, N. SOTER,

AND J. KINNEY. Permeability characteristics of the human small intestine. *J. Clin. Invest.* 44: 1935–1944, 1965.
120. FRIGERIO, B., M. RAVAZOLA, S. ITO, R. BUFFA, C. CAPELLA, E. SOLCIA, AND L. ORCI. Histochemical and ultrastructural identification of neurotensin cells in the dog ileum. *Histochemistry* 54: 123–131, 1977.
121. FRIZZELL, R. A., L. MARKSCHEID-KASPI, AND S. G. SCHULTZ. Oxidative metabolism of rabbit ileal mucosa. *Am. J. Physiol.* 226: 1142–1148, 1974.
122. FROMM, D., AND N. HALPERN. Effects of histamine receptor antagonists on ion transport by isolated ileum of the rabbit. *Gastroenterology* 77: 1034–1038, 1979.
123. FRONEK, K., AND A. FRONEK. Combined effect of exercise and digestion on hemodynamics in conscious dogs. *Am. J. Physiol.* 218: 555–559, 1970.
124. FRONEK, K., AND L. H. STAHLGREN. Systemic and regional hemodynamic changes during food intake and digestion in non-anesthetized dogs. *Circ. Res.* 23: 687–692, 1968.
125. FUMIA, F. D., D. I. EDELSTONE, AND I. R. HOLZMAN. Blood flow and oxygen delivery to fetal organs as functions of fetal hematocrit. *Am. J. Obstet. Gynecol.* 150: 274–282, 1984.
126. GAFFNEY, G. R., AND H. E. WILLIAMSON. Effect of indomethacin and meclofenamate on canine mesenteric and celiac blood flow. *Res. Commun. Chem. Pathol. Pharmacol.* 25: 165–168, 1979.
127. GALLAVAN, R. H., JR., M. H. CHEN, S. N. JOFFE, AND E. D. JACOBSON. Vasoactive intestinal polypeptide, cholecystokinin, glucagon, and bile-oleate-induced jejunal hyperemia. *Am. J. Physiol.* 248 (*Gastrointest. Liver Physiol.* 11): G208–G215, 1985.
128. GALLAVAN, R. H., JR., AND C. C. CHOU. Carbohydrate metabolism during the postprandial intestinal hyperemia. *Proc. Soc. Exp. Biol. Med.* 171: 214–220, 1982.
129. GALLAVAN, R. H., JR., AND C. C. CHOU. Prostaglandin synthesis inhibition and postprandial intestinal hyperemia. *Am. J. Physiol.* 242 (*Gastrointest. Liver Physiol.* 5): G140–G146, 1982.
130. GALLAVAN, R. H., JR., AND C. C. CHOU. Possible mechanisms for the initiation and maintenance of postprandial intestinal hyperemia. *Am. J. Physiol.* 249 (*Gastrointest. Liver Physiol.* 12): G301–G308, 1985.
131. GALLAVAN, R. H., JR., C. C. CHOU, P. R. KVIETYS, AND S. P. SIT. Regional blood flow during digestion in the conscious dog. *Am. J. Physiol.* 238 (*Heart Circ. Physiol.* 7): H220–H225, 1980.
132. GALLAVAN, R. H., JR., J. D. FONDACARO, AND E. D. JACOBSON. Intestinal blood flow and oxygen consumption. *Proc. Soc. Exp. Biol. Med.* 174: 74–78, 1983.
133. GALLAVAN, R. H., JR., AND E. D. JACOBSON. Prostaglandins and the splanchnic circulation. *Proc. Soc. Exp. Biol. Med.* 170: 391–397, 1982.
134. GALLAVAN, R. H., JR., C. SHAW, R. F. MURPHY, S. V. JOFFE, AND E. D. JACOBSON. The lipid-induced jejunal hyperemia and neurotensin release (Abstract). *Dig. Dis. Sci.* 29: 295, 1984.
135. GANNON, B. The coexistence of fountain and tuft patterns of blood supply in individual intestinal villi of rabbit and man: resolution of an old controversy. *Bibl. Anat.* 20: 130–133, 1981.
136. GANNON, B., J. BROWNING, P. ROGERS, AND B. HARPER. Microvascular organization in the intestine. In: *Microcirculation of the Alimentary Tract-Physiology and Pathology*, edited by A. Koo, S. K. Lam, and L. H. Smaje. Singapore: World Scientific Publ., 1983, p. 39–52. (Proc. Symp. Hong Kong, March 28–30, 1983.)
137. GANNON, B., R. W. GORE, AND P. A. W. ROGERS. Is there an anatomical basis for a vascular countercurrent mechanism in rabbit and human intestinal villi? *Biomed. Res.* 2: 235–241, 1981.
138. GANROT, P. O., C. B. LAURELL, AND K. OHLSSON. Concentration of trypsin inhibitors of different molecular size and of albumin and haptoglobulin in blood and lymph of various organs in the dog. *Acta Physiol. Scand.* 79: 280–286, 1970.
139. GARLICK, D. G. Factors affecting the transport of extracellular molecules in skeletal muscle. In: *Capillary Permeability*, edited by C. Crone and N. A. Lassen. Copenhagen: Munksgaard, 1970, p. 228–238. (Alfred Benzoin Symp., 2nd., 1969.)
140. GELMAN, S. Effects of anesthetics on splanchnic circulation. In: *Cardiovascular Action of Anesthetics and Drugs Used in Anesthesia*, edited by B. M. Altura and S. Halevy. New York: Karger, 1987.
141. GELMAN, S., K. C. FOWLER, AND L. R. SMITH. Regional blood flow during isoflurane and halothane anesthesia. *Anesth. Analg.* 63: 557–565, 1984.
142. GIRAUD, G. D., AND K. L. MACCANNELL. Decreased nutrient blood flow during dopamine- and epinephrine-induced intestinal vasodilation. *J. Pharmacol. Exp. Ther.* 230: 214–220, 1984.
143. GORE, R. W. Fluid exchange across single capillaries in rat intestinal muscle. *Am. J. Physiol.* 242 (*Heart Circ. Physiol.* 11): H268–H287, 1982.
144. GORE, R. W., AND H. G. BOHLEN. Microvascular pressures in rat intestinal muscle and mucosal villi. *Am. J. Physiol.* 233 (*Heart Circ. Physiol.* 2): H685–H693, 1977.
145. GORE, R. W., W. SCHOKNECHT, AND H. G. BOHLEN. Filtration coefficients of single capillaries in rat intestinal muscle. In: *Microcirculation*, edited by J. Grayson and W. Zingg. New York: Plenum, 1976, p. 331–332.
146. GRANGER, D. N. Intestinal microcirculation and transmucosal fluid transport. *Am. J. Physiol.* 240 (*Gastrointest. Liver Physiol.* 3): G343–G349, 1981.
147. GRANGER, D. N., AND J. A. BARROWMAN. Microcirculation of the alimentary tract. I. Physiology of transcapillary fluid and solute exchange. *Gastroenterology* 84: 846–868, 1983.
148. GRANGER, D. N., J. A. BARROWMAN, S. L. HARPER, P. R. KVIETYS, AND R. J. KORTHUIS. Sympathetic stimulation and intestinal capillary fluid exchange. *Am. J. Physiol.* 247 (*Gastrointest. Liver Physiol.* 10): G279–G283, 1984.
149. GRANGER, D. N., B. H. COOK, H. J. GRANGER, AND A. E. TAYLOR. Histochemistry of microvascular smooth muscle in the gastrointestinal tract. *Microvasc. Res.* 12: 157–167, 1976.
150. GRANGER, D. N., B. H. COOK, AND A. E. TAYLOR. Structural locus of transmucosal albumin efflux in canine ileum: a fluorescence study. *Gastroenterology* 71: 1023–1027, 1976.
151. GRANGER, D. N., R. CROSS, AND J. A. BARROWMAN. Effects of various secretagogues and human carcinoid serum or lymph flow in the cat ileum. *Gastroenterology* 83: 896–901, 1982.
152. GRANGER, D. N., AND H. J. GRANGER. Systems analysis of intestinal hemodynamics and oxygenation. *Am. J. Physiol.* 245 (*Gastrointest. Liver Physiol.* 8): G786–G796, 1983.
153. GRANGER, D. N., J. P. GRANGER, R. A. BRACE, R. E. PARKER, AND A. E. TAYLOR. Analysis of the permeability characteristics of intestinal capillaries. *Circ. Res.* 44: 335–344, 1979.
155. GRANGER, D. N., S. L. HARPER, R. J. KORTHUIS, H. G. BOHLEN, AND P. R. KVIETYS. Intestinal vasoregulation in spontaneously hypertensive rats. *Am. J. Physiol.* 249 (*Gastrointest. Liver Physiol.* 12): G786–G791, 1985.
156. GRANGER, D. N., AND P. R. KVIETYS. The splanchnic circulation: intrinsic regulation. *Annu. Rev. Physiol.* 43: 409–418, 1981.
157. GRANGER, D. N., AND P. R. KVIETYS. Digestive system: small and large intestines. F. Lymphatic system. In: *Blood Vessels and Lymphatics in Organ Systems*, edited by D. I. Abramson and P. B. Dorbin. Orlando, FL: Academic, 1984, chapt. 13, p. 450–455.
158. GRANGER, D. N., P. R. KVIETYS, D. MAILMAN, AND P. D. I. RICHARDSON. Intrinsic regulation of functional blood flow and water absorption in canine colon. *J. Physiol. Lond.* 307: 443–451, 1980.
159. GRANGER, D. N., P. R. KVIETYS, N. A. MORTILLARO, AND A. E. TAYLOR. Effect of luminal distension on intestinal transcapillary fluid exchange. *Am. J. Physiol.* 239 (*Gastrointest. Liver Physiol.* 2): G516–G523, 1980.
160. GRANGER, D. N., P. R. KVIETYS, D. A. PARKS, AND J. N. BENOIT. Intestinal blood flow: relations to function. *Surv. Dig.*

*Dis.* 1: 217–228, 1983.
161. GRANGER, D. N., P. R. KVIETYS, AND M. A. PERRY. Role of exchange vessels in the regulation of intestinal oxygenation. *Am. J. Physiol.* 242 (*Gastrointest. Liver Physiol.* 5): G570–G574, 1982.
162. GRANGER, D. N., P. R. KVIETYS, M. A. PERRY, J. A. BARROWMAN. The microcirculation and intestinal transport. In: *Physiology of the Gastrointestinal Tract* (2nd ed.), edited by L. R. Johnson. New York: Raven, 1987, vol. 2, chapt. 62, p. 1671–1697.
163. GRANGER, D. N., P. R. KVIETYS, M. A. PERRY, AND A. E. TAYLOR. Relationship between intestinal volume secretion and oxygen uptake. *Dig. Dis. Sci.* 27: 42–48, 1982.
164. GRANGER, D. N., P. R. KVIETYS, W. H. WILBORN, N. A. MORTILLARO, AND A. E. TAYLOR. Mechanism of glucagon-induced intestinal secretion. *Am. J. Physiol.* 239 (*Gastrointest. Liver Physiol.* 2): G30–G38, 1980.
165. GRANGER, D. N., N. A. MORTILLARO, P. R. KVIETYS, G. RUTILI, J. C. PARKER, AND A. E. TAYLOR. Role of the interstitial matrix during intestinal volume absorption. *Am. J. Physiol.* 238 (*Gastrointest. Liver Physiol.* 1): G183–G189, 1980.
166. GRANGER, D. N., N. A. MORTILLARO, P. R. KVIETYS, AND A. E. TAYLOR. Regulation of interstitial fluid volume in the small bowel. In: *Tissue Fluid Pressure and Composition*, edited by A. R. Hargens. Baltimore, MD: Williams & Wilkins, 1981, p. 171–183.
167. GRANGER, D. N., N. A. MORTILLARO, M. A. PERRY, AND P. R. KVIETYS. Autoregulation of intestinal capillary filtration rate. *Am. J. Physiol.* 243 (*Gastrointest. Liver Physiol.* 6): G475–G483, 1982.
168. GRANGER, D. N., N. A. MORTILLARO, AND A. E. TAYLOR. Interactions of intestinal lymph flow and secretion. *Am. J. Physiol.* 232 (*Endocrinol. Metab. Gastrointest. Physiol.* 1): E13–E18, 1977.
169. GRANGER, D. N., N. A. MORTILLARO, AND A. E. TAYLOR. Effects of various secretagogues on ileal lymph flow (Abstract). *Gastroenterology* 76: 123, 1979.
170. GRANGER, D. N., R. E. PARKER, E. W. QUILLEN, R. A. BRACE, AND A. E. TAYLOR. Lymph flow transients. In: *Lymphology*, edited by P. Malek. Stuttgart, FRG: Thieme, 1977, p. 61–63.
171. GRANGER, D. N., M. A. PERRY, P. R. KVIETYS, D. A. PARKS, AND J. N. BENOIT. Metabolic, myogenic and hormonal factors in local regulation of alimentary tract blood flow. In: *Microcirculation of the Alimentary Tract-Physiology and Pathology*. Singapore: World Scientific Publ., 1983, p. 131–142. (Proc. Symp. Hong Kong, March 28–30, 1983.)
172. GRANGER, D. N., M. A. PERRY, P. R. KVIETYS, AND A. E. TAYLOR. Interstitium-to-blood movement of macromolecules in the absorbing small intestine. *Am. J. Physiol.* 241 (*Gastrointest. Liver Physiol.* 4): G31–G36, 1981.
173. GRANGER, D. N., M. A. PERRY, P. R. KVIETYS, AND A. E. TAYLOR. Permeability of intestinal capillaries: effects of fat absorption and gastrointestinal hormones. *Am. J. Physiol.* 242 (*Gastrointest. Liver Physiol.* 5): G194–G201, 1982.
174. GRANGER, D. N., M. A. PERRY, P. R. KVIETYS, AND A. E. TAYLOR. A new method for estimating intestinal capillary pressure. *Am. J. Physiol.* 244 (*Gastrointest. Liver Physiol.* 7): G341–G344, 1983.
175. GRANGER, D. N., M. A. PERRY, P. R. KVIETYS, AND A. E. TAYLOR. Capillary and interstitial forces during fluid absorption in the cat small intestine. *Gastroenterology* 86: 262–273, 1984.
175a. GRANGER, D. N., A. J. PREMEN, AND P. R. KVIETYS. Effects of intestinal hormones on jejunal blood flow (Abstract). *Federation Proc.* 44: 445, 1985.
176. GRANGER, D. N., P. D. I. RICHARDSON, P. R. KVIETYS, AND N. A. MORTILLARO. Intestinal blood flow. *Gastroenterology* 78: 837–863, 1980.
177. GRANGER, D. N., P. D. I. RICHARDSON, AND A. E. TAYLOR. The effects of isoprenaline and bradykinin on capillary filtration in the cat small intestine. *Br. J. Pharmacol.* 67: 361–366, 1979.
178. GRANGER, D. N., P. D. I. RICHARDSON, AND A. E. TAYLOR. Volumetric assessment of the capillary filtration coefficient in the cat small intestine. *Pfluegers Arch.* 381: 25–33, 1979.
179. GRANGER, D. N., G. RUTILI, AND J. M. MCCORD. Superoxide radicals in feline intestinal ischemia. *Gastroenterology* 81: 22–29, 1981.
180. GRANGER, D. N., M. SENNETT, P. MCELEARNEY, AND A. E. TAYLOR. Effect of local arterial hypotension on cat intestinal capillary permeability. *Gastroenterology* 79: 474–480, 1980.
181. GRANGER, D. N., J. S. SHACKLEFORD, AND A. E. TAYLOR. Prostaglandin $E_1$-induced filtration secretion in the feline ileum. *Am. J. Physiol.* 236 (*Endocrinol. Metab. Gastrointest. Physiol.* 5): E788–E798, 1979.
182. GRANGER, D. N., AND A. E. TAYLOR. Effects of solute-coupled transport on lymph flow and oncotic pressures in cat ileum. *Am. J. Physiol.* 235 (*Endocrinol. Metab. Gastrointest. Physiol.* 4): E429–E436, 1978.
183. GRANGER, D. N., AND A. E. TAYLOR. Intestinal secretagogues: effects on in vivo and in vitro oxygen consumption (Abstract). *Federation Proc.* 38: 952, 1979.
184. GRANGER, D. N., AND A. E. TAYLOR. Permeability of intestinal capillaries to endogenous macromolecules. *Am. J. Physiol.* 238 (*Heart Circ. Physiol.* 7): H457–H464, 1980.
185. GRANGER, D. N., AND A. E. TAYLOR. Permselectivity of intestinal capillaries. *Physiologist* 23: 47–52, 1980.
186. GRANGER, D. N., M. ULRICH, D. A. PARKS, AND S. L. HARPER. Transcapillary exchange during intestinal fluid absorption. In: *Physiology of the Intestinal Circulation*, edited by A. P. Shepherd and D. N. Granger. New York: Raven, 1984, p. 211–221.
187. GRANGER, D. N., J. VALLEAU, R. PARKER, R. LANE, AND A. TAYLOR. Effects of adenosine on intestinal hemodynamics, oxygen delivery, and capillary fluid exchange. *Am. J. Physiol.* 235 (*Heart Circ. Physiol.* 4): H707–H719, 1978.
188. GRANGER, H. J. Role of the interstitial matrix and lymphatic pump in regulation of transcapillary fluid balance. *Microvasc. Res.* 18: 209–216, 1979.
189. GRANGER, H. J. Physicochemical properties of the extracellular matrix. In: *Tissue Fluid Pressure and Composition*, edited by A. R. Hargens. Baltimore, MD: Williams & Wilkins, p. 51–61.
190. GRANGER, H. J., J. L. BORDERS, G. A. MENINGER, A. H. GOODMAN, AND G. E. BARNES. Microcirculatory control systems. In: *The Physiology and Pharmacology of the Microcirculation*, edited by N. A. Mortillaro. Orlando, FL: Academic, 1983, vol. 1, chapt. 5, p. 209–236.
191. GRANGER, H. J., A. H. GOODMAN, AND D. N. GRANGER. Role of resistance and exchange vessels in local microvascular control of skeletal muscle oxygenation in the dog. *Circ. Res.* 38: 379–385, 1976.
192. GRANGER, H. J., AND C. P. NORRIS. Intrinsic regulation of intestinal oxygenation in the anesthetized dog. *Am. J. Physiol.* 238 (*Heart Circ. Physiol.* 7): H836–H843, 1980.
193. GRANGER, H. J., AND C. P. NORRIS. Role of adenosine in local control of intestinal circulation in the dog. *Circ. Res.* 46: 764–770, 1980.
194. GRANGER, H. J., AND R. A. NYHOF. Dynamics of intestinal oxygenation: interactions between oxygen supply and uptake. *Am. J. Physiol.* 243 (*Gastrointest. Liver Physiol.* 6): G91–G96, 1982.
195. GRANGER, H. J., AND A. P. SHEPHERD. Dynamics and control of the microcirculation. In: *Advances in Biomedical Engineering*, edited by J. Brown. New York: Academic, 1979, vol. 7, p. 1–63.
196. GRAY, G. M., AND H. L. COOPER. Protein digestion and absorption. *Gastroenterology* 61: 535–544, 1971.
197. GRAYSON, J. The gastrointestinal circulation. In: *Gastrointestinal Physiology*, edited by E. D. Jacobson and L. L. Shanbour. Baltimore, MD: University Park, 1974, vol. 4, p. 105–138.
198. GROSZMANN, R. J., A. T. BLEI, E. H. STORER, AND H. O. CONN. Intestinal $O_2$ consumption during mechanical and

pharmacological reduction in portal pressure. *Am. J. Physiol.* 238 (*Gastrointest. Liver Physiol.* 1): G502–G508, 1980.
199. GUTH, P. H., AND E. SMITH. Histamine receptors in mesenteric circulation of the cat and rat. *Am. J. Physiol.* 234 (*Endocrinol. Metab. Gastrointest. Physiol.* 3): E370–E374, 1978.
200. GUYTON, A. C., K. SCHEEL, AND D. MURPHIES. Interstitial fluid pressure. III. Its effect in resistance to tissue fluid mobility. *Circ. Res.* 19: 412–419, 1966.
201. GUYTON, A. C., A. E. TAYLOR, AND H. J. GRANGER. *Circulatory Physiology II. Dynamics and Control of the Body Fluids.* Philadelphia, PA: Saunders, 1975.
202. HADDY, F. J., C. C. CHOU, J. B. SCOTT, AND J. M. DABNEY. Intestinal vascular responses to naturally occurring vasoactive substances. *Gastroenterology* 52: 444–451, 1967.
203. HADDY, F. J., AND J. B. SCOTT. Metabolically linked vasoactive chemicals in local regulation of blood flow. *Physiol. Rev.* 48: 688–707, 1968.
204. HADDY, F. J., AND J. B. SCOTT. Metabolic factors in peripheral circulatory regulation. *Federation Proc.* 34: 2006–2011, 1975.
205. HAINSWORTH, R., AND R. J. LINDEN. Reflex control of vascular capacitance. In: *Cardiovascular Physiology III*, edited by A. C. Guyton and D. B. Young. Baltimore, MD: University Park, 1979, p. 67–124.
206. HAKIM, A. A., AND N. LIFSON. Effects of pressure on water and solute transport by dog intestinal mucosa in vitro. *Am. J. Physiol.* 216: 276–286, 1969.
207. HALJAMAE, H., M. JODAL, AND O. LUNDGREN. Countercurrent multiplication of sodium in intestinal villi during absorption of sodium chloride. *Acta Physiol. Scand.* 89: 580–593, 1973.
208. HALLBACK, D. A., L. HULTEN, M. JODAL, J. LINDHAGEN, AND O. LUNDGREN. Evidence for the existence of a countercurrent exchanger in the small intestine in man. *Gastroenterology* 74: 683–690, 1978.
209. HALLBACK, D. A., M. JODAL, AND O. LUNDGREN. Importance of sodium and glucose for the establishment of a villous tissue hyperosmolality by the intestinal countercurrent multiplier. *Acta Physiol. Scand.* 107: 89–96, 1979.
210. HALLBACK, D. A., M. JODAL, AND O. LUNDGREN. Effects of cholera toxin on villous tissue osmolality and fluid and electrolyte transport in the small intestine of the cat. *Acta Physiol. Scand.* 107: 239–249, 1979.
211. HANSON, K. M. Hemodynamic effects of distension of the dog small intestine. *Am. J. Physiol.* 225: 456–460, 1973.
212. HANSON, K. M. Splanchnic vascular response to infusion of prostaglandins $A_1$, $A_2$, and $B_2$. *Pharmacology* 14: 166–172, 1976.
213. HANSON, K. M., AND P. C. JOHNSON. Evidence for local arteriovenous reflex in intestine. *J. Appl. Physiol.* 17: 509–513, 1962.
214. HANSON, K. M., AND P. C. JOHNSON. Pressure-flow relationships in isolated dog colon. *Am. J. Physiol.* 212: 574–579, 1967.
215. HANSON, K. M., AND F. T. MOORE. Effects of intraluminal pressure in the colon on its vascular pressure-flow relationships. *Proc. Soc. Exp. Biol. Med.* 131: 373–376, 1969.
216. HARDY, J. D., AND P. BARD. Body temperature regulation. In: *Medical Physiology*, edited by V. B. Mountcastle. St. Louis, MO: Mosby, 1974, vol. II, p. 1305–1342.
217. HARGENS, A. R., AND B. W. ZWEIFACH. Contractile stimuli in collecting lymph vessels. *Am. J. Physiol.* 233 (*Heart Circ. Physiol.* 2): H57–H65, 1977.
218. HARPER, S. L., J. A. BARROWMAN, P. R. KVIETYS, AND D. N. GRANGER. Effect of neurotensin on intestinal capillary permeability and blood flow. *Am. J. Physiol.* 247 (*Gastrointest. Liver Physiol.* 10): G161–G166, 1984.
219. HERNANDEZ, L. A., P. R. KVIETYS, AND D. N. GRANGER. Postprandial hemodynamics in the conscious rat. *Am. J. Physiol.* 251 (*Gastrointest. Liver Physiol.* 14): G117–G123, 1986.
220. HERRICK, J. F., H. E. ESSEX, F. C. MANN, AND E. J. BALDES. The effect of digestion on blood flow on certain blood vessels of the dog. *Am. J. Physiol.* 108: 621–628, 1934.
221. HINSHAW, L. B. Arterial and venous pressure-resistance relationships in perfused leg and intestine. *Am. J. Physiol.* 203: 271–274, 1962.
222. HOFFMAN, W. E., D. J. MILETICH, AND R. F. ALBRECHT. Cardiovascular and regional blood flow changes during halothane anesthesia in the aged rat. *Anesthesiology* 56: 444–448, 1982.
223. HOFMANN, A. F., AND B. BORGSTROM. The intraluminal phase of fat digestion in man: the lipid content of the micellar and oil phases of intestinal content obtained during fat digestion and absorption. *J. Clin. Invest.* 43: 247–257, 1964.
224. HOLZMAN, I. R., B. TABATA, AND D. I. EDELSTONE. Effects of varying hematocrit on intestinal oxygen uptake in neonatal lambs. *Am. J. Physiol.* 248 (*Gastrointest. Liver Physiol.* 11): G432–G436, 1985.
225. HOWLAND, R. D., AND S. SPECTOR. Disposition of histamine in mammalian blood vessels. *J. Pharmacol. Exp. Ther.* 182: 239–245, 1972.
226. HSIEH, C. P., AND C. C. CHOU. Role of humoral substances in increasing the duodenal blood flow and motility when the acid of food stuff is in the lumen (Abstract). *Federation Proc.* 31: 391, 1972.
227. HSIEH, C. P., J. M. DABNEY, W. T. CHEN, AND C. C. CHOU. Effect of lumen acidity and osmolarity on duodenal blood flow and motility (Abstract). *Physiologist* 13: 227, 1970.
228. IDVALL, J., K. F. ARONSEN, AND P. STENBERG. Tissue perfusion and distribution of cardiac output during ketamine anesthesia in normovolemic rats. *Acta Anaesthesiol. Scand.* 24: 257–263, 1980.
229. INBERG, M. V., T. HAVIA, AND M. AROLA. Effect of oxygen breathing on jejunal tissue gas tensions during superior mesenteric arterial occlusion. *Scand. J. Gastroenterol.* 9: 337–342, 1974.
230. JACOBSON, E. D., R. H. GALLAVAN, JR., AND J. D. FONDACARO. A model of the mesenteric circulation. *Am. J. Physiol.* 242 (*Gastrointest. Liver Physiol.* 5): G541–G546, 1982.
231. JÖBSIS, F. F. Basic processes in cellular respiration. In: *Handbook of Physiology. Respiration*, edited by W. O. Fenn and H. Rahn. Washington, DC: Am. Physiol. Soc., 1964, sect. 3, vol. 1, chapt. 2, p. 63–124.
232. JODAL, M. *The Significance of the Intestinal Countercurrent Exchanger for the Absorption of Sodium and Fatty Acids.* Goteborg, Sweden: Gotab, 1973.
233. JODAL, M. An autoradiographic study of the intestinal absorption of $^{22}$Na. *Acta Physiol. Scand.* 90: 79–85, 1974.
234. JODAL, M., U. HAGLUND, AND O. LUNDGREN. Countercurrent exchange mechanisms in the small intestine. In: *Physiology of the Intestinal Circulation*, edited by A. P. Shepherd and D. N. Granger. New York: Raven, 1984, p. 83–98.
235. JODAL, M., D. A. HALLBACK, AND O. LUNDGREN. Tissue osmolality in intestinal villi during luminal perfusion with isotonic electrolyte solutions. *Acta Physiol. Scand.* 102: 94–107, 1978.
236. JODAL, M., AND O. LUNDGREN. The distribution of absorbed $^3$H-palmitic acid in the intestinal villi of the cat during various circulatory conditions. *Acta Physiol. Scand.* 89: 318–326, 1973.
237. JODAL, M., AND O. LUNDGREN. Studies on the in vivo absorption of butyric acid in the small intestine of the cat. *Acta Physiol. Scand.* 89: 327–333, 1973.
238. JODAL, M., J. SVANVIK, AND O. LUNDGREN. The importance of the intestinal countercurrent exchanger for $^{85}$Kr absorption from the feline gut. *Acta Physiol. Scand.* 100: 412–423, 1977.
239. JOHNS, B. L., AND C. F. ROTHE. Delayed vascular compliance and fluid exchange in the canine intestine. *Am. J. Physiol.* 234 (*Heart Circ. Physiol.* 3): H660–H669, 1978.
240. JOHNSON, P. C. Myogenic nature of increase in intestinal vascular resistance with venous pressure elevation. *Circ. Res.* 6: 992–999, 1959.
241. JOHNSON, P. C. Autoregulation of intestinal blood flow. *Am. J. Physiol.* 199: 311–318, 1960.
243. JOHNSON, P. C. Origin, localization, and homeostatic significance of autoregulation in the intestine. *Circ. Res.* 14/15,

Suppl.: 225–233, 1964.
244. JOHNSON, P. C. Effect of venous pressure on mean capillary pressure and vascular resistance in the intestine. *Circ. Res.* 16: 294–300, 1965.
245. JOHNSON, P. C. The myogenic response. In: *Handbook of Physiology. The Cardiovascular System. Vascular Smooth Muscle*, edited by D. F. Bohr, A. P. Somlyo, and H. V. Sparks, Jr., Bethesda, MD: Am. Physiol. Soc., 1980, sect. 2, vol. II, chapt. 15, p. 409–442.
246. JOHNSON, P. C. Myogenic and venous-arteriolar responses in intestinal circulation. In: *Physiology of the Intestinal Circulation*, edited by A. P. Shepherd and D. N. Granger. New York: Raven, 1984, chapt. 4, p. 49–60.
247. JOHNSON, P. C., AND K. M. HANSON. Effect of arterial pressure on arterial and venous resistance of intestine. *J. Appl. Physiol.* 17: 503–508, 1962.
248. JOHNSON, P. C., AND K. M. HANSON. Relation between venous pressure and blood volume in the intestine. *Am. J. Physiol.* 204: 31–34, 1963.
249. JOHNSON, P. C., AND K. M. HANSON. Capillary filtration in the small intestine of the dog. *Circ. Res.* 19: 766–773, 1966.
250. JOLLIFFE, N., AND H. W. SMITH. The excretion of urine in the dog. II. The urea and creatinine clearance on cracker meal diet. *Am. J. Physiol.* 99: 101–107, 1931.
251. KAMPP, M., AND O. LUNDGREN. Evidence for countercurrent exchange in intestinal villi. *Acta. Physiol. Scand.* 68: 103–112, 1966.
252. KAMPP, M., AND O. LUNDGREN. Blood flow and flow distribution in the small intestine of the cat as analysed by the $Kr^{85}$ washout technique. *Acta. Physiol. Scand.* 72: 282–297, 1968.
253. KAMPP, M., O. LUNDGREN, AND N. J. NILSSON. Extravascular shunting of oxygen in the small intestine of the cat. *Acta Physiol. Scand.* 72: 396–403, 1968.
254. KAMPP, M., O. LUNDGREN, AND J. SJOSTRAND. On the components of the $Kr^{85}$ washout curves from the small intestine of the cat. *Acta Physiol. Scand.* 72: 257–281, 1968.
255. KAMPP, M., O. LUNDGREN, AND J. SJOSTRAND. The distribution of intravascularly administered lipid soluble and lipid insoluble substances in the mucosa and the submucosa of the small intestine of the cat. *Acta Physiol. Scand.* 72: 469–480, 1968.
256. KARNOVSKY, M. J. The ultrastructural basis of transcapillary exchanges. *J. Gen. Physiol.* 52: 641–696, 1968.
257. KATZ, J. A., L. SELLERS, G. BANORIS, AND S. GOLDEN. Studies on the extravascular albumin of rats. In: *Plasma Protein Metabolism*, edited by M. Rothschild and P. Waldmonn. New York: Academic, 1970, chapt. 8, p. 129–154.
258. KAUFFMAN, G. L., JR., D. AURES, AND M. I. GROSSMAN. Intravenous indomethacin and aspirin reduce basal gastric mucosal blood flow in dogs. *Am. J. Physiol.* 238 (*Gastrointest. Liver Physiol.* 1): G131–G134, 1980.
259. KAWAUE, Y., AND J. IRIUCHIJIMA. Changes in cardiac output and peripheral flows in pentobarbital anesthesia in the rat. *Jpn. J. Physiol.* 34: 283–294, 1984.
260. KELLUM, J. M., AND B. M. JAFFE. Release of immunoreactive serotonin following acid perfusion of the duodenum. *Ann. Surg.* 184: 633–636, 1976.
261. KELLUM, J. M., AND B. M. JAFFE. Validation and application of a radioimmunoassay for serotonin. *Gastroenterology* 70: 516–522, 1976.
262. KEUSCH, G. T., J. J. RAHAL, JR., L. WEINSTEIN, AND G. F. GRADY. Biochemical effects of cholera enterotoxin: oxidative metabolism in the infant rabbit. *Am. J. Physiol.* 218: 703–707, 1970.
263. KIEL, J. W., V. PITTS, J. N. BENOIT, D. N. GRANGER, AND A. P. SHEPHERD. Reduced vascular sensitivity to norepinephrine in portal-hypertensive rats. *Am. J. Physiol.* 248 (*Gastrointest. Liver Physiol.* 11): G192–G195, 1985.
264. KNAPP, H. R., O. OSWALD, B. J. SWEETMAN, AND J. A. OATES. Synthesis and metabolism of prostaglandins $E_2$, $F_{2\alpha}$, and $D_2$ by the rat gastrointestinal tract. Stimulation by a hypertonic environment in vitro. *Prostaglandins* 15: 751–757, 1978.
265. KOEHLER, R. C., B. W. McDONALD, AND J. A. KRASNEY. Influence of $CO_2$ on cardiovascular response to hypoxia in conscious dogs. *Am. J. Physiol.* 239 (*Heart Circ. Physiol.* 8): H545–H558, 1980.
266. KOKKO, J. P. Countercurrent exchanger in the small intestine of man: is there evidence for its existence? *Gastroenterology* 74: 791–793, 1978.
267. KONTUREK, S. J., J. JAWOREK, M. CIESZKOWSKI, W. PAWLIK, J. KANIA, AND S. R. BLOOM. Comparison of effects of neurotensin and fat on pancreatic stimulation in dogs. *Am. J. Physiol.* 244 (*Gastrointest. Liver Physiol.* 7): G590–G598, 1983.
268. KONTUREK, S. J., AND R. SIEBERS. Role of histamine $H_1$- and $H_2$-receptors in myoelectric activity of small bowel in the dog. *Am. J. Physiol.* 238 (*Gastrointest. Liver Physiol.* 1): G50–G56, 1980.
269. KOO, A., S. K. LAM, AND L. H. SMAJE (editors). *Microcirculation of the Alimentary Tract*. Singapore: World Scientific Publ. 1983.
270. KVIETYS, P. R.. Microcirculation of the large intestine. In: *The Physiology and Pharmacology of the Microcirculation*, edited by N. A. Mortillaro. Orlando, FL: Academic, 1984, p. 77–94.
271. KVIETYS, P. R., J. A. BARROWMAN, AND D. N. GRANGER. Effects of anesthetics and other experimental conditions on splanchnic blood flow. In: *The Measurement of Splanchnic Blood Flow*, edited by D. N. Granger and G. B. Bulkley. Baltimore, MD: Williams & Wilkins, 1981, p. 59–65.
272. KVIETYS, P. R., J. A. BARROWMAN, S. L. HARPER, AND D. N. GRANGER. Relations between canine intestinal motility, blood flow and oxygenation (Abstract). *Federation Proc.* 43: 1010, 1985.
273. KVIETYS, P. R., R. H. GALLAVAN, AND C. C. CHOU. Contribution of bile to postprandial intestinal hyperemia. *Am. J. Physiol.* 238 (*Gastrointest. Liver Physiol.* 1): G284–G288, 1980.
274. KVIETYS, P. R., AND D. N. GRANGER. Effect of volatile fatty acids on blood flow and oxygen uptake by the dog colon. *Gastroenterology* 80: 962–969, 1981.
275. KVIETYS, P. R., AND D. N. GRANGER. Effects of solute-coupled fluid absorption on blood flow and oxygen uptake in dog colon. *Gastroenterology* 81: 450–457, 1981.
276. KVIETYS, P. R., AND D. N. GRANGER. The colonic circulation. *Federation Proc.* 41: 2106–2110, 1982.
277. KVIETYS, P. R., AND D. N. GRANGER. Relation between intestinal blood flow and oxygen uptake. *Am. J. Physiol.* 242 (*Gastrointest. Liver Physiol.* 5): G202–G208, 1982.
278. KVIETYS, P. R., AND D. N. GRANGER. Vasoactive agents and splanchnic oxygen uptake. *Am. J. Physiol.* 243 (*Gastrointest. Liver Physiol.* 6): G1–G9, 1982.
279. KVIETYS, P. R., AND D. N. GRANGER. Physiology, pharmacology and pathology of the colonic circulation. In: *Physiology of the Intestinal Circulation*, edited by A. P. Shepherd and D. N. Granger. New York: Raven, 1984, p. 131–142.
281. KVIETYS, P. R., S. L. HARPER, R. J. KORTHUIS, AND D. N. GRANGER. Effects of temperature on ileal blood flow and oxygenation. *Am. J. Physiol.* 249 (*Gastrointest. Liver Physiol.* 12): G246–G249, 1985.
282. KVIETYS, P. R., J. M. McLENDON, AND D. N. GRANGER. Postprandial intestinal hyperemia: role of bile salts in the ileum. *Am. J. Physiol.* 241 (*Gastrointest. Liver Physiol.* 4): G469–G477, 1981.
283. KVIETYS, P. R., T. MILLER, AND D. N. GRANGER. Intrinsic control of colonic blood flow and oxygenation. *Am. J. Physiol.* 238 (*Gastrointest. Liver Physiol.* 1): G478–G484, 1980.
284. KVIETYS, P. R., C. A. NAVIA, A. J. PREMEN, AND D. N. GRANGER. Quantitative assessment of the two-component model of intestinal circulation. *Am. J. Physiol.* 251 (*Gastrointest. Liver Physiol.* 14): G446–G452, 1986.
285. KVIETYS, P. R., M. A. PERRY, AND D. N. GRANGER. Intestinal capillary exchange capacity and oxygen delivery-to-demand ratio. *Am. J. Physiol.* 245 (*Gastrointest. Liver Physiol.* 8):

G635–G640, 1983.
286. KVIETYS, P. R., R. PITTMAN, AND C. C. CHOU. Contribution of luminal concentration of nutrients and osmolality to postprandial hyperemia in dogs. *Proc. Soc. Exp. Biol. Med.* 152: 659–663, 1976.
287. KVIETYS, P. R., W. H. WILBORN, AND D. N. GRANGER. Effect of atropine on bile-oleic acid-induced alterations in dog jejunal hemodynamics, oxygenation, and net transmucosal water movement. *Gastroenterology* 80: 31–38, 1981.
288. KVIETYS, P. R., W. H. WILBORN, AND D. N. GRANGER. Effects of net transmucosal volume flux on lymph flow in the canine colon: structural-functional relationship. *Gastroenterology* 81: 1080–1090, 1981.
289. LAINE, G. A., AND H. J. GRANGER. Permeability of intestinal capillaries in chronic arterial hypertension. *Hypertension Dallas* 5: 722–727, 1983.
290. LARSSON, L. I., J. FAHRENKRUG, O. SCHAFFALITZKY DE MUCKADELL, F. SUNDLER, R. HAKANSON, AND J. F. REHFELD. Localization of vasoactive intestinal polypeptide (VIP) to central and peripheral neurons. *Proc. Natl. Acad. Sci. USA* 73: 3197–3200, 1976.
291. LAWRENCE, J. A., D. BRYAN, K. B. ROBERTS, AND J. A. BARROWMAN. Effect of secretin on intestinal lymph flow and composition in rat. *Q. J. Exp. Physiol. Cogn. Med. Sci.* 66: 297–305, 1981.
292. LEAK, L. V., AND J. F. BURKE. Ultrastructure studies on the lymphatic anchoring filaments. *J. Cell Biol.* 36: 129–149, 1968.
293. LEE, J. S. A micropuncture study of water transport by dog jejunal villi in vitro. *Am. J. Physiol.* 217: 1528–1533, 1969.
294. LEE, J. S. Contraction of villi and fluid transport in dog jejunal mucosa in vitro. *Am. J. Physiol.* 221: 488–495, 1971.
295. LEE, J. S. Lymph capillary pressure of rat intestinal villi during fluid absorption. *Am. J. Physiol.* 237 (*Endocrinol. Metab. Gastrointest. Physiol.* 6): E301–E307
296. LEE, J. S. Lymph flow during fluid absorption from rat jejunum. *Am. J. Physiol.* 240 (*Gastrointest. Liver Physiol.* 3): G312–G316, 1981.
297. LEE, J. S. Lymph pressure in intestinal villi and lymph flow during fluid secretion. In: *Tissue Fluid Pressure and Composition*, edited by A. R. Hargens. Baltimore, MD: Williams & Wilkins, 1981, p. 165–172.
298. LEE, J. S. Lymphatic contractility. In: *Physiology of the Intestinal Circulation*, edited by A. P. Shepherd and D. N. Granger. New York: Raven, 1984, p. 201–210.
299. LEE, J. S., AND K. M. DUNCAN. Lymphatic and venous transport of water from rat jejunum: a vascular perfusion study. *Gastroenterology* 54: 559–567, 1968.
300. LEE, K. E., AND R. A. SUMMERILL. Glomerular filtration rate following administration of individual amino acids in conscious dogs. *Q. J. Exp. Physiol. Cogn. Med. Sci.* 67: 459–465, 1982.
301. LEES, M. H., J. HILL, A. J. OCHSNER, AND C. THOMAS. Regional blood flows of the rhesus monkey during halothane anesthesia. *Anesth. Analg.* 50: 270–281, 1971.
302. LEHNINGER, A. L. *Biochemistry. The Molecular Basis of Cell Structure and Function* (2nd ed.). New York: Worth, 1975.
303. LEVINE, G. W. Anticoagulant, antithrombotic and thrombolytic drugs. In: *The Pharmacological Basis of Therapeutics*, edited by L. S. Goodman and A. Gilman. New York: Macmillan, 1975.
304. LEVINE, S. E., D. N. GRANGER, R. A. BRACE, AND A. E. TAYLOR. Effect of hyperosmolality on vascular resistance and lymph flow in the cat ileum. *Am. J. Physiol.* 234 (*Heart Circ. Physiol.* 3): H14–H20, 1978.
305. LEVITT, D. G., J. H. BOND, AND M. D. LEVITT. Use of a model of small bowel mucosa to predict passive absorption. *Am. J. Physiol.* 239 (*Gastrointest. Liver Physiol.* 2): G23–G29, 1980.
306. LEVITT, M. D., AND D. G. LEVITT. Use of inert gases to study the interaction of blood flow and diffusion during passive absorption from gastrointestinal tract of the rat. *J. Clin. Invest.* 52: 1852–1862, 1973.

307. LUNDEEN, G., M. MANOHAR, AND C. PARKS. Systemic distribution of blood flow in swine while awake and during 1.0 and 1.5 MAC isoflurane anesthesia with or without 50% nitrous oxide. *Anesth. Analg.* 62: 499–512, 1983.
308. LUNDGREN, O. Studies on blood flow distribution and countercurrent exchange in the small intestine. *Acta Physiol. Scand. Suppl.* 303: 1–42, 1967.
309. LUNDGREN. O. The alimentary canal. In: *Peripheral Circulation*, edited by P. C. Johnson. New York: Wiley, 1978, p. 255–283.
310. Lundgren, O. Role of splanchnic resistance vessels in overall cardiovascular homeostasis. *Federation Proc.* 42: 1673–1677, 1983.
310a. Lundgren. O. Countercurrent exchange mechanisms in the small intestine. In: *Physiology of the Intestinal Circulation*, edited by A. P. Shepherd and D. N. Granger. New York: Raven, 1984, p. 83–97.
311. LUNDGREN, O. Microcirculation of the gastrointestinal tract and pancreas. In: *Handbook of Physiology. The Cardiovascular System. Microcirculation*, edited by E. M. Renkin and C. C. Michel. Bethesda, MD: Am. Physiol. Soc., 1984, sect. 2, vol. IV, pt. 2, chapt. 17, p. 799–863.
312. LUNDGREN, O., AND U. HAGLUND. The pathophysiology of the intestinal countercurrent exchanger. *Life Sci.* 23: 1411–1422, 1978.
313. LUNDGREN, O., AND J. SVANVIK. Mucosal hemodynamics in the small intestine of the cat during reduced perfusion pressure. *Acta Physiol. Scand.* 88: 551–563, 1973.
314. LUNDGREN, O., AND J. SVANVIK. Gastrointestinal circulation. In: *Gastrointestinal Physiology II*, edited by R. K. Crane. Baltimore, MD: University Park, 1976, vol. 12, p. 1–33.
316. MACDONALD, J. M., M. M. WEBSTER, JR., AND C. H. TENNYSON. Serotonin and bradykinin in the dumping syndrome. *Am. J. Surg.* 117: 204–211, 1969.
317. MACFERRAN, S. N., AND D. MAILMAN. Effects of glucagon on canine intestinal sodium and water fluxes and regional blood flow. *J. Physiol. Lond.* 266: 1–12, 1977.
318. MAILMAN, D. Effects of vasoactive intestinal polypeptide on intestinal absorption and blood flow. *J. Physiol. Lond.* 279: 121–132, 1978.
319. MAILMAN, D. Effects of pentagastrin on intestinal absorption and blood flow in the anesthetized dog. *J. Physiol. Lond.* 307: 429–442, 1980.
320. MAILMAN, D. Blood flow and intestinal absorption. *Federation Proc.* 41: 2096–2100, 1982.
321. MAILMAN, D. Relationships between intestinal absorption and hemodynamics. *Annu. Rev. Physiol.* 44: 43–55, 1982.
322. MAILMAN, D. Morphine-neural interactions on canine intestinal absorption and blood flow. *Br. J. Pharmacol.* 81: 263–270, 1984.
323. MAILMAN, D. Tritiated water clearance as a measure of intestinal absorptive site and total blood flow. In: *Measurement of Blood Flow: Applications to the Splanchnic Circulation*, edited by D. N. Granger and G. B. Bulkley. Baltimore, MD: Williams & Wilkins, 1981, p. 338–361.
324. MAILMAN, D., AND K. JORDAN. The effect of saline and hyperoncotic dextran infusion on canine ileal salt and water absorption and regional blood flow. *J. Physiol. Lond.* 252: 97–113, 1975.
325. MAILMAN, D., W. PAWLIK, A. P. SHEPHERD, L. L. TAGUE, AND E. D. JACOBSON. Cyclic nucleotide metabolism and vasodilation in canine mesenteric artery. *Am. J. Physiol.* 232 (*Heart Circ. Physiol.* 1): H191–H196, 1977.
326. MALL, J. P. Die Blut-und Lymphwege im Dunndarm des Hundes. *Abh. Sachs. Ges. Wiss.* 14: 153–189, 1888.
327. MANDERS, W. T., AND S. F. VATNER. Effects of sodium pentobarbital anesthesia on left ventricular function and distribution of cardiac output in dogs, with particular reference to the mechanism for tachycardia. *Circ. Res.* 39: 512–517, 1976.
328. MANGINO, M. J., AND C. C. CHOU. Arachidonic acid and postprandial intestinal hyperemia. *Am. J. Physiol.* 246 (*Gas-

*trointest. Liver Physiol.* 9): G521–G527, 1984.
329. MATON, P. N., A. C. SELDON, AND V. S. CHADWICK. Large and small forms of cholecystokinin in human plasma: measurement using high pressure liquid chromatography and radioimmunoassay. *Regul. Pept.* 4: 251–260, 1982.
330. MATON, P. N., A. C. SELDON, M. L. FITZPATRICK, AND V. S. CHADWICK. Infusion of cholecystokinin octapeptide in man: relation between plasma cholecystokinin concentrations and gallbladder emptying rates. *Eur. J. Clin. Invest.* 14: 37–41, 1984.
331. MAYERSON, H. S., C. G. WOLFRAM, H. H. SHIRLEY, JR., AND K. WASSERMAN. Regional differences in capillary permeability. *Am. J. Physiol.* 198: 155–160, 1960.
332. MCCUSKEY, R. S., S. G. MCCLUGAGE, T. J. MOORE, AND M. L. MILLER. Responses of the fetal mesenteric microvascular system to maternal hypoxia. *Proc. Soc. Exp. Biol. Med.* 132: 636–639, 1969.
333. MCDONALD, G. B., D. R. SAUNDERS, M. WEIDMAN, AND L. FISHER. Portal venous transport of long-chain fatty acids absorbed from rat intestine. *Am. J. Physiol.* 239 (*Gastrointest. Liver Physiol.* 2): G141–G150, 1980.
334. MCNEILL, J. R. Intestinal vasoconstriction following diuretic-induced volume depletion: role of angiotensin and vasopressin. *Can. J. Physiol. Pharmacol.* 52: 829–839, 1974.
335. MCNEILL, J. R. Redundant nature of the vasopressin and renin-angiotensin systems in the control of mesenteric resistance vessels of the conscious, fasted cat. *Can. J. Physiol. Pharmacol.* 61: 770–773, 1983.
336. MCNEILL, J. R. Role of vasopressin in the control of arterial pressure. *Can. J. Physiol. Pharmacol.* 61: 1226–1235, 1983.
337. MCNEILL, J. R., AND C. C. Y. PANG. Effect of pentobarbital anesthesia and surgery on the control of arterial pressure and mesenteric resistance in cats: role of vasopressin and angiotensin. *Can. J. Physiol. Pharmacol.* 60: 363–368, 1982.
338. MCNEILL, J. R., R. D. STARK, AND C. V. GREENWAY. Intestinal vasoconstriction after hemorrhage: roles of vasopressin and angiotensin. *Am. J. Physiol.* 219: 1342–1347, 1970.
339. MCNEILL, J. R., W. C. WILCOX, AND C. C. Y. PANG. Vasopressin and angiotensin: reciprocal mechanisms controlling mesenteric conductance. *Am. J. Physiol.* 232 (*Heart Circ. Physiol.* 1): H260–H266, 1977.
340. MEININGER, G. A., L. K. ROUTH, AND H. J. GRANGER. Autoregulation and vasoconstriction in the intestine during acute renal hypertension. *Hypertension Dallas* 7: 364–373, 1985.
341. MICHEL, C. C. Measurement of permeability in single capillaries. *Arch. Int. Physiol. Biochim.* 86: 657–667, 1978.
342. MIZONISHI, T., AND T. SEMB. Effects of distension on mesenteric blood flow and $O_2$ saturation of venous blood in the dog intestinal loop. *Jpn. J. Physiol.* 29: 627–633, 1979.
344. MORTILLARO, N. A., AND R. ALLEN. Effects of venous pressure on intestinal metabolism (Abstract). *Federation Proc.* 39: 705, 1980.
345. MORTILLARO, N. A., D. N. GRANGER, P. R. KVIETYS, G. RUTILI, AND A. E. TAYLOR. Effects of histamine and histamine antagonists on intestinal capillary permeability. *Am. J. Physiol.* 240 (*Gastrointest. Liver Physiol.* 3): G381–G386, 1981.
346. MORTILLARO, N. A., AND H. J. GRANGER. Reactive hyperemia and oxygen extraction in the feline small intestine. *Circ. Res.* 41: 859–865, 1977.
347. MORTILLARO, N. A., AND S. J. MUSTAFA. Possible role of adenosine in intestinal reactive hyperemia (Abstract). *Federation Proc.* 37: 874, 1978.
348. MORTILLARO, N. A., AND A. E. TAYLOR. Interaction of capillary and tissue forces in the cat small intestine. *Circ. Res.* 39: 348–358, 1976.
349. NICOLL, P. A., AND A. E. TAYLOR. Lymph formation and flow. *Annu. Rev. Physiol.* 39: 73–95, 1977.
350. NIXON, S. E., AND G. E. MAWER. The digestion and absorption of protein in man. II. The form in which digested protein is absorbed. *Br. J. Nutr.* 24: 241–258, 1970.
351. NORRIS, C. P., G. E. BARNES, E. E. SMITH, AND H. J. GRANGER. Autoregulation of superior mesenteric flow in fasted and fed dogs. *Am. J. Physiol.* 237 (*Heart Circ. Physiol.* 6): H174–H177, 1979.
352. NOWAK, J., AND A. WENNONALM. Influence of indomethacin and of prostaglandin $E_1$ on total and regional blood flow in man. *Acta Physiol. Scand.* 102: 484–491, 1978.
353. NYHOF, R. A., AND C. C. CHOU. Absence of cholinergic or serotonergic mediation in food-induced intestinal hyperemia (Abstract). *Federation Proc.* 40: 491, 1981.
354. NYHOF, R. A., AND C. C. CHOU. Evidence against local neural mechanism for intestinal postprandial hyperemia. *Am. J. Physiol.* 245 (*Heart Circ. Physiol.* 14): H437–H446, 1983.
355. NYHOF, R. A., AND H. J. GRANGER. Acute local effects of angiotensin II on the intestinal vasculature. *Hypertension Dallas* 6: 13–19, 1984.
356. O'CONNOR, W. J., AND R. A. SUMMERILL. The effect of a meal of meat on glomerular filtration rate in dogs at normal urine flows. *J. Physiol. Lond.* 256: 81–91, 1976.
357. OHMAN, U. Blood flow and oxygen consumption in the feline small intestine: responses to artificial distention and intestinal obstruction. *Acta Chir. Scand.* 142: 329–333, 1976.
358. OLMSTEAD, W. W., E. S. NASSETT, AND M. I. KELLEY, JR. Amino acids in postprandial gut contents of man. *J. Nutr.* 90: 291–294, 1966.
359. ORMSBEE, H. S., AND J. D. FONDACARO. Minireview: action of serotonin on the gastrointestinal tract. *Proc. Soc. Exp. Biol. Med.* 178: 333–338, 1985.
360. OSTMAN, M., B. BIBER, J. MARTINER, AND S. REIZ. Effects of isoflurane on vascular tone and circulatory autoregulation. *Acta Physiol. Scand.* 29: 389–394, 1985.
361. PALADE, G. E., AND R. R. BRUNS. Structural modulations of plasmalemmal vesicles. *J. Cell Biol.* 37: 633–649, 1968.
362. PALADE, G. E., M. SIMIONESCU, AND N. SIMIONESCU. Structural aspects of the permeability of the microvascular endothelium. *Acta. Physiol. Scand. Suppl.* 463: 11–32, 1979.
363. PALS, D. T., AND F. R. STEGGERDA. Relation of intraintestinal carbon dioxide to intestinal blood flow. *Am. J. Physiol.* 210: 893–896, 1966.
364. PANG, C. C. Y. Effect of vasopressin antagonist and saralasin on regional blood flow following hemorrhage. *Am. J. Physiol.* 245 (*Heart Circ. Physiol.* 14): H749–H755, 1983.
365. PANG, C. C. Y. Vasopressin and angiotensin in the control of arterial pressure and regional blood flow in anesthetized, surgically stressed rats. *Can. J. Physiol. Pharmacol.* 61: 1494–1500, 1983.
366. PAPPENHEIMER, J. R., AND A. SOTO-RIVERA. Effective osmotic pressure of the plasma proteins and other quantities associated with the capillary circulation in the hindlimbs of cats and dogs. *Am. J. Physiol.* 152: 471–480, 1948.
367. PARKER, R. E., AND D. N. GRANGER. Effect of graded arterial occlusion on ileal blood flow distribution. *Proc. Soc. Exp. Biol. Med.* 162: 146–149, 1979.
368. PAWLIK, W. W., J. D. FONDACARO, AND E. D. JACOBSON. Metabolic hyperemia in the canine gut. *Am. J. Physiol.* 239 (*Gastrointest. Liver Physiol.* 2): G12–G17, 1980.
369. PAWLIK, W., AND E. D. JACOBSON. Effects of digoxin on the mesenteric circulation. *Cardiovasc. Res. Cent. Bull. Houston* 12: 80–84, 1974.
370. PAWLIK, W., A. P. SHEPHERD, AND E. D. JACOBSON. Effects of vasoactive agents on intestinal oxygen consumption and blood flow in dogs. *J. Clin. Invest.* 56: 484–490, 1975.
371. PAWLIK, W., L. L. TAGUE, B. L. TEPPERMAN, T. A. MILLER, AND E. D. JACOBSON. Histamine $H_1$- and $H_2$-receptor vasodilation of canine intestinal circulation. *Am. J. Physiol.* 233 (*Endocrinol. Metab. Gastrointest. Physiol.* 2): E219–E224, 1977.
372. PEETERS, L. L., R. E. SHELDON, M. D. JONES, E. L. MAKOWSKI, AND G. MESCHIA. Blood flow to fetal organs as a function of arterial oxygen content. *Am. J. Obstet. Gynecol.* 135: 637–646, 1979.
373. PERNOW, B. Substance P. *Pharmacol. Rev.* 35: 85–141, 1983.

374. PERRY, M. A., J. N. BENOIT, P. R. KVIETYS, AND D. N. GRANGER. Restricted transport of cationic macromolecules across intestinal capillaries. *Am. J. Physiol.* 245 (*Gastrointest. Liver Physiol.* 8): G568–G572, 1983.
375. PERRY, M. A., AND D. N. GRANGER. Permeability of intestinal capillaries to small molecules. *Am. J. Physiol.* 241 (*Gastrointest. Liver Physiol.* 4): G24–G30, 1981.
376. PERRY, M. A., A. P. SHEPHERD, P. R. KVIETYS, AND D. N. GRANGER. Effect of hypoxia on feline intestinal capillary permeability. *Am. J. Physiol.* 248 (*Gastrointest. Liver Physiol.* 11): G272–G276, 1985.
377. PITTS, R. F. The effect of protein and amino acid metabolism on the urea and xylose clearance. *J. Nutr.* 9: 657–666, 1935.
378. PITTS, R. F. The effects of infusing glycine and of varying the dietary protein intake on renal hemodynamics in the dog. *Am. J. Physiol.* 142: 355–365, 1944.
379. POLAK, J., S. SULLIVAN, S. BLOOM, A. BUCHAN, P. FACER, M. BROWN, AND A. PEARSE. Specific localisation of neurotensin to the N-cell in human intestine by radioimmunoassay and immunocytochemistry. *Nature Lond.* 270: 183–184, 1977.
380. POST, J. A., C. C. CHOU, AND P. R. KVIETYS. Possible mechanisms of postprandial intestinal hyperemia (Abstract). *Federation Proc.* 34: 459, 1975.
381. PREMEN, A. J. Importance of the liver during glucagon-mediated increases in canine renal hemodynamics. *Am. J. Physiol.* 249 (*Renal Fluid Electrolyte Physiol.* 18): F319–F322, 1985.
382. PREMEN, A. J., D. E. DOBBINS, C. Y. SOIKA, AND J. M. DABNEY. Relationship between substance P, intestinal wall compliance, and vascular resistance in the canine ileum. *Regul. Pept.* 9: 119–127, 1984.
383. PREMEN, A. J., J. E. HALL, AND M. J. SMITH, JR. Postprandial regulation of renal hemodynaimcs: role of pancreatic glucagon. *Am. J. Physiol.* 248 (*Renal Fluid Electrolyte Physiol.* 17): F656–F662, 1985.
384. PREMEN, A. J., P. R. KVIETYS, AND D. N. GRANGER. Postprandial regulation of intestinal blood flow: role of gastrointestinal hormones. *Am. J. Physiol.* 249 (*Gastrointest. Liver Physiol.* 12): G250–G255, 1985.
385. PREMEN, A. J., C. Y. SOIKA, J. M. DABNEY, AND D. E. DOBBINS. Effects of gastrointestinal hormones on ileal vascular and visceral smooth muscle. *Am. J. Physiol.* 246 (*Gastrointest. Liver Physiol.* 9): G1–G7, 1984.
386. PRIANO, L. L., AND S. F. VATNER. Generalized cardiovascular and regional hemodynamic effects on meperidine in conscious dogs. *Anesth. Analg.* 60: 649–654, 1981.
387. PRIANO, L. L., AND S. F. VATNER. Morphine effects on cardiac output and regional blood flow distribution in conscious dogs. *Anesthesiology* 55: 236–243, 1981.
388. PROCTOR, K. G. Contribution of hyperosmolality to glucose-induced intestinal hyperemia. *Am. J. Physiol.* 248 (*Gastrointest. Liver Physiol.* 11): G521–G525, 1985.
389. PROCTOR, K. G. Differential effect of cyclooxygenase inhibitors on absorptive hyperemia. *Am. J. Physiol.* 249 (*Heart Circ. Physiol.* 18): H755–H762, 1985.
390. PROCTOR, K. G. Possible role for adenosine on local regulation of absorptive hyperemia in rat intestine. *Circ. Res.* 59: 474–481, 1986.
391. PULLMAN, T. N., A. S. ALVING, R. J. DERN, AND M. LANDOWNE. The influence of dietary protein intake on specific renal functions in normal man. *J. Lab. Clin. Med.* 44: 320–332, 1954.
392. QUILLEN, E. W., D. N. GRANGER, AND A. E. TAYLOR. Effects of arginine vasopressin on capillary filtration in the cat ileum. *Gastroenterology* 73: 1290–1295, 1977.
393. REINHARDT, H. W., G. KACZMARCZYK, K. FARHRENHORST, I. BLENDINGER, M. GATZKA, U. KUHL, AND J. RIEDEL. Postprandial changes of renal blood flow: studies on conscious dogs on a high and low sodium intake. *Pfluegers Arch.* 354: 287–297, 1975.
394. RENKIN, E. M. Multiple pathways of capillary permeability. *Circ. Res.* 41: 735–743, 1977.
395. RENKIN, E. M. Relation of capillary morphology to transport of fluid and large molecules: a review. *Acta Physiol. Scand. Suppl.* 463: 81–91, 1979.
396. RENKIN, E. M., P. D. WATSON, C. H. SLOOP, W. L. JOYNER, AND F. E. CURRY. Transport pathways for fluid and large molecules in microvascular endothelium of the dog's paw. *Microvasc. Res.* 14: 205–214, 1977.
397. RICHARDSON, P. D. I., AND D. N. GRANGER. Capillary filtration coefficient as a measure of perfused capillary density. In: *Measurement of Blood Flow: Applications to the Splanchnic Circulation*, edited by D. N. Granger and G. B. Bulkley. Baltimore, MD: Williams & Wilkins, 1981, p. 319–335.
398. RICHARDSON, P. D. I., D. N. GRANGER, D. MAILMAN, AND P. R. KVIETYS. Permeability characteristics of colonic capillaries. *Am. J. Physiol.* 239 (*Gastrointest. Liver Physiol.* 2): G300–G305, 1980.
399. RICHARDSON, P. D. I., D. N. GRANGER, AND A. E. TAYLOR. Capillary filtration coefficient: the technique and its application to the small intestine. *Cardiovasc. Res.* 13: 547–561, 1979.
400. RIPPE, B., A. KAMIYA, AND B. FOLKOW. Transcapillary passage of albumin, effects of tissue cooling and of increases in filtration and plasma colloid osmotic pressure. *Acta Physiol. Scand.* 105: 171–187, 1979.
401. ROSS, G. The regional circulation. *Annu. Rev. Physiol.* 33: 445–478, 1971.
402. ROTHE, C. F. Venous system: physiology of the capacitance vessels. In: *Handbook of Physiology. The Cardiovascular System. Peripheral Circulation and Organ Blood Flow*, edited by J. T. Shepherd and F. M. Abboud. Bethesda, MD: Am. Physiol. Soc., 1983, sect. 2, vol. III, pt. 1, chapt. 13, p. 397–452.
403. ROTHE, C. F. Control of capacitance vessels. In: *Physiology of the Intestinal Circulation*, edited by A. P. Shepherd and D. N. Granger. New York: Raven, 1984, p. 73–81.
404. ROTHE, C. F., T. D. BENNETT, AND B. L. JOHNS. Linearity of the vascular pressure-volume relationship of the canine intestine. *Circ. Res.* 47: 551–558, 1980.
405. ROTHE, C. F., B. L. JOHNS, AND T. D. BENNETT. Vascular capacitance of dog intestine using mean transit time of indicator. *Am. J. Physiol.* 234 (*Heart Circ. Physiol.* 3): H7–H13, 1978.
406. RUF, W., G. T. SUEHIRO, A. SUEHIRO, V. PRESSLER, AND J. J. McNAMARA. Intestinal blood flow at various intraluminal pressures in the piglet with closed abdomen. *Ann. Surg.* 191: 157–163, 1980.
407. RUSZNYAK, I., M. FOLDI, AND G. SZABO. *Lymphatics and Lymph Circulation* (2nd ed.). Oxford, UK: Pergamon, 1967.
408. RYU, K. H., AND E. GRIM. Countercurrent exchange of water in canine jejunum. *Am. J. Physiol.* 249 (*Gastrointest. Liver Physiol.* 12): G377–G381, 1985.
409. SABESIN, S. M., AND S. FRASE. Electron microscopic studies of the assembly, intracellular transport, and secretion of chylomicrons by rat intestine. *J. Lipid. Res.* 18: 496–511, 1977.
410. SANDERS, K. M., AND G. ROSS. Effects of endogenous prostaglandin E on intestinal motility. *Am. J. Physiol.* 234 (*Endocrinol. Metab. Gastrointest. Physiol.* 3): E204–E208, 1978.
411. SAVOLAINEN, V. P. Splanchnic blood flow during anesthesia. *Int. Anesthesiol. Clin.* 7: 369–391, 1969.
412. SCHAYER, R. W., AND A. C. IVY. Release of $C^{14}$-histamine from stomach and intestine on feeding. *Am. J. Physiol.* 193: 400–402, 1958.
413. SCHEHADEH, Z., W. E. PRICE, AND E. D. JACOBSON. Effects of vasoactive agents on intestinal blood flow and motility on the dog. *Am. J. Physiol.* 216: 386–392, 1969.
414. SCHMITT, S. L., K. TAYLOR, R. SCHMIDT, D. VAN ORDEN, AND H. E. WILLIAMSON. The role of volume depletion, antidiuretic hormone and angiotensin II in the furosemide-induced decrease in mesenteric conductance in the dog. *J. Pharmacol. Exp. Ther.* 219: 407–414, 1981.
415. SCHRAUWEN, E., AND A. HOUVENAGHEL. A comparison of the threshold doses of various vasodilators in the pig mesenteric vascular bed. *Physiology* 8: 107, 1980.

416. SCHWAIGER, M., J. D. FONDACARO, AND E. D. JACOBSON. Effects of glucagon, histamine, and perhexiline on the ischemic canine mesenteric circulation. *Gastroenterology* 77: 730–735, 1979.
417. SCOTT, J. B., AND J. M. DABNEY. Relation of gut motility to blood flow in the ileum of the dog. *Circ. Res.* 14: 234–239, 1964.
418. SELKURT, E. E., C. F. ROTHE, AND D. RICHARDSON. Characteristics of reactive hyperemia in the canine intestine. *Circ. Res.* 15: 532–544, 1964.
419. SEYDE, W. C., L. MCGOWAN, N. LUND, B. DULING, AND D. E. LONGNECKER. Effects of anesthetics on regional hemodynamics in normovolemic and hemorrhaged rats. *Am. J. Physiol.* 249 (*Heart Circ. Physiol.* 18): H164–H173, 1985.
420. SHANNON, J. A., N. JOLLIFFE, AND H. W. SMITH. The excretion of urine in the dog. IV. The effect of maintenance diet, etc., upon the quantity of glomerular filtrate. *Am. J. Physiol.* 101: 625–638, 1932.
421. SHEPHERD, A. P. Myogenic responses of intestinal resistance and exchange vessels. *Am. J. Physiol.* 233 (*Heart Circ. Physiol.* 2): H547–H554, 1977.
422. SHEPHERD, A. P. Intestinal $O_2$ consumption and $^{86}Rb$ extraction during arterial hypoxia. *Am. J. Physiol.* 234 (*Endocrinol. Metab. Gastrointest. Physiol.* 3): E248–E251, 1978.
423. SHEPHERD, A. P. Effect of arterial pulse pressure and hypoxia on myogenic responses in the gut. *Am. J. Physiol.* 235 (*Heart Circ. Physiol.* 4): H157–H161, 1978.
424. SHEPHERD, A. P. Intestinal $O_2$ uptake during sympathetic stimulation and partial arterial occlusion. *Am. J. Physiol.* 236 (*Heart Circ. Physiol.* 5): H731–H735, 1979.
425. SHEPHERD, A. P. Intestinal capillary blood flow during metabolic hyperemia. *Am. J. Physiol.* 237 (*Endocrinol. Metab. Gastrointest. Physiol.* 6): E548–E554, 1979.
426. SHEPHERD, A. P. Intestinal blood flow autoregulation during foodstuff absorption. *Am. J. Physiol.* 239 (*Heart Circ. Physiol.* 8): H156–H162, 1980.
427. SHEPHERD, A. P. Metabolic control of intestinal oxygenation and blood flow. *Federation Proc.* 41: 2084–2089, 1982.
428. SHEPHERD, A. P. Role of capillary recruitment in the regulation of intestinal oxygenation. *Am. J. Physiol.* 242 (*Gastrointest. Liver Physiol.* 5): G435–G441, 1982.
429. SHEPHERD, A. P., AND D. N. GRANGER (editors). *Physiology of the Intestinal Circulation*. New York: Raven, 1984.
430. SHEPHERD, A. P., AND H. J. GRANGER. Autoregulatory escape in the gut: a systems analysis. *Gastroenterology* 65: 77–91, 1973.
431. SHEPHERD, A. P., W. PAWLIK, D. MAILMAN, T. F. BURKS, AND E. D. JACOBSON. Effects of vasoconstrictors on intestinal vascular resistance and oxygen extraction. *Am. J. Physiol.* 230: 298–305, 1976.
432. SHEPHERD, A. P., AND G. L. RIEDEL. Intestinal oxygen uptake versus blood flow relationship and optimal hematocrit for $O_2$ transport (Abstract). *Federation Proc.* 40: 491, 1981.
433. SHEPHERD, A. P., AND G. L. RIEDEL. Effects of pulsatile pressure and metabolic rate on intestinal autoregulation. *Am. J. Physiol.* 242 (*Heart Circ. Physiol.* 11): H769–H775, 1982.
434. SHEPHERD, A. P., AND G. L. RIEDEL. Optimal hematocrit for oxygenation of canine intestine. *Circ. Res.* 51: 233–240, 1982.
435. SHEPHERD, A. P., AND G. L. RIEDEL. Differences in reactive hyperemia between the intestinal mucosa and muscularis. *Am. J. Physiol.* 247 (*Gastrointest. Liver Physiol.* 10): G617–G622, 1984.
436. SHEPHERD, A. P., AND G. L. RIEDEL. Laser-Doppler blood flowmetry of intestinal mucosal hyperemia induced by glucose and bile. *Am. J. Physiol.* 248 (*Gastrointest. Liver Physiol.* 11): G393–G397, 1985.
437. SHEPHERD, A. P., G. L. RIEDEL, L. C. MAXWELL, AND J. W. KIEL. Selective vasodilators redistribute intestinal blood flow and depress oxygen uptake. *Am. J. Physiol.* 247 (*Gastrointest. Liver Physiol.* 10): G377–G384, 1984.
438. SHIKATA, J.-I., T. SHIDA, K. AMINO, AND K. ISHIOKA. Experimental studies on the hemodynamics of the small intestine following increased intraluminal pressure. *Surg. Gynecol. Obstet.* 156: 155–160, 1983.
439. SIDKY, M. M., AND J. W. BEAN. Local and general alterations of blood $CO_2$ and influence of intestinal motility in regulation of intestinal blood flow. *Am. J. Physiol.* 167: 413–425, 1951.
440. SIEPLER, J. K., H. J. AHLMAN, H. N. BHARGAVA, P. E. DONAHUE, AND L. M. NYHUS. A pharmacokinetic analysis of the vagal release of 5-hydroxytryptamine in the cat. *J. Neural Transm.* 47: 99–105, 1980.
441. SIMIONESCU. N., M. SIMIONESCU, AND G. PALADE. Permeability of intestinal capillaries. Pathway followed by dextrans and glycogens. *J. Cell Biol.* 53: 365–392, 1972.
442. SIMIONESCU, N., M. SIMIONESCU, AND G. E. PALADE. Structural-functional correlates in the transendothelial exchange of water soluble macromolecules. *Thromb. Res.* 8: 257–269, 1976.
443. SIMIONESCU, N., M. SIMIONESCU, AND G. E. PALADE. Differentiated microdomains on the luminal surface of the capillary endothelium. I. Preferential distribution of anionic sites. *J. Cell Biol.* 90: 605–613, 1981.
444. SIMON, G., M. B. PAMNANI, J. F. DUNKEL, AND H. W. OVERBECK. Mesenteric hemodynamics in early experimental renal hypertension in dogs. *Circ. Res.* 36: 791–798, 1975.
445. SIREGAR, H., AND C. C. CHOU. Relative contribution of fat, protein, carbohydrate, and ethanol to intestinal hyperemia. *Am. J. Physiol.* 242 (*Gastrointest. Liver Physiol.* 5): G27–G31, 1982.
446. SIT, S. P., AND C. C. CHOU. Time course of jejunal blood flow, $O_2$ uptake, and $O_2$ extraction during nutrient absorption. *Am. J. Physiol.* 247 (*Heart Circ. Physiol.* 16): H395–H402, 1984.
447. SIT, S. P., P. KVIETYS, R. GALLAVAN, AND C. C. CHOU. Postprandial intestinal hyperemia and oxygen consumption in dogs (Abstract). *Federation Proc.* 37: 653, 1978.
448. SIT, S. P., P. KVIETYS, R. GALLAVAN, C. C. CHOU, AND D. COLLINGS. Vascular effects of local i.a. infusion of micellar fatty acids and taurocholate (TCA) in the canine small intestine (Abstract). *Physiologist* 20: 88, 1977.
449. SIT, S. P., P. NYHOF, R. GALLAVAN, JR., AND C. C. CHOU. Mechanisms of glucose-induced hyperemia in the jejunum. *Proc. Soc. Exp. Biol. Med.* 163: 273–277, 1980.
450. SJOSTROM, B., AND K. E. WULFF. Influence of long-term anesthesia on regional blood flow distribution and hemodynamics in the dog. *Eur. Surg. Res.* 7: 1–9, 1975.
451. SJÖVALL, H., S. REDFORS, B. BIBER, J. MARTNER, AND O. WINSÖ. Evidence for cardiac volume-receptor regulation of feline jejunal blood flow and fluid transport. *Am. J. Physiol.* 246 (*Gastrointest. Liver Physiol.* 9): G401–G410, 1984.
452. SMAJE, L. H., AND J. R. HENDERSON. Microcirculation of the exocrine glands. In: *The Physiology and Pharmacology of the Microcirculation*, edited by N. A. Mortillaro. Orlando, FL: Academic, 1984, p. 325–385.
453. SNAPE, W. J., JR., S. H. WRIGHT, W. M. BATTLE, AND S. COHEN. The gastrocolic response: evidence for a neural mechanism. *Gastroenterology* 77: 1235–1240, 1979.
454. SOLOMON, A. K. Characterization of biological membranes by equivalent pores. *J. Gen. Physiol.* 51: 335–364, 1968.
455. STARLING, E. H. On the absorption of fluids from the connective tissue spaces. *J. Physiol. Lond.* 19: 312–326, 1896.
456. STEVENS, C. E. Physiological implications of microbial digestion in the large intestine of mammals: relation to dietary factors. *Am. J. Clin. Nutr.* 31: 5161–5168, 1978.
457. SVANVIK, J., J. TYLLSTROM, AND J. WALLENTIN. The effects of hypercapnia and hypoxia on the distribution of capillary blood flow in the denervated intestinal vascular bed. *Acta Physiol. Scand.* 74: 543–551, 1968.
458. SZWED, J. J., D. R. MAXWELL, R. ELLIOTT, AND L. R. REDLICH. Diuretics and small intestinal lymph flow in the dog. *J. Pharmacol. Exp. Ther.* 200: 88–94, 1977.
459. TAYLOR, A. E. Capillary fluid filtration. Starling forces and lymph flow. *Circ. Res.* 49: 557–575, 1981.
460. TAYLOR, A. E., AND D. N. GRANGER. Exchange of macromolecules across the microcirculation. In: *Handbook of Physiology.*

*The Cardiovascular System. Microcirculation*, edited by E. M. Renkin and C. C. Michel, Washington, DC: Am. Physiol. Soc., 1984, sect. 2, vol. IV, pt. 1, chapt. 11, p. 467–520.
461. TEPPERMAN, B. L., AND E. D. JACOBSON. Mesenteric circulation. In: *Physiology of the Gastrointestinal Tract* (1st ed.), edited by L. R. Johnson. New York: Raven, 1981, p. 1317–1336.
462. TEXTER, E. C., JR., H. C. LAURETA, E. D. FROHLICH, AND C.-C. CHOU. Effects of major cations on gastric and mesenteric vascular resistances. *Am. J. Physiol.* 212: 569–573, 1967.
463. TEXTER, E. C., JR., S. MERRILL, M. SCHWARTZ, G. VAN DERSTAPPEN, AND F. J. HADDY. Relationship of blood flow to pressure in the intestinal vascular bed of the dog. *Am. J. Physiol.* 202: 253–256, 1962.
464. TOROK, J. Influence of extravascular pressure on changes induced in vascular resistance in the small intestine by elevated venous pressure. *Physiol. Bohemoslov.* 29: 63–71, 1980.
465. TRANQUILLI, W. J., M. MANOHAR, C. M. PARKS, J. C. THURMAN, M. C. THEODORAKIS, AND J. BENSON. Systemic and regional blood flow distribution in unanesthetized swine and swine anesthetized with halothane and nitrous oxide, halothane, or enflurane. *Anesthesiology* 56: 369–379, 1982.
466. TURNER, S. G., AND J. A. BARROWMAN. Intestinal lymph flow and lymphatic transport of protein during fat absorption. *Q. J. Exp. Physiol. Cogn. Med. Sci.* 62: 175–180, 1977.
467. UDDMAN, R., J. ALUMETS, L. EDVINSSON, R. HAKANSON, AND F. SUNDLER. VIP nerve fibers around peripheral blood vessels. *Acta Physiol. Scand.* 112: 65–70, 1981.
468. VALLEAU, J. D., D. N. GRANGER, AND A. E. TAYLOR. Effect of solute-coupled volume absorption on oxygen consumption in cat ileum. *Am. J. Physiol.* 236 (*Endocrinol. Metab. Gastrointest. Physiol.* 5): E198–E203, 1979.
469. VAN HEERDEN, P. D., H. N. WAGNER, JR., AND S. KAIHARA. Intestinal blood flow during perfusion of the jejunum with hypertonic glucose in dogs. *Am. J. Physiol.* 215: 30–33, 1968.
470. VARGAS, F., AND J. A. JOHNSON. An estimate of reflection coefficient from rabbit heart capillaries. *J. Gen. Physiol.* 47: 667–677, 1964.
471. VARRO, V., G. BLAHO, L. CSERNEY, J. JUNG, AND F. SZARVAS. Effect of decreased local circulation on the absorptive capacity of the small intestine in the dog. *Am. J. Dig. Dis.* 10: 170–177, 1965.
472. VARRO, V., L. CSERNAY, F. SZARVAS, AND G. BLAHO. Effect of glucose and glycine solution on the circulation of the isolated jejunal loop in the dog. *Am. J. Dig. Dis.* 12: 60–64, 1967.
473. VATNER, S. F. Effects of exercise and excitement on mesenteric and renal dynamics in conscious, unrestrained baboons. *Am. J. Physiol.* 234 (*Heart Circ. Physiol.* 3): H210–H214, 1978.
474. VATNER, S. F., AND E. BRAUNWALD. Cardiovascular control mechanisms in the conscious state. *N. Engl. J. Med.* 293: 970–976, 1975.
475. VATNER, S. F., D. FRANKLIN, AND R. L. VAN CITTERS. Mesenteric vasoactivity associated with eating and digestion in the conscious dog. *Am. J. Physiol.* 219: 170–174, 1970.
476. VATNER, S. F., D. FRANKLIN, AND R. L. VAN CITTERS. Coronary and visceral vasoactivity associated with eating and digestion in the conscious dog. *Am. J. Physiol.* 219: 1380–1385, 1970.
477. VATNER, S. F., T. A. PATRICK, C. B. HIGGINS, AND D. FRANKLIN. Regional circulatory adjustments to eating and digestion in conscious unrestrained primates. *J. Appl. Physiol.* 36: 524–529, 1974.
478. VOGEL, G., AND I. MARTENSEN. The permeability of the plasma-lymph barrier of the small intestine of various species to macromolecules. *Lymphology* 15: 36–39, 1982.
479. VOROBIOFF, J., J. E. BREDFELDT, AND R. J. GROSZMANN. Hyperdynamic circulation in portal-hypertensive rat model: a primary factor for maintenance of chronic portal hypertension. *Am. J. Physiol.* 244 (*Gastrointest. Liver Physiol.* 7): G52–G57, 1983.
480. WALLENTIN, I. Importance of tissue pressure for the fluid equilibrium between the vascular and interstitial compartments in the small intestine. *Acta Physiol. Scand.* 68: 304–315, 1966.
481. WALUS, K. M., J. D. FONDACARO, AND E. D. JACOBSON. Hemodynamic and metabolic changes during stimulation of ileal motility. *Dig. Dis. Sci.* 26: 1069–1077, 1981.
482. WALUS, K. M., J. D. FONDACARO, AND E. D. JACOBSON. Effects of adenosine and its derivatives on the canine intestinal vasculature. *Gastroenterology* 81: 327–334, 1981.
483. WINNE, D. The influence of blood flow and water net flux on the absorption of tritiated water from the jejunum of the rat. *Naunyn-Schmiedeberg's Arch. Pharmacol.* 272: 417–436, 1972.
484. WINNE, D. The influence of blood flow and water net flux on the blood-to-lumen flux of tritiated water in the jejunum of the rat. *Naunyn-Schmiedeberg's Arch. Pharmacol.* 274: 357–374, 1972.
485. WINNE, D. The influence of blood flow on the absorption of L- and D-phenylalanine from the jejunum of the rat. *Naunyn-Schmiedeberg's Arch. Pharmacol.* 277: 113–138, 1973.
486. WINNE, D. The influence of villous countercurrent exchange on intestinal absorption. *J. Theor. Biol.* 53: 145–176, 1975.
487. WINNE, D. The vasculature of the jejunal villus. In: *Intestinal Permeation*, edited by M. Hoechst, D. Kramer, and F. Lauterbach. Amsterdam: Excerpta Med., 1975, p. 56–57. (Proc. 4th Workshop Conf., 19–22 October, 1975.)
488. WINNE, D. Influence of blood flow on intestinal absorption of drugs and nutrients. *Pharmacol. Ther.* 6: 333–393, 1979.
489. WINNE, D. Rat jejunum perfused in situ: effect of perfusion rate and intraluminal radius on absorption rate and effective unstirred layer thickness. *Naunyn-Schmiedeberg's Arch. Pharmacol.* 307: 265–274, 1979.
490. WINNE, D. Role of blood flow in intestinal permeation. In: *Handbook of Experimental Pharmacology*, edited by T. Z. Czaky. Berlin: Springer-Verlag, 1984, vol. 70, chapt. 23, p. 301–347.
491. WINNE, D. Models of the relationship between drug absorption and intestinal blood flow. In: *Physiology of Intestinal Circulation*, edited by A. P. Shepherd and D. N. Granger. New York: Raven, 1984, p. 289–304.
492. WINNE, D., AND J. REMISCHOVSKY. Intestinal blood flow and absorption of non-dissociable substances. *J. Pharm. Pharmacol.* 22: 640–641, 1970.
493. WITTE, M. H., C. L. WITTE, AND A. E. DUMONT. Estimates of net transcapillary water and protein flux in the liver and intestine of patients with portal hypertension from hepatic cirrhosis. *Gastroenterology* 80: 265–273, 1983.
494. WOLLIN, A., AND L. B. JACQUES. Plasma protein escape from the intestinal circulation to the lymphatics during fat absorption. *Proc. Soc. Exp. Biol. Med.* 142: 114–117, 1973.
495. WOLLIN, A., AND L. B. JAQUES. Blocking of olive oil induced plasma protein escape from the intestinal circulation by histamine antagonists and by a diamine oxidase releasing agent. *Agents Actions* 6: 589–592, 1976.
496. YABLONSKI, M. E., AND N. LIFSON. Mechanism of production of intestinal secretion by elevated venous pressure. *J. Clin. Invest.* 57: 904–915, 1976.
497. YOFFEY, J. M., AND F. C. COURTICE. *Lymphatics, Lymph and the Lymphomyeloid Complex*. New York: Academic, 1970.
498. YU, Y. M., L. C. YU, AND C. C. CHOU. Distribution of blood flow in the intestine with hypertonic glucose in the lumen. *Surgery St. Louis* 78: 520–525, 1975.
499. ZAWIEJA, D., AND B. J. BARBER. A comparison of protein concentration in villi and collecting lymphatics of rats. *Microvasc. Res.* 29: 262–263, 1985.

CHAPTER 40

# Gastrointestinal circulation and motor function

CHING CHUNG CHOU | *Departments of Physiology and Medicine, Michigan State University, East Lansing, Michigan*

## CHAPTER CONTENTS

History
Microvascular Anatomy
Anatomical and Methodological Considerations
Effects of Motility on Blood Flow in Small Intestine
   Rhythmic contractions
   Tonic contractions
   Blood flow distribution within gut wall
   Summary
Effects of Chemicals and Nerves on Blood Flow and Motility in Small Intestine
   Cholinergics
   Nerves
   Bradykinin
   Serotonin
   Other vasoactive drugs and gastrointestinal hormones
   Ions and hypertonicity
   Hypercapnia and hypoxemia
   Intestinal wall tension and blood flow
   Blood flow distribution within gut wall
   Summary
Motility and Blood Flow in Colon and Stomach
   Colon
   Stomach
   Summary
Effects of Intestinal Luminal Distension
   Effect on total blood flow
   Effect on compartmental blood flow, oxygen consumption, capillary filtration coefficient, and lymph flow
   Summary
Effect of Blood Flow and Hypoxia on Motor Function

THE RELATION BETWEEN intestinal motility and blood flow may be discussed from two points of view: the influence of motility and luminal pressure on blood flow and the effects of change in blood flow on motility.

Muscle contractions can affect blood flow by at least two mechanisms. An increase in contractions increases luminal pressure and exerts extravascular compression on the vessels encased within an organ, thereby interfering mechanically with its blood flow. An increase in contractions also increases the metabolic requirements of the contracting muscle, which in turn leads to an increase in blood flow to the muscle. These two mechanisms produce opposite effects on local blood flow, and the interplay of the two mechanisms is best demonstrated in the heart. As a result of mechanical compression, coronary blood flow during systole is 30% of that during diastole (86). An increase in cardiac contractions increases the mean coronary blood flow as a result of an increase in metabolic requirements; there is a linear correlation between coronary blood flow and myocardial $O_2$ consumption.

The effects of muscle contractions on gastrointestinal blood flow are much more complicated. The heart contracts en masse at a constant rhythm and with constant strength. Intestinal contractions, however, are usually random in time and space and vary in rhythm, strength, and duration. Segmental contractions are the most common type of contraction and involve only 1–2 cm of intestine, with a duration of 3–8 s. Therefore, unless blood flow is measured at the site of contraction, the compression effect of the contraction may be offset by relaxation of adjacent areas. This phenomenon was observed as early as 1934 by Anrep et al. (6), who stated that if the gut segment is longer than 6 cm, "part may contract while the other part relaxes, so that the blood flow may not represent the actual state of the circulation in the contracted part." Furthermore the inner circular muscle and external longitudinal muscle contract along different planes, and they may contract independently for a different duration and with different strength. Finally, the gut wall contains three main tissue layers. The compression effect of muscle contractions affects the blood flow of all three layers, but the metabolic hyperemia of muscle contractions occurs only in the muscle layer.

## HISTORY

Carl Ludwig, the inventor of the stromuhr in 1868 (cited in ref. 166), proposed that the small intestine might play the role of a peripheral heart. The intestinal peristaltic contractions therefore might influence the portal venous flow significantly. In 1931 Rein (cited in ref. 6) recorded the blood flow in the superior mesenteric vein with the thermostromuhr and observed that the blood flow exhibited characteristic undulations. The waves recurred at regular intervals of time and became more pronounced as the blood flow through the intestine became smaller. The pronounced waves and decreased flow were most likely the effects of intestinal contractions.

Anrep et al. (6) were probably the first group of investigators who clearly and definitely correlated the intestinal muscle contractions and blood flow. To obtain "a perfect synchronization between the contractions and the changes in blood flow," they used very short loops of canine intestine (4–6 cm). The arterial blood flow perfusing the entire loop was measured with a hot-wire anemometer. Both ends of the loop were tied, and one end of the segment was connected to a vertically placed glass tube partially filled with saline. Emptying of the segment was registered through the tube, a tambour, and a lever on recording paper, which also simultaneously registered blood flow via the hot wire. In this way they correlated the changes in blood flow and spontaneous contractions or a stronger contraction induced by vagal stimulation or pilocarpine injection. The recording showed that "the contractions of the intestine were invariably accompanied by a diminution of the arterial inflow and again, as in the striated muscle, the diminution became more pronounced as the contraction became stronger." They also observed that, as in the striated muscle, vigorous contractions of the intestine led to an increased blood flow during the periods intervening between the contractions. The mechanism underlying the increased blood flow was not given, but the authors did attribute the increased blood flow in the striated muscle to the vasodilator effect of "the chemical substances produced by the contracting muscles." They also used a microscope to observe the effect of contractions on small vessels. Obliteration of the vein started 1 s after the start of a contraction and was completed after 2 s. Obliteration of the artery occurred 3 s later, when the contraction was fully developed. Some blood was seen entrapped in the occluded superficial small vessels. During relaxation the artery opened up some time before the veins did. Contractions also caused displacement of different blood vessels in relation to each other. A moderately strong contraction produced a compression of capillaries but failed to compress the larger blood vessels.

Before 1940 several reports were published in clinical journals describing the effect of intestinal luminal distension on local blood flow and correlating the findings with pathophysiology of intestinal obstruction. Microscopic observations (186, 188) and measurements of blood flow (54, 77, 78) showed that passive distension of the intestinal wall by gas or fluid decreased local blood flow, and the ischemia was a significant mechanism for the development of necrosis. Van Zwalenburg (188) reported that, at lumen pressure of 30 mmHg, blood flow through the capillaries stopped; at 60 mmHg, arrest and slowing of flow in the small veins and arteries occurred; and at lumen pressure of 90 mmHg, there was almost complete cessation of flow. In 1940 Lawson and Chumley (122) showed that distension had more effect than just extravascular compression.

The relation between intestinal motility and blood flow was briefly described by Grim (87) in the 1963 edition of the *Handbook of Physiology* section on circulation. During the last 20 years several short reviews on this subject have been published (35, 40, 73, 93, 106, 194). Lundgren (127), in the 1984 edition of the *Handbook of Physiology* section on *the Cardiovascular System, Microcirculation*, devoted only a minor section of this topic in his comprehensive review on various aspects of microcirculation of the gastrointestinal tract and pancreas. This chapter therefore describes in more detail the works published after 1940 on the relation between gastrointestinal motor function and blood flow.

## MICROVASCULAR ANATOMY

Studies of microvascular anatomy have yielded measurements of the diameter and transmural pressures of the small vessels in the small intestinal wall in rats [Fig. 1; (20, 21, 80, 81)]. The intramural microcirculation begins as a first-order arteriole that is ~50 $\mu$m diameter and has a pressure of 44.8 mmHg at a systemic arterial pressure of 100–110 mmHg. The first-order arterioles (1A) penetrate both the longitudinal and circular muscle layers and run along the outer surface of the submucosa (80, 81). This vessel then gives rise to second- and third-order arterioles (2A, 3A) with transmural pressures of about 44.6 and 32.4 mmHg, respectively. The 2A may be regarded as arteriolar-arteriolar shunts, because they frequently join adjacent 1A. In large animals such as cats and dogs, the 1A course approximately radially around the circumference of the intestine, whereas the 2A lie along the longitudinal axis of the gut (18). The 3A penetrate through the submucosa to become the main arterioles (MA) of the villus. In small animals the 3A also give rise to fourth- and fifth-order arterioles (4A, 5A; 26.6 mmHg) in the circular and longitudinal muscle layers (CC and LC in Fig. 1A). In animals that have an adult body weight of more than 2 kg, the muscle layer is not perfused by vessels that eventually perfuse the mucosa (19). The muscle layer receives an independent vascular supply that branches from vessels analogous to the 1A and 2A described. Also the thick muscle layer of large animals has many large arterioles and an arteriolar branching pattern as complex as that of skeletal muscle. In rats the 5A run perpendicular to the muscle fibers and supply longitudinal and circular muscle capillaries (23.8 mmHg) that run parallel to the muscle fibers in each layer. Microcirculation of large and small animals therefore is distinctly different in terms of origin of perfusion,

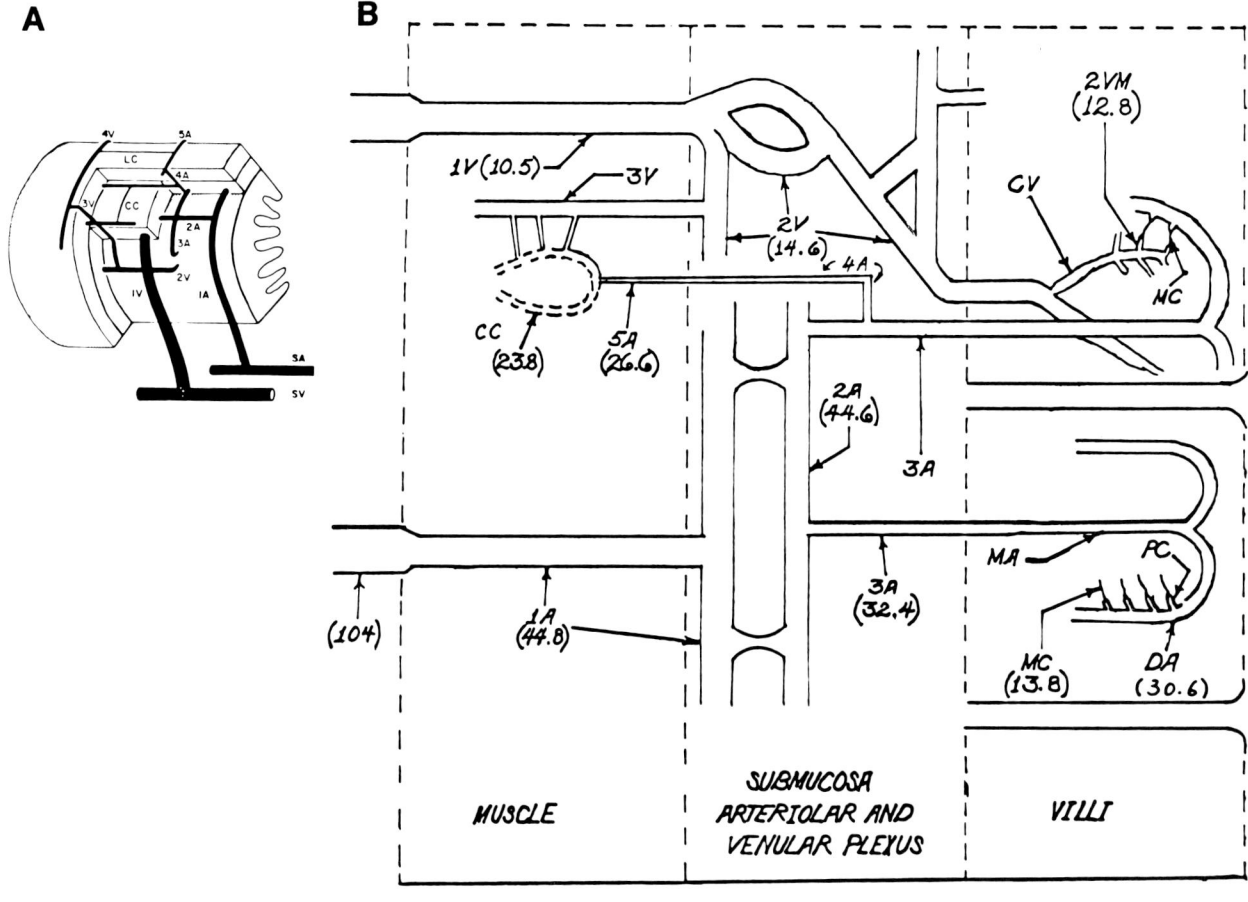

FIG. 1. Microvascular anatomy of rat intestine. 1A, first-order arteriole. [A from Gore and Bohlen (80). B from data of Gore and Bohlen (81).]

size of the arterioles, and complexity of the branching pattern (18, 19). How these differences affect the relationship between motility and blood flow is unknown; most studies have utilized large animals such as cats and dogs.

The pattern of perfusion within the villus is also different in various species but may be separated into two groups. In the first pattern, represented by rodents, cats, and dogs, a single MA runs through the center of the villus from its base to its tip (Fig. 1). At the tip of the villus, the MA branches into distributing arterioles (DA), from which the majority of capillaries are formed and cascade down the exterior surface of the villus (19). The capillaries form an extensive network just beneath the mucosal epithelium (81). Precapillary sphincters (PC) are present at the entrance of ~75% of the villus capillaries. The PC are single contractile cells that partially or completely encircle the initial segment of the capillaries and can alternately constrict and dilate independently of the DA that feeds the capillaries. In this pattern the flow of arterial and capillary blood is predominantly countercurrent. The second major pattern, represented by the rabbit and human, lacks anatomical conditions for countercurrent exchange; in fact there is no close proximity of all the subepithelial capillaries to the arteriole, and the flow of arterial and capillary blood is concurrent over 60% of the height of the villus (76).

The mucosal capillaries (13.8 mmHg) drain into the second-order mucosal venules (2VM; 12.8 mmHg), which in turn drain into one of two collecting venules (CV). The CV join to form a single main venule at the base of the villus. Blood returning from the villi drains into the second-order venules (2V) in the surface of the submucosa. The muscularis capillaries (23.8 mmHg) join fourth-order venules (4VM; 16.2 mmHg), which in turn form third-order venules (3V). The 3V descend through both muscle layers and enter the 2V (14.6 mmHg) in the submucosa. The submucosal 2V are a dense, interconnected network and can be considered a venous vascular pool that is drained by first-order venules (1V). The 1V, which carry blood from both the mucosa and muscularis, return the blood to the mesenteric veins.

The microcirculation of the stomach is different from that of the intestine. The small arteries supplying blood to the stomach pierce the muscle coat with large arterioles, which immediately provide the majority of arterioles to the muscle layer as well as second branches to the submucosa (90, 91). The arterioles in the submucosa anastomose to form large arteriolar arcades from which branches are sent to supply blood to the mucosal layer. Thus the submucosal and mucosal microvessels are connected in series, whereas the muscularis vascular bed is in parallel with the submucosal-mucosal vascular bed. Mucosal venules carry blood from the mucosa to the submucosa, where venules anastomose to form the venous submucosal plexus. In turn, this plexus drains into veins that pierce the muscle layer; just before the veins leave the muscle, they receive branches from venules draining the muscle layer. The difference in the arrangement of submucosal and muscularis microvessels between stomach and intestine (i.e., parallel vs. series) may influence the relation between motility and blood flow in these two organs.

## ANATOMICAL AND METHODOLOGICAL CONSIDERATIONS

A significant feature of the gastrointestinal circulation is the anatomical presence of anastomotic connections at several levels of vessel branching, from the main celiac and mesenteric arteries to the extensive submucosal vascular plexus. Each of these anastomoses provides a potential conduit for collateral blood flow. Although this arrangement protects tissues from complete ischemia in case of obstruction at any level of the arterial network, it constitutes a significant problem for investigators who attempt to determine the relationship between blood flow and motility. A recent study has shown that as much as 55% of the resting blood flow of an intestinal segment can be supplied by the collateral vessels from adjacent segments, when the blood supply to that section is completely abolished (27). Virtually all of the total collateral flow is derived from precapillary vessels and therefore is available for perfusing the capillaries. About two-thirds of the total collateral flow is derived from the extramural collaterals, whereas the remainder is supplied by intramural collaterals.

Most studies on the relationship between intestinal motility and blood flow have utilized a gut segment that is perfused by a single artery and drained by a single vein, the ends of which are usually separated from adjacent segments to avoid collateral blood flow. Some investigators used the entire small intestine while measuring blood flow through the superior mesenteric artery. The latter preparation is more physiological, but the results are complicated by the presence of collateral blood flow and the pattern of change in motor activity throughout the entire intestine. Intestinal contraction rarely involves the entire intestine at a given moment; contraction in one portion is usually accompanied by relaxation in other portions. The changes in blood flow measured at the superior mesenteric artery or even at an intestinal artery, therefore, are the net effect of contraction-relaxation activities of the entire intestinal tract or the entire loop under observation plus or minus collateral blood flow to or from other organs or adjacent loops. Because the difference in the gut preparation may influence the results of the study, the length of the gut segment used in most studies is described in the text.

The hemodynamic changes have been determined either by measuring blood flow under constant systemic arterial pressure (natural-flow preparation) or by measuring perfusion pressure under constant-flow conditions (constant-flow preparation). Under constant-flow conditions an increase or decrease in perfusion pressure indicates an increase (vasoconstriction) or decrease (vasodilation) in vascular resistance. Most studies used changes in luminal pressure, either via an intraluminally placed balloon or open-tipped tubing, as an indicator of changes in contraction-relaxation activities. Most studies from Sweden, however, used changes in lumen volume as indicators of contractile activity. Some used force transducers attached to the gut wall. The technique used in determining motor activities may also influence the results and should be considered in the analysis of motility-blood flow relationship. Because the contractile state of the intestine normally varies with time and space, and because the gut wall is composed of both contractile and noncontractile tissues, the ideal method to elucidate the relationship between blood flow and motility would simultaneously and continuously measure electrical and mechanical events associated with contractions and local tissue blood flow in multiple areas of the gastrointestinal tract.

## EFFECTS OF MOTILITY ON BLOOD FLOW IN SMALL INTESTINE

Rhythmic contractions are defined in this chapter as the segmental contractions that are reflected on the pressure recording as successive rhythmic oscillations of the luminal pressure, with a frequency equal to or less than the frequency of the slow waves of the gut segment under observation. The tonic contraction is the contraction that is reflected on the pressure recording by an increase in the basal luminal pressure. The tonic contraction usually lasts 1 min or longer and may appear successively for a period of time. Frequently the rhythmic contractions are superimposed on the tonic contraction. The strength of the contractions is defined as the amplitude of individual rhythmic contractions and the amplitude of the basal luminal pressure achieved at the height of the tonic contraction. Some reports called the rise in the basal lumen pressure an increase in tonus, tone, or tension (Fig. 2).

## Rhythmic Contractions

After Anrep et al. (6) reported the effect of motility on blood flow in 1934, no significant report appeared in the literature until the 1950s, when Sidky and Bean (12, 13, 134a, 174) performed a series of experiments to study the effect of rhythmic and tonic contractions on the arterial inflow and pressure, the venous outflow and pressure, and the volume of the jejunal loop (12–15 cm). The blood flow was determined by thermopile and the drop recorder. In one study (174) spontaneous motor activities and other variables were continuously observed for 3–4 h. Rhythmic segmental contractions produced a reciprocal periodicity in arterial and venous flows. During the contraction phase, the arterial flow decreased while the venous outflow increased, whereas during the relaxation phase the reverse took place (Fig. 2A). The magnitude of the flow changes was proportional to the strength of the individual contractions. Although arterial and venous flow showed reciprocal oscillation with each contraction and relaxation, the mean blood flow (ml/min) increased when the strength of rhythmic contractions increased (Fig. 2B). However, when the increased rhythmic contractions were accompanied by a simultaneous rise in the basal pressure (tonus), the mean blood flow decreased (Fig. 2A). The authors attributed the increased flow both to a pumping action of the rhythmic contractions and to an increase in release of metabolites or other vasodilators.

To demonstrate the effectiveness of pumping action of rhythmic contractions on blood flow, Sidky and Bean (174) occluded the venous outflow during the contractions. In 90 s after the occlusion, venous pressure rose to 70 mmHg, i.e., 28 mmHg above the perfusion pressure; the arterial perfusion pressure was 42 mmHg, which was unchanged throughout the occlusion period. They attributed the high venous pressure to the presence of valves in the venules, as de-

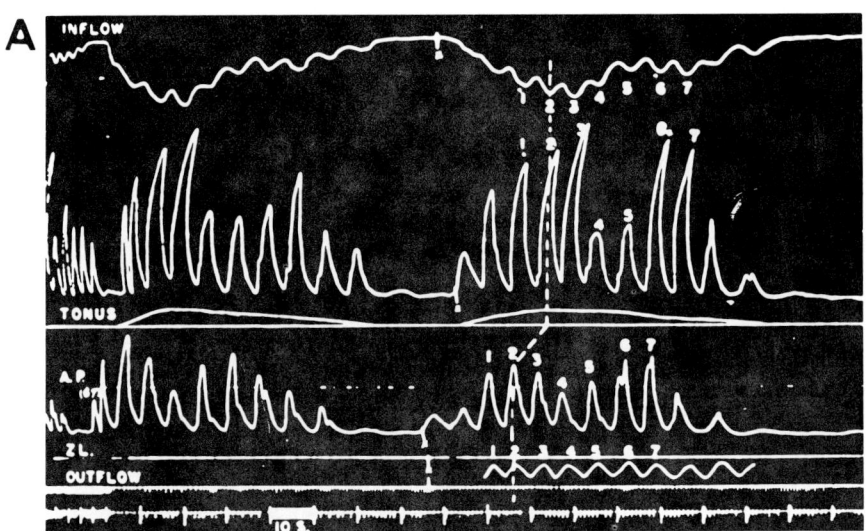

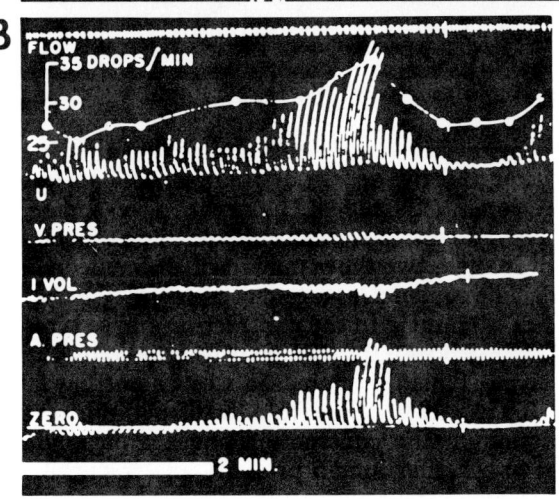

FIG. 2. *A*: effect of rhythmic segmental contractions on arterial inflow and venous outflow; numbers 1–7 indicate synchronous changes in intestinal movements and blood flow. Tonus of gut was plotted. *B*: effect of rhythmic segmental contractions on minute volume flow of blood (drops/min). Volume flow per minute is plotted. *Tracings* from *top* to *bottom* are flow, lumen pressure of upper end of gut loop, venous pressure, intestinal volume, arterial pressure, and lumen pressure at lower end of loop. [From Sidky and Bean (174).]

scribed by Mall (129). These venules carry blood from the submucosal venous plexes to the mesenteric veins (see 1V, Fig. 1). From this observation they concluded that "the rhythmical contractions are capable of pumping blood into the portal venous system against a pressure that is higher than that of the arterial inflow to the gut and thus contribute very importantly to the return of blood to the liver and to the dynamics of the general circulation." In the interpretation of their data one must consider their experimental preparation. The isolated intestinal loop was placed in an airtight container and perfused, at a pressure much lower than the aortic pressure, with blood in a reservoir. The blood was obtained from a donor dog and was diluted by the addition of normal saline and bubbled by a gas mixture of 30% $O_2$, 4% $CO_2$, and 66% $N_2$ in a reservoir (134a). Whether rhythmic contractions in the stomach, colon, and small intestine can act as a peristaltic pump to enhance venous return from the gut to the portal vein was also investigated by Semba et al. (165–169).

In the jejunal loop (6–9 cm in length) each individual spontaneous rhythmic contraction was accompanied by either an increase or decrease in venous outflow (166, 167). In one type, the contraction-phase type, each contraction was accompanied on the average by an increase in venous outflow from 0.042 to 0.068 ml·s$^{-1}$ and a decrease in arterial inflow from 0.058 to 0.049 ml·s$^{-1}$ (Fig. 3B). In another type, the relaxation-phase type, each contraction was accompanied by a decrease in both arterial inflow from 0.041 to 0.034 ml·s$^{-1}$ and venous outflow from 0.045 to 0.034 ml·s$^{-1}$ (Fig. 3A). The lumen pressures during relaxation for the contraction- and relaxation-phase types ranged from 3.3 to 28.8 mmHg ($n = 10$) and from 3.7 to 22.2 mmHg ($n = 5$), respectively. The lumen pressures achieved during each contraction ranged from 5.9 to 31.9 mmHg and from 6.8 to 22.9 mmHg for the contraction- and relaxation-phase types, respectively. Because the basal pressures, the frequencies of contractions (11.32 vs. 12.76 cycles/min), as well as the average amplitudes of each contraction (3.3 vs. 3.2 mmHg) in these two types do not appear to be different, it is difficult to attribute the difference in the pattern of changes in blood flow simply to difference in mechanical compression produced by the contractions. Because the changes in blood flow during contraction and relaxation were about the same in magnitude (Fig. 3), it appears that rhythmic contractions do not significantly alter the mean blood flow.

In the next study Semba et al. (167) correlated the changes in venous $O_2$ saturation with spontaneous rhythmic contractions. Each contraction was associated with either an increase or decrease in venous $O_2$ saturation in both contraction-phase type and relaxation-phase type; the arterial $O_2$ saturation was not altered by the contractions. The data of the venous $O_2$ saturation are difficult to interpret, because no corre-

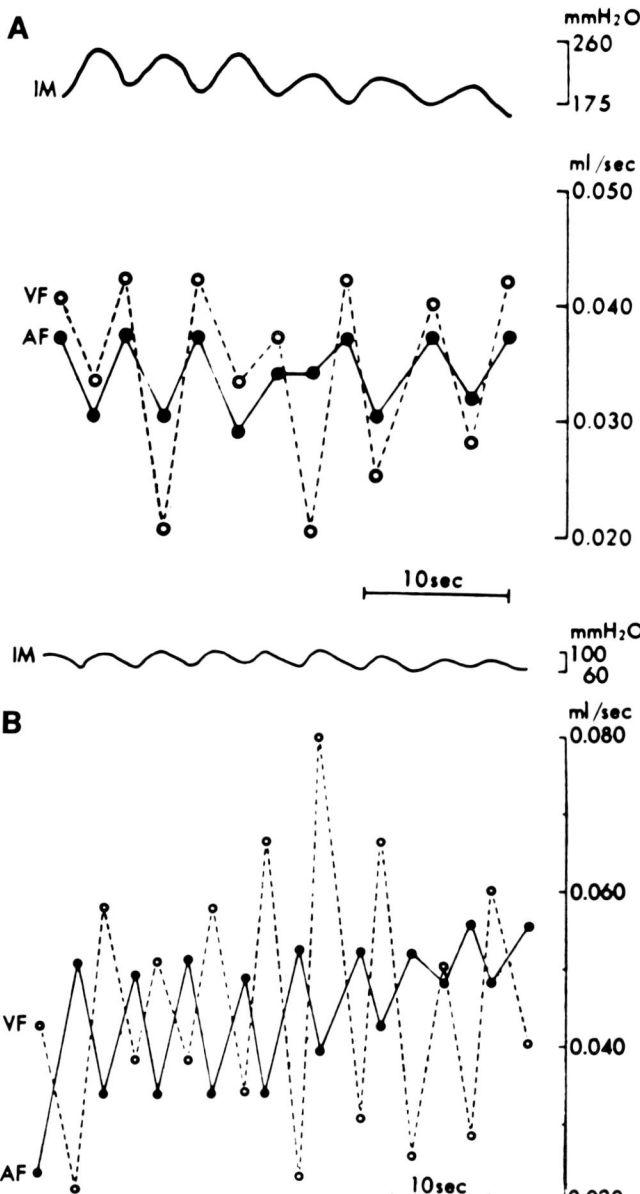

FIG. 3. Relation between lumen pressure (IM), arterial inflow (AF), and venous outflow (VF) during spontaneous rhythmic contractions. [From Semba et al. (166).]

lation can be made between the changes in the $O_2$ saturation and the degree of change in blood flow or contractions. This report, however, gave some data that may indicate that the difference in the blood flow pattern in these two types may result from mechanical factors. The lumen pressure increased from $14.8 \pm 3.7$ to $18.7 \pm 4.3$ mmHg in the contraction-phase type and from $3.6 \pm 0.8$ to $5.6 \pm 0.4$ mmHg in the relaxation-phase type. Thus the increased venous outflow (from $19.6 \pm 9.0$ to $24.6 \pm 8.3$ ml·min$^{-1}$·100 g$^{-1}$) during each contraction in the contraction-phase type might be related to a higher lumen pressure and higher amplitude of the contraction.

Other studies, which utilized the in situ jejunal loop of anesthetized (40, 79, 109) or conscious (155) dogs, also failed to demonstrate the pumping effect of spontaneous rhythmic contractions. Spontaneous rhythmic contractions produced concomitant changes in phasic instantaneous arterial inflow or venous outflow, but they did not alter mean blood flow. For each 1-mmHg increment in lumen pressure, venous outflow increased ~0.5 ml·min$^{-1}$, but an equivalent decrease in venous outflow took place during decreasing lumen pressure (109). In the isolated intestinal segment perfused in vitro with heparinized blood from a donor dog, Brobmann et al. (25) inflated the gut lumen rhythmically by a respirator pump to simulate rhythmic contractions. The arterial perfusion pressure was held constant at 80 mmHg. Oscillation of lumen pressure between 0 and 35 mmHg was accompanied by instantaneous reciprocal changes in arterial inflow and venous outflow. At the peak lumen pressure arterial inflow decreased while venous outflow increased, whereas the reverse occurred at low pressure; the mean blood flow did not change.

These recent studies have shown that the venous outflow increased (40, 79, 109, 155, 166, 167) or decreased (166, 167) during the contraction phase of spontaneous rhythmic contractions, but the rhythmic activity as a whole does not alter mean blood flow significantly. Nyhof and Chou (data presented in ref. 40), however, observed that blood flow (electromagnetic flowmeter) of the jejunal loop (15–20 cm long) did not change when weak rhythmic contractions (2–5 mmHg amplitude) appeared spontaneously, but stronger contractions (5–10 mmHg amplitude) were accompanied by an increase in flow and oxygen consumption. When the spontaneous rhythmic contractions were superimposed on an increase in basal luminal pressure, blood flow decreased. Thus spontaneous rhythmic contractions can be accompanied by no change, a decrease, or an increase in blood flow, depending on the strength and pattern of the contractions. These findings are similar to those of Sidky and Bean (174). The increased blood flow, however, does not appear to be due to pumping action of the contractions. The blood volume of the intestine is ~5–10 ml·100 g$^{-1}$ intestinal tissue (127). The pumping action may increase venous outflow for each contraction, but unless there is an active vasodilation to increase arterial inflow, venous outflow eventually returns to the levels of arterial inflow. The active vasodilation may result from the actions of vasodilators, metabolites, or other autacoids released during muscle contractions (see *Blood Flow Distribution Within Gut Wall*, p. 1483.)

Fioramonti and Bueno (70) found that the increase in the myoelectrical spiking activities during postprandial and interdigestive periods was accompanied by an increase in mean blood flow. With conscious dogs the investigators measured both the blood flow (by electromagnetic flowmeter) through a jejunal and an ileal artery and the myoelectric activities of the segments (6–9 cm of jejunum and 12–15 cm of ileum) perfused by the arteries for 24-h duration. Although the myoelectric activities may not accurately and quantitatively reflect the mechanical contractions and relaxations, this report provides valuable physiological information on the relationship between motor activity and blood flow throughout a 1-day period in the conscious animal. A daily meal consisting of a mixture of 200 g of canned food and 200 g of dry dog food was given at 11 A.M. The mean jejunal and ileal blood flow increased from 13.7 ± 3.4 and 15.1 ± 4.2 ml·min$^{-1}$ to 51.3 ± 9.4 and 55.2 ± 8.6 ml·min$^{-1}$ 20–60 min after the meal, respectively. The increased blood flow continued for 4–5 h in the jejunum and for 11 h in the ileum. During this postprandial period, spiking activities appeared irregularly and were accompanied by oscillations of 10–20 ml·min$^{-1}$ in jejunal blood flow. Blood flow was maximal during the periods of increased spiking activity and minimal during the periods of quiescence or reduced spiking activity. The myoelectrical spiking activities have been shown to be accompanied by rhythmic segmental contractions (50, 88, 180). This finding therefore suggests that an increase in rhythmic contractions during the postprandial period contributes to postprandial intestinal hyperemia, which has been well documented previously (45, 47, 75, 189).

Fioramonti and Bueno (70) also observed cyclic variations in blood flow accompanying the occurrence of the interdigestive migrating myoelectric complex (MMC). The blood flow was minimal during periods of quiescence (phase I) and increased during spiking activities. At the onset of phase II of the MMC, characterized by irregular spike activities, the mean blood flow increased progressively from 13.5 ± 2.9 to 31.5 ± 4.7 ml·min$^{-1}$ in the jejunum, and from 15.9 ± 4.2 to 26.9 ± 4.7 ml·min$^{-1}$ in the ileum. The maximal blood flow reached in the ileum was 53.2 ± 6.3 ml·min$^{-1}$, which was higher than that reached in the jejunum. Blood flow then returned to control level during the phase III of the MMC. If the intestinal chyme was prevented from reaching the segment by diverting the chyme through a T tube placed 20 cm above the segment under observation, the cyclic MMCs still appeared in the segment, but the concordant changes in blood flow were abolished. The cyclic changes in blood flow, therefore, appear to result from cyclic flow of intestinal content through the segment. It is unclear, however, whether the increase in blood flow results from the passage of the intestinal chyme through the lumen, distension of the lumen by the chyme, nutrient absorption, or from the chyme itself. The following factors have been shown to increase local intestinal blood flow: mechanical stimulation of the mucosal surface (15, 59, 107), a mild degree of distension (see EFFECTS OF INTESTINAL LUMINAL DIS-

TENSION, p. 1502), nutrient absorption (47, 49, 175), as well as the presence of digested products of food in the jejunum and that of bile in the ileum (45, 48). Infusion of 850 ml normal saline through the lumen of the small intestine induced rhythmic contractions (25–40 mmHg) and increased blood flow through the superior mesenteric artery (153).

*Tonic Contractions*

In contrast to the variable blood flow response to rhythmic contractions, blood flow decreases during the tonic contraction. Sidky and Bean (174) observed that spontaneous tonic contractions in the canine small intestine were accompanied by reciprocal changes in blood flow. The pattern of the accompanying changes in blood flow, however, differed from those that occurred during spontaneous rhythmic contractions. Each tonic contraction was accompanied by an abrupt decrease in both arterial inflow and venous outflow (Fig. 4). As the tonus started to fall, both the inflow and outflow started to rise, reaching their maximum when the lumen pressure reached precontraction levels. The posttonic hyperemia occurred whether or not rhythmic contractions were superimposed on the tonic contractions, and the magnitude of the hyperemia depended on the duration and the magnitude of the tonic contraction: the longer and stronger the contraction, the greater the hyperemia (Fig. 4). The posttonic hyperemia appears to represent a reactive hyperemia comparable to that seen in skeletal muscle following tetanic contraction (9). Sidky and Bean attributed the hyperemia to an increased production of metabolites and vasodilator substances during tonic contractions. A recent study further showed that $O_2$ consumption of the canine jejunal segment increased when the tonic contraction was superimposed on rhythmic contractions (40).

With the constant-flow preparation, Kachelhoffer et al. (109) correlated the strength of the spontaneous tonic contractions and the magnitude of the corresponding perfusion pressure. They found that the increases in lumen pressure were significantly related to the corresponding rise in perfusion pressure. Each 1-mmHg rise in lumen pressure was accompanied by an increase of 0.84 mmHg in perfusion pressure. Their finding therefore indicates that the tonic contraction increased local vascular resistance: the stronger the contraction, the greater the increased vascular resistance. The responses of blood flow to the tonic contraction induced by acetylcholine, physostigmine, bradykinin, and other stimuli are described in EFFECTS OF CHEMICALS AND NERVES ON BLOOD FLOW AND MOTILITY IN SMALL INTESTINE, p. 1486.

Coulic et al. (51) observed the microcirculatory event during spontaneous rhythmic contractions and the tonic contraction induced by the application of epinephrine on the mesentery. The intestinal microcirculatory responses to those contractions in rabbits, guinea pigs, and rats were similar. The spontaneous contraction and relaxation were accompanied by concomitant changes in the diameter of small vessels, particularly that of the venules. The venule diameter

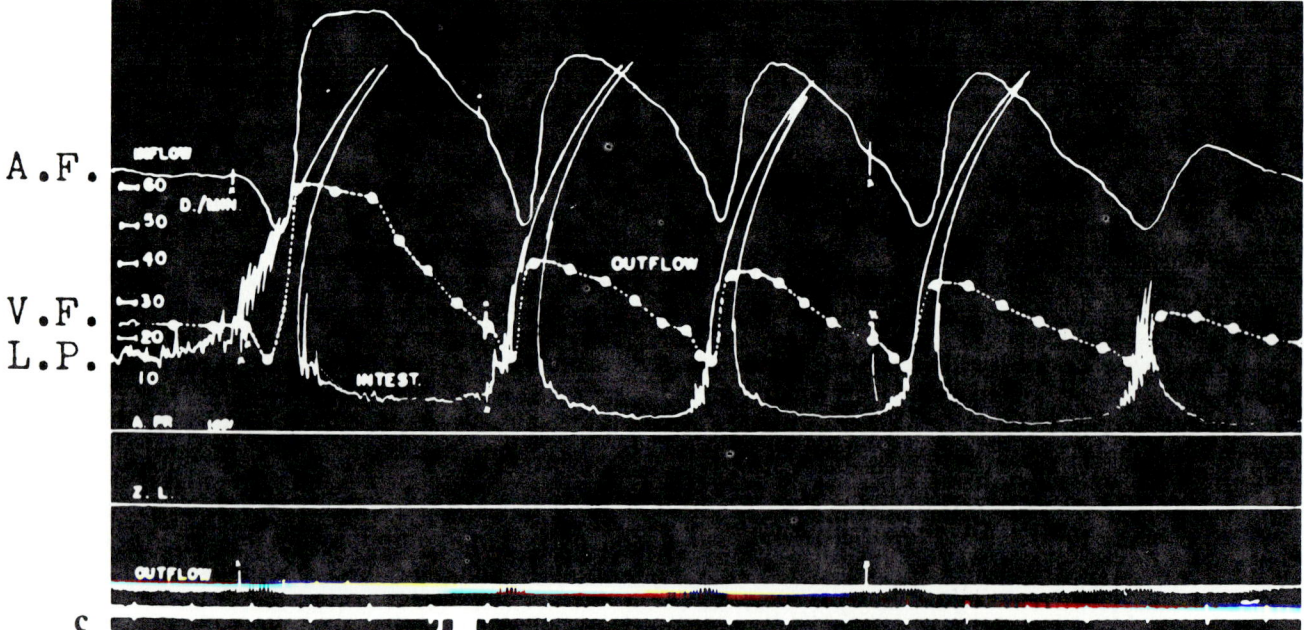

FIG. 4. Blood flow changes during and after tonic contractions. A.F., arterial inflow; V.F., venous outflow plotted on *dotted line*; L.P., lumen pressure. *Short vertical lines* indicate beginning of tonic contraction. [From Sidky and Bean (174).]

increased from ~85 μm during contraction to 125 μm during relaxation. The variation in small-vessel diameter depended more on the magnitude of the change in lumen pressure from contraction to relaxation than on the absolute levels of lumen pressure measured during contraction-relaxation activity. Tonic contraction (contraction tetanique) constricted primarily the venules, producing a plethora of the capillaries. The contour of the venules was irregular and uneven, and capillary stasis was observed. There was irregular dilation of the venules mainly at the postcapillary junction. At the same time previously unperfused venules and capillaries were now perfused. At the moment of relaxation the diameters of the arterioles and venules returned to control levels. The diameter of the arterioles was not significantly altered during the rhythmic or tonic contractions. This may indicate that these vessels are more resistant to compression than are the venules. Another possibility is that the arterioles may actively dilate to oppose the compression during contraction.

*Blood Flow Distribution Within Gut Wall*

The active hyperemia of muscle contractions (metabolic, functional, or work hyperemia) has been well documented in the heart and skeletal muscle. The muscle contractions increase oxygen consumption and requirements, which in turn lead to hyperemia by an increase in tissue vasodilatory metabolites and a decrease in tissue oxygen pressure ($P_{O_2}$). Rhythmic contractions can be accompanied by an increase in blood flow (40, 70, 153), and strong tonic contraction is accompanied by postcontraction hyperemia (6, 112, 162, 166, 168, 174). The increased flow during spontaneous contractions is accompanied by an increase in oxygen consumption (40). Kvietys and Granger (117) also reported that there was a linear relationship between $O_2$ consumption and the motility index during spontaneous rhythmic contractions: oxygen consumption ($\dot{V}_{O_2}$) = 0.99 + 0.01 motility index; $\dot{V}_{O_2}$ is expressed as a multiple of resting values and motility index as a mean of the pressure peaks per number of contractions per minute in mmHg. The active hyperemia of intestinal contractions, however, can be revealed only by the measurement of compartmental blood flow within the gut wall.

Chou and Grassmick (41) attempted to determine the existence of the active hyperemia in the muscle layer during rhythmic contractions, as induced by gentle manipulation of the gut wall or luminal distension, and during tonic contraction induced by physostigmine. In interpreting their data many factors must be considered (Fig. 5) that may be involved in the changes in blood flow induced by the three stimuli. Gently squeezing the wall of the jejunal loop (15–20 cm) between the thumb and forefinger for 1 min produced rhythmic contraction (12 cycles/min, 4–6 mmHg in amplitude) and significantly increased venous outflow. These effects of 1-min manipulation lasted for ~15 min (Fig. 6). Blood flow to the mucosal-submucosal layer was not significantly altered, but the flow to the muscularis increased from 0.30 ± 0.07 to 1.93 ± 0.05 ml·min$^{-1}$·g$^{-1}$. Moderate distension of the jejunal lumen with 15–20 ml normal saline increased the lumen pressure, which oscillated between 15 and 25 mmHg at 12–13 cycles/min. Total blood flow to the loop significantly increased, and the increased flow resulted primarily from an increase in flow to the muscularis layer (from 0.28 ± 0.08 to 1.24 ± 0.22 ml·min$^{-1}$·g$^{-1}$). The mucosal-submucosal flow was not significantly altered. The blood flow distribution within the gut wall was significantly altered in favor of the muscularis layer by both manipulation and distension (Fig. 7). The blood flow as well as the flow distribution within the gut wall of the stomach, small intestine, and colon that were left undisturbed within the abdominal cavity were not significantly altered by either manipulation or distension of the exteriorized segments. This finding indicates that the response to manipulation and distension was a local phenomenon. The manipulation and distension might stimulate local nerves or release vasodilator autacoids to increase blood flow. If this is true, the neurohumoral effect is confined to the muscularis layer alone. A vascular myogenic response may play a role in the distension-induced hyperemia (see EFFECTS OF INTESTINAL LUMINAL DISTENSION, p. 1502). If this is true, a similar response should occur in the mucosal-submucosal layer. The association of rhythmic contractions with hyperemia and confinement of the hyperemia to the muscularis layer suggest that the hyperemia results from intestinal contractions. Physostigmine (0.15–0.90 μg·kg$^{-1}$·min$^{-1}$ iv) increased basal lumen pressure of the small intestine to 37 ± 6 mmHg with little oscillation in the pressure, and decreased total blood flow to the gut wall of the stomach and small intestine as well as the colon (Figs. 6 and 8). The decrease in total flow to the gut wall was solely due to a decrease in blood flow to the mucosa-submucosal layer in all three organs (Fig. 8). Blood flow to the muscle layer was not significantly altered. The fraction of the total wall flow perfusing the mucosa-submucosa significantly decreased, while that perfusing the muscle layer significantly increased in the small intestine. This finding suggests that the physostigmine-induced tonic contraction decreased mucosal-submucosal blood flow by compressing the vessels of this compartment, but the compression effect was totally opposed by the contraction-induced active vasodilation occurring in the muscle layer.

A complete occlusion of the artery perfusing an ileal segment increases both lumen pressure and rhythmic contractions in dogs (34, 40, 162) and cats (146). (See also EFFECTS OF BLOOD FLOW AND HYPOXIA ON MOTOR FUNCTION, p. 1509.) When the occlusion is re-

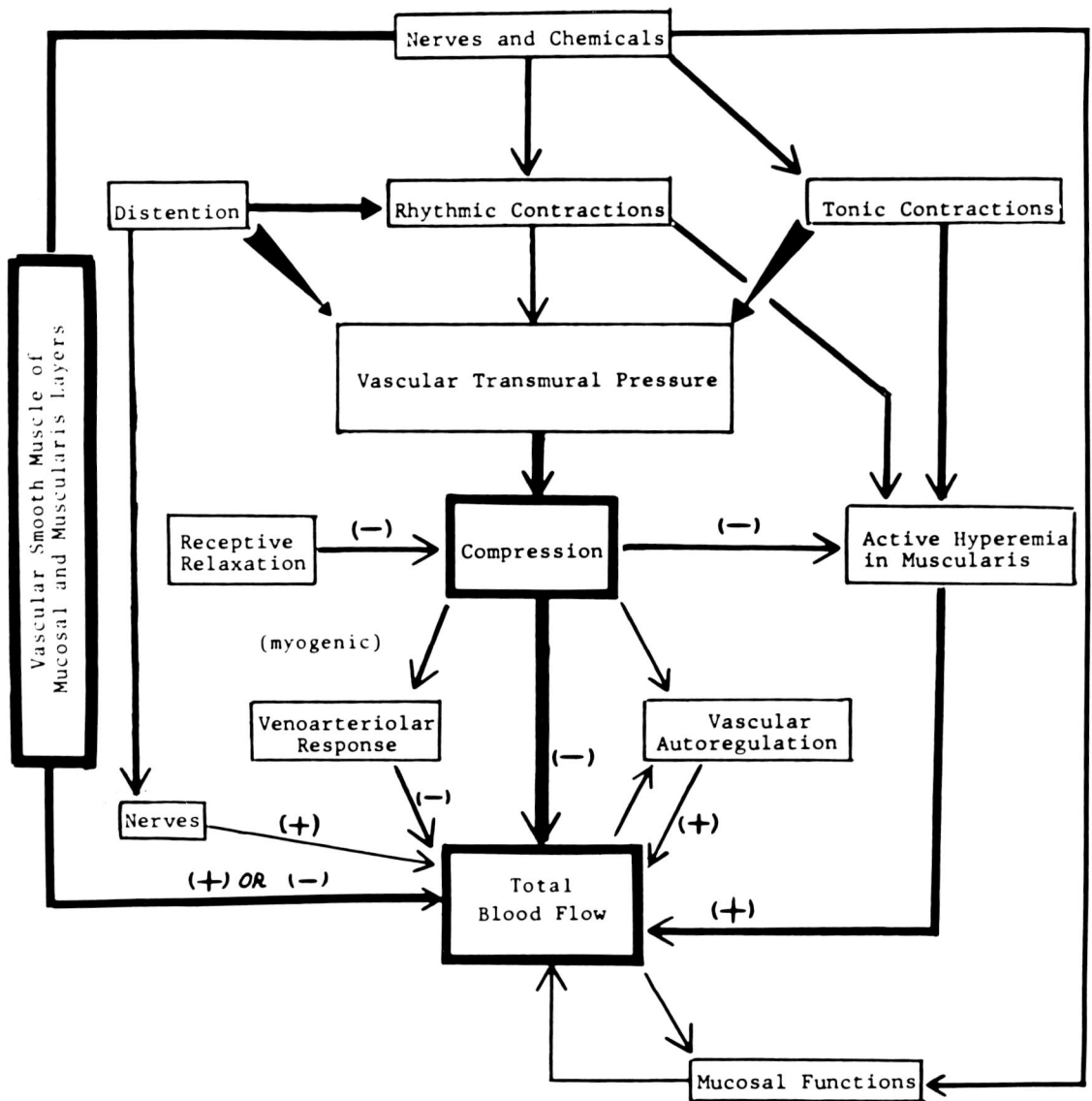

FIG. 5. Interplay of factors involved in relationship between intestinal distension, contractions, and blood flow.

leased, total blood flow increases; this phenomenon is called reactive hyperemia and has been used frequently to delineate the local mechanisms involved in the intrinsic regulation of intestinal blood flow. Parker and Granger (146) studied the effect of reactive hyperemia on blood flow to the mucosal-submucosal and muscularis layers. The levels of the reactive hyperemia following 1-min occlusion in the above two tissue layers were similar, that is, 2.1–3.6 times that of controls. The level of the reactive hyperemia following 2-min occlusion in the muscularis (6.30 ± 0.9 times control), however, was significantly greater than that in the mucosa-submucosa (2.48 ± 0.52 times control). Furthermore the rhythmic contractions that occurred during 2-min occlusion (7 ± 1.2 contractions/min) were significantly greater than those that occurred during 1-min occlusion (2.8 ± 0.6 contractions/min). The findings that the levels of the reactive hyperemia after 1-min and 2-min occlusion were similar in the mucosal-submucosal layer but different in the muscularis layer, and that the larger hyperemia in the muscularis layer was associated with the higher frequency of rhythmic contractions, suggest that the greater hyperemia in the muscularis may result from the active hyperemia of the contracting muscles.

Elevation of intestinal venous outflow pressure produces an increase in its vascular resistance (108, 164). According to the myogenic theory, the rise in intravascular and vascular transmural pressures as produced by the elevation of venous pressure induces

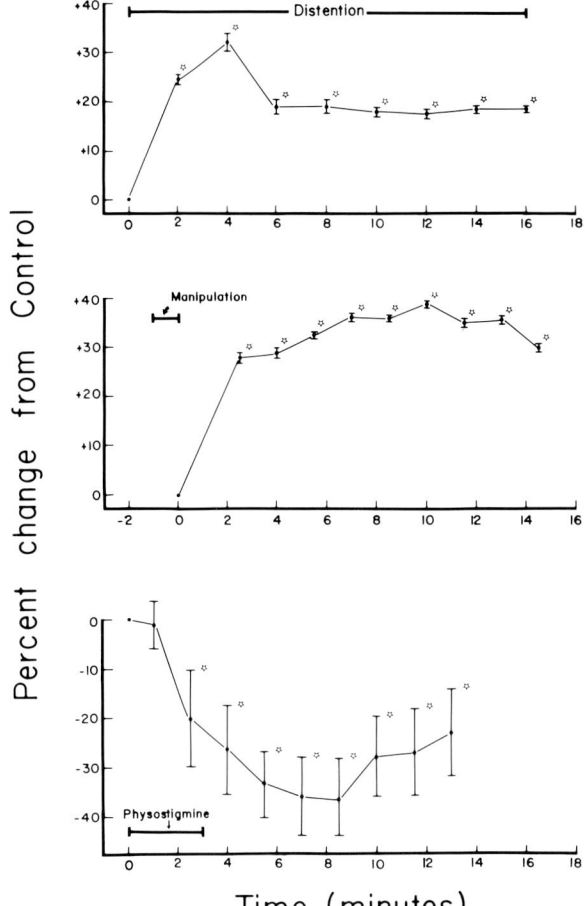

FIG. 6. Effects of luminal distension or manipulation of gut wall and infusion of physostigmine on venous outflow of jejunal segment. [From data of Chou and Grassmick (41).]

active contraction of the vascular smooth muscle, thereby increasing vascular resistance and decreasing total intestinal blood flow. This venoarteriolar response is independent of the gut wall tension (164). The response, however, can be modified by rhythmic contractions induced during elevation of venous pressure. Elevation of venous pressure to 20–30 mmHg has been shown to produce rhythmic contractions (82, 84, 135), an increase in $O_2$ consumption and glucose utilization (135), and an increase in blood flow to the muscularis while decreasing flow to the mucosa (84). This finding seems to suggest that the rhythmic contractions produce active vasodilation in the muscle layer that reverses the vasoconstriction of the venoarteriolar response; the vasoconstriction is still present in the noncontracting mucosal layer.

*Summary*

Spontaneous motor activity of the small intestine may increase, decrease, or have no effect on intestinal blood flow, depending on the pattern, strength, frequency, and duration of the contractions. Rhythmic contractions may be accompanied by corresponding oscillation of phasic instantaneous blood flow but may not alter mean blood flow (40, 79, 95, 109, 111, 143, 155, 166, 174, 197). A decrease in mean blood flow was observed when the rhythmic contractions were superimposed on the tonic contraction (40, 174). Rhythmic contractions, however, may be accompanied by an increase in flow (40, 70, 153, 166, 167, 174). A gentle manipulation of the gut wall (41), a moderate degree of distension of the gut lumen (41, 153), complete intestinal ischemia (34, 40, 146, 162), and elevation of venous pressure (82, 84, 135) often produce rhythmic contractions. These rhythmic contractions are accompanied by an increase in blood flow to the muscularis layer, whereas the vascular response in the mucosal layer is determined by the direct vascular effect of the stimulus (41, 84, 146). This seems to indicate that the active hyperemia of intestinal contractions does exist. The spontaneous tonic contraction is accompanied by a decrease in blood flow (109, 174). After each con-

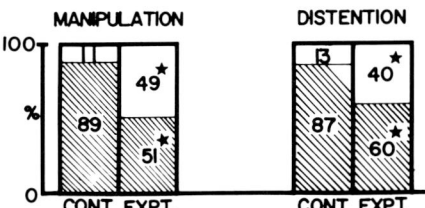

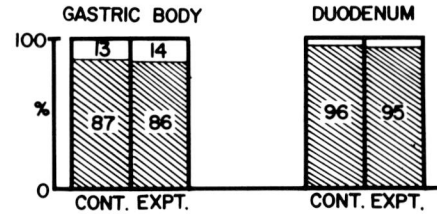

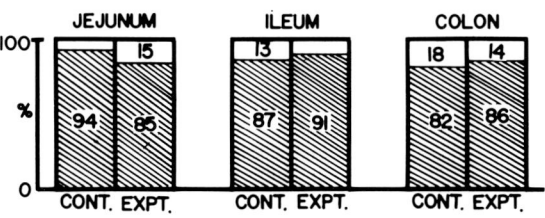

FIG. 7. Mean percentage distribution of blood flow within gut wall before (CONT) and after (EXPT) manipulation or during distension of exteriorized small intestine segments. Values of intact gastrointestinal tract were obtained from tissues left undisturbed within abdominal cavity. [From Chou and Grassmick (41).]

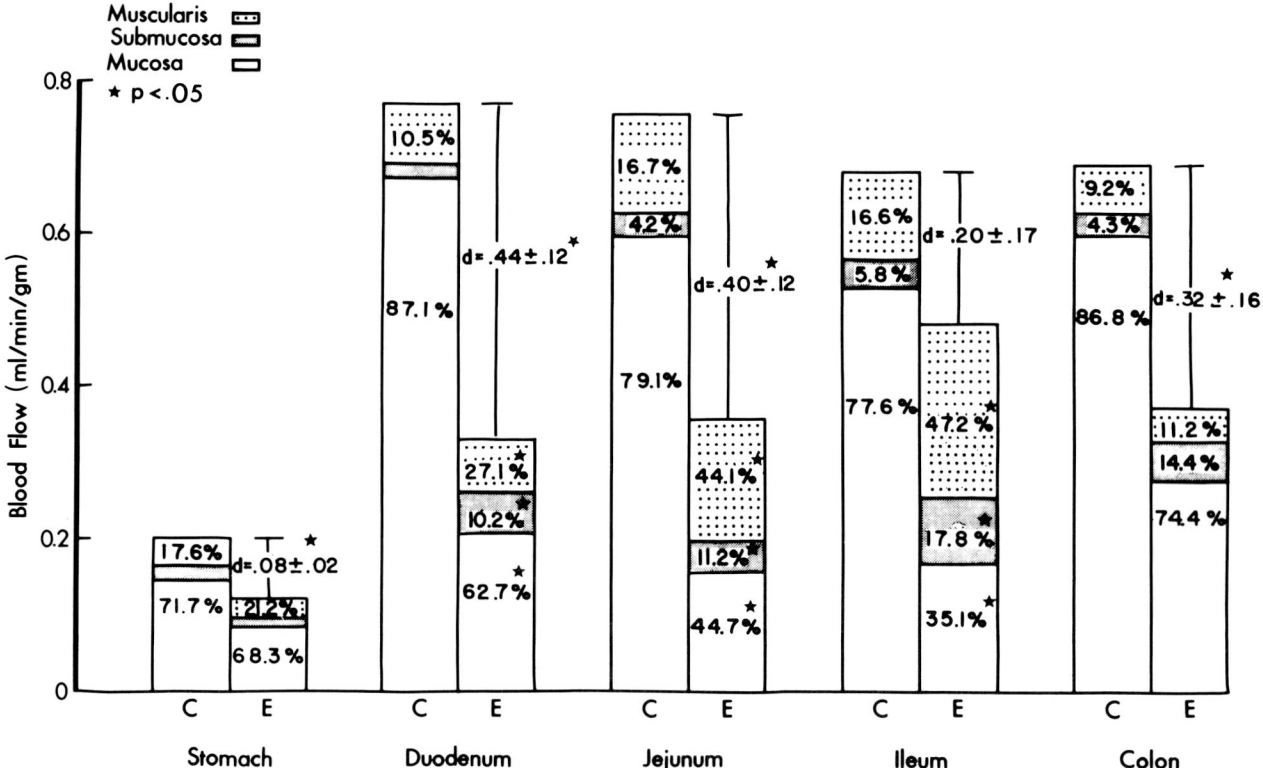

FIG. 8. Compartmental blood flow and percentage distribution of total wall flow to each compartment before (C) and after (E) intravenous infusion of physostigmine in gastrointestinal tract. [From data of Chou and Grassmick (41).]

traction the flow may increase if the contraction is strong (174). Thus in both spontaneous rhythmic and tonic contractions the mechanical compression effect as well as the active hyperemia of muscle contractions can be observed. In rhythmic contractions the active hyperemia occurs during the contractions, whereas in tonic contractions the hyperemia occurs after each contraction. The posttonic hyperemia repays the oxygen debt accumulated during the tonic contraction and is probably due to accumulation of vasodilator metabolites. The hyperemia, however, can be explained by the myogenic mechanism, that is, the contraction decreases the vascular transmural pressure, thereby initiating relaxation of the vascular smooth muscle. The other factors shown in Fig. 5 should also be included in the interpretation of the effects of intestinal contractions on blood flow.

EFFECTS OF CHEMICALS AND NERVES ON BLOOD FLOW AND MOTILITY IN SMALL INTESTINE

Many studies have utilized various stimuli that increase motor activities to determine the effect of motility on blood flow. Tables 1 and 2 show the effects of various neurotransmitters, hormones, and chemicals on blood flow and motor activity of the small intestine. Only the data resulting from simultaneous measurement of blood flow and motility are included in these tables. The preparations used are indicated by SS for the short segment, which is perfused by a single intestinal artery, and by LS for the long segment, which is perfused by more than one artery.

In interpreting the data one must consider the interplay of those factors shown in Figure 5. *1)* The sympathetic and parasympathetic nerves, as well as most chemicals, act not only on the visceral smooth muscle but also on the vascular smooth muscle. Some of these stimuli contract or relax both muscle types, but most stimuli contract intestinal muscle but relax vascular smooth muscle and vice versa. From the mechanical point of view, the net action of a stimulus on blood flow is the algebraic sum of the two additive or opposing effects, i.e., the magnitude and type (rhythmic or tonic) of the induced contractions and their potency as vasoactive agents. The additive effects, for example, vasodilation and relaxation of the intestinal muscle produced by $Mg^{2+}$, are usually difficult to demonstrate clearly, but the opposing effects, e.g., vasodilation and intestinal contraction produced by acetylcholine, can be more easily demonstrated. *2)* The vascular smooth muscle of the blood vessels in

TABLE 1. *Effects of Acetylcholine, Physostigmine, Bradykinin, and Serotonin on Intestinal Blood Flow and Motility*

| Stimuli | Lumen Pressure | Blood Flow | Gut | Ref. |
|---|---|---|---|---|
| Acetylcholine or pilocarpine | Unchanged | Increased | SS | 25, 79, 98,* 112, 154, 162, 174 |
| | | | LS | 170, 183* |
| | Minimal or rhythmic | Unchanged | SS | 25, 155 |
| | Increased | Increased | SS | 13, 26, 112, 162 |
| | | | LS | 153, 192 |
| | Increased | Decreased | SS | 6, 13, 16,* 25, 112, 154, 155, 174 |
| | | | LS | 98* |
| Physostigmine | Increased | Decreased | SS | 41, 79, 166 |
| Vagus efferents | Increased | Decreased | SS | 6 |
| Vagus afferents | Decreased | Decreased | SS | 111 |
| Sympathetic nerves | Decreased | Decreased | SS | 34,* 169 |
| Bradykinin | Unchanged | Increased | SS, LS | 39,* 66, 98,* 154, 170 |
| | Increased | Compromised | SS | 66, 154 |
| | Increased | Decreased | SS, LS | 39,* 154 |
| Serotonin | Unchanged | Increased | LS | 183* |
| | Increased | Unchanged | SS | 162 |
| | Increased | Increased | SS | 14, 79 |
| | Increased | Decreased | LS, SS | 79, 98* |

*Increased* indicates decreased vascular resistance and vice versa. SS, short segment; LS, long segment.    * Constant-flow preparation.

TABLE 2. *Effects of Various Vasoactive Chemicals and Gastrointestinal Hormones on Intestinal Blood Flow and Motility*

| | Lumen Pressure | Blood Flow | Gut | Ref. |
|---|---|---|---|---|
| Norepinephrine or epinephrine | Unchanged | Decreased | SS or LS | 16,* 162 |
| | | | LS | 98,* 170, 183* |
| Angiotensin II | Unchanged | Decreased | LS | 98,* 183* |
| | Increased | Decreased | LS | 170, 192 |
| $PGF_{2\alpha}$ | Increased | Decreased | LS | 170, 192 |
| Vasopressin | Unchanged | Decreased | LS | 170, 183* |
| Isoproterenol | Unchanged | Increased | LS | 98,* 154, 183* |
| Histamine | Increased | Increased | LS | 94, 98,* 149, 161, 170, 193 |
| | Unchanged | Increased | LS | 94, 183* |
| $PGE_1$ | Decreased | Increased | LS | 170 |
| Adenosine | Unchanged | Increased | SS, LS | 38,* 85, 98,* 190 |
| ATP | Increased | Increased | LS, SS | 38,* 98* |
| Morphine | Increased | Unchanged | LS | 98,* 192 |
| Gastrin | Increased | Increased | LS, SS | 14, 44,* 63, 147 |
| Cholecystokinin | Increased | Increased | LS, SS | 14, 44,* 61, 63, 147, 152,* 160 |
| Secretin | Decreased | Unchanged | SS | 147 |
| | Decreased | Increased | SS, LS | 61, 152* |
| | Unchanged | Increased | LS | 44,* 61 |
| Substance P | Increased | Increased | LS | 124, 159 |
| GIP | Decreased | Increased | SS, LS | 62, 152* |
| Neurotensin | Increased | Increased | LS | 8, 113 |

*Increased* indicates decreased vascular resistance and vice versa. SS, short segment; LS, long segment.    * Constant-flow preparation.

the mucosal and muscularis layers may respond differently to a stimulus. For example, adenosine increases total intestinal blood flow, but it decreases mucosal and increases muscularis blood flow (85, 172). It is still unclear, however, whether adenosine constricts mucosal vessels while dilating muscularis vessels or exerts a much greater vasodilation on the muscularis vasculatures than on the mucosal vasculatures. 3) The effect of a stimulus on blood flow may result from its effect on tissue activity. An increase in tissue activity (e.g., mucosal absorption and secretion and muscle contractions) increases tissue metabolism, thereby producing metabolic hyperemia in the tissue. This factor is difficult to evaluate, because a stimulus may increase mucosal functions while having little effect on muscle activities. In this case the stimulus is expected to increase mucosal blood flow more than muscularis blood flow, even if the stimulus relaxes equally the vascular smooth muscle of the mucosal and muscularis blood vessels. Finally, because mucosal and muscularis vascular beds are arranged in parallel (see Fig. 1), the change in blood flow measured at an intestinal artery or vein is the algebraic sum of the direct effect of a stimulus on the mucosal and muscularis vasculatures, its effect on mucosal and muscle activities and metabolism, and the mechanical compression effect of contractions. The physiological feedback systems, which are activated by changes in muscle tone and vascular transmural pressure, should also be considered (see Fig. 5). Included are such mechanisms as receptive relaxation of the visceral muscle, autoregulation of blood flow, venoarteriolar response, and stimulation of local nerves by the stimulus.

Figure 9 gives an example of how the motility can influence the direct vascular effect of a stimulus. An intra-arterial injection of 1 µg acetylcholine did not alter ileal intraluminal pressure but slightly lowered the perfusion pressure, indicating a fall in the vascular resistance. An injection of 10 µg acetylcholine, however, markedly raised the luminal pressure from 2 mmHg to 45–100 mmHg. Concomitantly perfusion pressure rose and fluctuated in rhythm with the fluctuation of the luminal pressure. Thus at low dosage the direct vasodilator action of acetylcholine was evident, but at high dosage the vasodilator action of acetylcholine was masked and overwhelmed by the compression effect of strong contractions; the vascular resistance doubled as a result of the contractions. The direct vasoconstrictor effect of epinephrine can also be reversed by its effect on ileal motility. When the ileal lumen pressure was high and displayed fluctuations, indicating an active ileal motility, an injection of 0.5 µg epinephrine lowered the lumen pressure from 30–50 mmHg to 5 mmHg and abolished fluctuations. Concomitantly the perfusion pressure fell. One minute later, when the lumen pressure was low and steady, the injection of the same dose of epinephrine produced a significant rise in perfusion pressure. Thus, depending on the state of intestinal motor activity, the same dose of epinephrine can increase or decrease intestinal vascular resistance.

## Cholinergics

The cholinergics are the drugs most commonly used to elucidate the relation between blood flow and motility, because they are powerful vasodilators as well as stimulators of intestinal contractions.

After observing that the intestinal blood flow is regulated not only by the vascular tone but also by spontaneous intestinal contractions (174), Bean and Sidky (13) studied the effect of acetylcholine. Acetylcholine increased arterial inflow and venous outflow of the intestinal loop, but whenever the tonic contraction appeared the increases in both flows were temporarily reduced for the duration of the contraction. Acetylcholine at higher doses produced strong tonic contractions that not only counteracted but also masked the vasodilator action of acetylcholine; both arterial inflow and venous outflow decreased well below preinjection levels. The conclusion was reached that acetylcholine can influence intestinal blood flow by at least four mechanisms. The blood flow is increased by *1*) its direct vasodilator action, *2*) release of metabolic vasodilator substances during muscle contractions, and *3*) propulsive pumping action of the rhythmic contractions, but *4*) blood flow is decreased by passive mechanical compression of the tonic contraction.

Subsequent studies have shown that acetylcholine can increase, decrease, or have no effect on blood flow, depending on the strength and type of intestinal contractions it produces (Table 1). Boatman and Brody (16) have attempted to determine whether the acetylcholine-induced decrease in blood flow is due to release of catecholamines. They found that acetylcholine (1–8 µg intra-arterial bolus injection) produced a biphasic effect on intestinal vascular resistance; an initial rise was followed by a fall in the resistance. The increased vascular resistance was always accompanied by a tonic

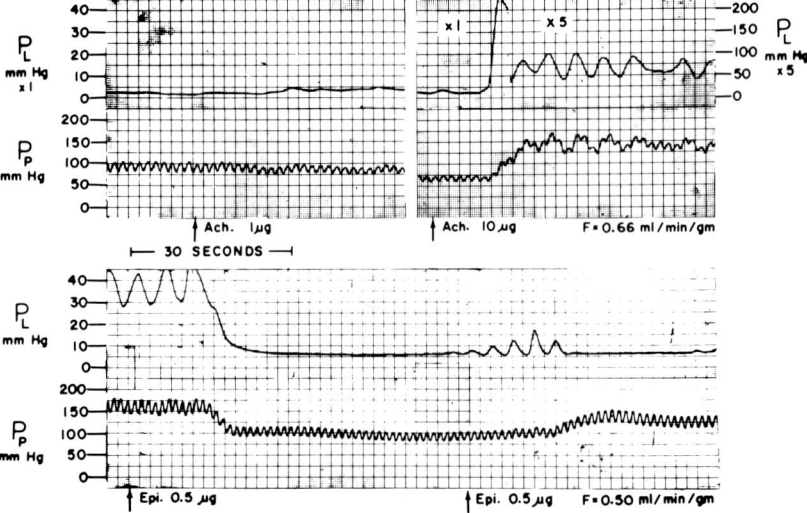

FIG. 9. Effects of acetylcholine (Ach) or epinephrine (Epi) injection on ileal perfusion pressure ($P_p$) and lumen pressure ($P_L$) in ileal segment perfused at constant blood flow rate (F). After injection of 10 µg acetylcholine, luminal pressure rose above 40 mmHg, so attenuation had to be increased to × 5. [From Chou and Dabney (38).]

contraction. Reserpine, which depletes the tissue stores of catecholamines, virtually abolished the vasoconstriction evoked by sympathetic nerve stimulation but had no effect on the acetylcholine-induced vasoconstriction or even served as an enhancer. From this observation the authors concluded that the acetylcholine-induced vasoconstriction does not result from liberation of catecholamines. The acetylcholine-induced increase in both intestinal contraction and vascular resistance was abolished by atropine but was attenuated by trimethylammonium chloride monohydrate ($\beta$TM10, SKF 6890-A, a drug that prevents the release of norepinephrine from nerve terminals) and phenoxybenzamine. A ganglionic blocking drug, hexamethonium, however, did not affect the acetylcholine actions. Application of an acetylcholine solution (1 mg·ml$^{-1}$) on the serosal surface produced contraction and increased vascular resistance. Distension of the gut lumen to increase lumen pressure to a level equal to or higher than that produced by acetylcholine produced only slight increase in resistance. From these two findings and the finding that the acetylcholine-induced vasoconstriction occurred mainly in the small vessels lying within the gut wall, the researchers concluded that the increased vascular resistance produced by acetylcholine was secondary to intestinal contraction, which compresses or distorts the vessels lying within the gut wall.

Scott and Dabney (162) found that acetylcholine increased intestinal blood flow at low dosages but decreased flow at high dosages. When the infusion was terminated, the blood flow rose to 246% of the control value, indicating that a part of the direct vasodilator effect of acetylcholine was masked by the increase in intestinal contraction. Kewenter (112) also reported similar findings in cats anesthetized with chloralose. Acetylcholine at low doses produced dose-dependent increases in intestinal blood flow, whereas at high doses it produced dose-dependent decreases in blood flow (Fig. 10). Intestinal motility increased (30–250 mmHg intraluminal pressure) proportionally to the acetylcholine doses. In some experiments marked blanching of the gut wall was observed. Intestinal volume also increased in a stepwise manner. The author postulated that the acetylcholine-induced increase in contractions compressed the intramural venules, which in turn increased capillary pressure, thereby producing an outward capillary filtration to increase intestinal volume. Acetylcholine or prostaglandin D$_2$ (PGD$_2$) infused intra-arterially at the dosages that markedly increased intestinal motility increased the permeability–surface area product (PS product) for rubidium (192). As Scott and Dabney had noticed (162), Kewenter also observed a large increase in blood flow on termination of the acetylcholine infusion, when the increase in motility had subsided (Fig. 10). This phase is probably equivalent to the posttonic hyperemia of the spontaneous tonic con-

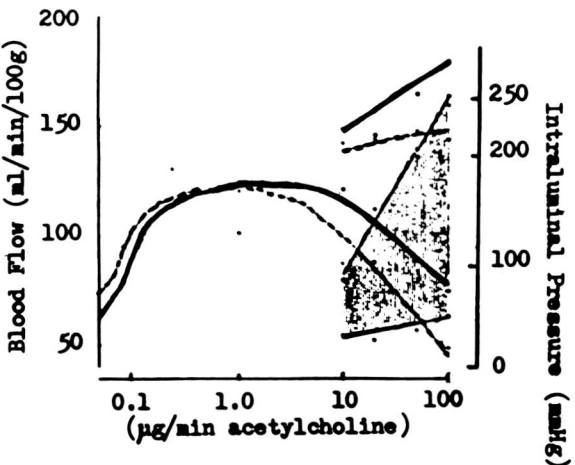

FIG. 10. Effects of intra-arterial infusions of acetylcholine on intestinal blood flow in denervated (*dashed line*) and innervated (*solid line*) jejunal loops. Lines in *upper right quadrant* show flow values obtained after cessation of acetylcholine infusion when motility increase had subsided. *Shaded area* indicates maximum and minimum intraluminal pressure changes induced by acetylcholine (10–100 μg/min). (From Kewenter (112). © 1971, reprinted by permission of Universitetsforlaget, Oslo.)

traction (see Fig. 4). Denervation of the intestinal segment did not significantly alter the vascular and motility responses to acetylcholine.

Pytkowski and Michalowski (155) attempted to correlate motility, blood flow, and the absorption rate of amino acids of jejunal loops (12–20 cm) in conscious as well as anesthetized dogs. In anesthetized dogs pilocarpine at low doses produced rhythmic contractions but did not significantly alter mean blood flow or amino acid absorption. Pilocarpine, 20–70 μg, or acetylcholine, 10–70 μg, produced dose-related increases in tonic contractions that were accompanied by a decrease in mean blood flow during contractions and an increase in the flow during relaxation. In conscious dogs, spontaneous tonic contractions or those induced by mechanical stimulation of the lumen by a balloon placed in the lumen also decreased blood flow. Significant negative correlations were observed between blood flow and motility and between amino acid absorption and the motility index in both conscious and anesthetized dogs (Fig. 11). To prove that the decreased absorption resulted from a decrease in blood flow, blood flow was decreased stepwise from 12.0 to 4.0 ml·min$^{-1}$·100 g$^{-1}$ by mechanically narrowing the intestinal artery in conscious and anesthetized dogs. A significant correlation existed between decreases in blood flow and amino acid absorption. The decreased amino acid absorption during tonic contractions therefore most likely resulted from contraction-induced decrease in blood flow. However, this phenomenon is unlikely to occur under physiological conditions for the following reasons. *1*) The intestinal motor activity after a meal consists primarily of rhythmic segmental contractions that are frequently accompanied by an increase in intestinal blood flow (40, 41). Fioramonti et al. (70, 71) have shown that postprandial rhythmic contractions increased intestinal blood flow and sugar absorption. The increased absorption may result mainly from the mixing action of the contractions. 2) The blood flow range studied, that is, 3 to 12 ml·min$^{-1}$·100 g$^{-1}$ (Fig. 11), is well below physiological range. The resting jejunal blood flow ranges from 30 to 100 ml·min$^{-1}$·100 g$^{-1}$ in anesthetized or conscious dogs (47, 48, 75, 127), and the blood flow after a meal is even higher (45, 47, 48, 75, 127, 189). It has been shown that glucose absorption is not altered by changes in blood flow within the physiological blood flow range (49, 175, 195). In intestinal ischemia, however, glucose and amino acid absorption may be compromised by tonic contractions.

Brobmann et al. (25) studied the effect of acetylcholine in in vitro intestinal segments that were perfused by heparinized blood from a donor dog. Acetylcholine increased blood flow if it did not significantly affect motility. If acetylcholine raised lumen pressure between 10 and 15 mmHg, blood flow did not change, but if the lumen pressure was increased above 15 mmHg, blood flow decreased. The difference in blood flow responses to acetylcholine thus results from interplay between direct vasodilator action and the compression effect of enhanced motility induced by acetylcholine.

All of these studies utilized small segments (10–20 cm in length) in attempting to determine the effect of intestinal contractions on local blood flow. Price et al. (153) measured blood flow through the superior mesenteric artery and correlated the change with changes in luminal pressure in the upper, middle, and lower small bowel. Acetylcholine, 14 μg·min$^{-1}$ for 7 min, did not significantly alter motility and increased, decreased, or did not alter the blood flow in 8 dogs. In another 7 dogs the infusion increased lumen pressure from 6 to 26 mmHg, with marked rhythmic contractions, and increased blood flow 28%. When the infusion was terminated, the contractions subsided before blood flow returned to control levels.

Cholinesterase inhibitors such as physostigmine also have been regularly used to determine the relation between intestinal blood flow and motility. Unlike acetylcholine, their action lasted longer. All studies to date showed that the cholinesterase inhibitors produced strong intestinal contractions while decreasing local blood flow [see Figs. 6, 8, 12; (41, 79, 166)].

*Nerves*

Kewenter (111) studied the vagal control of jejunal and ileal motility and blood flow. His major conclusion was that the vagal nerves do not carry any specific vasodilator fibers to the vessels of the small intestine. Whether or not the motor activities can influence blood flow was only marginally discussed in his report. A significant change in jejunal and ileal blood flow occurred only during activation of high-threshold fibers in the lower thoracic part or subdiaphragmatic portions of the vagus nerves. The activation induced by electrical stimulation at 8 V, 8 ms, and 4 Hz decreased jejunal and ileal motility, and it increased systemic arterial blood pressure as well as the intestinal vascular resistance. This response is the same as that to the sympathetic nerve stimulation, and it

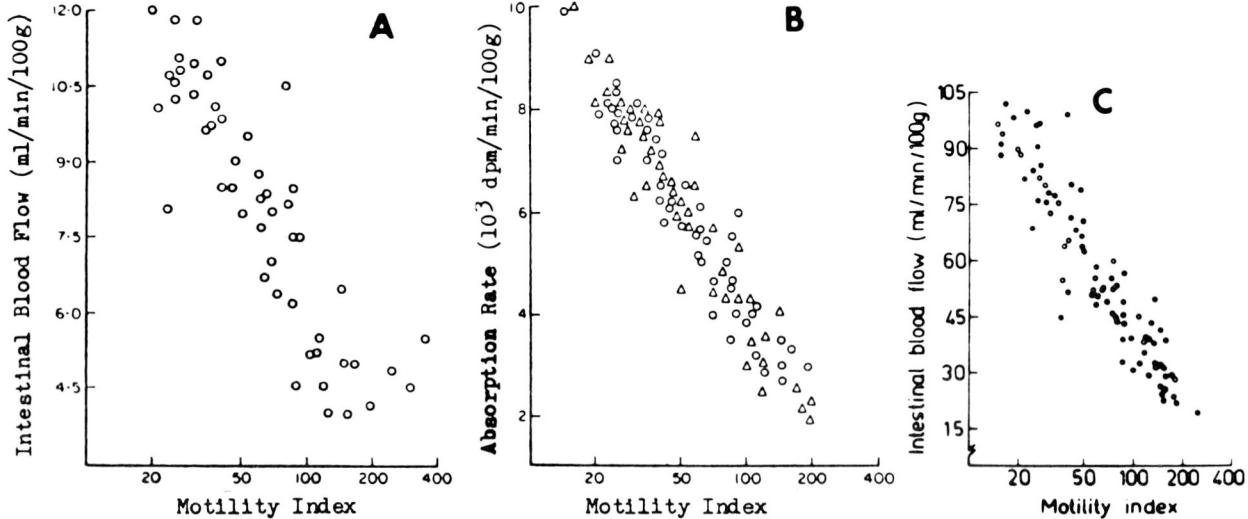

FIG. 11. *A*: relation between motility index and blood flow. *B*: relation between motility index and absorption rate of L-phenylalanine (*open circles*) and L-serine (*open triangles*). Values were obtained from jejunal loops of conscious dogs during spontaneous and mechanically induced tonic contractions. *C*: relation between motility index and intestinal blood flow after bradykinin or acetylcholine in anesthetized dogs. [*A*, *B* from Pytkowski and Michalowski (155); *C* from Pytkowski (154).]

appears to be a consequence of an antidromic activation of the afferent fibers involved in the intestinointestinal inhibitory reflex arc. Sympathetic activation by acute hemorrhagic hypotension or bilateral carotid artery occlusion has also been found to produce an increase in intestinal vascular resistance and a decrease in intestinal wall tension (34, 37).

Semba et al. (169) induced the intestinal inhibitory reflex by either electrical stimulation of the serosal surface of the loop under observation (120 cm in length) or luminal distension of the adjacent segment. The lumen pressure of the loop was maintained initially at 10–15 mmHg. The inhibitory reflex decreased lumen pressure 35%–45% and abolished the spontaneous rhythmic contractions. Blood flow decreased in the initial period 10%–15%, but returned to control levels within 30 s, even though the reflex inhibition of motility still remained. The blood flow then decreased again and eventually returned to control levels. A part of the change in blood flow resulted from corresponding changes in systemic arterial blood pressure. To avoid this effect the intestinal loop was perfused with blood from a donor dog, the blood pressure of which was unaffected by the inhibitory reflex. In these experiments the decrease in lumen pressure (36%) was accompanied by a decrease in blood flow and venous $O_2$ saturation. As the lumen pressure returned toward control levels, the flow and venous $O_2$ saturation returned toward controls, then increased above controls. In some experiments the pattern of the changes in the lumen pressure and flow was the same as has been described, but the venous $O_2$ saturation increased during the decrease in flow. Because arterial $O_2$ saturation remained constant, the increased venous $O_2$ saturation accompanying the decreased flow indicates a decrease in intestinal $O_2$ consumption, but the decreased venous $O_2$ saturation accompanying the decrease in flow does not indicate whether the $O_2$ consumption was changed. Thus reflex-induced inhibition of intestinal motility decreases intestinal blood flow and decreases or does not alter $O_2$ consumption. From a mechanical point of view the result is contrary to expectation. The decreased blood flow might be a direct vasoconstrictor effect of the adrenergic nerves that also inhibit intestinal motility. The association of decreased motility and $O_2$ consumption suggests that the decreased flow may be due in part to decrease in $O_2$ demand.

*Bradykinin*

In the small intestine and colon the threshold blood bradykinin concentration for inducing intestinal contraction (0.1 $\mu g \cdot ml^{-1}$ blood) was more than 10 times that for inducing vasodilation (66). Thus at low concentration (0.01 $\mu g \cdot ml^{-1}$ blood) bradykinin increased blood flow without altering intestinal motility, but at high concentrations (1 $\mu g \cdot ml^{-1}$ blood) the increased flow was compromised by a marked increase in tonic contraction. To determine whether the interference of blood flow resulted from mechanical compression of the contraction, Fasth and Hulten (66) compared the vascular response of the gut segment before and after extirpation of the gut wall. The latter preparation consisted mainly of lymphatic and adipose tissues. The minimal concentration of bradykinin at which blood flow was increased was the same in both preparations (0.001 $\mu g \cdot ml^{-1}$ blood), but the maximal increase in blood flow achieved in the intact preparation (100 $ml \cdot min^{-1} \cdot 100$ $g^{-1}$ tissue) was significantly smaller than that achieved in the preparation devoid of intestinal wall, that is, 150 $ml \cdot min^{-1} \cdot 100$ $g^{-1}$. The latter maximal blood flow value corresponds fairly well to maximal vasodilation as induced by supramaximal amounts of isoproterenol (128). Fasth and Hulten therefore concluded that the bradykinin-induced intestinal contraction can compromise its direct vasodilator action.

Chou et al. (39) studied the vascular and motility effects of bradykinin, kallidin, and eledoisin in the superior mesenteric vascular bed. Infusions of bradykinin, kallidin, and eledoisin at low doses (0.005–0.25 $\mu g \cdot min^{-1}$ ia) did not alter lumen pressure but significantly decreased the vascular resistance. A bolus intra-arterial injection of a large dose of bradykinin (5 $\mu g \cdot kg^{-1}$), kallidin (10 $\mu g \cdot kg^{-1}$), or eledoisin (0.5 $\mu g \cdot kg^{-1}$), however, produced a concurrent rise and fall in the lumen pressure and vascular resistance. Lumen pressure increased 60 mmHg at the height of the intestinal contraction, and during the period of tonic contraction marked blanching of the intestine was observed. During the contraction the vascular resistance of the small blood vessels within the gut wall markedly increased, while the vascular resistance of the artery and vein outside the gut wall decreased. The substantial increase in intramural vascular resistance appears to result from compression of the intramural blood vessels by the contracting muscles. The decrease in extramural arterial and venous resistance seems to result from passive distension of these arteries and veins, owing to the obstruction of arterial inflow and to the expulsion of venous outflow, respectively, by the strong tonic contraction.

Pytkowski (154) also found that the direct vasodilator effect of bradykinin could be reversed by its effect on motility in the jejunal segment. At low dosages (1–10 $nmol \cdot liter^{-1}$ blood) bradykinin increased flow without altering motility. At medium dosages (20–100 $nmol \cdot liter^{-1}$ blood) it caused segmental rhythmic contractions; blood flow decreased during contraction but increased during relaxation. At high dosages (0.2–10 $\mu mol \cdot liter^{-1}$ blood), bradykinin produced dose-dependent increases in the amplitude and duration of tonic contraction. The increases in motility index were significantly correlated with the decreases in blood flow, and the correlation is of the same character as that observed after acetylcholine infusion (Fig. 11C). Atropine blocked the vascular and motility effects of acetylcholine but did not affect those of bradykinin. Indomethacin blocked the vascular effect and attenuated the motility effect of bradykinin but did not influence those produced by acetylcholine, isoproterenol, or prostaglandin $E_2$ ($PGE_2$).

The results of the above three studies (39, 66, 154) appear to indicate that the intestinal muscle of the dog is more sensitive to bradykinin than is that of the cat. The threshold concentrations at which bradykinin stimulates motility were 100 $\mu g \cdot liter^{-1}$ and 10 $\mu g \cdot liter^{-1}$ in cats (66) and dogs (154), respectively. Consequently the effect of motility on blood flow appears to be greater in dogs than in cats. At high doses the bradykinin-induced tonic contractions attenuated the increased blood flow in cats (66) but reversed the increased flow in dogs (39, 154).

*Serotonin*

Serotonin is another vasodilator, the vascular effect of which may be compromised by the increase in motility that it produces. Thus at low dosage it produces vasodilation without altering lumen pressure (183), at medium dosage it increases motility without altering blood flow (162), and at high dosages it produces vigorous intestinal contraction and vasoconstriction (98). Geber (79) has reported that intra-arterial injection of 20 $\mu g$ serotonin increased intestinal motor activity in all 30 preparations, but blood flow increased in 60% of these preparations and decreased in 40%. Biber et al. (14), however, reported that serotonin increased blood flow and motility, and the vasodilation was not influenced by the increase in lumen pressure. Recent studies have shown that serotonin (3–6 $\mu g \cdot min^{-1}$ ia) increased blood flow as well as vasoactive intestinal polypeptide (VIP) release from the small intestine (15 cm in length) (107, 176). After intra-arterial infusion of apamin, a polypeptide from bee venom, serotonin decreased both the blood flow and VIP release. The authors proposed that the vasodilator action of serotonin (at low concentration) was due to release of VIP, and apamin inhibited the VIP release from the VIPergic neurons. The response of intestinal motility was not studied; all cats were atropinized. If VIP and the intramural nerves are involved in the vascular effects of serotonin, these factors should be included in the interpretation of data on serotonin-induced responses.

*Other Vasoactive Drugs and Gastrointestinal Hormones*

The vascular actions of almost all other vasoactive chemicals, autacoids, or gastrointestinal hormones are much more potent than their actions on the intestinal muscle. Furthermore, for those chemicals such as epinephrine, which relax the intestinal muscle, the effect of a decrease in intestinal contraction on blood flow is difficult to elucidate because the intestine does not frequently exhibit a state of sustained strong contraction. Thus the vasoconstrictors, such as angiotensin II, norepinephrine, epinephrine, prostaglandin $F_{2\alpha}$ ($PGF_{2\alpha}$), and vasopressin decreased intestinal blood flow and increased its vascular resistance, whereas the vasodilators such as isoproterenol, histamine, $PGE_1$, adenosine, adenosine 5'-triphosphate (ATP), gastrin, cholecystokinin, secretin, substance P, gastric inhibitory peptide (GIP), and neurotensin increased blood flow and decreased vascular resistance. The effects of these chemicals on intestinal luminal pressure and the sources of the information are listed in Table 2. Some chemicals require comments. At low dosages $PGE_2$ produced an increase in blood flow and rhythmic contractions, but at high dosages it produced tonic contractions and decreased blood flow (154). Glucagon increased systemic arterial pressure and intestinal blood flow while inhibiting motility (65). Of the three actions, the vasodilator effect is the only action of glucagon itself, because adrenalectomy abolished the other two effects. Cholecystokinin impeded duodenal and jejunal blood flow when strong contractions were induced (160).

*Ions and Hypertonicity*

Dabney et al. (52) studied the effect of intra-arterial infusions of isotonic NaCl, $MgCl_2$, KCl, or $CaCl_2$ solutions on ileal blood flow and lumen pressure. Magnesium chloride produced a dose-dependent increase in ileal blood flow but did not alter lumen pressure. Potassium chloride produced a biphasic effect on both blood flow and lumen pressure: at low infusion rates there was an increase in blood flow and decrease in lumen pressure, but at high infusion rates there was a decrease in flow and an increase in lumen pressure. Thus, in contrast to many stimuli that exert opposite effects on intestinal and vascular smooth muscles, $K^+$ relaxes both types of muscle at low infusion rates but contracts both types of muscle at high infusion rates. The effect of $K^+$ does not seem to be mediated by the intestinal nerves, because neither hexamethonium nor tetrodotoxin alters the biphasic vascular response (28). In the organ devoid of extravascular muscle, such as the kidney, $K^+$ still produces the biphasic vascular effect (74). This seems to indicate that the biphasic vascular response of the intestine is not secondary to the $K^+$-induced changes in motility. Calcium chloride did not significantly alter lumen pressure over the infusion range 0.012–0.5 $meq \cdot min^{-1}$ (52). Its effect on blood flow varied with dogs: blood flow increased markedly in 3, increased slightly in 5, and decreased markedly (almost stopped) in 2 dogs. Calcium chloride decreased ileal wall tension (52), produced a dose-dependent decrease in the vascular resistance of the stomach (184) but produced a dose-dependent increase in the vascular resistance of the kidney, heart, forelimb, and superior mesenteric vascular bed (74, 163, 184). Dabney et al. (52) therefore suggested that the variable blood flow response to $Ca^{2+}$ in the ileum might be due to the influence of the decreased ileal wall tension on its direct vasoconstrictor action.

Walus et al. (191), however, reported that intraarterial infusions of $CaCl_2$ produced a dose-dependent decrease in ileal blood flow and an increase in luminal pressure over the dosages 1.0–500 $\mu g \cdot kg^{-1} \cdot min^{-1}$. Calcium antagonists, nifedipine and diltiazem, on the other hand, produced a dose-dependent increase in ileal blood flow and a decrease in intraluminal pressure. A combined infusion of nifedipine (0.1 $\mu g \cdot kg^{-1} \cdot min^{-1}$) and $CaCl_2$ (500 $\mu g \cdot kg^{-1} \cdot min^{-1}$) increased blood flow to the same degree as did nifedipine, indicating that nifedipine blocked the vasoconstrictor effect of $CaCl_2$. Ileal blood flow and luminal pressure were significantly increased by $CaCl_2$ at 1 $mg \cdot kg^{-1} \cdot min^{-1}$; the increased flow was reversed to a significant decrease by digoxin, suggesting the involvement of $Na^+$-$K^+$-ATPase in the $CaCl_2$-induced vasodilation. However, because the osmolarity of the $CaCl_2$ solution used in this experiment was greater than the plasma osmolarity, the increased blood flow and luminal pressure might be partly due to the effect of hyperosmolarity per se. This study indicates that $Ca^{2+}$ ions at low infusion rates contract both vascular and intestinal smooth muscle, but at a high infusion rate they relax vascular smooth muscle and contract intestinal smooth muscle. The intestinal contractions, however, were of both rhythmic and tonic type and were observed mainly at the beginning of infusion of each dose. The reason for the discrepancy between this and other studies (52, 184) is unclear.

Application of a hypertonic NaCl solution (1%–5%) to the serosal surface or intravenous physostigmine produced tonic contraction and three types of blood flow response (Fig. 12). In two types, as the lumen pressure rose, venous outflow increased while arterial inflow decreased, but as the contraction was reaching its maximum, venous outflow decreased below control levels (166). In another type, both arterial inflow and venous outflow decreased during the tonic contraction. After the tonic contraction, both arterial inflow and venous outflow increased. The posttonic hyperemia depended on the magnitude and duration of the decreased blood flow occurring during the contraction. In another study Semba et al. (167) observed that the increased and decreased venous outflow were accompanied by a decrease and increase, respectively, in $O_2$ saturation of the venous blood. The $O_2$ saturation of the arterial blood remained constant. This indicates that the increase and decrease in blood flow were accompanied by an increase and decrease in intestinal $O_2$ consumption. The increase and decrease in $O_2$ consumption could well be due simply to the increase and decrease in blood flow, because the blood flow

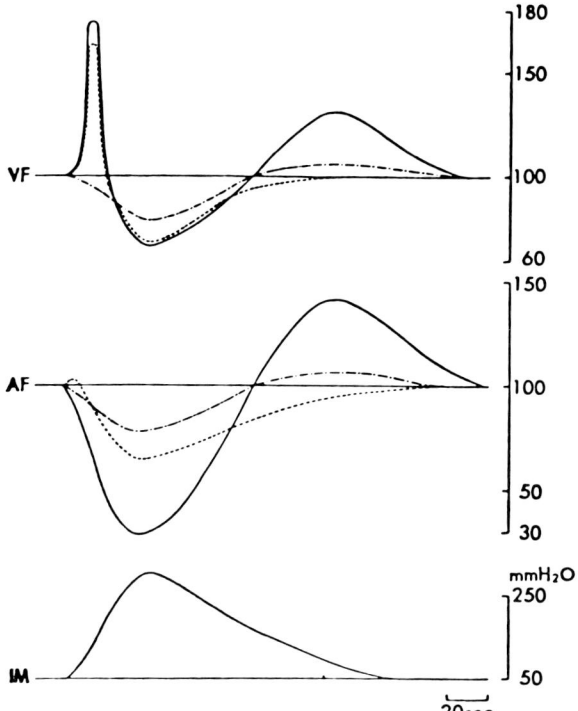

FIG. 12. Correlation between blood flow in vein (VF) and artery (AF) in tonic contraction induced by physostigmine or hypertonic NaCl solution. Control VF and AF were set at 100%. IM, intestinal intraluminal pressure. Three types of blood flow responses can be observed. [From Semba et al. (166).]

values in this study are in the range or at the margin of the levels (i.e., below 20 $ml \cdot min^{-1} \cdot 100$ $g^{-1}$) at which intestinal $O_2$ consumption can be decreased simply by a decrease in blood flow (118, 130). The increased $O_2$ consumption during posttonic hyperemia, however, may be a cause of the hyperemia (metabolic hyperemia).

Placement of a hypertonic (3,000 $mosmol \cdot kg^{-1}$) glucose or nonabsorbable polyethylene glycol into the jejunal lumen, however, produced rhythmic contractions and increased blood flow (36); the increased flow was confined only to the mucosal-submucosal layer (196). Both the motility and blood flow responses to the luminal placement of these hypertonic solutions were abolished after exposing the mucosa to a local anesthetic, suggesting that the responses were mediated by a local neural reflex initiated from the mucosa. Instillation of solutions with pH 1.5 or 2.0 into the duodenal lumen at 4 $ml \cdot min^{-1}$ increased duodenal blood flow and motility; pH 1.5 produced greater effects than did pH 2.0 (43). Duodenal instillation of 50% glucose produced vascular and motility responses similar to that of pH 2.0. Solutions with pH 2.5, 3.0, 8.0, 9.0, or 11.0 and solutions with osmolality 1,000–1,500 $mosmol \cdot kg^{-1}$, however, had no effect on duodenal blood flow or motility (42). Duodenal venous pH and osmolality were not altered significantly during instillation of any of these solutions.

## Hypercapnia and Hypoxemia

Hypercapnia, an increase in the blood $CO_2$, increases intestinal blood flow by direct vasodilatory action of $CO_2$ (or $H^+$), but it produced a triphasic action on intestinal motility: a transient increase in rhythmic contractions followed by an inhibition, then occasionally by sporadic tonic contractions (173). The responses of motility to $CO_2$ significantly affected its direct vasodilatory action. The gradual increase in blood flow induced by the direct vasodilatory action of $CO_2$ was abruptly augmented as soon as there was a pronounced increase in rhythmic contractions. The onset of strong tonic contractions then almost invariably decreased the intestinal blood flow and frequently nullified or reversed the preexisting vasodilating influence of high $CO_2$. In contrast to hypercapnemia, hypoxemia produced direct vasodilation and inhibited intestinal motility (12). Like epinephrine (see Fig. 9), the influence of reduction in motility on blood flow could be revealed only when strong contractions were present before the induction of hypoxemia. Thus hypoxemia increased blood flow and had little effect on intestinal motility when preexisting motility was low. However, if strong rhythmic contractions were present, the same level of hypoxemia inhibited the contractions and produced only a transient small increase in blood flow, which subsequently returned to control or below control levels. The researchers surmised that the failure of hypoxemia to produce a sustained increase in blood flow was due to the inhibition of rhythmic contractions; that is, the direct vasodilatory action of hypoxemia was offset by the decrease in blood flow accompanying the inhibition of rhythmic contractions. In an earlier study (174) they had shown that rhythmic contractions were accompanied by an increased flow in their experimental setting (see *Rhythmic Contractions*, p. 1479).

## Intestinal Wall Tension and Blood Flow

All of these studies described above measured changes in intestinal luminal pressure, and they frequently took the increase in the basal pressure as an indication of an increase in gut wall tension. Wall tension or intramural tension ($T$) is a mathematical function of the transmural pressure (P) and radius ($r$): $T = P \times r$ for the circumferential tension and $T = P \times r'/2$ for the longitudinal tension, where $r'$ is the average of the two principle radii of the curvature segment (156). Thus an increase in lumen pressure may not indicate an increase in wall tension if the wall diameter decreases. The wall diameter decreases during contraction. Evans (57) has suggested that the degree of tonus (tension) depends on the relation of a stretching force (F) applied to smooth muscle and the final length ($L$) that is attained (i.e., $T = F/L$). Chou and Dabney (34, 37, 38, 52) studied the relation between intestinal compliance (C) and vascular resistance ($R$) in the canine ileal segment perfused at constant blood flow. The compliance ($C = \Delta V/\Delta P$) was determined by measuring the changes in ileal intraluminal pressure ($\Delta P$) that were produced by infusions of warm water (37°C) at a constant rate into the flaccid balloon placed in the lumen to increase stepwise the balloon volume ($\Delta V$) to 10, 20, 30, and 40 ml (Fig. 13). The equation for the compliance has both components of the Laplace's and Evans' equations for wall tension. Fleischer (72) utilized a similar technique to determine the gut wall tension in vitro and found that tension (or contractile state) within the gut wall could be determined reliably by simultaneous measurement of intraluminal volume and pressure after distending the lumen at a constant rate.

Figure 14 shows an example of the experiments. Epinephrine at 0.2 $\mu g \cdot min^{-1}$ ia did not significantly alter either ileal perfusion pressure (and thus vascular resistance) or lumen pressure at zero intraluminal volume but did significantly increase the compliance from 0.88 to 2.15 $ml \cdot mmHg^{-1}$ (note the flatter slope of the pressure-volume ratio). This indicates that the measurement of compliance is a more sensitive technique than the recording of the lumen pressure for determining the effect of a stimulus on the intestinal contractile state. No change in vascular resistance may indicate that epinephrine at the dosage used had no vascular action. However, the result may stem from the interplay of vascular and intestinal muscle responses to epinephrine, i.e., the direct vasoconstrictor effect of epinephrine was offset by a decrease in the gut wall tension, which decompressed the blood vessels. This possibility is supported by the finding that the increase in vascular resistance (perfusion pressure) induced by distension was significantly lower during infusion of epinephrine than the controls (Fig. 14). In addition to intestinal wall tension and vascular resistance, the technique also can determine the effect of various stimuli on the rhythmic contractions appearing during distension and after deflation (Fig. 13). These contractions may be mediated by the intramural reflex (peristaltic reflex) (11, 58, 114). Table 3 shows the effects of various local and systemic stimuli on rhythmic contractions (as determined by the tracings of lumen pressure), wall tension (the opposite of compliance), and vascular resistance. All procedures affect wall tension and the rhythmic contractions in the same direction except adenosine, ATP, KCl at high concentration, and propranolol. These four chemicals at the dosages used appear to affect differentially the contractile state of the intestinal muscle and the neuromuscular mechanism involved in the initiation of rhythmic contractions. Adenosine or ATP increased the rhythmic contractions when the injec-

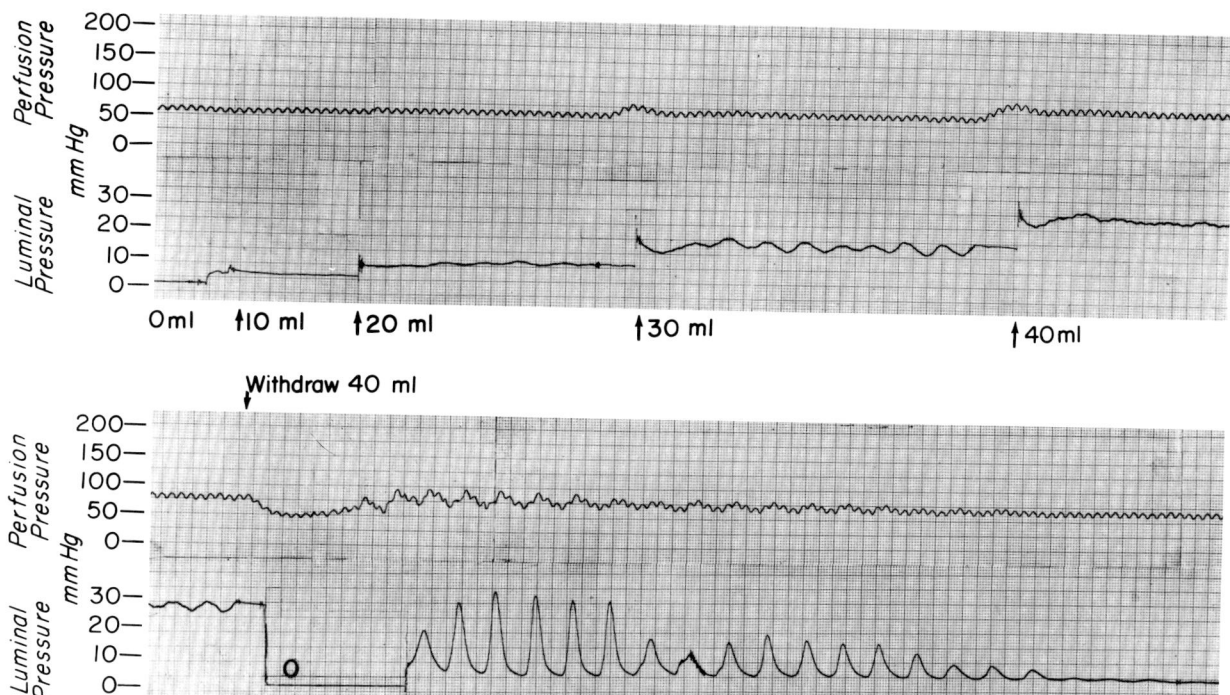

FIG. 13. Typical recording during measurement of ileal compliance. *Arrows* indicate infusions or withdrawal of water into or from balloon. Balloon volume increased in 10-ml steps to 40 ml, and total 40 ml was withdrawn in one step. Note that rhythmic segmental contractions appeared during distension and after withdrawal. [From Chou and Dabney (37).]

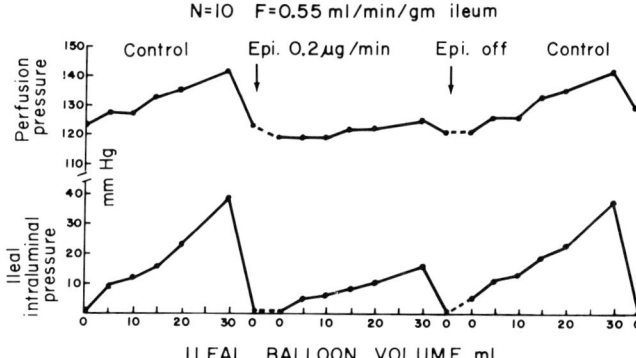

FIG. 14. Average effects of intra-arterial infusion of epinephrine on ileal perfusion and intraluminal pressures determined at various ileal balloon volumes. $N$, number of dogs tested; $F$, average blood flow, maintained constant by pump. [From Chou and Dabney (38).]

tion dose was 100 µg. None of the procedures significantly altered ileal basal luminal pressure at zero balloon volume, but all significantly altered intestinal wall tension (Fig. 14 is an example). This again indicates that the measurement of the compliance is a sensitive technique.

Table 3 also shows the effects of these stimuli on vascular resistance at zero balloon volume. At the dosages used, the direct vascular actions of these chemicals or procedures predominated, and the changes in wall tension were not strong enough to influence their vascular actions at lumen pressure below 5 mmHg. The resting vascular resistances, however, were significantly correlated with the resting gut wall tensions; the higher the wall tension, the higher was the vascular resistance (37, 52). Furthermore the distension-induced increase in vascular resistance was larger when the resting wall tension was higher, and vice versa [Fig. 14; (34, 37, 38, 39)]. (See EFFECTS OF INTESTINAL LUMINAL DISTENSION, p. 1502.) The vascular resistance is determined primarily by the vessel radius, which in turn is determined by the vascular transmural pressure. An increase or decrease in vascular extramural pressure by increasing or decreasing the gut wall tension decreases or increases the vessel radius, thereby increasing or decreasing the vascular resistance.

With the same technique Premen et al. (152) studied the effect of synthetic gastrin, secretin, GIP, and cholecystokinin octapeptide (CCK-8). At infusion rates that increased local arterial blood concentrations equivalent to those achieved after a meal, none of these hormones altered vascular resistance, but ileal compliance was increased by secretin and GIP, decreased by CCK-8, and unaffected by gastrin. At higher infusion rates both secretin and GIP decreased vascular resistance. At high infusion rates, CCK produced powerful phasic contractions, with concomitant

TABLE 3. *Effects of Various Chemicals on Ileal Motility, Wall Tension, and Vascular Resistance*

| | Doses/min, ia | Rhythmic Contractions* | Wall Tension | Vascular Resistance† |
|---|---|---|---|---|
| Local effect | | | | |
| Epinephrine | 0.2 µg | ↓ | ↓ | → |
| Acetylcholine | 0.4 µg | ↑ | ↑ | ↓ |
| Bradykinin | 0.1 µg | ↑ | ↑ | ↓ |
| Serotinin | 2.0 µg | ↑ | ↑ | → |
| Adenosine | 10.0 µg | → | ↑ | ↓ |
| Adenosine triphosphate | 10.0 µg | → | ↑ | ↓ |
| $CaCl_2$ | 0.12 meq | ↓ | ↓ | → |
| $MgCl_2$ | 0.12 meq | ↓ | ↓ | ↓ |
| KCl | 0.02 meq | → | → | ↓ |
| KCl | 0.07 meq | ↓ | ↓ | ↓ |
| KCl | 0.18 meq | ↓ | ↓ | ↓ |
| Phenoxybenzamine | 0.3 µg/kg | ↓ | ↓ | ↓ |
| Propranolol | 30.0 µg/kg | → | ↓ | ↑ |
| Systemic effect | | | | |
| Epinephrine, iv | 12.0 µg | ↓ | ↓ | → |
| Hemorrhage | | ↓ | | ↑ |
| Carotid occlusion | | → | ↓ or → | ↑ |

* Responses included spontaneous movements at zero balloon volume, and rhythmic activity during distension and after deflation.  † Resistance measured at zero balloon volume.   ↓, Decreases; ↑, increases; →, no change in variables measured.   [Data from Chou and Dabney (34, 37, 38) and Dabney et al. (52).]

large oscillation in luminal and perfusion pressures. The authors concluded that GIP, secretin, and CCK play an insignificant role in postprandial intestinal hyperemia but may play a role in stimulating intestinal motility after a meal.

## Blood Flow Distribution Within Gut Wall

The effect of physostigmine on blood flow distribution within the gut wall has been described (see Fig. 8). It was suggested from the study that the physostigmine-induced tonic contraction decreases mucosal-submucosal blood flow by mechanical compression, but it does not alter muscularis blood flow, because the contraction-induced vasodilation offsets the compression effect. Other investigators also produced evidence to support this thesis. Walus et al. (193) showed that at the beginning of intra-arterial infusion of histamine intestinal motility was unchanged and blood flow increased equally to both mucosal and muscle layers. As the infusion continued, intestinal motility increased, and the muscularis blood flow increased 230%, while mucosal blood flow returned to control levels. Furthermore $H_1$ receptor antagonist (tripelennamine) blocked both the increase in motility and the redistribution of blood flow. Methionine-enkephalin has little direct vascular action (192); but at doses of 0.03–1.0 $\mu g \cdot kg^{-1} \cdot min^{-1}$ intra-arterially, it produced dose-dependent increases in intestinal blood flow, $O_2$ consumption, and mean motility index (150). At 0.5 $\mu g \cdot kg^{-1} \cdot min^{-1}$, total intestinal flow increased 23%, while flow to the muscularis increased 50% and the motility index increased 107%. Neurotensin increased intestinal motility, blood flow, and $O_2$ consumption (113) and increased blood flow only to the muscle layer (300%) of the small and large intestine (8). The increase in intestinal $O_2$ consumption was significantly related to the increase in the motility index during intra-arterial infusion of acetylcholine and Met-enkephalin ($\dot{V}_{O_2}$ = 1.04 + 0.015 × motility index) (119). These studies thus showed the association of an increased motility and $O_2$ consumption, with a preferential increase in blood flow to the muscularis layer. This suggests that the increased muscularis flow is related to an active hyperemia of the contracting muscle. Glucagon decreased motility and redistributed blood flow away from the muscle layer, which may be related to decrease in muscle contractions (148). However, CCK, which increased intestinal motility and blood flow (see Table 2), increased mucosal blood flow more than muscularis blood flow (60). It is unclear whether this response results from the greater effect CCK has on the mucosal function and metabolism than on muscle contraction. Cholecystokinin produced a dose-dependent increase in intestinal $O_2$ consumption that is unrelated to the CCK-induced intestinal contraction (61).

Walus et al. (192) studied the effects of six drugs on motility, oxygen consumption, total blood flow, and distribution within the gut wall (Table 4). They concluded that increased motor activity has little influence on the intestinal circulation, because there was little consistent correlation between these two events during infusions of these drugs. They did, however, suggest that the direct vascular effects of the drugs on blood flow may be modified by mechanical and metabolic consequences of the drug-induced increase in motor activities. All six drugs increased both the basal

TABLE 4. *Comparison of Effects of Drugs on Various Hemodynamic and Metabolic Parameters*

| Drug* | Dose, µg· kg$^{-1}$·min$^{-1}$ | BF | MF | FBF | $\dot{V}_{O_2}$ | MMI |
|---|---|---|---|---|---|---|
| Acetylcholine | 1.0 | ++ | ++ | ++++ | 0 | +++++ |
| PGD$_2$ | 0.05 | + | ++ | +++ | + | +++++ |
| Met-enkephalin | 5.0 | + | + | + | + | ++++ |
| Morphine | 0.1 | 0 | 0 | − | 0 | +++++ |
| PGF$_{2\alpha}$ | 0.025 | − | + | 0 | + | +++++ |
| Angiotensin II | 0.025 | −− | − | −− | 0 | +++++ |

BF, blood flow to gut segment; MF, fraction of microspheres trapped in muscularis; FBF, fraction of blood flow to muscularis; $\dot{V}_{O_2}$, oxygen consumption; MMI, mean motility index; PGD$_2$, prostaglandin D$_2$; PGF$_{2\alpha}$, prostaglandin F$_{2\alpha}$. +, Increase; −, decrease; 0, no change. * Each drug was administered in a dose evoking comparable responses in intestinal motor activity. [Data from Walus et al. (192).]

lumen pressure and rhythmic contractions and increased equally the mean motility index (MMI, which is the sum of heights of all contractions during a 10-min period divided by the number of contractions in the same time). Acetylcholine and PGD$_2$ increased total wall flow with much of the increased flow going to the muscularis (FBF). Methionine-enkephalin produced a variable response of blood flow, but at 5 µg· kg$^{-1}$·min$^{-1}$ it increased MMI 250%, which was accompanied by a 28% increase in muscularis flow and only an 8% increase in total blood flow. Prostaglandin F$_{2\alpha}$, a mild vasoconstrictor, decreased total wall flow but increased oxygen consumption and did not significantly affect muscularis flow. The decreased total wall flow therefore was due to a decreased mucosal flow. These findings could be explained by the contraction-induced active hyperemia in the muscularis, which enhances the direct vasodilatory action or opposes the direct constrictor action of the drugs. Angiotensin II, a potent vasoconstrictor, however, equally decreased both the total and muscularis flow, whereas morphine, which increased motility, did not alter total flow or oxygen consumption but decreased flow to the muscle layer. The effect on intestinal oxygen consumption is difficult to interpret, because each drug may have different effects on mucosal and muscle metabolism, and the measured oxygen consumption is the sum of the responses in the functionally different tissues.

## Summary

The effect of chemically induced motility on intestinal blood flow depends on the sensitivity of vascular and intestinal smooth muscle to individual chemicals. The intestinal vascular smooth muscle is more sensitive than intestinal muscle to most chemicals. As a result, direct vascular action predominates at low infusion rates, but at high infusion rates the direct vascular action can be compromised or reversed by induced strong contractions. Rhythmic contractions are accompanied by cyclic changes in instantaneous blood flow, but the mean blood flow depends on the interplay of mechanical compression and the strength of the direct vasodilator action of individual chemicals. After tonic contractions, posttonic hyperemia occurs whether the blood flow is increased, decreased, or unchanged during the infusion. Furthermore, when the total wall blood flow is increased, the muscularis blood flow increases more than the mucosal-submucosal flow. When the total flow is decreased, the decreased flow occurs mainly in the mucosal-submucosal layer. These findings seem to indicate the existence of interplay between direct vascular action and mechanical compression and active hyperemia of intestinal contractions. In several experiments the contractions are accompanied by an increase in oxygen consumption. For the chemicals that inhibit motility, the effect of decreasing motility on blood flow can be revealed only when the preexisting motility is high. Intestinal compliance is more sensitive than lumen pressure in determining the effect of a stimulus on intestinal wall tension and the influence of the wall tension on intestinal vascular resistance.

## MOTILITY AND BLOOD FLOW IN COLON AND STOMACH

### Colon

There have been relatively few studies conducted to determine the effect of colonic motility on its blood flow in comparison with the numerous investigations of the small intestine. It is unclear whether the situation in the colon is similar to that in the small intestine. Fasth and Hulten (66) have shown that the effect of bradykinin on the relation between motility and blood flow in the colon was the same as that observed in the small intestine. On the other hand, as compared with their effect in the small intestine (Table 2), pentagastrin (64–4,096 ng/kg iv) decreased colonic blood flow without affecting motility, and CCK (1–4,096 mU·kg$^{-1}$ iv) affected neither colonic blood flow nor motility (160). Spontaneous contractions in the colon had no significant effect on its blood flow, but intense stimulation of the pelvic nerve increased motility in the distal colon and decreased blood flow (103). Spontaneous or distension-induced tonic contractions, however, decreased colonic blood flow (97).

Semba and Fujii (168) studied how intravenous injection of physostigmine (0.05 mg·kg$^{-1}$) or eserine sulfate (0.1–0.2 mg·kg$^{-1}$), stimulation of the pelvic nerve, and application of hypertonic salt solution on the colonic surface affected venous outflow and motility of the distal colon (15 cm long). All these stimulations produced tonic contraction lasting for at least 50 s (Fig. 15). Three types of venous outflow response were classified. Physostigmine and eserine sulfate produced contraction-phase (*open circles*) or relaxation-

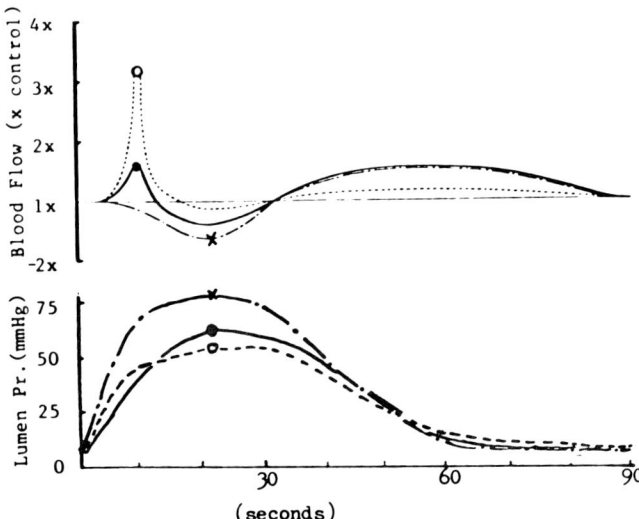

FIG. 15. Correlation between colonic motility and blood flow. *Open circles*, contraction type; ×, relaxation type; *filled circles*, combination type. [From Semba and Fujii (168). Lumen pressure tracings adapted by C. C. Chou according to description in text.]

phase (×) responses, whereas pelvic nerve stimulation or hypertonic solution produced a combination type of response (*closed circles*). Venous outflow increased during the initial tonic contraction 210% and 60% above controls in the contraction and combination types, respectively. As the tonic contraction reached its maximum, blood flow decreased below control levels. In the relaxation type, venous outflow decreased during the tonic contraction; the maximum lumen pressure achieved (70–100 mmHg) was greater than in the other two types. Thus tonic contraction in the distal colon can increase venous outflow transiently or produce a sustained decrease, depending on the strength of the contraction. In some cases the venous outflow stopped at the maximum contraction. During relaxation venous outflow started to increase, reaching above-control levels as the lumen pressure decreased to control levels. The hyperemia lasted for ~50 s, and the stronger the contraction, the greater was the posttonic hyperemia. The effect of tonic contraction on venous outflow is therefore similar to that in the small intestine. Physostigmine decreased colonic mucosal blood flow but did not significantly alter blood flow to the muscularis layer (41).

Serotonin increased both blood flow and motility in the proximal colon, in both cases mediated by local nerves, and the effects were similar to those evoked by pelvic nerve stimulation (64). However, only the vascular effect was blocked by dihydroergotamine, a serotonin-blocking drug. Vasoactive intestinal polypeptide produced a transient increase in the colonic blood flow and a delayed but sustained colonic contraction that persisted even after the end of the infusion (56). Whether the delayed colonic contraction caused transient nature of the hyperemia during VIP infusion is unclear. The vascular and motility effects of VIP in the colon were similar to those induced by pelvic nerve stimulation in atropinized cats (68).

Hulten (103) conducted a series of experiments to investigate the neural regulation of blood flow and motility in the colon in cats. The distribution of vasoconstrictor and vasodilator nerve fibers in the colon and the motility responses to stimulation of these nerves indicate that the colon is composed of two functionally different units (103, 104). The vagal and major splanchnic nerves supply the right colon, and the pelvic and lumbar sympathetic nerves supply the left colon and rectum. Electrical stimulation of the vagal nerves innervating the colon did not alter blood flow, apart from changes caused by an increase in colonic motility; the neurotransmitter is acetylcholine (105). Pelvic nerve stimulation, on the other hand, produced an increase in colonic secretion and motility, and a transient marked increase (~1 min) in blood flow (103). The transient increase in blood flow was followed by a more prolonged oscillation in blood flow. During oscillation, blood flow increased preferentially to the superficial mucosa, an effect that may be related to mucosal secretion. The muscularis blood flow also increased. The oscillation in total blood flow and the muscularis hyperemia may be related to the increased motility. Atropine abolished the increase in motility in the proximal colon, the colonic secretion, and the oscillation of the blood flow. The initial marked hyperemia and the increased motility in the distal colon were not affected by atropine.

Fasth et al. (68) measured the blood flow of the entire colon and rectum while recording changes in luminal volume (with rubber balloon) at the proximal and distal colon and the rectum. Pelvic nerve stimulation produced an immediate and sustained contraction of both the colon and rectum and a transient increase in the overall blood flow (Fig. 16). After atropine, pelvic nerve stimulation produced a delayed but sustained contraction of the proximal colon and a transient relaxation of the rectum. Concomitantly there was an immediate but transient hyperemia that was followed by recurrent increases in blood flow. The colonic hyperemia was prolonged, particularly during rectal relaxation (Fig. 16). Whether the relaxation was a cause of the prolongation of the hyperemia is unclear. The motility and vasodilator responses were not affected by adrenergic (phentolamine and propranolol) or by serotoninergic (dihydroergotamine) blockade. The authors suggested that the motility effect of pelvic nerve stimulation is mediated by cholinergic as well as noncholinergic, nonserotoninergic excitatory neurons and also by nonadrenergic, noncholinergic inhibitory neurons. The kallikrein-kinin system may be involved in the vasodilation and contractions induced by pelvic nerve stimulation.

Fasth et al. (67) found that in atropinized cats

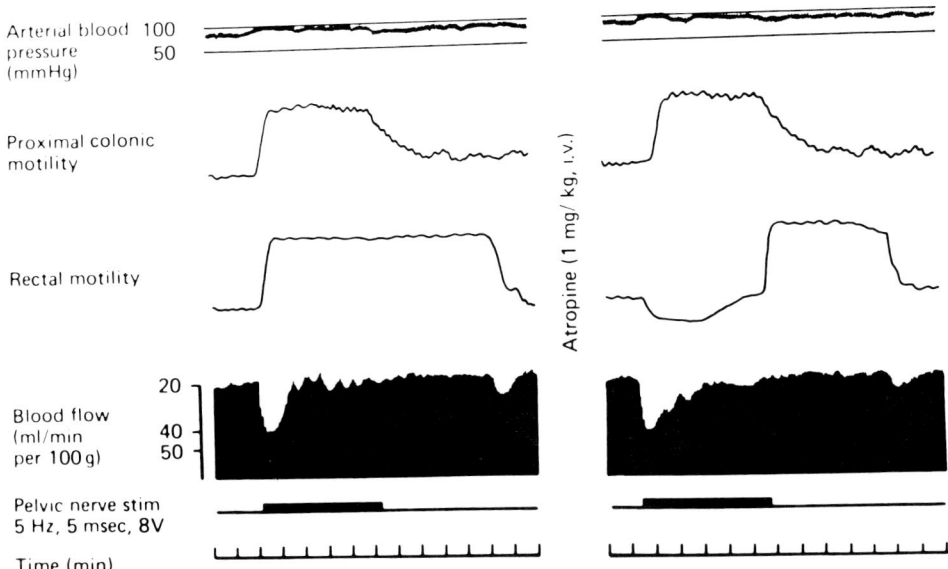

FIG. 16. Effects of pelvic nerve stimulation before (*left*) and after (*right*) atropine. [From Fasth et al. (68).]

colonic vasodilation and contraction induced by pelvic nerve stimulation were similar to effects produced by infusions of synthetic bradykinin and that after 2-h pelvic nerve stimulation the kallikrein levels in the colonic mucosa and muscle increased significantly. The increased tissue kallikrein appears to originate from plasma. Thus prolonged pelvic nerve stimulation causes extravasation of plasma kallikrein, forming kinin in the tissue and producing colonic vasodilation and contractions. In atropinized cats, trasylol® (which inhibits the kinin system) attenuated or blocked the initial vasodilation as well as the recurrent increases in blood flow (69). Trasylol, however, did not affect the proximal colon contraction and rectal relaxation. Thus the kinin system appears to play a role in the vasodilation but not in the motility response to pelvic nerve stimulation.

A substance P antagonist (D-Arg$^1$,D-Pro$^2$,D-Trp$^{7,9}$Leu$^{11}$)-substance P, or naloxone did not alter the colonic contraction and hyperemia in control cats, but in atropinized cats naloxone blocked the contraction without affecting vasodilation evoked by pelvic nerve stimulation (177). Sjöqvist et al. (177) proposed that there are at least three motoneuronal systems in the distal colon: one cholinergic and one enkephalinergic system mediating colonic contractions and one system mediating vasodilations with another transmitter. The vasodilation is not mediated by acetylcholine, substance P, or enkephalin but may be mediated by VIP (59, 107, 176). The transient vasodilation produced by pelvic nerve stimulation was accompanied by a significant increase in colonic venous plasma VIP concentration (59). Apamin either abolished or markedly attenuated the vasodilation but had no effect on colonic contraction induced by pelvic nerve stimulation (107). The blockade of the vasodilation was accompanied by an attenuation of VIP release from the colon. Apamin, however, did not alter VIP-induced vasodilation (107), suggesting that apamin may act to block the release of VIP from the VIPergic neurons.

From this description it is clear that the colonic contraction and the vasodilation induced by pelvic nerve stimulation are mediated by different mechanisms. This makes interpretation of data on the relation between motility and blood flow even more difficult and should be considered in addition to the factors shown in Figure 5. The vascular and motility responses to pelvic nerve stimulation also depend on pattern of the stimulation. Continuous stimulation produced both colonic contraction and a transient vasodilation, whereas burst stimulations produced only the vasodilation (4, 5). Both continuous and burst stimulations increased the output of VIP, and burst stimulations increased somatostatin output; substance P output was not altered by either stimulation (4).

Neural reflex can also produce accompanying changes in colonic motility and blood flow. Frictional stimulation of the rectal mucosa or distension of the rectal lumen produced a strong increase in the proximal colon motility and a concomitant transient increase in blood flow (103). These responses were somewhat similar to those produced by continuous stimulation of the efferent pelvic nerve. A strong distension of the rectal lumen sometimes produced straining movements, which were accompanied by an initial decrease in colonic blood flow and a delayed transient hyperemia. Mechanical stimulation of the sigmoid colon had little or no influence on colonic motility or blood flow, indicating that the receptors are present only in the rectum. The reflex responses described, however, were often difficult to reveal unless the sympathetic colonic nerve activity was abolished either by denervation or administration of guanethidine, and thus sympathetic inhibition on the parasympathetic reflex effects is indicated. The reflex responses were unaffected by vagotomy but were abolished by denervation of the pelvic nerves (pelvopelvic reflex). Repeated mechanical stimulation attenuated and eventually abolished the responses due to an "adaptation" of either the mechanoreceptors in the rectal wall or the effectors. Although the earlier study by Hulten (103) showed that atropine had no effect on the reflex-induced colonic contraction and vasodilation, a recent study by Sjöqvist et al. (177) has shown that atropine blocked the colonic contraction induced by distension of the rectum without affecting the hyperemic response. The atropine-resistant colonic vasodilation induced by mechanical stimulation of the rectal mucosa (stroking the surface with gauze for 5 min or distension) was accompanied by an increase in colonic venous plasma VIP concentration (59). Mechanical stimulation of the anal mucosa increased motility and blood flow of the distal colon, both of which were unaffected by either atropine or naloxone alone (Fig. 17). However, when naloxone was administered to previously atropinized cats, the colonic contraction was blocked, whereas the hyperemia was unaffected.

## Stomach

The relationship between gastric blood flow and secretion has been studied extensively. The studies on gastric blood flow and motility, however, are limited. Furthermore the proximal and distal portions of the stomach differ in motor function and also in their motility responses to various stimuli. As a result the effect of various stimuli on the relationship between blood flow and motility in the proximal and distal stomach may also differ. Schuurkes and Charbon (160) measured the motility of the antrum and corpus separately with strain gauges and found that pentagastrin (64–4,000 ng/kg iv) produced much stronger contractions and smaller increases in blood flow in the antrum than in the corpus. At antral contractions of $29 \pm 9$ g induced by 512 $ng \cdot kg^{-1}$ pentagastrin, antral blood flow was impeded $35\% \pm 5\%$. Thus, as in the small intestine, a strong gastric contraction can reverse the vasodilator action of a chemical. The increased corpus contractions did not affect the pentagastrin-induced vasodilation. Cholecystokinin slightly increased corpus tone and decreased its blood flow. It produced stronger antral contraction and increased, decreased, or had no effect on antral blood flow. Decreased flow was accompanied by strong contraction. Vasopressin did not alter motility but decreased blood flow equally to antrum and corpus. Other studies on the relation between blood flow and motility did not separate the responses for the antrum and corpus.

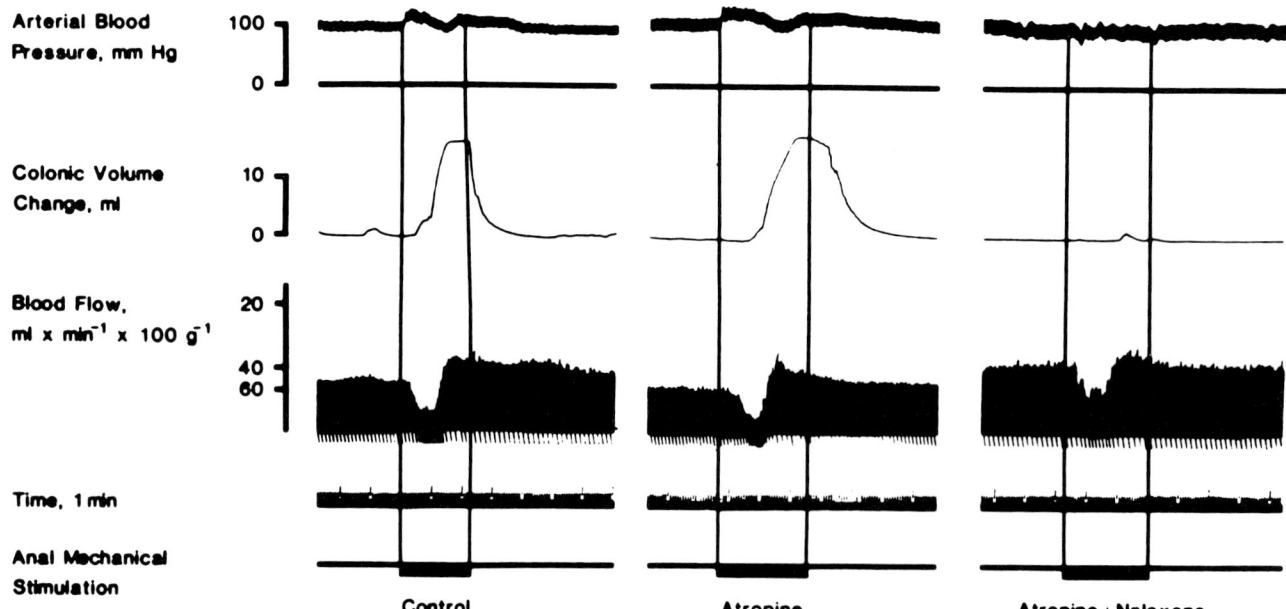

FIG. 17. Effect of mechanical stimulation of anal mucosa (indicated by *horizontal bars* and *vertical lines*) on colonic motility (volume change) and blood flow. [From Sjöqvist et al. (177).]

Semba et al. (165) observed three types of blood flow response (venous outflow through the gastrosplenic vein) to the gastric peristaltic contractions: contraction-phase, relaxation-phase, and combination types. The motility of the body and vestibular area of the stomach was measured by a balloon placed in the lumen. Each contraction in the contraction type lasted <20 s (mean, 13.1 s) and increased gastric body lumen pressure to 12 mmHg; the venous outflow increased 33% during contraction and decreased 9% during relaxation. Physostigmine produced tonic contractions, each contraction usually lasting longer than 40 s, with the mean amplitude of 33 mmHg; the venous outflow decreased 15% during contraction but increased 32% during relaxation. The combination type was produced by electrical stimulation of the vagus nerves at 2-30 V, 0.5 ms duration, and a frequency of 10-100 Hz. Each contraction lasted more than 50 s with the mean amplitude 8.8 mmHg. The venous outflow increased 25% during the initial phase of contraction, then decreased below control levels 19% at the maximal contraction; the flow then increased again (44% above control) during the relaxation period. The initial increase in blood flow may be due to an increase in gastric secretion or expulsion of venous blood by the contraction, but the decreased blood flow during the maximum contraction is most likely due to extravascular compression. Both physostigmine and vagal stimulation produced posttonic hyperemia similar to that observed in the small intestine and colon. The effect of physostigmine on gastric blood flow appears to result primarily from its effect on gastric motility. Physostigmine decreased blood flow to the gastric wall, but the decrease was confined to the mucosal layer (41). The mechanisms underlying this phenomenon have been discussed in EFFECTS OF CHEMICALS AND NERVES ON BLOOD FLOW AND MOTILITY IN SMALL INTESTINE, p. 1486.

Stimulation of the efferent high-threshold fibers increased gastric blood flow, and this increase was always accompanied by relaxation of the stomach (corpus and fundus) and stimulation of gastric acid and pepsinogen secretions (132). Gastric relaxation produced by either the vagal stimulation or distension of the esophagus was accompanied by an increase in VIP concentration in the gastric venous effluent (59), indicating that VIP may be involved in gastric relaxation and hyperemia. Vasoactive intestinal polypeptide infused intra-arterially at doses that resulted in plasma VIP concentrations between 0.2 and 3.0 $\mu$M·liter$^{-1}$ produced gastric relaxation and hyperemia (56). The increased blood flow returned to control levels soon after the infusion, but the gastric relaxation lasted 20-30 min after the infusion. Distension of the esophagus did not alter gastric blood flow but produced gastric relaxation similar to that produced by VIP infusion. Atropine did not alter VIP-induced responses. Serotonin decreased gastric mucosal blood flow but increased gastric motility; the decreased mucosal blood flow might be due to the enhanced motility (99). Serotonin at the same dosages, 5-80 mg·kg$^{-1}$ subcutaneously, also produced fibrinous thrombi in the mucosal vessels and mucosal erosion, which might result from serotonin-induced vascular and motility action. Prostaglandin $E_2$ increased the frequency of gastric slow waves and decreased both the antral motility and vascular resistance (115).

Distension of the canine stomach with air or balloon to intragastric pressure of 15 mmHg decreased gastric corpus blood flow 55% to 71% but did not alter gastric antrum blood flow (55). The decreased blood flow was mainly due to a decrease in blood flow to the mucosal and submucosal layers; the muscularis blood flow was unaffected by the distension. This response is similar to that occurring in the small and large intestine (41, 157). Gastric distension increased the surface area of the corpus 4.5 times but did not alter that of the antrum (55). The increased surface area could lengthen and narrow the submucosal and mucosal vessels, thereby decreasing blood flow.

In anesthetized cats, distension of the gastric balloon volume at 50 or 250 ml·min$^{-1}$ to increase intragastric pressure above 11-13 mmHg increased mean arterial blood pressure (20%-28%), myocardial contractility (16%-29%), and the total peripheral vascular resistance (23%-35%) without affecting the heart rate, aortic blood flow, and left ventricular end-diastolic pressure (126). The increased cardiac work should increase myocardial oxygen demand. This cardiovascular reflex therefore may play a role in the development of postprandial angina in humans. The reflex response to gastric distension was similar before and after laparotomy or section of the vagus nerve at the diaphragm. However, abdominal splanchnic nerve section significantly reduced the changes in blood pressure and myocardial contractility.

*Summary*

Changes in gastric and colonic motility can affect local blood flow in ways and by mechanisms similar to those observed in the small intestine. Semba et al. (165, 168) have found three types of blood flow response to changes in motility in both the stomach and colon. Vagal stimulation has a variable effect on gastric motility and blood flow and has little effect on the proximal colon. Pelvic nerve stimulation has significant effect on colonic motility or blood flow of the distal colon and rectum. The gastric and colonic responses can be elicited, respectively, by esophageal distension and rectal distension or mechanical stimulation of the anus. In addition to acetylcholine, the following chemicals have been proposed as neurotransmitters in the responses induced by nerve stimulation: VIP, kinins, and somatostatin. The vascular and motility responses, however, appear to be mediated by different neurotransmitters. As in the small intestine, drug-induced changes in blood flow depend on the potency of its action on vascular and visceral smooth muscle, but there is evidence that a significant change in motility can influence blood flow. Gastric distension can not only decrease gastric mucosal-submucosal blood flow but also can produce generalized cardiovascular response that is mediated by the splanchnic nerve. The effect of luminal distension in the colon is described next.

### EFFECTS OF INTESTINAL LUMINAL DISTENSION

Muscle contraction can decrease blood flow both by compressing the blood vessels adjacent to the muscle fibers and by increasing the lumen pressure. Luminal distension, on the other hand, can decrease blood flow only by increasing lumen pressure. The effect of luminal distension in decreasing blood flow is less than that of the contraction for the same increment in lumen pressure (16, 109). Kachelhoffer et al. (109) have shown that for each 1-mmHg rise in lumen pressure, the rise in vascular resistance produced by sustained spontaneous tonic contractions was 1.61 times that produced by luminal distension. There are other reasons for the more limited effect of luminal distension in decreasing total intestinal blood flow.

At lumen pressures between 0 and 25 mmHg, approximately 92% of lumen pressure is transmitted to the lymphatics and, presumably, to the interstitium of the intestinal wall (82). The interstitial fluid pressure of the gastric submucosa, as measured by Guyton's capsules, changes by exactly the same amount as lumen pressure in response to distension or infusion of cholinergic agents (2). The tissue pressure at different layers of the gut wall, however, may be different. In the heart there is an intramyocardial pressure gradient across the wall of the left ventricle during systole (136). The mean values of systolic intramural pressure at subepicardium (0% depth), 25%, 50%, 75%, and subendocardium (100% depth) were 6, 42, 80, 117, and 154 mmHg, respectively, whereas the average systolic left ventricular pressure was 132 mmHg. Thus the subendocardial tissue pressure is slightly higher than the ventricular pressure, but the subepicardial tissue pressure is only 5% of the ventricular pressure. The blood flow per tissue weight in the endocardium is about one-third of the epicardium during systole (100). If a similar situation occurs in the gut wall during an increase in lumen pressure, the tissue pressure of the outer layer of the gut wall will be <50% of the lumen pressure. The extravascular compression force will be small, and the resulting decrease in blood flow will be smaller than that predicted from the magnitude of the rise in lumen pressure. Additionally distension-induced rhythmic contractions (see Fig. 13) that increased blood flow in the muscle layer (see Fig. 7) and other factors shown in Figure 5 also act to reduce the effect of luminal distension in decreasing total intestinal blood flow. For example, distension stretches the gut wall but contractions do not. It has been proposed that stretching stimulates local neural reflexes to increase blood flow (120, 122).

Noer et al. (137) observed the vascular event occurring within the gut wall during luminal distension in rabbits and dogs with a wide-field binocular microscope placed above the serosa. Distension interrupted the blood flow through different segments of the microcirculation in a uniform order, the first change occurring in the venules (Fig. 18). At 30–40 mmHg, slowing or cessation of flow occurred in venules and slowing of flow started to appear in the arterioles and small veins. Many capillaries ceased functioning, reversal of flow appeared in certain segments, and intravascular clumping began to occur in both arteries and veins. At 50 mmHg, flow in the venous system, except in the large mural trunks, almost stopped while flow to the arterioles and small arteries began to slow down. At 80 mmHg and above, the blood flow in all vessels stopped, except in the largest arteries and in some larger veins, which showed oscillating flow. It was also noted that at 20 mmHg lumen pressure, tortuosity of the vessels decreased, and this condition was particularly apparent in dogs whose vessels normally show great tortuosity. A decrease in tortuosity, "gnarliness," as described by Burton and Patel (29), should decrease resistance to blood flow. The increase in blood flow during moderate distension (described in *Effect on Total Blood Flow*, p. 1503) may partly be due to this phenomenon.

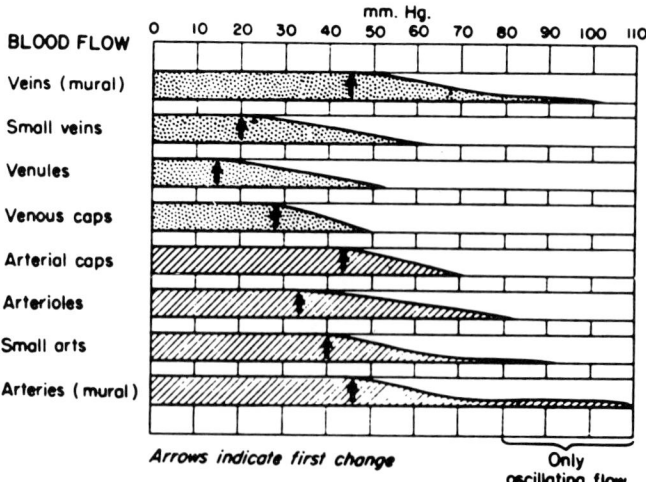

FIG. 18. Effect of varying levels of distending pressure on blood flow to various vascular segments within intestinal wall. [From Noer et al. (137).]

*Effect on Total Blood Flow*

Two procedures have been used to study the effects of luminal distension, that is, introduction of a certain volume of liquid or air into the lumen [constant volume; (37, 38, 95, 97, 153)] or continuous inflation to maintain a constant lumen pressure [constant pressure; (22, 25, 109, 122, 144, 157)]. Although the former is more physiological, the latter method is a better technique to elucidate the mechanical effects of distension.

Before 1940 it was reported that luminal distension decreased intestinal blood flow in proportion to the increment in lumen pressure (54, 77, 78). Lawson and Chumley (122), however, are the first researchers to report that luminal distension not only exerts extravascular compression but also induces other responses to produce variable changes in blood flow. Arterial blood flow to the ileal loop (6–12 cm) was measured by the differential manometry. Distension of the lumen with water produced five phases of blood flow response (Fig. 19A). Blood flow decreased when distension reached maximum within 8–10 s (phase I). The flow then returned to control levels within 1–3 min, even when lumen pressure was maintained constant at a level below 30 mmHg (phase II). In four animals, blood flow increased at the start and for the duration of distension (Fig. 19B). Two of these four animals had intact innervation, whereas the mesenteric nerves of the other two were cut an hour or more before the experiment. At deflation there was a sudden increase in flow above control levels. This deflation hyperemia (phase III) occurred whether blood flow decreased or increased during distension (Fig. 19A, B). Flow then returned to control values within 5–90 s, if distension was brief or if pressure was low. Longer and stronger distension (lumen pressure above 40 mmHg) prolonged the duration of deflation hyperemia, which lasted 6 min. In this situation the deflation hyperemia was interrupted by a period (10–50 s) of synchronous rhythmic oscillation in blood flow and intestinal contractions (phase IV); low flow accompanied the height of contraction. Phase 5 was the recovery of the hyperemia. The concordant oscillation of blood flow and gut contraction after deflation has also been observed by other investigators (see Fig. 13).

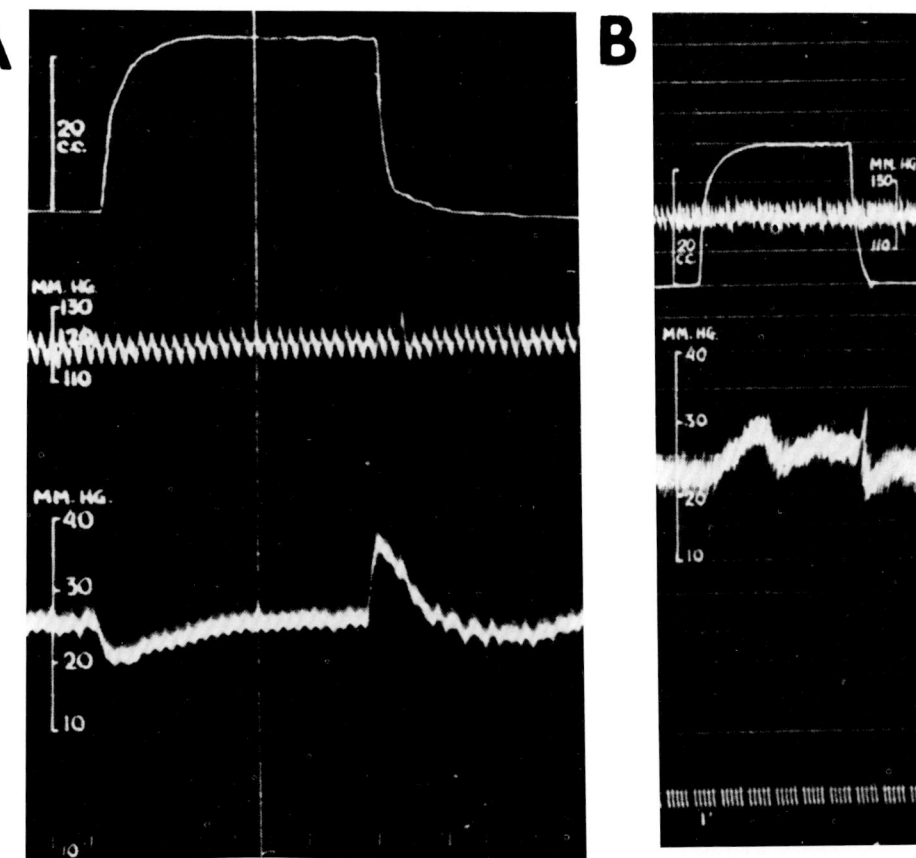

FIG. 19. Effect of luminal distension on blood flow. *Tracings from top down*: luminal volume, carotid artery pressure, and pressure difference between carotid and mesenteric arteries across constricting clamp, which indicates changes in blood flow. Time in intervals of 10 s (A) and 1 min (B). [From Lawson and Chumley (122).]

To determine the mechanism involved in the recovery of blood flow, the gut loop was encased in plaster of paris to prevent enlargement of the loop by distension (122). Under this condition distension produced a simple monophasic reduction in flow that persisted throughout the distension period. The encasement also abolished the deflation responses (phases III–V) if distending pressure was below 40 mmHg; the deflation hyperemia still occurred if the pressure was above 80 mmHg. The encased loop also showed a reactive hyperemia to occlusion of arterial blood flow, indicating that the vascular smooth muscle was unaffected by the encasement. Sectioning the mesenteric nerve had no effect on any phase of the response to distension. Application of cocaine to the mucosa, however, abolished or reduced the recovery of flow during phase II. The local anesthesia also abolished or attenuated the deflation hyperemia induced by moderate distension. The initial transient decrease in blood flow can be easily explained by extravascular compression of vessels by distension. The recovery of blood flow and hyperemia during distension appears to be related to stretching of the gut wall and the effect on local nerves, because prevention of the stretching and local mucosal anesthesia abolished or attenuated these two responses.

Lawson (120) subsequently investigated the possible mechanism of the deflation hyperemia that occurs after distending the lumen to a pressure below 40 mmHg for <2 min. In this study, changes in gut volume, arterial inflow, and venous outflow were measured. When the distended gut was deflated, venous outflow stopped briefly due to filling of decompressed vessels; flow then recovered or exceeded its control level within 2–8 s. Both arterial and venous flow then increased; the increased blood flow volume was considerably greater than the demonstrable volume reduction within the gut wall during distension. The authors concluded that only a small portion (<25%) of the deflation hyperemia can be attributed to refilling of decompressed vessels. From the following evidence, they also concluded that the remainder of the deflation hyperemia is not mediated by the mechanism(s) that induce reactive hyperemia. When the flow reduction produced by distension was duplicated by partial arterial occlusion, the hyperemia was always greater after the distension. Reactive hyperemia was proportional in magnitude to the duration of arterial occlusion, whereas deflation hyperemia did not increase with the duration of distension. Local mucosal anesthesia abolished the deflation hyperemia produced by moderate distension but had little or a lesser effect on reactive hyperemia as well as the deflation hyperemia produced by excessive distension (lumen pressure approaching systemic arterial pressure). It was surmised that the moderate distension does not reduce blood flow sufficiently to cause reactive hyperemia, if one assumes that distension exerts its compression effect equally on vessels of all tissue layers in the gut wall. That assumption is incorrect, however, because distension decreases blood flow only to the mucosa-submucosal layer (41, 55, 157), whereas arterial occlusion decreases blood flow to all tissue layers. It is therefore possible that the deflation hyperemia produced by excessive as well as by moderate distension is mediated by mechanisms that induce reactive hyperemia, particularly in the mucosal layer. The hyperemia that occurs after tonic contraction has been explained by the mechanisms that are involved in reactive hyperemia, based on either the metabolic or myogenic theory.

Hanson (95) was the next researcher to investigate the mechanism of distension-induced changes in blood flow. Ileal segments (mean wt, 193 g) were inflated and deflated in 50-ml steps with warmed mineral oil, whereas arterial inflow was measured with an electromagnetic flowmeter. Distension from zero lumen volume to 50 ml produced an initial increase in blood flow and lumen pressure, both of which returned to control levels in ~5 min (Fig. 20A). Distension from a lumen volume of 350–400 ml, however, produced an initial large increase in lumen pressure and decrease in blood flow, both of which returned toward control levels but never completely reached the control levels even 15 min after the inflation (Fig. 20B). The data were then analyzed according to lumen pressure. Significant decreases in blood flow occurred when lumen pressure was raised above 20 mmHg. There was a significant negative relationship between blood flow and lumen pressure; blood flow decreased from $37.8 \pm 4.8$ ml·min$^{-1}$·100 g$^{-1}$ at zero pressure to $23.4 \pm 3.0$ ml·min$^{-1}$·100 g$^{-1}$ at 50 mmHg. Deflation produced an initial increase in blood flow, which returned to control levels after 2–3 min. The researcher proposed that the initial vasodilation (Fig. 20A) was due to a de-

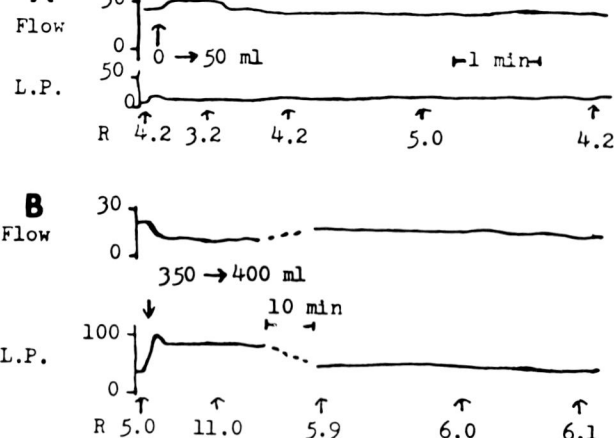

FIG. 20. Effects of distending canine ileal lumen from 0 to 50 ml lumen volume (A) and from 350 to 400 ml lumen volume (B). L.P., lumen pressure in mmHg; R, vascular resistance. Flow in ml·min$^{-1}$·100 g$^{-1}$. [From Hanson (95).]

crease in vascular transmural pressure (as a result of increasing extravascular pressure), which induced active relaxation of vascular smooth muscle (myogenic theory). The recovery of the flow during distension was due to stress relaxation of the intestinal smooth muscle that resulted in progressive decrease in lumen pressure and extravascular pressure. Papaverine, a smooth muscle relaxant, increased the distensibility (compliance) of the gut segment from 12.2 ± 1.8 to 17.7 ± 2.0 ml·mmHg$^{-1}$·100 g$^{-1}$. After papaverine, blood flow at each distension pressure was greater than that observed before the treatment, but the passive compression effect of distension was greater than that observed before the treatment. Papaverine also abolished the distension-induced initial vasodilation and abolished the autoregulation of blood flow. The researcher proposed that papaverine relaxed the vascular smooth muscle, rendering it incapable of responding to decreasing vascular transmural pressure with vasodilation. Thus, in contrast to Lawson's group (120, 122), who explained the hyperemia and recovery of blood flow during distension by neural mechanism, Hanson (95) explained it by the myogenic mechanism. The response can also be explained by the metabolic theory of autoregulation of blood flow.

In the colon, stepwise inflation decreased blood flow by an amount proportional to the lumen pressure (96, 97). The recovery pattern of both lumen pressure and blood flow toward control during distension and the occurrence of a transient hyperemia after deflation are similar to the observations made on the small intestine (95). Papaverine or distension to luminal pressure of 50 mmHg also abolished autoregulation of colonic blood flow or venoarteriolar response (96).

Brobmann et al. (25, 26) investigated the effect of distension on arterial inflow and venous outflow in vivo and in vitro. Sudden distension to a lumen pressure of 40 mmHg produced an initial decrease in both arterial inflow and venous outflow (26). Whereas venous outflow remained at the same level of decrease, arterial inflow returned toward control levels despite the fact that the gut lumen pressure was maintained at 40 mmHg. After deflation, arterial inflow increased for several minutes. The recovery of arterial inflow ("autoregulatory escape") during distension, however, was absent in the in vitro preparation (25).

With the constant-flow preparation, Kachelhoffer et al. (109) found that stepwise distension of the jejunal loops to a constant lumen pressure produced corresponding increases in perfusion pressure and that there was a linear relationship between the rises in distension pressure and the corresponding rises in perfusion pressure (Δ perfusion pressure, 0.57; Δ lumen pressure, 0.21). The study was performed with a basal lumen pressure of ~7 mmHg, and the increases in lumen pressure ranged between 2 and 15 mmHg. The researchers therefore claimed that the pressure changes are within the normal range, and thus the hemodynamic effects observed may occur in normal conditions.

The magnitude of the increase in gut lumen pressure and vascular resistance after distension can be influenced by preexisting gut wall tension and distensibility. Chou and Dabney (34, 37, 38, 52) have shown that when the ileal wall tension was increased as a result of infusion of acetylcholine, bradykinin, serotonin, or KCl (0.18 meq·min$^{-1}$), distension by the same volume of fluid increased lumen pressure and perfusion pressure to a greater level than before the infusions (Fig. 21). The opposite was true when the ileal wall tension was decreased by infusion of epinephrine, MgCl$_2$, and CaCl$_2$, or during hemorrhagic hypotension. This study was performed in the constant-flow preparation, and higher or lower perfusion pressure indicates higher or lower vascular resistance. The lumen was distended after the lumen and perfusion pressures had reached a steady state during infusions. The distensibility of the colon is greater than that of the ileum in dogs (46, 95, 97). As a result, colonic blood flow did not decrease significantly until the lumen volume was increased to and above 600 ml·100 g$^{-1}$ tissue weight; the ileal blood flow decreased significantly when the lumen volume was increased to and above 150 ml·100 g$^{-1}$ tissue weight (95, 97). Similarly distension of the small intestine to lumen pressure 30 mmHg decreased its blood flow 38%, but the same degree of distension in the colon did not alter colonic blood flow (157).

Most investigators (37, 41, 95, 97, 109, 122, 153) have observed the occurrence of rhythmic contractions during or after a moderate degree of distension. The contractions may be myogenic or induced by local nerves. Ohman (143) found that distension-induced rhythmic contractions occurred in innervated as well as denervated intestine. However, atropine abolished the contractions only in the denervated gut preparations. Some investigators found that these rhythmic contractions can mask or offset the extravascular compression effect of distension (41, 122, 153). Other investigators, however, found that these contractions had little or no influence on distension-induced decrease in blood flow (95, 109, 143). The differing findings probably result from variation in the strength and duration of the induced rhythmic contractions.

*Effect on Compartmental Blood Flow, Oxygen Consumption, Capillary Filtration Coefficient, and Lymph Flow*

The effect of a moderate distension (15–20 mmHg lumen pressure) on compartmental blood flow of the jejunum has been described (see Fig. 7). Ruf et al. (157) studied the effects in piglets of stepwise increases in lumen pressure to 15, 30, 45, and 60 mmHg by inflating 30-cm-long segments of small and large intestine with air. Flows were measured with microspheres after these pressures were maintained for 15

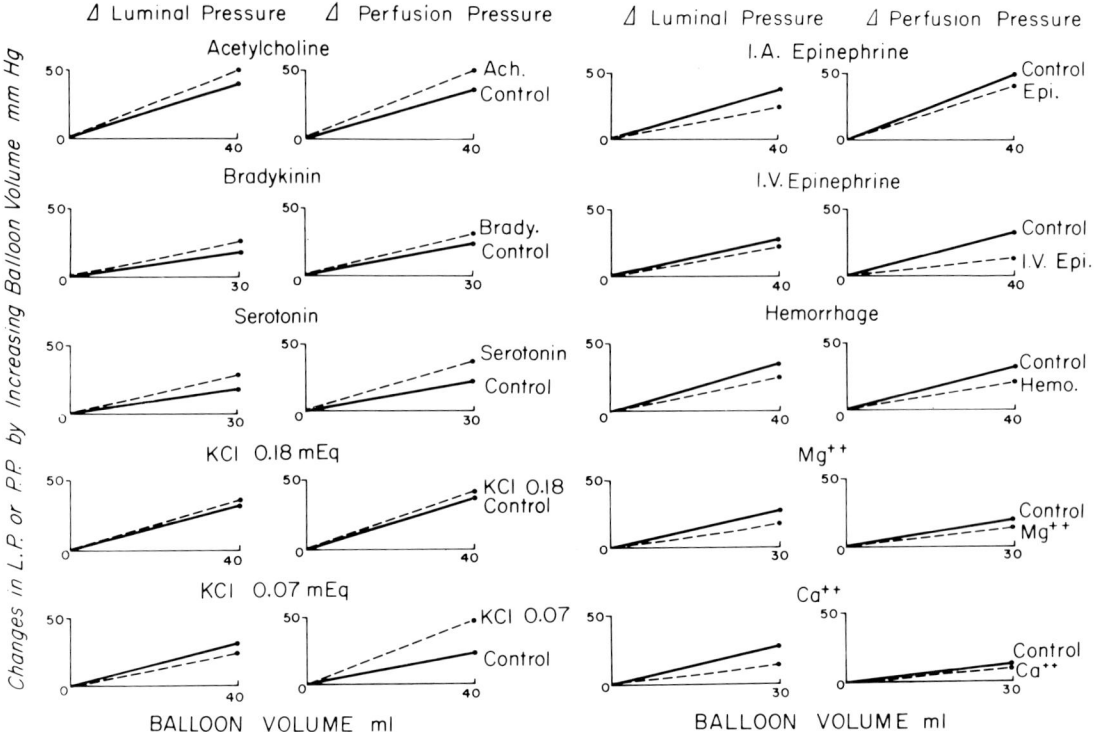

FIG. 21. Effects of various stimuli on distension-induced increments in luminal and perfusion pressures of ileal segments perfused at constant blood flow rate. *Ordinates* are increments in luminal or perfusion pressures resulting from increases in lumen volume from 0 to 30 ml or 0 to 40 ml. *Solid lines*, controls; *dotted lines*, experimental conditions. [Data from Chou and Dabney (34, 37, 38) and Dabney et al. (52).]

min. The total wall blood flow was not significantly changed at lumen pressures of 15 mmHg in the small intestine and 15–30 mmHg in the colon. However, at these pressures mucosal blood flow decreased significantly and muscularis flow increased significantly in both the small and large bowels. Distension to lumen pressure of 45 mmHg produced 24%–55% and 55%–72% decreases in total wall and mucosal flow in the small intestine and 13%–35% and 55%–69% decreases in the colon, respectively. Flows to the muscle layer of the small and large intestine, however, increased 118%, 83%, and 22%, and 161%, 149%, and 65% at lumen pressures of 15, 30, and 45 mmHg, respectively. The increased muscle blood flow might be related to muscle contractions (41). At 60 mmHg, total wall flow decreased to 25% of control and mucosal flow declined to ~20% of control, but muscle flow was reduced to only 75%–80% of control in both small and large intestine. Stepwise decreases in lumen pressure from 60 to 0 mmHg produced stepwise increases in blood flow of both small and large intestine; the increases in muscularis flow were greater than the corresponding increases in mucosal flow. Furthermore deflation hyperemia lasted only 15 min in the mucosa, whereas in the muscularis the hyperemia lasted >30 min. The greater and longer deflation hyperemia may be due to rhythmic contractions, an observation made earlier by Lawson and Chumley (122).

The effect of distension on intestinal oxygen consumption is difficult to analyze because distension produces not only a variable blood flow response but also diverse effects on intestinal motility (rhythmic contractions and receptive relaxation), absorption, and secretion (123, 125, 178, 179). Furthermore intestinal oxygen consumption is dependent on blood flow when the flow is <20 or 35 ml·min$^{-1}$·100 g$^{-1}$ (118, 130). If distension decreases blood flow below this level, the decreased oxygen consumption results from a decrease in oxygen delivery.

Lawson and Ambrose (121) found that distension to luminal pressure of 23 mmHg decreased oxygen consumption in all except 5 of their 32 experiments. The decreased oxygen consumption appeared to be due primarily to a decrease in the arteriovenous (AV) oxygen content difference. After the mucosal surface was anesthetized with cocaine, distension produced a greater reduction in blood flow, but the AV oxygen difference increased, resulting in a smaller decrease in oxygen consumption as compared with the untreated gut loops. They proposed that distension opens the AV shunts, thereby reducing oxygen consumption; local mucosal anesthesia prevents both events. In contrast to the observation made on the innervated gut, distension had no consistent effect on oxygen consumption in the denervated gut. Oxygen consumption increased in half of the 18 experiments and decreased in the other half. The failure of distension to reduce oxygen consumption was attributed to higher resting blood flow in the denervated gut. In the constant-flow preparation, distension to lumen pressures of below 25 mmHg (the level similar to that of the previous study) did not significantly alter intestinal oxygen consumption (109). These findings seem to indicate that the decreased oxygen consumption observed in the innervated gut (121) is secondary to distension-induced decrease in blood flow. A recent study (145) further showed that there was no significant relation between blood flow and oxygen consumption under resting conditions, but these two variables became significantly correlated when the intestine was distended to a lumen pressure of 20 mmHg for 10 min; a decrease in blood flow accompanied a decrease in oxygen consumption.

Recent studies have questioned the presence of anatomical AV shunts in the small intestine. The fraction of the total blood flow passing through the AV shunts >13 µm in diameter is 1% or less (127, 133) and the diameter of the arterioles perfusing the capillaries in the mucosal and muscularis layers is <13 µm (81). Furthermore various neural and chemical stimuli failed to alter the fraction of shunt blood flow (127). It is unlikely that distension opens the anatomical AV shunts.

Boley et al. (22), however, proposed that severe distension (60–210 mmHg) opens physiological AV shunts. The small intestine (12–18 inches) or colon (6–12 inches) was distended with air-to-lumen pressure of 210 mmHg in 30-mmHg increments; each pressure was maintained for 5 or 10 min. Distension below 30 mmHg produced no consistent changes in blood flow. Stepwise increases in lumen pressure from 30 to 120 mmHg resulted in corresponding decreases in flow. However, further increases in lumen pressure to 180 mmHg did not significantly decrease flow further; the flow was ~20%–35% of control. At these high pressures, venous $P_{O_2}$ almost equaled arterial $P_{O_2}$, indicating that tissue oxygen utilization was severely inhibited or that the residual flow was perfusing low- or nonnutritional vessels. It is unclear whether the decreased oxygen consumption was due to the decrease in flow, because the resting blood flow values were not shown in this report. Silicone rubber was injected intra-arterially during distension to determine the flow distribution within the gut wall. The submucosal and serosal vessels were filled with the injected silicone rubber at all lumen pressures, but the mucosal and muscularis vessels were partially filled at a lumen pressure of 30 mmHg and were devoid of silicone rubber at 60–90 mmHg. Although the $^{85}$Kr washout technique was also used to determine the compartmental blood flow within the gut wall, the data could suggest only that the decreased blood flow at a lumen pressure of 30–60 mmHg occurred mainly in the mucosal layer. This report concluded that distension to lumen pressure above 30 mmHg decreased total blood flow primarily because of a decrease in flow to the mucosal and muscularis layer. Oxygen consumption decreased because blood flow was shunted to functional arteriovenous communications or to low-resistance vascular beds that utilized little oxygen. The low- or nonnutritional vessels are located in the submucosa and serosa.

The finding of Boley et al. (22), however, is not entirely in agreement with the work of other investigators. As described previously, muscularis blood flow is increased by distension to lumen pressure at levels below 60 mmHg and is minimally decreased at the pressure of 60 mmHg (41, 157). Intestinal oxygen consumption does not significantly change until lumen pressure is increased to 80–100 mmHg in normal intestine [Fig. 22; (141, 142)]. The resting transmural pressures of the submucosal arterioles and venules (see 2A, 3A, and 2V in Fig. 1) are 32–45 mmHg. It is therefore somewhat difficult to comprehend how the submucosal vessels can escape compression from a lumen pressure equal to or higher than aortic pressure (120–210 mmHg). The serosal and marginal vessels may escape compression from this high pressure.

Ohman (144) conducted a series of experiments to investigate the effects of simple intestinal obstruction and acute distension in cats. After tying the terminal ileum, the lumen pressure proximal to the ligature was recorded for 72 h. Despite considerable intestinal distension, the lumen pressure was increased from 2–4 mmHg at zero time to only 5–10 mmHg (139). Subsequently Ohman compared the effect of acute distension on blood flow, oxygen consumption, and capillary filtration coefficient (CFC) of the normal (nonobstructed) and the previously obstructed small intestine. The entire small intestine from the ligament of Treitz to the ileocecal junction was denervated and isolated from the animal, placed in an organ chamber, and perfused with blood from the donor cat. Atropine was given to attenuate the distension-induced rhythmic contractions, because the contractions rendered CFC determinations impossible (143). The specimens were inflated with nitrogen gas in 20-mmHg increments from 0 to 100 mmHg lumen pressure. Stepwise increases in lumen pressure produced corresponding decreases in blood flow and increases in vascular resistance in both normal and previously obstructed specimens [Fig. 22; (141, 142)]. In the normal specimen neither CFC nor oxygen consumption was altered significantly at a lumen pressure of 20 mmHg. The CFC decreased significantly at a lumen pressure of 40 mmHg and above, and a significant decrease in oxygen consumption occurred only at lumen pressures of 80–100 mmHg. The decreased CFC

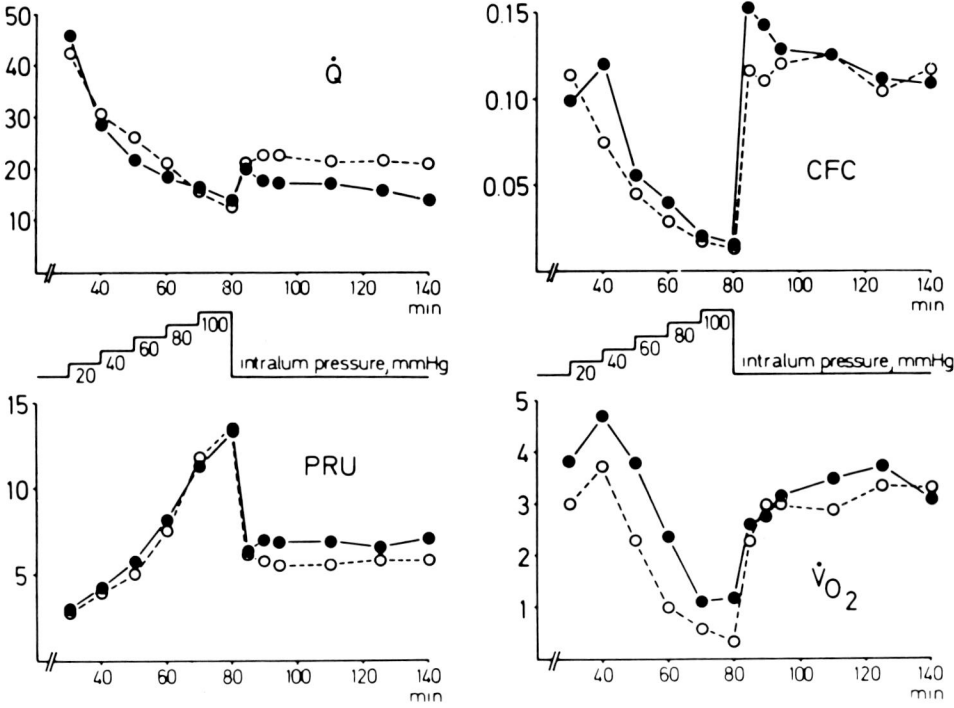

FIG. 22. Effects of stepwise distension to 100 mmHg lumen pressure and deflation on blood flow ($\dot{Q}$, ml·min$^{-1}$·100 g$^{-1}$), vascular resistance (PRU), capillary filtration coefficient (CFC, ml·min$^{-1}$·100 g$^{-1}$ dry wt), and oxygen consumption ($\dot{V}_{O_2}$, ml·min$^{-1}$·100 g$^{-1}$ dry wt) in denervated feline small bowel homologously perfused in vitro. *Filled circles*, nonobstructed intestine; *open circles*, previously obstructed intestine. [From Ohman (144).]

is most likely due to a decrease in blood flow. After deflation, CFC and oxygen consumption returned to control values, but blood flow and vascular resistance did not (Fig. 22). The low blood flow and high vascular resistance after the deflation resulted primarily from the duration of the experiment and the in vitro situation. In another series of experiments Ohman (143) found that blood flow decreased successively from 50–55 to 25 ml·min$^{-1}$·100 g$^{-1}$ over a 180-min experimental period, even when the intestine was not distended. The formation of edema during the 80-min period of distension may also contribute to the persistent reduction in flow. Other investigators have reported that blood flow does not return to control levels after prolonged, repeated, and intermittent distension to lumen pressures of 45–90 mmHg (185).

Because the lumen pressure of the small intestine subjected to simple obstruction is below 20 mmHg (140), and acute distension to 20 mmHg only decreased blood flow without affecting CFC and oxygen consumption (141), the intestine was distended to a lumen pressure of 20 mmHg for 60 min in the subsequent experiments (43). This prolonged distension produced a 50% decrease in blood flow (which never returned to control levels after deflation), a variable response of CFC, and no change in oxygen consumption. Ohman concluded that moderate distension does not significantly affect the microcirculation or "viability" of the intestine. The small intestine subjected to 72-h simple obstruction does not differ significantly from the nonobstructed normal intestine in resting blood flow, vascular resistance, CFC, and oxygen consumption (140). The obstructed bowel also responded normally to cholecystokinin with an increase in motility (139).

A mild luminal distension increases lymphatic pressure, lymph flow, and the rate of transmucosal fluid absorption (123, 125). Because fluid absorption per se can increase lymph flow, Granger et al. (82) utilized a nonabsorbable silicone solution to distend the gut lumen. At a venous pressure of 0 mmHg, luminal distension to a lumen pressure of 20 mmHg resulted in a progressive reduction in lymph oncotic pressure and lymph-to-plasma protein concentration ratio, while lymphatic flow and pressure progressively increased. However, when lumen pressure was further increased above 25 mmHg, lymphatic pressure and lymph flow decreased progressively. The authors also compared the effects of venous pressure elevation at 0 and 20 mmHg lumen pressure. At 0 mmHg lumen pressure, elevation of venous pressure to 30 mmHg resulted in a progressive increase in lymph flow and decrease in blood flow and lymph-to-plasma ratio. However, at lumen pressure of 20 mmHg, venous pressure elevation had no effect on lymph flow, lymph-to-plasma ratio, or blood flow until venous pressure exceeded the lumen pressure. Thus over a physiological range of luminal pressures (0–20 mmHg), lymph flow and lymphatic pressure parallel lumen pressure, whereas higher lumen pressures result in a progressive reduction in lymph flow. The decreased lymph flow might be due to lymphatic disruption or leakage, a greater increase in tissue pressure than capillary hydrostatic pressure (which reduces net capillary filtration pressure), or compression of the lymphatics. This report also indicated that for a given increase in lymph flow, luminal distension produces a smaller reduction in interstitial oncotic pressure than that produced by either venous pressure elevation or intestinal fluid absorption. The authors concluded that luminal distension not only mechanically increases capillary filtration but also increases capillary permeability.

*Summary*

Distension of the gut lumen can increase (41, 95, 120–122, 153), decrease (16, 22, 25, 54, 77, 78, 95–97, 120–122, 188), or not alter blood flow, depending on the magnitude and duration of the distension and preexisting gut wall tension. The decrease in blood flow has a linear relation to the distending luminal pressure. The decreased flow, however, is confined to the mucosal-submucosal layer. The muscularis flow may be increased or unchanged (41, 55, 157). The decreased flow is due to an increase in tissue pressure, which compresses the intramural vessels. The increased flow observed at a lumen pressure below 20–30 mmHg may be due to local neural reflex, autoregulation of blood flow by either myogenic or metabolic mechanism, a decrease in tortuosity of the vessels, and the distension-induced rhythmic contractions. Whether the blood flow is increased or decreased, the flow tends to return toward control levels during distension. The recovery may be due to autoregulation of blood flow or stretch-induced neural reflex. The interplay of these factors involved in the distension-induced changes in blood flow is shown in Figure 5. Deflation produces an increase in blood flow that may result from reactive hyperemia, neural reflex, and deflation-induced rhythmic contractions. A moderate degree of distension (20 mmHg or lower) does not significantly alter oxygen consumption and CFC, increases lymph flow, and induces rhythmic contractions.

The highest lumen pressure that can be achieved in pathological states is ~50 mmHg (discussion by E. T. Peter in ref. 22), whereas that produced by intestinal obstruction is usually below 20 mmHg (144). Thus, even in pathological states the effects of distension on intestinal blood flow, oxygen consumption, and CFC are probably minimal. In fact the mild and transient distension that occurs when chyme enters a gut segment benefits intestinal absorption. Rhythmic contractions induced by distension promote mixing and transport of chyme, and the increased metabolic demand for contractions is adequately met by an increase in flow to the muscles. A mild distension also increases CFC, capillary permeability, and lymph flow, all of which tend to enhance fluid and nutrient absorption.

### EFFECTS OF BLOOD FLOW AND HYPOXIA ON MOTOR FUNCTION

The muscle layer of the gastrointestinal wall comprises 22%–45% by weight and receives 5%–30% of the total gut wall blood flow (41). When calculated as flow per unit weight, muscularis blood flow is only ½ to ¹⁄₁₀ of mucosal flow, depending on the segment of the gastrointestinal tract and the condition of the gut preparation (23, 41, 75, 127, 161). The intestinal tissue $P_{O_2}$ at the muscle-submucosal interface is ~27 mmHg, whereas that at the villus apex is only 13 mmHg (17). Oxygen consumption by the muscularis is ¼ to ⅓ of mucosal oxygen consumption (131). Because of the difference in their demand for oxygen, mucosal and muscularis functions and viability will react differently to variation in blood flow.

Cassuto et al. (33) found that a 40%–60% reduction in total blood flow to the feline small intestine by partial occlusion of the superior mesenteric artery produced a reduction of 48%–70% and 31%–50% in muscularis and mucosal-submucosal flow, respectively. In spite of the greater ischemia in the muscularis, the study also showed that histologically the muscularis looked normal, whereas total destruction of the villi and various degrees of mucosal damage were observed. Probably the intestinal muscle is more resistant to ischemic hypoxia than is the mucosa because of its lower metabolic rate. A recent in vitro study supports this thesis. Anuras et al. (7) studied the effects of hypoxia on the electromyogram of the cat colon by altering the $O_2$ content of gases bubbling the muscle strip bath. Exposure to 75%, 55%, or 35% $O_2$ did not alter either the slow-wave frequency or the time occupied by the migrating spike bursts. With a gas mixture containing no oxygen, the slow-wave frequency decreased from ~5 to 3 cycles/min and the time occupied by migrating spike bursts decreased from 16.7% to 5.9%. Although the maximum changes occurred within 45 min of the exposure to 0% $O_2$, the two electrical events persisted for 3 h. Furthermore both the slow-wave frequency and the pattern of the migrating spike bursts returned to control states within 15 min on restoration of 95% $O_2$. The migrating spike bursts in the colon are related to prolonged contractions that occur independently of slow waves. Thus the frequency of colonic slow waves and contractions can be reduced by anoxia but not by hypoxia.

However, the persistence of the two events under anoxia for 3 h indicates that these events are not exclusively dependent on oxidative metabolism. Under in vivo conditions, the hypoxia-resistant muscle tissues are further protected by hemodynamic adjustments during hypoxia and ischemia. Reducing arterial $P_{O_2}$ to about 46 mmHg increased blood flow and capillary density, both of which tend to maintain oxygen delivery to the gut (171).

Bayliss and Starling (10) reported in 1898 that occlusion of the abdominal aorta abolished rhythmic contractions of the canine small intestine. The underlying mechanism may be stimulation of the sympathetic nervous system, because the same response was produced by splanchnic nerve stimulation. Others, however, found that occlusion of the mesenteric artery increased rhythmic contractions and lumen pressure (3, 198). Bean and Sidky (12) studied the effects of various hypoxic conditions on intestinal motility and blood flow. Perfusion of innervated or denervated intestinal segments with hypoxic blood (7% $O_2$) or ventilation with a gas mixture containing 7% $O_2$ for <5 min, a short period of asphyxia (tracheal occlusion for 2 min), or even intra-arterial injection of 0.3 ml of 1% sodium cyanide solution did not alter intestinal motility. Blood flow was increased by the perfusion of hypoxic blood or cyanide and was decreased by asphyxia. Perfusion of the hypoxic blood for a longer time period, however, reduced both the rhythmic contractions and the tonus of the gut, if strong rhythmic contractions were already present before the perfusion. If the preexisting motility was small, perfusion of the hypoxic blood produced an initial increase both in the rhythmic contractions and in basal luminal pressure, followed by marked decrease in basal pressure and absence of rhythmic activities. The response of the intestinal motility to ischemia and hypoxia, therefore, depends on extrinsic and intrinsic neural activities and the duration and severity of hypoxia. In general, ischemia and hypoxia produce a biphasic change in motility, that is, an initial transient increase, followed by a prolonged paralysis [Fig. 23; (31, 40, 89, 134, 187)]. Increasing blood flow to twice the resting levels, however, had no effect on spontaneous and distension-induced rhythmic contractions or intestinal wall tension (38).

In the constant-flow preparation, stopping or decreasing blood flow from 67 to 14 ml·min$^{-1}$·100 g$^{-1}$ did not significantly alter intestinal wall tension (38) but induced rhythmic contractions and enhanced distension-triggered rhythmic contractions (38, 162). In the naturally perfused gut segment, occlusion of the artery perfusing the segment produced intense rhythmic contractions lasting several minutes [Fig. 23; (31, 89)]. The enhanced rhythmic contractions are most likely due to stimulation of the intramural intrinsic nerves. Application of cocaine to the extrinsic intestinal nerve did not affect the ischemia-induced

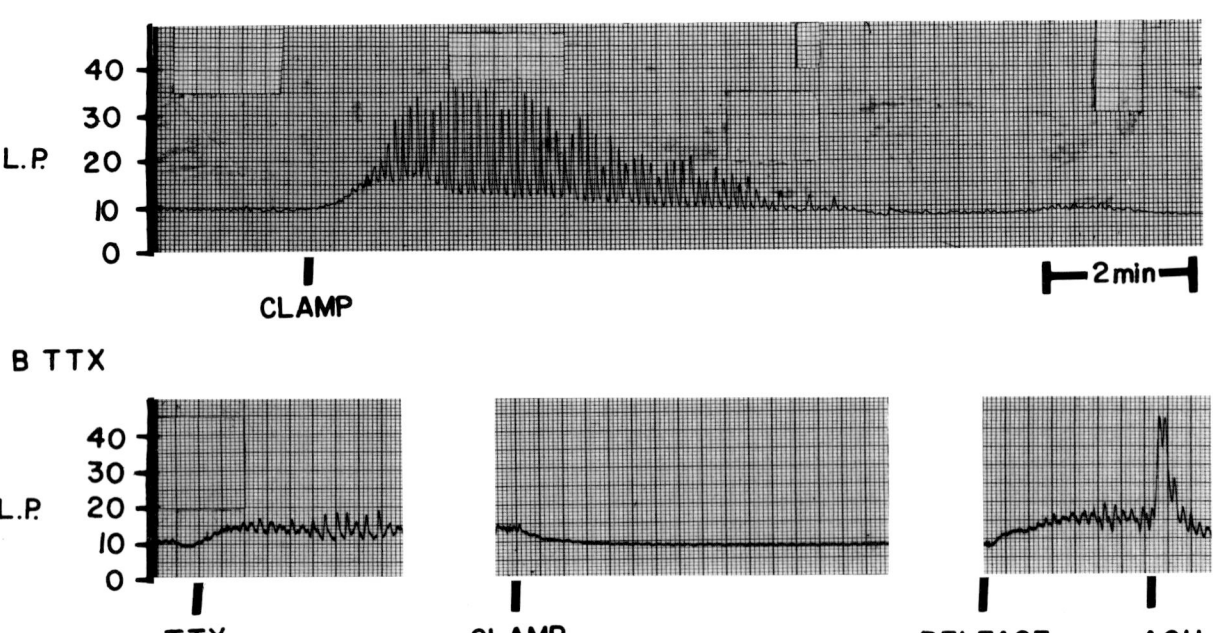

FIG. 23. Effect of occlusion of artery perfusing gut segment (CLAMP) before and after intra-arterial infusion of tetrodotoxin (TTX). [Adapted from Chou and Gallavan (40).]

contractions (151). Tetrodotoxin (ia) abolished the ischemia-induced increase in motility but did not affect acetylcholine-induced (ia) contractions (Fig. 23). One to fifteen minutes after ischemia or hypoxia is induced, the initial increase in contractile and electrical activities (31, 89, 134) progressively decreases, and the gut becomes quiescent with the disappearance of spike potentials. Some investigators (1, 134), however, found that contractile activities reappeared in the jejunum 30–60 min after occlusion of the superior mesenteric artery (SMA). The slow-wave frequency and the number of slow waves accompanied by spike potentials, however, were decreased.

Meissner et al. (134) compared the effect of 50% and 75% reduction in inhaled oxygen, occlusion of the SMA, and thrombin-induced mesenteric arterial and venous thrombosis on the contractile and electrical activities of the anesthetized canine upper jejunum. All four of these stimuli produced initial transient (2–5 min) intense rhythmic contractions, which were accompanied by the appearance of spike activity. After this initial excitatory response, the contractions returned to normal in dogs subjected to 50% reduction in inhaled oxygen (arterial $P_{O_2}$ 36 mmHg) but decreased slightly in the dogs subjected to SMA occlusion. The slow-wave frequency, however, remained unchanged in both groups throughout the 2-h experimental period (Fig. 24). The slow-wave frequency in the other two groups decreased progressively. The dogs subjected to 75% reduction of oxygen in inhaled gas mixture (arterial $P_{O_2}$ 16.8 mmHg) died ~30–50 min after the hypoxia, and during this period both contractile activity and spike potentials were absent. The slow waves persisted at a subnormal rate until the time of cardiac arrest. Superior mesenteric vein (SMV) and SMA thrombosis had an effect similar to that of 75% hypoxia. Slow waves disappeared in four of the five dogs 5–7 min after thrombin injection, although the waves persisted in one dog for 45 min. The slow waves therefore were highly resistant to hypoxia, whereas the spike potentials and contractile activity were more sensitive to hypoxia. The slow waves are myogenic in origin, whereas contractile activities depend on neural and humoral input. This study seems to suggest that the intestinal intrinsic nerves are more sensitive to reduction in arterial $P_{O_2}$ than are the intestinal muscles. The initial excitation and the subsequent changes in contractile and electrical activities after ischemia and hypoxia are most likely due to hypoxia-induced changes in the activity of intestinal neural plexuses.

In contrast, Abe et al. (1) found that SMA occlusion produced a progressive decrease in slow-wave frequency from 13.9 to 6.7 cycles/min at the end of a 2-h occlusion period. The slow-wave frequency returned to control levels, however, within 30 min after the release of the vascular occlusion. In the study of Meissner et al. (134) blood pressure in the SMA distal

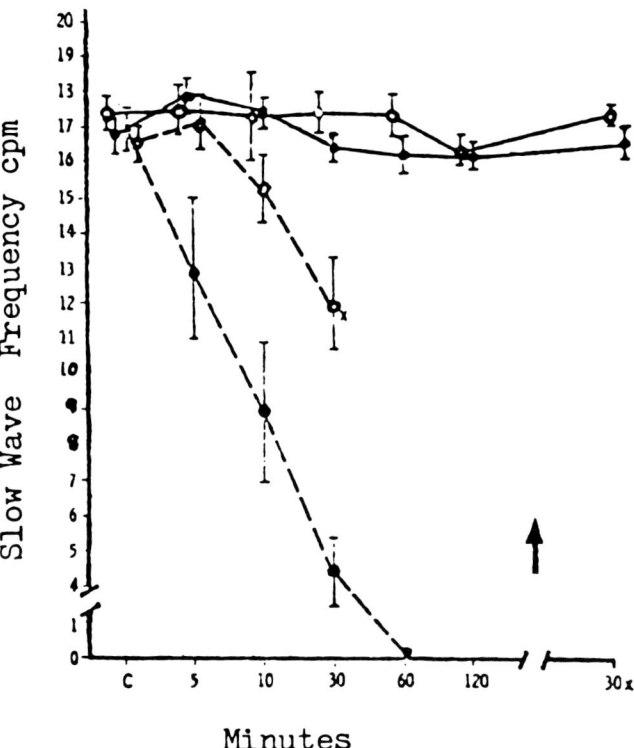

FIG. 24. Mean slow-wave frequency before (C) and after either hypoxia or occlusion of superior mesenteric artery (SMA). Arrow indicates termination of experimental perturbations. ○—○, 50% $O_2$ reduction; ○- - -○, 75% $O_2$ reduction; ●—●, SMA occlusion; ●- - -●, SMA + SMV thrombosis. [From Meissner et al. (134).]

to the occlusion was 15–20 mmHg. This indicates that there was substantial collateral circulation through the pancreaticoduodenal artery supplying blood to the jejunum. The unchanged slow-wave frequency in this study is probably due to smaller ischemic insult. Other investigators have shown that ligation of the artery perfusion the intestinal segments decreased the slow-wave frequency (31, 158) or abolished slow waves entirely (30, 110). In the case of decreasing frequency, slow waves were also present even after 18 h of complete ischemia (31, 158). The contractile activity and spike potentials, however, were absent, despite the presence of slow waves (31, 158). Asphyxia also progressively decreased slow-wave frequency (108).

The duration of ischemia determines whether or not the normal contractile and electrical activity recovers after revascularization. Guisan et al. (89) have shown that in conscious dogs the gut segment subjected to 1 h of complete ischemia exhibited more spontaneous rhythmic contractions and responded to application of 0.1 N HCl on the mucosa with more vigorous contractions during the initial 3 h of revascularization than did similarly treated control segments. The hypermotility and hyperexcitability occurred despite the fact that mucosal damage was observed microscopically in the biopsy specimen taken 1 h after the ischemia. The HCl application has been used to stimulate the intestinal intrinsic neural reflex. Acute ischemia of the 1-h duration, therefore, appears to produce hyperexcitability of the intestine after reestablishment of normal blood circulation.

Cabot and Kohatsu (31) determined the maximum duration of ischemia that allows the return of normal motility after reperfusion. The artery perfusing a gut segment midway between the ligament of Treitz and the ileocecal junction was occluded for 1–18 h. When circulation was restored within 1–3 h of ischemia, the slow waves, spike potentials, and spontaneous contractions returned to normal 1–13 min following revascularization. When the ischemia lasted >4 h, revascularization did not restore the spontaneous contractions and spike potentials, and the slow-wave frequency was irregular and subnormal. Furthermore the gut segments did not contract in response to mucosal mechanical (irritation or distension) and chemical (bethanechol) stimulation. The same observations were made 24–48 h after reperfusion. This study, as well as those described in this section, seems to indicate that normal contractile and electrical activities can be restored when the duration of ischemia and hypoxia is <4 h. The observations were made, however, ≤2 days after reperfusion.

Szurszewski and Steggerda (181, 182) studied the long-term effects of anoxia. The jejunal segments were subjected to anoxia by intravascular perfusion of Tyrode's solution for 4 h. Normal circulation was then restored and the electrical and contractile activities were observed in the conscious state. Although slow waves reappeared 7–10 days after the recirculation, the frequency was subnormal. Throughout the 30- to 90-day observation period the frequency of slow waves, as well as the frequency of contractile activities in both the longitudinal and transverse axes, were 14–15 times per minute, as compared with 17–18 times per minute in the adjacent normal segments. Furthermore the slow-wave activity from normal adjacent segments was conducted for only a short distance into the segment previously subjected to hypoxia. The contractions in the transverse muscle were not coordinated with those in the longitudinal muscle, and the contractions in the hypoxic segment were not coordinated with adjacent normal segments. Histological examination showed that the number of cells in the myenteric plexus was reduced, but the submucous plexus and the muscle layers appeared normal. The authors therefore concluded that the anoxia-induced changes in electrical and contractile activities were due to hypoxic insult on the myenteric plexus. In explanation of the results, they suggested that the myenteric plexus influences the rhythm of the myogenic system and coordinates the contractile patterns between muscle layers and between adjacent segments. Other investigators have also reported that 3–4 h of complete ischemia produced disappearance of ganglion cells (32, 102). The absence of the intrinsic intestinal reflex lasts for 49 days after the revascularization (102).

Kyi and Daniel (119), however, proposed that 4 h of ischemia produced acute damage to smooth muscle and acute and prolonged damage to intrinsic neural activity. Histologically only 25% of the ganglion cells were irreversibly changed by ischemia. They used two techniques to produce ischemic anoxia. After flushing out the blood from the vasculature of the isolated segments, the segments were either left in situ (102) or perfused with a physiological solution (181) for 4 h. In addition to the measurement of spontaneous electrical and contractile activities, the responses to various chemical, mechanical, and electrical stimuli were studied both shortly after 4 h of anoxia and 10–15 days after restoration of normal circulation. The responses to intra-arterial infusions of methacholine, nicotine, dimethylphenylpiperazinium (DMPP), and phenyldiguanide were reduced or absent after 4 h of ischemia. This indicates that ischemia affects both nerves and smooth muscle. The smooth muscle $Na^+$, $Ca^{2+}$, $Cl^-$, and water concentrations increased, while $K^+$ and $Mg^{2+}$ concentrations decreased, suggesting muscle damage. Muscle strips obtained from the ischemic segments showed no spontaneous rhythmic contractions and a reduced contractile response to methacholine, but exhibited normal responses to stimuli that act on nerves, i.e., DMPP, nicotine, and transmural electrical stimulation. The responses to these neural stimulants were reduced by hexamethonium and abolished by atropine. The acute in vitro study seems to suggest a more adverse effect of ischemic anoxia on muscle than on nerves. Similar pharmacological and chemical studies performed on the ischemic segments 10–15 days after revascularization indicated that muscle electrolyte concentrations were normal, and the contractile responses to the stimuli that act on nerves were also normal. The motility responses to luminal HCl or distension, however, were absent. Kyi and Daniel concluded that some intrinsic nerves were still functioning, and their histological examination revealed that 25% of the ganglion cells were normal, 50% had a varying degree of reversible changes, and 25% had irreversible changes. The pattern of change in the slow waves, i.e., decreased frequency and poor coupling in anoxic segments was similar to that observed by Szurszewski and Steggerda (181).

Ischemia produces similar effects on the electrical and contractile activities of the stomach (116). Spike potentials and spontaneous contractions disappeared 10–15 min after occlusion of the gastric artery and vein. The slow-wave frequency decreased progressively, and no slow waves were recorded 40 min after the ischemia. When the duration of ischemia was shorter than 2 h, slow waves reappeared within 10 min after recirculation but at a subnormal rate; no mechanical activity was present. Pentagastrin (5 mg ia) restored the slow-wave frequency to normal. After ischemia that lasted 2–4 h, recirculation of blood did not induce reappearance of slow waves, but pentagastrin restored the waves at a subnormal rate. When ischemia lasted longer than 4 h, neither recirculation nor pentagastrin could restore slow waves.

Ischemia changes the motility not only of the affected segment but of the remote segments of the gastrointestinal tract as well. In conscious dogs, ischemia in the distal ileum produced an immediate and prolonged (12 h) inhibition of proximal jejunal motility (53). The inhibition was prevented or relieved by the administration of phenoxybenzamine and propranolol. The inhibited jejunum still responded to methacholine with prompt contractions, indicating that the inhibition was mediated by an intestinointestinal reflex. In rats, ligation of 7–9 terminal vascular ramifications at the mesenteric border of the terminal ileum produced a transient increase in gastric emptying and intestinal transit, lasting 1 h (138). Ligation of 11–13 vascular ramifications, however, attenuated both gastric emptying and intestinal transit. The authors suggested that the effect of moderate ischemia is mediated by "ileogastric reflex" and speculated that the effect of the severe ischemia (11–13 vascular ligation) is due to ischemia-induced damage of the receptors responsible for the reflex. The changes in intestinal transit are secondary to changes in the rate of gastric emptying.

In summary, ischemia and hypoxia produced an immediate transient increase in contractile and electrical activities lasting for 1–5 min. After this transient increase, contractile activity and spike potentials decrease or disappear for as long as the hypoxia lasts. The slow waves are still present at normal or subnormal frequency, depending on the severity of the hypoxia and ischemia. These responses appear to be due to hypoxia-induced changes in intrinsic neural activities. Four hours is the critical duration of ischemia for irreversible depression of the contractile and electrical activities. Ischemia lasting longer than 4 h produces acute damage to both nerves and muscles. The smooth muscle, however, recovers to the level of normal function in about 2 wk after revascularization. When there is partial irreversible damage to intrinsic nerve plexuses, the slow-wave frequency of the affected gut is subnormal, and the coupling of slow waves, as well as intrinsic reflexes, are inhibited, probably permanently.

The author thanks Patricia Engelmann for her excellent secretarial help.

This work was supported in part by National Institutes of Health Grant HL-15231 and a grant from the American Heart Association of Michigan.

# REFERENCES

1. ABE, H., H. APPERT, J. CARBALLO, AND J. M. HOWARD. Nonmucosal serotonin in motility of the small bowel. *Arch. Surg.* 106: 183–187, 1973.
2. ALTAMIRANO, M., M. REQUENA, AND T. C. PÉREZ. Interstitial fluid pressure in canine gastric mucosa. *Am. J. Physiol.* 229: 1414–1420, 1975.
3. ALVAREZ, W. C. *Introduction to Gastroenterology.* New York: Hober, 1940, p. 199.
4. ANDERSSON, P. O., S. R. BLOOM, AND J. JARHULT. Colonic motor and vascular responses to pelvic nerve stimulation and their relation to local peptide release in the cat. *J. Physiol. Lond.* 334: 293–307, 1983.
5. ANDERSSON, P. O., AND J. JARHULT. Separation of colonic motor and blood flow responses to pelvic nerve stimulation in the cat. *Acta Physiol. Scand.* 113: 263–265, 1981.
6. ANREP, G. V., S. CERQUA, AND A. SAMANN. The effect of muscular contraction upon the blood flow in the skeletal muscle in the diaphragm and in the small intestine. *Proc. R. Soc. Lond. B. Biol. Sci.* 114: 245–257, 1934.
7. ANURAS, S., S. M. CHIEN, AND J. CHRISTENSEN. Metabolic dependence of the electromyogram of the cat colon. *Am. J. Physiol.* 239 (*Gastrointest. Liver Physiol.* 7): G173–G176, 1980.
8. BACA, I., V. MITTMANN, G. E. FEURLE, M. HASS, AND T. H. MULLER. The effect of neurotensin on regional intestinal blood flow in the dog. *Res. Exp. Med.* 179: 53–85, 1981.
9. BARCROFT, H. Circulation in skeletal muscle. In: *Handbook of Physiology. Circulation,* edited by W. F. Hamilton. Washington, DC: Am. Physiol. Soc., 1963, sect. 2, vol. II, chapt. 40, p. 1353–1385.
10. BAYLISS, W. M., AND E. H. STARLING. The influence of blood supply on intestinal movements. *J. Physiol. Lond.* 23: 34–35, 1898.
11. BAYLISS, W. M., AND E. H. STARLING. The movements and innervation of the small intestine. *J. Physiol. Lond.* 24: 99–143, 1899.
12. BEAN, J. W., AND M. M. SIDKY. Effects of low $O_2$ on intestinal blood flow, tonus and motility. *Am. J. Physiol.* 189: 541–547, 1957.
13. BEAN, J. W., AND M. M. SIDKY. Intestinal blood flow as influenced by vascular and motor reactions to acetycholine and carbon dioxide. *Am. J. Physiol.* 194: 512–518, 1958.
14. BIBER, B., J. FARA, AND O. LUNDGREN. Intestinal vascular responses to 5-hydroxytryptamine. *Acta Physiol. Scand.* 87: 526–534, 1973.
15. BIBER, B., O. LUNDGREN, AND J. SVANVIK. Studies on the intestinal vasodilatation observed after mechanical stimulation of the mucosa of the gut. *Acta Physiol. Scand.* 82: 177–190, 1971.
16. BOATMAN, D. L., AND M. J. BRODY. Effects of acetylcholine on intestinal vasculature of the dog. *J. Pharmacol. Exp. Ther.* 142: 185–191, 1963.
17. BOHLEN, H. G. Intestinal tissue $PO_2$ and microvascular responses during glucose exposure. *Am. J. Physiol.* 238 (*Heart Circ. Physiol.* 7): H164–H171, 1980.
18. BOHLEN, H. G. In vivo microscopy of the intestinal microcirculation. In: *Measurement of Blood Flow. Applications to the Splanchnic Circulation,* edited by D. N. Granger and G. B. Bulkley. Baltimore, MD: Williams & Wilkins, 1981, p. 91–104.
19. BOHLEN, H. G. Microvasculature structure and interaction in the wall of the small intestine. *Federation Proc.* 43: 7–9, 1984.
20. BOHLEN, H. G., AND R. W. GORE. Comparison of microvascular pressures and diameters in the innervated and denervated rat intestine. *Microvasc. Res.* 14: 251–264, 1977.
21. BOHLEN, H. G., AND R. W. GORE. Microvascular pressures in

rat intestinal muscle during direct nerve stimulation. *Microvasc. Res.* 17: 27–37, 1979.
22. BOLEY, S. J., G. P. AGRAWAL, A. R. WARREN, F. J. VEITH, B. S. LEVOWITZ, W. TREIBER, J. DOUGHERTY, S. S. SCHWARTZ, AND M. L. GLIEDMAN. Pathophysiologic effects of bowel distention on intestinal blood flow. *Am. J. Surg.* 117: 228–234, 1969.
23. BOND, J. H., R. A. PRENTISS, AND M. D. LEVITT. The effect of anesthesia and laparotomy on blood flow of the stomach, small bowel, and colon of the dog. *Surgery St. Louis* 87: 313–318, 1980.
24. BOWEN, J. C., W. PAWLIK, W. F. FANG, AND E. D. JACOBSON. Pharmacologic effects of gastrointestinal hormones on intestinal oxygen consumption and blood flow. *Surgery St. Louis* 78: 515–519, 1975.
25. BROBMANN, G. F., E. D. JACOBSON, AND G. A. BRECHER. Intestinal vascular responses to gut pressure and acetylcholine in vitro. *Angiologica Basel* 7: 129–139, 1970.
26. BROBMANN, G. F., E. D. JACOBSON, AND G. A. BRECHER. Effects of distension and acetylcholine on intestinal blood flow in vivo. *Angiologica Basel* 7: 140–146, 1970.
27. BULKLEY, G. B., W. A. WOMACK, J. M. DOWNEY, P. R. KVIETYS, AND D. N. GRANGER. Characterization of segmental collateral blood flow in the small intestine. *Am. J. Physiol.* 249 (*Gastrointest. Liver Physiol.* 12): G228–G235, 1985.
28. BURNS, T. D., AND J. M. DABNEY. Effects of hexamthonium ($C_6$) and tetrodotoxin (TTX) on the intestinal vascular response to local stimuli (Abstract). *Federation Proc.* 31: 391, 1972.
29. BURTON, A. C., AND D. J. PATEL. Effect on pulmonary vascular resistance of inflation of the rabbit lungs. *J. Appl. Physiol.* 12: 239–246, 1958.
30. BUSSEMAKER, J. B., AND J. LINDEMAN. Comparison of methods to determine viability of small intestine. *Ann. Surg.* 176: 97–101, 1972.
31. CABOT, R. M., AND S. KOHATSU. The effects of ischemia on the electrical and contractile activities of the canine small intestine. *Am. J. Surg.* 136: 242–246, 1978.
32. CANNON, W. B., AND I. R. BURKET. The endurance of anemia by nerve cells in the myenteric plexus. *Am. J. Physiol.* 32: 347–357, 1913.
33. CASSUTO, J., S. CEDGARD, J. HAGLUND, S. REDFORS, AND O. LUNDGREN. Intramural blood flows and flow distribution in the feline small intestine during arterial hypotension. *Acta Physiol. Scand.* 106: 335–342, 1979.
34. CHOU, C. C. The Role of Intestinal Wall Compliance in the Regulation of Intestinal Blood Flow. Norman: Univ. of Oklahoma, 1966. Dissertation.
35. CHOU, C. C. Relationship between intestinal blood flow and motility. *Ann. Rev. Physiol.* 44: 29–42, 1982.
36. CHOU, C. C., T. D. BURNS, C. P. HSIEH, AND J. M. DABNEY. Mechanisms of local vasodilation with hypertonic glucose in the jejunum. *Surgery St. Louis* 71: 380–387, 1972.
37. CHOU, C. C., AND J. M. DABNEY. Intestinal compliance. *Am. J. Dig. Dis.* 12: 1189–1197, 1967.
38. CHOU, C. C., AND J. M. DABNEY. Interrelation of ileal wall compliance and vascular resistance. *Am. J. Dig. Dis.* 12: 1198–1208, 1967.
39. CHOU, C. C., E. D. FROHLICH, AND E. C. TEXTER, JR. A comparative study of the effects of bradykinin, kallidin II and eledoisin on segmental superior mesenteric resistance. *J. Physiol. Lond.* 176: 1–11, 1965.
40. CHOU, C. C., AND R. H. GALLAVAN. Blood flow and intestinal motility. *Federation Proc.* 41: 2090–2095, 1982.
41. CHOU, C. C., AND B. GRASSMICK. Motility and blood flow distribution within the wall of the gastrointestinal tract. *Am. J. Physiol.* 235 (*Heart Circ. Physiol.* 4): H34–H39, 1978.
42. CHOU, C. C., C. P. HSIEH, T. D. BURNS, AND J. M. DABNEY. Effects of lumen pH and osmolarity on duodenal blood flow and motility. *Gastroenterology* 60: 648, 1971.
43. CHOU, C. C., C. P. HSIEH, AND J. M. DABNEY. Effects of acid and hyperosmolarity in the lumen of the canine duodenum on local blood flow and motility. *Gastroenterology* 58: 934, 1970.
44. CHOU, C. C., C. P. HSIEH, AND J. M. DABNEY. Comparison of vascular effects of gastrointestinal hormones on various organs. *Am. J. Physiol.* 232 (*Heart Circ. Physiol.* 1): H103–H109, 1977.
45. CHOU, C. C., C. P. HSIEH, Y. M. YU, P. KVIETYS, L. C. YU, R. PITTMAN, AND J. M. DABNEY. Localization of mesenteric hyperemia during digestion in dogs. *Am. J. Physiol.* 230: 583–589, 1976.
46. CHOU, C. C., D. H. KUIPER, AND C. P. HSIEH. Effects of diphenylhydantoin on motility and compliance of the canine ileum and colon. *Gastroenterology* 62: 734, 1972.
47. CHOU, C. C., AND P. R. KVIETYS. Physiological and pharmacological alterations in gastrointestinal blood flow. In: *Measurement of Blood Flow. Applications to the Splanchnic Circulation*, by D. N. Granger and G. B. Bulkley. Baltimore, MD: Williams & Wilkins, 1981, p. 475–509.
48. CHOU, C. C., P. KVIETYS, J. POST, AND S. P. SIT. Constituents of chyme responsible for postprandial intestinal hyperemia. *Am. J. Physiol.* 235 (*Heart Circ. Physiol.* 4): H677–H682, 1978.
49. CHOU, C. C., R. A. NYHOF, P. R. KVIETYS, S. P. SIT, AND R. H. GALLAVAN, JR. Regulation of jejunal blood flow and oxygenation during glucose and oleic acid absorption. *Am. J. Physiol.* 249 (*Gastrointest. Liver Physiol.* 12): G691–G701, 1985.
50. CODE, C. F., AND J. F. SCHLEGEL. The gastrointestinal interdigestive housekeeper: motor correlates of the interdigestive myoelectric complex of the dog. In: *Proceedings of the 4th International Symposium on Gastrointestinal Motility*, edited by E. E. Daniel, J. A. L. Gilbert, B. Schofield, T. K. Schnitka, and G. Scott. Banff, Canada: Vancouver Mitchell, 1974, p. 631–634.
51. COULIC, V., A. MAXIMENKOVA, AND L. FINIDOVA. Influence of the small bowel motility on its microcirculation. *Biol. Gastro-Enterol.* 9: 289–294, 1976.
52. DABNEY, J. M., J. B. SCOTT, AND C. C. CHOU. Effects of cations on ileal compliance and blood flow. *Am. J. Physiol.* 212: 835–839, 1967.
53. DIXON, J. A., C. G. HARMAN, R. L. NICHOLS, AND E. ENGLERT, JR. Intestinal motility following luminal and vascular occlusion of the small intestine. *Gastroenterology* 58: 673–678, 1970.
54. DRAGSTEDT, C. A., V. F. LANG, AND R. F. MILLET. The relative effects of distention on different portions of the intestine. *Arch. Surg.* 18: 2259–2263, 1929.
55. EDLICH, R. F., J. W. BORNER, J. KUPHAL, AND O. H. WANGENSTEEN. Gastric blood flow. 1. Its distribution during gastric distention. *Am. J. Surg.* 120: 35–37, 1970.
56. EKLUND, S., M. JODAL, O. LUNDGREN, AND A. SJÖQVIST. Effects of vasoactive intestinal polypeptide on blood flow, motility and fluid transport in the gastrointestinal tract of the cat. *Acta Physiol. Scand.* 105: 461–468, 1979.
57. EVANS, C. L. The physiology of plain muscle. *Physiol. Rev.* 6: 358–398, 1926.
58. EVANS, D. H. L., AND H. O. SCHILD. The reactions of plexus-free circular muscle of cat jejunum to drugs. *J. Physiol. Lond.* 119: 376–399, 1953.
59. FAHRENKRUG, J., U. HAGLUND, M. JODAL, O. LUNDGREN, L. OLBE, AND O. B. SCHAFFALITZKY DE MUCKADELL. Nervous release of vasoactive intestinal polypeptide in the gastrointestinal tract of cats: possible physiological implications. *J. Physiol. Lond.* 284: 291–305, 1978.
60. FARA, J. W., AND K. S. MADDEN. Effect of secretin and cholecystokinin on small intestinal blood flow distribution. *Am. J. Physiol.* 229: 1365–1370, 1975.
61. FARA, J. W., E. H. RUBINSTEIN, AND R. R. SONNENSCHEIN. Intestinal hormones in mesenteric vasodilation after intraduodenal agents. *Am. J. Physiol.* 223: 1058–1067, 1972.
62. FARA, J. W., AND A. M. SALAZER. Gastric inhibitory polypeptide increases mesenteric blood flow. *Proc. Soc. Exp. Biol. Med.*

158: 446–448, 1978.
63. FASTH, S., S. FILIPSSON, L. HULTEN, AND J. MARTINSON. The effect of the gastrointestinal hormones on small intestinal motility and blood flow. *Experientia Basel* 29: 982–984, 1973.
64. FASTH, S., H. HEDLUND, L. HULTEN, S. NORDGREN, AND T. ORESLAND. The effect of 5-hydroxytryptamine on large intestinal motility and blood flow in the cat. *Acta Physiol. Scand.* 118: 329–336, 1983.
65. FASTH, S., AND L. HULTEN. The effects of glucagon on intestinal motility and blood flow. *Acta Physiol. Scand.* 83: 169–173, 1971.
66. FASTH, S., AND L. HULTEN. The effect of bradykinin on intestinal motility and blood flow. *Acta Chir. Scand.* 139: 699–705, 1973.
67. FASTH, S., L. HULTEN, B. J. JOHNSON, S. NORDGREN, AND I. J. ZEITHIN. Mobilization of colonic kallikrein following pelvic nerve stimulation in the atropinized cat. *J. Physiol. Lond.* 285: 471–478, 1978.
68. FASTH, S., L. HULTEN, AND S. NORDGREN. Evidence for a dual pelvic nerve influence on large bowel motility in the cat. *J. Physiol. Lond.* 298: 159–169, 1980.
69. FASTH, S., L. HULTEN, S. NORDGREN, AND I. J. ZEITLIN. Studies on the atropine-resistant sacral parasympathetic vascular and motility responses in the cat colon. *J. Physiol. Lond.* 311: 421–429, 1981.
70. FIORAMONTI, J., AND L. BUENO. Relation between intestinal motility and mesenteric blood flow in the conscious dog. *Am. J. Physiol.* 246 (*Gastrointest. Liver Physiol.* 9): G108–G113, 1984.
71. FIORAMONTI, J., L. BUENO, AND M. RUCKEBUSCH. Blood sugar oscillations and duodenal migrating myoelectric complexes. *Am. J. Physiol.* 242 (*Gastrointest. Liver Physiol.* 5): G15–G20, 1982.
72. FLEISCHER, D. R. On the movement of intestinal tonus. *Gastroenterology* 58: 685–691, 1970.
73. FONDACARO, J. D. Intestinal blood flow and motility. In: *Physiology of the Intestinal Circulation*, edited by A. P. Shepherd and D. N. Granger. New York: Raven, 1984, p. 107–120.
74. FROHLICH, E. D., J. B. SCOTT, AND F. J. HADDY. Effect of cations on resistance and responsiveness of renal and forelimb vascular beds. *Am. J. Physiol.* 203: 583–587, 1962.
75. GALLAVAN, R. H., JR., C. C. CHOU, P. R. KVIETYS, AND S. P. SIT. Regional blood flow during digestion in the conscious dog. *Am. J. Physiol.* 238 (*Heart Circ. Physiol.* 7): H220–H225, 1980.
76. GANNON, B. J., R. W. GORE, AND P. A. W. ROGERS. Is there an anatomical basis for a vascular counter-current mechanism in rabbit and human intestinal villi? *Biomed. Res.* 2: 235–241, 1981.
77. GATCH, W. D., AND C. G. CULBERTSON. Circulatory disturbances caused by intestinal obstruction. *Ann. Surg.* 102: 619–635, 1935.
78. GATCH, W. D., H. M. TRUSLER, AND K. D. AYERS. Effects of gaseous distention on obstructed bowel. *Arch. Surg.* 14: 1215–1221, 1927.
79. GEBER, W. F. Intestinal blood flow-pressure responses during control and induced peristalsis. *Arch. Int. Pharmacodyn.* 157: 53–66, 1965.
80. GORE, R. W., AND H. G. BOHLEN. Pressure regulation in the microcirculation. *Federation Proc.* 34: 2031–2037, 1975.
81. GORE, R. W., AND H. G. BOHLEN. Microvascular pressures in rat intestinal muscle and mucosal villi. *Am. J. Physiol.* 233 (*Heart Circ. Physiol.* 6): H685–H693, 1977.
82. GRANGER, D. N., P. R. KVIETYS, N. A. MORTILLARO, AND A. E. TAYLOR. Effect of luminal distension on intestinal transcapillary fluid exchange. *Am. J. Physiol.* 239 (*Gastrointest. Liver Physiol.* 2): G516–G523, 1980.
83. GRANGER, D. N., P. D. I. RICHARDSON, P. R. KVIETYS, AND N. A. MORTILLARO. Intestinal blood flow. *Gastroenterology* 78: 837–863, 1980.
84. GRANGER, D. N., P. D. I. RICHARDSON, AND A. E. TAYLOR. Volumetric assessment of the capillary filtration coefficient in the cat small intestine. *Pfluegers Arch.* 381-25–33, 1979.
85. GRANGER, D. N., J. D. VALLEAU, R. E. PARKER, R. S. LANE, AND A. E. TAYLOR. Effects of adenosine on intestinal hemodynamics, oxygen delivery, and capillary fluid exchange. *Am. J. Physiol.* 235 (*Heart Circ. Physiol.* 4): H707–H719, 1978.
86. GREGG, D. E., E. M. KHOURI, AND C. R. RAYFORD. Systemic and coronary energetics in the resting unanesthetized dog. *Circ. Res.* 16: 102–113, 1965.
87. GRIM, E. The flow of blood in the mesenteric vessels. In: *Handbook of Physiology. Circulation*, edited by W. F. Hamilton. Washington, DC: Am. Physiol. Soc., 1963, sect. 2, vol. II, chapt. 42, p 1439–1456.
88. GRIVEL, M. L., AND Y. RUCKEBUSCH. The propagation of segmental contractions along the small intestine. *J. Physiol. Lond.* 227: 611–625, 1972.
89. GUISAN, Y. J., A. HRENO, AND F. N. GURD. Effect of acute ischemia on the motility of the small bowel in the awake dog. *Eur. Surg. Res.* 7: 23–33, 1975.
90. GUTH, P. H., T. MOLER, AND H. WAYLAND. Study of the gastric circulation by in vivo fluorescence microscopy. In: *Gastrointestinal Mucosal Blood Flow*, edited by L. P. Fielding. London: Churchill Livingstone, 1980, p. 17–25.
91. GUTH, P. H., AND A. ROSENBERG. In vivo microscopy of the gastric microcirculation. *Am. J. Dig. Dis.* 17: 391–398, 1972.
92. GUTH, P. H., AND E. SMITH. Histamine receptors in mesenteric circulation of the cat and rat. *Am. J. Physiol.* 234 (*Endocrinol. Metab. Gastrointest. Physiol.* 4): E370–E374, 1978.
93. HADDY, F. J., C. C. CHOU, J. B. SCOTT, AND J. M. DABNEY. Intestinal vascular responses to naturally occurring vasoactive substances. *Gastroenterology* 52: 444–451, 1967.
94. HAMILTON, T. C. Comparison of the vasodilator activity of acetylcholine, cholinomimetics and other vasodilators in two vascular beds of the cat. *Eur. J. Pharmacol.* 28: 11–17, 1974.
95. HANSON, K. M. Hemodynamic effects of distension of the dog small intestine. *Am. J. Physiol.* 225: 456–460, 1973.
96. HANSON, K. M., AND F. T. MOORE. Effects of intraluminal pressure in the colon on its vascular pressure-flow relationships. *Proc. Soc. Exp. Biol. Med.* 131: 373–376, 1969.
97. HANSON, K. M., AND F. T. MOORE. Pressure-volume relationships and blood flow in the distended colon. *Am. J. Physiol.* 217: 35–39, 1969.
98. HASHIMOTO, K., AND S. KUMAKURA. The pharmacological features of the coronary, renal, mesenteric and femoral arteries. *Jpn J. Physiol.* 15: 540–551, 1965.
99. HASHIZUME, T., K. HIROKAWA, S. AIBARA, H. OGAWA, AND A. KASAHARA. Pharmacological and histological studies of gastric mucosal lesion induced by serotonin in rats. *Arch. Int. Pharmacodyn. Ther.* 236: 96–108, 1978.
100. HESS, D. S., AND R. J. BACHE. Transmural distribution of myocardial blood flow during systole in the awake dog. *Circ. Res.* 38: 5–15, 1976.
101. HOLADAY, D. A., H. VOLK, AND J. MANDELL. Electrical activity of the small intestine with special reference to the origin of rhythmicity. *Am. J. Physiol.* 195: 505–515, 1958.
102. HUKUHARA, R. T., T. SUMI, AND S. KOTANI. Role of the ganglion cells in the small intestine taken in the intestinal intrinsic reflexes. *Jpn J. Physiol.* 11: 281–288, 1961.
103. HULTEN, L. Extrinsic nervous control of colonic motility and blood flow. *Acta Physiol. Scand. Suppl.* 335: 1–116, 1969.
104. HULTEN, L. Regulation of colonic motility and blood flow. *Nutr. Rev.* 35: 38–41, 1977.
105. HULTEN, L., M. JODAL, AND O. LUDGREN. Extrinsic nervous control of colonic blood flow. *Acta Physiol. Scand. Suppl.* 335: 39–50, 1969.
106. JACOBSON, E. D., G. F. BROBMANN, AND G. A. BRECKER. Intestinal motor activity and blood flow. *Gastroenterology* 58: 575–579, 1970.
107. JODAL, M., O. LUNDGREN, AND A. SJÖQVIST. The effect of apamin on nonadrenergic, noncholinergic vasodilator mechanism in the intestines of the cat. *J. Physiol. Lond.* 338: 207–219, 1983.

108. JOHNSON, P. C. Myogenic nature of increase in intestinal vascular resistance with venous pressure elevation. *Circ. Res.* 7: 992–999, 1959.
109. KACHELHOFFER, J., A. POUSSE, J. MARESCAUX, M. ITURIZAGA, AND J. F. GRENIER. Effects of motility and luminal distension on dog small intestine hemodynamics. *Eur. Surg. Res.* 10: 184–193, 1978.
110. KATZ, S., A. WAHAB, W. MURRAY, AND L. F. WILLIAMS. New parameters of viability in ischemic bowel disease. *Am. J. Surg.* 127: 136–141, 1974.
111. KEWENTER, J. The vagal control of the jejunal and ileal motility and blood flow. *Acta Physiol. Scand. Suppl.* 251: 1–68, 1965.
112. KEWENTER, J. Effects of graded acetylcholine infusions on intestinal motility, volume and blood flow. *Scand. J. Gastroenterol.* 6: 435–440, 1971.
113. KONTUREK, S. J., J. JAWOREK, M. CIESZKOWSKI, W. PAWLIK, J. KANIA, AND S. R. BLOOM. Comparison of effects of neurotensin and fat on pancreatic stimulation in dogs. *Am. J. Physiol.* 244 (*Gastrointest. Liver Physiol.* 7): G590–G598, 1983.
114. KOSTERITZ, H. W., V. W. PIRIE, AND J. A. ROBINSON. The mechanism of the peristaltic reflex in the isolated guinea-pig ileum. *J. Physiol. Lond.* 133: 681–694, 1956.
115. KOWALEWSKI, K., AND A. KOLODEJ. Effect of prostaglandin-$E_2$ on myoelectrical and mechanical activity of total isolated, ex-vivo-perfused, canine stomach. *Pharmacology* 13: 325–339, 1975.
116. KOWALEWSKI, K., S. ZAJAC, AND A. KOLODEJ. Effect of ischemic anoxia on electrical and mechanical activity of the totally isolated porcine stomach. *Eur. Surg. Res.* 8: 12–25, 1976.
117. KVIETYS, P. R., AND D. N. GRANGER. Vasoactive agents and splanchnic oxygen uptake. *Am. J. Physiol.* 243 (*Gastrointest. Liver Physiol.* 6): G1–G9, 1982.
118. KVIETYS, P. R., J. M. RUSSELL, AND D. N. GRANGER. Relationship between intestinal blood flow and oxygen uptake: effects of temperature, absorption and motility (Abstract). *Federation Proc.* 42: 340, 1983.
119. KYI, K. K. J., AND E. E. DANIEL. The effects of ischemia on intestinal nerves and electrical slow waves. *Am. J. Dig. Dis.* 15: 959–981, 1970.
120. LAWSON, H. The mechanism of deflation hyperemia in the intestine. *Am. J. Physiol.* 134: 147–156, 1941.
121. LAWSON, H., AND A. M. AMBROSE. The utilization of blood oxygen by the distended intestine. *Am. J. Physiol.* 135: 650–659, 1942.
122. LAWSON, H., AND J. CHUMLEY. The effect of distention on blood flow through the intestine. *Am. J. Physiol.* 131: 368–377, 1940.
123. LEE, J. S. Motility, lymphatic contractility, and distention pressure in intestinal absorption. *Am. J. Physiol.* 208: 621–627, 1965.
124. LEMBECK, F., AND R. HETTICH. Comparative study of the effects of substance P on blood pressure, salivatory functions and intestinal motility. *Naunyn-Schmiedebergs Arch. Pharmacol.* 265: 216–224, 1969.
125. LIFSON, N. Fluid secretion and hydrostatic pressure relationships in the small intestine. In: *Mechanisms of Intestinal Secretion*, edited by H. J. Binder. New York: Liss, 1979, vol. 12, p. 249–261 (Kroc Found. Ser.).
126. LONGHURST, J. C., H. L. SPILKER, AND G. A. ORDWAY. Cardiovascular reflexes elicited by passive gastric distension in anesthetized cats. *Am. J. Physiol.* 240 (*Heart Circ. Physiol.* 9): H539–H545, 1981.
127. LUNDGREN, O. Microcirculation of the gastrointestinal tract and pancreas. In: *Handbook of Physiology. The Cardiovascular System. Microcirculation*, edited by E. M. Renkin and C. C. Michel. Bethesda, MD: Am. Physiol. Soc., 1984, sect. 2, vol. IV, pt. 2, chapt. 17, p. 799–863.
128. LUNDGREN, O., AND I. WALLENTIN. Local chemical and nervous control of consecutive vascular sections in the mesenteric lymph nodes of the cat. *Angiologica Basel* 1: 284–296, 1964.
129. MALL, F. A study of the intestinal contraction. *Johns Hopkins Hosp. Rep.* 1: 37–75, 1896.
130. MANGINO, M. J., AND C. C. CHOU. Arachidonic acid and postprandial intestinal hyperemia. *Am. J. Physiol.* 246 (*Gastrointest. Liver Physiol.* 9): G521–G527, 1984.
131. MARTIN, A. W., AND F. A. FUHRMAN. The relationship between summated tissue respiration and metabolic rate in mouse and dog. *Physiol. Zool.* 28: 18–34, 1955.
132. MARTINSON, J. The effect of graded vagal stimulation on gastric motility, secretion, and blood flow in the cat. *Acta Physiol. Scand.* 65: 300–309, 1965.
133. MAXWELL, L. C., A. P. SHEPHERD, G. L. RIEDEL, AND M. D. MORRIS. Effect of microsphere size on apparent intramural distribution of intestinal blood flow. *Am. J. Physiol.* 241 (*Heart Circ. Physiol.* 10): H408–H414, 1981.
134. MEISSNER, A., K. L. BOWES, AND S. K. SARNA. Effects of ambient and stagnant hypoxia on the mechanical and electrical activity of the canine upper jejunum. *Can. J. Surg.* 19: 316–321, 1976.
134a. MOHAMED, M. S., AND J. W. BEAN. Local and general alterations of blood $CO_2$ and influence of intestinal motility in regulation of intestinal blood flow. *Am. J. Physiol.* 167: 413–425, 1951.
135. MORTILLARO, N. A., AND R. ALLEN. Effects of venous pressure on intestinal metabolism (Abstract). *Federation Proc.* 39: 705, 1980.
136. NEMATZADEH, D., P. A. KOT, J. C. ROSE, AND H. K. HUANG. Magnitude of the left ventricular intramyocardial pressure (IMP) gradient in the canine heart. *Physiologist* 19: 310, 1976.
137. NOER, R. J., H. J. ROBB, AND L. F. JACOBSON. Circulatory disturbances produced by acute intestinal distension in the living animal. *Arch. Surg.* 63: 520–528, 1951.
138. NYLANDER, G., AND S. WIKSTRÖM. Propulsive gastrointestinal motility in regional and graded ischemia of the small bowel. An experimental study in the rat. I. Immediate results. *Acta Chir. Scand. Suppl.* 385: 1–67, 1968.
139. OHMAN, U. Studies on small intestinal obstruction. I. Intraluminal pressure in experimental low small bowel obstruction in the cat. *Acta Chir. Scand.* 141: 413–416, 1975.
140. OHMAN, U. Studies on small intestinal obstruction. II. Blood flow, vascular resistance, capillary filtration, and oxygen consumption in denervated small bowel after obstruction. *Acta Chir. Scand.* 141: 417–423, 1975.
141. OHMAN, U. Studies on small intestinal obstruction. III. Circulatory effects of artificial small bowel distension. *Acta Chir. Scand.* 141: 536–544, 1975.
142. OHMAN, U. Studies on small intestinal obstruction. IV. Circulatory effects of artificial small bowel distension. *Acta Chir. Scand.* 141: 545–549, 1975.
143. OHMAN, U. Studies on small intestinal obstruction. V. Blood circulation in moderately distended small bowel. *Acta Chir. Scand.* 141: 763–770, 1975.
144. OHMAN, U. Studies on small intestinal obstruction. Blood circulation in obstructed and artificially distended small intestine in the cat. *Acta Chir. Scand. Suppl.* 452: 1–41, 1975.
145. OHMAN, U. Blood flow and oxygen consumption in the feline small intestine: responses to artificial distention and intestinal obstruction. *Acta Chir. Scand.* 142: 329–333, 1976.
146. PARKER, R. E., AND D. N. GRANGER. Effect of graded arterial occlusion on ileal blood flow distribution. *Proc. Soc. Exp. Biol. Med.* 162: 146–149, 1979.
147. PAWLIK, W., J. C. BOWEN, AND E. D. JACOBSON. Vasoactive and metabolic effects of gastrointestinal hormones in the intestine. *Mater. Med. Pol.* 31: 151–154, 1977.
148. PAWLIK, W. W., J. D. FONDACARO, AND E. D. JACOBSON. Metabolic hyperemia in the canine gut. *Am. J. Physiol.* 239 (*Gastrointest. Liver Physiol.* 2): G12–G17, 1980.
149. PAWLIK, W., L. L. TAGUE, B. L. TEPPERMAN, T. A. MILLER, AND E. D. JACOBSON. Histamine $H_1$- and $H_2$-receptor vasodilation of canine intestinal circulation. *Am. J. Physiol.* 233

(*Endocrinol. Metab. Gastrointest. Physiol.* 1): E219–E224, 1977.
150. PAWLIK, W. W., K. M. WALUS, AND J. D. FONDACARO. Effects of methionine-enkephalin on intestinal circulation and oxygen consumption. *Proc. Soc. Exp. Biol. Med.* 165: 26–31, 1980.
151. PERLMAN, D. M., AND J. W. COLE. A smooth muscle stimulating substance released from the intestine following acute arterial occlusion. *Surg. Forum* 9: 476–480, 1958.
152. PREMEN, A. J., C. Y. SOIKA, J. M. DABNEY, AND D. E. DOBBINS. Effects of gastrointestinal hormones on ileal vascular and visceral smooth muscle. *Am. J. Physiol.* 246 (*Gastrointest. Liver Physiol.* 9): G1–G7, 1984.
153. PRICE, W. E., Z. SHEHADEH, G. H. THOMPSON, L. D. UNDERWOOD, AND E. D. JACOBSON. Effects of acetylcholine on intestinal blood flow and motility. *Am. J. Physiol.* 216: 343–347, 1969.
154. PYTKOWSKI, B. On the contribution of prostaglandin-like substances to the action of bradykinin on intestinal motility and blood flow in canine jejunal loop in situ. *Eur. J. Clin. Invest.* 9: 391–396, 1979.
155. PYTKOWSKI, B., AND J. MICHALOWSKI. Motility- and blood flow-dependent absorption of amino acids in canine small intestine. *Eur. J. Clin. Invest.* 7: 79–86, 1977.
156. QUIGLEY, J. P., AND D. A. BRODY. Digestive tract: intraluminal pressures, gastrointestinal propulsion, gastric evacuation, pressure-wall tension relationships. In: *Medical Physics*, edited by O. Glasser. Chicago, IL: Yearbook, 1950, vol. II, p. 280.
157. RUF, W., G. T. SUEHIRO, A. SUEHIRO, V. PRESSLER, AND J. J. MCNAMARA. Intestinal blood flow at various intraluminal pressure in the piglet with closed abdomen. *Ann. Surg.* 191: 157–163, 1980.
158. SCHAMAUN, M. Electromyography to determine viability of injured small bowel segments; an experimental study with preliminary clinical observations. *Surgery St. Louis* 62: 899–909, 1967.
159. SCHRAUWEN, E., AND A. HOUVENAGHEL. Influence of substance P on mesenteric hemodynamics in the pig. *Arch. Int. Pharmacodyn. Ther.* 242: 315–317, 1979.
160. SCHUURKES, J. A. J., AND G. A. CHARBON. Motility and hemodynamics of the canine gastrointestinal tract. Stimulation by pentagastrin, cholecystokinin and vasopressin. *Arch. Int. Pharmacodyn. Ther.* 236: 214–227, 1978.
161. SCHWAIGER, M., J. D. FONDACARO, AND E. D. JACOBSON. Effects of glucagon, histamine and perheiline on the ischemic canine mesenteric circulation. *Gastroenterology* 77: 730–735, 1979.
162. SCOTT, J. B., AND J. M. DABNEY. Relation of gut motility to blood flow in the ileum of the dog. *Circ. Res.* 14, Suppl. 1: 235–239, 1964.
163. SCOTT, J. B., E. D. FROHLICH, R. A. HARDIN, AND F. J. HADDY. $Na^+$, $K^+$, $Ca^{++}$, and $Mg^{++}$ action on coronary vascular resistance in the dog heart. *Am. J. Physiol.* 201: 1095–1100, 1961.
164. SELKURT, E. E., AND P. C. JOHNSON. Effect of acute elevation of portal venous pressure on mesenteric blood volume, interstitial fluid volume, and hemodynamics. *Circ. Res.* 6: 592–599, 1958.
165. SEMBA, T., K. FUJII, AND Y. FUJII. Influence of peristaltic contraction of the stomach on blood flow through the gastrosplenic vein. *Hiroshima J. Med. Sci.* 19: 87–97, 1970.
166. SEMBA, T., K. FUJII, AND Y. FUJII. The influence of rhythmic and tonic contraction of the small intestine on blood flow through the intestinal segment. *Jpn. J. Physiol.* 21: 1–14, 1971.
167. SEMBA, T., K. FUJII, AND T. MIZONISHI. Relation of intestinal motility to venous outflow and saturation of blood $O_2$ through mesenteric blood vessels. *Jpn. J. Physiol.* 23: 541–557, 1973.
168. SEMBA, T., AND Y. FUJII. Relationship between venous flow and colonic peristalsis. *Jpn. J. Physiol.* 20: 408–416, 1970.
169. SEMBA, T., T. MIZONISHI, Y. IKEDA, AND Y. NAGAO. Influence of intestinal inhibitory reflex on mesenteric blood flow through an intestinal segment of the dog. *Jpn. J. Physiol.* 27: 439–450, 1977.
170. SHEHADEH, Z., W. E. PRICE, AND E. D. JACOBSON. Effects of vasoactive agents on intestinal blood flow and motility in the dog. *Am. J. Physiol.* 216: 386–392, 1969.
171. SHEPHERD, A. P. Intestinal $O_2$ consumption and $^{86}Rb$ extraction during arterial hypoxia. *Am. J. Physiol.* 234 (*Endocrinol. Metab. Gastrointest. Physiol.* 3): E248–E251, 1978.
172. SHEPHERD, A. P., G. L. RIEDEL, L. C. MAXWELL, AND J. W. KIEL. Selective vasodilators redistribute intestinal blood flow and depress oxygen uptake. *Am. J. Physiol.* 247 (*Gastrointest. Liver Physiol.* 10): G377–G384, 1984.
174. SIDKY, M., AND J. W. BEAN. Influence of rhythmic and tonic contraction of intestinal muscle on blood flow and blood reservoir capacity in dog intestine. *Am. J. Physiol.* 193: 386–392, 1958.
175. SIT, S. P., AND C. C. CHOU. Time course of jejunal blood flow, $O_2$ uptake, and $O_2$ extraction during nutrient absorption. *Am. J. Physiol.* 247 (*Heart Circ. Physiol.* 16): H395–H402, 1984.
176. SJÖQVIST, A., J. FAHRENKRUG, M. JODAL, AND O. LUNDGREN. Effect of apamin on release of vasoactive intestinal polypeptide (VIP) from the intestines of the cat. *Acta Physiol. Scand.* 119: 69–76, 1983.
177. SJÖQVIST, A., P. M. HELLSTRÖM, M. JODAL, AND O. LUNDGREN. Neurotransmitters involved in the colonic contraction and vasodilation elicited by activation of the pelvic nerves in the cat. *Gastroenterology* 86: 1481–1487, 1984.
178. SWABB, E. A., R. A. HYNES, AND M. DONOWITZ. Elevated intraluminal pressure alters rabbit small intestinal transport in vivo. *Am. J. Physiol.* 242 (*Gastrointest. Liver Physiol.* 5): G58–G64, 1982.
179. SWABB, E. A., R. A. HYNES, W. G. MARNANE, J. S. MCNEIL, R. A. DECKER, Y.-H. TAI, AND M. DONOWITZ. Intestinal filtration-secretion due to increased intraluminal pressure in rabbits. *Am. J. Physiol.* 242 (*Gastrointest. Liver Physiol.* 5): G65–G75, 1982.
180. SZURSZEWSKI, J. H. A migrating electric complex of the canine small intestine. *Am. J. Physiol.* 217: 1757–1763, 1969.
181. SZURSZEWSKI, J., AND F. R. STEGGERDA. The effect of hypoxia on the electrical slow wave of the canine small intestine. *Am. J. Dig. Dis.* 13: 168–177, 1968.
182. SZURSZEWSKI, J., AND F. R. STEGGERDA. The effect of hypoxia on the mechanical activity of the canine small intestine. *Am. J. Dig. Dis.* 13: 178–185, 1968.
183. TEXTER, E. C., JR., C. C. CHOU, S. L. MERRILL, H. C. LAURETA, AND E. D. FROHLICH. Direct effects of vasoactive agents on segmental resistance of the mesenteric and portal circulation. Studies with *l*-epinephrine, levarterenol, angiotensin, vasopressin, acetylcholine, metacholine, histamine, and serotonin. *J. Lab. Clin. Med.* 64: 624–633, 1964.
184. TEXTER, E. C., JR., H. C. LAURETA, E. D. FROHLICH, AND C. C. CHOU. Effects of major cations on gastric and mesenteric vascular resistances. *Am. J. Physiol.* 212: 569–573, 1967.
185. TUNICK, P. A., W. F. TREIBER, JR., M. FRANK, F. J. VEITH, M. L. GLIEDMAN, AND S. J. BOLEY. Pathophysiological effects of bowel distension on intestinal blood flow (II). *Curr. Top. Surg. Res.* 2: 59–69, 1970.
186. VAN BEUREN, F. T., JR. Relation between intestinal damage and delayed operation in acute mechanical ileus. *Ann. Surg.* 72: 610–615, 1920.
187. VAN LIERE, E. J. The effect of anoxia on the alimentary tract. *Physiol. Rev.* 21: 307–323, 1941.
188. VAN ZWALENBURG, C. Strangulation resulting from distention of hollow viscera. *Ann. Surg.* 46: 780–786, 1907.
189. VATNER, S. F., D. FRANKLIN, AND R. L. VAN CITTERS. Mesenteric vasoactivity associated with eating and digestion in the conscious dog. *Am. J. Physiol.* 219: 170–174, 1970.
190. WALUS, K. M., J. D. FONDACARO, AND E. D. JACOBSON. Effects of adenosine and its derivatives on the canine intestinal vasculature. *Gastroenterology* 81: 327–334, 1981.
191. WALUS, K. M., J. D. FONDACARO, AND E. D. JACOBSON. Effects of calcium and its antagonists on the canine mesenteric circulation. *Circ. Res.* 48: 692–700, 1981.

192. WALUS, K. M., J. D. FONDACARO, AND E. D. JACOBSON. Hemodynamic and metabolic changes during stimulation of ileal motility. *Dig. Dis. Sci.* 26: 1069–1077, 1981.
193. WALUS, K. M., J. D. FONDACARO, AND E. D. JACOBSON. A further characterization of histamine $H_1$ and $H_2$ effects and blockade in canine intestinal circulation. *Dig. Dis. Sci.* 26: 1542–1549, 1981.
194. WALUS, K. M., AND E. D. JACOBSON. Relation between small intestinal motility and circulation. *Am. J. Physiol.* 241 (*Gastrointest. Liver Physiol.* 4): G1–G15, 1981.
195. WILLIAMS, J. H., JR., M. MAGER, AND E. D. JACOBSON. Relationship of mesenteric blood flow to intestinal absorption of carbohydrates. *J. Lab. Clin. Med.* 6: 853–863, 1964.
196. YU, Y., M. LUKE, C. C. YU, AND C. C. CHOU. Distribution of blood flow in the intestine with hypertonic glucose in the lumen. *Surgery St. Louis* 78: 520–525, 1975.
197. ZEIGLER, M. G., R. W. BARTON, AND K. G. SWAN. Mesenteric blood flow and small intestinal motility in the dog. *Surgery St. Louis* 73: 649–656, 1973.
198. ZFASS, A. M., L. HOROWITZ, AND J. T. FARRAR. Effect of vascular occlusion on small-bowel intraluminal pressures in dogs. *Am. J. Dig. Dis.* 12: 154–161, 1967.

CHAPTER 41

# Hepatic circulation

CLIVE V. GREENWAY  
W. WAYNE LAUTT

Hepatorenal Research Unit, Department of Pharmacology and Therapeutics, University of Manitoba, Winnipeg, Canada

CHAPTER CONTENTS

Anatomy and Microcirculation
  Origin and distribution of hepatic blood supply
  Microcirculation
Blood Flows and Vascular Resistance
  Sinusoidal pressure
  Relation between portal flow and liver mass
  Intrinsic hepatic arterial flow regulation
    Metabolic control
    Hepatic arterial buffer response
    Autoregulation
    Other intrinsic responses
  Extrinsic hepatic arterial flow regulation
    Nervous control
    Autoregulatory escape
    Responses to humoral factors
    Blood gases and pH
    Other stimuli
Effects of Hepatic Blood Flow on Uptake of Substrates
  Goresky model
  Equilibrium model
  Parallel-tube model
  Comparison of models
  Measurement of hepatic blood flow by uptake
Hepatic Blood Volume
  Basic principles, terminology, and normal values
  Hepatic blood volume in perspective
  Passive changes in hepatic blood volume
    Flow and arterial resistance
    External pressure
    Redistribution of flows
    Hepatic venous resistance
  Active capacitance vessel constriction
    Sympathetic nerves and catecholamines
    Angiotensin
    Receptors in hepatic venous bed
  Reflex control of hepatic venous bed
    Reflex responses in anesthetized dogs
    Reflex responses in anesthetized cats
    General observations
  Control of cardiac preload and responses to drugs
  Other complex responses involving hepatic venous bed
    Hemorrhage and infusions
    Hypertension
    Shock and endotoxin
    Exercise
  Future prospects
Hepatic Fluid Exchange
  Sites of filtration and interstitial fluid
  Reabsorption of filtered fluid
  Effects of drugs on fluid exchange
  Effects of hepatic nerve stimulation on fluid exchange

*The liver is composed of two things: glandular acini and various branches of vessels. Hence if some common work is to result from them, there must be some commerce between the glands and the vessels.*

M. Malpighi, 1666 (268a)

THE LIVER IS SUPPLIED by the portal vein and hepatic artery. All parenchymal cells of the liver are perfused by mixed arterial and portal blood, and the distribution within and between liver lobes is uniform. Some features of the hepatic microcirculation are described in this chapter, including the role of the acinus. The liver receives a total blood flow of 100–130 ml·min$^{-1}$·100 g$^{-1}$ liver (30 ml·min$^{-1}$·kg$^{-1}$ body wt) in the dog, cat, and human, and the hepatic artery contributes 20%–33%. About 25% of the cardiac output perfuses the liver, although it constitutes only 2.5% of body wt. Extrahepatic vascular pressures are 80–120 mmHg in the hepatic artery and 7–10 mmHg in the portal vein. Changes in intrahepatic vascular resistance affect portal pressure but not portal flow, which is determined by arteriolar resistances in the splanchnic organs that drain into the portal vein. Sinusoidal pressure is almost equal to portal pressure. Intrahepatic resistance in the portal circuit is postsinusoidal and lies in lobar hepatic veins. The hepatic venous sphincters constrict in response to nerves and various blood-borne agents. The distensibility of these sphincters determines the nonlinear relationships between portal and inferior vena cava (IVC) pressure.

Some data indicate that portal flow and/or factors in portal blood exert a trophic effect that controls liver mass. Other data indicate chronic liver hypertrophy results in increased portal flow. These relationships between portal flow and liver mass require further study.

Intrinsic mechanisms in the hepatic arterial resistance vessels are reviewed. The hepatic arterial flow is neither controlled nor affected by parenchymal cell metabolism. The hepatic artery shows mild pressure-induced autoregulation that is dependent on a washout of locally produced adenosine, and the effects of portal flow on hepatic arterial resistance are mediated by washout of locally produced adenosine, which results in inverse changes in hepatic arterial flow. This latter mechanism, the hepatic arterial buffer response, is a major intrinsic mechanism that buffers the impact of portal flow changes on total hepatic flow.

Hepatic nerve stimulation and norepinephrine infusions produce constriction of the hepatic arterioles that is short-lived in cats due to autoregulatory escape but maintained in dogs. Constriction of the hepatic lobar venous resistance raises portal pressure, and this is maintained for the duration of stimulation. These neural effects are mediated by norepinephrine acting on $\alpha$-adrenoceptors. Cholinergic neural effects on the vasculature have not been proved. Autoregulatory escape is a puzzling phenomenon, and its mechanism and physiological significance are not yet understood. Interactions between neural, hormonal, and intrinsic control of hepatic arterial flow require further study. Although many vasoactive substances, nutrients, and intestinal hormones alter hepatic arterial flow when administered in pharmacological doses, only adenosine has so far been shown to have a physiologically significant role in the control of hepatic arterial flow. The hepatic arterial flow buffers changes in portal flow and maintains total hepatic flow as constant as possible.

The effects of hemodynamic changes on hepatic uptake of substrates and drugs are not well understood. The various models (the Goresky model, the equilibrium model, and the parallel-tube model) are described, and attempts to differentiate between them are discussed. Changes in hepatic blood flow would be expected to alter elimination of drugs with a high extraction more than those with a low extraction, but good experimental data are not available to critically test theoretical predictions. Although clearance techniques have been widely used to measure hepatic blood flow, the validity of these measurements has not been established over a wide range of flows and conditions. None of the substances used has been conclusively shown to be removed only by the liver and none is completely removed from the plasma during a single pass through the liver. Techniques in which hepatic extraction is assumed but not measured cannot be considered reliable. Basic animal studies are urgently needed to clarify these clearance and kinetic concepts and to find and validate appropriate methods that can be used to measure hepatic blood flow in humans.

Hepatic blood volume is large (35 ml/100 g liver; 12% of total blood volume), and the liver is an important blood volume reserve. The pressure-volume relationship, compliance, stressed volume, and unstressed volume are described and reviewed. Venoconstriction by the hepatic nerves and norepinephrine, mediated through $\alpha_2$-adrenoceptors, can mobilize up to 50% of hepatic blood volume, and this involves changes in unstressed volume with no change in compliance. The importance of the liver as a blood volume reserve is compared with that of the intestine, spleen, and other organs. Several mechanisms, especially changes in hepatic lobar venous resistance, tend to maintain portal pressure constant and to minimize passive changes in the hepatic blood volume. This allows control of the blood volume by the central nervous system (CNS).

Reflex control of hepatic and splanchnic venous beds by arterial baroreceptors and chemoreceptors has been demonstrated in dogs but not in cats. Anesthetics significantly depress venous reflex responses, and hepatic blood volume control cannot yet be studied in conscious animals or humans. The importance of simultaneous measurements of both blood volume and intrahepatic pressure in studies on reflex control is stressed.

The role of hepatic venous responses in control of cardiac preload and cardiac output is discussed. The actions of a variety of drugs on the hepatic venous bed and on cardiac output support the hypothesis that hepatic and splanchnic venoconstriction are important components in the actions of drugs that produce large sustained increases in cardiac output. Conversely, drugs that interfere with reflex control of the hepatic venous bed generally cause postural hypotension in clinical use. The importance of the hepatic venous system in hemorrhage, hypertension, shock, and exercise is reviewed. The splanchnic bed mobilizes or pools up to 60% of changes in total blood volume caused by hemorrhage or infusions, respectively, in cats, dogs, and humans, but the mechanisms of these effects have not yet been analyzed. Exciting new approaches to noninvasive measurements of hepatic and intestinal blood volume are described.

Fluid exchange in the liver is dependent on the classic Starling forces, but the colloid osmotic pressure gradient from sinusoid to lymphatic is small. During raised intrahepatic pressure, high-protein fluid is filtered from the sinusoids into lymphatics and peritoneal cavity. Protective mechanisms that limit filtration are not present in the liver, and fluid movements are large relative to those in other organs. The rate of filtration is directly proportional to sinusoidal pressure. Sympathetic nerve stimulation appears to reduce the filtration rate by an unknown mechanism.

In addition to the many reviews and articles cited here, a book resulting from a symposium in 1981 offers a review of many aspects of the hepatic circulation (218).

## ANATOMY AND MICROCIRCULATION

### Origin and Distribution of Hepatic Blood Supply

The common hepatic artery derives from the celiac artery (which also gives rise to the splenic and gastric arteries) and meets the portal vein near the hilum of the liver. It divides into the gastroduodenal artery and the hepatic artery proper, which passes to the liver adjacent to the portal vein. Frequently a gastroepiploic artery arises just distal to the T junction formed by the gastroduodenal and hepatic arteries. Portal blood flow derives from the spleen (10%), stomach (20%), pancreas (10%), and intestine (60%). Contributions of these organs vary widely, depending on the physiological state of the organism. The portal vein and the hepatic artery pass to the liver via the hilum along with lymphatics and anterior and posterior hepatic nerve plexuses. Flow is distributed to the parenchymal cell mass via the finest branches of the hepatic arterioles and portal venules, which drain into the acinus.

Studies of arterial and portal flow distribution with radioactive microspheres in anesthetized cats and dogs (130, 131) and anesthetized rats (22, 144) and also with $^{86}$Rb uptake in rats (281) show that streamlining of portal blood does not occur and that areas of the liver parenchyma are uniformly perfused by portal and arterial flow. Functional studies show that bile flow is equally stimulated by infusions of taurocholate into the hepatic artery or portal vein in cats (227). Indocyanine green (ICG) extraction (236), bromosulfophthalein (BSP) clearance (37), $^{85}$Kr extraction (24), and dilution curves for albumin and red cells (60) were similar after portal or hepatic arterial administration. Some earlier studies had suggested incomplete mixing of blood from portal and arterial sources in the sinusoids (21, 163), but these studies were repeated, and it was found that the difference could be accounted for by the presence of intact gastroduodenal arteries (24, 243).

Flow distribution is not altered by hepatic nerve stimulation, as shown by distribution of radioactive microspheres (130) and normal uptake of lidocaine (238) and $O_2$ (211). Raised hepatic venous pressure also does not cause redistribution of arterial or portal flow within the liver (131) or altered $O_2$ consumption (210). Norepinephrine and epinephrine did not alter $O_2$ consumption, ICG extraction, elimination of ethanol, or bile flow, indicating an absence of redistribution (203). Histamine caused some redistribution of portal blood flow toward the hilar regions in dogs (131).

Thus evidence obtained in vivo from normally perfused livers strongly indicates that, on average, all parenchymal cells of the liver are perfused by mixed arterial and portal blood and that distribution between and within liver lobes is uniform. Uneven flow distribution represents a perturbed hepatic perfusion and is frequently seen in isolated liver preparations.

*Microcirculation*

The acinus is the functional microvascular unit of the liver [Fig. 1; (293–295)]. It consists of a cluster of parenchymal cells, irregular in size (~2 mm diam) and shape, that is formed about an axis consisting of a terminal portal venule, a hepatic arteriole, a bile ductule, lymphatics, and nerves contained within a limiting plate of parenchymal cells. In a standard histological preparation, these vascular stalks appear as the portal triads located in hexagonal array around a terminal hepatic venule. Blood enters the acinus at its center, flows outward, and drains into terminal he-

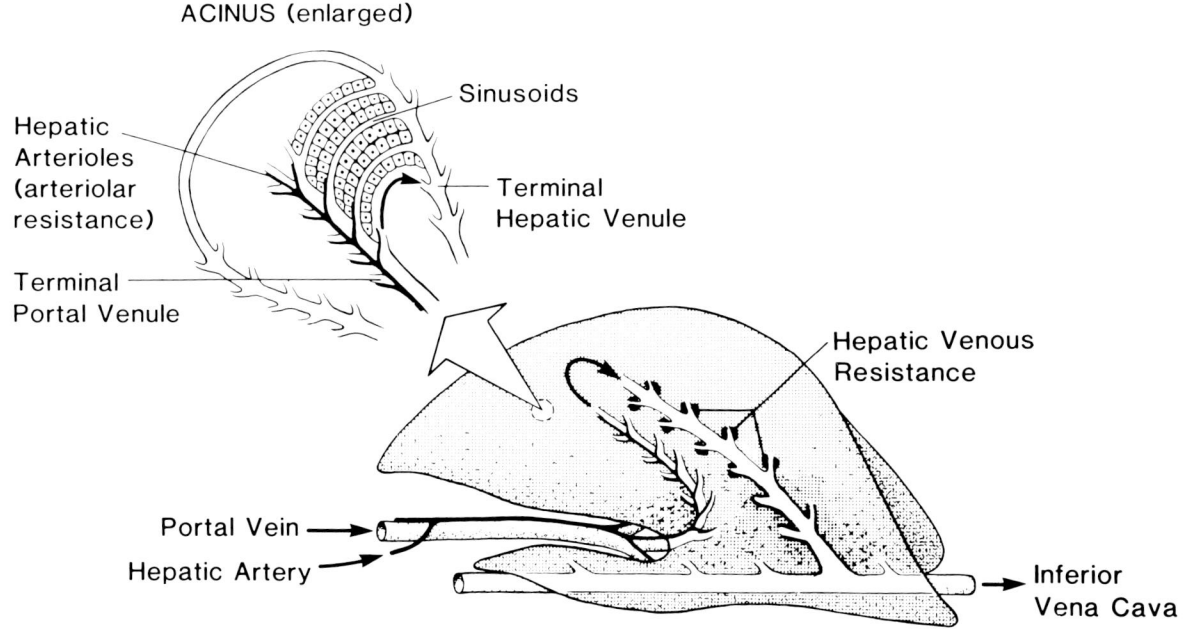

FIG. 1. Diagram of hepatic vascular bed.

patic venules at the periphery of the acinus. Arterial blood may enter the sinusoid directly or may first flow through the complex peribiliary plexus prior to entry into sinusoids. The functional significance of this peribiliary plexus is not known. Arterioportal anastomoses are seen only in the rat. In hamsters and humans, arteriolar and portal blood does not mix prior to entry into sinusoids (384).

Arterioles enter the acinus only in the central region or zone 1 (384). This region has the highest degree of oxygenation and the highest activity of respiratory enzymes. Zone 3 lies on the outer limits of the acinus and is supplied by blood that has already passed the parenchymal cells of zones 1 and 2. Zone 3 is supplied by the least-oxygenated blood and is rich in microsomal enzymes. Functional implications and distribution of enzymes in the various zones have been reviewed (145, 147, 293–295), and the classification of chemically induced liver injury has been discussed relative to the acinus and its zones (289). Rappaport (295) has strongly argued that the traditional description of hepatic hexagonal lobules should not be continued because there is "no structural, nor secretory unit in the imaginary hexagonal lobule," and we concur with this argument.

Discussions on hepatic uptake must take into account the unique microvascular arrangement of the acinus, which is ideally suited to the creation of high concentration gradients from zone 1 to zone 3. Flow in adjacent sinusoids is concurrent, and there is no opportunity within the hepatic structure for diffusible materials to short-circuit the vascular pathways (104). Oxygen cannot diffuse from arterial or portal blood to the venous compartment, and lack of significant intrahepatic shunts (24, 37, 60, 131, 144, 227, 236) indicates that hepatic venous levels of $O_2$ should be an index of the $O_2$ in blood leaving the sinusoids from zone 3. A similar statement is true for other compounds. This microvascular arrangement also precludes diffusion of substances from zone 3 back to the central region of the acinus where the inflow vessels are located. Metabolic by-products of hepatic parenchymal cells cannot influence the vascular smooth muscle that regulates hepatic arterial flow. Hepatic venous $O_2$ levels can be markedly depressed in situations of elevated $O_2$ extraction without resulting in arterial dilation (see *Intrinsic Hepatic Arterial Flow Regulation* p. 1524).

Microvascular dimensions for the human and rat liver have been summarized (293, 295). The mean diameter for terminal portal venules is ~47 μm in humans and ~15–20 μm in rats. Terminal hepatic arterioles are 24 μm and terminal hepatic venules 66 μm in diameter. The average acinus is 1.5 mm long and 0.8 mm wide with a volume of 1.26 mm³. Mean sinusoidal length was 330 μm (range 220–480 μm) in humans and 250 μm in rats. Blood passing along a sinusoid is sequentially distributed to ~20 hepatocytes (147), and individual hepatocytes may be in contact with plasma on two sides of the cell. (For a discussion of extracellular spaces, see HEPATIC FLUID EXCHANGE, p. 1551).

Sinusoids in zone 1 occupy a smaller volume fraction of liver space than sinusoids in zone 3, and plasma in zone 1 is more extensively in contact with parenchymal cell surfaces than plasma in zone 3 (264). Analysis of corrosion casts (159) and intravital microscopic analysis (145) shows that sinusoids of zone 1 are highly anastomotic, whereas sinusoids of zone 3 are straight and radially arranged. Endothelial fenestrations are also reported to be larger in zone 1 (140, 275). Red cell velocities vary in different sinusoids (200). The functional significance of these observations is not yet clear. Stimulation of the hepatic nerves caused a 50% reduction in total liver blood volume (see *Active Capacitance Vessel Constriction*, p. 1543) with little change in total blood flow (127, 211). Flow velocity must have increased considerably; however, hepatic uptake of $O_2$ (211) and lidocaine (238) were not altered. This indicates that lateral diffusion from plasma to hepatocyte is so fast that flow velocity may not be a limiting factor.

## BLOOD FLOWS AND VASCULAR RESISTANCE

The liver receives a total blood flow of 100–130 ml·min⁻¹·100 g⁻¹ liver (30 ml·min⁻¹·kg⁻¹ body wt) in the dog, cat, and human, and the hepatic artery contributes 20%–33% of the total. About 25% of the cardiac output perfuses the liver, although it constitutes only ~2.5% of body wt (136). Extrahepatic vascular pressures are ~100 mmHg for the hepatic artery and 7–10 mmHg for the portal vein. Changes in intrahepatic vascular resistance affect portal pressure but not portal flow, which is determined by arteriolar resistances in the splanchnic organs that drain into the portal vein.

### Sinusoidal Pressure

Previous reviewers (136, 213, 293) have concluded incorrectly that sinusoidal pressure is well below portal pressure and close to IVC pressure, based on one study in rats (271). Descriptions of portal resistance in the literature indicate that a presinusoidal resistance is assumed because portal flow rather than total hepatic flow was used in the calculations. The idea of a low sinusoidal pressure therefore appears to have been accepted by assumption and frequent repetition. However, many studies have provided direct and indirect evidence that sinusoidal pressure is close to portal pressure and that resistance in the portal circuit is postsinusoidal (114, 132, 134, 207, 231, 232, 265, 292). This pressure is significant because it relates to clinical interpretation of wedged venous pressure, ascites formation, control of hepatic blood volume, and fluid exchange and calculation of hepatic vascular resistances.

Greenway and Oshiro (132) passed a catheter from the jugular vein into the hepatic vein in dogs and found that hepatic lobar venous pressure approached portal pressure. Because these catheters were sealed at the tip and recorded side pressures and because cardiac venous pressure waves were clearly visible, they concluded that the catheters were not wedged. These data indicate that hepatic venous resistance accounted for the pressure drop across the portal circuit and that sinusoidal pressure was close to portal pressure. Similar data were obtained in cats (114). Stimulation of the hepatic nerves and norepinephrine infusions caused increases in portal and hepatic lobar venous pressures (114, 134). With chronically implanted capsules in dogs, Laine et al. (207) found portal pressures of 7.8 mmHg and interstitial pressures of 5.8 mmHg with venous pressures of 2 mmHg. Sinusoidal pressure was estimated to be only slightly lower than portal pressure. Mitzner (265) estimated sinusoidal pressure in the canine liver to be ~6.1 mmHg when portal pressure was 7 mmHg and hepatic venous pressure 1.6 mmHg. Additional evidence that portal and sinusoidal pressures are nearly equal is provided by recent studies on hepatic compliance [(134); see *Basic Principles, Terminology, and Normal Values*, p. 1537].

Thus the evidence indicates that hepatic lobar venous pressure is 80%–100% of portal pressure and that portal pressure or hepatic lobar venous pressure, but not large hepatic vein or IVC pressure, can be used as an estimate of sinusoidal pressure. Portal circuit resistance is largely postsinusoidal. One consequence of this is that calculation of hepatic arterial conductance or resistance should use hepatic arterial minus portal pressure as the pressure difference across the resistance vessels (118). This does not markedly alter the calculations, especially if the results are expressed as changes in resistance or conductance. However, previous calculations of portal resistance or conductance contain serious errors because they used portal flow instead of total hepatic flow. This necessitates reevaluation of the effects of pharmacological agents on portal resistance, and terminology must be clear in future studies so that "portal resistance," which implies presinusoidal resistance, is not confused with "hepatic lobar venous resistance," which is postsinusoidal.

In recent studies, we further validated the measurement of lobar venous pressures in cats, and we concluded that the postsinusoidal resistance site is located in lobar hepatic veins with a diameter of 1.5 to 2 mm over a length of <5 mm [Figs. 1–3; (231, 232)]. In dogs the resistance site has been localized to hepatic sphincters within 20 mm from the outlet of the hepatic veins into the IVC (234a, 242a). Pressure proximal to

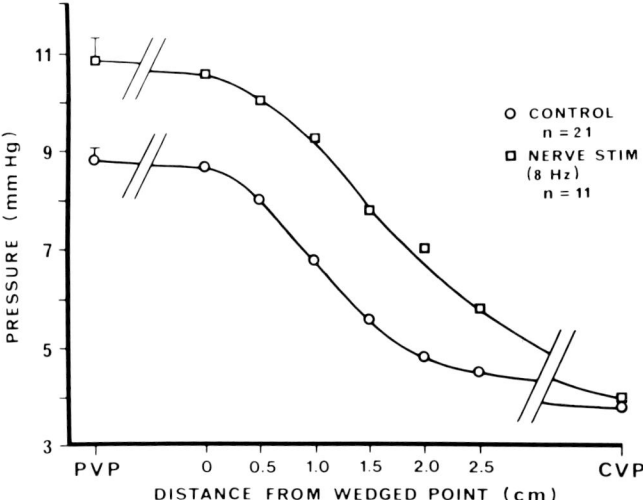

FIG. 2. Hepatic venous pressure profiles in basal state and at stable plateau phase during stimulation of hepatic nerves in cats. Portal venous pressure (PVP) and central venous pressure (CVP) were measured from stationary cannulas, whereas lobar venous profile was obtained by progressive withdrawal of lobar catheter. Pressures in portal vein and deep lobar venous pressures were not significantly different. Because pooled curves conceal steep contour of individual curves, data are recalculated in Fig. 3. [From Lautt et al. (232).]

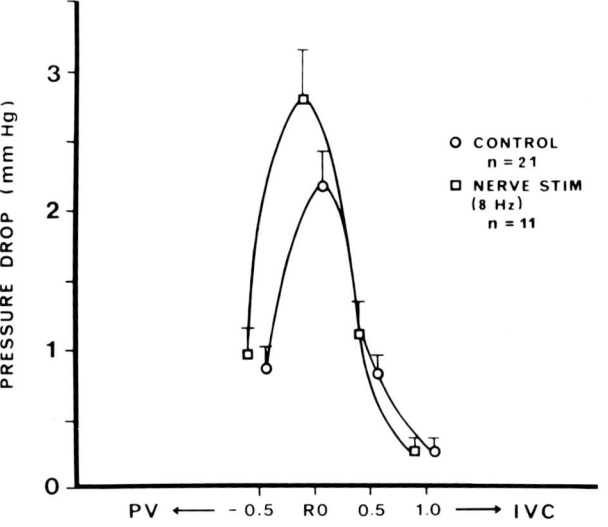

FIG. 3. Hepatic venous pressure profiles recalculated from Fig. 2. Steepest portion of each profile curve was identified (RO), and pressure drop proximal and distal to this position was calculated. Most postsinusoidal resistance occurs across a short segment of veins, and hepatic nerves cause constriction at this same site. Pressure gradient from portal vein (PV) to 5 mm proximal to hepatic venous sphincter is on left and pressure gradient between a site 10 mm distal to sphincter and inferior vena cava (IVC) is on right. [From Lautt et al. (232).]

this resistance site is equal to portal pressure, indicating that, in the control situation, presinusoidal and sinusoidal resistances are insignificant, and the entire pressure drop from portal vein to IVC occurs across the hepatic lobar venous resistance. However, during stimulation of the hepatic nerves and infusions of norepinephrine and angiotensin, some evidence for presinusoidal constriction was presented (231, 232, 234a, 242a).

When hepatic venous pressure is increased, the proportion of this pressure increment that is transmitted to the portal vein is less at low pressures and increases to ~75% at hepatic venous pressures >11 mmHg (123, 134, 158, 231). In one study, when hepatic venous pressure was >3.5 mmHg, pressure transmission to the portal vein was linear and almost 100% (18). Mitzner (265) suggested the postsinusoidal resistance site produced a waterfall effect whereby increases in central venous pressure were prevented from affecting sinusoidal pressure.

However, a true waterfall phenomenon does not exist, and even small increments in IVC pressure are partially transmitted upstream past the hepatic venous sphincters to the liver. The sphincters are distensible, and as IVC pressure rises, the proportion of this pressure transmitted to the liver increases (C. V. Greenway and W. W. Lautt, unpublished observations). This distensibility allows the large capacitance reservoir of the liver to protect the heart against acute large elevations in IVC pressure but minimizes changes in blood volume in the liver if the IVC pressure changes are small. The distensibility of the hepatic venous sphincters also explains how large changes in portal flow result in small changes in portal pressure.

Thus a variety of observations indicate that presinusoidal and postsinusoidal resistances in the portal circuit cannot be calculated by conventional methods, and these resistance values do not remain constant when pressures and flows are varied. This complex area requires much further study. Although the effects of many pharmacological agents on portal pressure have been studied (308, 309), these actions require reevaluation in the light of the previously mentioned considerations. (The physiological role of the postsinusoidal resistance site is further discussed in HEPATIC BLOOD VOLUME, p. 1537, and HEPATIC FLUID EXCHANGE, p. 1551).

Portal pressure increases induced by the hepatic nerves are mediated by $\alpha$-adrenergic receptors and can be blocked by phentolamine (214) and yohimbine (328). Increases produced by infusions of norepinephrine are less completely blocked by yohimbine (328). Whereas adenosine can abolish the constrictor effects of nerve stimulation, angiotensin, and norepinephrine on hepatic arterial resistance, no such block is seen for the portal pressure elevations produced by these stimuli (233). Most of the rise in portal pressure produced by nerve stimulation, norepinephrine, angiotensin (cats) and histamine (dogs) has been shown to be consequent to constriction of the hepatic venous sphincters (231, 232, 234a, 242a).

*Relation Between Portal Flow and Liver Mass*

The following discussion is speculative, but important mechanisms that require investigation are indicated by the data. After partial hepatectomy in pigs, portal blood flow initially increased both in absolute units and relative to the remaining liver mass. This increase preceded the maximum regeneration phase (181). Reduction of portal flow by shunts results in atrophy and failure of liver regeneration after partial hepatectomy (25). Studies where pancreatic and intestinal flow were diverted to different parts of the liver suggested that liver mass depends on hepatotrophic factors in pancreatic venous blood (252). These observations indicate that portal flow and/or factors in portal blood exert a trophic effect on the liver that controls liver mass. In contrast, other observations have been interpreted to indicate liver mass controls portal flow in some way. When a series of enzyme-inducing agents were tested for effects on hepatic blood flow, only phenobarbital increased liver mass. This increase was accompanied by an increase in portal flow, and there was no increase in flow expressed per unit liver weight (254, 273). Thus chronic changes in liver weight were associated with changes in portal flow, leading to the speculation that "total hepatic blood flow is influenced by the mass of the liver and the responsible, but as yet unknown, mechanism involves the portal circulation" (273). Similar conclusions were reached as a result of anticonvulsant therapy in epileptics (288). A relationship between liver mass and portal flow or composition is clear, whereas causality is not clear. A primary elevation in portal flow or trophic factors might induce liver growth, or hepatic hypertrophy may feed back to the splanchnic organs to increase portal flow. In addition, reduced portal flow to the liver leads to responses that tend to return portal flow to normal. Diversion of portal blood by portacaval shunting resulted in increased splanchnic blood flow and generally reduced peripheral vascular resistance (241, 368), possibly mediated by elevated plasma glucagon levels (20) or by reduced pressure sensed at some as yet unlocalized hepatic baroreceptors. Evidence for the existence of hepatic baroreceptors has been reported, but their physiological function has not been shown (for review see ref. 221).

*Intrinsic Hepatic Arterial Flow Regulation*

Intrinsic regulation refers to mechanisms that regulate hepatic arterial flow exclusive of nerves and blood-borne vasoactive compounds. This area has recently undergone some major conceptual changes. Previous views were that the hepatic arterial flow was controlled by metabolic demands of the parenchymal cell mass; the hepatic artery showed mild autoregulation in response to altered perfusion pressure, and this autoregulation was myogenic in origin; altered portal perfusion caused an inverse change in hepatic arterial flow that was mediated by a myogenic mechanism or was secondary to altered $O_2$ supply. Recent data disprove these earlier concepts and are consistent with three hypotheses: *1)* the hepatic artery is not controlled or affected by parenchymal cell metabolism, *2)* the hepatic artery shows mild autoregulation that is dependent on a washout of locally produced adenosine, *3)* the effect of portal flow on the hepatic arterial resistance is mediated by washout of locally produced adenosine, which results in inverse changes in hepatic arterial flow. This latter mechanism, the hepatic arterial buffer response, is a major intrinsic control that buffers the impact of portal flow changes on total hepatic flow.

METABOLIC CONTROL. The data showing lack of subservience of the hepatic arterial flow to hepatic $O_2$ or metabolic requirements have been reviewed (222). Alteration of hepatic $O_2$ supply was attained by isovolemic hemodilution with a large volume of 1:1 Ringers solution and Dextran 75 in anesthetized cats. Oxygen delivery decreased to 68% of control, and hepatic venous and portal $O_2$ content declined. The intestine responded with a vasodilation related to the $O_2$ deficit, but the hepatic artery did not show a dilation; it showed a small constriction, and total hepatic flow remained constant. The degree of arterial flow change correlated inversely with the portal flow change and provided the first clue that this was a flow regulation rather than an $O_2$ supply–based regulation (209). In a separate series of experiments, hepatic $O_2$ demand was altered either by dinitrophenol to increase $O_2$ demand or SKF 525A (2-diethylaminoethyl-2,2-diphenylvalerate HCl) to inhibit metabolism. The hepatic $O_2$ demands were maintained solely by altered hepatic extraction. Despite the fact that the intestinal blood supply showed metabolism-related changes in blood flow, the hepatic arterial flow showed no tendency to change in correlation with $O_2$ demand or blood gas levels in portal or hepatic venous blood (215).

One response that initially appeared to contradict this lack of hepatic metabolic control of arterial flow was the accepted fact that bile salts stimulate hepatic metabolism (as shown by increased bile flow) and they also cause hepatic arterial vasodilation. However, the vascular and metabolic responses of the liver to bile salts are independent and occur at different doses (227). Low doses of taurocholate (1 $\mu$M·min$^{-1}$·kg$^{-1}$ body wt) produce elevated bile flow but no arterial vasodilation. Higher doses given by close intra-arterial infusion produce dose-related vasodilator responses in both the superior mesenteric and hepatic arteries. The independence of vascular and metabolic effects was shown when the same dose of taurocholate, infused into either the portal vein or the hepatic artery, produced equal effects on bile flow, although the hepatic arterial vasodilation was two to three times greater during intra-arterial infusion than during intraportal infusion. These studies were done in cats. Lactic acidosis in dogs resulted in elevated portal flow, reduced arterial flow, and reduced $O_2$ delivery to the liver, and hepatic venous $O_2$ levels fell significantly (168). Chronic alcohol exposure in rats led to elevated $O_2$ demand by the liver, but the hepatic artery constricted (39).

Thus evidence from many sources supports the statement that hepatic arterial resistance is not controlled by hepatic parenchymal cell metabolism (212). This is further supported by the microcirculatory architecture described previously that precludes parenchymal cell metabolites reaching the hepatic arterioles.

HEPATIC ARTERIAL BUFFER RESPONSE. The earliest known studies reporting an effect of changes in portal perfusion on the hepatic arterial flow were by Betz (1863) and Gad (1873), and the term *hepatic arterial buffer response* was suggested for this intrinsic regulatory mechanism (219). Earlier work was reviewed by Greenway and Stark (136). Although it is clear that changes in portal flow cause inverse changes in hepatic arterial resistance, the mechanism of this response has remained elusive until recently. To study the mechanism, it was essential to have a preparation that shows reproducible responses that could then be manipulated according to the hypothesis being tested. A suitable model was proposed by Lautt et al. (235). Hepatic arterial flow and superior mesenteric arterial flow were measured with electromagnetic flowmeters after all other arteries supplying the portal flow were ligated. Although the responses produced were not quantitatively normal (223), the reproducibility of the response was well suited for pharmacological studies of the mechanism. The most consistent quantitative expression of the buffer response is the buffer capacity—the change in hepatic arterial flow divided by the change in portal flow expressed as a percentage.

Recent studies support the hypothesis that washout of locally produced adenosine can account for the hepatic arterial buffer response. Other factors, e.g., the hepatic nerves, myogenic responses, and systemic vasoactive compounds, may also significantly affect hepatic arterial flow and interact with the buffer response. Certain criteria have been demonstrated to support the hypothesis that adenosine mediates the buffer response: *1)* Adenosine must dilate the hepatic artery. *2)* Portal blood must have access to the arterial resistance vessels so that portal flow can wash away adenosine from the area of the resistance vessels. *3)* Potentiators of exogenous adenosine effects should potentiate the buffer response. *4)* Blockers of exogenous adenosine effects should inhibit the buffer response.

The first criterion that adenosine must fulfill as a candidate for the intrinsic regulator of the buffer response is to dilate the hepatic artery. Dose-response curves indicate that adenosine is an extremely effective dilator. A dose of 2 mg·min$^{-1}$·kg$^{-1}$ body wt into the hepatic artery doubles hepatic arterial conductance without systemic hemodynamic effects due to recirculation (235). The extreme lability of adenosine prevents any calculations of local adenosine concentrations from the rates of infusion. Maximal hepatic arterial vasodilation could not be obtained with adenosine without producing systemic vascular effects. However, kinetic analysis with a double reciprocal plot of dose and effect indicated a maximal dilation would be equivalent to an increase in conductance of 250% over basal level. The intra-arterial dose that produced a half-maximal dilation was 0.19 mg·min$^{-1}$·kg$^{-1}$ body wt (233). In contrast prostaglandin E$_2$ (PGE$_2$), secretin, isoproterenol, histamine, and glucagon produced calculated maximal increases in hepatic arterial conductance of <170% (126, 301). Thus adenosine causes the most dramatic dilation of the hepatic artery reported with any drug or stimulus.

For adenosine levels to be controlled in the area of the hepatic resistance vessels by washout into portal blood, it must be demonstrated that portal blood has access to the arterial resistance vessels. This was shown by the fact that vasoactive compounds infused into the portal blood produced vascular effects on the hepatic arterioles (227, 236, 309). If adenosine can diffuse from portal blood to arterial resistance vessels, it is reasonable to assume that diffusion can also occur in the opposite direction.

Regarding the third criterion, dipyridamole blocked uptake of adenosine into cells (267) and potentiated the dilator effects of exogenous adenosine. The buffer response was also potentiated, resulting in an increase in buffer capacity from 23% to 34% (235). The fourth criterion of correlating adenosine antagonism with blockade of the buffer response has been fulfilled with 3-isobutyl-1-methylxanthine (235), with the more consistent antagonist 8-phenyltheophylline (234), and with 8-sulfophenyltheophylline (83). These antagonists blocked the buffer response as well as the response to close-arterial infusions of adenosine. Dose-response relationships showed that the capacity of the buffer response and the dilator effect of exogenous adenosine were reduced in a parallel manner (233). The dilator effect of isoproterenol was not altered by 8-phenyltheophylline.

These data support the hypothesis that the local concentration of adenosine at the site of the hepatic arterial resistance vessels is controlled by washout into the portal vein. Alternate hypotheses not involving adenosine can be eliminated based on the complete abolition of the buffer response by adenosine antagonists, although the hepatic artery shows normal vascular responses to infusions of vasoconstrictors (W. W. Lautt, unpublished observations) and isoproterenol (234). [The development of this hypothesis with details of alternate hypotheses and implications can be followed in a series of reviews (212, 219, 222).]

Areas that require clarification include demonstration of the site of adenosine production and the site of hepatic arterial resistance. These sites may be localized within the portal triad, enclosed within the limiting plate that surrounds the hepatic arteriole, portal venule, and bile ductule in the space of Mall (Fig. 4). Although the data are consistent with the hypothesis that adenosine production is constant and local concentrations are regulated by washout, it is not clear if the basal production of adenosine can be altered by physiological factors.

The capacity of the hepatic arterial buffer response in the conscious animal has not been reported. Buffer capacities reported over the years vary greatly, depending on the methodology used. Isolated perfused livers (324) and livers perfused with arterial long circuits (158) show weak buffer capacities. Anesthetized, acute surgical preparations show a buffer capacity of ~25% in cats (219, 233, 235) and dogs (251). Other studies done for different purposes suggest buffer capacities of 61%–100% in rats (90) and dogs (143, 168). Problems of quantitation have been discussed in detail (223).

The physiological role of the buffer response has not yet been studied extensively. The original hypothesis relating the hepatic arterial buffer response to liver function proposed that the hepatic artery, rather than being subservient to hepatic metabolic demands, was the guardian of humoral clearance rates (212). Reduction of hepatic blood flow is known to decrease hepatic clearance of such compounds as BSP, ICG, colloidal gold, galactose, denatured albumin, lidocaine, oxyphenbutazone, colloidal chromic phosphate (for

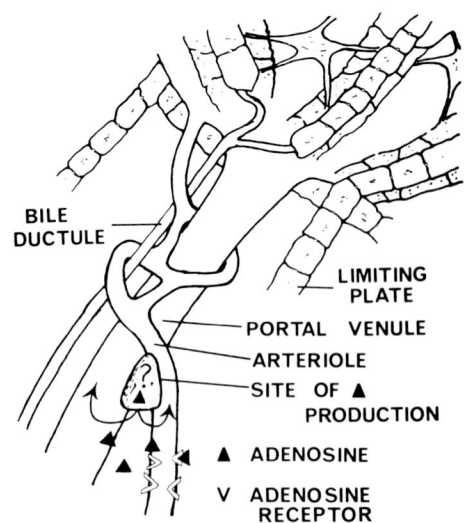

FIG. 4. Junctions of hepatic arterioles, portal venules, and sinusoids in the space of Mall showing postulated site of adenosine production. This adenosine concentration, which determines hepatic arteriolar tone, is regulated by production and washout into portal and hepatic arterial blood. [From Lautt et al. (235).]

review see ref. 223), and endogenous compounds, e.g., aldosterone, hydrocortisone, deoxycorticosterone, corticosterone, and progesterone (263). The hepatic arterial flow buffers changes in portal flow and tends to minimize the impact of these portal flow changes on hepatic clearances.

Other possible functions of the buffer response have been suggested. The consequences to total $O_2$ supply of portal flow reduction and arterial flow elevation protect against hypoxic damage induced by hypovolemia or other low-flow states. This function may only be of consequence for large portal flow reductions because the liver normally receives more $O_2$ than it requires and it can readily extract more $O_2$ to compensate for altered delivery (39, 209, 215). Oxygen delivery can be reduced to 60% with only a modest (<10%) decline in $O_2$ consumption (209, 245, 246). Blumgart et al. (24) calculated that the 24% buffer capacity in their preparations held total $O_2$ supply almost steady. Thus, although $O_2$ delivery per se is not regulated, the buffer mechanism assures hepatic priority in terms of $O_2$ supply in any situation where portal flow is restricted. However, in situations of elevated portal flow and compensatory decrease in arterial flow, total $O_2$ delivery to the liver can actually be reduced as a result of the buffer response (168).

The lack of ability of the liver to regulate its blood flow in accordance with the metabolic activity of the parenchymal cells is not disadvantageous to the liver under normal physiological conditions because of the excess $O_2$ delivered and the hepatic capacity to increase $O_2$ extraction. However, in some pathological states, this lack of metabolic control of blood flow can be detrimental. In situations where $O_2$ demand becomes excessive, i.e., during chronic alcohol exposure (174), the liver cannot protect itself by dilating the hepatic artery. It has been reported that chronic alcohol consumption leads to nearly doubling of hepatic $O_2$ use, and 60%–80% of this $O_2$ is used for metabolism of alcohol, primarily for mitochondrial reoxidation of NADH (174). Alcoholic liver damage can be augmented by keeping rats in an $O_2$-poor environment, and damage can be prevented by administration of the metabolic inhibitor propylthiouracil (173). Thus the evidence that alcohol-induced damage is hypoxic in nature is strongly but not universally (367) supported, and the utility of this evidence was shown in a clinical trial where alcohol-damaged livers in humans recovered significantly after propylthiouracil (282). Chronic alcohol dosing of rats led to elevated $O_2$ consumption with no dilation of the hepatic artery (39). The hepatic artery showed a mild constriction, probably in response to the mild elevation in portal flow that was seen in these animals.

Evidence for increased toxicity of other compounds in a relatively hypoxic liver was also reported. The formation of active toxic metabolites may occur to a greater extent, and the ability of glutathione to detoxify such metabolites may be reduced when the $NAD^+/NADH$ ratio is altered by hypoxia. This may occur with carbon tetrachloride (330) and halothane (257). Could hepatic arterial vasodilation protect the liver by providing a more aerobic environment? There are no data that provide answers to this question, but a recent review of the buffer response provides evidence to support this possibility (223). It is interesting that the most useful prognostic indicator for a successful portacaval shunt is the presence and magnitude of the buffer response (47).

A note of caution must be added to these speculations. After portacaval shunt in dogs, hepatic arterial vasodilation did not persist, and by 3 wk, hepatic arterial flow had returned to the control levels (148). The importance of the buffer response in chronic situations requires further study.

AUTOREGULATION. The term *autoregulation* has been used rather loosely, and in this chapter we use it specifically to describe the nonlinearity of the hepatic arterial pressure-flow relationship. It has been assumed that this response, where an increase in arterial perfusion pressure results in constriction of the hepatic artery, is due to a myogenic response of the arteriolar smooth muscle to stretch (136, 157, 158). However, a metabolic washout hypothesis is equally tenable. Recent studies show that, like the hepatic arterial buffer response where portal flow can wash out adenosine from the area of the hepatic arterial resistance vessels, flow in the hepatic artery can also wash out this endogenous adenosine to completely account for autoregulation of the hepatic artery (83). By this mechanism, increased arterial flow secondary to increased pressure results in a washout of adenosine from the space of Mall and leads to a constriction of the hepatic artery. The adenosine antagonists, 8-phenyltheophylline and 8-sulfophenyltheophylline, convert the typical pressure-flow curve from one that is convex to the pressure axis to one that is linear. Dose-related decreases in autoregulation, buffer response, and response to exogenous adenosine were reported (83).

OTHER INTRINSIC RESPONSES. After release of a complete occlusion of the hepatic artery, a brief but large hyperemic episode occurs—postocclusive hyperemia. In dogs the flow overshoot was related to the duration of the occlusion, and reduced portal flow inhibited the overshoot (157). We could not confirm this relationship to duration of occlusion in cats, and adenosine antagonists did not alter the postocclusive hyperemia (Lautt and Legare, unpublished observations). The mechanism of postocclusive hyperemia is unknown. A myogenic response has been suggested as the mechanism of both the hepatic arterial buffer response and pressure-induced autoregulation in the hepatic artery based on the ability of papaverine, a vasodilator, to inhibit the responses (157). However, any mechanism would be unable to further dilate a fully dilated artery, and this test is thus unable to differentiate mechanisms. Infusion of isoproterenol was also able to eliminate autoregulation by fully dilating the hepatic artery (83). The ability of adenosine antagonists to completely block the buffer response and autoregulation eliminates the role of myogenic mechanisms in these responses. One situation where myogenic effects are possible is the hepatic arterial vasoconstriction during raised hepatic venous pressure. This effect was seen when portal flow was held constant (18, 158) but was absent or small if portal flow was allowed to decline (210).

*Extrinsic Hepatic Arterial Flow Regulation*

NERVOUS CONTROL. Hepatic blood vessels receive a rich nerve supply from the anterior hepatic plexus (along the common hepatic artery) and the posterior hepatic plexus (along the portal vein). These plexuses meet at the junction of the hepatic artery and gastroduodenal artery and pass to the liver. The functions and effects of the hepatic nerves on the liver have been reviewed recently (216, 221). Direct stimulation of the mixed nerve bundle surrounding the hepatic artery produced a marked decrease in hepatic arterial flow and conductance (for review see ref. 136). The conductance changes were frequency dependent, reaching a maximum at 8–12 Hz in cats and dogs (127, 130). In cats the hepatic arterial flow begins to return to control levels despite continued nerve stimulation (Fig. 5). This phenomenon is called *autoregulatory escape*. On cessation of nerve stimulation, a period of hyperemia is seen in cats and dogs (130). The mechanism of this poststimulatory hyperemia is unknown but may be related to the mechanism of escape.

Hepatic arterial constriction induced by nerve stimulation can be reversed to a mild dilation after administration of α-adrenoceptor blockers (127). This dilation is blocked by β-adrenoceptor blockers (126). Yamaguchi and Garceau (382) showed a frequency-related elevation in hepatic venous norepinephrine levels that correlated with the changes in hepatic arterial conductance. Modulation of the constrictor effects of the hepatic nerves is seen with adenosine, but the inhibition is nonselective because the responses to norepinephrine, angiotensin, and vasopressin infusions are also inhibited (233). Glucagon infusions have been reported to depress neurogenic and norepinephrine-induced constriction in the canine hepatic artery (300). However, this did not occur in cats (112). Other potential neuromodulators have not been evaluated.

The hepatic arterial resistance vessels are probably not under tonic sympathetic nerve influence in anesthetized animals. Acute denervation produced no significant hemodynamic effects in cats (211) or dogs (61, 270). However, in these experiments only the

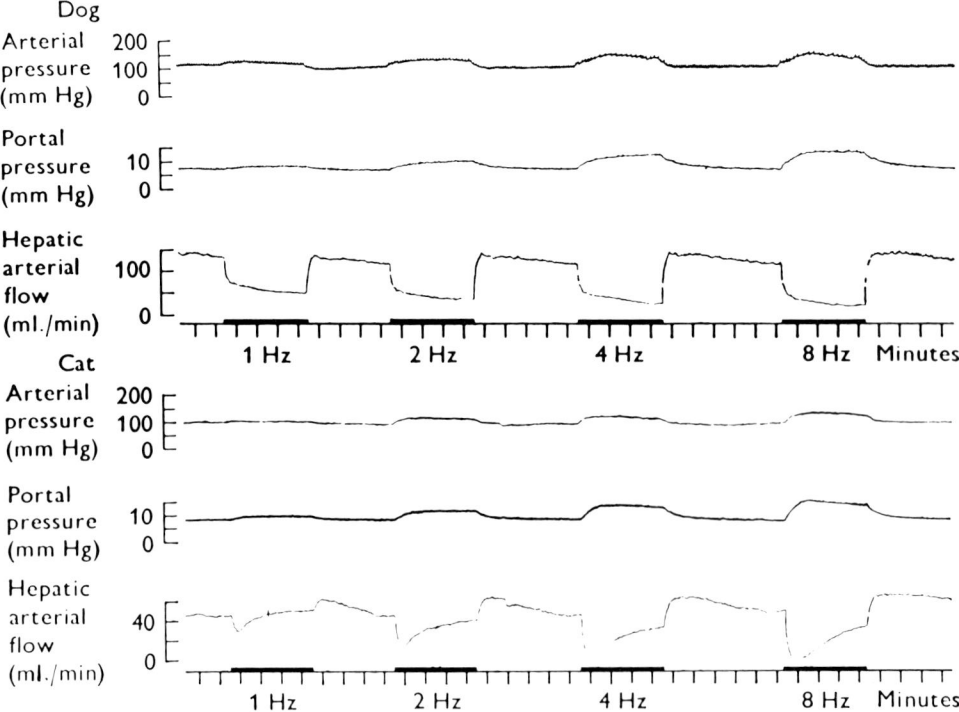

FIG. 5. Arterial pressure, portal pressure, and hepatic arterial flow responses to stimulation of hepatic nerves in 1 cat and 1 dog. Note occurrence of autoregulatory escape of flow response in cat but not in dog. [From Greenway and Oshiro (130).]

anterior nerve plexus was sectioned, and this produced a variable reduction in the reflex constriction (127, 217). Complete chronic (>2 wk) denervation of rapid onset (<20 min) can be obtained by painting phenol on the tissues at the hilum of the liver (225). Chronic sympathetic denervation by intraportal injection of 6-hydroxydopamine caused denervation supersensitivity in hepatic capacitance vessels (226), and this may also occur in resistance vessels. Reflex constriction of the hepatic artery occurs in response to bilateral occlusion of the carotid arteries (127, 220) and manipulation of the carotid baroreceptors (53, 362). Although reflex effects of the arterial baroreceptors and chemoreceptors on total splanchnic blood flow have been extensively studied, there have been surprisingly few studies on the hepatic arterial resistance and none in preparations where portal flow was controlled.

Cholinergic nervous effects have not been demonstrated in the liver vasculature. The anterior plexus is a mixed nerve bundle carrying parasympathetic as well as sympathetic fibers (240). Nevertheless a combination of $\alpha$- and $\beta$-adrenoceptor blockers completely prevents vascular responses to direct nerve stimulation (127). Vagal stimulation was reported to cause microvascular dilation (198, 199) or constriction (296) in transilluminated livers, but arterial flow was not measured.

AUTOREGULATORY ESCAPE. Autoregulatory escape is the failure of arteriolar smooth muscle to maintain a contraction in the presence of continued nerve stimulation. Escape was seen in mesenteric arterioles of cat, dog, and human, lymph glands, kidney, and spleen in cats, and stomach in rats (116, 119). The hepatic artery in cats shows classic escape, but in dogs escape did not occur [see Fig. 5; (130)], although others have reported some escape (156, 270). Because tachyphylaxis can occur in many situations and may appear similar to autoregulatory escape, several criteria have been suggested to differentiate true autoregulatory escape. The next discussion is based on recent reviews (116, 119), and specific reference is made only to recent or other work not cited in those reviews.

True autoregulatory escape has several characteristics. It occurs in arteriolar smooth muscle, whereas contraction is well maintained in postcapillary venous smooth muscle. In the liver, the hepatic arteriolar responses had undergone significant escape within 2 min, whereas portal pressure responses did not escape (127). However, a later study showed some escape in the portal pressure response (211). The mean escape in the hepatic artery to direct nerve stimulation was 83% compared with 37% escape in portal pressure response. The part of the portal pressure response that showed escape appeared to be presinusoidal constriction, whereas the maintained part of the portal pressure response was postsinusoidal (231). Hepatic blood volume responses were also well maintained with no escape (137). In a large series of animals, autoregulatory escape in the hepatic artery can vary greatly, indicating that some precondition may modulate the extent of the escape. Escape is also seen in response to close intra-arterial or intraportal infusions of norepinephrine in cats, thus eliminating depressed transmitter release or corelease of a dilator transmitter as possible mechanisms. Escape occurs during reflex as well as direct activation of the hepatic nerves. Escape occurred at all frequencies of stimulation and was proportionally as large at low as at high frequencies. In some cats, flow escaped to above the control prestimulation level, and cessation of stimulation was followed by a marked poststimulatory hyperemia, indicating that simple desensitization of receptors or failure of muscle contraction is not an adequate explanation of the phenomenon. Escape occurred during constant-flow perfusion as well as during constant-pressure perfusion, and a redistribution of flow within the liver did not occur. This eliminates accumulation of vasodilator metabolites as a mechanism and indicates that escape involves relaxation of the same vessels that originally constricted. Escape was unaltered after $\beta$-adrenoceptor antagonists, atropine, antihistamines, indomethacin, naloxone, or adenosine antagonists. The mechanism is still unknown. Release of some dilator not related to metabolism and not blocked by any of the blockers listed previously remains a possible mechanism, but it must be released by both nerve stimulation and infusions of norepinephrine. Failure to maintain arteriolar smooth muscle contraction due to accumulation of intracellular $Na^+$ is also possible. Either of these mechanisms could explain escape to above control and poststimulatory hyperemia if it is assumed that the vasodilator or the intracellular accumulation of $Na^+$ is removed more slowly than the norepinephrine.

Thus autoregulatory escape to sympathetic nerve stimulation occurs in the arterioles that supply the splanchnic circulation via both portal and hepatic arterial circuits in cats and via the portal circuit in dogs. This escape should minimize the impact of sympathetic activity on blood flow while allowing well-maintained blood volume and metabolic responses. However, the physiological importance and the ways in which this escape interacts with other mechanisms controlling hepatic arterial flow are not clear at present. It has also not yet been examined in the hepatic arterial bed of humans. If the variability of the escape is due to physiological modulatory mechanisms, these are still unknown.

RESPONSES TO HUMORAL FACTORS. Effects of vasoactive agents on hepatic arterial flow have been extensively reviewed (136, 299, 301, 302) and are discussed only briefly. Blood-borne agents can reach the liver either via the hepatic artery or the portal vein. Substances released locally into the portal blood from the splanchnic organs could serve subtle regulatory roles as modulators of hepatic arterial flow. Such substances comprise a rapidly expanding list, including all of the gut hormones, many autacoids, nutrients absorbed from the intestinal tract, and bile salts undergoing enterohepatic recirculation. Substances in portal blood are able to gain access to the hepatic arterial resistance vessels (227, 235, 236, 302).

Although the vasoactive gut hormones have frequently been tested for activity on the hepatic arterial resistance vessels, several factors limit the usefulness of most studies. Doses required for vasoactive effects seem well outside the physiological range (299), but most studies have not measured plasma concentrations. Most studies do not report portal flow, and none have controlled portal flow to prevent the hepatic arterial buffer response. Substances that change portal flow may produce indirect effects on hepatic arterial flow through this buffer response; e.g., vasopressin infused into the hepatic artery caused constriction, whereas intravenous infusion caused reduced portal flow and dilation of the hepatic artery (136). Similarly histamine directly dilated the hepatic artery but intravenously caused elevated portal flow and reduced hepatic arterial flow (204). Finally, many compounds were tested by administration of boluses. Bolus administration does not allow for steady-state concentrations or flows, and interpretation can be difficult.

Gut hormones reported to cause dilation of the hepatic artery include gastrin, pentagastrin, and secretin (290, 303) and vasoactive intestinal polypeptide [VIP; (309)], although the doses appear outside the physiological range. Cholecystokinin caused dilation in doses that may be attained during digestion (303). Bile salts were discussed previously.

It was reported that glucagon not only caused arterial dilation but also selectively antagonized arterial constriction induced by sympathetic nerve stimulation, norepinephrine, angiotensin, and vasopressin in dogs (300). This was not confirmed in cats (112). If endogenous physiological levels of glucagon can impair hepatic arterial constriction, this would indicate a function for glucagon not only as a dilator of the hepatic artery but also as a modulator of reflex mechanisms. Glucagon levels are partly regulated by hepatic clearance, and the reduced clearance after portacaval shunts has been proposed as a putative mechanism for elevated portal flow and reduced mesenteric arterial resistance (20). However, other studies have suggested physiological levels of plasma glucagon have no systemic effect on arterial blood flow (27), although the hepatic artery was not studied. Adenosine infusion also causes dilation of the hepatic artery and reduces hepatic arterial constriction caused by the sympathetic nerves, norepinephrine, angiotensin, and vasopressin (233). It is not yet clear whether the impairment of constrictor responses occurs with physiologically relevant doses of adenosine.

Increases in plasma tonicity due to glucose release from the liver occur during hemorrhage and trauma caused by hepatic nerve activation and adrenal medullary secretions (228). Plasma osmotic pressure is also elevated by a number of therapeutic or diagnostic measures, e.g., radiopaque angiographic compounds, blood volume expanders, osmotic diuretics, and intravenous alimentation (255). The hepatic artery dilates in a dose-dependent manner to intra-arterial, intravenous, and intraportal infusions of hypertonic saline and glucose (237, 307), and total hepatic blood flow increases during intravenous glucose infusions (26). The physiological role of osmotic pressure in control of hepatic arterial flow is unknown but may be significant; e.g., postprandial elevations of osmolarity in portal and systemic blood were estimated to increase hepatic arterial flow by ~10% (54).

Angiotensin constricted the hepatic, splenic, and mesenteric arteries (57) with the hepatic artery showing the least constriction, probably because reduced portal flow activated the buffer response. Angiotensin I constricted the hepatic artery only after local conversion to angiotensin II (71). Vasopressin constricted the hepatic artery on close intra-arterial or intraportal infusion, but intravenous infusion caused splenic and mesenteric constriction and hepatic arterial dilation or no change (57, 102, 155, 193, 304). Although this hepatic arterial dilation has been attributed to the buffer response, this may not be the case (50). Various hormones and autacoids have been shown to dilate the hepatic artery in pharmacological doses, e.g., parathyroid hormone (55), $PGE_2$, histamine, and bradykinin (301, 302). Prostaglandin $E_2$ is released into the portal blood from the spleen in response to nerve stimulation or adrenaline infusion (70, 103), but whether it reaches levels sufficient to dilate the hepatic artery is not known. Prostacyclin infusion in dogs increased portal flow with no change in hepatic arterial flow (78). Histamine acts on the hepatic artery predominantly through $H_1$ receptors in dogs (302). Redistribution of arterial flow does not occur, but portal flow is somewhat redistributed from peripheral to hilar regions of liver lobes in dogs (131). Intravenous histamine causes elevated portal flow and reduced arterial flow (204), another probable example of the buffer response overriding a direct effect on the hepatic artery. Dopamine causes constriction or dilation of the hepatic artery that may be due to stimulation of $\alpha$-adrenoceptors and dopamine receptors, respectively (305). In cats dopamine increases portal flow and decreases hepatic arterial flow (205), resembling the effects of epinephrine (136). Serotonin also causes a biphasic response, when given by bolus injection, with an initial dilation followed by a secondary constriction (306).

BLOOD GASES AND pH. Blood gas and pH effects on hepatic arterial resistance are difficult to interpret because systemic effects and changes in portal flow occur. However, in general systemic changes in blood gases do not produce marked effects on the hepatic circulation. Hypoxia [partial pressure of $O_2$ ($PO_2$) = 35–45 mmHg] caused no hepatic arterial resistance effect in cats or dogs in some studies (208, 325), whereas others reported mild hepatic arterial constriction that could be prevented by hepatic denervation (167, 250). Systemic hypoxia and hypercapnia, caused by increasing the dead space of the endotracheal catheter, caused elevated cardiac output, elevated portal flow (42%), and constriction of the hepatic artery. Total hepatic flow remained within 11% of control (253). Hyperoxia ($PO_2$ = 400 mmHg) did not alter hepatic blood flow (166). Hypercapnia produced a mild hepatic arterial dilation in cats, whereas hypocapnia induced a mild vasoconstriction (325). Severe hypercapnia [partial pressure of $CO_2$ ($PCO_2$) = 100 mmHg] raised portal flow and produced a mild constriction of the hepatic artery that could be prevented by hepatic denervation (250). Systemic acidosis caused elevated portal flow and reduced arterial flow with no change in total hepatic flow. Systemic alkalosis did not change hepatic arterial flow (168). Portal acidosis caused dilation, and portal hyperoxia caused constriction of the hepatic artery (101).

Many of these hepatic arterial responses may be secondary to portal flow changes and mediated by the hepatic arterial buffer response. Only studies comparing hepatic arterial flows when portal flow is allowed to change and when it is held constant can resolve these issues.

OTHER STIMULI. Postprandial elevation in hepatic flow occurs, but this is largely due to elevation of portal flow with little change in hepatic arterial flow (99, 366). Few data are available on hepatic arterial flow in exercise due to the technical difficulties of measuring this flow in conscious animals. In one study with microspheres, hepatic arterial flow decreased during steady-state exercise but increased during exhaustive exercise (322).

Hemorrhage results in reduced hepatic blood flow, but the proportion of the cardiac output to the liver is increased (4, 128, 136, 336). Dilation of the hepatic artery compensated for reduced portal flow early in the response, but both flows declined with increasingly severe hypovolemia. In cats the hepatic arterial flow did not decrease until systemic pressure was <80 mmHg, and portal flow was substantially reduced at this point (128). The response of the hepatic artery is affected by the nearly complete escape from neurogenic constriction coupled with the hepatic arterial buffer response to reduced portal flow. Thus, even when total flow was slightly reduced, $O_2$ delivery was well protected. The brain, heart, and hepatic artery increase their proportion of the cardiac output during hemorrhage, resulting in selective protection of these tissues from hypoxia (94). This protective hepatic arterial dilation was blocked during halothane anesthesia (4). Intrahepatic distribution of blood flow appeared normal, and liver functions were well maintained after hemorrhage equivalent to 25% of the blood volume (202). In dogs, hemorrhage reducing cardiac output to 50% led to some redistribution of intrahepatic flow toward the hilum (336). Portal pressure during hemorrhage was not notably depressed due to a balance between reduced portal flow and constrictor effects within the liver (202, 269). The hepatic microcirculation in transilluminated preparations shows a normal appearance until severe levels of hemorrhage are reached, when stagnation of flow and clumping of cells are seen (197, 365).

In circulatory shock many complex changes occur in the liver, and it is impossible to separate primary vascular and metabolic changes from changes secondary to effects elsewhere. Consideration of these complex changes is beyond the scope of this chapter.

### EFFECTS OF HEPATIC BLOOD FLOW ON UPTAKE OF SUBSTRATES

This topic, reviewed recently (272, 380), is important because it relates circulation to function. Changes in hepatic vascular parameters, pressures, flows, and volumes result in changes in hepatic uptake of metabolic substrates and drugs, and the results are of practical significance. However, it is very difficult to review this area and to separate fact from speculation. Several approaches to kinetic analysis of hepatic uptake of metabolic substrates and drugs have been developed in more than one hundred published papers. These approaches are highly mathematical but are based on inadequately validated premises. Many investigators ignore the possibility of alternate interpretations, and in those papers where the existence of other approaches is acknowledged, the discussion is often confined to demonstration of the inferiority of the other approaches. Many investigators use computer programs that are neither listed nor offered to other workers. In addition the experimental data used in these models is either generated by computer or derived from studies on isolated perfused rat livers. Only a small proportion of the work relates to studies in anesthetized animals with an intact hepatic vasculature.

Studies on the isolated perfused rat liver, because of their apparent technical simplicity, are convenient for determining kinetic parameters relating to hepatocyte uptake or plasma binding of substrates, but they are quite unsuitable for determining the effects of changes in hepatic hemodynamics on these kinetic parameters. Flows, pressures, distribution of flows, relations between portal and hepatic arterial flows, and $O_2$ supply are all abnormal in these preparations.

Important controls, e.g., verification of uniformity of perfusion at each of several flow rates, are usually not reported, and the apparent effects of increasing flow may be due to perfusion of previously poorly perfused areas of the liver. Thus the results may be due to increased liver mass rather than increased flow. In the previous sections, we have described the intricate interactions between portal and hepatic arterial flows, and various mechanisms that safeguard total hepatic flow and $O_2$ delivery. These mechanisms are entirely abolished in an isolated rat liver perfused only through the portal vein. Even when the hepatic artery is separately perfused, arterial and portal routes do not provide equal accessibility to parenchymal tissue (3) as they do in the anesthetized animal (see *Origin and Distribution of Hepatic Blood Supply*, p. 1520). Although extraction may appear high when a nonprotein perfusate is used, extraction of substances by the isolated perfused liver is much lower than in anesthetized animals or humans when the isolated liver perfusate contains normal levels of albumin. For example, BSP extraction in the presence of 1% and 4.5% albumin was only 22% and 8%, respectively, in the isolated perfused liver (146), in contrast to 36%–60% at normal albumin levels in vivo (8, 31, 381). We emphasize these problems in the hope that this chapter will stimulate wider discussion of the models and more varied experimental approaches. Some of the pitfalls of kinetic analysis have been examined (100).

The three major approaches that are discussed here are the Goresky model, the equilibrium model, and the parallel tube model. An attempt is made to give a brief overview of the concepts and assumptions of these models, but the reader is referred to the cited literature for details and mathematical derivations.

*Goresky Model*

One approach with multiple indicator dilution curves and a computer model has been extensively described and recently reviewed by Goresky (105, 106). With this technique in anesthetized dogs, the time of emergence in hepatic venous blood of substances injected into the portal vein is compared with that of substances with a known distribution in blood and extracellular and intracellular water. Kinetic parameters of uptake and exchange can be calculated with a sophisticated model. The technique involves anesthesia and minimal surgery, although 50 ml of blood are rapidly withdrawn from a hepatic vein for each measurement. Although many interesting aspects of hepatic uptake have been studied in these anesthetized animals, the effects of hemodynamic changes on the uptake process have not been examined. Luxon and Forker (247) have criticized the approach and discussed potential errors due to the technical difficulty of accurately measuring radioactivity in the tail of the outflow curves. They also point out that the inherent weakness of compartmental analysis is that errors arising from false assumptions are often not apparent from the data. They have proposed a modified approach with an isolated perfused liver (98), but this may not be as suitable for hemodynamic studies as the anesthetized dog. This approach has not been discussed as widely as other models, perhaps because it has not been related to commonly measured clinical pharmacokinetic parameters. In addition Goresky has made no attempt to relate his approach to the other models described next.

*Equilibrium Model*

Another approach has been a model based on the concept of hepatic clearance and its relation to hepatic blood flow (32, 317). It was reviewed and extended to incorporate drug binding in plasma by Wilkinson and Shand (380). This model has become known as the *venous equilibrium*, *equilibrium*, or *well-stirred* model. Hepatic clearance is the apparent volume of blood completely cleared of a drug or substrate by the liver per unit time. Clearance depends on blood flow and on the capacity of the liver to eliminate the drug. It is expressed as blood flow times extraction, and the extraction depends on both the blood flow and the maximum capacity of the liver to remove drug in the absence of any flow limitation. This maximum capacity was named *intrinsic clearance*. It was shown to equal flow times extraction divided by (1 − extraction) and to be analogous in enzyme kinetics to maximal velocity divided by the Michaelis constant ($V_{max}/K_m$). It was demonstrated that clearance, after an oral dose of a drug that is fully absorbed and only metabolized by the liver, is equal to intrinsic clearance.

The equilibrium model was compared with the classic pharmacokinetic linear two-compartment open model and claimed to give a more physiologically relevant interpretation (317). Clearance parameters are more obviously related to physiological factors than rate constants and apparent volumes of distribution (380), but these models are identical (370, 371), and the compartment model can give clinically relevant information (192). The equilibrium model is based on three important assumptions: *1*) Distribution of the substrate into the liver is perfusion-rate limited. *2*) Elimination by metabolism or biliary excretion is assumed to be a first-order process. *3*) The substrate in the liver water is in equilibrium with emergent venous blood. This last assumption has caused the greatest controversy. Wilkinson and Shand (380) suggested that this approach, with measurement of intrinsic clearance and drug binding, would allow prediction of the effects of changes in hepatic blood flow on the disposition of a variety of drugs. The predicted relationships between hepatic clearance, extraction, and hepatic blood flow are shown in Figure 6, and Wilkinson and Shand described the concepts.

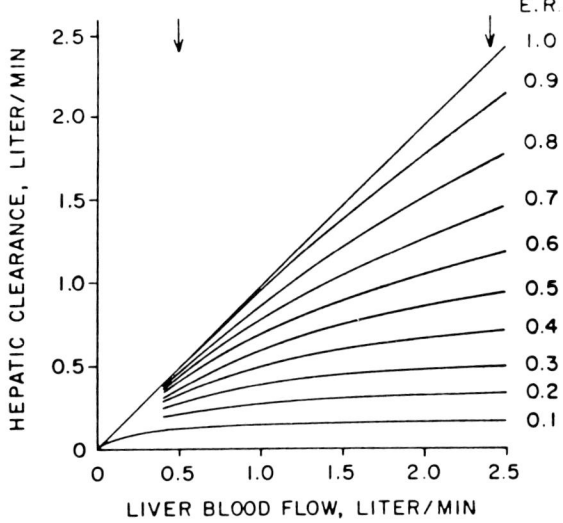
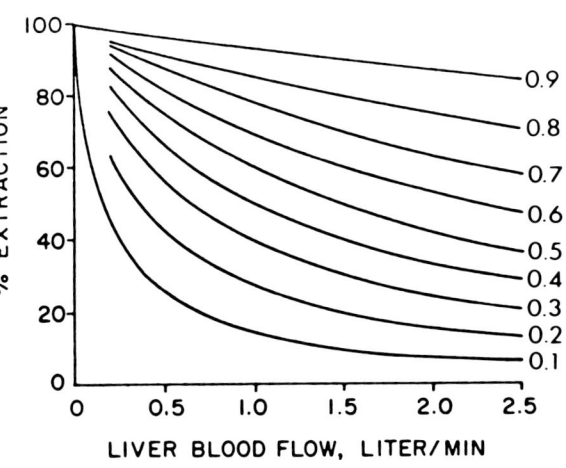

FIG. 6. *Left panel*: relationship between liver blood flow and total hepatic clearance for drugs with various extraction rates. *Arrows*, normal physiological range of liver blood flow in humans; extraction values (E.R.) refer to normal flow of 1.5 liters/min. *Right panel*: relationship between extraction and liver blood flow for drugs with varying extraction values at a normal flow of 1.5 liters/min. [From Wilkinson and Shand (380).]

If a drug has a low extraction due to a small intrinsic clearance relative to liver blood flow, hepatic clearance and elimination half-life will be independent of changes in liver blood flow but highly sensitive to the ability of the liver to metabolize the drug (intrinsic clearance). There will be only a small first-pass extraction after oral administration, and most of the drug will reach the systemic circulation. Variations in hepatic blood flow will not significantly affect this availability. On the other hand, for a drug with a high extraction due to a large intrinsic clearance relative to liver blood flow, hepatic clearance will predominantly reflect liver blood flow rather than drug-metabolizing activity. Consequently the clearance and half-life will be sensitive to changes in flow and insensitive to alterations in metabolic activity. This drug will exhibit significant first-pass hepatic elimination after an oral dose, and the availability will be readily affected by changes in intrinsic clearance but not by hepatic blood flow. When the hepatic extraction of total drug exceeds the free fraction in blood, systemic clearance of total drug will be unchanged by alterations in binding, and half-life will tend to decrease with increased binding due to reduction in volume of distribution. If the extraction of total drug is restricted to the free fraction in blood, total systemic clearance will be dependent on binding, and half-life will be prolonged as binding increases. Antipyrine was a prototype for the low-extraction group, whereas propranolol was a prototype of the high-extraction group (380). Thus the influence of blood flow on drug elimination depends markedly on the intrinsic ability of the liver to remove the drug. These considerations led to a method for measurement of hepatic blood flow in humans based on determination of blood concentration-time curves after oral and intravenous administration of the same dose of a drug with a high intrinsic clearance (380).

The validity of this model was tested in several situations in anesthetized animals. The effects of increased hepatic blood flow produced by two infusions of glucagon on propranolol clearance were examined in the monkey (33). Although the data were reported to conform to the model predictions, extraction of propranolol in this species was only 33%. The predictions for a very high or a very low intrinsic clearance could not be tested rigorously. Increases in hepatic blood flow of 26% and 113% with the two glucagon infusions produced identical increases in propranolol clearance of 15%, and calculated extraction decreased 7% and 44% respectively. Extraction of oxyphenbutazone also decreased as hepatic flow increased (379). In contrast to these effects of increased flow on extraction, no change in lidocaine extraction was reported when hepatic blood flow was reduced in cats (239) and dogs (34). In the cats, extraction of lidocaine was 34%, a value very similar to that of propranolol in monkeys. The differences could be due to decreased versus increased flow, different species, or different drugs. It was proposed that the reduction of lidocaine clearance by propranolol was due to decreased hepatic blood flow because hepatic extraction of lidocaine was not changed (34). However, in this study, hepatic blood flow was not measured independently but was calculated by the Fick principle with lidocaine as the indicator. A more recent study in humans suggested that the reduction in lidocaine clearance by propranolol was too large to be explained on the basis of the reduction in hepatic blood flow. Because propranolol also reduced clearance of theophylline and antipyrine, drugs whose clearance was not predicted to change with flow, effects of propranolol on hepatic uptake, or enzyme activities were postulated (65, 286). Clearances of morphine (high intrinsic clearance) and pentobarbital (low intrinsic clearance) were not significantly altered during hepatic venous congestion in rats that reduced hepatic blood flow to 50% control levels. Calculated extraction of morphine was 66% in control rats and 100% in rats with liver congestion. However, mean systemic availability after oral administration of morphine was unchanged during liver congestion (196). We have been unable to discern any consistent pattern in these results.

*Parallel-Tube Model*

A third theoretical approach to the interrelationships between blood flow and drug or substrate uptake by the liver was developed by Bass et al. (14). This model has been called the *sinusoidal-perfusion* or *parallel-tube* model. In this model, drugs or substrates are progressively eliminated as blood flows along the sinusoids, resulting in concentration gradients along the sinusoids that determine elimination rate. Thus, in the equilibrium model, the liver is regarded as a well-stirred compartment with the drug concentration in the liver in equilibrium with that in the emergent blood, whereas in the parallel-tube model, the liver is regarded as a parallel tube with enzymes distributed along the tube and the drug concentration declining along the length of the tube (284). The parallel-tube model, like the equilibrium model, predicts that at high substrate concentrations or low enzyme activities, uptake will be relatively independent of flow, whereas at low substrate concentrations and high enzyme activities, uptake will be highly flow dependent.

In the parallel-tube model a single parallel sinusoid is assumed. Lateral diffusion is fast enough to maintain a uniform lateral concentration with enzymatic elimination at the boundary. Convective flow transports the substrate or drug along the sinusoid. Elimination depends on the Michaelis-Menten relationship ($K_m$) with the substrate concentration being the logarithmic average of the concentrations entering and leaving the sinusoids. This is an important difference between the equilibrium and parallel-tube models. In the former model, the liver cells are in equilibrium with the outflow concentration, whereas in the latter model, they are in equilibrium with the logarithmic average of the inflow and outflow concentrations. The calculations for the parallel-tube model are independent of the spatial distribution of enzyme along the sinusoids, but if this is uniform, the concentration profile along the sinusoid varies from linear at high inflow concentrations relative to $K_m$ to exponential at low inflow concentrations relative to $K_m$. The prototype substance for this model was galactose.

The implications of this model, in terms of the effects of hepatic blood flow on elimination, were described further by Keiding (186). The relationships between elimination and flow are complex, but for a given elimination rate, the logarithmic mean sinusoidal concentration is independent of flow, whereas in the equilibrium model the hepatic outflow concentration is independent of flow. Keiding compared the definitions of the different clearances at low substrate concentrations much below $K_m$. Hepatic clearance equals elimination rate divided by inflow concentration for both models. Intrinsic clearance in the equilibrium model (380) equals elimination rate divided by outflow concentration. In the parallel-tube model, intrinsic clearance equals elimination rate divided by the logarithmic mean sinusoidal concentration (186).

*Comparison of Models*

The two models, equilibrium and parallel tube, have been compared mathematically (186, 284). Both models predicted similar hepatic drug clearances under a variety of conditions, and in many experimental situations data can be fitted equally well to either model (165, 187). Differences were described in regard to the effects of hepatic blood flow on hepatic venous compared with logarithmic mean sinusoidal concentrations, and in regard to the effects of hepatic blood flow on systemic availability after oral administration, area under the concentration-time curve after oral administration, and steady-state blood concentrations after oral administration of drugs with a high extraction. The equilibrium model predicts much less effect of flow on oral availability, whereas the parallel-tube model predicts increases in flow will markedly increase oral availability. Other differences between the models are seen when protein binding is altered (266).

McLean et al. (258) reported studies in humans that showed that the area under the concentration-time curve after oral administration was dependent on flow, but they still interpreted this in terms of the equilibrium model. A sustained increase in hepatic blood flow reduced the extent of first-pass metabolism but increased the rate at which the drug was subsequently cleared from plasma. These effects canceled out, giving no net effect of hepatic blood flow on the area under the arterial concentration-time curve. However, if the increase in hepatic blood flow was temporary, as happens after a meal, the decreased first-pass effect exceeded the later effect on drug clearance, resulting in an increased area under the concentration-time curve. They discussed other factors that might complicate interpretation and concluded that it was not possible to predict whether the bioavailability of a drug subject to first-pass metabolism would be affected by a meal. Others argued that the effect of a meal on bioavailability was too large to be due to increased hepatic blood flow (350, 351). In a recent study in anesthetized dogs (160), mesenteric blood flow measured by electromagnetic flowmeter was increased ~100% by administration of hydralazine. Hydralazine increased oral availability of propranolol by 443%, whereas systemic clearance of intravenous propranolol increased by 42%. Thus hydralazine produced a major change in first-pass hepatic clearance of propranolol, and the most likely explanation of this was increased hepatic blood flow. (The authors do not interpret these effects in terms of the available models, but the data appear more consistent with the parallel-tube model.)

During the late 1970s, each of the two groups that developed the models reported data supporting their own model. Keiding and Andreasen (187) reviewed the studies on isolated perfused livers. One study supported each model (189, 285), and two studies were unable to distinguish between the models. This situation, where two well-defined quantitative models were used side by side, although they contradicted each other in their basic hypotheses and quantitative predictions, was pointed out by Bass (11). The discrepancies in the reported data led Bass et al. (11–13, 15, 16) to reconsider the assumption in the parallel-tube model that all the sinusoids were identical, and the maximal arteriovenous concentration difference ($V_{max}$/flow for each sinusoid) was the same for each sinusoid. They suggested that the large variability in the flows and hepatocyte numbers along individual sinusoids must generate variability in this ratio. Intrahepatic shunts generated by sinusoids lined by dead hepatocytes would be an extreme example of this variability. Incorporation of this variability into the parallel-tube model led to the distributed-perfusion model. This more complex model has not yet been widely considered in the literature.

The controversy continues in recent studies of the isolated perfused rat liver. Keiding and Steiness (191) found that both inflow and outflow concentrations changed while the logarithmic mean sinusoidal concentration did not change during propranolol infusions at different flow rates, whereas Ahmad et al. (2) reported outflow concentration did not change at different flow rates during lidocaine and meperidine infusions. Ethanol elimination constants were more consistent with the parallel-tube model (190), whereas altered protein binding of propranolol caused changes that conformed precisely to the predictions of the equilibrium model (180). Recently the proponents of the equilibrium model presented data on diazepam elimination that were more consistent with the parallel-tube model (318). A theoretical attempt to relate the various models was made by Wagner et al. (370, 371).

Both models assume equilibrium occurs between free (unbound) drug or substrate across the hepatocyte membrane and that, at steady state, the elimination rate from blood equals the sum of the rates of metabolism and biliary excretion. These are clearly serious oversimplifications. Overwhelming evidence exists in favor of active transport across hepatocyte membranes and accumulation of some substances (e.g., ICG) inside the hepatocytes. The role of drug binding in hepatic uptake is complex (82, 358, 380). The concept of albumin receptors that may enhance drug and substrate uptake further complicates the situation (7, 96, 97, 146, 169, 280, 377). Further discussion of these important issues is beyond the scope of this chapter, but perhaps two comments are justified. First, the parallel-tube and distributed models are intuitively more appealing because they can be related to the known sinusoidal concentration gradients and non-homogeneity of hepatocytes (35, 145). The concept that all hepatocytes are in equilibrium with effluent hepatic blood clearly contradicts known facts. It seems unlikely that any one model will be found that will accommodate all drugs under all conditions because models are inherently oversimplifications of complex processes. Second, it would be worthwhile to add new dimensions to the experimental studies. The isolated rat liver model has many hemodynamic limitations. The human pharmacokinetic studies can never substantiate the concepts of hemodynamics on hepatic drug removal because they involve circular reasoning. The clearance concepts are used to calculate hepatic blood flow, and the measurements are then used to validate the clearance concepts. Although technically difficult and subject to an array of other complicating factors (e.g., anesthesia, surgery), studies in anesthetized animals with independent measurements of hemodynamic factors are needed to help resolve these controversies (119a).

*Measurement of Hepatic Blood Flow by Uptake*

In spite of our sketchy knowledge of the relationships between uptake of drugs and substrates and hepatic blood flow, attempts have been made for many years to measure hepatic blood flow in humans from the uptake of certain substances. The early work on these clearances and techniques based on the Fick principle was extensively reviewed in 1963 by Bradley (30), and the assumptions inherent in the methods have been discussed in many other papers (8, 29, 31, 161, 188, 242, 342, 364, 376, 381). Bradley (30) concluded that "suitable test substances have been found and adequate evidence of reliability has been forthcoming to warrant qualified acceptance of much of the data set out in the literature." This conclusion may have been premature. There are few studies where measurements of blood flow by clearance techniques have been compared with direct flow measurements (76, 276, 329, 331), and none of these studies examined a wide range of conditions or flows. In none of these studies was flow varied experimentally to show that direct and clearance methods remained in agreement. In many cases, verification of clearance techniques has depended on obtaining values for hepatic blood flow that fall within the accepted range, although in some cases two or more substances were compared simultaneously (364, 381). Although the mean values were similar in these comparisons, there was a large, apparently random variability in individual values. The accuracy, precision, and variability of the clearance measurements remain in doubt, especially under conditions other than normal flows in normal subjects. Validation of these techniques requires careful studies in anesthetized animals over a wide range of hepatic blood flows (48, 48a, 48b).

The approach most likely to give accurate estimates involves infusion of a test substance until a steady-state blood level is reached, followed by several measurements of arterial and mixed hepatic venous concentrations. Estimated flow then equals clearance divided by extraction, providing that four conditions are met in all the situations where flow is to be estimated:

1. The hepatic venous samples are representative of mixed hepatic venous blood and contain no refluxed IVC blood. Variations between samples taken simultaneously from two separate venous catheters ranged from 7% to 36% in one study (381) but were smaller in another (331).

2. The concentration of the substance in hepatic arterial and portal venous blood is equal, and no enterohepatic recirculation of the substance occurs.

3. The drug is removed exclusively by the liver. This is the most difficult assumption to verify, especially in humans. It has been approached by showing that arteriovenous differences across other organs are zero (but small differences are difficult to detect), and that the substance does not disappear from blood in hepatectomized animals. Although it is generally accepted that ICG is removed exclusively by the liver, in dogs there was an exponential decline in plasma ICG concentration at a time when hepatic venous concentration exceeded arterial concentration due to saturation of hepatic uptake (342). Stekiel et al. (342) did not comment on this, but the only explanation appears to be extrahepatic removal. In cats there is extrahepatic distribution of ICG (48b) and extrahepatic elimination of galactose (48).

4. The hepatic elimination rate must be constant so that arterial and hepatic venous concentrations remain constant over the sampling period. In the presence of even minor departures from steady state, the infusion rate will not equal the hepatic uptake. Several reports indicate that infusions of BSP and ICG never attain steady-state arterial levels (48a, 51, 194, 242, 378).

When the conditions of the measurements are modified to simplify the procedure, much larger errors become possible. Two major simplifications involve using a bolus dose instead of an infusion and assuming that hepatic venous concentration is zero to avoid hepatic venous catheterization. With a bolus injection there are three additional assumptions:

1. The hepatic elimination rate constant must not change over a wide range of blood concentrations.

2. Distribution equilibrium must be achieved very rapidly before sampling is begun. These two assumptions result in a blood concentration-time relationship that is described by a single exponential over the whole concentration range. Few if any of the relationships published in the papers cited in this section completely fulfill this requirement.

3. The extraction must be determined from the difference in concentration in the blood entering the hepatic sinusoids before extraction begins, and the concentration in the same blood after it leaves the sinusoids (242). Thus the hepatic venous sample must be taken one transit time later than the arterial sample. If the arterial concentration is falling rapidly, as it does with ICG, the intestinal transit time will result in different concentrations in portal and hepatic arterial blood flowing into the liver. Because hepatic blood volume varies markedly in different animals, the hepatic transit time is variable and unknown and varies with the flow. These problems give a variability in extraction of at least ± 10% (48b).

Measurement of hepatic blood flow by determination of systemic clearance with the assumption that hepatic venous concentration equals zero is subject to even greater errors, especially when hepatic disease is known to be present (142, 188). Extraction of ICG ranges from 15% to 77% and is usually ~65% in normal volunteers (8, 51, 59, 242, 344, 376, 381). Extraction of BSP ranges from 36% to 60% (8, 31, 329, 381), whereas extraction of galactose ranges from 78% to 95% (161, 364, 381). However, galactose may not give accurate estimates of hepatic blood flow (48, 188). A method for determination of extraction from a two-compartment analysis of the plasma ICG concentration-time curve has been proposed (107), but it has not been validated by comparison with direct measurements of extraction. A method with dynamic technetium-99m($^{99m}$Tc)–sulfur colloid scans relies on the same assumption of 100% elimination during passage through the liver (288).

The equilibrium model also predicts that hepatic blood flow can be calculated from the blood concentration-time curves after oral and intravenous administration of a drug with a high intrinsic clearance (380). This approach is only accurate with drugs with a high extraction ratio due to errors in measuring the area under the arterial concentration-time curve (343). These equations were applied to calculate apparent hepatic extraction of several substances, including ICG and rose bengal in rats (171). Calculated flow was not reported, but calculations from the data indicate that hepatic flow values were markedly different for the five test substances and much larger than normal values for hepatic blood flow in rats. Therefore the accuracy of this approach must be questioned, at least in rats.

The difficulties with these simplified methods are illustrated by the controversy over the mechanism of the interaction between propranolol and cimetidine. Cimetidine reduced the clearance of propranolol. Hepatic blood flow estimated from systemic ICG clearance after a bolus of ICG was reduced by 25% after a single dose of cimetidine and by 33% after a 7-day treatment with cimetidine. Hepatic blood flow estimated from oral and systemic clearances of propranolol also decreased by 36%. It was concluded that cimetidine reduced hepatic blood flow by $H_2$-receptor block, and this caused the decrease in propranolol clearance (87). The interaction between propranolol and cimetidine was confirmed, but ranitidine did not produce the same effects on propranolol clearance, and it reduced systemic ICG clearance by only 15%, suggesting the effect was not mediated by $H_2$-receptor block (298). In addition, a 25%–33% basal vasodilator tone mediated through $H_2$ receptors in the intestinal or hepatic arterial resistance vessels was not confirmed in animal studies [(56, 149); F. J. Burczynski and C. V. Greenway, unpublished observations]. Because cimetidine is known to interfere with hepatic metabolism of many drugs by interacting with the cytochrome *P*-450–phase I reactions, and because its effects on extraction of ICG are unknown, the conclusion that it reduced hepatic blood flow was not justified by the data. Direct measurements of hepatic blood flow during abdominal surgery in patients did not confirm this effect. Portal flow was unchanged, whereas hepatic arterial flow increased slightly (363). Other reports that failed to confirm a reduction in hepatic blood flow by cimetidine were cited by Groszmann (142). Subsequent studies on ICG clearance in humans could not confirm a reduction after cimetidine (69, 75). Other recent studies have used systemic clearance of ICG as a measure of hepatic blood flow in humans in relation to lidocaine clearance and postural changes (86), inhibitors of prostaglandin synthesis (88, 89), and the effects of food on propranolol availability (350). These reports must be interpreted cautiously (142).

## HEPATIC BLOOD VOLUME

Blood volume in mammals ranges from 60 to 85 ml/kg body wt. Of this ~20% is in the arterial system, ~10% is in the capillaries, and ~70% is in the venous system (93, 312). The venous bed has both resistance and capacitance functions, and some general principles were presented in 1964 by Folkow and Mellander (93). In the liver, the hepatic venous resistance, located in the lobar hepatic veins, plays an important role in control of sinusoidal pressure and hence in transsinusoidal fluid movements and passive capacitance effects. The capacitance function of the venous system serves to control the distribution of the blood volume and cardiac filling pressures (115, 117, 312). If the blood volume of an organ can be varied, the amount of blood that can be mobilized or stored serves as a blood volume reserve, and the organ serves as a blood reservoir. To carry out this blood reservoir function, an organ must contain a significant portion of the blood volume, it must be relatively insensitive to extraneous pressures that might cause inappropriate changes in its blood volume, and its blood content must be controlled by the CNS (117, 129). In this section we review the role of the liver as a blood reservoir and its importance in overall cardiovascular homeostasis.

### Basic Principles, Terminology, and Normal Values

The primary determinants of the volume of blood in an organ are the distending transmural pressure, the compliance of the vessels, and the unstressed volume. Relationships between pressure and volume can be illustrated with a pressure-volume graph (Fig. 7). The terms *capacitance, compliance,* and *stressed* and *unstressed volumes* are used here according to the definitions of Rothe (312, 313). The values discussed in this section are summarized in Table 1.

Compliance is the extent to which the volume of the vessel changes in response to a small change in transmural pressure, i.e., the slope of the pressure-volume curve. It is expressed in ml/mmHg per unit tissue or animal weight. Organ vascular compliance mainly reflects the most compliant structures, usually assumed to be the veins. However, in the liver, where the entire vascular bed is enclosed within the parenchyma of the organ, organ compliance may reflect tissue compliance rather than vascular compliance (134). Stressed volume is the volume of blood in the organ due to distension by the intravascular transmural pressure. If the pressure-volume relationship in the organ is linear over the physiological range, i.e., compliance is constant, stressed volume is transmural pressure times compliance. An early attempt to measure compliance in cat liver was made by Lautt and Greenway (230). In this study, hepatic volume was plotted against IVC pressure, and a nonlinear relationship with compliances of 1–3 ml·mmHg$^{-1}$·100 g$^{-1}$ liver was reported. This work was later confirmed in cats (261). In dogs, Bennett and Rothe (18) reported a linear pressure-volume relationship and an apparent compliance of 2 ml·mmHg$^{-1}$·100 g$^{-1}$ liver based on similar changes in hepatic outflow pressure beyond the hepatic venous resistance. These approaches were shown to be inaccurate after it was found that intrahepatic transmural pressure is close to portal pressure and not to IVC pressure. The nonlinear relationship in the cat was due to incomplete transmission of

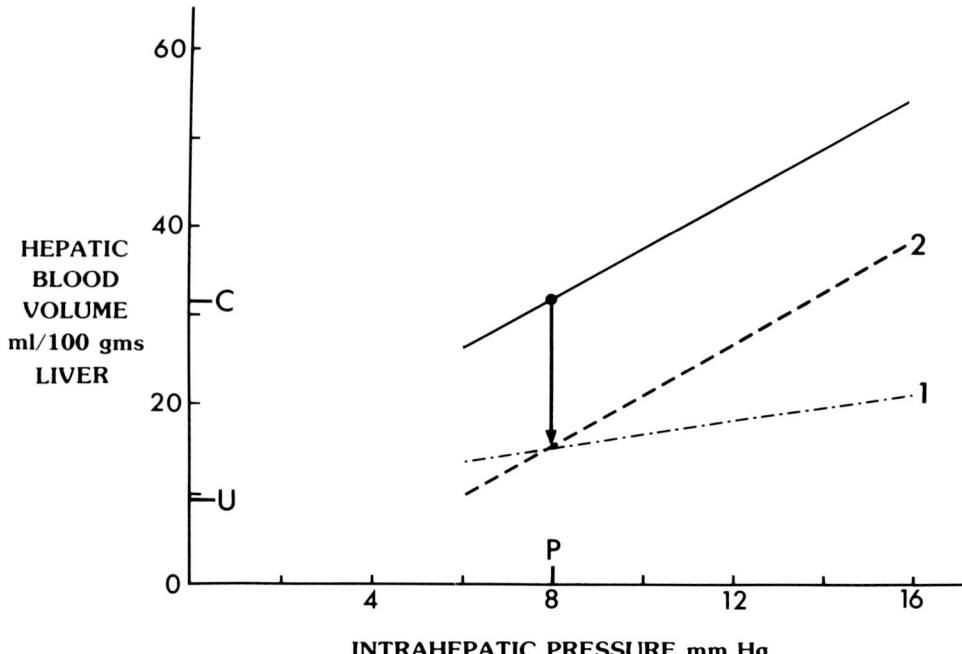

FIG. 7. Pressure-volume relationship in hepatic venous bed (*solid line*). At transmural pressure P, hepatic blood volume or capacitance is C, [unstressed volume (U) plus stressed volume]. Slope of *solid line*, compliance. Venoconstriction (*arrow*) could result from a change in compliance with no change in unstressed volume (*line 1*), a change in unstressed volume with no change in compliance (*line 2*), or a combination of changes in both compliance and unstressed volume.

pressure from the IVC to the intrahepatic venules. In a recent study intrahepatic pressure was recorded on both sides of the liver and was varied by changing portal flow and by changing IVC pressure. The results are shown in Figure 8. Linear pressure-volume relationships over the physiological range were reported with a calculated compliance of 2.5-3 ml·mmHg$^{-1}$·100 g$^{-1}$ liver or 0.6 ml·mmHg$^{-1}$·kg$^{-1}$ body wt (134). At a control portal pressure of 8 mmHg, stressed volume was 22 ml/100 g liver or 4.8 ml/kg body wt. No other values of compliance calculated with intrahepatic pressure have been reported at the present time. Hepatic pressure-volume relationships and calculated compliances were very similar when intrahepatic pressure was varied by changing both portal flow and outflow pressure (134). These observations provide strong evidence that sinusoidal pressure is close to portal pressure, and that resistance in the portal circuit is primarily postsinusoidal in the lobar hepatic veins. If resistance in the portal circuit were primarily presinusoidal, changes in hepatic flow would not cause passive changes in hepatic blood volume.

Oberg and Rosell (278) found that pressures in the range of 6-11 mmHg were required to keep veins in a fully circular shape. Below these pressures, volume changes occurred mainly by geometric changes as the veins collapsed and assumed an elliptical shape, and the pressure-volume relationships were nonlinear. Portal pressure is normally 8-10 mmHg, and an important function of the hepatic venous resistance may be to maintain this pressure and thus prevent passive collapse of the splanchnic venous bed. Because portal pressure does not usually fall below 6 mmHg, the pressure-volume relationships in both liver and intestine are linear over the physiological range.

Because hepatic blood volume is linearly related to intrahepatic pressure, and because intrahepatic pressure is linearly related to flow (134), blood volume is linearly related to flow (18, 67, 224). When flow changed by 1 ml·min$^{-1}$·100 g$^{-1}$ liver, blood volume changed by 0.09 ml/100 g liver (134) and 0.11 ml/100 g liver (224) in cats, and by 0.07 ml/100 g liver (18, 67) in dogs. However, in one of these studies (67), flow was not varied experimentally, and the control hepatic blood flow and volume in each of a group of dogs were correlated. Considering the different methods and species, these values are in good agreement. Because extrapolation of the intrahepatic pressure-flow relationship does not give zero pressure at zero flow (134), the apparent hepatic blood volume at zero flow obtained by extrapolation of the volume-flow relationship does not correspond to the unstressed volume.

When the linear pressure-volume relationship in the liver is extrapolated from the physiological range to zero pressure, a theoretical positive volume intercept is seen (see Figs. 7 and 8). This is the unstressed volume; the theoretical volume that would be contained within the vascular bed at zero pressure if all

TABLE 1. *Normal Values for Some Splanchnic Venous Parameters*

| Organ | Per 100 g Tissue | Per kg Body Wt |
|---|---|---|
| Liver | | |
| Compliance, ml/mmHg | 2.8 | 0.6 |
| Stressed volume, ml at 8 mmHg | 22 | 4.8 |
| Unstressed volume, ml | 15 | 3.4 |
| Capacitance, ml at 8 mmHg | | |
| Denervated | 37 | 8.2 |
| Denervated* | 30 | 9 |
| Innervated* | 20 | 6 |
| Change in volume per ml/min change in flow | | |
| Cat | 0.1 | |
| Dog | 0.07 | |
| Spleen | | |
| Compliance | ? | |
| Stressed volume | ? | |
| Unstressed volume, ml | | |
| Cat | | 9 |
| Dog | | 13 |
| Intestine | | |
| Compliance, ml/mmHg | 0.3 | 0.2 |
| Stressed volume, ml at 8 mmHg | 2.4 | 1.6 |
| Unstressed volume, ml | | |
| Cat | 4.6 | 2.6 |
| Dog | 7.6 | 4.4 |
| Capacitance, ml at 8 mmHg | | |
| Cat | 7 | 4.2 |
| Dog | 10 | 6 |
| Total Splanchnic | | |
| Compliance, ml/mmHg | | 0.8 |
| Stressed volume, ml at 8 mmHg | | 6.5 |
| Unstressed volume, ml | | |
| Cat | | 15 |
| Dog | | 20 |
| Capacitance, ml at 8 mmHg | | |
| Cat | | 21 |
| Dog | | 28 |

* Uncorrected for residual blood in liver.

the vessels remained circular and did not collapse. Unstressed volume cannot be measured directly. When the liver is removed from the animal and allowed to drain, variable degrees of vessel collapse occur, resulting in a variable residual volume that is less than the true unstressed volume. In anesthetized cats with denervated livers, unstressed volume is 12–15 ml/100 g parenchymal tissue or 3.4 ml/kg body wt (134). After death, drained liver contained a residual volume of 5–15 ml/100 g in cats (10, 134). Unless allowance is made for this substantial and variable residual blood volume, expression of hepatic parameters per unit liver weight can introduce substantial variability (134).

Capacitance is the total volume of blood contained in the liver at a given transmural pressure. It is the sum of the unstressed volume plus the stressed volume at that pressure. In anesthetized cats with denervated livers, total liver blood volume was 37 ml/100 g liver or 8.2 ml/kg body wt at a portal pressure of 8 mmHg (134). Values of 23–33 ml/100 g liver were reported in earlier studies where the liver weight was not corrected for the residual undrained blood volume (111, 130, 131, 137, 230, 326). The uncorrected volume was significantly smaller in innervated livers—20 ml/100 g (121, 327). Note that in these papers, capacitance was incorrectly referred to as compliance. In dogs with denervated livers not corrected for undrained residual blood, liver blood volumes were 31 ml/100 g liver, 11 ml/kg body wt at a portal pressure of 7.4 mmHg (130, 131) and 27 ml/100 g liver, 7.2 ml/kg body wt at an unrecorded portal pressure (52). In innervated livers, values of 18–20 ml/100 g liver were reported as the volumes between portal and hepatic venous catheters at unrecorded portal pressures (67, 68). Because total blood volume is 60 ml/kg body wt in cats (141, 388) and 85 ml/kg body wt in dogs (312), blood volume in the denervated liver is ~12% of total blood volume. In one study in humans, hepatic plasma volume was 12.6% of total plasma volume (59).

*Hepatic Blood Volume in Perspective*

In Tables 1 and 2, the values given for hepatic blood volume are compared with those for other vascular beds and earlier measurements (129, 130) are updated. Muscle, skin, and adipose tissue contain significant volumes of blood. Muscle contains ~3 ml/100 g tissue, adipose tissue ~5 ml/100 g tissue, and early work indicated ~33% of this could be expelled by sympathetic nerve stimulation (77, 259, 278). Although reflex increases in venous pressure were reported in isolated segments of human forearm veins (249, 262), recent studies have shown that blood volume changes in skeletal muscle are primarily passive changes secondary to changes in flow, and the muscle capacitance vessels do not respond directly to sympathetic nerve stimulation (244, 248) or to baroreceptor or chemoreceptor reflexes (40, 45, 80, 152, 154). From this and the other data reviewed by Rothe (312), it seems reasonable to conclude that mobilization of blood from skeletal muscle is usually passive. Capacitance vessels of skin are involved in the specialized function of temperature regulation. Measurements of compliance and stressed and unstressed volumes are not available for these beds.

Pulmonary blood volume has been reported to be 12% of total blood volume in rats and dogs, and 1% of total blood volume could be mobilized by sympathetic nerve stimulation. Hemorrhage mobilized 3% of total blood volume from the lungs, but pressures were not recorded (1). In other studies in dogs, pulmonary blood volume was 7%–15% of total blood volume, and pulmonary vascular compliance was 0.3–0.5 ml·mmHg$^{-1}$·kg$^{-1}$ body wt (332, 356, 357, 374).

Thus muscle, skin, adipose tissue, the cardiopulmonary region, and the kidneys contain 44% of the blood volume, but sympathetic nerve stimulation can

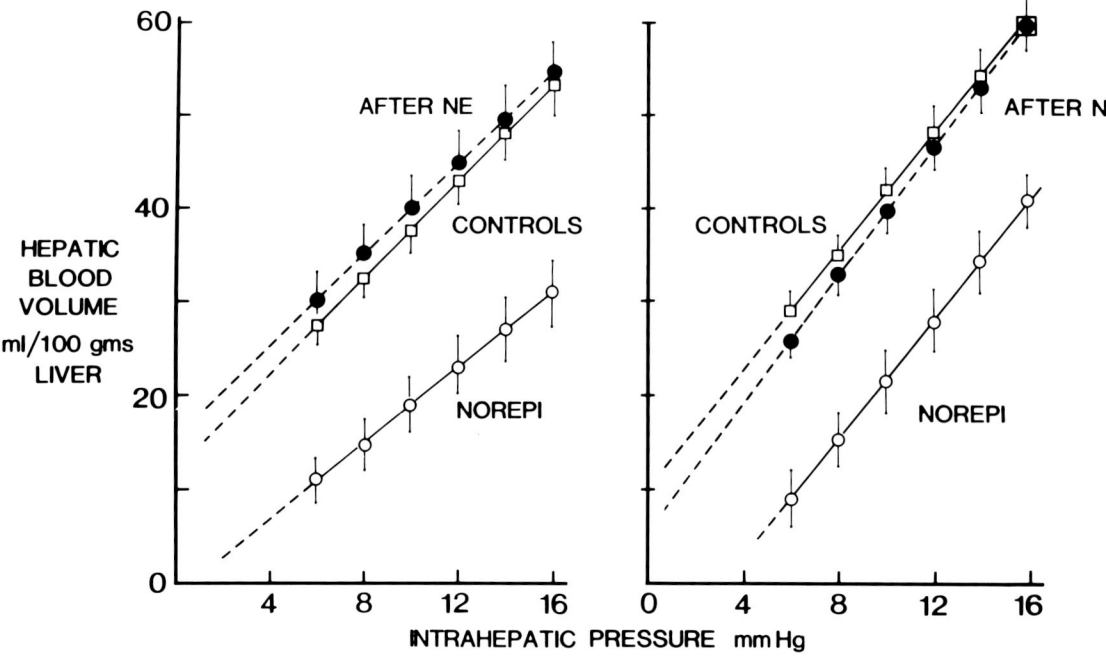

FIG. 8. Relationships between hepatic blood volume and intrahepatic pressure before, during, and after infusion of norepinephrine (NE), determined by varying portal flow (*left panel*) or by varying hepatic outflow pressure (*right panel*). Values are means ± SE; $n = 9$ for cats. [From Greenway et al. (134).]

TABLE 2. *Regional Distribution of Blood Volume and Mobilization by Sympathetic Nerve Stimulation*

| Organ | % Body Weight | % Total Blood Volume | % Total Blood Volume Mobilized |
|---|---|---|---|
| Splanchnic bed | | | |
|   Liver* | 2.5 | 12 | 6 |
|   Spleen | 1 | 14 | 12 |
|   Intestine | 6 | 7 | 3 |
|   Total | 9.5 | 33 | 21 |
| Skeletal muscle† | 45 | 17 | 5 |
| Adipose tissue† | 14 | 9 | 3 |
| Skin‡ | 3 | 2 | 1 |
| Lungs | 1.5 | 10 | 1 |
| Heart chambers | | 5 | |
| Kidneys | 0.5 | 1 | |
| Rest | 26.5 | 23 | |
| Totals | 100 | 100 | 31 |

* Parenchymal tissue excluding residual blood and bile. † Mobilization may be entirely passive secondary to flow change. ‡ Involved in temperature regulation. [Updated from Greenway and Lister (129).]

mobilize at most 10% of the blood volume from these regions (see Table 2). In contrast the splanchnic vascular bed contains ~33% of the blood volume—28 ml/kg body wt in dogs and 21 ml/kg body wt in cats (129). Early lower estimates were obtained with techniques that underestimated the splanchnic blood volume either because they measured the portion of the splanchnic blood volume that did not passively drain during arterial occlusion (164) or because the spleen was not included (63). Splanchnic blood volume was 21% and 28% of total blood volume in conscious and anesthetized rats (1), but it is not clear whether the technique would have included splenic red cell volume. In humans lower values for splanchnic blood volume have been reported—20%–25% of total blood volume (291, 369). The difference may be due to the absence of significant red cell storage in the human spleen. In cats and dogs splenic volume comprises 10%–16% of total blood volume, and most of this can be mobilized by sympathetic nerve stimulation (52, 74, 129, 201). Exercise in conscious beagles mobilized 12.7 ml/kg body wt from the spleen and this was 33% of total red cell volume. Passive changes in splenic volume in response to changes in flow are very small (135), but splenic compliance has not been reported. In humans the spleen is small, and no evidence of a significant reservoir function has been found (6, 359).

Values for intestinal blood volume are lower in cats than in dogs in accordance with the differences in total blood volumes in these species. In cats values of 6–9 ml/100 g tissue, 4.2 ml/kg body wt, 7% total blood volume have been reported (91, 287). In dogs values of 18 ml/100 g tissue, 6% total blood volume (74), 12 ml/100 g (52) and 8.5–10.4 ml/100 g (176, 314, 315) have been reported. If stomach and large intestine contain similar amounts of blood, then the gastrointestinal tract, which comprises 6% of body wt, contains 4.2 ml/kg body wt in cats and 6 ml/kg in dogs, ~7% of total blood volume in both species. These same studies showed that 40%–60% of this volume could be expelled by various stimuli. Intestinal compliance was linear over the range 0–20 mmHg with a value of 0.2–0.3 ml·mmHg$^{-1}$·100 g$^{-1}$ tissue. In another study (178), a linear pressure-volume curve over the same range was observed and compliance was 0.34 ml·mmHg$^{-1}$·100 g$^{-1}$ tissue. If the total gastrointestinal tract (6% body wt) is similar to the small intestine with a venous compliance of ~0.3 ml·mmHg$^{-1}$·100 g$^{-1}$ tissue, then compliance is 0.2 ml·mmHg$^{-1}$·kg$^{-1}$ body wt. Summing this intestinal compliance with the value of 0.6 ml·mmHg$^{-1}$·kg$^{-1}$ body wt for the liver gives a total splanchnic compliance of 0.8 ml·mmHg$^{-1}$·kg$^{-1}$ body wt. Direct measurements gave values of 0.75 ml·mmHg$^{-1}$·kg$^{-1}$ body wt (46) and 1.1 ml·mmHg$^{-1}$·kg$^{-1}$ body wt (42). At a portal pressure of 8 mmHg, intestinal stressed volume is 1.4–2.4 ml/100 g tissue if the pressure in the capacitance vessels is close to portal pressure, and unstressed volume is ~8 ml/100 g tissue in dogs. Unstressed volume appears to be a higher proportion of total volume in the intestine than it is in the liver.

These values are very variable because of a variety of factors. In any one animal, total blood volume, sympathetic tone, surgical stress, and depth of anesthesia all cause large variations in both stressed and unstressed volumes. Nevertheless the data clearly indicate the major importance of the intestine and liver as whole-blood reservoirs and the spleen as a red cell reservoir in species other than humans. If total splanchnic compliance is ~0.8 ml·mmHg$^{-1}$·kg$^{-1}$ body wt, then splanchnic stressed volume at a portal pressure of 8 mmHg is 6.4 ml/kg body wt. If the spleen is considered as unstressed volume, total splanchnic unstressed volume in dogs ≅21 ml/kg body wt or 75% of splanchnic blood volume. This value can be compared with the estimate that unstressed volume for the whole body is 70% of total blood volume (312).

*Passive Changes in Hepatic Blood Volume*

FLOW AND ARTERIAL RESISTANCE. Passive changes in stressed volume occur when intrahepatic pressure changes, causing distension or passive elastic recoil of the vessel walls. Intrahepatic pressure is close to portal pressure (see *Sinusoidal Pressure*, p. 1522). Although there have been several studies on the effects of mechanical reduction of blood flow on hepatic blood volume, intrahepatic pressure was measured in only one of them. As discussed earlier, hepatic blood volume is linearly related to hepatic blood flow with a slope of 0.07–0.1 ml/100 g liver for each ml·min$^{-1}$·100 g$^{-1}$ liver change in blood flow. Both Brooksby and Donald (42) and Bennett and Rothe (18) used these data to conclude that a significant part of the decrease in hepatic blood volume during sympathetic nerve stimulation was passive and secondary to decrease in blood flow. This argument is invalid and clearly indicates the importance of measuring intrahepatic pressure. When flow is reduced by mechanical reduction of hepatic inflow, intrahepatic pressure falls, and passive reduction in hepatic blood volume occurs. However, during sympathetic nerve stimulation, intrahepatic pressure rises in spite of decreased blood flow, so the resulting passive change in blood volume would be an increase, not a decrease. This increase in intrahepatic pressure occurs due to constriction of the hepatic venous resistance. Conversely, in cats epinephrine produces a marked increase in portal and hence hepatic blood flow, whereas norepinephrine has little effect on hepatic blood flow (136). However, both drugs produce equally large decreases in hepatic blood volume (125).

These considerations suggest an important concept. Blood flow in the portal vein is the sum of flows in the gastrointestinal and splenic circulations and is largely determined by arteriolar resistances in these organs. Changes in portal and intrahepatic pressures in response to these changes in portal blood flow are minimized by two important mechanisms: *1*) changes in hepatic lobar venous resistance and *2*) changes in hepatic arterial flow. The effect of hepatic venous resistance was shown in the experiments of Fasth et al. (84). Selective stimulation of the mesenteric nerves reduced portal pressure by 24%, whereas selective stimulation of the hepatic nerves increased portal pressure by 30%. Simultaneous stimulation of hepatic and mesenteric sympathetic nerves caused small and variable initial changes in portal pressure, and during steady-state stimulation, portal pressure was unchanged from the prestimulation control level. Changes in portal flow and changes in hepatic venous resistance were in balance. In addition changes in portal flow normally cause inverse changes in hepatic arterial flow, the hepatic arterial buffer response described earlier. This reduces the changes in total hepatic flow and therefore should minimize the changes in portal and intrahepatic pressures and hepatic blood volume. Autoregulatory escape in the mesenteric arterioles of cats and dogs and in the hepatic arterioles of cats but not dogs also minimizes blood flow changes during sympathetic activity (116, 119). These flow changes may play an important role in stabilizing portal pressure.

EXTERNAL PRESSURE. Another important stimulus that might be expected to cause changes in hepatic volume is external pressure on the splanchnic vessels. In most experimental preparations, the external pressure on the liver is constant and close to atmospheric pressure. However, the liver is normally enclosed in the peritoneal cavity, and intraperitoneal pressure varies widely in a mobile animal or human. It rises substantially during normal walking movements and can rise to 200 mmHg during straining (139). Such increases in external pressure would cause collapse of the splanchnic blood reservoir if protective mechanisms were not available. As Brauer (35) stated, collapse of vessels occurs at the point of lowest transmural pressure, and it is impossible to squeeze out the liver like a sponge by pressing on its surface. When intraperitoneal pressure increases, the IVC and hepatic veins are compressed, and hepatic venous pressure rises to the same extent as intraperitoneal pressure (35, 93, 389). Portal transmural pressure does not change and is relatively insensitive to changes in intraperitoneal pressure.

The data discussed in the previous sections indicate that an important aspect of the evolution of the splanchnic circulation was protection of the splanchnic blood reservoir against passive effects secondary to changes in flows or external pressures. The hepatic venous and arterial resistances tend to stabilize portal pressure in the face of portal flow changes, whereas the anatomical arrangement of the peritoneal cavity protects the blood reservoir against changes in external pressures during movement. These protective mechanisms are only seen when the splanchnic circulation is studied as a whole, and they are circumvented by experimental procedures that measure changes in one vascular parameter while holding the others constant. Protective features like these are not present in other venous beds such as skeletal muscle.

REDISTRIBUTION OF FLOWS. Because different venous beds have different venous compliances, a redistribution of blood flow should cause a redistribution of blood volume. If blood flow is redistributed from kidney to splanchnic bed, then portal pressure would be expected to increase, pooling blood in the splanchnic reservoir and reducing cardiac filling pressures. These possibilities have been discussed (62, 115, 312, 316). This mechanism could only cause a redistribution of stressed volume, and the previous discussion emphasizes the protective mechanisms in the splanchnic bed that minimize pressure changes. However, this mechanism does not explain the blood volume changes caused by the baroreceptor reflex (46), and although it needs further study, in particular with intrahepatic pressure measurements, it does not seem to be a major physiological control mechanism. The system seems designed to minimize the passive consequences of flow redistribution.

In a series of studies, Kiil's group (172, 345–347) have compared the effects on cardiac output of aortic occlusion close to the heart (when peripheral arterial pressure does not fall) and distal to the aortic arch (when splanchnic arterial pressure falls markedly). In the latter situation cardiac preload and cardiac output increased. Up to 70% of this effect was shown to be due to passive drainage of blood from the splanchnic area. Although they claimed this drainage was from intestine and spleen but not liver, this seems unlikely. Estimation of liver volume from a single dimension of one lobe may not be accurate. However, these studies indicate that, at least under rather unusual conditions (descending thoracic aortic occlusion), passive redistribution of blood volume can maintain cardiac filling and output.

HEPATIC VENOUS RESISTANCE. Early studies in the dog, reviewed by Greenway and Stark (136), had suggested that hepatic blood volume was controlled by an outflow sphincter in the hepatic venous system. This led to the concept that venoconstriction caused pooling of blood in the liver and decreased cardiac filling pressures (195). A variety of mechanisms usually associated with pathological conditions, e.g., anaphylaxis, endotoxin, extensive surgery and trauma, and blood transfusion reactions, can result in outflow block in dogs. Administration of histamine produces this response (132), but it is not clear whether endogenous histamine is a mediator in the pathological situations where outflow block occurs. However, in the 1960s, after studies in skeletal muscle (259), intestine (91), and liver (137), it became clear that venoconstriction caused a decrease in blood volume rather than an increase. It is now accepted that active contraction of capacitance vessels mobilizes blood and redistributes it to other organs (see *Active Capacitance Vessel Constriction*, p. 1543).

Nevertheless the possibility of hepatic pooling due to increased hepatic venous resistance should not be forgotten and merits serious study. At present the only proven example of this mechanism is this action of histamine in the dog's liver (17, 132, 234a, 372). This appears to be a selective effect of histamine on hepatic venous resistance without an action on the hepatic capacitance vessels. Norepinephrine and histamine caused similar increases in intrahepatic pressure. With histamine, this increase in intrahepatic pressure caused a passive distension of the liver, whereas with norepinephrine, this passive distension was overcome by an active contraction of the capacitance vessels (132). Histamine does not alter hepatic venous resistance in the cat (125), and the human liver has not been studied. Angiotensin, norepinephrine, and hepatic nerve stimulation all cause contraction of a short segment of lobar hepatic vein, leading to raised intrahepatic pressure (231, 234a). Active contraction of the blood vessels upstream from this sphincter must occur, because hepatic blood volume decreases despite the rise in intrahepatic pressure.

Green (110) and Rutlen et al. (319, 320) have recently explained the actions of isoproterenol, norepinephrine, and acetylcholine on hepatic blood volume by changes in hepatic venous resistance. They demonstrated that isoproterenol and norepinephrine caused a decrease in hepatic volume, a decrease in portal pressure, and a decrease in calculated hepatic venous resistance. These responses, which are contrary to those observed by others, may be due to development of outflow block during their surgical preparation because portal pressures were markedly elevated. Sympathomimetic amines are well known to antagonize mechanisms involving histamine and autacoid release (antiallergic action). In these experiments portal pressure decreased 7–10 mmHg, and this decrease, given a hepatic compliance of 0.6 ml·mmHg$^{-1}$·kg$^{-1}$ body wt in 20-kg dogs, would cause passive drainage of 80–120 ml blood from the liver. They observed 80 ml of blood displaced from the liver by isoproterenol. However, decreases in portal pressure of this magnitude cannot be produced starting at a normal portal pressure of ~8 mmHg, and isoproterenol and norepinephrine increase portal pressure in all other studies. In cats isoproterenol reduces hepatic blood volume despite an increase in intrahepatic pressure, and hepatic venous resistance does not change (326). Thus the effects of isoproterenol on cardiac filling in cats appear to be mediated by a mechanism that does not involve reduction in hepatic venous resistance and passive emptying of the liver.

Supple and Powell (349) showed acetylcholine increased splanchnic vascular capacity in dogs in association with an increased hepatic venous resistance. This response was mimicked by mechanical obstruction of outflow to produce the same rise in portal venous pressure and prevented by holding portal venous pressure constant by venting portal flow. Although they suggested this response may be part of a vagally mediated reflex, there is presently no evidence for a vagal innervation of the hepatic venous resistance site.

It therefore remains possible that drugs selective for the smooth muscle of the hepatic venous resistance site may be found. This area of control of hepatic venous resistance and outflow block merits study. Although it is claimed that outflow block occurs only in dogs, we have seen massive outflow block in cats as a blood transfusion reaction (C. V. Greenway, unpublished observations). Because the main resistance site in the portal circuit appears to be postsinusoidal in both cats and dogs, the major difference between cats and dogs now appears to be the sensitivity of this site to histamine.

### Active Capacitance Vessel Constriction

SYMPATHETIC NERVES AND CATECHOLAMINES. In 1929 Grab, Janssen, and Rein [cited by Knisely et al. (195)] demonstrated in dogs that epinephrine could induce expulsion of an amount of blood equivalent to >50% of the weight of the emptied liver, and Griffith and Emery (138) observed similar effects in cats. Other earlier studies were reviewed by Greenway and Stark (136). Recent studies have repeatedly demonstrated the important effects of the sympathetic nervous system and the catecholamines, norepinephrine and epinephrine, on splanchnic and hepatic blood volumes (17, 41, 42, 52, 53, 67, 68, 73, 125, 130, 137, 150, 151, 153, 183, 184, 319, 320), and these studies have been reviewed recently (117, 216, 312).

Figures 9 and 10 illustrate responses in cats and dogs (130). In these experiments, portal flow was unchanged, and portal pressure increased. In dogs 36% and in cats 47% of the total hepatic blood volume could be expelled, and the responses were essentially maximal at 4–6 Hz. These responses have been confirmed many times in our laboratory, and up to 50% of hepatic blood volume could be expelled by maximal nerve stimulation (111, 114, 137, 326, 327). Bennett et al. (17) reported a reduction in hepatic blood volume of 3.8 ml/kg body wt in dogs during hepatic nerve stimulation at 5 Hz. This represents ~40% of normal hepatic blood volume. When intrahepatic pressure was increased by raising IVC pressure, responses to sympathetic nerve stimulation were impaired at portal pressures >12 mmHg (114, 183), but the responses to norepinephrine were not impaired (224).

Capacitance responses at each frequency of nerve

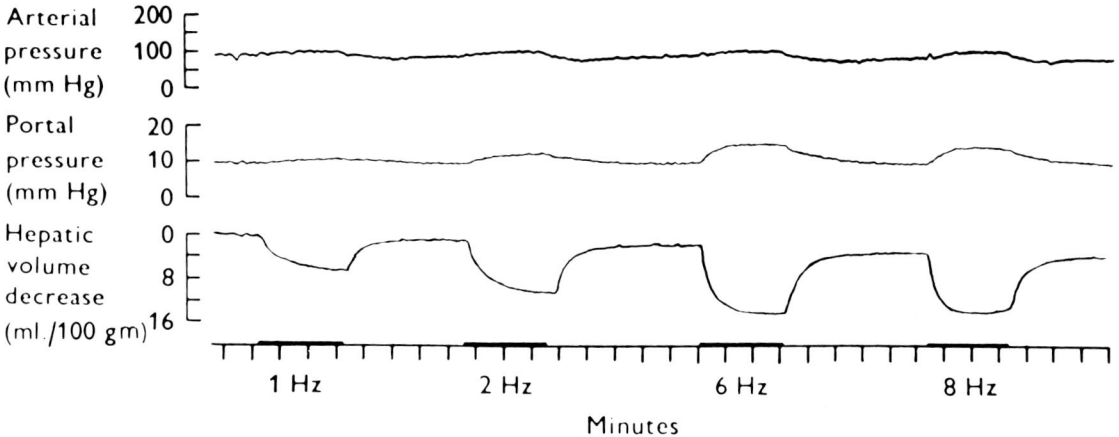

FIG. 9. Effects of hepatic nerve stimulation on hepatic volume recorded by plethysmography in 1 dog. [From Greenway and Oshiro (130).]

stimulation were greater, relative to the maximum response, than resistance responses (Fig. 11). Capacitance responses reached their maximum at lower frequencies than hepatic arterial resistance responses (137), although this may partly be a consequence of expressing flow responses as resistance (340). This has been confirmed for the entire splanchnic bed (183).

The importance of measuring intrahepatic pressure has been discussed. Because intrahepatic pressure increases during sympathetic nerve stimulation and during infusions of norepinephrine and epinephrine, these stimuli tend to cause a passive increase in hepatic volume, and the expulsion of up to 50% of total liver blood volume must be entirely an active contraction by the vessel walls. This raises the unanswered question concerning distribution of the blood volume within the liver, of which little new has been found since 1971 (136). Is >50% of the liver blood volume in the hepatic venous system, or do the sinusoids themselves contract? Transillumination-microscopy studies show that the sinusoids contract (297). Endothelial cells were seen to contract and their nuclei to bulge into the lumen. However, in this study the central and sublobular venules did not respond to nerve stimulation or catecholamines, and occlusion of flow did not cause passive decreases in microvascular calibers. No hemodynamic measurements of pressures, flows, and overall volume changes were made, and high concentrations of norepinephrine were applied locally. It is not possible at present to fit together the direct microscopic observations of the liver microcirculation and the overall hemodynamic measurements, but the magnitude of the hepatic-volume response to sympathetic nerve stimulation strongly indicates contraction of sinusoids must be involved as part of the capacitance response.

Active contraction of capacitance vessels could occur by two possible mechanisms, *1*) a decrease in compliance or *2*) a decrease in unstressed volume. The available evidence indicates that active venous changes occur mainly by a change in unstressed volume (312). Bennett et al. (17) reported a decrease in apparent hepatic compliance of 36% during hepatic nerve stimulation, but hepatic compliance was determined from increments in IVC pressure, and transmission of these increments to the intrahepatic vessels was not determined. The responses to norepinephrine infusions were recently studied in the cat liver (134). Intrahepatic pressure was varied by changing portal flow and by changing outflow pressure, and pressure-volume curves were determined before, during, and after norepinephrine infusion (see Fig. 8). It was shown that the volume response was entirely due to a reduction in unstressed volume. Compliance was unchanged. When these data are evaluated in conjunction with other data (312), it seems reasonable to conclude that active venoconstriction in the liver and other organs involves a decrease in unstressed volume. The concept of venoconstriction as a change in unstressed volume rather than a change in venous compliance has interesting physiological consequences. If venoconstriction occurred by a decrease in compliance, the amount of blood actively mobilized would become progressively smaller as the intrahepatic pressure decreased (see Fig. 7, line 1). This would mean that in those situations where mobilization of blood was most vital, e.g., after hemorrhage, the amount that could be mobilized by the sympathetic nervous system would become smaller as the hemodynamic status deteriorated. In contrast, when venoconstriction causes a change in unstressed volume with no change in compliance, the amount of blood mobilized by the sympathetic nervous system is independent of intrahepatic pressure (see Fig. 7, line 2). In this case, the volumes mobilized actively by the change in unstressed volume and passively by the decline in intrahepatic pressure are additive. This is illustrated in Figure 12. This would give the animal the best chance

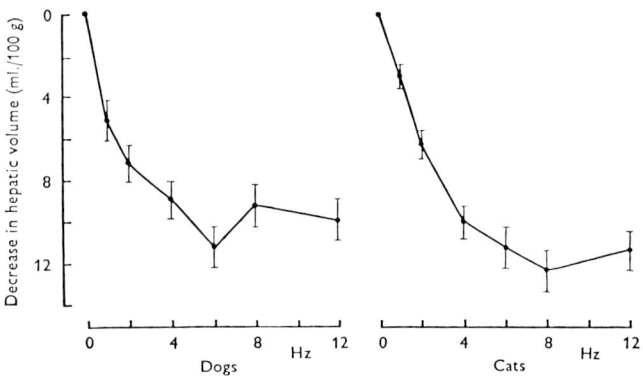

FIG. 10. Mean (± SE) changes in hepatic volume during hepatic nerve stimulation in 13 dogs and 15 cats. Mean control hepatic blood volume was 31 ml/100 g liver in dogs and 27 ml/100 g liver in cats. [From Greenway and Oshiro (130).]

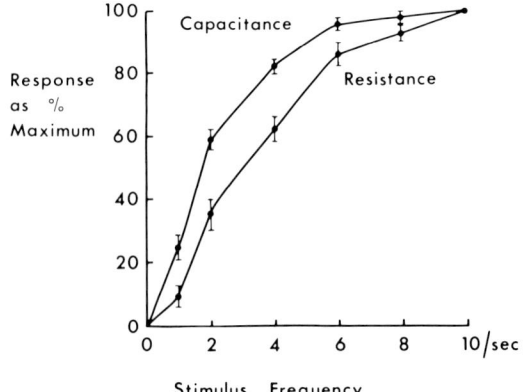

FIG. 11. Frequency-response curves for capacitance and resistance responses to hepatic nerve stimulation in cats. [From Greenway et al. (137).]

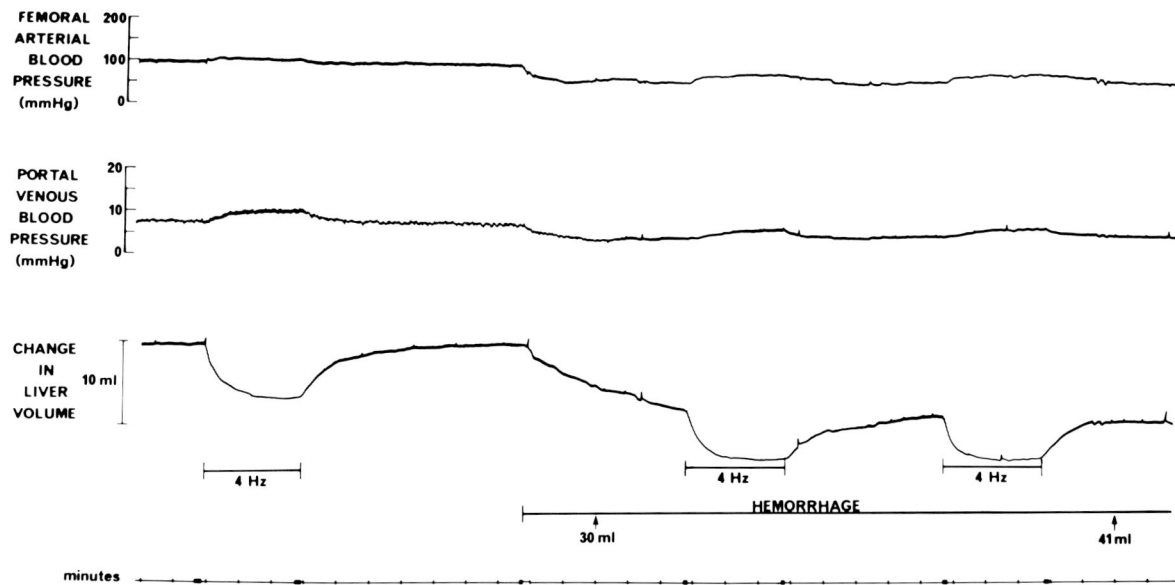

FIG. 12. Effects of hepatic nerve stimulation in 1 cat before and after hemorrhage. Note that in spite of the change in stressed volume after hemorrhage, change in unstressed volume produced by nerve stimulation is almost unchanged. Thus effects of passive and active mobilization of blood volume are additive.

of survival. Unstressed volume is hemodynamically inactive, and when venoconstriction changes unstressed volume into stressed volume, it is equivalent to a transfusion of a significant amount of blood. If all the blood mobilized by the sympathetic nervous system (31% blood volume, see Table 2) involves conversion of unstressed volume to stressed volume, then total stressed volume in the animal can be doubled from 30% to 60% of total blood volume.

ANGIOTENSIN. Although angiotensin has no significant effects on the capacitance vessels in skeletal muscle (28, 58, 85, 175), it appears to exert important effects on those of the splanchnic bed, including the liver. Greenway and Lautt (125) reported dose-response curves for hepatic arterial flow and volume in cats, and significant changes in hepatic blood volume occurred over the same range of doses that produced intestinal vasoconstriction and modest rises in arterial pressure. It was estimated that doses within the probable physiological range of endogenous production decreased hepatic blood volume by up to 20%.

More recently Stokland et al. (348) investigated the mechanism of the increase in arterial pressure during angiotensin infusion. They found that about half of the rise in arterial pressure was due to increased end-diastolic volume, and two-thirds of this increase in preload was due to active contraction of the splanchnic capacitance vessels, resulting in redistribution of blood volume. Nifedipine causes an unexpected contraction of the hepatic capacitance vessels (326). Recent work has shown that this was blocked by nephrectomy and was mediated through the renin-angiotensin system (328a).

Thus it seems clear that angiotensin can constrict hepatic capacitance vessels, but the importance of endogenous levels is not yet clear. It is not known whether angiotensin reduces unstressed volume or venous compliance, but because portal pressure rises substantially (125, 231), the effect must involve active contraction of the capacitance vessels.

RECEPTORS IN HEPATIC VENOUS BED. Hepatic capacitance responses to sympathetic nerve stimulation were blocked by phentolamine and phenoxybenzamine but not by prazosin (111). Phenylephrine had much weaker effects on hepatic blood volume than on arterial and portal pressures relative to norepinephrine, whereas $\alpha$-methylnorepinephrine produced marked responses that were blocked by yohimbine but not prazosin (328). These data indicate that hepatic blood volume responses to both sympathetic nerve stimulation and infusion of catecholamines are mediated through $\alpha_2$-receptors, whereas portal pressure responses (hepatic lobar venous resistance) are mediated through both $\alpha_1$- and $\alpha_2$-receptors. In contrast, the intestinal capacitance vessel responses were mediated through both $\alpha_1$- and $\alpha_2$-receptors, and both appear to be innervated in the intestine (287).

Intra-arterial infusions of isoproterenol had no effect on hepatic blood volume, indicating $\beta$-receptors were not present in the hepatic venous bed (125, 326). Angiotensin causes hepatic capacitance vessel constriction (see ANGIOTENSIN, this page), so the capacitance vessels presumably have angiotensin receptors. In the dog, histamine and acetylcholine receptors appear to be present in the hepatic venous resistance sites but not in the capacitance vessels (132, 349).

Vasopressin seems to have minor direct effects on hepatic blood volume or venous resistance in cats (125). However, studies on vasopressin in the absence of endogenous levels have not yet been done. No other receptors have yet been definitely shown to be present in the hepatic venous bed.

As in the portal vein, the lobar hepatic veins have both longitudinal and circular smooth muscle, and the amounts and distribution vary in different species (385). It is not clear whether these muscles differ in their sensitivity to drugs, although in the portal vein, differences have been shown (43). In rat portal vein, two adrenergic nerve plexuses are present, and substance P–immunoreactive substance is present in both plexuses and in both circular and longitudinal muscle layers. In contrast, VIP immunofluorescence is restricted to the adventitial plexus. Substance P stimulates, whereas VIP inhibits portal vein rhythmic activity, and these substances may modulate sympathetic nerve responses (9). This area has yet to be explored in the hepatic venous bed.

### Reflex Control of Hepatic Venous Bed

An excellent review of reflex control of the venous system has recently been published by Rothe (312). The very powerful sympathetic nervous control of the hepatic capacitance vessels described in the previous section has clearly evolved for some purpose, but the detailed mechanisms of this control remain obscure. Most reflexes produce complex responses in many vascular beds and interact with each other in complex ways. The precise role of the hepatic venous bed is not clear largely due to technical and surgical limitations. To record all the required hepatic vascular parameters (flows, pressures, and volume) is extremely difficult (17, 134). Precise control of stimulation of sensory receptors, e.g., carotid and aortic baroreceptors and chemoreceptors (150, 151, 153, 183, 184), cerebral $P_{CO_2}$ levels (95), or precise stimulation of CNS regions, e.g., the fastigial nucleus, is also extremely difficult. Attempts to combine the two preparations have inevitably simplified one or other aspect, making interpretation of the data difficult. Intrahepatic pressures have most frequently been neglected. Although a reflex venous response restricted to one organ may cause a clear redistribution of blood volume to or from that organ, a generalized venous response may be manifest as generalized changes in venous (or mean circulatory) pressures with little redistribution of blood volume. Thus accurate assessment of pressures is as important as measurements of regional blood volumes.

Furthermore the venous system reflexes are frequently invoked in complex situations, e.g., postural changes, temperature regulation, and muscular exercise. These situations are extremely difficult to study in anesthetized animals, and at present, hepatic venous responses cannot be studied in conscious animals. The responses to such stimuli, e.g., arterial pressure and cardiac output, seen in anesthetized animals strongly indicate that the venous component is blocked by the anesthetics. In anesthetized cats, tilting and exercise produced significant hypotension. Exercise produced by motor nerve stimulation failed to increase cardiac output, although $O_2$ consumption and $CO_2$ production increased significantly (C. V. Greenway, unpublished observations). These types of effects are seen after adrenergic block in humans. The responses to hemorrhage in conscious and anesthetized dogs were compared in a study by Zimpfer et al. (387). Arterial pressure and cardiac output fell much more in the anesthetized dogs. They concluded that pentobarbital did not change the control sympathetic tone but markedly blunted the sympathetic but not the renin-angiotensin system response to hemorrhage. In conscious dogs, mean arterial pressure was well maintained up to a blood loss of 15 ml/kg body wt, whereas in anesthetized dogs it had already fallen 12% after loss of 5 ml/kg body wt. On the other hand, it is hard to imagine that the direct responses to sympathetic nerve stimulation and catecholamines could be much larger in conscious animals than the 50% reduction in hepatic blood volume seen in anesthetized animals. These data strengthen the hypothesis that anesthesia significantly blunts the central nervous mechanisms that control the venous system, including the liver, and this explains the lack of understanding of these mechanisms.

REFLEX RESPONSES IN ANESTHETIZED DOGS. Hainsworth and Karim (150) examined total splanchnic capacitance changes in chloralose-anesthetized dogs in response to changes in carotid sinus pressure. Decreases in carotid sinus pressure increased splanchnic resistance by 67% and reduced splanchnic capacitance by 5 ml/kg body wt (25% splanchnic blood volume). These responses were abolished by crushing the splanchnic nerves. Changes in aortic baroreceptor pressure caused similar but smaller changes that were more variable from dog to dog (184). Stimulation of carotid chemoreceptors with venous blood increased arterial pressure by 38% and decreased splanchnic vascular capacitance by 1 ml/kg body wt. When carotid sinus perfusion pressure was high, stimulation of the chemoreceptors produced smaller resistance but larger capacitance responses than when the pressure was low. In this series, a decrease in carotid sinus pressure produced a decrease in splanchnic capacitance of 1.2 ml/kg body wt (151). Stimulation of aortic chemoreceptors by venous blood or cyanide increased splanchnic resistance and decreased splanchnic capacitance by 0.9–1.2 ml/kg body wt, and the responses were qualitatively similar to those to carotid chemoreceptor stimulation (153). When the cephalic circulation was perfused with blood equilibrated at different $CO_2$ levels, an increase in $P_{CO_2}$ increased splanchnic resistance and decreased splanchnic capacitance. The effect was reduced when carotid sinus pressure was high, but the reflex effects of changes in carotid sinus pressure were enhanced when cephalic $P_{CO_2}$ was raised (95). Portal and hepatic venous pressures were not reported in these studies and the mechanisms and sites of these splanchnic capacitance changes cannot be analyzed.

Brooksby and Donald (41) observed a 32% decrease in total splanchnic blood volume when carotid sinus pressure was changed from 200 to 40 mmHg (Fig. 13). This compared with a 48% decrease at 2 Hz and a 66% decrease at 15 Hz direct splanchnic nerve stimulation. Carneiro and Donald (53) observed a 16% decrease in hepatic blood volume when carotid sinus pressure was reduced from 144 to 40 mmHg and a 20% increase in hepatic blood volume when carotid sinus pressure was raised to 240 mmHg. Hepatic blood volume decreased by 42% when all carotid and cardiopulmonary afferent input to the CNS was interrupted. Maximum hepatic nerve stimulation decreased hepatic blood volume by 60%. Interruption of vagal afferent input from cardiopulmonary receptors alone decreased hepatic blood volume by 15% when carotid sinus pressure was 40 mmHg but had no effect at carotid sinus pressures >160 mmHg. In a further study comparing the intestine, spleen, and liver, bilateral carotid occlusion in vagotomized dogs mobilized 6%–30% of organ blood volume (52). Portal pressures were not reported, and the mechanisms of these volume changes cannot be analyzed. This work was reviewed by Donald (73).

In a series of studies on total vascular capacitance changes resulting from the baroreceptor reflex, Shoukas and co-workers (46, 333–335) concluded that most of the 7–8 ml blood/kg body wt mobilized when carotid sinus pressure was changed from 200 to 50 mmHg came from the splanchnic bed (6.6 ml/kg splanchnic, 1.0 ml/kg nonsplanchnic). Splanchnic venous compliance was estimated at 0.8 ml·mmHg$^{-1}$·kg$^{-1}$ body wt at 50 mmHg sinus pressure and 0.7 ml·mmHg$^{-1}$·kg$^{-1}$ body wt at 200 mmHg sinus pressure, and these values were not significantly different. However, because an increase in central venous pressure is only partially transmitted to the splanchnic bed, and because this transmission changes during hepatic venous constriction by norepinephrine (134), these measurements may underestimate the true splanchnic compliance.

Cousineau et al. (68) used indicator dilution techniques to measure hepatic blood volume in response to bilateral carotid occlusion. Arterial pressure rose from 112 to 167 mmHg, hepatic blood flow was unchanged, whereas hepatic blood volume decreased 40%.

Surprisingly, in the series of experiments discussed earlier by Kiil's group (172, 345, 346) where thoracic aortic occlusion produced large increases in pressures in the carotid sinus and aortic arch, no reflex component in the splanchnic capacitance vessels could be detected and the responses were interpreted as passive drainage due to decreased pressure.

REFLEX RESPONSES IN ANESTHETIZED CATS. Bilateral carotid occlusion had no effect on hepatic blood volume in cats (229), although hepatic arterial resistance responses could be demonstrated (127), and the reflex

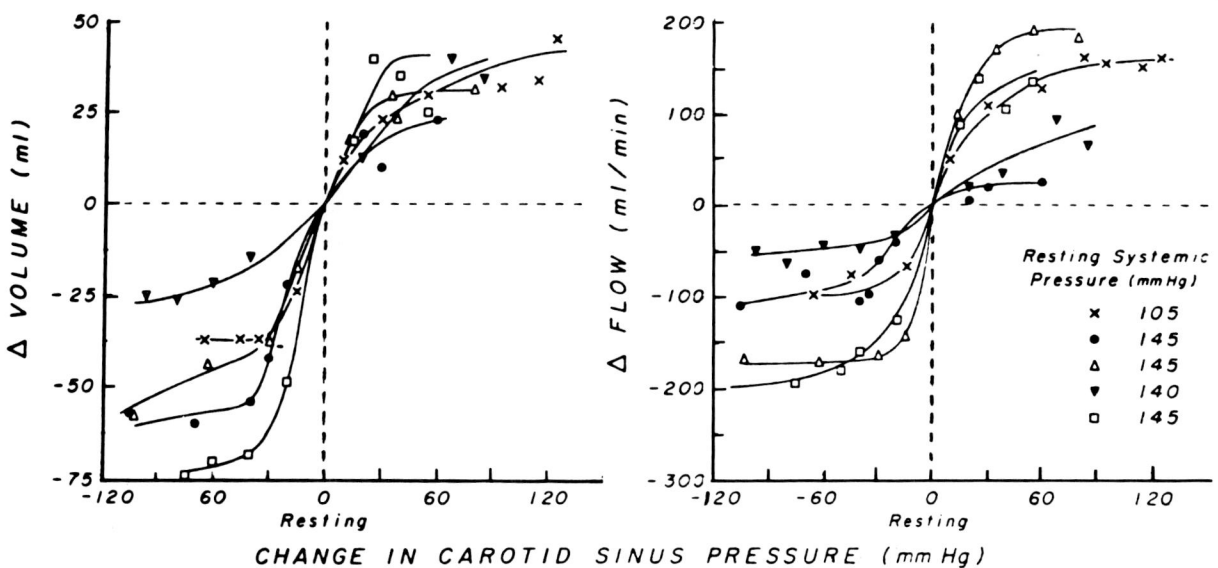

FIG. 13. Increases and decreases in splanchnic blood volume and flow in response to graded isolated changes in pressure in carotid sinus in 5 dogs. *Points* indicate response to increase or decrease in carotid sinus pressure from constant (windkessel-controlled) systemic arterial pressure. Control pressure for each dog is listed. [From Brooksby and Donald (41).]

was very effective in buffering responses to drugs (122). The lack of effect of the baroreceptor reflex on hepatic blood volume in cats was confirmed both by carotid occlusion and by changing pressure in isolated carotid sinus pouches with the vagi intact and cut (220). Attempts so far to elicit reflex hepatic venous responses in cats have been unsuccessful (C. V. Greenway, unpublished observations). Oberg and White (279) showed that the main effects of stimulation of vagal afferents in cats were elicited on the heart and renal vessels, and they found no evidence for a strong involvement of capacitance vessels in reflex patterns mediated by cardiac afferents. Although it has been suggested that venomotor reflexes may be less important in the cat because its small size reduces the gravitational effects of postural changes (117), the effects of direct stimulation of the hepatic nerves are as large in the cat as in the dog. Either reflex responses are blocked by anesthesia (185, 387), or the major reflex mechanisms in cats have not yet been discovered. However, responses to hemorrhage also showed no evidence of active-reflex hepatic venous responses (224).

GENERAL OBSERVATIONS. The role of the venous system in cardiovascular reflexes is controversial and has been discussed (312, 316). There is a large body of circumstantial evidence in favor of reflex control of the venous system, and of the splanchnic and hepatic venous beds in particular, in all species including humans, but direct evidence has been found only in dogs. The mechanisms, active or passive, have not been analyzed critically. The baroreceptor and cardiopulmonary reflexes appear to be inhibitory to sympathetic tone on the hepatic venous system, but the central nervous mechanisms responsible for this tone are unknown. Because hepatic blood volume is smaller in innervated livers than in denervated livers and increases after hexamethonium and nonselective $\alpha$-receptor blockers, sympathetic venous tone is present in anesthetized animals. It is not clear whether the CNS can produce selective venous responses, i.e., whether capacitance responses in the intestine, liver, and spleen can be activated individually and/or independently from resistance responses. Much remains to be done before the reflex and central nervous control of the hepatic venous bed are understood.

## Control of Cardiac Preload and Responses to Drugs

The role of the venous system in control of preload has been reviewed by Rothe (312) in relation to physiological responses, and by Greenway (115, 117) in relation to pharmacological responses. Cardiac output is controlled by contractility, heart rate, preload, and afterload. However, preload and afterload are not independent determinants of cardiac output; they are themselves altered by cardiac output. Stellate ganglion stimulation at a fixed heart rate in dogs caused only a modest sustained rise in cardiac output (323). As stroke volume rose due to increased contractility, preload decreased and afterload increased, limiting the increase in cardiac output. To produce a large sustained rise in cardiac output, cardiac stimulation must be accompanied by venoconstriction, which maintains preload and arteriolar vasodilatation, which prevents a rise in afterload. The response to infusion of epinephrine clearly illustrates this (Fig. 14, *left panel*). The primary action of epinephrine appears to be on the heart because preload, indicated by right atrial pressure, and afterload, indicated by arterial pressure, are unchanged. However, when we compare these responses with the effects of stellate ganglion stimu-

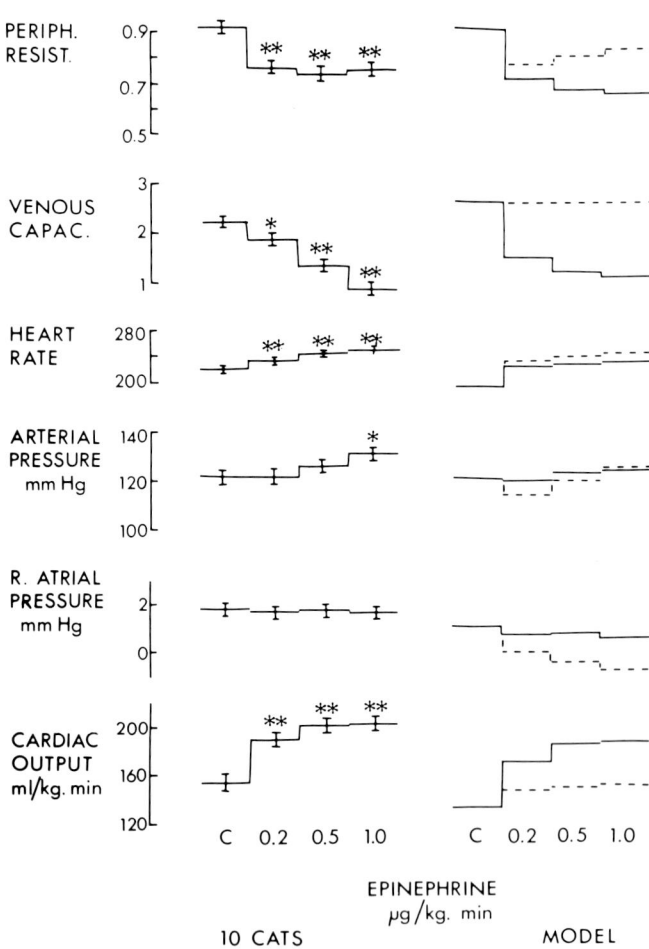

FIG. 14. Effects of intravenous epinephrine infusions on cardiac output and other variables in 10 cats (*left panel*) and effects of epinephrine predicted by computer model (*right panel*). Venous capacitance for cats is hepatic in ml·mmHg$^{-1}$·100 g$^{-1}$ liver and that for model is total splanchnic in ml·mmHg$^{-1}$·kg$^{-1}$ body wt. *Dashed lines*, predicted responses if epinephrine did not reduce splanchnic venous capacitance (cardiac preload falls, and increase in cardiac output is markedly attenuated). *, $P < 0.05$; **, $P < 0.01$. [From Greenway and Innes (117, 121).]

lation, it is clear that epinephrine has actions that maintain preload and prevent a rise in afterload. Measurement of total peripheral resistance and hepatic venous capacitance clearly substantiated this. How important is the venoconstriction in maintaining the increase in cardiac output? This is hard to test experimentally because there are no drugs that selectively block the venous responses. Computer models (see Fig. 14, *right panel*) suggest that if venoconstriction did not occur, preload would fall, and cardiac output would increase by <50% of that in the presence of venoconstriction (115, 117). From these considerations, we developed the hypothesis that all large sustained increases in cardiac output require either venoconstriction or blood volume expansion.

However, responses to isoproterenol appeared to contradict this hypothesis because isoproterenol caused a marked increase in cardiac output but did not contract the hepatic venous system (125). We therefore reexamined the venous responses to isoproterenol (111, 326). Whereas intra-arterial infusions of small doses of isoproterenol had no direct effects on hepatic blood volume, intravenous infusions caused a reduction in hepatic blood volume. This response was accompanied by increases in portal and hepatic lobar venous pressures with no change in hepatic venous resistance, indicating active contraction of the hepatic capacitance vessels. This response was still present after hepatic denervation, adrenalectomy, and nephrectomy. The mechanism remains unknown (326).

Nifedipine, a calcium-channel blocking agent, produced a similar hepatic venoconstriction that was mediated through the renin-angiotensin system (see ANGIOTENSIN, p. 1545), and hydralazine also produced an unexpected hepatic venoconstriction accompanied by a large sustained increase in cardiac output (121). Dopamine constricts the hepatic venous bed probably by acting on the $\alpha_2$-receptors (121). Thus all of the agents that caused hepatic venoconstriction with large decreases in hepatic capacitance also caused large increases in cardiac output (115). Conversely, arteriolar vasodilator drugs that did not produce hepatic venoconstriction, i.e., nitroprusside, diazoxide, and prazosin, did not increase cardiac output (115, 121). Nitroglycerine caused a decrease in portal pressure and a rise in hepatic blood volume, indicating hepatic venodilation (111).

These pharmacological studies thus support the hypothesis that drugs that produce large sustained increases in cardiac output produce hepatic venoconstriction, which serves to maintain cardiac preload. The effects of these vasodilators can be related to their effects on cardiac output and pulmonary congestion when they are used in the treatment of cardiac failure (115).

This approach, relating venous responses in the liver measured by plethysmography to cardiac output changes, accords well with another major approach to the venous system. When venous return is long-circuited through a reservoir and cardiac output is kept constant with a pump, the change in the level of the reservoir during administration of a drug reflects the volume of blood that has to be given to or removed from the animal to hold cardiac output constant (115). Thus venoconstriction, which would cause an increase in cardiac output in the intact animal, now causes a rise in reservoir volume at a constant cardiac output. Norepinephrine, epinephrine, and isoproterenol increase reservoir volume, whereas nitroglycerin decreases it (19, 38, 110, 182, 335). Of particular interest in view of the evidence that hepatic venous responses are mediated by $\alpha_2$-receptors was the absence of a response to phenylephrine except in high doses (19). However, others reported a venoconstrictor action of phenylephrine (5).

Another example of the complex interaction between the factors that affect cardiac output is the response to splanchnic nerve stimulation (120). If the adrenal glands are intact, splanchnic nerve stimulation gives responses similar to those during infusions of epinephrine. However, in adrenalectomized cats, splanchnic nerve stimulation causes marked increases in preload and afterload with no change in cardiac output. If the increase in afterload is prevented by an arteriovenous shunt or by infusion of an arteriolar vasodilator, e.g., nitroprusside, then cardiac output increases, and because more blood is pumped from the right atrium, preload increases to a smaller extent. Two mechanisms are probably involved in the failure of cardiac output to increase in response to the large increase in right atrial pressure. The increase in arterial pressure increases peak end-systolic left ventricular pressure, and this results in increased end-systolic volume at a constant contractility. The increased end-systolic volume compensates for the increased end-diastolic volume. In addition, left ventricular transmural pressure depends on pericardial pressure, which in turn depends on right ventricular pressure. A sudden increase in preload by splanchnic nerve stimulation raises right atrial, right ventricular, and pericardial pressures, and this reduces left ventricular transmural pressure. Thus left ventricular filling in a heart with an intact pericardium is impeded by increased filling of the right ventricle (338, 339, 361).

These examples illustrate some of the relationships between preload, afterload, and cardiac contractility. Venoconstriction is necessary to maintain preload in the presence of increased contractility and decreased afterload to produce a large sustained rise in cardiac output, but a large rise in preload alone may impede cardiac output through its effects on left ventricular filling and on afterload.

Some drugs may have little effect on the smooth muscle but may interfere with the normal innervation of the hepatic capacitance vessels. This may occur by $\alpha_2$-receptor blockade, e.g., yohimbine (328); presynaptic receptor blockade resulting in inhibition of norepinephrine release, e.g., clonidine and bromocryptine (C. V. Greenway, unpublished observations); depletion of transmitter, e.g., reserpine, guanethidine, and 6-hydroxydopamine (226); or sympathetic ganglionic block, e.g., hexamethonium (63) and trimethaphan camphorsulfonate. These drugs would be expected to have little effect on preload in situations where sympathetic tone on the hepatic vascular bed is minimal but to prevent compensatory responses involving the venous capacitance vessels. These drugs cause postural hypotension in clinical use, whereas drugs that dilate arterioles but do not block splanchnic venous responses are less likely to produce postural hypotension (e.g., prazosin, diazoxide, hydralazine, nifedipine). Therefore drugs that impair splanchnic and particularly hepatic venoconstriction mediated by the splanchnic nerves appear to cause postural hypotension. Because sympathetic venoconstriction in muscles now appears insignificant, it seems likely that on standing, blood pools in the legs, and this is largely compensated by sympathetic splanchnic venoconstriction. When this splanchnic venoconstriction is blocked, postural hypotension results. However, it should be noted that inhibition of venous responses is not the only mechanism involved in postural hypotension, and it does not appear to be involved in the vasovagal syncope that may follow the hypotension (81).

*Other Complex Responses Involving Hepatic Venous Bed*

HEMORRHAGE AND INFUSIONS. The venous system plays an important role in responses to changes in blood volume. There is convincing data that the entire splanchnic bed and each of its components, liver, intestine, and spleen, are involved. With moderate hemorrhages up to 15% total blood volume, 50%-65% of the blood removed comes from the splanchnic bed (41, 52, 129, 206). In cats (Fig. 15) the liver contributed 21%-25%, the gastrointestinal tract 22%, and the spleen 19% of the volume removed (129, 224), whereas in dogs the liver contributed 14%, the gastrointestinal tract 7%, and the spleen 35% (52). In humans, the splanchnic bed contributed 53% of the blood removed (291). During infusions of blood equivalent to 10%-34% of the blood volume, again the splanchnic bed pooled 66% of the infused volume with the liver pooling 20%, the gastrointestinal tract 40%, and the spleen only 6% of the total in cats (129). In rats, small hemorrhages decreased pulmonary blood volume more than splanchnic blood volume, but with larger hemorrhages, the limited compensatory ability of the lung

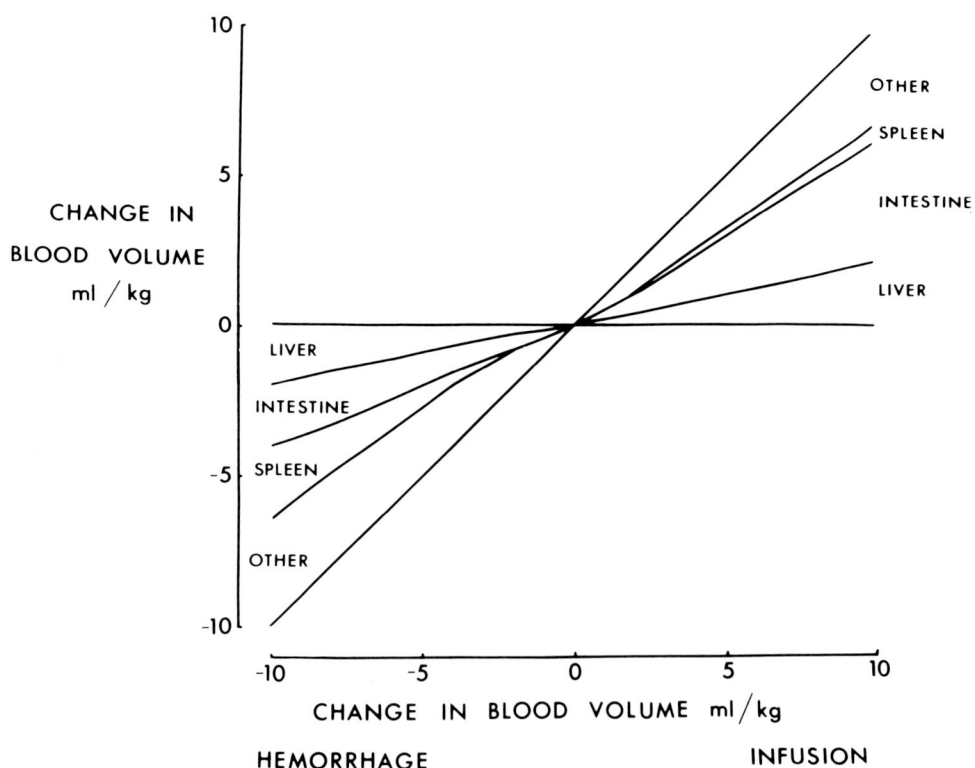

FIG. 15. Contribution of components of splanchnic reservoir when total blood volume was changed by hemorrhage or infusion of blood in cats. [From Greenway (117).]

was exceeded and the splanchnic bed played a more important role (1).

Thus some two-thirds of blood removed from or added to the circulation is mobilized from or pooled in the splanchnic bed. This confirms the importance of the splanchnic bed as a blood reservoir, with its large blood content and large compliance. Although these studies are clear on the role of the splanchnic venous bed, they give little information on the mechanisms involved. Portal and intrahepatic pressures and stressed and unstressed volumes were not recorded in any of these studies. Investigation of these responses is impeded by the depressant effect of anesthetics on the active responses. In conscious dogs, arterial pressure was well maintained up to a blood loss of 15 ml/kg body wt, whereas in anesthetized dogs, it had already fallen 12% after a blood loss of only 5 ml/kg body wt (287).

HYPERTENSION. In hypertension, arterial pressures are increased, while cardiac output is relatively normal, and this combination seems to require an increase in cardiac filling pressures. There is substantial evidence that cardiac filling pressure and mean circulatory pressure are increased in hypertensive animal models and that this is due to a decreased venous compliance rather than an increased stressed or total blood volume (49, 274, 283, 310, 352, 360, 383). The role of the liver in these changes is not clear and requires investigation. Some investigators assume that the significantly decreased venous compliance can be explained by increased sympathetic activity. However, the data presented earlier indicate that sympathetic venoconstriction occurs by a change in unstressed volume without a significant change in compliance. This means the venous compliance changes in hypertension cannot be due to increased sympathetic activity. Study of these aspects might provide significant evidence against the sympathetic-overactivity hypothesis for the pathogenesis of hypertension.

SHOCK AND ENDOTOXIN. Anaphylactic shock and the acute responses to endotoxin in dogs involve massive hepatic congestion due to increased hepatic venous resistance: outflow block (162, 355, 372). Although histamine injected into the portal or hepatic veins produced a similar response (18, 132), it is still not known whether histamine mediates these responses, and little new information has been reported recently. However, many shock conditions in other species, less acute and dramatic than outflow block, appear to be associated with reduced cardiac filling pressures, indicating a defect in venous responsiveness. Responses of the hepatic venous bed to endotoxin in cats were reported recently, and it was shown that endotoxin caused a markedly depressed responsiveness of the hepatic venous bed to sympathetic nerve stimulation, norepinephrine, and angiotensin and a modest pooling of blood in the liver probably due to impairment of preexisting sympathetic tone (327). As the condition of the animals deteriorates due to multiple other actions of endotoxin, the impaired ability to mobilize the hepatic venous reservoir may play an important role in the progressive decline of the cardiac output. However, this cannot be a major factor in the lethality of endotoxin because blood volume expansion does not overcome the lethal effects.

EXERCISE. If the hypothesis that large sustained increases in cardiac output require venoconstriction to maintain cardiac filling pressures is correct, then venoconstriction should play a major role in the cardiovascular changes accompanying muscular exercise. There is evidence for activity of the venous system (312). Splenic contraction occurs in dogs (201) and splanchnic blood volume decreases in humans (369). The problems of studying hepatic blood volume in conscious normal exercising mammals have not been solved. Blood-pool imaging with $^{99m}$Tc-labeled red cells demonstrated significant reduction (25%) in hepatic counts during exercise in patients without coronary artery disease (44).

*Future Prospects*

Knowledge of the splanchnic blood reservoir, its significance, and its control has increased over the past few years. Some hard knowledge and many questions and ideas have been raised for discussion. Many of these questions cannot be resolved until splanchnic blood volume and ultimately splanchnic venous compliance and unstressed volume can be measured without anesthesia and with minimal surgical intervention. New techniques are on the horizon, in particular blood-pool imaging with $^{99m}$Tc-labeled red cells, and a $\gamma$-camera is being increasingly used to study regional blood volumes. However, this noninvasive technique is hard to calibrate, and to be useful, it must be combined with pressure measurements. Only qualitative estimates of regional blood volume without pressure measurements have been reported (44, 268, 321, 337, 339, 353, 354, 375). Rothe (312) presents a long list of situations in which venoconstriction may occur in humans. Determining the sites and mechanisms involved by using new techniques promises to be an exciting experience for researchers in this field.

HEPATIC FLUID EXCHANGE

The first major study on the effects of increased hepatic venous pressure on transsinusoidal fluid movement in the liver was done in rats by Brauer et al. (36), and the area has been reviewed (35, 113, 136). Raised venous pressure caused increased hepatic lymph flow and transudation of fluid across the capsule of the liver. The basic factors controlling movement of fluid across capillary walls were delineated by Starling (341) and can be described in a simplified way by the following equation

$$J_d = K_{fc}[(P_c - P_i) - \sigma(P_{oc} - P_{oi})] \quad (1)$$

where $P_c$ and $P_i$ are the hydrostatic pressure in the capillary and interstitial fluid, respectively, and $P_{oc}$ and $P_{oi}$ are the colloid osmotic pressures in the capillary and interstitial fluid, respectively, $\sigma$ is the osmotic reflection coefficient for protein; $J_d$ is the net fluid movement across the vascular walls, and $K_{fc}$ is the capillary filtration coefficient—the product of capillary permeability and surface area. In a quantitative attempt to study fluid exchange in the liver, Greenway and Lautt (123, 137) used the technique for measuring $K_{fc}$ developed by Folkow's group for use in the intestine (92, 109, 133, 177, 178, 179, 259, 260, 373)

$$K_{fc} = \Delta J_d / \Delta P_c \text{ per unit tissue wt} \quad (2)$$

where $\Delta J_d$ is the change in filtration rate produced by an induced change in capillary pressure $\Delta P_c$. However, the response to an increase in venous pressure was different in the liver (Fig. 16). The slow outward fluid movement during raised venous pressure was maintained at a constant rate for at least 8 h, provided plasma volume was maintained. Thus the protective mechanisms that limit the filtration in the intestine and skeletal muscle were not present in the liver. The fluid was not accumulating in the extracellular space of the liver, and it could be quantitatively removed from the plethysmograph if the instrument was filled with mineral oil to prevent mixing. The fluid had a protein content of at least 80% that of plasma, indicating that hindrance to the passage of protein across the vascular walls was minimal at raised venous pressure. Conventional measurement of $K_{fc}$ in the liver overestimates the true values because venous distension is not complete in 30 s, and the first reported values of 0.3 ml·min$^{-1}$·mmHg$^{-1}$·100 g$^{-1}$ liver (137) were incorrect. Later, $K_{fc}$ was calculated from the filtration rate 20–30 min after raising the venous pressure, giving a $K_{fc}$ of 0.06 ml·min$^{-1}$·mmHg·100 g$^{-1}$ liver (123). When it became clear that pressure in the intrahepatic vessels was close to portal pressure, the data were recalculated with portal pressures as intrahepatic pressures (114). Because the transmission factor from hepatic vein to portal vein varies at different venous pressures (123, 134, 231), the $K_{fc}$ calculated with portal pressure is larger than that calculated with hepatic venous pressure. Thus the recalculation indicated that the hepatic $K_{fc}$ in the anesthetized cat was closer to 0.08 ml·min$^{-1}$·mmHg$^{-1}$·100 g$^{-1}$ liver, and the relationship between filtration rate and intrahepatic pressure was linear. Other recently reported data were obtained with different techniques. Laine et al. (207) studied the effects of raised venous pressure in the dog liver by using lymph flow as an index of filtration with measurement of interstitial pressure by a capsule technique. Sinusoidal pressure was close to portal pressure at 7 mmHg and capsular pressure was 5.8 mmHg, giving a filtration pressure of 1.2 mmHg. Calculated $K_{fc}$ was 0.08 ml·min$^{-1}$·mmHg$^{-1}$·100 g$^{-1}$ liver. Although these values for the cat and dog are very similar, the agreement appears fortuitous. One $K_{fc}$ value is calculated from measurements of total fluid filtration divided by the pressure gradient from blood vessel to peritoneal cavity. The other value is calculated from lymph flow in one major lymphatic divided by the pressure gradient from blood vessel to hepatic interstitial space (capsule). Both values probably underestimate the $K_{fc}$.

Bennett et al. (17, 18) recently attempted to assess fluid filtration in the dog liver during raised hepatic venous pressure by two methods. One involved hematocrit changes in hepatic venous outflow, whereas the other measured the slope of outflow minus inflow during the last few seconds of the period of raised hepatic venous pressure. They confirmed that fluid loss from the vascular system during raised hepatic venous pressure was large but again found it difficult to quantitate. In addition, there appeared to be a rapid increase in extravascular volume on raising IVC pressure, and this volume returned to the vascular system when the pressure was lowered. They were unable to quantitate this change or localize the site but suggested it may reflect expansion of the space of Disse. Steady-state filtration rates in the range 0.2–0.7 ml·min$^{-1}$·mmHg$^{-1}$·100 g$^{-1}$ tissue were calculated.

Thus measurements of fluid filtration from the plasma as lymph or transudate in response to raised intrahepatic pressure have proved difficult and given variable results. However, there seems no doubt that, in relation to other organs, such fluid movements are very large in the liver.

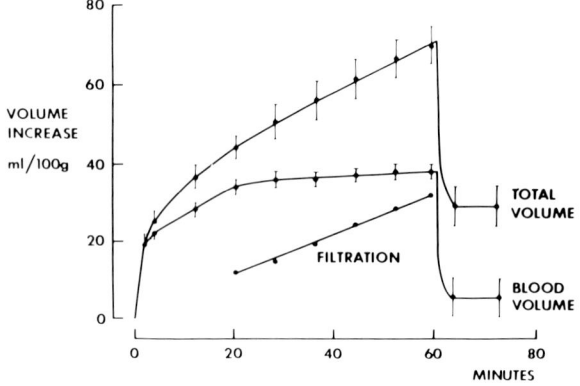

FIG. 16. Changes in total hepatic volume and blood volume (mean ± SE) in 5 cats when hepatic venous pressure was increased to 9.4 mmHg for 60 min. Transsinusoidal fluid filtration was calculated by subtracting mean values of two curves. [From Greenway and Lautt (123).]

## Sites of Filtration and Interstitial Fluid

On the basis of a series of studies with multiple-indicator dilution techniques, Goresky (105) has concluded that no continuous anatomic barrier exists between plasma and the space of Disse. The endothelial lining therefore serves to contain red cells, but virtually immediate lateral diffusion equilibrium is expected for most molecules within the space of Disse. Sinusoids in zone 1 of the acinus form richly anastomotic channels, whereas sinusoids in zone 3 are more radially arranged. There are fenestrations throughout the length of the sinusoids comprised of single large 3 $\mu$m holes and small clustered 1 $\mu$m holes surrounded by microfilaments (145). There are no lymphatics associated with the sinusoids. Lymph vessels appear to arise in the spaces of Mall around the portal tracts, forming extensive lymphatic plexuses that anastomose with other lymphatic plexuses on the surface of the liver underneath the capsule. These anastomoses thus provide a lymphatic pathway from deep in the liver to the surface. Other lymphatic plexuses are found around the larger hepatic veins (35, 64). When formation of lymph exceeds the capacity of the major lymph trunks, exudation of lymph on the surface of the liver occurs (35, 36, 123, 170). Morphological studies suggest that the sinusoidal lumen is 10.6%, the space of Disse is 5%, and the bile canaliculi comprise of 0.4% of parenchymal volume (23).

The picture that emerges from this anatomy is compatible with the physiological data on extracellular spaces in the liver. Sodium (8.9%), sucrose (8.8%), and inulin (7.7%) spaces were almost equal. Albumin extravascular space was 5.7% of liver weight and 64% of the Na$^+$ space (105). Extravascular sucrose spaces were 9.5 and 6.5 ml/100 g liver in other dogs, and these spaces were unchanged by bilateral carotid occlusion (67, 68). In cats a much larger interstitial volume of 23 ml/100 g liver was reported (10), and this high value requires confirmation. The albumin space was 59% of the interstitial space with cat albumin, and this increased to 66% when hepatic venous pressure was raised. The lymph to plasma concentration ratio varied only slightly with molecular size and was 1.0 for lactoglobulin, 0.88 for albumin, and 0.69 for $\gamma$-globulin. Protein content of lymph was 80-95% that of plasma, and hepatic lymph proteins originated from blood, not from new synthesis (35, 72, 108, 136, 207).

These data indicate that 60% of the interstitial space is accessible to albumin, and this presumably includes the spaces of Disse, the spaces of Mall, and the lymphatics. Lymph appears to be formed by filtration of high-protein fluid from the spaces of Disse across the limiting plate into the lymphatics in the spaces of Mall, and across the limiting plate into the tissue spaces and lymphatics around the hepatic veins. The limiting plate appears to represent a very minor barrier to passage of proteins, depending on their molecular weights (72, 108, 207). The site of the remaining 40% of the interstitial space that is normally inaccessible to albumin but becomes accessible to albumin when hepatic venous pressure is raised remains unknown. Hepatocytes are joined by tight junctions (79), and the volumes of any spaces beyond the tight junctions are not known. Brauer (35) estimated biliary spaces as 2% of liver weight. Spaces between hepatocytes beyond the tight junctions plus biliary spaces could represent the spaces normally inaccessible to albumin. Increased hepatic venous pressure could increase albumin-accessible space by disrupting the tight junctions and the canalicular system. Bile flow is markedly reduced by a short period of raised hepatic venous pressure, and on restoration of the venous pressure, bile flow does not recover over the following hours in anesthetized cats. The uptake of BSP from the plasma into the hepatocytes is unimpaired at this stage, but no BSP appears in the small residual bile flow. This may indicate disruption of the bile canaliculi and tight junctions, with passage of the canalicular bile into the plasma or lymph instead of into the bile ducts (113).

Total lymph flow from the liver has never been measured. Brauer (35) estimated it at 0.04-0.06 ml· min$^{-1}$· 100 g$^{-1}$ liver, whereas Laine et al. (207) reported 0.06 ml/min from one prenodal lymphatic in dogs. Lymph flow increased 63%/mmHg increment in interstitial pressure.

*Reabsorption of Filtered Fluid*

There is no evidence that reabsorption of fluid can occur from a plethysmograph or the peritoneal cavity into the hepatic vasculature. It is very difficult to reverse the hydrostatic pressure gradient across the small hepatic vessels because raising intraperitoneal or plethysmograph pressure compresses the large veins. Thus sinusoidal pressure increases by the same amount as extravascular pressure (389). It appears that protection of the liver against edema is achieved by lymphatic drainage and transudation across the capsule, rather than by mechanisms that limit filtration or that allow reabsorption of the fluid into the hepatic vessels (123, 207).

Zink (388) has studied the reabsorption of fluid from the peritoneal cavity by encasing the abdomen in a rigid plaster cast to form an abdominal plethysmograph. The rate of fluid absorption from the peritoneal cavity was directly proportional to the intraperitoneal pressure regardless of whether the intraperitoneal fluid was free from protein or contained a protein concentration equivalent to that of plasma. The relationship between absorption and intraperitoneal pressure was approximately linear with a rate of 0.02 ml· min$^{-1}$· mmHg$^{-1}$ in 2.5-kg cats. This would give a rate of 0.01 ml·min$^{-1}$·mmHg$^{-1}$·kg$^{-1}$ body wt or 0.04 ml· min$^{-1}$·mmHg$^{-1}$·100 g$^{-1}$ liver. Thus removal from the peritoneal cavity per unit pressure appears to be substantially slower than formation, and this may explain the occurrence of ascites in some pathological situations. Further studies with $^{131}$I-labeled albumin showed that protein was absorbed from the peritoneal cavity in equal proportion to the absorption of fluid, and the fractional rates of protein absorption were never significantly different from the fractional rates of fluid absorption. Both fractional rates were independent of the protein concentration in the peritoneal cavity, and this indicated that the removal process involved lymphatic absorption rather than transcapillary absorption (256). Earlier Courtice and co-workers (66, 386) suggested that this reabsorption was restricted to the diaphragmatic lymphatics, but this conclusion requires confirmation. Zink (389) went on to examine the relationships between formation and removal of peritoneal fluid by simultaneously varying hepatic venous and intraperitoneal pressures. With a hepatic venous pressure of 12 mmHg and an intraperitoneal pressure of zero, filtration of fluid occurred into the peritoneal cavity from the liver. As intraperitoneal pressure was increased, net filtration decreased, then stopped and then reversed to a net absorption. This was caused by two processes: increasing intraperitoneal pressure increased reabsorption from the peritoneal cavity, and it reduced filtration from the liver by reducing the pressure gradient across the vascular walls within the liver. Thus the pathogenesis of ascites can be viewed as a dynamic state determined by filtration from the hepatic vasculature, hepatic lymphatic drainage, and reabsorption from the peritoneal cavity (207, 389). The various factors present in pathological situations that influence this balance are beyond the scope of this chapter.

*Effects of Drugs on Fluid Exchange*

Various sphincters have been postulated in the hepatic vascular bed (79, 136), and it seemed possible that $K_{fc}$ would be variable under different conditions as it is in other vascular beds (260). This problem was examined by Greenway and Lautt (124). Because a change in $K_{fc}$ would not be apparent unless there was an ongoing filtration, a steady-state filtration was induced by raising hepatic venous pressure, and the effects of drug infusions on this filtration were assessed. Infusions of epinephrine, isoproterenol, and histamine had no effect on the steady-state filtration produced by the increased hepatic venous pressure, and it was concluded that these drugs did not modify either surface area or permeability within the liver. In contrast to these results in cats, a large filtration with histamine and a smaller filtration with epinephrine was seen in dogs (17). Because histamine produces outflow block in dogs but not in cats, this difference would be expected for histamine, but the difference for epinephrine cannot at present be explained.

*Effects of Hepatic Nerve Stimulation on Fluid Exchange*

Stimulation of the hepatic nerves causes an increase in portal pressure and a maintained decrease in hepatic volume. On cessation of stimulation, these variables recovered to the control values (see *Active Capacitance Vessel Constriction*, p. 1543). These responses presented no problem when it was believed that sinusoidal pressure was low and portal pressure was increased by a presinusoidal portal constriction (136, 216). However, when data indicated that the sympathetic nerves produced an increase in intrahepatic pressure that was at least 80% of the increase in portal pressure, the response became unexplainable. The rise in intrahepatic vascular pressure should have caused a substantial filtration during the period of nerve stimulation, and Bennett et al. (17) reported increased filtration in dogs during hepatic nerve stimulation with constant flow perfusion. We therefore reexamined the problem in cats (113). The venous pressure was increased to induce a steady filtration that was recorded for at least 20 min. The nerve stimulation was then carried out, and after cessation the hepatic volume was followed until the control slope had again been recorded for at least 10 min. This slope was then extrapolated back to the point when the stimulation was terminated. The net effect of the stimulation on the filtration could then be determined independent of the blood volume changes during the stimulation. It was clear that when venous pressure was increased sufficiently to raise portal pressure by a moderate amount, the resulting filtration rate was significantly reduced during hepatic nerve stimulation lasting 3–10 min despite the increase in intravascular distending pressure (Fig. 17). However, when venous pressure was markedly increased, the filtration rate was not significantly altered during nerve stimulation. Thus the effect of hepatic nerve stimulation on filtration rate was abolished at high distending pressures, resembling the abolition of the blood volume response (113, 114). There are at least two possible explanations for the inhibition of filtration by sympathetic nerve stimulation. First, the sympathetic nerves reduce sinusoidal surface area. Greenway and Oshiro (131) demonstrated that hepatic nerve stimulation does not cause a gross redistribution of flow within the liver, but this does not exclude the possibility of a general reduction in the number of open sinusoids, thus a

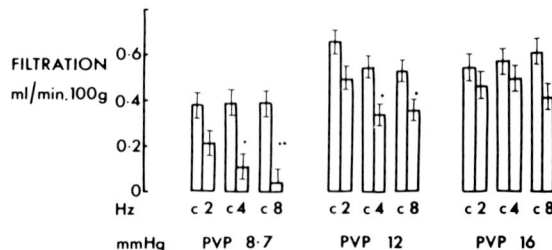

FIG. 17. Filtration rates induced by 3 levels of increased hepatic venous pressure during control periods (C) and during hepatic nerve stimulation at frequencies of 2, 4, and 8 Hz in 6 cats (means ± SE; *, $P < 0.05$; **, $P < 0.01$). Control portal pressure was 6.7 mmHg. [From Greenway (113).]

reduction in surface area. Although changes in $O_2$ delivery occurred during the first 3 min of hepatic nerve stimulation, $O_2$ uptake then returned to normal (216), and lidocaine clearance was not altered (238). Thus it is unlikely that reduction in sinusoidal surface area can explain the absence of filtration during nerve stimulation. Second, the sympathetic nerves reduce sinusoidal permeability. Effects of sympathetic nerves on vascular permeability have been reported, and it is possible that vascular permeability may be increased in adipose tissue and brain by sympathetic stimulation (311). In the liver, the nerves would have to decrease an already high permeability (108) to explain our results (113). Decreased sinusoidal permeability or permeability of the limiting plate separating the spaces of Disse and Mall are possible explanations for the absence of filtration during hepatic nerve stimulation.

It is clear that quantitative studies on hepatic fluid exchange and lymph flow have proved difficult, and much remains to be done. All of the studies have major technical problems, and many quantitative discrepancies between the results are not yet explainable.

None of this work could have been done without the enthusiastic help of our graduate students and technicians.

This study was supported by grants from the Medical Research Council of Canada, the Manitoba and Saskatchewan Heart Foundations, and the Canadian Liver Foundation.

REFERENCES

1. AARSETH, P. The effects of intraperitoneally and intravenously administered pentobarbitone anesthesia on pulmonary and splanchnic blood volumes in rats. *Acta Physiol. Scand.* 85: 270–276, 1972.
2. AHMAD, A. B., P. N. BENNETT, AND M. ROWLAND. Models of hepatic drug clearance: discrimination between the "well stirred" and "parallel tube" models. *J. Pharm. Pharmacol.* 35: 219–224, 1983.
3. AHMAD, A. B., P. N. BENNETT, AND M. ROWLAND. Influence of route of hepatic administration on drug availability. *J. Pharmacol. Exp. Ther.* 230: 718–725, 1984.
4. ANDREEN, M., L. IRESTEDT, AND B. ZETTERSTRÖM. The different responses of the hepatic arterial bed to hypovolemia and to halothane anesthesia. *Acta Anaesthesiol. Scand.* 21: 457–469, 1977.
5. APPLETON, C., M. OLAJOS, E. MORKIN, AND S. GOLDMAN. $\alpha$-1 adrenergic control of the venous circulation in intact dogs. *J. Pharmacol. Exp. Ther.* 233: 729–734, 1985.
6. AYERS, A. B., B. N. DAVIES, AND P. G. WITHRINGTON. Responses of the isolated, perfused human spleen to sympathetic nerve stimulation, catecholamines and polypeptides. *Br. J. Pharmacol.* 44: 17–30, 1972.
7. BAKER, K. J., AND S. E. BRADLEY. Binding of sulfobromophthalein (BSP) sodium by plasma albumin. Its role in hepatic BSP extraction. *J. Clin. Invest.* 45: 281–287, 1966.
8. BANASZAK, E. F., W. J. STEKIEL, R. A. GRACE, AND J. J. SMITH. Estimation of hepatic blood flow using a single injection dye clearance method. *Am. J. Physiol.* 198: 877–880, 1960.
9. BARJA, F., AND R. MATHISON. Adrenergic and peptidergic (substance P and vasoactive intestinal polypeptide) innervation of the rat portal vein. *Blood Vessels* 19: 263–272, 1982.
10. BARROWMAN, J. A., M. A. PERRY, P. R. KVIETYS, AND D. N. GRANGER. Exclusion phenomenon in the liver interstitium. *Am. J. Physiol.* 243 (*Gastrointest. Liver Physiol.* 6): G410–G414, 1982.
11. BASS, L. Current models of hepatic elimination. *Gastroenterology* 76: 1504–1505, 1979.
12. BASS, L. Flow dependence of first-order uptake of substances by heterogeneous perfused organs. *J. Theor. Biol.* 86: 365–376, 1980.
13. BASS, L. Models of hepatic drug elimination. *J. Pharm. Sci.* 72: 1229, 1983.
14. BASS, L., S. KEIDING, K. WINKLER, AND N. TYGSTRUP. Enzymatic elimination of substrates flowing through the intact liver. *J. Theor. Biol.* 61: 393–409, 1976.
15. BASS, L., AND P. J. ROBINSON. Effects of capillary heterogeneity on rates of steady uptake of substances by the intact liver. *Microvasc. Res.* 22: 43–57, 1981.
16. BASS, L., P. ROBINSON, AND A. J. BRACKEN. Hepatic elimination of flowing substrates: the distributed model. *J. Theor. Biol.* 72: 161–184, 1978.
17. BENNETT, T. D., C. L. MACANESPIE, AND C. F. ROTHE. Active hepatic capacitance responses to neural and humoral stimuli in dogs. *Am. J. Physiol.* 242 (*Heart Circ. Physiol.* 11): H1000–H1009, 1982.
18. BENNETT, T. D., AND C. F. ROTHE. Hepatic capacitance responses to changes in flow and hepatic venous pressure in dogs. *Am. J. Physiol.* 240 (*Heart Circ. Physiol.* 9): H18–H28, 1981.
19. BENNETT, T. D., C. R. WYSS, AND A. M. SCHER. Changes in vascular capacity in awake dogs in response to carotid sinus occlusion and administration of catecholamines. *Circ. Res.* 55: 440–453, 1984.
20. BENOIT, J. N., J. A. BARROWMAN, S. L. HARPER, P. R. KVIETYS, AND D. N. GRANGER. Role of humoral factors in the intestinal hyperemia associated with chronic portal hypertension. *Am. J. Physiol.* 247 (*Gastrointest. Liver Physiol.* 10): G486–G493, 1984.
21. BIRTCH, A. G., B. H. CASEY, AND R. M. ZAKHEIM. Hepatic blood flow measured by the krypton-85 clearance technique. *Surgery St. Louis* 62: 174–180, 1967.
22. BLEI, A. T., D. J. O'REILLY, J. GOTTSTEIN, W. W. HAUCK, AND M. ZIMMER. Distribution of portal blood flow in the liver of the rat: a microsphere study. *J. Lab. Clin. Med.* 104: 404–413, 1984.
23. BLOUIN, A., R. P. BOLENDER, AND E. R. WEIBEL. Distribution of organelles and membranes between hepatocytes and nonhepatocytes in the rat liver parenchyma. *J. Cell Biol.* 72: 441–455, 1977.
24. BLUMGART, L. H., A. M. HARPER, D. P. LEIBERMAN, AND R. T. MATHIE. Liver blood flow measurement with [85]krypton clearance by portal venous and hepatic arterial routes of injection (Abstract). *Br. J. Pharmacol.* 60: 278P, 1977.
25. BOLLMAN, J. L. The animal with an Eck fistula. *Physiol. Rev.* 41: 607–621, 1961.
26. BOR, N. M., M. ALVUR, M. ERCAN, AND C. F. BEKDIK. Hepatic blood flow during rapid intravenous glucose tolerance test. *Res. Exp. Med.* 177: 159–165, 1980.
27. BORNHOF, C., P. O. SCHWILLE, H. J. BEIJER, AND G. A. CHARBON. Hemodynamic splanchnic and renal changes associated with administration of arginine-hydrochloride in dogs. *Res. Exp. Med.* 177: 57–70, 1980.
28. BORUCKI, L. J., D. LEVENSON, AND N. K. HOLLENBERG. Cardiovascular responses to blockade of angiotensin and $\alpha$-adrenergic receptors. *Am. J. Physiol.* 235 (*Renal Fluid Electrolyte Physiol.* 4): F199–F202, 1978.
29. BRADLEY, E. L. Measurement of hepatic blood flow in man. *Surgery* 75: 783–789, 1974.
30. BRADLEY, S. E. The hepatic circulation. In: *Handbook of Physiology. Circulation*, edited by W. F. Hamilton. Bethesda, MD: Am. Physiol. Soc., 1963, sect. 2, vol. 2, chapt. 41, p. 1387–1438.

31. BRADLEY, S. E., F. J. INGELFINGER, AND G. P. BRADLEY. Hepatic circulation in cirrhosis of the liver. *Circulation* 5: 419–429, 1952.
32. BRANCH, R. A., A. S. NIES, AND D. G. SHAND. The disposition of propranolol. VIII. General implications of the effects of liver blood flow on elimination from the perfused rat liver. *Drug Metab. Dispos.* 1: 687–690, 1973.
33. BRANCH, R. A., D. G. SHAND, AND A. S. NIES. Increase in hepatic blood flow and D-propranolol clearance by glucagon in the monkey. *J. Pharm. Exp. Ther.* 187: 581–587, 1973.
34. BRANCH, R. A., D. G. SHAND, G. R. WILKINSON, AND A. S. NIES. The reduction of lidocaine clearance by DL-propranolol: an example of hemodynamic drug interaction. *J. Pharm. Exp. Ther.* 184: 515–519, 1973.
35. BRAUER, R. W. Liver circulation and function. *Physiol. Rev.* 43: 115–213, 1963.
36. BRAUER, R. W., R. J. HOLLOWAY, AND G. F. LEONG. Changes in liver function and structure due to experimental passive congestion under controlled hepatic vein pressures. *Am. J. Physiol.* 197: 681–692, 1959.
37. BRAUER, R. W., O. S. SHILL, AND J. S. KREBS. Studies concerning functional differences between liver regions supplied by the hepatic artery and by the portal vein. *J. Clin. Invest.* 38: 2202–2214, 1959.
38. BRAUNWALD, E., J. ROSS, R. L. KAHLER, T. E. GAFFNEY, A. GOLDBLATT, AND D. T. MASON. Reflex control of the systemic venous bed. Effects on venous tone of vasoactive drugs and of baroreceptor and chemoreceptor stimulation. *Circ. Res.* 12: 539–550, 1963.
39. BREDFELDT, J. E., E. M. RILEY, AND R. J. GROSZMANN. Compensatory mechanism in response to an elevated hepatic oxygen consumption in chronic ethanol-fed rats. *Am. J. Physiol.* 248 (*Gastrointest. Liver Physiol.* 11): G507–G511, 1985.
40. BRITTON, S. L., AND D. E. DONALD. Response of large hindlimb veins of dog to aortic arch chemoreceptor stimulation. *Am. J. Physiol.* 242 (*Heart Circ. Physiol.* 11): H1050–H1055, 1982.
41. BROOKSBY, G. A., AND D. E. DONALD. Dynamic changes in splanchnic blood flow and blood volume in dogs during activation of sympathetic nerves. *Circ. Res.* 29: 227–238, 1971.
42. BROOKSBY, G. A., AND D. E. DONALD. Release of blood from the splanchnic circulation in dogs. *Circ. Res.* 31: 105–118, 1972.
43. BROWN, B. P., S. ANURAS, AND D. D. HEISTAD. Responsiveness of longitudinal and circular muscle layers in the portal vein. *Am. J. Physiol.* 242 (*Gastrointest. Liver Physiol.* 5): G498–G503, 1982.
44. BROWN, K. A., R. D. OKADA, C. A. BOUCHER, J. A. ROTHENDLER, H. W. STRAUSS, AND G. H. POHOST. Exercise induced changes in hepatic blood volume measured during cardiac equilibrium cineangiography. *J. Am. Coll. Cardiol.* 2: 514–521, 1983.
45. BROWSE, N. L., D. E. DONALD, AND J. T. SHEPHERD. Role of the veins in the carotid sinus reflex. *Am. J. Physiol.* 210: 1424–1434, 1966.
46. BRUNNER, M. J., A. A. SHOUKAS, AND C. L. MACANESPIE. The effect of the carotid sinus baroreceptor reflex on blood flow and volume redistribution in the total systemic vascular bed of the dog. *Circ. Res.* 48: 274–285, 1981.
47. BURCHELL, A. R., A. H. MORENO, W. F. PANKE, AND T. F. NEALON. Hepatic artery flow improvement after portocaval shunt: a single hemodynamic clinical correlate. *Ann. Surg.* 184: 289–300, 1976.
48. BURCZYNSKI, F. J., AND C. V. GREENWAY. Hepatic blood flow: accuracy of estimation from galactose clearances in cats. *Can. J. Physiol. Pharmacol.* 64: 1310–1315, 1986.
48a. BURCZYNSKI, F. J., C. V. GREENWAY, AND D. S. SITAR. Hepatic blood flow: accuracy of estimation from infusions of indocyanine green in anesthetized cats. *Br. J. Pharmacol.* 91: 651–659, 1987.
48b. BURCZYNSKI, F. J., K. L. PUSHKA, D. S. SITAR, AND C. V. GREENWAY. Hepatic plasma flow: accuracy of estimation from bolus injections of indocyanine green. *Am. J. Physiol.* 252 (*Heart Circ. Physiol.* 21): H953–H962, 1987.
49. BURKE, M. J., W. J. STEKIEL, AND J. H. LOMBARD. Reduced venoconstrictor reserve in spontaneously hypertensive rats subjected to hemorrhagic states. *Circ. Shock* 14: 25–37, 1984.
50. BYNUM, T. E., AND J. W. FARA. Hepatic artery response to vasopressin. *Am. J. Physiol.* 239 (*Gastrointest. Liver Physiol.* 2): G378–G381, 1980.
51. CAESAR, J., S. SHALDON, L. CHIANDUSSI, L. GUEVARA, AND S. SHERLOCK. The use of indocyanine green in the measurement of hepatic blood flow and as a test of hepatic function. *Clin. Sci.* 21: 43–57, 1961.
52. CARNEIRO, J. J., AND D. E. DONALD. Blood reservoir function of dog spleen, liver, and intestine. *Am. J. Physiol.* 232 (*Heart Circ. Physiol.* 1): H67–H72, 1977.
53. CARNEIRO, J. J., AND D. E. DONALD. Change in liver blood flow and blood content in dogs during direct and reflex alteration of hepatic sympathetic nerve activity. *Circ. Res.* 40: 150–158, 1977.
54. CARR, D. H., AND D. A. TITCHEN. Postprandial changes in parotid salivary secretion and plasma osmolality and the effects of intravenous infusions of saline solutions. *Q. J. Exp. Physiol. Cogn. Med. Sci.* 63: 1–21, 1978.
55. CHARBON, G. A., AND P. F. HULSTAERT. Augmentation of arterial hepatic and renal flow by extracted and synthetic parathyroid hormone. *Endocrinology* 95: 621–626, 1974.
56. CHOU, C. C., AND H. SIREGAR. Role of histamine $H_1$- and $H_2$-receptors in postprandial intestinal hyperemia. *Am. J. Physiol.* 243 (*Gastrointest. Liver Physiol.* 6): G248–G252, 1982.
57. COHEN, M. M., D. S. SITAR, J. R. MCNEILL, AND C. V. GREENWAY. Vasopressin and angiotensin on resistance vessels of spleen, intestine, and liver. *Am. J. Physiol.* 218: 1704–1706, 1970.
58. COHN, J. N. Relationship of plasma volume changes to resistance and capacitance vessel effects of sympathomimetic amines and angiotensin in man. *Clin. Sci.* 30: 267–278, 1966.
59. COHN, J. N., I. M. KHATRY, AND R. J. GROSZMANN. Hepatic blood flow in alcoholic liver disease measured by an indicator dilution technique. *Am. J. Med.* 53: 704–714, 1972.
60. COHN, J. N., AND A. L. PINKERSON. Intrahepatic distribution of hepatic arterial and portal venous flows in the dog. *Am. J. Physiol.* 216: 285–289, 1969.
61. COHN, R., AND S. KOUNTZ. Factors influencing control of arterial circulation in the liver of the dog. *Am. J. Physiol.* 205: 1260–1264, 1963.
62. COLEMAN, T. G., R. D. MANNING, R. A. NORMAN, AND A. C. GUYTON. Control of cardiac output by regional blood flow distribution. *Ann. Biomed. Eng.* 2: 149–163, 1974.
63. COMBES, B., J. R. PREEDY, H. O. WHEELER, R. M. HAYS, AND S. E. BRADLEY. The hemodynamic effects of hexamethonium bromide in the dog with special reference to "splanchnic pooling." *J. Clin. Invest.* 36: 860–865, 1957.
64. COMPARINI, L. Lymph vessels in the liver in man. *Angiologica Basel* 6: 262–274, 1969.
65. CONRAD, K. A., J. M. BYERS, P. R. FINLEY, AND L. BURNHAM. Lidocaine elimination: effects of metoprolol and of propranolol. *Clin. Pharmacol. Ther.* 33: 133–138, 1983.
66. COURTICE, F. C., AND A. W. STEINBECK. The effects of lymphatic obstruction and of posture on the absorption of protein from the peritoneal cavity. *Aust. J. Exp. Biol. Med. Sci.* 29: 451–458, 1951.
67. COUSINEAU, D., C. A. GORESKY, AND C. P. ROSE. Blood flow and norepinephrine effects on liver vascular and extravascular volumes. *Am. J. Physiol.* 244 (*Heart Circ. Physiol.* 13): H495–H504, 1983.
68. COUSINEAU, D., C. A. GORESKY, C. P. ROSE, AND S. LEE. Reflex sympathetic effects on liver vascular space and liver perfusion in dogs. *Am. J. Physiol.* 248 (*Heart Circ. Physiol.* 17): H186–H192, 1985.
69. DANESHMEND, T. K., M. D. ENE, G. PARKER, AND C. J. ROBERTS. Effects of chronic oral cimetidine on apparent liver

blood flow and hepatic microsomal enzyme activity in man. *Gut* 25: 125–128, 1984.
70. DAVIES, B. N., E. W. HORTON, AND P. G. WITHRINGTON. The occurrence of prostaglandin E2 in splenic venous blood of the dog following splenic nerve stimulation. *Br. J. Pharmacol.* 32: 127–135, 1968.
71. DI SALVO, J., S. BRITTON, P. GALVAS, AND T. W. SANDERS. Effects of angiotensin I and angiotensin II on canine hepatic vascular resistance. *Circ. Res.* 32: 85–92, 1973.
72. DIVE, C., A. C. NADALINI, AND J. F. HEREMANS. Origin and composition of hepatic lymph proteins in the dog. *Lymphology* 4: 133–139, 1971.
73. DONALD, D. E. Mobilization of blood from the splanchnic circulation. In: *Hepatic Circulation in Health and Disease*, edited by W. W. Lautt. New York: Raven, 1981, p. 193–201.
74. DONALD, D. E., AND L. L. AARHUS. Active and passive release of blood from canine spleen and small intestine. *Am. J. Physiol.* 227: 1166–1172, 1974.
75. DONN, K. H., J. R. POWELL, J. F. ROGERS, AND J. R. PLACHETKA. Lack of effect of histamine H$_2$-receptor antagonists on indocyanine green disposition measured by two methods. *J. Clin. Pharmacol.* 24: 360–370, 1984.
76. DRAPANAS, T., D. N. KLUGE, AND W. G. SCHENK. Measurement of hepatic blood flow by bromsulphalein and by the electromagnetic flowmeter. *Surgery St. Louis* 48: 1017–1021, 1960.
77. ECKSTEIN, J. W., AND W. K. HAMILTON. The pressure-volume responses of human forearm veins during epinephrine and norepinephrine infusions. *J. Clin. Invest.* 36: 1663–1671, 1957.
78. EINZIG, S., G. H. RAO, AND J. G. WHITE. Differential sensitivity of regional vascular beds in the dog to low-dose prostacyclin infusion. *Can. J. Physiol. Pharmacol.* 58: 940–946, 1980.
79. ELIAS, H., AND J. C. SHERRICK. *Morphology of the Liver.* New York: Academic, 1969.
80. EPSTEIN, S. E., G. D. BEISER, M. STAMPFER, AND E. BRAUNWALD. Role of the venous system in baroreceptor-mediated reflexes in man. *J. Clin. Invest.* 47: 139–152, 1968.
81. EPSTEIN, S. E., M. STAMPFER, AND G. D. BEISER. Role of the capacitance and resistance vessels in vasovagal syndrome. *Circulation* 37: 524–533, 1968.
82. EVANS, G. H., AND SHAND, D. G. Disposition of propranolol. VI. Independent variations in steady-state circulating drug concentrations and half-life as a result of plasma drug binding in man. *Clin. Pharmacol. Ther.* 14: 494–500, 1973.
83. EZZAT, W. R., AND W. W. LAUTT. An adenosine mediated mechanism of hepatic arterial pressure-flow autoregulation. *Am. J. Physiol.* 252 (*Heart Circ. Physiol.* 21): H836–H845, 1987.
84. FASTH, S., L. HULTÉN, AND S. NORDGREN. Adjustments of hepatic and small intestine blood flow on selective vasoconstrictor fibre stimulation. *Acta Physiol. Scand.* 110: 343–350, 1980.
85. FAXON, D. P., M. A. CREAGER, J. L. HALPERIN, H. GAVRAS, J. D. COFFMAN, AND T. J. RYAN. Central and peripheral hemodynamic effects of angiotensin inhibition in patients with refractory congestive heart failure. *Circulation* 61: 925–930, 1980.
86. FEELY, J., D. WADE, C. B. MCALLISTER, G. R. WILKINSON, AND D. ROBERTSON. Effect of hypotension on liver blood flow and lidocaine disposition. *N. Engl. J. Med.* 307: 866–869, 1982.
87. FEELY, J., G. R. WILKINSON, AND A. J. WOOD. Reduction of liver blood flow and propranolol metabolism by cimetidine. *N. Engl. J. Med.* 304: 692–695, 1981.
88. FEELY, J., AND A. J. WOOD. Effect on apparent liver blood flow of histamine-receptor blockers and inhibition of prostaglandin synthesis. *Clin. Pharmacol. Ther.* 33: 91–94, 1983.
89. FEELY, J., AND A. J. WOOD. Effects of inhibitors of prostaglandin synthesis on hepatic drug clearance. *Br. J. Clin. Pharmacol.* 15: 109–111, 1983.
90. FERNANDEZ-MUÑOZ, D., C. CARAMELO, J. C. SANTOS, A. BLANCHART, L. HERNANDO, AND J. M. LÓPEZ-NOVOA. Systemic and splanchnic haemodynamic disturbances in conscious rats with experimental liver cirrhosis without ascites. *Am. J. Physiol.* 249 (*Gastrointest. Liver Physiol.* 12): G316–G320, 1985.
91. FOLKOW, B., D. H. LEWIS, O. LUNDGREN, S. MELLANDER, AND I. WALLENTIN. The effect of graded vasoconstrictor fibre stimulation on the intestinal resistance and capacitance vessels. *Acta Physiol. Scand.* 61: 445–457, 1964.
92. FOLKOW, B., D. H. LEWIS, O. LUNDGREN, S. MELLANDER, AND I. WALLENTIN. The effect of the sympathetic vasoconstrictor fibres on the distribution of capillary blood flow in the intestine. *Acta Physiol. Scand.* 61: 458–466, 1964.
93. FOLKOW, B., AND S. MELLANDER. Veins and venous tone. *Am. Heart J.* 68: 397–408, 1964.
94. FOLKOW, B., AND E. NEIL. Hemorrhage. In: *Circulation*, edited by B. Folkow and E. Neil. New York: Oxford Univ. Press, 1971, p. 548–555.
95. FORD, R., R. HAINSWORTH, A. J. RANKIN, AND A. O. SOLADOYE. Abdominal vascular responses to changes in carbon dioxide tension in the cephalic circulation of anesthetized dogs. *J. Physiol. Lond.* 358: 417–431, 1985.
96. FORKER, E. L., AND B. A. LUXON. Albumin binding and hepatic uptake: the importance of model selection. *J. Pharm. Sci.* 72: 1232–1233, 1983.
97. FORKER, E. L., AND B. A. LUXON. Albumin-mediated transport of rose bengal by perfused rat liver. *J. Clin. Invest.* 72: 1764–1771, 1983.
98. FORKER, E. L., AND B. A. LUXON. Analyzing tracer disappearance curves to study hepatic transport kinetics. *Am. J. Physiol.* 244 (*Gastrointest. Liver Physiol.* 7): G573–G577, 1983.
99. GALLAVAN, R. H., C. C. CHOU, P. R. KVIETYS, AND S. P. SIT. Regional blood flow during digestion in the conscious dog. *Am. J. Physiol.* 238 (*Heart Circ. Physiol.* 7): H220–H225, 1980.
100. GARDNER, M. L., AND G. L. ATKINS. Kinetic analysis of transport processes in the intestine and other tissues. *Clin. Sci.* 63: 405–414, 1982.
101. GELMAN, S., AND E. A. ERNST. Role of pH, P$_{CO_2}$, and O$_2$ content of portal blood in hepatic circulatory autoregulation. *Am. J. Physiol.* 233 (*Endocrinol. Metab. Gastrointest. Physiol.* 2): E255–E262, 1977.
102. GELMAN, S., AND E. A. ERNST. Nitroprusside prevents adverse hemodynamic effects of vasopressin. *Arch. Surg.* 113: 1465–1471, 1978.
103. GILMORE, N., J. R. VANE, AND J. H. WYLLIE. Prostaglandins released by the spleen. *Nature Lond.* 218: 1135–1140, 1968.
104. GORESKY, C. A. The lobular design of the liver: its effect on uptake process. In: *Regulation of Hepatic Metabolism*, edited by F. Lundquist and N. Tygstrup. New York: Academic, 1974, p. 808–819.
105. GORESKY, C. A. Cell membrane transport processes: their role in hepatic uptake. In: *The Liver: Biology and Pathobiology*, edited by I. Aries, H. Popper, D. Schacter, and D. A. Shafritz. New York: Raven, 1982, p. 581–599.
106. GORESKY, C. A. Kinetic interpretations of hepatic multiple-indicator dilution studies. *Am. J. Physiol.* 245 (*Gastrointest. Liver Physiol.* 8): G1–G12, 1983.
107. GRAINGER, S. L., P. W. KEELING, I. M. BROWN, J. H. MARIGOLD, AND R. P. THOMPSON. Clearance and non-invasive determination of the hepatic extraction of indocyanine green in baboons and man. *Clin. Sci.* 64: 207–212, 1983.
108. GRANGER, D. N., T. MILLER, R. ALLEN, R. E. PARKER, J. C. PARKER, AND A. E. TAYLOR. Permselectivity of cat liver blood-lymph barrier to endogenous macromolecules. *Gastroenterology* 77: 103–109, 1979.
109. GRANGER, D. N., P. D. RICHARDSON, AND A. E. TAYLOR. Volumetric assessment of the capillary filtration coefficient in the cat small intestine. *Pfluegers Arch.* 381: 25–33, 1979.
110. GREEN, J. F. Mechanism of action of isoproterenol on venous return. *Am. J. Physiol.* 232 (*Heart Circ. Physiol.* 1): H152–H156, 1977.
111. GREENWAY, C. V. Effects of sodium nitroprusside, isosorbide

dinitrate, isoproterenol, phentolamine and prazosin on hepatic venous responses to sympathetic nerve stimulation in the cat. *J. Pharmacol. Exp. Ther.* 209: 56–61, 1979.
112. GREENWAY, C. V. Discussion. In: *Hepatic Circulation in Health and Disease*, edited by W. W. Lautt. New York: Raven, 1981, p. 224.
113. GREENWAY, C. V. Hepatic fluid exchange. In: *Hepatic Circulation in Health and Disease*, edited by W. W. Lautt. New York: Raven, 1981, p. 153–167.
114. GREENWAY, C. V. Hepatic plethysmography. In: *Hepatic Circulation in Health and Disease*, edited by W. W. Lautt. New York: Raven, 1981, p. 41–54.
115. GREENWAY, C. V. Mechanisms and quantitative assessment of drug effects on cardiac output using a new model of the circulation. *Pharmacol. Rev.* 33: 213–251, 1981.
116. GREENWAY, C. V. Autoregulatory escape in arteriolar resistance vessels. In: *Smooth Muscle Contraction*, edited by N. Stephens. New York: Dekker, 1984, p. 473–484.
117. GREENWAY, C. V. Role of splanchnic venous system in overall cardiovascular homeostasis. *Federation Proc.* 42: 1678–1684, 1983.
118. GREENWAY, C. V. Liver. Physiology and pharmacology of blood circulation. In: *Blood Vessels and Lymphatics in Organ Systems*, edited by D. I. Abramson and P. B. Dobrin. Orlando, FL: Academic, 1984, p. 477–489.
119. GREENWAY, C. V. Neural control and autoregulatory escape. In: *Physiology of the Intestinal Circulation*, edited by A. P. Shepherd and D. N. Granger. New York: Raven, 1984, p. 61–71.
119a. GREENWAY, C. V., AND F. J. BURCZYNSKI. Effects of liver blood flow on hepatic uptake kinetics of galactose in anesthetized cats: parallel tube model. *Can. J. Physiol. Pharmacol.* 65: 1193–1199, 1987.
120. GREENWAY, C. V., AND I. R. INNES. Effects of splanchnic nerve stimulation on cardiac preload, afterload and output in cats. *Circ. Res.* 46: 181–189, 1980.
121. GREENWAY, C. V., AND I. R. INNES. Effects of arteriolar vasodilators on hepatic venous compliance and cardiac output in anesthetized cats. *J. Cardiovasc. Pharmacol.* 3: 1321–1331, 1981.
122. GREENWAY, C. V., AND I. R. INNES. Effects of carotid sinus baroreceptor reflex on responses to phenylephrine and nitroprusside in anesthetized cats. *J. Cardiovasc. Pharmacol.* 3: 169–177, 1981.
123. GREENWAY, C. V., AND W. W. LAUTT. Effects of hepatic venous pressure on transsinusoidal fluid transfer in the liver of the anesthetized cat. *Circ. Res.* 26: 697–703, 1970.
124. GREENWAY, C. V., AND W. W. LAUTT. Effects of adrenaline, isoprenaline and histamine on transsinusoidal fluid filtration in the cat liver. *Br. J. Pharmacol.* 44: 185–191, 1972.
125. GREENWAY, C. V., AND W. W. LAUTT. Effects of infusions of catecholamines, angiotensin, vasopressin and histamine on hepatic blood volume in the anaesthetized cat. *Br. J. Pharmacol.* 44: 177–184, 1972.
126. GREENWAY, C. V., AND A. E. LAWSON. Beta-adrenergic receptors in the hepatic arterial bed of the anesthetized cat. *Can. J. Physiol. Pharmacol.* 47: 415–419, 1969.
127. GREENWAY, C. V., A. E. LAWSON, AND S. MELLANDER. The effects of stimulation of the hepatic nerves, infusions of noradrenaline and occlusion of the carotid arteries on liver blood flow in the anaesthetized cat. *J. Physiol. Lond.* 192: 21–41, 1967.
128. GREENWAY, C. V., A. E. LAWSON, AND R. D. STARK. The effect of haemorrhage on hepatic artery and portal vein flows in the anesthetized cat. *J. Physiol. Lond.* 193: 375–379, 1967.
129. GREENWAY, C. V., AND G. E. LISTER. Capacitance effects and blood reservoir function in the splanchnic vascular bed during non-hypotensive haemorrhage and blood volume expansion in anaesthetized cats. *J. Physiol. Lond.* 237: 279–294, 1974.
130. GREENWAY, C. V., AND G. OSHIRO. Comparison of the effects of hepatic nerve stimulation on arterial flow, distribution of arterial and portal flows and blood content in the livers of anaesthetized cats and dogs. *J. Physiol. Lond.* 227: 487–501, 1972.
131. GREENWAY, C. V. AND G. OSHIRO. Intrahepatic distribution of portal and hepatic arterial blood flows in anaesthetized cats and dogs and the effects of portal occlusion, raised venous pressure and histamine. *J. Physiol. Lond.* 227: 473–485, 1972.
132. GREENWAY, C. V., AND G. OSHIRO. Effects of histamine on hepatic volume (outflow block) in anaesthetized dogs. *Br. J. Pharmacol.* 47: 282–290, 1973.
133. GREENWAY, C. V., G. D. SCOTT, AND J. ZINK. Sites of autoregulatory escape of blood flow in the mesenteric vascular bed. *J. Physiol. Lond.* 259: 1–12, 1976.
134. GREENWAY, C. V., K. L. SEAMAN, AND I. R. INNES. Norepinephrine on venous compliance and unstressed volume in cat liver. *Am. J. Physiol.* 248 (*Heart Circ. Physiol.* 17): H468–H476, 1985.
135. GREENWAY, C. V., AND R. D. STARK. Vascular responses of the spleen to rapid haemorrhage in the anaesthetized cat. *J. Physiol. Lond.* 204: 169–179, 1969.
136. GREENWAY, C. V., AND R. D. STARK. Hepatic vascular bed. *Physiol. Rev.* 51: 23–65, 1971.
137. GREENWAY, C. V., R. D. STARK, AND W. W. LAUTT. Capacitance responses and fluid exchange in the cat liver during stimulation of the hepatic nerves. *Circ. Res.* 25: 277–284, 1969.
138. GRIFFITH, F. R., JR., AND F. E. EMERY. The vasomotor control of the liver circulation. *Am. J. Physiol.* 95: 20–34, 1930.
139. GRILLNER, S., J. NILSSON, AND A. THORSTENSSON. Intraabdominal pressure changes during natural movements in man. *Acta Physiol. Scand.* 103: 275–283, 1978.
140. GRISHAM, J. W., W. NOPANITAYA, J. COMPAGNO, AND A. E. NAGEL. Scanning electron microscopy of normal rat liver: the surface structure of its cells and tissue components. *Am. J. Anat.* 144: 295–322, 1975.
141. GROOM, A. C., S. ROWLANDS, AND H. W. THOMAS. Some circulatory responses to haemorrhage in the cat. *Q. J. Exp. Physiol.* 50: 385–405, 1965.
142. GROSZMANN, R. J. The measurement of liver blood flow using clearance techniques. *Hepatology Baltimore* 3: 1039–1040, 1983.
143. GROSZMANN, R. J., A. T. BLEI, J. L. KNIAZ, E. H. STORER, AND H. O. CONN. Portal pressure reduction induced by partial mechanical obstruction of the superior mesenteric artery in the anaesthetized dog. *Gastroenterology* 75: 187–192, 1978.
144. GROSZMANN, R. J., J. VOROBIOFF, AND E. RILEY. Splanchnic hemodynamics in portal-hypertensive rats: measurements with γ-labelled microsphere. *Am. J. Physiol.* 242 (*Gastrointest. Liver Physiol.* 5): G156–G160, 1982.
145. GUMUCIO, D. L. Functional and anatomic heterogeneity in the liver acinus: impact on transport. *Am. J. Physiol.* 244 (*Gastrointest. Liver Physiol.* 7): G578–G582, 1983.
146. GUMUCIO, D. L., J. J. GUMUCIO, J. A. WILSON, C. CUTTER, M. KRAUSS, R. CALDWELL, AND E. CHEN. Albumin influences sulfobromophthalein transport by hepatocytes of each acinar zone. *Am. J. Physiol.* 246 (*Gastrointest. Liver Physiol.* 9): G86–G95, 1984.
147. GUMUCIO, J. J., AND D. L. MILLER. Functional implications of liver cell heterogeneity. *Gastroenterology* 80: 393–403, 1981.
148. GURLL, N. J., D. G. REYNOLDS, D. COON, AND S. S. SHIRAZI. Acute and chronic splanchnic blood flow responses to portacaval shunt in the normal dog. *Gastroenterology* 78: 1432–1436, 1980.
149. GUTH, P. H., AND E. SMITH. Histamine receptors in mesenteric circulation of the cat and rat. *Am. J. Physiol.* 234 (*Endocrinol. Metab. Gastrointest. Physiol.* 3): E370–E374, 1978.
150. HAINSWORTH, R., AND F. KARIM. Responses of abdominal vascular capacitance in the anaesthetized dog to changes in carotid sinus pressure. *J. Physiol. Lond.* 262: 659–677, 1976.
151. HAINSWORTH, R., F. KARIM, K. H. MCGREGOR, AND A. J. RANKIN. Effects of stimulation of aortic chemoreceptors on abdominal vascular resistance and capacitance in anaesthe-

tized dogs. *J. Physiol. Lond.* 334: 421–431, 1983.
152. HAINSWORTH, R., F. KARIM, K. H. MCGREGOR, AND L. M. WOOD. Hind limb vascular capacitance responses in anaesthetized dogs. *J. Physiol. Lond.* 337: 417–428, 1983.
153. HAINSWORTH, R., F. KARIM, K. H. MCGREGOR, AND L. M. WOOD. Responses of abdominal vascular resistance and capacitance to stimulation of carotid chemoreceptors in anaesthetized dogs. *J. Physiol. Lond.* 334: 409–419, 1983.
154. HAINSWORTH, R., F. KARIM, AND J. B. STOKER. The influence of aortic baroreceptors on venous tone in the perfused hind limb of the dog. *J. Physiol. Lond.* 244: 337–351, 1975.
155. HANSON, K. M. Vascular response of intestine and liver to intravenous infusion of vasopressin. *Am. J. Physiol.* 219: 779–784, 1970.
156. HANSON, K. M. Escape of the liver vasculature from adrenergic vasoconstriction. *Proc. Soc. Exp. Biol. Med.* 141: 385–390, 1972.
157. HANSON, K. M. Dilator responses of the canine hepatic vasculature. *Angiologica Basel* 10: 15–23, 1973.
158. HANSON, K. M., AND P. C. JOHNSON. Local control of hepatic arterial and portal venous flow in the dog. *Am. J. Physiol.* 211: 712–720, 1966.
159. HASE, T., AND J. BRIM. Observations on microcirculatory architecture of rat liver. *Anat. Rec.* 156: 157–174, 1966.
160. HEINZOW, B., H. CORBETT, S. CONSTANTINIDES, R. BOURNE, AND A. J. MCLEAN. Interaction between oral hydralazine and propranolol. I. Changes in absorption, presystemic clearance and splanchnic blood flow. *J. Pharmacol. Exp. Ther.* 229: 509–514, 1984.
161. HENDERSON, J. M., AND S. S. HANNA. Effective liver blood flow: determination by galactose clearance. *Can. J. Surg.* 26: 129–132, 1983.
162. HINSHAW, L. B., D. A. REINS, AND R. J. HILL. Responses of isolated liver to endotoxin. *Can. J. Physiol. Pharmacol.* 44: 529–541, 1966.
163. HOLLENBERG, M., AND J. DOUGHERTY. Liver blood flow measured by portal venous and hepatic arterial routes with $Kr^{85}$. *Am. J. Physiol.* 210: 926–932, 1966.
164. HORVATH, S. M., T. KELLY, G. E. FOLK, JR., AND B. K. HUTT. Measurement of blood volumes in the splanchnic bed of the dog. *Am. J. Physiol.* 189: 573–575, 1957.
165. HUET, P., AND J. VILLENEUVE. Determinants of drug disposition in patients with cirrhosis. *Hepatology Baltimore* 3: 913–918, 1983.
166. HUGHES, R. L., R. T. MATHIE, D. CAMPBELL, AND W. FITCH. Effect of hypercarbia on hepatic blood flow and oxygen consumption in the greyhound. *Br. J. Anaesth.* 51: 289–296, 1979.
167. HUGHES, R. L., R. T. MATHIE, D. CAMPBELL, AND W. FITCH. Systemic hypoxia and hyperoxia, and liver blood flow and oxygen consumption in the greyhound. *Pfluegers Arch.* 381: 151–157, 1979.
168. HUGHES, R. L., R. T. MATHIE, W. FITCH, AND D. CAMPBELL. Liver blood flow and oxygen consumption during metabolic acidosis and alkalosis in the greyhound. *Clin. Sci.* 60: 355–361, 1980.
169. HUTTER, J. F., H. M. PIPER, AND P. G. SPIECKERMANN. Kinetic analysis of myocardial fatty acid oxidation suggesting an albumin receptor mediated uptake process. *J. Mol. Cell. Cardiol.* 16: 219–226, 1984.
170. HYATT, R. E., G. H. LAWRENCE, AND J. R. SMITH. Observations on the origin of ascites from experimental hepatic congestion. *J. Lab. Clin. Med.* 45: 274–280, 1955.
171. IGA, T., AND C. D. KLAASSEN. Hepatic extraction of nonmetabolizable xenobiotics in rats. *J. Pharmacol. Exp. Ther.* 211: 690–697, 1979.
172. ILEBEKK, A., J. THORVALDSON, AND F. KIIL. Left ventricular function during acute elevation of aortic blood pressure in dogs. *Am. J. Physiol.* 231: 1476–1484, 1976.
173. ISRAEL, Y., H. KALANT, H. ORREGO, J. M. KHANNA, L. VIDELA, AND J. M. PHILLIPS. Experimental alcohol-induced hepatic necrosis: suppression by propylthiouracil. *Proc. Natl. Acad. Sci. USA* 72: 1137–1141, 1975.
174. ISRAEL, Y., AND H. ORREGO. Hepatocyte demand and substrate supply as factors in the susceptibility to alcoholic injury: pathogenesis and prevention. *Clin. Gastroenterol.* 10: 355–373, 1981.
175. JÄRHULT, J. Comparative effects of angiotensin and noradrenaline on resistance, capicitance, and precapillary sphincter vessels in cat skeletal muscle. *Acta Physiol. Scand.* 81: 315–324, 1971.
176. JOHNS, B. L., AND C. F. ROTHE. Delayed vascular compliance and fluid exchange in the canine intestine. *Am. J. Physiol.* 234 (*Heart Circ. Physiol.* 3): H660–H669, 1978.
177. JOHNSON, P. C. Effect of venous pressure on mean capillary pressure and vascular resistance in the intestine. *Circ. Res.* 16: 294–300, 1965.
178. JOHNSON, P. C., AND K. M. HANSON. Relation between venous pressure and blood volume in the intestine. *Am. J. Physiol.* 204: 31–34, 1963.
179. JOHNSON, P. C., AND K. M. HANSON. Capillary filtration in the small intestine of the dog. *Circ. Res.* 19: 766–773, 1966.
180. JONES, D. B., D. J. MORGAN, G. W. MIHALY, L. K. WEBSTER, AND R. A. SMALLWOOD. Discrimination between the venous equilibrium and sinusoidal models of hepatic drug elimination in the isolated perfused rat liver by perturbation of propranolol protein binding. *J. Pharmacol. Exp. Ther.* 229: 522–526, 1984.
181. KAHN, D., R. VAN HOORN-HICKMAN, AND J. TERBLANCHE. Liver blood flow after partial hepatectomy in the pig. *J. Surg. Res.* 37: 290–294, 1984.
182. KAISER, G. A., J. ROSS, AND E. BRAUNWALD. α- and β-adrenergic receptor mechanisms in the systemic venous bed. *J. Pharmacol. Exp. Ther.* 144: 156–162, 1964.
183. KARIM, F., AND R. HAINSWORTH. Responses of abdominal vascular capacitance to stimulation of splanchnic nerves. *Am. J. Physiol.* 231: 434–440, 1976.
184. KARIM, F., R. HAINSWORTH, AND R. P. PANDEY. Reflex responses of abdominal vascular capacitance from aortic baroreceptors in dog. *Am. J. Physiol.* 235: (*Heart Circ. Physiol.* 4): H488–H493, 1978.
185. KAUFMAN, M. P., K. J. RYBICKI, T. G. WALDROP, AND J. H. MITCHELL. Effect on arterial pressure of rhythmically contracting the hindlimb muscles of cats. *J. Appl. Physiol.: Respirat. Environ. Exercise Physiol.* 56: 1265–1271, 1984.
186. KEIDING, S. Hepatic elimination kinetics: the influence of hepatic blood flow on clearance determinations. *Scand. J. Clin. Lab. Invest.* 36: 113–118, 1976.
187. KEIDING, S., AND P. B. ANDREASEN. Hepatic clearance measurements and pharmacokinetics. *Pharmacology Basel* 19: 105–110, 1979.
188. KEIDING, S., AND L. BASS. Galactose clearance as a measure of hepatic blood flow. *Gastroenterology* 85: 986–987, 1983.
189. KEIDING, S., AND E. CHIARANTINI. Effect of sinusoidal perfusion on galactose elimination kinetics in perfused rat liver. *J. Pharmacol. Exp. Ther.* 205: 465–470, 1978.
190. KEIDING, S., AND K. PRIISHOLM. Current models of hepatic pharmacokinetics: flow effects on kinetic constants of ethanol elimination in perfused rat liver. *Biochem. Pharmacol.* 20: 3209–3212, 1984.
191. KEIDING, S., AND E. STEINESS. Flow dependence of propranolol elimination in perfused rat liver. *J. Pharmacol. Exp. Ther.* 230: 474–477, 1984.
192. KELLER, F., AND J. SCHOLLE. Criticism of pharmacokinetic clearance concepts. *Int. J. Clin. Pharmacol. Ther. Toxicol.* 21: 563–568, 1983.
193. KERR, J. C., R. W. HOBSON, R. F. SEELIG, AND K. G. SWAN. Vasopressin: route of administration and effects on canine hepatic and superior mesenteric arterial blood flows. *Ann. Surg.* 187: 137–142, 1978.
194. KLAASSEN, C. D., AND G. L. PLAA. Plasma disappearance and biliary excretion of indocyanine green in rats, rabbits and dogs. *Toxicol. Appl. Pharmacol.* 15: 374–384, 1969.
195. KNISELY, M. H., F. HARDING, AND H. DEBACKER. Hepatic

sphincters. *Science Wash. DC* 125: 1023–1026, 1957.
196. KNODELL, R. G., R. M. FARLEIGH, N. M. STEELE, AND J. H. BOND. Effects of liver congestion on hepatic drug metabolism in the rat. *J. Pharmacol. Exp. Ther.* 221: 52–57, 1982.
197. KOO, A., AND I. Y. LIANG. Blood flow in hepatic sinusoids in experimental hemorrhagic shock in the rat. *Microvasc. Res.* 13: 315–325, 1977.
198. KOO, A., AND I. Y. LIANG. Microvascular filling pattern in rat liver sinusoids during vagal stimulation. *J. Physiol. Lond.* 295: 191–199, 1979.
199. KOO, A., AND I. Y. LIANG. Vagus-mediated vasodilator tone in the rat terminal liver microcirculation. *Microvasc. Res.* 18: 413–420, 1979.
200. KOO, A., I. Y. LIANG, AND K. K. CHENG. The terminal hepatic microcirculation in the rat. *Q. J. Exp. Physiol.* 60: 261–266, 1975.
201. KRAAN, W. J., G. H. HUISMAN, AND J. VELTHUIZEN. Splenic storage volume in the unanesthetized resting beagle. *Eur. J. Appl. Physiol.* 38: 197–206, 1978.
202. KRARUP, N. The effect of hemorrhage on hepatosplanchnic hemodynamics, liver function and hepatic metabolism. *Acta Physiol. Scand.* 89: 269–277, 1973.
203. KRARUP, N. The effects of noradrenaline and adrenaline on hepatosplanchnic hemodynamics, functional capacity of the liver and hepatic metabolism. *Acta Physiol. Scand.* 87: 307–319, 1973.
204. KRARUP, N. Effects of histamine, vasopressin and angiotensin II on hepatosplanchnic hemodynamics, liver function and hepatic metabolism in cats. *Acta Physiol. Scand.* 95: 311–317, 1975.
205. KULLMANN, R., W. R. BREULL, K. WASSERMANN, AND A. KONOPATZKI. Blood flow redistribution by dopamine in the feline gastrointestinal tract. *Naunyn-Schmiedeberg's Arch. Pharmacol.* 323: 145–148, 1983.
206. LACROIX, E., AND I. LEUSEN. Splanchnic and general hemodynamics after acute hemorrhage in the anaesthetized dog. *Arch. Int. Physiol. Biochim.* 75: 12–26, 1967.
207. LAINE, G. A., J. T. HALL, S. H. LAINE, AND H. J. GRANGER. Transsinusoidal fluid dynamics in canine liver during venous hypertension. *Circ. Res.* 45: 317–323, 1979.
208. LARSEN, J. A., N. KRARUP, AND A. MUNCK. Liver hemodynamics and liver function in cats during graded hypoxic hypoxemia. *Acta Physiol. Scand.* 98: 257–262, 1976.
209. LAUTT, W. W. Control of hepatic and intestinal blood flow: effect of isovolemic haemodilution on blood flow and oxygen uptake in the intact liver and intestines. *J. Physiol. Lond.* 265: 313–326, 1977.
210. LAUTT, W. W. Effects of acute, passive hepatic congestion on blood flow and oxygen uptake in the intact liver of the cat. *Circ. Res.* 41: 787–790, 1977.
211. LAUTT, W. W. Effect of stimulation of hepatic nerves on hepatic $O_2$ uptake and blood flow. *Am. J. Physiol.* 232 (*Heart Circ. Physiol.* 1): H652–H656, 1977.
212. LAUTT, W. W. The hepatic artery: subservient to hepatic metabolism or guardian of normal hepatic clearance rates of humoral substances. *Gen. Pharmacol.* 8: 73–78, 1977.
213. LAUTT, W. W. Hepatic vasculature: a conceptual review. *Gastroenterology* 73: 1163–1169, 1977.
214. LAUTT, W. W. Neural activation of α-adrenoreceptors in glucose mobilization from the liver. *Can. J. Physiol. Pharmacol.* 57: 1037–1039, 1979.
215. LAUTT, W. W. Control of hepatic arterial blood flow: independence from liver metabolic activity. *Am. J. Physiol.* 239 (*Heart Circ. Physiol.* 8): H559–H564, 1980.
216. LAUTT, W. W. Hepatic nerves: a review of their functions and effects. *Can. J. Physiol. Pharmacol.* 58: 105–123, 1980.
217. LAUTT, W. W. Evaluation of surgical denervation of the liver in cats. *Can. J. Physiol. Pharmacol.* 59: 1013–1016, 1981.
218. LAUTT, W. W. (editor) *Hepatic Circulation in Health and Disease.* New York: Raven, 1981.
219. LAUTT, W. W. Role and control of the hepatic artery. In: *Hepatic Circulation in Health and Disease*, edited by W. W. Lautt. New York: Raven, 1981, p. 203–226.
220. LAUTT, W. W. Carotid sinus baroreceptor effects on cat livers in control and hemorrhaged states. *Can. J. Physiol. Pharmacol.* 60: 1592–1602, 1982.
221. LAUTT, W. W. Afferent and efferent neural roles in liver function. *Prog. Neurobiol. Oxford* 21: 323–348, 1983.
222. LAUTT, W. W. Relationship between hepatic blood flow and overall metabolism: the hepatic arterial buffer response. *Federation Proc.* 42: 1662–1666, 1983.
223. LAUTT, W. W. Mechanism and role of intrinsic regulation of hepatic arterial blood flow: the hepatic arterial buffer response. *Am. J. Physiol.* 249 (*Gastrointest. Liver Physiol.* 12): G549–G556, 1985.
224. LAUTT, W. W., L. C. BROWN, AND J. S. DURHAM. Active and passive control of hepatic blood volume responses to hemorrhage at normal and raised hepatic venous pressures in cats. *Can. J. Physiol. Pharmacol.* 58: 1049–1057, 1980.
225. LAUTT, W. W., AND A. M. CARROLL. Evaluation of topical phenol as a means of producing autonomic denervation of the liver. *Can. J. Physiol. Pharmacol.* 62: 849–853, 1984.
226. LAUTT, W. W., AND M. G. CÔTÉ. Functional evaluation of 6-hydroxy-dopamine-induced sympathectomy in the liver of the cat. *J. Pharmacol. Exp. Ther.* 198: 562–567, 1976.
227. LAUTT, W. W., AND T. R. DANIELS. Differential effect of taurocholic acid on hepatic arterial resistance vessels and bile flow. *Am. J. Physiol.* 244 (*Gastrointest. Liver Physiol.* 7): G366–G369, 1983.
228. LAUTT, W. W., P. D. DWAN, AND R. R. SINGH. Control of the hyperglycemic response to hemorrhage in cats. *Can. J. Physiol. Pharmacol.* 60: 1618–1623, 1982.
229. LAUTT, W. W., AND C. V. GREENWAY. Hepatic capacitance vessel responses to bilateral carotid occlusion in anesthetized cats. *Can. J. Physiol. Pharmacol.* 50: 244–247, 1972.
230. LAUTT, W. W., AND C. V. GREENWAY. Hepatic venous compliance and role of liver as a blood reservoir. *Am. J. Physiol.* 231: 292–295, 1976.
231. LAUTT, W. W., C. V. GREENWAY, AND D. J. LEGARE. Effect of hepatic nerves, norepinephrine, angiotensin, elevated central venous pressure on postsinusoidal resistance sites and intrahepatic pressures. *Microvasc. Res.* 33: 50–61, 1987.
232. LAUTT, W. W., C. V. GREENWAY, D. J. LEGARE, AND H. WEISMAN. Localization of intrahepatic portal vascular resistance. *Am. J. Physiol.* 251 (*Gastrointest. Liver Physiol.* 14): G375–G381, 1986.
233. LAUTT, W. W., AND D. J. LEGARE. Adenosine modulation of hepatic arterial but not portal venous constriction induced by sympathetic nerves, norepinephrine, angiotensin and vasopressin. *Can. J. Physiol. Pharmacol.* 64: 449–454, 1986.
234. LAUTT, W. W., AND D. J. LEGARE. The use of 8-phenyltheophylline as a competitive antagonist of adenosine and inhibitor of the intrinsic regulatory mechanism of the hepatic artery. *Can. J. Physiol. Pharmacol.* 63: 717–722, 1985.
234a. LAUTT, W. W., AND D. J. LEGARE. Effect of histamine, norepinephrine and nerves on vascular resistance and pressures in dog liver. *Am. J. Physiol.* 252 (*Gastrointest. Liver Physiol.* 15): G472–G478, 1987.
235. LAUTT, W. W., D. J. LEGARE, AND M. S. D'ALMEIDA. Adenosine as putative regulator of hepatic arterial flow (the buffer response). *Am. J. Physiol.* 248 (*Heart Circ. Physiol.* 17): H331–H338, 1985.
236. LAUTT, W. W., D. J. LEGARE, AND T. R. DANIELS. The comparative effect of administration of substances via the hepatic artery or portal vein on hepatic arterial resistance, liver blood volume, and hepatic extraction in cats. *Hepatology Baltimore* 4: 927–932, 1984.
237. LAUTT, W. W., T. L. MACLACHLAN, AND L. C. BROWN. The effect of hypertonic infusions on hepatic blood flows and liver volume in the cat. *Can. J. Physiol. Pharmacol.* 55: 1339–1344, 1977.
238. LAUTT, W. W., AND F. S. SKELTON. Effect of hepatic nerve

stimulation on hepatic uptake of lidocaine in the cat. *Life Sci.* 19: 433–436, 1976.
239. LAUTT, W. W., AND F. S. SKELTON. The effect of SKF-525A and of altered hepatic blood flow on lidocaine clearance in the cat. *Can. J. Physiol. Pharmacol.* 55: 7–12, 1976.
240. LAUTT, W. W., AND C. WONG. Hepatic parasympathetic neural effect on glucose balance in the intact liver. *Can. J. Physiol. Pharmacol.* 56: 679–682, 1978.
241. LEBREC, D., AND L. BLANCHET. Effect of two models of portal hypertension on splanchnic organ blood flow in the rat. *Clin. Sci.* 68: 23–28, 1985.
242. LEEVY, C. M., C. L. MENDENHALL, W. LESKO, AND M. M. HOWARD. Estimation of hepatic blood flow with indocyanine green. *J. Clin. Invest.* 41: 1169–1179, 1962.
242a. LEGARE, D. J., AND W. W. LAUTT. Hepatic venous resistance site in the dog: localization and validation of intrahepatic pressure measurements. *Can. J. Physiol. Pharmacol.* 65: 352–359, 1987.
243. LEIBERMAN, D. P., R. T. MATHIE, A. M. HARPER, AND L. H. BLUMGART. The hepatic arterial and portal venous circulations of the liver studied with krypton-85 clearance technique. *J. Surg. Res.* 25: 154–162, 1978.
244. LESH, T. A., AND C. F. ROTHE. Sympathetic and hemodynamic effects on capacitance vessels in dog skeletal muscle. *Am. J. Physiol.* 217: 819–827, 1969.
245. LUTZ, J., H. HENRICH, AND E. BAUEREISEN. Oxygen supply and uptake in the liver and intestine. *Pfluegers Arch.* 360: 7–15, 1975.
246. LUTZ, J., AND H. SCHULTZE. Oxygen consumption and oxygen extraction of the feline liver under different types of induced hypoxia. In: *Oxygen Transport to Tissue*, edited by I. A. Silver, M. Erecinska, and H. I. Bicher. New York: Plenum, 1978, vol. 3, p. 537–543.
247. LUXON, B. A., AND E. L. FORKER. Simulation and analysis of hepatic indicator dilution curves. *Am. J. Physiol.* 243 (*Gastrointest. Liver Physiol.* 6): G76–G89, 1982.
248. MARSHALL, J. M. The influence of the sympathetic nervous system on individual vessels of the microcirculation of skeletal muscle of the cat. *J. Physiol. Lond.* 332: 169–186, 1982.
249. MASON, D. T., AND E. BRAUNWALD. Effects of guanethidine, reserpine and methyldopa on reflex venous and arterial constriction in man. *J. Clin. Invest.* 43: 1449–1463, 1964.
250. MATHIE, R. T., AND L. H. BLUMGART. Effect of denervation on the hepatic haemodynamic response to hypercapnia and hypoxia in the dog. *Pfluegers Arch.* 397: 152–157, 1983.
251. MATHIE, R. T., AND L. H. BLUMGART. The hepatic haemodynamic response to acute portal venous blood flow reductions in the dog. *Pfluegers Arch.* 399: 223–227, 1983.
252. MATHIE, R. T., D. P. LEIBERMAN, A. M. HARPER, AND L. H. BLUMGART. The role of blood flow in the control of liver size. *J. Surg. Res.* 27: 139–144, 1979.
253. MATSUNO, H. Study on the hepatic circulation. *Jpn. Circ. J.* 33: 387–397, 1969.
254. MCDEVITT, D. G., A. S. NIES, AND G. R. WILKINSON. Influence of phenobarbital on factors responsible for hepatic clearance of indocyanine green in the rat: relative contributions of induction and altered liver blood flow. *Biochem. Pharmacol.* 26: 1247–1250, 1977.
255. MCGRATH, M. A., AND J. T. SHEPHERD. Hyperosmolarity: effects on nerves and smooth muscle of cutaneous veins. *Am. J. Physiol.* 231: 141–147, 1976.
256. MCKAY, T., J. ZINK, AND C. V. GREENWAY. Relative rates of absorption of fluid and protein from the peritoneal cavity in cats. *Lymphology* 11: 106–110, 1978.
257. MCLAIN, G. E., I. G. SIPES, AND B. B. BROWN. An animal model of halothane hepatotoxicity. *Anesthesiology* 51: 321–326, 1979.
258. MCLEAN, A. J., P. J. MCNAMARA, P. DUSOUICH, M. GIBALDI, AND D. LALKA. Food, splanchnic blood flow, and bioavailability of drugs subject to first-pass metabolism. *Clin. Pharmacol. Ther.* 24: 5–10, 1978.

259. MELLANDER, S. Comparative studies on the adrenergic neurohormonal control of resistance and capacitance vessels in the cat. *Acta Physiol. Scand. Suppl.* 176: 1–86, 1960.
260. MELLANDER, S., AND B. JOHANSSON. Control of resistance, exchange and capacitance functions in the peripheral circulation. *Pharmacol. Rev.* 20: 117–196, 1968.
261. MENDOZA, A. E., C. C. GENSTLER, R. D. GILBERT, AND G. G. POWER. Vascular compliance in the adult cat liver (Abstract). *Clin. Res.* 29: 15, 1981.
262. MERRITT, F. L., AND A. M. WEISSLER. Reflex venomotor alterations during exercise and hyperventilation. *Am. Heart J.* 58: 382–387, 1959.
263. MESSERLI, F. H., W. NOWACZYNSKI, M. HONDA, J. GENEST, R. BOUCHER, O. KUCHEL, AND J. M. ROJO-ORTEGA. Effects of angiotensin II on steroid metabolism and hepatic blood flow in man. *Circ. Res.* 40: 204–207, 1977.
264. MILLER, D. L. Quantitative morphological assessment of the sinusoids of the hepatic acinus. In: *Hepatic Circulation in Health and Disease*, edited by W. W. Lautt. New York: Raven, 1981, p. 111–135.
265. MITZNER, W. Hepatic outflow resistance, sinusoidal pressure, and the vascular waterfall. *Am. J. Physiol.* 227: 513–519, 1974.
266. MORGAN, D. J., AND K. RAYMOND. Use of the unbound drug concentration in blood to discriminate between two models of hepatic drug elimination. *J. Pharm. Sci.* 71: 600–602, 1982.
267. MORITOKI, H. Possible mechanism of potentiation of the action of adenosine by some vasodilators. In: *Physiology and Pharmacology of Adenosine Derivatives*, edited by J. W. Daly, Y. Kuroda, J. W. Phillis, H. Shimizu, and M. Ui. New York: Raven, 1983, p. 197–207.
268. MOSTBECK, A., H. PARTSCH, AND L. PESCHL. Investigations on peripheral blood distribution. In: *Third Adalat Symposium*, edited by A. D. Jatene and P. R. Lichtlen. Amsterdam: Excerpta Medica, 1976, p. 91–97.
269. MOTOOKA, T. Influence of bleeding and acetylcholine on the hepatic circulation. *Jpn. Circ. J.* 33: 95–104, 1969.
269a. MOTTA, P., M. MUTO, AND T. FUJITA. *The Liver: An Atlas of Scanning Electron Microscopy*. Tokyo: Igaku Shoin, 1978.
270. MUNDSCHAU, G. A., S. W. ZIMMERMAN, J. W. GILDERSLEEVE, AND Q. R. MURPHY. Hepatic and mesenteric artery resistances after sinoaortic denervation and hemorrhage. *Am. J. Physiol.* 211: 77–82, 1966.
271. NAKATA, K., G. F. LEONG, AND R. W. BRAUER. Direct measurement of blood pressures in minute vessels of the liver. *Am. J. Physiol.* 199: 1181–1188, 1960.
272. NIES, A. S., D. G. SHAND, AND G. R. WILKINSON. Altered hepatic blood flow and drug disposition. In: *Handbook of Clinical Pharmacokinetics*, edited by L. F. Prescott and M. Gibaldi. Auckland, New Zealand: Adis, 1983, p. 75–96.
273. NIES, A. S., G. R. WILKINSON, B. D. RUSH, J. T. STROTHER, AND D. G. MCDEVITT. Effects of alteration of hepatic microsomal enzyme activity on liver blood flow in the rat. *Biochem. Pharmacol.* 25: 1991–1993, 1976.
274. NILSSON, H., AND B. FOLKOW. Structurally reduced compliance of the venous capacitance vessels in spontaneously hypertensive rats (SHR). *Acta Physiol. Scand.* 110: 215–217, 1980.
275. NOPANITAYA, W., J. C. LAMB, J. W. GRISHAM, AND J. L. CARSON. Effect of hepatic venous outflow obstruction on pores and fenestration in sinusoidal endothelium. *Br. J. Exp. Path.* 57: 604–609, 1976.
276. NXUMALO, J. L., M. TERANAKA, AND W. G. SCHENK. Hepatic blood flow measurement. *Arch. Surg.* 113: 169–172, 1978.
277. OBERG, B. The relationship between active constriction and passive recoil of the veins at various distending pressures. *Acta Physiol. Scand.* 71: 233–247, 1967.
278. OBERG, B., AND S. ROSELL. Sympathetic control of consecutive vascular sections in canine subcutaneous adipose tissue. *Acta Physiol. Scand.* 71: 47–56, 1967.
279. OBERG, B., AND S. WHITE. Circulatory effects of interruption and stimulation of cardiac vagal afferents. *Acta Physiol. Scand.*

80: 383–394, 1970.
280. OCKNER, R. K., R. A. WEISIGER, AND J. L. GOLLAN. Hepatic uptake of albumin-bound substances: albumin receptor concept. *Am. J. Physiol.* 245 (*Gastrointest. Liver Physiol.* 8): G13–G18, 1983.
281. OHNHAUS, E. E. The distribution of $Rb^{86}$ in different parts of the liver. *Pfluegers Arch.* 346: 157–161, 1974.
282. ORREGO, H., H. KALANT, Y. ISRAEL, J. BLAKE, A. MEDLINE, J. G. RANKIN, A. ARMSTRONG, AND B. KAPUR. Effect of short-term therapy with propylthiouracil in patients with alcoholic liver disease. *Gastroenterology* 76: 105–115, 1975.
283. PAMNANI, M. B., G. SIMON, AND H. W. OVERBECK. Increased mesenteric blood flow and decreased mesenteric venous compliance in dogs with chronic perinephritic hypertension. *Proc. Soc. Exp. Biol. Med.* 161: 397–401, 1979.
284. PANG, K. S., AND M. ROWLAND. Hepatic clearance of drugs. I. Theoretical considerations of a "well-stirred" model and a "parallel tube" model. Influence of hepatic blood flow, plasma and blood cell binding and the hepatocellular enzymatic activity on hepatic drug clearance. *J. Pharmacokinet. Biopharm.* 5: 625–653, 1977.
285. PANG, K. S., AND M. ROWLAND. Hepatic clearance of drugs. II. Experimental evidence for acceptance of the "well-stirred" model over the "parallel tube" model using lidocaine in the perfused rat liver in situ preparation. *J. Pharmacokinet. Biopharm.* 5: 655–680, 1977.
286. PARKER, G., T. K. DANESHMEND, AND C. J. ROBERTS. Do β-blockers differ in their effects on hepatic microsomal enzymes and liver blood flow? *J. Clin. Pharmacol.* 24: 493–499, 1984.
287. PATEL, P., D. BOSE, AND C. V. GREENWAY. Effects of prazosin and phenoxybenzamine on α- and β-receptor-mediated responses in intestinal resistance and capacitance vessels. *J. Cardiovasc. Pharmacol.* 3: 1050–1059, 1981.
288. PIRTTIAHO, H. I., E. A. SOTANIEMI, R. O. PELKONEN, AND U. PITKANEN. Hepatic blood flow and drug metabolism in patients on enzyme-inducing anticonvulsants. *Eur. J. Clin. Pharmacol.* 22: 441–445, 1982.
289. PLAA, G. L. Toxicology of the liver. In: *Toxicology: The Basic Science of Poisons*, edited by L. J. Casarett and J. Doull. New York: Macmillan, 1975, p. 170–189.
290. POST, J. A., AND K. M. HANSON. Hepatic vascular and biliary responses to infusion of gastrointestinal hormones and bile salts. *Digestion* 12: 65–77, 1975.
291. PRICE, H. L., S. DEUTSCH, B. E. MARSHALL, G. W. STEPHEN, M. G. BEHAR, AND G. R. NEUFELD. Hemodynamic and metabolic effects of hemorrhage in man, with particular reference to the splanchnic circulation. *Circ. Res.* 18: 469–474, 1966.
292. PRICE, J. B., P. W. MCFATE, AND R. F. SHAW. Dynamics of blood flow through the canine liver. *Surgery* 56: 1109–1120, 1964.
293. RAPPAPORT, A. M. The microcirculatory hepatic unit. *Microvasc. Res.* 6: 212–228, 1973.
294. RAPPAPORT, A. M. The microcirculatory hepatic unit. In: *Drugs and the Liver*, edited by F. K. Schuttauer. New York: Springer-Verlag, 1975, p. 425–434.
295. RAPPAPORT, A. M. The acinus-microvascular unit of the liver. In: *Hepatic Circulation in Health and Disease*, edited by W. W. Lautt. New York: Raven, 1981, p. 175–192.
296. REILLY, F. D., R. V. DIMLICH, E. V. CILENTO, AND R. S. MCCUSKEY. Hepatic microvascular regulatory mechanisms. II. Cholinergic mechanisms. *Hepatology Baltimore* 2: 230–235, 1982.
297. REILLY, F. D., R. S. MCCUSKEY, AND E. V. CILENTO. Hepatic microvascular regulatory mechanisms. I. Adrenergic mechanisms. *Microvasc. Res.* 21: 103–116, 1981.
298. REIMANN, I. W., U. KLOTZ, AND J. C. FROLICH. Effects of cimetidine and ranitidine on steady-state propranolol kinetics and dynamics. *Clin. Pharmacol. Ther.* 32: 749–757, 1982.
299. RICHARDSON, P. D., AND D. N. GRANGER. Microcirculation of the liver and spleen. In: *The Physiology and Pharmacology of the Microcirculation*, edited by N. A. Mortillaro. Orlando, FL: Academic, 1984, vol. 8, p. 95–131.
300. RICHARDSON, P. D., AND P. G. WITHRINGTON. The inhibition by glucagon of the vasoconstrictor actions of noradrenaline, angiotensin and vasopressin on the hepatic arterial vascular bed of the dog. *Br. J. Pharmacol.* 57: 93–102, 1976.
301. RICHARDSON, P. D., AND P. G. WITHRINGTON. The vasodilator actions of isoprenaline, histamine, prostaglandin E2, glucagon and secretin on the hepatic arterial vascular bed of the dog. *Br. J. Pharmacol.* 57: 581–588, 1976.
302. RICHARDSON, P. D., AND P. G. WITHRINGTON. A comparison of the effects of bradykinin, 5-hydroxytryptamine and histamine on the hepatic arterial and portal venous vascular beds of the dog: histamine H1 and H2 receptor populations. *Br. J. Pharmacol.* 60: 123–133, 1977.
303. RICHARDSON, P. D., AND P. G. WITHRINGTON. The effects of glucagon, secretin, pancreozymin and pentagastrin on the hepatic arterial vascular bed of the dog. *Br. J. Pharmacol.* 59: 147–156, 1977.
304. RICHARDSON, P. D., AND P. G. WITHRINGTON. The effects of intraportal injections of noradrenaline, adrenaline, vasopressin and angiotensin on the hepatic portal vascular bed of the dog: marked tachyphylaxis to angiotensin. *Br. J. Pharmacol.* 59: 293–301, 1977.
305. RICHARDSON, P. D., AND P. G. WITHRINGTON. Responses of the canine hepatic arterial and portal venous vascular beds to dopamine. *Eur. J. Pharmacol.* 48: 337–349, 1978.
306. RICHARDSON, P. D., AND P. G. WITHRINGTON. Responses of the simultaneously-perfused hepatic arterial and portal venous vascular beds of the dog to histamine and 5-hydroxytryptamine. *Br. J. Pharmacol.* 64: 581–588, 1978.
307. RICHARDSON, P. D., AND P. G. WITHRINGTON. Effects of intraportal infusions of hypertonic solutions on hepatic haemodynamics in the dog. *J. Physiol. Lond.* 301: 82–83, 1979.
308. RICHARDSON, P. D., AND P. G. WITHRINGTON. Liver blood flow. I. Intrinsic and nervous control of liver blood flow. *Gastroenterology* 81: 159–173, 1981.
309. RICHARDSON, P. D., AND P. G. WITHRINGTON. Liver blood flow. II. Effects of drugs and hormones on liver blood flow. *Gastroenterology* 81: 356–375, 1981.
310. RICKSTEN, S. E., T. YAO, AND P. THOREN. Peripheral and central vascular compliances in conscious normotensive and spontaneously hypertensive rats. *Acta Physiol. Scand.* 112: 169–177, 1981.
311. ROSELL, S. Neuronal control of microvessels. *Annu. Rev. Physiol.* 42: 359–371, 1980.
312. ROTHE, C. F. Reflex control of veins and vascular capacitance. *Physiol. Rev.* 63: 1281–1342, 1983.
313. ROTHE, C. F. Properties of veins. In: *Blood Vessels and Lymphatics in Organ Systems*, edited by D. I. Abramson and P. B. Dobrin. Orlando, FL: Academic, 1984, p. 85–96.
314. ROTHE, C. F., T. D. BENNETT, AND B. L. JOHNS. Linearity of the vascular pressure-volume relationship of the canine intestine. *Circ. Res.* 47: 551–558, 1980.
315. ROTHE, C. F., B. L. JOHNS, AND T. D. BENNETT. Vascular capacitance of dog intestine using mean transit time of indicator. *Am. J. Physiol.* 234 (*Heart Circ. Physiol.* 3): H7–H13, 1978.
316. ROWELL, L. B. Reflex control of regional circulation in humans. *J. Auton. Nerv. Syst.* 11: 101–114, 1984.
317. ROWLAND, M., L. Z. BENET, AND G. G. GRAHAM. Clearance concepts in pharmacokinetics. *J. Pharmacokinet. Biopharm.* 1: 123–136, 1973.
318. ROWLAND, M., D. LEITCH, G. FLEMING, AND B. SMITH. Protein binding and hepatic clearance: discrimination between models of hepatic clearance with diazepam, a drug of high intrinsic clearance, in the isolated perfused rat liver preparation. *J. Pharmacokinet. Biopharm.* 12: 129–147, 1984.
319. RUTLEN, D. L., E. W. SUPPLE, AND W. J. POWELL. The role of the liver in the adrenergic regulation of blood flow from the splanchnic to the central circulation. *Yale J. Biol. Med.* 52: 99–106, 1979.

320. RUTLEN, D. L., E. W. SUPPLE, AND W. J. POWELL. Adrenergic regulation of total systemic distensibility. *Am. J. Cardiol.* 47: 579–588, 1981.
321. RUTLEN, D. L., F. J. WACKERS, AND B. L. ZARET. Radionuclide assessment of peripheral intravascular capacity: a technique to measure intravascular volume changes in the capacitance circulation in man. *Circulation* 64: 146–152, 1981.
322. SANDERS, T. M., R. A. WERNER, AND C. M. BLOOR. Visceral blood flow distribution during exercise to exhaustion in conscious dogs. *J. Appl. Physiol.* 40: 927–931, 1976.
323. SARNOFF, S. J., J. P. GILMORE, AND A. G. WALLACE. The influence of autonomic nerve activity on adaptive mechanisms in the heart. In: *Nervous Control of the Heart*, edited by W. C. Randall. Baltimore: Williams and Wilkins, 1965, p. 54–129.
324. SATO, T., M. SHIRATAKA, N. IKEDA, AND F. S. GRODINS. Steady-state systems analysis of hepatic hemodynamics in the isolated perfused canine liver. *Am. J. Physiol.* 233 (*Regulatory Integrative Comp. Physiol.* 2): R188–R197, 1977.
325. SCHOLTHOLT, J., AND T. SHIRAISHI. The reaction of liver and intestinal blood flow to a general hypoxia, hypocapnia and hypercapnia in the anesthetized dog. *Pfluegers Arch.* 318: 185–201, 1970.
326. SEAMAN, K., AND C. V. GREENWAY. Hepatic venoconstrictor effects of isoproterenol and nifedipine in anesthetized cats. *Can. J. Physiol. Pharmacol.* 62: 665–672, 1984.
327. SEAMAN, K. L., AND C. V. GREENWAY. Loss of hepatic venous responsiveness after endotoxin in anesthetized cats. *Am. J. Physiol.* 246 (*Heart Circ. Physiol.* 15): H658–H663, 1984.
328. SEGSTRO, R., AND C. V. GREENWAY. Alpha-adrenoceptor subtypes mediating sympathetic mobilization of blood from the hepatic venous system in anesthetized cats. *J. Pharmacol. Exp. Ther.* 236: 224–229, 1986.
328a. SEGSTRO, R., K. L. SEAMAN, I. R. INNES, AND C. V. GREENWAY. Effects of nifedipine on hepatic blood volume in cats: indirect venoconstriction and absence of inhibition of postsynaptic α-2 adrenoceptor responses. *Can. J. Physiol. Pharmacol.* 64: 615–620, 1986.
329. SELKURT, E. E. Comparison of the bromosulphalein method with simultaneous direct hepatic blood flow. *Circ. Res.* 2: 155–159, 1954.
330. SHEN, E. S., V. F. GARRY, AND M. W. ANDERS. Effect of hypoxia on carbon tetrachloride hepatotoxicity. *Biochem. Pharmacol.* 31: 3787–3793, 1982.
331. SHOEMAKER, W. C. Measurement of hepatic blood flow in the unanesthetized dog by a modified bromsulphalein method. *J. Appl. Physiol.* 15: 473–478, 1960.
332. SHOUKAS, A. A. Carotid sinus baroreceptor reflex control and epinephrine. Influence on capacitive and resistive properties of the total pulmonary vascular bed of the dog. *Circ. Res.* 51: 95–101, 1982.
333. SHOUKAS, A. A., AND M. C. BRUNNER. Epinephrine and the carotid sinus baroreceptor reflex. Influence on capacitive and resistive properties of the total systemic vascular bed of the dog. *Circ. Res.* 47: 249–257, 1980.
334. SHOUKAS, A. A., AND K. SAGAWA. Total systemic vascular compliance measured as incremental volume-pressure ratio. *Circ. Res.* 28: 277–289, 1971.
335. SHOUKAS, A. A., AND K. SAGAWA. Control of total systemic vascular capacity by the carotid sinus baroreceptor reflex. *Circ. Res.* 33: 22–33, 1973.
336. SLATER, G., B. C. VLADECK, R. BASSIN, AND W. C. SHOEMAKER. Sequential changes in hepatic blood flows during hemorrhagic shock. *Am. J. Physiol.* 223: 1428–1432, 1972.
337. SMISETH, O. A., I. KINGMA, D. E. MANYARI, E. R. SMITH, AND J. V. TYBERG. Mechanism of nitroglycerin-induced blood volume redistribution (Abstract). *J. Am. Coll. Cardiol.* 5: 553, 1985.
338. SMISETH, O. A., H. REFSUM, AND J. V. TYBERG. Pericardial pressure assessed by right atrial pressure: a basis for calculation of left ventricular transmural pressure. *Am. Heart J.* 108: 603–605, 1984.
339. SMITH, E. R., O. A. SMISETH, I. KINGMA, D. MANYARI, I. BELENKIE, AND J. V. TYBERG. Mechanism of action of nitrates. Role of changes in venous capacitance and in the left ventricular diastolic pressure-volume relations. *Am. J. Med.* 76: 14–21, 1984.
340. STARK, R. D. Conductance or resistance? *Nature Lond.* 217: 779, 1968.
341. STARLING, E. H. On the absorption of fluids from the connective tissue spaces. *J. Physiol. Lond.* 19: 312–326, 1896.
342. STEKIEL, W. J., J. P. KAMPINE, E. F. BANASZAK, AND J. J. SMITH. Hepatic clearance of indocyanine in the dog. *Am. J. Physiol.* 198: 881–885, 1960.
343. STELLA, V. J., K. YAMAOKA, AND R. H. LEVY. An added complication in the estimation of apparent hepatic blood flow in vivo by pharmacokinetic parameters. *Drug Metab. Dispos.* 9: 172–173, 1981.
344. STENSON, R. E., R. T. CONSTANTINO, AND D. C. HARRISON. Interrelationships of hepatic blood flow, cardiac output and blood levels of lidocaine in man. *Circulation* 43: 205–211, 1971.
345. STOKLAND, O., M. M. MILLER, A. ILEBEKK, AND F. KIIL. Mechanism of hemodynamic responses to occlusion of the descending thoracic aorta. *Am. J. Physiol.* 238 (*Heart Circ. Physiol.* 7): H423–H429, 1980.
346. STOKLAND, O., M. MOLAUG, J. THORVALDSON, A. ILEBEKK, AND F. KIIL. Cardiac effects of splanchnic and non-splanchnic blood volume redistribution during aortic occlusions in dogs. *Acta Physiol. Scand.* 113: 139–146, 1981.
347. STOKLAND, O., J. THORVALDSON, A. ILEBEKK, AND F. KIIL. Contributions of blood drainage from the liver, spleen and intestines to cardiac effects of aortic occlusion in the dog. *Acta Physiol. Scand.* 114: 351–362, 1982.
348. STOKLAND, O., J. THORVALDSON, A. ILEBEKK, AND F. KIIL. Mechanism of blood pressure elevation during angiotensin infusion. *Acta Physiol. Scand.* 115: 455–465, 1982.
349. SUPPLE, E. W., AND W. J. POWELL. Effect of acetylcholine on vascular capacity in the dog. *J. Clin. Invest.* 68: 64–74, 1981.
350. SVENSSON, C. K., D. J. EDWARDS, P. M. MAURIELLO, S. H. BARDE, A. C. FOSTER, R. A. LANC, E. MIDDLETON, AND D. LALKA. Effect of food on hepatic blood flow: implications in the "food effect" phenomenon. *Clin. Pharmacol. Ther.* 34: 316–323, 1983.
351. SVENSSON, C. K., P. M. MAURIELLO, S. H. BARDE, E. MIDDLETON, AND D. LALKA. Effect of carbohydrates on estimated hepatic blood flow. *Clin. Pharmacol. Ther.* 35: 660–665, 1984.
352. TAKESHITA, A., AND A. L. MARK. Decreased venous distensibility in borderline hypertension. *Hypertension Dallas* 1: 202–206, 1979.
353. TEULE, G. J., W. DEN HOLLANDER, W. BRONSVELD, A. VAN LAMBALGEN, G. A. HEIDENDAL, AND L. G. THIJS. Non-invasive detection of blood volume redistribution in canine endotoxin shock. *Circ. Shock* 8: 627–634, 1981.
354. TEULE, G. J., A. VAN LINGEN, M. A. VERWAY VAN VUGHT, A. D. KESTER, R. C. MACKAAY, P. D. BEZEMER, G. A. HEIDENDAL, AND A. D. THIJS. Role of peripheral pooling in porcine *Escherichia coli* sepsis. *Circ. Shock* 12: 115–123, 1984.
355. THOMAS, W. D., AND H. E. ESSEX. Observations on the hepatic venous circulation with special reference to the sphincteric mechanism. *Am. J. Physiol.* 158: 303–310, 1949.
356. THORVALDSON, J., A. ILEBEKK, S. LERAAND, AND F. KIIL. Determinants of pulmonary blood volume. Effects of acute changes in pulmonary vascular pressures and flow. *Acta Physiol. Scand.* 121: 45–56, 1984.
357. THORVALDSON, J., O. STOKLAND, M. MOLAUG, AND A. ILEBEKK. Cardiopulmonary blood volume during acute blood pressure elevations in dog. *Acta Physiol. Scand.* 122: 137–144, 1984.
358. TILLEMENT, J., G. HOUIN, R. ZINI, S. URIEN, E. ALBENGRES, J. BARRE, M. LECOMTE, P. D'ATHIS, AND B. SEBILLE. The binding of drugs to blood plasma and macromolecules: recent advances and therapeutic significance. *Adv. Drug Res.* 13: 59–94, 1984.
359. TOGHILL, P. J., AND B. N. C. PRICHARD. A study of the action

of noradrenaline on the splenic red cell pool. *Clin. Sci.* 26: 203–212, 1964.
360. TRIPPODO, N. C., J. YAMAMOTO, AND E. D. FROHLICH. Whole-body venous capacitance and effective total tissue compliance in SHR. *Hypertension Dallas* 3: 104–112, 1981.
361. TYBERG, J. V. Ventricular interaction and the pericardium. In: *The Ventricle: Basic and Clinical Aspects*, edited by H. J. Levine and W. H. Gaasch. Boston: Nijhoff, 1985, p. 171–184.
362. TYDÉN, G., H. SAMNEGÅRD, AND L. THULIN. The effects of changes in the carotid sinus baroreceptor activity on splanchnic blood flow in anesthetized man. *Acta Physiol. Scand.* 106: 187–189, 1979.
363. TYDEN, G., L. THULIN, AND B. NYBERG. The effect of cimetidine on liver blood flow in anesthetized man. *Acta Chir. Scand.* 149: 303–305, 1983.
364. TYGSTRUP, N., AND K. WINKLER. Galactose blood clearance as a measure of hepatic blood flow. *Clin. Sci.* 17: 1–9, 1958.
365. VANECKO, R. M., P. B. SZANTO, AND W. C. SHOEMAKER. Microcirculatory changes in primate liver during shock. *Surg. Gynec. Obstet.* 129: 995–1004, 1969.
366. VATNER, S. F., T. A. PATRICK, C. B. HIGGINS, AND D. FRANKLIN. Regional circulatory adjustments to eating and digestion in conscious unrestrained primates. *J. Appl. Physiol.* 36: 524–529, 1974.
367. VILLENEUVE, J. P., G. POMIER, AND P. M. HUET. Effect of ethanol on hepatic blood flow in unanesthetized dogs with chronic portal and hepatic vein catheterization. *Can. J. Physiol. Pharmacol.* 59: 598–603, 1981.
368. VOROBIOFF, J., J. E. BREDFELDT, AND R. J. GROSZMANN. Hyperdynamic circulation in portal-hypertensive rat model: a primary factor for maintenance of chronic portal hypertension. *Am. J. Physiol.* 244 (*Gastrointest. Liver Physiol.* 7): G52–G57, 1983.
369. WADE, O. L., B. COMBES, A. W. CHILDS, H. O. WHEELER, A. COURNAND, AND S. E. BRADLEY. The effect of exercise on the splanchnic blood flow and splanchnic blood volume in normal man. *Clin. Sci.* 15: 457–463, 1956.
370. WAGNER, J. G. Relationships among the venous equilibrium ("well-stirred") model, the sinusoidal perfusion ("parallel-tube") model and a specific two-compartment open model. *Drug Metab. Dispos.* 13: 119–120, 1985.
371. WAGNER, J. G., G. J. SZPUNAR, AND J. J. FERRY. Exact mathematical equivalence of the venous equilibrium ("well-stirred") model, the sinusoidal perfusion ("parallel-tube") model and a specific two-compartment open model. *Drug Metab. Dispos.* 12: 385–388, 1984.
372. WALKER, W. F., J. S. MACDONALD, AND C. PICKARD. Hepatic sphincter mechanism in the dog. *Br. J. Surg.* 48: 218–220, 1960.
373. WALLENTIN, I. Importance of tissue pressure for the fluid equilibrium between the vascular and interstitial compartments in the small intestine. *Acta Physiol. Scand.* 68: 304–315, 1966.
374. WANNER, A., R. BEGIN, M. COHN, AND M. A. SACKNER. Vascular volumes of the pulmonary circulation in intact dogs. *J. Appl. Physiol.: Respirat. Environ. Exercise Physiol.* 44: 956–963, 1978.
375. WATHEN, C. G., W. J. HANNAN, C. J. ADIE, AND A. L. MUIR. A radionuclide method for the simultaneous study of the effects of drugs on central and peripheral haemodynamics. *Br. J. Clin. Pharmacol.* 16: 45–50, 1983.
376. WEIGAND, B. D., S. G. KETTERER, AND E. RAPAPORT. The use of indocyanine green for the evaluation of hepatic function and blood flow in man. *Am. J. Digest. Dis.* 5: 427–436, 1960.
377. WEISIGER, R., J. GOLLAN, AND R. OCKNER. Receptors for albumin on the liver cell surface may mediate uptake of fatty acids and other albumin-bound substances. *Science Wash. DC* 211: 1048–1051, 1981.
378. WHEELER, H. O., R. M. EPSTEIN, R. R. ROBINSON, AND E. S. SNELL. Hepatic storage and excretion of sulfobromophthalein sodium in the dog. *J. Clin. Invest.* 39: 236–247, 1960.
379. WHITSETT, T. L., P. G. DAYTON, AND J. L. MCNAY. The effect of hepatic blood flow on the hepatic removal rate of oxyphenbutazone in the dog. *J. Pharmacol. Exp. Ther.* 177: 246–255, 1971.
380. WILKINSON, G. R., AND D. G. SHAND. A physiological approach to hepatic drug clearance. *Clin. Pharmacol. Ther.* 18: 377–390, 1975.
381. WINKLER, K., J. A. LARSEN, T. MUNKNER, AND N. TYGSTRUP. Determination of the hepatic blood flow in man by simultaneous use of five test substances measured in two parts of the liver. *Scand. J. Clin. Lab. Invest.* 17: 423–432, 1965.
382. YAMAGUCHI, N., AND D. GARCEAU. Correlations between hemodynamic parameters of the liver and norepinephrine release upon hepatic nerve stimulation in the dog. *Can. J. Physiol. Pharmacol.* 58: 1347–1355, 1980.
383. YAMAMOTO, J., N. C. TRIPPODO, A. A. MACPHEE, AND E. D. FROHLICH. Decreased total venous capacity in Goldblatt hypertensive rats. *Am. J. Physiol.* 240 (*Heart Circ. Physiol.* 9): H487–H492, 1981.
384. YAMAMOTO, K., I. SHERMAN, J. M. PHILLIPS, AND M. M. FISHER. Three-dimensional observations of the hepatic arterial terminations in rat, hamster and human liver by scanning electron microscopy of microvascular casts. *Hepatology Baltimore* 5: 452–456, 1985.
385. YEAGER, V. L., D. J. ANDERSON, AND J. J. TAYLOR. Smooth muscle in the hepatic artery, portal vein and hepatic vein within the liver of the raccoon and guinea pig. *Experientia* 41: 262–265, 1985.
386. YOFFEY, J. M., AND F. C. COURTICE. *Lymphatics, Lymph and the Lymphomyeloid Complex.* New York: Academic, 1970, p. 206–320.
387. ZIMPFER, M., W. T. MANDERS, A. C. BARGER, AND S. F. VATNER. Pentobarbital alters compensatory neural and humoral mechanisms in response to hemorrhage. *Am. J. Physiol.* 243 (*Heart Circ. Physiol.* 12): H713–H721, 1982.
388. ZINK, J., AND C. V. GREENWAY. Control of ascites absorption in anesthetized cats: effects of intraperitoneal pressure, protein and furosemide diuresis. *Gastroenterology* 73: 1119–1124, 1977.
389. ZINK, J., AND C. V. GREENWAY. Intraperitoneal pressure in formation and reabsorption of ascites in cats. *Am. J. Physiol.* 233 (*Heart Circ. Physiol.* 2): H185–H190, 1977.

CHAPTER 42

# Circulation of the pancreas and salivary glands

PETER R. KVIETYS
D. NEIL GRANGER

Department of Physiology and Biophysics, Louisiana State University Medical Center, Shreveport, Louisiana

SCOT L. HARPER

Department of Physiology, College of Medicine, University of South Alabama, Mobile, Alabama

## CHAPTER CONTENTS

Anatomical Considerations
  Blood vessels
    Extraglandular
    Intraglandular
  Lymph vessels
    Extraglandular
    Intraglandular
  Nerves
    Sympathetic
    Parasympathetic
Basal Hemodynamics and Oxygenation
Intrinsic Regulation of Blood Flow and Oxygenation
  Metabolic regulation
  Myogenic regulation
  Kallikrein-kinin regulation
  Evidence for intrinsic vasoregulation
    Pressure-flow autoregulation
    Reactive hyperemia
    Hypoxic vasodilation
    Venous pressure elevation
Functional Hyperemia
  Characteristics of functional hyperemia
  Mediators of functional hyperemia
    Intrinsic factors
    Extrinsic factors
Circulatory Adjustments to Hyperplasia
Transcapillary Fluid and Solute Exchange
  Ultrastructural basis of capillary exchange
  Transcapillary fluid exchange
    Net capillary filtration rate
    Capillary filtration coefficient
    Capillary pressure
    Interstitial fluid pressure
    Osmotic reflection coefficient
    Transcapillary oncotic pressure gradient
  Interaction of capillary and interstitial forces during stimulated secretion
  Microvascular permeability
    Small solutes
    Macromolecules
Extrinsic Regulation of Blood Flow
  Sympathetic nerve stimulation
    Pancreas
    Salivary gland
  Pharmacology
Summary

THE PANCREAS AND SALIVARY GLANDS are capable of secreting large volumes of fluid. When maximally stimulated, these glands can secrete their weight in juice in less than 30 min. The electrolytes, water, and $O_2$ required for exocrine secretion are ultimately derived from the blood. Thus it is not surprising that the major focus of studies on the exocrine circulations has been on the circulatory adjustments that occur during enhanced secretory activity. Several important advances have been made in understanding the interactions between the microcirculation and exocrine secretion since the chapter by Jacobson in the 1967 edition of the *Handbook* section on the alimentary canal (111). The major objective of this chapter is to summarize these new contributions and place them in perspective with earlier work. After a brief description of the pertinent vascular anatomy, the evidence for intrinsic regulation of blood flow in the salivary glands and pancreas is reviewed. This is followed by an assessment of the mechanisms that mediate the hyperemia associated with enhanced glandular secretion. The available information on transcapillary fluid and solute exchange in these glands is summarized, and a working hypothesis regarding the role of the microcirculation in providing the fluid for secretion is presented. Finally, the influence of the autonomic nervous system and various circulating substances on the glandular circulations is summarized. The reader should also refer to other recent reviews of salivary and pancreatic circulations (76, 77, 126, 148, 149, 168, 219, 220).

## ANATOMICAL CONSIDERATIONS

### Blood vessels

EXTRAGLANDULAR. A brief description of the major blood vessels and lymphatics of the salivary glands and pancreas of humans (199, 239–241) is presented, and the interested reader should refer to other treatises for corresponding descriptions of the vascular anatomy in other species (32, 40, 52, 79, 156, 220, 240).

*Salivary glands.* The arterial supply of the salivary glands is derived from various branches of the external carotid artery. The parotid gland is perfused by small branches of the posterior auricular artery. The superficial temporal artery supplies the parotid gland by way of parotid vessels and small branches of the transverse facial arteries. The submandibular gland is supplied by the glandular branches of the facial artery and small vessels of the lingual artery. The sublingual gland is perfused by the sublingual branch of the lingual artery and the submental branch of the facial artery.

The venous drainage of the salivary glands is provided by tributaries of the external and internal jugular veins. The parotid gland is drained by the parotid vein, which empties into the facial vein, a tributary of the internal jugular vein. In addition, small veins leaving the gland drain into the superficial temporal vein, which drains into the retromandibular vein. The retromandibular vein subsequently divides into two branches, an anterior branch, which unites with the facial vein (supplying the internal jugular vein) and a posterior branch, which joins the posterior auricular vein to form the external jugular vein. The submandibular gland is drained by the submandibular branch of the facial vein, branches of the anterior jugular vein, and the lingual vein. Subsequently the facial and lingual veins enter the internal jugular vein, whereas the anterior jugular vein empties into the external jugular vein. The venous drainage of the sublingual gland involves the submental and sublingual veins, the former emptying into the facial vein and the latter joining the lingual vein. Both the facial and lingual veins subsequently enter the internal jugular vein.

*Pancreas.* The human pancreas derives its arterial supply from the celiac and superior mesenteric arteries. The splenic branch of the celiac artery gives rise to numerous small vessels that supply the body and tail of the pancreas. The hepatic branch of the celiac artery gives rise to the gastroduodenal artery, which in turn gives off the anterior and posterior superior pancreaticoduodenal arteries. The superior pancreaticoduodenal vessels anastomose with their corresponding inferior pancreaticoduodenal vessels, which arise from the superior mesenteric artery. Branches of the inferior and superior pancreaticoduodenal vessels supply the head and body of the pancreas.

The venous drainage of the pancreas is provided by tributaries of the portal vein. The pancreatic veins drain the body and tail of the pancreas and empty into the splenic vein. The superior and inferior pancreaticoduodenal veins, which accompany their corresponding arteries, drain the head and neck of the pancreas and drain into the superior mesenteric vein. The superior mesenteric and the splenic veins join to form the portal vein.

INTRAGLANDULAR. The following description of the intraglandular microcirculation is based on scanning electron microscopic studies of corrosion casts of rat salivary glands (164, 168, 169) and rat and rabbit pancreas (28, 163, 165–168, 170).

*Salivary glands.* In all three salivary glands (parotid, submandibular, and sublingual), the arterioles course along the inter- and intralobular ducts to supply the capillary plexi surrounding the acini and ducts. The terminal branches of the intralobular arterioles supply the capillary plexus surrounding the acini and initial portions of the duct system (i.e., the intercalated and convoluted ducts). From this plexus arise venules that either enter the venous drainage running along the ducts or supply the capillary plexus surrounding the more distal portion of the intralobular duct system (i.e., the striated duct). The intralobular veins join to form the interlobular veins that exit the gland. The capillary network around the interlobular excretory ducts is supplied by terminal branches of interlobular arterioles. Thus the vascular supply of the acini and interlobular ducts is arranged in parallel, whereas that of the acini and intralobular ducts is in series, with the flow through the portal system being concurrent with salivary flow (Fig. 1A). The capillary networks of the ducts are much more dense than those of the acini. Although no arteriovenous anastomoses are present within the gland, arterioarterial and venovenous anastomoses are plentiful around the ducts.

This description differs from that presented in a previous chapter by Leeson in the 1967 edition of the *Handbook* section on the alimentary canal (131). In that chapter the intraglandular vascular arrangement was characterized by the presence of arteriovenous anastomoses and a portal circulation with blood flowing countercurrent to salivary flow (i.e., portal vessels from the ductular plexus supply the acinar plexus). Although a few studies have indicated that arteriovenous anastomoses are present in the salivary microcirculation, the bulk of both anatomical and physiological studies do not support their existence (220). The existence of a countercurrent portal system was based on physiological studies utilizing iodide clearance into the ducts to estimate salivary blood flow (30). The assumptions of this study have been criticized as being both qualitatively and quantitatively erroneous (220). Even the existence of a series arrangement of the salivary vasculature has been questioned by results of physiological studies (64). However, an adequate explanation has been offered to reconcile the physiological data and anatomical findings (166).

*Pancreas.* The interlobular arteries of the pancreas course along the ducts and give rise to the intralobular arteries. The intralobular arteries divide into arteriolar branches that directly supply *1*) the glomuslike capillary network of the islets (insular arterioles), *2*) the capillary plexus of the acini (acinar arterioles), and *3*) the periductular capillary plexus (periductular arterioles). Efferent vessels from the islet capillary network either enter the acinar capillary plexus (via insuloacinar portal vessels) or the periductular capillary plexus (via the insuloductular route) or drain directly into intralobular veins. Efferent vessels from the acinar capillary network either enter the ductular capillary plexus or drain directly into the intralobular veins. Efferent vessels from the ductular plexus drain directly into the intralobular veins. The intralobular veins join to form the interlobular veins, which run along with the corresponding arterioles and exit the gland. Thus the microvascular arrangement of the exocrine pancreas is remarkably similar to that of the salivary gland (Fig. 1*B*). In both glands the vascular supply to the acini and ducts are arranged both in series and in parallel. The series arrangement between the acinar and ductular capillary networks is concurrent with the flow of pancreatic juice. The presence of an endocrine (islets) circulation in the pancreas is the feature that most distinguishes the pancreas from the salivary gland.

In general the results of other anatomical and physiological studies support the previous description of the pancreatic microcirculation (2, 35, 89, 137, 138). There seems to be universal agreement on the existence of an insuloacinar portal system. The only points of contention are the existence of *1*) an insuloductal portal system, *2*) a direct arterial supply to the ductal capillaries, and *3*) a direct venous drainage from the islets to intralobular veins (63, 137, 138). The basis for these discrepancies may be that the vascular channels in question are of small caliber and rather infrequent. Inasmuch as only the islets in close apposition to the ducts have efferent vessels that communicate with the ductal capillary plexus (163, 164, 166), it would be expected that some investigators do not refer to this portal system (138). Not only have electron microscopic analyses of corrosion casts revealed the presence of such channels, but intravital microscopic studies of the in situ pancreas have demonstrated the movement of fluorescent tracer molecules from the capillary plexus of an islet to an adjacent ductular plexus (163). Some investigators, using latex casts of the pancreatic vessels, claim that there is neither a direct arterial supply to the ducts nor a direct venous drainage from the islet capillary plexus to intralobular veins (138). However, most of the evidence supports the existence of such vascular connections (2, 28, 164, 168).

In conclusion, the intraglandular pancreatic circulation can be described as consisting of three portal systems. One portal system, the acinoductular route, is very similar to that seen in the salivary gland. The other two portal systems, the insuloacinar and insuloductular routes, provide vascular connections between the endocrine and exocrine portions of the pancreas. It is believed that these channels provide a means by which the hormones of the islet cells can reach the acini or ducts in high concentrations and regulate their activity (89, 90). The control of blood flow, and thereby delivery of hormones, from the endocrine to exocrine portions of the pancreas is believed to be a function of the tone of precapillary sphincters situated between the islet and exocrine circulations (2, 155).

*Lymph Vessels*

EXTRAGLANDULAR. A brief description of the major lymph vessels draining the salivary glands and pan-

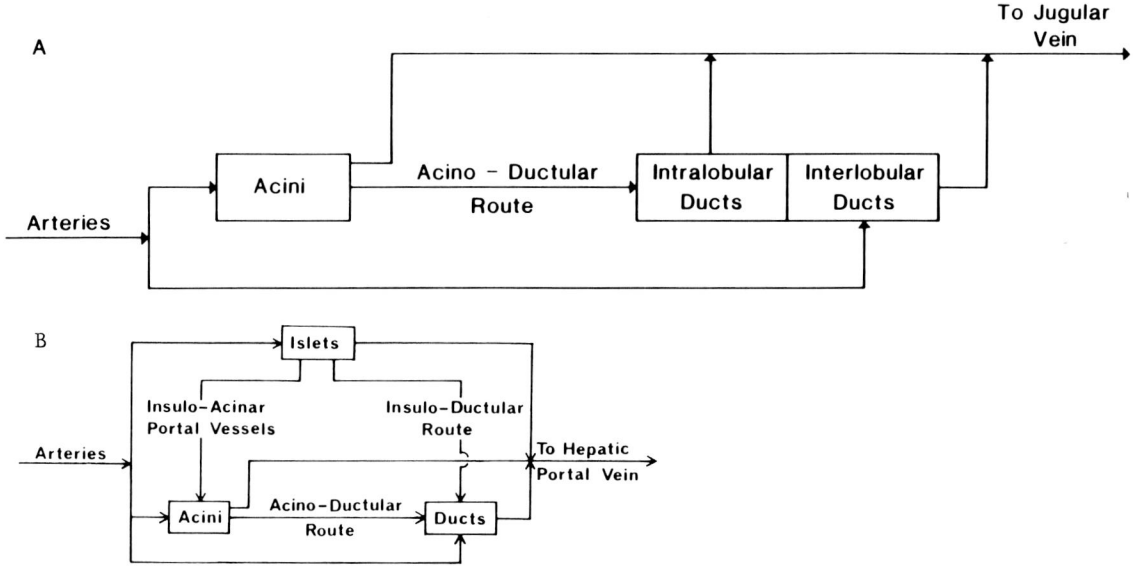

FIG. 1. Schematic representation of intraglandular portal circulations of salivary gland (*A*) and pancreas (*B*). [From Ohtani et al. (168).]

creas of humans (184, 199, 241) is presented here, and the interested reader should also refer to other reviews for descriptions of the lymphatic vessels in other species (40, 52, 79).

*Salivary glands.* The lymph vessels draining the parotid gland pass through several lymph nodes located within or on the surface of the gland and enter the deep cervical lymph nodes. The lymph vessels draining the submandibular gland pass through the submandibular lymph nodes before entering the deep cervical lymph nodes. The efferent lymph vessels draining the deep cervical lymph nodes form the jugular trunk, which in turn subdivides into the left and right trunks. The left trunk empties into the general circulation via the thoracic duct, whereas the right lymphatic trunk terminates at the junction of the right subclavian and internal jugular veins.

*Pancreas.* Most of the lymph vessels draining the pancreas end in the pancreatic, splenic, and hepatic lymph nodes, which eventually drain to the celiac lymph nodes. Some lymphatics from the head of the pancreas drain directly into the superior mesenteric lymph nodes. Efferents from the superior mesenteric and celiac nodes join other preaortic lymph nodes to form the intestinal lymph trunks, which enter the cisterna chyli of the thoracic duct.

INTRAGLANDULAR. There is very little information available on the intraglandular lymphatic vessels of the pancreas and salivary gland (11, 12, 73, 201).

*Salivary glands.* Valved lymphatic vessels have been seen that course along the blood vessels and ducts. Initial lymph vessels lie in very close apposition to acinar cells in dogs and humans, whereas they are found near the initial ducts in the rabbit.

*Pancreas.* Initial lymphatics have been observed near the acinar and islets cells (73, 201). However, it is generally believed that lymphatic vessels do not penetrate the islets (73).

## Nerves

SYMPATHETIC. *Salivary glands.* The preganglionic sympathetic fibers are derived from the first two thoracic segments and enter the superior cervical ganglion. The postganglionic fibers leaving the superior cervical ganglion pass through the carotid plexi and course along arteries supplying each gland. The catecholamine-containing postganglionic fibers terminate around acini, ducts, and blood vessels. The density of adrenergic innervation of blood vessels is greatest in the arterioles and least in the venules (115, 199, 200, 241).

*Pancreas.* Preganglionic sympathetic fibers are derived from the fifth to tenth thoracic segments and synapse with postganglionic fibers in the celiac plexus and its derivatives the superior mesenteric and hepatic plexi. The postganglionic fibers leaving the plexi course along with the arteries supplying the pancreas.

Nerve terminals in close apposition to arterioles are adrenergic (134, 199, 241).

PARASYMPATHETIC. *Salivary glands.* The preganglionic parasympathetic fibers are derived from the salivary nuclei. Preganglionic fibers from the superior salivatory nucleus pass in the facial nerve to the chorda tympani and subsequently to the lingual nerve, which enters the submandibular ganglion. Postganglionic fibers from the submandibular ganglion innervate the acini, ducts, and arterioles of the submandibular and sublingual glands. Preganglionic fibers from the inferior salivatory nuclei course along the glossopharyngeal nerve to the otic ganglion. Postganglionic fibers from the otic ganglion pass in the auricular temporal nerve to the ducts, acini, and arterioles of the parotid gland. The parotid gland is also supplied by facial parasympathetic fibers (199, 241). Acetylcholine is present in the postganglionic nerve terminals near arterioles (115, 200). There is also evidence for nerve terminals containing vasoactive intestinal polypeptide (VIP) (139) and substance P (47, 181). Whether acetylcholine and VIP coexist in the same nerve terminals or are confined to separate nerve fibers remains uncertain (139).

*Pancreas.* The preganglionic parasympathetic fibers originate in the dorsal nucleus of the vagus in the medulla oblongata. The fibers enter the abdomen via the anterior and posterior vagal trunks. A branch of the posterior trunk passes through the celiac plexus without synapsing, and its fibers course along with the arteries to the pancreas. The major vagal supply to the pancreas is via the posterior trunk, with relatively few branches of the anterior vagal trunk reaching the pancreas. The vagal fibers synapse on cell bodies of postganglionic fibers within the substance of the gland (134, 199, 241). As in the salivary gland, there is evidence that nerve terminals containing acetylcholine (134), VIP (139), and substance P (18) are present in close apposition to the blood vessels and secretory elements.

## BASAL HEMODYNAMICS AND OXYGENATION

A variety of techniques have been employed to measure blood flow in the salivary gland and pancreas. Table 1 presents basal values for various hemodynamic and oxygenation parameters in salivary glands and pancreas of several species. Because it is relatively simple to measure salivary blood flow via the external jugular vein, the venous outflow technique has been widely used to estimate blood flow and $O_2$ uptake in this organ. Direct measurement of blood flow by venous collection is more difficult and less desirable in the pancreas, because of the multiple venous drainage and admixture with duodenal venous blood. Thus other methods (e.g., microsphere, electromagnetic probes) are more commonly used in the pancreas.

The resting rates of blood flow and $O_2$ uptake in the

TABLE 1. *Basal Values of Hemodynamic and Oxygenation Parameters in the Salivary Gland and Pancreas*

| | Salivary Gland | Ref. | Pancreas | Ref. |
|---|---|---|---|---|
| Blood flow, ml·min$^{-1}$·100 g$^{-1}$ | 16–50 | 225, 233 | 35–173 | 3, 126, 174 |
| Total vascular resistance, mmHg·(ml$^{-1}$·min$^{-1}$·100 g$^{-1}$) | 2.0–6.25 | 225, 233 | 0.58–2.86 | 3, 174 |
| Precapillary resistance, mmHg·(ml$^{-1}$·min$^{-1}$·100 g$^{-1}$) | 2.25 | 48 | 1.56 | 125 |
| Postcapillary resistance, mmHg·(ml$^{-1}$·min$^{-1}$·100 g$^{-1}$) | 0.25 | 48 | 0.05 | 125 |
| Capillary filtration coefficient, ml·min$^{-1}$·mmHg$^{-1}$·100 g$^{-1}$ | 0.10–0.30 | 48, 151 | 0.10–0.30 | 48, 125 |
| Capillary pressure, mmHg | 9–11 | 48 | 8.0–13.0 | 48, 125 |
| Arteriovenous O$_2$ difference, ml/100 ml blood | 6.6–15.5 | 225, 233 | 2.6–8.3 | 3, 125 |
| O$_2$ uptake, ml·min$^{-1}$·100 g$^{-1}$ | 1.6–3.6 | 225, 233 | 1.5–4.0 | 3, 125 |

pancreas and salivary glands generally fall within the ranges reported for gastrointestinal organs of the same species (126, 148, 149, 220). The very wide range of blood flows reported for the pancreas presumably results from differences in species, anesthesia, and techniques used to measure blood flow. For example, pancreatic blood flow is significantly lower in anesthetized animals (174). The available data indicate that blood flow, O$_2$ uptake, and tissue O$_2$ tension are similar in the head, body, and tail of the pancreas (1, 7, 84). Whether differences exist between the various salivary glands remains uncertain inasmuch as virtually all studies in this area have employed the submandibular (submaxillary) gland.

Arteriolar tone and precapillary sphincter tone are the major determinants of the rate of nutrient and O$_2$ delivery to the parenchyma. Changes in arteriolar tone modify the resistance to the total flow of blood through the tissue, whereas the tone of precapillary sphincters determines the density of capillaries open to perfusion of blood. Because the delivery of O$_2$ and nutrients to the parenchyma is controlled by both arteriolar and precapillary sphincter tone, concomitant determinations of blood flow and capillary exchange capacity have proved useful in interpretation of results on the effects of various physiological perturbations on O$_2$ and nutrient exchange in both the pancreas and salivary glands. The capillary filtration coefficient ($K_f$) is a measurement of the hydraulic conductivity of exchange vessels in a tissue; as such, it provides a useful index of the functional exchange capacity of the circulation in that tissue (197). Estimates of $K_f$ in the pancreas and salivary glands under resting conditions generally range between 0.10 and 0.30 ml·min$^{-1}$·mmHg$^{-1}$·100 g$^{-1}$, which is similar to resting values reported for the stomach and intestine (48, 125, 151, 197). The $K_f$ can increase by four to five times during maximal vasodilation in both pancreas and salivary glands (48, 125, 151), indicating that only one-fourth to one-fifth of the capillaries are perfused under resting conditions.

## INTRINSIC REGULATION OF BLOOD FLOW AND OXYGENATION

There is much evidence indicating that gastrointestinal tissues possess an intrinsic ability to regulate blood flow and O$_2$ uptake during a variety of physiological stresses. Intrinsic regulation is generally considered to result from metabolic or mechanical changes in the parenchyma and/or vascular smooth muscle that ultimately lead to arteriolar and precapillary sphincter dilation or constriction. Three mechanisms are commonly invoked to explain intrinsic regulation of pancreatic and salivary gland blood flow and oxygenation, i.e., metabolic, kallikrein-kinin, and myogenic mechanisms.

### Metabolic Regulation

According to the metabolic theory of intrinsic vasoregulation, vascular resistance and precapillary sphincter tone are linked to the metabolic state of the tissue. Any condition that produces an imbalance between tissue O$_2$ supply and O$_2$ demand results in a reduction in tissue O$_2$ tension (P$_{O_2}$) and an accumulation of vasodilator metabolites in the interstitial fluid. The fall in tissue P$_{O_2}$ and/or accumulation of vasodilator metabolites cause relaxation of arteriolar and precapillary sphincter smooth muscle. The resulting increase in blood flow and/or O$_2$ extraction restores the O$_2$ supply to a level that is compatible with tissue O$_2$ demand. Therefore the metabolic model of intrinsic vasoregulation predicts that the rate of O$_2$ delivery to the parenchyma, rather than blood flow per se, is the controlled variable (75, 221).

Although there is little direct evidence supporting a role for tissue P$_{O_2}$ in the control of pancreatic and salivary gland blood flows, the results of a recent report indicate that pancreatic tissue P$_{O_2}$ decreases significantly from a control value of 25 mmHg when either blood flow is reduced or secretion is stimulated by cholecystokinin (CCK) (84). Purine compounds (117), K$^+$ (41), and hyperosmolality (150) have been proposed as metabolic mediators of blood flow in the pancreas and salivary glands. These substances are known to accumulate in the stimulated gland and produce vasodilation when infused into the blood supply of the resting gland (41, 117, 150).

### Myogenic Regulation

The myogenic theory of intrinsic vasoregulation is based on the assumption that vascular wall tension is a controlled variable (114). According to this concept, tension receptors modulate vascular smooth muscle tone in response to changes in microvascular transmural pressure. Thus, in accordance with Laplace's law, resistance vessels should dilate when vascular transmural pressure is decreased and constrict when it is increased. In many respects the predicted effects of a myogenic mechanism are very similar to those of a metabolic mechanism. For instance, both theories predict a reduced vascular resistance in response to a fall in arterial pressure, the myogenic theory because of a fall in vascular transmural pressure and the metabolic theory because of a reduction in tissue $P_{O_2}$ or an accumulation of vasodilator metabolites. One experimental perturbation that allows for clear differentiation between the two mechanisms is acute venous pressure elevation (78). The myogenic theory predicts an increased vascular resistance in response to the increased transmural pressure, whereas the metabolic theory predicts a fall in vascular resistance in response to the reduction in blood flow and $O_2$ supply to the tissue.

### Kallikrein-Kinin Regulation

The salivary gland and pancreas are the richest sources of serine proteases called kallikreins (23). The kallikreins react with plasma substrates called kininogens to generate kinins (e.g., bradykinin), which are potent vasodilator peptides. Glandular kallikreins have been implicated in the regulation of blood flow in both salivary glands (92, 94, 136) and pancreas (20a, 56, 95, 96, 190). Kallikrein is stored in the ductal system where it is secreted into the interstitial fluid in response to specific stimuli that usually produce vasodilation. Such stimuli include parasympathetic and sympathetic activation in the salivary glands (94, 190) and CCK and acetylcholine in the pancreas (95, 96). Once within the interstitium, the kallikrein can release kinins from substrates before it is inactivated by plasma protease inhibitors. Kininlike substances can be detected in the venous effluent and the tissue content of kallikrein increases during parasympathetic and sympathetic stimulation in the salivary glands (56, 95).

### Evidence for Intrinsic Vasoregulation

There are several experimental perturbations that are used to establish the existence of intrinsic vascular control mechanisms. These include pressure-flow autoregulation, reactive hyperemia, hypoxic vasodilation, and response to acute venous pressure elevation (78). Although all of these perturbations have been applied to the pancreas, intrinsic vasoregulation studies in the salivary glands have focused only on pressure-flow autoregulation.

PRESSURE-FLOW AUTOREGULATION. Autoregulation is defined as the ability of an organ to maintain a relatively constant blood flow (or $O_2$ uptake) during alterations in arterial pressure. Graded decrements in arterial pressure lead to progressive reductions in pancreatic blood flow [Fig. 2; (125)]. Because vascular resistance also decreases as perfusion pressure is reduced, blood flow appears to be actively autoregulated. The degree of flow autoregulation is such that blood flow falls by 70% of the decrement of pressure. This response is comparable to results reported for other splanchnic organs. The extent of flow autoregulation in the pancreas is highly dependent on the initial (or resting) vascular resistance, i.e., the autoregulatory ability is greater if the initial vascular resistance is high.

In contrast to the active flow autoregulation observed in the pancreas, the salivary gland behaves like a passive vascular bed. Fazekas et al. (54) have demonstrated that blood flow (measured by $H_2$ gas clearance) in the rabbit submandibular gland is linearly related to arterial pressure. Vascular resistance remained constant when arterial pressure was varied between 130 and 22 mmHg. The reason for the absence of pressure-flow autoregulation in the salivary glands is not readily apparent; however, the fact that the experiments were performed with sympathetically innervated preparations and that arterial pressure was altered via the carotid artery may have some bearing.

In the pancreas, the arteriovenous $O_2$ difference increases progressively as arterial pressure is reduced [Fig. 2; (125)]. This rise in tissue $O_2$ extraction is sufficient to compensate for the reduction in blood flow so that pancreatic $O_2$ uptake remains at the control level until arterial pressure is reduced below 20 mmHg. The rise in $O_2$ extraction produced by a reduction in arterial pressure is associated with a concomitant increase in $K_f$. The capillary recruitment that occurs when arterial pressure is reduced may be important in maintaining tissue oxygenation.

Both myogenic and metabolic theories predict decreases in vascular resistance and increases in capillary exchange capacity during reductions in arterial pressure. Therefore it is difficult to attribute the pancreatic vascular responses to either mechanism based only on blood flow and $K_f$ data. However, because the $O_2$ delivery version of the metabolic theory predicts that tissue $O_2$ delivery (not blood flow per se) is the regulated variable, the ability of the pancreas to maintain its $O_2$ uptake during reductions in perfusion pressure to 20 mmHg suggests that a metabolic mechanism may be operative in the pancreas. An alternate explanation is that the responses of resistance and exchange vessels to pressure alterations are of little consequence in the regulation of pancreatic $O_2$ uptake and that the large margin of safety against hypoxia observed when pressure is reduced can be attributed to a low critical $P_{O_2}$ (minimal cell $P_{O_2}$ for normal oxidative metabolism) in the pancreas. Kvietys et al. (126) have assessed the quantitative significance of blood flow autoregulation and capillary recruitment in maintaining a constant pancreatic $O_2$ uptake when arterial pressure is reduced. Their analysis was based on a mathematical model (75) and data obtained from the dog pan-

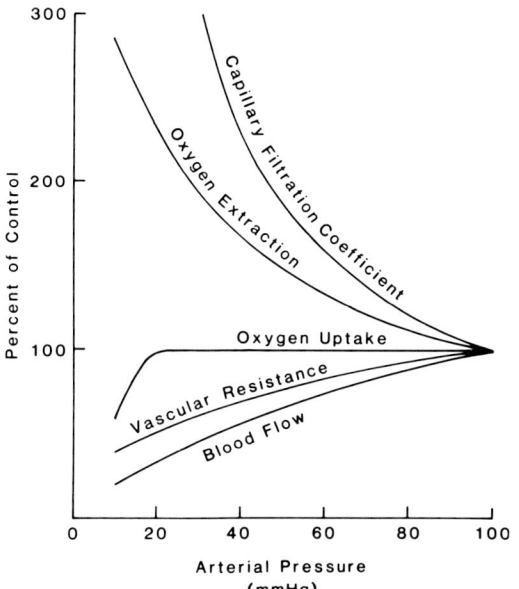

FIG. 2. Effects of reducing arterial pressure on pancreatic hemodynamics and oxygenation. [From Kvietys et al. (126).]

creas (125). The model predicted that, in the absence of flow autoregulation and capillary recruitment, tissue hypoxia (and a reduction in $O_2$ uptake) should occur only when arterial pressure falls below 50 mmHg. With regulation of both resistance and exchange vessels, arterial pressure must be reduced to below 15 mmHg before the tissue becomes hypoxic. Recruitment of capillaries appears to be of slightly greater quantitative importance than autoregulation of blood flow in maintaining tissue $P_{O_2}$ above the critical level. Thus the vascular readjustments that occur in the pancreas when arterial pressure is reduced provide about a 35 mmHg margin of safety against tissue hypoxia (126).

REACTIVE HYPEREMIA. The responses of the pancreatic vasculature to 15-, 30-, and 60-s arterial occlusions are summarized in Figure 3. The magnitude and duration of the reactive hyperemic responses are directly related to the duration of the arterial occlusion. The volume flow debt incurred during the arterial occlusion is completely repaid after a 15-s occlusion; however, the percent repayment falls to 75% and 55% after release of 30- and 60-s occlusions, respectively. For a given duration of occlusion the percent repayment of the flow debt is inversely related to the preocclusion flow, i.e., the lower the preocclusion blood flow the greater the percentage repayment. Both metabolic and myogenic mechanisms can explain the active vasodilation during arterial occlusion; however, only metabolic factors can account for the direct relationship between the duration of occlusion and the magnitude of the reactive hyperemia.

Although the reactive hyperemic response has not been systematically studied in salivary glands, Rabito et al. (190) have obtained evidence that indicates that the kallikrein-kinin system does not play a role in the reactive hyperemia. They observed an abrupt increase in glandular blood flow (11-fold) and kallikrein secretion rate (57-fold) after termination of a 1-min sympathetic stimulation. In contrast, arterial occlusion for 1 min did not alter glandular kallikrein output in the postischemic period.

HYPOXIC VASODILATION. Arterial hypoxemia and hypercapnia both elicit vasodilation in the intestines (78), findings consistent with metabolic vasoregulation. Broadie and co-workers (29) have examined the effect of systemic hypoxia and hypercapnia on pancreatic blood flow, measured by $^{86}$Rb clearance. Both conditions reduced pancreatic blood flow to about one half the resting level. These findings may be explained by the fact that the experiments were performed with intact sympathetic innervation. Thus any tendency for metabolic factors to produce vasodilation may have been overridden by chemoreceptor-activated sympathetic vasoconstriction.

VENOUS PRESSURE ELEVATION. Figure 4 illustrates the effects of acute venous pressure elevation (from 2.2 to 12.4 mmHg) on pancreatic hemodynamics and oxygenation (125). In the pancreas, venous pressure elevation reduces blood flow and increases vascular resistance. These changes are associated with a rise in both the arteriovenous $O_2$ difference and $K_f$ coefficient, whereas $O_2$ uptake remains at the control value. The changes produced by venous pressure elevation are consistent with myogenic constriction of resistance vessels and metabolic dilation of precapillary sphincters. The capillary recruitment resulting from precapillary sphincter dilation appears to play a significant role in preventing tissue hypoxia in the face of a fall in blood flow. Kvietys et al. (126) have shown, using a mathematical model based on hemodynamic

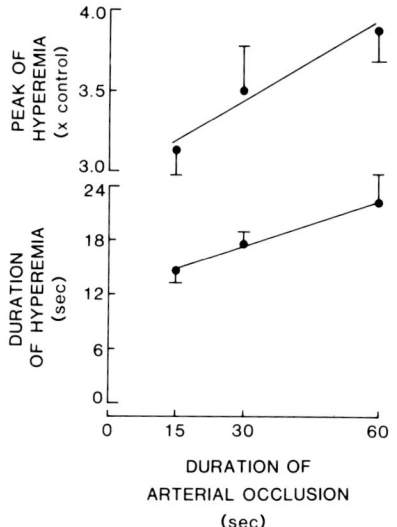

FIG. 3. Effects of graded arterial occlusions on magnitude and duration of postocclusion hyperemic response. [From Kvietys et al. (125).]

and $O_2$-exchange data from the dog pancreas, that the myogenic constriction of resistance vessels during acute venous hypertension predisposes the pancreas to tissue hypoxia at lower venous pressures than if the pancreatic circulation were a purely passive system. The model also predicts that in the absence of exchange vessel regulation, the myogenic response would cause pancreatic $O_2$ uptake to decrease when venous pressure is elevated to 15 mmHg. With exchange vessel regulation, however, venous pressure would have to exceed 40 mmHg before the pancreas becomes hypoxic.

## FUNCTIONAL HYPEREMIA

### Characteristics of Functional Hyperemia

Bernard (22) first described the basic characteristics of the functional hyperemia in salivary glands. He showed that instillation of vinegar into the mouth of a dog elicits an increase in secretion and blood flow from the submandibular gland. The enhanced salivation and associated hyperemia were due to a gustatory reflex having an efferent pathway in the chorda tympani, inasmuch as both of these responses were abolished after section of the nerve. Stimulation of the distal end of the cut nerve produced changes in salivary secretion rate and blood flow similar to placement of vinegar in the mouth. Since the epochal studies of Bernard, electrical stimulation of the parasympathetic fibers has been the model of choice for studying functional hyperemia in the salivary glands (Table 2).

As a matter of convenience, constant rates of stimulation at different frequencies have been used to determine the relationship between salivary secretion and blood flow. The threshold stimulation frequency

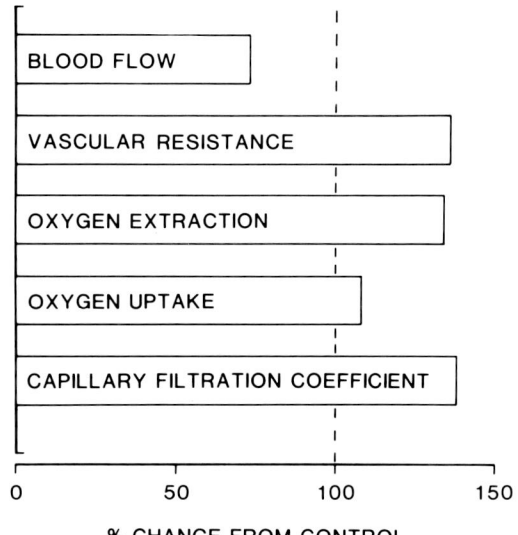

FIG. 4. Effects of venous pressure elevation (from 2.2 to 12.4 mmHg) on pancreatic hemodynamics and oxygenation. [From Kvietys et al. (125).]

for increasing salivary flow and blood flow is 0.3–0.5 Hz (71). Further increases in stimulation frequency increase both salivation rate and blood flow in a frequency-dependent manner to a maximum of 10–20 Hz (41, 71, 232). As shown in Figure 5, the blood flow response to low-frequency continuous stimulation (<5 Hz) is characterized by a transient, intense hyperemia followed by a lower steady-state hyperemia. At higher stimulation frequencies (>5 Hz) the initial transient overshoot in blood flow is absent. Stimulation of the chorda tympani at a constant frequency of 7–8 Hz in the anesthetized animal can produce secretion rates equivalent to the maximum rates observed during feeding (50). A quantitatively different response is

TABLE 2. *Effects of Autonomic Nerve Stimulation on Salivary Blood Flow*

|  | Stimulation Frequency, Hz | Change in Blood Flow, % |  | Ref. |
|---|---|---|---|---|
| Parasympathetic stimulation | 0.5 | +109 |  | 71, 232 |
|  | 1 | +100 to +259 |  | 150, 217 |
|  | 2 | +67 to +300 |  | 41, 56, 70, 118, 143, 144, 150, 212, 217 |
|  | 4 | +480 to +647 |  | 117, 217 |
|  | 5 | +200 to +441 |  | 41, 71, 132 |
|  | 10 | +160 to +900 |  | 41, 71, 118, 136, 149, 190, 209, 228 |
|  | 15 | +263 to +606 |  | 140, 141, 143 |
|  | 20 | +328 to +1,480 |  | 19, 24, 27, 41, 69, 118, 119 |
|  | 25 | +391 to +1,150 |  | 187 |
|  |  | During stimulation | Post-stimulation |  |
| Sympathetic stimulation | 0.5 | −42 |  | 71 |
|  | 2–4 | −55 | +177 | 102 |
|  | 5 | −49 to −95 | +75 | 71, 205, 212 |
|  | 6 | −20 to −68 | +200 to +260 | 102, 141, 145 |
|  | 10 | −50 | +300 to +991 | 68, 190 |
|  | 16 | −74 | +519 | 102 |
|  | 20 | −75 | +300 | 68 |
|  | 25 | −60 to −84 | +20 | 24, 158 |

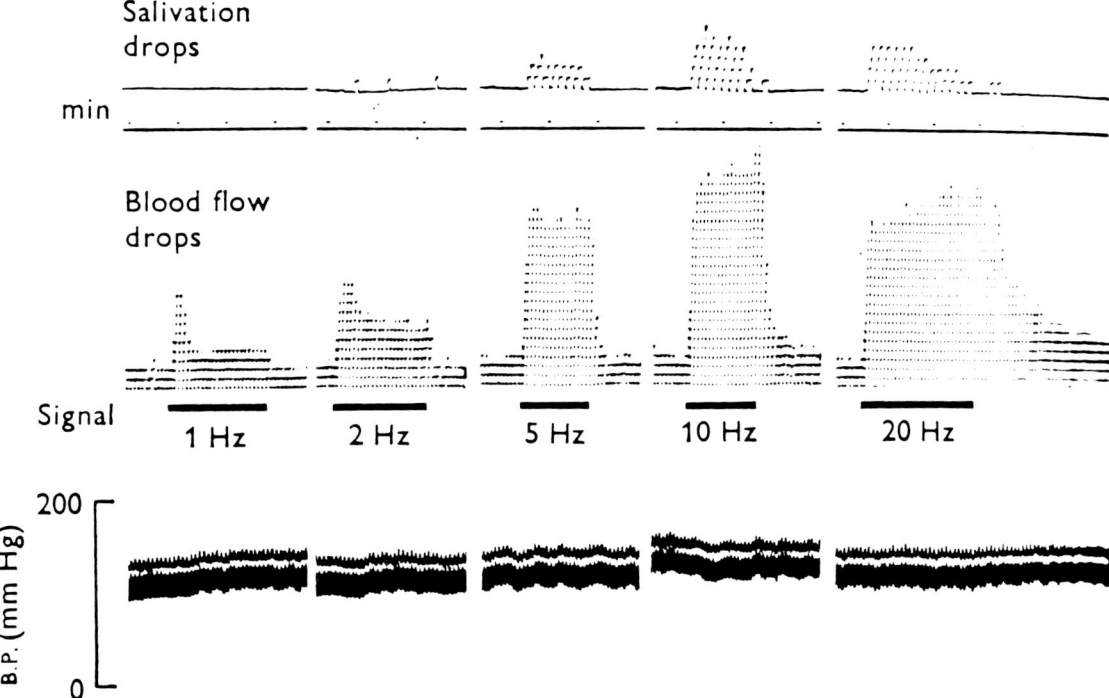

FIG. 5. Effect of chorda stimulation on salivary gland secretion rate and blood flow. [From Darke and Smaje (41).]

obtained if the nerve is stimulated intermittently (4). Intermittent stimulation of the chorda tympani at different frequencies with 1-s bursts at 10-s intervals results in a frequency-dependent increase in salivary secretion and decrease in vascular resistance that do not reach maximum values until 40–60 Hz frequencies are applied (Fig. 6). High-frequency (25-Hz) continuous chorda stimulation applied for brief periods (<5 s) results in a slowly developing hyperemia that becomes evident after cessation of nerve stimulation (187). This poststimulation hyperemia appears to be associated with cation transport in the glands.

The functional hyperemia in the salivary glands has received a great deal of attention since the observation by Heidenhain (85) that atropine can abolish the secretory response to parasympathetic nerve stimulation without altering the hyperemic response. Most investigators have confirmed this phenomenon; however, in some instances atropine has been shown to block both the hyperemia and secretory response to nerve stimulation (111, 220). The ability of atropine to prevent the hyperemia and enhanced secretion produced by nerve stimulation is dependent on the stimulation frequency (4, 41). The vasodilation is abolished or attenuated at the low stimulation frequencies. Only at high stimulation frequencies does atropine fail to modify the hyperemic response to nerve stimulation (Fig. 6). Inasmuch as ganglionic blockade can prevent the vasodilatory response in atropinized animals (226), the parasympathetic nerves may be releasing a noncholinergic, vasodilator substance. The poststimulation hyperemia is also drastically reduced in the presence of atropine (187).

Activation of the sympathetic nervous system also stimulates salivary secretion. However, a role for sympathetic nerves in the functional hyperemia seems unlikely, inasmuch as adrenergic stimulation leads to a significant reduction in salivary gland blood flow (Table 2).

Bernard (21) was the first to provide evidence, albeit indirect, of a functional hyperemia in the pancreas. He noted that the canine pancreas changed in color from white to red and appeared engorged after feeding. It has since been reported that pancreatic blood flow increases after feeding (67, 124), duodenal acidification (20), or intraluminal placement of oil (53) or glucose (57). The postprandial pancreatic hyperemia appears to be linked to secretory activity (53, 124). The pancreatic secretory response to a meal is mediated primarily by the parasympathetic nervous system (vagus) during the cephalic phase and by hormones (e.g., secretin and CCK) during the intestinal phase. Electrical stimulation of the vagus as well as exogenous administration of secretin and CCK have been shown to increase pancreatic exocrine secretion and blood flow (Table 3).

The functional hyperemia in the pancreas is not as well characterized as that of the salivary glands. The available evidence indicates that the functional vasodilation in response to nerve-induced pancreatic secretion is similar in some respects to that observed in the salivary glands. Atropine can substantially reduce

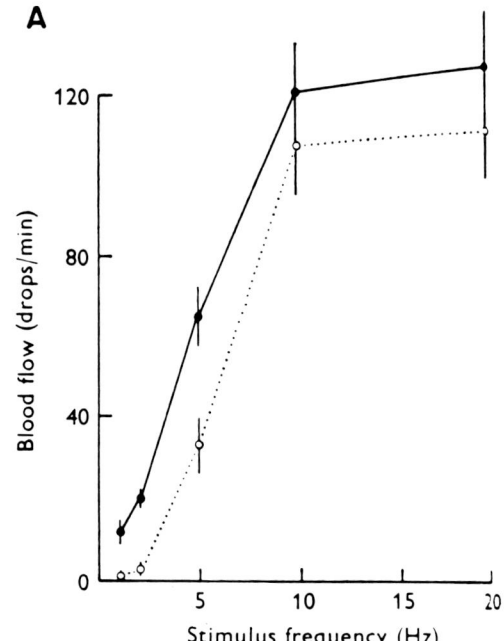

FIG. 6. *A*: relationship between steady-state salivary blood flow and frequency of stimulation of the chorda lingual nerve with continuous mode of nerve stimulation. *Solid line*, before atropine; *dashed line*, after atropine. *B*: relationship between steady-state salivary vascular resistance and frequency of stimulation of chorda tympani nerve with intermittent mode of nerve stimulation. *Open bars*, before atropine; *solid bars*, after atropine; *n*, number of observations. [*A* from Darke and Smaje (41); *B* from Andersson et al. (4).]

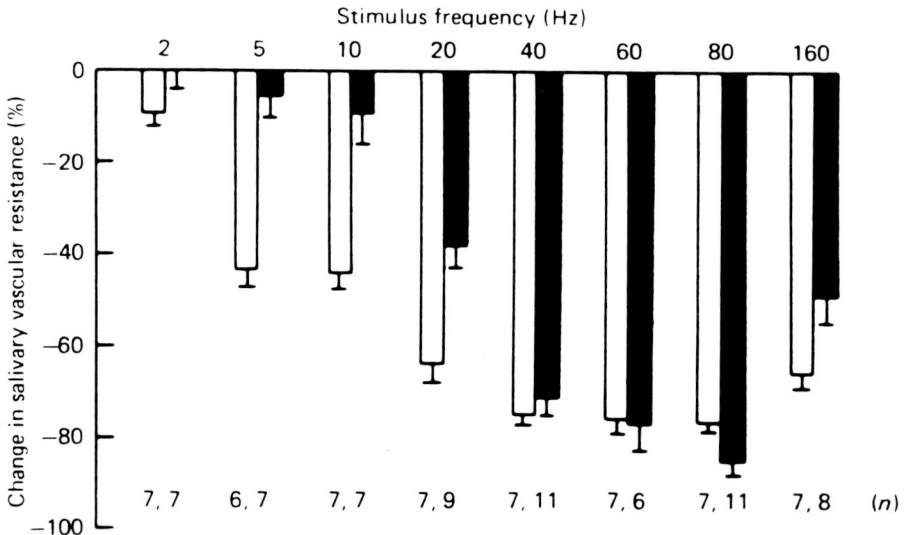

amylase output without altering the pancreatic hyperemic response to parasympathetic nerve (vagus) stimulation in the pig (91), a phenomenon not confirmed in the dog (96). There is even evidence that the pancreas may not require a functional hyperemia to meet the demands of enhanced secretory activity, inasmuch as secretin can induce almost maximal secretory responses without altering pancreatic blood flow (16, 44).

*Mediators of Functional Hyperemia*

Both intrinsic (metabolic and kallikrein-kinin system) and extrinsic (nerves and hormones) mechanisms have been invoked to explain how glandular blood flow and functional activity are coupled. This section presents evidence that argues for and against each of these mechanisms.

INTRINSIC FACTORS. *Metabolic.* A direct linear relationship between the rate of exocrine secretion and $O_2$ consumption has been demonstrated in the submaxillary gland (225, 233) and pancreas (6, 121, 126, 180). In both glands, the magnitude of the functional hyperemia is proportional to the increment in $O_2$ consumption [Fig. 7; (121, 233)]. There is also evidence that enhanced glandular activity is associated with capillary recruitment. The $K_f$ in the submandibular gland increases up to threefold during secretion induced by chorda stimulation (151). In vivo microscopy

TABLE 3. *Effects of Vagal Stimulation and Gastrointestinal Hormones on Pancreatic Blood Flow*

| Condition or Hormone | Stimulation Frequency or Dose | Change in Blood Flow, % | Ref. |
|---|---|---|---|
| Vagal stimulation | 10 Hz | +25 to +125 | 95, 113 |
| Cholecystokinin (CCK) | 1–2 IU/kg, ia | +10 | 113 |
| | 0.125 U/kg, ia | +130 | 178 |
| | 0.1–1.0 U, ia | +21 to +85 | 112 |
| | 2 U·kg$^{-1}$·min$^{-1}$, iv | +87 to 150 | 235 |
| | 0.3–2 U/kg, iv | +15 to +118 | 44, 72 |
| | 2 CU/kg, iv | +11 | 42 |
| | 5 IU/kg, iv | +213 | 7 |
| | 5–100 U, iv | +89 to +400 | 66, 95 |
| CCK-8 | 50 µg/kg, ia | +10 | 175 |
| | 4 µg/kg, iv | +9 | 84 |
| Caerulein | 240 µg/min, ia | +100 | 161 |
| | 2–100 µg/kg, ia | +14 to +35 | 44, 100, 175 |
| Secretin | 0.05–0.2 U/kg, ia | −10 to +22 | 100, 178 |
| | 0.01–0.3 U, ia | 0 to +19 | 110, 112 |
| | 0.1–0.5 U·kg$^{-1}$·min$^{-1}$, iv | +8 to −13 | 14 |
| | 0.1–0.3 IU·kg$^{-1}$·min$^{-1}$, iv | 0 to +5 | 113 |
| | 20 U/h, iv | +200 | 6 |
| | 0.06–5 U/kg, iv | −10 to +188 | 16, 17, 46, 72, 186 |
| | 0.08–2.0 CU/kg, iv | +5 to +300 | 37, 42, 44, 84 |
| | 10 IU/kg, iv | +119 | 7 |
| | 10 µg/100 g, iv | +29 to +63 | 120 |
| | 5–75 U, iv | 0 to +50 | 113 |
| Secretin + CCK | 0.1–0.3 IU/kg, iv (secretin) 1.0–2.0 IU/kg, ia (CCK) | +50 to +100 | 113 |

ia, Intra-arterial; iv, intravenous.

studies have demonstrated an increase in perfused capillary density in the pancreas during secretion induced by secretin and CCK (87). These findings suggest that the oxidative requirements of enhanced secretory activity can be met by an increase in glandular blood flow and/or capillary surface area. In support of this contention is the observation that in the secretin-stimulated pancreas the increased O$_2$ demand is met by an increase in O$_2$ extraction when a hyperemia does not occur (17). These observations are in accord with the metabolic model of intrinsic vasoregulation, which predicts that O$_2$ delivery to the parenchyma, rather than blood flow per se, is the controlled variable. Mediators of the vascular adjustments to enhanced metabolic demands of secretory activity may be either a direct effect of decreased tissue P$_{O_2}$, release of vasodilator metabolites (e.g., K$^+$, purine compounds) or increased interstitial osmolality.

A continuous measurement of interstitial P$_{O_2}$ has been obtained in the pancreas. When nonvasoactive doses of CCK are used to increase pancreatic enzyme secretion, tissue P$_{O_2}$ in the vicinity of the acinar cells decreases by as much as 45% (84). The changes in tissue P$_{O_2}$ paralleled the changes in enzyme output; i.e., when enzyme output was at its peak, tissue P$_{O_2}$ reaches its lowest value.

The vasodilators K$^+$ and adenosine have been implicated in the functional hyperemia of the exocrine glands (34, 117). There is a direct linear relationship between the rate of saliva formation and the amount of K$^+$ lost from the secretory units to the local circulation (129). The rise in venous K$^+$ concentration parallels the increase in venous outflow from the gland

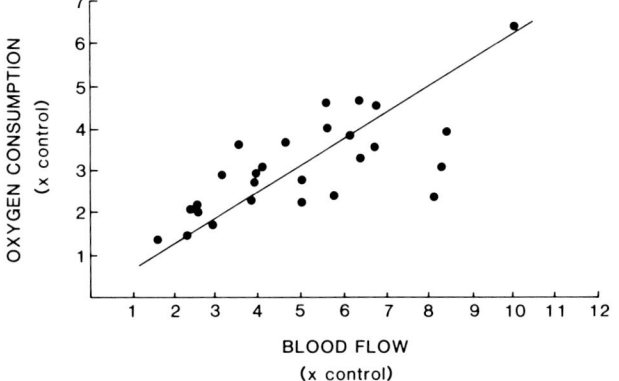

FIG. 7. Relationship between salivary O$_2$ consumption and blood flow during salivary secretion. [Adapted from Terroux et al. (233).]

during secretion induced by acetylcholine (129) and chorda stimulation (41, 187). At low stimulation frequencies (2 Hz) the hyperemic response rises and wanes concomitant to the initial increase and subsequent decline in venous K$^+$ concentration (41). However, with higher stimulation frequencies (>10 Hz) the hyperemic response is maintained despite a return of venous K$^+$ concentration to basal values (41, 187).

The rate of K$^+$ uptake by the gland may play an important role in the poststimulation hyperemia. There is a direct linear relationship between the magnitude of the poststimulation phase of vasodilation and the amount of K$^+$ taken up actively by the gland (187). Furthermore oubain prevents the reuptake of K$^+$ and the vasodilation without altering K$^+$ loss or salivary secretion in response to chorda stimulation.

Although adenosine is a vasodilator in both pancreas and salivary glands (see Tables 5 and 6), there is relatively little evidence that supports a role for purine compounds in the functional hyperemia. Dipyridamole, which prevents the uptake of adenosine, potentiates the hyperemic response to chorda stimulation (117), indicating that adenosine may play a role in the functional hyperemia.

Hyperosmolality, resulting from enhanced functional activity, has been implicated in the functional hyperemia in the salivary glands. Chorda stimulation (0.25–20 Hz) increases the osmolality of venous blood draining the submandibular gland by as much as 35 mosmol/kgH$_2$O (150). The magnitude of the hyperemia induced by nerve stimulation at low frequencies (up to 4–10 Hz) is directly related to the venous osmolality. At higher stimulation frequencies the magnitude of the hyperemic response increases further without a concomitant increases in venous osmolality. Infusion of hypertonic solutions increases submandibular blood flow. The relationship between the magnitude of the hyperemic response and venous osmolality is similar to that observed with low-frequency chorda stimulation. Thus, as in the absorbing small intestine (78), tissue hyperosmolality may be an important contributing factor in the functional hyperemia of the salivary gland. In the pancreas, intravascular administration of hypertonic solutions also produces a hyperemic response whose magnitude is directly related to local venous osmolality (59, 113). However, vagal stimulation (10 Hz) or infusions of secretin and/or CCK increases pancreatic secretion and blood flow without altering local venous osmolality. Thus it is unlikely that tissue hyperosmolality contributes to the functional hyperemia in the pancreas.

*Kallikrein-kinin system.* The early studies of Hilton et al. (92, 94–96) supported the hypothesis that the kallikrein-kinin system plays a role in the functional hyperemia in the salivary glands and pancreas. Stimulation of the parasympathetic nerves supplying the submandibular gland and pancreas produces a glandular hyperemia that is associated with the release of kallikrein (or precursor) from glandular cells into the local circulation as well as into the juice (56, 92, 94, 96). In the pancreas, CCK initiates a hyperemia that is associated with increased levels of kallikrein in the venous outflow (95, 96). On the other hand, secretin neither produces a hyperemia nor releases kallikrein from the gland (95). Thus it appears that only those secretagogues that induce a functional hyperemia release kallikrein.

A considerable amount of evidence has also been presented that argues against a role for kinins in the functional hyperemia in the salivary glands. Studies in which salivary secretion, kallikrein release from the gland, and vasodilation were assessed at different frequencies of chorda stimulation indicate that although secretion rate and the magnitude of dilation is directly related to the frequency of nerve stimulation, the amount of kallikrein released is not (19, 56). If tachyphylaxis to the vasodilator actions of bradykinin is induced, the hyperemic response to chorda stimulation is not abolished (206). Glands perfused with either kininogen-free solutions (187) or perfusates from which kinins cannot be generated (24) still exhibit the maximal vascular response to chorda stimulation. Pretreatment with carboxypeptidase B (a bradykinin-degrading enzyme) at doses sufficient to prevent bradykinin-induced vasodilation does not affect the hyperemia produced by chorda stimulation (218).

*Histamine and prostaglandins.* Both histamine and prostaglandins have been implicated in the functional vasodilation in the salivary glands. Histamine can increase salivary secretion and blood flow (209, 211). The secretory response is due to H$_2$-receptor activation, whereas the vasodilation is attributed to activation of both H$_1$ and H$_2$ receptors (209). The H$_2$-receptor antagonist metiamide reduces the secretory and vascular responses to chorda stimulation (223). Although prostaglandin F$_{2\alpha}$ increases both salivary secretion and blood flow (228), the evidence in favor of a role for prostaglandins in the hyperemia induced by chorda stimulation is weak. Prostaglandins cannot be detected in the venous effluent from the submandibular gland during nerve stimulation (56). The effects of prostaglandin-synthesis inhibition on the hyperemic response to chorda stimulation are equivocal; i.e., indomethacin has been shown to decrease (55) or not affect (56) the secretory and vascular responses.

EXTRINSIC FACTORS. *Neural.* The parasympathetic nerve terminals in the salivary glands and pancreas contain acetylcholine and VIP. These vasodilators are released into the circulation of the salivary glands during parasympathetic nerve stimulation (27, 101, 139, 142–144, 146). Thus both acetylcholine and VIP have been proposed as mediators of the functional hyperemia in the salivary glands. Very little information is available on the potential role of these neurotransmitters in the pancreatic hyperemia induced by vagal stimulation.

Several lines of evidence support a role for acetylcholine in the functional hyperemia in the salivary glands. The administration of atropine (4, 41, 118) or acetylcholinesterase (217) abolishes or attenuates the hyperemic response to low-frequency chorda stimulation. Similarly, depletion of acetylcholine stores from postganglionic neurons completely abolishes the vasodilator effect of stimulation (118). Administration of eserine, a potentiator of acetylcholine's actions, enhances the hyperemic response to chorda stimulation (118).

The major argument against a role for acetylcholine in the functional hyperemia is the atropine-resistant vasodilation observed during high-frequency nerve stimulation (Fig. 6). Pretreatment with atropine, at doses that can abolish the secretory and vascular effects of exogenous acetylcholine, prevents the secretory response but not the hyperemic response to chorda stimulation at frequencies >10 Hz (4, 23, 41, 220). Indeed the hyperemic response to high-frequency stimulation is actually enhanced (139). Inasmuch as there is no ongoing secretory activity after atropine administration, the atropine-resistant vasodilation observed during high-frequency nerve stimulation cannot be considered a functional hyperemia. Furthermore the maximal secretory responses to meals can be mimicked by using stimulation frequencies <10 Hz, i.e., 4–8 Hz (50). Nonetheless the atropine resistant vasodilation observed during high-frequency stimulation has provided the impetus for the search for noncholinergic vasodilator fibers in parasympathetic nerves.

There is evidence that supports a role for VIP in the atropine-resistant vasodilation and in the functional hyperemia. Not only is VIP output increased during chorda stimulation, but its release is augmented in atropinized animals in which the hyperemic response is enhanced (141, 144, 146). Some investigators have noted that intra-arterial infusion of VIP (to achieve blood levels comparable to those produced by nerve stimulation) produces a hyperemia of the same order of magnitude as that observed with chorda stimulation (27). Others, however, claim that several hundredfold higher blood levels of VIP must be achieved with intra-arterial infusion than observed during nerve stimulation in order to mimic the neurally mediated vasodilation (142). Infusion of VIP antiserum reduces the secretory and vascular responses to low-frequency (2-Hz) chorda stimulation (141, 143). Pretreatment with avian pancreatic polypeptide, at doses that block the vascular actions of exogenous VIP, prevents the vasodilation associated with chorda stimulation (139). However, this has not been confirmed by others (118). A serious objection to the VIP hypothesis is the fact that desensitization (tachyphylaxis) of the submandibular vasculature to VIP does not alter the hyperemic response to chorda stimulation (118).

It has also been proposed that VIP and acetylcholine work in concert to elicit the functional hyperemia (139). Both neurotransmitters are released simultaneously during activation of the chorda lingual nerve (144) and may even be located in the same nerve terminals (139). Although VIP potentiates the secretory responses to acetylcholine, their effects on blood flow are only additive (139, 142). The proponents of the dual mediator hypothesis contend that acetylcholine may be more important at low stimulation frequencies, whereas VIP plays a more important role during high-frequency stimulation.

Substance P–containing neurons have also been demonstrated in the pancreas and salivary glands. Although substance P can increase both salivary secretion and blood flow (132), its vasodilator properties are neither as consistent nor as potent as those of VIP or acetylcholine (118, 142). Although purinergic nerves in the alimentary tract have been implicated in the noncholinergic responses to parasympathetic nerve activation (31), little information is available on the intraglandular distribution or potential role for ATP in the functional vasodilation. Although ATP is a weak vasodilator in the salivary glands and pancreas (see Tables 5 and 6), there is no evidence to suggest that ATP is released during chorda stimulation.

*Humoral.* The major regulators of pancreatic secretion are hormones such as secretin and CCK. Both hormones dilate pancreatic blood vessels (Table 4) and have been implicated in the postprandial hyperemia. Their potential role in the functional hyperemia is based on studies in which infusion of secretin or CCK increased both pancreatic secretion rate and blood flow (6, 7, 53, 72, 91). However, the magnitude of the vasodilation is not well correlated with the secretion rate (7, 16). Indeed, both secretin and CCK octapeptide (CCK-8) can increase pancreatic exocrine secretions without altering blood flow (16, 84) (Fig. 8). Thus it appears that the minimal concentration of secretin and CCK-8 required to induce pancreatic secretion is much lower than that required for vasodilation. Although it is possible that secretin and CCK may potentiate each other's action on pancreatic blood vessels, this seems unlikely in light of a recent study of the intestinal vascular responses to secretin and/or CCK in which no evidence for potentiation was obtained (188).

### CIRCULATORY ADJUSTMENTS TO HYPERPLASIA

Recent studies have examined the acute and chronic effects of raw soya flour (RSF)- and CCK-8–induced pancreatic growth on blood flow. Raw soya flour feeding induces pancreatic growth, presumably by increasing the release of endogenous CCK via a trypsin inhibitor, and a parallel increase in total pancreatic blood flow after 4 wk of RSF feeding (160). However, when normalized per 100 g pancreatic weight, blood flow in RSF-fed rats was not different from control, suggesting that blood flow increases in proportion to increments in organ mass. These results are confirmed by a study involving repeated subcutaneous injections

TABLE 4. *Capillary Permeability–Surface Area Products and Calculated Equivalent Pore Radii in Salivary Gland and Pancreas*

| | Salivary Gland | Pancreas |
|---|---|---|
| Permeability–surface area product values, ml·min$^{-1}$·100 g$^{-1}$ | | |
| EDTA ($r = 5.3$ Å) | >800 | 110 |
| Cyanocobalamin ($r = 5.7$ Å) | 411 | |
| Inulin ($r = 12.0$ Å) | 180 | 23.2 |
| β-Lactoglobulin A ($r = 27$ Å) | | 4.9 |
| Equivalent pore radius, Å | 120 | 68 |

$r$, Radius. Data from refs. 82, 127, 153.

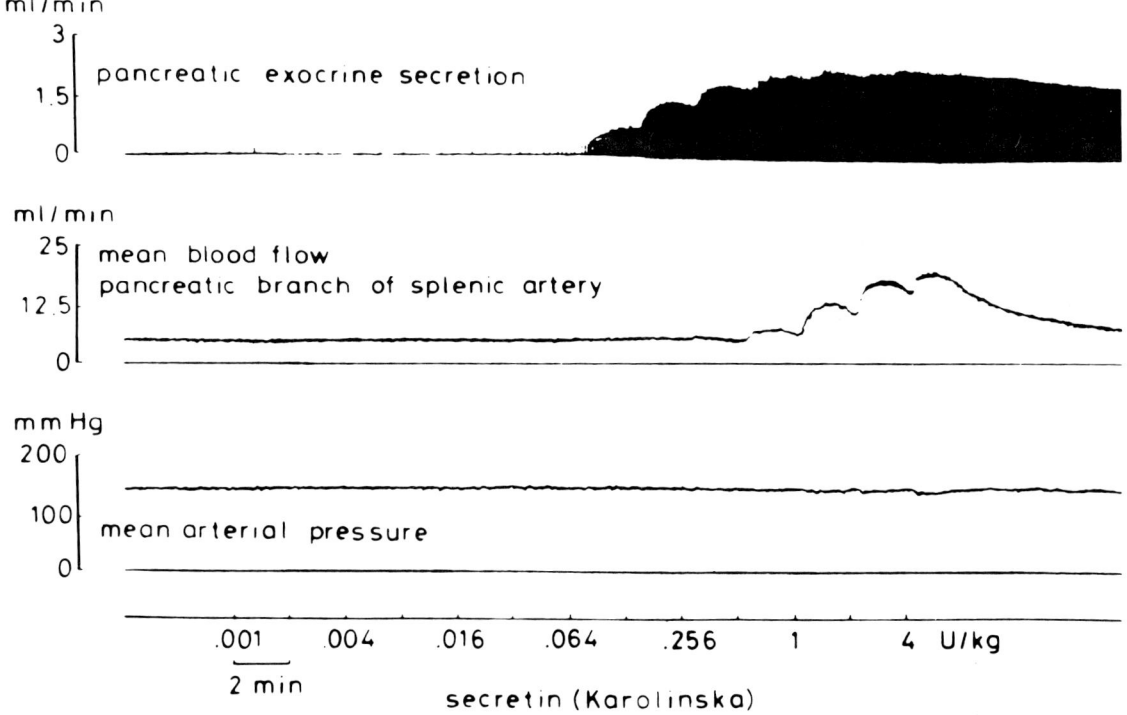

FIG. 8. Effects of intravenous secretin on pancreatic secretion rate and blood flow. [From Beijer et al. (16).]

of CCK-8 in which long-term (7- and 14-day) injections were characterized by parallel increases in pancreatic weight and blood flow in rats (83). However, this study also documented short-term increases in blood flow (at 2 days of treatment) that were not accompanied by significant organ growth (Fig. 9). The short-term pancreatic hyperemia was attributed to vasodilator metabolite accumulation, because the time course of the hyperemic response closely parallels growth-induced increases in DNA synthesis. The contributions of vasodilator metabolites, other vasoactive agents, and vascular proliferation to this response warrant further investigation.

### TRANSCAPILLARY FLUID AND SOLUTE EXCHANGE

#### Ultrastructural Basis of Capillary Exchange

There are several special characteristics of pancreatic and salivary capillaries that account for their unique permeability properties. Both tissues are richly vascularized; therefore, the total surface area available for transcapillary exchange is high. Estimates of capillary surface area in salivary glands range between 228 and 1,280 $cm^2/g$ of tissue (38, 64, 86). This compares with smaller values reported for the intestinal mucosa (125 $cm^2/g$) and skeletal muscle (70 $cm^2/g$) (194). Ligation of the salivary duct for 2 wk reduces the total capillary surface area by approximately 35% (38). Capillary surface area estimates for the pancreas have not been reported. However, some physiological evidence suggests that there are fewer capillaries per gram of tissue in the pancreas compared with the salivary gland (183). Within the pancreas, the density of capillaries appears to be greater in the islets of Langerhans than in the exocrine tissue (220).

Another feature of capillaries in the salivary gland and pancreas is that they are fenestrated. The fenestrae are circular openings in the endothelial cytoplasm with an average diameter ranging between 500 Å and 800 Å (38, 172). The dimensions and numbers of fenestrae generally increase along the length of the capillaries (172, 229). A large proportion of the fenestrae are covered by thin diaphragms with a central knob. The fenestrae are generally distributed in clusters that are small yet clearly outlined in the pancreas and salivary gland (38, 213). In the pancreas, fenestrae account for ~6% of the total endothelial surface (213), whereas a value of 0.6% has been reported for the salivary gland (38). The capillaries perfusing salivary acini have fewer and smaller fenestrae than do ductal capillaries (202). In the pancreas, the endocrine capillaries are about 10 times more fenestrated than the exocrine capillaries (88, 90a).

There are several ultrastructural studies that address the permeability of fenestrae in pancreatic and salivary capillaries to electron-dense markers (60, 106, 157, 238). The results of these studies are often inconsistent. However, the data as a whole indicate that all

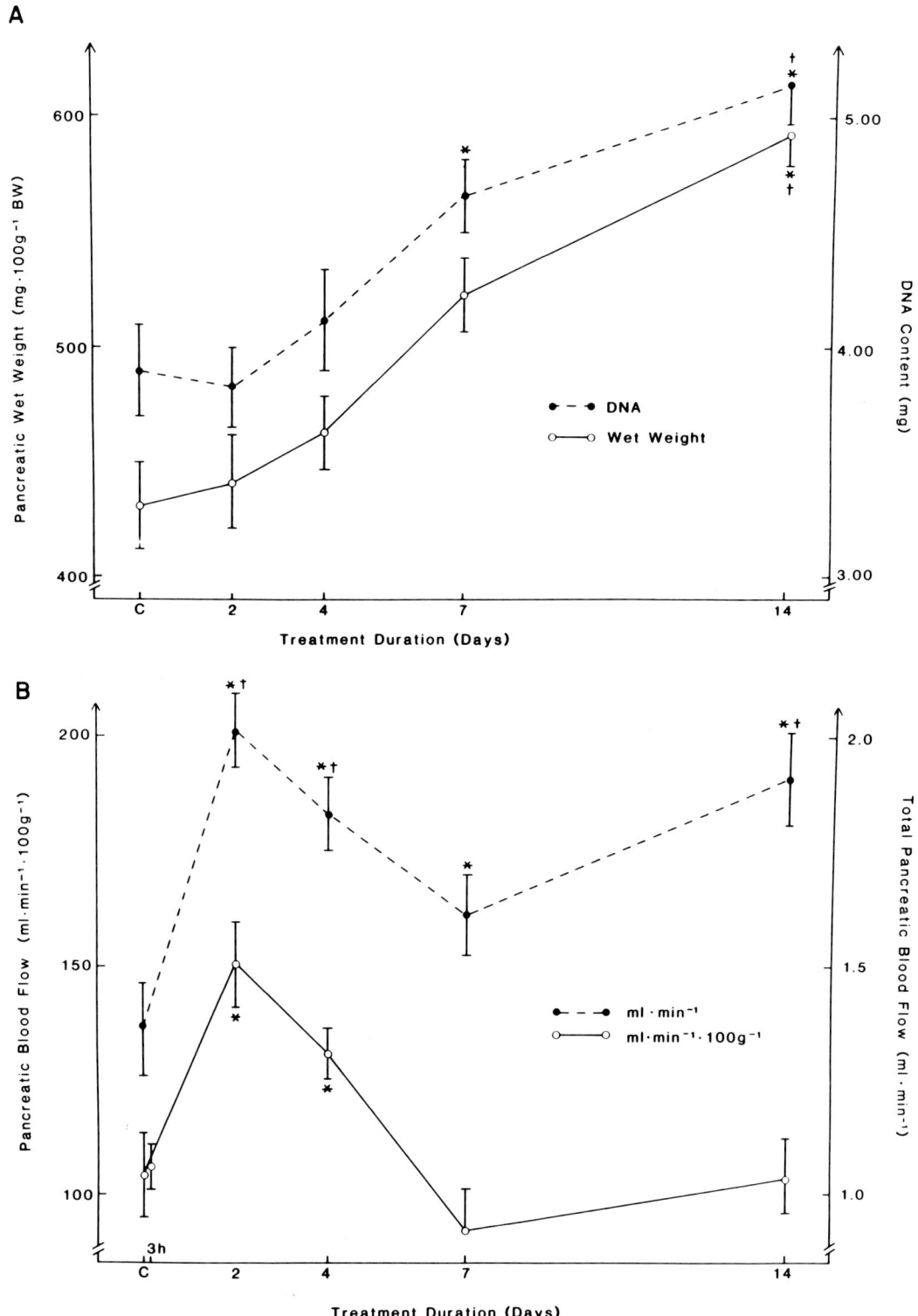

FIG. 9. Effect of CCK-OP stimulation on pancreatic growth (*A*) and on tissue blood flow (*B*). Cholecystokinin octapeptide was administered for 2, 4, 7, and 14 days. BW, body weight. [From Harper et al. (83).]

fenestrae are easily permeated by small tracer molecules such as horseradish peroxidase (solute diam = ~50 Å), whereas tracers of 100 Å diameter or larger exit only through a relatively small fraction of the entire population (60, 157, 172). The diaphragms appear to be the rate-limiting structures that account for restriction of large solute movement at fenestrae.

Other structural features of pancreatic and salivary gland capillaries that account for their permeability properties are the intercellular junctions, plasmalemmal vesicles, and the basement membrane. Although it is rather clear that the intercellular junctions in fenestrated capillaries are impermeable to large molecules such as ferritin, there are contradictory reports regarding the ease with which smaller tracers (e.g., horseradish peroxidase) cross the intercellular junctions (172, 238). Nonetheless it would appear that the intercellular junctions play a less significant role in transcapillary exchange of both water and solutes than the fenestrae because the frequency and dimensions of the latter far exceed the former in both pancreatic and salivary gland capillaries. In the pancreas, the intercellular spaces account for 0.08% of the endothelial surface (213).

Plasmalemmal vesicles are scattered throughout the endothelial cytoplasm in pancreatic and salivary gland capillaries (157, 238). These small spherical vesicles of an outer diameter of ~700 Å are surrounded by a unit membrane. The vesicles appear either as isolated single units in the cytoplasmic matrix, as chains of fused vesicles, or as vesicles opened on either the blood or tissue front of the endothelial cells. The vesicles are able to fuse with the plasmalemma as well as detach from it, and the free-floating vesicles found in the cytoplasm are considered to be in transit from a previous detachment to a future fusion point. Inasmuch as large particles and molecules gain access to the vesicle lumen and are shuttled between blood and tissue fronts of the endothelial cell, vesicular exchange is often considered as a pathway for transcapillary exchange of macromolecules. Data obtained from studies of pancreatic and salivary gland capillaries are consistent with this notion because a variety of electron-dense tracers (horseradish peroxidase, ferritin, thorotrast) gain access to the interstitium via the vesicular pathway (60, 157, 172, 238). The relative importance of vesicular exchange in macromolecule transport is difficult to assess; the amount transported is probably small relative to that occurring across open fenestrae because the latter are numerous and afford a pathway for both diffusive and convective exchange (vesicular exchange behaves as a purely diffusive pathway). Studies on other tissues indicate that vesicular exchange plays a relatively minor role in transcapillary exchange of macromolecules (231).

The basement membrane surrounding fenestrated capillaries is formed by a layer of fine fibrillar material similar to that surrounding other capillaries. Although there are no structurally recognizable pathways across the basement membrane, there is evidence that this structure reduces the rate of transport of large tracer particles. Tracer particles [radius ($r$) = 62–150 Å] transiently accumulate in the subendothelial space against the basement membrane to form small clusters opposite permeable fenestrae. Particles ranging in radius between 25 and 55 Å are not temporarily retained by the basement membrane (157, 172).

In most capillary permeability studies, the molecular probes and capillary pores are treated as rigid structures exhibiting no net electrical charge. Recent ultrastructural studies (38, 159, 173, 214–216) suggest that solute charge is also an important determinant of transcapillary exchange in the pancreas and salivary gland. The distribution of anionic sites on the blood front of the fenestrated endothelium of pancreatic capillaries has been assessed by using cationized ferritin (159, 173, 214–216). From the pattern of binding of cationized ferritin to the capillary surface, a high density of anionic sites was demonstrated on the fenestral diaphragms. Binding could not be demonstrated on the membrane of vesicles and transendothelial channels. These studies suggest that the fenestral diaphragms of pancreatic capillaries will discriminate against anionic molecules, whereas vesicles and transendothelial channels may favor the penetration of anionic molecules and discriminate against cationic molecules. Cationized ferritin also binds to the surface of fenestrae and the luminal surface of endothelium in capillaries of the submandibular gland [Fig. 10; (38)].

*Transcapillary Fluid Exchange*

In comparison to other organs in the alimentary tract relatively little is known about the factors that govern transcapillary fluid exchange in the salivary glands and pancreas. However, there is sufficient information to gain an understanding of what may be the major determinants of the rate of fluid exchange in these tissues. Fluid exchange across pancreatic and salivary gland capillaries can be described in terms of the Starling hypothesis (224), i.e.,

$$J_v = K_f[(P_c - P_t) - \sigma_d(\pi_p - \pi_t)]$$

where $J_v$ is the net capillary fluid filtration rate; $K_f$ is the capillary filtration coefficient; $P_c$ is the capillary hydrostatic pressure; $P_t$ is the interstitial fluid pressure; $\sigma_d$ is the capillary osmotic reflection coefficient for total plasma proteins; $\pi_p$ is the plasma oncotic pressure; and $\pi_t$ is the interstitial oncotic pressure.

NET CAPILLARY FILTRATION RATE. In tissues that produce a basal secretion, such as salivary glands and pancreas, $J_v$ is equal to the sum of lymph flow and fluid secretion rate when the tissue is neither gaining nor losing weight. Basal lymph flow values of 0.14 ml·min$^{-1}$·100 g$^{-1}$ and 0.009 ml·min$^{-1}$·100 g$^{-1}$ have been reported for salivary gland (122) and pancreas (77,

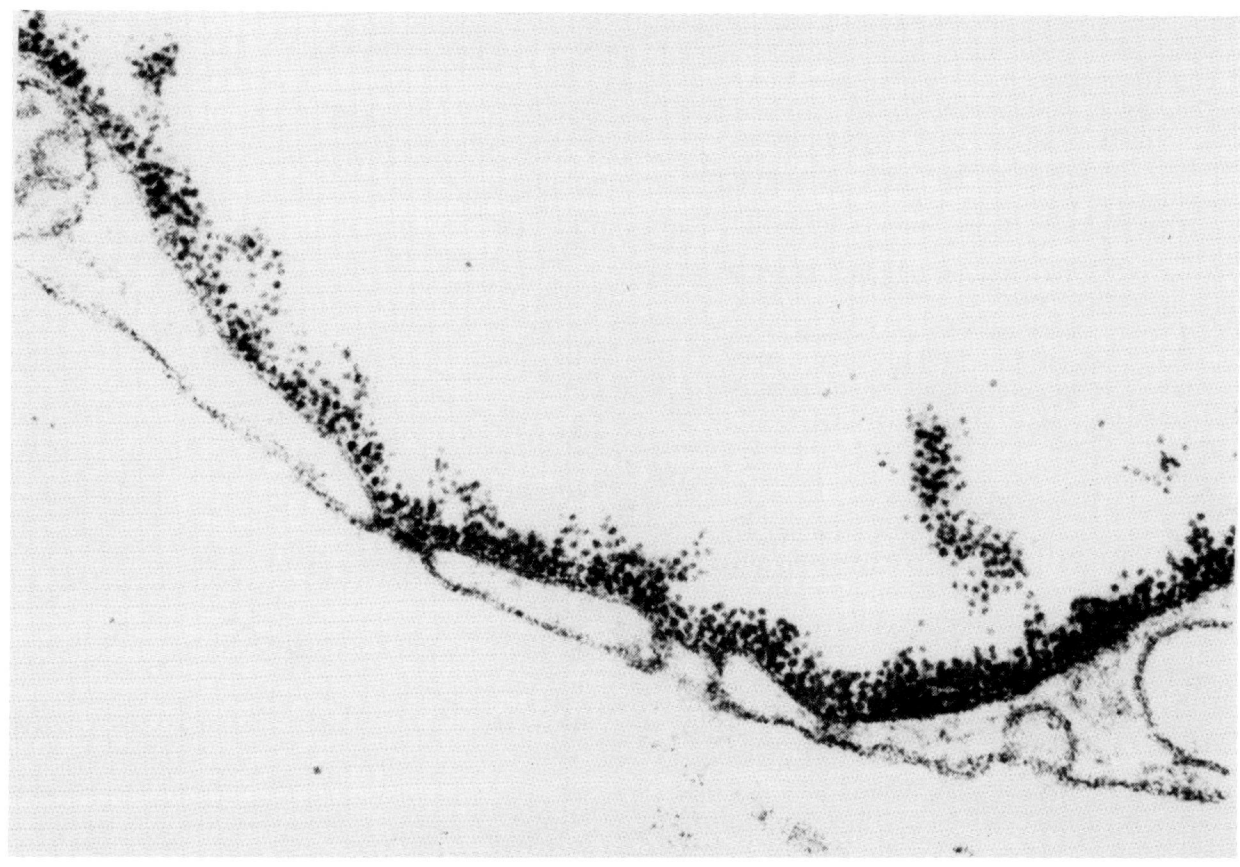

FIG. 10. Binding of cationized ferritin to endothelial surface of capillary in rabbit submandibular gland. × 148,000. [From Smaje (219).]

176), respectively. These values probably underestimate lymph flow inasmuch as only one of several lymphatics draining the tissues were cannulated. Basal pancreatic secretion rate generally ranges between 0.008 and 0.060 ml·min$^{-1}$·100 g$^{-1}$, whereas 0.10–2.0 ml·min$^{-1}$·100 g$^{-1}$ is generally reported for basal salivary secretion rate. Thus $J_v$ in the pancreas is roughly comparable to values reported for other organs in the digestive system, whereas the values in salivary gland are much higher.

Capillary filtration rate can be increased by a variety of conditions, including venous obstruction (8), intravenous saline infusion (176), and experimental pancreatitis (74). However, the most potent physiological stimulus for enhanced pancreatic and salivary gland capillary fluid filtration is an increased glandular secretion rate. Inasmuch as the salivary gland can secrete as much as 30 ml·min$^{-1}$·100 g$^{-1}$ (233), $J_v$ increases by at least that amount (because salivary lymph flow also rises). Fluid extraction from the vasculature of the maximally stimulated gland is ~15% of blood flow, thereby leading to a significant increase in venous hematocrit (148). The effects of enhanced glandular secretion on $J_v$ are not as impressive in the pancreas, although $J_v$ can increase 30-fold when the gland is maximally stimulated with secretin (77).

CAPILLARY FILTRATION COEFFICIENT. The $K_f$ is a measure of the hydraulic conductance of the microvascular barrier and, as such, is influenced by the size and number of pores in each capillary and by the number of them being perfused (surface area). The $K_f$ has been measured in the pancreas and salivary glands by using volumetric or gravimetric techniques. Resting values ranging between 0.10 and 0.35 ml·min$^{-1}$·mmHg$^{-1}$·100 g$^{-1}$ have been reported for pancreas (48, 125) and salivary gland (48, 151). These values are comparable to those usually measured in the small intestine (196). Inasmuch as capillary surface area is four to five times greater in salivary gland than intestine, the pore area for water exchange per capillary is roughly four to five times higher in intestinal capillaries.

Agents and conditions that cause vasodilation lead to an increased $K_f$ in both pancreas and salivary gland. Maximal vasodilation with papaverine produces a 2- to 10-fold increase in $K_f$, whereas maximal vasodilation with bradykinin produces a 5- to 20-fold increase (48). The rise in $K_f$ produced by papaverine is assumed to reflect capillary recruitment, whereas the greater effect of bradykinin presumably reflects a combination of capillary recruitment and an increased capillary permeability. Parasympathetic nerve stimulation in the submandibular gland produces a threefold increase in $K_f$ (151), presumably because of capillary recruitment. Reductions in pancreatic blood flow, produced either by lowering local arterial pressure or increasing venous pressure, lead to significant increases in $K_f$ (125). The latter responses are considered to result from metabolic relaxation of precapillary sphincters that control perfused capillary density.

CAPILLARY PRESSURE. Volumetric and gravimetric techniques have been used to measure capillary hydrostatic pressure in the salivary gland and pancreas (48, 125, 151). Eliassen et al. (48) reported a mean $P_c$ ranging between 9 and 11 mmHg in the submandibular gland that increased to a value exceeding 40 mmHg during maximal vasodilation. Other investigators (151) measured a $P_c$ of ~20 mmHg in the resting gland that subsequently increased to 38 mmHg during maximal vasodilation produced by chorda stimulation.

Kvietys et al. (125) obtained a highly significant correlation between pancreatic $P_c$ and portal venous pressure (Fig. 11). Their results indicate that pancreatic $P_c$ is 8–13 mmHg at normal portal pressures (5–10 mmHg). When portal pressure is elevated, ~90% of the increment in venous pressure is transmitted to the capillaries. The relatively low $P_c$ measured in pancreas reflects a precapillary to postcapillary resistance ratio ($R_a/R_v$) of ~30. The unusually high $R_a/R_v$ may be explained by the existence of portal circulations between islets and acini, and acini and ducts. The relative importance of each capillary bed (islet, acinar, and ductal) in the whole-organ estimate of $P_c$ remains unclear.

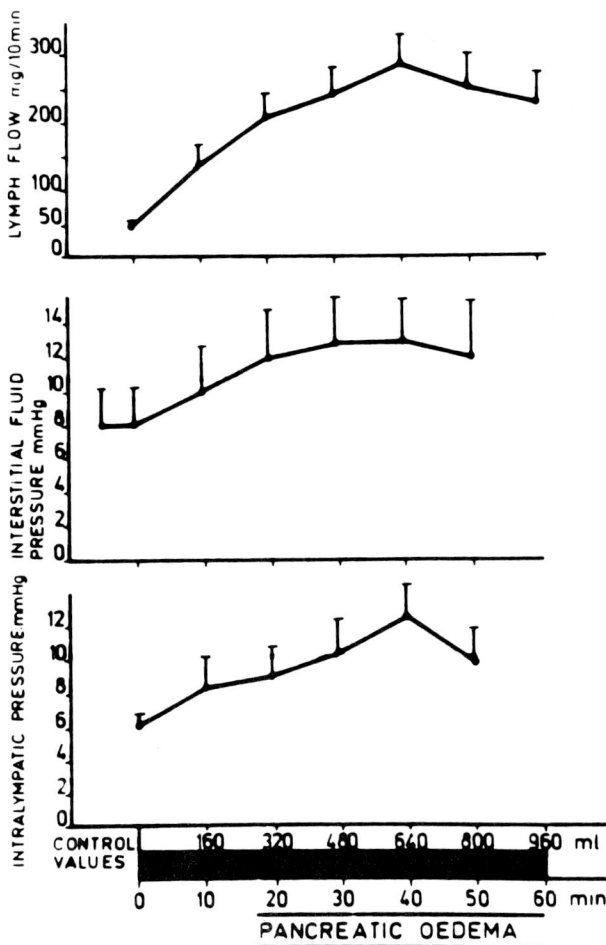

FIG. 12. Effect of intra-arterial saline load on pancreaticoduodenal lymph flow and intralymphatic pressure and on pancreatic interstitial fluid pressure in the dog. *Solid bar*, period of saline infusion. [From Papp et al. (176).]

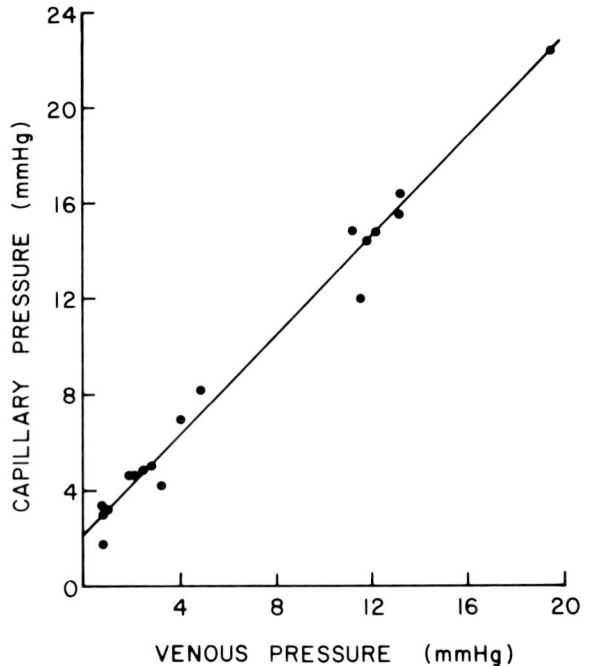

FIG. 11. Relationship between pancreatic capillary pressure and portal venous pressure. [From Kvietys et al. (125).]

INTERSTITIAL FLUID PRESSURE. Estimates of $P_t$ have been obtained for the pancreas by using capsule (176) and microcatheter (45) techniques. Papp and co-workers (176) implanted perforated hollow capsules into the pancreas of dogs and measured intracapsular pressure 14–16 days thereafter. Mean pressure in the lumen of the implanted capsule was ~8 mmHg under resting conditions. Intravenous saline loading caused $P_t$ to rise to 13 mmHg. The time course of the rise in $P_t$ was well correlated to the concomitant elevations in pancreaticoduodenal lymph flow and intralymphatic pressure, supporting the contention that capsule pressure reflects interstitial fluid pressure (Fig. 12).

Pancreatic tissue pressure has been recently measured by insertion of a tiny transducer-connected cannula into the pancreas of control patients and patients with chronic pancreatitis (45). A mean value of 7.3 mmHg was measured in normal pancreas, whereas a mean value of 20 mmHg was obtained in the inflamed pancreas. The microcatheter estimates of $P_t$ were virtually identical to simultaneously measured ductal pressures.

The estimates of basal pancreatic $P_t$ obtained with the capsule and microcatheter techniques are substantially larger than values reported for stomach (0.50 mmHg) and small intestine (−2.0 mmHg) yet similar to values obtained in encapsulated organs such as liver (6.0 mmHg) and kidney (6.0 mmHg) (74). Although the latter observation lends some credibility to the pancreatic measurements, the high values measured in the pancreas may reflect interstitial edema induced by autodigestion initiated by inserting the pressure measuring devices into the parenchyma. The microcatheter technique can also be criticized on the grounds that such a device measures total tissue pressure rather than $P_t$ (230). It is also important to note that pancreatic $P_t$ calculated from $J_v$ and the balance of the other Starling parameters is approximately −6 mmHg. When the measured value of $P_t$ (7 mmHg) is incorporated into the Starling equation, net capillary fluid absorption is predicted, an unlikely possibility.

OSMOTIC REFLECTION COEFFICIENT. The capillaries in the salivary gland and pancreas are permeable to plasma proteins, therefore only part of the oncotic pressure generated by plasma proteins is exerted across these capillaries. The $\sigma_d$ describes that fraction of the total oncotic pressure generated across the capillary wall. Despite the importance of this parameter in determining the rate of capillary fluid movement, there is little information regarding it in the pancreas and salivary gland. Based on basal lymph-to-plasma protein concentration ratios (L/P) reported by Koo et al. (122) one would predict a minimal $\sigma_d$ for total plasma proteins of ~0.80 in salivary gland. Smaje (219) has predicted, using a mathematical model based on albumin clearance data, that $\sigma_d$ for albumin may be as high as 0.95 in salivary gland capillaries. A value of 0.85 has been reported for $\sigma_d$ in the dog pancreas (77). The latter estimate was based on L/P ratios measured at a high $J_v$ in a single animal. This small amount of data indicates that $\sigma_d$ for total proteins in pancreatic and salivary gland capillaries is comparable to values reported for other tissues in the digestive system (183).

TRANSCAPILLARY ONCOTIC PRESSURE GRADIENT. If one assumes that lymph provides a valid reflection of interstitial fluid, the transcapillary oncotic pressure can be estimated from lymph and plasma by using either an oncometer or equations that relate protein concentration to oncotic pressure. The data in the literature suggest that the resting transcapillary oncotic pressure gradient in pancreas (11.3 mmHg) is comparable to values reported for stomach (11.5 mmHg), small intestine (13.0 mmHg), and colon (12.8 mmHg) (77). The salivary gland exhibits a slightly larger gradient (15.9 mmHg) than all of the aforementioned tissues.

*Interaction of Capillary and Interstitial Forces During Stimulated Secretion*

Inasmuch as the microcirculation is responsible for providing the fluid for salivary and pancreatic secretions, the additional fluid required during periods of stimulated secretion must result from alterations in forces and membrane parameters governing transcapillary fluid exchange. Enhanced salivary secretion is usually associated with intense vasodilation, which can lead to an increase of 18 mmHg in $P_c$ (151). The increased $P_c$, coupled to a threefold rise (to 1.0 ml·min$^{-1}$·mmHg$^{-1}$·100 g$^{-1}$) in capillary hydraulic conductance ($K_{fc}$), could allow for increased $J_v$ approaching 18.0 ml·min$^{-1}$·100 g$^{-1}$ (151). If these changes are not sufficient to meet the fluid requirements for salivation, then interstitial fluid volume will fall (197) and ultimately lead to alterations in the interstitial forces. With interstitial dehydration, $P_t$ falls and $\pi_t$ rises. These changes in interstitial forces could greatly increase the net capillary filtration pressure, thereby providing more fluid for salivation via the vasculature.

The pancreas is capable of secreting ~0.4 ml·min$^{-1}$·100 g$^{-1}$ of juice during maximal stimulation with secretin (125). Although this rate of secretion represents a 30-fold increase in $J_v$ (assuming lymph flow is unchanged), little is known of the adjustments that occur in the Starling forces to accommodate such massive fluid movement from blood to acini and ducts. Inasmuch as pancreatic blood flow can double after a meal (36), it is possible that an increase in $P_c$ may provide the driving force for the enhanced $J_v$. However, because pancreatic secretion can increase to near maximum without any change in pancreatic blood flow (16), an increased $P_c$ is not necessary to drive fluid from the vasculature to the acini and ducts. The $K_f$ has been shown to increase fourfold during stimulation with kinins (substances released during vagal-induced pancreatic secretion); therefore it is likely that an increase in capillary surface area contributes to the transfer of fluid across the microvasculature (48). Nonetheless $K_f$ would have to increase eightfold to account entirely for the increased $J_v$ during secretion, an unlikely possibility. Another mechanism by which fluid can be removed from the vasculature during secretion is via changes in interstitial forces. In the absence of changes in $P_c$ or $K_f$, an alteration in interstitial forces (decreased $P_t$ and/or increased $\pi_t$) of <1.5 mmHg would be more than sufficient to provide the driving force for the enhanced capillary filtration observed during maximal pancreatic secretion.

*Microvascular Permeability*

SMALL SOLUTES. Two experimental approaches have been used to study the permeability of salivary gland and pancreatic capillaries to small solutes: the osmotic transient method (219) and the indicator-diffusion technique (82, 127, 153). Results from osmotic tran-

TABLE 5. *Effects of Vasoactive Agents on Salivary Gland Blood Flow*

| Drug/Agent | Dose | Change in Blood Flow,% | Ref. |
|---|---|---|---|
| Cholinergic agonists and antagonists | | | |
| Acetylcholine | 5–20 pmol/min, ia | +75 to +150 | 142, 143 |
| | 0.1–10 µg/min, ia | +200 to +500 | 55, 145, 217 |
| | 27 pM, ia | +200 | 118 |
| | 30 nmol, ia | +150 to +317 | 210, 228 |
| | 0.01–10 µg, ia | +200 to +525 | 24, 203, 204 |
| | 200 mg/min, iv | +343 | 27 |
| Bethanechol | 0.1–3 µg, ia | +75 | 204 |
| Methacholine | 0.1–3 µg, ia | +100 | 204 |
| Carbachol | 0.01–1 µg, ia | +100 | 204 |
| Pilocarpine | 1–10 µg, ia | +50 | 204 |
| Physostigmine | 1–100 µg, ia | +10 to +50 | 204 |
| Neostigmine | 1–10 µg, ia | +5 | 204 |
| Nicotine | 1–30 µg, ia | +125 | 204 |
| 1,1-Dimethyl-4-phenylpiperzinium iodide | 1–30 µg, ia | +150 | 204 |
| Lobeline | 1–30 µg, ia | +60 | 204 |
| Tetramethylammonium chloride | 1–30 µg, ia | +75 | 204 |
| 4-*m*-Chlorophenylcarbamoyloxy-2-butynyltrimethylammonium chloride | 1–30 µg, ia | +40 | 204 |
| Tetraethylammonium bromide | 0.3–10 µg, ia | −5 | 204 |
| 4-*m*-Chlorophenylcarbamoyloxy-2-butymyltrimethylammonium chloride | 0.3 µg, ia | +50 | 203 |
| 1,1-Dimethyl-4-phenylpiperazinium | 10 µg | +275 | 203 |
| Acetylcholine (0.05 µg) + atropine | 5 µg, ia | +283 | 24 |
| Adrenergic agonists and antagonists | | | |
| L-Glutamate stimulation of A5 catecholamine nucleus | | −19 | 222 |
| Isoproterenol | 5 × 10$^{-10}$ mol/min, ia | +300 | 142 |
| | 0.03–3 µg, ia | +190 to +350 | 68, 204 |
| Norepinephrine | 0.03–1 µg, ia | −54 to −90 | 135, 204 |
| L-Epinephrine | 0.03–1 µg, ia | −90 | 204 |
| Dopamine | 1–30 µg, ia | −80 | 204 |
| Tyramine | 3–100 µg, ia | −83 | 204 |
| Phenylephrine | 0.3–10 µg, ia | −80 | 204 |
| Methoxamine | 3–10 µg, ia | −80 | 204 |
| Autacoids | | | |
| Dihydroergotamine with sympathetic nerve stimulation | 2.0–4.0 mg/kg | no change | 232 |
| Phenethylamine | 10 nmol–1 µmol, ia | +63 to +229 | 234 |
| Histamine | 1–100 nmol, ia | +125 to +360 | 210, 234 |
| | 0.01–10 µg, ia | +300 to +425 | 204 |
| Metiamide | 1 µmol/ml blood | −32 | 224 |
| Bradykinin | 1.5–10 µg/min, ia | +361 to +400 | 27, 218 |
| | 0.01–1,850 µg, ia | +75 to +400 | 24, 204 |
| Bradykinin potentiating factor | 1–2 mg/kg, iv | +80 | 205 |
| 5-Hydroxytryptamine creatinine sulfate | 0.1–30 µg, ia | +67 to +150 | 204 |
| Active polypeptides | | | |
| Secretin | 10$^{-8}$ mol, ia | +280 | 210 |
| | 0.1–3 µg, ia | +220 | 204 |
| Glucagon | 10$^{-8}$ mol, ia | +33 | 210 |
| Vasoactive intestinal polypeptide | 20–100 pmol/min, ia | +133 to +600 | 142, 143 |
| | 0.1 µg/min, ia | +180 | 145 |
| | 10$^{-14}$ M, ia | 0 | 142 |
| | 6 pM, ia | +600 | 118 |
| | 6–100 pmol, ia | +320 to +600 | 118, 210 |
| | 20 mg/min, iv | +417 | 27 |
| Angiotensin II | 0.1–3 µg, ia | −50 | 204 |
| Oxytocin | 0.01–0.3 µg, ia | −60 | 204 |
| Lysine vasopressin | 0.01–0.03 µg, ia | −80 | 204 |
| Gastrin tetrapeptide | 0.3–3 µg, ia | +67 | 204 |
| Cholecystokinin | 0.1–3 µg, ia | −180 | 204 |
| Kallikrein | 0.01 ± 1 µg, ia | +133 | 204 |
| Avian pancreatic polypeptide | 1,000 pmol/min, ia | −26 | 147 |
| Bovine pancreatic polypeptide | 1,000 pmol/min, ia | −28 | 147 |
| Neuropeptide Y | 100 pmol/min, ia | −50 | 147 |
| Peptide YY | 10 pmol/min, ia | −50 | 147 |

TABLE 5—Continued

| Drug/Agent | Dose | Change in Blood Flow, % | Ref. |
|---|---|---|---|
| Adenyl compounds | | | |
| cAMP | 10 mM, ia | +260 | 117 |
| Dibutyryl cAMP | 10 mM, ia | +100 | 117 |
| 3-Isobutyl-1-methylxanthine | 0.5 mM, ia | +160 | 117 |
| cGMP | 10 mM, ia | +100 | 117 |
| Dibutyryl cGMP | 10 mM, ia | +160 | 117 |
| Adenosine | 1–30 µg, ia | +133 | 204 |
| | 10 mM, ia | +400 | 117 |
| ATP | 0.1–30 µg, ia | +300 | 204 |
| | 1 mM, ia | +500 | 117 |
| AMP | 1–30 µg, ia | +75 | 204 |
| ADP | 1–30 µg, ia | +75 | 204 |
| Uridine | 10–100 µg, ia | +10 | 204 |
| UMP | 10–100 µg, ia | +50 | 204 |
| UDP | 10–100 µg, ia | +100 | 204 |
| UTP | 1–100 µg, ia | +125 | 204 |
| Triphosphopyridine nucleotide | 10–30 µg, ia | +75 | 204 |
| Diphosphopyridine nucleotide | 10–30 µg, ia | +75 | 204 |
| Prostaglandins | | | |
| Prostaglandin $F_{2\alpha}$ | 10–100 pmol, ia | +42 to +254 | 228 |
| Indomethacin | 4 mg/kg, iv | −3 to −15 | 55 |
| Miscellaneous compounds | | | |
| Dimaprit | 3 µmol, ia | +135 | 234 |
| Quinine | 10 µmol, ia | +180 | 117 |
| Papaverine | 10 µmol, ia | +690 | 117 |
| | 1–30 µg, ia | +225 | 204 |
| Nitroglycerin | 1–30 µg, ia | +200 | 204 |
| Dipyridamole | 10–300 µg, ia | +125 | 204 |
| Verapamil | 10–100 µg, ia | +167 | 204 |
| Hydralazine | 10–300 µg, ia | +75 | 204 |
| Caffeine | 0.1–1 µg, ia | +100 | 204 |
| Theophylline ethylenediamine | 0.1–1 µg, ia | +25 | 204 |
| Theophylline | 10 µmol, ia | +190 | 117 |
| Theobromine | 0.1–1 µg, ia | +33 | 204 |
| Captopril | 10 mg, iv | +142 | 20a |
| Hypertonic infusion | 8–27 mosmol/kg | +145 to +470 | 102 |
| Hypertonic glucose | 600–1,200 mosmol/kgH$_2$O | | 150 |
| | +4 mosmol | +44 | |
| | +12 mosmol | +129 | |
| | +23 mosmol | +178 | |
| | +35 mosmol | +452 | |
| Cocaine | 3–100 µg, ia | −30 | 204 |
| Procaine | 3–100 µg, ia | +10 | 204 |
| Ergotamine | 1–30 µg, ia | −60 | 204 |
| Tolazoline | 10–30 µg, ia | +80 | 204 |
| Morphine | 10–100 µg, ia | +125 | 204 |

ia, Intra-arterial; iv, intravenous.

sient studies in rabbit submandibular gland indicate that $\sigma_d$ of salivary capillaries for raffinose ($r = 5.7$ Å) and inulin ($r = 12$ Å) are 0.013 and 0.24, respectively (219). The $\sigma_d$ values for raffinose and inulin are consistent with equivalent pores of radii of 110 Å and 55 Å, respectively. Both pore size estimates are significantly smaller than ultrastructural predictions of fenestral dimensions ($r = \sim250$–400 Å), indicating that a barrier other than the fenestral opening is rate limiting in terms of solute restriction.

The indicator-dilution principle has been used to obtain estimates of the permeability–surface area product ($PS$) for small tracer molecules in both pancreas (82, 127) and salivary gland (153). Table 4 summarizes the PS values for $^{51}$Cr-labeled EDTA, cyanocobalamin, inulin, and β-lactoglobulin A measured in salivary gland and pancreas. At high plasma flow rates the $PS$ values measured in pancreas are similar to values reported for the small intestine (182), whereas the salivary gland values are about eight times larger than in the small intestine. The equivalent pore size predicted from the $PS$ data is significantly smaller in the pancreas ($r = 68$ Å) than salivary gland ($r = 120$ Å). Because some of the tracers used in these studies appeared to be flow limited, even during maximal vasodilation, both pore sizes may be an overestimate.

In salivary glands perfused at constant flow, parasympathetic stimulation leads to a decrease in $PS$ for $^{51}$Cr-EDTA, cyanocobalamin, and insulin (154). It is suggested that this may be the result of a redistribu-

TABLE 6. *Effects of Vasoactive Agents on Pancreatic Blood Flow*

| Drug/Agent | Dose | Change in Blood Flow, % | Ref. |
|---|---|---|---|
| **Cholinergic agonists and antagonists** | | | |
| Acetylcholine | 10–100 µg, ia | +92 to +174 | 110, 112, 113, 133 |
| | 1 mg/kg, iv | +60 | 95 |
| 1,1-Dimethyl-4-phenylpiperazinium | 100 µg, ia | +25 to −26 | 110, 112 |
| | 300 µg, ia | −29 to +37 | 110 |
| Decholin | 3.72 mg/min, ia | +63 | 191 |
| | 10 mg, ia | +20 | 178 |
| | 10%, iv | +68 to +140 | 177 |
| Methacholine | 10 µg, ia | +340 | 112 |
| Carbachol | 10 µg, ia | +285 | 112 |
| Bethanechol | 10–100 µg, ia | +213 to +310 | 112 |
| Pilocarpine | 30 µg, ia | +51 | 112 |
| Physostigmine | 100 µg, ia | −27 | 112 |
| Neostigmine | 100 µg, ia | +33 | 112 |
| Lobeline | 100 µg, ia | +122 | 112 |
| Nicotine | 100 µg, ia | +37 | 112 |
| Tetramethylammonium | 100 µg, ia | +84 | 112 |
| 4-*m*-Chlorophenylcarbamoyloxy-2-butynyltrimethylammonium chloride | 10 µg, ia | +77 | 112 |
| Carbamylcholine + atropine 10 mg | 100 µg, ia | +33 | 236 |
| Urecholine | 4 mg, iv | +129 | 72 |
| **Adrenergic agonists and antagonists** | | | |
| Epinephrine | 0.006 µg/min, ia | −3 | 191 |
| | 0.3 µg, ia | −37 | 112 |
| | 1 µg·kg$^{-1}$·min$^{-1}$, iv | −33 to −55 | 42, 186 |
| | 10 µg, iv | +250 | 9 |
| | 25 µg, iv | −10 | 108 |
| Norepinephrine | 6 µg/min, ia | −86 | 191 |
| | 0.3–200 µg, ia | −51 to −97 | 112, 236 |
| | 2 µg·kg$^{-1}$·min$^{-1}$, iv | +2 to +31 | 42, 195 |
| | 10 µg, iv | +75 | 9 |
| Dopamine | 500 µg/kg, ia | +25 | 108 |
| | 1–10 µg, ia | −6 to −41 | 112 |
| | 6–25 µg·kg$^{-1}$·min$^{-1}$, iv | −13 to +22 | 123, 198 |
| L-Dopa | 1 mg, ia | 0 | 112 |
| Isoproterenol | 15 µg/kg, ia | +110 to +150 | 113 |
| | 3 µg, ia | +88 | 112 |
| | 0.06–0.90 µg·kg$^{-1}$·min$^{-1}$, iv | −3 to −4 | 97 |
| | 2 µg/min, iv | −4 | 128 |
| Phenylephrine | 1 µg, ia | −41 | 112 |
| Dibenzyline | 8 µg·kg$^{-1}$·min$^{-1}$, iv | −25 | 42 |
| Phenoxybenzamine | 5 mg/kg, iv | −2 | 198 |
| Methoxamine | 10 µg, ia | −38 | 112 |
| Ephedrine | 100 µg, ia | −28 | 112 |
| Tyramine | 10 µg, ia | −29 | 112 |
| **Autacoids** | | | |
| Histamine | 0.5–10 µg, ia | +25 to +285 | 112, 178 |
| | 1 µg·kg$^{-1}$·min$^{-1}$, iv | −15 | 42 |
| | 1 µg, iv | +75 | 177 |
| 5-Hydroxytryptamine | 10 µg, ia | −32 | 112 |
| Bradykinin | 2–4 µg/kg, ia | +200 to +300 | 113 |
| | 0.3 µg, ia | +275 | 112 |
| | 25 µg·kg$^{-1}$·min$^{-1}$, iv | −3 | 5 |
| **Active polypeptides** | | | |
| Vasopressin | 0.1 µg, ia | −76 | 112 |
| | 0.01 CU·kg$^{-1}$·min$^{-1}$, iv | −82 | 236 |
| | 2.05–131 mU/kg, iv | −17 to −80 | 18 |
| | 0.1–4.5 U/kg, iv | −38 to −46 | 179, 236 |
| Vasoactive intestinal polypeptide (VIP) | 20–400 µg/min, ia | 0 | 162 |
| | 128 ng/kg, iv | +100 | 26 |
| Synthetic chicken VIP | 2 µg/kg, iv | +50 | 107 |
| Insulin | 2 mU/min, ia | −34 | 192 |
| | 10 U, ia | +15 | 112 |
| Oxytocin | 0.1 µg, ia | −18 | 112 |
| Eledoisin | 0.1 µg, ia | +217 | 112 |
| Kallikrein | 0.1 µg, ia | +200 | 112 |
| Angiotensin II | 0.1 µg, ia | −45 | 112 |
| Gastrin | 1 µg, ia | +47 | 112 |
| Pentagastrin | 0.2 µg/kg, ia | +81 | 72 |
| | 64 ng/kg, iv | +124 | 104 |
| Glucagon | 1 µg/kg BW, ia | +8 | 175 |
| | 10 µg, ia | +33 | 112 |
| | 8–50 µg/kg BW, iv | 0 to −27 | 179, 186 |
| | 0.5 U/100 g BW, iv | +6 to −2 | 120 |

TABLE 6—*Continued*

| Drug/Agent | Dose | Change in Blood Flow, % | Ref. |
|---|---|---|---|
| Somatostatin | 3.3 $\mu$g·kg$^{-1}$ BW·min$^{-1}$, iv | +31 | 43 |
| | 200 $\mu$g/kg·min$^{-1}$, iv | −49 | 189 |
| | 50–100 $\mu$g/min, iv | −8 to −29 | 14 |
| | 100 mg/min, iv | −56 | 191 |
| Neurotensin | 25–50 pmol·kg$^{-1}$·min$^{-1}$, ia | +27 to +36 | 121 |
| Adenyl compounds | | | |
| Adenosine | 100 $\mu$g, ia | +152 | 112 |
| AMP | 100 $\mu$g, ia | +120 | 112 |
| ADP | 100 $\mu$g, ia | +185 | 112 |
| ATP | 100 $\mu$g, ia | +271 | 112 |
| Uridine | 100 $\mu$g, ia | +10 | 112 |
| UMP | 100 $\mu$g, ia | −9 | 112 |
| UDP | 100 $\mu$g, ia | +77 | 112 |
| UTP | 100 $\mu$g, ia | +222 | 112 |
| Diphosphopyridine nucleotide | 100 $\mu$g, ia | +19 | 112 |
| Triphosphopyridine nucleotide | 100 $\mu$g, ia | +14 | 112 |
| cAMP | 1 mg, ia | +75 | 112 |
| Dibutyryl cAMP | 1–3 mg, ia | +15 to +83 | 112 |
| Prostaglandins | | | |
| Prostacyclin | 0.3 $\mu$g·kg$^{-1}$·min$^{-1}$, iv | −12 to −25 | 207 |
| PGE$_1$ | 5 $\mu$g, ia | −41 | 33 |
| | 125 $\mu$g/kg, ia | +14 | 175 |
| PGE$_2$ | 100–300 $\mu$g/kg, ia | +17 to +28 | 99, 110 |
| | 100 ng/kg, ia | +21 | 99 |
| PGI$_2$ | 100–300 $\mu$g/kg, ia | +16 to +26 | 99, 100 |
| | 100 ng/kg, ia | +17 | 99 |
| PGF$_{2\alpha}$ | 300 $\mu$g/kg, ia | −3 | 99 |
| | 100 ng/kg, ia | −6 to +4 | 99 |
| PGD$_2$ | 100 $\mu$g/kg, ia | −15 | 99 |
| | 30 ng/kg, ia | −11 to +8 | 99 |
| Thromboxane B$_2$ | 300 $\mu$g/kg, ia | +21 | 99 |
| | 100 ng/kg, ia | +13 | 99 |
| Indomethacin | 20 $\mu$g·kg$^{-1}$·min$^{-1}$, iv | −24 | 99 |
| | 10 $\mu$g/kg, iv | −37 | 108 |
| | 5 mg/kg, iv | +12 | 227 |
| Meclofenamate | 20 $\mu$g·kg$^{-1}$·min$^{-1}$, iv | −27 | 99 |
| Arachidonic acid | 5–10 $\mu$g/kg, ia | +20 to +49 | 99, 108 |
| Miscellaneous | | | |
| Minoxidil | 2 mg/kg, iv | +43 | 198 |
| | 1–30 mg/kg, po | +86 to +119 | 105 |
| Nitroprusside | 10 $\mu$g·kg$^{-1}$·min$^{-1}$, iv | −32 | 198 |
| Nitroglycerin | 10 $\mu$g, ia | +120 | 112 |
| Hydralazine | 100 $\mu$g, ia | −14 | 112 |
| Papaverine | 0.01–100 mg, ia | +30 to +59 | 112, 133 |
| | 10–30 mg/kg, ia | +300 to +400 | 113 |
| Aminophylline | 8 mg/min, ia | +200 to +310 | 39 |
| Caffeine | 3 mg, ia | +221 | 112 |
| Theophylline | 1–10 mg, ia | +133 to +396 | 112 |
| Theobromine | 3 mg, ia | +101 | 112 |
| Dipyridamole | 100 $\mu$g, ia | +52 | 112 |
| Verapamil | 10 $\mu$g, ia | +236 | 112 |
| Nicardipine | 1–100 $\mu$g, ia | 0 to +114 | 109 |
| Galactose | 7.2 mg/min, ia | +12 | 39 |
| Cortisone | 200 mg/day for 1 mo, iv | +59 | 42 |
| Furosemide | 1.2–9.6 mg/kg, iv | −28 to +35 | 98, 237 |
| Ethacrynic acid | 2 mg/kg, iv | −25 | 98 |
| Diazoxide | 10 mg/kg, iv | +85 | 98 |
| Tetraethylammonium | 100 $\mu$g, ia | +7 | 112 |
| Cocaine | 100 $\mu$g, ia | −36 | 112 |
| Procaine | 100 $\mu$g, ia | +70 | 112 |
| Tolazoline | 10 $\mu$g, ia | +31 | 112 |
| Morphine | 30 $\mu$g, ia | 0 | 112 |
| Ergotamine | 10 $\mu$g, ia | −27 | 112 |
| Ouabain | 10 $\mu$g, ia | −34 | 112 |
| Strospeside | 100 $\mu$g, ia | −42 | 112 |
| Xenopsin | 2 $\mu$g·kg$^{-1}$·h$^{-1}$, iv | +297 | 242 |
| Pentobarbital | 25–30 mg/kg, iv | −30 to −69 | 7, 15, 51, 65 |
| $\alpha$-Chloralose | 2% (0.5 ml/kg), iv | −86 | 15 |
| Ethanol | 0.5–1.5 g/kg, iv | −10 to −37 | 103, 193 |
| | 106 mg/dl, blood conc. | −22 | 65 |
| Hypertonic glucose | 0.7–5.56 mM/kg, iv | +6 to +50 | 59 |
| | 15%–30% glucose, ia | +167 to +250 | 113 |
| | 0.5–1.0 g/kg, iv | +26 to +43 | 57, 58 |

BW, body weight; ia, intra-arterial; iv, intravenous; po, by mouth.

tion of flow from the acinar microcirculation to the less permeable ductal vasculature. Ligation of the submandibular duct for 3–12 days also significantly reduces the PS for small lipid-insoluble molecules (154).

MACROMOLECULES. Relatively little is known about the permeability of salivary gland and pancreatic capillaries to macromolecules. Studies employing lymph protein concentration (122), radiolabeled-albumin clearance (81), and indicator-diffusion techniques (219) indicate that the permeability of salivary gland capillaries to albumin is comparable to that reported for the small intestine. It should be noted that these studies do not provide quantitative estimates of reflection coefficients or permeability coefficients. However, a single estimate of $\sigma_d$ for total proteins in the pancreas (77) suggests that these purely fenestrated tissues exhibit permeability characteristics for macromolecules that are comparable to values reported for other organs of the digestive system (183).

### EXTRINSIC REGULATION OF BLOOD FLOW

It is well recognized that the autonomic nervous system exerts a significant influence on pancreatic and salivary blood flows. This section describes the role of the sympathetic nervous system in the regulation of blood flow in these exocrine tissues. The influence of parasympathetic nerves on the exocrine circulations is discussed in *Mediators of Functional Hyperemia*, p. 1574.

### Sympathetic Nerve Stimulation

PANCREAS. Relatively few studies have addressed the responses of the pancreatic circulation to sympathetic nerve stimulation. In general, sympathetic stimulation results in an initial decrease in blood flow due to vasoconstriction (10, 61, 80) followed by vasodilation after the stimulation ceases (10). The time course of this sympathetic postdilation is directly related to both the duration and frequency of nerve stimulation. The sympathetic vasoconstriction is due to $\alpha$-adrenoceptor stimulation, inasmuch as the effect can be blocked by infusion of $\alpha$-receptor blocking agents (10). There appears to be no cholinergic element to the response, because atropine pretreatment has no effect on the vascular response to nerve stimulation (61). The sympathetic postdilation is at least partially due to $\beta$-receptor stimulation (10), although other factors such as vasodilator metabolite accumulation may play a role. In the isolated, perfused rat pancreas, prostaglandin $E_1$ ($PGE_1$) and $PGE_2$ reduced the vasoconstrictor responses to periarterial sympathetic nerve stimulation, although it is still unclear to what extent prostaglandins may modulate adrenergic responses in pancreatic vessels (80). Administration of prostaglandin synthetase inhibitors also reduced the vasoconstrictor responses to adrenergic stimulation, suggesting that prostaglandins directly affect the neuroeffector junction (80). The role of endogenous prostaglandins in the regulation of pancreatic blood flow, especially during sympathetic stimulation, remains to be established.

SALIVARY GLAND. The vasculature of the salivary gland generally exhibits a biphasic response to sympathetic stimulation, characterized by sustained vasoconstriction during the stimulation and vasodilation when the stimulation ceases. A wide variety of stimulation frequencies have been employed in several species. For example, stimulation at 5–6 Hz in rats reduces salivary blood flow by 49%–100% (190, 212, 232) while inducing a poststimulation hyperemia as high as 991% above control blood flow (190). In the rabbit, stimulation at 3–25 Hz reduces salivary blood flow by 29%–95% (70, 71, 158), whereas stimulation at 25 Hz results in only a 20% poststimulation hyperemia (158). In the cat, sympathetic stimulation at 5–25 Hz results in flow decrements ranging from 20% to 75% (24, 68, 102, 117, 140, 145, 205), usually in a frequency-dependent fashion. The poststimulation hyperemia ranges from 75% to 366% above control levels. There appears to be little correlation between stimulus frequency and the magnitude of poststimulation flow increments.

The mechanism(s) accounting for the poststimulation hyperemia has been the subject of numerous investigations. A role for adrenoreceptors is supported by a study showing that reserpine blocks all vascular responses to sympathetic stimulation (205). Hilton and Lewis (93) suggested that kallikrein, known to be released by sympathetic stimulation, induces vasodilation after cessation of stimulation. Additionally, recent experiments in the rat (190) demonstrated a 57-fold increase in kallikrein secretion rate after sympathetic stimulation, and this was associated with an 11-fold increase in salivary blood flow. Pretreatment with $\alpha$-adrenergic blocking agents (phentolamine, prazosin) blocked the sympathetic stimulation-induced increment in kallikrein. Phentolamine blocked the poststimulation hyperemia, whereas prazosin attenuated it by approximately one half (190). Earlier studies did not demonstrate blockade of the response with the $\alpha$-antagonist tolazoline (24). Thus kallikreins acting via $\alpha_1$-adrenoreceptors (68, 190) may be responsible for the reactive vasodilation seen after sympathetic stimulation. $\beta$-Receptor activation has also been implicated as playing a major role in the poststimulation hyperemia because several studies demonstrated attenuation of the dilator response with $\beta$-blockers such as propranolol (212) or pronethalol (24). However, other studies (68, 158, 190) do not present convincing evidence that $\beta$-receptors are involved in the vasodilation, because the phenomenon largely persists after receptor blockade. Whether there is a causal link between postulated $\beta$-receptor activation and cAMP release (117) remains to be established.

Other studies (102, 150) have suggested that an

increment in tissue osmolality might account for vasodilation after sympathetic stimulation. Significant increases in tissue osmolality are associated with the hyperemia after sympathetic stimulation (102). Furthermore infusions of hypertonic solutions increase blood flow by roughly the same magnitude when poststimulation venous blood levels are achieved (102, 150). Although the available evidence is circumstantial, tissue osmolality cannot be ruled out as a mediator of poststimulation hyperemia.

PHARMACOLOGY

The vasculature of the exocrine glands is sensitive to many drugs and hormones. Tables 5 and 6 summarize the available data regarding the effects of various vasoactive agents on blood flow in the salivary gland and pancreas. In general the qualitative responses of the exocrine glands to vasoactive substances are similar to those reported for the gastrointestinal tract (36, 77). Although several naturally occurring substances are vasoactive in the exocrine glands, caution must be exercised in extrapolating the data listed in Tables 5 and 6 to normal physiological processes, inasmuch as the concentration of drugs used in most studies appear to be outside of the physiological range.

SUMMARY

Since the last *Handbook* coverage of the circulation of the exocrine glands 20 years ago (111), many significant advances have been made in the understanding of this area (239). Scanning electron microscopic observations of vascular corrosion casts of the pancreas and salivary glands have led to a substantial revision of views regarding the intraglandular vascular anatomy. These studies have revealed striking similarities between the portal circulations of the exocrine pancreas and salivary glands. Progress in understanding the intrinsic regulation of the blood flow and oxygenation has been limited to the pancreas. Enough data have been obtained to allow for quantitation of the relative roles of resistance and exchange vessels in maintaining constant pancreatic oxygenation in the face of alterations in arterial and venous pressures. Similar studies in the salivary gland are warranted.

The relationship between exocrine secretion and glandular blood flow has captured the imagination of many investigators. Stimulation of parasympathetic nerves is the most frequently used model for assessing the mechanisms involved in the functional hyperemia in the salivary gland. As a matter of convenience, continuous nerve stimulation has been widely employed. In many cases the stimulation frequencies far exceed those required to mimic the maximal response to gustatory stimuli during a meal. A variety of intrinsic and extrinsic factors have been implicated in the functional hyperemia observed at stimulation frequencies <10 Hz. These include metabolic factors ($K^+$, osmolality), kinins, and vasodilator neurotransmitters (acetylcholine, VIP). There is compelling evidence both for and against a role for most of these factors in the functional hyperemia, and it's quite likely that no single factor is entirely responsible for the vasodilation that accompanies enhanced salivation. When high-frequency stimulation is used (10–20 Hz), an atropine-resistant vasodilation is observed. The atropine-resistant vasodilation has been attributed to noncholinergic vasodilator parasympathetic fibers. Recent evidence implicates VIP as the neurotransmitter of these noncholinergic vasodilator fibers. Although the use of continuous nerve stimulation has provided a great deal of information, intermittent stimulation (bursts) may be a more appropriate means of mimicking physiological events. The few studies employing intermittent stimulation suggest that the responses elicited by this mode of stimulation are quantitatively different from those observed with continuous stimulation.

Intravascular administration of secretin and CCK has been the model of choice for studying the relationship between pancreatic secretion and blood flow. In general these hormones have been administered at doses that lead to blood concentrations of secretin and CCK that are substantially greater than those observed postprandially. Nonetheless it is apparent that when these hormones are given individually near-maximal secretion rates can be obtained in the absence of vasodilation.

There are several characteristic features of the microcirculation of pancreas and salivary glands that optimize the ability of these exocrine glands to move large amounts of fluid and electrolytes from the blood to the transporting epithelia. In comparison to skeletal muscle and the intestine, the exocrine glands have a high capillary density and consequently a large capillary surface area for secretion. The capillaries are of the fenestrated type. These fenestrations greatly enhance the hydraulic conductivity of the capillaries and provide an enormous area for solute exchange. The capillaries of the pancreas and salivary glands are highly permeable to small solutes, yet are relatively impermeable to macromolecules. This allows for the maintenance of a constant interstitial fluid volume by restricting colloids to the intravascular compartment yet facilitates the transport of secreted solutes from the intravascular to extravascular spaces. Although there is quantitative information on the membrane parameters, forces, and flows that govern transcapillary fluid exchange, very little is known about the changes in all these factors during enhanced secretory activity.

We are grateful for the clerical assistance of Sandy Worley and Ursula Romano. We also thank Penny Cook for preparing the illustrations and Beth Granger for arranging the references.

The research of Dr. Kvietys was supported by the National Institute of Diabetes and Digestive and Kidney Diseases Grant DK-33548.

## REFERENCES

1. ADAMS, H. W., AND P. D. WEBSTER. A study of synthesis of DNA, RNA and oxygen uptake in segments of the rat pancreas. *Dig. Dis. Sci.* 22: 898–901, 1977.
2. ALI, S. S. Angioarchitecture of the pancreas of the cat. Light-scanning-, and transmission-electron microscopy. *Cell Tissue Res.* 235: 675–682, 1984.
3. ALTEVEER, R. J., M. J. JAFFE, AND J. VAN DAM. Hemodynamics and metabolism of the in vivo vascularly isolated canine pancreas. *Am. J. Physiol.* 236 (*Endocrinol. Metab. Gastrointest. Physiol.* 5): E626–E632, 1979.
4. ANDERSSON, P.-O., S. R. BLOOM, A. V. EDWARDS, AND J. JÄRHULT. Effects of stimulation of the chorda tympani in bursts on submaxillary responses in the cat. *J. Physiol. Lond.* 322: 469–483, 1982.
5. ARCIDIACONO, F. G., E. J. REININGER, AND L. A. SAPIRSTEIN. Effect of bradykinin on total peripheral resistance and regional vascular resistance in the rat. *Bibl. Anat.* 9: 29–32, 1967.
6. AUGIER, D., J. P. BOUCARD, J. P. PASCAL, A. RIBET, AND N. VAYSSE. Relationships between blood flow and secretion in the isolated perfused canine pancreas. *J. Physiol. Lond.* 221: 55–69, 1972.
7. AUNE, S., AND L. S. SEMB. The effect of secretin and pancreozymin on pancreatic blood flow in the conscious and anesthetized dog. *Acta Physiol. Scand.* 76: 406–414, 1969.
8. BAINBRIDGE, F. A. Observations on the lymph from the submaxillary gland of the dog. *J. Physiol. Lond.* 26: 79–91, 1900.
9. BARLOW, T. E., J. R. GREENWELL, A. A. HARPER, AND T. SCRATCHERD. The effect of adrenaline and noradrenaline on the blood flow, electrical conductance and external secretion of the pancreas. *J. Physiol. Lond.* 217: 665–678, 1971.
10. BARLOW, T. E., J. R. GREENWELL, A. A. HARPER, AND T. SCRATCHERD. The influence of the splanchnic nerves on the external secretion, blood flow, and electrical conductance of the cat pancreas. *J. Physiol. Lond.* 236: 421–433, 1974.
11. BARROWMAN, J. A. *Physiology of the Gastro-Intestinal Lymphatic System.* Cambridge, UK: Cambridge Univ. Press, 1978.
12. BARROWMAN, J. A., P. TSO, P. R. KVIETYS, AND D. N. GRANGER. Gastrointestinal lymph and lymphatics. In: *Experimental Biology of the Lymphatic Circulation,* edited by M. G. Johnston. Amsterdam: Elsevier, 1985, p. 327–354.
13. BARTON, S., C. KARPINSKI, C. MORIVAKI, AND M. SCHACHTER. Sialotonin: vasopressor substance in saliva and submandibular gland of the cat. *J. Physiol. Lond.* 261: 523–533, 1975.
14. BECKER, R. H. A., J. SCHOLTHOLT, B. A. SCHOELKENS, W. JUNG, AND O. SPETH. A microsphere study on the effects of somatostatin and secretin on regional blood flow in anesthetized dogs. *Regul. Pept.* 4: 341–351, 1982.
15. BEDRAN DE CASTRO, M. T. B., H. F. DOWNEY, G. J. CRYSTAL, AND F. A. BASHOUR. Effect of controlled ventilation on renal and splanchnic blood flows during nicotine. *Am. J. Physiol.* 248 (*Heart Circ. Physiol.* 17): H360–H365, 1985.
16. BEIJER, H. J. M., F. A. S. BROUWER, AND G. A. CHARBON. Time course and sensitivity of secretin-stimulated pancreatic secretion and blood flow in the anesthetized dog. *Scand. J. Gastroenterol.* 14: 295–300, 1979.
17. BEIJER, H. J. M., A. H. J. MAAS, AND G. A. CHARBON. Pancreatic $O_2$ consumption and $CO_2$ output during secretin-induced, exocrine secretion from the pancreas in the anesthetized dog. *Pfluegers Arch.* 400: 318–323, 1984.
18. BEIJER, H. J. M., A. H. J. MAAS, AND G. A. CHARBON. A vasopressin-induced decrease in pancreatic blood flow and in pancreatic exocrine secretion in the anesthetized dog. *Pfluegers Arch.* 400: 324–328, 1984.
19. BEILENSON, S., M. SCHACTER, AND L. H. SMAJE. Secretion of kallikrein and its role in vasodilation in the submaxillary gland. *J. Physiol. Lond.* 199: 303–317, 1968.
20. BENYO, I., A. FAZEKAS, E. POSCH, L. ROSEVALLI, AND G. SZABO. Circulatory effects of intraduodenal acidification in the rat. *Res. Exp. Med.* 177: 221–226, 1980.
20a. BERG, T., T. B. ORSTAVIK, O. A. CARRETERO, AND G. SCICLI. Kallikrein-kinin system in the regulation of submandibular gland blood flow. *Am. J. Physiol.* 242 (*Heart Circ. Physiol.* 11): H1010–H1014, 1982.
21. BERNARD, C. Memoires sur le pancreas. *CR Seances Acad Sci. Ser. III Sci. Vie, Suppl.,* 1: 379–563, 1856.
22. BERNARD, C. De l'influence de deux ordres de nerfs qui determinent les variations de couleur du sang veineux dans les organes glandulaires. *CR Acad. Sci. Ser. III Sci. Vie,* 47: 245–253, 1858.
23. BHOOLA, K. D., M. LEMON, AND R. MATHEWS. Kallikrein in exocrine glands. In: *Handbook of Experimental Pharmacology. Bradykinin, Kallidin and Kallikrein,* edited by E. G. Erdos. Berlin: Springer-Verlag, 1979, vol. 25, p. 489–523.
24. BHOOLA, K. D., J. MORLEY, M. SCHACHTER, AND L. H. SMAJE. Vasodilatation in the submaxillary gland of the cat. *J. Physiol. Lond.* 179: 172–184, 1965.
25. BLAIR-WEST, J. R., J. P. COGHLAN, D. A. DENTON, J. NELSON, R. D. WRIGHT, AND A. YAMAUCHI. Ionic, histological and vascular factors in the reaction of the sheep's parotid to high and low mineralocorticoid status. *J. Physiol. Lond.* 205: 563–579, 1969.
26. BLITZ, W., AND G. A. CHARBON. Regional vascular influence of vasoactive intestinal polypeptide. *Scand. J. Gastroenterol.* 18: 755–763, 1983.
27. BLOOM, S. R., AND A. V. EDWARDS. Vasoactive intestinal peptide and relation to atropine resistant vasodilatation in the submaxillary gland of the cat. *J. Physiol. Lond.* 300: 41–53, 1980.
28. BONNER-WEIR, S., AND L. ORCI. New perspectives on the microcirculature of the islets of Langerhans in the rat. *Diabetes* 31: 883–889, 1982.
29. BROADIE, T. A., M. DEVEDAS, J. RYSAVY, A. S. LEONARD, AND J. P. DELANEY. The effect of hypoxia and hypercapnia on canine pancreatic blood flow. *J. Surg. Res.* 27: 114–118, 1979.
30. BURGEN, A. S. U., AND P. SEEMAN. The role of the salivary duct system in the formation of saliva. *Can. J. Biochem. Physiol.* 36: 119–143, 1958.
31. BURNSTOCK, G. Purinergic nerves. *Pharmacol. Rev.* 24: 509–581, 1972.
32. CADETE-LEITE, A. The arteries of the pancreas of the dog. An injection-corrosion and microangiographic study. *Am. J. Anat.* 137: 151–157, 1913.
33. CASE, R. M., AND T. SCRATCHERD. Prostaglandin action on pancreatic blood flow and on electrolyte and enzyme secretion by exocrine pancreas in vivo and in vitro. *J. Physiol. Lond.* 226: 393–405, 1972.
34. CHAPAL, J., AND M.-M. LOUBATIERES-MARIANI. Evidence for purinergic receptors on vascular smooth muscle in rat pancreas. *Eur. J. Pharmacol.* 87: 423–430, 1983.
35. CHILVERS, E. R., AND N. W. THOMAS. The blood supply of the islets of Langerhans in the Mongolian gerbil. *J. Anat.* 136: 339–347, 1983.
36. CHOU, C. C., AND P. R. KVIETYS. Physiological and pharmacological alterations in gastrointestinal blood flow. In: *Measurement of Blood Flow: Application to the Splanchnic Circulation,* edited by D. N. Granger and G. B. Bulkley. Baltimore, MD: Williams & Wilkins, 1981, p. 477–507.
37. CHUNG, R. S., AND S. SAFAIE-SHIRAZI. The effect of secretin on pancreatic blood flow in the awake and anesthetized dog. *Proc. Soc. Exp. Biol. Med.* 173: 620–625, 1983.
38. CLOUGH, G., AND L. H. SMAJE. Exchange area and surface properties of the microvasculature of the rabbit submandibular gland following duct ligation. *J. Physiol. Lond.* 354: 445–456, 1984.
39. CODDLING, J. A., M. A. ASHWORTH, J. HUNTER, AND R. E. HAIST. Effect on pancreatic blood flow and insulin output of infusions of aminophylline, galactose and galactose plus ami-

nophylline into an isolated in situ portion of pancreas. *Horm. Metab. Res.* 9: 261–266, 1977.
40. CROUCH, J. E. *Text-Atlas of Cat Anatomy.* Philadelphia, PA: Lea & Febiger, 1969.
41. DARKE, A. C., AND K. H. SMAJE. Dependence of functional vasodilation in the submandibular gland upon stimulation frequency. *J. Physiol. Lond.* 226: 191–203, 1972.
42. DELANEY, J. P., AND E. GRIM. Influence of hormones and drugs on canine pancreatic blood flow. *Am. J. Physiol.* 211: 1398–1402, 1966.
43. DOERTENBACH, J. G., C. HOTTENROTT, U. SCHWEDES, K. H. USADEL, AND A. ENCKE. Haemodynamic effects of somatostatin in acute gastrointestinal hemorrhage in dogs. *Resuscitation* 10: 57–61, 1982.
44. DORIGOTTI, L., AND H. GLASSER. Comparative effects of caerulein, pancreoxymin and secretin on pancreatic blood flow. *Experientia Basel* 24: 806–807, 1968.
45. EBBEHAJ, N., L. B. SVENDSEN, AND P. MADSEN. Pancreatic tissue pressure: techniques and pathophysiological aspects. *Scand. J. Gastroenterol.* 19: 1066–1068, 1984.
46. EICHELTER, P., AND W. G. SCHENK. Hemodynamics of pancreatic secretion. *Arch. Surg.* 93: 200–207, 1966.
47. EKSTROM, J., E. BRODIN, R. EKMAN, R. HAKANSON, AND F. SUNDLER. Vasoactive intestinal peptide and substance P in salivary glands of the rat following denervation or duct ligation. *Regul. Pept.* 10: 1–10, 1984.
48. ELIASSEN, E., B. FOLKOW, AND S. HILTON. Blood flow and capillary filtration capacities in salivary and pancreatic glands as compared with skeletal muscle. *Acta. Physiol. Scand.* 87: 11A–12A, 1973.
50. EMMELIN, N., AND J. HOLMBERG. Impulse frequency in secretory nerves of salivary glands. *J. Physiol. Lond.* 191: 205–214, 1967.
51. ERICSSON, B. F. Effect of pentobarbital sodium anesthesia, as judged with aid of radioactive carbonized microspheres, on cardiac output and its fractional distribution in the dog. *Acta Chir. Scand.* 137: 613–620, 1971.
52. EVANS, H. E., AND G. C. CHRISTENSEN. *Miller's Anatomy of the Dog* (2nd ed.). Philadelphia, PA: Saunders, 1979.
53. FARA, J. W., E. H. RUBINSTEIN, AND R. R. SONNENSCHEIN. Intestinal hormones in mesenteric after intraduodenal agents. *Am. J. Physiol.* 223: 1058–1067, 1972.
54. FAZEKAS, A., E. POSCH, AND T. ZELLES. Pressure-flow relations in the vascular bed of the rat submandibular gland. *J. Dent. Res.* 61: 66–68, 1982.
55. FAZEKAS, A., E. POSCH, AND T. ZELLES. Effect of indomethacin on the blood flow of the rat submandibular gland. *J. Dent. Res.* 62: 537–539, 1983.
56. FERREIRA, S. H., AND L. H. SMAJE. Bradykinin and functional vasodilatation in the slivary gland. *Br. J. Pharmacol.* 58: 201–209, 1976.
57. FISCHER, U., H. HOMMEL, AND E. SALZSIEDER. Pancreatic blood flow in conscious dogs after oral administration of glucose. *Diabetologia* 12: 133–136, 1976.
58. FISCHER, U., H. HOMMEL, AND E. SCHMID. Continuous registration of the pancreatic blood flow after intravenous application of glucose. *Experientia Basel* 29: 884–885, 1973.
59. FISCHER, U., H. HOMMEL, AND E. SCHMID. Dynamics of canine pancreatic blood flow and of insulin secretion during an intravenous glucose load. *Pfluegers Arch.* 358: 89–100, 1975.
60. FLOREY, H. W. The missing link. The structure of capillaries. *Q. J. Exp. Physiol.* 53: 1–5, 1968.
61. FORSYTH, R. P. Sympathetic nervous system control of distribution of cardiac output in unanesthetized monkeys. *Federation Proc.* 31: 1240–1244, 1972.
62. FRANSDEN, E. K., G. A. KRISHNA, AND S. I. SAID. Vasoactive intestinal polypeptide promotes cyclic adenosine 3',5'-monophosphate accumulation in guinea-pig trachea. *Br. J. Pharmacol.* 62: 367–369, 1978.
63. FRASER, P. A., AND J. R. HENDERSON. The arrangement of endocrine and exocrine pancreatic microcirculation observed in the living rabbit. *Q. J. Exp. Physiol.* 65: 151–158, 1980.
64. FRASER, P. A., AND L. H. SMAJE. The organization of the salivary gland microcirculation. *J. Physiol. Lond.* 272: 121–136, 1977.
65. FRIEDMAN, H. S., R. LOWERY, E. SHAUGHNESSY, AND J. SCORZA. The effects of ethanol on pancreatic blood flow in awake and anesthetized dogs. *Proc. Soc. Exp. Biol. Med.* 174: 377–382, 1983.
66. FROGGE, J. D., A. S. HERMRECK, AND A. P. THAL. Metabolic and hemodynamic effects of secretin and pancreozymin on the pancreas. *Surgery* 68: 498–502, 1970.
67. GALLAVAN, R. H., C. C. CHOU, P. R. KVIETYS, AND S. P. SIT. Regional blood flow during digestion in the conscious dog. *Am. J. Physiol.* 238 (*Heart Circ. Physiol.* 7): H220–H225, 1980.
68. GAUTVIK, K., M. KRIZ, K. LUND-LARSEN, AND B. A. WAALER. Sympathetic vasodilatation, kallikrein release and adrenergic receptors in the cat submandibular salivary gland. *Acta Physiol. Scand.* 90: 438–444, 1974.
69. GAUTVIK, K. M., K. NUSTAD, AND J. VYSTYD. Kininogenase activity in the stimulated submandibular salivary gland in cats. *Acta Physiol. Scand.* 85: 438–445, 1972.
70. GJORSTRUP, P. Effects of sympathetic nerve stimulation in the presence of a flow parasympathetic secretion in the parotid and submaxillary glands of the rabbit. *Acta Physiol. Scand.* 101: 211–218, 1977.
71. GJORSTRUP, P. Blood flow and secretion in submaxillary gland of the rabbit during stimulation of the autonomic nerves. *Acta Physiol. Scand.* 115: 91–95, 1982.
72. GOODHEAD, B., H. S. HIMAL, AND J. ZANBILOWICZ. Relationship between pancreatic secretion and pancreatic blood flow. *Gut* 11: 62–68, 1970.
73. GRANGER, D. N., AND J. A. BARROWMAN. Microcirculation of the alimentary tract. I. Physiology of transcapillary fluid and solute exchange. *Gastroenterology* 84: 846–868, 1983.
74. GRANGER, D. N., AND J. A. BARROWMAN. Gastrointestinal and liver edema. In: *Edema*, edited by N. C. Staub and A. E. Taylor. New York: Raven, 1984, p. 615–656.
75. GRANGER, D. N., AND H. J. GRANGER. Systems analysis of intestinal hemodynamics and oxygenation. *Am. J. Physiol.* 245 (*Gastrointest. Liver Physiol.* 8): G786–G796, 1983.
76. GRANGER, D. N., P. R. KVIETYS, M. A. PERRY, D. A. PARKS, AND J. N. BENOIT. Metabolic, myogenic and humoral factors in local regulation of alimentary tract blood flow. In: *Microcirculation of the Alimentary Tract*, edited by A. Koo, S. K. Lam, and L. H. Smaje. Singapore: World Scientific, 1983, p. 131–142.
77. GRANGER, D. N., M. A. PERRY, AND P. R. KVIETYS. The microcirculation and fluid transport in digestive organs. *Federation Proc.* 42: 1667–1672, 1983.
78. GRANGER, D. N., P. D. I. RICHARDSON, P. R. KVIETYS, AND N. A. MORTILLARO. Intestinal blood flow. *Gastroenterology* 78: 837–863, 1980.
79. GREENE, E. C. *Anatomy of the Rat.* New York: Hafner, 1935, vol. 27.
80. HAMAMDŽIC, M., AND K. U. MALIK. Prostaglandins in adrenergic transmission of isolated perfused rat pancreas. *Am. J. Physiol.* 232 (*Endocrinol. Metab. Gastrointest. Physiol.* 1): E201–E209, 1977.
81. HARALDSSON, B., L. REGNER, R. HULTBORN, L. WEISS, AND B. RIPPE. Transcapillary passage of albumin in mammary tumours and in normal lactating mammary glands of the rat. *Acta Physiol. Scand.* 122: 497–505, 1984.
82. HARALDSSON, B., B. RIPPE, B. J. MOXHAM, AND B. FOLKOW. Permeability of fenestrated capillaries in the isolated pig pancreas, with effects of bradykinin and histamine, as studied by simultaneous registration of filtration and diffusion capacities. *Acta Physiol. Scand.* 114: 67–74, 1982.
83. HARPER, S. L., D. N. GRANGER, J. A. BARROWMAN, P. R. KVIETYS, AND M. G. ULRICH. Relation between pancreatic growth and blood flow. *Am. J. Physiol.* 248 (*Gastrointest. Liver Physiol.* 11): G61–G67, 1985.

84. HARPER, S. L., V. H. PITTS, D. N. GRANGER, AND P. R. KVIETYS. Pancreatic tissue oxygenation during secretory stimulation. *Am. J. Physiol.* 250 (*Gastrointest. Liver Physiol.* 13): G316–G322, 1986.
85. HEIDENHAIN, R. Ueber die Wirkung einiger Gifte auf die Nerven der glandula submaxillaris. *Arch. Gesamte. Physiol. Mens. Tiere Pfluegers* 5: 309–318, 1872.
86. HEINS, P., AND A. TAMARIN. Response of the rat submaxillary gland to pilocarpine: a quantitative analysis of gross and microscopic changes. *J. Dent. Res.* 47: 575–579, 1968.
87. HEISIG, N. Pancreatic microcirculation under the influence of adequate secretory stimulation. *Bibl. Anat.* 9: 176–180, 1967.
88. HENDERSON, J. R. The role of the islet of Langerhans in exocrine function of the pancreas. In: *Microcirculation of the Alimentary Tract*, edited by A. Koo, S. K. Lam, and L. H. Smaje. Singapore: World Scientific, 1983, p. 235–239.
89. HENDERSON, J. R., AND P. M. DANIEL. A comparative study of the portal vessels connecting the endocrine and exocrine pancreas, with a discussion of some functional implication. *Q. J. Exp. Physiol.* 64: 267–275, 1979.
90. HENDERSON, J. R., AND P. M. DANIEL. Capillary beds and portal circulations. In: *Handbook of Physiology. The Cardiovascular System. Microcirculation*, edited by E. M. Renkin and C. C. Michel. Bethesda, MD: Am. Physiol. Soc., 1984, sect. 2, vol. IV, pt. 2, chapt. 25, p. 1035–1046.
90a. HENDERSON, J. R., AND M. C. MOSS. A morphometric study of the endocrine and exocrine capillaries of the pancreas. *Q. J. Exp. Physiol.* 70: 347–356, 1985.
91. HICKSON, J. C. D. The secretory and vascular response to nervous and hormonal stimulation in the pancreas of the pig. *J. Physiol. Lond.* 206: 299–322, 1970.
92. HILTON, S. M., AND G. P. LEWIS. The cause of the vasodilatation accompanying activity in the submandibular salivary gland. *J. Physiol. Lond.* 128: 235–248, 1955.
93. HILTON, S. M., AND G. P. LEWIS. The mechanism of the functional hyperemia in the submandibular salivary gland. *J. Physiol. Lond.* 129: 253–271, 1955.
94. HILTON, S. M., AND G. P. LEWIS. The relationship between glandular activity, bradykinin formation and functional vasodilatation in the submandibular salivary gland. *J. Physiol. Lond.* 134: 471–483, 1956.
95. HILTON, S. M., AND M. JONES. Plasma kinin and functional vasodilation in the pancreas. *J. Physiol. Lond.* 165: 35P–36P, 1963.
96. HILTON, S. M., AND M. JONES. The role of plasma kinin in functional vasodilation in the pancreas. *J. Physiol. Lond.* 195: 521–533, 1968.
97. HOFFBRAND, B. I., R. P. FORSYTH, AND K. L. MELMON. Dose-related effects of isoprenaline on the distribution of cardiac output and myocardial blood flow in conscious monkeys. *Cardiovasc. Res.* 7: 664–669, 1973.
98. HOLLAND, S. D., AND H. E. WILLIAMSON. Acute effects of high cailing diuretics on pancreatic blood flow and function. *J. Pharmacol. Exp. Ther.* 229: 440–446, 1984.
99. HOMMA, T., AND K. U. MALIK. Effect of prostaglandins on pancreatic circulation in anesthetized dogs. *J. Pharmacol. Exp. Ther.* 222: 623–628, 1982.
100. HOMMA, T., AND K. U. MALIK. Effect of secretin and caerulein in canine pancreas: relation to prostaglandins. *Am. J. Physiol.* 244 (*Gastrointest. Liver Physiol.* 7): G660–G667, 1983.
101. HOLMBERG, J. Release of acetylcholine in the parotid gland of the dog during stimulation of postganglionic nerves. *Acta Physiol. Scand.* 86: 115–119, 1972.
102. HOLMBERG, J., AND L. LUNDVALL. Tissue hyperosmolality as a causal factor in vasodilatation following sympathetic stimulation of the submandibular gland. *Acta Physiol. Scand.* 98: 400–406, 1976.
103. HOWITZ, L. D., AND J. H. MYERS. Ethanol-induced alterations in pancreatic blood flow in conscious dogs. *Circ. Res.* 50: 250–256, 1982.
104. HULSTAERT, P. F., W. J. C. GEURTS, F. A. S. BROUWER, H. J. M. BEIJER, AND G. A. CHARBON. Hemodynamic actions of pentagastrin. *Scand. J. Gastroenterol.* 15: 7–15, 1980.
105. HUMPHREY, S. J., AND G. R. ZINS. Whole body and regional hemodynamic effects of minoxidil in the conscious dog. *J. Cardiovasc. Pharmacol.* 6: 979–988, 1984.
106. HURLEY, J. V., AND N. E. W. MCCALLUM. The degree of functional significance of the escape of marker particles from small blood vessels with fenestrated endothelium. *J. Pathol.* 113: 183–196, 1974.
107. INOUE, K., T. KAWANO, K. SHIMA, T. KIM, T. SUZUKI, T. TOBE, M. TAKEYAMA, AND H. YAJIMA. Effect of synthetic chicken vasoactive intestinal peptide on pancreatic blood flow and on exocrine and endocrine secretions of the pancreas in dogs. *Dis. Dis. Sci.* 28: 724–732, 1983.
108. IWATSUKI, K., T. HOMMA, AND K. U. MALIK. Contribution of prostaglandins to dopamine actions in the pancreas of anesthetized dogs. *Am. J. Physiol.* 248 (*Gastrointest. Liver Physiol.* 11): G110–G117, 1985.
109. IWATSUKI, K., F. IIJIMA, AND S. CHIBA. Secretory and vascular effects of the optical isomers of nicardipine. *Clin. Exp. Pharmacol. Physiol.* 11: 1–5, 1984.
110. IWATSUKI, K., K. IKEDA, F. IIJIMA, AND S. CHIBA. Secretory and vascular responses to 1,1-dimethyl-4-phenylpiperazinium (DMPP) of the blood-perfused canine pancreas. *Arch. Int. Pharmacodyn.* 256: 283–291, 1982.
111. JACOBSON, E. D. Secretion and blood flow in the gastrointestinal tract. In: *Handbook of Physiology. Alimentary Canal. Secretion*, edited by C. F. Code. Washington, DC: Am. Physiol. Soc., 1967, sect. 6, vol. II, chapt. 59, p. 1043–1062.
112. JAKEUCHI, O., S. SATOH, AND K. HASHIMOTO. Secretory and vascular response to various biogenic and foreign substances of the perfused canine pancreas. *Jpn. J. Pharmacol.* 24: 57–73, 1974.
113. JÄRHULT, J., AND A. THULIN. Hyperosmolality and pancreatic blood flow. *Pfluegers Arch.* 370: 127–130, 1977.
114. JOHNSON, P. C. The myogenic response. In: *Handbook of Physiology. Cardiovascular System. Vascular Smooth Muscle*, edited by D. F. Bohr, A. T. Somlyo, and H. V. Sparks, Jr. Bethesda, MD: Am. Physiol. Soc., 1980, section 2, vol. II, chapt. 15, 409–442.
115. JONES, C. J. Perivascular nerves in the rat submandibular salivary gland. *Neurosci. Lett.* 13: 19–23, 1979.
116. JONES, C. J., AND G. E. MANN. A possible role for adenosine 3′:5′-cyclic monophosphate in nerve-mediated vasodilatation. *Biochem. Soc. Trans.* 5: 428–430, 1977.
117. JONES, C. J., G. E. MANN, AND L. H. SMAJE. The role of cyclic nucleotides and related compounds in nerve-mediated vasodilation in the cat submandibular gland. *Br. J. Pharmacol.* 68: 485–497, 1980.
118. KARPINSKI, E., S. BARTON, D. LONGRIDGE, AND M. SCHACHTER. A study of vasoactive intestinal peptide and acetylcholine as possible mediators of vasodilation in the cat submandibular gland. *Can. J. Physiol. Pharmacol.* 62: 650–653, 1984.
119. KARPINSKI, C., S. BARTON, AND M. SCHACHTER. Vasodilator nerve fibers to the submaxillary gland of the cat. *Nature Lond.* 232: 122–124, 1971.
120. KITANI, K., Y. SUZUKI, AND R. MIURA. Differences in the effects of secretin and glucagon on the blood circulation of unanesthetized rats. *Acta Hepato-Gastroenterol.* 25: 470–473, 1978.
121. KONTUREK, S. J., J. JAWOREK, M. CIESZKOWSKI, W. PAWLIK, J. KANIA, AND S. R. BLOOM. Comparison of effects of neurotensin and fat on pancreatic stimulation in dogs. *Am. J. Physiol.* 244 (*Gastrointest. Liver Physiol.* 7): G590–G598, 1983.
122. KOO, A., L. H. SMAJE, AND P. D. SPENCER. Low permeability to macromolecules of the fenestrated capillaries in the cat submandibular gland. *Bibl. Anat.* 20: 301–304, 1981.
123. KULLMANN, R., W. R. BREULL, J. REINSBERG, K. WASSERMANN, AND A. KONOPATZKI. Dopamine produces vasodilation in specific regions and layers of the rabbit gastrointestinal tract. *Life Sci.* 32: 2115–2122, 1983.

124. KUZNETSOVA, E. K. Characteristics of blood supply of the pancreas during different phases of its activity. *Fiziol. Z. Kiev* 48: T99–T104, 1962.
125. KVIETYS, P. R., J. M. MCLENDON, G. B. BULKLEY, M. A. PERRY, AND D. N. GRANGER. Pancreatic circulation: intrinsic regulation. *Am. J. Physiol.* 242 (*Gastrointest. Liver Physiol.* 5): G596–G602, 1982.
126. KVIETYS, P. R., W. G. PATTERSON, AND D. N. GRANGER. Intrinsic and extrinsic regulation of the pancreatic microcirculation. In: *Progress in Microcirculation Research II*, edited by F. C. Courtice, D. G. Garlick, and M. A. Perry. Sydney, Australia: Univ. of New South Wales Press, 1984, p. 243–252.
127. KVIETYS, P. R., M. A. PERRY, AND D. N. GRANGER. Permeability of pancreatic capillaries to small molecules. *Am. J. Physiol.* 245 (*Gastrointest. Liver Physiol.* 8): G519–G524, 1983.
128. LABORSKY, G. J., AND J. W. ENSINCK. Contribution of the pancreas to circulating somatostatin-like immunoreactivity in the normal dog. *J. Clin. Invest.* 73: 216–223, 1984.
129. LANGESEN, L. P., J. O. D. NIELSEN, AND J. H. POULSEN. Partial dissociation between salivary secretion and active potassium transport in the perfused cat submandibular gland. *Pflueger Arch.* 364: 167–173, 1976.
130. LARSSON, L.-I., J. FAHRENKRUG, J. J. HOLST, AND O. B. SCHAFFALITZKY DE MUCKADELL. Innervation of the pancreas by vasoactive intestinal polypeptide (VIP) immunoreactive nerves. *Life Sci.* 22: 773–780, 1978.
131. LEESON, C. R. Structure of salivary glands. In: *Handbook of Physiology. Alimentary Canal. Secretion,* edited by C. F. Code. Washington, DC: Am. Physiol. Soc., 1967, sect. 6, vol. II, chapt. 32, p. 463–495.
132. LEMBECK, F., AND R. HEITTICH. Comparative study of the effects of substance P on blood pressure, salivatory functions and intestinal motility. *Naunyn-Schmiedebergs Arch. Pharmacol.* 265: 216–224, 1969.
133. LENNINGER, S. Effects of acetylcholine and papaverine on the secretion and blood flow from the pancreas of the cat. *Acta Physiol. Scand.* 89: 260–268, 1973.
134. LENNINGER, S. The autonomic innervation of the exocrine pancreas. *Med. Clin. North Am.* 58: 1310–1318, 1974.
135. LEWIS, G. P. The role of plasma kinins as mediator of functional vasodilation. *Gastroenterology* 52: 406–413, 1967.
136. LEWIS, G. P. Role of kinins and prostaglandins as mediators of functional hyperemia. *Proc. R. Soc. Med.* 64: 6–9, 1971.
137. LIFSON, N., K. G. KRAMLINGER, R. R. MAYRAND, AND E. J. LENDER. Blood flow is the rabbit pancreas with special reference to the islets of langerhans. *Gastroenterology* 79: 466–473, 1980.
138. LIFSON, N., AND C. U. LASSA. Note on the blood supply of the ducts of the rabbit pancreas. *Microvasc. Res.* 22: 171–176, 1981.
139. LUNDBERG, J. M. Evidence for coexistence of vasoactive intestinal polypeptide and acetylcholine in neurons of cat exocrine glands. Morphological, biochemical and functional studies. *Acta. Physiol. Scand. Suppl.* 496: 1–57, 1981.
140. LUNDBERG, J. M., A. ANGGÅRD, AND J. FAHRENKRUG. Complementary role of vasoactive intestinal polypeptide (VIP) and acetylcholine for cat submandibular gland blood flow and secretion. I. VIP release. *Acta Physiol. Scand.* 113: 317–327, 1981.
141. LUNDBERG, J. M., A. ANGGÅRD, AND J. FAHRENKRUG. Complementary role of vasoactive intestinal polypeptide (VIP) and acetylcholine by cat submandibular gland blood flow and secretion. II. Effects of cholinergic antagonists and VIP antiserum. *Acta Physiol. Scand.* 113: 329–336, 1981.
142. LUNDBERG, J. M., A. ANGGÅRD, AND J. FAHRENKRUG. Complementary role of vasoactive intestinal polypeptide (VIP) and acetylcholine for cat submandibular gland blood flow and secretion. III. Effects of local infusions. *Acta Physiol. Scand.* 114: 329–337, 1982.
143. LUNDBERG, J. M., A. ANGGÅRD, J. FAHRENKRUG, T. HOKFELT, AND V. MUTT. Vasoactive intestinal polypeptide in cholinergic neurons of exocrine glands: functional significance of coexisting transmitters for vasodilation and secretion. *Proc. Natl. Acad. Sci. USA* 77: 1651–1655, 1980.
144. LUNDBERG, J. M., A. ANGGÅRD, J. FAHRENKRUG, G. LUNDGREN, AND B. HOLMSTEDT. Corelease of VIP and acetylcholine in relation to blood flow and salivary secretion in cat submandibular salivary gland. *Acta Physiol. Scand.* 115: 525–528, 1982.
145. LUNDBERG, J. M., A. ANGGÅRD, T. HÖKFELT, AND J. KIMMEL. Avian pancreatic polypeptide (APP) inhibits atropine resistant vasodilation in cat submandibular salivary gland and nasal mucosa: possible interaction with VIP. *Acta Physiol. Scand.* 110: 199–201, 1980.
146. LUNDBERG, J. M., J. FAHRENKRUG, O. LARSSON, AND A. ANGGÅRD. Corelease of vasoactive intestinal polypeptide and peptide histidine isoleucine in relation to atropine-resistant vasodilation in cat submandibular salivary gland. *Neurosci. Lett.* 52: 34–42, 1984.
147. LUNDBERG, J. M., AND K. TATEMOTO. Pancreatic polypeptide family (APP, BPP, NPY and PYY) in relation to sympathetic vasoconstriction resistant to α-adrenoceptor blockade. *Acta Physiol. Scand.* 116: 393–402, 1981.
148. LUNDGREN, O. The alimentary canal. In: *Peripheral Circulation,* edited by P. C. Johnson. New York: Wiley, 1978, p. 255–283.
149. LUNDGREN, O. Microcirculation of the gastrointestinal tract and pancreas. In: *Handbook of Physiology. The Cardiovascular System. Microcirculation,* edited by E. M. Renkin and C. C. Michel. Bethesda, MD: Am. Physiol. Soc., 1984, sect. 2, vol. IV, pt. 2, chapt. 17, p. 799–863.
150. LUNDVALL, J., AND J. HOLMBERG. Role of tissue hyperosmolality in functional vasodilatation in the submandibular gland. *Acta Physiol. Scand* 92: 165–174, 1974.
161. LUNDVALL, J., AND J. HOLMBERG. Mechanisms involved in transcapillary fluid movement into the secreting cat submandibular (Abstract). *Acta Physiol. Scand.* 102: 16A, 1978.
152. LUNDVALL, J., AND J. HOLMBERG. Dynamics of saliva secretion and tissue volume changes during parasympathetic stimulation in the constant flow perfused cat submandibular gland. *Acta Physiol. Scand.* 102: 382–384, 1978.
153. MANN, G. E., L. H. SMAJE, AND D. L. YUDILEVICH. Permeability of the fenestrated capillaries of the cat submandibular gland to lipid-insoluble molecules. *J. Physiol. Lond.* 297: 335–354, 1979.
154. MANN, G. E., L. H. SMAJE, AND D. L. YUDILEVICH. Transcapillary exchange in the cat salivary gland during secretion, bradykinin infusion and after chronic duct ligation. *J. Physiol. Lond.* 297: 355–367, 1979.
155. MCCUSKEY, R. S., AND T. M. CHAPMAN. Microscopy of the living pancreas in situ. *Am. J. Anat.* 126: 395–407, 1969.
156. MIA, M. A., AND R. F. SIS. The arterial supply to the salivary glands of the cat. *Arch. Oral Biol.* 15: 1–10, 1970.
157. MOHAMED, A. H. Ultrastructural permeability studies in capillaries of rabbit oral mucosa and salivary glands. *Microvasc. Res.* 9: 287–303, 1975.
158. MORENO, M., E. MARTÍNEZ DE VICTORIA, AND M. A. LÓPEZ. Effect of sympathetic stimulation on salivary secretion in submandibular gland in the rabbit stimulated by pilocarpine. *Rev. Esp. Fisiol.* 40: 15–18, 1984.
159. MURESAN, V., AND M. C. CONSTANTINESCU. Distribution of sialoglycoconjugates on the luminal surface of the endothelial cell in the fenestrated capillaries of the pancreas. *J. Histochem. Cytochem.* 33: 474–476, 1985.
160. OATES, P. S., N. W. BRUCE, AND R. G. H. MORGAN. Pancreatic blood flow in the rat during enlargement, involution, and cholecystokinin treatment. *Am. J. Physiol.* 247 (*Gastrointest. Liver Physiol.* 10): G457–G462, 1984.
161. OHNEDA, A., K. HORIGOME, S. ISHII, Y. KAI, AND M. CHIBA. Effect of caerulein upon insulin and glucagon secretion in dogs. *Horm. Metab. Res.* 10: 7–11, 1978.
162. OHNEDA, A., S. ISHII, K. HORIGOME, M. CHIBA, T. SAKAI, Y. KAI, K. WANTANABE, AND S. YAMAGATA. Effect of intrapan-

creatic administration of vasoactive intestinal peptide upon the release of insulin and glucagon in dogs. *Horm. Metab. Res.* 9: 447–452, 1977.

163. OHTANI, O. Microcirculation of the pancreas: a correlative study of intravital microscopy with scanning electron microscopy of vascular corrosion casts. *Arch. Histol. Jpn.* 46: 315–325, 1983.

164. OHTANI, O. Microvascular organization of the salivary glands as visualized by scanning electron microscopy of microvascular corrosion casts. In: *Microcirculation of the Alimentary Tract*, edited by A. Koo, S. K. Lam, and L. H. Smaje. Singapore: World Scientific, 1983, p. 11–16.

165. OHTANI, O. Review of scanning electron and light microscopic methods in microcirculation research and their application in pancreatic studies. *Scanning Electron Micros.* 2: 653–661, 1984.

166. OHTANI, O., AND T. FUJITA. Microcirculation of the pancreas with special reference to periductular circulation. A scanning electron microscope study of vascular casts. *Biomed. Res.* 1: 130–140, 1980.

167. OHTANI, O., AND T. FUJITA. Insulo-acinar portal system of the pancreas. A scanning electron microscope study of corrosion casts. In: *Progress in Clinical Biological Research. Advances in the Morphology of Cells and Tissues*, edited by E. A. Vidrio and M. A. Galina. New York: Liss, 1981, vol. 59B, p. 111–120.

168. OHTANI, O., A. KIKUTA, A. OHTSUKA, T. TAGUCHI, AND T. MURAKAMI. Microvasculature as studied by the microvascular corrosion casting/scanning electron microscope method. I. Endocrine and digestive system. *Arch. Histol. Jpn.* 46: 1–42, 1983.

169. OHTANI, O., A. OHTSUKA, J. LIPSETT, AND B. GANNON. The microvasculature of rat salivary glands. A scanning electron microscopic study. *Acta. Anat.* 115: 345–356, 1983.

170. OHTANI, O., A. OHTSUKA, AND T. MURAKAMI. Microvascular organization of the pancreas. In: *Microcirculation of the Alimentary Tract*, edited by A. Koo, S. K. Lam, and L. H. Smaje. Singapore: World Scientific, 1983, p. 29–38.

171. BERG, T., ORSTAVIK, T. B., O. A. CARRETERO, AND G. SCICLI. Kallikrein-kinin system in the regulation of submandibular gland blood flow. *Am. J. Physiol.* 242 (*Heart Circ. Physiol.* 11): H1010–H1014, 1982.

172. PALADE, G. E., M. SIMIONESCU, AND N. SIMIONESCU. Structural aspects of the permeability of the microvascular endothelium. *Acta. Physiol. Scand. Suppl.* 463: 11–32, 1979.

173. PALADE, G. E., M. SIMIONESCU, AND N. SIMIONESCU. Differentiated microdomains on the luminal surface of the capillary endothelium. *Biorheology* 17: 563–568, 1981.

174. PAPP, M. Role of the circulation in acute pancreatitis. In: *Pathophysiology of the Splanchnic Circulation*, edited by P. R. Kvietys, J. A. Barrowman, and D. N. Granger. Boca Raton, FL: CRC, 1987, vol. 2, p. 119–135.

175. PAPP, M., S. FEHER, B. VARGA, AND G. FOLLY. Humoral influences on local blood flow and external secretion of the resting dog pancreas. *Acta Med. Acad. Sci. Hung.* 34: 185–198, 1977.

176. PAPP, M., G. B. MAKARA, AND G. FOLLY. Impeded interstitial fluid movement: a factor in pancreatic edema. *Lymphology* 8: 148–153, 1975.

177. PAPP, M., B. VARGA, Z. S. ACS, I. KRASZNAI, AND J. FOELDES. Pharmacological effects on pancreatic blood flow. *Arch. Int. Pharmacodyn.* 161: 61–67, 1966.

178. PAPP, M., B. VARGA, AND G. FOLLY. Effects of secretin, pancreozymin, histamine and decholin and canine pancreatic blood flow. *Pfluegers Arch.* 340: 349–360, 1973.

179. PAPP, M., B. VARGA, G. VARGA, AND G. FOLLY. Pancreatic Secretion: I. Effects of vasopressin and glucagon on pancreatic blood flow and secretion. *Mt. Sinai J. Med.* 50: 439–440, 1983.

180. PASCAL, J. P., P. ROUX, N. VAYSSE, A. LACROIX, C. MARTINEL, AND A. RIBET. Respiratory exchanges and acid-base balance during perfusion of ex vivo isolated pancreas. *Dig. Dis. Sci.* 21: 381–388, 1976.

181. PERNOW, B. Substance P: its distribution, pharmacological actions and possible physiological role in sensory neurons. *Clin. Physiol.* 1: 235–251, 1981.

182. PERRY, M. A., AND D. N. GRANGER. Permeability of intestinal capillaries to small molecules. *Am. J. Physiol.* 241 (*Gastrointest. Liver Physiol.* 4): G24–G30, 1981.

183. PERRY, M. A., AND D. N. GRANGER. Permeability of intestinal capillaries to small solutes and to plasma proteins. In: *Microcirculation of the Alimentary Tract*, edited by A. Koo, S. K. Lam, and L. H. Smaje. Singapore: World Scientific, 1983, p. 179–196.

184. PISSAS, A. Anatomoclinical and anatomosurgical essay on the lymphatic circulation of the pancreas. *Anat. Clin.* 6: 255–280, 1984.

185. PISSIOTIS, C. A., R. E. CONDON, AND L. M. NYHUS. Effect of vasopressin on pancreatic blood flow in acute hemorrhagic pancreatitis. *Am. J. Surg.* 123: 203–208, 1972.

186. POLANSKY, D. B., AND S. SAFAIE-SHIRAZI. Simultaneous measurements of pancreatic blood flow, endocrine, and exocrine secretion in conscious dogs. *Surg. Forum* 28: 91–93, 1977.

187. POULSEN, J. H. Two phases of chorda-lingual induced vasodilation in the cat's submandibular gland during prolonged perfusion with Locke solution. *J. Physiol. Lond.* 253: 79–94, 1975.

188. PREMEN, A. J., P. R. KVIETYS, AND D. N. GRANGER. Postprandial regulation of intestinal blood flow: role of gastrointestinal hormones. *Am. J. Physiol.* 249 (*Gastrointest. Liver Physiol.* 12): G250–G255, 1985.

189. PRICE, B. A., B. M. JAFFE, AND M. J. ZINNER. Effect of exogenous somatostatin infusion on gastrointestinal blood flow and hormones in the conscious dog. *Gastroenterology* 88: 80–85, 1985.

190. RABITO, S. F., T. B. ORSTAVIK, A. G. SCICLI, A. SCHORK, AND O. A. CARRETERO. Role of the autonomic nervous system in the release of rat submandibular gland kallikrein into the circulation. *Circ. Res.* 52: 635–641, 1983.

191. RAPPAPORT, A. M., T. KAWAMURA, J. K. DAVIDSON, B. J. LIN, S. OHIRA, M. ZEIGLER, J. A. CODDLING, J. HENDERSON, AND R. E. HAIST. Effects of hormones and of blood flow on insulin output of isolated pancreas in situ. *Am. J. Physiol.* 221: 343–348, 1971.

192. RAPPAPORT, A. M., S. OHIRA, J. A. CODDLING, G. EMPEY, A. KALNINS, B. J. LIN, AND R. E. HAIST. Effects on insulin output and on pancreatic blood flow of exogenous insulin infusion into an in situ isolated portion of the pancreas. *Endocrinology* 91: 168–176, 1972.

193. REGAN, T. J. Regional circulatory responses to alcohol and its congeners. *Federation Proc.* 41: 2438–2442, 1982.

194. RENKIN, E. M., AND F. E. CURRY. Transport of water and solutes across capillary endothelium. *Membrane Transport in Biology. Transport Organs*, edited by G. Giebisch, D. C. Tosteson, and H. H. Ussing. Berlin: Springer-Verlag, 1978, vol 4, p. 1–45.

195. RIBES, G., E. R. SRIMBLE, J. BLAYAC, C. B. WOLLHEIM, AND M. LOUBATIERES-MARIANI. In vivo stimulation of pancreatic hormone secretion by norepinephrine infusion in the dog. *Am. J. Physiol.* 246 (*Endocrinol. Metab.* 9): E339–E343, 1984.

196. RICHARDSON, P. D. I., AND D. N. GRANGER. Capillary filtration coefficient as a measure of perfused capillary density. In: *Measurement of Blood Flow: Applications to the Splanchnic Circulation*, edited by D. N. Granger and G. B. Bulkley. Baltimore, MD: Williams & Wilkins, 1981, p. 321–336.

197. RICHARDSON, P. D. I., D. N. GRANGER, AND A. E. TAYLOR. Capillary filtration coefficient: The technique and its application to the small intestine. *Cardiovasc. Res.* 13: 547–561, 1979.

198. ROBIE, N. W., AND J. L. MCNAY. Comparative splanchnic blood flow effects of various vasodilator compounds. *Circ. Shock* 4: 69–78, 1977.

199. ROMANES, G. J. (editor). *Cunningham's Textbook of Anatomy* (12th ed.). London: Oxford Univ. Press, 1972.

200. ROSSINI, R. B., A. B. MACHADO, AND C. R. S. MACHADO. A histochemical study of catecholamines and cholinesterases in the autonomib nerves of the human minor salivary glands. *Histochem. J.* 11: 661–668, 1979.

201. RUSZNYAK, I., M. FOLDI, AND G. SZABO. *Lymphatics and*

*Lymph Circulation. Physiology and Pathology.* Oxford, UK: Pergamon, 1967. [Transl. by A. Deak and J. Fesus.]
202. RUTBERG, U. Ultrastructure and secretory mechanisms of the parotid gland. *Acta Odontol. Scand.* 19, Suppl. 30: 7–69, 1961.
203. SATOH, S., N. TAIRA, AND K. HASHIMOTO. Absence of a neurally-mediated process in salivation and vasodilation caused by McN-A-343 in the dog submaxillary gland. *Jpn. J. Pharmacol.* 23: 581, 1973.
204. SATOH, S., O. TAKEUCHI, AND K. HASHIMOTO. Pharmacological behavior of the submaxillary gland and its vasculature of the dog. *Tohoku J. Exp. Med.* 108: 377–388, 1972.
205. SCHACHTER, M., S. BARTON, AND E. KARPINSKI. Sympathetic vasodilatation in the submaxillary gland and its enhancement after chronic parasympathetic denervation. *Experientia Basel* 29: 1498–1499, 1973.
206. SCHACTER, M., AND S. BEILENSON. Kallikrein and vasodilation in the submaxillary gland. *Gastroenterology* 52: 401–405, 1967.
207. SEELIG, R. F., J. C. KERR, R. W. HOBSON II, AND G. W. MACHIEDO. Prostacyclin (epoprostenol): its effect on canine splanchnic blood flow during hemorrhagic shock. *Arch. Surg.* 116: 428–430, 1981.
208. SHAPIRO, H., AND L. G. BRITT. The action of vasopressin on the gastrointestinal tract. *Dig. Dis. Sci.* 17: 649–667, 1972.
209. SHIMIZU, T., K. NUNOKI, AND N. TAIRA. Characterization of neuronal and vascular histamine receptors mediating the salivary and vasodilator responses to histamine of the dog submandibular gland. *Tohoku J. Exp. Med.* 134: 1–8, 1981.
210. SHIMIZU, T., AND N. TAIRA. Assessment of the effects of vasoactive intestinal peptide (VIP) on blood flow through and salivation of the dog salivary gland in comparison with those of secretin, glucagon, and acetylcholine. *Br. J. Pharmacol.* 65: 683–687, 1979.
211. SHIMIZU, T., AND N. TAIRA. Pharmacological analysis of salivary and blood flow responses to histamine of the submandibular gland of the dog. *Br. J. Pharmacol.* 68: 651–661, 1980.
212. SHULIN, A. Blood flow changes in the submaxillary gland of the rat on parasympathetic and sympathetic nerve stimulation. *Acta Physiol. Scand.* 97: 104–109, 1976.
213. SIMIONESCU, M., N. SIMIONESCU, AND G. E. PALADE. Morphometric data on the endothelium of blood capillaries. *J. Cell Biol.* 60: 128–152, 1974.
214. SIMIONESCU, M., N. SIMIONESCU, AND G. E. PALADE. Preferential distribution of anionic sites on the basement membrane and the abluminal aspect of the endothelium in fenestrated capillaries. *J. Cell Biol.* 95: 425–434, 1982.
215. SIMIONESCU, M., N. SIMIONESCU, AND G. E. PALADE. Partial chemical characterization of the anionic sites in the basal lamina of fenestrated capillaries. *Microvasc. Res.* 28: 352–367, 1984.
216. SIMIONESCU, N., M. SIMIONESCU, AND G. E. PALADE. Differentiated microdomains on the luminal surface of the capillary endothelium. I. Preferential distribution of anionic sites. *J. Cell Biol.* 90: 605–613, 1981.
217. SKINNER, N. S., JR., J. C. COSTIN, AND M. E. WEBSTER. Acetylcholine and functional vasodilation in the submaxillary gland of the cat. *Eur. J. Pharmacol.* 12: 271–275, 1970.
218. SKINNER, N. S., JR., AND M. E. WEBSTER. Kinins, beta-adrenergic receptors and functional vasodilatation in the submaxillary gland of the cat. *J. Physiol. Lond.* 195: 505–519, 1968.
219. SMAJE, L. H. Permeability of salivary gland capillaries. In: *Microcirculation of the Alimentary Tract,* edited by A. Koo, S. K. Lam, and L. H. Smaje. Singapore: World Scientific, 1983, p. 167–177.
220. SMAJE, L. H., AND J. R. HENDERSON. Microcirculation of the exocrine glands. In: *The Physiology and Pharmacology of the Microcirculation,* edited by N. A. Mortillaro. Orlando, FL: Academic, 1984, vol. 2, p. 325–385.
221. SPARKS, H. V., JR. Effects of local metabolic factors on vascular smooth muscle. In: *Handbook of Physiology. Cardiovascular System. Vascular Smooth Muscle,* edited by D. F. Bohr, A. T. Somlyo, and H. V. Sparks, Jr. Bethesda, MD: Am. Physiol. Soc., 1980, sect. 2, vol. II, chapt. 17, p. 475–513.
222. STANEK, K. A., J. J. NEIL, W. B. SAWYER, AND A. D. LOEWY. Changes in regional blood flow and cardiac output after L-glutamate stimulation of A5 cell group. *Am. J. Physiol.* 246 (*Heart Circ. Physiol.* 15): H44–H51, 1984.
223. STANOVNIK, L., AND F. ERJAVEC. The inhibition of salivary secretion by histamine $H_2$-antagonists: a study on the cat submandibular gland. *Agents Actions* 13: 196–199, 1983.
224. STARLING, E. H. On the absorption of fluid from the connective tissue spaces. *J. Physiol. Lond.* 19: 312–326, 1896.
225. STROMBLAD, B. C. R. Gaserous metabolism of the normal and denervated submandibular gland of the cat. *J. Physiol. Lond.* 145: 551–561, 1959.
226. STROMBLAD, B. C. R., AND P. E. DRESSEL. Experiments on atropine-resistant vasodilation in salivary glands. *Can. J. Biochem. Physiol.* 41: 519–524, 1963.
227. STUDLEY, J. G. N., J. B. LEE, AND W. G. SCHENK, JR. Effects of indomethacin on blood flow in the normal pancreas in conscious dogs. *J. Surg. Res.* 37: 464–466, 1984.
228. TAIRA, N., A. NARIMATSU, AND S. SATOH. Differential block by 1-hyoscyamine of the salivary and vascular responses of the dog mandibular gland to prostaglandin $F_{2\alpha}$. *Life Sci.* 17: 1869–1875, 1975.
229. TAKADA, M. Fenestrated venules of the large salivary glands. *Anat. Rec.* 166: 605–610, 1970.
230. TAYLOR, A. E. Capillary fluid filtration: Starling forces and lymph flow. *Circ. Res.* 49: 557–575, 1981.
231. TAYLOR, A. E., AND D. N. GRANGER. Exchange of macromolecules across the circulation. In: *Handbook of Physiology. The Cardiovascular System. Microcirculation,* edited by E. M. Renkin and C. C. Michel. Bethesda, MD: Am. Physiol. Soc., 1984, sect. 2, vol. IV, pt. 1, chapt. 11, p. 467–520.
232. TEMPLETON, D., AND A. THULIN. Secretory, motor and vascular effects in sublingual gland of the rat caused by autonomic nerve stimulation. *Q. J. Exp. Physiol.* 63: 59–66, 1978.
233. TERROUX, K. G., P. SEKELJ, AND A. S. V. BURGEN. Oxygen consumption and blood flow in the submaxillary gland of the dog. *Can. J. Biochem. Physiol.* 37: 5–15, 1959.
234. TETSUO, S., K. NUNOKI, AND N. TAIRA. Characterization of neuronal and vascular histamine receptors mediating the salivary and vasodilator responses to histamine of the dog submandibular gland. *Tohoku J. Exp. Med.* 134: 1–8, 1981.
235. THULIN, L., AND P. OLSSON. Effects of pure natural cholecystokinin on splanchnic circulation in the dog. *Acta Chir. Scand.* 139: 681–686, 1973.
236. VAYSSE, N., M. J. BASTIE, J. P. PASCAL, C. MARTINEL, G. FOURTANIER, AND A. RIBET. Effects of catecholamines and their inhibitors on the isolated canine pancreas. I. Noradrenaline and isoprenaline. *Gastroenterology* 72: 711–718, 1977.
237. WALLACH, S., G. A. CHARBON, H. J. M. BEIJER, H. J. ENDEMAN, J. O. O. HOEKE, J. SCHRIJVER, AND A. STRUYVENBERG. Effects of furosemide on biliary secretion, pancreatic blood flow, and pancreatic exocrine secretion. *J. Clin. Pharmacol.* 23: 401–413, 1983.
238. WALTERS, M. N., J. M. PAPADIMITRIOCE, T. A. ROBERTSON, AND J. M. ARCHER. Permeability of pancreatic endothelium to horseradish peroxidase. *J. Pathol.* 100: 31–37, 1970.
239. WARNER, N. E. Blood vessels and lymphatics of the pancreas. In: *Blood Vessels and Lymphatics in Organ Systems,* edited by D. I. Abramson and P. B. Dobrin. Orlando, FL: Academic, 1984, p. 296–304.
240. WHEATON, L. G., M. G. SAAR, L. SCHLOSSBERG, AND G. B. BULKLEY. Gross anatomy of the splanchnic vasculature. In: *Measurement of Blood Flow: Applications to the Splanchnic Circulation,* edited by D. N. Granger and G. B. Bulkley. Baltimore, MD: Williams & Wilkins, 1981, p. 9–45.
241. WILLIAMS, P. L., AND R. WARWICK. *Gray's Anatomy* (36th ed.). Philadelphia, PA: Saunders, 1980.
242. ZINNER, M. J., F. KASHER, I. M. MODLIN, AND B. M. JAFFE. Effect of xenopsin on blood flow, hormone release, and acid secretion. *Am. J. Physiol.* 243 (*Gastrointest. Liver Physiol.* 6): G195–G199, 1982.

CHAPTER 43

# Neonatal intestinal circulation

PHILIP T. NOWICKI | *Department of Pediatrics, Ohio State University and Children's Hospital Research Foundation, Columbus, Ohio*

CHAPTER CONTENTS

Hemodynamics and Oxygenation of Fasting Neonatal Intestine
Neural Regulation of Neonatal Intestinal Circulation
   Transection of splanchnic nerve
   Direct stimulation of splanchnic nerve
   Reflex control of neonatal intestinal circulation
Intrinsic Regulation of Neonatal Intestinal Circulation
   Response to feeding
   Response to hypoxemia
   Response to hypotension
Summary

UNTIL RECENTLY a paucity of data existed on neonatal intestinal circulation. Recent work, however, has begun to characterize the physiology of the intestinal circulation during fetal and postnatal life. Initial investigations focused primarily on the response of the neonatal intestinal circulation to physiological perturbations common to human neonates, such as asphyxia, because this response was considered germane to the pathogenesis of several neonatal diseases, including necrotizing enterocolitis (16, 28). More recent studies, however, have begun to explore regulation of intestinal hemodynamics and oxygenation in the perinatal period.

Porcine and ovine species have been the most widely used animals for studying the neonatal intestinal circulation because the newborn of these species are sufficiently large to permit surgical instrumentation. The lamb offers the advantage of adaptability to chronic instrumentation during both fetal and neonatal life. However, the piglet shares more physiological similarities with the human infant, particularly as regards developmental, nutritional, and digestive physiology (3); thus they may be more suited for these investigations.

## HEMODYNAMICS AND OXYGENATION OF FASTING NEONATAL INTESTINE

At birth the neonatal gastrointestinal tract becomes solely responsible for assimilation of water and nutrients. The functional activities of the intestine, including absorption, secretion, and motility, increase significantly in the immediate postnatal period. Concurrent with this increase in intestinal function is a phase of rapid intestinal growth. Swine intestinal weight increases fourfold in the first 9 postnatal days (29), whereas lamb intestine doubles in weight every 2 wk for the first 2 mo after birth (8). The intense anabolic activity of the postnatal intestine suggests that the oxidative requirements of the fasting neonatal intestine may be greater than those of adult intestine. Therefore, it might be anticipated that the neonatal intestinal circulation is specifically adapted to meet these increased oxidative demands and that the fasting conditions of the neonatal intestinal circulation might be dissimilar from those described in the adult intestine.

Intestinal circulation during fasting has been investigated in chronically catheterized fetal (6, 27) and neonatal (5, 8) lambs (Table 1). During fetal life, intestinal blood flow increased from ~40 $ml \cdot min^{-1} \cdot 100\ g^{-1}$ at midgestation (27) to 100 $ml \cdot min^{-1} \cdot 100\ g^{-1}$ at term gestation (6). Following birth, intestinal blood flow increased to ~200 $ml \cdot min^{-1} \cdot 100\ g^{-1}$ and intestinal oxygen uptake also increased significantly (5, 8). Edelstone and Holzman (5) speculated that these changes reflect an adaptation to the different metabolic requirements of fetal and postnatal intestine.

Fasting values for gastrointestinal blood flow and oxygen uptake have also been determined in chronically catheterized, conscious swine [Table 1; (25)]. The gastrointestinal tract received 12% of the cardiac output in neonatal swine. Blood flow to the stomach, jejunum, ileum, and colon averaged 120, 145, 95, and 75 $ml \cdot min^{-1} \cdot 100\ g^{-1}$, respectively. Within the jejunum and ileum, the mucosa and submucosa received 85% of the total intestinal blood flow. Values for intestinal blood flow and oxygen uptake in neonatal swine were lower than those observed in lambs. The discrepancy between fasting circulatory conditions in neonatal lamb and swine intestine may be due, in part, to the digestive physiology of these species. The lamb is a ruminant species, and although true ruminant digestive physiology may not commence for several weeks after birth, it is conceivable that the ruminant newborn may never be in a true fasting or preprandial state (25). By contrast, the swine is a nonruminant species, and the gastric emptying and intestinal tran-

TABLE 1. *Intestinal Hemodynamics and Oxygenation in Fasting Neonatal Intestine*

|  | Swine | Lamb |
|---|---|---|
| Age, days | 2 | 7 |
| Arterial blood pressure, mmHg | 58 | 60 |
| Intestinal blood flow, ml·min$^{-1}$·100 g$^{-1}$ | 135 | 214 |
| Intestinal vascular resistance, mmHg·ml$^{-1}$·min·100 g$^{-1}$ | 0.43 | 0.27 |
| Intestinal oxygen extraction, % | 18 | 21 |
| Intestinal oxygen uptake, ml O$_2$·min$^{-1}$·100 g$^{-1}$ | 1.99 | 5.60 |
| Hematocrit, % | 27 | 27 |
| Arterial oxygen content, ml O$_2$/dl | 10.4 | 12.6 |
| Arterial P$_{O_2}$, mmHg | 83 | 83 |

Mean values of chronically catheterized, conscious animals. [Data for lambs from Edelstone and Holzman (7); data for swine from Nowicki et al. (25).]

sit times of newborn swine closely approximate those in human infants. Although fasting blood flow and oxygen uptake were lower in neonatal swine than in lambs, these values were still considerably higher than those reported for the intestinal circulations of adult cats and dogs (11, 19).

The hemodynamic conditions in the fasting intestine change in the first postnatal month (2, 20). In anesthetized (pentobarbital) swine, Buckley et al. (2) demonstrated that mesenteric artery blood flow increased from 32 ml·min$^{-1}$ to 123 ml·min$^{-1}$ from birth to 4 wk of age. This increase was associated with a reduction in mesenteric artery resistance from 2.4 pressure resistance units (PRU) to 1.1 PRU and an increase in mean aortic blood pressure from 68 mmHg to 95 mmHg. In extrinsically denervated loops of swine intestine, Nowicki (20) observed a decrease in intestinal blood flow from 60 ml·min$^{-1}$·100 g$^{-1}$ to 27 ml·min$^{-1}$·100 g$^{-1}$ in the first postnatal month. Because these data were expressed per unit of tissue weight, direct comparison with the data of Buckley et al. (2) is not feasible. The data of Nowicki (20) indicate that circulatory conditions within the fasting intestine undergo a postnatal transition, so that by 1 mo after birth these conditions are similar to those previously reported in adult canine intestine (11).

## NEURAL REGULATION OF NEONATAL INTESTINAL CIRCULATION

The effect of transection and direct and reflex stimulation of the splanchnic nerve on intestinal hemodynamics has been investigated in swine of various postnatal ages. These experiments were performed in animals anesthetized with pentobarbital, and the intestines were in situ (and thus autoperfused) during data collection. For transection and direct nerve-stimulation studies, the left splanchnic nerve was instrumented in the retroperitoneal space just rostral to the diaphragm.

### Transection of Splanchnic Nerve

Transection of the splanchnic nerve resulted in a 13% decrease in mesenteric artery vascular resistance in 1-day-old swine but did not significantly affect mesenteric artery blood flow. At 2–4 days old, however, splanchnic nerve transection resulted in a 14% increase in mesenteric artery blood flow. By 2 wk old, splanchnic nerve transection resulted in a 22% increase in mesenteric artery blood flow and a 16% reduction in mesenteric artery vascular resistance. These data indicate that sympathetic innervation contributes to mesenteric artery tone in the immediate postnatal period and that this contribution increases with advancing postnatal age (2).

### Direct Stimulation of Splanchnic Nerve

Constant-current stimulation of the splanchnic nerve (0.5–1.0 mA, 3 Hz, 1.2-ms pulse duration for 20 s) resulted in a significant reduction in mesenteric artery blood flow and an increase in mesenteric artery vascular resistance in neonatal swine. This effect of splanchnic nerve stimulation was blocked by prior administration of phentolamine (0.25–0.75 mg/kg iv). The magnitude of mesenteric artery vasoconstriction during splanchnic nerve stimulation was age dependent. Constant-current stimulation (0.5–1.0 mA, 15 Hz, 1.2-ms pulse duration for 20 s) increased mesenteric vascular resistance by 18%, 29%, and 65% in 1-day-old, 2-wk-old, and 1-mo-old animals, respectively. The latency between nerve stimulation and mesenteric artery vasoconstriction was significantly shorter in older animals (2).

### Reflex Control of Neonatal Intestinal Circulation

Carotid sinus inhibition by bilateral carotid artery occlusion was accompanied by a 6%–10% increase in mesenteric artery vascular resistance in neonatal swine, and the magnitude of this vasoconstriction was similar in 1-mo-old animals (2). Although the baroreceptor response is immature in neonatal swine, this response did include vasoconstriction of the mesenteric artery (9). The role of intestinal circulation in the systemic cardiovascular response to the stress of hemorrhagic hypotension or hypoxemia has also been determined in neonatal swine. Rapid hemorrhage (5–15 ml/kg) resulted in mesenteric artery vasoconstriction and decreased mesenteric artery blood flow in animals 2–7 days old (10). The effect of hypoxemia was dependent on the degree to which P$_{O_2}$, and thus arterial oxygen content, was lowered. Moderate hypoxemia (P$_{O_2}$ = 50 mmHg) resulted in mesenteric artery vasodilation and increased mesenteric artery blood flow. By contrast, severe hypoxemia (P$_{O_2}$ = 25 mmHg) resulted in mesenteric artery vasoconstriction and intestinal ischemia (10). Prior administration of phentolamine (1.5 mg/kg) or surgical denervation of the intestine eliminated the mesenteric artery vasoconstriction observed during severe hypoxemia in neonatal swine (21).

Extrinsic neurohumoral regulation facilitates integration of intestinal circulation into systemic cardiovascular responses. The aforementioned data indicate that functional sympathetic innervation of intestinal circulation is present, but relatively immature, in the neonatal period and that rapid postnatal maturation of sympathetic innervation occurs. Although it is clear that extrinsic neural regulation of intestinal circulation is present in the postnatal period, numerous aspects of this regulation remain to be elucidated. The studies of Buckley et al. (2) did not include observation of the effect of sympathetic stimulation on intestinal oxygen uptake, nor were the nerve-stimulation periods of sufficient duration to determine if "autoregulatory escape" from sympathetic stimulation (26) occurs in the neonatal intestinal circulation. Furthermore, the role of humoral factors in the extrinsic regulation of the neonatal intestinal circulation is virtually unexplored.

## INTRINSIC REGULATION OF NEONATAL INTESTINAL CIRCULATION

Studies in adult animals have determined that intrinsic, or local, control of the intestinal circulation plays a major role in regulation of intestinal hemodynamics and oxygenation (11, 12). Intrinsic regulation is totally independent of extrinsic nervous activity. Of the several mechanisms hypothesized to explain intrinsic regulation, the myogenic hypothesis (14) and the metabolic hypothesis (12) have received the most experimental support. The myogenic hypothesis is based on the ability of vascular smooth muscle within the microcirculation to alter its tone in response to

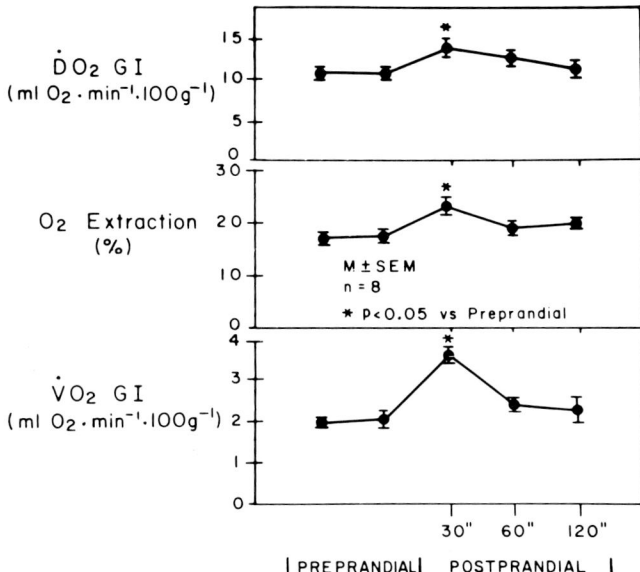

FIG. 2. Effect of feeding on $O_2$ delivery, extraction, and uptake by gastrointestinal tract in neonatal swine fasted for 8 h prior to feeding. Oxygen delivery was calculated as the product of blood flow and arterial $O_2$ content; $O_2$ extraction, as the ratio of arteriovenous $O_2$ difference ($a - v\ O_2$) to arterial $O_2$ content; and $O_2$ uptake, as the product of blood flow and $a - v\ O_2$. $\dot{D}_{O_2}$, oxygen delivery; $\dot{V}_{O_2}$, oxygen uptake. [From Nowicki et al. (25).]

changes in transmural pressure (14). The myogenic mechanism serves to regulate capillary pressure; thus, according to the myogenic hypothesis, blood-tissue fluid exchange is the principal variable controlled at the local (tissue) level (17). By contrast, the metabolic hypothesis postulates that tissue oxygen uptake is the principal variable controlled by intrinsic vascular regulation (11). According to the metabolic hypothesis, a feedback signal is produced by the intestinal parenchyma in proportion to the oxidative requirements of the tissue. This signal interacts with vascular elements within the microcirculation (resistance vessels and precapillary sphincters) to regulate local oxygen-transport processes. In this fashion the metabolic feedback signal couples intestinal oxidative requirements with the actions of the intestinal microcirculation and so maintains tissue oxygen uptake at a level consistent with the metabolic activity of the tissue (11).

Most studies of the neonatal intestinal circulation have employed chronically catheterized animal preparations or preparations in which the intestinal circulation was innervated during data collection. This experimental design eliminates the confounding variables of anesthesia and recent surgical trauma but simultaneously limits delineation between neural and intrinsic regulation of the intestinal circulation. Therefore, evidence for intrinsic regulation of the neonatal intestinal circulation is primarily indirect. Evidence for intrinsic metabolic regulation of the neo-

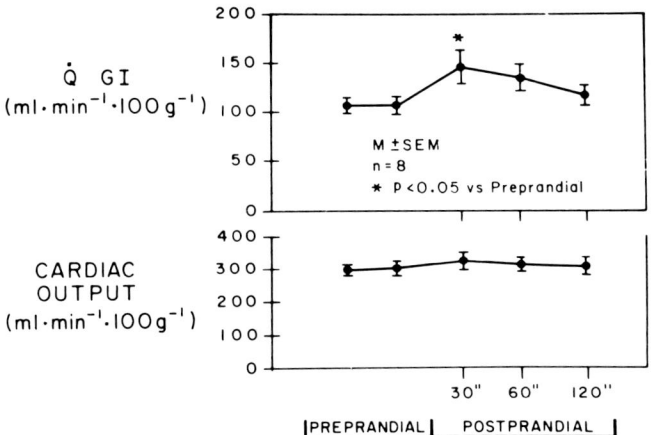

FIG. 1. Effect of feeding on total gastrointestinal blood flow and cardiac output in neonatal swine fasted for 8 h prior to feeding. $\dot{Q}$, perfusion; GI, gastrointestinal system. [From Nowicki et al. (25).]

natal intestinal circulation is derived from studies in which tissue oxygen uptake was quantified during imposed changes in the availability-to-demand ratio of oxygen. Feeding (increased oxygen requirements) and hypoxemia or hypotension (decreased oxygen supply) have been used to alter the oxygen–availability-to-demand ratio in the neonatal intestine. At present no experimental data exists to support the presence of a myogenic response in the neonatal intestinal circulation.

*Response to Feeding*

The phenomenon of postprandial hyperemia has been studied in chronically catheterized, conscious neonatal lambs (4) and swine [Fig. 1; (25)]. In lambs the total gastrointestinal blood flow increased by 23% 1 h after feeding, and this postprandial hyperemia was localized to the stomach. Oxygen extraction by the intestine increased by 41% and 45% at 1 and 2 h after feeding, respectively; oxygen uptake by the entire gastrointestinal tract increased by 65% and 51% at 1 and 2 h after feeding (4). The relatively small degree of postprandial hyperemia and its localization to the stomach might be the consequence of the ruminant digestive physiology of the ovine species (25). Nowicki et al. (25) fasted 2-day-old swine for 8 h prior to orogastric gavage feeding with artificial sow milk. Total gastrointestinal blood flow increased 35% 30 min after feeding, but then rapidly returned to preprandial levels (Fig. 2). This increase in gastrointestinal blood flow was not accompanied by an increase in cardiac output. The postprandial hyperemia was localized to the small intestine, primarily the mucosal layer of the jejunum. Oxygen extraction by the intestine increased 33% 30 min after feeding, and total gastrointestinal oxygen uptake increased 72% at that time (Fig. 3). Using intravital microscopy, Meller et al. (18) also noted an increase in jejunal blood flow in neonatal swine intestine after instillation of glucose into the jejunum. Ileal blood flow did not change when glucose was instilled into the jejunal segment, and no change in jejunal or ileal blood flow was noted when water or a hypertonic mannitol solution was infused into the jejunum. Yao et al. (30) demonstrated that the magnitude and duration of the postprandial hyperemia was dependent on postnatal age. These investigators measured mesenteric artery flow in anesthetized (pentobarbital) 2-day-old and 2-wk-old swine before and after feeding. Neonatal animals demonstrated a 16% increase in mesenteric artery flow 30 min after feeding. By contrast, older animals demonstrated a 38% increase in mesenteric artery flow 30 min after feeding, and this postprandial hyperemia lasted 120 min. This increase in mesenteric artery flow was due to a concomitant reduction in mesenteric vascular resistance, not an increase in cardiac output or systemic blood pressure.

*Response to Hypoxemia*

The effect of hypoxic hypoxemia on intestinal hemodynamics and oxygenation has been evaluated

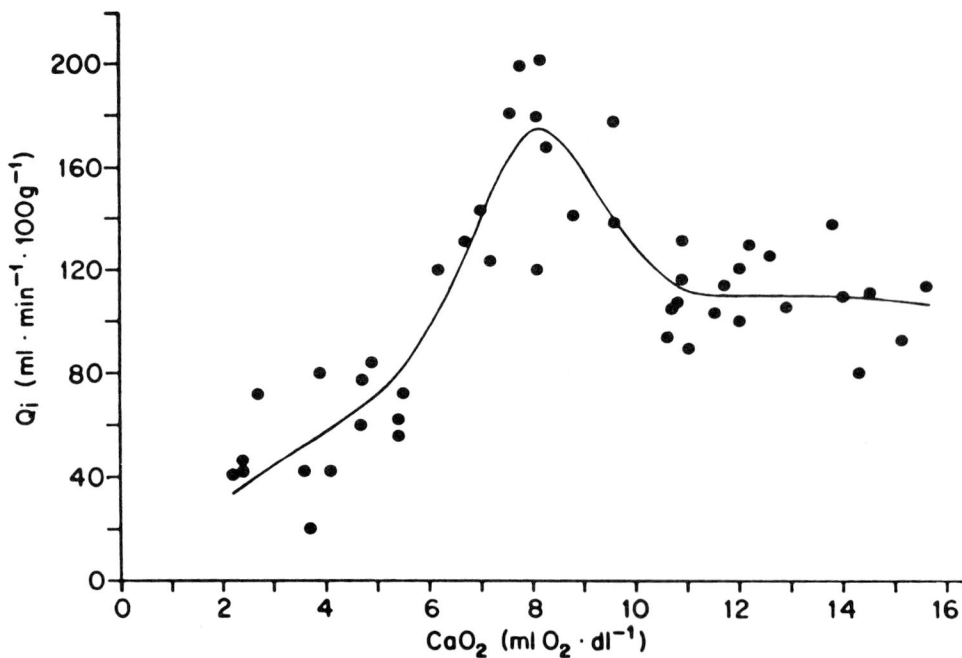

FIG. 3. Intestinal blood flow ($\dot{Q}_i$) as a function of arterial $O_2$ content ($Ca_{O_2}$) in neonatal swine. *Curve*, 46 measurements in 23 animals: $y = 0.135e^{[-0.34(x-8.08)^2]} + 16x - 0.64x^2$. [From Nowicki et al. (22).]

in neonatal swine (15, 22) and lambs (8). In swine mild hypoxic hypoxemia ($P_{O_2}$ = 50–60 mmHg, arterial oxygen content = 7–9 ml $O_2$/dl) resulted in an increase in intestinal blood flow; however, severe hypoxic hypoxemia ($P_{O_2}$ < 30 mmHg, arterial oxygen content < 5 ml $O_2$/dl) resulted in a decrease in intestinal blood flow (Fig. 3). These changes in intestinal blood flow were mediated primarily by changes in intestinal vascular resistance, not by changes in cardiac output. Oxygen uptake by the intestine was unaffected by reduction of arterial oxygen content until the latter was decreased below 4.5 ml $O_2$/dl, at which point oxygen uptake decreased (Fig. 4). Nowicki et al. (22) postulated that intestinal vasodilation during moderate hypoxemia was mediated by intrinsic vascular regulation, whereas vasoconstriction during severe hypoxemia was mediated by neural regulation of the intestinal circulation. This hypothesis was supported by the observation that intestinal vascular resistance remained unchanged during severe hypoxemia following surgical denervation of the intestine (21). In lambs, Edelstone et al. (8) did not observe intestinal vasodilation during moderate degrees of hypoxic hypoxemia but did note intestinal vasoconstriction during severe hypoxemia. Oxygen extraction by the intestine increased as $P_{O_2}$ was reduced. Consequently intestinal oxygen uptake was preserved until arterial oxygen content was reduced below 6.5 ml $O_2$/dl.

The effect of anemic hypoxemia on intestinal hemodynamics and oxygenation has also been studied. In chronically catheterized neonatal lambs, hematocrit and arterial oxygen content were decreased from 32% and 13 ml $O_2$/dl to 20% and 8 ml $O_2$/dl over a period of 2 days. This degree of anemic hypoxemia did not significantly affect intestinal blood flow, oxygen extraction, or oxygen uptake (24). Holzman et al. (13) varied the hematocrit in chronically catheterized, conscious lambs (hematocrit range: 8–54%). These investigators observed no change in intestinal blood flow in response to changes in hematocrit; however, oxygen extraction by the intestine increased as hematocrit was reduced, and intestinal oxygen uptake was independent of hematocrit over the hematocrit range studied.

*Response to Hypotension*

The effect of perfusion-pressure reductions on intestinal hemodynamics and oxygenation has been determined in neonatal swine (1, 23). Nowicki et al. (23) decreased intestinal perfusion pressure by means of an aortic screw clamp in anesthetized (pentobarbital)

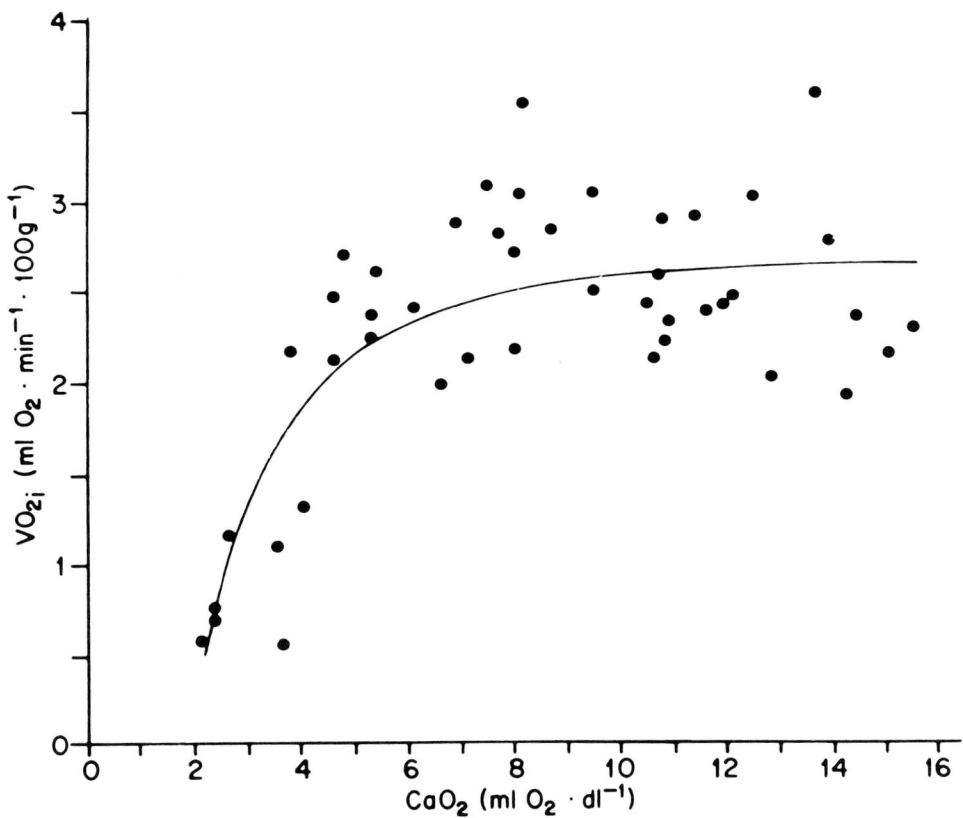

FIG. 4. Intestinal $O_2$ uptake ($V_{O_{2i}}$) as a function of arterial $O_2$ content ($Ca_{O_2}$) in neonatal swine. *Curve*, 46 measurements in 23 animals. $y = (4.905 \ln x - 3.14)^{x^{1/2}}$. [From Nowicki et al. (22).]

5-day-old animals. Each step reduction in perfusion pressure resulted in a decrease in intestinal blood flow that was quantitatively greater than the concomitant reduction in pressure (Fig. 5). Stated otherwise, pressure-flow regulation was not observed in neonatal intestinal circulation. However, oxygen extraction by the intestine increased as perfusion pressure was reduced (Fig. 6). Consequently tissue oxygen uptake was maintained at >95% of its base-line value until perfusion pressure was reduced to <70% of its base-line value (Fig. 7). Similar findings were reported by Buckley et al. (1).

Recent observations indicate that the response of intestinal circulation to perfusion-pressure reduction is dependent, in part, on postnatal age (1, 20). Buckley et al. (1) reported that pressure-flow regulation was present in the intestinal circulation of 1-mo-old swine. Nowicki (20) also observed that pressure-flow regulation was present in 1-mo-old animals. In addition these investigators reported that tissue oxygen uptake was more effectively maintained during perfusion-pressure reductions in 1-mo-old than in 3-day-old swine.

The responses to feeding, hypoxemia, and hypotension all suggest that intrinsic metabolic regulation of the intestinal circulation is present in neonates. In each instance tissue oxygen uptake, the variable postulated as the principal variable controlled by intrinsic metabolic regulation, was preserved despite minor fluctuations in the oxygen–availability-to-demand ratio. In addition the data of Yao et al. (30), Buckley et al. (1), and Nowicki (20) could be interpreted to indicate that the efficacy of intrinsic metabolic regulation of the intestinal circulation improves with advancing postnatal age. Much additional work is necessary, however, to confirm these observations. In particular

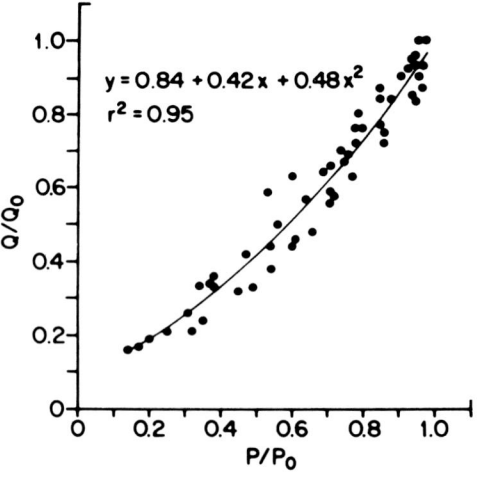

FIG. 5. Relationship between normalized intestinal blood flow ($\dot{Q}/\dot{Q}_0$) and normalized perfusion pressure ($P/P_0$) in neonatal swine. Curve, 6 measurements in each of 9 animals. [From Nowicki et al. (23).]

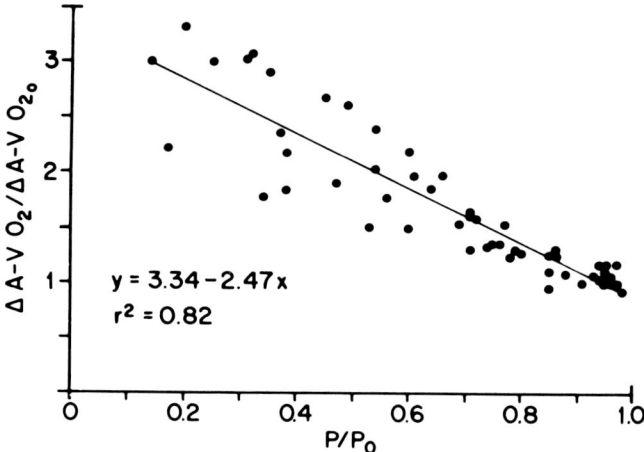

FIG. 6. Relationship between normalized arteriovenous $O_2$ difference ($a - v\ O_2 / a - v\ O_{2_0}$) and normalized perfusion pressure ($P/P_0$) in neonatal swine. Curve, 6 measurements from each of 9 animals. [From Nowicki et al. (23).]

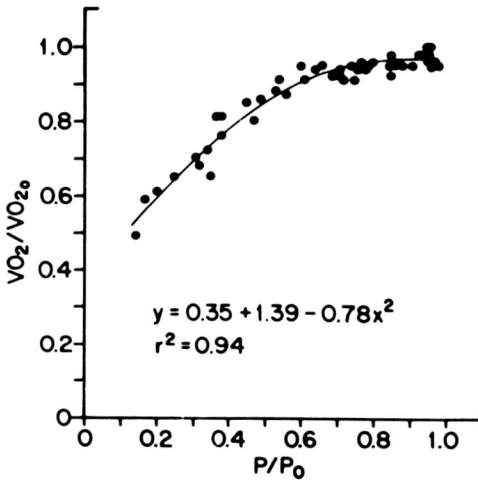

FIG. 7. Relationship between normalized intestinal $O_2$ uptake ($V_{O_2}/V_{O_{2_0}}$) and intestinal perfusion pressure ($P/P_0$) in neonatal swine. Curve, 6 measurements from each of 9 animals. [From Nowicki et al. (23).]

it is mandatory that the presence of intrinsic regulation be confirmed in denervated intestine. Assessment of the developmental changes in the efficacy of intrinsic regulation of the intestinal circulation requires strict control of other factors that might influence tissue oxygenation, such as hemoglobin concentration and hemoglobin oxygen-binding affinity. Evaluation of the myogenic response in the neonatal intestinal circulation also remains to be performed.

## SUMMARY

Regulation of intestinal hemodynamics and oxygenation is clearly present in the neonatal intestine. Existing data confirm that extrinsic neural regulation of the intestinal circulation is present immediately after birth and suggest that intrinsic vascular regulation is also present in the perinatal period. Several studies have indicated that the efficacy of extrinsic and intrinsic regulation of the intestinal circulation is dependent, in part, on postnatal age. Much additional work, however, is necessary, particularly to clarify the efficacy of intrinsic control of the developing postnatal intestinal circulation.

REFERENCES

1. BUCKLEY, N. M., P. BRAZEAU, AND I. D. FRASIER. Intestinal and femoral blood flow autoregulation in developing swine. *Biol. Neonate* 49: 229–240, 1986.
2. BUCKLEY, N. M., P. BRAZEAU, I. D. FRASIER, AND P. M. GOOTMAN. Circulatory effects of splanchnic nerve stimulation in developing swine. *Am. J. Physiol.* 248 (*Heart Circ. Physiol.* 17): H69–H74, 1985.
3. DOUGLAS, W. R. Of pigs and men and research. *Space Life Sci.* 3: 226–234, 1972.
4. EDELSTONE, D. I., AND I. R. HOLZMAN. Gastrointestinal tract $O_2$ uptake and regional blood flows during digestion in conscious newborn lambs. *Am. J. Physiol.* 241 (*Gastrointest. Liver Physiol.* 4): G289–G293, 1981.
5. EDELSTONE, D. T., AND I. R. HOLZMAN. Oxygen consumption by the gastrointestinal tract and liver in conscious newborn lambs. *Am. J. Physiol.* 240 (*Gastrointest. Liver Physiol.* 3): G297–G304, 1981.
6. EDELSTONE, D. I., AND I. R. HOLZMAN. Fetal intestinal oxygen consumption at various levels of oxygenation. *Am. J. Physiol.* 242 (*Heart Circ. Physiol.* 11): H50–H54, 1982.
7. EDELSTONE, D. I., AND I. R. HOLZMAN. Fetal and neonatal intestinal circulation. In: *Physiology in the Intestinal Circulation*. New York: Raven, 1984, p. 179.
8. EDELSTONE, D. I., D. R. LATTANZI, M. E. PAULONE, AND I. R. HOLZMAN. Neonatal intestinal oxygen consumption during arterial hypoxemia. *Am. J. Physiol.* 244 (*Gastrointest. Liver Physiol.* 7): G278–G283, 1983.
9. GOOTMAN, P. M., N. GOOTMAN, AND B. J. BUCKLEY. Maturation of central autonomic control of the circulation. *Federation Proc.* 42: 1648–1655, 1983.
10. GOOTMAN, P. M., N. GOOTMAN, P. TURLAPATY, A. C. YAO, B. J. BUCKLEY, AND B. M. ALTURA. Autonomic nervous regulation of cardiovascular function in neonates. *Ciba Found. Symp.* 83: 70–93, 1981.
11. GRANGER, D. N., AND H. J. GRANGER. Systems analysis of intestinal hemodynamics and oxygenation. *Am. J. Physiol.* 245 (*Gastrointest. Liver Physiol.* 8): G786–G796, 1983.
12. GRANGER, H. J., AND A. P. SHEPHERD. Intrinsic microvascular control of tissue oxygen delivery. *Microvasc. Res.* 5: 49–72, 1973.
13. HOLZMAN, I. R., B. TABATA, AND D. I. EDELSTONE. Effects of varying hematocrit on intestinal oxygen uptake in neonatal lambs. *Am. J. Physiol.* 248 (*Gastrointest. Liver Physiol.* 11): G432–G436, 1985.
14. JOHNSON, P. C. Review of previous studies and current theories of autoregulation. *Circ. Res.* 15 Suppl. 1: 2–9, 1964.
15. KARNA, P., A. SENAGORE, AND C. C. CHOU. Comparison of the effect of asphyxia, hypoxia, and acidosis on intestinal blood flow and $O_2$ uptake in newborn piglets. *Pediatr. Rev.* 20: 929–932, 1986.
16. KLIEGMAN, R. M., AND A. A. FANAROFF. Necrotizing enterocolitis. *N. Engl. J. Med.* 310: 1095–1103, 1984.
17. MELLANDER, S., AND B. JOHANSSON. Control of resistance, exchange, and capacitance functions in the peripheral circulation. *Pharmacol. Rev.* 20: 117–196, 1968.
18. MELLER, J. L., S. A. WOLF, M. K. FERGUSON, R. L. C. REPLOGLE, AND D. W. SHERMETA. The microvascular response of the neonatal mesentery to hypertonic feedings. *Pediatr. Res.* 20: 1136–1138, 1986.
19. MORTILLARO, N. A., AND H. J. GRANGER. Reactive hyperemia and oxygen extraction in the feline small intestine. *Circ. Res.* 41: 859–865, 1977.
20. NOWICKI, P. T. Autoregulation of blood flow and oxygen uptake in the developing intestinal circulation (Abstract). *Pediatr. Res.* 21: 371A, 1987.
21. NOWICKI, P. T., D. A. CANIANO, AND K. SZANISZLO. Effect of intestinal denervation on intestinal vascular response to severe arterial hypoxia in newborn swine. *Am. J. Physiol.* 253: (*Gastrointest. Liver Physiol.* 16): G201–G205, 1987.
22. NOWICKI, P. T., N. B. HANSEN, J. R. HAYES, J. A. MENKE, AND R. R. MILLER. Intestinal blood flow and $O_2$ uptake during hypoxemia in the newborn piglet. *Am. J. Physiol.* 251 (*Gastrointest. Liver Physiol.* 14): G19–G24, 1986.
23. NOWICKI, P. T., N. B. HANSEN, AND J. A. MENKE. Intestinal blood flow and oxygen uptake in the neonatal piglet during reduced perfusion pressure. *Am. J. Physiol.* 251 (*Gastrointest. Liver Physiol.* 15): G190–G194, 1987.
24. NOWICKI, P. T., N. B. HANSEN, W. OH, AND B. S. STONESTREET. Gastrointestinal blood flow and oxygen consumption in the newborn lamb: effect of chronic anemia and acute hypoxia. *Pediatr. Res.* 18(5): 420–425, 1984.
25. NOWICKI, P. T., B. S. STONESTREET, N. B. HANSEN, A. C. YAO, AND W. OH. Gastrointestinal blood flow and oxygen consumption in awake newborn piglets: effect of feeding. *Am. J. Physiol.* 245 (*Gastrointest. Liver Physiol.* 8): G697–G702, 1983.
26. ROSS, G. Escape of mesenteric vessels from adrenergic and nonadrenergic vasoconstriction. *Am. J. Physiol.* 221: 1217–1222, 1971.
27. RUDOLPH, A. M., AND M. A. HEYMANN. Circulatory changes during growth in the fetal lamb. *Circ. Res.* 26: 289–299, 1970.
28. TOULOUKIAN, R. J., J. N. POSCH, AND R. SPENCER. The pathogenesis of ischemic gastroenterocolitis of the neonate: selective gut mucosal ischemia in asphyxiated neonatal piglets. *J. Pediatr. Surg.* 7(2): 194–204, 1972.
29. WIDDOWSON, E. M., V. E. COLOMBO, AND C. A. ARTAVANIS. Changes in the organs of pigs in response to feeding for the first 24 hours after birth. *Biol. Neonate* 28: 272–281, 1976.
30. YAO, A. C., P. M. GOOTMAN, P. P. FRANKFURT, AND S. M. DIRUSSO. Age-related superior mesenteric arterial flow changes in piglets: effects of feeding and hemorrhage. *Am. J. Physiol.* 251 (*Gastrointest. Liver Physiol.* 14): G718–G723, 1986.

CHAPTER 44

# Electrophysiological and neuromuscular relationships in extramural blood vessels

D. L. KREULEN  
K. D. KEEF

Department of Pharmacology, University of Arizona Health Sciences Center, Tucson, Arizona

## CHAPTER CONTENTS

Innervation of Mesenteric Circulation
  Anatomy
    Density
    Depth of innvervation
    Junctional cleft width
    Functional ramifications
Mesenteric Artery
  Resting membrane potential
  Cell coupling
  Active membrane properties
    Membrane rectification
    Action potentials
  Responses to addition of autonomic neurotransmitters
    Norepinephrine
    Acetylcholine
  Responses to nerve stimulation
    Excitatory junction potentials
    Dependence on calcium
    Facilitation and summation
    Spontaneous excitatory junction potentials
    Neurally evoked action potentials
    Slow depolarization
    Slow hyperpolarization
  Pharmacology of neuroeffector transmission
    Excitatory junction potentials
    Slow depolarization
    Slow hyperpolarization
  Prejunctional effects on neuromuscular transmission
    Adrenergic Agents
    Cholinergic agents
    Prostaglandins
    Purinergic agents
    Nonadrenergic noncholinergic transmission
Neuromuscular Relationships in Nonmammalian Artery
Mesenteric Vein
  Resting membrane potential
  Action potentials
  Passive membrane properties
  Response to autonomic transmitter substances
    Norepinephrine
    Acetylcholine
  Response to nerve stimulation
    Excitatory junction potentials
    Action potentials
    Slow depolarization
  Pharmacology of neuroeffector transmission
    Excitatory junction potentials
    Slow depolarization
Portal Vein
  Spontaneous action potentials
  Cell coupling
  Response to nerve stimulation
  Response to neurotransmitters
    Norepinephrine
    Acetylcholine
Functional Implications of Neuromuscular Differences Between Artery and Vein
Conclusions

THE SPLANCHNIC CIRCULATION consists of the blood supply to the entire abdominal portion of the digestive system including the liver; it receives 25%–30% of the cardiac output, with 60% of this output going to the superior mesenteric artery and inferior mesenteric artery, the vessels that supply the intestines (121, 188). The splanchnic circulation is also a major reservoir, containing up to 38% of whole-body blood volume, with ~80% of this contained in the venous or capacitance vessels (71). Because it comprises such a large proportion of the cardiac output and blood volume, the splanchnic circulation is generally assumed to play an important part in overall cardiovascular homeostasis, in addition to providing adequate perfusion in the gastrointestinal system (70, 159, 188).

The blood supply to the gastrointestinal tract is divided into two circuits that are in series with one another: the extramural and the intramural blood vessels. The extramural or mesenteric circulation is composed of those blood vessels that are outside of the tract and that course in the mesentery. These arteries are the branches of the abdominal aorta that divide to distribute blood to the different parts of the tract: the celiac, superior mesenteric, and inferior mesenteric arteries. The mesenteric arteries also branch to capillary networks within the mesentery itself (58, 66). Veins accompany most of the branches of these major vessels and ultimately form the portal vein, which carries all intestinal blood to the liver. The mesenteric arteries distribute blood flow among the different abdominal organs and thereby contribute to the control of blood volume in the splanchnic circulation as well as affecting systemic blood pressure. The mesenteric veins represent a significant blood reservoir, and their state of contraction can alter the volume of blood in the splanchnic circuit. The portal vein has a particularly important function: control of the pressure in a segment of the hepatic circulation [see the chapter by Greenway and Lautt in this *Handbook*; (72)].

The intramural blood vessels consist of the blood vessels within the intestinal wall that distribute the blood supply between the mucosal-submucosal and muscular layers and provide the exchange capacity required for the large secretory and absorptive loads of the intestine. Like the mesenteric vessels, the intramural vessels are innervated by the sympathetic nervous system that is extrinsic to the wall of the intestines. In addition the intramural vessels are probably influenced by the enteric nervous system that is intrinsic to the intestinal tract as well as by changes in the environment within the wall of the intestine. By virtue of their intimate relationship with intrinsic nerves and the "intrinsic reflexes" that are known to alter blood flow (14, 15), it is likely that the intramural blood vessels are controlled by a subset of different control mechanisms than the extramural blood vessels (see the chapter by Hirst in this *Handbook*.)

The splanchnic blood vessels are controlled by both systemic and local factors, including the sympathetic division of the autonomic nervous system, the intrinsic properties of vascular smooth muscle, circulating neurohumoral factors, and local metabolic factors (121). The splanchnic blood vessels, arteries as well as veins, are innervated, and the sympathetic nervous system is perhaps the most important factor for adjustments in resistance and capacitance within the splanchnic bed (27, 55, 56, 71, 192). Sympathetic nerves also tonically activate splanchnic blood vessels (sympathetic tone); systemic blood pressure decreases after section of splanchnic nerves (120, 141).

Anatomic, neurochemical, and functional properties of the autonomic nervous system govern the manner in which it modulates the mesenteric circulation. The segmental origin of preganglionic fibers within the central nervous system, the distribution of fibers to neurons in sympathetic ganglia, the factors affecting ganglionic transmission, the distribution patterns of postganglionic fibers to the mesenteric blood vessels, the structure of the neuromuscular junction, and the neurotransmitter(s) utilized by the nerves are all important aspects of the neural control of blood vessels. The vascular neuroeffector junction is the last point in the neural control pathway where signals from the nervous system to blood vessels are modified. These signals are modified by the factors that affect neurotransmitter release: the anatomical characteristics of the neuroeffector junction, the interactions of neurotransmitters with vascular smooth muscle as well as with each other, the state of the vascular smooth muscle, substances derived from the endothelial lining of the vessels, and circulating hormones. This chapter discusses the relationship of sympathetic nerves with the smooth muscle of mesenteric arteries and veins, emphasizing the electrophysiology of neuromuscular transmission. We review recent knowledge concerning the transmission of signals from sympathetic nerves to mesenteric blood vessels and the relationship of the characteristics of this transmission to the function of the mesenteric circulation. Neuromuscular transmission in arteries has been reviewed elsewhere (146, 183, 226).

## INNERVATION OF MESENTERIC CIRCULATION

### Anatomy

The sympathetic innervation of the mesenteric blood vessels is supplied by the lumbosacral outflow of the spinal cord. Preganglionic fibers from several segmental levels join to form the splanchnic nerves, of which there are usually four groups: the greater, lesser, and least splanchnic nerves that innervate the celiac and superior mesenteric ganglia, and the lumbar splanchnic nerves that supply preganglionic fibers to the inferior mesenteric ganglion (144, 171). In the dog some of the nerves from the lumbosacral spinal cord do not pass in the splanchnic nerves to innervate ganglionic neurons; thus section of splanchnic nerves does not completely denervate the splanchnic circulation in this species (26).

Mesenteric blood vessels are innervated by the axons of the sympathetic ganglionic neurons emanating from the prevertebral ganglia (celiac, superior mesenteric, and inferior mesenteric). The mesenteric nerve fibers course with the mesenteric blood vessels and enter the gastrointestinal tract with them. The macroscopic fibers that lie alongside the blood vessels, both within and outside of the adventitia, are termed *paravascular nerves*; from these nerves, branches enter the adventitia of the mesenteric arteries and veins, divide, and form the *terminal ground plexus* (34, 44, 45, 64). Nerve bundles that course in the adventitia and in the superficial aspects of the smooth muscle with the terminal plexus surround the blood vessels and are termed the *perivascular nerves*.

As the terminal axons branch, they lose their Schwann cell sheath and form varicosities in the region of the smooth muscle cells. It is generally accepted that the storage, release, and reuptake of neurotransmitter occur at the varicosities of the terminal axons (8, 34).

The neuromuscular junctions of smooth muscle have been classified based on the structure of the terminal axons and the varicosity–muscle cell junction. *Small axon bundles* consist of groups of terminal axons enveloped in a Schwann cell sheath. The Schwann cell covering is interrupted only at intervals, and the varicosities, when exposed, do not make close contact with the muscle cells. Close-contact varicosities, on the other hand, consist of axons without Schwann cell covering that come into close apposition with muscle cells. Often the varicosities are indented into the surface of smooth muscle cells. In mesenteric blood vessels, although the small axon bundles coursing in the adventitial-medial border predominate (8, 11), there are reports of close-contact varicosities (44).

Several characteristics of the innervation of mesenteric blood vessels are important determinants of the physiological properties of the mesenteric circulation. These characteristics include the density of nerve fibers and varicosities, the depth of the innervation into the medial layer of the vessels, the distance between the varicosities and smooth muscle cells, and the amount of tissue between the varicosities and the smooth muscle cells.

DENSITY. In mesenteric blood vessels, as in all blood vessels, the catecholaminergic innervation (as revealed by catecholamine fluorescence) is most dense at the adventitial-medial border (8, 34, 64). Generally the principal mesenteric arteries are densely innervated and the accompanying veins are usually less densely innervated. The portal vein is as densely innervated as most other extracranial veins (107). The precapillary arterioles and collecting venules are not innervated, and small veins >30 μm diam have one or more nerve fibers running with them, but the nerves do not form a plexus (Fig. 1). Some studies report no correlation between the density of the nerve fibers and the size of the principal arteries or veins [rat (64)], whereas others show that the density of innervation decreases from primary to tertiary branches of the mesenteric arteries [rabbit (79)]. Hejtmancik and Su (79) also report that the periarterial plexus branches more extensively in primary arteries than it does in tertiary arteries.

In both arteries and veins the magnitude of the contractile response to nerve stimulation is correlated with the density of the innervation (10). In the guinea pig, Cowen (44) found that varicosities are more dense in the mesenteric artery, which is most responsive to nerve stimulation, than they are in the carotid and renal arteries, which are less responsive. However, there must be other factors governing the responsiveness to norepinephrine (NE) because the concentration required to cause 50% of maximum effect ($EC_{50}$) of NE for veins is less than that for arteries (221), but the latter are more densely innervated (11, 64).

DEPTH OF INNERVATION. The degree to which nerve fibers invade the muscular elements of blood vessels is variable, depending on the type and size of the vessel as well as the species; however, compared with densely innervated tissues such as the vas deferens, the number of nerve fibers among muscle cells is relatively sparse in vascular smooth muscle (34). Although the innervation of vascular smooth muscle is most dense at the adventitial-medial border (11, 63,

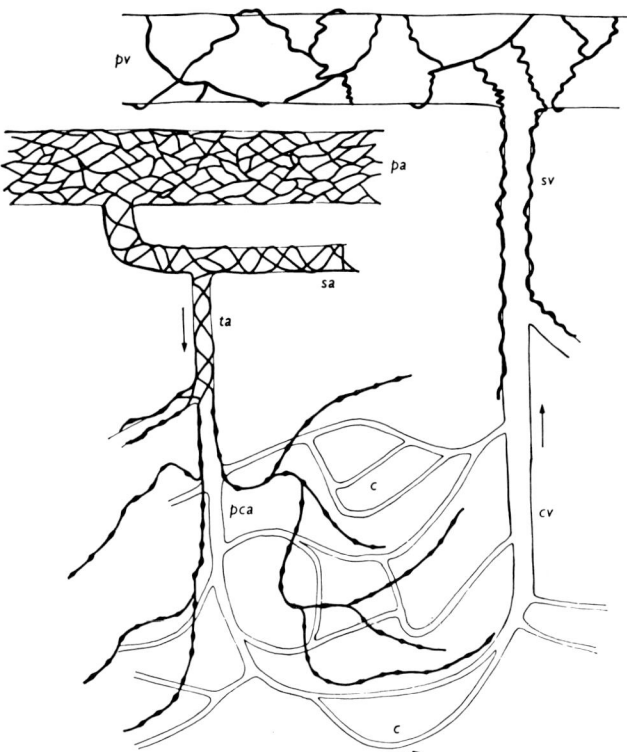

FIG. 1. Representation of relationship between adrenergic nerves and mesenteric blood vessels of the rat. c, Capillary; cv, collecting venule; pa, principal artery; pca, precapillary arteriole; pv, principal vein; sa, small artery of microvasculature; sv, small vein; ta, terminal arteriole; *Heavy lines*, adrenergic nerves; *arrows*, direction of blood flow. Precapillary arterioles and collecting venules are not innervated. [From Furness and Marshall (64).]

226), fibers penetrate into the media of mesenteric arteries of several species, including the dog, rat, and guinea pig (173).

JUNCTIONAL CLEFT WIDTH. A related structural aspect of the innervation of vascular smooth muscle is the relationship of nerve varicosities to smooth muscle cells. The distance between varicosities and vascular smooth muscle varies among and within vessels; generally the smaller the vessel, the smaller the distance. In a study of mesenteric artery of the guinea pig, Cowen (44) found that the distance between nerve varicosities and muscle cells was small when compared with the distance in the renal and carotid arteries. He also found occasional outpocketings or projections of muscle cells in close proximity to nerve varicosities (44). In mesenteric vessels several average junctional widths have been reported: rat portal vein, 100 nm (25); rat mesenteric arteries, 500 nm (48) and 200 nm (51); and guinea pig mesenteric artery, 900 nm (44). These distances are compared with 20 nm in the guinea pig vas deferens (169) and 1,900 nm in the rabbit pulmonary artery (227).

FUNCTIONAL RAMIFICATIONS. The magnitude of the responses of blood vessels to nerve stimulation or application of NE is related to the structural characteristics of the innervation. Generally the greater the density of sympathetic nerve terminals, the greater the response of the vessel to nerve stimulation. In addition, the smaller the gap in the neuromuscular junction, the larger the $EC_{50}$ for exogenous NE (10). These findings imply that a denser innervation releases more NE from nerve terminals and that the close proximity of varicosities to vascular smooth muscle restricts access of exogenous NE to the effector sites. Ljung et al. (155) compared the responses of different arteries and veins to transmural nerve stimulation. The small saphenous vein, which has an innervation that penetrates into the media, has a steeper frequency-response relationship than the anterior mesenteric vein, which has an innervation limited to the adventitial-medial border. Cowen (44) compared the neuromuscular distances in mesenteric, carotid, and renal arteries of the guinea pig. Not only is the distance between varicosities and muscle cells least in the mesenteric vessels but there is less connective, fibroblast, and Schwann cell tissue interposed between the nerve and muscle. The junctional cleft width averages 900 nm in the mesenteric, 4,200 nm in the carotid, and 4,700 nm in the renal arteries. These characteristics of the mesenteric artery explain its greater responsiveness to nerve stimulation compared with the responsiveness of other arteries.

The mesenteric blood vessels must be equipped to respond not only to the local demands of the abdominal organs but also to the systemic demands of the whole organism. This involves both afferent and efferent pathways throughout the autonomic nervous system. The final common pathway in blood vessel control is the sympathetic neuron and the neuromuscular junction. Transmission along postganglionic sympathetic neurons and at the neuroeffector junction is the subject of this chapter. Knowledge about the transmission of impulses to individual smooth muscle cells from sympathetic neurons helps to explain the mechanisms of vasoconstriction in both arteries and veins. Chemical transmission of information from sympathetic nerves involves NE as a neurotransmitter and postjunctional adrenergic receptors; other neurotransmitters and receptors are probably also involved. Furthermore the differences in the neuromuscular junction in artery and vein may be the basis of the functional differences between the responses of these two vessels. Finally, many questions regarding the cellular mechanisms of neural control of mesenteric vascular smooth muscle and their relationship to the physiology of the mesenteric circulation remain unanswered.

## MESENTERIC ARTERY

### Resting Membrane Potential

The potential difference recorded across the membrane of vascular smooth muscle is the result of a selectively permeable cell membrane and an unequal distribution of various ionic species. This unequal distribution of ions is maintained by energy-dependent ion-pumping mechanisms. The level of the resting membrane potential in vascular smooth muscle depends on the relative permeability of the cell to $K^+$, $Cl^-$, and $Na^+$, as well as the distribution of these ions across the membrane. If the relative permeabilities of these three ions (i.e., $P_K$, $P_{Na}$, and $P_{Cl}$) are known, as well as their intracellular (i) and extracellular (o) concentrations, the membrane potential ($E_m$) can be predicted from the constant field equation derived by Goldman, Hodgkin, and Katz (69, 92)

$$E_m = -60 \log \frac{P_{K^+}[K^+]_i + P_{Na^+}[Na^+]_i + P_{Cl^-}[Cl^-]_o}{P_{K^+}[K^+]_o + P_{Na^+}[Na^+]_o + P_{Cl^-}[Cl^-]_i} \quad (1)$$

In vascular smooth muscle $E_m$ predicted from this equation is often less negative than the measured $E_m$. This difference has been attributed to the additional contribution of an electrogenic $Na^+$-$K^+$ pump, although in the guinea pig mucosal arterioles, ouabain and $K^+$-free solution can affect membrane conductance in a manner that could account for the changes in $E_m$ (91). A detailed discussion of the studies that have contributed to the understanding of membrane permeation and ionic content in vascular smooth muscle is beyond the scope of this chapter (for additional information see ref. 124).

The resting $E_m$ reported for various mesenteric arteries ranges from −39 to −73 mV (Table 1). Although some of this variation undoubtedly reflects differences in experimental approach adopted by various investigators, there is also evidence that $E_m$ may vary along different portions of the arterial tree. In the guinea pig mesentery, $E_m$ of the jejunal artery (−52 mV) is significantly less than that recorded in either the cranial mesenteric artery (−60 mV) or a branch of the jejunal artery (−68 mV). The regional differences in $E_m$ were attributed to different values in the $P_{Na^+}/P_{K^+}$ ratio (217).

### Cell Coupling

Like most visceral smooth muscles, vascular smooth muscle behaves as an electrical syncytium in that an electrical signal in one part of the tissue is conducted to other parts through low-resistance connections between adjacent smooth muscle cells [Table 2 (219, 220)]. The structural substrate of this low-resistance pathway, often termed the *nexus* or *gap junction*, is the region of close apposition between adjacent muscle cells (20, 43, 187, 222, 227). These connections are studied electrophysiologically by injecting current into one or more cells and recording the spread of current into other cells in the tissue. Experiments involving injection of current have taken several forms.

TABLE 1. *Electrophysiological Characteristics of Mammalian Blood Vessels*

| | MP | EJP | SDP | AP | Phentolamine | | Prazosin | | Yohimbine | | Ref. |
|---|---|---|---|---|---|---|---|---|---|---|---|
| | | | | | EJP | SDP | EJP | SDP | EJP | SDP | |
| Guinea pig artery | | | | | | | | | | | |
| Mesenteric, in vivo | −39 | + | + | +(24) | | | | | | | 198 |
| Mesenteric, 200 μm | −72 | + | | +(50) | | | | | | | 3 |
| Jejunal mesenteric, 100 μm | −69 | + | − | * | $10^{-7}$ ↑ | $10^{-7}$ 0 | | | $5 \times 10^{-7}$ ↑ | | 117 |
| Jejunal mesenteric, 120–200 μm | −69 | + | | | $10^{-7}$ ↑f ↑s | $10^{-7}$ 0f 0s | | | $10^{-7}$ ↓f ↑s | | 148 |
| Jejunal mesenteric, 150–200 μm | −70 | + | | +(35) | | | | | | | 153 |
| Jejunal mesenteric, 100–150 μm | −50 | + | | +(45) | | | | | | | 233 |
| Jejunal mesenteric, 120–200 μm | −69 | + | | | $10^{-7}$ ↑f ↑s | | | | $10^{-7}$ ↓f ↑s | | 149 |
| Ileal mesenteric, 100 μm | −70 | + | | +(65) | | | | | | | 213 |
| Ileal mesenteric, 250–500 μm | −73 | + | + | − | | $10^{-6}$ ↓ | $5 \times 10^{-7}$ 0 | $5 \times 10^{-7}$ ↓ | | | 104 |
| Colonic mesenteric, 100–500 μm | −74 | + | + | − | | $10^{-6}$ ↓ | | | | | 143 |
| Superior mesenteric | −68 | + | | +(50) | | | | | | | 206 |
| Renal | −67 | +● | | − | $10^{-7}$ ↑ | | $5 \times 10^{-7}$ ↑ | | $5 \times 10^{-7}$ ↑ | | 161 |
| Guinea pig arterioles | | | | | | | | | | | |
| Mucosal | −65 to −75 | + | | +(55) | | | | | | | 83 |
| Rabbit artery | | | | | | | | | | | |
| Mesenteric, 100–150 μm | −70 | + | | +(50) | | | | | | | 162 |
| Mesenteric | −54 | + | | − | | | | | | | 198 |
| Mesenteric | −70 | + | + | +(45) | $10^{-7}$ ↑s | $10^{-6}$ ↓ | $10^{-5}$ 0s | $10^{-6}$ ↓ | $10^{-7}$ ↑s | $10^{-6}$ 0 | 170 |
| Jejunal mesenteric, 120–200 μm | −72 | + | | | $10^{-7}$ 0s 0f | | | | $10^{-7}$ 0s 0f | | 149 |
| Rat artery | | | | | | | | | | | |
| Ileal mesenteric, 60–150 μm | −69 | + | | +(70) | | | | | | | 82 |
| Cat arterioles | | | | | | | | | | | |
| Mucosal | −64 | + | | +(40) | | | $3 \times 10^{-6}$ ↓ | | | | 175 |
| Dog artery | | | | | | | | | | | |
| Jejunal mesenteric | −68 | + | | +(28) | $10^{-7}$ ↓f ↑s | $10^{-6}$ 0f 0s | | | | | 140 |
| Pig artery | | | | | | | | | | | |
| Mesenteric, 300 μm | −53 | +● | | | | | | | | | 115 |
| Guinea pig vein | | | | | | | | | | | |
| Colonic mesenteric, 200–500 μm | −71 | − | + | | $10^{-6}$ ↓ | | $5 \times 10^{-7}$ ↓ | | | | 104 |
| Colonic mesenteric, 100–500 μm | −71 | − | + | +(44) | $10^{-6}$ ↓ | | $10^{-6}$ ↓ | | | | 143 |
| Ileal mesenteric | −63 | − | + | R +(20) | $10^{-6}$ ↓ | | | | | | 209 |
| Renal | −47 | − | − | − | | | | | | | 161 |
| Dog vein | | | | | | | | | | | |
| Mesenteric, 300–500 μm | −65 to −75 | + | + | +(35) | $10^{-7}$ ↑ | $10^{-7}$ ↓ | $3 \times 10^{-7}$ ↑ | $10^{-6}$ ↓ | $10^{-7}$ 0 | $10^{-7}$ ↓ | 211 |
| Cat venules | | | | | | | | | | | |
| Mucosal | −51 | − | + | R | | | $3 \times 10^{-6}$ ↓ | | | | 174 |

MP, membrane potential in mV; EJP, excitatory junction potential; SDP, slow depolarization potential; AP, action potential (value in parentheses in mV); EJP, excitatory junction potential; +, yes; −, no; *, rarely; 0, no effect; s, facilitated; f, first; ↓, decreased; ↑, increased; R, rhythmic potential changes. ● With repetitive stimulation.

The clearest demonstration of current spread in vascular smooth muscle was performed in the submucosal arterioles with two independent microelectrodes: one to pass current into one cell, the other to record membrane potential in another cell. In this preparation, current injected in one branch of an arteriole can be recorded as a voltage deflection in an adjoining branch of the arteriole. The most plausible explanation of the spread of current over distances of several cell lengths is that current spreads via low-resistance intercellular connections (84).

Low-resistance coupling between adjacent vascular

TABLE 2. *Summary of Some Cable Constants in Mammalian Blood Vessels*

| | $\lambda$, mm | $\tau_m$, ms | $\tau_f$, ms | Ref. |
|---|---|---|---|---|
| **Rabbit** | | | | |
| Main pulmonary artery | 1.48[a] | 182 | | 39 |
| | 1.90[a,b] | | | |
| | 1.7[a] | | | 112 |
| | 0.8[a,c] | | | |
| | 1.86[d] | 208 | | 73 |
| | 3.44[b,d] | | | |
| Common carotid artery | 1.13[a] | 212 | | 166 |
| Aorta | 2.1[d] | 433 | | 167 |
| Saphenous artery | 0.54[e] | 174 | 175 | 100 |
| **Guinea pig** | | | | |
| Mesenteric artery | 0.81[e] | 129 | 206 | 153 |
| | | 181[f] | 426[f] | |
| | | | 113 | 143 |
| Portal vein | 0.52[e,g] | 330 | | 110 |
| | 0.61[e] | 240 | | 150 |
| | 0.71[e] | | | 77 |
| Mucosal arterioles | 1.46[h] | 375 | 310 | 81 |
| Ear artery | 1.03[e] | 410 | | 126 |
| Abdominal aorta | 0.66[a] | 180 | | 125 |
| Pulmonary artery | 1.22[a] | | | 77 |
| Basilar artery | 0.78[e] | | | 129 |
| Renal artery | 0.54[a] | 240 | | 161 |
| Renal vein | 0.43[a] | 98 | | 161 |
| **Dog** | | | | |
| Coronary artery | 0.83[a] | 410 | | 109 |
| **Rat** | | | | |
| Pulmonary artery | 1.4[a] | 238 | | 152 |
| Portal vein | 1.22[e] | 190 | | 152 |
| **Fowl** | | | | |
| Mesenteric artery | 2.8[e] | 257 | | 20 |
| | 2.8[e,f] | 466[f] | | |
| **Pig** | | | | |
| Coronary artery | 0.67[e] | 290 | | 108 |

$\lambda$, Length constant; $\tau_m$, membrane time constant; $\tau_f$, muscle fiber time constant. [a] Helical measurement. [b] 10 mM tetraethylammonium added. [c] 59 mM potassium in the perfusing medium. [d] Circular measurement. [e] Longitudinal measurement. [f] 30°C–31°C. [g] Hypertonic solution. [h] Short cable, 2 microelectrodes.

Although there is still some disagreement as to the extent of coupling between smooth muscle cells, the general consensus is that all vascular smooth muscles are to some degree electrically coupled: all of the measurements of space constant ($\lambda$) yield values that are more than several cell lengths (Table 2). The most widely used method for measuring coupling in smooth muscle is the partition-stimulation method of Abe and Tomita (1). With this method, current is applied to the smooth muscle cells with two large silver plates. Responses are recorded in an extrapolar region separated from the stimulation site by an insulating partition. By recording at varying distances from the site of stimulation, the cable properties of the tissue can be determined. These properties include the length constant ($\lambda$) and the membrane time constant ($\tau_m$). The length constant is the distance (in mm) that an applied signal will travel before declining in amplitude to $1/e$ (~37%) of its initial amplitude and is an indication of the longitudinal resistance of the tissue. The membrane time constant is a measure of the time course (in ms) of electrotonic potentials; in smooth muscle this is determined by measuring the time taken for electrotonic potentials to reach half their maximum amplitude at different distances from the stimulating plate. The relationship between these times and distances is linear, with a slope of $\tau_m/2\lambda$ (93).

If internal resistance is less than either the junctional resistance or the membrane resistance, the measured value for $\lambda$ would be expected to depend on the orientation of the smooth muscle cells. That is, $\lambda$ is longer in the long orientation of the smooth muscle cells than at a 90° angle to their long orientation. Thus measurements made on arterial preparations in which the smooth muscle cells are oriented helically or circularly yield values of $\lambda$ that are longer than those obtained from measurements made along the long axis of the vessel and therefore across the long axis of the smooth muscle cells. The cable constants measured in several vascular tissues are compared in Table 2. The values obtained for the guinea pig jejunal artery measured in the longitudinal direction [$\lambda = 0.81$ mm; $\tau_m = 129$ ms (153)] are comparable with these values in the saphenous artery [$\lambda = 0.54$ mm; $\tau_m = 174$ ms (100)] but somewhat less than that in the guinea pig ear artery [$\lambda = 1.03$ mm; $\tau_m = 410$ ms (126)].

One splanchnic vessel, which differs markedly from mammalian mesenteric arteries, is the fowl anterior mesenteric artery (17–20); $\lambda$ in this vessel measured in the longitudinal direction is 2.8 mm (20). This is the largest value of $\lambda$ reported for either arteries or veins and far exceeds other measurements made in the longitudinal direction. A partial explanation for this large value of $\lambda$ is that, unlike most splanchnic arteries, there is a distinct longitudinally oriented layer of smooth muscle cells in the fowl anterior mesenteric artery (5).

smooth muscle cells is also suggested by the values of input resistance obtained by injecting current into a cell in a blood vessel with an intracellular microelectrode and recording the resulting voltage deflection in that same cell. With this method, the references obtained for input resistance range from 3 to 21 M$\Omega$ [aorta (167), mesenteric artery (78)]. These values are much lower than values obtained in cells that have been isolated. In short segments (200 $\mu$m) of cerebral arterioles in which current spread is limited, the input resistance is 102 M$\Omega$ (90). All of these values are small compared with the 5,000-M$\Omega$ measured in individual cells dissociated from the guinea pig mesenteric artery (7) or the 3,600 M$\Omega$ measured in individual cells dissociated from the azygous vein (204). The discrepancies between these different values of input resistance can be explained if one assumes that cells are electrically coupled to one another; the input resistance measured in cells within tissue is actually a measure of "tissue input resistance."

*Active Membrane Properties*

The active properties of mesenteric vascular smooth muscle include the voltage-dependent conductances that are activated by directly changing the membrane potential, by the action of neurotransmitters released from nerves, or by the application of neurotransmitter substances. Neurally evoked action potentials are considered in *Responses to Nerve Stimulation*, p. 1614.

MEMBRANE RECTIFICATION. In vascular smooth muscle (including mesenteric vessels) the relationship between current and voltage is linear at moderate membrane hyperpolarization, indicating that membrane resistance does not change at voltages more negative than the resting membrane potential (39, 73, 108, 152, 153, 161, 212). On the other hand, in the depolarizing direction, more and more current is required to attain a given amount of depolarization; this signifies a change in the resistance of the membrane and is called *rectification*. Rectification in vascular smooth muscle is attributed to a voltage-dependent increase in conductance of $K^+$ channels and has been demonstrated in a number of different arteries (23, 39, 73, 108, 112, 115, 152, 153, 161, 212).

ACTION POTENTIALS. Nearly all in vitro preparations of mesenteric blood vessels are electrically quiescent in the absence of any external stimulus. The most notable exception to this in mammals is the portal vein (see PORTAL VEIN, p. 1625; Table 1). However, action potentials have been recorded in the guinea pig mesenteric artery in an ex vivo preparation in which the nerve and blood supply of the mesentery was maintained attached to the animal (198). Contrary to other studies in vitro, Zelcer and Sperelakis (233) recorded spontaneous action potentials in the distended guinea pig mesenteric artery, which were abolished by lowering the temperature to 35°C from 37°C. In several other studies of these same blood vessels (117, 148, 149, 155), including two studies performed at 37°C (104, 143), no spontaneous action potentials were reported. Furthermore pressurization of the mesenteric arteries, even at 38°C, produced no action potentials (K. D. Keef and D. L. Kreulen, unpublished observations). The relatively low resting membrane potentials recorded by Zelcer and Sperelakis (233) may account for the presence of action potentials. In summary, it may be that under specific conditions in vitro spontaneous action potentials occur in the mesenteric artery; whether these conditions can occur in the unanesthetized animal is not known.

Although spontaneous action potentials are rare in mammalian mesenteric blood vessels, action potentials can be induced by direct depolarization or by blockade of $K^+$ currents with drugs such as tetraethylammonium (TEA). Because of cell-to-cell coupling it is usually not possible to evoke action potentials in large blood vessels by injection of current into a single cell through an intracellular microelectrode. However, in smaller diameter vessels that have been cut to short segments it is possible to evoke action potentials in this manner (82, 90). For example, a 57-mV action potential can be evoked by injection of 1.1 nA of depolarizing current in a cell in a short segment of the 2-day-old rat mesenteric arteriole (82). In this preparation the relatively small number of cells distributed within a thin medial layer increases the tissue input resistance and enables the small amount of current to produce a greater depolarization of the cell membrane.

In larger mesenteric blood vessels it is difficult to evoke action potentials with depolarizing current even if the current is applied to the entire vessel with the use of a partition-stimulation chamber (118, 155); instead, small active responses graded in amplitude with the stimulus strength are obtained. These are similar to the responses recorded in other arteries with the same method of stimulation [pulmonary artery (39), aorta (167), saphenous artery (100)]. In the presence of TEA, which reduces resting and voltage-dependent $K^+$ conductance ($G_{K^+}$) in smooth muscle (39, 73, 166), depolarizing currents applied by the partition-stimulation method or into a single cell give rise to large-amplitude action potentials (3, 73, 78, 118, 213). This suggests that rectification of the membrane as a result of the opening of voltage-dependent $K^+$ channels occurs to such an extent that only small abortive action potentials are obtained. Application of TEA also gives rise to spontaneous action potentials or membrane fluctuations in the mesenteric artery [Fig. 2; (78, 213, 217)]. Similar behavior is observed when $BaCl_2$ is applied to mesenteric artery (18, 78).

Application of NE produces action potentials in some mesenteric arteries and arterioles (23, 119, 127, 183). In gastric arterioles the $\alpha$-agonist phenylephrine also produces action potentials (175). In mesenteric artery the action potentials are typically superimposed on a membrane depolarization and vary considerably both in amplitude and duration (Fig. 3). The action potentials are in some way related specifically to the addition of NE and not just to the depolarization, because an equal amount of depolarization with $K^+$ does not initiate action potentials (23, 176, 217).

Voltage-clamp analysis of the currents underlying the action potential obtained in TEA in cerebral arterioles has demonstrated two distinct inward $Ca^{2+}$ currents that are associated with regenerative responses: a transient, rapidly inactivating current and a plateau, noninactivating current. Both of these currents are diminished by replacing $Ca^{2+}$ in the bathing medium with $Co^{2+}$ or by the addition of the $Ca^{2+}$ antagonists nifedipine or verapamil (90). Two inward $Ca^{2+}$ currents have also been demonstrated in isolated single cells dissociated from the azygous vein (204). An inward $Na^+$ current is also found in the azygous vein cells.

## Responses to Addition of Autonomic Neurotransmitters

The literature as it relates to electrophysiological experiments investigating the actions of NE and acetylcholine (ACh) in mesenteric vessels is reviewed in this section. For more comprehensive reviews of the actions of drugs in vascular smooth muscle the reader is referred to references 21, 28, 146, 185, 196, 230.

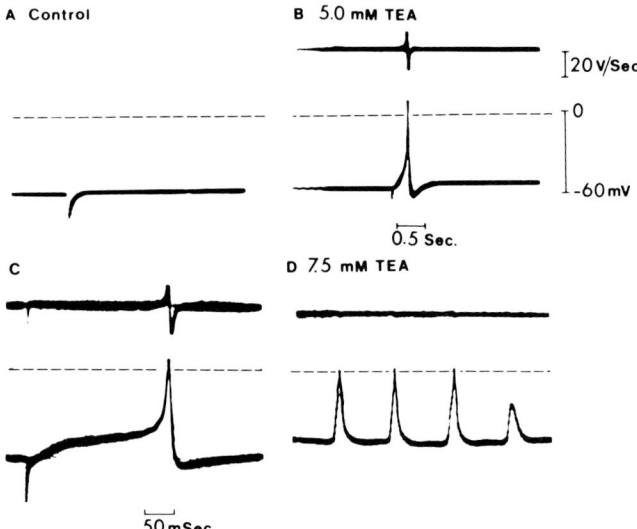

FIG. 2. Induction of excitability by tetraethylammonium ion (TEA) in the normally inexcitable vascular smooth muscle from guinea pig superior mesenteric artery. *A*: control shows resting potential of approx. −58 mV and lack of spontaneous action potentials or responses to intense external electrical stimulation (1-shock artifact depicted). *B*: record from same cell impaled in *A* 5 min after addition of 5 mM TEA, illustrates a large overshooting action potential produced in response to electrical stimulation. *C*: record from another cell shown at a faster sweep speed. *D*: record from another muscle exposed to 7.5 mM TEA illustrates partial depolarization and production of spontaneous action potentials. Time scale in *B* applies to all panels except *C*; voltage calibration in *B* applies to all panels; dV/dt calibration in *B* applies to *B–D*. [From Harder and Sperelakis (78).]

NOREPINEPHRINE. Addition of NE to the mesenteric artery of the rat, rabbit, or guinea pig leads to depolarization and contraction (23, 106, 117, 119, 127, 148, 170, 176, 217). The excitatory action of NE on the mesenteric artery is due to stimulation of $\alpha$-receptors, because both contraction and depolarization are blocked by phentolamine (119, 148, 176). The responses appear to be due to the $\alpha_1$-receptor subtype, because depolarization and contraction are also suppressed by the $\alpha_1$-receptor antagonist prazosin (117, 119, 148).

Several splanchnic vessels contain both $\alpha$- and $\beta$-adrenergic receptors. In the rat mesenteric artery, the NE-induced depolarization is converted to a hyperpolarization in the presence of phentolamine (176). This hyperpolarization is blocked by propranolol, indicating that it is the result of $\beta$-receptor stimulation. Furthermore the $\beta$-receptor agonist isoproterenol initiates hyperpolarization in the rat mesenteric artery (176) as well as in several guinea pig mesenteric arteries of varying sizes (217). Isoproterenol relaxes the mesenteric artery that has been contracted with excess $K^+$ (116, 217).

The mechanism of action of NE on splanchnic arteries is not known in detail. A change in membrane resistance is indicated by the change in the amplitude of the electrotonic potential (partition-stimulation method) in the presence of high concentrations of NE ($>10^{-5}$ M). In mesenteric arteries of the guinea pig and rabbit, the changes in membrane resistance vary with the laboratory in which the studies are performed. Both a decrease (23, 119, 148) and an increase (127) in the amplitude of the electrotonic potential have been reported. However, depolarization alone can produce changes in the membrane conductance due to the rectifying properties of the membrane (23). The reduction in electrotonic potential is considered to be indicative of an increase in membrane conductance. In the rabbit main pulmonary artery, NE increases membrane permeability for $K^+$, $Cl^-$, and $Na^+$ (39). Possibly a similar mechanism of excitation occurs in

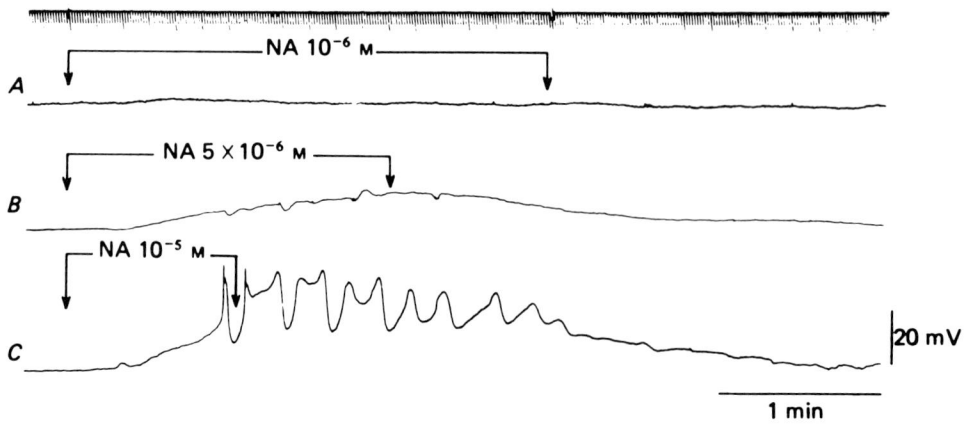

FIG. 3. Effects of noradrenaline (NA) on membrane potential of single smooth cell of rabbit mesenteric artery. NA was applied between *arrows*. [From Itoh et al. (119).]

the mesenteric artery with addition of NE. However, Takata (217) suggests that NE decreases $K^+$ permeability in the guinea pig jejunal artery because the NE-induced depolarization is increased by decreasing extracellular $K^+$. Norepinephrine has a similar effect in mesenteric vein (209).

The contraction associated with the administration of NE to mesenteric blood vessels in vitro appears to be the result of both the depolarization produced and an action of NE not mediated by depolarization. This is apparent from a comparison of the voltage-contraction relationships produced by $K^+$ and NE (23). Although maximum contraction is obtained after NE has depolarized the cells by ~13 mV, contraction with elevated $K^+$ does not begin until the cells have depolarized by $\geq 15$ mV, and even a 50-mV depolarization with $K^+$ produces only ~60% of the maximum NE contraction (Fig. 4). Thus NE apparently elevates intracellular $Ca^{2+}$ by a mechanism that is partially voltage independent. Another manifestation of this phenomenon is that vessels contracted with 179 mM $K^+$ can be further contracted with epinephrine (197). The disparity between the voltage-contraction relationships for NE and $K^+$ is also seen in rat mesenteric arteries (176), as well as in vessels from other vascular beds (39, 42, 50, 117, 125, 168, 205).

In some blood vessels NE initiates rhythmic potential changes that are superimposed on the depolarization (23, 119, 129, 176, 183). In small segments of rat mesenteric artery, these rhythmic potential changes appear to initiate the rhythmic contractions because they precede the contractions by ~1.2 s (176). A similar relationship between phenylephrine-initiated rhythmic contractions and rhythmic potential changes occurs in cat gastric arterioles (170). However, in the guinea pig jejunal artery, rhythmic potential changes are not essential for rhythm generation because rhythmic contractions are observed in the majority of preparations, whereas rhythmic changes in membrane potential are seen infrequently (119). These differences may reflect species differences or, alternatively, may be related to differences in the techniques used for measuring contraction.

ACETYLCHOLINE. Functional cholinergic innervation of mesenteric blood vessels has not been demonstrated. Despite this, ACh has excitatory and inhibitory actions on mesenteric blood vessels that are mediated through muscarinic receptors on the smooth muscle and endothelial cells, respectively. Studies on the importance of the endothelium and the "endothelium-derived relaxation factor" in mediating the effects of ACh are rather recent (23, 62) and have made the interpretation of earlier studies difficult because the integrity of the endothelium was not assessed.

In the guinea pig mesenteric artery in which the endothelium is intact, carbachol produces a dose-dependent membrane hyperpolarization. If the endothelium is removed, carbachol produces a membrane depolarization (23). Both of these actions of carbachol are blocked by the muscarinic antagonist atropine.

Cholinergic agonists hyperpolarize some guinea pig and rabbit mesenteric vessels [see Fig. 9 for an example; (22, 23, 151, 217)]. This hyperpolarization has been attributed to an increase in $K^+$ conductance for several reasons: 1) the hyperpolarization is associated with a reduction in the amplitude of electrotonic potentials (23); 2) the amplitude of the hyperpolarization is greater in reduced $[K^+]$ (1.2 mM) and smaller or abolished in elevated $[K^+]$ (25 mM) (151, 217); 3) the reversal potential ($E_{rev}$) for hyperpolarization is approximately equal to the $K^+$ equilibrium potential [$E_{rev}$ = $-70$ mV (217)]; and 4) the amount of hyperpolarization is not affected by reducing $[Na^+]_o$ (152). Thus the relationship of the resting membrane potential to the $K^+$ equilibrium potential would be expected to affect the amplitude of the hyperpolarization. For example, in guinea pig jejunal artery, ACh (up to $5 \times 10^{-5}$ M) does not change membrane potential in normal $K^+$ medium (153, 217) but results in a hyperpolarization in low $K^+$ medium, presumably because in low $K^+$ medium the $E_K$ becomes more negative than the resting membrane potential (217).

Cholinergic agonists can contract or relax mesenteric blood vessels, although relaxation is the most common observation and has been reported for previously contracted (NE- or $K^+$-induced contraction) mesenteric arteries of the dog, cat, guinea pig, and rabbit (23, 62, 151, 217). In other arteries, such as the rabbit aorta, muscarinic relaxation is strictly dependent on the presence of an intact endothelium (62). However, in the guinea pig mesenteric artery, some relaxation persists in the absence of endothelium,

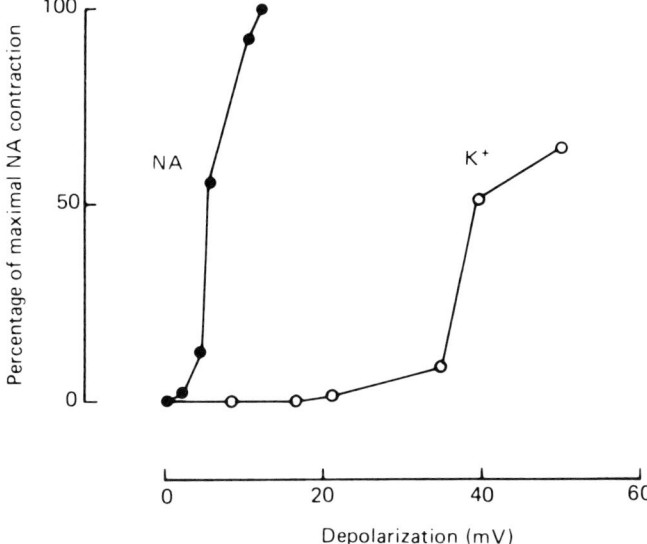

FIG. 4. Relationship between contraction and depolarization produced by noradrenaline (NA) and raised external $K^+$ in guinea pig mesenteric artery. Potassium contractions were expressed as percentage of the maximal contraction to NA. [From Bolton et al. (23).]

which suggests that there are inhibitory muscarinic receptors on the smooth muscle cells (23). There are also excitatory muscarinic receptors on the smooth muscle cells in this tissue, because carbachol enhances the contractions produced with threshold concentrations of $K^+$ in the absence of endothelium (23).

There is an apparent dissociation between the electrical and mechanical effects of cholinergic agonists. In the guinea pig and rabbit mesenteric arteries contracted with NE or $K^+$, cholinergic relaxation can occur in the absence of a change in membrane potential (23, 151, 217). Similarly, ACh contracts and at the same time hyperpolarizes mesenteric artery (151). Because the contractile response to ACh is not abolished in $Ca^{2+}$-free solution, Kuriyama and Suzuki (151) suggested that ACh not only hyperpolarized the smooth muscle but also initiated the release of intracellular sequestered $Ca^{2+}$ by a membrane-potential–independent mechanism. It is not known how muscarinic activation induces relaxation in the absence of a change in membrane potential. Bolton et al. (23) stated the problem clearly: "The main mechanism of carbachol's inhibitory action is at present obscure, especially as it inhibits both $[K]_o$ and NE contractions which we believe utilize $Ca^{2+}$ from different sources."

*Responses to Nerve Stimulation*

The electrophysiology of neuroeffector transmission in mesenteric arteries, the pharmacology of that transmission, and the relationship of electrophysiological responses to the function of the mesenteric circulation are reviewed in this section. Many in vivo studies have demonstrated that when the splanchnic nerves are stimulated electrically there is a decrease in both volume and flow in the splanchnic circulation. The means by which nerve activation results in a change in blood vessel diameter has been studied in detail in recent years, with the use of intracellular microelectrode recordings in vascular smooth muscle. The study of these events reveals much about the mechanism of smooth muscle control by nerves but also raises many interesting questions concerning the relationship of neurotransmitter action and membrane electrical events to blood vessel contractility.

Two different types of nerve stimulation are used in vitro: paravascular (nerve trunk) and perivascular (transmural). Paravascular nerve stimulation involves drawing the macroscopic nerve bundles coursing alongside blood vessels into stimulating electrodes that are located some distance from the recording site (104, 143). Perivascular nerve stimulation involves placing stimulating electrodes on either side of the blood vessel at or near the recording site. A variant of perivascular stimulation makes use of suction electrodes into which the end of a segment of vessel is drawn. Perivascular stimulation has been employed most frequently in vitro because small dissected preparations have not enabled lengths of paravascular nerves to be retained with the vessels.

One tacit assumption of nerve stimulation is that the electrical activation of autonomic nerve fibers initiates an action potential that propagates from the site of initiation along the terminal axons, releasing neurotransmitter from varicosities where the depolarization leads to $Ca^{2+}$ influx. With perivascular stimulation, electrical activation of nerves probably involves not only depolarization of terminal axons but also of varicosities directly. This direct activation is manifested by the inability of tetrodotoxin (TTX) to completely abolish the responses to perivascular nerve stimulation (103, 134, 181).

The nature of the postjunctional electrical and mechanical events associated with nerve stimulation depends on the parameters of nerve stimulation, including intensity, frequency, duration, and the pattern in which these variables are combined. The single transient depolarization associated with application of a single nerve shock is called an excitatory junction potential (EJP), which was first described in the guinea pig mesenteric artery in vivo (198) and has since been described in many mesenteric blood vessels. However, the EJP is not found in the mesenteric veins of the guinea pig (104, 143, 209). Repetitive electrical stimulation of nerves can lead to an increase in the amplitude of individual EJPs (facilitation), summation of EJPs, slow depolarization, and/or hyperpolarization of the vascular smooth muscle membrane. Each of these phenomena may under certain circumstances be an expression of a different neuromuscular event in the mesenteric neurovascular system and therefore is considered separately.

EXCITATORY JUNCTION POTENTIALS. Nerve stimulation in vitro evokes synchronous firing of all axons, whereas the natural firing of sympathetic nerves in vivo is asynchronous. Based on this difference Neild (179) predicted that nervous activity in vivo would not give rise to discrete EJPs but rather to irregularly shaped slow depolarizations. In guinea pig and rat mesenteric arteries (198, 200), as well as in guinea pig and rabbit ear arteries (180), discrete EJPs are not recorded in vivo, although they can be generated by electrical nerve stimulation. Despite its possible nonphysiologic nature, the EJP is a convenient experimental phenomenon that provides us with a discrete, reproducible electrical event related to the release of neurotransmitter. This response can be subjected to experimental interventions that are directed at understanding neuromuscular transmission in blood vessels.

The EJP is a transient depolarization with a rapid onset (30–100 ms to peak) and a duration of 0.3–1.5 s, which has been recorded in all of the in vitro arterial smooth muscle preparations that have been tested and in the dog mesenteric vein (211). In mesenteric arteries tested, EJPs have been reported in large and small extramural arteries of the guinea pig, rabbit, dog, pig, and rat (115, 140, 143, 153, 162, 206, 232) and in intramural arterioles of the cat and guinea pig [Table 1; (83, 174)]. They have also been recorded in vivo in guinea pig and rabbit mesenteric arteries (198, 200). Inhibitory postjunctional potentials, with a time course similar to the EJP, have not been recorded in mesenteric vessels.

The transmitter-initiated membrane depolarization in smooth muscle has been referred to as the EJP, to distinguish it from the electrical response occurring at the more specialized skeletal neuromuscular junction [end-plate potential (EPP)]. The mechanism for initiation of an EJP differs from that of the skeletal muscle EPP in that the EJP is the result of transmitter release from multiple dispersed sites with a syncytially arranged target, whereas the EPP is the result of transmitter release from a single nerve terminal onto the highly specialized end plate of a single-cell cable.

In some vascular preparations there are "stepped" increases in EJP amplitude in response to continuously increased stimulus voltage (40, 83, 147, 153). Figure 5 shows an example of the plateaus in the intensity-amplitude relationship in guinea pig mesenteric artery. It has been suggested that this stepwise relationship is due to progressive recruitment of higher threshold nerve fibers.

If the membrane current associated with the EJP is brief in duration then the decline of the EJP should simply reflect the passive properties of the smooth muscle membrane. Ideally when the muscle is uniformly activated, the decline of the EJP should be exponential and the time constant ($\tau_f$) should be equivalent to the muscle fiber membrane time constant ($\tau_m$). This is what is experimentally observed in mucosal arterioles (54, 84) and in the rabbit saphenous artery (100). However, in the guinea pig mesenteric artery Kuriyama and Suzuki (153) reported that $\tau_m$ was considerably shorter than $\tau_f$. Furthermore $\tau_m$ was unaffected by reducing temperature from 35°C to 30°C, whereas $\tau_f$ was markedly prolonged (Table 2). This group suggested several factors that might explain the differences in $\tau_m$ and $\tau_f$, including 1) diffuse innervation with nerves of different excitabilities and 2) the possibility that NE release from nerve terminals is not brief.

An EJP can be obtained with a single brief (0.02-0.5 ms) stimulus pulse applied with transmural stimulating electrodes. Although both smooth muscle and nerves are present in the field of stimulation, nerves are preferentially excited because of their shorter $\tau_m$. This is usually confirmed by demonstrating that the neural responses are abolished by the application of TTX (126, 148, 153, 210, 214). However, the sensitivity to TTX of EJPs evoked with perivascular nerve stimulation depends on the intensity of the nerve stimulation. Small amplitude (3-4 mV) "test" EJPs evoked with perivascular nerve stimulation are eliminated in the presence of TTX; nevertheless EJPs can be obtained in the guinea pig mesenteric artery (104) and the rat tail artery (182) in the presence of TTX by increasing the stimulus voltage. Reduced but recognizable EJPs were also obtained by Itoh et al. (117) in the rat tail artery in the presence of TTX. In the guinea pig ear artery, EJPs and action potentials can still be recorded near the stimulating electrodes in the presence of TTX (134), whereas EJPs recorded at a distance from the stimulating electrode are abolished (Fig. 6). The shape of the TTX-insensitive membrane responses in the guinea pig ear artery are identical with responses that are TTX sensitive. Similarly EJPs evoked with paravascular nerve stimulation (where stimulation is distant from recording site) are sensitive to TTX, and this block cannot be overwhelmed with higher stimulus intensities (103). One interpretation of these findings is that the nerve terminals are directly depolarized with perivascular (but not paravascular) nerve stimulation. Nerve terminals are known to release transmitter in response to direct depolarization (49, 133). These observations call into question the assumed differentiation that is typically made between neural TTX-sensitive responses and direct muscle stimulation TTX-insensitive responses in studies utilizing transmural nerve stimulation.

DEPENDENCE ON CALCIUM. Release of transmitter is dependent on the presence of $Ca^{2+}$ in the extracellular solution [e.g., motor terminal (132), sympathetic nerve to spleen (135), mouse vas deferens (9)]. This dependence on $[Ca^{2+}]_o$ is because $Ca^{2+}$ enters the nerve terminal during the action potential and in some way signals the cell to release transmitter. Because the size of the EJP is dependent on the amount of transmitter

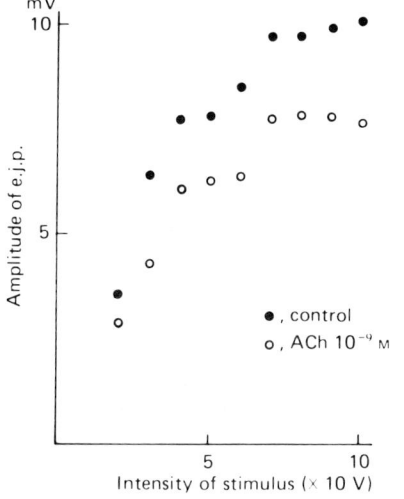

FIG. 5. Effect of acetylcholine (ACh) on amplitude of excitatory junction potentials (EJP) in guinea pig jejunal mesenteric artery induced by increasing stimulus intensity. In absence of ACh, amplitude of EJPs increased with 4 steps as stimulus intensity was increased; with ACh ($10^{-9}$ M), amplitude of EJPs decreased but continued to show stepwise increase in amplitude with increasing stimulus intensity. [From Kuriyama and Suzuki (153).]

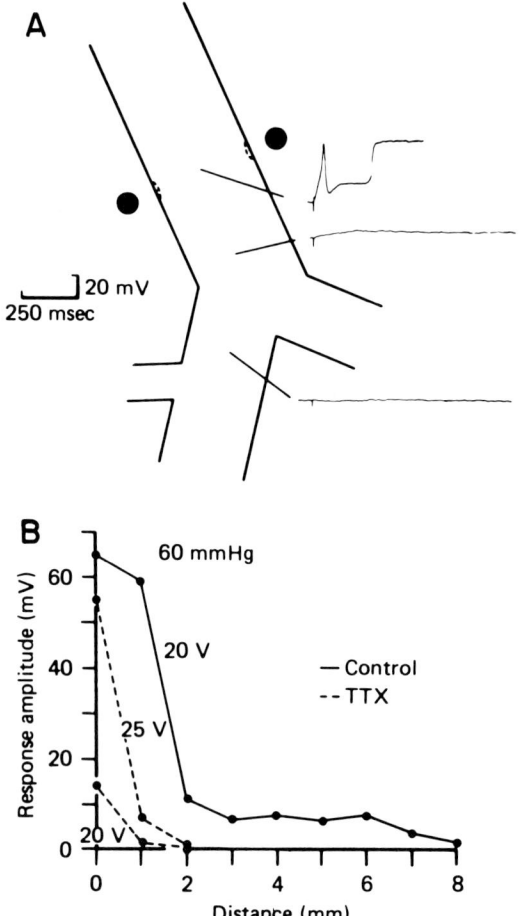

FIG. 6. Responses to single perivascular nerve stimulus in presence of $3 \times 10^{-6}$ M tetrodotoxin (TTX) in guinea pig ear artery. A: responses obtained between stimulating electrodes and at distances of 1 and 2 mm from them. Although an action potential is recorded at stimulating electrode, only small slow potential change is observed at 1 mm distance. B: peak amplitude of response against distance from stimulating electrodes in presence and absence of TTX. After exposure to TTX, responses are only obtained near stimulating electrodes. [From Keef and Neild (134).]

uted to a gradual increase of $Ca^{2+}$ in the nerve terminal (8, 132). In mesenteric arteries and mucosal arterioles of the guinea pig and rabbit, facilitation occurs at frequencies of stimulation >0.1–0.2 Hz (83, 117, 143, 148, 153, 162, 232). In the guinea pig mesenteric artery (3, 148, 160) facilitation in response to frequencies <1 Hz is accurately predicted by equations derived for the neuromuscular junction of the frog (164). This suggests that facilitation in the mesenteric artery is governed by the same processes that occur in the frog neuromuscular junction: processing involving $Ca^{2+}$ mobilization. With longer periods of repetitive nerve stimulation, the amplitude of successive EJPs is less than that predicted, particularly at frequencies >0.5 Hz. In addition, the selective $\alpha_2$-antagonist yohimbine enhances facilitation in the guinea pig mesenteric artery. These results suggest that presynaptic autoinhibition limits facilitation at higher frequencies (148).

In the dog mesenteric artery there is also a logarithmic relationship between the amplitude of the first and second EJP when plotted against the time interval between them, as predicted by Mallart and Martin (164). However, beyond two EJPs, amplitude cannot be predicted by these equations, and a depression phenomenon is often apparent (140). The erratic nature of successive EJPs in the dog mesenteric artery more closely resembles the responses to repetitive stimulation observed in the guinea pig ear artery (126) than that of other mesenteric arteries that have been studied.

As the frequency of stimulation is increased there is also a second interaction that takes place between successive EJPs, i.e., summation. When the stimulus interval is decreased to less than the duration of an individual EJP, the membrane does not entirely repolarize from one EJP before the next arrives; the result is that the membrane progressively depolarizes until a steady state of depolarization is obtained. The level of steady-state depolarization is related to the frequency of stimulation and is a function of both facilitation and summation. In some cases the degree of depolarization is sufficient to elicit an action potential. Summation can be demonstrated in all mesenteric vessels in which an EJP occurs. The depolarization due to summation must be differentiated from the slow depolarization in arteries that persists for several seconds after the end of stimulation and in veins persists in the absence of EJPs (see SLOW DEPOLARIZATION, p. 1618).

released, the effect of $[Ca^{2+}]_o$ on transmission is often studied by measuring the amplitude of the EJP at various $[Ca^{2+}]_o$. In the guinea pig jejunal artery there is a logarithmic relationship between EJP amplitude and $[Ca^{2+}]_o$ (147–149, 232). The same relationship occurs in the guinea pig vas deferens (113). On the other hand, in the mouse vas deferens EJP amplitude is dependent on $[Ca^{2+}]_o^2$ (9). What these differing relationships imply in terms of the mechanism of action of $Ca^{2+}$ is unclear.

FACILITATION AND SUMMATION. When the nerves to blood vessels are stimulated repetitively, there is often a progressive increase in the amplitude of successive EJPs until a final steady-state amplitude is obtained. This facilitation presumably represents an increased release of neurotransmitter with successive stimuli. This increased release of transmitter has been attrib-

SPONTANEOUS EXCITATORY JUNCTION POTENTIALS. In 1962 Burnstock and Holman (36) described small spontaneous depolarizing potentials that occurred in the absence of nerve stimulation in the guinea pig vas deferens. These spontaneous excitatory junction potentials (SEJPs) were similar to the EJP but of shorter duration and have subsequently been recorded in a number of different blood vessels, including the guinea pig jejunal artery (147, 153, 232), mucosal arterioles (86), ear artery (126), and uterine artery (6); the rabbit saphenous artery (100); and the rat tail artery (40). The origin of these SEJPs is presumed to be leakage of transmitter from nerve terminals similar to leakage at the skeletal neuromuscular junction (8, 132). Because this leakage occurs randomly, individual SEJPs probably originate from a point source of junctional current, whereas the evoked EJP is the result of simultaneous release from multiple sites. In the vas deferens the time course of the SEJP approximates the time course of the junctional current (36, 38, 96).

The amplitude histograms of SEJPs plotted for a number of different vessels are skewed toward lower amplitudes [e.g., guinea pig mesenteric artery (153), guinea pig mucosal arterioles (86), guinea pig ear artery (126), rat tail artery (40)]. This distribution is typical of junction potentials recorded from systems with distributed innervation (8, 29, 68). A detailed analysis to determine whether these events are indeed related to quantal release of transmitter (132) is not possible in most of these preparations, because the SEJPs are attenuated by the passive membrane properties of the smooth muscle (99). The one exception is a study of SEJPs in guinea pig mucosal arterioles that demonstrated the quantal nature of release (86).

The frequency of SEJPs in the guinea pig mesenteric artery ($\leq 1$ event/min) is less than that in the guinea pig ear artery (126) or in the rat tail artery (40). This frequency is increased markedly by removal of $K^+$ from the medium (215). The electrical recordings of SEJPs in this study nicely complement the work of Bonaccorsi et al. (24), in which large quantities of [$^3$H]NE release were associated with exposure of arteries to $K^+$-free medium. Frequency of SEJPs can also be increased in the guinea pig mesenteric artery by adding TEA (147, 217) or 2-nicotinamidoethyl nitrate (115). Hypertonicity (10 g/100 ml sucrose in Krebs solution) increases SEJP frequency in guinea pig mucosal arterioles (86).

In the guinea pig renal artery, SEJPs recorded in normal $K^+$ medium are not abolished in the presence of TTX but are eliminated by treatment with guanethidine. Thus the SEJPs are probably a result of spontaneous release from sympathetic nerves (161). In the guinea pig mesenteric artery TTX reduces the frequency of SEJPs induced in $K^+$-free medium (215). This suggests that the release of neurotransmitter is dependent on fast $Na^+$ action potentials in the nerves rather than spontaneous release. Thus the small depolarizations in $K^+$-free medium may be more appropriately termed *miniature excitatory junction potentials*.

NEURALLY EVOKED ACTION POTENTIALS. Reports of all-or-none action potentials in blood vessels are rare, whether neurally or directly evoked. Rather, responses to nerve stimulation are graded in a peculiar way. If the peak of the EJP reaches a "critical" potential either through summation, facilitation, or increased stimulus intensity, its shape changes. Usually this takes the form of a small peak on top of the EJP. These kinds of changes can be graded (41, 134, 140, 206, 210) and are termed *active responses* (206). In guinea pig inferior mesenteric artery, paravascular nerve stimulation (up to 30 Hz) does not elicit action potentials or active responses, and contraction of the vessels is correlated with the degree of membrane depolarization (104, 143).

Table 1 indicates in which blood vessels action potentials have been recorded. Action potentials are consistently elicited in submucosal arterioles of the guinea pig (83); however, there is some disagreement as to the ability to elicit action potentials in larger mesenteric vessels. Earlier studies (153, 198, 232) suggest that action potentials of 35–45 mV can be elicited, whereas a later study by Itoh et al. (117) reports that they were rarely obtained. Kreulen and co-workers (104, 143) have not been able to evoke action potentials in branches of the inferior mesenteric artery of the guinea pig.

The ability to generate an action potential probably depends not only on the vessel tested but also on the way the vessel is prepared and the method of stimulation. Action potential generation may also depend on the degree of stretch on the vessel. Keef and Neild (134) have shown that distension of the guinea pig ear artery converts this tissue from one that produces graded active responses dependent on stimulus voltage to one that produces an all-or-none action potential. This behavior is also observed in the guinea pig saphenous artery (K. D. Keef, unpublished observations). Furthermore, helically cutting a vessel or dissecting off a portion of the adventitia has the potential of damaging nerves and thereby compromising responses to nerve stimulation.

The method of nerve stimulation will also probably affect the responses evoked in blood vessels. In the guinea pig inferior mesenteric artery, transmural stimulation produces only a local 3- to 5-mm contraction in the region of the stimulating electrodes, whereas stimulation of the nerve trunks exiting from the inferior mesenteric ganglion (paravascular) produces a contraction along the entire 30-mm length of the artery (K. D. Keef, O. D. Hottenstein, and D. L. Kreulen, unpublished observations). Perivascular stimulation can evoke TTX-insensitive responses (see *Responses to Nerve Stimulation*, p. 1614). It may also produce more intense local stimulation of nerve terminals. For example, in the ear artery, action potentials are generated in the region of the transmural stimulating electrodes but do not propagate away from the stimulated region in the presence of TTX (Fig. 6).

Transmembrane flux of $Ca^{2+}$ is important for the vascular smooth muscle action potential because the maximum rate of rise of the action potential is reduced in low-$Ca^{2+}$ medium, whereas the spike amplitude and maximum rate of rise are unaffected in a solution in which all NaCl is replaced with choline chloride (232). Furthermore the action potential in the guinea pig and rabbit mesenteric artery is suppressed by diltiazem, nifedipine, or verapamil (162, 213, 232). The nerve-evoked action potentials in the rat tail artery are resistant to the $Ca^{2+}$ antagonist nifedipine, although the contractions associated with nerve stimulation are abolished (207). Furthermore TEA increases the amplitude of the nerve-evoked action potential—this TEA component of the action potential is abolished with nifedipine.

SLOW DEPOLARIZATION. Membrane depolarizations that are evoked by repetitive nerve stimulation have been recorded in several arteries (6, 41, 104, 143, 171, 198, 210, 214). These have been termed *slow depolarizations* because of their relatively long duration compared with EJP duration and because they seem to be generated by a separate mechanism from that of the EJP. The amplitude and duration of slow depolarizations are dependent on the frequency, intensity, and duration of nerve stimulation. Slow depolarizations were first reported in the in vivo guinea pig inferior mesenteric artery (198) and the in vitro uterine artery (6). They also have been reported in the rat tail artery (41), the rabbit ear artery (214), and the guinea pig main pulmonary artery (210). In the rabbit mesenteric artery, 100 or more stimuli produce a maximum depolarization of 8–10 mV at 10 Hz (171). In the guinea pig inferior mesenteric artery, slow depolarizations, evoked with paravascular nerve stimulation of 1–10 Hz, range in amplitude from 0.5 to 4.5 mV and have durations of 5–10 s (104, 143). However, repetitive nerve stimulation does not evoke a slow depolarization in the guinea pig jejunal artery (117). These differences may be related to regional variation in membrane properties of guinea pig mesenteric vessels (217).

The duration of the slow depolarization varies widely among different arteries. Those recorded in the inferior mesenteric artery are much shorter (5–10 s) than those recorded in the rat tail and guinea pig pulmonary arteries (1–3 min). The development of the slow depolarization is correlated with contraction; both the depolarization and the contraction associated with repetitive stimulation are antagonized by the $\alpha_1$-antagonist prazosin (104). The rate of onset of the slow depolarization is slower in arteries than in veins, and at a given frequency of nerve stimulation, both the contraction and the slow depolarization are proportionally less in arteries than in veins (see SLOW DEPOLARIZATION, p. 1624). It has been suggested that slow depolarization represents the diffusion of transmitter away from the junctional region to extrajunctional receptors. The pharmacology leading to this hypothesis is discussed in *Pharmacology of Neuroeffector Transmission*, p. 1625.

SLOW HYPERPOLARIZATION. Repetitive nerve stimulation can evoke a membrane hyperpolarization that has a 10- to 20-s latency to onset and a duration of 20–80 s (143). In the guinea pig inferior mesenteric artery the hyperpolarization is not blocked by adrenergic or cholinergic antagonists (143). Blockade of $\alpha_1$-adrenergic receptors with prazosin blocks the slow depolarization and enhances the slow hyperpolarization (105). Similarly if the nerves are stimulated at frequencies >5 Hz and longer than 5–10 s, only a slow depolarization of the membrane is evoked: apparently the slow depolarization masks the slow hyperpolarization (105). A nerve-evoked membrane hyperpolarization has not been reported in other arteries. This hyperpolarization is also apparently different from the hyperpolarization elicited in mesenteric arteries of the rat (176) and guinea pig (217) by stimulation of $\beta$-adrenergic receptors.

*Pharmacology of Neuroeffector Transmission*

Vasoconstriction elicited with either electrical or reflex nerve activation is attenuated by $\alpha$-adrenergic antagonists as well as by compounds that deplete NE from sympathetic nerves (for review see ref. 11). The contractile responses to nerve stimulation are not as easily antagonized as responses to the addition of NE (13, 101, 145). Furthermore the junctional depolarization (i.e., EJP) is not blocked by $\alpha$-receptor antagonists, whereas the extrajunctional depolarization (i.e., slow depolarization) is (35, 41, 104, 117, 171, 181, 210, 216). Pharmacologic studies of neuroeffector transmission in mesenteric arteries have raised interesting questions regarding the role of NE as a neurotransmitter as well as introduced the possibility that other substances might also function as sympathetic neurotransmitters.

EXCITATORY JUNCTION POTENTIALS. The EJPs evoked with transmural, suction, or nerve-trunk stimulation are not blocked by either $\alpha$- or $\beta$-adrenergic antagonists [see Table 1 and Table 1 of ref. 183)]; however, they are attenuated by compounds that deplete NE from sympathetic nerves such as guanethidine (41, 100, 117, 148, 162, 170, 172, 206, 210, 214, 216) and 6-hydroxydopamine (41, 148). In vivo reserpinization also diminishes the response to perivascular nerve stimulation. However, EJPs can still be obtained with increased stimulus voltages after reserpinization, although catecholamine fluorescence has been eliminated (41) and NE content is reduced to 1% of control (216). Although the EJP is resistant to reserpinization, the slow depolarization is readily abolished (see SLOW DEPOLARIZATION, p. 1619).

Two alternative hypotheses have been proposed to explain the inability of adrenergic antagonists to suppress EJPs. The first hypothesis suggests that there are specialized junctional receptors for NE that are insensitive to the conventional α-receptor antagonists in the concentration range used to block extrajunctional α-receptors (85, 87–89). The second hypothesis suggests that another substance (perhaps ATP) is coreleased with NE and that the EJP is the result of this second transmitter combining with a nonadrenergic postjunctional receptor (35, 194, 195).

The junctional adrenergic receptor hypothesis is based on the observation that ionophoretically applied NE evoked an EJP-like depolarization only in certain locations in the submucosal arterioles. These "hot spots" correlate with the position of nerve varicosities and therefore are considered to be neuromuscular junctions (85). Because these junctional adrenergic receptors are activated by NE but not blocked by conventional α-receptor antagonists, they are given the unique designation of γ-receptors (87).

No other laboratory has repeated these experiments, correlating sites of NE depolarization with the position of sympathetic nerves. However, in the rabbit ear artery, NE or ATP ionophoretically placed at random sites on the artery evokes transient depolarizations from all sites (216). The response to ATP is more rapid than the response to NE and thus more closely resembles the time course of the EJP. Similarly the NE depolarization is blocked by prazosin, but the ATP depolarization is not. One difficulty with ionophoretic application of NE in the rabbit ear artery is that unlike in the guinea pig mucosal arterioles, iontophoretic application of NE depolarizes the cells by stimulating α-receptors. This depolarization might mask γ-receptor–mediated depolarization.

Results that contradict the special junctional adrenergic receptor hypothesis come from studies of the effects of reserpinization on the EJP and the slow depolarization (216). The EJPs and slow depolarizations apparently are evoked by transmitters released from the same nerves, because their amplitudes are correlated when the intensity of nerve stimulation is graded. However, reserpinization abolishes the slow depolarization but not the EJP. It would not be possible to dissociate these two potentials from one another if they both were mediated by NE.

A recently developed adrenergic antagonist, 3,4-dihydro-8-(2-hydroxy-3-isopropylamino-propoxy)-3-nitroxy-2H-1-benzopyran (K-351), appears to act at both junctional and extrajunctional adrenergic receptors. It reduces the amplitude of the EJP, as well as the contractile responses associated with nerve stimulation or addition of NE, in both the guinea pig and the canine mesenteric artery (3, 140). Because the facilitation process is unaltered in either of these vessels, an effect on prejunctional α-receptors is discounted. The adrenergic antagonist K-351 appears specific for adrenergic receptors because the ACh-induced contraction is unaltered and the K$^+$-induced contraction is only slightly reduced in the presence of K-351. Furthermore K-351 does not alter the Ca$^{2+}$-tension relationship in skinned fibers (3). The ability of a compound with adrenergic-antagonist properties to reduce the amplitude of EJPs is strong pharmacological support for the hypothesis that EJPs are produced when NE acts on junctional adrenergic receptors at the neuromuscular junction of vascular smooth muscle. In the dog mesenteric vein, K-351 does not reduce the amplitude of the EJP, which suggests K-351 may act at some point other than the junctional adrenergic receptor in arteries or, alternatively, that the transmitter generating the EJP in veins is different from that in arteries.

The alternate transmitter hypothesis for the resistance of EJPs to adrenergic antagonists is based on the observation that desensitization of purinergic receptors with α,β-methylene ATP abolishes the EJP [rat tail artery (35, 182, 193); guinea pig and rabbit mesenteric artery (106)]. This hypothesis actually has its basis in experiments in the vas deferens where the purinergic-receptor antagonist arylazido aminopropionyl ATP (ANAPP$_3$) has been shown to block EJPs as well as the rapid contraction evoked with nerve stimulation (53, 194, 195). In the rabbit mesenteric artery, α,β-methylene ATP (0.1 μM) appears to act postjunctionally because it decreases the amplitude of EJPs to 30% of control but does not affect the overflow of NE measured with liquid chromatography (106). The contractile response to nerve stimulation in the rabbit mesenteric artery is also reduced by α,β-methylene ATP, whereas the release of [$^3$H]NE is unaltered (145). In studies of the rat tail artery, Neild and Kotecha (182) point out that although α,β-methylene ATP reduces the EJP it has yet to be determined, whether this effect is on a specific receptor or on the conductance changes that give rise to the excitatory junctional current. The depolarization produced by NE in the rat basilar artery, an artery that lacks α- and β-adrenergic receptors, is abolished by α,β-methylene ATP (37, 89).

Presently neither of these two hypotheses completely explains all the data. What they share is the idea that NE is released from sympathetic nerve terminals. Furthermore the concept of stimulation of extrajunctional α-receptors by diffusion of NE away from the junctional region is compatible with both. The idea that ATP, functioning as a cotransmitter, elicits junctional responses is attractive because of the profound effects of purinergic-receptor desensitization on EJPs, the parallels with the vas deferens, and the costorage of purines with catecholamines in sympathetic nerve vesicles (16, 31, 52, 138). The resolution of the discrepancies between these two hypotheses awaits the confirmation in other laboratories of junctional adrenergic receptors and a more detailed investigation of the role of purines in vascular neuroeffector transmission.

SLOW DEPOLARIZATION. The slow membrane depolarization and associated constriction that are evoked with repetitive nerve stimulation are reduced or abolished by α-adrenergic antagonists. Both are also diminished by guanethidine, 6-hydroxydopamine, or reserpine (41, 171, 210, 216). In the guinea pig mesenteric artery there is a shift of the frequency–slow depolarization relationship in the presence of 0.5 µM prazosin (104). In the rat tail artery the junctional depolarizations and contractions induced junctionally can be separated from those induced extrajunctionally with the $\alpha_1$-antagonist prazosin (42, 181). That is, the extrajunctional slow depolarization and associated contraction are inhibited by prazosin, whereas the junctionally induced action potential and associated contraction are not (Fig. 7). These pharmacologic studies suggest that the contractile response to nerve stimulation in arteries is the sum of the responses to junctional receptor stimulation (non-α) and extrajunctional receptor stimulation (α).

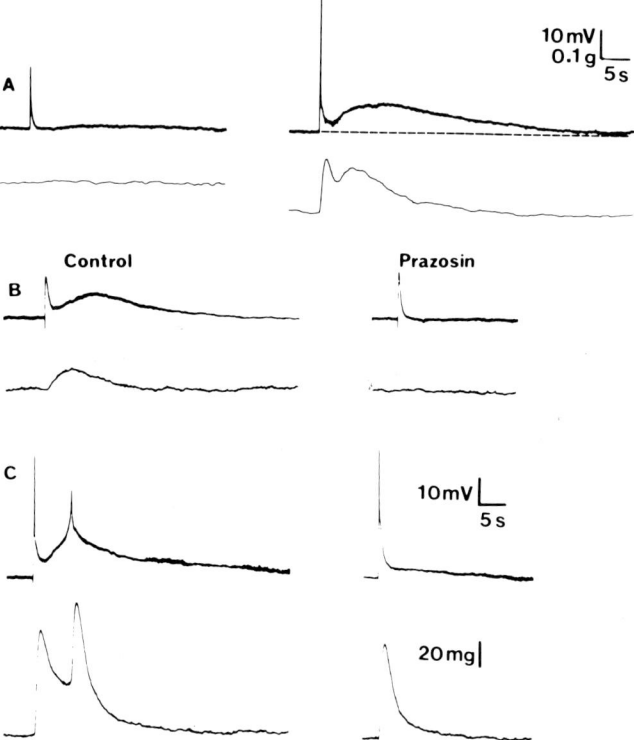

FIG. 7. Simultaneous recordings of electrical (*top tracing*) and mechanical (*bottom tracing*) activities of rat tail artery induced by stimulation of perivascular nerves with single 0.05-ms pulse. *A*: stimulation at 40 V produced excitatory junction potential (EJP) and no contraction (*left panel*). Increasing the stimulus strength to 120 V induces active response on EJP and long sustained depolarization; fast phasic and slow sustained contraction were also observed (*right panel*). *B*: in another preparation, stimulation at 88 V elicited slow depolarization and slow contraction that were abolished by prazosin ($5 \times 10^{-9}$ g/ml). EJP was subthreshold and was not affected by prazosin. *C*: increasing stimulus strength to 90 V initiated fast phasic contraction associated with action potential arising from EJP; a second fast contraction was triggered when slow depolarization reached threshold. Prazosin abolished only second fast contraction. [From Cheung (42).]

SLOW HYPERPOLARIZATION. The slow hyperpolarization evoked in guinea pig inferior mesenteric artery is not blocked by prazosin, phentolamine, propranalol, or atropine (143). However, the artery exhibits desensitization as the slow hyperpolarization is attenuated by applying stimulus trains at <2-min intervals (105).

## Prejunctional Effects on Neuromuscular Transmission

A large variety of vasoactive substances may exert their effects either partially or completely by modulating adrenergic neuromuscular transmission. These substances include (but are not limited to) bradykinin, adenosine, ATP, prostaglandins, and ACh. Prejunctional receptors, thought to exist on the sympathetic nerve terminals, mediate changes in the amount of neurotransmitter released as a result of nerve activation. The evidence for adrenergic prejunctional receptors is extensive and is discussed in several reviews (154, 199, 202, 226, 231). Prejunctional receptors on nerve terminals for neurotransmitters that are released from those same terminals are often called "autoreceptors." Many extrinsic substances also affect neurotransmitter release from sympathetic nerve terminals in mesenteric blood vessels.

ADRENERGIC AGENTS. Prejunctional autoreceptors in blood vessels are of the $\alpha_2$-subtype. Adding NE to the perfusion medium reduces the amplitude of the EJP in the guinea pig mesenteric artery (148). Similarly the selective $\alpha_2$-receptor agonist clonidine decreases the amplitude of the EJP, and the selective $\alpha_2$-receptor antagonist yohimbine enhances the amplitude of the facilitated EJP (142, 148, 149). However, there is disagreement as to the presence of presynaptic $\alpha_2$-receptors in rabbit mesenteric artery. In one study neither phentolamine nor yohimbine affected the amplitude of EJPs (149), whereas in another study both these drugs increased the amplitude of the EJP [see Table 1 (170)]. Although yohimbine is more effective than phentolamine in increasing the amplitude of EJPs, there is a larger increase in the overflow of NE with phentolamine than there is with yohimbine. This suggests that yohimbine may have effects on the smooth muscle in addition to its prejunctional effects (170).

CHOLINERGIC AGENTS. Many studies have verified the inhibitory actions of ACh or other cholinergic agonists on neurotransmitter release from sympathetic nerves (30, 142, 153, 157, 163, 186, 191, 201, 203, 224, 225). These actions are at muscarinic cholinergic receptors because they are antagonized by atropine. However, there is no evidence that atropine alone increases the amplitude of EJPs. In the rabbit mesenteric artery, atropine ($10^{-6}$ M) does not alter the contractile response to nerve stimulation (145).

PROSTAGLANDINS. Various prostaglandins, including

PGE$_1$, PGE$_2$, PGF$_{2\alpha}$, PGI$_2$, and thromboxane A$_2$ (cTxA$_2$) attenuate the release of neurotransmitter (for review see refs. 2, 178). In the mesenteric arteries the prostaglandins reduce the amplitude of the EJP (147, 149, 160), presumably by inhibition of transmitter release, because the same concentrations of prostaglandins do not affect the vascular smooth muscle membrane potential or resistance (147, 160). Indomethacin, a cyclooxygenase inhibitor, increases the amplitude of EJPs in guinea pig and rabbit mesenteric artery (147, 160). In light of this observation Kuriyama and Makita (147, 149) have speculated that prostaglandins may be synthesized in the mesenteric artery and act as local neuromodulator substances. Indomethacin enhances neuromuscular transmission in the mesenteric vasculature but not in guinea pig vas deferens (113) or canine bronchial muscle (114).

The actions of ACh and the prostaglandins resemble one another in that they both decrease the amplitude of the EJP without changing the number of nerve fibers activated by a given level of stimulus (see Fig. 5). However, the actions of ACh differ from those of the prostaglandins in that the prostaglandins have very little effect on the smooth muscle membrane potential or resistance with concentrations of $10^{-6}$ M or below (147, 160), whereas ACh in concentrations >$10^{-8}$ M results in vascular smooth muscle hyperpolarization and a decrease in membrane resistance (23). The actions of ACh also differ from those of the prostaglandins in that ACh enhances facilitation (153), whereas the prostaglandins have no effect on facilitation (147, 160). Finally, the actions of prostaglandin on EJP amplitude are reversed by increasing the [Ca$^{2+}$] in solution (147). These observations led Kuriyama and Makita (147) to speculate that ACh may act on the nerve terminal to modulate both Ca$^{2+}$ entry and Ca$^{2+}$ mobilization, whereas the prostaglandins act on Ca$^{2+}$ entry alone.

PURINERGIC AGENTS. Adenosine and adenine nucleotides inhibit presynaptically NE release from sympathetic neurons in vascular tissues (30, 33). Purinergic receptors can be divided into two subtypes (P$_1$ and P$_2$) depending on the relative potency of various adenine nucleotides and the actions of antagonists. The P$_1$ receptors are blocked by the methylxanthines, and adenosine is the most potent in producing effects at these receptors, with AMP, ADP, and ATP being progressively less potent. The P$_2$ receptors are blocked by quinidine as well as by 2-imidazole and 2,2′ pyridilsatogen. The order of potency of compounds for these receptors is the reverse of that for P$_1$ receptors: ATP, ADP, AMP, and adenosine in order of decreasing potency. Finally, P$_1$-receptor stimulation is associated with the production of cAMP, whereas P$_2$-receptor stimulation is associated with prostaglandin synthesis (30).

The EJP amplitude is effectively reduced by ATP in jejunal arteries of guinea pig and rabbit (106, 149). Adenosine, however, reduces EJP amplitude only in the rabbit (149). The interpretation of the effects of purines on arterial preparations is complicated by the fact that these compounds have both pre- and postjunctional effects. In the rabbit mesenteric artery, high concentrations of ATP ($10^{-4}$ M) result in a small but significant reduction in the overflow of NE. However, this same concentration of ATP nearly abolishes the EJP, depolarizes the smooth muscle, and increases membrane conductance (106). In this same tissue, $\alpha,\beta$-methylene ATP does not affect the overflow of NE but reduces the amplitude of the EJP to 20% of control. Facilitation of EJPs is also reduced by these agents, suggesting that they may inhibit mobilization of cytoplasmic Ca$^{2+}$ in nerve terminals. In the guinea pig mesenteric artery $\alpha,\beta$-methylene ATP produces a pronounced depolarization and reduces the amplitude of the EJP (106; O. D. Hottenstein and D. L. Kreulen, unpublished observations). In contrast, Kuriyama and Makita reported no effect of ATP or adenosine in the guinea pig jejunal artery (149).

NONADRENERGIC NONCHOLINERGIC TRANSMISSION. Neurons in sympathetic ganglia, and especially in the prevertebral ganglia, contain several neuroactive substances that in some cases are costored with NE. These substances include the neuropeptides vasopressin (76), neuropeptide Y (158), somatostatin (95, 158), the enkephalins (190), and vasoactive intestinal polypeptide (94). Substance P–like immunoreactivity is found in association with sensory nerves in the mesenteric blood vessels of the guinea pig (65). Very little is known about the effects of these substances on neuroeffector transmission in mesenteric blood vessels, but they could be neurotransmitters themselves and/or modulate the effects of other neurotransmitters. Few studies have investigated the effects of any of these substances on neuroeffector transmission in mesenteric blood vessels—either as transmitters or as modulators of transmission. (For effects of peptides on vascular smooth muscle see ref. 189; for further review see refs. 30, 32.)

## NEUROMUSCULAR RELATIONSHIPS IN NONMAMMALIAN ARTERY

The fowl mesenteric artery differs from the mammalian mesenteric artery in its anatomy, physiology, and pharmacology (17–20). Neuroeffector transmission in this vessel is also exceptional. Large phasic contractions associated with bursts of action potentials are observed both in vitro and in vivo. The pharmacology of neural responses and the orientation of the smooth muscle cells also differ from those in other arteries. Where an EJP can be recorded in most mesenteric arteries in response to transmural stimulation, none is reported for the fowl mesenteric artery. Instead stimulation of nerves leads to either action

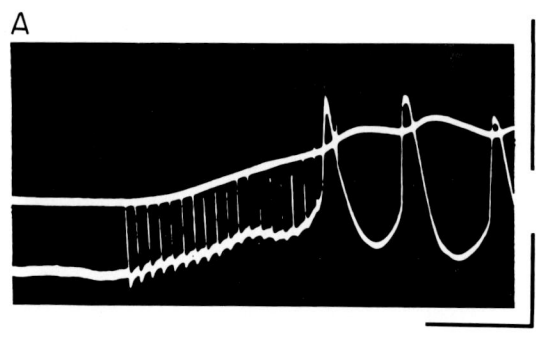
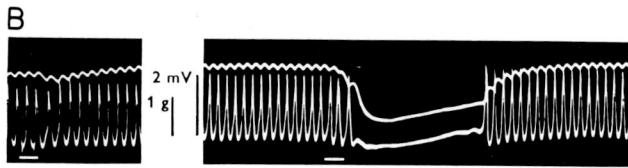

FIG. 8. Effects of brief electrical stimuli on longitudinal muscle of anterior mesenteric artery of domestic fowl measured by sucrose-gap method. *A*: depolarization without action potentials (*lower trace*) accompanies smooth rise in tension (*upper trace*) with repetitive stimulation at 5 Hz; action potentials are associated with small rapid contractions. Upper vertical bar, 1-g calibration; *lower vertical bar*, 2-mV calibration; *horizontal calibration*, 2 s. *B*: effects of brief electrical stimuli on preparation in which tone was raised by adding 0.2 mg/ml BaCl$_2$ to physiological saline in presence of hyoscine (10 ng/ml). *Upper trace*, contractile response. *Lower trace*, membrane potential response. Electrical stimulation at supramaximal strength was applied for 5 s at 1 Hz (*left panel*) or 10 Hz (*right panel*). Complete inhibition of action potentials occurs at the higher frequency of stimulation. [From Bolton (18)].

potential generation at higher frequencies of stimulation or to an initial slow depolarization followed by action potentials at low frequency stimulation (Fig. 8). Furthermore this excitatory response is cholinergic, since it is blocked by hyoscine. Adrenergic neurons appear to exert an effect on this vessel, because transmural stimulation of the contracted blood vessel results in the presence of hyoscine in relaxation. Relaxation is associated with a cessation of action potentials and is blocked by the β-receptor antagonist propranolol. From these observations Bolton (18) concludes that the fowl mesenteric artery is innervated by excitatory cholinergic neurons and inhibitory adrenergic neurons.

## MESENTERIC VEIN

There are relatively few electrophysiological studies of mesenteric veins, with the exception of the portal-anterior mesenteric vein. The portal vein differs from other mesenteric veins anatomically and electrophysiologically; therefore it is considered separately. Because of the relatively large splanchnic blood volume and the large reflex changes in that volume, understanding the neuromuscular relationships in the mesenteric veins will probably improve understanding of the neural control of the splanchnic circulation. Just as the function of mesenteric veins differs from that of mesenteric arteries, so too there are compelling differences in neuromuscular transmission between these two kinds of vessels.

### Resting Membrane Potential

Generally the membrane potentials of quiescent mesenteric veins are greater (more negative) than those recorded in the portal vein. Furthermore the resting membrane potential of mesenteric vein is generally less than that of mesenteric arteries. In a comparison of five mesenteric vessels of the guinea pig, Takata (217) obtained the following order for the magnitude of potential: branch jejunal artery (−68 mV) > cranial mesenteric artery (−60 mV) > jejunal artery (−52 mV) ≥ jejunal vein (−50 mV) = portal vein (−48 mV). These regional differences in membrane potential may be attributable to differences in the $P_{Na}/P_K$ ratio in the different vessels. The membrane potentials of adjacent sections of the guinea pig inferior mesenteric artery and vein differ by only 3 mV [−74 mV vs. −71 mV (104)]. In the intramural gastric vessels of the cat the arterioles are 13 mV more polarized than the venules [−64 mV vs. −51 mV (174)]; likewise the guinea pig renal vein (−46.8 mV) is depolarized compared with the renal artery [−66.8 mV (161)]. In the gastric submucosal vessels this difference in membrane potential may explain why venules contract more than arterioles in response to small depolarizing stimuli; i.e., venules are less polarized and thus closer to the voltage threshold for contraction. In the guinea pig inferior mesenteric vessels, however, the difference in membrane potential is too small to explain the difference in reactivity of these vessels to nerve stimulation; therefore other mechanisms related to neuroeffector transmission underlie the difference in responsiveness of these two vessels (104).

### Action Potentials

Spontaneous electrical activity is not observed in the vena cava (46) nor in more distal veins of the mesentery (104, 143, 128, 209, 217). However, in guinea pig jejunal vein in vitro, rhythmic potential changes of 1- to 20-mV amplitude, 0.1- to 1.5-s duration occurring over 5–20 min can be evoked by a brief nerve stimulation (20 Hz for 1 s). This activity is myogenic because it is not blocked by TTX or phentolamine.

### Passive Membrane Properties

The current-voltage relationship of the guinea pig mesenteric vein is linear in the hyperpolarizing direction and exhibits nonlinearities or rectification in the depolarizing direction (3, 77, 110, 130, 209). The amplitude of nerve-evoked depolarization is enhanced by TEA, and the occurrence of oscillatory potentials is increased. Both of these observations are compatible with a reduction in rectification by TEA.

Several studies have addressed coupling in the portal vein; however, no measurements of cable constants have been reported for other mesenteric veins. In a helically cut preparation of the guinea pig renal vein, the length constant is 0.43 mm and the membrane time constant is 98 ms (161). The functional characteristics of mesenteric veins suggest that venous cells are electrically coupled. Electrotonic potentials can be recorded in venous smooth muscle if current is applied to the tissue with the partition-stimulation method (209). Mesenteric veins respond more rapidly to nerve stimulation than do arteries (104) and yet contain a lower density of innervation (64). It seems probable that excitation due to neurotransmitter release is conducted through the tissue via low-resistance electrical pathways.

*Response to Autonomic Transmitter Substances*

NOREPINEPHRINE. Norepinephrine elicits a dose-dependent depolarization and contraction in electrically quiescent mesenteric veins of the dog (139, 211) and guinea pig (128, 209). At high doses ($>10^{-6}$ M), slow waves or action potentials are often superimposed on the depolarization. The NE-induced depolarization is associated with a reduction in the $K^+$ conductance (209). Although the depolarization elicited in guinea pig mesenteric vein is not affected by changing the extracellular concentrations of $Na^+$ or $Cl^-$, the NE-induced depolarization in portal vein is mediated by an increase in $Cl^-$ conductance (229). In the dog mesenteric vein the depolarization is abolished by the $\alpha_2$-antagonist yohimbine but not the $\alpha_1$-antagonist prazosin (139, 211). Isoproterenol hyperpolarizes the smooth muscle membrane of jejunal mesenteric veins; in contracted veins the hyperpolarization is associated with relaxation (217).

ACETYLCHOLINE. The electrical response of extramural veins to ACh varies depending on the vein studied. Acetylcholine hyperpolarizes and contracts guinea pig jejunal veins through an action on muscarinic receptors (128, 217). In contrast, the portal vein depolarizes and contracts. The responses are shown in Figure 9. This means that the jejunal vein contracts in the face of membrane hyperpolarization. This dissociation between electrical and contractile events with ACh is also seen in the rabbit mesenteric artery (152) and the guinea pig coronary artery (136). The contraction can therefore be attributed to voltage-independent mechanisms: either an increase in $Ca^{2+}$ conductance or a release of $Ca^{2+}$ from storage sites.

The guinea pig jejunal artery and vein hyperpolarize in the presence of ACh when the $[K^+]_o$ concentration is normal (5.9 mM). However, when $[K^+]_o$ is increased to 118 mM, ACh does not hyperpolarize either vessel, although it contracts the vein and relaxes the artery (217). The basis for the differences in the action of ACh in the vein and artery is not known.

*Response to Nerve Stimulation*

EXCITATORY JUNCTION POTENTIALS. The EJP cannot be evoked in the guinea pig mesenteric veins of the ileum (209), the distal colon (104, 143), or the rabbit portal vein (97). The dog mesenteric vein is the only mesenteric vein in which EJPs have been reported (211). The characteristics of the EJPs of the dog mesenteric vein resemble EJP characteristics recorded in mesenteric arteries in that they have a similar time course, their amplitude is stimulus strength dependent, and repetitive nerve stimulation leads to facilitation.

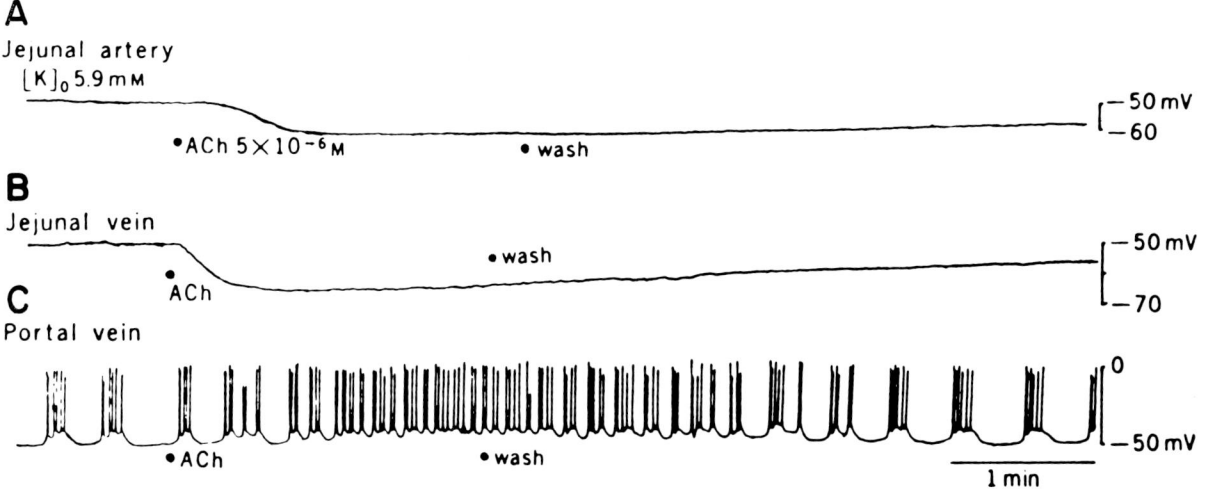

FIG. 9. Effects of acetylcholine (ACh) on various splanchnic vessels in guinea pig. Although ACh initiates a hyperpolarization in both jejunal mesenteric artery and vein, it depolarizes the portal vein. $[K]_o$, extracellular potassium concentration. [Adapted from Takata (217).]

ACTION POTENTIALS. Repetitive nerve stimulation in mesenteric veins without EJPs elicits a slow depolarization on which action potentials of variable amplitude (10-40 mV) and slow time course (3- to 5-s duration) are often superimposed [Fig. 10; (143, 209)]. As in many arteries, these action potentials are graded in amplitude (Fig. 11). In the inferior mesenteric vein and its branches, larger amplitude action potentials are obtained from smaller diameter veins than from the larger veins (O. D. Hottenstein and D. L. Kreulen, unpublished observations). The ionic basis of these neurally induced vein action potentials is not known.

In the dog mesenteric vein, EJPs that reach threshold give rise to an action potential that is graded in amplitude with stimulus strength (139, 209). This is similar to the response in some arteries (41, 134, 140, 206, 210).

SLOW DEPOLARIZATION. Repetitive nerve stimulation gives rise to a slow depolarization in all mesenteric veins studied. These include the jejunal vein

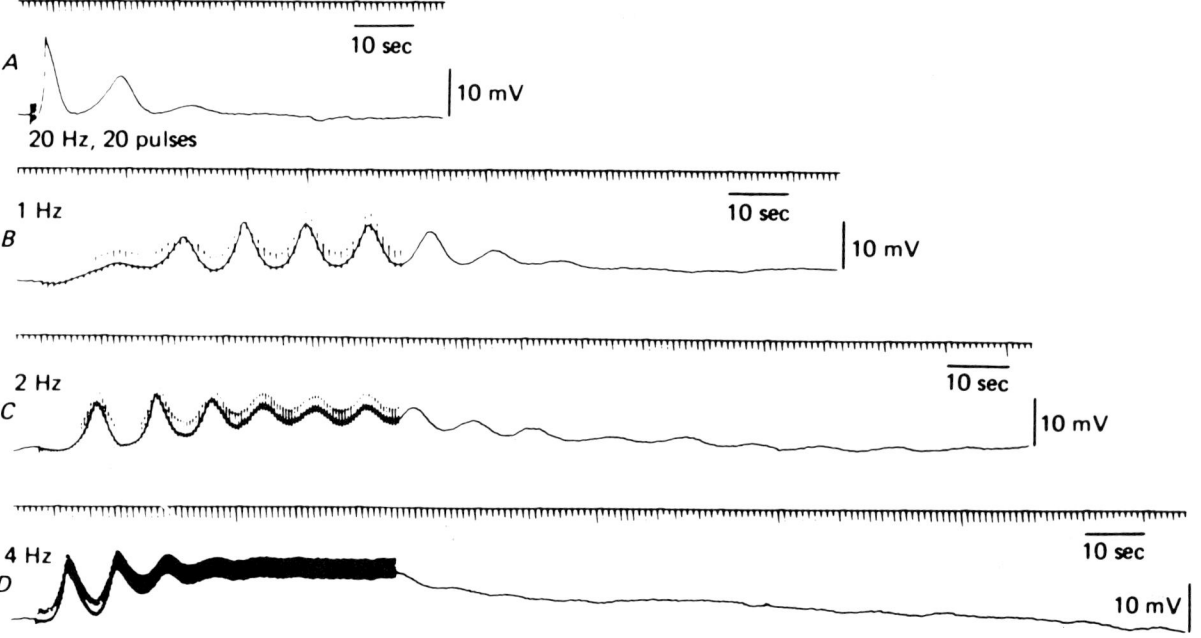

FIG. 10. Action potentials and slow waves induced by nerve stimulation, recorded from smooth muscle cells of guinea pig mesenteric vein. A: nerve stimulation (20 Hz, 1 s) induced action potential and slow waves. Train of pulses at 1 Hz (B), 2 Hz (C), or 4 Hz (D) was applied for 1 min. Upper trace in each record, time scale of 1 s. [From Suzuki (209).]

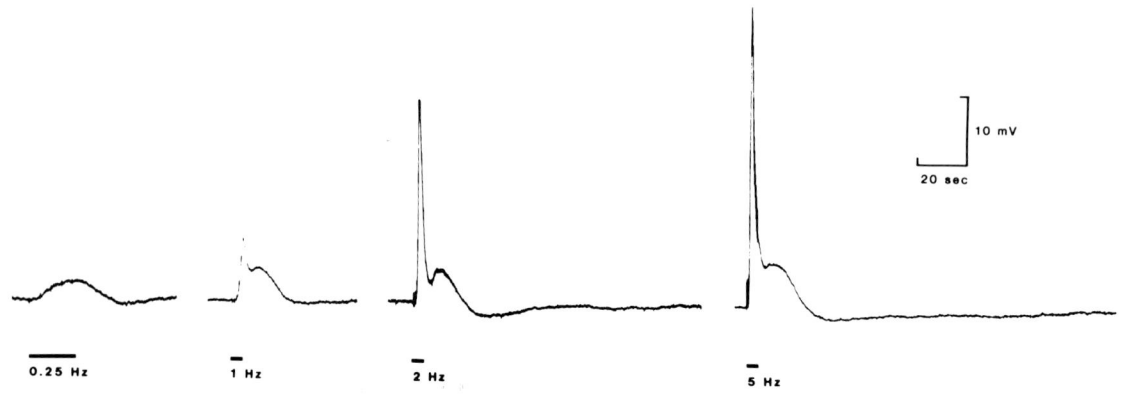

FIG. 11. Action potentials and slow depolarization, recorded in small (tertiary) mesenteric vein of distal colon in guinea pig with repetitive stimulation of lumbar colonic nerves. Note increasing amplitude action potentials recorded with higher frequencies. Resting membrane potential −70 mV; stimuli 10 V, 0.2 ms. (O. D. Hottenstein and D. L. Kreulen, unpublished observations.)

(209); the inferior mesenteric vein (104, 143); the dog mesenteric vein, which also exhibits EJPs (139, 211); and the spontaneously active portal vein (97). The amplitude of the slow depolarization is dependent on the frequency, duration, and strength of the stimulus until a maximum depolarization of 5–12 mV is obtained. Sometimes slow oscillations are superimposed on the depolarization (209). Action potentials are often superimposed on larger depolarizations evoked at frequencies >5 Hz [Figs. 10, 11; (143, 209)]. Both the slow depolarizations and action potentials are association with contraction (104, 143).

The slow depolarization appears to be mediated by NE acting on postjunctional $\alpha$-receptors. The long latency (up to 2 s) of the slow depolarization and its slow time course (compared with arterial EJPs, for example) support the explanation that it is due to the diffusion of NE away from the nerve terminals to extrajunctional $\alpha$-receptors. Furthermore the response to nerve stimulation in the guinea pig mesenteric vein closely resembles the depolarization and oscillations obtained with exogenous NE (209).

The intramural venules of the cat stomach also produce a slow depolarization in response to repetitive nerve stimulation (174). The venules differ from extramural veins in that in some venule cells repetitive nerve stimulation evokes a slow hyperpolarization or biphasic response. In the gastric submucosal venules the slow depolarization is blocked by prazosin, whereas the slow hyperpolarization is blocked by propranolol (174).

*Pharmacology of Neuroeffector Transmission*

EXCITATORY JUNCTION POTENTIALS. The only vein in which EJPs can be evoked with nerve stimulation is the dog mesenteric artery (139, 211). The EJP recorded in the dog mesenteric vein is suppressed by guanethidine or TTX; thus it appears to be due to release of transmitter from sympathetic nerves (139, 211). The pharmacology of the dog mesenteric vein EJP resembles that of the guinea pig mesenteric artery EJP in that *1*) vein EJPs are not blocked by $\alpha$-receptor antagonists, *2*) vein EJPs are reduced in amplitude by NE, and *3*) yohimbine or phentolamine enhances facilitation of venous EJPs. The pharmacology of the venous EJP is subject to the same controversies as those surrounding the transmitter responsible for the arterial EJP (see *Pharmacology of Neuroeffector Transmission*, p. 1618).

SLOW DEPOLARIZATION. The nerve-induced slow depolarization in the guinea pig jejunal vein (59, 209), guinea pig inferior mesenteric vein (104, 143), dog mesenteric vein (211), and rabbit portal vein (97) is abolished by phentolamine or TTX; thus it appears to be due to the action of neurally released NE on $\alpha$-adrenergic receptors. In this way the venous slow depolarization resembles the arterial slow depolarization (35, 41, 104, 143, 171, 181, 210, 214, 216).

The slow depolarization of the guinea pig inferior mesenteric vein appears to be mediated by stimulation of both $\alpha_1$- and $\alpha_2$-adrenergic receptors, because complete inhibition is not achieved until the vessel is exposed to both antagonists simultaneously (O. D. Hottenstein and D. L. Kreulen, unpublished observations). However, the slow depolarization in the dog mesenteric vein appears to be mediated by $\alpha_2$-receptors because it is blocked by yohimbine but not by prazosin (211).

PORTAL VEIN

The portal vein is unique among mesenteric vessels of mammals because it has a relatively thick medial layer of longitudinally oriented smooth muscle (97) and because it has spontaneous electrical and mechanical activity. Probably it is these interesting properties that account for the portal vein being the most studied mesenteric blood vessel. The portal vein and its distal branch the anterior mesenteric vein have similar properties and are subsequently referred to as the portal vein. To facilitate comparison, the properties of the portal vein are reviewed in the same manner used for other mesenteric vessels.

*Spontaneous Action Potentials*

The presence of spontaneous slow waves and action potentials makes the portal vein unique among mammalian mesenteric blood vessels. This electrical activity is associated with irregular contractions. Spontaneous activity has been reported in the in vitro portal vein of the dog (53); guinea pig (70, 128, 150, 177, 217, 228), rat (4, 54, 61, 80, 122, 152, 156), sheep (98), baboon (46), and rabbit [Fig. 12; (46, 47, 97, 197)]. Spikes can also be generated in the portal vein by application of inward or outward current with the partition-stimulation method (1). Outward current initiates a spike by depolarizing the tissue to threshold, and inward current by anode-break excitation (110, 152).

Portal vein spontaneous activity is myogenic (as opposed to neurogenic) because it is not blocked by phentolamine (97, 208, 228), phenoxybenzamine (123, 228), atropine (208), hexamethonium (208), or TTX (97, 110), but it can be reduced or abolished by membrane hyperpolarization (3). Portal vein action potentials are insensitive to reduced $[Na^+]_o$ but are blocked by $Mn^{2+}$ and verapamil (70) or by removal of extracellular $Ca^{2+}$ (4, 47, 208, 223). These results suggest that the inward current is carried predominantly by $Ca^{2+}$.

Spontaneous action potentials of the portal vein are variable in amplitude (maximum amplitude 50–60 mV) and time course (maximum rise of spike 11.6 V/s) (81, 97, 128, 150, 152, 177). Variability can even be recorded from a single cell (3, 81). Three types of spontaneous action potentials have been described for the guinea pig portal vein: *1*) pacemaker-type action potentials with prepotentials resembling the pacemaker potential of cardiac muscle, *2*) spikes with a rapid repolarization phase, and *3*) spikes with a hump during the repolarization phase (110).

Action potentials typically occur in bursts superimposed on a slow depolarization (Fig. 12). Bursts of action potentials may vary in duration from 2 to 30 s and occur at a rate of 1–27 per min. Each burst of electrical activity is typically associated with contraction of the tissue (123). Under some circumstances continuous discharge of action potentials predominates (81, 150, 152). Increasing $[K^+]_o$ from 4.7 mM to 30 mM converts activity in the rat portal vein from burst activity to continuous activity, with low-amplitude contractions occurring at the same frequency as the spikes (81). When $[K^+]$ is raised above 40–50 mM, a "depolarization block" of spike generation occurs (81, 152).

Spontaneous activity originates from pacemaker sites within the tissue. Conduction of the action potential through the tissue is decremental and nonuniform, with activity from a single pacemaker conducting 2–5 mm from the site of origin (80). In several different preparations the conduction velocity ranges from 0.5 to 3 cm/s (61, 110, 156). Pacemaker activity from one site will affect the activity generated at another (80, 156); thus the overall contractile response of the tissue depends on the extent of pacemaker site synchronization, the number of active pacemakers, and the configuration of electrical activity (i.e., burst duration, rate, frequency).

Some degree of rectification appears to be present in portal vein in the depolarizing direction. Hara et al. (77) report that both procaine and 4-aminopyridine (compounds with actions similar to TEA on $K^+$ conductance) reduce rectification in the guinea pig portal vein.

*Cell Coupling*

Cable constants of the portal vein have been reported for the guinea pig and rat. The length constant ($\lambda$) of the guinea pig (range: 0.52–0.71 mm) measured in the direction of cell orientation (longitudinally) is shorter than the length constant of the rat portal vein (1.2 mm) or of the majority of helically cut arteries (see Table 2). Because $\lambda = \sqrt{R_m/R_i}$, a small $\lambda$ will be obtained if either the membrane resistance ($R_m$) is low or the internal resistance ($R_i$) including coupling resistance is high.

Coupling in the guinea pig portal vein has also been examined by measuring electrical activity simultaneously from two or more points in the preparation. With two intracellular microelectrodes placed from 0.13 to 2 mm apart, there is a constant delay between the action potentials measured at each electrode for a given impalement, which suggests that activity originates from pacemaker regions and conducts outward into nonpacing regions. There is a linear relationship between the delay and the distance between the recording electrodes; the conduction velocity (slope) is 0.58 cm/s (110). This is considerably less than the conduction velocity in rat portal vein [1.7–3 cm/s (61, 156)]. The difference is probably related to the longer length constant of rat portal vein (Table 2).

In the rat portal vein, action potentials recorded with multiple extracellular electrodes at 1-mm intervals reveal multiple pacemaker sites. Within a pacemaker area, spikes fire at the same frequency but differ in amplitude. Electrodes placed in different pacemaker areas record spikes of different frequencies. The conclusions of this study are *1*) action potentials conduct over only a limited distance (2–5 mm), *2*) this conduction is decremental, and *3*) rat portal vein is controlled by multiple pacing regions (80).

*Response to Nerve Stimulation*

Single nerve shocks do not evoke EJPs in portal vein; repetitive nerve stimulation evokes a slow depolarization accompanied by an increase in the frequency of action potential burst [Fig. 12; (96)]. In separate experiments measuring the contractile response of the portal vein, nerve stimulation elicits an increase in the tone and the frequency of rhythmic contractions [Fig. 13; (123)].

*Response to Neurotransmitters*

NOREPINEPHRINE. Norepinephrine depolarizes the portal vein of a number of different species, including rat (123, 152), guinea pig (70, 128, 228), rabbit (46, 97, 197), and dog (197). This depolarization is associated with an increase in the frequency of spikes and spike

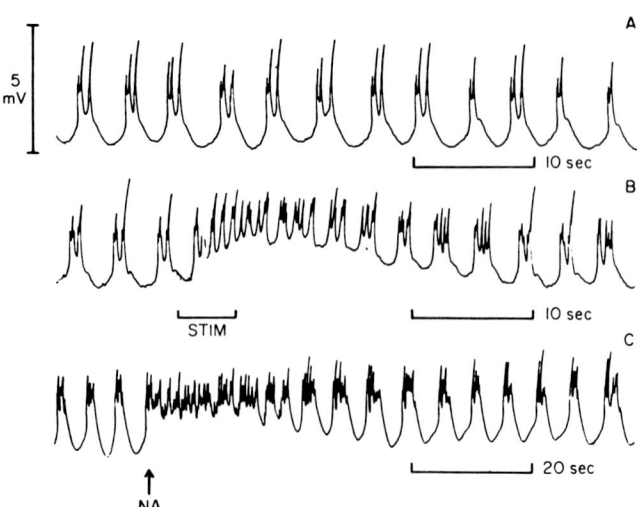

FIG. 12. Spontaneous and evoked activity in strip of rabbit portal vein, recorded with sucrose-gap technique. *A*: normal ongoing spontaneous activity; *B*: response to stimulation of intramural noradrenergic nerves; *C*: response to 0.1 µg/ml of noradrenaline (NA). [From Holman (96).]

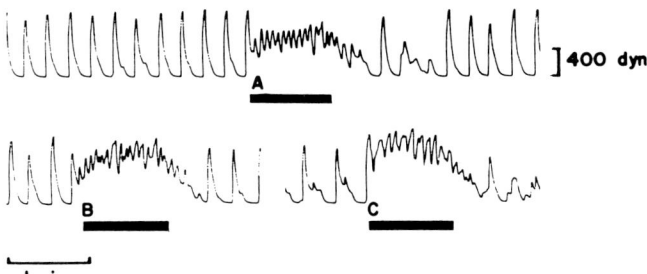

FIG. 13. Contractile responses of innervated strip of rabbit portal vein to postganglionic nerve stimulation in vitro. A: 4 Hz; B: 8 Hz; C: 16 Hz. Increase in contraction frequency produced by nerve stimulation in this regularly contracting muscle. *Heavy bar*, stimulation time. [From Johansson and Ljung (122).]

bursts (Fig. 12). The increase in electrical activity also corresponds to an increase in the frequency and force of contractions (47, 70, 97, 122, 156, 197, 217). As the membrane depolarizes, the amplitude of spikes progressively decreases until, under some circumstances, action potentials are completely eliminated and the muscle is tonically contracted (122). Epinephrine (61, 177) and phenylephrine (217, 228) produce effects similar to those of NE. The excitatory actions of these agonists are due to $\alpha$-receptor stimulation, because the responses are blocked by phentolamine.

When NE is added to the rabbit or guinea pig portal vein in the presence of phenoxybenzamine, spontaneous activity is inhibited, an action that is antagonized by the $\beta$-receptor antagonist propranolol (123, 228). Similarly in portal veins of rabbit, rat, and guinea pig, isoproterenol decreases the frequency of spontaneous action potentials and burst duration (46, 47, 97, 122, 151, 208, 217, 228).

ACETYLCHOLINE. Acetylcholine depolarizes the portal vein through an atropine-sensitive mechanism [see Fig. 9; (128, 217)]. Several studies have reported that ACh initially hyperpolarizes the portal vein before depolarization (60, 61, 177).

## FUNCTIONAL IMPLICATIONS OF NEUROMUSCULAR DIFFERENCES BETWEEN ARTERY AND VEIN

Several anatomical and functional differences between arterial and venous neuromuscular apparatus have been described. These include the greater density of the perivascular nerve supply in arteries than in veins, the presence of EJPs in arteries but not in veins (with one exception), a slow depolarization with a more rapid onset in veins than in arteries, a slow depolarization with a lower half-maximal nerve stimulation frequency in veins than in arteries, and a more rapid onset of nerve-evoked contraction in veins than in arteries.

The more rapid response of the venous or capacitance side of the splanchnic circulation compared with the arterial or resistance side has been reported in several species. In humans moderate hemorrhage results in decreases in splanchnic blood volume without significant arterial constriction (184). In experimental animal preparations the volume changes occur before and at lower frequencies than the resistance changes, whether the innervation of the splanchnic circulation is activated reflexly or stimulated directly (57, 67, 71, 74, 131, 218). These resistance-capacitance differences are not universal because they do not occur in the skeletal muscle vasculature (75, 165).

Neuromuscular transmission in guinea pig inferior mesenteric artery and vein has been compared in vitro, and relationships between nerve stimulation frequency and vessel responses were found to correspond to the physiological differences between artery and vein (104, 143). The more rapid onset of contraction and lower frequency for half-maximal contraction is correlated with a more rapid and greater slow depolarization in veins than in arteries (Fig. 14). The smaller proportional response of arteries to nerve stimulation at lower frequencies may be a consequence of the presence of inhibitory neurotransmitter(s); i.e., the slow hyperpolarizations that occur in the guinea pig inferior mesenteric artery but not in the vein may be the reason why the frequency-response relationship for constriction of artery is shifted to higher frequencies compared with constriction of vein (Fig. 15). It seems that the depolarization and contraction recorded in the artery are the sum of inhibitory and excitatory influences. For example, the hyperpolarizations are more apparent at low frequencies or in the presence of prazosin. At high frequencies in the absence of an $\alpha$-antagonist, the hyperpolarization is masked by the excitatory $\alpha$-adrenergic depolarization, but the underlying presence of the putative inhibitory neurotransmitter decreases the excitatory response. Perhaps, because the vein has no inhibitory potentials, it depolarizes proportionally more than the artery (Fig. 15). Thus the functional differences between the resistance and capacitance circulation may have their bases in the differences in the mechanism of neuromuscular transmission.

When compared directly, the NE concentration-response relationship for veins is to the left of that for arteries; i.e., NE is more potent in veins than in arteries (221). A suggested explanation of this difference is that there are more postjunctional $\alpha_2$-receptors in mesenteric vein than in artery. This might also be the case in the guinea pig, because the $\alpha_1$-antagonist prazosin is not as effective against slow depolarizations and contractions in inferior mesenteric vein as it is in the corresponding artery (104). These kinds of differences could also reflect differences in the structure of the innervation, although these have not been investigated in the guinea pig inferior mesenteric artery and vein. Understanding the basis of the functional differences between mesenteric artery and vein will require knowledge of the neuromuscular relationships in these blood vessels.

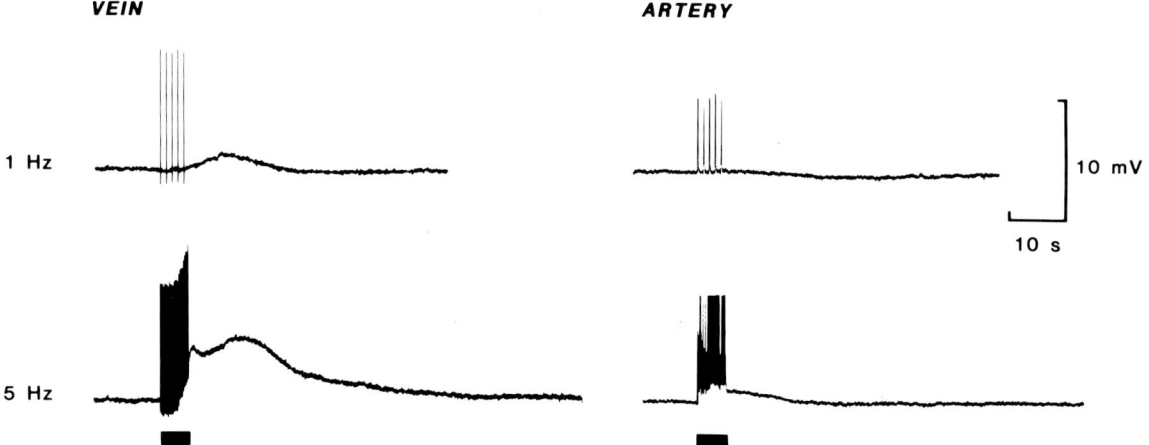

FIG. 14. Comparison of membrane potential responses of mesenteric vein and artery to repetitive lumbar colonic nerve stimulation (supramaximal). Greater slow depolarizations occur at both frequencies in vein. Vertical deflections in venous tracing during stimulation are stimulus artifacts; in artery, vertical deflections at 1 Hz are excitatory junction potentials (EJP), whereas at 5 Hz, stimulus artifacts are superimposed upon EJP. Bar, period of stimulation. [Adapted from Hottenstein and Kreulen (104).]

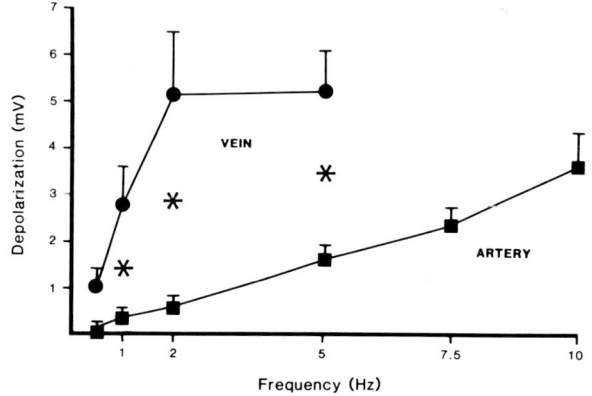

FIG. 15. Frequency dependence of the amplitude of slow depolarization in vein and artery of distal colonic mesentery of guinea pig. Seven artery cell and 11 vein cell responses were compared by unpaired $t$ test ($P < 0.01$). [Adapted from Hottenstein and Kreulen (104).]

## CONCLUSIONS

This review has dealt with the structure and function of the neuromuscular junction of mesenteric artery. Neuromuscular transmission in the mesenteric blood vessels is a multifaceted process that depends on the anatomy of the innervation, the functional characteristics of the vascular smooth muscle, and the ability of various humoral factors to interact with nerve and muscle. Many of the properties of the neuromuscular apparatus of mesenteric blood vessels are similar to other vascular beds as well as other smooth muscle organs. However, there is great structural and functional variety among the many different species and smooth muscle organs that have been studied. The mesenteric vasculature seems to share in this variety.

Two kinds of neural signals from sympathetic nerves have been recorded in the mesenteric vasculature—fast and slow. There is controversy regarding the mechanism of the mediation of these signals, but they appear to be mediated by more than one neurotransmitter, perhaps several. Each kind of signal may also reflect a neuromuscular junction of a particular structure. Constriction of blood vessels may depend on both the fast and slow signals, but the slow excitatory signals are most closely associated with contraction of the smooth muscle and with the release of NE. Neural signals can be modulated by substances that modify the release of neurotransmitter from nerve terminals and/or alter the responsiveness of the vascular smooth muscle cells. Finally, the physiological differences between the arterial and venous sides of the mesenteric circulation may be based on the degree to which each kind of neural signal predominates in veins and arteries. Elucidating structural and functional details of the mesenteric blood vessel neuromuscular junction should continue to contribute to our understanding of the mechanisms underlying the neural control of the splanchnic circulation.

We express our sincere appreciation to Drs. M. Holman, T. Neild, and H. Suzuki for reading a preliminary version of this review and offering many helpful comments and suggestions and to Rita Wedell for editorial and secretarial assistance.

Research was supported by the National Institutes of Health grant HL-27781, a Research Career Development Award HL-01136 (D. L. Kreulen), and a New Investigator Research Award HL-34449 (K. D. Keef).

# REFERENCES

1. ABE, Y., AND T. TOMITA. Cable properties of smooth muscle. *J. Physiol. Lond.* 196: 87–100, 1968.
2. ARMSTRONG, J. M., AND A. F. GREEN. Evaluation of agents that release or modify release of adrenergic transmission. In: *Adrenergic Activators and Inhibitors*, edited by L. Szekeres. Berlin: Springer-Verlag, 1980, p. 135–221.
3. ASADA, H., T. NANJO, T. ITOH, H. SUZUKI, AND H. KURIYAMA. Effects of 3,4-dihydro-8-(2-hydroxy-3-isopropylaminopropoxy)-3-nitroxy-2H-1-benzopyran (K-351) on smooth muscle cells and neuromuscular transmission in guinea-pig vascular tissues. *J. Pharmacol. Exp. Ther.* 223: 560–572, 1982.
4. AXELSSON, J., B. WAHLSTROM, B. JOHANSSON, AND O. JONSSON. Influence of the ionic environment on spontaneous electrical and mechanical activity of the rat portal vein. *Circ. Res.* 21: 609–618, 1967.
5. BALL, R. A., J. H. SAUTTER, AND M. S. KATTER. Morphological characteristics of the anterior mesenteric artery of the fowl. *Anat. Rec.* 146: 251–255, 1963.
6. BELL, C. Transmission from vasoconstrictor and vasodilator nerves to single smooth muscle cells of the guinea-pig uterine artery. *J. Physiol. Lond.* 205: 695–708, 1969.
7. BENHAN, C. D., T. B. BOLTON, R. J. LANG, AND T. TAKEWAKI. Calcium-activated potassium channels in single smooth muscle cells of rabbit jejunum and guinea-pig mesenteric artery. *J. Physiol. Lond.* 371: 45–67, 1986.
8. BENNETT, M. R. *Autonomic Neuromuscular Transmission*. Cambridge, UK: Cambridge Univ. Press, 1972.
9. BENNETT, M. R., AND T. FLORRIN. An electrophysiological analysis of the effects of $Ca^{2+}$ ions on neuromuscular transmission in the mouse vas deferens. *Br. J. Pharmacol.* 55: 97–104, 1975.
10. BEVAN, J. A. Some functional consequences of variation in adrenergic synaptic cleft width and in nerve density and distribution. *Federation Proc.* 36: 2439–2443, 1977.
11. BEVAN, J. A., R. D. BEVAN, AND S. P. DUCKLES. Adrenergic regulation of vascular smooth muscle. In: *Handbook of Physiology. The Cardiovascular System. Vascular Smooth Muscle*, edited by D. F. Bohr, A. P. Somlyo, and H. V. Sparks, Jr. Bethesda, MD: Am. Physiol. Soc., 1980, sect. 2, vol. II, chapt. 18, p. 515–566.
12. BEVAN, J. A., D. W. HOSMER, B. LJUNG, B. L. PEGRAN, AND C. SU. Innervation pattern and neurogenic response of rabbit veins. *Blood Vessels* 11: 172–182, 1974.
13. BEVAN, J. A., AND C. SU. Distribution theory of resistance of neurogenic vasoconstriction to alpha-receptor blockade in the rabbit. *Circ. Res.* 28: 179–187, 1971.
14. BIBER, B., J. FARA, AND O. LUNDGREN. A pharmacological study of intestinal vasodilator mechanisms in the cat. *Acta Physiol. Scand.* 90: 673–683, 1974.
15. BIBER, B., O. LUNDGREN, AND J. SVANVIK. Studies on the intestinal vasodilatation observed after mechanical stimulation of the mucosa of the gut. *Acta Physiol. Scand.* 82: 177–190, 1971.
16. BLASCHKO, H., G. V. R. BORN, A. D'IORIO, AND N. R. EADE. Observations on the distribution of catecholamines and adenosine triphosphate in the bovine adrenal medulla. *J. Physiol. Lond.* 133: 548–557, 1956.
17. BOLTON, T. B. Studies of the longitudinal muscle of the anterior mesenteric artery of the domestic fowl. *J. Physiol. Lond.* 196: 273–281, 1968.
18. BOLTON, T. B. Electrical and mechanical activity of the longitudinal muscle of the anterior mesenteric artery of the domestic fowl. *J. Physiol. Lond.* 196: 283–292, 1968.
19. BOLTON, T. B. Spontaneous and evoked release of neurotransmitter substances in the longitudinal muscle of the anterior mesenteric artery of the domestic fowl. *Br. J. Pharmacol.* 35: 112–120, 1969.
20. BOLTON, T. B. Electrical properties and constants of longitudinal muscle from the avian anterior mesenteric artery. *Blood Vessels* 11: 65–78, 1974.
21. BOLTON, T. B. Mechanisms of action of transmitters and other substances on smooth muscle. *Physiol. Rev.* 59: 609–718, 1979.
22. BOLTON, T. B., AND L. H. CLAPP. Endothelial-dependent relaxant actions of carbachol and substance P in arterial smooth muscle. *Br. J. Pharmacol.* 87: 713–723, 1986.
23. BOLTON, T. B., R. J. LANG, AND T. TAKEWAKI. Mechanism of action of noradrenaline and carbachol on smooth muscle of guinea-pig anterior mesenteric artery. *J. Physiol. Lond.* 351: 549–572, 1984.
24. BONACCORSI, A., K. HERMSMEYER, O. APRIGLIANO, C. B. SMITH, AND D. F. BOHR. Mechanism of potassium relaxation of arterial muscle. *Blood Vessels* 14: 261–276, 1977.
25. BOOZ, K. H. Zur Innervation der Autonom pulsie-renden Vena Portae der weissen Ratte. Einehistochemishe und electronenmikroskopische Untersuchung. *Z. Zellforsch. Mikrosk. Anat.* 117: 394–418, 1971.
26. BROOKSBY, G. A., AND D. E. DONALD. Sympathetic outflow from spinal cord to splanchnic circulation of the dog. *Am. J. Physiol.* 219: 1429–1433, 1970.
27. BROOKSBY, G. A., AND D. E. DONALD. Dynamic changes in splanchnic blood flow and blood volume in dogs during activation of sympathetic nerves. *Circ. Res.* 29: 227–238, 1971.
28. BULBRING, E., H. OHASHI, AND T. TOMITA. Adrenergic mechanisms. In: *Smooth Muscle*, edited by E. Bulbring, A. F. Brading, A. W. Jones, and T. Tomita. Baltimore, MD: Williams & Wilkins, 1981, p. 219–248.
29. BURKE, W. Spontaneous potentials in slow muscle fibres of the frog. *J. Physiol. Lond.* 135: 511–521, 1957.
30. BURNSTOCK, G. Cholinergic and purinergic regulation of blood vessels. In: *Handbook of Physiology. The Cardiovascular System. Vascular Smooth Muscle*, edited by D. F. Bohr, A. P. Somlyo, and H. V. Sparks, Jr. Bethesda, MD: Am. Physiol. Soc., 1980, sect. 2, vol. II, chapt. 19, p. 567–612.
31. BURNSTOCK, G. The co-transmitter hypothesis, with special reference to the storage and release of ATP with noradrenaline and acetylcholine. In: *Co-Transmission*, edited by A. C. Cuello. London: Macmillan, 1982, p. 151–163.
32. BURNSTOCK, G. The changing face of autonomic neuromuscular transmission. *Acta Physiol. Scand.* 126: 67–91, 1986.
33. BURNSTOCK, G. (editor). *Purinergic Receptors*. London: Chapman & Hall, 1981.
34. BURNSTOCK, G., AND M. COSTA. *Adrenergic Neurons: Their Organization, Function & Development in the Peripheral Nervous System*. New York: Wiley, 1975, p. 225.
35. BURNSTOCK, G., S. G. GRIFFITH, AND P. SNEDDON. Autonomic nerves in the precapillary vessel wall. *J. Cardiovasc. Pharmacol.* 6, Suppl. 2: S344–S353, 1984.
36. BURNSTOCK, G., AND M. E. HOLMAN. Spontaneous potentials at sympathetic nerve endings in smooth muscle. *J. Physiol. Lond.* 160: 446–460, 1962.
37. BYRNE, N. G., AND W. A. LARGE. The effect of $\alpha,\beta$-methylene ATP on the depolarization evoked by noradrenaline ($\gamma$-adrenoceptor response) and ATP in the immature rat basilar artery. *Br. J. Pharmacol.* 88: 6–8, 1986.
38. BYWATER, R. A. R., AND G. S. TAYLOR. The passive membrane properties and excitatory junction potentials of the guinea-pig vas deferens. *J. Physiol. Lond.* 300: 303–316, 1980.
39. CASTEELS, R., K. KITAMURA, H. KURIYAMA, AND H. SUZUKI. The membrane properties of the smooth muscle cells of the rabbit main pulmonary artery. *J. Physiol. Lond.* 271: 41–61, 1977.
40. CHEUNG, D. W. Spontaneous and evoked excitatory junction potentials in rat tail arteries. *J. Physiol. Lond.* 328: 449–459, 1982.
41. CHEUNG, D. W. Two components in the cellular response of rat tail arteries to nerve stimulation. *J. Physiol. Lond.* 328: 461–468, 1982.

42. CHEUNG, D. W. Neural regulation and mechanical activities in the rat tail artery. *Pfluegers Arch.* 400: 335–337, 1984.
43. CLIFF, W. J., AND D. PHIL. The aortic tunica media in growing rats studied with the electron microscope. *Lab. Invest.* 17: 599–615, 1967.
44. COWEN, T. An ultrastructural comparison of neuromuscular relationships in blood vessels with functional and "non-functional" neuromuscular transmission. *J. Neurocytol.* 13: 369–392, 1984.
45. COWEN, T., D. E. MACCORMICK, W. D. TOFF, G. BURNSTOCK, AND J. S. LUMLEY. The effect of surgical procedures on blood vessel innervation. A fluorescence histochemical study of degeneration and regrowth of perivascular adrenergic nerves. *Blood Vessels* 19: 65–78, 1982.
46. CUTHBERT, A. W. Electrical activity in mammalian veins. *Bibl. Anat.* 8: 11–15, 1966.
47. CUTHBERT, A. W., AND M. C. SUTTER. The effects of drugs on the relation between the action potential discharge and tension in a mammalian vein. *Br. J. Pharmacol.* 25: 592–601, 1965.
48. DEVINE, C. E., AND F. O. SIMPSON. The fine structure of vascular sympathetic neuromuscular contacts in the rat. *Am. J. Anat.* 121: 153–174, 1967.
49. DRAPEAU, P., AND M. BLAUSTEIN. Calcium and neurotransmitter release. In: *Trends in Autonomic Pharmacology*, edited by S. Kalsner. Munich, FRG: Urban & Schwarzeuberg, 1982.
50. DROOGMANS, G., L. RAEYMAEKERS, AND R. CASTEELS. Electro- and pharmacomechanical coupling in the smooth muscle cells of the rabbit ear artery. *J. Gen. Physiol.* 70: 129–148, 1977.
51. ESTERHUIZEN, A. C., J. D. P. GRAHAM, J. D. LEVER, AND T. L. B. SPRIGGS. Catecholamine and acetylcholinesterase distribution in relation to noradrenaline release. *Br. J. Pharmacol.* 32: 46–56, 1968.
52. FALCK, B., N. A. HILLARP, AND B. HOGBERG. Content and intracellular distribution of adenosine triphosphate in cow adrenal medulla. *Acta Physiol. Scand.* 36: 360–376, 1956.
53. FEDAN, J. S., G. K. HOGABOOM, J. P. O'DONNELL, J. COLBY, AND D. P. WESTFALL. Contribution by purines to the neurogenic response of the vas deferens of the guinea pig. *Eur. J. Pharmacol.* 69: 41–53, 1981.
54. FINKEL, A. S., G. D. S. HIRST, AND D. F. VAN HELDEN. Some properties of excitatory junction currents recorded from submucosal arterioles of guinea-pig ileum. *J. Physiol. Lond.* 351: 87–98, 1984.
55. FOLKOW, B., D. H. LEWIS, O. LUNDGREN, S. MELLANDER, AND I. WALLENTIN. The effect of graded vasoconstrictor fibre stimulation on the intestinal resistance and capacitance vessels. *Acta Physiol. Scand.* 61: 445–457, 1964.
56. FOLKOW, B., AND E. NEIL. *Circulation.* New York: Oxford Univ. Press, 1971.
57. FORD, R., R. HAINSWORTH, A. J. RANKIN, AND A. O. SOLADOYE. Abdominal vascular responses to changes in carbon dioxide tension in the cephalic circulation of anaesthetized dogs. *J. Physiol. Lond.* 358: 417–431, 1985.
58. FRASHER, W. G., AND H. WAYLAND. Repeating modular organization of the microcirculation of cat mesentery. *Microvasc. Res.* 4: 62–76, 1972.
59. FUJIOKA, M., AND H. SUZUKI. Effect of amosulalol on the electrical responses of guinea-pig vascular smooth muscle to adrenoceptor activation. *Br. J. Pharmacol.* 84: 489–497, 1985.
60. FUNAKI, S. Electrical and mechanical activity of isolated smooth muscle from the portal vein of the rat. *Bibl. Anat.* 8: 5–10, 1966.
61. FUNAKI, S., AND D. F. BOHR. Electrical and mechanical activity of isolated vascular smooth muscle of the rat. *Nature Lond.* 203: 192–194, 1964.
62. FURCHGOTT, R. F. Role of the endothelium in responses of vascular smooth muscle. *Circ. Res.* 53: 557–573, 1983.
63. FURNESS, J. B. The adrenergic innervation of the vessels supplying and draining the gastrointestinal tract. *Z. Zellforsch. Mikrosk. Anat.* 113: 67–82, 1971.
64. FURNESS, J. B., AND J. M. MARSHALL. Correlation of the directly observed responses of mesenteric vessels of the rat to nerve stimulation and noradrenaline with the distribution of adrenergic nerves. *J. Physiol. Lond.* 239: 75–88, 1974.
65. FURNESS, J. B., R. E. PAPKA, N. G. DELLA, M. COSTA, AND R. L. ESKAY. Substance P-like immunoreactivity in nerves associated with the vascular system of guinea-pigs. *Neuroscience* 7: 447–459, 1982.
66. GANNON, B. J., S. M. ROSENBERGER, T. D. VERSLUIS, AND P. C. JOHNSON. Autoregulatory patterns in the arteriolar network of cat mesentery. *Microvasc. Res.* 26: 1–14, 1983.
67. GERO, J., AND M. GEROVA. In vivo studies of sympathetic control of vessels of different function. In: *Physiology and Pharmacology of Vascular Neuroeffector Systems*, edited by J. A. Bevan, R. F. Furchgott, R. A. Maxwell, and A. P. Somylo. New York: Karger, 1971, p. 86–94.
68. GINSBORG, B. L. Spontaneous activity in muscle fibres of the chick. *J. Physiol. Lond.* 150: 707–717, 1960.
69. GOLDMAN, D. E. Potential, impedance and rectification in membranes. *J. Gen. Physiol.* 27: 37–60, 1944.
70. GOLENHOFEN, K., N. HERMSTEIN, AND E. LAMMEL. Membrane potential and contraction of vascular smooth muscle (portal vein) during application of noradrenaline and high potassium, and selective inhibitory effects of iproveratril (verapamil). *Microvasc. Res.* 5: 73–80, 1973.
71. GREENWAY, C. V. Role of splanchnic venous system in overall cardiovascular homeostasis. *Federation Proc.* 42: 1678–1684, 1983.
72. GREENWAY, C. V., AND R. D. STARK. Hepatic vascular bed. *Physiol. Rev.* 51: 23–65, 1971.
73. HAEUSLER, G., AND S. THORENS. Effects of tetraethyl-ammonium chloride on contractile, membrane and cable properties of rabbit artery muscle. *J. Physiol. Lond.* 303: 203–224, 1980.
74. HAINSWORTH, R., AND F. KARIM. Responses of abdominal vascular capacitance in the anaesthetized dog to changes in carotid sinus pressure. *J. Physiol. Lond.* 262: 659–677, 1976.
75. HAINSWORTH, R., F. KARIM, K. H. MCGREGOR, AND L. M. WOOD. Hind-limb vascular-capacitance responses in anaesthetized dogs. *J. Physiol. Lond.* 337: 417–428, 1983.
76. HANLEY, M. R., H. P. BENTON, S. L. LIGHTMAN, K. TODD, E. A. BONE, P. FRETTEN, AND S. PALMER. A vasopressin-like peptide in the mammalian sympathetic nervous system. *Nature Lond.* 309: 258–261, 1984.
77. HARA, Y., K. KITAMURA, AND H. KURIYAMA. Actions of 4-aminopyridine on vascular smooth muscle tissues of the guinea-pig. *Br. J. Pharmacol.* 68: 99–106, 1980.
78. HARDER, D. R., AND N. SPERELAKIS. Membrane electrical properties of vascular smooth muscle from the guinea pig superior mesenteric artery. *Pfluegers Arch.* 378: 111–119, 1978.
79. HEJTMANCIK, M., JR., AND C. SU. Segmental variation of adrenergic innervation in rabbit mesenteric vasculature. *J. Cardiovasc. Pharmacol.* 3: 1141–1151, 1981.
80. HERMSMEYER, K. Multiple pacemaker sites in spontaneously active vascular muscle. *Circ. Res.* 33: 244–251, 1973.
81. HERMSMEYER, K. $Ba^{2+}$ and $K^+$ alteration of $K^+$ conductance in spontaneously active vascular muscle. *Am. J. Physiol.* 230: 1031–1036, 1976.
82. HILL, C. E., G. D. S. HIRST, AND D. F. VAN HELDEN. Development of sympathetic innervation to proximal and distal arteries of the rat mesentery. *J. Physiol. Lond.* 338: 129–147, 1983.
83. HIRST, G. D. S. Neuromuscular transmission in arterioles of guinea-pig submucosa. *J. Physiol. Lond.* 273: 263–275, 1977.
84. HIRST, G. D. S., AND T. O. NEILD. An analysis of excitatory junctional potentials recorded from arterioles. *J. Physiol. Lond.* 280: 87–104, 1978.
85. HIRST, G. D. S., AND T. O. NEILD. Evidence for two populations of excitatory receptors for noradrenaline on arteriolar smooth muscle. *Nature Lond.* 283: 767–768, 1980.

86. HIRST, G. D. S., AND T. O. NEILD. Some properties of spontaneous excitatory junction potentials recorded from arterioles of guinea-pigs. *J. Physiol. Lond.* 303: 43–60, 1980.
87. HIRST, G. D. S., AND T. O. NEILD. Noradrenergic transmission—reply to McGrath (Letter to the editor). *Nature Lond.* 288: 301–302, 1980.
88. HIRST, G. D. S., AND T. O. NEILD. Localization of specialized noradrenaline receptors at neuromuscular junctions on arterioles of the guinea-pig. *J. Physiol. Lond.* 313: 343–350, 1981.
89. HIRST, G. D. S., T. O. NEILD, AND G. D. SILVERBERG. Noradrenaline receptors on the rat basilar artery. *J. Physiol. Lond.* 328: 351–360, 1982.
90. HIRST, G. D. S., G. D. SILVERBERG, AND D. F. VAN HELDEN. The action potential and underlying ionic currents in proximal rat middle cerebral arterioles. *J. Physiol. Lond.* 371: 289–304, 1986.
91. HIRST, G. D. S., AND D. F. VAN HELDEN. Ionic basis of the resting potential of submucosal arterioles in the ileum of the guinea-pig. *J. Physiol. Lond.* 333: 53–67, 1982.
92. HODGKIN, A. L., AND B. KATZ. The effect of sodium ions on the electrical activity of the giant axon of the squid. *J. Physiol. Lond.* 108: 37–77, 1949.
93. HODGKIN, A. L., AND W. A. H. RUSHTON. The electrical constants of a crustacean nerve fibre. *Proc. R. Soc. Lond. B Biol. Sci.* 133: 444–479, 1946.
94. HOKFELT, T., L.-G. ELFVIN, M. SCHULTZBERG, R. ELDE, M. GOLDSTEIN, AND R. LUFT. Occurrence of somatostatin-like immuno-reactivity in some peripheral sympathetic noradrenergic neurons. *Proc. Natl. Acad. Sci. USA.* 74: 3587–3591, 1977.
95. HOKFELT, T., L.-G. ELFVIN, M. SCHULTZBERG, K. FUXE, S. I. SAID, V. MUTT, AND M. GOLDSTEIN. Immunohistochemical evidence of vasoactive intestinal polypeptide-containing neurons and nerve fibers in sympathetic ganglia. *Neuroscience* 2: 885–896, 1977.
96. HOLMAN, M. E. Junction potentials in smooth muscle. In: *Smooth Muscle*, edited by E. Bulbring, A. F. Brading, A. W. Jones, and T. Tomita. Baltimore, MD: Williams & Wilkins, 1970, p. 244–288.
97. HOLMAN, M. E., C. B. KASBY, M. B. SUTHERS, AND J. A. F. WILSON. Some properties of the smooth muscle of rabbit portal vein. *J. Physiol. Lond.* 196: 111–132, 1968.
98. HOLMAN, M. E., AND A. MCLEAN. The innervation of sheep mesenteric veins. *J. Physiol. Lond.* 190: 55–69, 1967.
99. HOLMAN, M. E., AND T. O. NEILD. Membrane properties. *Br. Med. Bull.* 35: 235–241, 1979.
100. HOLMAN, M. E., AND A. M. SUPRENANT. Some properties of the excitatory junction potentials recorded from saphenous arteries of rabbits. *J. Physiol. Lond.* 287: 337–351, 1979.
101. HOLMAN, M. E., AND A. M. SUPRENANT. Effects of tetraethylammonium chloride on sympathetic neuromuscular transmission in saphenous artery of young rabbits. *J. Physiol. Lond.* 305: 451–465, 1980.
102. HOLMAN, M. E., AND A. M. SUPRENANT. An electrophysiological analysis of the effects of noradrenaline and α-receptor antagonists on neuromuscular transmission in mammalian muscular arteries. *Br. J. Pharmacol.* 71: 651–661, 1980.
103. HOTTENSTEIN, O. D., AND D. L. KREULEN. Comparison of intracellular electrical responses in mesenteric artery to para- and perivascular nerve stimulation (Abstract). *Blood Vessels* 21: 190, 1984.
104. HOTTENSTEIN, O. D., AND D. L. KREULEN. Frequency dependence of guinea-pig inferior mesenteric artery and vein responses to repetitive lumbar colonic nerve stimulation. *J. Physiol. Lond.* 384: 153–167, 1987.
105. HOTTENSTEIN, O. D., AND D. L. KREULEN. Nonadrenergic hyperpolarization of arterial smooth muscle produced by repetitive sympathetic nerve stimulation in mesenteric arteries (Abstract). *Federation Proc.* 45: 745, 1986.
106. ISHIKAWA, S. Actions of ATP and α,β-methylene ATP on neuromuscular transmission and smooth muscle membrane of the rabbit and guinea-pig mesenteric arteries. *Br. J. Pharmacol.* 86: 777–787, 1985.
107. ITAKURA, T., K. NAKAKITA, I. KAMEI, Y. NAKA, K. NAKAI, N. KOMAI, H. YOKOI, O. NISHIMURA, AND N. OKADA. Aminergic innervation of cerebral veins. *J. Neurosurg.* 60: 140–144, 1984.
108. ITO, Y., K. KITAMURA, AND H. KURIYAMA. Effects of acetylcholine and catecholamines on the smooth muscle cell of the porcine coronary artery. *J. Physiol. Lond.* 294: 595–611, 1979.
109. ITO, Y., K. KITAMURA, AND H. KURIYAMA. Nitroglycerine and catecholamine actions on smooth muscle cells of the canine coronary artery. *J. Physiol. Lond.* 309: 171–183, 1980.
110. ITO, Y., AND H. KURIYAMA. Membrane properties of the smooth-muscle fibres of the guinea-pig portal vein. *J. Physiol. Lond.* 214: 427–441, 1971.
111. ITO, Y., H. SUZUKI, AND H. KURIYAMA. Effects of caffeine and procaine on the membrane and mechanical properties of the smooth muscle cells of the rabbit main pulmonary artery. *Jpn. J. Physiol.* 27: 467–481, 1977.
112. ITO, Y., H. SUZUKI, AND H. KURIYAMA. On the roles of calcium ion during potassium-induced contracture in the smooth muscle cells of the main pulmonary artery. *Jpn. J. Physiol.* 27: 755–770, 1977.
113. ITO, Y., AND K. TAJIMA. An electrophysiological analysis of the actions of prostaglandins on neuromuscular transmission in the guinea-pig vas deferens. *J. Physiol. Lond.* 297: 521–537, 1979.
114. ITO, Y., AND K. TAJIMA. Actions of indomethacin and prostaglandins on neuroeffector transmission in the dog trachea. *J. Physiol. Lond.* 319: 379–392, 1981.
115. ITOH, T., K. FURUKAWA, M. KAJIWARA, K. KITAMURA, H. SUZUKI, AND H. KURIYAMA. Effects of 2-nicotinamidoethyl nitrate on smooth muscle cells and on adrenergic transmission in the guinea-pig and porcine mesenteric arteries. *J. Pharmacol. Exp. Ther.* 218: 260–270, 1981.
116. ITOH, T., H. IZUMI, AND H. KURIYAMA. Mechanisms of relaxation induced by activation of β-adrenoceptors in smooth muscle cells of the guinea-pig mesenteric artery. *J. Physiol. Lond.* 326: 475–493, 1982.
117. ITOH, T., K. KITAMURA, AND H. KURIYAMA. Roles of extrajunctional receptors in the response of guinea-pig mesenteric and rat tail arteries to adrenergic nerves. *J. Physiol. Lond.* 345: 409–422, 1983.
118. ITOH, T., H. KURIYAMA, AND H. SUZUKI. Excitation-contraction coupling in smooth muscle cells of the guinea-pig mesenteric artery. *J. Physiol. Lond.* 321: 513–535, 1981.
119. ITOH, T., H. KURIYAMA, AND H. SUZUKI. Differences and similarities in the noradrenaline- and caffeine-induced mechanical responses in the rabbit mesenteric artery. *J. Physiol. Lond.* 337: 609–629, 1983.
120. IZQUIERDO, J. J., AND I. KOCH. Uber den Einfluss der Nervi splanchnici auf den arteriellen Blutdruck des Kaninchens. *Z. Kreislaufforsch.* 22: 735–743, 1930.
121. JACOBSON, E. D. Physiology of the mesenteric circulation. *Physiologist* 25: 439–443, 1982.
122. JOHANSSON, B., O. JOHSSON, J. AXELSSON, D. PHIL, AND B. WAHLSTROM. Electrical and mechanical characteristics of vascular smooth muscle response norepinephrine and Isoproterenol. *Circ. Res.* 21: 619–633, 1967.
123. JOHANSSON, B., AND B. LJUNG. Sympathetic control of rhythmically active vascular smooth muscle as studied by a nerve-muscle preparation of portal vein. *Acta Physiol. Scand.* 70: 299–311, 1967.
124. JONES, A. W. Content and fluxes of electrolytes. In: *Handbook of Physiology. The Cardiovascular System. Vascular Smooth Muscle*, edited by D. F. Bohr, A. P. Somlyo, and H. V. Sparks, Jr. Bethesda, MD: Am. Physiol. Soc., 1980, sect. 2, vol. II, chapt. 11, p. 253–299.
125. KAJIWARA, M. General features of electical and mechanical properties of smooth muscle cells in the guinea-pig abdominal aorta. *Pfluegers Arch.* 393: 109–117, 1982.
126. KAJIWARA, M., K. KITAMURA, AND H. KURIYAMA. Neuromus-

cular transmission and smooth muscle membrane properties in the guinea-pig ear artery. *J. Physiol. Lond.* 315: 283–302, 1981.
127. KARASHIMA, T. Effects of vasopressin on smooth muscle cells of guinea-pig mesenteric vessels. *Br. J. Pharmacol.* 72: 673–684, 1981.
128. KARASHIMA, T., T. ITOH, AND H. KURIYAMA. Effects of 2-nicotinamidoethyl nitrate on smooth muscle cells of the guinea-pig mesenteric and portal veins. *J. Pharmacol. Exp. Ther.* 221: 472–480, 1982.
129. KARASHIMA, T., AND H. KURIYAMA. Electrical properties of smooth muscle cell membrane and neuromuscular transmission in the guinea-pig basilar artery. *Br. J. Pharmacol.* 74: 495–504, 1981.
130. KARASHIMA, T., AND Y. TAKATA. The effects of ATP related compounds on the electrical activity of the rat portal vein. *Gen. Pharmacol.* 10: 477–487, 1979.
131. KARIM, F., AND R. HAINSWORTH. Responses of abdominal vascular capacitance to stimulation of splanchnic nerves. *Am. J. Physiol.* 231: 434–440, 1976.
132. KATZ, B. *The Release of Neural Transmitter Substances*. Liverpool, UK: Univ. Press, 1969.
133. KATZ, B., AND R. MILEDI. A study of synaptic transmission in the absence of nerve impulses. *J. Physiol. Lond.* 192: 407–436, 1967.
134. KEEF, K., AND T. O. NEILD. Modification of the response to nerve stimulation in small arteries of guinea-pig caused by distension of the artery. *J. Physiol. Lond.* 331: 355–365, 1982.
135. KIRPEKER, S., AND Y. MISU. Release of noradrenaline by splenic nerve stimulation and its dependence on calcium. *J. Physiol. Lond.* 188: 219–234, 1967.
136. KITAMURA, K., AND H. KURIYAMA. Effects of acetylcholine on the smooth muscle cell of isolated main coronary artery of the guinea pig. *J. Physiol. Lond.* 293: 119–133, 1979.
137. KITAMURA, K., H. SUZUKI, AND H. KURIYAMA. Prostaglandin action on the main pulmonary artery and portal vein of the rabbit. *Jpn. J. Physiol.* 26: 681–692, 1976.
138. KLEIN, R. L. Chemical composition of the large noradrenergic vesicles. In: *Neurotransmitter Vesicles*, edited by R. L. Klein, H. Lagercrantz, and H. Zimmerman. London: Academic, 1982, p. 133–174.
139. KOU, K., J. IBENGWE, AND H. SUZUKI. Effects of alpha-adrenoceptor antagonists on electrical and mechanical responses of the isolated dog mesenteric vein to perivascular nerve stimulation and exogenous noradrenaline. *Naunyn-Schmiedebergs Arch. Pharmakol.* 326: 7–13, 1984.
140. KOU, K., H. KURIYAMA, AND H. SUZUKI. Effects of 3,4-dihydro-8-(2-hydroxy-3-isopropylaminopropoxy)-3-nitroxy-2H-1-benzopyran (K-351) on smooth muscle cells and neuromuscular transmission in the canine mesenteric artery. *Br. J. Pharmacol.* 77: 679–689, 1982.
141. KREMER, M., AND S. WRIGHT. The effects of blood pressure of section of the splanchnic nerves. *Q. J. Exp. Physiol.* 21: 319–335, 1932.
142. KREULEN, D. L. Clonidine and carbachol inhibit neurotransmission to mesenteric arteries in the guinea pig. *Proc. West. Pharmacol. Soc.* 25: 369–372, 1982.
143. KREULEN, D. L. Activation of mesenteric arteries and veins by preganglionic and postganglionic nerves. *Am. J. Physiol.* 251 (*Heart Circ. Physiol.* 20): H1267–H1275, 1986.
144. KREULEN, D. L., AND J. H. SZURSZEWSKI. Nerve pathways in celiac plexus of the guinea pig. *Am. J. Physiol.* 237 (*Endocrinol. Metab. Gastrointest. Physiol.* 6): E90–E97, 1979.
145. KUGELGEN, I. V., AND K. STARKE. Noradrenaline and adenosine triphosphate as co-transmitters of neurogenic vasoconstriction in rabbit mesenteric artery. *J. Physiol. Lond.* 367: 435–455, 1985.
146. KURIYAMA, H., Y. ITO, H. SUZUKI, K. KITAMURA, AND T. ITOH. Factors modifying contraction-relaxation cycle in vascular smooth muscles. *Am. J. Physiol.* 243 (*Heart Circ. Physiol.* 12): H641–H662, 1982.
147. KURIYAMA, H., AND Y. MAKITA. Modulation of neuromuscular transmission by endogenous and exogenous prostaglandins in the guinea-pig mesenteric artery. *J. Physiol. Lond.* 327: 431–448, 1982.
148. KURIYAMA, H., AND Y. MAKITA. Modulation of noradrenergic transmission in the guinea-pig mesenteric artery: an electrophysiological study. *J. Physiol. Lond.* 335: 609–627, 1983.
149. KURIYAMA, H., AND Y. MAKITA. The presynaptic regulation of noradrenaline release differs in mesenteric arteries of the rabbit and guinea-pig. *J. Physiol. Lond.* 351: 379–396, 1984.
150. KURIYAMA, H., K. OSHIMA, AND Y. SAKAMOTO. The membrane properties of the smooth muscle of the guinea-pig portal vein in isotonic and hypertonic solutions. *J. Physiol. Lond.* 217: 179–199, 1971.
151. KURIYAMA, H., AND H. SUZUKI. The effects of acetylcholine on the membrane and contractile properties of smooth muscle cells of the rabbit superior mesenteric artery. *Br. J. Pharmacol.* 64: 493–501, 1978.
152. KURIYAMA, H., AND H. SUZUKI. Electrical property and chemical sensitivity of vascular smooth muscles in normotensive and spontaneously hypertensive rats. *J. Physiol. Lond.* 285: 409–424, 1978.
153. KURIYAMA, H., AND H. SUZUKI. Adrenergic transmissions in the guinea-pig mesenteric artery and their cholinergic modulations. *J. Physiol. Lond.* 317: 383–396, 1981.
154. LANGER, S. Z. Presynaptic receptors and their role in the regulation of transmitter release. *Br. J. Pharmacol.* 60: 481–497, 1977.
155. LJUNG, B., J. A. BEVAN, B. L. PEGRAM, R. E. PURDY, AND M. SU. Vasomotor nerve control of isolated arteries and veins. *Acta Physiol. Scand.* 94: 506–516, 1975.
156. LJUNG, B., AND L. STAGE. Adrenergic excitatory influences on initiation and conduction of electrical activity in the rat portal vein. *Acta Physiol. Scand.* 80: 131–141, 1970.
157. LOFFELHOLZ, K., AND E. MUSCHOLL. A muscarinic inhibition of noradrenaline release evoked by post-ganglionic sympathetic stimulation. *Naunyn-Schmiedebergs Arch. Pharmakol.* 265: 1–15, 1969.
158. LUNDBERG, J. M., T. HÖKFELT, A. ANGGÅRD, L. TERENIUS, R. ELDE, K. MARKEY, M. GOLDSTEIN, AND J. KIMMEL. Organizational principles in the peripheral sympathetic nervous system: subdivision by coexisting peptides (somatostatin-, avian pancreatic polypeptide-, and vasoactive intestinal polypeptide-like immunoreactive materials). *Proc. Natl. Acad. Sci. USA.* 79: 1303–1307, 1982.
159. LUNDGREN, O. Role of splanchnic resistance vessels in overall cardiovascular homeostasis. *Federation Proc.* 42: 1673–1677, 1983.
160. MAKITA, Y. Effects of prostaglandin $I_2$ on smooth muscle cells and neuromuscular transmission in the guinea-pig mesenteric artery. *Br. J. Pharmacol.* 78: 517–527, 1983.
161. MAKITA, Y. Effects of adrenoceptor agonists and antagonists on smooth muscle cells and neuromuscular transmission in the guinea-pig renal artery and vein. *Br. J. Pharmacol.* 80: 671–679, 1983.
162. MAKITA, Y., Y. KANMURA, T. ITOH, H. SUZUKI, AND H. KURIYAMA. Effects of nifedipine derivatives on smooth muscle cells and neuromuscular transmission in the rabbit mesenteric artery. *Naunyn-Schmiedebergs Arch. Pharmakol.* 324: 302–312, 1983.
163. MALIK, K. U., AND G. M. LING. Modification by acetylcholine of the response of rat mesenteric arteries to sympathetic stimulation. *Circ. Res.* 25: 1–9, 1969.
164. MALLART, A., AND A. R. MARTIN. An analysis of facilitation of transmitter release at the neuromuscular junction of the frog. *J. Physiol. Lond.* 193: 679–694, 1967.
165. MARSHALL, J. M. The influence of the sympathetic nervous system on individual vessels of the microcirculation of skeletal muscle of the rat. *J. Physiol. Lond.* 332: 169–186, 1982.
166. MEKATA, F. Electrophysiological studies of the smooth muscle cell membrane of the rabbit common carotid artery. *J. Gen.*

*Physiol.* 57: 738–751, 1971.
167. MEKATA, F. Current spread in the smooth muscle of the rabbit aorta. *J. Physiol. Lond.* 242: 143–155, 1974.
168. MEKATA, F., AND H. NIU. Biophysical effects of adrenaline on the smooth muscle of the rabbit common carotid artery. *J. Gen. Physiol.* 59: 92–102, 1972.
169. MERRILLEES, N. C. R., G. BURNSTOCK, AND M. E. HOLMAN. Correlation of fine structure and physiology of the innervation of smooth muscle in the guinea pig vas deferens. *J. Cell Biol.* 19: 529–550, 1963.
170. MISHIMA, S., H. MIYAHARA, AND H. SUZUKI. Transmitter release modulated by α-adrenoceptor antagonists in the rabbit mesenteric artery: a comparison between noradrenaline outflow and electrical activity. *Br. J. Pharmacol.* 83: 537–547, 1984.
171. MITCHELL, G. A. G. *Anatomy of the Autonomic Nervous System.* Edinburgh, UK: Livingstone, 1953.
172. MIYAHARA, H., AND H. SUZUKI. Effects of tyramine on noradrenaline outflow and electrical responses induced by field stimulation in the perfused rabbit ear artery. *Br. J. Pharmacol.* 86: 405–416, 1985.
173. MOHRI, K., N. OHGUSHI, M. IKEDA, K. YAMAMOTO, K. TSUNEKAWA, M. FUJIWARA, AND T. MURYOBAYASHI. Histochemical demonstration of adrenergic fibers in the smooth muscle layer of media of arteries supplying abdominal organs. *Arch. Jpn. Chir.* 38: 236–248, 1969.
174. MORGAN, K. G. Comparison of membrane electrical activity of cat gastric submucosal arterioles and venules. *J. Physiol. Lond.* 345: 135–147, 1983.
175. MORGAN, K. G. Electrophysiological differentiation of α-receptors on arteriolar smooth muscle. *Am. J. Physiol.* 244 (*Heart Circ. Physiol.* 13): H540–H545, 1983.
176. MULVANY, M. J., H. NILSSON, AND J. A. FLATMAN. Role of membrane potential in the response of rat small mesenteric arteries to exogenous noradrenaline stimulation. *J. Physiol. Lond.* 332: 363–373, 1982.
177. NAKAJIMA, A., AND L. HORN. Electrical activity of single vascular smooth muscle fibers. *Am. J. Physiol.* 213: 25–30, 1967.
178. NEEDLEMAN, P., AND P. C. ISAKSON. Intrinsic prostaglandin biosynthesis in blood vessels. In: *Handbook of Physiology. The Cardiovascular System. Vascular Smooth Muscle*, edited by D. F. Bohr, A. P. Somlyo, and H. V. Sparks, Jr. Bethesda, MD: Am. Physiol. Soc., 1980, sect. 2, vol. II, chapt. 20, p. 613–633.
179. NEILD, T. O. The relation between the structure and innervation of small arteries and arterioles and the smooth muscle membrane potential changes expected at different levels of sympathetic nerve activity. *Proc. R. Soc. Lond. B Biol. Sci.* 220: 237–249, 1983.
180. NEILD, T. O., AND K. KEEF. Measurements of the membrane potential of arterial smooth muscle in anesthetized animals and its relationship to changes in artery diameter. *Microvasc. Res.* 30: 19–28, 1985.
181. NEILD, T. O., AND N. KOTECHA. Two-component responses to sympathetic nerve stimulation in the rat tail artery. *Comp. Biochem. Physiol. C Comp. Pharmacol. Toxicol.* 81: 311–317, 1985.
182. NEILD, T. O., AND N. KOTECHA. Effects of α,β-methylene ATP on membrane potential, neuromuscular transmission and smooth muscle contraction in the rat tail artery. *Gen. Pharmacol.* 17: 461–464, 1986.
183. NEILD, T. O., AND E. ZELCER. Noradrenergic neuromuscular transmission with special reference to arterial smooth muscle. *Prog. Neurobiol. Oxf.* 19: 141–158, 1982.
184. PRICE, H. L., S. DEUTSCH, B. E. MARSHALL, G. W. STEPHEN, M. G. BEHNER, AND G. R. NEUFELD. Hemodynamic and metabolic effect of hemorrhage in man, with particular reference to the splanchnic circulation. *Circ. Res.* 18: 469–474, 1966.
185. PROSSER, C. L. Smooth muscle. *Annu. Rev. Physiol.* 36: 503–535, 1974.
186. RAND, M. J., AND B. VARMA. The effects of cholinomimetic drugs on responses to sympathetic nerve stimulation and noradrenaline in the rabbit ear artery. *Br. J. Pharmacol.* 38: 758–770, 1970.
187. RHODIN, J. A. G. The ultrastructure of mammalian arterioles and precapillary sphincters. *J. Ultrastruct. Res.* 18: 181–223, 1967.
188. ROWELL, L. B., AND J. M. JOHNSON. Role of the splanchnic circulation in reflex control of the cardiovascular system. In: *Physiology of the Intestinal Circulation*, edited by A. P. Shepard and D. N. Granger. New York: Raven, 1984, p. 153–163.
189. SCHMID, P. G., F. M. SHARABI, AND M. I. PHILLIPS. Peptides and blood vessels. In: *Handbook of Physiology. The Cardiovascular System. Peripheral Circulation and Organ Blood Flow*, edited by J. T. Shepherd and F. M. Abboud. Bethesda, MD: Am. Physiol. Soc., 1983, sect. 2, vol. III, pt. 2, chapt. 22, p. 815–835.
190. SCHULTZBERG, M., J. M. LUNDBERG, T. HOKFELT, L. TERENIUS, J. BRANDT, R. EDLE, AND M. GOLDSTEIN. Enkephalin-like immunoreactivity in gland cells and nerve terminals of the adrenal medulla. *Neuroscience* 3: 1169–1186, 1978.
191. SHEPHERD, J. T., R. R. LORENZ, G. M. TYCE, AND P. M. VANHOUTTE. Acetylcholine—inhibition of transmitter release from adrenergic nerve terminals mediated by muscarinic receptors. *Federation Proc.* 37: 191–194, 1978.
192. SHEPHERD, J. T., AND P. M. VANHOUTTE. *The Human Cardiovascular System: Facts and Concepts.* New York: Raven, 1979.
193. SNEDDON, P., AND G. BURNSTOCK. ATP as a co-transmitter in rat tail artery. *Eur. J. Pharmacol.* 106: 149–152, 1985.
194. SNEDDON, P., AND D. P. WESTFALL. Pharmacological evidence that adenosine triphosphate and noradrenaline are cotransmitters in guinea-pig vas deferens. *J. Physiol. Lond.* 347: 561–580, 1984.
195. SNEDDON, P., D. P. WESTFALL, AND J. S. FEDAN. Cotransmitters in the motor nerves of the guinea pig vas deferens: electrophysiological evidence. *Science Wash. DC* 218: 693–695, 1982.
196. SOMLYO, A. P., AND A. V. SOMLYO. Vascular smooth muscle. II. Pharmacology of normal and hypertensive vessels. *Pharmacol. Rev.* 22: 249–353, 1970.
197. SOMLYO, A. V., AND A. P. SOMLYO. Electromechanical and pharmacomechanical coupling in vascular smooth muscle. *J. Pharmacol. Exp. Ther.* 159: 129–145, 1968.
198. SPEDEN, R. N. Electrical activity of single smooth muscle cells of the mesenteric artery produced by splanchnic nerve stimulation in the guinea pig. *Nature Lond.* 202: 193–194, 1964.
199. STARKE, K. Regulation of noradrenaline release by presynaptic receptor systems. *Rev. Physiol. Biochem. Pharmacol.* 77: 1–124, 1977.
200. STEEDMAN, W. M. Microelectrode studies on mammalian vascular smooth muscle. *J. Physiol. Lond.* 186: 382–400, 1966.
201. STEINSLAND, O. D., R. F. FURCHGOTT, AND S. M. KIRPEKER. Inhibition of adrenergic neurotransmission by parasympathomimetics in the rabbit ear artery. *J. Pharmacol. Exp. Ther.* 184: 346–356, 1973.
202. STJARNE, L. Adrenoceptor mediated positive and negative feedback control of noradrenaline secretion from human vasoconstrictor nerves (Abstract). *Acta Physiol. Scand.* 95: 18A–19A, 1975.
203. STORY, D. F., G. S. ALLEN, A. B. GLOVER, W. HOPE, M. W. MCCULLOCH, M. J. RAND, AND C. SARANTOS. Modulation of adrenergic transmission by acetylcholine. *Clin. Exp. Pharmacol. Physiol. Suppl.* 2: 27–33, 1975.
204. STUREK, M., AND K. HERMSMEYER. Calcium and sodium channels in spontaneously contracting vascular muscle cells. *Science Wash. DC* 233: 475–478, 1986.
205. SU, C., J. A. BEVAN, AND R. C. URSILLO. Electrical quiescence of pulmonary artery smooth muscle during sympathomimetic stimulation. *Circ. Res.* 15: 20–27, 1964.
206. SURPRENANT, A. M. A comparative study of neuromuscular transmission in several mammalian arteries. *Pfluegers Arch.*

386: 85-91, 1980.
207. SURPRENANT, A. M., T. O. NEILD, AND M. E. HOLMAN. Effects of nifedipine on nerve-evoked action potentials and consequent contractions in rat tail artery. *Pfluegers Arch.* 396: 342-349, 1983.
208. SUTTER, M. C. The pharmacology of isolated veins. *Br. J. Pharmacol.* 24: 742-751, 1965.
209. SUZUKI, H. Effects of endogenous and exogenous noradrenaline on the smooth muscle of guinea-pig mesenteric vein. *J. Physiol. Lond.* 321: 495-512, 1981.
210. SUZUKI, H. An electrophysiological study of excitatory neuromuscular transmission in the guinea-pig main pulmonary artery. *J. Physiol. Lond.* 336: 47-59, 1983.
211. SUZUKI, H. Adrenergic transmission in the dog mesenteric vein and its modulation by alpha-adrenoceptor antagonists. *Br. J. Pharmacol.* 81: 479-489, 1984.
212. SUZUKI, H. Electrical responses of smooth muscle cells of the rabbit ear artery to adenosine triphosphate. *J. Physiol. Lond.* 359: 401-415, 1985.
213. SUZUKI, H., T. ITOH, AND H. KURIYAMA. Effects of diltiazem on smooth muscles and neuromuscular junction in the mesenteric artery. *Am. J. Physiol.* 242 (*Heart Circ. Physiol.* 11): H325-H336, 1982.
214. SUZUKI, H., AND K. KOU. Electrical components contributing to the nerve-mediated contractions in the smooth muscle of the rabbit ear artery. *Jpn. J. Physiol.* 33: 743-756, 1983.
215. SUZUKI, H., AND H. KURIYAMA. Observation of quantal release of noradrenaline from vascular smooth muscle in potassium-free solution. *Jpn. J. Physiol.* 30: 665-670, 1980.
216. SUZUKI, H., S. MISHIMA, AND H. MIYAHARA. Effects of reserpine on electrical responses evoked by perivascular nerve stimulation in the rabbit ear artery. *Biomed. Res.* 5: 259-266, 1984.
217. TAKATA, Y. Regional differences in electrical and mechanical properties of guinea-pig mesenteric vessels. *Jpn. J. Physiol.* 30: 709-728, 1980.
218. TKANCHENKO, B. I. Comparison of response characteristics in resistance and capacitance vessels. In: *Regulation of Capacitance Vessels*, edited by A. M. Chernukh, B. I. Tkatchenko, A. G. B. Kovách and S. Biró. Budapest: Akad. Kiado, 1978, p. 103-132.
219. TOMITA, T. Electrical properties of mammalian smooth muscle. In: *Smooth Muscle*, edited by E. Bulbring, A. F. Brading, A. W. Jones, and T. Tomita. London: Edward Arnold, 1970, p. 197-243.
220. TOMITA, T. Electrophysiology of mammalian smooth muscle. *Prog. Biophys. Mol. Biol.* 30: 185-203, 1975.
221. TORNEBRANDT, K., A. NOBIN, AND C. OWMAN. Pharmacological characterization of alpha-adrenergic receptor subtypes mediating contraction in human mesenteric arteries and veins. *Blood Vessels* 22: 179-195, 1985.
222. UEHARA, Y., AND G. BURNSTOCK. Demonstration of "gap junctions" between smooth muscle cells. *J. Cell Biol.* 44: 215-217, 1970.
223. UVELIUS, B., S. B. SIGURDSSON, AND B. JOHANSSON. Strontium and barium as substitutes for calcium on electrical and mechanical activity in rat portal vein. *Blood Vessels* 11: 245-259, 1974.
224. VANHOUTTE, P. M. Inhibition by acetylcholine of adrenergic neurotransmission in vascular smooth muscle. *Circ. Res.* 34: 317-326, 1974.
225. VANHOUTTE, P. M., R. R. LORENZ, AND G. M. TYCE. Inhibition of norepinephrine-$^3$H release from sympathetic nerve endings in veins by acetylcholine. *J. Pharmacol. Exp. Ther.* 185: 386-394, 1973.
226. VANHOUTTE, P. M., T. J. VERBEUREN, AND R. C. WEBB. Local modulation of adrenergic neuroeffector interaction in the blood vessel wall. *Physiol. Rev.* 61: 151-247, 1981.
227. VERITY, M. A., AND J. A. BEVAN. Fine structural study of the terminal effector plexus, neuromuscular relationships in the pulmonary artery. *J. Anat.* 103: 49-63, 1968.
228. VON LOH, D. The effect of adrenergic drugs on spontaneously active vascular smooth muscle studied by long-term intracellular recording of membrane-potential. *Angiologica Basel* 8: 144-155, 1971.
229. WAHLSTROM, B. A. A study on the action of noradrenaline on ionic content and sodium potassium and chloride effluxes in the rat portal vein. *Acta Physiol. Scand.* 89: 522-530, 1973.
230. WEISS, G. B. Calcium and contractility in vascular smooth muscle. In: *Advances in General and Cellular Pharmacology*, edited by T. Narahashi and C. P. Bianchi. Plenum, 1977, vol. 2.
231. WESTFALL, T. C. Local regulation of adrenergic neurotransmission. *Physiol. Rev.* 57: 659-728, 1977.
232. ZELCER, E., AND N. SPERELAKIS. Ionic dependence of electrical activity in small mesenteric arteries of guinea-pigs. *Pfluegers Arch.* 392: 72-78, 1981.
233. ZELCER, E., AND N. SPERELAKIS. Spontaneous electrical activity in pressurized small mesenteric arteries. *Blood Vessels* 19: 301-310, 1982.

CHAPTER 45

# Neuromuscular transmission in intramural blood vessels

G. D. S. HIRST | *Department of Zoology, University of Melbourne, Parkville, Victoria, Australia*

CHAPTER CONTENTS

Organization and Structure of Intramural Blood Vessels
Innervation of Intramural Blood Vessels
Passive Electrical Properties of Submucosal Arterioles
    Resting potential
    Electrical coupling between arteriolar smooth muscle cells
    Summary
Neuromuscular Transmission in Arterioles
Responses of Submucosal Arterioles to Sympathetic
        Nerve Stimulation
Analysis of Excitatory Junction Potentials
    Time course
    Quantal content
    Summary
Initiation of Contraction in Submucosal Arterioles
    Potential-dependent calcium entry
    Receptor-activated tension development
    Summary
Integration in Submucosal Arterioles
Pharmacology of Excitatory Junction Potentials
    Identity of transmitter responsible for initiation of excitatory
        junction potentials
        Norepinephrine
        Cotransmission
Summary and Future Directions

---

THIS CHAPTER DISCUSSES electrophysiological studies on the process of synaptic transmission between sympathetic nerves and the vascular smooth cells that form a part of the wall of the intramural blood vessels of the intestine. The only data available on this topic have been obtained from submucosal arterioles of the guinea pig small intestine (74, 80, 81, 83) and the cat stomach and from the venules of the cat stomach (127). Comparative studies are needed to know if the phenomena reviewed in this chapter are relevant to intramural vessels in other regions of the intestine and in other species. Nevertheless many of the phenomena that occur in submucosal arterioles and venules do occur in systemic arteries and veins of various vascular beds of different species. Rather than restrict this review to data on intramural vessels, the subject matter has been extended to highlight the similarities and dissimilarities between these and other vascular tissues. In an attempt to prevent overlap with other chapters in this *Handbook*, data from other vessels are not exhaustively reviewed. Omissions reflect a desire to prevent duplication rather than to ignore the importance of such work. Where possible, reference is made to a number of excellent reviews available in the expanding literature based on vascular research.

The intramural blood vessels form a part of the splanchnic circulation. A detailed description of this region of the circulation and the factors influencing its resistance are found both in another volume of the *Handbook* (41) and a recent text (141). At rest, about one-fourth of the cardiac output is directed to the splanchnic circulation. Of this, about one-third passes through the hepatic artery to the liver; the bulk of the remainder is distributed to the stomach and small and large intestines by the mesenteric circulation. As with other vascular beds, the resistance offered by the splanchnic circulation is modified by sympathetic nerve activity, circulating vasoactive agents, and local metabolic products.

The blood flow to the stomach and intestines can be further compartmentalized (see ref. 50). The largest proportion, ~70%–80%, of blood in the mesenteric circulation passes to the submucosal and mucosal layers where it provides for the secretory and absorptive roles of the intestine. The remaining smaller proportion of blood is distributed to the longitudinal and circular smooth muscle layers of the intestine and the myenteric plexus.

Stimulation of the sympathetic nerves to the intestinal vasculature results in an abrupt increase in vascular resistance. The increased resistance is often not well maintained, and "escape" appears to result from blood flow redistribution within the intramural vessels (65). There are suggestions that, in addition to the sympathetic innervation, the intramural vessels of the cat receive an intrinsic dilator innervation (11; see, however, ref. 51). The correlates of this innervation have not been detected in electrophysiological studies on isolated intramural vessels of the guinea pig or cat. Whereas exercise and increased body temperature lead

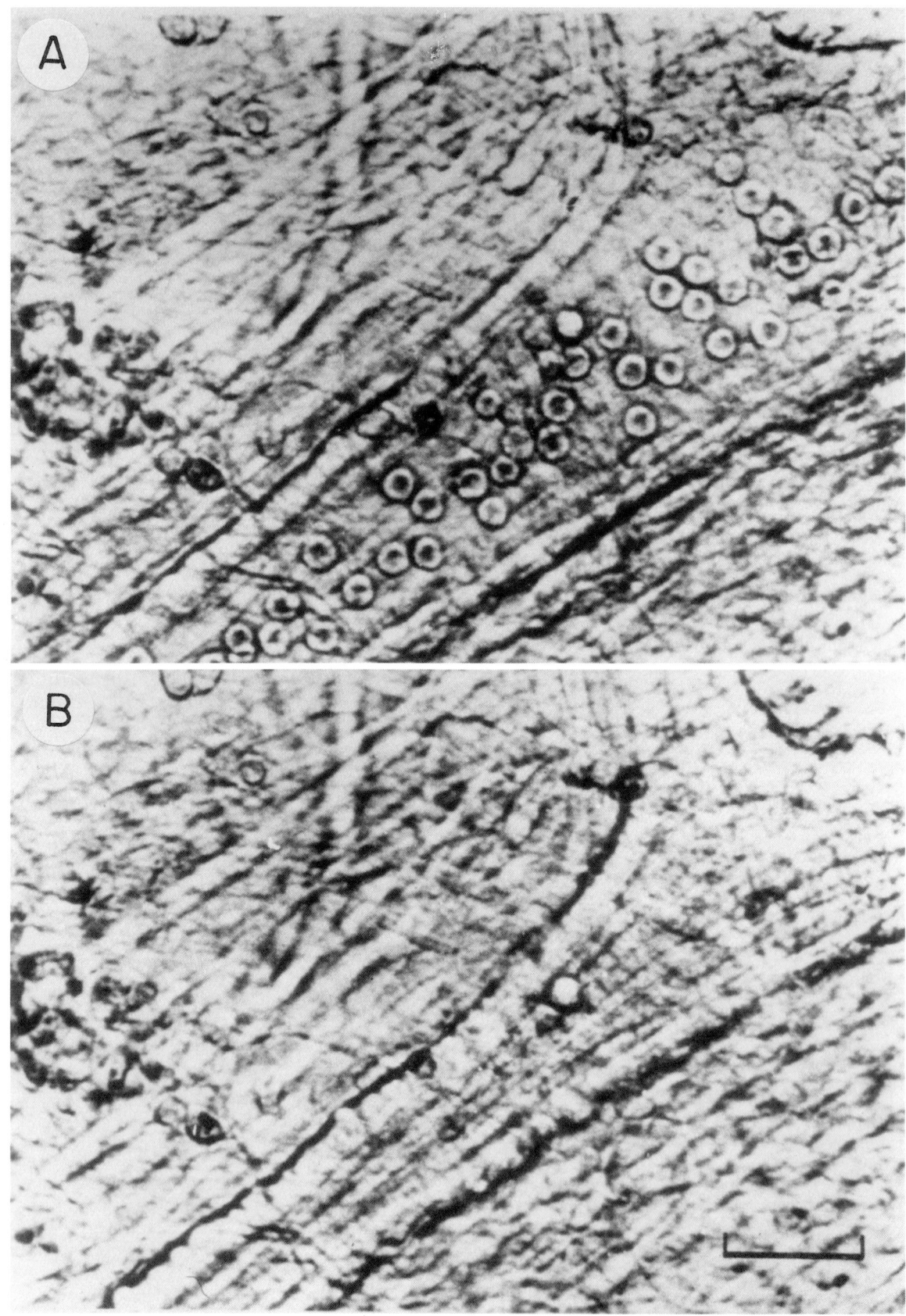

to sympathetic vasoconstriction of the intraluminal vessels, feeding results in vasodilation. Although the removal of sympathetic nervous tone may play a role in the postprandial increase in blood flow, such vascular responses are also thought to be in part mediated by the changed levels of circulating gastrointestinal hormones (45).

The following sections deal with the structure of the intraluminal vasculature and its innervation, the passive electrical properties of arterioles, and the responses of these vessels to sympathetic nerve activity. Finally, because there is an intense debate over the nature of the sympathetic transmitter released by sympathetic nerves innervating arteries, the arguments for and against norepinephrine being the sole transmitter and the alternative proposal, cotransmission where norepinephrine and another substance are released together, are presented.

## ORGANIZATION AND STRUCTURE OF INTRAMURAL BLOOD VESSELS

Blood reaches the small and large intestine via the superior and inferior mesenteric arteries. These distributing arteries give rise to arcades of mesenteric arteries that divide into two branches as they reach the intestine. Each branch runs longitudinally along the gut in the mesenteric border, one in an oral direction and the other in an aboral direction. At intervals the arterial branches lying in the mesenteric border give rise to pairs of fine arterial branches, each of which penetrates the serosal surface of the intestine on different sides of the mesenteric border. The arteries running along the mesenteric border often link with those derived from adjacent mesenteric arcades.

Immediately after penetrating the serosal surface of the intestine, the intramural arteries often give off finer arteriolar branches, from which originates a capillary network supplying the myenteric plexus and smooth muscle layers. The more prominent arterial branches pass through both the longitudinal and circular smooth muscle layers to form an extensive branching network of arterioles, with numerous arteriolar-arteriolar anastomoses, in the submucosa. Twigs of arteriole originating from this network course at right angles down into the mucosa and give rise to a capillary network in the villi (28). Blood is returned to the circulation by way of collecting venules lying in the villi and submucosa. The intramural venules are thin walled and, in the small intestine, may be devoid of smooth muscle cells. The venules converge and form individual mesenteric veins leaving the intestine near the entry points of arteries of the mesenteric border. Ultimately blood flows into the hepatic circulation.

The intramural arterioles have thin walls (wall thickness 4–10 $\mu$m) that can readily be visualized without staining. An example of a submucosal arteriole from guinea pig small intestine is shown in Figure 1. The walls of the arterioles are composed of an adventitial layer containing sympathetic axons, a single layer of smooth muscle cells, and an inner thin endothelial cell layer. In submucosal arterioles, as in most arteries, individual smooth muscle cells have an elongated shape and are 20–60 $\mu$m in length (94) with a diameter of ~4 $\mu$m at their thickest part. The cells are organized almost at right angles, pitch angle 80°–84°, to the pathway of the arteriole. Thus a 100-$\mu$m length of arteriole of external diameter of 30 $\mu$m contains ~50–70 individual smooth muscle cells. In finer arterioles individual smooth muscle cells may completely wrap around an arteriole (94).

The smooth muscle cells of the arteriolar wall each have a nucleus, mitochondria, and sarcoplasmic reticulum (139). The arteriolar muscle membrane shows many invaginations called caveolae that in mesenteric arteries are loosely arranged into rows (60). The muscle membrane is wrapped by basal lamina that does not penetrate down into the caveolae (60). The basal lamina does not appear to form a diffusional barrier, since large extracellular markers can penetrate it and fill caveolae (40, 60). Areas of the membranes of adjacent smooth muscle cells lie close to each other and form gap junctions. These have been reported to occupy a relatively large proportion of the surface area of arterioles (139). It is generally assumed that such structures are the sites where intercellular communication between smooth muscle cells occurs.

## INNERVATION OF INTRAMURAL BLOOD VESSELS

The sympathetic innervation of intramural blood vessels of the guinea pig small intestine is limited to arterioles. The collecting venules in the small intestine have very fine walls. After appropriate fixation to demonstrate the localization of catecholamines with the Falck-Hillarp technique (44), the venules appear devoid of innervation. Occasionally sympathetic nerve fibers pass in relative proximity, but these fibers appear to be en route to other targets. A very similar paucity of innervation has been described for the collecting venules of rat mesentery (56). In contrast,

FIG. 1. Micrographs of submucosal arteriole of guinea pig ileum viewed with conventional optics showing submucosal arterioles that were dissected from a segment of guinea pig ileum. An arteriole with ~50-$\mu$m diam runs diagonally across micrographs; finer branch at proximal end is visible in *right corner*. Arteriole has wall thickness of ~5 $\mu$m, which is less than that of red blood cells remaining in vessel lumen in *A*. *B* shows the same vessel during maintained sympathetic nerve stimulation. *Calibration bar*, 30 $\mu$m. [From Hirst (74).]

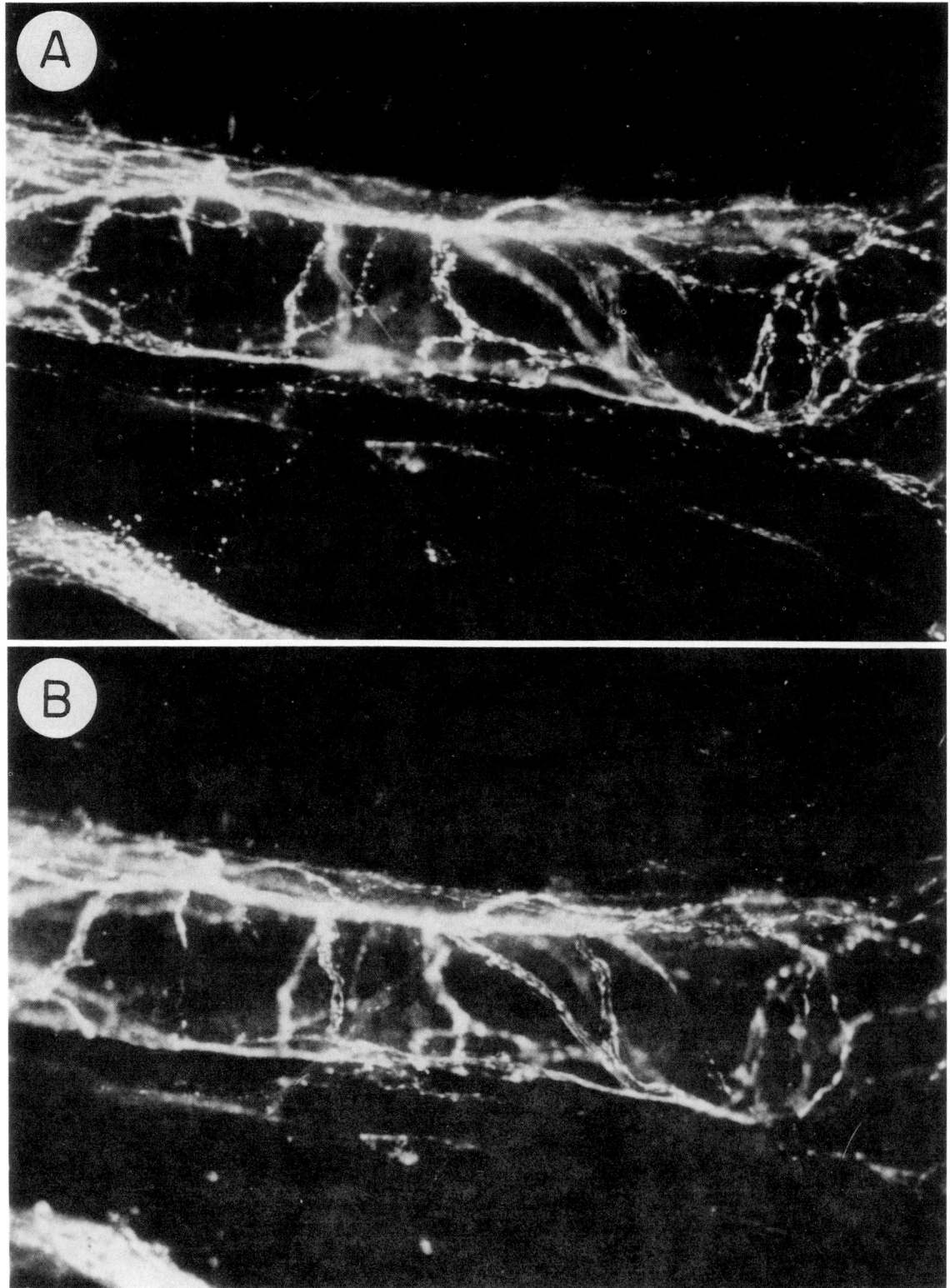

FIG. 2. Micrographs showing sympathetic innervation of submucosal arteriole of guinea pig. Preparation was fixed and viewed with Falck-Hillarp technique, which demonstrates catecholamine-containing nerves. Two plates are of same segment of arteriolar tree: one is focused on luminal surface and other on inner surface of arteriole. Bundles of brightly fluorescent axons and single beaded axons can be seen wrapped around arteriole. *Calibration bar*, μm. 50 μm. (Micrography courtesy of E. M. MacLachlan.)

electrophysiological data suggest that venules of cat stomach receive a sympathetic innervation (127).

The fluorescence histochemistry technique demonstrates an abundant network of fluorescent fibers ramifying over the surface of submucosal arterioles [Fig. 2; (81)]. Very similar innervation patterns have been described from many other arterial preparations (20, 134). Sympathetic nerve fibers run in loose bundles along the mesenteric arteries and follow their pathway into the intestine. The individual axons give rise to numerous fine branches of varicose terminal axons. The varicosities are separated by lengths (8–10 $\mu$m) of fine axon; individual varicosities have lengths of ~2 $\mu$m and diameters of 1 $\mu$m. Counts of varicosity density indicate that submucosal arterioles are very densely innervated: there are ~150 varicosities/300 $\mu$m of arteriole (81). This figure may be an underestimate since it was derived from light microscopy, a procedure that would not have allowed two or more adjacent varicosities to be distinguished (119). The sympathetic fibers do not penetrate into the smooth muscle layer.

The extent of vascular territory innervated by an individual fiber is not known. However, studies of the innervation pattern to the iris suggest that individual sympathetic fibers innervate a restricted area extending for ~200–400 $\mu$m and that the territories of individual axons overlap (8). Certainly in the mesenteric circulation the number of fibers innervating a given region of artery is restricted to a few fibers (<10), and the number decreases with decreased arteriolar diameter (see RESPONSES OF SUBMUCOSAL ARTERIOLES TO SYMPATHETIC NERVE STIMULATION, p. 1645). During development, ingrowing axons do not innervate the more proximal vascular tissue but preferentially innervate the finer distal vessels. Axons, arriving subsequently, innervate the proximal vascular tissue. The early arriving axons do not lay down collaterals to innervate these proximal structures (72). Thus discrete axons innervate discrete regions of a vascular bed. Clearly the entire bed may be activated in unison if appropriate central nervous processing occurs during reflex activity. It would be of great interest to know if there were any preferred sympathetic pathways to peripheral arterioles.

At the ultrastructural level, individual terminal axons have a characteristic appearance. Fine axons (diam 0.1—0.5 $\mu$m) are interrupted at regular intervals by varicosities that contain small granular vesicles, a lesser number of large granular vesicles, and mitochondria [Fig. 3; (89)]. The sympathetic transmitter is stored in both vesicle types, with a small amount free in the cytosol (52, 62, 113). Whereas the bundles of preterminal axons are wrapped by Schwann cells, the finer intervaricose axons often lose part of this wrap. The terminal varicosities are usually partly enveloped in Schwann cells.

There is said to be a large diversity of separations between the membranes of varicosities of the nearest vascular smooth muscle effector cell (140). The basis for this idea has been extensively reviewed (10, 39). In most studies on arteries and arterioles, the ultrastructural organization has been examined by taking random sections through a tissue. With this approach the separation between neuronal tissue containing vesicles and the nearest arterial smooth muscle has been found to vary between 0.05 and 10 $\mu$m (10). Taking the same approach, a similar diversity of neuromuscular separations is found in submucosal arterioles (119). However, in the latter study serial sections were also taken and the entire orientation of individual varicosities was reconstructed. It was found that a very high proportion (between 85% and 91%) of individual varicosities form intimate contact with the smooth muscle surface. This area of contact was associated with a fusion of the basal laminae of the arteriolar smooth muscles and the varicosity (Fig. 3). The separation between varicosity membrane and arteriolar membrane, in the region where the basal lamina was fused, was ~35–75 nm in preparations perfused at physiological pressures. There was considerable variation in size between the areas of contact, and in general the larger the varicosity the larger the area of contact and the greater the number of vesicles (Fig. 4). The reconstructions also indicated that a definite streaming of small granular vesicles toward the area of contact occurred (Fig. 5). None of the other traditional presynaptic or postsynaptic specializations found at many other synapses were detected. Similar specialized neuroeffector arrangements have been described for a number of other arterial vessels, but their frequency has not been determined with the serial sectioning technique (10, 20, 39). In the vas deferens similar neuroeffector arrangements have been described (8).

The sympathetic fibers to submucosal arterioles, in addition to containing norepinephrine, as do other sympathetic nerve fibers to vascular tissues, contain the peptide neuropeptide Y (NPY) (57). The subcellular location of this peptide has not been defined. At present there is no reason to believe that this substance acts as the major transmitter substance in intestinal vessels. The effects of sympathetic nerve stimulation are not mimicked in the mesenteric circulation by NPY (108). This clearly does not preclude either a more long-term role for this agent in modifying vascular reactivity or its involvement as a developmental marker. Interestingly the sympathetic nerve fibers that innervate the enteric nervous system are devoid of NPY (57).

Thus the nerves that innervate intramural arterioles contain norepinephrine, and they are restricted to the adventitial surface. The light-microscopic studies suggest that there are many varicosities from which transmitter release may occur along the surface of the arterioles. The ultrastructural studies indicate that virtually all of these varicosities form close appositions with arteriolar smooth muscle. In the areas of prox-

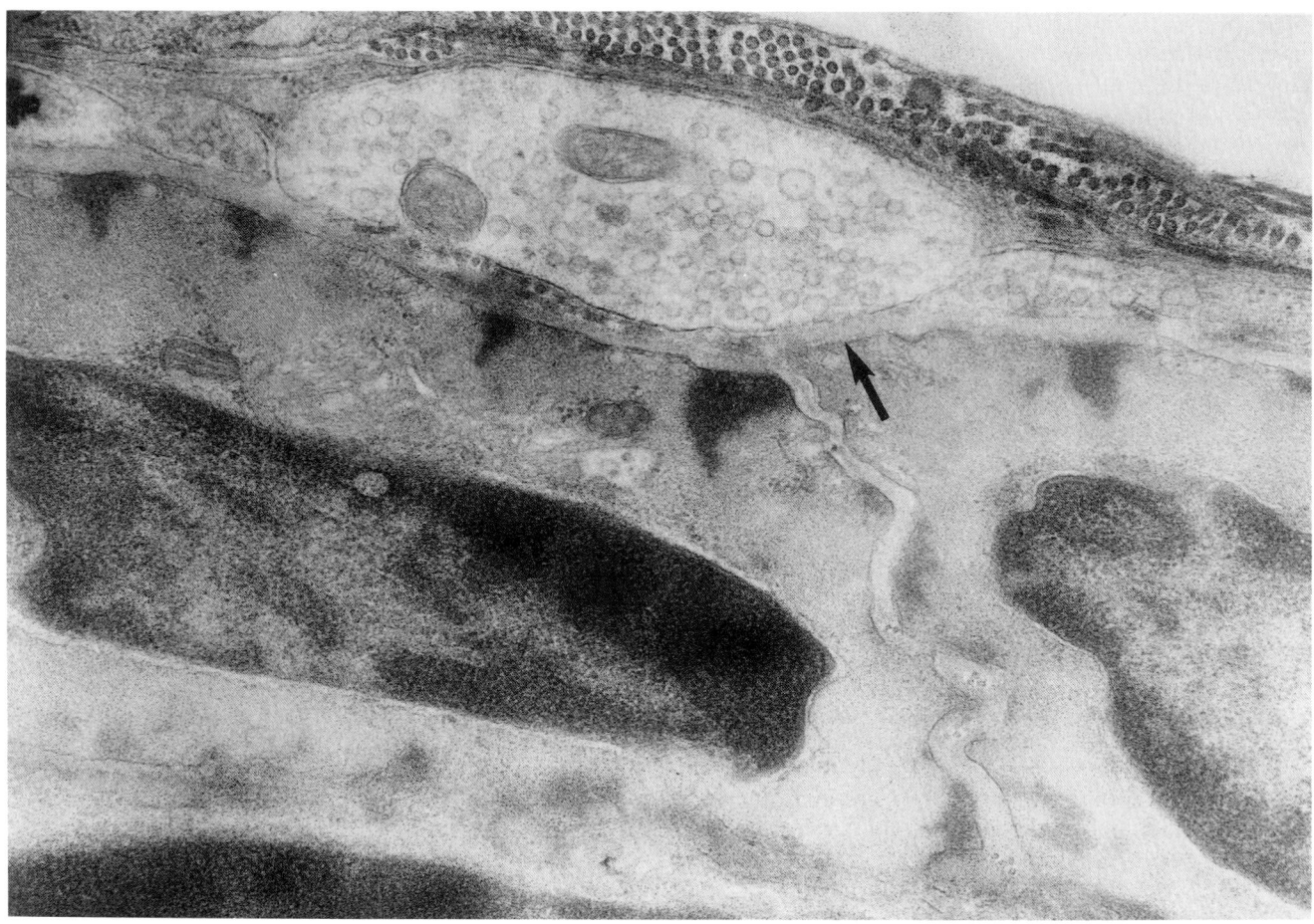

FIG. 3. Electron micrograph of sympathetic nerve varicosity. Figure shows varicosity in apposition with 2 submucosal arteriolar smooth muscle cells. *Arrow*, basal laminae of 1 smooth muscle cell and varicosity are fused. In this section and adjacent ones separation between nerve and muscle was 60 μm. Note abundant small granular vesicles, mitochondria, and occasional large granular vesicle. *Calibration bar*, 0.5 μm. (Micrograph courtesy of S. Luff.)

imity the presynaptic terminals contain many small granular vesicles.

## PASSIVE ELECTRICAL PROPERTIES OF SUBMUCOSAL ARTERIOLES

All excitable cells at rest have a potential difference between the inside of the cell and the extracellular fluid. The potential difference is typically approximately −60 to −90 mV, internal negative, and is called the resting potential. Resting potentials result from an asymmetric distribution of individual ion concentrations on either side of the cell membrane; the gradients are maintained by ion-specific energy-requiring transport systems. Most excitable cells (e.g., individual skeletal muscle fiber, neurons) are not electrically connected to adjacent cells. This does not appear to be the case for most target organs of the autonomic nervous system. For example, individual cardiac muscle cells are connected to neighboring cells by structures that allow ion movement between the endoplasm of these cells. Excitation of one cell results in the flow of excitatory current into adjacent cells (98). Autonomic end organs (e.g., intestine, bladder, blood vessels) contain large numbers of individual smooth muscle cells. These cells, like cardiac muscle cells, are electrically connected to their neighboring cells to form syncytia. To understand the processes underlying induced membrane potential changes in these organs, it is essential to understand how currents can flow passively through the syncytia. Clearly what is of interest are the passive electrical properties of the syncytia, not those of the individual cells in isolation.

### Resting Potential

When a submucosal arteriole is impaled with an intracellular recording electrode, a resting potential of

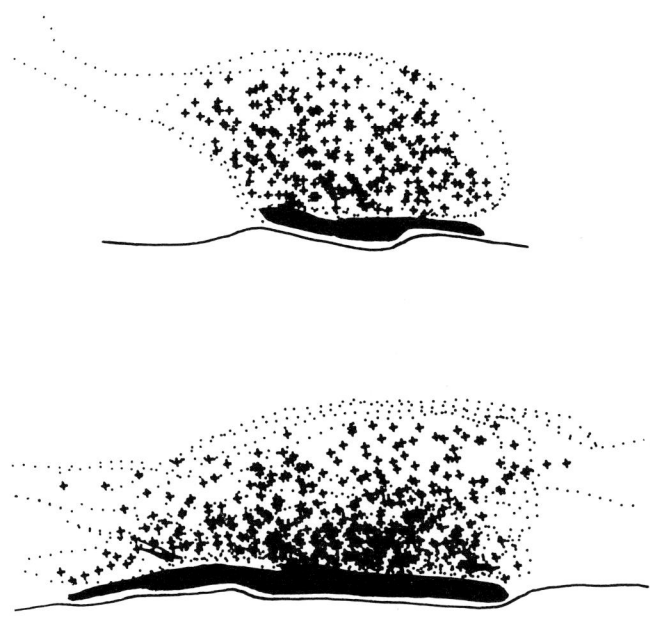

FIG. 4. Reconstruction of 2 different varicosities. Figure illustrates small (*upper*) and averaged-sized (*lower*) varicosity. Figure prepared by computer superimpositions of successive electron micrographs. *Dotted lines*, membranes of varicosities seen in sequential sections; *crosses*, positions of synaptic vesicles; *solid shading*, areas of fusion of basal laminae, where thickening of these areas reflect undulations in areas of contact rather than variations in cleft width; *solid lines*, sections of arteriolar muscle membrane. Larger varicosity has a larger area of contact and contains more vesicles. In both, vesicles are concentrated toward regions of apposition with underlying smooth muscle layer. *Calibration bar*, 1.0 µm. (Micrograph courtesy of S. Luff and E. M. MacLachlan.)

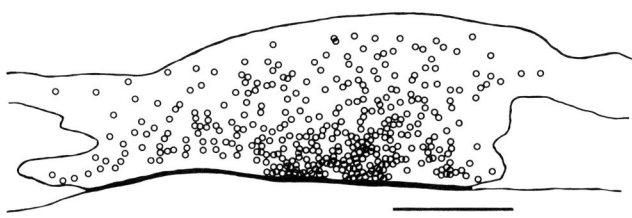

FIG. 5. Drawing of lower varicosity shown in Fig. 4. For clarity only 1 neuronal membrane has been shown. *Open circles*, small granular vesicles. Vesicles are connected toward region of fused basal lamellae. Varicosity is en passant; terminal axons can be seen originating on either side of junctional swelling. *Calibration bar*, 0.5 µm.

−70 mV is detected (74, 86, 127). Similar values of resting potential are found in arterioles and arteries of a variety of vascular beds taken from a variety of species (5, 15, 30–32, 53, 72, 91, 92, 101, 110, 112, 124, 154). These values are ∼20 mV more negative than those reported for recordings of arterial resting potential in vivo (147, 148, 150). The reason for the difference is not known, but if it does not reflect ongoing sympathetic nerve activity, it will have a profound effect on the reactivity of vascular tissue. Voltage-dependent calcium channels are first activated at membrane potentials near −50 mV (85). Reported in vivo resting potentials are very close to this potential; evidently only small depolarizations are required to trigger calcium entry. In virtually all reports, arterial resting membrane potentials, recorded in vitro, were stable, other than for occasional, transient, small-amplitude depolarizing potentials that result from the spontaneous release of quanta of sympathetic transmitter (32, 74, 81, 92, 112). Thus there is little to suggest that arterial smooth muscle cells in vitro generate myogenic activity. This is in clear contrast to many intestinal smooth muscle preparations (162) and to some venous smooth muscle preparations (90).

The ionic basis of the resting potential of intestinal arterioles has been examined in only one species [guinea pig (86)]. Much of these data and interpretation are similar to that obtained from other arteries. However, differences exist that may result from technical matters. Therefore it is perhaps appropriate to briefly comment on the methods of analysis applied in determining the ionic basis of resting membrane potentials. The most direct method is to measure the flux of ions across a cell membrane after loading the tissue with the appropriate radioactive ion. Under a variety of conditions the amount of the specific ion leaving a cell can then be estimated. If the initial starting concentration gradients, intracellular volume, and extracellular space are known, then the rate of appearance of the marked ion in extracellular fluid provides a measure of the permeability of that ion across the cell membrane (see refs. 17, 29). With smooth muscle preparations these conditions are difficult to achieve. The preparations are multicellular with a complex structural organization that often results in restricted diffusion paths from the surface of the muscle cells to the bulk extracellular compartment. Unfortunately where this limitation is least likely to occur, i.e., in arterioles that are structurally less complex and have only a monolayer of smooth muscle cells, albeit with attached supportive cells, ion flux studies have not been attempted. An alternative method is to measure the resting membrane potential in solutions where the concentrations of specific ions are systematically varied. The changes in potential are then related to the resting conductances of those ions (73). This method carries the assumptions that changes in the external concentration of an ion do not change either the internal concentration of that ion or that of others and that the conductance of specific ion channels is only changed in a predictable manner (64, 73, 87). Perhaps because of the large ratio of surface area to volume of smooth muscle cells, the first condition is not always met. For example, with ion-sensitive electrodes it has been shown in the ureter that a change in the external concentration of some ions leads to a change in the internal concentration of other ions (2).

To minimize these problems, segments of submucosal arteriole were subjected to rapid, transient (~1 min) changes in the ionic composition of the extracellular fluid. Both the resting membrane potential and input resistance of the arterioles were measured (86). Because large changes in the external concentration of either sodium or chloride ions had little effect on the resting potential, it was concluded that the contribution of these ions was slight (86). These observations contrast with intestinal muscle where appreciable chloride permeability has been demonstrated at rest (136). The observation that the resting sodium permeability is low also indicates that unless sodium is entering cells in a "nonelectrical" manner, the instantaneous contribution to the resting potential of an electrogenic sodium-pump current must be small (86, 160). Clearly at rest the outward pump current could only equal the current resulting from the passive inward leakage of sodium. If, as is generally held to be the case, sodium extrusion is linked to potassium uptake in a 3:2 ratio (160), the pump current will be that much smaller.

The relationship between external potassium concentration and resting potential was complex. As the external potassium concentration $[K^+]_o$ was increased, the resting membrane potential depolarized. Initially

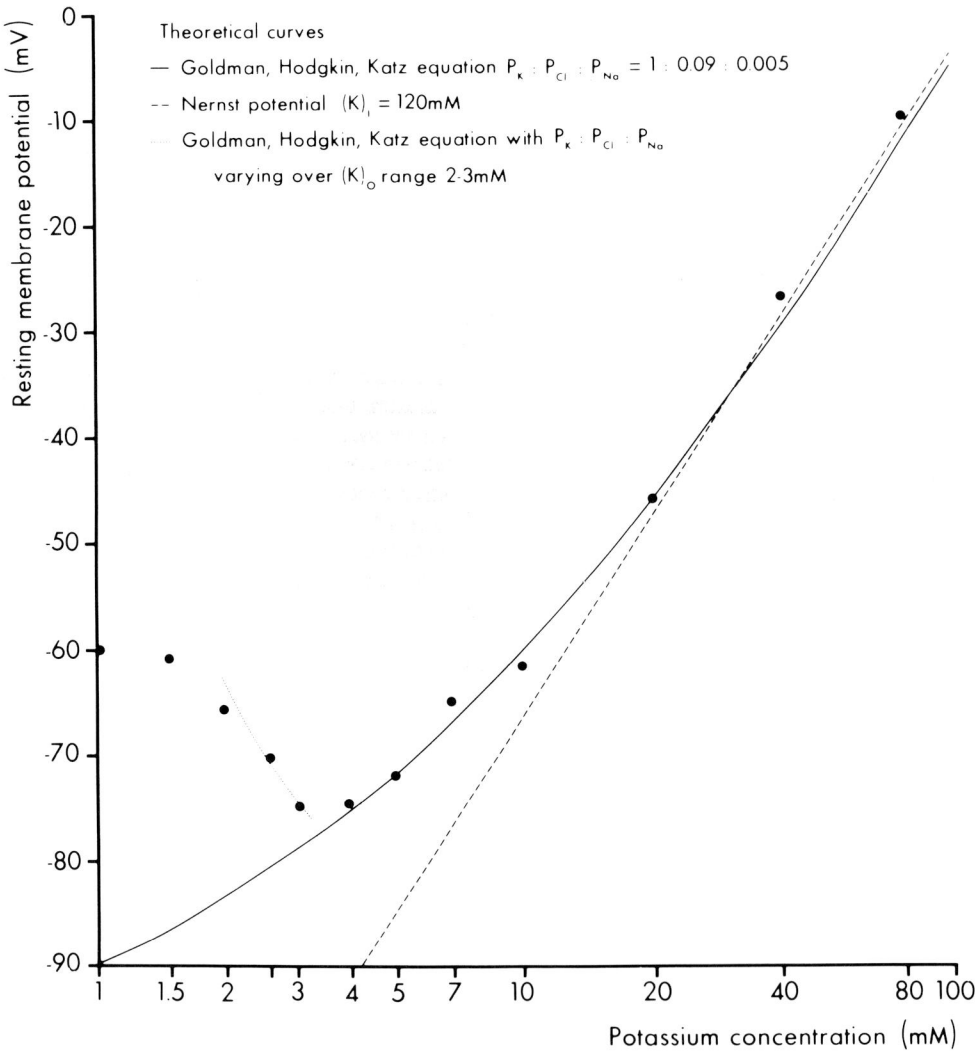

FIG. 6. Relationship between membrane potential of submucosal arterioles and external potassium concentration. *Closed circles*, membrane potentials of submucosal arterioles measured in different extracellular potassium concentrations; *solid line*, relationship between membrane potential and potassium concentration predicted by Goldman-Hodgkin-Katz equation with permeability ratios $P_{K^+}:P_{Cl^-}:P_{Na^+}$ assumed to be 1:0.09:0.005; *dashed line*, Nernst prediction for relationship with an intracellular potassium concentration of 120 mM. Fit between Goldman-Hodgkin-Katz prediction and experimental data is good for external potassium concentrations in range of 4 to 80 mM. At concentrations <4 mM a marked difference between predicted and observed relationships is apparent. [From Hirst and van Helden (86).]

the relationship between $[K^+]_o$ and membrane potential was less steep than predicted by the Nernst equation {internal $[K^+]$ being assumed to be 130 mM (29, 86)}. Above a $[K^+]_o$ of 20 mM, the relationship was well described by the Nernst equation (Fig. 6). These data were well fitted by the Goldman-Hodgkin-Katz equation (64, 73, 87) when the relative permeabilities of sodium, chloride, and potassium were assumed to be 0.005:0.09:1 (Fig. 6). Similarly an important contribution to the resting membrane potential is made by a relatively high potassium conductance in a number of other systemic arteries (31, 42, 69). When $[K^+]_o$ was reduced, the membrane potential initially hyperpolarized, but at external potassium concentrations of <2 mM, the membrane was depolarized. This was not directly attributable to inhibition of a sodium-potassium electrogenic transport system. The depolarization was associated with a dramatic increase in membrane resistance, far greater than can be accounted for by the Goldman-Hodgkin-Katz equation (Fig. 7). This observation was taken to mean that the resting potassium permeability of these arterioles is in some way sensitive to $[K^+]_o$. As $[K^+]_o$ is reduced, the equilibrium potential for potassium ($E_{K+}$) will become more negative and tend to cause an increase in resting potential; conversely, as the resting potassium conductance ($g_K$) is reduced by reducing $[K^+]_o$, the resting conductances of other ions will become more dominant. Although the mechanism is not fully understood, the observations provide an experimental basis for the known profound effects of hypokalemia on vascular reactivity. A further and also unexplained observation made in this study was that other procedures that inhibited the activity of sodium-potassium ion transport systems also increased membrane resistivity and frequently induced myogenic activity. In contrast to these views on the ionic basis of submucosal resting potential, a number of researchers have presented data that imply that a substantial contribution to the resting potential of arteries is made by the ongoing activity of an electrogenic sodium-potassium transport system (29, 69). Unfortunately in these studies the effect of ion changes and other experimental procedures on membrane resistance was not determined.

Thus it appears that the resting potential of arterioles is largely determined by their relatively high conductance to potassium ions with both sodium and chloride ions making only minor contributions. The role of active sodium transport systems in the regulation of cell resting potential and hence vascular reactivity requires further study.

### Electrical Coupling Between Arteriolar Smooth Muscle Cells

Electrical coupling between smooth muscle cells of vascular preparations has been demonstrated with the extracellular polarization technique first described by Hodgkin and Rushton (88) and modified by Abe and Tomita (1, 161) for smooth muscle. These experiments showed that potential changes occurred several hundred smooth muscle cell diameters from a pair of fixed polarizing plates (53, 66, 91, 112, 124, 125). Electrical coupling between individual arteriolar cells of submucosal arterioles has been demonstrated directly. Two intracellular recording electrodes were inserted into the smooth muscle layer of the same arteriolar tree (80, 81). The electrodes were separated by up to several hundred smooth muscle cell diameters. When a small current was passed through one electrode, a membrane potential change was detected at the second electrode (Fig. 8). If the current-passing electrode was withdrawn and the same current passed, no membrane potential change occurred. These results could only have been obtained if at least some of the current was able to flow from the site of injection to neighboring cells via intercellular couplings. Thus a proportion of the current entering a cell flows to a neighboring cell, the remaining proportion leaking across the cell membrane resistance to give a membrane potential change. If the sympathetic transmitter, released at a neuroeffector junction, induces a junctional current, that current will leak similarly through the syncytium to change the membrane potential of the syncytium. If transmitter is only released at a single point, for example, the spontaneous release of a quantum of transmitter, the current will be rapidly dissipated and the potential change will be restricted in area. If transmitter is released at a number of spatially separated points, then the potential of the whole syncytium will change.

Branching arteriolar trees, consisting of large num-

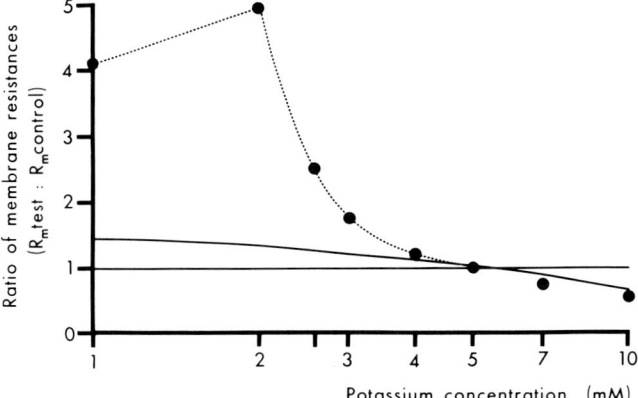

FIG. 7. Relationship between membrane resistance and external potassium concentration. *Closed circles*, membrane resistances ($R_m$) of submucosal arterioles [expressed as a ratio of resistance in test potassium to resistance in control potassium (5 mM)], which were determined in different extracellular potassium concentrations. *Dashed line*, crossing a ratio of unity (*solid line*), is relationship between membrane resistance and potassium concentration predicted by Goldman-Hodgkin-Katz equation. Similar to Fig. 6 there is a marked divergence between predicted and observed curves at extracellular potassium concentrations <4 mM. [From Hirst and van Helden (86).]

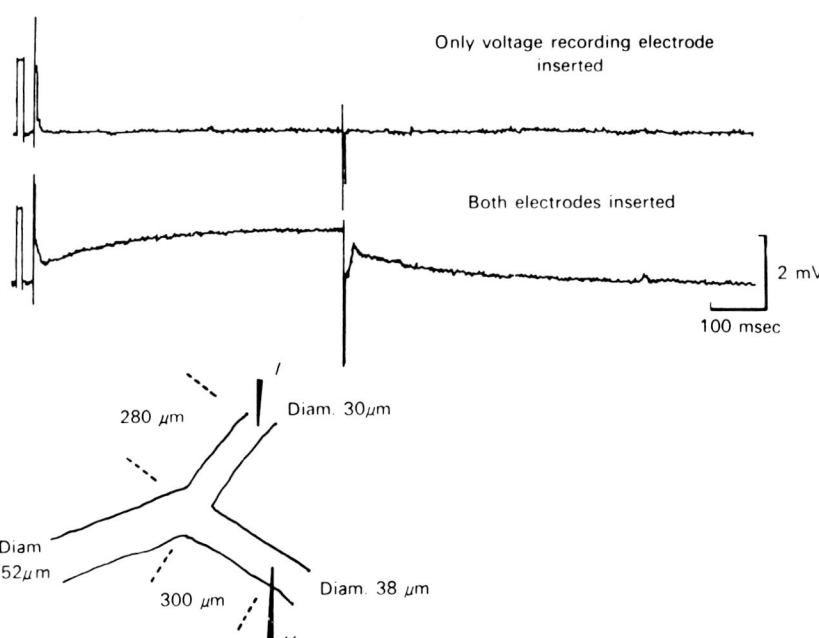

FIG. 8. Electrical coupling between arteriolar smooth muscle cells. Two independent intracellular recording electrodes were inserted into separate branches of same arteriolar tree with total separation of 580 μm. When current (1 nA) was passed through 1 electrode a membrane potential change was detected at other electrode. Potential change (*upper trace*) was not detected if same current was passed through current-passing electrode after just withdrawing it from arteriolar smooth muscle layer. [From Hirst and Neild (80).]

bers of interconnected smooth muscle cells, are difficult to analyze electrically. Their description is analogous to that of the complex dendritic trees associated with central neurones (98). Consequently the electrical properties of arteriolar smooth muscle were analyzed with nonbranching lengths of arteriole cut from an arteriolar tree. The cut muscle layers at the ends of these lengths seal so as to offer a very high resistance to the extracellular fluid (80, 81). Thus these preparations, or segments of arteriole, can be treated as short electrical cables with sealed ends (98). Again with paired intracellular recording techniques, currents were passed through one electrode, and both the amplitude and time course of the induced potential change were recorded with the second electrode (see Fig. 11 for examples). Because the physical length of arteriolar segments and the separation and positioning of electrodes could be determined with a microscope, the electrical length constant, the input resistance, and the membrane time constant could be estimated. The values for length constant were in the range of 1.4–1.5 mm and those for time constant were in the range of 300–700 ms. Values similar to this have been obtained for other arterial preparations with the external polarization technique (91, 112, 124).

After making assumptions about the shape of smooth muscle cells and their organization (see refs. 80, 94) and knowing the intensity of current injected, values of specific membrane resistance and capacitance can be calculated. The average values were 66 $k\Omega \cdot cm^2$ and 5 $\mu F \cdot cm^{-2}$, respectively. This value of specific membrane resistance is extremely high when compared with that of other excitable cells (98). This presumably reflects the paucity of resting ion channels that might be expected for cells with such high ratio of surface area to volume. If it is further assumed that the specific membrane capacitance of these cells is 1 $\mu F \cdot cm^{-2}$, as appears to be for most excitable cells (35), the error reflecting inaccuracies in the estimates of cell surface area, the value of specific membrane resistance, rises by a factor of 5. In low extracellular potassium concentrations or after exposure to ouabain, the values of specific membrane resistance rise toward the values determined for bimolecular lipid layers devoid of membrane channels. This is also consistent with the view that smooth muscle cells are only slightly permeant to any ion species at rest (86).

## Summary

Submucosal arterioles share many properties with other arteries and other smooth muscles. Their resting potential is largely determined by their relatively high permeability to potassium ions. Individual arteriolar smooth muscles are coupled to their neighbors; a group of cells rather than a single cell forms the target for nervous influences. The high specific membrane resistance measured favors current flow between individual cells via low-resistance couplings rather than escape across the cell membrane and also enables those cells that have high ratios of surface area to volume to maintain their ionic gradients with relatively little energy expenditure.

## NEUROMUSCULAR TRANSMISSION IN ARTERIOLES

At all synapses examined so far, invasion of the presynaptic terminal by an action potential causes a part of the terminal to become permeable to calcium ions. The resulting increase in intracellular calcium concentration facilitates transmitter release from a large store of preformed packets or quanta of transmitter. In the absence of stimulation, transmitter is released spontaneously, usually in the form of single quanta of transmitter; occasionally the leak of small quantities of nonpackaged transmitter has been detected (103). After release, whether evoked or occurring spontaneously, transmitter diffuses across the synaptic cleft and binds to postsynaptic receptors that are specific for that chemical. At most synapses, occupation of a synaptic receptor by one or more molecules of transmitter promotes a conformational change in the receptor so that associated structures in the membrane become permeable to specific ions. These ions diffuse down their concentration gradients and lead to a membrane potential change, unless the null potential of the specific ion is the same as the resting potential. At some synapses, rather than opening channels, transmitters activate a complex series of intracellular changes that may manifest themselves as conductance increases or decreases or alternatively as a changed metabolic status of the cell. It is apparent that in some vessels transmission results from a mixture of postsynaptic phenomena, one involving the rapid opening of membrane channels and the other involving more complex intracellular events (see refs. 14, 16).

## RESPONSES OF SUBMUCOSAL ARTERIOLES TO SYMPATHETIC NERVE STIMULATION

Stimulation of the nerves to submucosal arterioles causes a transient depolarization of the arteriolar smooth muscle membrane potential [Fig. 9; (74, 127)]. Such a depolarization is known as an excitatory junction potential (EJP). When initiated by a single stimulus an EJP has a slow time course compared with most synaptic potentials recorded from neuronal or skeletal synapses. Its time course is, however, faster than that of other junction potentials recorded from smooth muscle preparations. The time to peak membrane potential change (~10 mV) is ~100 ms; thereafter the potential decays with a time course that can be described by a single exponential function (range of time constants 300–700 ms). Excitatory junction potentials result from nerve activation: they are not detected after degeneration of the perivascular nerves, and they are prevented by tetrodotoxin (TTX) or by elevated extracellular magnesium concentrations (74, 81, 133).

Excitatory junction potentials similar to those recorded from submucosal arterioles had been previously recorded from vasa deferentia of a number of species (20, 21, 109) and from mesenteric and uterine arteries (5, 147, 148). Subsequently, all the mammalian systemic arteries that have been examined have been shown to generate this characteristic EJP in response to sympathetic nerve stimulation (16, 32, 33, 72, 91, 95, 96, 101, 102, 112, 154). In contrast, low-pressure vessels, i.e., pulmonary arteries and many venous preparations, do not generate EJPs with this

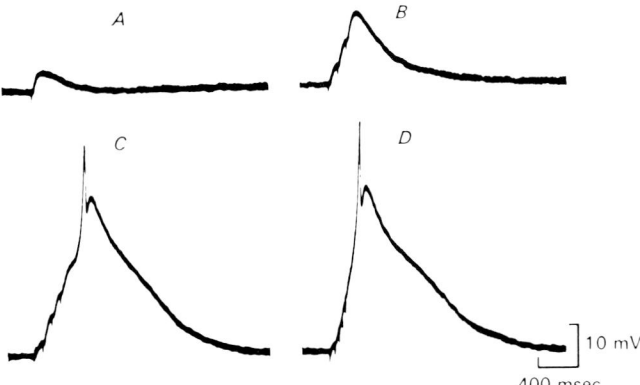

FIG. 9. Membrane potential changes recorded from submucosal arteriole in responses to perivascular nerve stimulation. *Traces* show membrane potential changes produced by 1, 3 (10 Hz), 4 (10 Hz), and 5 stimuli (20 Hz). Excitatory junction potential, initiated by single stimulus, has time to peak of ~100 ms and total duration of ~1 s. With large number of stimuli, junctional depolarization exceeded threshold and initiated action potentials with rapid and plateau components. Arteriolar constriction was only detected if an action potential had been first initiated. [From Hirst (74).]

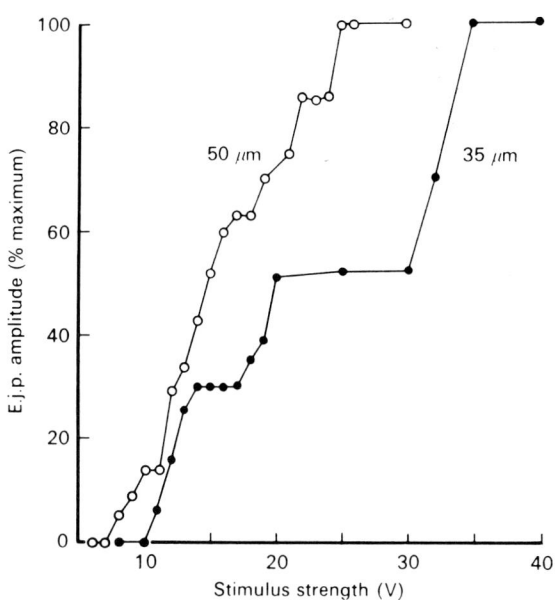

FIG. 10. Relationship between amplitude of excitatory junction potentials (EJPs) recorded from 2 different arterioles and stimulus strength applied to perivascular nerves. As strength is increased, amplitude of EJPs increases up to a maximum value. Relationships are not smooth, indicating that each arteriole is innervated by a number of fibers, each of a different threshold. Presumably finer vessel was innervated by 3 fibers and larger by 5 fibers. [From Hirst (74).]

characteristic time course. In these vessels repetitive sympathetic nerve stimulation initiates much slower and much smaller membrane depolarizations with times to peak of ~1–2 s and total durations of tens of seconds (16, 90, 127, 153, 155, 156; see, however, ref. 106). These slow junctional responses may be further distinguished from arterial EJPs, because unlike the latter, they are abolished by α-adrenoreceptor antagonists. Arteries with a thermoregulatory function generate a two-component membrane potential change in response to sympathetic nerve stimulation. There is an antagonist resistant EJP with a duration of ~1 s; this is followed by a slow α-antagonist–sensitive depolarization (32, 33, 96, 101).

The amplitude of the EJP recorded from submucosal arterioles and other systemic arteries can be varied by varying the strength of stimulus applied to the perivascular nerves. As the strength is increased, the amplitude increases up to a maximum. In submucosal arterioles the relationship between stimulus strength and EJP amplitude is not smooth; rather it is interrupted by a variable number of plateaus [Fig. 10; (74)]. This means that a given area of the arteriolar tree syncytium is innervated by a restricted number of nerve fibers of differing threshold. Taking the examples shown in Figure 10, the finer vessel was innervated by three fibers and the larger vessel by five fibers. Qualitatively similar observations have been made on uterine arteries (5).

During a train of perivascular low-frequency stimuli (~1 Hz), successive EJPs recorded from submucosal arterioles and other systemic arteries increase in amplitude to reach a stable amplitude; that is, they facilitate. After a brief train of stimuli, facilitation decays with a time constant of ~2–4 s (74). A similar value for the decay of facilitation has been reported for sympathetic transmission in the guinea pig vas deferens (8).

Individual EJPs, because they are too small, do not initiate constriction of submucosal arterioles. Rather the sympathetic nerves must be stimulated repetitively at frequencies >2 Hz so that successive EJPs sum to give a larger depolarization. At a critical depolarization of ~15–20 mV (absolute membrane potentials of about −50 mV), a regenerative membrane potential change occurs (Fig. 9). This regenerative membrane potential change invariably triggers constriction. Similar observations have been made from other arteries (e.g., see ref. 91). The ionic events underlying these regenerative membrane potential changes are described in *Potential-Dependent Calcium Entry*, p. 1650. However, this sequence of events, transmitter-induced membrane depolarization followed by potential-dependent increases in postjunctional membrane permeability, is not a prerequisite for tension generation in all vascular beds. In the low-pressure vessels and in "thermoregulatory" arteries, the slow, α-antagonist–sensitive membrane depolarizations that follow sympathetic nerve stimulation are, without reinforcement, associated with constriction.

## ANALYSIS OF EXCITATORY JUNCTION POTENTIALS

### Time Course

Excitatory junction potentials recorded from submucosal arterioles have rise times of 100 ms and decay with time constants of ~500 ms. The passive electrical membrane time constant of a given preparation and time constant of decay of its EJP have been measured and found to be identical (Fig. 11). With these data the time course of junctional current flow can be calculated (Fig. 12). It can be seen that the peak junctional current occurs ~10–20 ms after the start of current flow and that the current is complete after ~200 ms. Thus the current is brief compared with the membrane time constant. Similar observations and deductions have been made for EJPs recorded from rabbit saphenous artery (91) and from guinea pig vas deferens (27). Similarly at many peripheral and central synapses the time course of excitatory synaptic current flow is brief when compared with their postsynaptic membrane time constants (48, 138).

A more direct measure of the time course and intensity of synaptic currents can be obtained with voltage-clamp techniques (47). Excitatory junctional currents (EJCs) have been measured in submucosal arterioles by a single-electrode voltage-clamp technique (Figs. 13, 14). Electrically short segments of arterioles (length <0.1 of an electrical length constant) were used to ensure isopotentiality during voltage clamping. The currents had time courses identical to those predicted from cable analyses, with times to peak of 10 ms followed by an exponential decay [time constants ~50 ms (Fig. 13)]. Like many other excitatory synaptic currents, the amplitudes of EJCs decreased as the arteriole was depolarized and increased when the arteriole was hyperpolarized (Fig. 14). The null potential, determined by extrapolation, was 0 mV. Unlike most other excitatory synaptic currents, the time course of decay of EJCs was not voltage sensitive (Fig. 14). It is not known if this lack of voltage sensitivity is a property of the individual junctional channels activated by transmitter or if it means that the decay of junctional current reflects a persistent stay of transmitter in a junctional cleft.

Large changes in extracellular chloride concentration had no effect on EJCs; this suggests the chloride permeability is not changed during sympathetic transmission in these vessels. The substitution of sodium chloride by sucrose dramatically reduced the amplitude of EJCs, suggesting that the inward current detected at resting potential was largely carried by sodium ions. The determination of a null potential in control solution near 0 mV implies that potassium conductance also increases during an EJC.

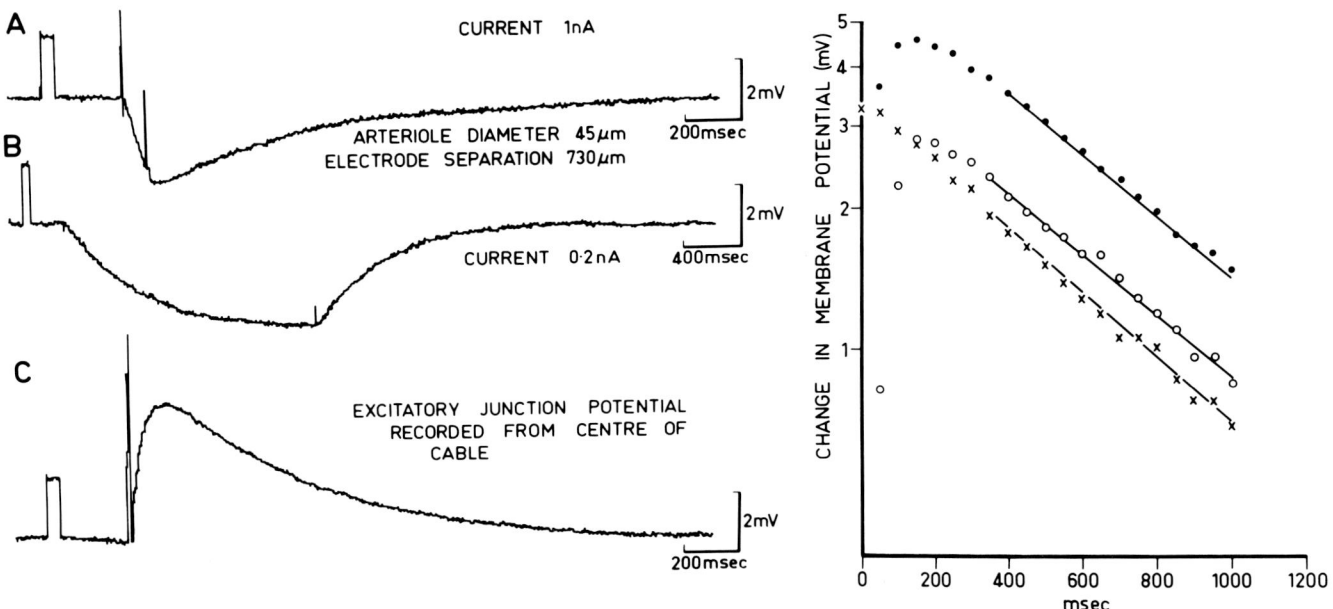

FIG. 11. Passive electrical properties of 1.4-mm segment of arteriole. One electrode, used to inject current, was inserted in center of preparation and second electrode, used for recording membrane potential, was inserted toward one end of arteriole. Short and long current pulses were injected and resultant membrane potential changes, along with excitatory junction potentials evoked by transmural stimulation, were recorded. Data are plotted in the *right half* of figure. Time course of decay of 3 potential changes is the same, and each can be described by a single exponential. These data can be used to determine passive electrical properties of arteriole (for further details, see ref. 80). [From Hirst and Neild (80).]

These observations are qualitatively the same as those made at the skeletal neuromuscular junction but are to be contrasted with the junctional potentials recorded from a number of other smooth muscle preparations where norepinephrine is known to be the transmitter. For example, in rat anococcygeus muscle, sympathetic nerve activity results in a membrane depolarization that is sensitive to $\alpha$-blockade and has a time course slower than the EJP recorded from systemic arteries. Experimental data indicate that the slow junctional potential results solely from an increase in chloride permeability (116–118). Similarly in uterine muscle, $\alpha$-adrenoreceptor activation results in an increased permeability to chloride ions (18, 19).

*Quantal Content*

It is generally accepted that arteries are innervated by many sympathetic nerve fibers, each having several hundred varicosities. Because many ultrastructural studies failed to detect a high proportion of appositions between nerve and smooth muscle, it was assumed that on stimulation each varicosity released either a vesicle of transmitter or a fraction of a vesicle (8, 10, 140), and the artery was bathed in transmitter. The transmitter thus diffused from the adventitial surface into the artery wall to cause vasoconstriction (10). Intramural arterioles are also densely innervated by varicose sympathetic nerve fibers. In these preparations most of the varicosities form appositions with the postjunctional smooth muscle membrane. The varicosities contain numerous vesicles that are concentrated toward the region of junctional contact.

However, electrophysiological data from submucosal arterioles suggest that when a large number of varicosities are stimulated, only a few release transmitter per impulse. Spontaneous excitatory junction potentials (SEJPs) can be recorded from submucosal arterioles. Like spontaneous quantal potentials recorded from other synapses, they persist in TTX. Both SEJPs and EJPs recorded from electrically short segments of arteriole have identical time courses (Fig. 15), which suggest that EJPs result from the synchronous release of SEJPs. Unlike SEJPs recorded from electrically more complex smooth muscle preparations (22), the entire amplitude distribution curve could be readily distinguished from the background recording noise (81). The SEJPs had a unimodal distribution that was well described by a gamma function (122), suggesting that they result from the release of transmitter from a pool or pools of preformed packages of transmitter. The SEJPs had mean amplitudes of 1–3 mV and as such were only smaller than the mean amplitude of the evoked potentials by factors 2 to 5 (Fig. 15). This indicates that not many quanta must be released to make up an evoked response.

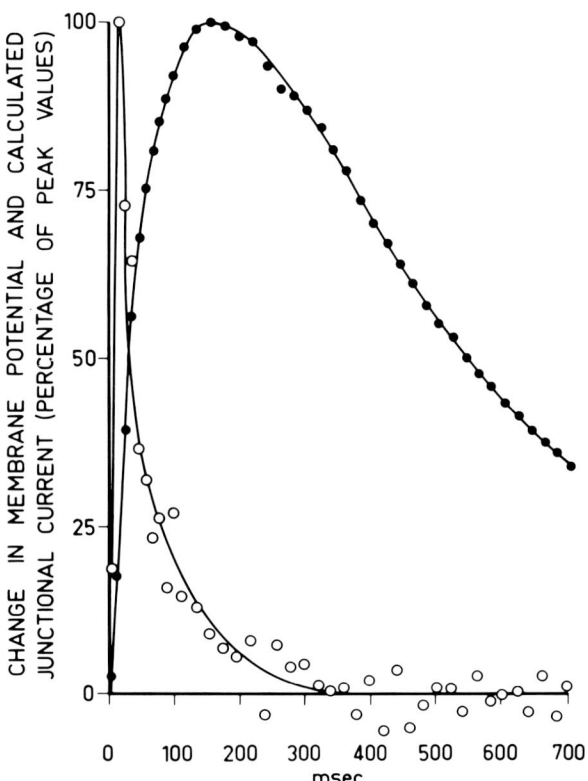

FIG. 12. Time course of junctional current (*open circles*) derived from time course of excitatory junction potential (*closed circles*) and arteriolar passive electrical properties. Current time was calculated using equation suggested by Curtis and Eccles (37), which assumes that the segment of arteriole is isopotential during current flow. Current reaches peak after 10 ms and then decays to 0 within a further 200 ms. More prolonged time course of excitatory junction potential reflects long membrane time constant of arteriolar smooth muscle membrane. [From Hirst and Neild (80).]

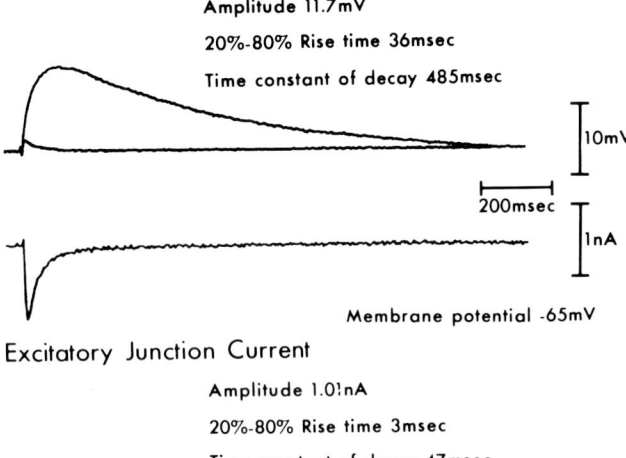

FIG. 13. Comparison between excitatory junctional current (EJC) and excitatory junction potential (EJP) that it produces. EJP was recorded in voltage-recording mode; EJC was recorded in single-electrode voltage-clamp mode. Decay of both can be described by single exponentials: time constant of decay of EJP was 485 ms and that of EJC was 47 ms. [From Hirst et al. (76).]

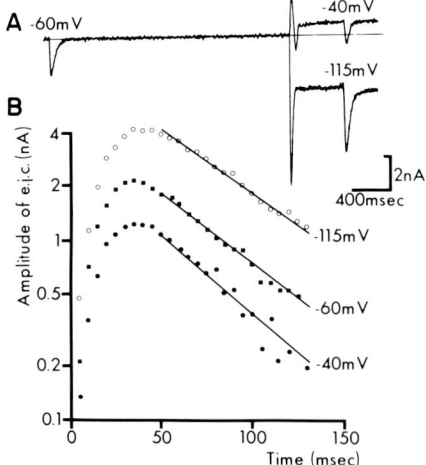

FIG. 14. Effect of membrane potential on excitatory junctional current (EJC) amplitude and time course. *A*: current records allow comparison between amplitude of EJC recorded at holding potential of −60 mV with those recorded during voltage-clamp steps to −40 mV and −115 mV. At depolarized potential, current amplitude is reduced, and at hyperpolarized level, amplitude is increased. *B*: plots of time courses of these 3 junctional currents: time course of decay of each is very similar. Rise time of EJC is slowed because of filtering (100 Hz) to improve signal-to-noise ratio. [From Finkel et al. (47).]

When the number of sympathetic varicosities in the preparations was counted from fluorescence micrographs; the preparations were found to contain ~100–200 varicosities. Evidently the likelihood of a varicosity releasing transmitter per nerve impulse is very low, being 1 in 50 or lower (81, 119).

Even with supramaximal perivascular nerve stimuli, successive EJPs recorded from the short segments of arteriole fluctuated in amplitude; release of a quantum occasionally failed to occur. This is also consistent with the view that the probability of release at each neuroeffector junction is very low. This observation is quantitatively different from most mammalian synapses. At most, release occurs with a much higher probability than 0.02 when normal calcium is present. Only when the extracellular calcium concentration is lowered does such a low probability of release usually occur (120, 122). As a check of the hypothesis that EJPs were made up from the synchronous release of a number of SEJPs, the amplitude distributions of both EJPs and SEJPs in a given tissue were determined. It was possible to simulate the distribution curve of EJPs by adding together small numbers of multiples of the SEJP amplitude distribution curves (81). Thus only a few restricted and spatially separate areas of arteriolar surface are exposed to transmitter during a single excitation of many varicosities.

Spontaneous EJPs have been recorded from other arterial preparations and also from the vasa deferentia of a number of species (13, 20, 22, 27, 32, 36, 91, 112, 151). Unlike those recorded from short segments of arteriole, the SEJPs in these tissues have faster time

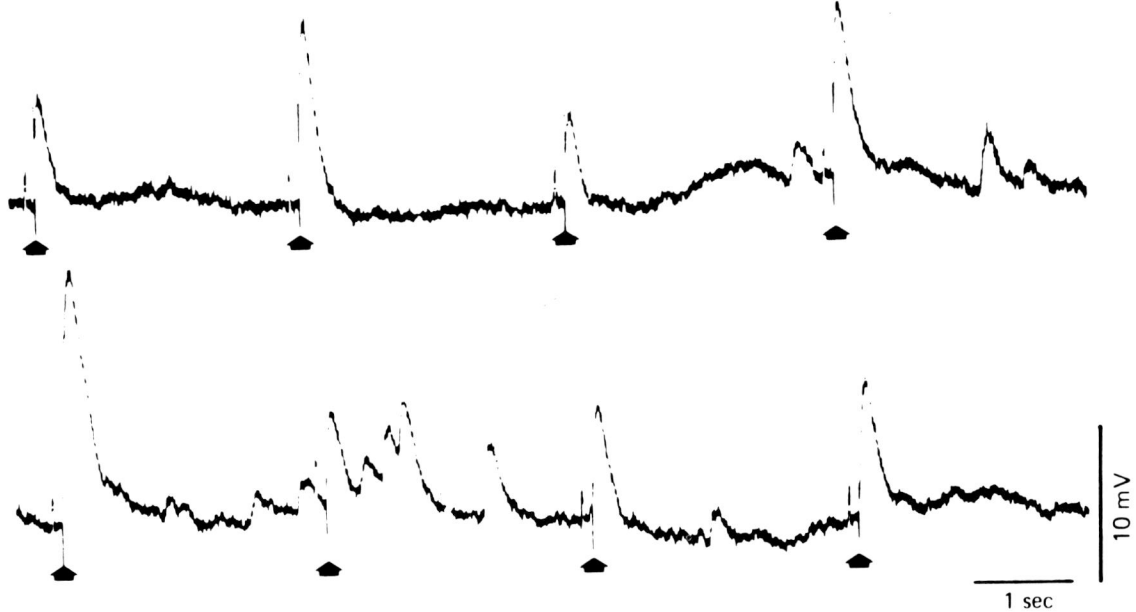

FIG. 15. Recordings from short segment of arteriole during train of low-frequency, supramaximal transmural stimuli. *Arrows*, successive excitatory junction potentials (EJPs) fluctuate in amplitude but not time course. Spontaneous EJPs (SEJPs), with a similar time course, occurred at irregular intervals during recording period. Only a few SEJPs would have to be released synchronously to generate an EJP [From Hirst and Neild (81).]

courses than those of EJPs. This reflects the differing electrical properties of the target tissues. Arteries and vasa deferentia have muscular walls that consist of many layers of smooth muscle cells. Because the cells are electrically coupled to form multidimensional syncytia, the time course of a potential change initiated by a point current, i.e., the junctional current from a single quantum of transmitter, more closely reflects the time course of that current (8). Making use of this property of syncytia, the evoked release of sympathetic transmitter from restricted numbers of varicosities have been studies in guinea pig vas deferens. Again the conclusion was reached that the probability of release from a given neuroeffector junction was extremely low (13, 36).

The junctional currents that underlie SEJPs have been recorded with a voltage clamp (47). Again spontaneous excitatory junctional currents (SEJCs) had the same time courses as evoked junctional currents and again the amplitudes of EJCs and SEJCs differed by a factor of <5. Of particular interest are the peak amplitudes of SEJCs. These were in the range of 0.1–0.2 nA (Fig. 16). This value is very similar to that of spontaneous excitatory synaptic current recorded from both parasympathetic and sympathetic ganglion cells (79, 137). It is also similar to that of a unitary synaptic current recorded from cat motor neurons (48, 99), but it is ~10 times smaller than that of a miniature end-plate current recorded from skeletal muscle (61). The amplitude of current flowing through a single transmitter-activated channel at submucosal arteriole

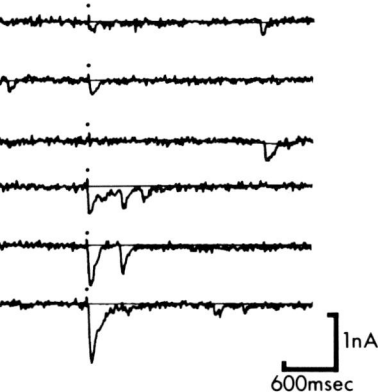

FIG. 16. Voltage-clamp recording from short segment of arteriole during train of low-frequency, supramaximal transmural stimuli; 6 successive records of membrane current (holding potential −60 mV) are shown. *Closed circles*, stimuli were given. Successive excitatory junctional currents (EJCs) fluctuated in amplitude and on one occasion failed to release. Spontaneous EJCs (SEJCs) are also shown as irregularly occurring inward currents; again their amplitudes are only slightly smaller than those evoked currents. SEJCs had peak amplitudes of 0.1–0.2 nA. [From Finkel et al. (47).]

neuroeffector junctions is not known. However, at many other excitatory synapses, including both ganglion cells and the skeletal neuromuscular junction, a single channel activated by transmitter generate ~1 pA at resting potential (61). This suggests that a quantum of transmitter in a ganglion cell opens ~100–200 individual channels. This is far less than the number of molecules of acetylcholine, the transmitter at these synapses, present in a presynaptic vesicle

(107, 137). This either suggests that there are a restricted number of synaptic channels under an individual release point or alternatively that the synaptic receptors can only be activated by the high local concentration of transmitter that occurs very close to the point of vesicular release. Whatever the explanation, a similar phenomenon must occur at sympathetic neuroeffector junctions on submucosal arterioles if the sympathetic transmitter is norepinephrine. The number of molecules of norepinephrine in a vesicle obtained from sympathetic nerves is calculated to be ~1,000–10,000 (8, 20, 42, 113). If, however, the transmitter is ATP, all the 20–50 molecules of ATP present in a sympathetic vesicle (52) must bind and even then open very large channels. This problem requires further study.

*Summary*

The data reviewed suggest that transmission between sympathetic nerve fibers and submucosal arterioles utilizes the same mechanisms as other synapses. Stimulation of sympathetic nerves results in a calcium-dependent release of transmitter from a preformed store of quanta of transmitter. However, the probability of release from a given varicosity is extremely low; transmission proceeds without hindrance because of the many varicosities present. After release, quanta produce discrete conductance changes, allowing inward current flow. Because of the syncytial properties of arterioles, excitatory current flows through each individual smooth muscle cell and depolarization is detected throughout the arteriole.

INITIATION OF CONTRACTION IN SUBMUCOSAL ARTERIOLES

Smooth muscle cells generate tension when the concentration of free calcium around their contractile proteins is increased (38, 43, 146). In arteries, the intracellular concentration of calcium can be increased by two different mechanisms, which can be distinguished. One mechanism requires depolarization of the smooth muscle membrane. This activates voltage-dependent calcium channels and allows calcium entry to occur. The other mechanism does not require a membrane potential change; rather an agonist occupies a receptor on the smooth muscle membrane and in some way causes the release of calcium from a bound store. The distinction between the two mechanisms is illustrated by the following observations. Pulmonary arteries generate tension after exposure to increased $[K^+]_o$ only when the membrane has been depolarized to beyond −50 mV (31). In contrast, superfusion of this same artery with norepinephrine produces a maximal contraction without a detectable membrane potential change (31, 42); this process, called pharmacomechanical coupling, has been reviewed (146). As a further distinction, the potential-dependent constrictions of arteries produced by increasing $[K^+]_o$ are readily inhibited by the calcium antagonist nitrendipine, whereas those caused by superfused norepinephrine (receptor activated) are more resistant (4).

*Potential-Dependent Calcium Entry*

This mechanism is of prime importance in the generation of constriction by submucosal arterioles after sympathetic nerve activity. Constriction of these arterioles is only observed when EJPs sum to reduce the membrane potential to below an absolute value of −50 mV. At membrane potentials near this value, regenerative potential changes are superimposed on the junction potentials and constriction occurs. The regenerative potentials frequently have two components: a rapid transient component and a more prolonged plateau component (see Fig. 9). On occasions only the slower plateau component is detected, and this alone is sufficient to trigger constriction (74). The ionic currents that underlie the rapid and plateau components of the regenerative responses generated in submucosal arterioles have not been examined in full but have been studied sufficiently (G. D. S. Hirst and D. F. van Helden, unpublished observations) to be confident that they are similar to those activated in rat cerebral arterioles by depolarization (71, 85). In cerebral arterioles, membrane depolarization produced by injection of constant currents evokes small-amplitude regenerative responses (Fig. 17) that in turn trigger vasoconstriction. When tetraethylammonium chloride (TEA) was included in the perfusion fluid to prevent activation of delayed rectifiers (66), pronounced regenerative responses were recorded. These had configurations similar to the action potentials superimposed on large-amplitude EJPs of submucosal arterioles (cf. Fig. 9 with Fig. 17). Both components of the directly initiated responses persisted in the presence of TTX, but both were abolished by substituting manganese ions for the extracellular calcium ions (Fig. 17). Both components of regenerative responses were also reduced by the calcium antagonists verapamil and nifedipine. Action potentials with similar configurations are generated by a number of vascular smooth preparations when TEA is present (42, 92).

With a single-electrode voltage clamp, two distinct inward currents were recorded when arteriolar membrane potential was stepped over a range of depolarized levels. One current had a threshold for activation of −50 mV: it had a small amplitude and never generated a net inward current. In the range of membrane potentials studied (up to −20 mV), the amplitude of this current increased as the depolarization increased; the current did not inactivate over 1 s. The second current was not detected until the membrane potential was depolarized to potentials less negative than −40

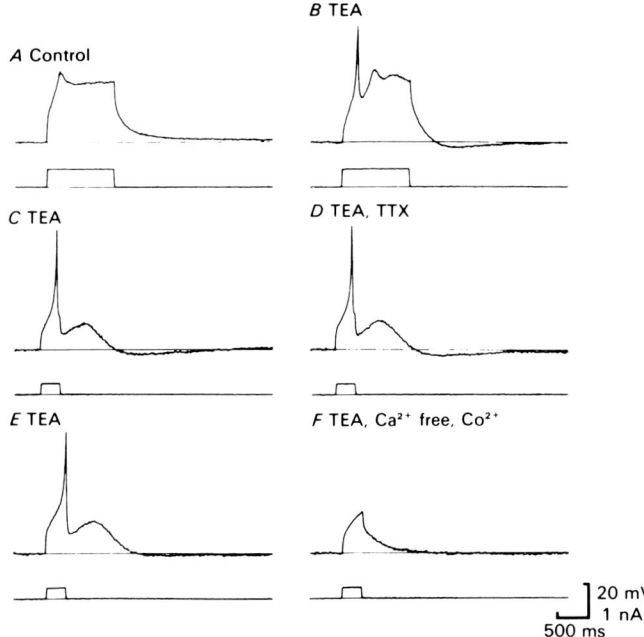

FIG. 17. Regenerative membrane potential changes initiated in rat cerebral arterioles. Each record was made from same short segment of arteriole and shows membrane potential changes produced by injecting depolarizing currents. A: control solution; a small regenerative potential change is superimposed on depolarizing potential change. B: after addition of tetraethylammonium chloride (TEA; 10 mM), depolarization now produced larger amplitude regenerative potential changes. C: duration of depolarizing pulse was shortened and 2-component action potential was readily distinguished. D: action potential had rapid component and slower plateau component each of which persisted in presence of tetrodotoxin (TTX; $1 \times 10^{-6}$ M). E: control response obtained before addition of manganese ions. F: both components were abolished by substitution of calcium ions by manganese ions. [From Hirst et al. (85).]

mV. This current had a large peak-current amplitude and could be readily distinguished from the first current because it inactivated with time. When the membrane was held steadily depolarized, after an initial peak the current decayed with a time constant of 20 ms. As both currents are abolished by manganese ions or nifedipine, both presumably result from an increase in calcium conductance.

By taking the integrals of the inward currents as a function of membrane potential (Fig. 18), the amount of charge, i.e., calcium, entering through each channel can be estimated. For sustained depolarizations, which will occur during tonic sympathetic nerve activity, the bulk of calcium entry will be via the low-threshold noninactivating channel. After an estimation of the arteriolar smooth muscle volume, and with the assumption that no calcium is bound or expelled during the depolarizing step, the increase in internal calcium concentration can be calculated. Such calculations indicate that as the amplitude of the depolarizing step is varied, the internal calcium concentration is also smoothly varied, and sufficient calcium enters to trigger constriction. For example, 1-s depolarization to a

potential of −30 mV causes the internal calcium concentration to rise to $1 \times 10^{-5}$ M. This concentration produces a maximal constriction of skinned smooth muscle fibers (43) and is far in excess of that required to initiate constriction in other vascular muscles (38).

These data suggest that regenerative responses of arterioles result solely from voltage-dependent increases in calcium permeability. A similar role for calcium ions in action potential generation has been suggested for a number of other smooth preparations (162), including other arteries (104, 105). It is still not clear, however, what role, if any, sodium ions play in action potential generation. Under certain conditions some smooth muscles can generate action potentials in the absence of calcium, provided that sodium is present (162). Whether this reflects the normal selectivity of smooth muscle calcium channels or a loss of selectivity of calcium channels to calcium when exposed to calcium-free solutions is not clear.

### Receptor-Activated Tension Development

Many vascular smooth muscle preparations generate tension when exposed to norepinephrine with

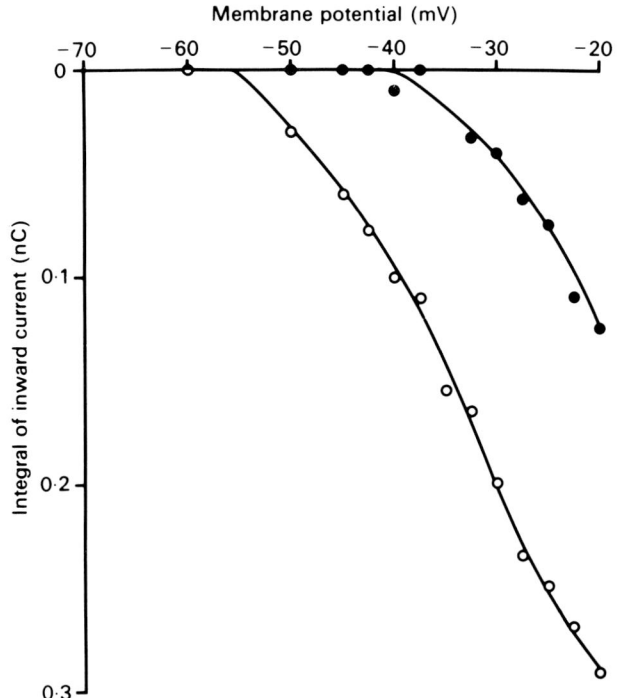

FIG. 18. Integrals of inward calcium currents in cerebral arterioles. When segments of arteriole were voltage clamped and their potentials stepped to depolarized potentials, 2 distinct inward currents were detected. Small depolarizations resulted in a small-amplitude, noninactivating current; with larger depolarizations a rapidly inactivating component was superimposed on noninactivating current. Integrals of current flowing through low-threshold, noninactivating current (*open circles*) and high-threshold, inactivating current (*closed circles*) are plotted as function of membrane potential. Charge increases smoothly as function of depolarization. [From Hirst et al. (85).]

either a small or even a nondetectable membrane potential change (146). These responses result from the activation of α-adrenoreceptors. Initially the responses are not dependent on the presence of extracellular calcium. That is, the first exposure to norepinephrine in the absence of extracellular calcium produces a constriction. However, successive constrictions only occur if calcium is present in the extracellular fluid. These and other observations have led to the view that α-adrenoreceptor activation in some way displaces calcium from a membrane-bound site and so increases its free intracellular concentration. For successive contractions to occur, the membrane site must be refilled with calcium from the extracellular fluid.

In arteries where membrane potential changes do occur after α-adrenoreceptor activation (15, 32, 33, 95, 128), it is not clear whether the membrane potential change is a prerequisite for contraction or whether it occurs as a consequence of other cellular changes brought about by receptor activation. In the rat tail artery, constriction resulting from α-adrenoreceptor activation precedes the associated membrane potential change (33).

Submucosal arterioles, like other arteries, when exposed to superfused norepinephrine, constrict. The constrictions, initiated by a threshold concentration of norepinephrine, are not associated with a marked membrane potential change, but rather the membrane potential record becomes unstable (Fig. 19). However, with higher concentrations of norepinephrine, large membrane potential changes are detected. All the membrane potential changes produced by concentrations of norepinephrine $<1 \times 10^{-4}$ M are blocked by the α-antagonists prazosin and phentolamine. They therefore result from the activation of α-adrenoreceptors. When small amounts of norepinephrine are applied with an ionophoretic electrode to areas of arteriole devoid of sympathetic nerve endings, only the area of tissue near the ionophoretic electrode constrict, and no membrane potential change is detected (82). When large amounts of norepinephrine are applied to the same areas a larger constriction is observed, and this may be associated with a long-latency, small-amplitude depolarization (latency ~1 s, amplitude ~10 mV). Again these types of responses are abolished by α-adrenoreceptor antagonists. Evidently if sufficient α-adrenoreceptors are activated they cause membrane depolarization.

Membrane depolarizations in response to superfused norepinephrine have also been detected from rabbit saphenous artery preparations and from those of rat or guinea pig mesentery (15, 93, 128). No consistent change in membrane resistance was detected during the norepinephrine-induced depolarization of

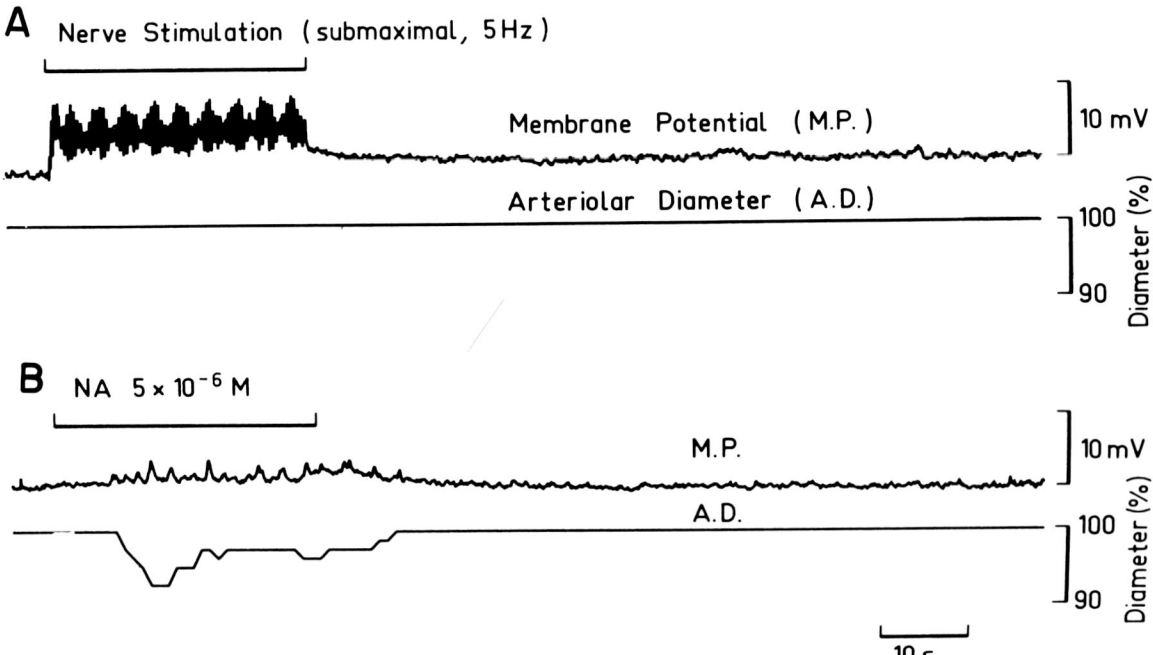

FIG. 19. Comparison between membrane potential changes and arteriolar diameter changes produced by repetitive nerve stimulation and superfusion of norepinephrine [noradrenaline (NA)]. *A*: perivascular nerves were stimulated repetitively to produce maintained depolarization of ~7 mV; stimulus strength was adjusted so only 1 or 2 nerve fibers were stimulated and to prevent initiation of suprathreshold membrane potential change. This potential change did not lead to constriction. *B*: in contrast, a threshold concentration of norepinephrine ($1 \times 10^{-6}$ M) caused membrane potential to become "noisy" but produced a constriction. Both responses to norepinephrine unlike responses to sympathetic nerve stimulation, were abolished by phentolamine or prazosin.

guinea pig mesentery (15); a similar observation has been made on submucosal arterioles (G. D. S. Hirst, unpublished observations).

A high concentration of norepinephrine is required to activate $\alpha$-adrenoreceptors on submucosal arterioles. The concentration for a threshold response is always in excess of $1 \times 10^{-6}$ M (76). Above threshold the dose-response curve is steep; maximal rhythmical responses are produced by concentrations $\sim 3$ times higher than threshold concentrations. The threshold concentrations when compared with those required to first initiate contraction of veins, pulmonary arteries, and large distributing arteries differ by several orders of magnitude (31, 90). For example, responses are generated by pulmonary arteries exposed to norepinephrine concentrations of $1 \times 10^{-8}$ M. The threshold concentrations for contraction of mesenteric arteries of guinea pigs and rabbits are also $\sim 1 \times 10^{-6}$ M (78). Moreover fine arteries have a low $\alpha$-adrenoreceptor reserve in vivo, since injection of an irreversible antagonist has a far more dramatic effect on finer vessels than on larger vessels (77). These observations suggest that as the diameter of an artery decreases, as a result of branching in the periphery, the sensitivity of that artery for $\alpha$-adrenoreceptor activation falls. The physiological significance of these observations is not clear. It is generally held that major sites of peripheral resistance in the circulation lie in fine arteries and arterioles (external diam 20–200 $\mu$m) and that peripheral resistance is changed when both circulating factors and neuronal influences act on these fine vessels. If the in vitro sensitivities of arteries and arterioles are indeed representative of their sensitivities in vivo, it is difficult to see how the concentration of circulating catecholamines can rise to levels where arteriolar constriction will be triggered.

*Summary*

Submucosal arterioles may generate tension by two distinct cellular mechanisms. When an arteriole is depolarized its membrane becomes permeable to calcium ions and constriction occurs. In contrast, when exposed to norepinephrine a constriction results that does not seem to require a membrane potential change. There is no evidence, despite their ability to release norepinephrine that sympathetic nerves to submucosal arterioles when stimulated cause the activation of the $\alpha$-adrenoreceptors present on these vessels. The nervous responses of this tissue are resistant to $\alpha$-blockade (see PHARMACOLOGY OF EXCITATORY JUNCTION POTENTIALS, p. 1654). Constriction appears to result from membrane depolarization triggering voltage-dependent calcium entry. These observations are in direct contrast to responses recorded from veins and pulmonary arteries. In those vessels, the small-amplitude slow depolarizations recorded after sympathetic nerve stimulation are abolished by $\alpha$-adrenoreceptor blockade; concurrent with this, the mechanical responses are abolished. In cutaneous arteries with a thermoregulatory function, the responses to nerve stimulation are biphasic. The slower component of the responses in these tissues does result from receptor activation, but there is controversy as to whether the receptor type is $\alpha_1$ or $\alpha_2$ (32, 96). Evidently the importance of both $\alpha$-adrenoreceptors in neuronal control must vary from vascular bed to vascular bed.

INTEGRATION IN SUBMUCOSAL ARTERIOLES

Many neurons (e.g., motoneurons and sympathetic ganglion cells) generate an output after integrating the responses of several synaptic inputs that have been activated either synchronously or asynchronously (138, 142). Individual presynaptic terminals release one or a few quanta of transmitter; release often occurs with a high probability after the invasion of the terminal by an action potential (103, 120). The resulting synaptic current is usually brief, but the time course of the consequential synaptic potential is prolonged because of the displacement of charge on the postsynaptic membrane. If sufficient charge is displaced to cause an appropriate depolarization at some site on the postsynaptic neuron, for example, the axon hillock of motoneurons, then the cell generates an action potential. The action potential is conducted by the axon to the subsequent target tissue. In the examples cited, the motorneuron innervates a number of skeletal muscle fibers in a muscle block; the axon of the sympathetic ganglion cell innervates an involuntary organ such as an artery. At an individual skeletal neuromuscular junction, there is an extensive presynaptic terminal containing many release sites. As the release sites are sequentially invaded by the presynaptic action potential, a large proportion of each release site releases single quanta of transmitter. This ensures that the end-plate potential is suprathreshold for the initiation of a muscle action potential and hence muscle contraction.

In contrast to skeletal muscle fibers, when a single sympathetic nerve fiber innervating an arteriole or artery is activated, vasoconstriction does not occur. Rather a process of integration occurs in the end organ. Several nerve fibers must be activated within a short period of time or individual fibers must generate bursts of impulses. Moreover the output of a vascular bed, i.e., the resistance offered, is smoothly varied with the frequency of sympathetic nerve traffic. Over a limited range, as the frequency of stimulation rises, the peripheral resistance increases, with stimulation frequencies of $\sim 10$ Hz causing a cessation of flow. When recordings have been made from preganglionic neurons (123), from sympathetic ganglion cells (142), or from single isolated sympathetic nerves (100) in vivo, an ongoing discharge of action potentials has usually been detected. Many of these pathways are thought to be vasoconstrictor, because the appropriate manipulation of sensory inputs varies the rate of action-potential discharge and the vascular resistance in parallel. The range of frequencies encountered in such studies is from <1 Hz to, under conditions of extreme stimulation, 20 Hz. Clearly the arrival of impulses in a vascular bed will be asynchronous, and since in a given bed each sympathetic neuron only innervates a restricted territory, the final area activated will vary. This section discusses how the data from electrophysiological studies can be incorporated into a description of the neural control of arterioles in vivo. This somewhat speculative approach is being taken because there are few data available about the membrane potential events that occur in vivo during either ongoing or changed sympathetic nerve activity (148, 150). A description that is limited to membrane potential changes of arterioles does not preclude the existence of vasomotor control mechanisms that are voltage independent or nonneuronal control mechanisms, for example, hormonal influences or local metabolite production that may sometimes be dominant in the control of the circulation to viscera and other organs (see ref. 141).

Fine arterioles are functionally innervated by two of five individual axons (see Fig. 6). Each axon appears to lay down a terminal ground plexus that covers ~200- to 400-μm length of arteriole, with overlap between innervative fields. The terminal ground plexus of each individual fiber gives rise to several hundred varicosities, each of which is likely to release transmitter but does so only with a very low probability (1 in 50) per nerve impulse. These data suggest that a single axon when excited will release ~5-10 quanta of transmitter, and this release will occur over one-third to one-half of an electrical length constant. These conditions have been simulated by Neild (132). The computations showed that at low frequency (2 Hz) asynchronous firing of all the axons to a given region of tissue will produce a small and irregular but essentially maintained depolarization. As the mean frequency of sympathetic discharge increases, so the level of depolarization increases. With fine arterioles a frequency of 4 Hz produces a depolarization of 10 mV and 8 Hz a depolarization of 20 mV (Fig. 20). The simulations are characterized by their noisiness rather than by the presence of discrete EJPs (Fig. 20). Further increases give rise to larger and larger depolarizations. These conditions would be entirely appropriate to allow sustained and frequency-dependent calcium entry through the noninactivating voltage-dependent pathway for calcium. Thus the constriction of a given length of arteriole will vary as a function of the mean frequency of tonic discharge in the sympathetic nerves.

Each vascular bed is made up of fine arterioles that originate from progressively thicker-walled vessels. As either the diameter of the artery or the wall thickness increases, the surface area of the smooth muscle per unit length will increase. Under these conditions more and more transmitter must be released to discharge the membrane capacity. Thus a second integrative feature of a vascular bed will be the ability of the sympathetic nerves to "recruit" more of the arterial vasculature in that bed. This model for integration depends then on the presence of a potential-dependent mechanism to allow calcium entry and in turn provides an explanation for the effectiveness of calcium antagonists in reducing peripheral resistance. It also depends on arterioles having the long values of membrane time constant determined experimentally (80). Integration in submucosal arterioles could not occur with the frequencies of sympathetic nerve firing that have been found in vivo without these values of membrane time constant.

## PHARMACOLOGY OF EXCITATORY JUNCTION POTENTIALS

The traditional view of sympathetic nerve transmission in arteries and arterioles is that sympathetic nerves release norepinephrine; after release the norepinephrine diffuses to the arterial smooth muscles and activates α-adrenoreceptors. This is the case for veins and pulmonary arteries where the nerve responses have a characteristically slow time course

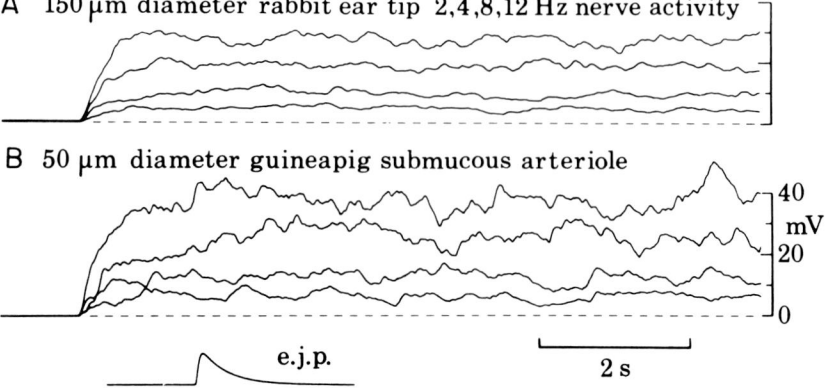

FIG. 20. Calculations of membrane potential changes that occur in blood vessels of different sizes during repetitive asynchronous sympathetic nerve activity. A: rabbit ear artery (diam 150 μm); B: arteriole of guinea pig submucosa (diam 50 μm). Sustained but irregular potential changes occur in both vessels and in finer vessel, at a given frequency of stimulation, membrane potential change is larger. [From Neild (132).]

(total duration >10 s, latency >500 ms). The nervous responses in these tissues and the slow component of the nervous response of thermoregulatory arteries are abolished by $\alpha$-adrenoreceptor antagonists (33, 89, 96, 101, 155, 156, 158). Similar observations have been made on rat anococcygeous muscle where the sympathetic nerve responses are also slow (116, 117). In contrast, EJPs of submucosal arterioles, even though abolished by guanethidine or sympathetic denervation, persist in the presence of very high concentrations of a great variety of $\alpha$-adrenoreceptor antagonists (75, 82, 133). Excitatory junction potentials are also unaffected by $\alpha$-adrenoreceptor blockade, nicotinic-receptor blockade, and muscarinic-receptor blockade (82, 133). Identical observations have also been made on a number of different arterial preparations with a variety of competitive and irreversible $\alpha$-adrenoreceptor antagonists (16, 32, 53, 54, 72, 84, 93, 95, 96, 101, 102, 110, 111, 143). During trains of stimuli many of these agents potentiate the amplitude of EJPs (93). These reports closely parallel the insensitivity of EJPs of vasa deferentia of a number of species to many $\alpha$-adrenoreceptor antagonists (9, 24). The EJPs are abolished by superfusing the preparations with norepinephrine. This effect is prevented by prior treatment of the tissue with $\alpha_2$-adrenoreceptor antagonists (93). This observation, along with the potentiation of EJPs by $\alpha_2$-antagonists, is most readily explained on the basis that the sympathetic nerves have autoinhibitory catecholamine receptors (115, 149).

It could be argued that the failure of $\alpha$-adrenoreceptor antagonists to block transmission arises because although an $\alpha$-adrenoreceptor is activated, neuronally released norepinephrine is present in high local concentrations (7). The sympathetic nerves innervating submucosal arterioles form many close appositions with the smooth muscle layer (see Figs. 3–5) with vesicles concentrated toward the regions of contact. A calculation of the concentration profile of norepinephrine around the release site of a vesicle containing norepinephrine has been made with the assumption that diffusion can occur in three dimensions (10). Even under these conditions the initial starting concentrations near the point of release are very high, on the order of 10 mM. With the neuronal structures described for the innervation of submucosal arterioles, such concentrations can reasonably be expected to persist for a few milliseconds and then drop either because of diffusion along the junctional cleft or as a result of neuronal uptake (97). Similar high local concentrations of acetylcholine are predicted to occur at the skeletal neuromuscular junction, which shares many of the structural features of sympathetic nerves on arterioles (107, 119).

However, none of these arguments would preclude $\alpha$-adrenoreceptor antagonists from abolishing EJPs unless they could not gain access to the neuroeffector junction. Most potent antagonists dissociate from receptors with a dissociation constant of several minutes. If one takes the duration of EJCs in submucosal arterioles as a measure of the persistence of transmitter in the subsynaptic region (i.e., 200 ms), it is apparent that the chance of total receptor antagonist dissociation occurring in this time is negligible. Thus a competitive antagonist must appear as an irreversible entity in the nonequilibrium conditions occurring during the neuronal release of transmitter. Moreover even more complex arguments would have to be marshalled to explain the failure of irreversible antagonists to prevent EJPs if the receptor activated were of the $\alpha$-type.

Thus it is unequivocable that the receptor activated by transmitter released from sympathetic nerves to produce EJPs is not a conventional adrenoreceptor. Two hypotheses have been put forward to explain these findings. The first is that the transmitter released by the sympathetic nerves, norepinephrine, activates specialized junctional receptors called $\gamma$-receptors. The second is that the EJP results from the release of a different substance, a purine derivative such as ATP.

The view is often taken that because it is clear that stimulated sympathetic nerves release norepinephrine and that norepinephrine applied to arterioles produces vasoconstriction by activating $\alpha$-receptors, an $\alpha$-resistant component will be of no significance. Support for this view has been found in the observation that $\alpha$-receptor antagonists interfere with neuronally induced constrictions of rat tail artery. It has been pointed out that some arteries generate tension by two distinct mechanisms after sympathetic nerve activation: a potential-dependent mechanism and a receptor-activated mechanism (16). The balance between the two mechanisms in the rat tail artery can be altered by varying the stimulus parameters (33). Thus a dominant role for $\alpha$-receptors in these tissues is likely. When hindlimb resistance changes after sympathetic nerve stimulation in the dog were determined, it was found that these responses were abolished by phentolamine (6). This was again taken to mean that neuronal responses in vivo were mediated entirely via receptor activation. There are, however, doubts that the action of phentolamine is limited to $\alpha_1$- and $\alpha_2$-blockade. In both dogs (163) and rabbit (77) this compound causes a marked vasoconstriction, an effect presumably masked by compensatory reflex changes in nonganglion-blocked animals (6).

Conversely there are a number of reports that suggest that in some vascular beds neuronally induced vasoconstriction, at least in part, does not involve $\alpha$-adenoreceptor activation. In many isolated arterial preparations, nervous responses are largely unaffected by $\alpha$-blockade (108, 129, 130; G. D. S. Hirst and M. J. Lew, unpublished observations). In dogs, reflex changes in blood pressure after baroreceptor occlusion are attenuated but not abolished by chronic administration of the irreversible $\alpha$-adrenoreceptor antagonist phenoxybenzamine (63). In rats, direct sympathetic stimulation of the sympathetic outflow produces responses that are only in part reduced by $\alpha$-blockade (49). In this study the $\alpha_1$-antagonist prazosin was used. This compound has direct effects on the voltage sensitivity of calcium entry, raising the threshold for the initiation of regeneration arteriolar responses (76). With the irreversible $\alpha$-adrenoreceptor antagonist benextramine (126), no component attributable to $\alpha$-receptor activation could be found in the responses of rabbit hindlimb vasculature to postganglionic sympathetic nerve stimulation (77). Similarly $\alpha$-resistant reflex increases in blood pressure could be detected in conscious rabbits (77).

These data suggest that $\alpha$-antagonist–resistant neuronal responses do occur in vivo, and they are important in some vascular beds.

*Identity of Transmitter Responsible for Initiation of Excitatory Junction Potentials*

A compound can be accepted as a transmitter if it fulfills two criteria. A specific amount of the substance must be shown to be released from a nerve terminal by an action potential. Replacing the same amount of transmitter in the same area or areas of the postsynaptic membrane, as is present during activation by neuronally released transmitter, must produce a response identical to that produced by the presynaptic stimulus. In practice, experimental limitations have prevented rigorous testing of these criteria at most synapses. The amounts of transmitter released are small, and the substance is rapidly inactivated; hence the substance is frequently difficult to detect, let alone quantitate, its concentration. The presynaptic terminal accomplishes release with extreme brevity, applying locally high concentrations to small and often spatially separated areas. Only at a few synapses has it been possible to introduce transmitters with the same degree of localization and with the same rapidity.

Thus a number of less rigorous criteria have been defined. *1*) A storage mechanism, usually in the form of vesicles, must be present; *2*) the synthetic apparatus for transmitter synthesis must be present; *3*) release from a preformed store must occur and if the storage is impaired then transmission would be expected to be impaired; *4*) a local inactivation mechanism for the transmitter should exist; and *5*) application of the transmitter should produce responses qualitatively the same as the responses to nerve stimulation. Conviction on this point is usually sought from the availability of an appropriate specific antagonist.

This section deals with the nature of the transmitter released by sympathetic nerves. The data considered relate to the two alternate hypotheses, norepinephrine as the sole transmitter and cotransmission. It is hoped that the reader will ignore the author's bias and realize that the argument is unresolved.

NOREPINEPHRINE. All systemic arteries and arterioles are wrapped with sympathetic nerve fibers that contain norepinephrine stored in vesicles. The localization and nature of the synthetic apparatus for norepinephrine production has been described and reviewed (62). Although norepinephrine release has not been measured directly from submucosal arterioles, it has been measured from mesenteric arteries that give rise to the mucosal vasculature (108) and from many other arterial preparations. Depletion of norepinephrine stores by reserpine causes a reduction, but not an abolition, in the amplitude of vasoconstrictor responses produced by sympathetic nerve stimulation (62). There are arguments as to whether the responses and the stores should be reduced in parallel and whether this would be expected (20). Thus norepinephrine in part fulfills the first three criteria as a transmitter substance.

Similarly there is abundant evidence that sympathetic nerves may inactivate norepinephrine by neuronal uptake (97). However, although uptake is prevented by cocaine and desmethylimipramine, the time course of submucosal EJPs is unaffected by either of these substances (unpublished observations). Similarly the time course of EJPs recorded from mesenteric arteries and vasa deferentia is little affected by cocaine (9, 111). This suggests that removal of transmitter is not the rate-limiting factor in termination of the junctional conductance change, as one would expect diffusion to clear a synaptic cleft in a shorter time than the duration of an EJC (47). Alternatively, the transmitter is not norepinephrine.

There are many reports that show that applied norepinephrine does not at a cellular level mimic the responses to sympathetic nerve stimulation (16). Norepinephrine, applied by superfusion, activates receptors; EJPs do not involve the activation of $\alpha$-adrenoreceptors. For the transmitter to be norepinephrine an alternative receptor must exist. Evidence for the existence of an alternative receptor comes from a number of studies. The first evidence came from studies on distributing arteries. Furchgott (55) and subsequently Bevan et al. (10) pointed out that some arteries had populations of excitatory receptors that were resistant to $\alpha$-adenoreceptor blockade. These receptors were characterized as having a low affinity for norepinephrine and lacking the selectivity normally associated with catecholamine receptors. Electrophysiological studies have confirmed that norepinephrine can depolarize a number of arteries by activating a receptor that is not blocked by either $\alpha$- or $\beta$-adrenoreceptor antagonists (25, 82–84, 119). Clearly the presence of such a receptor does not necessarily imply a role in junctional transmission, but its absence would negate a role for norepinephrine in junctional transmission.

Norepinephrine receptors ($\gamma$-receptors), which are resistant to adrenoreceptor blockade, have been demonstrated on submucosal arterioles (Fig. 21). These receptors, when activated by ionophoretically applied norepinephrine, caused a short-latency (<10 ms), rapid membrane depolarization similar to that produced by nerve stimulation (83). Such responses were only detected from areas that were subsequently shown by histochemical techniques to be close to sympathetic nerves [Fig. 22; (83)]. Thus submucosal arterioles on a microscale possess a population of norepinephrine receptors that are restricted to regions appropriate for neuroeffector transmission and that produce a response when exposed to norepinephrine

similar to that from nerve stimulation. In contrast, many other regions of the arteriole could be shown to possess $\alpha$-receptors which when activated cause a localized constriction without a detectable membrane potential change. This nonelectrical response was readily abolished by $\alpha$-adrenoreceptor antagonists. These areas would be targets for superfused norepinephrine.

The $\gamma$-receptors on submucosal arterioles can be activated by superfusing high concentrations (1–10 mM) of norepinephrine. These responses are initially masked by the membrane potential changes that result from high concentrations of norepinephrine activating extrajunctional receptors but are detected after $\alpha$-blockade (Fig. 23). Very similar observations were subsequently made on rat basilar arteries, a tissue that at maturity lacks $\alpha$-adrenoreceptors (25, 84).

Perhaps more convincing evidence in favor of a role of norepinephrine activating $\gamma$-receptors to produce EJPs comes from studies where the larger scale distribution of $\gamma$-receptors has been examined. These receptors are absent on pulmonary arteries and veins but present on cerebral arteries and systemic arteries (J. A. Bevan, personal communication). The former tissues do not generate rapid EJPs in response to nerve stimulation but generate only slow $\alpha$-sensitive depolarizations; in the latter two studies, EJPs with the same characteristics as those in submucosal arterioles are detected.

Thus it would seem there are few grounds to doubt

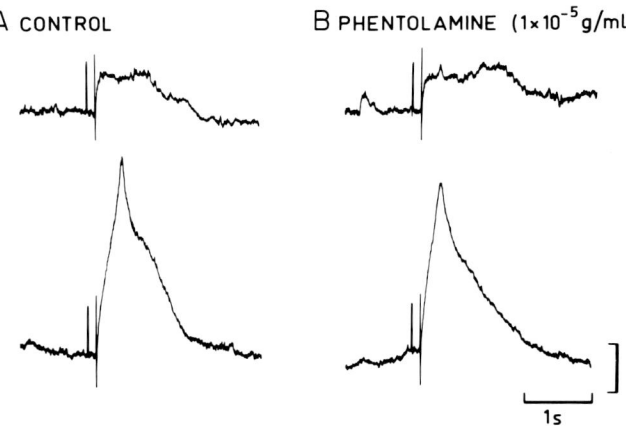

FIG. 21. Membrane potential changes produced by ionophoretic application of norepinephrine. A: records were produced by 2 pulses of norepinephrine (duration 10 ms, 40 and 50 nA, respectively); B: records produced by similar pulses after adding phentolamine (3 × $10^{-5}$ M) to physiological saline. Both responses persist and a spontaneous excitatory junction potential is also seen.

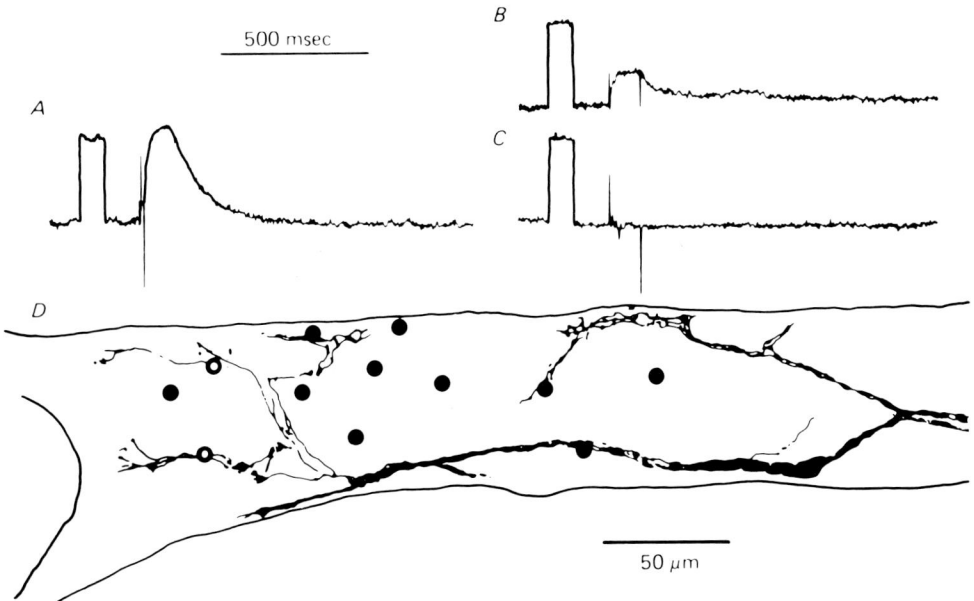

FIG. 22. Junctional localization of positions where norepinephrine produces receptor activation. Trace A shows membrane potential response produced by ionophoretic application of norepinephrine. Traces B and C show lack of membrane potential changes when electrode position was varied. D: map of distribution of sympathetic nerve fibers. Open circles, positions at which depolarizing responses were detected; closed circles, points where membrane potential changes were not detected. All "hot spots" were subsequently found to be within 10 μm of a fluorescent nerve. [From Hirst and Neild (83).]

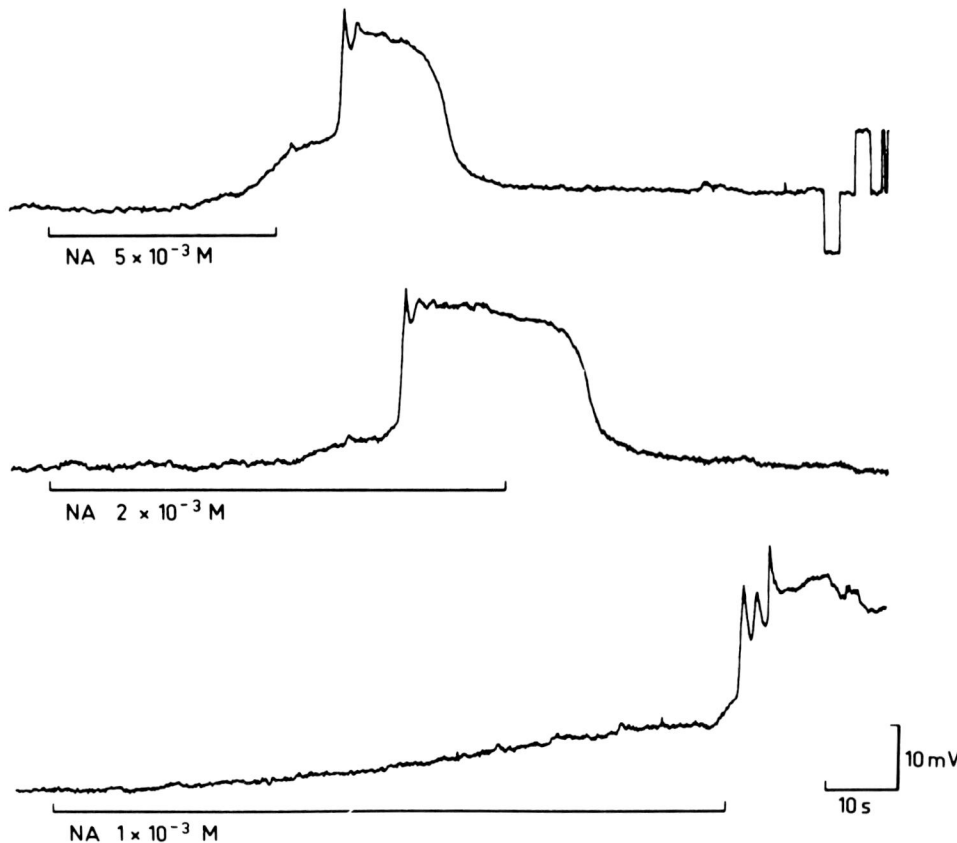

FIG. 23. Activation of γ-receptors by bath-applied norepinephrine [noradrenaline (NA)]. Records were made from a submucosal arteriole in presence of prazosin ($1 \times 10^{-6}$ M). Norepinephrine was applied by superfusion. Note high concentration of norepinephrine required to activate receptors; similar responses were detected in lower concentrations of prazosin, suggesting that responses do not result from activation of receptors.

the role of norepinephrine as a sympathetic transmitter: sympathetic nerves synthesize, store, and release norepinephrine, and norepinephrine applied to the regions near sympathetic nerves produces a response similar to those produced by stimulating those nerves. A major criticism of the hypothesis is that a specific antagonist to γ-receptors and EJPs does not exist. Although both are blocked by desensitization by α, β-methylene-ATP, this substance also blocks the responses of vascular tissues to ATP (26).

COTRANSMISSION. The concept that sympathetic nerve transmission in arteries utilize two different transmitter substances is an extension of the idea that cotransmission occurs in other sympathetically innervated tissues (131). In the vas deferens, sympathetic nerve stimulation produces a contraction with two components. There is a rapid transient phase of contraction that is followed by a slower more sustained phase (3, 121, 159). Whereas both phases are abolished by guanethidine, only the second slower phase is abolished by α-adrenoreceptor blockade; the initial phase persisted or was even potentiated (121). Conversely, the initial rapid phase is reduced or abolished by both nifedipine, a voltage-dependent calcium antagonist, and by a photoactivated ATP antagonist [arylazido aminoproprionyl adenosine triphosphate (ANAPP$_3$)] (144). When tissues are taken from animals that have been pretreated with reserpine to reduce the neuronal norepinephrine content to very low levels (4), the contractile responses to a given set of stimulation parameters are greatly reduced (4). However, after an appropriate increase in stimulus strength, contractile responses can be initiated (4, 121). Under these conditions only the initial resistant component is detected (121). These observations have been taken to mean that during transmission a sympathetic nerve releases vesicles containing both ATP and norepinephrine. Thus ATP produces membrane depolarization, thereby triggering voltage-dependent calcium entry to cause the rapid initial contraction: norepinephrine activates α-adrenoreceptors and leads to the more sustained secondary contraction.

Electrophysiological data consistent with this hypothesis have been reported. Sympathetic nerve stimulation initiates an EJP that, if of sufficient amplitude, triggers an action potential and a rapid contraction; the action potential is selectively abolished by the calcium antagonist nifedipine (12). The second slower phase of contraction is not associated with a detectable membrane potential change and presumably results from a voltage-independent receptor mechanism. Adenosine triphosphate causes depolarization, whereas norepinephrine causes little or no membrane potential change. Both the depolarization produced by ATP and the EJP are abolished by ANAPP$_3$, whereas the contractile effects of norepinephrine are unimpaired (145).

Very similar observations have been made on the rat tail artery. Sympathetic nerve stimulation produces a two-component contraction (32). Membrane potential records show that these arteries generate an EJP that is very similar to that detected in submucosal arterioles. If the EJP is of sufficient amplitude it initiates a regenerative membrane potential change and rapid constriction. This is followed by a second slower phase of contraction that precedes a small, slow depolarization (33). Whereas the slow components of the sympathetic nerve response are abolished by $\alpha$-adrenoceptor blockade, the EJP-associated regenerative membrane changes and rapid constriction persist. The application of ATP by ionophoresis produces a membrane depolarization that is a little slower than the EJP (157); this is perhaps surprising if ATP were the transmitter, because when applied at a point the transmitter would be expected to produce a response faster than the EJP and have a time course similar to an SEJP. Both the EJP and the depolarization produced by ATP are not detected in tissues that have been desensitized by the stable ATP analogue $\alpha,\beta$-methylene-ATP (143; see also refs. 108, 129, 130). Moreover purines are released by sympathetic nerves to the vasculature (152). All of these observations are explicable by the hypothesis that sympathetic nerves release vesicles containing ATP and norepinephrine.

By analogy the EJPs recorded from other arteries should result from ATP release. This suggestion implies that in the few arteries that are devoid of receptors (84), norepinephrine released by sympathetic nerves serves no vasomotor role. Moreover cotransmission does not appear to occur in a number of systemic arteries that do possess adrenoreceptors. In submucosal arterioles, constriction only occurs if a regenerative membrane potential change is detected (74). It has been pointed out that in a number of vascular beds, nervously induced vasoconstriction is not impaired by $\alpha$-adenoreceptor blockade. Evidently if norepinephrine does not initiate the EJP then it must have no role in the control of arteriolar tone. Clearly, however, these arguments do not preclude ATP being the primary transmitter; there are numerous other biologically active substances present in nerves that have no known function (58). It is unusual, however, for them to be released with such ease as is norepinephrine.

Perhaps the greatest difficulty faced by the purinergic hypothesis relates to the storage and release of this substance. All excitable cells are readily able to synthesize and accumulate ATP. Whereas in catecholamine-containing cells of the adrenal medulla, ATP and norepinephrine are costored in vesicles with a ratio of 1:4, this does not seem to be the case in vesicles of peripheral sympathetic nerves. After purification, ratios of much less than 1:30 (ATP: norepinephrine) are found (52, 113, 151). It has been argued that even this residual amount of ATP reflects mitochondrial contamination (34). Release of ATP from sympathetic nerves after electrical stimulation has not been detected. Transmurally stimulated vas deferens does release detectable quantities of ATP, but unlike the EJP and the mechanical responses associated with the stimuli, the release is not suppressed by TTX (165). A further differentiation is that the release of norepinephrine from synaptasomes but not that of ATP is suppressed by $\alpha_2$-adrenoreceptor activation (T.D. White, personal communication). Furthermore, although the release of label has been detected after the incubation of innervated vasa deferentia in radioactively labeled adenosine, this release persists in hypertonic solution (164). Because EJPs are prevented by hypertonic solutions and SEJPs persist, the labeled material cannot be involved in the generation of EJPs.

During the development of the sympathetic innervation to rat mesentery and vas deferens, the earliest responses attributable to nerve activation result from $\alpha$-receptor activation. After maturation of the sympathetic innervation, the $\alpha$-resistant responses are initiated (59, 72). This would suggest that the transmitter being released changes, because immature arteries possess ATP receptors (26). Where such a change in transmitter identity has been shown to occur during development, the sympathetic nerves lose their ability to store and release norepinephrine (114). This is not the case for sympathetic nerves innervating arteries. Moreover, adrenal medullary vesicles, which may not be a good model for peripheral sympathetic vesicles, contain high proportions of ATP and low proportions of norepinephrine at birth (135). This developmental change is in the opposite direction to that expected if ATP was the mature transmitter substance. Similarly it has been pointed out that in some vascular tissues sympathetic nerve transmission fails to initiate EJPs; rather only a slow response is initiated. Certainly in one of these tissues, the pulmonary artery, ATP is excitatory. This would impose certain constraints on the sympathetic nerves in these tissues. Either they must selectively fail to release ATP or the local concentration of ATP in the neuroeffector region must be low. Alternatively, ATP receptors must be selectively excluded from neuroeffector regions.

The most compelling data in support of a role for ATP come from experiments involving purine antagonists. Their selectivity has only been checked against agonists used in concentrations that do not cause rapid conductance changes (143–145). Thus α,β-methylene-ATP does not prevent the depolarization that may accompany α-adrenoceptor activation (95). However, in a recent study where the effects of α,β-methylene-ATP on depolarizations produced by receptor activation and ATP were compared, both responses were abolished (26). This indicates that α,β-methylene-ATP cannot be used as a selective antagonist. Nevertheless, at this stage, the best hope of distinguishing the two hypotheses seems to lie in the discovery of specific antagonists to γ-receptors and ATP.

SUMMARY AND FUTURE DIRECTIONS

This chapter indicates that the information about the membrane events that are associated with the sympathetic control of intramural intestinal blood vessels is limited. The data available describe a process of transmission that is different to that generally held to occur in other smooth muscles. The essential features of the neural control system are illustrated in Figure 24. Sympathetic postganglionic axons give rise to fine-branched terminal axons, a few of which innervate restricted areas of a given vascular bed. Individual terminal axons give rise to many specialized presynaptic structures, i.e., varicosities (see Fig. 2). The individual varicosities form well-organized contacts with the arterial smooth muscle layer; each contact has an area of apposition between the presynaptic terminal and the smooth muscle membrane (Fig. 24, shaded area). These varicosities contain transmitter that is stored predominantly in small granular vesicles (Fig. 24, open circles); the vesicles are concentrated toward the area of apposition (see Figs. 3–5). When the sympathetic nerves are stimulated, transmitter is released from this preformed store as quanta (see Figs. 15, 16). However, release only occurs at a few discrete points over the surface of the arteriole. At the points of release, brief discrete EJCs are initiated (see Figs. 12, 13). The junctional current results from an increase in both sodium and potassium conductance; thus at resting potential the predominant ion movement is that of inward sodium (Fig. 24). The depolarization resulting from this current is not restricted to the activated smooth muscle cell but is detected along the arteriole because of efficient intercellular electrical couplings (see Figs. 8, 11; illustrated as a gap junction in Fig. 24). Although submucosal arterioles have α-adrenoreceptors distributed over their surface (Fig. 24), these do not appear to be activated by neuronally released norepinephrine. When activated by superfused norepinephrine, α-adrenoreceptors lead to an increase in internal calcium concentration that initially is not dependent on free external calcium ions. Constriction after sympathetic nerve stimulation results from the involvement of a different membrane mechanism, i.e., the activation of voltage-dependent calcium conductances (see Figs. 9, 17, 18). Excitatory junction potentials are long lasting because of the long membrane time constant of arterioles (see Fig. 11). If

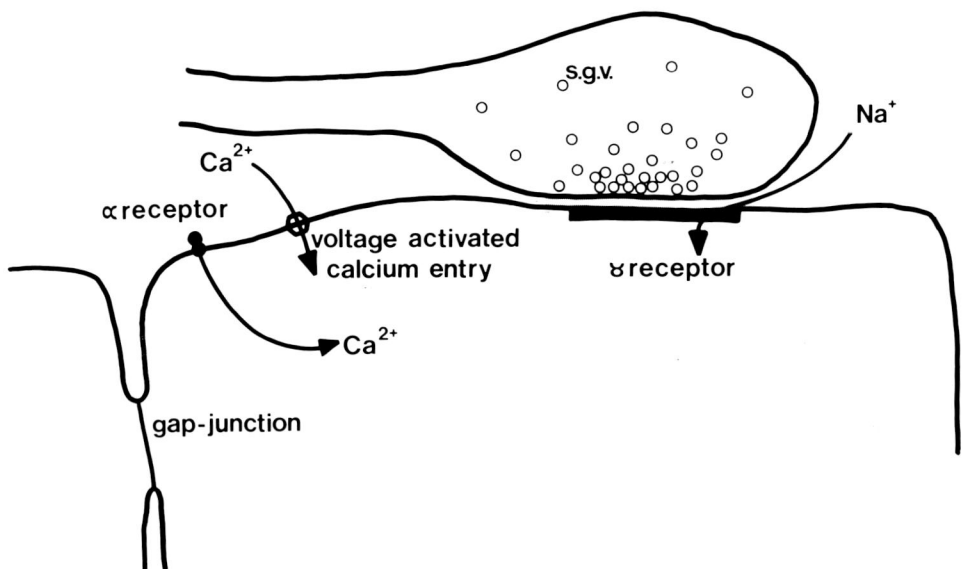

FIG. 24. Diagram of neural control system in submucosal arteriole. Figure shows sympathetic varicosity containing small granular vesicles (open circles; s.g.v.); vesicles are concentrated toward region of apposition (shaded area) between varicosity and underlying smooth muscle cell. Individual smooth muscle cells are electrically coupled to neighboring cells by low-resistance electrical contacts (gap junction); resulting syncytium forms neuroeffector target. In junctional cleft, specialized receptors to norepinephrine are located (γ-receptors), which when activated allow an influx of sodium ions and an efflux of potassium ions. Resulting depolarization causes opening of voltage-dependent calcium channels (hexagon), leading to calcium entry from extracellular fluid. In contrast, α-receptors, which have an extrajunctional location, when activated by norepinephrine, lead to increase in internal calcium concentration by discharging a bound store.

there is ongoing sympathetic nerve activity the membrane depolarizations will be persistent. Such potential changes then allow sustained calcium entry (see Fig. 18).

This description of neuromuscular transmission avoids many of the controversies relating to arterial smooth muscle. Perhaps there are more controversies than accepted ideas about the mechanisms involved in neuronal control of blood vessels. These will only be resolved by further studies. Obvious examples of areas of argument raised by this article are Is norepinephrine the transmitter released by sympathetic nerves causing the EJP? Are there specialized receptors to norepinephrine in regions near the sympathetic nerve terminals? Do the $\alpha$-receptors on fine arteriolar vessels have no physiological role? Is the transmitter released by sympathetic nerves a purine, and does a change occur during development? Do nonadrenoceptors mechanisms matter? Do electrogenic currents contribute directly to resting membrane potentials? Are all individual arterial smooth muscle cells coupled together into syncytia? Research in this area over the new few years will provide answers to many of these questions and may challenge many of the existing concepts of neural regulation in the autonomic nervous system.

REFERENCES

1. ABE, Y., AND T. TOMITA. Cable properties of smooth muscle. *J. Physiol. Lond.* 214: 173–190, 1968.
2. AICKIN, C. C., A. F. BRADING, AND T. V. BURGYGA. Evidence for sodium-calcium exchange on the guinea-pig ureter. *J. Physiol. Lond.* 347: 411–430, 1984.
3. AMBACHE, N., AND M. A. ZAR. Evidence against adrenergic motor transmission in the guinea-pig vas deferens. *J. Physiol. Lond.* 216: 359–389, 1971.
4. ANGUS, J. A., AND R. M. BRAZENOR. Relaxation of large coronary artery by verapamil, D600 and nifedipine is constrictor sensitive: comparison with glycerol trinitrate. *J. Cardiovasc. Pharmacol.* 5: 321–328, 1983.
5. BELL, C. Transmission from vasoconstrictor and vasodilator nerves to single muscle cells of the guinea-pig uterine artery. *J. Physiol. Lond.* 205: 695–708, 1969.
6. BELL, C. Comparison of the antagonist effects of phentolamine on vasoconstrictor responses to exogenous and neurally released noradrenaline in vivo. *Br. J. Pharmacol.* 85: 249–253, 1985.
7. BELL, C., AND M. VOGT. Release of endogenous noradrenaline from an isolated muscular artery. *J. Physiol. Lond.* 215: 509–520, 1971.
8. BENNETT, M. R. *Autonomic Neuromuscular Transmission.* Cambridge, UK: Cambridge Univ. Press, 1972.
9. BENNETT, M. R., AND J. MIDDLETON. An electrophysiological analysis of the effects of amine-uptake blockers and $\alpha$-adrenoceptor blockers on adrenergic neuromuscular transmission. *Br. J. Pharmacol.* 55: 87–95, 1975.
10. BEVAN, J. A., R. D. BEVAN, AND S. P. DUCKLES. Adrenergic regulation of vascular smooth muscle. In: *Handbook of Physiology. The Cardiovascular System. Vascular Smooth Muscle*, edited by D. F. Bohr, A. P. Somlyo, and H. V. Sparks, Jr. Bethesda, MD: Am. Physiol. Soc., 1980, sect. 2, vol. II, chapt. 18, p. 515–566.
11. BIBER, B., J. FARA, AND O. LUNDGREN. Intestinal vasodilation response to transmural electrical stimulation. *Acta. Physiol. Scand. Suppl.* 87: 277–282, 1973.
12. BLAKELEY, A. G. H., D. A. BROWN, T. C. CUNNANE, A. M. FRENCH, J. C. MCGRATH, AND N. C. SCOTT. Effects of nifedipine on electrical and mechanical responses of rat and guinea-pig vas deferens. *Nature Lond.* 294: 759–761, 1981.
13. BLAKELEY, A. G. H., AND T. C. CUNNANE. The packeted release of transmitter from the sympathetic nerves of the guinea-pig vas deferens: an electrophysiological study. *J. Physiol. Lond.* 296: 85–96, 1979.
14. BOLTON, T. B. Mechanisms of action of transmitters and other substances on smooth muscle. *Physiol. Rev.* 59: 606–718, 1979.
15. BOLTON, T. B., R. J. LANG, AND T. TAKEWAKI. Mechanisms of action of noradrenaline and carbachol on myometrial smooth muscle of guinea-pig anterior mesenteric artery. *J. Physiol. Lond.* 351: 549–572, 1981.
16. BOLTON, T. B., AND W. A. LARGE. Are junction potentials essential? Dual mechanism of smooth muscle cell activation by transmitter released from autonomic nerves. *Q. J. Exp. Physiol. Cogn. Med. Sci.* 71: 1–28, 1986.
17. BRADING, A. F. Ionic distribution and mechanisms of transmembrane ion movements in smooth muscle. In: *Smooth Muscle: An Assessment of Current Knowledge*, edited by E. Bülbring, A. F. Brading, A. W. Jones, and T. Tomita. London: Arnold, 1981, p. 65–92.
18. BÜLBRING, E., H. OHASHI, AND T. TOMITA. Adrenergic mechanisms. In: *Smooth Muscle: An Assessment of Current Knowledge*, edited by E. Bülbring, A. F. Brading, A. W. Jones, and T. Tomita. London: Arnold, 1981, p. 219–248.
19. BÜLBRING, E., AND J. H. SZURSZEWSKI. The stimulant action of noradrenaline ($\alpha$-action) on guinea-pig myometrium compared with that of acetylcholine. *Proc. R. Soc. Lond. B Biol. Sci.* 185: 225–262, 1974.
20. BURNSTOCK, G., AND M. COSTA. *Adrenergic Neurones.* London: Chapman & Hall, 1975.
21. BURNSTOCK, G., AND M. E. HOLMAN. The transmission of excitation from autonomic nerve to smooth muscle. *J. Physiol. Lond.* 155: 115–133, 1961.
22. BURNSTOCK, G., AND M. E. HOLMAN. Spontaneous potentials at sympathetic nerve endings in smooth muscle. *J. Physiol. Lond.* 160: 446–460, 1962.
23. BURNSTOCK, G., AND M. E. HOLMAN. Effect of denervation and of reserpine treatment on transmission at sympathetic nerve endings. *J. Physiol. Lond.* 160: 461–469, 1962.
24. BURNSTOCK, G., AND M. E. HOLMAN. An electrophysiological investigation of the actions of some autonomic blocking drugs on transmission in the guinea-pig vas deferens. *Br. J. Pharmacol.* 23: 600–612, 1964.
25. BYRNE, N. G., G. D. S. HIRST, AND W. A. LARGE. Electrophysiological analysis of adrenoceptors in the rat basilar artery during development. *Br. J. Pharmacol.* 86: 217–227, 1985.
26. BYRNE, N. G., AND W. A. LARGE. The effect of $\alpha,\beta$-methylene ATP on the depolarizations evoked by noradrenaline ($\gamma$-response) and ATP in the immature rat basilar artery. *Br. J. Pharmacol.* 88: 6–8, 1986.
27. BYWATER, R. A. R., AND G. S. TAYLOR. The passive membrane properties and excitatory junction potentials of the guinea-pig vas deferens. *J. Physiol. Lond.* 300: 303–316, 1980.
28. CASLEY-SMITH, J. R., AND B. J. GANNON. Intestinal microcirculation: spatial organization and fine structure. In: *Physiology of the Intestinal Circulation*, edited by A. P. Shepherd and D. N. Granger. New York: Raven, 1984, p. 9–32.
29. CASTEELS, R. Membrane potential in smooth muscle cells. In: *Smooth Muscle: An Assessment of Current Knowledge*, edited by E. Bülbring, A. F. Brading, A. W. Jones, and T. Tomita. London: Arnold, 1981, p. 105–126.
30. CASTEELS, R., K. KITAMURA, H. KURYAMA, AND H. SUZUKI. The membrane properties of the smooth muscle cells of the

rabbit main pulmonary artery. *J. Physiol. Lond.* 271: 41–61, 1979.
31. CASTEELS, R., K. KITAMURA, H. KURYAMA, AND H. SUZUKI. Excitation-contraction coupling in the smooth muscle cells of the rabbit main pulmonary artery. *J. Physiol. Lond.* 271: 62–79, 1979.
32. CHEUNG, D. W. Two components in the cellular response of the rat tail artery to nerve stimulation. *J. Physiol. Lond.* 328: 461–468, 1982.
33. CHEUNG, D. W. Neural regulation of electrical and mechanical activities in the rat tail artery. *Pfluegers Arch.* 400: 335–357, 1984.
34. CHUBB, I. W. In: *Synapses*, edited by G. A. Cotterell and P. N. R. Usherwood. London: Blackie, 1977, p. 269–290.
35. COLE, K. S. *Membranes, Ions and Impulses: A Chapter of Classical Biophysics*. Berkeley: Univ. of California Press, 1968.
36. CUNNANE, T. C., AND L. STJARNE. Secretion of transmitter from individual varicosities of guinea-pig and mouse vas deferens: all-or-none and extremely intermittent. *Neuroscience* 7: 2565–2576, 1982.
37. CURTIS, D. R., AND J. C. ECCLES. The time course of excitatory and inhibitory synaptic actions. *J. Physiol. Lond.* 145: 529–546, 1959.
38. DE FEO, T. T., AND K. G. MORGAN. Calcium force relationships as detected with aequorin in two different vascular smooth muscles of the ferret. *J. Physiol. Lond.* 369: 269–282, 1985.
39. DEVINE, C. E., AND F. O. SIMPSON. The fine structure of vascular sympathetic neuromuscular contacts in the rat. *Am. J. Anat.* 121: 153–174, 1967.
40. DEVINE, C. E., A. V. SOMLYO, AND A. P. SOMLYO. Sarcoplasmic reticulum and excitation-contraction coupling in mammalian smooth muscles. *J. Cell Biol.* 52: 690–718, 1972.
41. DONALD, D. E. Splanchnic circulation. In: *Handbook of Physiology. The Cardiovascular System. Peripheral Circulation*, edited by J. T. Shepherd and F. M. Abboud. Bethesda, MD: Am. Physiol. Soc., 1983, sect. 2, vol. III, chapt. 7, p. 219–240.
42. DROOGMANS, G., L. RAEYMAEKERS, AND R. CASTEELS. Electro- and pharmacochemical coupling in the smooth muscle cells of the rabbit ear artery. *J. Gen. Physiol.* 70: 129–148, 1977.
43. ENDO, M., T. KITAZAWA, S. YAGI, M. IINO, AND Y. KIKUTA. Some properties of chemically skinned smooth muscle fibres. In: *Excitation-Contraction Coupling in Smooth Muscle*, edited by R. Casteels, T. Godfraind, and J. C. Ruegg. Amsterdam: Elsevier/North-Holland, 1984, p. 199–209.
44. FALCK, B., N.-A. HILLARP, G. THIEME, AND TORP. Fluorescence of catecholamines and related compounds condensed with formaldehyde. *J. Histochem. Cytochem.* 10: 348–354, 1962.
45. FARA, J. W. Post prandial mesenteric hyperemia. In: *Physiology of the Intestinal Circulation*, edited by A. P. Shepherd and D. N. Granger. New York: Raven, 1984, p. 99–106.
46. FEDAN, J. S., G. K. HOGABOOM, J. P. O'DONNELL, J. COLBY, AND D. P. WESTFALL. Contribution by purines to the neurogenic response of the vas deferens of the guinea-pig. *Eur. J. Pharmacol.* 69: 41–53, 1981.
47. FINKEL, A. S., G. D. S. HIRST, AND D. F. VAN HELDEN. Some properties of excitatory junction currents recorded from submucosal arterioles of guinea-pig ileum. *J. Physiol. Lond.* 351: 87–98, 1984.
48. FINKEL, A. S., AND S. J. REDMAN. The synaptic current evoked by impulses in single group 1a axons. *J. Physiol. Lond.* 342: 615–632, 1983.
49. FLAVAHAN, N. A., T. L. GRANT, J. GREIG, AND J. C. MCGRATH. Analysis of alpha-receptor mediated, and other, components in the sympathetic vasopressor responses of the pithed rat. *Br. J. Pharmacol.* 86: 265–274, 1985.
50. FOLKOW, B., AND E. NEIL. *Circulation*. Oxford, UK: Oxford Univ. Press, 1971.
51. FONDACARO, J. D. Intestinal blood flow and motility. In: *Physiology of the Intestinal Circulation*, edited by A. P. Shepherd, and D. N. Granger. New York: Raven, 1984, p. 107–120.
52. FRIED, G., H. LAGERCRANTZ, R. KLEIN, AND A. THURESON-KLEIN. Large and small noradrenergic vesicles—origin, contents and functional significance. In: *Catecholamines: Basic and Peripheral Mechanisms*, edited by E. Usdin, A. Carlson, A. Dahlstrom, and J. Engel. New York: Liss, 1984, p. 45–53.
53. FUJIWARA, S., T. ITOH, AND H. SUZUKI. Membrane properties and excitatory neuromuscular transmission in the smooth muscle of dog cerebral arteries. *Br. J. Pharmacol.* 77: 447–455, 1982.
54. FUJIWARA, S., AND H. KURIYAMA. Nicardipine actions on smooth muscle cells and excitatory neuromuscular transmission in the guinea-pig basilar artery. *J. Pharmacol. Exp. Ther.* 225: 447–455, 1983.
55. FURCHGOTT, R. F. The classification of adrenoceptors (adrenergic receptors). An evaluation from the stand point of receptor theory. In: *Handbuch der Experimentellen Pharmakologie. Catecholamines*, edited by H. Blaschko and H. Muscholl. New York: Springer-Verlag, 1972, vol. 33, p. 283–335.
56. FURNESS, J. B. Arrangement of blood vessels and their relation with adrenergic nerves in the rat mesentry. *J. Anat.* 115: 347–364, 1973.
57. FURNESS, J. B., M. COSTA, P. C. EMSON, R. HÅKANSON, E. MOGHIMZADEH, F. SUNDLER, I. L. TAYLOR, AND R. E. CHANCE. Distribution, pathways and reactions to drug treatment of nerves with neuropeptide Y and pancreatic polypeptide-like immunoreactivity in the guinea-pig digestive tract. *Cell Tissue Res.* 234: 71–92, 1983.
58. FURNESS, J. B., M. COSTA, I. J. GIBBINS, I. J. LLEWELLYN-SMITH, AND J. R. OLIVER. Neurochemically similar myenteric and submucous neurons directly tracted to the mucosa of the small intestine. *Cell Tissue Res.* 241: 155–163, 1985.
59. FURNESS, J. B., J. MCLEAN, AND G. BURNSTOCK. Distribution of adrenergic nerves and changes in neuromuscular transmission in the mouse vas deferens during post-natal development. *Dev. Biol.* 21: 491–505, 1970.
60. GABELLA, G. Structure of smooth muscles. In: *Smooth Muscle: An Assessment of Current Knowledge*, edited by E. Bülbring, A. F. Brading, A. W. Jones, and T. Tomita. London: Arnold, 1981, p. 1–46.
61. GAGE, P. W. Generation of end-plate potentials. *Physiol. Rev.* 56: 177–247, 1976.
62. GEFFEN, L., AND B. JARROTT. Cellular aspects of catecholaminergic neurons. In: *Handbook of Physiology. The Nervous System, Cellular Biology of Neurons*, edited by E. R. Kandell. Bethesda, MD: Am. Physiol. Soc., 1977, sect. 1, vol. 1, pt. 1, chapt. 15, p. 521–571.
63. GLICK, G., S. E. EPSTEIN, A. S. WECHSLER, AND E. BRAUNWALD. Physiological differences between the effects of neuronally released and bloodborne norepinephrine on beta adrenergic receptors in the arterial bed of the dog. *Circ. Res.* 21: 217–227, 1985.
64. GOLDMAN, D. E. Potential, impedance and rectification in membranes. *J. Gen. Physiol.* 27: 37–60, 1968.
65. GREENWAY, C. V. Neural control and autoregulatory escape. In: *Physiology of the Intestinal Circulation*, edited by A. P. Shepherd and D. N. Granger. New York: Raven, 1984, p. 61–72.
66. HAEUSLER, G., AND S. THORENS. Effects of tetraethylammonium chloride on contractile, membrane and cable properties of rabbit artery muscle. *J. Physiol. Lond.* 303: 203–224, 1980.
68. HENDRICKX, H., AND R. CASTEELS. Electrogenic sodium pump in arterial smooth muscle cells. *Pfluegers Arch.* 346: 299–306, 1974.
69. HERMSMEYER, K. Electrogenesis of increased norepinephrine sensitivity of arterial vascular muscle in hypertension. *Circ. Res.* 38: 362–367, 1976.
70. HILL, C. E., G. D. S. HIRST, M. C. NGU, AND D. F. VAN HELDEN. Sympathetic postganglionic reinnervation of mesenteric arteries and enteric neurones of the ileum of the rat. *J. Auton. Nerv. Syst.* 14: 317–334, 1985.

71. HILL, C. E., G. D. S. HIRST, G. D. SILVERBERG, AND D. F. VAN HELDEN. Sympathetic innervation and excitability of arterioles originating from the rat middle cerebral artery. *J. Physiol. Lond.* 371: 305–316, 1986.
72. HILL, C. E., G. D. S. HIRST, AND D. F. HELDEN. Development of the sympathetic innervation to proximal and distal arteries of the rat mesentry. *J. Physiol. Lond.* 338: 129–147, 1983.
73. HILLE, B. Ionic basis of resting and action potentials. In: *Handbook of Physiology. The Nervous System. Cellular Biology of Neurons*, edited by E. R. Kandell. Bethesda, MD: Am. Physiol. Soc. 1977, sect. 1, vol. 1, pt. 1, chapt. 4, 99–136.
74. HIRST, G. D. S. Neuromuscular transmission in arterioles of guinea-pig submucosa. *J. Physiol. Lond.* 273: 87–104, 1977.
75. HIRST, G. D. S. Identification of transmitters in the autonomic nervous system. *Proc. Aust. Physiol. Pharmacol. Soc.* 9: 91–93, 1978.
76. HIRST, G. D. S., S. DE GLARIA, AND D. F. VAN HELDEN. Neuromuscular transmission in arterioles. *Experientia Basel* 41: 874–879, 1985.
77. HIRST, G. D. S., AND M. J. LEW. Lack of involvement of alpha-adrenoceptors in sympathetic neural vasoconstriction in the hindquarters of the rabbit. *Brit. J. Pharmacol.* 90: 51–60, 1987.
79. HIRST, G. D. S., AND E. M. MCLACHLAN. Post-natal development of ganglia in the lower lumbar sympathetic chain of the rat. *J. Physiol. Lond.* 349: 119–134, 1984.
80. HIRST, G. D. S., AND T. O. NEILD. An analysis of excitatory junctional potentials recorded arterioles. *J. Physiol. Lond.* 280: 87–104, 1978.
81. HIRST, G. D. S., AND T. O. NEILD. Some properties of spontaneous excitatory junction potentials recorded from arterioles of guinea-pigs. *J. Physiol. Lond.* 303: 43–60, 1980.
82. HIRST, G. D. S., AND T. O. NEILD. Evidence for two populations of excitatory receptors for noradrenaline on arteriolar smooth muscle. *Nature Lond.* 283: 767–768, 1980.
83. HIRST, G. D. S., AND T. O. NEILD. Localization of specialized noradrenaline receptors at neuromuscular junctions on arterioles of the guinea-pig. *J. Physiol. Lond.* 313: 343–350, 1981.
84. HIRST, G. D. S., T. O. NEILD, AND G. D. SILVERBERG. Noradrenaline receptors on the rat basilar artery. *J. Physiol. Lond.* 328: 351–360, 1982.
85. HIRST, G. D. S., G. D. SILVERBERG, AND D. F. VAN HELDEN. The action potential and underlying ionic currents in proximal rat middle cerebral arterioles. *J. Physiol. Lond.* 371: 289–304, 1986.
86. HIRST, G. D. S., AND D. F. VAN HELDEN. Ionic basis of the resting potential of submucosal arterioles in the ileum of the guinea-pig. *J. Physiol. Lond.* 333: 53–67, 1982.
87. HODGKIN, A. L., AND B. KATZ. The effect of sodium ions on the electrical activity of the giant axon of the squid. *J. Physiol. Lond.* 148: 37–77, 1949.
88. HODGKIN, A. L., AND W. A. H. RUSHTON. The electrical constants of a crustacean nerve fibre. *Proc. R. Soc. Lond. B Biol. Sci.* 133: 444–479, 1946.
89. HÖKFELT, T. Distribution of noradrenaline storing particles in peripheral neurons as revealed by electron microscopy. *Acta Physiol. Scand.* 76: 427–440, 1969.
90. HOLMAN, M. E., C. B. KASBY, M. B. SUTHERS, AND J. A. F. WILSON. Some properties of the smooth muscle of rabbit portal vein. *J. Physiol. Lond.* 196: 111–132, 1968.
91. HOLMAN, M. E., AND A. M. SURPRENANT. Some properties of the excitatory junction potentials recorded from saphenous arteries of rabbits. *J. Physiol. Lond.* 287: 337–351, 1979.
92. HOLMAN, M. E., AND A. M. SURPRENANT. Effects of tetraethylammonium chloride on sympathetic neuromuscular transmission in saphenous artery of young rabbits. *J. Physiol. Lond.* 305: 451–465, 1980.
93. HOLMAN, M. E., AND A. M. SURPRENANT. An electrophysiological analysis of the effects of noradrenaline and receptor antagonists on neuromuscular transmission in mammalian muscular arteries. *Br. J. Pharmacol.* 71: 337–351, 1980.
94. HUA, C., AND B. CRAGG. Measurements of smooth muscle cells in arterioles of guinea-pig ileum. *Acta Anat.* 107: 224–230, 1980.
95. ISHIKAWA, S. Actions of ATP and $\alpha,\beta$-methylene ATP on neuromuscular transmission and smooth muscle membranes of the rabbit and guinea-pig mesenteric arteries. *Br. J. Pharmacol.* 86: 777–787, 1985.
96. ITOH, T., K. KITAMURA, AND H. KURIYAMA. Roles of extrajunctional receptors in the response of guinea-pig mesenteric and rat tail arteries to adrenergic nerves. *J. Physiol. Lond.* 345: 409–422, 1983.
97. IVERSEN, L. L. The Uptake and Storage of Noradrenaline in Sympathetic Nerves. London: Cambridge Univ. Press, 1967.
98. JACK, J. J. B., D. NOBLE, AND R. W. TSIEN. *Electrical Current Flow in Excitable Cells.* Oxford, UK: Clarendon, 1975.
99. JACK, J. J. B., S. J. REDMAN, AND K. WONG. The components of synaptic potentials evoked in cat spinal motoneurons by impulses in single 1a afferents. *J. Physiol. Lond.* 321: 65–96, 1981.
100. JANIG, W. Organization of the lumbar sympathetic outflow to skeletal muscle and skin of the cat hind limb and tail. *Rev. Physiol. Biochem. Pharmacol.* 102: 121–213, 1985.
101. KAJIWARA, M., K. KITAMURA, AND H. KURIYAMA. Neuromuscular transmission and smooth muscle membrane properties in the guinea-pig ear artery. *J. Physiol. Lond.* 315: 283–302, 1981.
102. KANMURA, Y., T. ITOH, H. SUZUKI, Y. ITO, AND H. KURIYAMA. Effects of nifedipine on smooth muscle cells of the rabbit mesenteric artery. *J. Pharmacol. Exp. Ther.* 226: 238–248, 1983.
103. KATZ, B. The Release of Neural Transmitter Substances. The Sherrington Lectures X, Liverpool, UK: Liverpool University, 1969.
104. KEATINGE, W. R. Ionic requirements for arterial action potential. *J. Physiol. Lond.* 194: 168–182, 1968.
105. KEATINGE, W. R. Mechanism of slow discharge of sheep carotid artery. *J. Physiol. Lond.* 279: 275–289, 1978.
106. KOU, K., J. IBENGE, AND H. SUZUKI. Effects of alpha-adrenoceptor antagonists on electrical and mechanical responses of the isolated dog mesenteric vein to perivascular nerve stimulation and exogenous noradrenaline. *Naunyn-Schmiedeberg's Arch. Pharmacol.* 326: 7–13, 1984.
107. KUFFLER, S. W., AND J. G. NICHOLLS. *From Neuron to Brain.* Sunderland, MA: Sinauer, 1976.
108. KUGELGEN, I. V., AND K. STARKE. Noradrenaline and adenosine triphosphate as co-transmitters of neurogenic vasoconstriction in rabbit mesenteric arteries. *J. Physiol. Lond.* 367: 435–455, 1985.
109. KURIYAMA, H. Electrophysiological observations on the motor innervation of the smooth muscle cells of the guinea-pig vas deferens. *J. Physiol. Lond.* 169: 213–228, 1963.
110. KURIYAMA, H., AND Y. MAKITA. Modulation of noradrenergic transmission in the guinea-pig mesenteric artery: an electrophysiological study. *J. Physiol. Lond.* 335: 609–627, 1983.
111. KURIYAMA, H., AND A. SUYAMA. Multiple actions of cocaine on neuromuscular transmission and smooth muscle cells of the guinea-pig mesenteric artery. *J. Physiol. Lond.* 337: 631–654, 1983.
112. KURIYAMA, H., AND H. SUZUKI. Adrenergic transmission in the mesenteric artery and their cholinergic modulations. *J. Physiol. Lond.* 317: 383–396, 1981.
113. LAGERECRANTZ, H. On the consumption and function of large dense cored vesicles in sympathetic nerves. *Neuroscience* 1: 81–92, 1976.
114. LANDIS, S. C., AND D. KEEFE. Evidence for neurotransmitter plasticity in vivo: developmental changes in properties of cholinergic sympathetic neurones. *Dev. Biol.* 98: 349–372, 1983.
115. LANGER, S. Z. Presynaptic receptors and their role in regulation of transmitter release. *Br. J. Pharmacol.* 60: 481–497, 1977.
116. LARGE, W. A. Membrane potential responses of the mouse

anococcygeus muscle to ionophoretically applied noradrenaline. *J. Physiol. Lond.* 326: 385–400, 1982.
117. LARGE, W. A. Membrane potential responses to ionophoretically applied adrenoceptor agonists in the mouse anococcygeus muscle. *Br. J. Pharmacol.* 79: 233–243, 1983.
118. LARGE, W. A. The effect of chloride removal on the responses of the isolated rat anococcygeus muscle to $\alpha_1$-adrenoceptor stimulation. *J. Physiol. Lond.* 352: 17–29, 1984.
119. LUFF, S. E., E. M. MCLACHLAN, AND G. D. S. HIRST. An ultrastructural analysis of the sympathetic neuromuscular junctions on arterioles of the submucosa of the guinea pig ileum. *J. Comp. Neurol.* 257: 578–594, 1987.
120. MARTIN, A. R. Quantal nature of synaptic transmission. *Physiol. Rev.* 46: 51–66, 1966.
121. MCGRATH, J. C. Adrenergic and 'non-adrenergic' components in the contractile response of the vas deferens to a single indirect stimulus. *J. Physiol. Lond.* 283: 23–39, 1978.
122. MCLACHLAN, E. M. The statistics of transmitter release at chemical synapses. In: *Neurophysiology III*, edited by R. Porter. Baltimore, MD: University Park, 1978, vol. 17, p. 49–117. (Int. Rev. Physiol. Ser.)
123. MCLACHLAN, E. M., AND G. D. S. HIRST. Some properties of preganglionic neurons in upper thoracic spinal cord of the cat. *J. Neurophysiol.* 43: 1251–1265, 1980.
124. MEKATA, F. Current-spread in the smooth muscle of the rabbit aorta. *J. Physiol. Lond.* 242: 143–155, 1974.
125. MEKATA, F. Rectification in the smooth muscle cell membrane of rabbit aorta. *J. Physiol. Lond.* 258: 269–278, 1976.
126. MELCHIORRE, C., M. S. YONG, B. G. BENFEY, AND B. BELLEAU. Molecular properties of the adrenergic $\alpha$-receptor. 2. Optimal covalent inhibition by two different prototypes of polyamine disulphides. *J. Med. Chem.* 21: 1126–1128, 1978.
127. MORGAN, K. G. Comparison of membrane electrical activity of cat gastric submucosal arterioles and venules. *J. Physiol. Lond.* 345: 135–147, 1983.
128. MULVANY, M. J., H. NILSSON, AND J. A. FLATMAN. Role of membrane potential in the response of rat small mesenteric arteries to exogenous noradrenaline stimulation. *J. Physiol. Lond.* 332: 539–551, 1982.
129. MURUMATSU, I., M. FUJIWARA, A. MIURA, AND Y. SAKAKIBARA. Possible involvement of adenine nucleotides in sympathetic neuroeffector mechanisms of dog basilar artery. *J. Pharmacol. Exp. Ther.* 216: 401–409, 1981.
130. MURUMATSU, I., S. KIGOSHI, AND M. OSHITA. Nonadrenergic nature of prazosin-resistant sympathetic contraction in the dog mesenteric artery. *J. Pharmacol. Exp. Ther.* 229: 532–538, 1984.
131. NAKANISHI, H., AND H. TAKEDA. The possible role of adenosine triphosphate in chemical transmission between the hypogastric nerve terminal and seminal vesicle. *Jpn. J. Pharmacol.* 23: 479–483, 1973.
132. NEILD, T. O. The relation between the structure and innervation of small arteries and arterioles and the smooth muscle membrane potential changes expected at different levels of sympathetic nerve activity. *Proc. R. Soc. Lond. B Biol. Sci.*: 237–249, 1983.
133. NEILD, T. O., & E. ZELCER. Noradrenergic neuromuscular transmission with special reference to arterial smooth muscle. *Prog. Neurobiol.* 19: 141–158, 1982.
134. NORBERG, K. A., AND B. HAMBERGER. The sympathetic adrenergic neuron. Some characteristics revealed by histochemical studies on the intraneuronal distribution of the transmitter. *Acta Physiol. Scand. Suppl.* 238: 1–42, 1964.
135. O'BRIEN, R. A., M. DA PRADA, AND A. PLETSCHER. The ontogenesis of catecholamines and adenosine-5'-triphosphate in the adrenal medulla. *Life Sci.* 11: 749–759, 1972.
136. OHASHI, H. An estimate of the proportion of the resting membrane conductance of the smooth muscle of taenia coli to chloride. *J. Physiol. Lond.* 210: 405–419, 1970.
137. RANG, H. P. The characteristics of synaptic current and responses to acetylcholine of rat submandibular ganglion cells. *J. Physiol. Lond.* 311: 23–55, 1981.
138. REDMAN, S. J. Synaptic transmission in the central nervous system. *Prog. Neurobiol.* 12: 33–83, 1979.
139. RHODIN, J. A. G. The ultrastructure of mammalian arterioles and precapillary sphincters. *J. Ultrastruct. Res.* 18: 181–223, 1967.
140. ROWAN, R. A., AND J. A. BEVAN. Distribution of adrenergic synaptic cleft width in vascular and nonvascular smooth muscle. In: *Vascular Neuroeffector Mechanisms*, edited by J. A. Bevan. New York: Raven, 1983, p. 75–83. (4th Int. Symp.)
141. SHEPHERD, A. P., AND D. N. GRANGER. *Physiology of the Intestinal Circulation*. New York: Raven, 1984.
142. SKOK, V. I. *Physiology of Autonomic Ganglia*. Tokyo: Igaku Shoin, 1975.
143. SNEDDON, P., AND G. BURNSTOCK. ATP as a co-transmitter in rat tail artery. *Eur. J. Pharmacol.* 106: 149–152, 1984.
144. SNEDDON, P., AND D. P. WESTFALL. Pharmacological evidence that adenosine triphosphate and noradrenaline are co-transmitters in the guinea-pig vas deferens. *J. Physiol. Lond.* 347: 561–580, 1984.
145. SNEDDON, P., D. P. WESTFALL, AND J. S. FEDAN. Cotransmitters in the motor nerves of the guinea-pig vas deferens: electrophysiological evidence. *Science Wash. DC* 218: 693–694, 1982.
146. SOMLYO, A. P., AND A. V. SOMLYO. Vascular smooth muscle. 1. Normal structure, pathology, biochemistry and biophysics. *Pharmacol. Rev.* 20: 197–272, 1968.
147. SPEDEN, R. N. Electrical activity of single smooth muscle cells of the mesenteric artery produced by splanchnic nerve stimulation in the guinea-pig. *Nature Lond.* 202: 193–194, 1964.
148. SPEDEN, R. N. Excitation of vascular smooth muscle. In: *Smooth Muscle*, edited by E. Bülbring, A. F. Brading, A. W. Jones, and T. Tomita. London: Arnold, 1970, p. 558–588.
149. STARKE, K. Regulation of noradrenaline release by presynaptic receptor systems. *Rev. Physiol. Biochem. Pharmacol.* 77: 1–124, 1977.
150. STEEDMAN, W. A. Micro-electrode studies on mammalian vascular muscle. *J. Physiol. Lond.* 186: 382–400, 1966.
151. STJÄRNE, L., AND P. ASTRAND. Relative pre- and postjunctional roles of noradrenaline and adenosine-5'-triphosphate as neurotransmitters of the sympathetic nerves of guinea-pig vas deferens. *Neuroscience* 14: 929–946, 1985.
152. SU, C. Neurogenic release of purine compounds in blood vessels. *J. Pharmacol. Exp. Ther.* 195: 159–166, 1975.
153. SU, C., J. A. BEVAN, AND R. C. URSILLO. Electrical quiescence of pulmonary artery smooth muscle during sympathomimetic stimulation. *Circ. Res.* 15: 20–27, 1964.
154. SUPRENANT, A. A comparative study of neuromuscular transmission in several mammalian muscular arteries. *Pfluegers Arch.* 396: 85–91, 1980.
155. SUZUKI, H. Effects of endogenous and exogenous noradrenaline on the smooth muscle of guinea-pig mesenteric vein. *J. Physiol. Lond.* 321: 495–512, 1981.
156. SUZUKI, H. An electrophysiological study of excitatory neuromuscular transmission in the guinea-pig main pulmonary artery. *J. Physiol. Lond.* 336: 47–59, 1983.
157. SUZUKI, H. Electrical responses of smooth muscle cells of the rabbit ear artery to adenosine triphosphate. *J. Physiol. Lond.* 359: 401–416, 1985.
158. SUZUKI, H., AND K. KOU. Electrical components contributing to the nerve-mediated contractions in the smooth muscles of the rabbit ear artery. *Jpn. J. Physiol.* 33: 743–756, 1983.
159. SWEDIN, G. Biphasic mechanical response of the isolated vas deferens to nerve stimulation. *Acta Physiol. Scand.* 81: 574–576, 1971.
160. THOMAS, R. C. Electrogenic sodium pump in nerve and muscle cells. *Physiol. Rev.* 52: 563–594, 1972.
161. TOMITA, T. Electrical properties of mammalian smooth muscle. In: *Smooth Muscle*, edited by E. Bülbring, A. F. Brading, A. W. Jones, and T. Tomita. London: Arnold, 1970, p. 197–243.

162. TOMITA, T. Electrical activity (spikes and slow waves) in gastro-intestinal smooth muscle. In: *Smooth Muscle: an Assessment of Current Knowledge,* edited by E. Bülbring, A. F. Brading, A. W. Jones, and T. Tomita. London: Arnold, 1981, p. 127–156.

163. VATNER, S. F., D. R. KNIGHT, AND T. H. HINTZE. Norepinephrine-induced beta-1 adrenergic peripheral vasodilation in conscious dogs. *Am. J. Physiol.* 249: 49–56, 1985.

164. WESTFALL, D. P., R. E. STITZEL, AND J. N. ROWE. The postjunctional effects and neural release of purine compounds in the guinea-pig vas deferens. *Eur. J. Pharmacol.* 50: 27–38, 1978.

165. WHITE, T., P. POTTER, C. MOODY, AND G. BURNSTOCK. Tetrodoxin resistant release of ATP from guinea-pig taenia coli and vas deferens during electrical field stimulation in the presence of luciferin-luciferase. *Can. J. Physiol. Pharmacol.* 59: 1094–1100, 1981.

CHAPTER 46

# Neurohormonal control of gastrointestinal blood flow

MATS JODAL
OVE LUNDGREN

*Department of Physiology, University of Göteborg, Göteborg, Sweden*

CHAPTER CONTENTS

Established Neurotransmitters
  Acetylcholine
  Norepinephrine
    General aspects of adrenergic vascular innervation
    Physiology: in vitro studies
    Physiology: in vivo studies
Neurotransmitter Candidates
  Enkephalins
  Neuropeptide Y
  Peptide histidine isoleucine
  Substance P
  Vasoactive intestinal polypeptide
Hormones
  Angiotensin
  Antidiuretic hormone
  Epinephrine
  Gastrin and pentagastrin
  Glucagon and enteroglucagon
  Secretin
Hormone Candidates
  Motilin
  Peptide YY
Neurotransmitters and/or Hormones
  Cholecystokinin
  5-Hydroxytryptamine (serotonin)
  Neurotensin
  Somatostatin
Integrated Responses
  High-pressure baroreceptors
  Cardiac mechanoreceptors
  Arterial chemoreceptors
  Hemorrhagic hypotension
    Resistance vessels
    Precapillary sphincters
    Exchange vessels
    Capacitance vessels
  Postprandial hyperemia

FIFTEEN YEARS AGO it would have been a limited task to review the neurohormonal control of the gastrointestinal circulation. At that time, three peptide hormones of gastrointestinal origin were known, i.e., gastrin, cholecystokinin (CCK), and secretin, and the neurotransmitters of the enteric nervous system were believed to be two, acetylcholine and norepinephrine. Since then a truly revolutionary development has occurred: the isolation and characterization of several peptides that presumably act as hormones and/or neurotransmitters in the gastrointestinal tract. This development has made our task difficult not only because it implies a larger field of literature to cover but also because it is presently impossible to present a coherent picture of the field that integrates morphological and physiological observations. This is mainly due to a lack of knowledge of the physiology of the various peptides. The field of the gastrointestinal peptides is characterized by a large body of morphological (i.e., immunohistochemical) studies with few physiological studies that clearly indicate the function of the peptide under study.

Some of the compounds (peptides and amines) that are of interest with regard to the neurohormonal control of the gastrointestinal circulation seem to exist in both enteric nerves and epithelial cells. The latter localization suggests a hormonal function. This makes it difficult to organize this chapter according to function. We have therefore chosen to discuss our topic primarily based on the different substances that are of interest. These compounds have been divided into groups, i.e., established neurotransmitters and hormones, candidate neurotransmitters and hormones, and compounds that may be both hormones and neurotransmitters. In the final part of this chapter, we discuss some integrated responses, i.e., postprandial hyperemia and some cardiovascular reflexes.

ESTABLISHED NEUROTRANSMITTERS

The classic view of neuronal function implies that each neuron releases one transmitter substance (e.g., norepinephrine or acetylcholine). This view has lately been challenged, because the application of various histochemical techniques to the study of the autonomic nervous system has revealed that two or more putative neurotransmitters may coexist in the same neuron (cf. ref. 179). The functional implications of such findings are not known and understood with regard to the vascular control or the control of any other organ function. Some possible consequences are described here in connection with neuropeptide Y (NPY), which exists with norepinephrine in many adrenergic fibers innervating vascular smooth muscles.

*Acetylcholine*

Acetylcholine is one of the two classic transmitters within the autonomic nervous system. It is known to be a neurotransmitter in autonomic ganglia and at certain effector cells. Receptor antagonists exist that are more or less specific for both sites of release. However, until recently, specific staining methods for cholinergic neurons were lacking. The most commonly used histochemical method, which traces acetylcholinesterase, is considered to stain also noncholinergic neurons. There are few, if any, observations on the vascular innervation of nerve fibers containing cholinesterase (cf. ref. 360).

A more specific immunohistochemical method is the one mapping the distribution of choline acetyltransferase (ChAt) in nerves. Applying this technique to the submucosal plexus of the small intestine of the guinea pig reveals three types of ChAt neurons (133, 135): *1*) neurons that, in addition to acetycholine, contain immunoreactivity for each of the peptides, cholecystokinin, somatostatin, and NPY; *2*) neurons that also contain substance P (SP); and *3*) neurons that do not contain any detectable amounts of the peptides studied by Furness et al. (135), i.e., besides those already mentioned, they do not contain vasoactive intestinal polypeptide (VIP). Hence no coexistence of acetylcholine and VIP could be demonstrated in this study on the guinea pig. The extent to which the different types of ChAt neurons innervate vascular smooth muscle cannot be judged from the published reports.

Acetylcholine is in vivo a vascular smooth muscle relaxant in most tissues, including the gastrointestinal tract (17, 175, 220, 351, 370, 401). However, in vitro acetylcholine constricts vascular smooth muscles, and the same response is seen in vivo if the endothelium is damaged. Such observations lead Furchgott (130) to propose that the vasodilatation induced by acetylcholine is induced through an endothelial mechanism, possibly involving the release of some messenger substance. The vasodilatation evoked by close intra-arterial infusion of acetylcholine in vivo seems to be more pronounced in the muscle layer, because ileal muscle blood flow is increased to a greater extent than total blood flow (428). Concomitantly, an increased number of capillaries are recruited, as judged by an augmented $^{86}$Rb clearance (428). However, when acetylcholine is given in high enough doses [>10 µg (55 nmol)/min to a 15-g segment of feline small intestine], motility in the alimentary canal may increase to such an extent as to decrease intestinal blood flow (220, 351).

In the stomach (denervated sympathetically), a vasodilatation is seen on stimulating vagal nerves concomitant to an increase of gastric acid secretion (184, 277). These nervous effects are markedly influenced by atropine. In a dose that completely blocks the secretory response in a cat, atropine abolishes 70%–90% of the vasodilatation (277). These observations may be taken as evidence for the existence of cholinergic vasodilator fibers in the stomach, but the increased blood flow may also reflect a "work hyperemia" secondary to the augmented secretion and/or motility. Inhibiting secretion by atropine then also abolishes the vasodilatation. The onset of the vascular response on vagal stimulation is very fast, occurring within 10–20 s (277). Such a fast vascular response suggests a direct cholinergic vascular innervation, but admittedly this argument gives only an indirect support for such an innervation.

Stimulating the vagal nerves to the feline small intestine does not evoke any vasodilatation, even when stimulus parameters change widely (219). On the other hand, electrical stimulation of the main parasympathetic outflow to the cat colon (pelvic nerves) evokes in the sympathetically denervated colon a vasodilatation that consists of two phases (188, 189). Immediately upon the start of the stimulation, a marked transient vasodilatation is apparent. This is followed by an oscillating blood flow concomitant to colonic secretion of fluid and/or mucus. The blood flow oscillations may be secondary to colonic motility. After atropinization, only the initial increase of flow is observed, whereas the flow oscillations and secretion are abolished. It was concluded from such experiments that two vasodilator mechanisms are involved in the pelvic nerve response in the colon: an initial noncholinergic hyperemia and an atropine-sensitive flow increase that may be secondary to a net colonic secretion. However, as in the stomach, it is uncertain whether there is a direct cholinergic innervation of the colonic vessels.

It has been claimed by Fasth and co-workers (119, 121) that atropine has no effect on the colonic vasodilatation elicited via the pelvic nerves. However, the illustrations presented by these authors clearly show that atropine does reduce the vasodilatation in the way described in the previous paragraph (see Fig. 1 in ref. 119). Colonic secretion was not recorded in these experiments.

To summarize, both in the stomach and in the colon there are nervous vasodilator mechanisms that are abolished by atropine, suggesting the involvement of cholinergic nerves. However, presently it is not possible to establish whether the observed nervous effects are caused by a direct vascular innervation of cholinergic nerve fibers or secondary to a cholinergic innervation of the gastric and/or colonic epithelium and muscular layer. To answer the question of a possible cholinergic innervation of the gastrointestinal vasculature, the distribution of cholinergic fibers within the alimentary canal needs to be investigated with a specific histochemical technique that puts special emphasis on the vascular innervation. Furthermore experimental approaches (physiological and/or pharmacological), designed to discriminate between cholinergic vascular responses and cholinergic effects on other gastrointestinal functions, have to be developed.

This discussion assumes that cholinergic effects exist on different types of smooth muscles and/or epithelium. There are, however, reports that suggest that cholinergic receptors on adrenergic neurons inhibit the release of norepinephrine (232, 414). Such a mechanism should be borne in mind when interpreting the effects of cholinergic agonists on innervated vascular beds in vivo.

*Norepinephrine*

According to classic concepts, the sympathetic innervation reaching the gastrointestinal tract consists of postganglionic fibers releasing norepinephrine (possibly together with a peptide NPY, as discussed in *Neuropeptide Y*, p. 1678) upon activation. The presence of norepinephrine in histological sections can be visualized by the fluorescent histochemical method of Falck-Hillarp, which reveals an extensive adrenergic innervation of the two nerve plexuses of the alimentary tract (131, 295, 329, 363, 374). The epithelium is also innervated, particularly in the crypts, whereas the direct adrenergic innervation of the smooth muscle layers is rather sparse. The blood vessels are also densely innervated (374).

GENERAL ASPECTS OF ADRENERGIC VASCULAR INNERVATION. The structure of the sympathetic adrenergic vascular innervation is well investigated in the peripheral autonomic nervous system, and it is probable that the cholinergic and peptidergic innervation of the vascular smooth muscles is arranged in principle like that of the adrenergic nerves. This innervation is therefore described here in some detail [for a more thorough review, see Bevan et al. (22)]. The adrenergic nerves reaching the vessels are nonmyelinated and they usually form two plexuses in the vascular adventitia: an outer plexus in the middle or outer one-third of the adventitia and an inner plexus, situated at the adventitiomedial junction, forming a ground plexus of the type usually found in autonomically innervated tissues. The axons, 0.25–0.5 $\mu$m in diameter, exhibit periodic swellings or varicosities, 1.5–2 $\mu$m in diameter, at intervals of 3–10 $\mu$m. In these varicosities or nodes, a large number of comparatively small storage vesicles (diam 35–60 nm) are found, containing norepinephrine, as revealed by the fluorescence histochemical technique. Electromicrographs also reveal the presence of large granular vesicles (diam 60–120 nm). These vesicles seem to contain NPY and, possibly, norepinephrine (263). It is apparent from this arrangement that a nerve impulse passing along an axon can successively depolarize a series of varicosities.

This description indicates that the terminal branches of sympathetic nerves only make contact with the outer layer of the muscular layer in the media, whereas the rest of the smooth muscle cells is controlled indirectly via low-resistance intercellular bridges, or nexa. The distance between the sympathetic nerves and the vascular smooth muscles ("synaptic cleft") varies between vessels, which gives the impression that the smaller the blood vessels, the narrower the cleft. The range of distances reported for various vessels varies from 4 $\mu$m in conduit arteries to $\leq$60 nm in the smallest vessels. In the rat mesenteric artery, the distance has been measured to 500 nm (88). The density of the nerve plexus varies also along the vascular tree and is more closely meshed in arteries than in veins (293).

The vesicles and their enzymes for norepinephrine synthesis are synthesized by the smooth endoplasmic reticulum in the cell soma. By ligating the axon it can be shown that norepinephrine, vesicles, and enzymes accumulate above the nervous constriction, reflecting the axonal transport occurring from cell soma along the axon. Norepinephrine can be synthesized in the peripheral varicosities, whereas the peptidergic neurotransmitters are assumed to be produced in the ribosomes in the cell soma (179).

The depolarization of the membrane varicosity represents the stimulus for transmitter release, an influx of $Ca^{2+}$ linking in an unknown way the depolarization to the transmitter release. Exocytosis is the most likely mechanism for the release of the transmitter(s) (22). Two major hypotheses have been discussed with regard to the so-called quantal release of transmitter, i.e., the amount of transmitter release by one action potential. According to one hypothesis, only part of the total transmitter content of each vesicle (granule) can be released, whereas the other hypothesis infers that the entire content of one vesicle (granule) is always emptied and therefore represents the quantal release. In the second case, it is necessary to assume that the depolarization of each varicosity is followed by transmitter release only now and then, because all authors agree that the total amount of transmitter released per impulse is considerably less than the total amount of neurotransmitter in one varicosity.

The norepinephrine released from nerve varicosities into the synaptic cleft diffuses toward its receptor on the plasma membrane of the effector cell: the vascular smooth muscle. The norepinephrine that does not reach a postsynaptic receptor is inactivated in various ways. At least three mechanisms exist: *1*) an extracellular breakdown by specific enzymes (monoamine oxidase and catechol-$O$-methyltransferase), 2) a reuptake into the varicosity, and 3) a diffusion of norepinephrine into the blood circulation. Finally, it is generally believed that there exist presynaptic adrenergic receptors that exert a negative feedback influence on the transmitter release.

PHYSIOLOGY: IN VITRO STUDIES. The intestinal circulation offers the experimental advantage that small mesenteric vessels can be isolated and studied in vitro. This experimental approach has been used particularly in the rat. The proximal part of the superior mesenteric artery of this species has a diameter of ~1.2 mm at a distending pressure of ~100 mmHg. The arteries located in the mesentery close to the intestinal wall have a corresponding diameter of 150–200 μm (292). At that level, resistance to flow becomes prominent, as also shown in vivo by direct pressure measurements. In the rat, approximately one-half of the total resistance in the intestinal vascular bed resides in the vessels in the mesentery (142). Thus these vessels are well suited for studies of the nervous control of the resistance vessels. It has been shown that the nerves exert most of their control on the proximal resistance vessels [for references, see Nilsson (292)], which makes the mesenteric resistance vessels even more suitable for investigations of nervous control.

The adrenergic nervous control of the mesenteric vessels of the rat has been the subject of a series of reports by Nilsson and co-workers (291–294). They studied both mesenteric resistance and capacitance vessels in vitro under nervous influence. The vascular nerves were activated by electrical field stimulation. A single electrical stimulus induces very weak contractions in the superior mesenteric artery (diam 1.16 ± 0.03 mm), whereas clear-cut contractions are seen in the small arteries (diam 192 ± 8 μm). On the other hand, stimulation of the vascular smooth muscle directly evokes a response in all vessels, regardless of size (Fig. 1). Repetitive stimulation of the nerves at a frequency >4–6 Hz evokes a two-phase response in the small-size artery. First, a quick contraction is observed within 2 s after beginning the stimulation, corresponding to ~10–20% of the maximal response seen as a result of prolonged stimulation. Then a gradual increase in tension is seen, reaching a stable level after 1–3 min (Fig. 2). The veins contract more quickly and within seconds reach their maximal response, which is maintained throughout the stimulation period. In view of the fact that the constriction of the resistance vessels "fades" in vivo when the electrical stimulation of the splanchnic nerves is prolonged for more than 1–2 min (autoregulatory escape response), it is interesting to note that the arterial response to nerve stimulation is maintained even at prolonged stimulation in vitro. Only the small veins under the influence of norepinephrine exhibit a fading vasoconstriction (Fig. 2). However, a sustained venous vasoconstriction is seen after administration of a β-

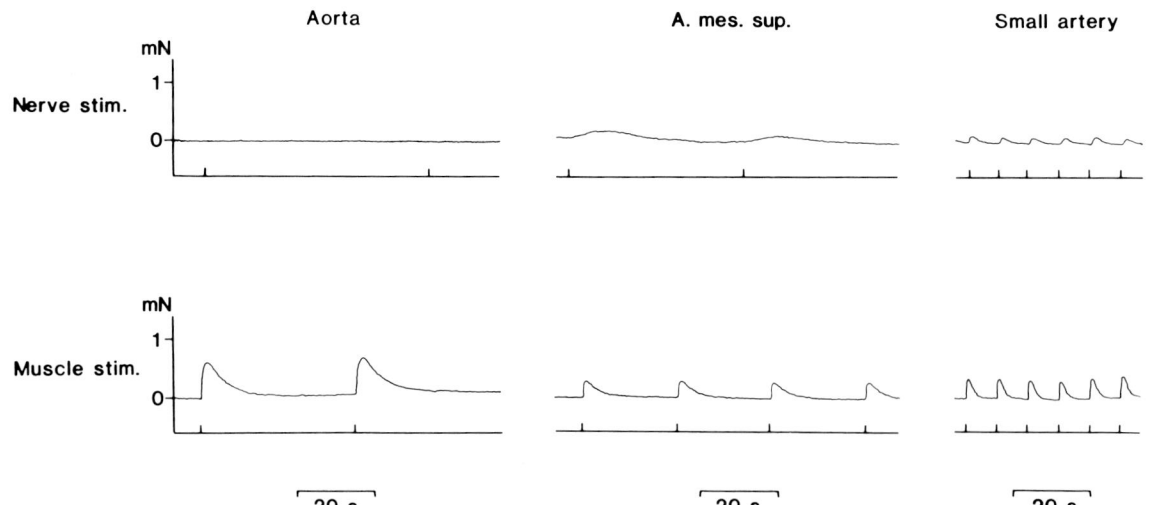

FIG. 1. Effect of electrical field stimulation (single pulses, 2-ms duration) on 3 different types of vascular smooth muscle preparations (*upper panels*) from rat. Experiments were performed in vitro, with tension measured between 2 metal rods introduced into vascular lumen. Electrical parameters were chosen so as to simulate only nervous tissue, as indicated by abolishment of response by tetrodotoxin. *Lower panels*, effect of single electrical pulses of long enough (100 ms) duration to stimulate directly vascular smooth muscles. Experiment was performed in presence of 0.1 μM tetrodotoxin in organ bath. Note large difference in nervous effects on different vessels. [From Nilsson (291).]

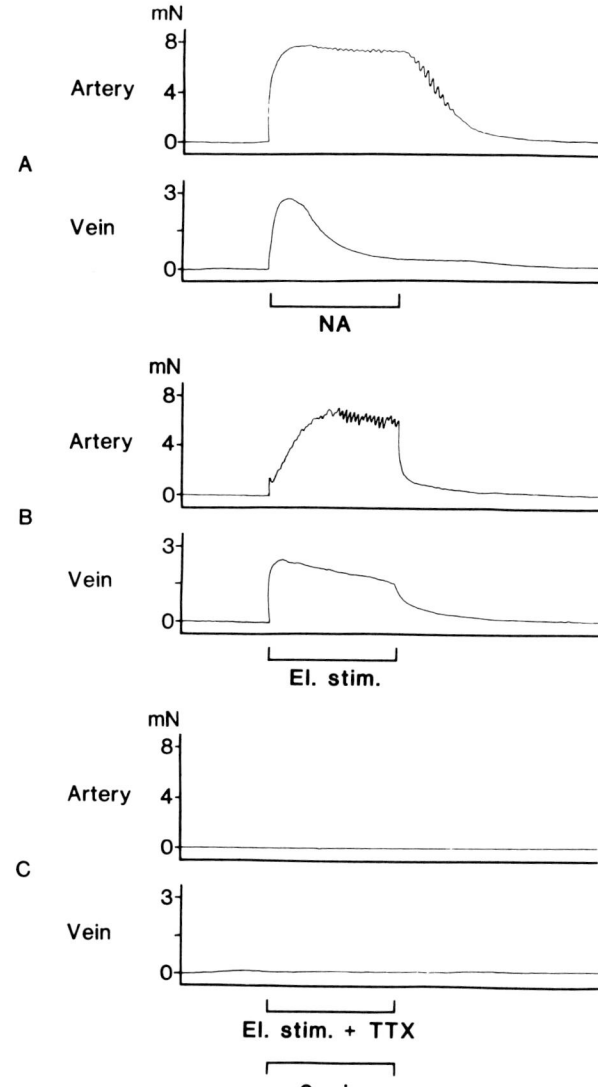

FIG. 2. *A*: responses of rat isolated small mesenteric artery and vein to exogenous norepinephrine (NA). *B*: corresponding responses to transmural electrical field stimulation at 16 Hz and supramaximal intensity of electrical stimulation. *C*: lack of responses to transmural field stimulation of type used in *B* after exposure to tetrodotoxin (TTX, 0.1 µM). [From Nilsson et al. (294).]

adrenergic receptor blocker (293), whereas an α-adrenergic blocker inhibits all effects (291).

The failure by Nilsson et al. (291–294) to demonstrate any fading response to norepinephrine in their in vitro system is at variance with the findings reported by Fara and Ross (113). They showed an escape to norepinephrine when studying the feline superior mesenteric artery in vitro. The escape phenomenon was demonstrated also in vessels taken from vascular beds known to show no autoregulatory escape in vivo during electrical stimulation of the vasoconstrictor fibers [e.g., the femoral artery (113)]. Furthermore Fara (109) stimulated large and small mesenteric vessels electrically in vitro and observed an escape that was more sluggish and less pronounced than after norepinephrine. The in vitro experiments suggest that the vessels in the mesentery exhibit an escape to norepinephrine, whereas no or little escape is observed when stimulating the adrenergic nerves electrically.

An interesting observation was reported by Nilsson et al. (294) regarding the importance of the firing pattern for the response of the vascular smooth muscles. Stimulation at a constant rate of 1.8 Hz evokes a very weak response of the small artery, whereas the vein shows a more pronounced contraction. When the same average rate of stimulation is delivered in bursts in a way that it is recorded from a cutaneous nerve of a human subject, pronounced contractions of both the small artery and veins are observed. Similar observations have been made in vivo when stimulating the pelvic nerves (12), although quantitatively not as pronounced as in the experiments by Nilsson et al. (294). The difference between the responses of the artery and the vein can be explained by the different frequency-response curves for the two types of mesenteric vessels. The response of the artery to stimulation frequencies <2 Hz is quite small, whereas a considerable contraction of the vein occurs at the same rate of stimulation. Hence only during the bursts of nervous activity is the artery stimulated to contraction (294).

PHYSIOLOGY: IN VIVO STUDIES. The studies of the sympathetic adrenergic control of the gastrointestinal tract have been most detailed with regard to the intestinal vascular beds, particularly the small intestine vascular bed. Therefore the description that follows is first devoted to intestinal studies and followed by a review of the studies on the stomach.

*Intestines.* Pflüger (319) was the first to demonstrate that the intestinal vessels are innervated by sympathetic fibers that produce vasoconstriction when electrically stimulated. The early animal studies were mainly attempting to confirm the observations by Pflüger with plethysmography and other indirect flow methods (for a survey of the very early investigations see ref. 53). The presence of adrenergic receptors on the smooth muscles of the resistance vessels was also demonstrated in some reports (29, 55, 148). With the advent of more sophisticated methods, it became possible to study the adrenergic control in more detail, and the following discussion is mainly based on these studies.

The renewed interest in the sympathetic nervous control of the gastrointestinal tract was initiated by the investigations of Folkow et al. (125, 126), who studied the effects of the vasoconstrictor fibers on the consecutive intestinal vascular sections with a plethysmographic method. This technique allows one to follow reactions within the resistance vessels (reflected as changes in blood flow), capacitance vessels (estimated as alterations in tissue volume), and precapillary sphincters [measured in terms of capillary filtration coefficient ($K_{f,c}$)]. The studies by Folkow and co-workers, made on the feline small intestine, showed that a continuous graded activation of the splanchnic nerves constricted the resistance and capacitance vessels as well as precapillary sphincters (Fig. 3). Within 2–4 min of the onset of stimulation of the constrictor fibers, blood flow increased (autoregulatory escape from the influence of vasoconstrictor fibers), and flow reached a new steady-state level moderately below control. The neurogenic effect on the capacitance vessels and on the precapillary sphincters remained largely unaltered throughout a stimulation period of 10–20 min. In the studies by Folkow et al. (125), mean capillary pressure seemed to stay fairly constant during the phase of steady-state flow, as judged by a constant tissue volume. Although blood flow was only slightly reduced during the steady-state phase of vasoconstriction, a pronounced reactive hyperemia was regularly seen on cessation of the stimulation.

It is apparent from Figure 3 that the response of the resistance vessels can be divided into two major phases: 1) autoregulatory escape from vasomotor fiber influence after the initial pronounced vasoconstriction and 2) the steady-state phase of nervous vasoconstriction. Our discussion is organized under these two subheadings and is based on the unproven assumption that the intra-arterial infusion of norepinephrine mimics in all hemodynamic respects the sympathetic nervous effects on the intestinal circulation. The recent demonstration of a peptide, NPY, in the adrenergic nerves of the gastrointestinal tract suggests that vasoconstrictor substances other than norepinephrine may also contribute to the sympathetic nervous vasoconstriction.

*Autoregulatory escape.* The presence of an autoregulatory escape from adrenergic influence has been shown in rats (188, 348), rabbits (348), cats (93, 94, 125, 126, 188, 191, 269, 270, 348), dogs (392, 393), and humans (191). It seems to be absent in baboons [(*Papia anubis*; (217)] but present in *Macaca mulatta* and *Aotus trivirgatus* (348).

The autoregulatory escape is not an experimental artifact caused by a depletion of the neurotransmitter(s) involved. This conclusion is based on several observations. The escape occurs at physiological rates of stimulation and can be seen on repeated electrical stimulations of the vasoconstrictor nerves (125, 126, 269, 270). Furthermore the escape is confined to the resistance vessels in the face of a well-maintained sympathetic influence on the precapillary sphincters and the capacitance vessels. Finally the response may also be evoked reflexly, e.g., by unloading the baroreceptors (298).

The first question to be discussed in regard to the autoregulatory escape in the small intestine is where does the escape occur. The original idea proposed by Folkow et al. (126) and Wallentin (427) was that the escape depends, at least in part, on the opening of

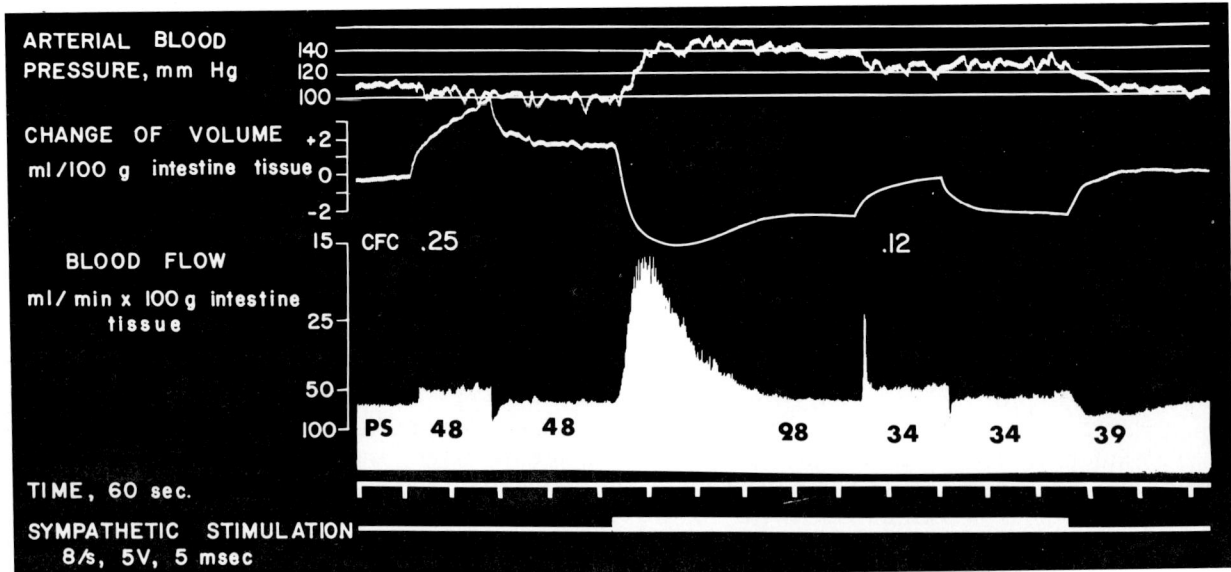

FIG. 3. Effect of electrical stimulation of splanchnic nerves (*signal*) on arterial pressure, tissue volume, intestinal blood flow, capillary filtration coefficient (CFC, $K_{f,c}$), and permeability–surface area product (PS) for $^{86}$Rb in feline small intestine. PS values were determined at regular intervals as indicated on figure. CFC was estimated from slow, continuous increase of tissue volume while increasing venous outflow pressure. Blood flow was measured with drop counter coupled to ordinate writer, implying that ordinate height is inversely proportional to rate of blood flow. Note that vasoconstriction of veins (estimated from decrease of tissue volume) and precapillary sphincters (measured with CFC and PS) is maintained in the face of decreasing flow resistance. [From Dresel et al. (93).]

submucosal vascular shunts. This conclusion was based on determinations of $K_{f,c}$ (Fig. 3) and on studies of the distribution of intra-arterially injected India ink, which suggested that blood flow in the mucosa is lowered during nervous vasoconstriction. Folkow and co-workers (126) proposed that the *Venenbällchen* described by Spanner (385) in the submucosa represent such shunts. A redistribution of blood flow explains why $K_{f,c}$ remains low when total intestinal blood flow increases. However, the studies by Dresel et al. (93) using $^{86}$Rb exclude the involvement of true shunts. In his thesis, Wallentin (427) summarized his own and Folkow's work on the escape and concluded that the escape reflects a relaxation of previously constricted vessels, leading to a physiological shunting of blood through capillaries. This opinion was later supported by other researchers (241, 372), who observed a decline of oxygen consumption when activating the vasoconstrictor fibers also during constant-flow conditions. This was interpreted as a closing of some of the intestinal precapillary sphincters.

The proposal that a redistribution of blood flow from the mucosa to the submucosa occurs during sympathetic nervous stimulation has not been confirmed by researchers using the $^{86}$Rb-clearance technique (93, 348), microspheres (152), in vivo microscopy (41), indicator-dilution methods (389), or carbon monoxide uptake (382) as a measure of mucosal blood flow. None of these studies demonstrated that mucosal blood flow decreased proportionally more than total intestinal blood flow during nervous stimulation. In two studies, one of which attempted to estimate submucosal blood flow (152, 348), no vasodilatation was observed in this wall layer. In humans, the flow distribution to the mucosa-submucosa and to the muscular layer has been investigated (191). A slight redistribution of flow from the muscle layer to the superficial parts of the intestinal wall seems to occur, but the technique used could not measure blood flow in the submucosa selectively.

From this discussion one may conclude that the escape seems to be explained by a physiological shunting of blood flow in the intestinal tissue through previously nervously constricted vessels. The location of this event is not fully established. One possibility is that it occurs throughout the whole intestinal wall. However, observations made in our laboratory, where two techniques based on two entirely different physical principles were used, suggest that the autoregulatory escape reflects a flow redistribution within the mucosa.

Svanvik (389) recorded plasma flow in the intestinal villi using a technique based on the indicator-dilution principle involving the recording of the passage of an intravascular tracer ($^{198}$Au-labeled colloids) through the superficial parts of the mucosa. During the stimulation of the sympathetic nerves, a villus vasoconstriction was seen concomitant to the initial decrease of total intestinal blood flow (Fig. 4). The escape of total blood flow was accompanied by an escape of the villus vessels. In fact villus plasma flow (and villus plasma volume) increased to a level that was slightly higher than control, despite continued sympathetic nerve activation. Svanvik proposed that the vessels supplying the intestinal crypts—less sensitive to vasodilator metabolites—are dominated by sympathetic fibers. The tone of the villus arterial vessels, on the other hand, is largely determined by the chemical environment surrounding them as they pass between the crypts. On nerve stimulation both types of vessels constrict, and the escape is explained largely by the dilatation of the villus vessels, when metabolites accumulate in the crypt region.

Svanvik's results (389) were confirmed in an indirect way by the results reported by Sjövall et al. (382). They studied the steady-state phase of sympathetic vasoconstriction using a combination of methods (inert-gas elimination from the muscle layer and carbon monoxide uptake from the lumen) to estimate what they called absorptive site (mainly villus) blood flow, nonabsorptive site (mainly crypt) blood flow, and muscle layer blood flow. After they allowed total intestinal blood flow to decrease (i.e., by keeping arterial pressure constant) during the nervous vasoconstriction, they observed a marked vasoconstriction of the nonabsorptive site blood flow, whereas blood flow in the villi remained largely unchanged. The fraction of total blood flow distributed to the muscle layer was not influenced by sympathetic nerves. The results of these two studies are also consistent with the findings of an unchanged blood flow distribution between mucosa, submucosa, and muscle reported during nervous vasoconstriction by Ross (348).

Several explanations for the reopening of the nervously vasoconstricted vessels have been proposed. Svanvik's hypothesis (389) infers the involvement of metabolites accumulating in the intestinal wall during the initial nervous vasoconstriction. Granger and Shepherd (147, 371) also proposed a model for the autoregulatory escape and suggested that tissue metabolites, partial pressure of $O_2$ ($P_{O_2}$) in particular, are fully responsible for the escape from the adrenergic influence. There are few, if any, experimental observations that directly infer the participation of metabolites in the escape phenomenon. However, the vasodilatation seen on cessation of the nervous stimulation clearly suggests the presence of vasodilating metabolites in the tissue. Furthermore the slow onset of the escape is compatible with a metabolite accumulation. Keeping blood flow constant through the intestine with a pump during the nervous stimulation does not abolish the escape phenomenon (94, 152, 241), and a decrease in oxygen consumption still occurs (372). The latter observation suggests that even during constant-flow conditions a vasoconstriction may occur in some part of the intestinal wall, leading to an accumulation of metabolites.

Based on their in vitro work summarized earlier (see

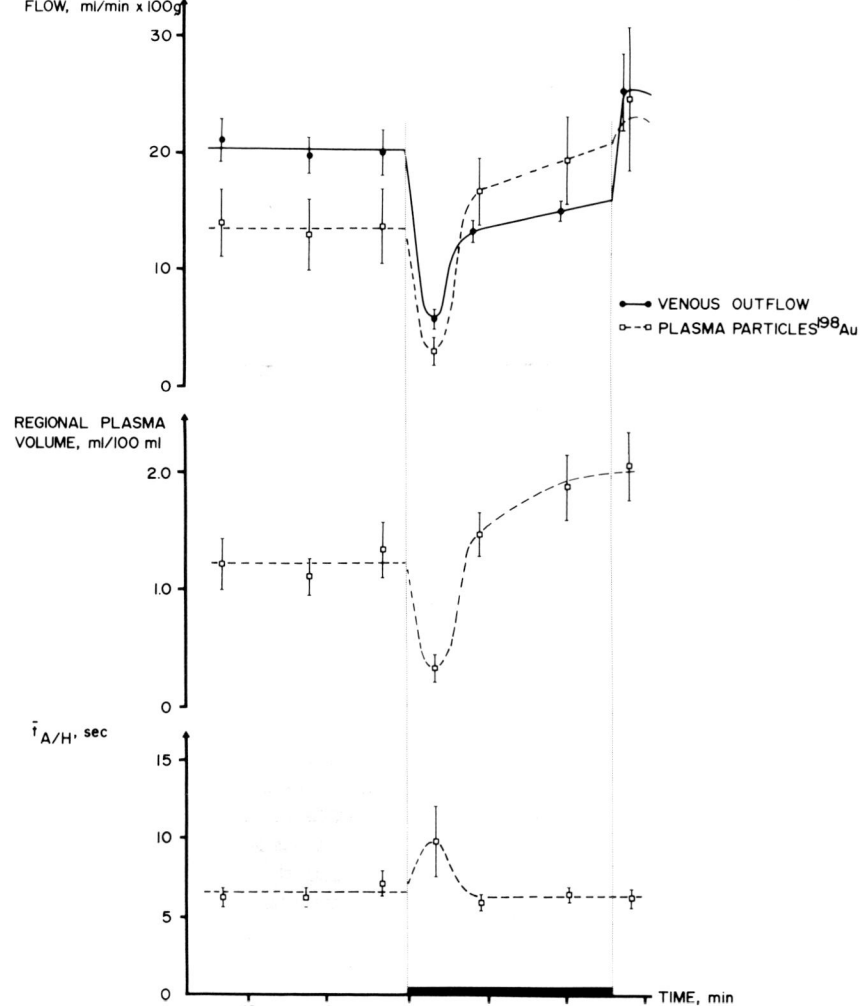

FIG. 4. Effect of electrical stimulation of periarterial nerves (signal) on venous outflow and on flow, volume, and mean transit time ($t_{A/H}$) for plasma in villi. Experiment was performed in cat small intestine, and electrical stimulation was performed at 8 Hz, 10 V, 5 ms. [From Svanvik (389).]

PHYSIOLOGY: IN VITRO STUDIES, p. 1670), Fara and Ross (109, 113, 352) suggested another mechanism for the autoregulatory escape. They proposed that the escape to norepinephrine may be due to an inherent property of the vascular smooth muscle cells and is not dependent on any external influence such as an accumulation of dilating metabolites. The same conclusion was reached by Henrich (173). According to Ross (352), the escape is due to a fading of the propagated electrical activity of the vascular smooth muscle as a response to continuous stimuli, a mechanism similar to the more general phenomenon of adaptation. According to Richardson and Johnson (337), the myogenic properties underlying the autoregulatory escape are not identical to those explaining the autoregulation of intestinal blood flow.

An involvement of $\beta$-adrenergic receptors in the autoregulatory escape was proposed by Ross (349). This may be the explanation to the escape seen during infusion of norepinephrine in cats and rats, although Henrich et al. (176) could not demonstrate any corresponding phenomenon in rats. Similarly, Ross (352) was unable to demonstrate any effect of a $\beta$-blocking agent on isolated strips of mesenteric vessels. Furthermore the nervously elicited escape has not been shown to be influenced significantly by $\beta$-adrenergic receptor blockers (349, 373). Thus the available experimental evidence suggests that the escape seen after a nervous vasoconstriction is not mediated via $\beta$-adrenergic receptors.

Finally Shanbour and Jacobson (369) proposed two other mechanisms for the escape, i.e., a refractoriness of the adrenergic receptors on the vascular smooth muscle cells and/or a release of undefined dilator substances. According to the authors, the mechanisms function independent of a possible accumulation of metabolites. The evidence for the proposals is largely circumstantial, but the histochemical investigations demonstrating several putative neurotransmitters in the same neuron suggest that a release of an undefined dilator substance is a viable hypothesis.

In summary, a number of mechanisms have been

proposed for the vascular escape from adrenergic influence. The nervous escape is apparently an adjustment occurring in the intestinal wall, possibly a relaxation of the villus arterial vessels in response to an accumulation of vasodilating metabolites. The available evidence suggests that norepinephrine does not in all details mimic the nervously evoked autoregulatory escape. Finally the latter phenomenon seems not to reflect any inherent property of the vessels in the mesentery.

The physiological importance of the escape phenomenon is not known. It should be pointed out, however, that some observations made by Henrich and Lutz (174) suggest that the initial strong vasoconstriction is more or less absent when the infused dose of norepinephrine is slowly increased, simulating the changes occurring during more physiological conditions. Similarly one would assume that the rate of firing in the splanchnic nerves seldom increase from 0 to 8 Hz (the firing rate at which the most pronounced escape is observed) within 1–2 s in the intact organism. Hence the initial vasoconstriction is in a sense an experimental artifact, and the steady-state phase probably represents a more physiological hemodynamic situation.

Steady state of nervous vasoconstriction. There are several reports concerning the reactions of the resistance vessels during adrenergic influence (15, 93, 94, 125, 126, 137, 148, 152, 176, 241, 270, 337, 348, 372, 373, 375, 392, 393). Most of the observations were made during the intravascular infusion of catecholamines, although the direct nervous influence on the vascular smooth muscles plays a much more important quantitative role in vivo. Nervous vasoconstriction evokes a comparatively moderate blood flow decrease, in contrast to the findings seen, e.g., in skeletal muscle. Most studies of the intestinal vascular bed report resistance increases not exceeding 100%, even at stimulation rates in the upper range of the physiological values (~10 Hz). In contrast, stimulation of the sympathetic vasoconstrictor fibers to the hindlimb skeletal muscles of the cat increases flow resistance 5–8 times at corresponding rates of stimulation (284, 285).

The pharmacological analysis of the sympathetic vasoconstriction in the small intestine has shown that the sympathetic effect is more or less completely abolished by $\alpha$-adrenergic receptor antagonists (51, 86, 310, 350). In an attempt to differentiate between $\alpha_1$- and $\alpha_2$-effects, Patel et al. (310) showed that both receptor types probably participate in the intestinal sympathetic vasoconstriction. In the colonic vascular bed, $\alpha$-adrenergic blocking agents only reduce the sympathetic vasoconstriction (172). This has been explained by the concomitant release of NPY, as discussed in *Neuropeptide Y*, p. 1678.

The blood flow distribution within the intestinal wall during adrenergic influence has mostly been studied in cats. All quantitative studies in this species suggest that there is virtually no redistribution between the mucosa-submucosa and the muscularis layers (152, 191, 349). However, there is experimental evidence for a redistribution within the mucosa during nervous stimulation in such a way that blood flow in the villi is maintained during the nervous influence, whereas a vasoconstriction occurs in the crypts. The findings by Svanvik (389, 390) and Sjövall et al. (382), supporting this view, were reviewed in some detail above. The results from the report by Sjövall et al. are summarized in Table 1. As shown in Table 1, the maintenance of blood flow in the villi during nervous vasoconstriction infers that the fraction of total blood flow distributed to that part of the intestine increases from 30% to 50%.

Bohlen et al. (41) reported observations on rats that may be interpreted to mean that flow resistance in the villi decreases during nervous vasoconstriction also in that species. Bohlen and co-workers used the methods of in vivo microscopy to measure red cell velocities, vessel diameters, and microvascular pressures. At a stimulation rate of 16 Hz, flow resistance in the villous circulation is only one-half of that of control in the presence of an unchanged resistance in the muscle layer.

One study has been devoted to the sympathetic nervous control of the human intestinal circulation. Hultén et al. (191) showed that a larger fraction of total blood flow is distributed to the mucosa-submucosa during the steady-state phase of nervous vasoconstriction than during control studies. The comparison of the flow distribution at equal total blood flows makes the difference particularly pronounced. At a total blood flow of ~20 ml·min$^{-1}$·100 g$^{-1}$, ~60% of

TABLE 1. *Effect of Sympathetic Nerve Stimulation on Total Blood Flow, Intramural Flows, and Flow Distribution in Cat Small Intestine*

| | Total Intestinal Blood Flow | Absorptive Site | | Nonabsorptive Site | | Muscle Layer | |
|---|---|---|---|---|---|---|---|
| | | F | D | F | D | F | D |
| Control | 24.8 ± 3.2 | 6.4 ± 0.6 | 28.4 ± 3.1 | 12.3 ± 3.1 | 43.1 ± 6.5 | 6.1 ± 0.6 | 28.8 ± 4.2 |
| Stimulation | 14.5 ± 1.6 | 6.8 ± 0.6 | 50.1 ± 5.4 | 4.1 ± 1.8 | 21.4 ± 8.2 | 4.5 ± 0.6 | 30.7 ± 5.0 |
| Control | 25.0 ± 3.2 | 7.3 ± 1.0 | 33.1 ± 6.4 | 12.4 ± 3.8 | 39.6 ± 8.8 | 6.6 ± 0.7 | 27.6 ± 4.0 |

Values are means ± SE of 11 observations. Arterial blood pressure was kept constant during 4-Hz stimulation. Blood flow expressed in ml × min$^{-1}$ × 100 g$^{-1}$ intestine; flow distribution (D) measured in percent of total blood flow; F, intramural flows. [From Sjövall et al. (382).]

total blood flow is diverted to the mucosa-submucosa during control conditions and ~90% during sympathetic nerve activation.

One important hemodynamic observation made by Folkow et al. (126) was that $K_{f,c}$ is markedly reduced during the nervous vasoconstriction, as is $^{86}$Rb clearance. It was concluded that these observations reflected a nervously induced reduction of perfused capillaries as a consequence of a constriction of precapillary sphincters, leading to a physiological shunting of blood flow in parts of the mucosa. In agreement with this, several researchers have reported that oxygen uptake decreases during nervous vasoconstriction, an observation that has been interpreted to mean that the mean distance for blood-tissue oxygen delivery is so increased that oxygen delivery becomes diffusion limited. Quantitatively $K_{f,c}$ decreases to approximately one-half of control when the sympathetic fibers are stimulated at 8 Hz (Fig. 3). Oxygen uptake decreases by 60%–70% of control in the same experimental situation (372, 373).

Folkow et al. (126) observed that the intestinal tissue volume stayed constant during stimulation of the sympathetic nerves after the initial constriction of the capacitance vessels. This observation indicates that mean hydrostatic capillary pressure in the whole small intestine remains constant during sympathetic nervous vasoconstriction. One cannot exclude, however, the possibility that mean capillary pressure does change in the different layers of the intestinal wall in such a way that the overall effect is an unchanged tissue volume. Bohlen and Gore (39) measured pressures in the microvessels of the intestinal wall layers of innervated and denervated intestines without finding any difference in mean capillary pressure between the two groups. Because firing rate in the innervated rat intestines is probably fairly low (≤3 Hz), higher rates of stimulation may influence mean capillary pressure. In another study by Bohlen and Gore (40), it was also shown that electrical stimulation of the splanchnic nerves at frequencies >4 Hz lowers pressures in small arterioles in the muscle layer, at least during the first 2 min of stimulation. The short observation period implies that the measured pressures may not be representative for the steady-state phase of vasoconstriction. Finally Granger et al. (143) attempted to estimate mean capillary pressure with a method involving the occlusion of the venous outflow from an intestinal segment and recording the changes in tissue volume. With this indirect method, they estimated that postganglionic sympathetic nerve stimulation at 4 Hz decreases intestinal mean capillary hydrostatic pressure to ~1.75 mmHg. It is obvious that to resolve the question of the sympathetic influence on capillary pressure in the gut studies have to be performed in which direct pressure measurements in capillaries of the different vascular circuits of the intestinal wall are made during prolonged nerve activation.

A venous constriction that expels blood from the intestines is also induced by the sympathetic influence. The maximal reduction of regional blood volume induced by the sympathetic nerves is ~40% in cats (125), which is seen at the highest rate of nervous firing. The corresponding figure for dogs is ~60% (48, 90, 91). The sympathetic effect is in part passive because of a decrease in transmural pressure. It has been demonstrated that the greater the active part of this nervous vasoconstriction, the larger the venous transmural pressure. At a venous pressure of 0 cmH$_2$O, ~25% of the capacitance response to sympathetic stimulation in the feline small intestine is active, whereas the corresponding figure at 20 cmH$_2$O is 75% (299). Similar findings have been reported for dogs (49, 90, 91).

The relative and absolute amounts of blood that can be mobilized from the intestines by sympathetic nerve stimulation can be calculated from the intestinal blood content and from the figures given for nervously induced constriction of the intestinal capacitance vessels. In all species where such a calculation can be performed (humans, dogs, cats), it can be estimated that 1.5%–2% of the total body blood volume can be mobilized on maximal activation of the sympathetic vasoconstrictor fibers. This corresponds to the following absolute volumes: humans 50–170 ml (310); dogs (10 kg body wt) ~29 ml (90); cats (3 kg body wt) ~4 ml (125).

The vascular response pattern evoked by sympathetic activation has been studied mostly in the small intestine. The colonic vascular bed is in this respect much less investigated. The results available from experiments on cats (189) and humans (191) suggest that the vascular response is generally the same as that of the small intestine. This is particularly true for the response of the consecutive vascular sections (189). Thus an autoregulatory escape phenomenon is seen, and $K_{f,c}$ is markedly lowered during the steady-state phase of vasoconstriction. The flow distribution is poorly investigated. A nervous vasoconstriction is seen in both the mucosa and the muscle layer in the two species studied, i.e., humans and cats. In humans, the vasoconstriction seems to be more pronounced in the muscle layer, leading to a certain redistribution of flow toward the mucosa (191). This is not seen in cats (190).

One can only speculate on the significance for intestinal functions of the neurally induced vasoconstriction. The studies of the flow distribution within the mucosa of the small intestine show that the vasoconstriction occurs almost exclusively in the crypts, whereas villus blood flow remains unchanged as compared with control. Hence the absorption occurring in the villi is probably not influenced by the reduction of total intestinal blood flow occurring on sympathetic nerve activation. The reduction of crypt blood flow may, on the other hand, inhibit secretory mechanisms in that part of the gut. In line with this, we have shown that sympathetic stimulation diminishes tissue-to-lumen flux of water and as a result net fluid uptake increases (382) However, our results are not consistent with the view that the sympathetic control of intestinal fluid transport is entirely secondary to intestinal hemodynamic changes (382).

*Stomach.* The presence of adrenergic receptors in the gastric vascular bed has been demonstrated in several studies by intravascular administration of adrenergic drugs (35, 55, 82, 83, 129, 160, 161, 199, 290, 368, 440, 443). Oren-Wolman and Guth (302) made a detailed investigation of these receptors by studying the sensitivity of submucosal gastric arterioles of different sizes to norepinephrine in rat experiments where the submucosal vasculature was exposed in vivo. They were unable to demonstrate any difference in adrenergic sensitivity between different-sized arterial vessels in the submucosa. In this respect, the gastric submucosal vessels differ from those of the mesentery where a difference in sensitivity has been demonstrated (9).

The sympathetic nervous influence on the gastric circulation has also been investigated by many other researchers (158, 160, 161, 200, 201); all these reports consistently show a vascular constriction during sympathetic activation. The response pattern evoked by the vasoconstrictor fibers is in principle similar to that described in some detail for the small intestine, i.e., a transient vasoconstriction of the resistance vessels (autoregulatory escape from vasoconstrictor fiber influence), a constriction of the precapillary sphincters as reflected by a lowered $K_{f,c}$, and an expelling of blood from the stomach as a consequence of the constriction of the capacitance vessels. Mean capillary pressure remains at the control level, as judged by a constant volume during the sympathetic vasoconstriction. On cessation of stimulation, tissue volume, blood flow, and $K_{f,c}$ return to control levels within 2–3 min. Thus the vascular response pattern on sympathetic activation is similar in the stomach and in the small intestine. Quantitative differences may exist, but this question has not been studied experimentally.

With regard to parallel-coupled vascular circuits, it has been shown that splanchnic nerve stimulation at 10 Hz in dogs decreases corpus mucosal blood flow to 25% of control in the face of a 60% reduction of total gastric blood flow (184).

The stomach differs functionally from the small intestines in that the mucosa of the stomach is in principle a secretory structure, whereas the intestinal mucosa is mainly absorptive. The preceding paragraphs described the vascular response to sympathetic nervous activation seen during nonsecretory conditions. During the stimulation of the splanchnic nerves during gastric secretion, induced by, e.g., pentagastrin, a vasoconstriction is also seen. However, the response of the resistance vessels is more pronounced during the second than during the first 10-min period of sympathetic stimulation (158). This observation may be explained by the presence of dilating metabolites in the secreting tissue counteracting the constrictor influence of norepinephrine released by the nervous system during the first 10-min observation period, whereas during the second period the vasoconstriction has diminished acid secretion and hence also the concentration of vasodilating metabolites.

The latter proposal is supported by observations made on flow distribution within the gastric wall, which has been studied mostly with the aminopyrine technique of Jacobson and his co-workers (see ref. 199 and refs. 158, 183, 332, 333). Most of these studies have been devoted to an investigation of the effects of sympathetic nerve activation during enhanced gastric secretion evoked by gastrin infusion or vagal nerve stimulation. These studies showed that mucosal blood flow decreases to ~30% of control on stimulation of the vasoconstrictor fibers at 10 Hz. Similar observations were made by Semb (368) on conscious cats during intravenous infusion of norepinephrine at a rate of 1 $\mu g \cdot min^{-1} \cdot kg^{-1}$, with the use of a hydrogen-clearance technique to measure gastric mucosal flow. The rate of norepinephrine infusion used by Semb is within the physiological range of release from the adrenals. Concomitantly, gastric secretion of both $H^+$ and pepsinogen decreased strongly, an effect that may be secondary to a flow-induced deprivation of nutrients. This conclusion is also supported by the observation that the nervously induced secretion is more pronounced when blood pressure is prevented from increasing, i.e., when the mucosal vasoconstriction is most pronounced.

There are, however, observations that are more consistent with the hypothesis that the decrease of acid secretion on sympathetic nerve stimulation is not caused by the nervous vasoconstriction but by a direct effect of the adrenergic influence on the secreting cells. Two reports by Yokotani et al. (436, 437) support this hypothesis by showing an inhibition of vagally or betanechol-induced (cholinergic agonist) acid secretion by postganglionic splanchnic nerve stimulation in the face of a largely unchanged gastric mucosal blood flow. The experiments were performed on rats with the aminopyrine technique for measuring mucosal blood flow. Indirect support for a direct adrenergic influence on the parietal cell was also reported by Grund et al. (158), who found that oxygen extraction was unchanged before and during sympathetic nerve stimulation, despite the reduction of acid secretion. However, to our knowledge there are no reports demonstrating adrenergic receptors on the parietal cell.

The aminopyrine technique only allows investigation of the secretory portion of the gastric wall. Few studies have been devoted to investigations of changes of mucosal blood flow in relation to blood flow in the other parts of the gastric wall. Delaney and Grim (87), using the potassium-clearance technique, estimated that the amount of blood distributed to the mucosa was ~72% during control and 64% during norepinephrine infusion. A similar redistribution of blood flow was reported by Grund et al. (158) in cats during sympathetic nervous vasoconstriction and by Zinner et al. (442) in the baboon during epinephrine infusion.

### NEUROTRANSMITTER CANDIDATES

The peptides listed as neurotransmitter candidates represent substances that in the great majority of immunohistochemical investigations have been found exclusively in enteric nerves. Some early reports on the localization of SP and VIP suggested that these compounds also existed in epithelial cells, but subsequent investigations have failed to confirm this view.

### Enkephalins

The naturally occurring opiate receptor agonists Met- and Leu-enkephalin were isolated, characterized, and synthetized in 1975 (185) and a year later reported to be present in the myenteric plexus in gastrointestinal tract (102). From a series of morphological studies we now know that numerous nerve cell bodies containing Met- and Leu-enkephalins are present in the myenteric plexus throughout the gastrointestinal tract (136, 222, 363, 394). However, in the submucous plexus, a small number of immunoreactive cell bodies are found only in the duodenum and colon (rat) and in cecum (guinea pig). Nerve fibers containing enkephalin are abundant in the myenteric plexus and in the circular muscle layer, whereas the submucous plexus is less densely innervated. Only single fibers are seen around some blood vessels in the basal parts of the mucosa and the submucosa. At the mucosa, a few single fibers are occasionally found along the epithelium. In the epithelial cells, enkephalin-immunoreactive material seems only to be present in some species in specific areas of the gastrointestinal tract, e.g., in the pylorus and the duodenum of dogs. The morphological observations strongly indicate that the physiological role of the enkephalins in the gastrointestinal tract is that of neurotransmitters and not of blood-borne hormones.

The distribution of the enkephalins within the gastrointestinal wall indicates that a possible involvement of enkephalins in the control of gastrointestinal blood flow must primarily engage indirect mechanisms through a release of the peptide from interneurons that in turn influence the vascular innervation. It is well known that the enkephalins both hyperpolarize myenteric neurons, indicating an inhibition of neuronal activity (296), and elicit contractions of the muscularis propria through a direct action on receptors on the effector cell (31). The vascular effect on intravenous or intra-arterial administration of Met-enkephalin (dogs) or morphine (humans) is an increase of blood flow to the gastrointestinal tract (227, 229, 243, 315, 428). In dogs, Konturek et al. (229) and Walus et al. (428) have shown that the vasodilatation is selectively localized to the gastric mucosa and to the intestinal muscle layer, respectively. Concomitantly, the gastric acid secretion and intestinal motility are stimulated, favoring an effect of the opioid peptide on the vasculature that is secondary to metabolic events in the tissue. It is unknown whether there are opioid receptors on vascular smooth muscles.

### Neuropeptide Y

Neuropeptide Y belongs to the pancreatic polypeptide family of peptides (Table 2) containing 36 amino acid residues. Its name refers to its localization to nervous tissue and to the fact that tyrosine residues are located at both the $NH_2$- and the COOH-terminals, Y being the abbreviation for tyrosine in the single-letter amino acid code. The NPY was isolated from the porcine brain by Tatemoto et al. (397) after the demonstration of pancreatic polypeptide-like material in the mammalian brain. With immunohistochemical techniques, NPY-like material has been demonstrated in both central and peripheral nerves (for review see ref. 103). In the gastrointestinal tract, the number of NPY-positive nerves found is even greater than that of nerves containing dopamine β-hydroxylase, an enzyme present in adrenergic nerves (263). The NPY immunoreactivity is found in the ganglion cells of the myenteric and submucous nervous plexuses and in nerves making contact with vascular smooth muscles (263, 264). In the nerves controlling vascular smooth muscles, NPY coexists with norepinephrine. This has been demonstrated in several tissues in all species studied, including humans [gastrointestinal tract, heart, lung, pancreas, urogenital tract (263, 264)]. The vascular innervation of NPY-containing neurons seems to be organized in the same way as is the adrenergic innervation described for norepinephrine. A typical ground plexus is found on the outer surface of the muscle media (103, 410), the plexus being more dense on arteries than on veins (410).

In the autonomic innervation of the gut, the coex-

TABLE 2. *Families of Hormones in Gastrointestinal Tract*

| Family | Substances |
|---|---|
| Gastrin | Cholecystokinin |
|  | Gastrin |
| Pancreatic polypeptide | Neuropeptide Y |
|  | Pancreatic polypeptide |
|  | Peptide YY |
| Secretin | Enteroglucagon (glicantin) |
|  | Gastric inhibitory peptide |
|  | Glucagon |
|  | Peptide histidine isoleucine |
|  | Secretin |
|  | Vasoactive intestinal polypeptide |

istence between NPY and norepinephrine is found in three locations: in sympathetic ganglia, in the pelvic plexus, and in the vascular innervation (263). The NPY nerve cell bodies in the nerve plexuses do not contain any norepinephrine. Treatment of the guinea pig with the catecholamine neurotoxin 6-hydroxydopamine or with reserpine, which depletes cathecholamine stores, also depletes NPY-containing sympathetic neurons of their peptide immunoreactivity in many tissues. For that reason, the NPY immunoreactivity is absent in the vascular innervation of the gut wall after reserpine but present in the submucosal nerve cell bodies where NPY does not coexist with norepinephrine (103, 264). Abdominal sympathectomy causes the disappearance of some NPY fibers, notably those around blood vessels (99, 134, 387), suggesting that these adrenergic nerves are extrinsic.

The effects of NPY on several rabbit arteries and veins were studied in vitro by Edvinsson et al. (97). They found that NPY in a 30 nM concentration rarely causes a contraction of any of the arteries tested. A weak contraction was seen in four of six experiments on the gastroepiploic artery at an NPY concentration of 300 nM. The veins showed even weaker responses than the arteries. On the other hand, Edvinsson and his co-workers demonstrated that NPY potentiates the vascular response to norepinephrine without affecting maximum response. The constriction of the gastroepiploic artery evoked by 10 $\mu$M norepinephrine is enhanced almost 300% by the presence of 10 nM NPY in the organ bath (97). Similar results were reported by Ekblad et al. (99) and Lundberg et al. (258). Lundberg et al. (84, 260) also showed that NPY enhances the contractile force of the rat portal vein.

The vascular effects of NPY in vivo have been investigated mainly in the submandibular gland (261) and in the colon (172). The circulatory studies have only been concerned with the reactions of total organ blood flow, and no detailed hemodynamic analysis of the type described earlier for the sympathetic influence has been performed. Both in the submandibular gland and in the colon, NPY (infused close intra-arterially) evokes a vasoconstriction that is more sluggish in onset than that seen with norepinephrine. In the colon, the NPY vasoconstriction has been estimated to be ~25 times more pronounced than that induced by norepinephrine when compared at the same molar concentrations. The threshold response to NPY was seen at a plasma concentration of 10 nM. This observation seems surprising in view of the quite weak vascular responses that were seen by Edvinsson et al. (97) in vitro. It suggests that most of the vascular effects of NPY in vivo is on vessels smaller than those studied by Edvinsson and co-workers.

The NPY-evoked vasoconstriction is not influenced by $\alpha$- or $\beta$-adrenergic receptor blocking agents (172). It has been suggested that the colonic vasoconstriction seen on electrical stimulation of the sympathetic nerves after blocking adrenergic receptors on the vascular smooth muscle cells is mediated by the release of NPY from the sympathetic nerves (172). In line with this, it has been found that guanethidine, which completely abolishes the colonic sympathetic vasoconstriction, also depletes the tissues of their NPY contents.

The coexistence of NPY and norepinephrine in the vascular innervation of the gastrointestinal tract represents an example of a peptide and a nonpeptide as cotransmitters. In other neurons, two peptides or two nonpeptides may coexist. The functional implications for nervous vascular smooth muscle control of the coexistence of NPY and norepinephrine are still obscure. The NPY is preferentially released at high frequencies, whereas norepinephrine is released at low, continuous frequencies of nerve stimulation (259). The effects may be pre- and postsynaptic, and in the case of NPY both types of actions have been demonstrated. Neuropeptide Y has been shown to inhibit the neurally induced release of norepinephrine through a presynaptic action in the portal vein (84) and in the femoral (258) and submandibular artery (265), whereas the same could not be demonstrated in the gastroepiploic artery (99). In the same preparations, an enhanced vascular contraction to norepinephrine or transmural electrical field stimulation is seen in vitro when NPY is present in the organ bath, suggesting a postsynaptic effect of NPY (84, 97, 99, 258). The latter effect has been suggested to reflect an unmasking of adrenergic receptors by NPY increasing the number of available $\alpha$-adrenoreceptor sites (2, 97). Another proposed mechanism for the enhanced vascular smooth muscle contraction in the face of decreased release of norepinephrine is that NPY facilitates excitation-contraction coupling in the muscles by increasing the availability to $Ca^{2+}$. This proposal is based on the observation that the NPY-induced contraction is blocked by $Ca^{2+}$-entry antagonist (258, 265).

*Peptide Histidine Isoleucine*

Peptide histidine isoleucine (PHI) is a peptide isolated in 1981 by Tatemoto and Mutt (399) that shows a striking sequence homology with the peptides within the secretin-glucagon family (Table 2), particularly with VIP. Furthermore VIP and PHI are derived from the same precursor molecule (67, 434). No PHI has been found in the intestinal epithelial cells (68), but PHI coexists with VIP in some neurons of the enteric nervous system. The pharmacological characteristics of PHI are similar to those of VIP. Thus intra-arterial infusion causes a vasodilatation in the submandibular gland of the cats, but PHI is much less potent than VIP when compared on a molar basis (262). To our knowledge no investigation has been performed on the effects of PHI on gastrointestinal blood flow.

## Substance P

Substance P is a polypeptide composed of 11 amino acid residues. The peptide was first isolated in a semipure form by von Euler and Gaddum (105) as an alcohol tissue extract lowering arterial pressure. It was found to be particularly abundant in the gastrointestinal tract and in the brain. It was later purified and characterized by Chang et al. (62).

Immunohistochemical studies have revealed that SP is mainly localized to nervous tissue. Cell bodies containing SP are present in nervous plexuses in almost all parts of the gastrointestinal tract (for details see refs. 213, 363). A dense SP innervation has been demonstrated in the muscular layer of the gastrointestinal tract of all species studied. The SP innervation of the mucosa is moderately dense in most species except in chicken and humans, where a dense SP innervation is observed (47, 213). The SP-immunoreactive fibers innervating vessels are present in the basal part of the mucosa and in the submucosa in all species studied, including humans (73, 213, 363).

The functional importance of the SP-containing fibers is unknown. The abundance of SP fibers in the muscular layers clearly indicates a controlling function of gastrointestinal motility by these nerves. It has also been proposed that SP fibers in the enteric nervous system are sensory in nature, based on the proposal that SP is the neurotransmitter in primary sensory neurons (318). The vascular innervation of SP fibers suggests that SP also controls blood flow, but it should be pointed out that a sensory function of the fibers making contact with the vasculature cannot be excluded.

The early observation by von Euler and Gaddum (105) that SP had hypotensive effects suggested that SP was a dilator agent, and this has been shown later to be the case. Löfström et al. (256), using a partially pure SP preparation showed a vasodilation in skin and muscle in humans. Intravenous (54, 168) or close intra-arterial (283, 322, 361) infusions of SP evoke vasodilatations in the superior mesenteric artery in the face of lowered perfusion pressure. Nerve-conduction blocking agents (tetrodotoxin) and various neurotransmitter receptor antagonists do not influence the vasodilatation evoked by SP (256, 361), suggesting that SP exerts its effect directly on the vascular smooth muscles. Substance P is a very potent vasodilator evoking its effects in pigs and dogs on intravenous infusion at a rate of $<1$ ng·min$^{-1}$·kg$^{-1}$ (i.e., $<1$ pmol·min$^{-1}$·kg$^{-1}$). As with many other vasodilator agents, SP causes contraction of vessels in vitro. This has been shown on the mesenteric and portal vein of rats (79, 205).

In one study on rats, SP given intravenously caused a decrease of gastric mucosal blood flow concomitant to an inhibition of the gastric acid secretion evoked by bethanechol or vagal stimulation (435). It is probable that the effect of SP on blood flow is secondary to its inhibitory effect on the secreting epithelium rather than a direct effect on the vascular smooth muscles.

There is scant evidence that SP is involved in any vasodilator mechanisms in the gastrointestinal tract. Stimulations of the vagal, splanchnic, and pelvic nerves have failed to evoke any increase in the release of SP-immunoreactive substances into the bloodstream (3, 11, 236). Furthermore the colonic vasodilatation evoked by electrical stimulation of the pelvic nerves is not influenced by a SP receptor antagonist (378). Therefore the available experimental evidence does not argue that SP-containing neurons are of any physiological importance in the control of gastrointestinal blood flow.

Although no studies indicate that electrical stimulation of nerves cause any release of SP into the blood stream, there is evidence for its release into the intestinal lumen (3, 411). This observation has prompted an investigation into the question whether luminal SP may evoke any change of intestinal blood flow. In such studies, Zinner et al. (155, 433, 444) have observed a doubling of mucosal blood flow of the feline small bowel when perfusing the lumen with a solution containing 1–2 nM SP. This effect was not influenced by hexamethonium, atropine, tetrodotoxin, or lidocaine. No change of portal venous SP immunoreactivity could be demonstrated. The authors concluded that the vascular SP effect is mediated through a nonneural mechanism of unknown nature. The concentration of SP in the intestinal perfusate used by Zinner and co-workers is several orders of magnitude higher than that observed in the gut, even during maximal electrical stimulation of the vagal nerves.

## Vasoactive Intestinal Polypeptide

Vasoactive intestinal polypeptide was isolated by Said and Mutt (356, 357) and shown to be a 28–amino acid residue (289) requiring the whole sequence for full biological activity (34). Initially VIP was believed to be located in epithelial cells in the gastrointestinal tract, but it is now generally agreed that VIP is almost exclusively localized to nerves (237, 238, 240).

The distribution of the VIP-containing nerves within the gastrointestinal wall has been studied in humans and in most laboratory animals (75, 76, 213, 237, 238, 240, 363). Generally the VIP-containing nerves are the major component of the peptidergic innervation of the gastrointestinal wall, and the fibers are extensively distributed in all parts of the alimentary canal. Numerous VIP-immunoreactive cell bodies are found particularly in the submucous plexus but also in the myenteric plexus. The VIP-immunoreactive nerve fibers, all of intrinsic origin (75), richly supply most effector cell types in the gastrointestinal wall, including the blood vessels. This indicates that

VIP may be involved in the nervous regulation of most gastrointestinal functions either directly at the effector cell or indirectly via VIP interneurons (75).

The vascular smooth muscle VIP innervation is found in all vessels of the gastrointestinal tract, including the large conduit arteries in the mesentery (409). The arterial innervation is more dense in the mucosa than in the submucosa (213). The veins are generally less innervated by VIP fibers than the arteries. After studying the vascular VIP innervation in more detail, Uddman et al. (410) reported that it is organized in the same manner as the adrenergic innervation in alimentary canal. Hence the peptide-containing nerve fibers are seen at the outer boundary of the smooth muscle media, suggesting that the released transmitter controls the outer smooth muscle layer directly and the rest of the muscle cells via low-resistance nexuses (cf. description of innervation of norepinephrine).

Vasoactive intestinal polypeptide was originally isolated from a fraction with vasoactive properties obtained during the purification of secretion, and it is now well established that VIP potently relaxes vascular smooth muscles in the gastrointestinal tract in vivo (11, 101, 138, 208, 356, 357). Furthermore Andersson et al. (11) investigated the relative sensitivity to VIP in the colonic and rectal vascular beds. They showed the intra-arterial infusions of VIP dose-dependently enhance the blood flow in both organs, the rectal vasculature being 50–100 times more sensitive. A vascular smooth muscle relaxation also occurs in vitro (205), which indicates that VIP acts directly on the vascular smooth muscles and not indirectly via a second messenger produced in the endothelium (cf. ref. 130).

It is well established that VIP evokes intestinal secretion (101), and therefore it seems most likely that the intestinal vasodilatation induced by VIP is mainly confined to the mucosa. This has also been confirmed in in vivo microscopy studies (181). On the other hand, Mailman (272) found that, besides eliciting an intestinal secretion, VIP reduced blood flow in the absorptive parts of the mucosa (i.e., in villi). The estimation of blood flow was, however, based in this study on the clearance of tritiated water from the small intestinal lumen, a method that has been questioned on theoretical grounds (266).

Vasoactive intestinal polypeptide has been proposed to be engaged as a neurotransmitter in the control of blood flow in all the segments of the gastrointestinal tract. It is well known that the acid secretion in the stomach, evoked by vagal stimulation, is accompanied by a mucosal vasodilatation that is usually considered to be secondary to the metabolism of the parietal cells (cf. discussion in *Acetylcholine*, p. 1668). However, an involvement of vasodilator nerve fibers cannot be excluded (266). Vagal activation of those nerve fibers in cats (so-called high-threshold fibers that evoke the acid secretion) and the vasodilatation result in an increased release of VIP into the venous drainage, which may indicate an involvement of vasodilator VIPergic neurons in the response (107). However, in dogs, intravascular infusions of VIP decrease gastric blood flow and pentagastrin-induced acid secretion (225), whereas the opposite effects are seen in cats (412).

During digestion, the blood flow in the small intestine increases markedly in those areas that are exposed to the chyme, i.e., a local mechanical or chemical stimulation seems to be necessary. The involvement of mechanical factors in the control of the intestinal circulation was suggested in a study by Fioramonti and Bueno (123). They demonstrated in conscious dogs that every migrating myelectric complex is accompanied by an intestinal hyperemia, provided the intestinal contents were not diverted in the orad direction. Furthermore, in anesthetized cats, Biber and co-workers (27, 28) showed that gentle mechanical stimulation of the intestinal mucosa elicits a local mucosal vasodilatation mediated via an intramural nervous reflex involving a serotonergic receptor. The mechanically induced vasodilatation is, however, not influenced by nicotinic-receptor blockade. A hyperemia with similar pharmacological characteristics as just described is also seen upon transmural electrical field stimulation of the feline small intestine (24).

Sjöqvist et al. (377) produced evidence supporting the hypothesis that VIP may be the transmitter substance at the vascular smooth muscles in the reflex studied by Biber et al. (24, 27, 28). This conclusion is based on the observations that mechanical activation, electrical field stimulation, or close intra-arterial infusions of serotonin [5-hydroxytryptamine (5-HT)] increase the VIP release into the venous effluent concomitantly with the vasodilatation (101, 107, 377). Furthermore, tetrodotoxin, a nerve-conduction blocker, inhibits both the VIP release and the vasodilatation (101). A concomitant inhibition of VIP release and hyperemia is also seen when giving apamin, a polypeptide isolated from bee venom (205, 377). Since apamin does not antagonize the VIP effect on the vascular smooth muscle either in vivo or in vitro, it was proposed that apamin acts through a presynaptic inhibition of VIP release (377). Also the chemically induced postprandial hyperemia seems to be accompanied by a release of VIP (138), which suggests that chemical stimuli may work via the same mechanisms as the mechanical ones.

It has also been proposed that VIP may be involved in the intense mucosal vasodilatation in the colon and rectum after activation of the defecation reflex. Direct electrical stimulation of the efferent fibers or reflex activation of these fibers in the pelvic nerves increase the VIP release into the venous effluent concomitantly with the vasodilatation in both colon and rectum (11, 12, 107, 377). Administration of apamin blocks both the colonic vasodilatation and the VIP release but leaves the nerve-induced motility and vasoconstrictor response unaffected (377).

In the discussed vasodilatator mechanisms in the small and large intestines, strong evidence favors the hypothesis that VIP is the neurotransmitter that relaxes the vascular smooth muscles. Vasoactive intestinal polypeptide fullfills most of the criteria for a substance to be accepted as a neurotransmitter (196). However, a specific VIP-receptor blocker is not yet at hand, and until such a substance is found and tested, VIP has to wait for a full acceptance as a neurotransmitter involved in the control of gastrointestinal blood flow.

## HORMONES

One of the five hormones discussed here, i.e., gastrin, has also been inferred to be localized in nervous tissue after Vanderhaeghen et al. (413) demonstrated that brain contains gastrinlike immunoreactivity. Because the bulk of this immunoreactivity has been found to be a molecule closely related to gastrin, i.e., cholecystokinin COOH-terminal octapeptide (CCK-8), we discuss gastrin as a "pure" hormone in this review. (For discussion of CCK see NEUROTRANSMITTERS AND/OR HORMONES, p. 1687.) One major problem that needs to be faced when reviewing hormonal effects is to establish the physiological plasma concentration of the hormones and, hence, to know whether the observed vascular effects are only induced by pharmacological plasma concentrations. Unfortunately, only few studies discussed in this review address this question.

There is, however, another way (other than through blood) in which hormones, secreted at the basolateral membrane of cells located in the intestinal epithelial layer, may influence the submucosal blood vessels controlling mucosal blood flow: namely, through the lymphatics. This is suggested by the morphological studies by Ohtani and Ohtsuka (301) who demonstrated that each submucosal arterial vessel is running in close contact with two lymphatic vessels, which drain the lymph from the lacteals in the villi. Hence lymph represents another vehicle for transporting substances from the villi to the submucosal arteries. When fluid absorption increases in connection with a meal, lymph flow via the lacteals also increases. Substances in the interstitial space of the villi may then very quickly be transported to the submucosa. The proposed mechanism has been demonstrated for $Na^+$, the concentration of which increases at the villus tip because of a countercurrent multiplication of this solute. Within minutes, an increased $Na^+$ concentration in the villi is reflected as an increased concentration also in the submucosa (38).

*Angiotensin*

There are three types (I–III) of angiotensin, with angiotensin II being the most important for cardiovascular control. This octapeptide is formed from angiotensin I by splitting off two amino acids. Angiotensin I, in turn, is formed from a plasma glycoprotein by renin, which is an acid protease released from the kidneys. The prime physiological role of the renin-angiotensin system and thus of angiotensin is to control the balance of $Na^+$ in the body (32).

It is well established that angiotensin is a very potent vasoconstrictor substance (cf. ref. 316). This property of angiotensin is supposed to be physiologically most important in the regulation of the transcapillary exchange in the renal glomeruli. However, in situations where $Na^+$ depletion is connected with a decrease in blood volume (e.g., in hemorrhage), angiotensin also seems to play an important role in the regulation of the systemic arterial pressure (128, 279, 281, 282). This observation is also supported by the finding that intravenous or intra-arterial infusions of angiotensin, resulting in plasma concentrations in the upper physiological or in pharmacological ranges, increase the resistance in the splanchnic vascular beds (127, 163, 313, 401).

There is a cooperation between angiotensin and the sympathetic nervous system that takes place at several different levels (for references see ref. 316). Thus angiotensin can induce pressure responses through central activation of the sympathetic nervous system by catecholamine release from the adrenal medulla, by nervous activation at the ganglionic level, and finally by facilitation of the norepinephrine release from peripheral sympathetic nerve endings. The last mentioned effect seems to be most pronounced at low physiological firing rates in sympathetic nerves. In line with this, it has been shown in the intestinal vascular bed that $\alpha$-adrenoreceptor partially inhibits the angiotensin-induced increase in vascular resistance (231, 249).

The constriction of the resistance vessels, induced by physiological plasma concentrations of angiotensin, seems to be well maintained (338), which contrasts with the response elicited by the adrenergic agonists (Fig. 3). However, at higher angiotensin concentrations, the response shows a tendency to fade (280) or exhibits tachyphylaxis (207). The number of capillaries open to perfusion is diminished by angiotensin, as judged by changes in $K_{f,c}$ (338) and oxygen consumption (313). No study of the angiotensin effect on mean hydrostatic capillary pressure in the gastrointestinal tract seems to have been published. On the other hand, there are several observations that indicate a negligible effect of angiotensin on the veins in the gastrointestinal tract (163, 401).

The vasoconstriction evoked by angiotensin is relatively more pronounced in the muscle layer than in the mucosa-submucosa, inferring a redistribution of blood flow to the latter layer (428). However, it is not known whether the vascular effect of angiotensin varies within the mucosa and is more pronounced in, for example, the intestinal crypt region as has been proposed for the adrenergic mechanisms.

*Antidiuretic Hormone*

The antidiuretic hormone (ADH) is a novapeptide, first isolated and characterized by du Vigneaud. It is synthesized in the cell soma of neurons in the supraoptic and paraventricular nuclei of the hypothalamus. The main function of ADH is to participate in the regulation of the osmolality in the body fluids. The osmolality of blood is the most important factor in the regulation of ADH release.

The nonosmotic control mechanisms of ADH release, e.g., the release via the sympathetic system, mainly exert their effects by lowering the threshold of the osmoregulatory system. However, at severe hypovolemia or hypotension, the nonosmotic control system can enhance the ADH plasma levels exponentially to reach concentrations in which it may exert potent vasoconstrictor influence (343, 362). Thus there are some observations indicating that ADH is of importance for the control of arterial pressure (80, 242) as well as of intestinal flow resistance (279, 281, 282) during hemorrhagic hypotension.

Intra-arterial or intravenous administration of ADH evokes a sustained reduction of the total blood flow to the whole splanchnic area (359, 364), to the small intestine (72, 170, 218, 349, 373), and to the colon (216). The escape phenomenon seen when the sympathetic nerves are activated (see *Norepinephrine*, p. 1669; Fig. 3) does not occur during the ADH infusion, and on its cessation blood flow gradually returns to the control values without any poststimulatory reactive hyperemia. However, villus blood flow shows a prominent reactive hyperemia on stopping the ADH infusion when studied with in vivo microscopy (181). This indicates that the different parallel-coupled vascular circuits within the intestinal wall react differently to ADH.

The capacitance vessels constrict on ADH infusion but to a much smaller degree than seen on activation of sympathetic nerves (116, 327). In in vitro experiments on isolated mesenteric vessels (210), ADH fails to influence the tonus of the smooth muscles of the portal and mesenteric veins. This supports the view that the capacitance response in vivo is mainly a passive phenomenon following a fall of transmural pressure, secondary to a constriction of the precapillary vessels (299). This property of ADH has been extensively used in the clinical treatment of bleeding varicose veins in the esophagus.

The effect of ADH on capillary fluid exchange has been studied by two groups. Granger and co-workers (327, 341) found that ADH markedly reduced the capillary surface area available for solute and fluid exchange as estimated by the $K_{f,c}$. The reduction in $K_{f,c}$ was more pronounced in the dog colon than in the cat ileum when compared at resistance responses of a similar magnitude. In the cat ileum, ADH was also reported to increase the precapillary-to-postcapillary resistance ratio, resulting in a fall of the mean capillary pressure and a net fluid transport from tissue to blood. However, this effect was apparently small, since in the only original recording shown in the report tissue volume reaches an isovolumetric state as soon as 3 min after the start of the ADH infusion. In the study of dog colon by Richardson et al. (341), the effects of ADH on mean capillary pressure were not reported.

The other group (116) found no change in $K_{f,c}$ or in mean capillary pressure after close intra-arterial ADH infusions in the small intestine of the cat. However, the increase in arterial resistance evoked by ADH in this study was only ~30%, i.e., a reduction of the flow resistance that in the study by Quillen et al. (327) only elicited a small decrease of $K_{f,c}$. Thus the findings of Fasth et al. (116) are the same as those reported by Quillen et al. (327) when comparisons are made at similar changes of flow resistance. Furthermore it seems clear from the studies on $K_{f,c}$ and capillary fluid exchange summarized here that the ADH plasma concentration needed to influence these variables is so high that it is doubtful whether the ADH effects on transcapillary exchange play any pathophysiological role even in severe hemorrhage.

*Epinephrine*

The catecholamines epinephrine and norepinephrine are released from the adrenal glands to act as hormones. The relative amounts of the two substances vary from species to species. Norepinephrine induces vasoconstriction via $\alpha$-adrenergic receptors as described in more detail in *Norepinephrine*, p. 1669.

Epinephrine is generally considered to differ from norepinephrine in that epinephrine more effectively stimulates $\beta$-adrenergic receptors. This seems also to be the case in the gastrointestinal tract. For example, close intra-arterial injections or infusions of epinephrine into the canine gastric circulation evoke an initial vasoconstriction (blocked by $\alpha$-adrenergic agents) followed by vasodilatation [$\beta$-adrenergic effect (192, 440, 441)], whereas norepinephrine only induces a vasoconstrictor response on intra-arterial infusion (440, 441). On the other hand, in the baboon, epinephrine causes a "pure" $\alpha$-adrenergic vasoconstriction (443). Two studies on dogs suggest that the effect of epinephrine may differ in different parts of the gastric microcirculation, causing a vasodilatation in one and a vasoconstriction in another part (192, 440, 441). The mechanism underlying this effect is unknown.

In quantitative terms, the gastric blood flow in the baboon was approximately halfed on intra-arterial infusion of 0.05 µg (0.03 nM)·min$^{-1}$·kg$^{-1}$ (443). The same dose in the dog, which is within the physiological range (60, 276), caused after a transient constriction an approximate doubling of mesenteric blood flow. However, the release of norepinephrine from nerve endings is of more quantitative importance for the control of blood flow than the release of the blood-borne catecholamines (60). This is explained by the fact that the neurotransmitter concentration that can be reached in the synaptic cleft is considerably higher than that in plasma (22, 60).

Intravenous infusions of epinephrine also cause both vasoconstrictor and vasodilator responses in the stomach (50, 82, 192, 290, 419, 440), although the vasodilator response seems to be more frequent on intravenous than on intra-arterial administration. This may be due to the fact that an intravenous infusion causes a more pronounced vasopressor response than the close intra-arterial infusion. This, in turn, may inhibit a sympathetic nervous vasoconstriction through an activation of vascular baroreceptors and/or volume receptors. Hence the effects seen on intravenous infusions of epinephrine may be reflecting not only the direct vascular effect of epinephrine.

Walder (426) reported from studies on excised human stomachs that epinephrine opens up arteriovenous shunts and allows 100-µm glass spheres to pass through the gastric vasculature. Zinner et al. (442) were unable to confirm any such effect in baboons with microspheres of 15-µm average diameter. This conclusion is in line with that reached by Lundgren (266), who after reviewing the literature on arteriovenous shunting in the gastrointestinal tract concluded that such shunts, if they exist, are of minor functional importance.

In the small intestine, the vascular response to intra-arterial and intravenous administration of epinephrine is qualitatively similar. Some vasoconstriction is reported by all researchers, who administered epinephrine in close intra-arterial infusion to the canine or rat gut (174, 176, 313, 314, 373, 392, 393, 401, 432), whereas an epinephrine infusion in the baboon evokes a vasodilatation (217). The investigations on the cat by Greenway and Lawson (149, 150) indicate that epinephrine given intravenously causes a vasodilatation in low doses but a vasoconstriction at high doses. Also in the dog, it can be shown that epinephrine stimulates β-adrenergic receptors, because the vasoconstrictor effect is potentiated after α-adrenergic blockade (313, 314, 373, 392, 393, 432). An autoregulatory escape reaction of the type described for the intestinal vasoconstriction after sympathetic nerve activation or infusion of norepinephrine has been observed by some investigators (173, 174, 392, 393). The doses used in the infusions experiments were the same as those used in the gastric experiments, i.e., within the physiological range.

Intra-arterial or intravenous injections evoke varying responses. Clark (69), Folkow et al. (124), and Binet et al. (29) observed vasoconstrictions recording venous outflow, whereas Bülbring and Burns (52) recorded an increased intestinal volume, which they interpreted as caused by vasodilatation. In two more recent studies (192, 392) an α-adrenergic vasoconstriction followed by a β-adrenergic vasodilatation was observed. No apparent explanation exists for these different results.

Most of the investigations summarized here have been devoted to studies of total organ blood flow. In a few studies, intramural blood flow has been recorded. Zinner et al. (442), using microspheres in the baboon, showed that epinephrine induces no major redistribution of blood flow between the different gastric wall layers during resting conditions. Jacobson et al. (199) measured gastric mucosal blood flow with the aminopyrine-clearance technique. The administration of epinephrine close intra-arterially during gastrin-induced acid secretion in the dog stomach diminished acid secretion and mucosal blood flow in the face of a largely unchanged celiac artery blood flow, implying a marked redistribution of flow caused by epinephrine. The different results obtained by Zinner et al. (442) and Jacobson et al. (199) are, at least in part, explained by the fact that the studies were performed during different functional states of the stomach.

The reactions of the consecutive vascular sections (resistance, exchange, and capacitance vessels) to epinephrine have been monitored by some researchers. Shepherd et al. (373) estimated the number of capillaries open to perfusion by determining $^{86}$Rb clearance and oxygen extraction in the small intestine of the dog. The results with both techniques suggested that a low dose of epinephrine relaxed the precapillary sphincters, whereas a higher dose induced sphincter vasoconstriction, diminishing the number of perfused capillaries. The authors attribute these effects to the action of epinephrine on different types of adrenergic receptors and/or metabolic effects of the catecholamine. Texter et al. (401) obtained experimental evidence for a venous vasoconstriction induced by epinephrine in the canine intestine.

## Gastrin and Pentagastrin

Gastrin is a polypeptide hormone found in the so-called G cells in the gastric antrum and the duodenum. Chemically gastrin exists in several forms, the most common ones being G-17 and G-4, consisting of 17 and 4 amino acid residues, respectively. The G-4 is considered to be most common in nervous tissue, as described in connection with CCK. Gastrin has a well-established hormonal function controlling gastric acid secretion. Its control of blood flow is closely coupled to the gastric acid production, as has been shown in several studies in which gastrin or its biological analogue pentagastrin was used.

Two studies have been devoted to the general hemodynamic effects of pentagastrin administered intravenously (187, 383). At the doses given, gastric blood flow increased, in one of the studies concomitant to an increase in duodenal-pancreatic blood flow. All other vascular beds were unaffected, implying that the vascular effects of gastrin are limited to the upper parts of the gastrointestinal tract (187, 273, 383). Very high doses of pentagastrin may, however, increase blood flow in other parts of the gastrointestinal tract (108).

It has been demonstrated repeatedly that gastrin and pentagastrin in doses that increase gastric acid secretion increase gastric mucosal blood flow (162, 183, 198, 199, 248, 274, 286, 304, 334, 354, 367, 383, 400, 417–419). This effect has also been shown in humans with pentagastrin (159). Many of these studies were performed with the clearance method originally described by Jacobson et al. (199) in which aminopyrine or a similar tracer was used. Total blood flow to the stomach may in some instances be constant in the face of a clear-cut increase of mucosal blood flow upon giving gastrin and pentagastrin. This was, for example, shown by Swan and Jacobson (391), who performed experiments on Heidenhahn pouches in dogs. Acid secretory rate increased in a dose-dependent manner when gastrin was given. Mucosal blood flow increased concomitantly, whereas total blood flow to the pouch measured with an electromagnetic flowmeter remained constant.

The observations by Swan and Jacobson (391) strongly suggest that an increasing fraction of total gastric blood flow is distributed to the mucosa during acid secretion. This has also been demonstrated in the corpus of the human stomach with an inert-gas clearance method (194). In the resting state, ~75% of total gastric blood flow is diverted to the mucosa-submucosa. The increase in total gastric blood flow from an average value of 13 to 53 ml·min$^{-1}$·100 g$^{-1}$ after giving pentagastrin subcutaneously [6 μg (8 μmol)/kg body wt] increased the fraction diverted to the mucosa-submucosa to >95%. Similar observations were made with the microsphere technique by Skarstein et al. (383) and Varhaug et al. (417, 418) on the feline stomach.

The aminopyrine-clearance method used in several studies of the hemodynamic effects of gastrin and pentagastrin is based on the fact that weak bases, lipophilic at a normal pH, become ionized and lipophobic in an acid environment such as the gastric lumen. Hence the aminopyrine cleared from plasma into the gastric lumen is trapped by the low pH of the gastric juice. The methods based on such principles can only measure blood flow in the acid-secreting parts of the gastric mucosa. To study the distribution of blood flow between the different parts of the stomach (antrum, corpus, fundus) other techniques must be used, such as the microsphere method and inert-gas clearance techniques. Studies with such methods show both in humans and in animals that pentagastrin increases blood flow only in corpus, i.e., where the acid is secreted (194, 355). This observation indicates that gastrin's vascular effects are mainly secondary to its effects on secretion through an accumulation of metabolites and/or hypoxia. This conclusion is also supported by the investigations showing that the vasodilatation in the gastric wall on pentagastrin infusion is confined to the mucosa.

*Glucagon and Enteroglucagon*

Glucagon, a 29–amino acid residue polypeptide, is secreted by the α-cells of the pancreatic islets and is primarily involved in the regulation of plasma glucose concentration. Biochemically it resembles gastric inhibitory peptide (GIP), secretin, and VIP (Table 2). A glucagon-like peptide (enteroglucagon) is present in some intestinal epithelial cells (L cell) and is, in contrast to the pancreatic glucagon, released in connection with a meal (395). The function of enteroglucagon is unknown, and to our knowledge it has not been examined with regard to its cardiovascular effects.

The normal glucagon concentration in plasma is between 50 and 150 pg (15–45 fmol)/ml (202a), but at stress situations in conscious monkeys the plasma concentration may reach values ≦2 ng (0.5 pmol)/ml (33). The peripheral vascular effects of glucagon are mainly localized to the mesenteric and hepatic vascular beds (45, 223, 347). Intra-arterial fusions of glucagon in doses that probably correspond to plasma concentrations of ~20–40 ng (5–10 pmol)/ml induce a sustained and significant vasodilatation in the superior mesenteric and hepatic arteries of cats (144, 347), whereas blood flow in the femoral and renal arteries is unaltered (347). Intravenous infusions at rates of ≧1 μg (300 pmol)·min$^{-1}$·kg$^{-1}$ cause a similar response in dogs (186, 271, 342, 406) and in monkeys (45), whereas an enhanced jejunal blood flow is reported in cats at a dose of 0.25 μg (70 pmol)·min$^{-1}$·kg$^{-1}$. These observations strongly indicate that the plasma concentration of glucagon, necessary to dilate the mesenteric resistance vessels, is at or above the maximal physiological level.

The peripheral vascular effect of glucagon is not influenced by extrinsic denervation or β-adrenergic blockade (347). Furthermore, it is not related to changes in plasma glucose levels (405).

In the small intestine, glucagon seems to elicit an increased villus blood flow even when the superior mesenteric blood flow is unchanged, suggesting a particular sensitivity to glucagon of the vessels controlling the villus circulation (181). In contrast, the submucosal (cats) and mucosal (rats) arterioles of the stomach are not affected by intra-arterial infusions of glucagon in doses ≦27 μg (8 nmol)·min$^{-1}$·kg$^{-1}$ (162).

In the dog ileum, close intra-arterial administration of glucagon [50 pg (15 fmol)·min$^{-1}$·kg$^{-1}$] significantly increases $K_{f,c}$ and mean capillary pressure (144). The latter effect of glucagon reflects a decrease of the precapillary-to-postcapillary resistance ratio. Furthermore measurements of lymph-to-plasma protein concentrations suggest that glucagon also increases capillary hydraulic conductivity. These vascular effects were proposed to be responsible for the intestinal secretion induced during the glucagon infusion, which, according to Granger et al. (144), is further facilitated by a disruption of the mucosal epithelium. An enhancement of $K_{f,c}$ was also reported by Richardson (339) in the cat jejunum when giving glucagon intravenously [0.25 $\mu$g (70 pmol)$\cdot$min$^{-1}\cdot$kg$^{-1}$] but only after $\alpha$-adrenoceptor blockade. This can be explained by the finding that glucagon releases catecholamines from the adrenal glands (118).

*Secretin*

Secretin, discovered in 1902 by Bayliss and Starling, is a polypeptide containing 27 amino acids (288) and localized only to the intestinal epithelial cells (56, 320). Chemically secretin is related to VIP (Table 2). Secretin is believed to be released from the duodenum and the upper part of the small intestine in response to an acid environment in the gut lumen, controlling pancreatic secretion.

Porcine secretin given close intra-arterially or intravenously in doses believed to be physiological evokes a dilatation of the resistance vessels in the small intestine of cats (26, 112, 114, 115, 340, 346), rabbits (89), and dogs (64) as well as an increase of $K_{f,c}$ (26, 340). However, most studies on the gastric circulation have failed to demonstrate any gastric vascular response (19, 87, 115), except in one study where vasoconstriction was observed, probably secondary to an inhibition of gastric acid secretion (199).

In experiments with synthetic secretin it has not been possible to reproduce the observations on the small intestine made with porcine secretin and summarized in the preceding paragraph. No vascular response is seen in either the gastric or the intestinal vascular beds (44, 162), suggesting that porcine secretin contains an impurity (possibly VIP) that causes the vascular effects. Thus there seems to be no evidence favoring a role for secretin in the physiological regulation of gastrointestinal blood flow.

## HORMONE CANDIDATES

Most of the peptides isolated from the gastrointestinal tract have originally been proposed to be hormones. Subsequent investigations have often shown that many of the newly discovered compounds are possible neurotransmitters or may function as both neurotransmitters and hormones. However, GIP, motilin, pancreatic polypeptide, and peptide YY (PYY) are examples of peptides generally believed to function only as hormones. These proposals are usually based on at least two types of observations: the immunohistochemical demonstration of the peptide in certain epithelial cells and the release of the compound into blood in connection with a meal. To our knowledge, there are no studies that show that GIP or pancreatic polypeptide influence gastrointestinal blood flow. A few studies of motilin and PYY are reviewed in this chapter.

*Motilin*

Motilin is a 22–amino acid polypeptide originally isolated from the porcine gut. It has been shown to lower blood pressure in a dose-dependent manner in the pithed rat without changing heart rate. This effect was seen when giving motilin intravenously in doses ranging from 30 to 300 nmol/kg body wt (98). It was suggested in that study that motilin lowers blood pressure via a direct action on the vascular smooth muscles. Konturek et al. (224) studied the effect of a synthetic analogue to motilin on the gastric secretion of acid and pepsinogen and on the mucosal hyperemia evoked by pentagastrin or histamine. Motilin inhibited the secretion and reduced mucosal blood flow. Konturek and collaborators concluded that the vasoconstriction evoked by motilin is secondary to its action on gastric secretion. The contradictory results of these two studies clearly indicate that we do not know whether motilin is of any importance for cardiovascular control.

*Peptide YY*

Peptide YY is a 36–amino acid residue polypeptide recently isolated from the porcine small intestine by Tatemoto and Mutt (396, 398). Like NPY, PYY belongs to the pancreatic polypeptide family of peptides (Table 2), and its name refers to the fact that there are tyrosine residues at both ends of the PYY molecule. The peptide has been localized to epithelial cells, particularly in the distal part of the small intestine and in the colon. Some cells are provided with a process in the basal region, suggesting a paracrine action of PYY when released. It is released by the presence of fatty acids in the intestinal lumen (12a, 306, 307). Peptide YY is presumably a hormone, but its physiological functions are not known. It has been suggested that it inhibits pancreatic secretion (193, 306, 307, 396).

The vascular effects in the gastrointestinal tract have been investigated in the feline small intestine. There PYY was shown to cause vasoconstriction in a dose of 150 pm/kg body wt given close intra-arterially. The vascular effect was unaffected by guanethidine (261). Similar observations have been reported in the pancreas (193) and in the submandibular gland (261,

262). It is not known whether the observed vascular effects are of physiological importance.

## NEUROTRANSMITTERS AND/OR HORMONES

### Cholecystokinin

Cholecystokinin is one of the classic intestinal hormones first isolated and characterized by Mutt and Jorpes (287). It is a polypeptide consisting of 33 amino acid residues. The biological activity resides in the 8 amino acids in the carboxylic end of the molecule. Chemically it is related to gastrin, and the 4 amino acids at the carboxylic end are identical to that of gastrin (Table 2). Cholecystokinin immunoreactivity has been demonstrated in epithelial cells in the intestinal tract, presumed to have a hormonal function (I cells), and in nerves in the central and peripheral nervous systems. The CCK located in nerves is the 8- or 4-amino acid carboxylic end of the hormone (CCK-8, CCK-4). Because the 4-amino acid sequence is identical to that of gastrin, the nervously situated CCK is sometimes referred to as gastrin/CCK.

The nervous distribution of CCK has been most thoroughly studied in the guinea pig and the rat. The number of cell bodies and nerve fibers showing immunoreactivity to gastrin/CCK is much smaller than that of SP, VIP, enkephalins, and somatostatin. Cell bodies staining for gastrin/CCK immunoreactivity are only present in the colon of rats and guinea pigs. Immunoreactive nerve fibers are seen in all parts of the gastrointestinal tract but mostly in small numbers and not in all layers (for a detailed description see ref. 363). Immunoreactive fibers are observed around blood vessels in the basal part of the mucosa and in the submucosa of all parts of the alimentary canal of the rat but only occasionally in the guinea pig. The physiological function of these nerves is not known.

The established physiological role of CCK is that of controlling the enzyme-rich secretion from the pancreas and the tonus of the smooth muscles in the gallbladder. The role of CCK in the control of gastrointestinal blood flow is less clearly established. Intra-arterial or intravenous infusions of CCK in amounts assumed to be physiological cause a vasodilatation in the small intestine of cats (26, 112, 114, 115) and dogs (64). Within the physiological range no vasodilatation or a very small one is seen in the large intestine, the stomach, the hindlimb, the heart, and the kidneys (19, 64, 112, 115). The vasodilatation induced by CCK occurs throughout the intestinal wall in such a way that a larger fraction than usual is distributed to the mucosa (112).

Perfusing a duodenal segment in the cat with an isotonic solution of L-phenylalanine causes a jejunal vasodilatation within 10 min (26, 115). Simultaneously with the relaxation of the resistance vessels, $K_{f,c}$ increases, sometimes even before any effect on intestinal blood flow is apparent. The $K_{f,c}$ probably mainly reflects a relaxation of the precapillary sphincters (26). The vascular effects evoked by luminal perfusion with L-phenylalanine were at the time (in 1973) attributed to CCK released from the gut. However, since then a large number of hormone candidates have been demonstrated in the gut, some of which may participate in the observed vascular response.

The mechanisms by which CCK influences smooth muscle vascular tone have in part been investigated in vitro. Physiological concentrations of CCK cause a muscular relaxation, suggesting that CCK receptors are present on the smooth muscle plasma membranes (109a). Experiments in vivo suggest that CCK may also act by increasing metabolism (115).

Nervous mechanisms (including the participation of CCK-containing neurons) may also be involved in certain vascular effects of CCK. Thus atropine partially blocks the CCK vasodilatation induced by pharmacological (44) but not by physiological (115) doses. Furthermore the vascular effects induced by L-phenylalanine are completely abolished by atropine (115).

### 5-Hydroxytryptamine (Serotonin)

Serotonin was isolated independently by Page and Erspamer (305). It is found in most mammalian tissues and its concentration in the gastrointestinal tract is very high (74). With the Falck-Hillarp technique, 5-HT in the alimentary canal was localized to the enterochromaffin (EC) cells; however, it was not possible to demonstrate 5-HT in nerves in the gut with the fluorescence method (4, 5). Not until an immunohistochemical technique had been developed could 5-HT be shown in the enteric nervous system (77, 132). However, the total amount of 5-HT in nerves amounts to <5% of the total 5-HT content in the intestinal wall (74).

The morphology of the 5-HT–containing enteric neurons differs between species. In the guinea pig, most of the neurons seem to be confined to the enteric nervous system (77, 132), whereas the 5-HT innervation in the rat may be at least in part extrinsic (85). The cell bodies in the guinea pig are located in the myenteric plexus exclusively. Nerve fibers are found in both the myenteric and submucosal nerve plexuses. In both rat and guinea pig some, although not particularly dense, vascular innervation has been reported.

The systemic hemodynamic response to intravenous infusion of 5-HT has been investigated in dogs (439). In these experiments, the gastrointestinal vascular bed was innervated, implying that the observed vascular responses represent the net effect of a direct action of the infused drug and possible changes in the extrinsic neural (mainly sympathetic) influence on the vascular smooth muscles, elicited from cardiovascular receptor stations (e.g., baroreceptors, volume receptors). With the radioactive microsphere technique, Zinner and co-workers (439) found that graded infusion of 5-HT (4–10 $\mu g \cdot min^{-1} \cdot kg^{-1}$) caused an increased cardiac output and decreased systemic vascular resistance with redistribution of regional blood flow. Thus the blood flow to the heart, adrenals, fundus, and antrum parts of the stomach increased while a decreased flow to the spleen, pancreas, and skin was observed. When the mucosal and muscular layers of the gastrointestinal tract were compared, 5-HT given intravenously was found to selectively increase blood flow to the muscularis, particularly in the upper part of the small intestine.

When Page isolated 5-HT (305) he was searching for the serum vasoconstrictor, using the vascular bed of the rabbit ear as bioassay. However, the vascular response of 5-HT has been shown to be rather complex (for reviews see refs. 415 and 416), involving a direct action of the compound on the vascular smooth muscles together with action on nerves. This complex action is clearly demonstrated in the gastrointestinal tract, mostly in studies on the feline small and large intestines (25, 117). A comparatively small dose of 5-HT in the superior mesenteric artery (20 $\mu g/min$, i.e., 50 nmol/min, in a 15-g segment of small intestine) evokes a dilatation of the resistance vessels and the precapillary sphincters that is apparently secondary to an activation of vasodilator nerves, since the dilator response is abolished by giving tetrodotoxin but uninfluenced by muscarinic, nicotinic, or adrenergic receptor-blocking agents (25, 110). It is possible that the nerves involved are VIPergic, because we have shown that VIP is released from the gut when infusing 5-HT close intra-arterially (100, 377).

A nervous involvement in vascular effects of 5-HT in the cat colon was also demonstrated by Fasth et al. (117). A small dose of 5-HT evokes, as in the small bowel, a vasodilatation that is absent after giving the ganglionic blocking agent hexamethonium. At a higher infusion rate of 5-HT (50 $\mu g/min$, i.e., $\geq 120$ nmol/min), vasoconstriction is seen, which is blocked by phentolamine but not by hexamethonium. These experiments suggest that in the colon the infused 5-HT activated both pre- and postganglionic nerves, evoking vasodilatation and vasoconstriction, respectively.

The physiological importance of 5-HT in the control of the intestinal vasculature cannot be determined from the experiments described in the preceeding paragraphs. However, there is one vascular mechanism that is influenced by some 5-HT–receptor blockers as reported by Biber et al. (28). These authors described vasodilatation that is seen after a slight mechanical stimulation of the intestinal mucosa. A similar mechanism was also observed in the proximal but not in the distal colon of the cat (120) and in the jejunum of the rat (21). The mechanically induced vasodilatation is abolished by, e.g., tetrodotoxin but is not influenced by adrenergic or cholinergic blocking agents. On the other hand, 5-HT–receptor blockade (5-HT tachyphylaxis, D-2-bromolysergic acid diethylamide, dihydroergotamine) abolishes the reflex vasodilatation (28). From these experiments Biber et al. (28) concluded that mechanical mucosal stimulation elicits a local nervous reflex dilatation in which 5-HT plays a role. The same mechanism is apparently stimulated electrically by field stimulation across the intestinal wall (24).

The interaction between nerves and 5-HT can be explained by at least two mechanisms based on the morphological localization of 5-HT in the intestines. *1*) Serotonin may be a neurotransmitter of a neuron in the proposed reflex (Fig. 5). Because the direct muscular action of 5-HT most probably is vasoconstrictory, the hypothetical 5-HT neuron is probably not making direct contact with the vascular smooth muscle but may rather be the transmitter of an interneuron, the nerve cell making contact with the VIPergic vasculature. This proposal is also substantiated by the scant vascular 5-HT innervation reported by all morphologists. The VIPergic vascular innervation, on the other hand, is dense (363, 409). *2*) Mechanical stimulation of the mucosa may cause the release of 5-HT from the EC cells, which activates dendrites situated adjacent to the intestinal epithelium. In this way the reflex is elicited (Fig. 5). In the colon, the experimental evidence favors the presence of a cholin-

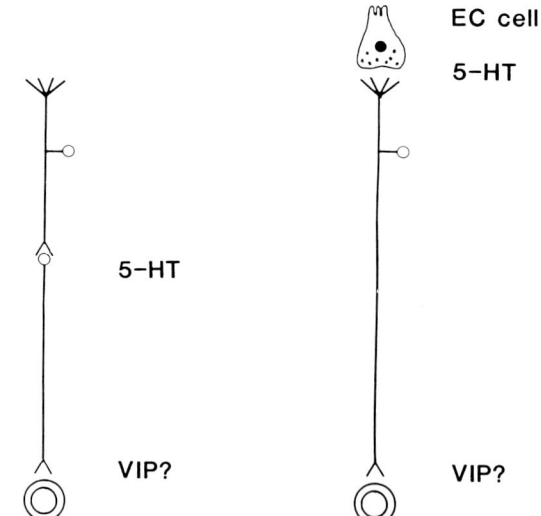

FIG. 5. Hypothetical arrangements of nervous reflex underlying vasodilator response to mechanical stimulation of small intestine mucosa. Two possible mechanisms are presented. *Left*, reflex arrangement with mechanical receptor in tissue being activated, which in turn activates via serotonin (5-HT) synapse a 2nd neuron releasing vasoactive intestinal polypeptide (VIP) at vascular smooth muscle cells. According to reflex arrangement on *right*, enterochromaffin (EC) cell acts as mechanoreceptor activating a VIPergic neuron. In the colon, reflex arrangements may be similar, although a cholinergic neuron may be included in reflex.

ergic neuron in the nervous reflex dilatation, which otherwise may be organized like in the small intestine.

An endoluminal release of mucosal 5-HT has been demonstrated morphologically and biochemically in perfused segments of the rat and cat small intestines (3, 6, 153). Serotonin is released constantly into the gut lumen at a low rate that seems to be enhanced by vagal nerve stimulation. Pretreatment with atropine or hexamethonium abolishes vagally induced endoluminal release of 5-HT, indicating involvement of cholinergic receptors (154, 438). It has been suggested that the endoluminally released 5-HT participates in the physiological control of intestinal blood flow. Thus luminal perfusion of the cat small intestine with 5-HT in concentrations in the upper range of that seen on vagal activation causes a hyperemia in the muscle layer of the perfused segment. The 5-HT–induced regional hyperemia of the muscular layer is prevented by blockade of muscarinic receptors or by local anesthesia of the gut segment, thus indicating either the activation of a local nervous reflex involving cholinergic neurotransmissions or secondary effects due to 5-HT–induced motility.

## Neurotensin

Neurotensin is a 13–amino acid peptide that originally was isolated and characterized by Carraway and Leeman (59). In the gastrointestinal tract, the neurotensin-like immunoreactivity is located in endocrine cells of the open type (N cells), particularly in the distal part of the small intestine (92, 182, 386). Nerve fibers containing neurotensin immunoreactivity have also been observed but in low numbers within the smooth muscles and the myenteric plexus of the gastrointestinal tract (244, 363). No observations of any vascular neurotensin innervation have been reported.

The plasma concentration of neurotensin-like immunoreactivity is markedly increased in the venous blood after a meal and after ingestion of fat (cf. ref. 344). The major part of this immunoreactivity, however, comprises biologically inactive metabolites with the $NH_2$-terminal of the neurotensin molecule. The biologically active form that has to be measured with a COOH-terminally directed antibody is not enhanced at all (169) or only constitutes a smaller fraction of the neurotensin-like material released into the plasma after a meal (95, 122, 245, 278, 402). In these types of experiments, the maximal concentration of neurotensin in venous plasma is 20–30 pM.

Intravenous infusions of neurotensin, resulting in an estimated plasma concentration of neurotensin significantly higher than that measured after a meal, induce usually a 20%–30% increase in ileal blood flow in several species (14, 171, 226, 303, 345). In most of the studies only total intestinal blood flow was measured, but Baca et al. (14), using the microsphere technique, found that the vasodilatation is confined to the muscularis layer. This observation is consistent with the findings of Thor et al. (403) that neurotensin augments intestinal motility, changing it from a fasting to a postprandial pattern. On the other hand, an intra-arterial infusion of neurotensin in the dose, similar to that used in the previously cited studies, failed to enhance jejunal blood flow in the dog (323). Thus if neurotensin exerts its biological effect via blood, i.e., as a hormone, the quantitative importance of this peptide in the direct regulation of gastrointestinal blood flow is small.

In 1982 Leeman and Carraway (246) proposed that neurotensin might mainly act as a local hormone, i.e., diffusion to neighboring cells should be the major mechanism responsible for the biological effects of neurotensin. Such a mechanism may explain the observations on the neurotensin effect on capillary permeability by Harper et al. (171). These authors showed that neurotensin increases capillary hydraulic permeability to the same extent as seen during fat absorption.

A paracrine mechanism cannot, however, explain the possible involvement of neurotensin in the postprandial hyperemia, because the resistance vessels controlling mucosal blood flow are located too far away from the villus epithelium and capillary network. A lymphatic transport of neurotensin may, as proposed in HORMONES, p. 1682, be one way in which neurotensin, released in the villi, reaches the smooth muscle cells of the submucosal arterioles. Finally, an intestinal vasodilatation may be evoked by neurotensin activating local nerve reflexes in the enteric nervous system, as proposed for 5-HT in Fig. 5.

## Somatostatin

Somatostatin is a polypeptide consisting of 14 amino acid residues. It was isolated as the compound inhibiting the release of growth hormone from the pituitary gland (46). Subsequently somatostatin was found in nervous tissue in the gastrointestinal tract (78, 212, 213, 363) where it is also found in epithelial endocrine-like cells throughout the gastrointestinal tract (213, 321).

Cell bodies of neurons containing somatostatin are located in both myenteric and submucosal plexuses in the intestines, whereas they are absent in the stomach (212, 213, 363). Nerve fibers are distributed to all wall layers of the intestines, but they are particularly numerous in nerve plexuses (363). There are only a few nerve fibers seen in the stomach. No somatostatin innervation to the gastrointestinal vasculature has been reported. Morphological and neurophysiological evidence suggests that somatostatin nerves function as inhibitory interneurons in the enteric nervous system (131a, 431).

Somatostatin is found in the endocrine cells (the so-called D cells) that are distributed throughout the gastrointestinal tract (78, 213, 321). The appearance of these epithelial cells has been studied particularly in the antral mucosa of the stomach, where the somatostatin cells are provided with long processes on the side facing the tissue, as described in detail by Larsson et al. (239). The processes extend along the basement membrane of the epithelium and make contact with several other epithelial cells. In the stomach, the somatostatin-containing processes often make contact with the epithelial cells containing gastrin (the G cell). This morphological arrangement suggests that the major action of somatostatin is of paracrine type, and it has also been demonstrated that somatostatin inhibits the release of gastrin. However, a humoral function cannot be ruled out, as the circulating somatostatin levels increase after a meal (422).

The infusion of somatostatin into animals and humans causes vasoconstriction in the gastrointestinal vascular beds. Thus portal blood flow is reduced to 40%–55% of control in dogs after an intravenous bolus injection of 25–200 µg (15–120 nmol) somatostatin (202), with the effect mainly confined to the gastric and pancreatic vascular circuits (18). Similar results were obtained also in humans (425). In the canine intestines, Konturek et al. (230) demonstrated a 15% reduction of blood flow when giving close intra-arterially 0.25 or 0.5 $nmol \cdot h^{-1} \cdot kg^{-1}$. Human blood flow in the ileocolic and left colic artery is diminished to ~65% of control during a 1-min intravenous infusion [1 µg (600 pmol)$\cdot min^{-1} \cdot kg^{-1}$] (408). Total gastric blood flow is decreased on somatostatin intravenous infusion in dogs [0.5–4 µg (0.3–2.4 nmol)$\cdot h^{-1} \cdot kg^{-1}$] (228) and also in humans after an intravenous bolus injection [170 µg (100 nmol)] (195) when gastric acid secretion had been increased by pentagastrin. Concomitantly gastric acid secretion is reduced. A vasoconstriction is seen in the secreting parts of the human gastric mucosa, as revealed by aminopyrine-clearance and inert-gas clearance techniques (195, 228, 384). In a study on the canine stomach, it was shown that the reduction of blood flow in the fundus was confined to the mucosa, whereas this was not the case in the antrum (325). In contrast to all these studies that have demonstrated a decrease of total and/or regional blood flow on giving somatostatin to the acid secreting stomach, Leung and Guth (247) recorded an increased mucosal blood flow when inhibiting acid secretion in the rat stomach with intravenous somatostatin [16 µg (9.6 nmol)$\cdot h^{-1} \cdot kg^{-1}$]. There is no obvious explanation why their results differ from those of the other investigators. The amounts of somatostatin infused in most of the experiments described here produce plasma concentrations of somatostatin that are within the physiological range (311).

The exact mode of vascular action of somatostatin is unknown. The vasoconstrictor effect in the stomach on somatostatin infusion might be secondary to its effect on acid secretion, as judged by the different effects on antral and fundic mucosal blood flow. Any direct effect of somatostatin on vascular smooth muscles seems less likely, because no such effect can be demonstrated by the polypeptide in vitro (71).

## INTEGRATED RESPONSES

In the final part of this review we describe and discuss some integrated effects on the gastrointestinal circulation that involve the participation of the nervous and hormonal control systems. The topics covered here are the reflex nervous control and the vascular response during hemorrhage and digestion. The reflex studies of the gastrointestinal tract have mainly been devoted to the reflexes elicited from cardiovascular receptors: the high-pressure baroreceptors, the volume receptors, and the chemoreceptors. These reflexes are described first.

### High-Pressure Baroreceptors

The baroreceptors, located in the carotid arteries and the aortic arch, are stretch receptors not excited by pressure per se but by the expansion of the arterial wall. In the normal pressure ranges, these receptors exert an inhibitory influence on the bulbar vasopressure center, thereby maintaining arterial pressure within the normal range. Most studies of the baroreceptor function have been performed by withdrawing the baroreceptor constraint. In experiments on anesthetized animals, this is usually accomplished by occluding the carotid arteries or by perfusing the isolated carotid sinus or aortic arch at known pressures. In humans, such studies cannot be performed for obvious reasons, and indirect methods such as neck suction are applied that mimic an increased stimulation of the baroreceptors. The same effect can also be accomplished by afferent electrical stimulation of the nerves to the carotid sinus or the aortic arch. Bleeding is another procedure that influences baroreceptor function. However, bleeding evokes a complex reflex adjustment elicited from baroreceptors, volume receptors, and eventually also chemoreceptors. Hemorrhage is therefore described separately.

There are several early reports describing the cardiovascular effects of afferent stimulation of the so-called depressor nerve believed to contain the fibers from the baroreceptors in the aortic arch. For example, Bayliss (16) reported an intestinal vasodilatation on stimulation of this nerve. However, it seems likely that the depressor nerve also contains fibers from the heart and its volume receptors; therefore these studies are not included in this review.

Afferent stimulation of the carotid sinus nerve represents a pure simulation of an activation of the carotid baroreceptors. Vatner and co-workers (420, 421) performed such studies on conscious and anesthetized dogs provided with flowmeter probes on the superior mesenteric, renal, and ilial arteries. The electrical stimulation lowers perfusion pressure and regional flow resistance in the vascular beds studied. The decrease of flow resistance is most pronounced in the vascular circuit of the iliac artery (mainly skeletal muscles), with flow resistance ~40% of control during carotid sinus stimulation. The corresponding value for the renal and mesenteric vascular beds is ~80% of control. The decrease observed in skeletal muscles undoubtedly reflects a withdrawal of nervous vasoconstrictor influence, whereas the decrease of flow resistance in the two other vascular beds may simply reflect a change of flow resistance accompanying a lowered perfusion pressure (so-called autoregulation of blood flow). It can be concluded from these studies that the nerves from the carotid sinus exert a more pronounced inhibitory influence on the bulbar neurons controlling the skeletal muscle circulation than on those controlling the circulation of the kidney or the intestines.

Most studies of the effects of unloading of the high-pressure baroreceptors have been devoted to the reflex control of either the resistance or the capacitance vessels. The animal studies have been performed almost exclusively on the small intestine or on the whole splanchnic area.

The most thorough investigation of the consecutive sections of the intestinal vascular bed was performed by Öberg (298), who studied simultaneously the reactions within several of the consecutive sections of the intestinal vascular bed in cats. Figure 6 is taken from his study. In this experiment, the pressure in the isolated right carotid sinus was suddenly lowered to 0 mmHg. In addition to a transient vasoconstriction of the resistance vessels, an expulsion of blood from the intestines is apparent (abrupt decrease of tissue volume) as well as a constriction of the precapillary sphincters as recorded by a decrease of the $K_{f,c}$ (not shown in Fig. 6). The mean hydrostatic capillary pressure remains largely unchanged, as judged from the constant intestinal tissue volume after the initial changes of the capacitance vessels tone. This response pattern is in all respects similar to that seen on direct electrical stimulation of the sympathetic vasoconstrictor fibers of the gut (for more details see *Norepinephrine*, p. 1669). There are no published reports on the effect of carotid sinus unloading on blood flow in the different layers of the intestinal wall.

The intestinal vascular reactions in Figure 6 are different from those seen in the skeletal muscle vascular bed, as also shown on the same Figure 6. In the muscle vascular bed, the nervous vasoconstriction of the resistance vessels is maintained and there is a pronounced decrease of mean hydrostatic capillary pressure secondary to an increase of the precapillary-to-postcapillary resistance ratio. The latter response pattern is similar to that recorded when stimulating the regional vasoconstrictor fibers to a skeletal muscle (70, 284).

The constriction of the intestinal resistance vessels observed by Öberg (298) has been reported by several

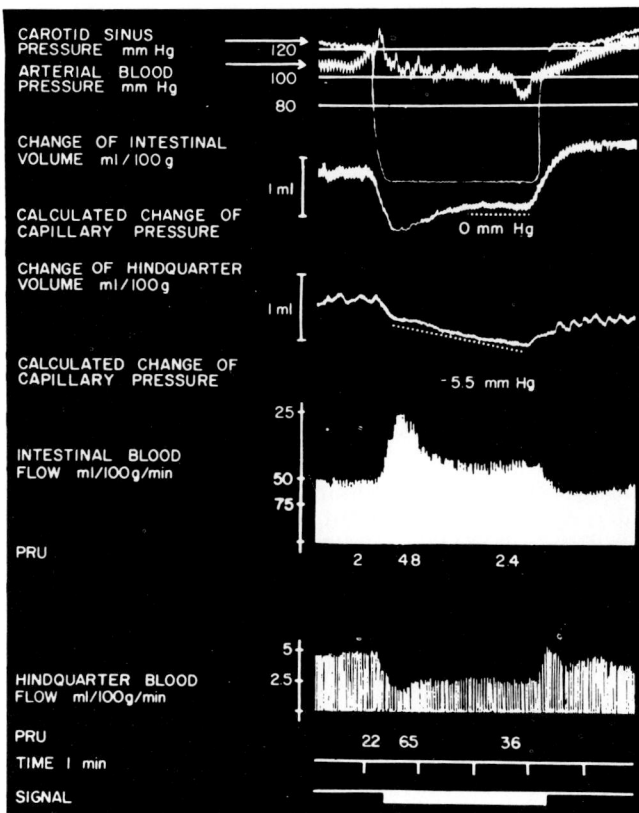

FIG. 6. Effects of reduction of pressure and pulsations in perfused right carotid sinus on resistance and capacitance vessels and net transcapillary fluid transfer in feline hindquarters and intestine. Cat was anesthetized with chloralose, curarized, atropinized, and kept under artificial ventilation. Vagal nerves had been cut in the neck. Intestinal blood flow was measured in such a way that height of ordinate writer was inversely proportional to rate of blood flow, whereas there was a direct relation between height and flow rate when recording hindquarter blood flow. Note continuous decrease in hindquarter volume on lowering carotid sinus pressure, whereas intestinal tissue volume after a transient decrease stays more or less constant. Peripheral resistance units (PRU) were calculated by dividing arterial pressure (in mmHg) by regional blood flow (in ml· 100 g$^{-1}$·min$^{-1}$). [From Öberg (298).]

authors using different techniques. In early studies, it was common to study indirectly the importance of the splanchnic vessels for the baroreceptor control by cutting the splanchnic nerves and observing the effects on arterial pressure (for a review of very early literature see ref. 197). Izquierdo and Koch (197) showed in anesthetized rabbits that severing the splanchnic nerves acutely lowered arterial pressure by ~30% of control, observations that have been confirmed in more recent studies (429). The more direct demonstration of a reduced blood flow in the whole splanchnic area or in the intestines when varying baroreceptor stimulation has been made in several animal studies (e.g., see refs. 215, 298, 380).

The constriction of the capacitance vessels on lowering carotid sinus pressure, illustrated in Figure 6 as a rapid decrease of tissue volume, has been shown in several studies (7, 96, 141, 178, 292, 298). Heymans et al. (178) observed that perfusion pressure through an isolated, innervated mesenteric vein is increased on carotid occlusion. Using a similar experimental approach Eckstein et al. (96) failed to demonstrate any constriction of the colonic veins of the dog when unloading the carotid baroreceptors. Alexander (7) studied the capacitance response in another indirect way by determining pressure-volume diagrams from the intestinal venous bed. Pressure decrease in an isolated carotid sinus preparation changes the shape of the venous distensibility curve of the intestinal veins, which suggests a vasoconstriction.

Although the approaches used in the studies cited in the preceding paragraph only provide qualitative information, studies with concomitant measurements of inflow and outflow of blood, plethysmography, or indicator-dilution techniques give a more quantitative picture of the baroreceptor control of the gastrointestinal capacitance vessels. Quantitatively carotid occlusion decreases regional blood volume ~6% in the dog (57, 58) and 10%–15% in the cat (164). The change in intestinal volume, illustrated on Figure 6, where carotid sinus pressure on one side was lowered to zero, corresponds to a 10%–15% decrease of intestinal blood volume. These results should be compared with the reduction of blood volume in the intestine during hemorrhage, which amounts to 40%–50% and ~60% of the resting regional blood volume in the cat (165, 166, 298) and in the dog (57), respectively. Hemorrhage apparently evokes larger decreases of blood volume than deloading of the high-pressure baroreceptors alone. The difference is due to the fact that hemorrhage not only influences the baroreceptor but also the volume and chemoreceptor control of circulation.

It is generally believed that the vascular effects of unloading the baroreceptors are induced through an increased firing in the regional sympathetic vasoconstrictor fibers. Based on such assumptions, Kendrick et al. (215) estimated rate of firing in the vasoconstrictor nerves by comparing the vascular effects seen when eliciting the baroreceptor reflex with those seen on direct electrical stimulation of the splanchnic nerves. Decreasing carotid sinus pressure from 175 to 135 mmHg increased the rate of fiber discharge to ~1 Hz. A further reduction to 100 mmHg increases firing rate 0.5 Hz. At the very lowest intrasinus pressures, a firing rate of 6–7 Hz was calculated. The magnitude of the resistance and capacitance responses suggests that the firing rate to the two consecutive sections of the intestinal vasculature is the same, whereas a similar analysis in the skeletal muscle vascular bed indicated that the firing rate to the resistance vessels is higher than that to the capacitance vessels. One report (407) indicates the action potentials to the resistance vessels are larger than those controlling the capacitance vessels.

The experimental approach used by Öberg et al. to estimate rate of firing in sympathetic fibers implies that the baroreceptor effect is more or less exclusively mediated via nerves. There are few experiments that attempted to elucidate that question. Theoretically circulating epinephrine, norepinephrine, and angiotensin may be involved in the response to baroreceptor unloading. Sjövall et al. (380) showed that the vasoconstrictor response to carotid occlusion in the feline small intestine is markedly reduced but not totally abolished by cutting the splanchnic nerves. Approximately one-third of the vascular response persists after sympathetic denervation. On the other hand, Karim et al. (210a) reported that all the reflex adjustments evoked from the aortic arch are abolished by crushing the sympathetic trunks and the splanchnic nerves below the diaphragm.

The studies summarized here were all performed on animals. It is not possible to selectively unload the baroreceptors in humans. Instead, the baroreceptors are investigated during stretch, which is achieved by neck suction increasing the transmural pressure gradient across the wall of the carotid sinus. Furthermore, in these studies, splanchnic blood flow instead of intestinal blood flow has been studied, because no technique is yet available to investigate quantitatively intestinal blood flow in awake humans. Neck suction during resting control conditions lowers arterial pressure but has no effect on splanchnic or forearm vascular resistance (1). This may be explained by one of two hypotheses: 1) the baroreceptors do not exert any influence on the splanchnic vasculature; 2) there is no resting firing in the splanchnic vasoconstrictor fibers that can be inhibited upon increasing the transmural pressure at the baroreceptors. The second hypothesis was tested by Abboud et al. (1), who lowered the intrathoracic blood volume by applying a subatmospheric pressure on the lower body, which evokes a prompt constriction of the forearm vessels and, with a certain time lag, also a vasoconstriction in the splanchnic region. Neck suction application in this experimental situation causes a vasodilatation of the splanchnic but not of the forearm vessels. These observations suggest that the baroreceptors exert a control of the splanchnic but not of the forearm resistance vessels. These findings are at variance with the observations made in animals (cf. Fig. 6).

Some observations reported by Rowell et al. (353) and Johnson et al. (206) in experiments with lower body suction also suggest that the baroreceptors influence splanchnic blood flow. In both reports it was found that the forearm blood flow decreases immediately on applying the suction, probably through an unloading of the thoracic volume receptors, whereas a splanchnic vasoconstriction is seen first when the aortic pulse pressure is lowered, i.e., when the baroreceptors are unloaded. This is illustrated in Figure 7.

*Cardiac Mechanoreceptors*

The receptors acting as volume receptors within the cardiovascular system are mainly located in the heart,

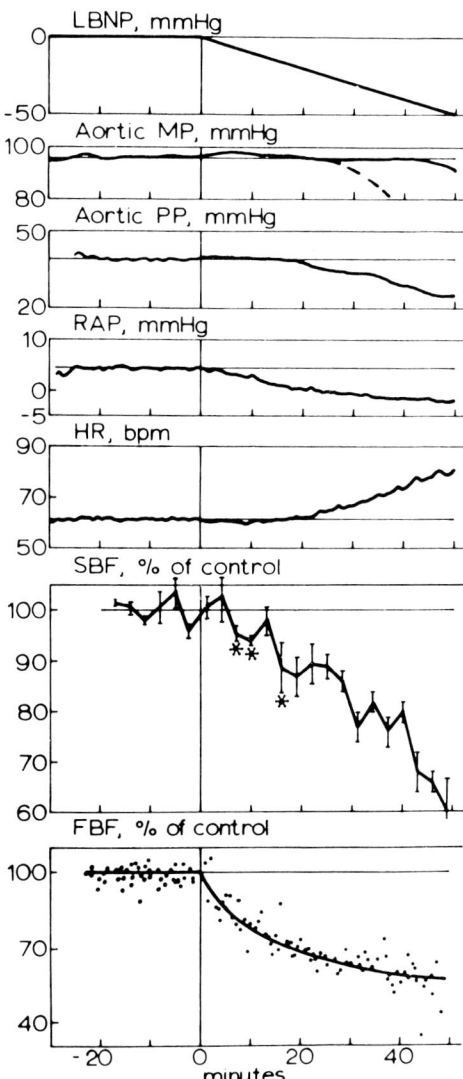

FIG. 7. Average response to lower body negative pressure (LBNP) of 9 subjects. MP, mean pressure; PP, pulse pressure; RAP, right atrial pressure; HR, heart rate; SBF, splanchnic blood flow; FBF, forearm blood flow. *Broken line* for aortic MP shows response of 2 subjects, who had a marked fall at LBNP of −35 mmHg; *solid line* thereafter shows average aortic MP for remaining 4 subjects. *Asterisk* denotes first 3 significant decrements ($P < 0.05$) in splanchnic blood flow beyond control. [From Johnson et al. (206).]

which is provided with a population of mechanoreceptors. This low-pressure part of the cardiovascular system is particularly sensitive to volume changes because of its high distensibility. The afferent pathways run in the vagal nerves mainly of the unmyelinated type. The volume receptors are believed to exert their vascular effects via a restraining influence on the bulbar pressure center. (For recent reviews see refs. 30, 404.)

Although it is fairly easy to isolate and specifically stimulate the carotid baroreceptors, the cardiac mechanoreceptors are much more difficult to study in an appropriate manner. Attempts have been made to distend the atria with a balloon. Such experimental procedures, however, influence venous return to the heart and, secondarily, lower arterial pressure. Therefore, in animal experiments, indirect techniques have been used, such as electrical stimulation of the vagal afferents or the vagal fibers from the heart (the cardiac vagal nerves). Other indirect methods involve the use of positive pressure ventilation and inspiratory resistance breathing (IRB), which influences the stretch of the intrathoracic mechanoreceptors through changes of pleural pressures.

There exists a fairly large number of reports concerning the cardiovascular effects elicited from the cardiac mechanoreceptors. However, most studies have been interested in the blood flow through skeletal muscles and kidneys. A few studies have been devoted to the circulation of the intestinal tract. It was shown early with qualitative techniques that stimulating the so-called depressor nerve causes a vasodilatation of the intestinal vascular bed of cats (16). Using more quantitative techniques, Öberg and White (300) studied the effects on the intestinal resistance and capacitance vessels of stimulating the cardiac vagal fibers in the cat. The responses seen reach a maximum at a stimulation rate of 8–12 Hz. The stimulation evokes a complex cardiovascular response that includes a decreased heart rate and a vasodilatation in all the vascular beds studied (skeletal muscle, kidney, and small intestine). The reduction in flow resistance is more pronounced in the skeletal muscles and in the kidneys than in the intestinal vascular bed. Concomitant to the lowered flow resistance a venous vasodilatation is seen, whereas no change of mean capillary pressure is observed. The reflex effects elicited from baroreceptors and from cardiac receptors are quantitatively the same on the intestinal resistance and capacitance vessels.

The observations made on the resistance vessels by Öberg and White were confirmed in a study by Sjövall (379) primarily devoted to the reflex nervous control of fluid transport in the small intestine. He observed that stimulating the cardiac nerves at 1 Hz evokes no intestinal vasodilatation, whereas it is apparent at a stimulation rate of 4 Hz. On the other hand, an increased fluid uptake is seen already at stimulation rates <1 Hz. Sjövall also reported that cutting the vagal nerves at rest does not change intestinal flow resistance. This is consistent with the findings of Thorén (404) that the resting rate of firing in the atrial C fibers is ~1.4 Hz, which implies that the cardiac mechanoreceptors do not exert any influence on the intestinal vasculature at rest.

Stimulating the cardiac nerves mimics activation of receptors throughout the cardiac wall. These receptors can be directly activated by giving a veratrum alkaloids intravascularly, as was demonstrated already by von Bezold and Hirt (23) in 1867. In his thesis work, Öberg (298) injected protoveratrine into the right atrium of cats and followed the reactions of the consecutive vascular section in the small intestine. The same response as that described in the preceding paragraph is seen, i.e., a vasodilatation of resistance and capacitance vessels. Flow resistance decreases to ~75% of control, and the venous dilatation increases regional blood volume ~15% of control. Precapillary-to-postcapillary resistance ratio is not changed by the drug-induced reflex, which was abolished by cutting the vagal nerves.

Sjövall et al. (381) varied the intrathoracic blood volume by two noninvasive techniques, positive-pressure ventilation (PPV) and IRB. A very good correlation was seen between change of central blood volume (measured with an indicator dilution method) and change of intestinal vascular resistance (Fig. 8). A decrease of blood volume increases flow resistance and vice versa. A similar correlation is seen between decrease of transmural central venous pressure (difference between central venous pressure and esophageal pressure) and increase of intestinal vascular resistance. Vagotomy largely eliminates these effects.

To summarize, the observations made on animals (mainly cats) strongly suggest that deloading the volume receptors in the heart causes a vasoconstriction of the intestinal resistance and capacitance vessels without influencing mean capillary hydrostatic pressure, mainly through an activation of the sympathetic nervous system. Quantitatively, these effects are similar to those observed when unloading the baroreceptors in the carotid arteries. During normal resting conditions, the cardiac volume receptors do not exert any influence on the intestinal resistance vessels. The physiological significance of this reflex vasoconstriction of the intestinal vascular bed (and presumably other splanchnic vascular beds) is to help to maintain a sufficient arterial blood pressure during, e.g., hemorrhage.

In humans lower body suction has been used in studies of the intrathoracic volume receptor control of the splanchnic circulation; [see Fig. 7; (1, 206, 353)]. These studies were commented on earlier, when discussing the baroreceptor control of gastrointestinal blood flow. It was then concluded that deloading the volume receptor causes no or little change of splanchnic blood flow, whereas deloading the baroreceptors markedly diminishes blood flow in the splanchnic organs. This species difference may be related to the fact that humans are posturally upright animals.

*Arterial Chemoreceptors*

The arterial chemoreceptors are located in the neck region (glomus caroticum and glomus aorticum). They are extremely well vascularized and provided with cells that may sense the partial pressures of oxygen and carbon dioxide in blood. Hypercapnia and hypoxia increase the rate of firing in the afferent nerves from the chemoreceptors, the two stimuli potentiating each other at certain pressures, as discussed in detail in a recent review by Eyzaguirre et al. (106). The aortic chemoreceptor seems to be less sensitive to hypoxia

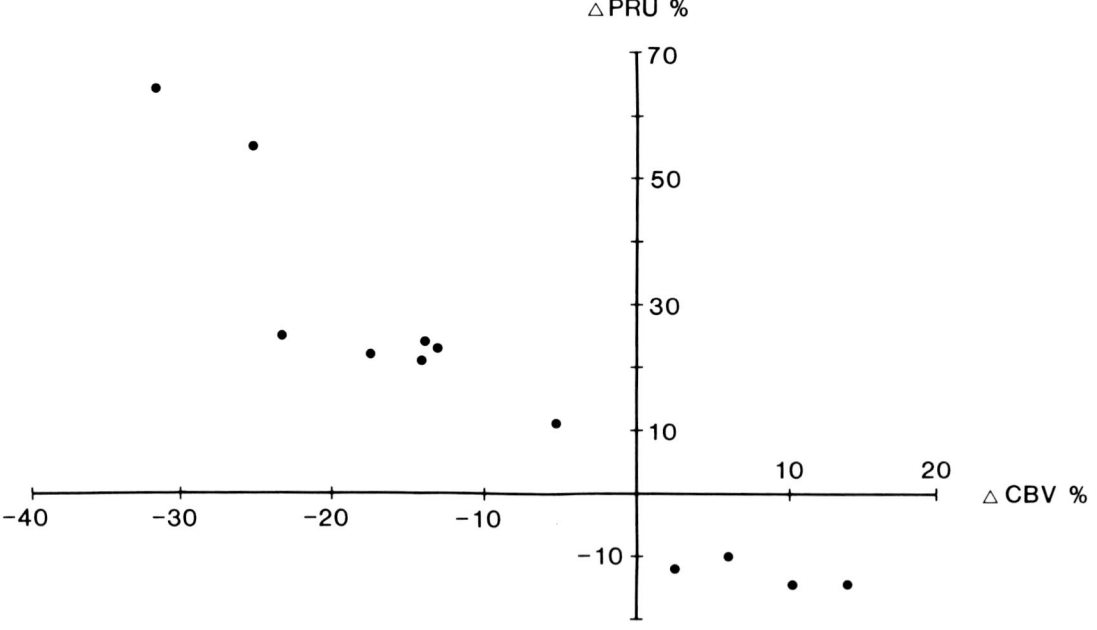

FIG. 8. Relative change of central blood volume ($\Delta$CBV) as related to relative change of intestinal flow resistance (peripheral resistance units, $\Delta$PRU) in cats. CBV was changed by positive pressure ventilation and estimated by an indicator-dilution technique. Decrease of CBV is accompanied by increased PRU, probably reflecting decreased inhibition of bulbar vasopressor center through deloading of intrathoracic volume receptors. [From Sjövall et al. (381).]

than the carotid one. Afferent nervous impulses evoke reflexes that influence respiratory and cardiovascular functions.

In experimental animals, the most common technique for studying the role of the chemoreceptors has been to perfuse the isolated carotid receptor with venous blood or to inject some compound (e.g., sodium cyanide) close to the receptor to be stimulated. This evokes a vasoconstriction in all vascular beds studied, including the intestinal ones. As with all the other vascular reflexes reviewed by us, the resistance vessels are the best studied ones (20, 255, 298). The initial peak effect corresponds to a 30%–60% increase of flow resistance in the small intestine of the cat. During the steady-state phase, the flow reduction amounts to ~20% of control flow as reported by Öberg (298).

The vasoconstriction of the intestinal resistance vessels has been compared with the vascular response evoked in skeletal muscle by the same stimulation of the arterial chemoreceptors. In all reports where this question has been studied, the intestinal vasoconstrictor response has been smaller than the skeletal muscle one (20, 255, 298). Little and Öberg (255) reported that the skeletal muscle vasoconstriction is on an average 2.5 times greater than that of the intestine. However, this calculation is based on the peak response of the intestinal resistance vessels, implying that the intestinal resistance response would have been considerably smaller had the calculations been made on the steady-state phase effects (cf. Fig. 3).

The precapillary sphincters become constricted on chemoreceptor activation, as judged by a decrease of $K_{f,c}$ (298). The capacitance vessels also constrict (96, 298) corresponding to ~10% of regional blood volume (298). Eckstein et al. (96) studied the constriction of the capacitance vessels by determining the perfusion pressure necessary to maintain a constant flow through an isolated segment of the colonic vein. With this method they failed to show any venous response on stimulating the carotid chemoreceptor, whereas a clear-cut reflex response was seen when stimulating the aortic chemoreceptor. This observation is at variance with findings of Öberg (298). These two observations may be reconciled if the venous constriction seen by Öberg primarily was caused by a passive decrease of venous volume, secondary to a decrease of transmural pressure. Alternatively, the technique used by Eckstein et al. (96) cannot detect capacitance changes as small as those evoked by chemoreceptor activation.

*Hemorrhagic Hypotension*

Bleeding evokes complex compensatory mechanisms involving the nervous and hormonal control systems. These, in turn, may be responsible for, e.g., morphological and/or biochemical changes of great importance for the survival of the organism. Therefore a very large body of knowledge could be reviewed here. This review makes no claim to cover all these various aspects of the subject. Instead, we focus our interest on the hemodynamic changes occurring in the gastrointestinal tract initially after a bleeding. Even within this restricted field we do not claim to review all the pertinent publications.

RESISTANCE VESSELS. There are many studies showing that the resistance vessels of the gastrointestinal tract constrict during bleeding (61, 81, 165, 166, 252, 253, 257, 298, 317, 330, 331, 335, 336, 365, 366, 388). This vascular response is, however, not as pronounced as that seen in the skeletal muscle vascular bed, at least in most experimental animals. Quantitatively, a reduction by bleeding of the estimated blood volume by ~35% in a cat increases intestinal resistance 20%–30% when arterial pressure falls from 140 to 70 mmHg (165, 166), whereas flow resistance in the skeletal muscle vascular bed increases ≧100%–150% (267). Reduction of the circulating blood volume in humans by lower body suction reduces splanchnic blood flow by ~30% in the face of 10% reduction of blood pressure. Forearm blood flow decreases ~45% during the same experimental conditions. When it is taken into account that different fractions of cardiac output are distributed to the splanchnic organs and to the skeletal muscles, it can be calculated that these two vascular regions account for about one-third each of the increase of total peripheral resistance seen when simulating a hemorrhage in humans.

The comparatively small vascular response in the gastrointestinal tract is due to several mechanisms. *1)* The smooth muscles of the gastrointestinal vasculature can adjust its tone depending on the transmural pressure gradient (myogenic phenomenon) and thus maintain flow rate despite reductions in perfusion pressure. During prolonged periods of low perfusion pressure, an accumulation of dilating metabolites also contributes to the autoregulation of blood flow. This type of vascular adjustments is more pronounced in the intestines than in skeletal muscle, at least as judged from animal experiments. *2)* The sympathetic nervous vasoconstriction of the various part of the gastrointestinal tract is small compared with the one observed in a skeletal muscle vascular bed. *3)* The difference between the vascular reactions in skeletal muscle and gastrointestinal tract may be due to different rates of firing in the regional sympathetic fibers. However, observations made on stimulating carotid baroreceptors do not substantiate this view (215).

During the course of hemorrhagic hypotension, gastrointestinal vascular resistance decreases steadily (165, 166, 330, 331). This response is usually ascribed to a fading sympathetic vasoconstrictor response explained in terms of an accumulation of vasodilating local metabolites. However, it could also reflect a depletion of neurotransmitter(s).

The distribution of blood flow among the different vascular circuits of the gastrointestinal wall has not been studied as extensively as the overall resistance response. In our laboratory, we have investigated the flow distribution during hemorrhagic hypotension with a combination of techniques (330). Muscle layer blood flow was estimated from the elimination of $^{85}$Kr, as recorded by a detector placed outside the intestinal wall at the antimesenteric border, whereas villous red cell flow was calculated from the disappearance rate of carbon monoxide. The loss of ~30% of the animal's estimated blood volume lowers blood pressure from 140 to 80 mmHg. Total blood flow decreases to approximately one-half of control values. Flow distribution between the different parts of the intestinal wall, i.e., absorptive site (villi), nonabsorptive site (crypts), or muscle layer, is largely unchanged, particularly in those intestines that do not develop villous intestinal lesions after a 2-h period of arterial hypotension. In the animals that do develop lesions, a certain redistribution of flow toward the villi is observed.

A sympathetic influence on the resistance vessels during hemorrhage is clearly demonstrated in experimental animals, because the vasoconstriction cannot be seen in animals in which the splanchnic nerves have been cut, interfering with the preganglionic nerve supply to the splanchnic organs, including the kidney and adrenal glands (331). This observation suggests that the importance of vasopressin for the control of intestinal blood flow is small, at least in anesthetized cats, although one cannot entirely exclude the ADH release is indirectly reduced by severing the splanchnic nerves, since angiotensin may control the release of ADH (43, 328). The sympathetic influence can theoretically be exerted through a direct nervous action on the vascular smooth muscles or through a release of circulating vasoconstrictor agents such as epinephrine, norepinephrine, and angiotensin. These compounds are released in hemorrhage via an unloading of the baroreceptor and volume receptors. The catecholamine release is completely abolished by cutting the splanchnic nerves, whereas the renin release only in part is mediated via an activation of nerve fibers in the splanchnic nerves.

Experiments in which the sympathetic nerve fibers were cut pre- or postganglionically suggest that the sympathetic influence on the intestinal resistance vessels is mainly exerted through circulating vasoconstrictor agents (282, 330). In line with this, McNeil and co-workers (279–282) have provided evidence that angiotensin plays an important role in the control of the resistance vessels in hemorrhage. It is also possible that the nervous and humoral influences potentiate each other in the control of the resistance vessels in the same way in which they do when controlling net fluid transport (249).

In some investigations, attempts have been made to elucidate the receptor stations involved in the vascular adjustments in the intestinal vascular beds caused by hemorrhage. Pelletier et al. (317) performed studies in which the chemoreceptor influence had been eliminated by ventilating the dogs with pure oxygen. The aortic nerves were cut to eliminate any influence from the receptors located to the aortic arch. Furthermore, during the experiments the effects elicited from the cardiopulmonary and carotid sinus receptors were abolished. A vasoconstriction of the superior mesenteric artery was seen upon hemorrhage (10% of the estimated blood volume), quantitatively similar when either one or both of the receptor stations in the cardiopulmonary area and in the carotid sinus were intact. The intestinal vascular bed therefore seems to be controlled to approximately the same extent from both receptors upon bleeding in dogs. In fact, the results suggest that one receptor station can take over from the other. In contrast, the constriction of the skeletal muscle vascular bed was predominantly mediated through an unloading of the carotid sinus baroreceptors in the dog during hemorrhage. However, the experiments simulating bleeding in humans (lower body suction) clearly suggest that the carotid sinus baroreceptors are more important than the cardiac mechanoreceptors for the control of the resistance vessels in the splanchnic area. (For the discussion see *High-Pressure Baroreceptors*, p. 1690, and *Cardiac Mechanoreceptors*, p. 1692; Fig. 7.)

PRECAPILLARY SPHINCTERS. The number of perfused intestinal capillaries, as reflected by changes in $K_{f,c}$, seems to increase slightly or remain within the control range when the small intestine is subjected to hemorrhagic hypotension (165, 166). This observation is rather surprising in view of the fact that the sympathetic influence on $K_{f,c}$ is to reduce its magnitude (126). The unchanged $K_{f,c}$, however, may be explained by at least two mechanisms: *1*) an augmented number of pores per unit area of capillary wall and/or an increased pore size, secondary to hypoxic damage, and *2*) a relaxation of precapillary sphincters, caused by a decrease of the transmural pressure and/or accumulation of vasodilating metabolites.

Granger and co-workers (145, 146, 308, 309) have reported observations that suggest that capillary permeability increases when the intestine has been exposed to a 1-h period of arterial hypotension. They showed that the estimated osmotic reflection coefficient for plasma proteins is decreased in the "shocked" intestine as compared with control, probably because of increased size of the capillary pores. The increase of capillary permeability may be caused by the formation of free superoxide radicals in the tissue, particularly when restoring blood flow after the ischemia (308, 309). Therefore this mechanism can hardly explain the increase of $K_{f,c}$ seen almost immediately upon inducing the hemorrhage (165, 166). In experiments in which villous plasma flow was determined with a method based on the indicator-dilution principle, it was shown that villous plasma flow stays constant when the perfusion pressure decreased within quite wide limits (268). Furthermore the number of blood-perfused villi seems to increase at low perfusion pressure, presumably secondary to a relaxation of precapillary sphincters. These observations made on cats suggest that the unchanged or increased $K_{f,c}$ during hemorrhage may, at least in part, reflect a reduction of the number of perfused capillaries in nonvillous tissue and a concomitant increase in the number of blood-perfused villi.

EXCHANGE VESSELS. The plethysmographic method makes it possible to estimate changes in the Starling equilibrium across the capillary wall as changes in tissue volume. Such studies indicate that hemorrhage does not influence to any large extent the fluid equilibrium across the intestinal capillaries (165, 166). This conclusion is based mainly on experiments performed on the feline small bowel. The response may be different in the dog, since observations suggest that mean capillary pressure is increased in that species during shock (252, 253). Furthermore, in the rat, direct pressure measurements in the different parts of the intestinal vascular tree have been made by Bohlen et al. (39, 40, 42). Measurements in the muscle and submucosal layers at various arterial pressures demonstrate that pressure in the muscle capillaries is linearly correlated with arterial pressure. The latter findings may be reconciled with our observations on the cat gut, if one assumes that autoregulation of mean capillary pressure occurs mainly in the extensive capillary network in the gastrointestinal mucosa.

CAPACITANCE VESSELS. Severe bleeding (~35% of the estimated total blood volume) causes a rapid reduction of the intestinal blood volume amounting to 3–4 ml/100 g tissue in the cat (164, 165) and ~8 ml/100 g in the dog (57). The decrease of volume reflects both a passive change caused by decrease of the transmural venous pressure and an active constriction of the vascular smooth muscle cells under the influence of nerves and hormones. In experiments on cats, the component ascribed to nerves and hormones has been estimated to account for ~70% of the observed decrease of blood volume, based on experiments with cut splanchnic nerves (165, 166). The relative importance of nerves and hormones in the control of the capacitance vessels in hemorrhage is unknown.

The sympathetic influence on the capacitance vessels declines during the course of a hemorrhagic hypotension in the same fashion as observed for the resistance vessels (165, 166). The mechanism underlying this response pattern is unknown, but an accumulation of metabolites and/or a failure of neurotransmission may be involved. The decreased sympathetic influence on the capacitance vessels during a prolonged hemorrhagic hypotension leads to an increased blood volume in the gastrointestinal organs. Lillehei et al. (252, 253) proposed that such a "pooling" of blood in the splanchnic organs was of great importance in explaining so-called irreversible shock. However, a simple calculation makes it clear that the increase of blood in the splanchnic capacitance vessel seen in hemorrhage represents only 3%–4% of the total blood volume at most, a decrease of circulating blood volume that hardly can explain the irreversibility of shock (165, 166).

*Postprandial Hyperemia*

The aim of this section is to discuss the possible mechanisms behind the postprandial vasodilatation in the small intestine. For a full review of this subject, including the vascular events in the other parts of the gastrointestinal tract as well as the relation between the luminal contents and the gastrointestinal vasodilatation, see recent reviews (65, 111, 139). From these reviews it can be summarized that the blood flow to the gastrointestinal tract increases ~50%–100% of control after a meal. The hyperemia is mainly localized to the mucosa and seems to occur only in those parts of the gastrointestinal tract that is exposed to the chyme. Furthermore, the luminal contents that produce the intestinal vasodilatation are digested food products, particularly micellar solutions of fatty acids.

Direct measurements of microvascular pressures within the vasculature in the intestinal wall of the rat (142) indicate that ~70% of the intravascular pressure drop occurs upstream to the mucosal arterioles. Furthermore the arterioles supplying the villi lose their smooth muscle coat when they reach the basal part of the villus (203, 275). These observations strongly suggest that the control of the blood flow to the intestinal mucosa, including the villi, is exerted by resistance vessels at a comparatively large distance from the absorbing epithelium in the villi (142). Furthermore such a morphology strongly suggests that absorbed solutes as well as any metabolite released from the absorbing enterocytes probably will have great difficulty reaching and controlling precapillary resistance vessels, if the solutes are absorbed via the veins.

Another way to reach the resistance vessels would be via the lymph vessels in the villous core, an effect that is further facilitated by the close proximity of the lymph and arteriolar vessels in the submucosa (301). The vasoactive substances have then to pass unabsorbed through the dense capillary network situated between the villus epithelium and lymph vessel. Because most absorbed substances, except for the chylomicrones, are mainly drained from the mucosa via the blood, it seems unlikely that a significant transport occurs to the lymph vessel, unless special mechanisms are involved such as an accumulation of a solute at the villous tip due to "trapping" in the villous countercurrent exchanger. A considerable lymph transport may also occur if the compound is water soluble with a large molecular mass (i.e., with low capillary permeability).

From this discussion it seems clear that the mechanisms underlying the functional hyperemia in the intestine are more complex than, for example, in the skeletal muscle and ought to involve remote working systems such as nervous and/or hormonal mechanisms. On the other hand, the regulation of the villous capillary surface area available for transcapillary exchange is probably controlled by local mechanism(s), because the precapillary sphincters are localized in close proximity to the villous epithelium, at least in the rat (142).

The luminal stimuli that induce the postprandial hyperemia may either be mechanical, as evoked by motility, or chemical. In the latter case, food constituents may principally affect the intestinal resistance vessels through a direct effect on the vascular smooth muscles or indirectly through metabolic, neuronal, or hormonal mechanisms. When investigating the involvement of these different mechanisms in the postprandial hyperemia, it is necessary to keep in mind that it is difficult to differentiate between a direct effect of a substance and an effect secondary to a metabolic change caused by the active transport of the substance.

A prerequisite for a direct mechanism is that the absorbed substance per se exhibits vasodilator properties. One group of substances that fulfill these criteria is the bile acids, because these agents, infused intra-arterially and dose-dependently, increase ileal blood flow, as shown by Kvietys et al. (234). In this study, the arterial bile salt concentration was calculated to correspond to the concentrations normally reached in the vessels draining the ileal mucosa. Intraluminal administration of physiological concentrations of bile or bile acids in the ileum, but not in the jejunum, also increase intestinal blood flow (66, 233, 234, 376). This may indicate that absorbed bile acids reach the mucosal resistance vessels in concentrations needed to elicit vasodilatation. However, an indirect mechanism is also quite possible, since it is well established that bile salts are only actively absorbed in the ileum but not in the jejunum.

The linkage between active transport of digested food products and intestinal hyperemia is likely to be mediated either through a decrease of oxygen tension in the tissue and/or through a release of vasoactive metabolites into the interstitial space. With regard to the role of $P_{O_2}$ Svanvik et al. (390a) showed that hypoxia induced a vascular response that mimics the postprandial hyperemia, i.e., an increase of both intestinal blood flow and $K_{f,c}$. However, as the arterial $P_{O_2}$ had to be reduced to 55 mmHg to elicit a significant intestinal vasodilatation, the authors consider it unlikely that a reduction in tissue $P_{O_2}$ can be of any physiological importance in the postprandial hyperemia.

The importance of tissue $P_{O_2}$ in the intestinal hyperemia evoked in the rat by placing glucose in the intestinal lumen was studied by Bohlen (36). In these investigations, changes in $P_{O_2}$ and vascular diameters at different levels of the intestinal wall were directly measured during glucose absorption. Luminal glucose concentrations of 1.5–30 mM induced a dilatation of all submucosal arterioles, resulting in a doubling of calculated blood flow. Concomitantly, the tissue $P_{O_2}$ in the villous apex, normally ~15 mmHg, was decreased to 6–8 mmHg during the glucose exposure irrespective of the glucose concentration used. The submucosal $P_{O_2}$, on the other hand, showed a tendency to increase despite a marked relaxation of the submucosal resistance vessels. These results indicate that the increase in villous capillary surface area, which occurs during the absorption, may be due to a direct effect of a reduced oxygen tension, whereas the observed intestinal hyperemia is not caused by hypoxia per se. In another series of experiments, Bohlen (37) investigated the effect of luminal $P_{O_2}$ on the glucose-induced intestinal hyperemia. Also in this study, the $P_{O_2}$ surrounding the submucosal arterioles was almost unaffected during glucose absorption, even with luminal $P_{O_2}$ varying between 5 and 75 mmHg. Together, these observations suggest that it is the oxygen tension within the villous epithelium rather than the $P_{O_2}$ around the submucosal arterioles that is of importance for the postprandial hyperemia. Thus, even if part of the functional hyperemia may be induced by a direct effect on the arterioles by a reduced $P_{O_2}$ in the villous and crypt region, the major part of the vasodilatation seems to be caused by some other mechanism, possibly triggered by metabolic changes in the villi.

The role of metabolites from ATP, particularly adenosine, in the postprandial hyperemia has been investigated by several researchers (146a, 146b, 427a). Adenosine always dose-dependently increases total intestinal blood flow, but in two studies this vasodilatation occurred mainly in the muscularis (146a), whereas Walus et al. (427a) found a redistribution of the blood flow toward the mucosa-submucosa. Furthermore, the adenosine antagonist theophylline did not inhibit the postprandial hyperemia (146b). These observations strongly indicate that these substances are of minor importance in the local control of mucosal blood flow.

Intestinal hyperosmolality, secondary either to an increased metabolism or to an enhanced luminal osmolality, is another mechanism that has been suggested to be responsible for the postprandial hyperemia. Intravascular infusions of hyperosmolar glucose and sodium chloride solutions also reduce the intestinal vascular resistance. This effect seems to be more pronounced in the small intestine than in other vascular beds (63, 250). However, an enhanced luminal osmolality per se, even reaching values as high as 3,000 mosmol/kg $H_2O$, has a very limited effect on the intestinal flow resistance (63, 235, 315, 326) or on the perfused capillary surface area measured as the permeability surface product for $^{86}Rb$ (315), although Hallbäck et al. (167) showed with a cryoscopic technique that augmenting luminal osmolality with mannitol to 600 mosmol/kg H$_2$O created a significant tissue hyperosmolality in the upper parts of the villi. However, tissue osmolality at the villous base was close or equal to isotonicity in the studies by Hallbäck et al. (167), probably because of the presence of the villous countercurrent exchanger (204). These findings agree with the observations made by Chou et al. (63), who showed that placing a hyperosmolar solution (1,200 mosmol/kg H$_2$O) of glucose or polyethylene glycol in the intestinal lumen enhances osmolality only 10–12 mosmol/kg H$_2$O in the venous effluent from the gut.

From the observations just described, one is tempted to draw the conclusion that tissue hyperosmolality is not of any functional importance in explaining postprandial hyperemia in the gut. However, Bohlen (38) showed that adding glucose to an isotonic electrolyte solution in the intestinal lumen of a rat augments both osmolality at the villous tip (probably because of a countercurrent multiplication in the villus) and also evokes a hyperosmolality in the vicinity of the submucosal arterioles, probably secondary to a transport of hyperosmolar solution from the villous to the submucosal compartment. Bohlen proposed that the increased osmolality in the submucosa is responsible at least in part for the hyperemia that is simultaneously observed. One major difference between the experiments with luminal hypertonic and isotonic solutions is that the small intestine is secreting fluid in the former case, whereas a net fluid absorption occurs with an isotonic electrolyte-glucose solution in the lumen. This difference may explain the results just described, because a net fluid absorption also elicits an increase in lymph flow. The hypertonic fluid in the absorbing villi may in this situation be transported via the lymphatics from the villi to the submucosa, whereas such a fluid transport is not occurring in the experiments with a hypertonic luminal solution.

The involvement of the enteric nervous system in the postprandial hyperemia has been studied by several authors. Thus mechanical stimulation of the intestinal mucosa induces a local increase in mucosal blood flow that is blocked by nerve-blocking agents. The organization of this reflex, including the possibility of 5-HT and VIP participating in this mechanism, is thoroughly discussed in *Vasoactive Intestinal Polypeptide*, p. 1680 and in *5-Hydroxytryptamine (Serotonin)*, p. 1687 (see also Fig. 5). Such a mechanism may in part explain the hyperemia accompanying every migrating myoelectric complex observed in conscious dogs (123). This hyperemia is not observed if the luminal contents are drained out in the cephalad direction, suggesting the possibility that some luminal factor must also be present to evoke the mechanically induced intestinal hyperemia.

The possible engagement of local nervous reflexes in the nutrient-induced intestinal hyperemia has also been investigated, but the results are more contradictory. The jejunal vasodilatation after glucose or oleic acid absorption is not blocked by tetrodotoxin, hexamethonium, methysergide (297), or atropine (36, 177, 234). This implies that neither nerves carrying Na$^+$-dependent action potentials nor nicotinic, serotonergic, or muscarinic receptors seem to be involved. On the other hand, the vascular response to the luminal nutrients is attenuated by intraluminal administration of a local anesthetic (63, 292), but this effect can, at least partly, be explained by an inhibition of the active transport processes in the epithelium (292). Perfusing a jejunal segment with an isotonic solution of L-phenylalanine evokes a vasodilatation that is blocked by atropine (115). Similarly, atropine blocks the intestinal vascular response during digestion in conscious dogs (420a). Furthermore, the oleate-induced hyperemia is accompanied by a release of VIP (138), which indicates that VIPergic enteric nerves are activated. Finally, a further indirect support for the involvement of a noncholinergic nerves in postprandial hyperemia are the findings by Fara et al. (115) and Hernandez et al. (177) that vagotomy attenuates the postprandial hyperemia, a finding that lead Hernandez et al. to propose that the hyperemic response is mediated by the vagus nerves. From this review, it seems clear that the question of a possible involvement of nervous mechanism in the intestinal work hyperemia evoked by certain luminal nutrients is unsettled.

With regard to the question of a possible hormonal involvement in postprandial hyperemia, some early observations made by Fara et al. (115) suggest that hormones are of importance in this response. These authors showed that installing into the duodenum solutions with corn oil, L-phenylalanine (127 mM), or hydrochloric acid (127 mM) induces, with a certain time lag, an increase of blood flow in the superior mesenteric artery. Furthermore, intraduodenal administration of corn oil also elicits an increased blood flow in an adjacent jejunal segment. Cross-perfusion experiments demonstrated that venous blood from a duodenal segment containing corn oil increases blood flow in the small intestine of a recipient cat. These interesting experiments can be criticized on the grounds that the luminal stimuli were more pharmacological than physiological in the sense that meals do not usually contain only one substance but a mixture of nutrients.

In subsequent investigations of intraluminal factors of importance for the postprandial hyperemia, the intestinal mucosa has been exposed to solutions containing several food constituents. In most of these studies, the authors have tried to link the postprandial hyperemia to a release into blood of a vasoactive hormone or hormone candidate. The hormones most often discussed are CCK, gastrin, GIP, glucagon, neurotensin, and secretin (138, 323, 324). The effects of the individual substances are discussed in respective sections of this chapter. From experiments in which these different hormones have been given in amounts that correspond to the concentrations seen in blood after a meal, it can be concluded that physiological concentrations of these substances are not able to relax the intestinal resistance vessels (324). This seems also to be true when secretin, neurotensin, and CCK-8 are simultaneously infused close intra-arterially in doses calculated to give postprandial plasma concentrations (323). On the other hand, pharmacological concentrations of some of these peptide hormones increase intestinal blood flow, as has been discussed at length in this chapter.

In summary, the postprandial hyperemia in the small intestine seems to be caused by several factors working in concert. Part of the vasodilatation may be explained by mechanisms coupled to changes in tissue metabolism (tissue $P_{O_2}$ and hyperosmolality), whereas, at least during mechanical stimulation of the mucosa, local nervous reflexes are also involved. On the other hand, there is conflicting evidence with regard to a possible role for gastrointestinal hormones.

The authors gratefully acknowledge the excellent secretarial help of Eva Bengtsson.
Research in our laboratory was supported by Grant 2855 from the Swedish Medical Research Council.

REFERENCES

1. ABBOUD, F. M., D. L. ECKBERG, U. J. JOHANNSEN, AND A. L. MARK. Carotid and cardiopulmonary baroreceptor control of splanchnic and forearm vascular resistance during venous pooling in man. *J. Physiol. Lond.* 286: 173–184, 1979.
2. AGNATI, L. F., K. FUXE, F. BENFENATI, N. BATTISTINI, A. HÄRFSTRAND, K. TATEMOTO, T. HÖKFELT, AND V. MUTT. Neuropeptide Y in vitro selectively increases the number of $\alpha_2$-adrenergic binding sites in membranes of the medulla oblongata of the rat. *Acta Physiol. Scand.* 118: 293–295, 1983.
3. AHLMAN, H., L. DEMAGISTRIS, M. ZINNER, AND B. M. JAFFE. Release of immunoreactive serotonin into the lumen of the feline gut in response to vagal nerve stimulation. *Science Wash. DC* 213: 1254–1255, 1981.
4. AHLMAN, H., AND L. ENERBÄCK. A cytofluorimetric study of the myenteric plexus in the guinea pig. *Cell Tissue Res.* 153: 419–434, 1974.
5. AHLMAN, H., L. ENERBÄCK, J. KEWENTER, AND B. STORM. Effects of extrinsic denervation on the fluorescences of monoamines in the small intestine of the cat. *Acta Physiol. Scand.* 89: 429–435, 1973.
6. AHLMAN, H., K. GRÖNSTAD, O. NILSSON, AND A. DAHLSTRÖM. Biochemical and morphological studies on the secretion of 5-HT into the gut lumen of the rat. *Biogenic Amines* 1: 63–73, 1984.
7. ALEXANDER, R. S. The participation of the venomotor system in pressor reflexes. *Circ. Res.* 2: 405–409, 1954.
8. ALTURA, B. M. Chemical and humoral regulation of blood flow through the precapillary sphincters. *Microvasc. Res.* 3: 361–384, 1971.
9. ALUMETS, J., R. HÅKANSON, F. SUNDLER, AND K.-J. CHANG. Leu-enkephalin-like material in nerves and enterochromaffin cells in the gut. *Histochemistry* 56: 187–196, 1978.
10. ANDERSSON, P.-O. Adrenergic, Cholinergic, and Vipergic Neuro-Effector Control. With Special Reference to High-Frequency Burst Excitation Patterns. Lund: Univ. of Lund, 1983. PhD Thesis.
11. ANDERSSON, P.-O., S. R. BLOOM, A. V. EDWARDS, J. JÄRHULT, AND S. MELLANDER. Neural vasodilator control in the rectum of the cat and its possible mediation by vasoactive intestinal polypeptide. *J. Physiol. Lond.* 344: 49–67, 1983.
12. ANDERSSON, P.-O., S. R. BLOOM, AND J. JÄRHULT. Colonic motor and vascular responses to pelvic nerve stimulation and their relation to local peptide release in the cat. *J. Physiol. Lond.* 334: 293–307, 1983.
12a. APONTE, G. W., A. S. FINK, J. H. MEYER, K. TATEMOTO, AND I. L. TAYLOR. Regional distribution and release of peptide YY with fatty acids of different chain length. *Am. J. Physiol.* 249 (*Gastrointest. Liver Physiol.* 12): G745–G750, 1985.
13. AUDEN, R. M., AND D. E. DONALD. Reflex responses of the isolated in situ portal vein of the dog. *J. Surg. Res.* 18: 35–42, 1975.
14. BACA, I., U. MITTMANN, G. E. FEURLE, M. HAAS, AND T. MÜLLER. Effect of neurotensin on regional intestinal blood flow in the dog. *Res. Exp. Med.* 179: 53–58, 1981.
15. BAKER, R., AND D. MENDEL. Some observation on "autoregulatory escape" in cat intestine. *J. Physiol. Lond.* 190: 229–240, 1967.
16. BAYLISS, W. M. On the physiology of the depressor nerve. *J. Physiol. Lond.* 14: 303–325, 1893.
17. BEAN, J. W., AND M. M. SIDKY. Intestinal blood flow as influenced by vascular and motor reactions to acetylcholine and carbon dioxide. *Am. J. Physiol.* 194: 512–518, 1958.
18. BECKER, R. H. A., J. SCHOLTHOLT, B. A. SCHÖLKENS, W. JUNG, AND O. SPETH. A microsphere study on the effects of somatostatin and secretin on regional blood flow in anesthetized dogs. *Regul. Pept.* 4: 341–351, 1982.
19. BENYO, I., AND G. SZABO. The effect of intestinal hormones on splanchnic circulation. *Res. Exp. Med.* 173: 301–306, 1978.
20. BERNTHAL, T., AND F. J. SCHWIND. A comparison in intestine and leg of the reflex vascular response to carotid-aortic chemoreceptor stimulation. *Am. J. Physiol.* 143: 361–372, 1945.
21. BEUBLER, E., AND H. JUAN. PGE-release, blood flow and transmucosal water movement after mechanical stimulation of the rat jejunal mucosa. *Naunyn-Schmiedebergs Arch. Exp. Pathol. Pharmakol.* 305: 91–95, 1978.
22. BEVAN, J. A., R. D. BEVAN, AND S. P. DUCKLES. Adrenergic regulation of vascular smooth muscle. In: *Handbook of Physiology. The Cardiovascular System. Vascular Smooth Muscle*, edited by D. F. Bohr, A. P. Somlyo, and H. V. Sparks, Jr. Bethesda, MD: Am. Physiol. Soc., 1980, sect. 2, vol. II, chapt. 18, p. 515–566.
23. BEZOLD, A. VON, AND L. HIRT. Über die physiologischen Wirkungen des essigsauren Veratrins. *Unters. Physiol. Lab. Würtzburg* 1: 75–156, 1867.
24. BIBER, B., J. FARA, AND O. LUNDGREN. Intestinal vasodilatation in response to transmural electrical field stimulation. *Acta Physiol. Scand.* 87: 277–282, 1973.
25. BIBER, B., J. FARA, AND O. LUNDGREN. Intestinal vascular responses to 5-HT. *Acta Physiol. Scand.* 87: 526–534, 1973.
26. BIBER, B., J. FARA, AND O. LUNDGREN. Vascular reactions in the small intestine during vasodilatation. *Acta Physiol. Scand.* 89: 449–456, 1973.
27. BIBER, B., J. FARA, AND O. LUNDGREN. A pharmacological study of intestinal vasodilator mechanisms in the cat. *Acta Physiol. Scand.* 90: 673–683, 1974.
28. BIBER, B., O. LUNDGREN, AND J. SVANVIK. Studies on the intestinal vasodilatation observed after mechanical stimulation of the mucosa of the gut. *Acta Physiol. Scand.* 82: 177–190, 1971.
29. BINET, L., M. BURSTEIN, AND D. COULLAUD. Sur les réactions vasomotrices au niveau de l'intestin grêle. *C. R. Seances Soc. Biol. Fil.* 148: 1954–1958, 1954.
30. BISHOP, V., A. MALLIANI, AND P. THORÉN. Cardiac mechanoreceptors. In: *Handbook of Physiology. The Cardiovascular System. Peripheral Circulation and Organ Blood Flow*, edited by J. T. Shepherd and F. M. Abboud. Bethesda, MD: Am.

Physiol. Soc., 1983, sect. 2, vol. III, pt. 2, chapt. 15, p. 497–555.
31. BITAR, K. N., AND G. M. MAKHLOUF. Specific opiate receptors on isolated mammalian gastric smooth muscle cells. *Nature Lond.* 297: 72–74, 1982.
32. BLAIR-WEST, J. R. Renin-angiotensin system and sodium metabolism. In: *Kidney and Urinary Tract Physiology*, edited by K. Thurau. Baltimore, MD: University Park, 1976, vol. II, p. 95–143.
33. BLOOM, S. R., P. M. DANIEL, D. I. JOHNSTON, O. OGAWA, AND O. E. PRATT. Release of glucagon, induced by stress. *Q. J. Exp. Physiol. Cogn. Med. Sci.* 58: 99–108, 1973.
34. BODANZKY, M., Y. S. KLAUSNER, AND S. I. SAID. Biological activities of synthetic peptides corresponding to fragments of and to the entire sequence of the vasoactive intestinal peptide. *Proc. Natl. Acad. Sci. USA* 70: 382–384, 1973.
35. BOENHEIM, F. Über das Minutenvolumen des Magens und seine Beeinflussing durch Blutdruck, durch Vagusreizung, durch Histamin und durch Organextrakte. *Z. Gesamte Exp. Med.* 71: 185–191, 1930.
36. BOHLEN, H. G. Intestinal tissue $P_{O_2}$ and microvascular responses during glucose exposure. *Am. J. Physiol.* 238 (*Heart Circ. Physiol.* 7): H164–H171, 1980.
37. BOHLEN, H. G. Intestinal mucosal oxygenation influences absorptive hyperemia. *Am. J. Physiol.* 239 (*Heart Circ. Physiol.* 8): H489–H493, 1980.
38. BOHLEN, H. G. $Na^+$-induced intestinal interstitial hyperosmolality and vascular responses during absorptive hyperemia. *Am. J. Physiol.* 242 (*Heart Circ. Physiol.* 11): H785–H789, 1982.
39. BOHLEN, H. G., AND R. W. GORE. Comparison of microvascular pressures and diameters in the innervated and denervated rat intestine. *Microvasc. Res.* 14: 251–264, 1977.
40. BOHLEN, H. G., AND R. W. GORE. Microvascular pressures in rat intestinal muscle during direct nerve stimulation. *Microvasc. Res.* 17: 27–37, 1979.
41. BOHLEN, H. G., H. HENRICH, R. W. GORE, AND P. C. JOHNSON. Intestinal muscle and mucosal blood flow during direct sympathetic stimulation. *Am. J. Physiol.* 235 (*Heart Circ. Physiol.* 4): H40–H45, 1978.
42. BOHLEN, H. G., P. M. HUTCHINS, C. E. RAPELA, AND H. D. GREEN. Microvascular control in intestinal mucosa of normal and hemorrhaged rats. *Am. J. Physiol.* 229: 1159–1164, 1975.
43. BONJOUR, J. P., AND R. L. MALVIN. Stimulation of ADH release by the renin-angiotensin system. *Am. J. Physiol.* 218: 1555–1559, 1970.
44. BOWEN, J. C., W. PAWLIK, W.-F. FANG, AND E. D. JACOBSON. Pharmacologic effects of gastrointestinal hormones on intestinal oxygen consumption and blood flow. *Surgery St. Louis* 78: 515–519, 1975.
45. BRANCH, R. A., D. G. SHAND, AND A. S. NIES. Increase in hepatic blood flow and d-propranolol clearance by glucagon in the monkey. *J. Pharmacol. Exp. Ther.* 187: 581–587, 1973.
46. BRAZEAU, P., W. VALE, R. BURGUS, N. LING, M. BUTCHER, J. RIVIER, AND R. GUILLEMIN. Hypothalamic polypeptide that inhibits the secretion of immunoreactive growth hormone. *Science Wash. DC* 179: 77–79, 1973.
47. BRODIN, E., K. SJÖLUND, R. HÅKANSON, AND F. SUNDLER. Substance P-containing nerve fibers are numerous in human but not in feline intestinal mucosa. *Gastroenterology* 85: 557–564, 1983.
48. BROOKSBY, G. A., AND D. E. DONALD. Dynamic changes in splanchnic blood flow and blood volume in dogs during activation of sympathetic nerves. *Circ. Res.* 29: 227–238, 1971.
49. BROOKSBY, G. A., AND D. E. DONALD. Release of blood from the splanchnic circulation of dogs. *Circ. Res.* 31: 105–118, 1972.
50. BRUN, G. C. Variations in the diameter of abdominal arteries after intravenous injection of adrenaline. *Acta Pharmacol.* 1: 403–419, 1946.
51. BRUNSSON, I., S. EKLUND, M. JODAL, O. LUNDGREN, AND H. SJÖVALL. The effect of vasodilatation and sympathetic nerve activation on net water absorption in the cat's small intestine. *Acta Physiol. Scand.* 106: 61–68, 1979.
52. BÜLBRING, E., AND J. H. BURNS. Sympathetic vaso-dilation in the skin and the intestine of the dog. *J. Physiol. Lond.* 87: 254–274, 1936.
53. BUNCH, J. L. On the vaso-motor nerves of the small intestine. *J. Physiol. Lond.* 24: 72–98, 1899.
54. BURCHER, E., J. H. ATTERHÖG, B. PERNOW, AND S. ROSELL. Cardiovascular effects of SP: effects on the heart and regional blood flow in the dog. In: *Substance P*, edited by U. S. von Euler and B. Pernow. New York: Raven, 1977, p. 261. (Nobel Symp. Ser. no. 37.)
55. BURTON-OPITZ, R. Uber die Strömung des Blutes in dem Gebiete der Pfortader. III. Das Stromvolum der Vena lienalis. *Pfluegers Arch. Gesamte Physiol. Menschen Tiere* 135: 205–244, 1910.
56. BUSSOLATI, G., C. CAPELLA, E. SOLCIA, AND P. VEZZADINI. Ultrastructural and immunofluorescent investigations on the secretin cell in the dog intestinal mucosa. *Histochemie* 26: 218–227, 1971.
57. CARNEIRO, J. J., AND D. E. DONALD. Blood reservoir function of dog spleen, liver, and intestine. *Am. J. Physiol.* 232 (*Heart Circ. Physiol.* 1): H67–H72, 1977.
58. CARNEIRO, J. J., AND D. E. DONALD. Change in liver blood flow and blood content in dogs during direct and reflex alteration of hepatic sympathetic nerve activity. *Circ. Res.* 40: 150–158, 1977.
59. CARRAWAY, R., AND S. E. LEEMAN. The isolation of a new hypotensive peptide, neurotensin, from bovine hypothalami. *J. Biol. Chem.* 248: 6854–6861, 1973.
60. CELANDER, O. The range of control exercised by the "sympathico-adrenal system." *Acta Physiol. Scand.* 116: 1–132, 1954.
61. CHALMERS, J. P., P. J. KORNER, AND S. W. WHITE. Effects of haemorrhage on the distribution of peripheral blood flow in the rabbit. *J. Physiol. Lond.* 192: 561–574, 1967.
62. CHANG, M. M., S. E. LEEMAN, AND H. D. NIALL. Amino-acid sequence of substance P. *Nat. New Biol.* 232: 86–87, 1971.
63. CHOU, C.-C., T. D. BURNS, C. P. HSIEH, AND J. M. DABNEY. Mechanisms of local vasodilation with hypertonic glucose in the jejunum. *Surgery St. Louis* 71: 380–387, 1972.
64. CHOU, C. C., C. P. HSIEH, AND J. M. DABNEY. Comparison of vascular effects of gastrointestinal hormones in various organs. *Am. J. Physiol.* 232 (*Heart Circ. Physiol.* 1): H103–H109, 1977.
65. CHOU, C.-C., AND P. R. KVIETYS. Physiological and pharmacological alterations in gastrointestinal blood flow. In: *Measurements of Blood Flow. Applications to the Splanchnic Circulation*, edited by D. N. Granger and G. B. Bulkley. Baltimore, MD: Williams & Wilkins, 1981, p. 475–509.
66. CHOU, C.-C., P. KVIETYS, J. POST, AND S. P. SIT. Constituents of chyme responsible for postprandial intestinal hyperemia. *Am. J. Physiol.* 235 (*Heart Circ. Physiol.* 4): H677–H682, 1978.
67. CHRISTOFIDES, N. D., J. M. POLAK, AND S. R. BLOOM. Studies on the distribution of PHI in mammals. *Peptides NY* 5: 261–266, 1984.
68. CHRISTOFIDES, N. D., Y. YIANGOU, E. AARONS, G.-L. FERRI, K. TATEMOTO, J. M. POLAK, AND S. R. BLOOM. Radioimmunoassay and intramural distribution of PHI-IR in human intestine. *Dig. Dis. Sci.* 28: 507–512, 1983.
69. CLARK, G. A. The vaso-dilator action of adrenaline. *J. Physiol. Lond.* 80: 429–440, 1934.
70. COBBOLD, A., B. FOLKOW, I. KJELLMER, AND S. MELLANDER. Nervous and local chemical control of pre-capillary sphincters in skeletal muscle as measured by changes in filtration coefficient. *Acta Physiol. Scand.* 57: 180–192, 1963.
71. COHEN, M. L., E. ROSLING, K. WILEY, AND I. H. SLATER. Somatostatin inhibits adrenergic and cholinergic neurotransmission in smooth muscle. *Life Sci.* 23: 1659–1664, 1978.
72. COHEN, M. M., D. S. SITAR, J. R. MCNEILL, AND C. V. GREENWAY. Vasopressin and angiotensin on resistance vessels of spleen, intestine, and liver. *Am. J. Physiol.* 218: 1704–1706, 1970.
73. COSTA, M., A. C. CUELLO, J. B. FURNESS, AND R. FRANCO.

Distribution of enteric neurons showing immunoreactivity for substance P in the guinea-pig ileum. *Neuroscience* 5: 323–331, 1980.

74. COSTA, M., AND J. B. FURNESS. On the possibility that an indoleamine is a neurotransmitter in the gastrointestinal tract. *Biochem. Pharmacol.* 28: 565–571, 1979.

75. COSTA, M., AND J. B. FURNESS. The origins, pathways and terminations of neurons with VIP-like immunoreactivity in the guinea-pig small intestine. *Neuroscience* 8: 665–676, 1983.

76. COSTA, M., J. B. FURNESS, R. BUFFA, AND S. I. SAID. Distribution of enteric nerve cell bodies and axons showing immunoreactivity for vasoactive intestinal polypeptide in the guinea-pig intestine. *Neuroscience* 5: 587–596, 1980.

77. COSTA, M., J. B. FURNESS, A. C. CUELLO, A. A. J. VERHOFSTAD, H. W. J. STEINBUSCH, AND R. P. ELDE. Neurons with 5-hydroxytryptamine-like immunoreactivity in the enteric nervous system: their visualization and reactions to drug treatment. *Neuroscience* 7: 351–363, 1982.

78. COSTA, M., J. B. FURNESS, I. J. LLEWELLYN SMITH, B. DAVIES, AND J. OLIVER. An immunohistochemical study of the projections of somatostatin-containing neurons in the guinea-pig intestine. *Neuroscience* 5: 841–852, 1980.

79. COUTURE, R., AND D. REGOLI. Mini review: smooth muscle pharmacology of substance P. *Pharmacology Basel:* 24: 1–25, 1982.

80. COWLEY, A. W., JR., S. J. SWITZER, AND M. M. GUINN. Evidence and quantification of the vasopressin arterial pressure control system in the dog. *Circ. Res.* 46: 58–67, 1980.

81. CULL, T. E., M. P. SCIBETTA, AND E. E. SELKURT. Arterial inflow into the mesenteric and hepatic vascular circuits during hemorrhagic shock. *Am. J. Physiol.* 185: 365–371, 1956.

82. CUMMING, J. D., A. L. HAIGH, E. H. L. HARRIES, AND M. E. NUTT. A study of gastric secretion and blood flow in the anaesthetized dog. *J. Physiol. Lond.* 168: 219–233, 1963.

83. CURWAIN, B. P., AND P. HOLTON. The effects of isoprenaline and noradrenaline on pentagastrin-stimulated gastric acid secretion and mucosal blood flow in the dog. *Br. J. Pharmacol.* 46: 225–233, 1972.

84. DAHLÖF, C., P. DAHLÖF, K. TATEMOTO, AND J. M. LUNDBERG. Neuropeptide Y (NPY) reduces field stimulation-evoked release of noradrenaline and enhances force of contraction in the rat portal vein. *Naunyn-Schmiedeberg's Arch. Pharmacol.* 328: 327–330, 1985.

85. DAHLSTRÖM, A., AND H. AHLMAN. Immunocytochemical evidence for the presence of tryptaminergic nerves of blood vessels, smooth muscle and myenteric plexus in the rat small intestine. *Acta Physiol. Scand.* 117: 589–591, 1983.

86. DALE, H. H. On the action of ergotoxine; with special reference to the existence of sympathetic vasodilators. *J. Physiol. Lond.* 46: 291–300, 1913.

87. DELANEY, J. P., AND E. GRIM. Experimentally induced variations in canine gastric blood flow and its distribution. *Am. J. Physiol.* 208: 353–358, 1965.

88. DEVINE, C. E., AND F. O. SIMPSON. The fine structure of vascular sympathetic neuromuscular contacts in the rat. *Am. J. Anat.* 121: 153–174, 1967.

89. DIECKHOFF, D., K. HALL, AND U. RITTER. Einfluss des Sekretins auf die arteriellen und venösen Drücke im Mesenterialkreislauf des Kaninchens. *Res. Exp. Med.* 162: 75–81, 1974.

90. DONALD, D. E. Splanchnic circulation. In: *Handbook of Physiology. The Cardiovascular System. Peripheral Circulation and Organ Blood Flow*, edited by D. F. Bohr, A. P. Somlyo, and H. V. Sparks, Jr. Bethesda, MD: Am. Physiol. Soc., 1980, sect. 2, vol. III, pt. 1, chapt. 7, p. 219–240.

91. DONALD, D. E., AND L. L. AARHUS. Active and passive release of blood from canine spleen and small intestine. *Am. J. Physiol.* 227: 1166–1172, 1974.

92. DOYLE, H., G. H. GREELEY, JR., L. MATE, T. SAKAMOTO, C. M. TOWNSEND, JR., AND J. C. THOMPSON. Distribution of neurotensin in the canine gastrointestinal tract. *Surgery St. Louis* 97: 337–341, 1985.

93. DRESEL, P., B. FOLKOW, AND I. WALLENTIN. Rubidium[86] clearance during neurogenic redistribution of intestinal blood flow. *Acta Physiol. Scand.* 67: 173–184, 1966.

94. DRESEL, P., AND I. WALLENTIN. Effects of sympathetic vasoconstrictor fibres, noradrenaline and vasopressin on the intestinal vascular resistance during constant blood flow or blood pressure. *Acta Physiol. Scand.* 66: 427–436, 1966.

95. EAVES, E. R., J. HANSKY, AND M. G. KORMAN. The effect of atropine and vagal stimulation on the release of neurotensin-like immunoreactivity in man. *Regul. Pept.* 11: 1–10, 1985.

96. ECKSTEIN, J. W., A. L. MARK, P. G. SCHMID, T. IIZUKA, AND M. G. WENDLING. Responses of capacitance vessels to physiologic stimuli. *Trans. Am. Clin. Climatol. Assoc.* 81: 57–64, 1970.

97. EDVINSSON, L., E. EKBLAD, R. HÅKANSON, AND C. WAHLESTEDT. Neuroeptide Y potentiates the effect of various vasoconstrictor agents on rabbit blood vessels. *Br. J. Pharmacol.* 83: 519–525, 1984.

98. EIMERL, J., M. A. BAYORH, Z. ZUKOWSKA-GRÓJEC, AND G. FEUERSTEIN. Motilin effects on the heart and blood vessels of the pithed rat. *Neuropeptides* 6: 157–165, 1985.

99. EKBLAD, E., L. EDVINSSON, C. WAHLESTEDT, R. UDDMAN, R. HÅKANSON, AND F. SUNDLER. Neuropeptide Y co-exists and co-operates with noradrenaline in perivascular nerve fibers. *Regul. Pept.* 8: 225–235, 1984.

100. EKLUND, S., J. FAHRENKRUG, M. JODAL, O. LUNDGREN, O. B. SCHAFFALITZKY DE MUCKADELL, AND A. SJÖQVIST. Vasoactive intestinal polypeptide, 5-hydroxytryptamine and reflex hyperaemia in the small intestine of the cat. *J. Physiol. Lond.* 302: 549–557, 1980.

101. EKLUND, S., M. JODAL, O. LUNDGREN, AND A. SJÖQVIST. Effects of vasoactive intestinal polypeptide on blood flow, motility and fluid transport in the gastrointestinal tract of the cat. *Acta Physiol. Scand.* 105: 461–468, 1979.

102. ELDE, R., T. HÖKFELT, O. JOHANSSON, AND L. TERENIUS. Immunohistochemical studies using antibodies to leucine-enkephalin: initial observations on the nervous system of the rat. *Neuroscience* 1: 349–351, 1976.

103. EMSON, P. C., AND M. E. DE QUIDT. NPY—a new member of the pancreatic polypeptide family. *Trends Neurosci.* 5: 31–35, 1984.

104. ESTENSEN, R. D., AND R. P. GILBERT. Response of ileal segment weight to prolonged levarterenol infusion. *Am. J. Physiol.* 201: 628–630, 1961.

105. EULER, U. S. VON, AND J. H. GADDUM. An unidentified depressor substance in certain tissue extracts. *J. Physiol. Lond.* 72: 74–87, 1931.

106. EYZAGUIRRE, C., R. FITZGERALD, S. LAHIRI, AND P. ZAPATA. Arterial chemoreceptors. In: *Handbook of Physiology. The Cardiovascular System. Peripheral Circulation and Organ Blood Flow*, edited by J. T. Shepherd and F. M. Abboud. Bethesda, MD: Am. Physiol. Soc., 1983, sect. 2, vol. III, pt. 2, chapt. 16, p. 557–621.

107. FAHRENKRUG, J., U. HAGLUND, M. JODAL, O. LUNDGREN, L. OLBE, AND O. B. SCHAFFALITZKY DE MUCKADELL. Nervous release of vasoactive intestinal polypeptide in the gastrointestinal tract of cats. Possible physiological implications. *J. Physiol. Lond.* 284: 291–305, 1978.

108. FANG, W.-F., AND H. W. STROBEL. Stimulation of colonic blood flow by pentagastrin (41392). *Proc. Soc. Exp. Biol. Med.* 170: 35–38, 1982.

109. FARA, J. W. Escape from tension induced by noradrenaline or electrical stimulation in isolated mesenteric arteries. *Br. J. Pharmacol.* 43: 865–867, 1971.

110. FARA, J. W. Mesenteric vasodilator effect of 5-hydroxytryptamine: possible enteric neuron mediation. *Arch. Int. Pharmacodyn. Ther.* 221: 235–249, 1976.

111. FARA, J. W. Postprandial mesenteric hyperemia. In: *Physiology of the Intestinal Circulation*, edited by A. P. Shepherd and D. N. Granger. New York: Raven, 1984, p. 99–106.

112. FARA, J. W., AND K. S. MADDEN. Effect of secretin and cholecystokinin on small intestinal blood flow distribution. *Am. J. Physiol.* 229: 1365–1370, 1975.

113. FARA, J. W., AND G. ROSS. Escape from drug-induced constriction of isolated arterial segments from various vascular beds. *Blood Vessels* 9: 27–33, 1972.
114. FARA, J. W., E. H. RUBINSTEIN, AND R. R. SONNENSCHEIN. Visceral and behavioral responses to intraduodenal fat. *Science Wash. DC* 166: 110–111, 1969.
115. FARA, J. W., E. H. RUBINSTEIN, AND R. R. SONNENSCHEIN. Intestinal hormones in mesenteric vasodilation after intraduodenal agents. *Am. J. Physiol.* 223: 1058–1067, 1972.
116. FASTH, S., U. HAGLUND, AND L. HULTÉN. Effects of regional vasopressin infusion on intestinal series-coupled vascular sections. *Acta Chir. Scand.* 147: 577–581, 1981.
117. FASTH, S., H. HEDLUND, L. HULTÉN, S. NORDGREN, AND T. ÖRESLAND. The effects of 5-hydroxytryptamine on large intestinal motility and blood flow in the cat. *Acta Physiol. Scand.* 118: 329–336, 1983.
118. FASTH, S., AND L. HULTÉN. The effect of glucagon on intestinal motility and blood flow. *Acta Physiol. Scand.* 83: 169–173, 1971.
119. FASTH, S., L. HULTÉN, B. J. JOHNSSON, S. NORDGREN, AND I. J. ZEITLIN. Mobilization of colonic kallikrein following pelvic nerve stimulation in the atropinized cat. *J. Physiol. Lond.* 285: 471–478, 1978.
120. FASTH, S., L. HULTÉN, O. LUNDGREN, AND S. NORDGREN. Vascular responses to mechanical stimulation of the mucosa of the cat colon. *Acta Physiol. Scand.* 101: 98–104, 1977.
121. FASTH, S., L. HULTÉN, S. NORDGREN, AND J. ZEITLIN. Studies on the atropine-resistant sacral parasympathetic vascular and motility responses in the cat colon. *J. Physiol. Lond.* 311: 421–429, 1981.
122. FERRIS, C. F., M. J. ARMSTRONG, J. K. GEORGE, C. A. STEVENS, R. E. CARRAWAY, AND S. E. LEEMAN. Alcohol and fatty acid stimulation of neurotensin release from rat small intestine. *Endocrinology* 116: 1133–1138, 1985.
123. FIORAMONTI, J., AND L. BUENO. Relation between intestinal motility and mesenteric blood flow in the conscious dog. *Am. J. Physiol.* 246 (*Gastrointest. Liver Physiol.* 9): G108–G113, 1984.
124. FOLKOW, B., J. FROST, AND B. UVNÄS. Action of adrenaline, nor-adrenaline and some other sympathomimetic drugs on the muscular, cutaneous and splanchnic vessels of the cat. *Acta Physiol. Scand.* 15: 412–420, 1948.
125. FOLKOW, B., D. H. LEWIS, O. LUNDGREN, S. MELLANDER, AND I. WALLENTIN. The effect of graded vasoconstrictor fibre stimulation on the intestinal resistance and capacitance vessels. *Acta Physiol. Scand.* 61: 445–457, 1964.
126. FOLKOW, B., D. H. LEWIS, O. LUNDGREN, S. MELLANDER, AND I. WALLENTIN. The effect of the sympathetic vasoconstrictor fibres on the distribution of capillary blood flow in the intestine. *Acta Physiol. Scand.* 61: 458–466, 1964.
127. FORSYTH, R. P., B. I. HOFFBRAND, AND K. L. MELMON. Hemodynamic effects of angiotensin in normal and environmentally stressed monkeys. *Circulation* 44: 119–129, 1971.
128. FREEMAN, R. H., J. O. DAVIS, J. A. JOHNSON, W. S. SPIELMAN, AND M. L. ZATZMAN. Arterial pressure regulation during hemorrhage: homeostatic role of angiotensin II (38735). *Proc. Soc. Exp. Biol. Med.* 149: 19–22, 1975.
129. FRIESEN, S. R., AND A. HEMINGWAY. The vascular response of the stomach to experimental alterations in the autonomic nervous system of the dog. *Am. J. Surg.* 18: 195–200, 1952.
130. FURCHGOTT, R. F. Role of endothelium in responses of vascular smooth muscle. *Circ. Res.* 53: 557–573, 1983.
131. FURNESS, J. B. The adrenergic innervation of the vessels supplying and draining the gastrointestinal tract. *Z. Zellforsch. Mikrosk. Anat.* 113: 67–82, 1971.
131a. FURNESS, J. B., AND M. COSTA. Types of nerves in the enteric nervous system. *Neuroscience* 5: 1–20, 1980.
132. FURNESS, J. B., AND M. COSTA. Neurons with 5-hydroxytryptamine-like immunoreactivity in the enteric nervous system: their projections in the guinea-pig small intestine. *Neuroscience* 7: 341–349, 1982.
133. FURNESS, J. B., M. COSTA, AND F. ECKENSTEIN. Neurones localized with antibodies against choline acetyltransferase in the enteric nervous system. *Neurosci. Lett.* 40: 105–109, 1983.
134. FURNESS, J. B., M. COSTA, P. C. EMSON, R. HÅKANSON, E. MOGHIM-ZADEH, F. SUNDLER, I. L. TAYLOR, AND R. E. CHANCE. Distribution, pathways and reactions to drug treatment of nerves with neuropeptide Y- and pancreatic polypeptide-like immunoreactivity in the guinea-pig digestive tract. *Cell Tissue Res.* 234: 71–92, 1983.
135. FURNESS, J. B., M. COSTA, AND J. R. KEAST. Choline acetyltransferase- and peptide immunoreactivity of submucous neurons in the small intestine of the guinea-pig. *Cell Tissue Res.* 237: 329–336, 1984.
136. FURNESS, J. B., M. COSTA, AND R. J. MILLER. Distribution and projections of nerves with enkephalin-like immunoreactivity in the guinea-pig small intestine. *Neuroscience* 8: 653–664, 1983.
137. FURNESS, J. B., AND J. M. MARSHALL. Correlation of the directly observed responses of mesenteric vessels of the rat to nerve stimulation and noradrenaline with the distribution of adrenergic nerves. *J. Physiol. Lond.* 239: 75–88, 1974.
138. GALLAVAN, R. H., JR., M. H. CHEN, S. N. JOFFE, AND E. D. JACOBSON. Vasoactive intestinal polypeptide, cholecystokinin, glucagon, and bile-oleate-induced jejunal hyperemia. *Am. J. Physiol.* 248 (*Gastrointest. Liver Physiol.* 11): G208–G215, 1985.
139. GALLAVAN, R. H., JR., AND C.-C. CHOU. Possible mechanisms for the initiation and maintenance of postprandial intestinal hyperemia. *Am. J. Physiol.* 249 (*Gastrointest. Liver Physiol.* 12): G301–G308, 1985.
140. GIRAUD, G. D., AND L. MACCANNELL. Decreased nutrient blood flow during dopamine- and epinephrine-induced intestinal vasodilation. *J. Pharmacol. Exp. Ther.* 230: 214–220, 1984.
141. GOLLWITZER-MEIER, K., AND H. SCHULTE. Der Einfluss der Sinusnerven auf Venensystem und Herzminutenvolumen. *Pluegers Arch. Gesamte Physiol. Menschen Tiere* 229: 264–277, 1931.
142. GORE, R. W., AND H. G. BOHLEN. Microvascular pressures in rat intestinal muscle and mucosal villi. *Am. J. Physiol.* 233 (*Heart Circ. Physiol.* 2): H685–H693, 1977.
143. GRANGER, D. N., J. A. BARROWMAN, S. L. HARPER, P. R. KVIETYS, AND R. J. KORTHUIS. Sympathetic stimulation and intestinal capillary fluid exchange. *Am. J. Physiol.* 247 (*Gastrointest. Liver Physiol.* 10): G279–G283, 1984.
144. GRANGER, D. N., P. R. KVIETYS, W. H. WILBORN, N. A. MORTILLARO, AND A. E. TAYLOR. Mechanism of glucagon-induced intestinal secretion. *Am. J. Physiol.* 239 (*Gastrointest. Liver Physiol.* 2): G30–G38, 1980.
145. GRANGER, D. N., G. RUTILI, AND J. M. MCCORD. Superoxide radicals in feline intestinal ischemia. *Gastroenterology* 81: 22–29, 1981.
146. GRANGER, D. N., M. SENNETT, P. MCELEARNEY, AND A. E. TAYLOR. Effect of local arterial hypotension on cat intestinal capillary permeability. *Gastroenterology* 79: 474–480, 1980.
146a. GRANGER, D. N., J. D. VALLEAU, R. E. PARKER, R. S. LANE, AND A. E. TAYLOR. Effects of adenosine on intestinal hemodynamics, oxygen delivery, and capillary fluid exchange. *Am. J. Physiol.* 235 (*Heart Circ. Physiol.* 4): H707–H719, 1978.
146b. GRANGER, H. J., AND C. P. NORRIS. Role of adenosine in local control of intestinal circulation in the dog. *Circ. Res.* 46: 764–770, 1980.
147. GRANGER, H. J., AND A. P. SHEPHERD. Dynamics and control of the microcirculation. In: *Advances in Biomedical Engineering*, edited by J. H. U. Brown. New York: Academic, 1979, vol. 7, p. 1–63.
148. GREEN, H. D., C. P. DEAL, JR., S. BARDHANABAEDYA, AND A. B. DENISON, JR. The effects of adrenergic substances and ischemia on the blood flow and peripheral resistance of the canine mesenteric vascular bed before and during adrenergic blockade. *J. Pharmacol. Exp. Ther.* 113: 115–123, 1955.
149. GREENWAY, C. V., AND A. E. LAWSON. The effects of adrenaline and noradrenaline on venous return and regional blood

flows in the anesthetized cat with special reference to intestinal blood flow. *J. Physiol. Lond.* 186: 579–595, 1966.
150. GREENWAY, C. V., AND A. E. LAWSON. Effects of adrenaline and propranolol on the superior mesenteric artery blood flow. *Can. J. Pharmacol.* 46: 906–908, 1968.
151. GREENWAY, C. V., AND G. E. LISTER. Capacitance effects and blood reservoir function in the splanchnic vascular bed during non-hypotensive hemorrhage and blood volume expansion in anesthetized cats. *J. Physiol. Lond.* 237: 279–294, 1974.
152. GREENWAY, C. V., G. D. SCOTT, AND J. ZINK. Sites of autoregulatory escape of blood flow in the mesenteric vascular bed. *J. Physiol. Lond.* 259: 1–12, 1976.
153. GRÖNSTAD, K. O., A. DAHLSTRÖM, L. FLORENCE, M. J. ZINNER, H. AHLMAN, AND B. M. JAFFE. Regulatory mechanisms in the endoluminal release of serotonin and substance P from the feline jejunum. *Dig. Dis. Sci.* 32: 393–400, 1987.
154. GRÖNSTAD, K. O., A. DAHLSTRÖM, B. M. JAFFE, AND H. AHLMAN. Regional and selective changes in blood flow of the feline small intestine induced by endoluminal serotonin. *Acta Physiol. Scand.* 127: 207–213, 1986.
155. GRÖNSTAD, K. O., A. DAHLSTRÖM, B. M. JAFFE, M. J. ZINNER, AND H. AHLMAN. Studies on the mucosal hyperemia of the feline small intestine observed at endoluminal perfusion with substance P. *Acta Physiol. Scand.* 128: 97–108, 1986.
156. GRÖNSTAD, K. O., A. DEMAGISTRIS, A. DAHLSTRÖM, O. NILSSON, B. PRICE, M. J. ZINNER, B. M. JAFFE, AND H. AHLMAN. The effects of vagal nerve stimulation on endoluminal release of serotonin and substance P into the feline small intestine. *Scand. J. Gastroenterol.* 20: 163–169, 1985.
158. GRUND, E. R., J. D. REED, AND D. J. SANDERS. The effect of sympathetic nerve stimulation on acid secretion, regional blood flows and oxygen usage by stomachs of anaesthetized cats. *J. Physiol. Lond.* 248: 639–647, 1975.
159. GUTH, P. H., H. BAUMANN, M. I. GROSSMAN, D. AURES, AND J. ELASHOFF. Measurement of gastric mucosal blood flow in man. *Gastroenterology* 74: 831–834, 1978.
160. GUTH, P. H., AND E. SMITH. Vasoactive agents and the gastric microcirculation. *Microvasc. Res.* 8: 125–131, 1974.
161. GUTH, P. H., AND E. SMITH. Escape from vasoconstriction in the gastric microcirculation. *Am. J. Physiol.* 228: 1893–1895, 1975.
162. GUTH, P. H., AND E. SMITH. The effect of gastrointestinal hormones on the gastric microcirculation. *Gastroenterology* 71: 435–438, 1976.
163. HADDY, F. J., J. I. MOLNAR, C. W. BORDEN, AND E. C. TEXTER, JR. Comparison of direct effects of angiotensin and other vasoactive agents on small and large blood vessels in several vascular beds. *Circulation* 25: 239–246, 1962.
164. HADJIMINAS, J., AND B. ÖBERG. Effects of carotid baroreceptor reflexes on venous tone in skeletal muscle and intestine of the cat. *Acta Physiol. Scand.* 72: 518–532, 1968.
165. HAGLUND, U. Vascular reactions in the small intestine of the cat during hemorrhage. *Acta Physiol. Scand.* 89: 129–141, 1973.
166. HAGLUND, U. The small intestine in hypotension and hemorrhage. An experimental cardiovascular study in the cat. *Acta Physiol. Scand. Suppl.* 387: 1–37, 1973.
167. HALLBÄCK, D.-A., M. JODAL, AND O. LUNDGREN. Villous tissue osmolality, water and electrolyte transport in the cat small intestine at varying luminal osmolalities. *Acta Physiol. Scand.* 110: 95–100, 1980.
168. HALLBERG, D., AND B. PERNOW. Effect of subsance P on various vascular beds in the dog. *Acta Physiol. Scand.* 93: 277–285, 1975.
169. HAMMER, R. A., R. E. CARRAWAY, AND S. E. LEEMAN. Elevation of plasma neurotensinlike immunoreactivity after a meal. *J. Clin. Invest.* 70: 74–81, 1982.
170. HANSSON, K. M. Vascular response of intestine and liver to intravenous infusion of vasopressin. *Am. J. Physiol.* 219: 779–784, 1970.
171. HARPER, S. L., J. A. BARROWMAN, P. R. KVIETYS, AND D. N. GRANGER. Effect of neurotensin on intestinal capillary permeability and blood flow. *Am. J. Physiol.* 247 (*Gastrointest. Liver Physiol.* 10): G161–G166, 1984.
172. HELLSTRÖM, P. M., O. OLERUP, AND K. TATEMOTO. Neuropeptide Y may mediate effects of sympathetic nerve stimulations on colonic motility and blood flow in the cat. *Acta Physiol. Scand.* 124: 613–624, 1985.
173. HENRICH, H. Adjustment behavior of adrenergic-induced vasoconstriction in the intestinal circulation of the cat. *Angiologica Basel* 10: 233–247, 1973.
174. HENRICH, H., AND J. LUTZ. Das vasculäre Escape-Phänomen am Intestinalkreislauf und seine Auslösung durch unterschiedliche vasoconstrictorische Substanzen. *Pfluegers Arch.* 329: 82–94, 1971.
175. HENRICH, H., AND G. SINGBARTL. Vascular adjustments in dilatory reactions. Effect of acetylcholine, isoproterenol and propranolol. *Angiologica Basel* 10: 185–197, 1973.
176. HENRICH, H., G. SINGBARTL, AND J. BIESTER. Adrenergic-induced vascular adjustments—initial and escape reactions. I. Influence of β-adrenergic blocking agents on the intestinal circulation of the rat (in vivo). *Pfluegers Arch.* 346: 1–12, 1974.
177. HERNANDEZ, L. A., P. R. KVIETYS, AND D. N. GRANGER. Postprandial hemodynamics in the conscious rat. *Am. J. Physiol.* 251 (*Gastrointest. Liver Physiol.* 14): G117–G123, 1986.
178. HEYMANS, C., J.-J. BOUCKAERT, AND L. DAUTREBANDE. Sinus carotidien et reflexes venomoteurs mesenteriques. *C. R. Seances Soc. Biol. Fil.* 105: 217–219, 1930.
179. HÖKFELT, T., O. JOHANSSON, Å. LJUNGDAL, J. M. LUNDBERG, AND M. SCHULTZBERG. Peptidergic neurons. *Nature Lond.* 284: 515–521, 1980.
180. HÖKFELT, T., J. F. REFELD, B. IVEMARK, M. GOLDSTEIN, AND K. MARKEY. Evidence for coexistence of dopamine and CCK in mesolimbic neurones. *Nature Lond.* 285: 476–478, 1980.
181. HOLLIGER, C., M. RADZYNER, AND M. KNOBLAUCH. Effects of glucagon, vasoactive intestinal peptide, and vasopressin on villous microcirculation and superior mesenteric artery blood flow of the rat. *Gastroenterology* 85: 1036–1043, 1983.
182. HOLZER, P., A. BUCSICS, A. SARIA, AND F. LEMBECK. A study of the concentrations of substance P and neurotensin in the gastrointestinal tract of various mammals. *Neuroscience* 7: 2919–2924, 1982.
183. HOOPER, R., J. D. REED, AND J. SANDERS. Pepsin secretion in the anaesthetized cat and the effect of sympathetic nerve stimulation. *J. Physiol. Lond.* 260: 609–627, 1976.
184. HOTTENROTT, C., R. SEUFERT, J. DOERTENBACH, AND G. BUCKBERG. The influence of autonomous nervous activity on total and regional gastric blood flow. *Scand. J. Gastroenterol.* 19, Suppl. 89: 37–39, 1984.
185. HUGHES, J., T. W. SMITH, H. W. KOSTERLITZ, L. A. FOTHERGILL, B. A. MORGAN, AND H. R. MORRIS. Identification of two related pentapeptides from the brain with potent opiate agonist activity. *Nature Lond.* 258: 577–579, 1975.
186. HULSTAERT, P. F., H. J. M. BEIJER, F. A. S. BROUWER, A. J. TEUNISSEN, AND G. A. CHARBON. Glucagon: hemodynamic action related to the effect on $K^+$ and $Na^+$ metabolism. *J. Appl. Physiol.* 37: 556–561, 1974.
187. HULSTAERT, P. F., W. J. C. GEURTS, F. A. S. GROUWER, H. J. M. BEIJER, AND G. A. CHARBON. Hemodynamic actions of pentagastrin. *Scand. J. Gastroenterol.* 15: 7–15, 1980.
188. HULTÉN, L., M. JODAL, AND O. LUNDGREN. Extrinsic nervous control of colonic blood flow. *Acta Physiol. Scand. Suppl.* 335: 39–49, 1969.
189. HULTÉN, L., M. JODAL, AND O. LUNDGREN. Local and nervous control of the consecutive vascular sections of the colon. *Acta Physiol. Scand. Suppl.* 335: 51–64, 1969.
190. HULTÉN, L., M. JODAL, AND O. LUNDGREN. Nervous control of blood flow in the parallel-coupled vascular sections of the colon. *Acta Physiol. Scand. Suppl.* 335: 65–76, 1969.
191. HULTÉN, L., J. LINDHAGEN, AND O. LUNDGREN. Sympathetic nervous control of intramural blood flow in the feline and human intestines. *Gastroenterology* 72: 41–48, 1977.
192. IMMINK, W. F. G. A., G. H. OUWEJAN, AND G. A. CHARBON.

Vasoactivity of adrenaline in regions covering the canine gastrointestinal tract. *Arch. Int. Pharmacodyn. Ther.* 268: 75–87, 1984.
193. INOUE, K., R. HOSOTANI, K. TATEMOTO, V. MUTT, AND T. TOBE. Effect of PYY on blood flow and exocrine secretion of the pancreas in dogs (Abstract). *Gastroenterology* 88: 1427–1985.
194. IVARSSON, L. E., N. DARLE, L. HULTEN, J. LINDHAGEN, AND O. LUNDGREN. Gastric blood flow and distribution: the effect of pentagastrin in anesthetized cat and man as studied by an inert gas elimination method. *Scand. J. Gastroenterol.* 17: 1037–1048, 1982.
195. IVARSSON, L. E., N. DARLE, AND O. LUNDGREN. The effects of somatostatin on blood flow in the secretory part of the human stomach. *Surg. Gastroenterol.* 1: 29–34, 1982.
196. IVERSEN, L. L. Non-adrenergic, non-cholinergic autonomic neurotransmission mechanisms—putative transmitters. In: *Neuroscience Research Program Bulletin*, edited by G. Burnstock, M. D. Gershon, T. Hökfelt, L. L. Iversen, H. W. Kosterlitz, and J. H. Szurszewski. Cambridge, MA: MIT Press, 1979, vol. 17, p. 406–459.
197. IZQUIERDO, J. J., AND E. KOCH. Über den Einfluss der Nervi Splanchnici auf den arteriellen Blutdruck des Kaninchens. *Z. Kreislaufforsch.* 22: 735–743, 1930.
198. JACOBSON, E. D., AND A. C. K. CHANG. Comparison of gastrin and histamine on gastric mucosal blood flow. *Proc. Soc. Exp. Biol. Med.* 130: 484–486, 1969.
199. JACOBSON, E. D., R. H. LINFORD, AND M. I. GROSSMAN. Gastric secretion in relation to mucosal blood flow studied by a clearance technic. *J. Clin. Invest.* 45: 1–13, 1966.
200. JANSSON, G., M. KAMPP, O. LUNDGREN, AND J. MARTINSON. Studies on the circulation of the stomach (Abstract). *Acta Physiol. Scand. Suppl.* 277: 91, 1966.
201. JANSSON, G., O. LUNDGREN, AND J. MARTINSON. Neurohormonal control of gastric blood flow. *Gastroenterology* 58: 425–429, 1970.
202. JASPAN, J., K. POLONSKY, M. LEWIS, AND A. R. MOOSSA. Reduction in portal vein blood flow by somatostatin. *Diabetes* 28: 888–891, 1979.
202a. JASPAN, J. B., AND H. RUBENSTEIN. Circulating glucagon. *Diabetes* 26: 887–902, 1977.
203. JODAL, M., U. HAGLUND, AND O. LUNDGREN. Countercurrent exchange mechanisms in the small intestine. In: *Physiology of the Intestinal Circulation*, edited by A. P. Shepherd and D. N. Granger. New York: Raven, 1984, p. 83–97.
204. JODAL, M., AND O. LUNDGREN. Countercurrent mechanisms in the mammalian gastrointestinal tract. *Gastroenterology* 91: 225–241, 1986.
205. JODAL, M., O. LUNDGREN, AND A. SJÖQVIST. The effect of apamin on non-adrenergic, non-cholinergic vasodilator mechanisms in the intestines of the cat. *J. Physiol. Lond.* 338: 207–219, 1983.
206. JOHNSON, J. M., L. B. ROWELL, M. NIEDERBERGER, AND M. M. EISMAN. Human splanchnic and forearm vasoconstrictor responses to reductions of right atrial and aortic pressures. *Circ. Res.* 34: 515–524, 1974.
207. JONSSON, O., J. SVANVIK, AND P. VIKGREN. Regional differences in vascular tachyphylaxis to angiotensin in the cat. *Angiologica Basel* 4: 299–309, 1967.
208. KACHELHOFFER, J., M. R. ELOY, A. POUSSE, D. HOHMATTER, AND J. F. GRENIER. Mesenteric vasomotor effects of vasoactive intestinal polypeptide. Study on perfused isolated canine jejunal loops. *Pfluegers Arch.* 352: 37–46, 1974.
209. KAPITOLA, J., O. KUCHEL, O. SCHREIBEROVA, AND I. JAHODA. Blood flow through organs of the rat after an intravenous injection of angiotensin. *Physiol. Bohemoslov.* 17: 437–443, 1968.
210. KARASHIMA, T. Effects of vasopressin on smooth muscle cells of guinea-pig mesenteric vessels. *Br. J. Pharmacol.* 72: 673–684, 1981.
210a. KARIM, F., R. HAINSWORTH, AND R. P. PANDEY. Reflex responses of abdominal vascular capacitance from aortic baroreceptors in dogs. *Am. J. Physiol.* 235 (*Heart Circ. Physiol.* 4): H488–493, 1978.
211. KARLSTRÖM, L. Mechanisms in bile salt-induced secretion in the small intestine. *Acta Physiol. Scand.* 126, Suppl. 549: 1–48, 1986.
212. KEAST, J. R., J. B. FURNESS, AND M. COSTA. Somatostatin in human enteric nerves. Distribution and characterization. *Cell Tissue Res.* 237: 299–308, 1984.
213. KEAST, J. R., J. B. FURNESS, AND M. COSTA. Distribution of certain peptide-containing nerve fibres and endocrine cells in the gastrointestinal mucosa in five mammalian species. *J. Comp. Neurol.* 236: 403–422, 1985.
214. KELLER, U., A. PERRUCHOUD, L. KAYASSEH, AND N. GYR. Effect of therapeutic doses of somatostatin (SST) on splanchnic blood flow in man (Abstract). *Eur. J. Clin. Invest.* 8: 335, 1978.
215. KENDRICK, E., B. ÖBERG, AND G. WENNERGREN. Vasoconstrictor fiber discharge to skeletal muscle, kidney, intestine and skin at varying levels of arterial baroreceptor activity in the cat. *Acta Physiol. Scand.* 85: 464–476, 1972.
216. KERR, J. C., R. W. HOBSON, R. F. SEELIG, AND K. G. SWAN. Influence of vasopressin on colon blood flow in monkeys. *Gastroenterology* 72: 474–478, 1977.
217. KERR, J. C., D. G. REYNOLDS, AND K. G. SWAN. Adrenergic stimulation and blockade in mesenteric circulation of the baboon. *Am. J. Physiol.* 234 (*Endocrinol. Metab. Gastrointest. Physiol.* 3): E457–E462, 1978.
218. KERR, J. C., D. G. REYNOLDS, AND K. G. SWAN. Vasopressin and blood flow to the canine small intestine. *J. Surg. Res.* 25: 435–441, 1978.
219. KEWENTER, J. The vagal control of the jejunal and ileal motility and blood flow. *Acta Physiol. Scand. Suppl.* 251: 1–68, 1965.
220. KEWENTER, J. Effects of graded acetylcholine infusions on intestinal motility, volume and blood flow. *Scand. J. Gastroenterol.* 6: 435–440, 1971.
221. KHUGAEVA, V. K., V. V. SUCHOW, AND M. I. TITOV. Effect of leu-enkephalin and tyrosine on lymphatic and blood microvessels. *Kardiologiya* 22: 83–86, 1982.
222. KOBAYASHI, S., M. SUZUKI, T. UCHIDA, AND N. YANAIHAR. Enkephalin neurons in the guinea pig duodenum: a light and electron microscopic immunocytochemical study using an antiserum to methionine-enkephalin-Arg[6]-Gly[7]-Leu[8]. *Biomed. Res.* 5: 489–506, 1984.
223. KOCK, N. G., S. TIBBLIN, AND W. G. SCHENK, JR. Hemodynamic response to glucagon: an experimental study of central, visceral and peripheral effects. *Ann. Surg.* 171: 373–379, 1970.
224. KONTUREK, S. J., A. DEMBIŃSKI, R. KRÓL, AND E. WUNSCH. Effect of 13-NLE-motilin on gastric secretion, serum gastrin level and mucosal blood flow in dogs. *J. Physiol. Lond.* 264: 665–672, 1977.
225. KONTUREK, S. J., A. DEMBIŃSKI, P. THOR, AND R. KRÓL. Comparison of vasoactive intestinal peptide (VIP) and secretin in gastric secretion and mucosal blood flow. *Pfluegers Arch.* 361: 175–181, 1976.
226. KONTUREK, S. J., J. JAWOREK, M. CIESZKOWSKI, W. PAWLIK, J. KANIA, AND S. R. BLOOM. Comparison of effects of neurotensin and fat on pancreatic stimulation in dogs. *Am. J. Physiol.* 244 (*Gastrointest. Liver Physiol.* 7): G590–G598, 1983.
227. KONTUREK, S. J., W. PAWLIK, K. M. WALUS, D. H. COY, AND A. V. SCHALLY. Methionine-enkephalin stimulates gastric secretion and gastric mucosal blood flow (40161). *Proc. Exp. Biol. Med.* 158: 156–160, 1978.
228. KONTUREK, S. J., J. TASLER, M. CIESZKOWSKI, D. H. COY, AND A. V. SCHALLY. Effect of growth hormone release-inhibiting hormone on gastric secretion, mucosal blood flow, and serum gastrin. *Gastroenterology* 70: 737–741, 1976.
229. KONTUREK, S. J., J. TASLER, M. CIESZKOWSKI, E. MIKOS, D. H. COY, AND A. V. SCHALLY. Comparison of methionine-enkephalin and morphine in the stimulation of gastric acid

secretion in the dog. *Gastroenterology* 78: 294–300, 1980.
230. KONTUREK, S. J., J. TASLER, J. JAWOREK, W. PAWLIK, K. M. WALUS, V. SCHUSDZIARRA, C. A. MEYERS, D. H. COY, AND A. V. SCHALLY. Gastrointestinal secretory, motor, circulatory, and metabolic effects of prosomatostatin. *Proc. Natl. Acad. Sci. USA* 78: 1967–1971, 1981.
231. KRASNEY, J. A. Effects of angiotensin on stroke volume and regional blood flow and resistance. *Am. J. Physiol.* 215: 1454–1461, 1968.
232. KURIYAMA, H., AND H. SUZUKI. Adrenergic transmissions in the guinea-pig mesenteric artery and their cholinergic modulations. *J. Physiol. Lond.* 317: 383–396, 1981.
233. KVIETYS, P. R., R. H. GALLAVAN, AND C.-C. CHOU. Contribution of bile to postprandial intestinal hyperemia. *Am. J. Physiol.* 238 (*Gastrointest. Liver Physiol.* 1): G284–G288, 1980.
234. KVIETYS, P. R., J. M. MCLENDON, AND D. N. GRANGER. Postprandial intestinal hyperemia: role of bile salts in the ileum. *Am. J. Physiol.* 241 (*Gastrointest. Liver Physiol.* 4): G469–G477, 1981.
235. KVIETYS, P. R., R. P. PITTMAN, AND C.-C. CHOU. Contribution of luminal concentration of nutrients and osmolality to postprandial intestinal hyperemia in dogs. *Proc. Soc. Exp. Biol. Med.* 152: 659–663, 1976.
236. LARSSON, I., H. AHLMAN, H. N. BHARGAVA, A. DAHLSTRÖM, G. PETTERSSON, AND J. KEWENTER. The effects of splanchnic nerve stimulation on the plasma levels of serotonin and substance P in the portal vein of the cat. *J. Neural Transm.* 46: 105–112, 1979.
237. LARSSON, L.-I. Ultrastructural localization of a new neuronal peptide (VIP). *Histochemistry* 54: 173–176, 1977.
238. LARSSON, L.-I., J. FAHRENKRUG, O. SCHAFFALITZKY DE MUCKADELL, F. SUNDLER, R. HÅKANSON, AND J. F. REHFELD. Localization of vasoactive intestinal polypeptide (VIP) to central and peripheral neurons. *Proc. Natl. Acad. Sci. USA* 73: 3197–3200, 1976.
239. LARSSON, L.-I., N. GOLTERMANN, L. DE MAGISTRIS, J. F. REHFELD, AND T. W. SCHWARTZ. Somatostatin cell processes as pathways for paracrine secretion. *Science Wash. DC* 205: 1393–1395, 1979.
240. LARSSON, L.-I., J. M. POLAK, R. BUFFA, F. SUNDLER, AND E. SOLCIA. On the immunocytochemical localization of the vasoactive intestinal polypeptide. *J. Histochem. Cytochem.* 27: 936–938, 1979.
241. LAUTT, W. W., AND S. A. GRAHAM. Effect of nerve stimulation on precapillary sphincters, oxygen extraction, and hemodynamics in the intestines of cats. *Circ. Res.* 41: 1805–1812, 1977.
242. LAYCOCK, J. F., W. PENN, D. G. SHIRLEY, AND S. J. WALTER. The role of vasopressin in blood pressure regulation immediately following acute haemorrhage in the rat. *J. Physiol. Lond.* 296: 267–275, 1979.
243. LEAMAN, D. M., L. LEVENSON, R. ZELIS, AND R. SHIROFF. Effect of morphine on splanchnic blood flow. *Br. Heart J.* 40: 569–571, 1978.
244. LEANDER, S., R. EKMAN, R. UDDMAN, F. SUNDLER, AND R. HÅKANSON. Neuronal cholecystokinin, gastrin-releasing peptide, neurotensin, and β-endorphin in the intestine of the guinea pig. *Cell Tissue Res.* 235: 521–531, 1984.
245. LEE, Y. C., J. M. ALLEN, L. O. UTTENTHAL, P. M. ROBERTS, S. S. GILL, AND S. R. BLOOM. Quantitation and characterization of human plasma neurotensin-like immunoreactivity in response to a meal. *Dig. Dis. Sci.* 30: 129–133, 1985.
246. LEEMAN, S. E., AND R. E. CARRAWAY. Neurotensin discovery, isolation, characterization, synthesis and possible physiological roles. *Ann. NY Acad. Sci.* 400: 1–16, 1982.
247. LEUNG, F. W., AND P. H. GUTH. Dissociated effects of somatostatin on gastric acid secretion and mucosal blood flow. *Am. J. Physiol.* 248 (*Gastrointest. Liver Physiol.* 11): G337–G341, 1985.
248. LEUNG, F. W., P. H. GUTH, O. U. SCREMIN, E. M. GOLANSKA, AND G. L. KAUFFMAN, JR. Regional gastric mucosal blood flow measurements by hydrogen gas clearance in the anesthetized rat and rabbit. *Gastroenterology* 87: 28–36, 1984.
249. LEVENS, N. R. Control of intestinal absorption by the renin-angiotensin system. *Am. J. Physiol.* 249 (*Gastrointest. Liver Physiol.* 12): G3–G15, 1985.
250. LEVINE, S. E., D. N. GRANGER, R. A. BRACE, AND A. E. TAYLOR. Effect of hyperosmolality on vascular resistance and lymph flow in the cat ileum. *Am. J. Physiol.* 234 (*Heart Circ. Physiol.* 3): H14–H20, 1978.
251. LILLEHEI, R. C. The intestinal factor in irreversible hemorrhagic shock. *Surgery St. Louis* 42: 1043–1054, 1957.
252. LILLEHEI, R. C., J. K. LONGERBEAM, J. H. BLOCH, AND W. G. MANAX. The nature of irreversible shock: experimental and clinical observations. *Ann. Surg.* 160: 682–708, 1964.
253. LILLEHEI, R. C., J. K. LONGERBEAM, J. H. BLOCH, AND W. G. MANAX. The modern treatment of shock based on physiologic principles. *Clin. Pharmacol. Ther.* 5: 63–101, 1964.
254. LIN, T.-M., D. C. EVANS, C. J. SHAAR, AND M. A. ROOT. Action of somatostatin on stomach, pancreas, gastric mucosal blood flow, and hormones. *Am. J. Physiol.* 244 (*Gastrointest. Liver Physiol.* 7): G40–G45, 1983.
255. LITTLE, R., AND B. ÖBERG. Circulatory responses to stimulation of the carotid body chemoreceptors in the cat. *Acta Physiol. Scand.* 93: 34–51, 1975.
256. LÖFSTRÖM, B., B. PERNOW, AND J. WAHREN. Vasodilating action of substance P in the human forearm. *Acta Physiol. Scand.* 63: 311–324, 1965.
257. LONGERBEAM, J. K., R. C. LILLEHEI, W. R. SCOTT, AND J. C. ROSENBERG. Visceral factors in shock. *J. Am. Med. Assoc.* 181: 878–883, 1962.
258. LUNDBERG, J. M., J. PERNOW, K. TATEMOTO, AND C. DAHLÖF. Pre- and postjunctional effects of NPY on sympathetic control of rat femoral artery. *Acta Physiol. Scand.* 123: 511–513, 1985.
259. LUNDBERG, J. M., A. RUDEHILL, A. SOLLEVI, E. THEODORSSON-NORHEIM, AND B. HAMBERGER. Frequency- and reserpine-dependent chemical coding of sympathetic transmission: differential release of noradrenaline and neuropeptide Y from pig spleen. *Neurosci. Lett.* 63: 96–100, 1986.
260. LUNDBERG, J. M., A. SARIA, A. ÄNGGÅRD, T. HÖKFELT, AND L. TERENIUS. Neuropeptide Y and noradrenaline interaction in peripheral cardiovascular control. *Clin. Exp. Hypertens. Part A Theory Pract.* 6: 1961–1972, 1984.
261. LUNDBERG, J. M., AND K. TATEMOTO. Pancreatic polypeptide family (APP, BPP, NPY and PYY) in relation to sympathetic vasoconstriction resistant to α-adrenoreceptor blockade. *Acta Physiol. Scand.* 116: 393–402, 1982.
262. LUNDBERG, J. M., AND K. TATEMOTO. Vascular effects of the peptides PYY and PHI: comparison with APP and VIP. *Eur. J. Pharmacol.* 83: 143–146, 1982.
263. LUNDBERG, J. M., L. TERENIUS, T. HÖKFELT, AND M. GOLDSTEIN. High levels of neuropeptide Y in peripheral noradrenergic neurons in various mammals including man. *Neurosci. Lett.* 42: 167–172, 1983.
264. LUNDBERG, J. M., L. TERENIUS, T. HÖKFELT, C. R. MARTLING, K. TATEMOTO, V. MUTT, J. POLAK, S. BLOOM, AND M. GOLDSTEIN. Neuropeptide Y (NPY)-like immunoreactivity in peripheral noradrenergic neurons and effects of NPY on sympathetic function. *Acta Physiol. Scand.* 116: 477–480, 1982.
265. LUNDBERG, J. M., L. TORSSELL, A. SOLLEVI, J. PERNOW, E. THEODORSSON-NORHEIM, A. ÄNGGÅRD, AND B. HAMBERGER. Neuropeptide Y and sympathetic vascular control in man. *Regul. Pept.* 13: 41–52, 1985.
266. LUNDGREN, O. Microcirculation of the gastrointestinal tract and pancreas. In: *Handbook of Physiology. The Cardiovascular System. Microcirculation*, edited by E. M. Renkin and C. C. Michel. Bethesda, MD: Am. Physiol. Soc., 1984, sect. 2, vol. IV, pt. 2, chapt. 17, p. 799–864.
267. LUNDGREN, O., J. LUNDVALL, AND S. MELLANDER. Range of sympathetic discharge and reflex vascular adjustments in skeletal muscle during hemorrhagic hypotension. *Acta Physiol. Scand.* 62: 380–390, 1964.

268. LUNDGREN, O., AND J. SVANVIK. Mucosal haemodynamics in the small intestine of the cat during reduced perfusion pressure. *Acta Physiol. Scand.* 88: 551–563, 1973.
269. LUTZ, J., AND H. HENRICH. Gefässkontraktionen in situ bei druck- und stromkonstanter Perfusion der intestinalen Strombahn und ihre Abhängigkeit vom Ausgangsdruck. *Pfluegers Arch.* 319: 68–81, 1970.
270. LUTZ, J., AND H. HENRICH. Vergleich des vasculären Escape-Phänomens an der intestinalen und renalen Strombahn bei nervaler sowie humoraler Auslösung. *Pfluegers Arch.* 339: 37–48, 1973.
271. MACFERRAN, S. N., AND D. MAILMAN. Effects of glucagon on canine intestinal sodium and water fluxes and regional blood flow. *J. Physiol. Lond.* 266: 1–12, 1977.
272. MAILMAN, D. Effects of vasoactive intestinal polypeptide on intestinal absorption and blood flow. *J. Physiol. Lond.* 279: 121–132, 1978.
273. MAILMAN, D. Effects of pentagastrin on intestinal absorption and blood flow in the anaesthetized dog. *J. Physiol. Lond.* 307: 429–442, 1980.
274. MAIN, I. H. M., AND B. J. R. WHITTLE. Gastric mucosal blood flow during pentagastrin- and histamine-stimulated secretion in the rat. *Br. J. Pharmacol.* 49: 534–542, 1973.
275. MALL, J. P. Die Blut- und Lymphwege im Dünndarm des Hundes. *Abh. Sächs. Ges. Wiss.* 14: 153–189, 1888.
276. MARLEY, E., AND G. I. PROUT. Physiology and pharmacology of the splanchnic-adrenal medullary junction. *J. Physiol. Lond.* 180: 483–513, 1965.
277. MARTINSON, J. The effect of graded vagal stimulation on gastric motility, secretion and blood flow in the cat. *Acta Physiol. Scand.* 65: 300–309, 1965.
278. MATSUMURA, M., M. OHNO, M. OHURA, I. SHIMIZU, S. KISHI, AND S. SAITO. Postprandial release of neurotensin-like immunoreactivity and its mechanism. *Gastroenterol. Jpn.* 19: 543–549, 1984.
279. MCNEILL, J. R. Role of vasopressin and angiotensin in response of splanchnic resistance vessels to hemorrhage. *Adv. Exp. Med. Biol.* 23: 127–144, 1971.
280. MCNEILL, J. R. Escape of intestinal resistance vessels to angiotensin II. *Can. J. Physiol. Pharmacol.* 52: 458–464, 1974.
281. MCNEILL, J. R. Intestinal vasoconstriction following diuretic-induced volume depletion: role of angiotensin and vasopressin. *Can. J. Physiol. Pharmacol.* 52: 829–839, 1974.
282. MCNEILL, J. R., R. D. STARK, AND C. V. GREENWAY. Intestinal vasoconstriction after hemorrhage: roles of vasopressin and angiotensin. *Am. J. Physiol.* 219: 1342–1347, 1970.
283. MELCHIORRI, P., F. TONELLI, AND L. NEGRI. Comparative circulatory effects of SP, eledoisin and physalemin in the dog. In: *Substance P*, edited by U. S. von Euler and B. Pernow. New York: Raven, 1977, p. 311–319. (Nobel Symp. Ser. no. 37.)
284. MELLANDER, S. Comparative studies on the adrenergic neurohormonal control of resistance and capacitance blood vessels in the cat. *Acta Physiol. Scand. Suppl.* 176: 1–86, 1960.
285. MELLANDER, S., AND B. JOHANSSON. Control of resistance, exchange, and capacitance functions in the peripheral circulation. *Pharmacol. Rev.* 30: 117–196, 1968.
286. MURAKAMI, M., M. MORGIA, T. MIYAKE, AND H. UCHINO. Contact electrode method in hydrogen gas clearance technique: a new method for determination of regional gastric mucosal blood flow in animals and humans. *Gastroenterology* 82: 457–467, 1982.
287. MUTT, V., AND J. E. JORPES. Structure of porcine cholecystokinin-pancreozymin. Cleavage with thrombin and with trypsin. *Eur. J. Biochem.* 6: 156–162, 1968.
288. MUTT, V., S. MAGNUSSON, J. E. JORPES, AND E. DAHL. Structure of porcine secretin. I. Degradation with trypsin and thrombin. Sequence of the trypsine peptides. The C-terminal residue. *Biochemistry* 4: 2358–2362, 1965.
289. MUTT, V., AND S. I. SAID. Structure of the porcine vasoactive intestinal octacosapeptide. The amino-acid sequence. Use of kallikrein in its determination. *Eur. J. Biochem.* 42: 581–589, 1974.
290. NICOLOFF, D. M., E. T. PETER, N. H. STONE, AND O. H. WANGENSTEEN. Effect of catecholamines on gastric secretion and blood flow. *Ann. Surg.* 159: 32–36, 1964.
291. NILSSON, H. Different nerve responses in consecutive sections of the arterial system. *Acta Physiol. Scand.* 121: 353–361, 1984.
292. NILSSON, H. Adrenergic nervous control of resistance and capacitance vessels. *Acta Physiol. Scand.* 124, Suppl. 541: 1–34, 1985.
293. NILSSON, H., M. GOLDSTEIN, AND O. NILSSON. Adrenergic innervation and neurogenic response in large and small arteries and veins from the rat. *Acta Physiol. Scand.* 126: 121–133, 1986.
294. NILSSON, H., B. LJUNG, N. SJÖBLOM, AND G. WALLIN. The influence of the sympathetic impulse pattern on contractile responses of rat mesenteric arteries and veins. *Acta Physiol. Scand.* 123: 303–309, 1985.
295. NORBERG, K.-A. Adrenergic innervation of the intestinal wall studied by fluorescence microscopy. *Int. J. Neuropharmacol.* 3: 379–382, 1964.
295a.NORDGREN, S. Neurohumoral Mechanisms Controlling Large Intestinal Blood Flow and Motility. Partille, Sweden: Uno Lundgren Tryckeri AB, 1980. PhD Thesis.
296. NORTH, R. A., Y. KATAYAMA, AND J. T. WILLIAMS. On the mechanism and site of action of enkephalin on single myenteric neurons. *Brain Res.* 165: 67–77, 1979.
297. NYHOF, R. A., AND C.-C. CHOU. Evidence against local neural mechanism for intestinal postprandial hyperemia. *Am. J. Physiol.* 245 (*Heart Circ. Physiol.* 14): H437–H446, 1983.
298. ÖBERG, B. Effects of cardiovascular reflexes on net capillary fluid transfer. *Acta Physiol. Scand. Suppl.* 229: 1–98, 1964.
299. ÖBERG, B., AND S. WHITE. Relation between active constriction and passive recoil of the veins at various distending pressures. *Acta Physiol. Scand.* 71: 233–247, 1967.
300. ÖBERG, B., AND S. WHITE. Circulatory effects of interruption and stimulation of cardiac vagal afferents. *Acta Physiol. Scand.* 80: 383–394, 1970.
301. OHTANI, O., AND A. OHTSUKA. Three-dimensional organization of lymphatics and their relationship to blood vessels in rabbit small intestine. A scanning electron microscopic study of corrosion casts. *Arch. Histol. Jpn.* 48: 255–268, 1985.
302. OREN-WOLMAN, N., AND P. H. GUTH. Adrenergic sensitivity of different-size gastric submucosal arterioles. *Microvasc. Res.* 28: 345–351, 1984.
303. ORNARHEIM, J., K. B. HELLE, AND G. JÖRGENSEN. Neurotensin induced increase in intestinal blood flow in the anesthetized rat. *Acta Physiol. Scand.* 114: 505–511, 1982.
304. ÖZTURKCAN, O., G. DE SAINT-BLANQUAT, AND R. DERACHE. Gastrine et flux sanguin de la muqueuse gastrique chez le rat. *Biol. Gastro-Enterol.* 6: 151–156, 1973.
305. PAGE, I. H. *Serotonin.* Chicago, IL: Year Book, 1968.
306. PAPPAS, T. N., H. T. DEBAS, Y. GOTO, AND I. L. TAYLOR. Peptide YY inhibits meal-stimulated pancreatic and gastric secretion. *Am. J. Physiol.* 248 (*Gastrointest. Liver Physiol.* 11): G118–G123, 1985.
307. PAPPAS, T. N., H. T. DEBAS, AND I. L. TAYLOR. Peptide YY: metabolism and effect on pancreatic secretion in dogs. *Gastroenterology* 89: 1387–1392, 1985.
308. PARKS, D. A., AND D. N. GRANGER. Ischemia-induced vascular changes: role of xanthine oxidase and hydroxyl radicals. *Am. J. Physiol.* 245 (*Gastrointest. Liver Physiol.* 8): G285–G289, 1983.
309. PARKS, D. A., A. K. SHAH, AND D. N. GRANGER. Oxygen radicals: effects on intestinal vascular permeability. *Am. J. Physiol.* 247 (*Gastrointest. Liver Physiol.* 10): G167–G170, 1984.
310. PATEL, P., D. BOSE, AND C. GREENWAY. Effects of prazosin and phenoxybenzamine on $\alpha$- and $\beta$-receptor-mediated responses in intestinal resistance and capacitance vessels. *J. Cardiovasc. Pharmacol.* 3: 1050–1059, 1981.

311. PATEL, Y. C., H. H. ZINGG, D. FITZ-PATRICK, AND C. B. SRIKANT. Somatostatin: some aspects of its physiology and pathophysiology. In: *Gut Hormones*, edited by S. R. Bloom and J. M. Polak. New York: Churchill Livingstone, 1981, p. 339–349.
312. PAWLIK, W. W., J. D. FONDACARO, AND E. D. JACOBSON. Metabolic hyperemia in canine gut. *Am. J. Physiol.* 239 (*Gastrointest. Liver Physiol.* 2): G12–G17, 1980.
313. PAWLIK, W. W., A. P. SHEPHERD, AND E. D. JACOBSON. Effects of vasoactive agents on intestinal oxygen consumption and blood flow in dogs. *J. Clin. Invest.* 56: 484–490, 1975.
314. PAWLIK, W. W., A. P. SHEPHERD, D. MAILMAN, L. L. SHANBOUR, AND E. D. JACOBSON. Effects of dopamine and epinephrine on intestinal blood flow and oxygen uptake. *Adv. Exp. Med. Biol.* 75: 511–516, 1976.
315. PAWLIK, W. W., K. M. WALUS, AND J. D. FONDACARO. Effects of methionine-enkephalin on intestinal circulation and oxygen consumption (40928). *Proc. Soc. Exp. Biol. Med.* 165: 26–31, 1980.
316. PEACH, M. J. Renin-angiotensin system: biochemistry and mechanisms of action. *Physiol. Rev.* 57: 313–370, 1977.
317. PELLETIER, C. L., A. J. EDIS, AND J. T. SHEPHERD. Circulatory reflex from vagal afferents in response to hemorrhage in the dog. *Circ. Res.* 29: 626–634, 1971.
318. PERNOW, B. Substance P. *Pharmacol. Rev.* 35: 86–141, 1982.
319. PFLÜGER, E. Zweite vorläufige Mitteilung über die Einwirkung der vorderen Rückenmarkswurzeln auf das Lumen der Gefässe. *Allg. Med. Central-Zeitung Berlin* 24: 601, 1855.
320. POLAK, J. M., I. COULLING, S. BLOOM, AND A. G. E. PEARSE. Immunofluorescent localization of secretin and enteroglucagon in human intestinal mucosa. *Scand. J. Gastroenterol.* 6: 739–744, 1971.
321. POLAK, J. M., A. G. E. PEARSE, L. GRIMELIUS, AND S. R. BLOOM. Growth-hormone release-inhibiting hormone in gastrointestinal and pancreatic D cells. *Lancet* 1: 1220–1222, 1975.
322. PREMEN, A. J., D. E. DOBBINS, C. Y. SOIKA, AND J. M. DABNEY. Relationship between substance P, intestinal wall compliance and vascular resistance in the canine ileum. *Regul. Pept.* 9: 119–127, 1984.
323. PREMEN, A. J., P. R. KVIETYS, AND D. N. GRANGER. Postprandial regulation of intestinal blood flow: role of gastrointestinal hormones. *Am. J. Physiol.* 249 (*Gastrointest. Liver Physiol.* 12): G250–G255, 1985.
324. PREMEN, A. J., C. Y. SOIKA, J. M. DABNEY, AND A. E. DOBBINS. Effects of gastrointestinal hormones on ileal vascular and visceral smooth muscle. *Am. J. Physiol.* 246 (*Gastrointest. Liver Physiol.* 9): G1–G7, 1984.
325. PRICE, B. A., B. M. JAFFE, AND M. J. ZINNER. Effect of exogenous somatostatin infusion on gastrointestinal blood flow and hormones in the conscious dog. *Gastroenterology* 88: 80–85, 1985.
326. PROCTOR, K. G. Contribution of hyperosmolality to glucose induced intestinal hyperemia. *Am. J. Physiol.* 248 (*Gastrointest. Liver Physiol.* 11): G521–G525, 1985.
327. QUILLEN, E. W., D. N. GRANGER, AND A. E. TAYLOR. Effects of arginine vasopressin on capillary filtration in the cat ileum. *Gastroenterology* 73: 1290–1295, 1977.
328. RAMSAY, D. J., L. C. KEIL, M. C. SHARPE, AND J. SHINSAKO. Angiotensin II infusion increases vasopressin, ACTH and 11-hydroxycorticosteroid secretion. *Am. J. Physiol.* 234 (*Regulatory Integrative Comp. Physiol.* 3): R66–R71, 1978.
329. READ, J. B., AND G. BURNSTOCK. Comparative histochemical studies of adrenergic nerves in the enteric plexuses of vertebrate large intestine. *Comp. Biochem. Physiol.* 27: 505–517, 1968.
330. REDFORS, S., D.-A. HALLBÄCK, H. SJÖVALL, M. JODAL, AND O. LUNDGREN. Effects of hemorrhage on intramural blood flow distribution, villous tissue osmolality and fluid and electrolyte transport in the cat small intestine. *Acta Physiol. Scand.* 121: 211–222, 1984.
331. REDFORS, S., AND H. SJÖVALL. The importance of nervous and humoral factors in the control of vascular resistance, blood flow distribution and net fluid absorption in the cat small intestine during hemorrhage. *Acta Physiol. Scand.* 121: 305–315, 1984.
332. REED, J. D., AND D. J. SANDERS. Splanchnic nerve inhibition of gastric acid secretion and mucosal blood flow in anaesthetized cats. *J. Physiol. Lond.* 219: 555–570, 1971.
333. REED, J. D., D. J. SANDERS, AND V. THORPE. The effect of splanchnic nerve stimulation on gastric acid secretion and mucosal blood flow in the anaesthetized cat. *J. Physiol. Lond.* 214: 1–13, 1971.
334. REED, J. D., AND J. R. SMY. Mechanisms relating gastric acid secretion and mucosal blood flow during gastrin and histamine stimulation. *J. Physiol. Lond.* 219: 571–585, 1971.
335. REIN, H. VON, AND R. RÖSSLER. Die Abhängigkeit der vasomotorischen Blutdruckregulation bei akuten Blutverlusten von den thermoregulatorischen Blutverschiebungen im Gesamtkreislaufe. *Z. Biol.* 89: 237–248, 1929.
336. REYNELL, P. C., P. A. MARKS, C. CHIDSEY, AND S. E. BRADLEY. Changes in splanchic blood volume and splanchnic blood flow in dogs after haemorrhage. *Clin Sci.* 14: 407–419, 1955.
337. RICHARDSON, D. R., AND P. C. JOHNSON. Comparison of autoregulatory escape and autoregulation in the intestinal vascular bed. *Am. J. Physiol.* 217: 586–590, 1969.
338. RICHARDSON, P. D. I. Drug-induced changes in capillary filtration coefficient and blood flow in the innervated small intestine of the anaesthetized cat. *Br. J. Pharmacol.* 52: 481–498, 1974.
339. RICHARDSON, P. D. I. The effects of glucagon and pentagastrin on capillary filtration coefficient in the innervated jejunum of the anaesthetized cat (Abstract). *Br. J. Pharmacol.* 54: 225P, 1975.
340. RICHARDSON, P. D. I. The actions of natural secretin on the small intestinal vasculature of the anaesthetized cat. *Br. J. Pharmacol.* 58: 127–135, 1976.
341. RICHARDSON, P. D. I., D. N. GRANGER, AND P. R. KVIETYS. Effects of norepinephrine, vasopressin, isoproterenol, and histamine on blood flow, oxygen uptake, and capillary filtration coefficient in the colon of the anesthetized dog. *Gastroenterology* 78: 1537–1544, 1980.
342. RICHARDSON, P. D. I., AND P. G. WITHRINGTON. The effects of intraportal infusions of glucagon on the hepatic arterial and portal venous vascular beds of the dog: inhibition of hepatic arterial vasoconstrictor responses to noradrenaline. *Pfluegers Arch.* 378: 135–140, 1978.
343. ROBERTSON, G. L. The regulation of vasopressin function in health and disease. In: *Recent Progress in Hormone Research*, edited by G. Pincus. New York: Academic, 1977, vol. 23, p. 333–385.
344. ROSELL, S. The role of neurotensin in the uptake and distribution of fat. *Ann. NY Acad. Sci.* 400: 183–197, 1982.
345. ROSELL, S., E. BURCHER, D. CHANG, AND K. FOLKERS. Cardiovascular and metabolic actions of neurotensin and (Gln$^4$)-neurotensin. *Acta Physiol. Scand.* 98: 484–491, 1976.
346. ROSS, G. Carviovascular effects of secretin. *Am. J. Physiol.* 218: 1166–1170, 1970.
347. ROSS, G. Regional circulatory effects of pancreatic glucagon. *Br. J. Pharmacol.* 38: 735–742, 1970.
348. ROSS, G. Effects of norepinephrine infusions on mesenteric arterial blood flow and its tissue distribution. *Proc. Soc. Exp. Biol. Med.* 137: 921–924, 1971.
349. ROSS, G. Escape of mesenteric vessels from adrenergic and nonadrenergic vasoconstriction. *Am. J. Physiol.* 221: 1217–1222, 1971.
350. ROSS, G. Vascular effects of periarterial mesenteric nerve stimulation after adrenergic neurone blockade. *Experientia Basel* 29: 289–290, 1973.
351. ROSS, G. Cholinergic responses and adrenergic-cholinergic interactions in the mesenteric vascular bed. *Arch. Int. Pharmacodyn. Ther.* 205: 114–123, 1975.
352. ROSS, G. Norepinephrine vasoconstrictor escape in isolated mesenteric arteries. *Am. J. Physiol.* 228: 1652–1655, 1975.
353. ROWELL, L. B., J.-M. R. DETRY, J. R. BLACKMON, AND C.

Wyss. Importance of the splanchnic vascular bed in human blood pressure regulation. *J. Appl. Physiol.* 32: 213–220, 1972.
354. Rudick, J., L. S. Semb, W. G. Guntheroth, G. L. Mullins, H. N. Harkins, and L. M. Nyhus. Gastric blood flow and acid secretion in the conscious dog under various physiological and pharmacological stimuli. *Surgery St. Louis* 58: 47–57, 1965.
355. Rudick, J., J. L. Werther, M. L. Chapman, D. A. Dreiling, and H. D. Janowitz. Mucosal blood flow in canine antral and fundic pouches. *Gastroenterology* 60: 263–271, 1971.
356. Said, S. I., and V. Mutt. Polypeptide with broad biological activity: isolation from small intestine. *Science Wash. DC* 169: 1217–1218, 1970.
357. Said, S. I., and V. Mutt. Potent peripheral and splanchnic vasodilator peptide from normal gut. *Nature Lond.* 225: 863–864, 1970.
358. Samnegård, H., L. Thulin, M. Andreen, G. Tyden, D. Hallberg, and S. Efendic. Circulatory effects of somatostatin in anaesthetized dogs. *Acta Chir. Scand.* 145: 209–212, 1979.
359. Schmid, P. G., Jr., F. M. Abboud, M. G. Wendling, E. S. Ramberg, A. L. Mark, D. D. Heistad, and J. W. Eckstein. Regional vascular effects of vasopressin: plasma levels and circulatory responses. *Am. J. Physiol.* 227: 998–1004, 1974.
360. Schofield, C. G. Anatomy of muscular and neural tissues in the alimentary canal. In: *Handbook of Physiology. Alimentary Canal. Motility*, edited by C. F. Code. Washington, DC: Am. Physiol. Soc., 1968, sect. 6, vol. IV, chapt. 80, p. 1579–1627.
361. Schrauwen, E., and A. Houvenaghel. Substance P: a powerful intestinal vasodilator in the pig. *Pfluegers Arch.* 386: 281–284, 1980.
362. Schrier, R. W., T. Berl, and R. J. Anderson. Osmotic and nonosmotic control of vasopressin release. *Am. J. Physiol.* 236: (*Renal Fluid Electrolyte Physiol.* 5): F321–F332, 1979.
363. Schultzberg, M., T. Hökfelt, G. Nilsson, L. Terenius, J. F. Rehfeld, M. Brown, R. Elde, M. Goldstein, and S. Said. Distribution of peptide- and catecholamine-containing neurons in the gastro-intestinal tract of rat and guinea-pig: immunohistochemical studies with antisera to substance P, vasoactive intestinal polypeptide, enkephalins, somatostatin, gastrin/cholecystokinin, neurotensin and dopamine β-hydroxylase. *Neuroscience* 5: 689–744, 1980.
364. Schuurkes, J. A. J., H. A. A. Brouwers, H. J. M. Beijer, G. A. Charbon, and H. Schapiro. Lysine-vasopressin: hemodynamic effects in the anesthetized dog. *Dig. Dis. Sci.* 21: 1012–1019, 1976.
365. Selkurt, E. E., R. S. Alexander, and M. B. Patterson. The role of the mesenteric circulation in the irreversibility of hemorrhagic shock. *Am. J. Physiol.* 149: 732–743, 1947.
366. Selkurt, E. E., and G. A. Brecher. Splanchnic hemodynamics and oxygen utilization during hemorrhagic shock in the dog. *Circ. Res.* 9: 693–704, 1956.
367. Semb, B. K. H. Effect of pentagastrin on regional gastric blood flow in conscious cats. *Scand. J. Gastroenterol.* 17: 425–428, 1982.
368. Semb, B. K. H. The effect of catecholamines on gastric mucosal flow. *Scand. J. Gastroenterol.* 17: 663–670, 1982.
369. Shanbour, L. L., and E. D. Jacobson. Autoregulatory escape in the gut. *Gastroenterology* 60: 145–148, 1971.
370. Shehadeh, Z., W. E. Price, and E. D. Jacobson. Effects of vasoactive agents on intestinal blood flow and motility in the dog. *Am. J. Physiol.* 216: 386–392, 1969.
371. Shepherd, A. P., and H. J. Granger. Autoregulatory escape in the gut: a system analysis. *Gastroenterology* 65: 77–91, 1973.
372. Shepherd, A. P., D. Mailman, T. F. Burks, and H. J. Granger. Effects of norepinephrine and sympathetic stimulation on extraction of oxygen and $^{86}$Rb in perfused canine small bowel. *Circ. Res.* 33: 166–174, 1973.
373. Shepherd, A. P., W. Pawlik, D. Mailman, T. F. Burks, and E. D. Jacobson. Effects of vasoconstrictors on intestinal vascular resistance and oxygen extraction. *Am. J. Physiol.* 230: 298–305, 1976.
374. Silva, D. G., G. Ross, and L. W. Osborne. Adrenergic innervation of the ileum of the cat. *Am. J. Physiol.* 220: 347–352, 1971.
375. Singbartl, G., and H. Henrich. Adrenergic-induced vascular adjustments—initial and escape reactions. II. Role of adrenergic receptors within different sections of the isolated intestinal vascular bed. *Pfluegers Arch.* 346: 13–24, 1974.
376. Sit, S. P., and C.-C. Chou. Time course of jejunal blood flow, $O_2$ uptake, and $O_2$ extraction during nutrient absorption. *Am. J. Physiol.* 247 (*Heart Circ. Physiol.* 16): H395–H402, 1984.
377. Sjöqvist, A., J. Fahrenkrug, M. Jodal, and O. Lundgren. Effect of apamin on release of vasoactive intestinal polypeptide (VIP) from the cat intestines. *Acta Physiol. Scand.* 119: 69–76, 1983.
378. Sjöqvist, A., P. M. Hellström, M. Jodal, and O. Lundgren. Neurotransmitters involved in the colonic contraction and vasodilatation elicited by activation of the pelvic nerves in the cat. *Gastroenterology* 86: 1481–1487, 1984.
379. Sjövall, H. Afferent vagal control of fluid absorption in the feline jejunum. *Acta Physiol. Scand.* 125: 125–133, 1985.
380. Sjövall, H., M. Jodal, S. Redfors, and O. Lundgren. The effect of carotid occlusion on the rate of net fluid absorption in the small intestine of rats and cats. *Acta Physiol. Scand.* 115: 447–453, 1982.
381. Sjövall, H., S. Redfors, B. Biber, J. Martner, and O. Winsö. Evidence for cardiac volume-receptor regulation of feline jejunal blood flow and fluid transport. *Am. J. Physiol.* 246 (*Gastrointest. Liver Physiol.* 9): G401–G410, 1984.
382. Sjövall, H., S. Redfors, D.-A. Hallbäck, S. Eklund, M. Jodal, and O. Lundgren. The effect of splanchnic nerve stimulation on blood flow distribution, villous tissue osmolality and fluid and electrolyte transport in the small intestine of the cat. *Acta Physiol. Scand.* 117: 359–365, 1983.
383. Skarstein, A., K. Svanes, O. Söreide, and J. E. Varhaug. Effect of pentagastrin on blood flow distribution in the stomach of cats with gastric ulcer. *Scand. J. Gastroenterol.* 12: 71–76, 1977.
384. Sonnenberg, A., and C. West. Somatostatin reduces gastric mucosal blood flow in normal subjects but not in patients with cirrhosis of the liver. *Gut* 24: 148–153, 1983.
385. Spanner, R. Neue Befunde über die Blutwege der Darmwand und ihre funktionelle Bedeutung. *Morph. Jb.* 69: 394–454, 1932.
386. Sundler, F., R. Håkanson, S. Leander, and R. Uddman. Light and electron microscopic localization of neurotensin in the gastrointestinal tract. *Ann. NY Acad. Sci.* 400: 94–104, 1982.
387. Sundler, F., E. Moghimzadeh, R. Håkanson, M. Ekelund, and P. Emson. Nerve fibers in the gut and pancreas of the rat displaying neuropeptide-Y immunoreactivity. *Cell Tissue Res.* 230: 487–493, 1983.
388. Svanes, K., J. E. Varhaug, P. Holm, A. Bakke, and I. Romslo. Effects of hemorrhagic shock on gastric blood flow and acid secretion in cats. *Acta Chir. Scand.* 147: 81–88, 1981.
389. Svanvik, J. Mucosal hemodynamics in the small intestine of the cat during regional sympathetic vasoconstrictor activation. *Acta Physiol. Scand.* 89: 19–29, 1973.
390. Svanvik, J. The effect of reduced perfusion pressure and regional sympathetic vasoconstrictor activation on the rate of absorption of $^{85}$Kr from the small intestine of the cat. *Acta Physiol. Scand.* 89: 239–248, 1973.
390a. Svanvik, J., J. Tyllström, and I. Wallentin. The effects of hypercapnia and hypoxia on the distribution of capillary blood flow in the denervated intestinal vascular bed. *Acta Physiol. Scand.* 74: 543–551, 1968.
391. Swan, K. G., and E. D. Jacobson. Gastric blood flow and secretion in conscious dogs. *Am. J. Physiol.* 212: 891–896, 1967.
392. Swan, K. G., and D. G. Reynolds. Adrenergic mechanisms in the canine mesenteric circulation. *Am. J. Physiol.* 220: 1779–1785, 1971.
393. Swan, K. G., and D. G. Reynolds. Effects of intra-arterial catecholamine infusions on blood flow in the canine gut.

*Gastroenterology* 61: 863–871, 1971.
394. TANGE, A. Distribution of peptide-containing endocrine cells and neurons in the gastrointestinal tract of the dog: immunohistochemical studies using antisera to somatostatin, substance, P, vasoactive intestinal polypeptide, met-enkephalin, and neurotensin. *Biomed. Res.* 4: 9–24, 1983.
395. TASAKA, Y., M. SEKINE, M. WAKATSUKI, H. OHGAWARA, AND K. SHIZUME. Levels of pancreatic glucagon, insulin and glucose during twenty-four hours of the day in normal subjects. *Horm. Metab. Res.* 7: 205–206, 1975.
396. TATEMOTO, K. Isolation and characterization of peptide YY (PYY), a candidate gut hormone that inhibits pancreatic exocrine secretion. *Proc. Natl. Acad. Sci. USA* 79: 2514–2518, 1982.
397. TATEMOTO, K., M. CARLQUIST, AND V. MUTT. Neuropeptide Y—a novel brain peptide with structural similarities to peptide YY and pancreatic polypeptide. *Nature Lond.* 296: 659–660, 1982.
398. TATEMOTO, K., AND V. MUTT. Isolation of two novel candidate hormones using a chemical method for finding natural occurring polypeptides. *Nature Lond.* 285: 417–418, 1980.
399. TATEMOTO, K., AND V. MUTT. Isolation and characterization of the intestinal peptide porcine PHI (PHI-27), a new member of the glucagon-secretin family. *Proc. Natl. Acad. Sci. USA* 78: 6603–6607, 1981.
400. TAYLOR, T. V., B. R. PULLAN, J. B. ELDER, AND B. TORRANCE. Effect of secretagogues on mucosal blood flow in the antrum and corpus of the stomach. *Gut* 19: 14–18, 1978.
401. TEXTER, E. C., C. C. CHOU, S. L. MERRILL, H. C. LAURETA, AND E. D. FROHLICH. Direct effects on vasoactive agents on segmental resistance of the mesenteric and portal circulation. Studies with L-epinephrine, levarterenol, angiotensin, vasopressin, acetylcholine, metacholine, histamine, and serotonin. *J. Lab. Clin. Med.* 64: 624–633, 1964.
402. THEODORSSON-NORHEIM, E., AND S. ROSELL. Characterization of human plasma neurotensin-like immunoreactivity after fat ingestion. *Regul. Pept.* 6: 207–218, 1983.
403. THOR, K., S. ROSELL, Å. RÖKAEUS, AND L. KAGER. (Gln$^4$)-neurotensin changes the motility pattern of the duodenum and proximal jejunum from a fasting-type to a fed-type. *Gastroenterology* 83: 569–574, 1982.
404. THORÉN, P. Role of cardiac vagal C-fibres in cardiovascular control. *Rev. Physiol. Biochem. Pharmacol.* 86: 1–94, 1979.
405. TIBBLIN, S., N. G. KOCK, AND W. G. SCHENK, JR. Dissociation of the hyperglycemic and vascular effects of glucagon. *Surgery St. Louis* 67: 816–825, 1970.
406. TIBBLIN, S., N. G. KOCK, AND W. G. SCHENK, JR. Splanchnic hemodynamic responses to glucagon. *Arch. Surg.* 100: 84–89, 1970.
407. TKACHENKO, B. I., M. I. VINOGRADOVA, AND V. A. MAKOVSKAJA. A correlation of responses of the resistance and capacitance vessels of the intestine and kidney to changes of impulse in postganglionic nerves under pressor reflexes. *Experientia Basel* 34: 1298–1299, 1978.
408. TYDÉN, G., H. SAMNEGÅRD, L. THULIN, O. MUHRBECK, AND S. EFENDIC. Circulatory effects of somatostatin in anesthetized man. *Acta Chir. Scand.* 145: 443–446, 1979.
409. UDDMAN, R., J. ALUMETS, L. EDVINSSON, R. HÅKANSON, AND F. SUNDLER. VIP nerve fibres around peripheral blood vessels. *Acta Physiol. Scand.* 112: 65–70, 1981.
410. UDDMAN, R., E. EKBLAD, L. EDVINSSON, R. HÅKANSON, AND F. SUNDLER. Neuropeptide Y-like immunoreactivity in perivascular nerve fibres of the guinea-pig. *Regul. Pept.* 10: 243–257, 1985.
411. UVNÄS-WALLENSTEN, K. Release of substance P-like immunoreactivity into the antral lumen of cats. *Acta Physiol. Scand.* 104: 464–468, 1978.
412. VAGNE, M., S. J. KONTUREK, AND J. A. CHAYVIALLE. Effect of vasoactive intestinal peptide on gastric secretion in the cat. *Gastroenterology* 83: 250–255, 1982.
413. VANDERHAEGHEN, J.-J., J. C. SIGNEAU, AND W. GEPTS. New peptide in the vertebrate CNS reacting with gastrin antibodies.

*Nature Lond.* 257: 604–605, 1975.
414. VAN HEE, R. H., AND P. M. VANHOUTTE. Cholinergic inhibition of adrenergic neurotransmission in the canine gastric artery. *Gastroenterology* 74: 1266–1270, 1978.
415. VANHOUTTE, P. M. Introductory remarks: why 5-hydroxytryptamine? *Federation Proc.* 42: 211–212, 1983.
416. VANHOUTTE, P. M. The elusory role of serotonin in vascular function and disease. *Biochem. Pharmacol.* 32: 3671–3674, 1983.
417. VARHAUG, J. E., K. SVANES, AND J. LEKVEN. Regional gastric blood flow and acid secretion during histamine $H_2$ receptor blockade in cats. *Scand. J. Gastroenterol.* 18: 977–986, 1983.
418. VARHAUG, J. E., K. SVANES, C. SVANES, AND J. LEKVEN. Gastric blood flow determination: intramural distribution and arteriovenous shunting of microspheres. *Am. J. Physiol.* 247 (*Gastrointest. Liver Physiol.* 10): G468–G479, 1984.
419. VARRO, V., Z. DÖBRÖNTE, AND I. SAGI. Interrelation between gastric blood flow and HCl secretion in dogs. *Acta Med. Acad. Sci. Hung.* 35: 1–20, 1978.
420. VATNER, S. F., D. FRANKLIN, AND E. BRAUNWALD. Effects of anesthesia and sleep on circulatory response to carotid sinus nerve stimulation *Am. J. Physiol.* 220: 1249–1255, 1971.
420a. VATNER, S. F., D. FRANKLIN, AND R. L. VAN CITTERS. Mesenteric vasoactivity associated with eating and digestion in the conscious dog. *Am. J. Physiol.* 219: 170–174, 1970.
421. VATNER, S. F., D. FRANKLIN, R. L. VAN CITTERS, AND E. BRAUNWALD. Effects of carotid sinus nerve stimulation on blood-flow distribution in conscious dogs at rest and during exercise. *Circ. Res.* 27: 495–503, 1970.
422. VINIK, A. I., B. SHAPIRO, B. GLASER, AND L. WAGNER. Circulating somatostatin in primates. In: *Gut Hormones*, edited by S. R. Bloom and J. M. Polak. New York: Churchill Livingstone, 1981, p. 370–375.
423. WAHLESTEDT, C., L. EDVINSSON, E. EKBLAD, AND R. HÅKANSON. Neuropeptide Y potentiates noradrenaline-evoked vasoconstriction: mode of action. *J. Pharmacol. Exp. Ther.* 234: 735–741, 1985.
424. WAHLESTEDT, C., N. YANAIHARA, AND R. HÅKANSON. Evidence for different pre- and post-junctional receptors for neuropeptide Y and related peptides. *Regul. Pept.* 13: 307–318, 1986.
425. WAHREN, J., S. EFENDIC, R. LUFT, L. HAGENFELDT, O. BJÖRKMAN, AND P. FELIG. Influence of somatostatin on splanchnic glucose metabolism in postoperative and 60-hour fasted humans. *J. Clin. Invest.* 59: 299–307, 1977.
426. WALDER, D. N. Arteriovenous anastomoses of the human stomach. *Clin. Sci.* 11: 57–71, 1952.
427. WALLENTIN, I. Studies on intestinal circulation. *Acta Physiol. Scand.* 279: 1–38, 1966.
427a. WALUS, K. M., J. D. FONDACARO, AND E. D. JACOBSON. Effects of adenosine and its derivatives on the canine intestinal vasculature. *Gastroenterology* 81: 327–334, 1981.
428. WALUS, K. M., W. PAWLIK, S. J. KONTUREK, AND A. V. SCHALLY. Effect of met-enkephalin and morphine on gastric secretion and blood flow. *Acta Physiol. Pol.* 32: 383–392, 1981.
429. WANG, H.-H., C. Y. CHAI, J. S. KUO, AND S. C. WANG. Participation of cardiac and peripheral sympathetics in carotid occlusion response. *Am. J. Physiol.* 218: 1548–1554, 1970.
430. WEISSMAN, M. L., E. H. RUBINSTEIN, AND R. R. SONNENSCHEIN. Vascular response to short-term systemic hypoxia, hypercapnia, and asphyxia in the cat. *Am. J. Physiol.* 230: 595–601, 1976.
431. WILLIAMS, J. T., AND R. A. NORTH. Inhibition of firing of myenteric neurones by somatostatin. *Brain Res.* 155: 165–168, 1978.
432. WILSON, S. E., G. BENNETT, M. A. WINSTON, AND A. JABOUR. Potentiation of epinephrine-induced mesenteric vasoconstriction with β-blockade. *J. Surg. Res.* 23: 274–278, 1977.
433. YEO, C. J., B. M. JAFFE, AND M. J. ZINNER. Local regulation of blood flow in the feline jejunum. *J. Clin. Invest.* 70: 1329–1333, 1982.
434. YIANGOU, Y., N. D. CHRISTOFIDES, M. A. BLANK, N. YANAI-

HARA, K. TATEMOTO, A. E. BISHOP, J. M. POLAK, AND S. R. BLOOM. Molecular forms of peptide histidine isoleucine-like immunoreactivity in the gastrointestinal tract. *Gastroenterology* 89: 516–524, 1985.
435. YOKOTANI, K., AND M. FUJIWARA. Effects of substance P on cholinergically stimulated gastric acid secretion and mucosal blood flow in rats. *J. Pharmacol. Exp. Ther.* 232: 826–830, 1985.
436. YOKOTANI, K., I. MURAMATSU, AND M. FUJIWARA. Effects of the sympathetic nervous system on bethanechol-induced elevation of gastric acid secretion and mucosal blood flow in rats. *J. Pharmacol. Exp. Ther.* 227: 478–483, 1983.
437. YOKOTANI, K., I. MURAMATSU, M. FUJIWARA, AND Y. OSUMI. Effects of the sympathoadrenal system on vagally induced gastric acid secretion and mucosal blood flow in rats. *J. Pharmacol. Exp. Ther.* 224: 436–442, 1983.
438. ZINNER, M. J., B. M. JAFFE, L. DEMAGISTRIS, A. DAHLSTRÖM, AND H. AHLMAN. The effect of cervical and thoracic vagal stimulation on luminal serotonin release and regional blood flow in cats. *Gastroenterology* 82: 1403–1408, 1982.
439. ZINNER, M. J., F. KASHER, AND B. M. JAFFE. The hemodynamic effects of intravenous infusions of serotonin in conscious dogs. *J. Surg. Res.* 34: 171–178, 1983.
440. ZINNER, M. J., J. C. KERR, AND D. G. REYNOLDS. Adrenergic mechanisms in canine gastric circulation. *Am. J. Physiol.* 229: 977–982, 1975.
441. ZINNER, M. J., J. C. KERR, AND D. G. REYNOLDS. Hemodynamic effects of intra-arterial infusions of catecholamines on the canine gastric circulation. *Surgery St. Louis* 78: 381–388, 1975.
442. ZINNER, M. J., J. C. KERR, AND D. G. REYNOLDS. Distribution and arteriovenous shunting of gastric blood flow in the baboon: effect of epinephrine and vasopressin infusions. *Gastroenterology* 71: 299–302, 1976.
443. ZINNER, M. J., J. C. KERR, AND D. G. REYNOLDS. Primate gastric circulation: effects of catecholamines and adrenergic blockade. *Am. J. Physiol.* 230: 346–350, 1976.
444. ZINNER, M. J., C. J. YEO, K. O. GRONSTAD, AND B. M. JAFFE. Endoluminal substance P as a cause of mucosal hyperemia in the feline gut by a nonneural mechanism. *Surgery St. Louis* 94: 166–171, 1983.

CHAPTER 47

# Pathophysiology of gastrointestinal circulation

ROBERT H. GALLAVAN, JR. | United States Department of Agriculture, Agriculture Research Service, El Reno, Oklahoma

DALE A. PARKS | Departments of Anesthesiology and Physiology, University of Alabama at Birmingham, Birmingham, Alabama

EUGENE D. JACOBSON | Department of Physiology, School of Medicine, University of Kansas, Kansas City, Kansas

## CHAPTER CONTENTS

Pathophysiology of Ischemic Injury
    Nonocclusive intestinal ischemia
        Mechanisms
            Therapeutic implications
    Occlusive disease
Shock and Intestinal Circulation
Portal Hypertension
Inflammatory Bowel Disease
Ulcers
Other Diseases
    Hypertension
    Diabetes mellitus
    Arteriovenous malformations
    Dumping syndrome and secretory disorders
    Miscellaneous disorders

THE CIRCULATION OF AN ORGAN is essential for its survival. Blood provides critical substrates for cellular metabolism, such as oxygen, nutrients, ions, and water. The blood also dissipates potentially toxic residues of cellular metabolism, such as carbon dioxide, organic metabolites, heat, ions, and water. It seems logical, therefore, in divining the etiology of a disease, particularly a disorder whose cause is uncertain, to consider a circulatory basis for the pathology. A vascular pathogenesis as an explanation appears even more tempting if the disease involves widespread morphological alterations of the blood vessels. The case for a circulatory factor becomes almost airtight when functional evidence of tissue ischemia is unearthed during the course of illness.

The problem with the preceding line of etiologic exploration is that a profound disease is likely to affect many aspects of the life of an organ, including its circulation. The key question, which usually goes unasked and therefore unanswered, is whether the circulatory deficit was the initial event in the pathogenesis of the illness or was a later and secondary effect of the disease. The importance of the question and its answer is more than academic because there are pharmacological and surgical interventions available to treat various types of circulatory disease. Curative or preventive treatment of an illness with such drugs or operations would require that the etiology of the illness be circulatory; otherwise such treatment would be palliative at best.

In this chapter we consider several disease processes in which the circulatory factor has been implicated or strongly suggested. We have attempted to maintain a balance between fair presentation and scholarly skepticism. The reader may also wish to consult earlier treatments of this subject (1, 94, 112, 113, 123, 154, 155, 157, 186, 251, 278, 298).

## PATHOPHYSIOLOGY OF ISCHEMIC INJURY

### Nonocclusive Intestinal Ischemia

MECHANISMS. Two major pathophysiological mechanisms have been suggested for mucosal injury associated with ischemia of the small intestine: tissue hypoxia (countercurrent mechanism) and oxygen free radicals (OFR).

Several lines of evidence suggest that hypoxia of the terminal villi is responsible for the mucosal injury produced by intestinal ischemia. Thus intraluminal perfusion of the intestinal lumen with oxygenated saline during ischemia significantly improved the microscopic and macroscopic appearance of the intestinal mucosa, which was evaluated 1 h posthypotensively (3, 126). Perfusion with nitrogenated saline or a stagnant solution containing glucose did not significantly alleviate mucosal injury (126). Intraluminal perfusion with oxygenated perfluorochemicals (12, 57) and gaseous oxygen (263, 282) were also beneficial.

It has been suggested that tissue hypoxia results

from extravascular shunting of oxygen from the central arterial vessel to a subepithelial capillary network (128). The existence of a countercurrent exchange mechanism is based on the anatomical arrangement of the vasculature within the villus. The shape of the intestinal villus of different species varies from a broad-based leaflike appearance to a slender fingerlike structure; however, the vascular architecture is similar in most of the species studied (50). In general, the arterial supply to the villus consists of a single arteriole that branches from the submucosal plexus. The arteriole ascends through the central stroma of the villus, losing its smooth muscle coat just beyond the base. The arteriole remains unbranched until it reaches the distal villus and arborizes into a complicated network of subepithelial capillaries. The latter vessels eventually converge and drain into a central vein. The three minimal anatomical requirements for the existence of a vascular countercurrent exchange mechanism in the villus are *1)* the presence of two blood vessels close together that comprise the limbs of a hairpin loop, *2)* the flow of blood that is in opposite directions in the parallel limbs, and *3)* the permeability of the vessel walls that allows the diffusion of a solute from the blood of one limb to the other in response to a concentration gradient. Clearly blood flow through the central arterial vessel is opposite to that in the subepithelial capillary network. The artery and vein of the villus are close, being ~15–20 μm apart in the cat (200), and the walls are highly permeable to many lipid soluble substances, including oxygen (167). Functionally it is important to note that the transit time of blood through the hairpin vascular loop of the resting villus is more than adequate to allow significant diffusion of oxygen across the 20-μm intervascular distance (161). Indicator dilution studies used to determine plasma transit times at various levels of blood flow yielded a mean transit time of 4–8 s at resting total intestinal blood flow (23, 201). Transit time decreased to ~1 s with maximum vasodilation and increased to 20–30 s when blood flow was reduced to 75% of control. Assuming free diffusion in water, it was calculated that a 75% concentration equilibrium was reached across the 20-μm distance in 0.1 s or less (128). Therefore mean transit time through the villus is more than adequate to allow substantial intervascular diffusion of oxygen under resting conditions. The increased efficiency of the countercurrent exchanger during low flow conditions could produce nearly anoxic conditions in the region of the villus tip. The exchanger therefore functions as a complex shunt that permits a portion of the arterial oxygen to diffuse into the nearby capillary network without first reaching the tips of the villi. Shunting of oxygen in the countercurrent exchanger implies that the partial pressure of oxygen ($P_{O_2}$) in the tissue would decrease from the base toward the tip of the villus. The existence of the postulated oxygen gradient was confirmed with oxygen microelectrodes in rat small intestine (27).

This hypothesis would also predict that the vast majority of the mucosal injury observed in the small intestine after ischemia would occur during the ischemic period when time available for diffusion of oxygen is maximal. However, recent studies have demonstrated that most of the injury observed with ischemia occurs on reperfusion of ischemic small bowel and not during the ischemic period (239). These results are not inconsistent with the view that the countercurrent exchange mechanism is responsible for the injury that occurs during the ischemic period. However, another mechanism, probably OFR, is responsible for most of the injury, i.e., the injury that occurs on reperfusion of ischemic tissues.

Oxygen free radicals are highly reactive and cytotoxic reduction products of molecular oxygen that may be responsible for the mucosal injury associated with ischemia in the small intestine (114, 236, 237, 241). By definition OFR are molecules or molecular fragments with one or more unpaired electrons in their outer orbital. The unpaired electron(s) makes OFR positively or negatively charged or electrically neutral, and endows OFR with very characteristic chemical reactivity and physical properties. In biological systems, the radical species tend to be found in derivatives of molecular oxygen, polyunsaturated fatty acids, sulfhydryl compounds, quinones, flavins, and certain other compounds that transfer electrons readily (252). The OFR are probably the most important radicals in aerobic systems. In humans ~95%–98% of all molecular oxygen is tetravalently reduced (addition of four electrons) by the cytochrome oxidase system to form water. The remaining 2%–5% of the oxygen can form cytotoxic OFR. Addition of a single electron to molecular oxygen forms superoxide anion, a second electron forms hydrogen peroxide, a third electron forms hydroxyl radical, and a fourth electron forms the final reduction product, water.

The cytotoxicity of these OFR probably results from their ability to degrade the lipid components of cellular, mitochondrial, and lysosomal membranes (171, 172). The membranes of mammalian cells contain considerable amounts of polyunsaturated fatty acids that are very susceptible to peroxidative injury (219). The OFR may react with the unsaturated lipids of the membranes, resulting in the formation of lipid peroxide radicals, lipid hydroperoxides, and fragmentation products such as malondialdehyde (172). If the peroxidative injury to the membranes is extensive, lipid peroxide products will be released into the extracellular space (219), thereby increasing vascular permeability (75, 192), altering leukocyte chemotaxis (214), forming various prostanoids (9), liberating histamine (88), and degrading collagen and hyaluronic acid—the constituents of basement membrane and the extracellular matrix (213).

A delicate balance exists between the cellular systems that generate OFR and the antioxidant mechanisms that have evolved to defend against radical injury. Three intracellular enzymes constitute the first line of defense against the toxic effects of OFR: superoxide dismutases (SOD), catalase, and glutathione peroxidase (GPO). The SOD are metalloproteins that catalyze the dismutation of superoxide radical. The Cu-Zn SOD is cytoplasmic, and the Mn SOD is chiefly mitochondrial; neither form is found in the extracellular fluid in high concentrations (210). Catalase, a cytoplasmic heme protein, is found in the mitochondria and certain organelles (e.g., peroxisomes); it reduces hydrogen peroxide to water. The GPO is a selenium-dependent enzyme found in high concentrations in the cytoplasm; it reduces hydrogen and organic peroxides to water and alcohols, respectively. Glutathione peroxidase is much more effective than catalase in the reduction of low concentrations of hydrogen peroxide, whereas catalase is more effective at high concentrations of hydrogen peroxide (87). In addition to the antioxidant enzymes, many water and lipid soluble substances serve as antioxidants by reducing reactive radical species to less active radical forms. The water soluble antioxidants include ascorbic acid (vitamin C), reduced glutathione, cysteine, ceruloplasmin, transferrin, and L-methionine. Lipid-soluble antioxidants include $\alpha$-tocopherol (vitamin E) and $\alpha$- and $\beta$-carotenes. In brief, OFR can attack most biological substrates and thereby result in structural and metabolic changes that jeopardize the viability of tissues. There exists an antioxidant defense system that protects against oxidant injury under normal conditions. The tissue injury that results from ischemia-reperfusion of the small intestine represents OFR overwhelming the cellular defense systems, and it is conceivable that supplemental antioxidants may be beneficial in intestinal ischemia.

Despite intense interest in the mechanisms by which gastric mucosal integrity is maintained or lost, there is surprisingly little evidence involving the role of OFR during damage to the mucosa. Recent studies indicate that OFR may play a role in the development of stress ulcers. These gastric ulcers are most commonly observed in patients who have sustained an episode of circulatory shock associated with severe trauma, brain injury, or burns. Experimental studies suggest that formation of stress ulcers is associated with a significant reduction in gastric blood flow (153, 293). It was found that SOD and allopurinol protected rats from gastric ulcers induced by hemorrhagic shock, whereas intravenously administered dimethyl sulfoxide (DMSO), a hydroxyl radical scavenger, failed to protect against the formation of these lesions (153). Conversely, gastric ulcers produced by cold stress were significantly reduced by a 5-day feeding with DMSO. The apparent discrepancy between the results with DMSO may be related to the dose and/or route of administration of the DMSO or to differences in mechanisms involved in these two forms of ulcers. Micrographs of the gastric mucosa exposed to the damaging effects of absolute ethanol exhibit edema, vacuolization, and necrosis of the luminal epithelial cells, lesions that bear some resemblance to those resulting from ischemia-reperfusion in the intestine. The application of necrotizing agents influences the activity of SOD in the gastric mucosa (224). Furthermore the severity of the ethanol-induced gastric lesions is greatly reduced by vitamin E (82), catalase (82), carotenes (82, 223), and the hydroxyl radical scavengers mannitol and sodium benzoate (82). The phenomenon of gastric mucosal cytoprotection by prostaglandins may provide fertile ground for further investigations of the role of OFR in gastric mucosal injury.

It is unlikely that hypoxia produced by a countercurrent mechanism is of great importance in ischemic damage of the gastric mucosa. This mechanism requires that oxygen diffuse between the arterial and venous arms of a vascular loop, thereby establishing a decreasing gradient of oxygen from base to tip of the villus. The vascular architecture of the gastric mucosa is such that countercurrent exchange of oxygen would be minimal.

The colon, like the stomach, has a vascular anatomy inconsistent with countercurrent exchange of oxygen. There are no villi in the colon, so the effects of countercurrent exchange would be minimal and would not account for the injury to the colonic mucosa observed with ischemia-reperfusion. Considerable evidence indicates that xanthine oxidase is the source of OFR produced in the ischemic small bowel; by contrast the colon contains considerably less xanthine oxidase activity (5). This finding does not preclude the production of OFR by another enzymatic mechanism during ischemia. The colonic mucosa is a relatively rich source of aldehyde oxidase, an enzyme that also produces OFR (180).

THERAPEUTIC IMPLICATIONS. Time is a critical factor in the management of intestinal ischemia. Patient management is successful when the onset of therapy occurs within 6–12 h after onset of the initial symptoms. Delay beyond this very narrow therapeutic window assures an almost certain fatal outcome for the patient (32). Good patient management necessitates extensive supportive therapy usually including antibiotics for infection and intravenous electrolyte solutions to correct hypovolemia and electrolyte imbalance. Oral cardiac glycosides may be needed to improve cardiac output and maintain blood pressure, although these agents are vasoconstrictors in the gut (45, 47). Surgery is a life-threatening procedure in nonocclusive intestinal ischemia because the low flow state has not resulted from a resectable thromboembolic obstruction of large vessels, and the patient is usually in too poor a state to tolerate the stress of major abdominal surgery. For these reasons, it is desirable to develop a less traumatic means of reversing the mesenteric ischemia before irreversible intestinal injury occurs. Several noninvasive approaches to management of mesenteric ischemia have been proposed, including anticoagulants (32, 178, 187), $\alpha$-adrenergic blocking agents (11, 228), corticosteroids (13, 25, 109, 129, 140, 146, 214), and vasodilator drugs (31, 34, 72, 99, 122, 179, 185, 207, 229, 273, 279, 303, 304). It is also possible that oxygen radical scavengers may be of benefit in nonocclusive mesenteric ischemia.

The use of anticoagulants in the management of mesenteric ischemia is controversial. Ischemic injury to the small intestine has been attributed to formation of microthrombi resulting from vasospasm and hemostasis. Consequently, anticoagulation with heparin has been proposed as an adjunct to supportive therapy, although there is no conclusive evidence to support the dissolution of previously formed clots by heparin. Liberal use of heparin has, however, resulted in significant intestinal bleeding and may convert an area of simple bowel infarction into an area of hemorrhagic infarction (32, 178, 187). Thromboses do occur in the late postoperative period and some form of anticoagulation may be introduced safely 48 h postoperatively (32).

Nonocclusive intestinal ischemia is believed to be a result of microvascular vasospasm. The vasospasm could result from either neurogenic mechanisms, e.g., increased sympathetic tone, or by the release of vasoconstrictor agents from the ischemic region of the small bowel. Phenoxybenzamine, an $\alpha$-adrenergic blocking agent, has been proposed as an adjunct to therapy for intestinal ischemia (11). In experimental animals it was found that preoperative treatment with phenoxybenzamine increased circulation in the ischemic region, whereas postoperative treatment was of little benefit (228). Blockade of $\alpha$-adrenergic receptors, like anticoagulants, may be of benefit in limiting secondary hemodynamic changes resulting from intestinal ischemia.

There is also more controversy than definitive data about the value of glucocorticosteroids and/or other steroids, e.g., mineralocorticosteroids, estrogens, and androgens, in treating mesenteric ischemia. Corticosteroids may be useful on theoretical grounds because they stabilize lysosomal and endothelial membranes and inhibit the release of mediators from endothelial and mast cells (129). Pharmacological doses of glucocorticosteroids and estrogens can act directly on the vascular smooth muscle of the microcirculation to inhibit the effects of many vasoconstrictor substances released during ischemia. The probable mechanism for inhibition of the constrictor effects involves prevention of the uptake and utilization of calcium ions essential for contraction of vascular smooth muscle. Steroids have been shown to be beneficial only if administered early in ischemia and in very high doses (129, 140, 146). Delayed treatment, at least in animal models, resulted in diminished perfusion and a high occurrence of secondary infections (146). Unfortunately, the probability of identifying a patient with intestinal ischemia during this narrow time frame is low (25), thereby severely limiting the usefulness of steroids. The seemingly paradoxical effect of steroids—beneficial if administered early and detrimental if not—has been explained in terms of OFR (140). High doses of steroids have been shown to inhibit generation of OFR from leukocytes (109). Generation of OFR would normally increase leukocyte activity through elaboration of a chemotactic substance (214). The initial response of the steroid would then be anti-inflammatory. The OFR are also instrumental in the killing of bacteria by phagocytes (13). Delayed or continued treatment with steroids would result in the loss of a significant defense mechanism and would allow secondary bacterial infections.

The advent of intra-arterial vasodilator therapy was a significant addition to the therapeutic armamentarium against mesenteric ischemia. A number of vasodilators have been suggested as possible candidates for use in ischemic disorders of the gut. An optimal agent should be selective, with minimal $\alpha$-adrenergic action or antagonism of other cardiovascular functions. The agent should have high potency as a local vasodilator drug without affecting systemic arterial blood pressure. There should be a rapid onset of effect of the intra-arterially administered dilator with rapid degradation so that there is no vasodilation beyond the mesenteric circulation. Another beneficial feature of the agent would be antagonism of platelet aggregation, which would limit disseminated intravascular coagulation. It would also be advantageous if the agent stabilized lysosomal membranes and increased capillary surface area, thereby enhancing the accessibility of oxygen to hypoxic tissues.

Papaverine has been infused intra-arterially to successfully treat nonocclusive mesenteric ischemia and is currently considered the drug of choice (31, 34). Papaverine is a fairly potent vasodilator and has minimal side effects because ~90% of the drug is inactivated with each circulation through the liver (72). However, even if small amounts of papaverine escape degradation, the drug may accumulate sufficiently to dilate precapillary resistance elements of the general circulation and cause hypotension. Papaverine is also a potent inhibitor of nucleotide phosphodiesterases and, therefore, prevents the normal metabolism of cAMP (279). However, it has been reported that patients who were administered intra-arterial papaverine for over 5 days suffered no significant systemic depressor effects (32).

Prostaglandin $E_1$ ($PGE_1$) has many of the characteristics of an ideal vasodilator agent and has been available for clinical use as an intra-arterial dilator (303). It has theoretical advantages over papaverine; thus papaverine, in the experimental animal, decreases intestinal oxygen consumption (185), whereas $PGE_1$ does not (44, 122). Prostaglandin $E_1$ is a very potent mesenteric dilator, is rapidly inactivated, stabilizes lysosomal membranes, and antagonizes aggregation of platelets. On the negative side, in theory, $PGE_1$ interacts with a number of endogenous vasoactive substances and potentiates the release of a number of vasoconstrictors, e.g., norepinephrine, epinephrine, and angiotensin II (207). Clinically, the only major side effect appears to be diarrhea, the severity of which is dose related (303).

Dopamine has also been advocated for amelioration of mesenteric ischemia. Dopamine is a moderately potent mesenteric vasodilator, although increases in mesenteric blood flow were observed only when the agent was given in low doses and in combination with volume replacement (229, 304). Dopamine also has $\alpha$-adrenergic properties that become evident with high doses of dopamine when vasoconstriction predominates and, even when administered in combination with volume replacement, leads to deterioration of mesenteric blood flow (229).

Glucagon is a vasodilator that also prompts a positive ionotropic effect on the heart (179). Infusions of glucagon increase splanchnic blood flow, increase oxygen consumption, and decrease mesenteric vascular resistance in the normal and ischemic small bowel (99, 273). Unfortunately, the dilation of the mesenteric circulation resulting from glucagon infusion is not sustained (185).

Other drugs that have been used as mesenteric dilators include gastrointestinal hormones (185, 304), acetylcholine (185), isoproterenol (304), and perhexiline (99, 273).

Despite significant advances in diagnosis and the success of vasodilator therapy, nonocclusive intestinal ischemia remains a challenging clinical problem and a cause of morbidity and mortality among aging patients (34, 36). There is considerable evidence in the literature to suggest that OFR scavengers may be of considerable benefit in nonocclusive ischemia. The normal delicate balance between the cellular systems that generate OFR and the antioxidant mechanisms that inactivate these radicals is upset in nonocclusive intestinal ischemia, leading to OFR-mediated injury. Antioxidant therapy, which might preserve the viability of ischemic gut, could involve administration of three intracellular enzymes that comprise the first line of defense against toxic OFR, namely, SOD, catalase, and GPO. Catalase and SOD have been demonstrated to attenuate the vascular permeability changes and morphological alterations (236, 271) associated with ischemia in experimental animals and to decrease mortality (69). The enzymatic source of the OFR produced in ischemic small intestine appears to be xanthine oxidase. Administration of allopurinol, a competitive inhibitor of xanthine oxidase, dramatically reduced the permeability changes (237) and morphological alterations associated with experimental ischemia (236). The hydroxyl radical scavengers DMSO and glycerol are effective in reducing ischemic injury (76, 237) and increasing survival (254). Evidence suggests that marked lipid peroxidation occurs with ischemia-reperfusion in the feline small intestine (329). Vitamin E ($\alpha$-tocopherol) limits lipid peroxidation (103, 212) and may be effective in preventing ischemic injury. Administration of antioxidants, either alone or in combination with vasodilator drugs, may become clinically acceptable for treatment of intestinal ischemia. However, the timeliness of instituting any therapy after the onset of ischemia remains a major limitation for outcome.

*Occlusive Disease*

Severe intestinal ischemia causes ~3% of American deaths, and more than half of the cases involve obstruction of the superior mesenteric artery or one of its major branches (158, 251). The immediate cause of the occlusion is an embolus or a thrombus, often at a site of an atheroma. Predisposing diseases and those disorders commonly associated with occlusive intestinal ischemia include widespread atherosclerosis, cardiac arrhythmias, dissecting aortic aneurysm, subendothelial hemorrhage, a growing tumor, vasculitides, irradiation injury, inadvertent ligation of an artery during abdominal surgery, and congestive cardiac failure (44, 240).

Abrupt cessation of blood flow to the gut produces intestinal gangrene in which necrosis spreads across the mucosal surface and penetrates the entire thickness of the bowel wall. Once the necrotic area has extended to the serosal surface of the intestinal wall, peritonitis ensues. Unless this inexorable sequence is interrupted early by surgical resection of dead bowel and supportive therapy with antibiotics and fluid/electrolyte replacement, the patient or the experimental animal will surely die.

The mucosa perishes quickly because of its higher resting demand for oxygen and nutrients. As this tissue succumbs to hypoxia is loses its ability to contain lumenal contents outside the tissue; these contents include proteolytic enzymes and bacteria, which invade the dying mucosa to hasten its destruction. Cellular lysosomes also release their damaging enzymes to further assure the demise of mucosal cells. Fluid and blood leak out of the mucosa into the lumen, where gas-forming microorganisms cause distension of the affected bowel wall. The second major intramural component is smooth muscle, which responds more slowly because of its lower metabolic rate. Initially after vascular occlusion the muscularis is spastic, but with death of this tissue the wall becomes flaccid.

The major symptom of occlusion is unremitting abdominal pain prompted by intramural muscle spasm initially and by bowel distension and peritonitis later in the course of this catastrophic disorder. A definitive diagnosis can be made angiographically by the demonstration of failure of the injected radiopaque solution to perfuse the blocked vessel.

Early diagnosis of mesenteric occlusion and institution of appropriate surgical and supportive therapy offer the only hope for survival. However, the state and age of the patient with serious coexistent cardiovascular disease contribute to the grim outlook in mesenteric occlusion even with early diagnosis and treatment.

## SHOCK AND INTESTINAL CIRCULATION

The degree to which the gastrointestinal tract contributes to or is affected by the circulatory derangements of shock depends on the type of shock and the animal model studied. In this section four common types of shock are discussed: hypovolemic, cardiogenic, septic, and anaphylactic. Attention is directed to changes in mesenteric blood flow associated with each form of shock, as well as to effects on gastrointestinal function.

During hypovolemic shock after either extensive burns or hemorrhage there are decreases in venous return, cardiac output, and systemic arterial blood pressure (136). These hemodynamic deficits initiate a chain of compensatory reactions, mediated primarily by the sympathetic nervous system (SNS), which serve to increase total peripheral resistance (TPR), restore blood pressure, and preserve blood flow to the heart, lungs, and brain (49, 56). Activation of the SNS is the result of changes in baroreceptor (141), chemoreceptor (96), low-pressure receptor (105, 141), and in some cases nociceptor activity (309).

Hemorrhage has been shown to increase the rate of firing of splanchnic nerve fibers (20, 107, 110) and to increase circulating catecholamine levels (136, 310, 311). Studies in dogs have shown 10- and 50-fold increases in plasma concentrations of epinephrine and norepinephrine, respectively, when arterial blood pressure was reduced to 40 mmHg. Furthermore systemic plasma concentrations of catecholamines correlate well with the severity of both the hemorrhage and the hypotension (196, 310).

The gastrointestinal circulation has a limited ability to maintain normal blood flow in the face of decreasing perfusion pressure (164, 165). A reduction in blood pressure from 100 mmHg to 40 mmHg results in a 45% decrease in mesenteric blood flow. In comparison, renal blood flow decreases only 15% under the same conditions (116). The degree to which increased adrenergic activity increases the magnitude of this ischemic insult to the small intestine is unclear. Some investigators believe that changes in mesenteric vascular resistance are mediated by circulating angiotensin II and vasopressin (218). However, even though vasopressin and angiotensin are vasoconstrictors in the intestinal circulation and have been shown to enhance catecholamine activity (7, 81, 226, 281), most studies in which hemorrhage has been reported to increase intestinal vascular resistance implicate the SNS as the primary mediator (17, 29, 125, 127, 159, 230, 291, 331).

In two studies in cats (118, 218), in one study in baboons (17), and in several canine studies (159, 197, 198a, 230), hemorrhage resulted in a sustained vasoconstriction of the intestinal circulation such that blood flow was less than expected after a decrease in perfusion pressure alone. In the rat, severing the sympathetic nerves to the small intestine converted a sustained increase in mucosal vascular resistance after hemorrhage to a vasodilation and preserved mucosal integrity (29). However, in another study, no significant change in total gastrointestinal vascular resistance occurred in rats after 30% of the blood volume had been removed (275).

Other studies (125, 127, 231) have indicated that hemorrhage elicits a transient increase in mesenteric vascular resistance followed by either a gradual return of resistance to values near control levels or active vasodilation during prolonged hypovolemia. This fading of the intestinal vasoconstrictor response may be due to the natural ability of local vasoregulatory mechanisms in the small intestine to escape the effects of the SNS on intestinal blood flow (97) or to a decrease in sympathetic nerve activity (20, 66, 67, 90, 265) and circulatory catecholamine levels (196, 310) during sustained hypotension; decline in SNS activity could result from insufficient blood flow in the central nervous system (57). Acidosis has also been shown to inhibit catecholamine activity (124). Finally, studies in the cat (15) and rhesus monkeys (101, 267) have been reported in which intestinal vascular resistance did not change during hemorrhagic shock.

In all the studies discussed, hemorrhage resulted in a significant decrease in gastrointestinal blood flow with a corresponding decrease in mucosal flow (60, 100, 326). This ischemic insult is the primary cause of the pathological changes in the gastrointestinal tract during hemorrhagic shock. Although the canine response to endotoxic shock also includes an increase in portal vascular resistance (84, 181) and a subsequent pooling of blood and edema formation in the splanchnic organs, this response is unique to that species (156, 295).

Cardiogenic shock is similar to hypovolemic shock in that hypotension is the direct result of a decrease in cardiac output, although the decrease in cardiac output in cardiogenic shock is due to impaired cardiac performance rather than to a decrease in venous return (6, 234, 317). As with hemorrhagic shock, a decrease in systemic arterial blood pressure elicits an increase in SNS activity. However, in cardiogenic shock, receptors located in the heart are activated that have opposite effects on the SNS. Some afferent nerve fibers from the heart appear to increase SNS activity during coronary ischemia (92, 206a). Furthermore, left circumflex coronary artery occlusion has been shown to increase the rate of firing of splanchnic nerve fibers (182). Other afferent fibers appear to inhibit SNS activity reflexly in an attempt to decrease the demand on the failing heart (2, 10, 65, 91, 102, 203).

As in studies in hemorrhagic shock, some authors feel that increased circulatory levels of vasopressin and angiotensin II rather than increased SNS activity are responsible for increased vascular resistance in the splanchnic circulation during cardiogenic shock (14, 43, 269). Vasopressin and angiotensin II have been shown to selectively reduce mesenteric arterial blood flow at plasma concentrations reported in the systemic circulation during cardiogenic shock (269). Furthermore cardiac tamponade produced a decrease in cardiac output and a selective increase in mesenteric and celiac artery resistance (26–13 × TPR) in dogs and pigs. This selective increase in resistance was mimicked by angiotensin II (14). In the colon, decreases in blood flow during cardiac tamponade were linearly correlated with pericardial pressure and mimicked by administration of angiotensin (43).

As a result of decreased perfusion pressure and increased mesenteric vascular resistance, gastrointestinal blood flow decreases during cardiogenic shock. However, exogenous factors also contribute to this ischemia. Digitalis is a drug commonly used in the treatment of chronic heart failure and is also a vasoconstrictor in the peripheral vascular bed (46–48, 276, 277). Cardiac glycosides have been found to decrease intestinal blood flow in dogs (302), monkeys (277), and humans (45, 70, 244). Use of catecholamines as part of drug therapy during heart failure will also compromise the gastrointestinal circulation. As in hemorrhagic shock, ischemia, and related events, OFR are responsible for pathological changes in the splanchnic organs during cardiogenic shock.

Septic shock is the result of the presence in the systemic circulation of either live gram-negative bacteria or their endotoxins, which consist of a lipopolysaccharide component of the gram-negative bacterial cell wall (204, 319). The most common bacteria associated with this condition is *Escherichia coli* (308, 319). Septic shock is characterized by systemic hypotension; however, the underlying mechanisms vary among species (38, 181) and depend on the agent used (live *E. coli* or endotoxin) (147, 149), the route of administration (42, 160), the dose and potency of the agent (39, 142), and the method of administration (bolus, infusion, septic focus) (37, 139).

In humans, septic shock has been reported to be associated with an increased cardiac output and decreased TPR (61, 62, 283) or a decreased cardiac output and increased TPR (313). The direction of change in TPR is apparently determined by predisposing factors (204). In unanesthetized (267, 328) and anesthetized (145) nonhuman primates, both cardiac output and TPR were reduced, whereas in the cat, cardiac output decreased but TPR did not change (84). A decrease in cardiac output and increase in TPR were reported in the dog (126, 131).

Endotoxin has been shown to increase SNS activity in cats (130) and to increase plasma catecholamine levels in cats and dogs (131). However, the effect of this sympathoadrenal axis activation on the intestinal circulation may be offset in part by the release of large amounts of vasoactive substances into the circulation such as bradykinin, histamine, and serotonin (242). Local autoregulatory mechanisms may also be involved.

In dogs, infusion of endotoxin or live *E. coli* into the systemic circulation has been reported to decrease mesenteric blood flow (38, 197, 198, 294) and to increase portal venous pressure (24, 39, 312, 328). The net effect is massive pooling of blood in the splanchnic vascular bed (108, 198, 312, 314). The increase in portal pressure is believed to be the result of constriction of the hepatic veins (120, 121, 148) and appears unique to dogs and rats (315).

The importance of splanchnic pooling in the pathophysiology of septic shock has been questioned because it has not been proven in other species (156, 294). Primates and cats show only moderate increases in portal venous pressure when challenged with either *E. coli* or endotoxin (38, 39, 149, 294), and there has been no indication of splanchnic pooling in past studies (39, 312). A recent study in cats demonstrated a 30% increase in hepatic blood volume in response to *Salmonella enteritidis* endotoxin, which, however, was associated with a decrease in portal venous tone (274).

The effects of live *E. coli* and endotoxin on intestinal blood flow vary in other species. In cats both agents cause an initial vasoconstriction and a decrease in intestinal blood flow (84, 119). Although feline mesenteric vascular resistance gradually returned to control, this effect was offset by a steady decline in blood pressure so that intestinal blood flow remained below control levels (84, 119). In nonhuman primates, on the other hand, endotoxin and *E. coli* infusions evoked a splanchnic vasodilation (38, 56, 101, 156, 267, 294–296, 328), which was apparently sufficient to maintain intestinal blood flow at control levels (38, 137, 294). Therefore, although septic shock can result in ischemia of the canine and feline gastrointestinal tract, it apparently has no significant effect on gastrointestinal blood flow in the nonhuman primates.

Anaphylaxis is an abrupt, immediate allergic reaction that frequently results in shock. As with other forms of circulatory shock, the pathology varies among different species. In the human and guinea pig, death results from asphyxia and respiratory distress (21). Death in the rabbit and monkey is apparently due to right heart failure after pulmonary venous constriction (165, 246, 275, 289, 290). Monkeys that survive the initial anaphylactic response may have a complicated recovery because of intestinal ischemia, because splanchnic blood flows are reduced 40%–90% within 30 min after the challenge (275).

In the dog, death can result from either respiratory distress during the initial anaphylactic response (168) or as a result of pathological changes in the splanchnic circulation after the challenge. As in other forms of shock, the canine anaphylactic response is associated with a histamine-mediated increase in hepatic venous resistance (21, 245) and splanchnic pooling. At 3 h after challenge, splanchnic arterial blood flow is still 43% below control (125) and animals frequently exhibit vomiting, bloody diarrhea, and severe liver damage (73, 74, 248). Consequently the recovery from a severe anaphylactic challenge in dogs is complicated by hemorrhagic and septic shock.

## PORTAL HYPERTENSION

In 1945, Whipple (314a) proposed that portal hypertension was the result of increased resistance to portal venous blood flow. This proposal was based on the observation that patients with portal vein thrombosis, as well as those with cirrhosis of the liver, demonstrated increased portal venous pressure, splenomegaly, and esophageal varices. The increased vascular resistance in cirrhosis is due to diffuse hepatic fibrosis (217) with compression displacement of hepatic venous channels by regenerating nodules (173) and an overall decrease in the number of hepatic venous channels (206).

This "backward theory" of portal hypertension predicts a progressive decrease in the contribution of the portal circulation to total hepatic blood flow, which is indeed the case (321). However, the model also predicts a decrease in arterial blood flow and a decrease in portal venous $P_{O_2}$. In fact, portal venous hypertension is usually accompanied by an increase in arterial inflow and an increase in portal venous $P_{O_2}$.

These findings led some to propose the "forward theory" of portal venous hypertension; i.e., portal hypertension is due to direct arterial-venous malformations with a hyperdynamic gut (321). Although closure of arteriovenous fistulas relieved ascites and variceal hemorrhage in cases where they were present, increasing blood flow with vasodilators did not reproduce the condition nor did vasoconstrictor or arterial ligation control portal hypertension in patients with cirrhosis (322). Therefore, active congestion has been implicated as the cause of portal hypertension (322, 323). Supporting this proposal is evidence that a combination of increased portal inflow, by either mechanical or pharmacological means, and increased portal resistance resulted in hemodynamic changes similar to those seen in chronic portal hypertension.

Normally an increase in intestinal venous pressure elicits the venous-arteriolar response, a myogenic reflex unique to the intestinal circulation (163). This response involves a reflex arteriolar vasoconstriction when venous pressure is elevated such that capillary pressure and consequently fluid filtration are maintained at normal levels. Although there is experimental evidence that indicates that the initial hemodynamic consequences of increased portal resistance are an increase in portal venous pressure and a decrease in intestinal blood flow (284), chronic portal hypertension is characterized by increased blood flow to the stomach (175, 176, 307), small intestine (22, 26, 284, 307), and ascending colon (111).

The increase in splanchnic blood flow associated with chronic portal hypertension is most likely due to the accumulation of vasodilators in the systemic circulation. As much as 95% of total portal inflow is shunted away from the liver via collateral veins. This shunting allows nutrients, gastrointestinal peptides, and metabolic by-products to escape metabolic conversion by the liver. Both chronic portal hypertension and experimentally induced portacaval shunting result in increased levels of prostacyclin (134) and glucagon (85, 170, 208, 209) in humans and animals. Secretion of pancreatic glucagon also appears to be directly stimulated in animals with portacaval shunts (85, 115, 208, 249, 280). Furthermore circulating glucagon levels are sufficient to account for 40% of the total increase in gastrointestinal blood flow in rats with chronically elevated portal venous pressure (22).

The intestinal circulation in patients with chronic portal hypertension is characterized by increased splanchnic arterial inflow, increased capillary and portal pressures, and significant portal systemic shunting (22). Pathological changes associated with these conditions include formation of varices with bleeding and increased filtration of capillary fluid.

Varices form as a result of venous distension due to the increased portal pressure and are usually found among the gastric coronary, diaphragmatic, esophageal, and superior and inferior hemorrhoidal veins. The increased diameter and pressure in these veins cause a marked increase in wall tension, and the walls of both the portal veins and the varices become fibrotic. Rupture usually occurs in the submucosa of the esophagus, possibly as a result of erosion of the mucosa from mechanical and chemical stresses (reflux of gastric juice). Exposure of the vessels to the esophageal lumen containing acid and the elevated lumen pressure and wall tension make it difficult to stop the bleeding. Therefore torrential hemorrhage of esophageal varices is a frequent cause of death in these patients (104).

The intestinal vasculature is highly permeable to water but relatively impermeable to high-molecular-weight molecules such as proteins (320). The increase in capillary pressure that develops in chronic portal hypertension results in the movement of large amounts of fluid into the splanchnic interstitial space. This movement is determined solely by the capillary hydrostatic pressure gradient. Although plasma protein levels fall in chronic liver disease, the high level of fluid filtration results in low interstitial fluid protein levels such that the net oncotic pressure gradient is either unchanged or favors filtration (325). In rare cases in which elevated posthepatic venous resistance is the cause of increased venous pressure, large amounts of protein-rich fluid move across the highly permeable sinusoids to form a protein-rich lymph (151).

The consequences of this increased formation of lymph depend on the rate of formation and the ability of first the gastrointestinal and then the abdominal lymphatics to return this fluid to the systemic circulation. As lymph formation exceeds the capacity of the gastrointestinal lymphatics to return fluid centrally, edema occurs (321) and fluid begins to move into the abdominal cavity. When the capacity of the abdominal lymphatics is exceeded, ascites occurs.

This loss of plasma fluid into the abdominal cavity is associated with renal-endocrine adjustments that serve to retain sodium and consequently water. This plasma expansion aggravates the situation and a vicious cycle of filtration–plasma expansion–filtration begins. Peritoneovenous shunts return ascitic fluid to the systemic circulation and lead to a rapid natriuresis, diuresis, and a decrease in renin and aldosterone levels (322, 324, 325). Diuretics are also used in the treatment of ascites (324, 325).

## INFLAMMATORY BOWEL DISEASE

Certain diseases of the colon are characterized by inflammation with dilated blood vessels and edema. In some of these disorders there are ulcerations of the mucosa, a process in which ischemia may play a role. In this section those colonic mucosal disorders in which the circulation has been implicated are discussed.

Ischemia of the colon can result in different levels of tissue injury, depending on the severity and duration of the reduction in blood flow and the nature of the microbial flora (33, 211, 268). In mild cases, ischemic colitis develops with transient ulcerative hemorrhagic lesions that are limited to the mucosa and submucosa. In some severe cases the result is necrosis and gangrene.

Ulcerative colitis and Crohn's disease are similar in nature and difficult to differentiate accurately. In both inflammatory bowel diseases (IBD) the etiology is unknown; genetics, environment, and the immune system have been proposed as contributory factors. The IBD are characterized by mucosal and submucosal ulcerations and increased vascularity (250). In the early stages of each disease the blood vessels of the mucosa and submucosa are dilated, blood flow is increased, and the tissue is edematous (111, 150). These pathological findings have been attributed to the release of endogenous substances such as histamine, prostaglandins, and kinins by inflamed tissue (138, 162, 169, 194, 253, 288), to the presence of bacterial endotoxins (169), and to OFR from invading leukocytes (169).

Ischemia per se can cause a form of colitis similar to IBD (33, 52, 91, 205, 211, 268). Furthermore the norepinephrine content of the rectal mucosa is increased in IBD, suggesting a possible mechanism in which stress might play a role in colonic pathology (183). A role for the colonic circulation in the pathogenesis of ulcerative colitis has been proposed (83), but there is little evidence to directly link these diseases with a vascular pathology.

## ULCERS

More than a century ago two great European pathologists, Virchow and Rokitansky, expressed their convictions that ischemia was the major etiological factor in peptic ulcers (264, 306). Virchow conceived of the initiating event as local vasospasm in the mucosal circulation. Subsequently, there were reports of a greater prevalence of peptic ulcers in patients suffering from cardiovascular diseases (30, 272). More than a half century ago Harvey Cushing reported the occurrence of gastrointestinal mucosal ulceration and bleeding in patients who had undergone brain surgery (154). He attributed a circulatory basis to these consequences of his operations. There were subsequent reports of morphological abnormalities in the mucosal vasculature of ulcer patients (256, 327), as well as intravascular agglutination and stasis (174) and early hemorrhages preceding ulceration (270). Later work failed to substantiate these findings (154, 266). Thus, for example, acute ulceration of the intestinal mucosa produced by indomethacin is strikingly different histologically from the acute mucosal lesion produced by drastic reduction in blood flow to the gut (86).

Another set of observations that lent weight to the circulatory hypothesis in ulcerogenesis came from pharmacological investigations. Experimental erosions or ulcers of the gastrointestinal mucosa were produced by chronic administration of vasoconstrictor drugs such as vasopressin (225) and sympathomimetic agents (202). However, investigators were also able to produce ulcers with vasodilator interventions such as sympathectomy (195), acetylcholine (154), and histamine (154).

There are several problems with the line of reasoning that postulates a simple circulatory explanation for the origins of peptic ulcer disease, namely, that the common disorder is a local vascular response of the mucosa to life-threatening diseases. The first difficulty is that the average patient with peptic ulcer disease has no other known illness. Furthermore this vascular hypothesis requires the intermediacy of another abnormally functioning system, such as the SNS, circulating vasoactive agents, paracrine constrictors, or metabolites that enhance capillary permeability. Abnormalities in important systems of the body would not only adversely affect the mucosal circulation of the stomach or duodenum but would also directly damage other tissues. The circulatory hypothesis fails to explain the specific localization of ulcers to certain mucosal sites where the lesions occur; a circulatory deficit should affect mucosal areas in which the ulcers do not form as well as the ulcerated mucosa. There may be only one lesion in the entire mucosal surface of the stomach or bowel in response to a life-threatening stress that, presumably, should have decreased mucosal blood flow or increased capillary permeability throughout the lining of the enteric canal. Because of the lack of specificity of the circulatory hypothesis in the older literature and its unanswered questions, the explanation had gained little credence until recently (123, 298).

A more sophisticated approach to a possible link between mucosal circulatory insufficiency and ulcerogenesis has surfaced in recent reports (123, 298). One feature of these more insightful studies has been the use of better clinical and experimental models.

Circulatory shock is ulcerogenic in humans and in laboratory animals. Under these conditions it is easier to visualize a sequence of demonstrable events that include hypotension, mucosal ischemia, and ulcer formation. A second feature of recent investigations has been a serious effort to discover metabolic and biophysical mechanisms involved in ischemic ulcers. The shock state evokes gastric mucosal ulceration and aggravates the ulcerogenic effects of topical damaging agents whose ulcerogenicity is antagonized by vasodilator agents (53, 188, 190, 221, 259, 262).

The rate of backdiffusion of secreted hydrogen ion from the gastric lumen may be used as an indicator of the integrity of the gastric epithelium. Agents that damage the mucosa and are ulcerogenic increase the rate of permeation of hydrogen ion into the tissue. Thus backdiffusion of hydrogen ion was accelerated during experimental hemorrhagic shock in both undamaged and damaged mucosae (287, 292). Other responses to gastric ischemia included reductions in tissue $P_{O_2}$, the transepithelial cell potential difference (PD) (35), and the transmucosal electrical PD (55), all suggestive signs of devitalization of the mucosal epithelium, which is the tissue most vulnerable to ulcer formation in shock. Several topical damaging agents were found to reduce gastric mucosal blood flow (232, 259), and vasodilator drugs prevented ulceration produced by topical damaging agents (215, 262). Several antiulcer drugs, namely cimetidine, carbenoxolone, and PGE, have been shown to prevent reduction in gastric mucosal blood flow evoked by ulcerogenic interventions (191, 286, 316).

Although the focusing of investigations on those forms of ulcerogenesis clearly associated with mucosal ischemia, as in shock, has produced a more credible experimental model, this selection has also removed inquiry somewhat from the etiology of commonplace peptic ulcers. The vast majority of patients suffering from peptic ulcers are not in a state of circulatory shock. It is possible that most peptic ulcers have a noncirculatory etiology. We are still ignorant of the etiology of usual ulcer disease in humans.

Findings also cast some doubt on a vascular etiology in other types of experimental ulceration. A frequently used ulcerogenic model involves application of a topical damaging agent to the gastric mucosa. Such agents increase the backdiffusion of hydrogen ion from the lumen into the tissue and, if left in contact with the mucosa for long, prompt the appearance of erosions and ulcers. Commonly used topical damaging agents include aspirin, ethanol, and taurocholate. Several investigators have shown that exposure of the gastric mucosa to these agents causes an increase in gastric mucosal blood flow (41, 54). This augmentation of blood flow has been interpreted as a secondary effect of the backdiffusion of hydrogen ion into the tissue, which is said to have a local vasodilator effect. One wonders what the interpretation of a decrease in mucosal blood flow would have been, had such occurred. It has also been reported that vasoconstrictor drugs and mucosal ischemia evoked by shock did not increase the backdiffusion of hydrogen ion from the gastric lumen (53, 71, 261).

There is some doubt about attributing the protective effects of certain antiulcer agents to their vasodilator properties alone. Isoproterenol and prostaglandins of the E and I series protected the mucosa against ulcers in shock states; these agents are vasodilator drugs. They are also antisecretory drugs in the stomach that reduce gastric acid production, a pharmacological effect that protects the mucosa against ulcer formation independent of coincident vascular effects. Furthermore in a recent report it was shown that 16,16-dimethyl-$PGE_2$ protected the rat gastric mucosa against much of the damaging action of topical absolute ethanol but did not increase gastric mucosal blood flows in so doing (189).

These findings suggest that mucosal ischemia may not be the initial event in the formation of some types of experimental ulcer. However, the lowering of blood flow to the mucosa may still be involved in other forms of mucosal ulceration. Left open is the question of the next step in the pathogenetic sequence of ischemic ulceration. This line of inquiry has led investigators into an exploration of the metabolic and other cellular consequences of mucosal ischemia. There is evidence suggesting that reduced blood flow during shock increases mucosal acidity, either through increasing the backdiffusion of lumenal hydrogen ion or by a direct action on local metabolism (177, 260). These findings have led to the hypothesis that impaired mucosal buffering ability, because of the low flow state, leads to damage by tissue hydrogen ion, which would otherwise be neutralized or carried off to the lungs and kidneys for disposition. Another mechanism that may be involved in the injury caused by mucosal ischemia is a decrease in intracellular high-energy compounds (220). Other studies have focused on maintenance of tissue $P_{O_2}$ and normal electrophysiological characteristics, rather than on enhancement of blood flow, during protection against shock-induced ulcers (247, 255). Finally, evidence from studies of intestinal ischemia suggests that mucosal damage may be mediated through accumulation of OFR (114). A similar mechanism may operate in the case of ischemic ulcers of the gastric mucosa (152).

In summary, the most common forms of peptic ulcers are of unknown origin. There is no definitive evidence for a circulatory etiology in these disorders. In the next most prevalent group of people suffering from peptic diseases, there is evidence for causation by topical damaging agents, such as aspirin and ethanol. Evidence for the mucosal circulation as the immediate target of these damaging agents is far from convincing. Ischemia does not appear to be the critical first step in damage caused by aspirin or ethanol. Finally, there are people who suffer erosions and ulceration during the course of circulatory shock. In these cases it is likely that mucosal ischemia plays a critical role. The steps that lead from reduced blood flow to the formation of an ulcer in the mucosa are speculative.

## OTHER DISEASES

### Hypertension

Arterial hypertension can be the result of an increase in cardiac output, an increase in TPR, or both. In the most common variety, namely essential hypertension, the cause is an increase in TPR (40, 63, 93). In humans, blood flow to the splanchnic organs appears to be the same in both normal and hypertensive patients, although in one report splanchnic blood flow was lower in hypertensive patients (40, 68, 143, 297, 318). In spontaneously hypertensive rats, the percent blood flow distribution to the splanchnic vascular bed was the same as in normotensive rats (227, 300, 301). Neurogenic hypertension has been shown to decrease splanchnic blood flow (4) and the effects of renovascular hypertension are variable (Table 1).

Within the splanchnic circulation, individual organs appear to respond to hypertension with parallel changes in vascular resistance (63, 95, 222, 227). However, in one study in dogs there was at least an initial difference among organ resistance changes, with the gastric and hepatic vasculature showing a selective increase in resistance (193). Neither total nor segmental vascular resistances changed in the ileal circulation of chronic, one-kidney, one-wrap perinephritic hypertensive dogs (235, 285), although there was an increase in small artery resistance in dogs with two-kidney, one-clip Goldblatt hypertension (117).

In general, blood vessels of the small intestine are more responsive to vasoconstrictor agents in hypertensive animals (64, 117, 132, 216) and, therefore, could be more susceptible to ischemia under conditions of stress. There is also an increase in intestinal vascular permeability to proteins in one-kidney, one-clip hypertensive dogs (184) and a total body loss of plasma albumin in subjects with essential hypertension (243, 305). However, no gastrointestinal pathology has been linked to hypertension.

### Diabetes Mellitus

The intestinal circulation in diabetes is characterized by atrophy of the smooth muscle layer of the intestinal vessels (8, 28), dilated arterioles (28), increased blood flow (199), and a decrease in capillary density (28). The decrease in capillary density is due to a loss of capillaries, which is rapid in the early stages of the disease and then declines in rate (28). The degree to which changes in the intestinal vasculature contribute to diabetic changes in gastrointestinal structure and motor function is unknown. Diabetes-induced formation of atherosclerotic plaques in large vessels could result in intestinal ischemia.

### Arteriovenous Malformations

Congenital and trauma-induced arteriovenous malformations may result in portal venous hypertension (321). These malformations are also the site of both

TABLE 1. *Hemodynamic Changes in Small Intestine During Acute and Chronic Phases of Experimental and Genetic Hypertension*

| Model | Duration, days | Blood Pressure, % | Blood Flow, % | Resistance, % | Ref. |
|---|---|---|---|---|---|
| Salt loading (dog) | 1 | +26 | | NS* | 193 |
| | 5 | +34 | | NS | 193 |
| One-kidney, one-wrap (dog) | 11 | +5 | +10 | NS | 285 |
| | 28–35 | +27 | +18 | NS | 235 |
| Two-kidney, one-wrap (dog) | 28 | +25 | +21 | NS | 285 |
| Two-kidney, one-clip (dog) | 32 | +35 | NS | +35 | 117 |
| Genetic (rat)† | 147 | +50 | NS | +50 | 227 |
| | 140–224 | +93 | NS | +120 | 300 |

* NS, no significant change.  † Wistar-Kyoto rats served as control for spontaneously hypertensive rats.  [From Nyhof et al. (230a).]

acute and chronic intermittent bleeding (258). Elderly patients sometimes acquire arteriovenous communications in the right colon, which are referred to as angiodysplasia (89). These are believed to be the result of ischemic large bowel disease subsequent to chronically elevated lumen pressure. It has been proposed that they form as a result of decreased mucosal blood flow and increased submucosal arteriovenous shunting (18).

*Dumping Syndrome and Secretory Disorders*

The sudden presentation of a hyperosmotic fluid into the small intestine, such as occurs after gastrectomy or a gastrojejunostomy, often results in a sudden movement of fluid into the intestinal lumen. In severe cases, cardiovascular collapse occurs (51). This increase in fluid flux into the intestinal lumen is associated with an increase in intestinal mucosal blood flow (330), which is apparently mediated by intrinsic neural reflexes (59). This increase in intestinal blood flow would seem to be necessary to maintain the fluid flux, but it is not known if similar results would be obtained if blood flow were held constant.

In general, the intestinal circulation serves a permissive role in intestinal secretory disorders. The circulation provides the necessary nutrients, oxygen, and fluid to support active secretory processes; however, simply increasing blood flow does not lead to intestinal secretion. Portal venous hypertension appears to be unique in that the intestinal circulation plays a direct role in the intestinal fluid disorder associated with the disease, i.e., ascites.

*Miscellaneous Disorders*

Esophageal achalasia and atresia may be due to ischemia of the lower esophagus during embryonic development. Transient ischemia may result from rotational stress, leading to necrosis of the neural tissue (79) and impaired motor function (achalasia). Embryonic intestinal ischemia may be the cause of intestinal stenosis and atresia and may also be responsible for esophageal atresia (16, 78).

It has been proposed that reflux esophagitis may be due to a malfunctioning lower esophageal sphincter that has been damaged because of ischemia (80). It has also been proposed that the susceptibility of the esophagus to acid injury is due to the relatively low blood flow to this region as opposed to the stomach. There is some evidence of neovascularization in patients with reflux esophagitis in which an increase in blood vessel diameter occurred with the growth of capillaries into the squamous cell layer (106).

Vasculitis is an inflammation of blood vessels that may be due to a variety of systemic diseases (primary) or may be the result of a local inflammation of the parenchymal tissue (secondary). Vasculitides can cause rupture of blood vessels, formation of aneurysms, fibrosis of the vessel wall, or the formation of thrombi in the vessel lumen. These sequelae would result in ischemia or hemorrhage (135).

Aneurysms are found in the splenic artery but rarely occur in the celiac and mesenteric arteries. Mesenteric aneurysms that have been reported are due to trauma, mycosis, or a leakage of pancreatic enzymes in pancreatitis. Celiac artery occlusion has also been reported to lead to aneurysms of the pancreaticoduodenal arteries as the result of increased turbulent flow through these collateral vessels (19).

Studies of the effects of intestinal obstruction and distention on mesenteric blood flow are extensive and have been reviewed recently (233). Although distending pressures of 20 mmHg or more have been shown to impair intestinal blood flow, oxygen uptake, and capillary perfusion, lumenal pressures in patients with intestinal obstruction rarely exceed 15 mmHg.

REFERENCES

1. ABRAMSON, D. I., AND P. B. DORBIN. *Blood Vessels and Lymphatics in Organ Systems.* New York: Academic, 1984.
2. AGRESS, C. M., H. F. GLASSNER, M. J. BINDER, AND J. FIELDS. Hemodynamic measurements in experimental coronary shock. *J. Appl. Physiol.* 10: 469–475, 1957.
3. AHREN, C., AND U. HAGLUND. Mucosal lesions in the small intestine of the cat during low flow. *Acta Physiol. Scand.* 88: 541–548, 1973.
4. ALEXANDER, N., AND V. DEQUATTRO. Regional and systemic hemodynamic patterns in rabbits with neurogenic hypertension. *Circ. Res.* 35: 636–645, 1974.
5. AL-KHALIDI, U. A. S., AND T. H. CHAGLASSIAN. The species distribution of xanthine oxidase. *Biochem. J.* 97: 318–321, 1965.
6. ALONSO, D. R., S. SCHEIDT, M. POST, AND T. K. KILLIP. Pathophysiology of cardiogenic shock. Quantification of myocardial necrosis, clinical, pathologic and electrocardiographic correlations. *Circulation* 48: 588–596, 1973.
7. ALTURA, B. M. Humoral, hormonal and myogenic mechanisms in microcirculatory regulation. In: *Microcirculation,* edited by G. Kaley and B. M. Altura. Baltimore, MD: University Park, 1977, vol. 2, p. 431–502.
8. ANGERWALL, L., AND J. SOVE SODENBERGH. Microangiography in the digestive tract in subjects with diabetes of early onset and long duration. *Diabetologia* 2: 117–122, 1966.
9. ARFORS, K. E., G. ARTURSON, D. BERGQVIST, AND E. SVENSJO. The effect of inhibition of prostaglandin synthesis on microvascular haemostasis and micromolecular leakage. *Thromb. Res.* 8: 393–402, 1976.
10. ASCANIO, G., F. BARRERA, E. V. LAUTSCH, AND M. J. OPPENHEIMER. Role of reflexes following myocardial necrobiosis. *Am. J. Physiol.* 209: 1081–1088, 1965.
11. ATHANASOULIS, C. A., J. WITTENBERG, AND R. BERNSTEIN. Vasodilatory drugs in the management of nonocclusive bowel ischemia. *Gastroenterology* 68: 146–150, 1975.
12. BABA, S., AND K. MIZUTANI. The intraluminal administration of perfluorochemicals to the ischemic gastrointestinal tract. *Aust. NZ J. Surg.* 51: 468–475, 1981.
13. BABIOR, B. M., R. S. KIPNES, AND J. T. CURNETTE. Biological defense mechanisms. The production of leukocytes of super-

oxide, a potential bactericidal agent. *J. Clin. Invest.* 52: 741–744, 1973.
14. BAILEY, R. W., G. B. BULKLEY, K. I. LEVY, J. H. ANDERSON, AND G. D. ZUIDEMA. Pathogenesis of nonocclusive mesenteric ischemia: studies in a porcine model induced by pericardial tamponade. *Surg. Forum* 33: 194–196, 1982.
15. BAKER, R., AND D. MENDEL. Some observations on 'autoregulatory escape' in cat intestine. *J. Physiol. Lond.* 190: 229–240, 1967.
16. BARNARD, C. The genesis of intestinal atresia. *Surg. Forum* 7: 393–396, 1956.
17. BARTON, R. W., D. A. REYNOLDS, AND K. G. SWAN. Mesenteric circulatory responses to hemorrhagic shock in the baboon. *Ann. Surg.* 175: 204–209, 1972.
18. BAUM, S., C. ATHANASOULIS, A. WALTMAN, J. GOLDABINI, R. SHAPIRO, A. WARSHAW, AND L. OTTINGER. Angiodysplasia of the right colon: a cause of gastrointestinal bleeding. *Am. J. Roentgenol.* 129: 789–794, 1977.
19. BAUM, S., AND H. A. JORDON. Angiography in vascular disorders of the gut. In: *Bockus Gastroenterology* (4th ed.), edited by J. E. Berk. Philadelphia, PA: Saunders, 1984, vol. 3, p. 1937–1982.
20. BECK, L., AND A. S. DANTAS. Vasomotor activity in hemorrhagic shock (Abstract). *Federation Proc.* 14: 318, 1955.
21. BECKER, E. L., AND K. F. AUSTIN. Anaphylaxis. In: *Textbook of Immunopathology* (2nd ed.), edited by P. A. Miescher and H. T. Mueller-Eberhard. New York: Grune & Stratton, 1976, p. 117–135.
22. BENOIT, J. N., J. A. BARROWMAN, S. L. HARPER, P. R. KVIETYS, AND D. N. GRANGER. Role of humoral factors in the intestinal hyperemia associated with chronic portal hypertension. *Am. J. Physiol.* 247 (*Gastrointest. Liver Physiol.* 10): G486–G493, 1984.
23. BIBER, B., O. LUNDGREN, AND J. SVANVIK. Intramural blood flow and blood volume in the small intestine of the cat analyzed by an indicator-dilution technique. *Acta Physiol. Scand.* 87: 391–403, 1973.
24. BIRGENS, H. S., J. HENRIKSEN, P. MATZEN, AND H. POULSEN. The shock liver. *Acta Med. Scand.* 204: 417–421, 1978.
25. BLAISDELL, F. W. The role of steroids in septic shock. *Circ. Shock* 8: 673–682, 1981.
26. BLANCHET, L., AND D. LEBREE. Changes in splanchnic blood flow in portal hypertensive rats. *Eur. J. Clin. Invest.* 12: 327–330, 1982.
27. BOHLEN, H. G. Intestinal tissue $P_{O_2}$ and microvascular responses during glucose exposure. *Am. J. Physiol.* 238 (*Heart Circ. Physiol.* 7): H164–H171, 1980.
28. BOHLEN, H. G., AND K. D. HANKINS. Early arteriolar and capillary changes in streptozotocin-induced diabetic rats and intraperitoneal hyperglycaemic rats. *Diabetologia* 22: 344–348, 1982.
29. BOHLEN, H. G., P. M. HUTCHINS, C. E. RAPELA, AND H. D. GREEN. Microvascular control in intestinal mucosa of normal and hemorrhaged rats. *Am. J. Physiol.* 229: 1159–1164, 1975.
30. BOLES, R. S., H. E. RIGGS, AND J. D. GRIFFITHS. The role of the circulation in the production of peptic ulcer. *Am. J. Dig. Dis.* 6: 632–640, 1939.
31. BOLEY, S. J., L. J. BRANDT, AND F. J. VEITH. Ischemic disorders of the intestines. *Curr. Probl. Surg.* 15: 1–85, 1978.
32. BOLEY, S. J., F. R. FEINSTEIN, R. SAMMARTANO, L. J. BRANDT, AND S. SPRAYREGEN. New concepts in the management of emboli of the superior mesenteric artery. *Surgery St. Louis* 153: 561–569, 1981.
33. BOLEY, S. J., S. SCHWARTZ, AND L. LASH. Reversible vascular occlusion of the colon. *Surg. Gynecol. Obstet.* 116: 53–60, 1963.
34. BOLEY, S. J., AND S. SPRAYREGEN. Treatment of mesenteric embolization. *Surg. Gynecol. Obstet.* 152: 165–170, 1980.
35. BOWEN, J. C., D. K. GARG, P. SALVATO, AND E. D. JACOBSON. Differential oxygen utilization in the stomach during vasopressin and tourniquet ischemia. *J. Surg. Res.* 25: 15–20, 1978.
36. BOWEN, J. C., W. PAWLIK, W. F. FANG, AND E. D. JACOBSON. Pharmacologic effects of gastrointestinal hormones on intestinal oxygen consumption and blood flow. *Surgery St. Louis* 78: 515–519, 1975.
37. BREDENBERG, C. E., G. A. TAYLOR, AND W. R. WEBB. The effect of thrombocytopenia on the pulmonary and systemic hemodynamics of canine endotoxin shock. *Surgery St. Louis* 87: 59–68, 1980.
38. BROBMANN, G. F., H. B. ULANO, L. B. HINSHAW, AND E. D. JACOBSON. Mesenteric vascular responses to endotoxin in the monkey and dog. *Am. J. Physiol.* 219: 1464–1467, 1970.
39. BROCKMAN, S. K., AND C. S. THOMAS, JR. The effect of *Escherichia coli* endotoxin on the circulation. *Surg. Gynecol. Obstet.* 125: 763–774, 1967.
40. BROD, J. Haemodynamic basis of acute pressor reactions and hypertension. *Br. Heart J.* 25: 227–245, 1963.
41. BRUGGEMAN, T. M., J. G. WOOD, AND H. W. DAVENPORT. Local control of blood flow in the dog's stomach: vasodilation caused by acid back-diffusion following topical application of salicyclic acid. *Gastroenterology* 77: 736–744, 1979.
42. BRUNGARDT, J. M., D. G. REYNOLDS, AND K. G. SWAN. Route of endotoxin delivery: effects of canine mesenteric hemodynamics. *Am. J. Physiol.* 223: 565–568, 1972.
43. BULKLEY, G. B., P. R. KVIETYS, M. A. PERRY, AND D. N. GRANGER. Effects of cardiac tamponade on colonic hemodynamics and oxygen uptake. *Am. J. Physiol.* 244 (*Gastrointest. Liver Physiol.* 7): G604–G612, 1983.
44. BYNUM, T. E., R. H. GALLAVAN, JR., AND E. D. JACOBSON. The pathophysiology of nonocclusive intestinal ischemia. In: *Physiology of the Intestinal Circulation*, edited by A. P. Shepherd and D. N. Granger. New York: Raven, 1984, p. 369–376.
45. BYNUM, T. E., AND H. G. HANLEY. Effect of digitalis on estimated splanchnic blood flow. *J. Lab. Clin. Med.* 19: 84–91, 1982.
46. BYNUM, T. E., H. HANLEY, AND J. S. COLE. Effect of digitalis glycosides on splanchnic blood flow in man (Abstract). *Clin. Res.* 21: 509, 1973.
47. BYNUM, T. E., AND E. D. JACOBSON. Shock, intestinal ischemia and digitalis. *Circ. Shock* 2: 235–237, 1975.
48. BYNUM, T. E., AND E. D. JACOBSON. Nonocclusive intestinal ischemia. *Arch. Int. Med.* 139: 281–282, 1979.
49. CANNON, W. B. *Traumatic Shock.* New York: Appleton, 1923.
50. CASLEY-SMITH, J. R., AND B. J. GANNON. Intestinal microcirculation: spatial organization and fine structure. In: *Physiology of the Intestinal Circulation*, edited by A. P. Shepherd and D. N. Granger. New York: Raven, 1984, p. 9–32.
51. CASTENFORS, H., H. ELLIASCH, AND E. HULTMAN. Effects of ingestion of hyperosmotic glucose solution on the splanchnic circulation in normal subjects and in partially gastrectomized patients reacting with circulatory collapse. *Scand. J. Clin. Lab. Invest.* 13: 512–524, 1961.
52. CAVE, D. R., AND J. B. KEISNER. Animal models of inflammatory bowel disease. *Z. Gastroenterol.* 17, Suppl.: 125–135, 1979.
53. CHEUNG, L. Y., AND N. CHANG. The role of gastric mucosal blood flow and $H^+$ back-diffusion in the pathogenesis of acute gastric erosions. *J. Surg. Res.* 22: 357–361, 1977.
54. CHEUNG, L. Y., F. G. MOODY, AND R. S. REESE. Effect of aspirin, bile salt, and ethanol on canine gastric mucosal blood flow. *Surgery St. Louis* 77: 786–792, 1975.
55. CHEUNG, L. Y., R. S. REESE, AND F. G. MOODY. Direct effect of endotoxin on the gastric mucosal microcirculation and electrical gradient. *Surgery St. Louis* 79: 564–568, 1976.
56. CHIEN, S. Role of the sympathetic nervous system in hemorrhage. *Physiol. Rev.* 47: 214–288, 1967.
57. CHIEN, S., AND M. I. GREGERSON. Hemorrhage and shock. In: *Medical Physiology* (12th ed.), edited by V. B. Mountcastle. St. Louis, MO: Mosby, 1968, p. 262–282.
59. CHOU, C. C., T. D. BURNS, C. P. HSIEH AND J. M. DABNEY. Mechanisms of local vasodilation with hypertonic glucose in the jejunum. *Surgery St. Louis* 71: 380–387, 1972.
60. CHOU, C. C., L. C. YU, AND Y. M. YU. Effects of acute hemorrhage and carotid artery occlusion on blood flow and its distribution in the wall of the gastrointestinal tract. In: *Micro-

*circulation*, edited by J. Grayson and W. Zinng. New York: Plenum, 1976, vol. 1, p. 343–345.
61. CLOWES, J. G., N. VUCINIE, AND N. WEIDNER. Circulatory and metabolic alterations associated with survival or death in peritonitis. *Ann. Surg.* 163: 866–885, 1966.
62. COHN, J. D., M. GREENSPAN, C. R. GOLDSTEIN, A. L. GUDWIN, J. H. SIEGEL, AND L. R. M. DEL GUERCIO. Arteriovenous shunting in high cardiac output shock syndromes. *Surg. Gynecol. Obstet.* 127: 282–288, 1968.
63. COLEMAN, T. G., H. J. GRANGER, AND A. C. GUYTON. Whole-body circulatory autoregulation and hypertension. *Circ. Res.* 29, Suppl. 2: 78–86, 1971.
64. COLLIS, M. G., AND B. J. ALPS. Vascular reactivity to noradrenaline, potassium chloride and angiotensin II in the rat perfused mesenteric vasculature preparation, during the development of renal hypertension. *Cardiovasc. Res.* 9: 118–126, 1975.
65. CONSTANTER, L. Extracardiac factors contributing to hypotension during coronary occlusion. *Am. J. Cardiol.* 11: 205–217, 1963.
66. CORAZZA, R., L. MANFREDIA, AND F. RASCHI. Attività elettrica delle fibre nervose simpatiche vasomotrici nell'emorragic prottrata fino alla morte, nel getto. *Minerva Med.* 54: 1691–1694, 1963.
67. CORAZZA, R., O. PINOTTI, AND F. RASCHI. Attività simpatica vasomotoria nello shock emorragico. *Arch. Sci. Biol.* 47: 275–286, 1963.
68. CULBERTSON, J. W., R. W. WILKINS, F. J. INGELFINGER, AND S. E. BRADLEY. The effect of the upright posture upon hepatic blood flow in normotensive and hypertensive subjects. *J. Clin. Invest.* 30: 305–311, 1951.
69. DALSING, M. C., J. L. GROSFELD, M. A. SHIFFLER, D. W. VANE, M. HULL, R. L. BAEHNER, AND T. R. WEBER. Superoxide dismutase: a cellular protective enzyme in bowel ischemia. *J. Surg. Res.* 34: 589–596, 1983.
70. DANFORD, R. O. The splanchnic vasoconstrictive effect of digoxin and its reversal by glucagon. In: *Vascular Disorders of the Intestine*, edited by S. J. Boley, S. S. Schwartz, and L. F. Williams, Jr. New York: Appleton-Century-Crofts, 1971, p. 421–435.
71. DAVENPORT, H. W., AND L. L. BARR. Failure of ischemia to break the dog's gastric mucosal barrier. *Gastroenterology* 65: 619–624, 1973.
72. DAVIS, L. J., J. ANDERSON, S. WALLACE, C. GIANTURCO, AND E. D. JACOBSON. The use of prostaglandin E1 to enhance the angiographic visualization of the splanchnic circulation. *Radiology* 114: 281–286, 1974.
73. DEAN, H. R., AND R. A. WEBB. The morbid anatomy and histology of anaphylaxis in the dog. *J. Pathol. Bacteriol.* 27: 51–64, 1924.
74. DEAN, H. R., AND R. A. WEBB. The blood changes in anaphylactic shock in the dog. *J. Pathol. Bacteriol.* 27: 65–78, 1924.
75. DEL MAESTRO, R. F., J. BJÖRK, AND K. E. ARFORS. Increase in microvascular permeability induced by enzymatically generated free radicals. II. Role of superoxide anion radical, hydrogen peroxide, and hydroxyl radical. *Microvasc. Res.* 22: 255–270, 1981.
76. DEMETRIOU, A. A., P. K. KAGOMA, S. KAISER, E. SEIFLER, X. T. NIU, AND S. M. LEVENSON. Effect of dimethyl sulfoxide and glycerol on acute bowel ischemia in the rat. *Am. J. Surg.* 149: 91–94, 1985.
77. DIETZMAN, R. H., L. H. ROMERO, C. B. BICKMAN, C. H. SHATNEY, AND R. C. LILLEHEI. The influence of the sympathetic nervous system during cardiogenic shock. *Surg. Gynecol. Obstet.* 137: 773–783, 1973.
78. EARLHAM, R. J. A study of the etiology of congenital stenosis of the gut. *Ann. R. Coll. Surg. Engl.* 51: 126–130, 1972.
79. EARLHAM, R. J. A vascular cause for aganglionic bowel. *Am. J. Dig. Dis.* 17: 255–261, 1972.
80. EARLHAM, R. J., J. F. SCHLEGEL, AND F. H. ELLIS. Effect of ischemia of lower esophagus and esophagastric junction on canine esophageal motor function. *J. Thorac. Cardiovasc. Surg.* 54: 822–831, 1967.
81. ERRINGTON, M. L., AND M. R. SILVA. On the role of vasopressin and angiotensin in the development of irreversible haemorrhagic shock. *J. Physiol. Lond.* 242: 119–141, 1974.
82. EVANGELISTA, S., AND A. MELI. Influence of antioxidants and radical scavengers on ethanol-induced gastric ulcers in the rat. *Gen. Pharmacol.* 16: 285–286, 1985.
83. FAIRBURN, R. A. On the aetiology of ulcerative colitis: a vascular hypothesis. *Lancet* 1: 697–699, 1973.
84. FALK, A., B. KAIJSER, H. E. MYRVOLD, AND U. HAGLUND. Intestinal vascular and central hemodynamic responses in the cat following i.v. infusion of live *E. coli* bacteria. *Circ. Shock* 7: 239–250, 1980.
85. FALLUCA, F., N. ZIPARO, L. GIANGRANDE, G. MENZINGER, AND S. STEPA. Exaggerated glucagon secretion in diabetic and non-diabetic subjects with surgical portacaval anastomosis. *Horm. Metab. Res.* 13: 545–547, 1981.
86. FANG, W. F., A. G. BROUGHTON, AND E. D. JACOBSON. Indomethacin induced intestinal inflammation. *Am. J. Dig. Dis.* 22: 749–760, 1977.
87. FANTONE, J. C., AND P. A. WARD. Oxygen-derived radicals and their metabolites: relationship to tissue injury. In: *Current Concepts*. Kalamazoo, MI: Upjohn, 1985, p. 1–51. (Upjohn Publ. No. 8800-67.)
88. FANTOZZI, R., S. BRUNELLESCHI, L. GIULIATTINI, P. BLANDINA, E. MASISI, G. CAVALLO, AND P. F. MANNAIONI. Mast cell and neutrophil interactions: a role for superoxide anion and histamine. *Agents Actions* 16: 260–264, 1985.
89. FATAAR, S., P. MORTON, AND A. SCHULMAN. Arteriovenous malformation of the gastrointestinal tract. *Clin. Radiol.* 32: 623–630, 1981.
90. FEDINA, L., M. KALLAI, AND A. G. B. KOVACH. Sympathetic nervous activity after hemorrhage. *Adv. Exp. Biol. Med.* 33: 473–480, 1973.
91. FELDER, R. F., AND M. D. THAMES. Interaction between cardiac receptors and sinoaortic baroreceptors in the control of efferent cardiac sympathetic nerve activity during myocardial ischemia in dogs. *Circ. Res.* 45: 728–736, 1979.
92. FEOLA, M., E. R. ARBEL, AND G. GLICK. Attenuation of cardiac sympathetic drive in experimental myocardial ischemia in dogs. *Am. Heart J.* 93: 82–88, 1977.
93. FERRARIO, C. M. Contribution of cardiac output and peripheral resistance to experimental renal hypertension. *Am. J. Physiol.* 226: 711–714, 1974.
94. FIELDING, L. P. *Gastrointestinal Mucosal Blood Flow*. London: Churchill Livingstone, 1980.
95. FLOHR, H., W. BRUELL, H. W. DAHNERS, D. REDEL, H. CONRADI, AND K. STOEPEL. Regional distribution of vascular resistance in two models of experimental renovascular hypertension. *Pfluegers Arch.* 362: 157–164, 1976.
96. FLOYD, N. F., AND E. NEIL. The influence of the sympathetic innervation of the carotid bifurcation on chemoceptor and baroceptor activity in the cat. *Arch. Int. Pharmacodyn.* 91: 230–239, 1952.
97. FOLKOW, B., D. H. LEWIS, O. LUNDGREN, S. MELLANDER, AND I. WALLENTIN. The effect of graded vasoconstrictor fibre stimulation on the intestinal resistance and capacitance vessels. *Acta Physiol. Scand.* 61: 445–457, 1964.
98. FOLKOW, B., AND E. NEIL. *Circulation*. London: Oxford Univ. Press, 1971.
99. FONDACARO, J. D., M. SCHWAIGER, AND E. D. JACOBSON. Effects of vasodilators on mesenteric ischemia and hypoxia induced by hemorrhage. *Circ. Shock* 6: 255–260, 1979.
100. FORSYTHE, R. P. Sympathetic nervous system control of distribution of cardiac output in unanesthetized monkeys. *Federation Proc.* 31: 1240–1244, 1972.
101. FORSYTHE, R. P., B. I. HOFFBRAND, AND K. MELMON. Redistribution of cardiac output during hemorrhage in the unanesthetized monkey. *Circ. Res.* 27: 311–320, 1970.
102. FREIS, E. D., H. W. SCHNAPER, R. L. JOHNSON, AND G. E. SCHREINER. Hemodynamic alterations in acute myocardial infarction. I. Cardiac output, mean arterial pressure, total

peripheral resistance, "central" and total blood volumes, venous pressure and average circulation time. *J. Clin. Invest.* 31: 131–140, 1952.
103. FUKUZAWA, K., S. TAKASE, AND H. TSUKATANI. The effect of concentration on the antioxidant effectiveness of tocopherol in lipid peroxidation induced by superoxide free radicals. *Arch. Biochem. Biophys.* 240: 117–120, 1985.
104. GAGOR, S. Digestive system: liver, pathophysiology, pathogenesis and pathology of blood circulation. In: *Blood Vessels and Lymphatics in Organ Systems,* edited by D. I. Abramson and P. B. Dorbin. New York: Academic, 1984, p. 489–496.
105. GAUER, O. H., AND J. P. HENRY. Circulatory basis of fluid volume control. *Physiol. Rev.* 43: 423–481, 1963.
106. GEBOES, K., V. DESMET, G. VANTRAPPEN, AND J. MEBIS. Vascular changes in the esophageal mucosa. *Gastrointest. Endosc.* 26: 29–32, 1980.
107. GERNANDT, B., G. LILJESTRAND, AND Y. ZOTTERMAN. Efferent impulses in the splanchnic nerve. *Acta Physiol. Scand.* 11: 231–247, 1946.
108. GILBERT, R. P. Mechanisms of the hemodynamic effects of endotoxin. *Physiol. Rev.* 40: 245–279, 1960.
109. GOLDSTEIN, I. M., D. ROOS, G. WEISSMANN, AND H. B. KAPLAN. Influence of corticosteroids on human polymorphonuclear leukocyte function in vitro. *Inflammation* 1: 305–315, 1976.
110. GOOTMAN, P. M., AND M. I. COHEN. Efferent splanchnic activity and systemic arterial pressure. *Am. J. Physiol.* 219: 897–903, 1970.
111. GRANGER, D. N., AND J. A. BARROWMAN. Microcirculation of the alimentary tract. II. Pathophysiology of edema. *Gastroenterology* 84: 1035–1049, 1983.
112. GRANGER, D. N., AND G. B. BULKLEY. *The Measurement of Splanchnic Blood Flow.* Baltimore, MD: Williams & Wilkins, 1981.
113. GRANGER, D. N., P. R. KVIETYS, AND J. A. BARROWMAN (editors). *Pathophysiology of the Splanchnic Circulation.* Boca Raton, FL: CRC, 1987.
114. GRANGER, D. N., G. RUTILI, AND J. M. MCCORD. Superoxide radicals in feline intestinal ischemia. *Gastroenterology* 81: 22–29, 1981.
115. GRECO, A. V., F. CRUCITTI, G. GHIRLANDA, R. MANNA, L. ALTOMONTE, A. G. REBUZZI, AND A. BERTOLI. Insulin and glucagon concentration in portal and peripheral veins in patients with hepatic cirrhosis. *Diabetologia* 17: 23–28, 1979.
116. GREEN, H. D., R. F. BOND, C. E. RAPELA, H. E. SCHMID, E. MANLEY, AND J. D. FARRAR. Competition between intrinsic and extrinsic controls of resistance vessels of major vascular beds during hemorrhagic hypotension and shock. In: *Advances in Shock Research,* edited by A. M. Lefer and L. M. Mela. New York: Liss, 1980, vol. 3, p. 77–104.
117. GREENBERG, S. Vascular responses of the perfused intestine to reactive agents during the development of two-kidney, one-clip Goldblatt hypertension in dogs. *Circ. Res.* 48: 895–906, 1981.
118. GREENWAY, C. V., A. E. LAWSON, AND R. D. STARK. The effect of haemorrhage on hepatic artery and portal vein flows in the anaesthetized cat. *J. Physiol. Lond.* 193: 375–379, 1967.
119. GREENWAY, C. V., AND V. S. MURTHY. Mesenteric vasoconstriction of endotoxin administration in cats pretreated with aspirin. *Br. J. Pharmacol.* 43: 259–269, 1971.
120. GREENWAY, C. V., AND G. OSHIRO. Effects of histamine on hepatic volume (outflow block) in anaesthetized dogs. *Br. J. Pharmacol.* 47: 282–290, 1973.
121. GREENWAY, C. V., AND R. D. STARK. Hepatic vascular bed. *Physiol. Rev.* 51: 23–65, 1971.
122. GROSFELD, J. L., K. KAMMAN, K. GROSS, D. CIKRIT, D. ROSS, M. WOLFE, S. KATZ, AND T. R. WEBER. Comparative effects of indomethicin, prostaglandin E1, and ibuprofen on bowel ischemia. *J. Pediat. Surg.* 18: 738–742, 1983.
123. GUTH, P. H., AND F. W. LEUNG. Physiology of the gastric circulation. In: *Physiology of the Gastrointestinal Tract* (2nd ed.), edited by L. R. Johnson. New York: Raven, 1987, vol. 2, p. 1031–1053.
124. HADDY, F. J. Local regulation of the peripheral vascular system. In: *Shock and Hypotension,* edited by L. C. Mills and J. H. Moyer. New York: Grune & Stratton, 1965, p. 111–117.
125. HAGLUND, U. Vascular reactions in the small intestine of the cat during hemorrhage. *Acta Physiol. Scand.* 89: 129–141, 1973.
126. HAGLUND, U., T. ABE, C. AHREN, I. BRAIDE, AND O. LUNDGREN. Intestinal mucosal lesions in shock. I. Studies on the pathogenesis. *Eur. Surg. Res.* 8: 435–447, 1976.
127. HAGLUND, U., AND O. LUNDGREN. The effects of vasoconstrictor fibre stimulation on the consecutive vascular sections of cat small intestine during hemorrhagic hypotension. *Acta Physiol. Scand.* 88: 95–108, 1973.
128. HAGLUND, U., AND O. LUNDGREN. Intestinal ischemia and shock factors. *Federation Proc.* 37: 2729–2731, 1978.
129. HALEVY, S., B. T. ALTURA, AND B. M. ALTURA. Pathophysiological basis for the use of steroids in the treatment of shock and trauma. *Klin. Wochenschr.* 60: 1021–1030, 1982.
130. HALINEN, M. O., M. O. K. HAKUMAKI, AND H. S. S. SARAJAS. Circulatory reflex responses during the initial stage of feline endotoxin shock. *Acta Physiol. Scand.* 101: 264–269, 1977.
131. HALL, R. C., AND R. L. HODGE. Vasoactive hormones in endotoxin shock: a comparative study in cats and dogs. *J. Physiol. Lond.* 213: 69–84, 1971.
132. HALLBACK, M., Y. LUNDGREN, AND L. WEISS. Reactivity of noradrenaline on aortic strips and portal veins from spontaneously hypertensive and normotensive rats. *Acta Physiol. Scand.* 81: 176–181, 1971.
134. HAMILTON, G., R. C. F. PHING, R. A. HUTTON, P. DANDONA, AND K. E. F. HOBBS. The relationship between prostacyclin activity and pressure in the portal vein. *Hepatology Baltimore* 2: 236–242, 1982.
135. HANAUER, S. B., AND S. C. KRAFT. Gastrointestinal manifestations of the vasculitis syndromes. In: *Bockus Gastroenterology* (4th ed.), edited by J. E. Berk. Philadelphia, PA: Saunders, 1984, vol. 7, p. 4525–4544.
136. HANQUET, M., A. CESSION-FASSION, AND J. LECOMTE. Changes in catecholamine levels during shock in man. *Can. Anaesth. Soc. J.* 17: 208–212, 1970.
137. HARRISON, L. H., JR., L. B. HINSHAW, J. J. COALSON, AND L. J. GREENFIELD. Effects of *E. coli* septic shock on pulmonary hemodynamics and capillary permeability. *J. Thorac. Cardiovasc. Surg.* 61: 795–803, 1971.
138. HAWKEY, C. J., AND S. C. TRUELOVE. Effect of prednisolone on prostaglandin synthesis by rectal mucosa in ulcerative colitis: investigation by laminar flow bioassay and radioimmunoassay. *Gut* 22: 190–193, 1981.
139. HERMRECK, A. S., AND A. P. THAL. Mechanisms for the high circulatory requirements in sepsis and septic shock. *Ann. Surg.* 170: 677–695, 1969.
140. HESS, M. L., AND N. H. MANSON. The paradox of steroid therapy: inhibition of oxygen free radicals. *Circ. Shock* 10: 1–5, 1983.
141. HEYMANS, C., AND E. NEIL. *Reflexogenic Areas of the Cardiovascular System.* Boston, MA: Little, Brown, 1958.
142. HILDEBRAND, G. J., J. NG, Y. SEYS, AND S. H. MADIN. Differentiation between pathogenic mechanisms of early and late phase of endotoxin shock. *Am. J. Physiol.* 210: 1451–1460, 1966.
143. HILEY, C. R., AND M. S. YATES. The distribution of cardiac output in the anesthetized spontaneously hypertensive rat. *Clin. Sci. Mol. Med.* 55: 317–320, 1970.
145. HINSHAW, L. B. Comparison of responses of canine and primate species to bacteria and bacterial endotoxin. In: *Shock in Low- and High-Flow States,* edited by B. Forscher, R. C. Lillehei, and S. S. Stubbs. Amsterdam: Excerpta Med., 1980, p. 126–136.
146. HINSHAW, L. B., L. T. ARCHER, B. K. BELLER-TODD, B. BENJAMIN, D. J. FLOURNOY, AND R. PASSEY. Survival of primates in lethal septic shock following delayed treatment with steroid. *Circ. Shock* 8: 291–300, 1981.
147. HINSHAW, L. B., B. BENJAMIN, D. D. HOLMES, B. BELLA, S.

T. ARCHER, J. J. COALSON, AND T. WHITSETT. Responses of the baboon to live *Escherichia coli* organisms and endotoxin. *Surg. Gynecol. Obstet.* 145: 1–11, 1977.
148. HINSHAW, L. B., D. A. REINS, AND R. J. HILL. Response of isolated liver to endotoxin. *Can. J. Physiol. Pharmacol.* 44: 529–541, 1966.
149. HINSHAW, L. B., L. A. SOLOMON, D. D. HOLMES, AND L. J. GREENFIELD. Comparison of canine responses to *Escherichia coli* organisms and endotoxin. *Surg. Gynecol. Obstet.* 127: 981–988, 1968.
150. HULTEN, L., J. LINDHAGEN, O. LUNDGREN, S. FASTH, AND C. AHREN. Regional intestinal blood flow in ulcerative colitis and Crohn's disease. *Gastroenterology* 72: 388–396, 1977.
151. HYATT, R. E., G. H. LAWRENCE, AND J. R. SMITH. Observations on the origin of ascites from experimental hepatic congestion. *J. Lab. Clin. Med.* 45: 274–280, 1955.
152. ITOH, M., AND P. H. GUTH. Role of oxygen-derived free radicals in hemorrhagic shock-induced gastric lesions in the rat. *Gastroenterology* 88: 1162–1167, 1985.
153. ITOH, M., F. W. LEUNG, K. HIRABAYASHI, AND P. H. GUTH. Role of blood flow in hemorrhagic shock-induced gastric injury. *Gastroenterology* 86: 1122–1130, 1984.
154. JACOBSON, E. D. The circulation of the stomach. *Gastroenterology* 48: 85–109, 1965.
155. JACOBSON, E. D. Secretion and blood flow in the gastrointestinal tract. In: *Handbook of Physiology. Alimentary Canal. Secretion*, edited by C. F. Code. Washington, DC: Am. Physiol. Soc., 1967, sect. 6, vol. II, chapt. 59, p. 1043–1062.
156. JACOBSON, E. D. Are adrenergic overactivity and splanchnic vasoconstriction the prime pathophysiological events in shock? In: *The Fundamental Mechanisms of Shock*, edited by L. B. Hinshaw and B. G. Cox. New York: Plenum, 1972, 109–112.
157. JACOBSON, E. D. Special aspects of endotoxin shock. In: *Shock, Metabolic Disorders and Therapy*, edited by E. D. Zimmerman, I. Staib, and E. D. Jacobson. New York: Schattauer, 1972. (Engl. ed.)
158. JACOBSON, E. D. *Report to the Congress of the United States of the National Commission on Digestive Diseases*. Washington, DC: US Govt. Printing Office, 1979, vol. IX, pt. 4, p. 27 (Table 3). [DHEW Publ. No. (NIH) 79-1878.]
159. JACOBSON, E. D., AND G. F. BROBMANN. The "adrenergic theory" of shock revisited. *Med. Counter Point* 2: 15–27, 1970.
160. JACOBSON, E. D., AND W. E. FARRAR, JR. Influence of route of administration on hemodynamic effects of endotoxin. *Am. J. Physiol.* 205: 799–802, 1963.
161. JODAL, M., U. HAGLUND, AND O. LUNDGREN. Countercurrent exchange mechanisms in the small intestine. In: *Physiology of the Intestinal Circulation*, edited by A. P. Shepherd and D. N. Granger. New York: Raven, 1984, p. 83–98.
162. JOHANSSON, C., B. KOLLBERG, R. NORDEMAR, K. SAMUELSON, AND S. BERKSTRÖM. Protective effect of prostaglandin $E_2$ in the gastrointestinal tract during indomethacin treatment of rheumatic disease. *Gastroenterology* 78: 479–483, 1980.
163. JOHNSON, P. C. Myogenic nature of increase in intestinal vascular resistance with venous pressure elevation. *Circ. Res.* 7: 992–999, 1959.
164. JOHNSON, P. C. Autoregulation of intestinal blood flow. *Am. J. Physiol.* 199: 311–318, 1960.
165. JOHNSON, P. C. Origin, localization and homeostatic significance of autoregulation in the intestine. *Circ. Res.* 15, Suppl. 1: I225–I232, 1964.
166. KALIMA, T. V., H. SALONIEMI, AND T. RAHKO. Experimental regional enteritis in pigs. *Scand. J. Gastroenterol.* 11: 353–362 1976.
167. KAMP, M., O. LUNDGREN, AND N. J. NILSSON. Extravascular shunting of oxygen in the small intestine of the cat. *Acta Physiol. Scand.* 72: 396–406, 1968.
168. KAPIN, M. A., AND J. L. FERGUSON. Hemodynamic and regional circulatory alterations in dog during anaphylactic challenge. *Am. J. Physiol.* 249 (*Heart Circ. Physiol.* 18): H430–H437, 1985.

169. KEISNER, J. B. Observations on the etiology and pathogenesis of inflammatory bowel disease. In: *Bockus Gastroenterology* (4th ed.), edited by J. E. Berk. Philadelphia, PA: Saunders, 1984, vol. 1, p. 521–539.
170. KELLER, V., C. E. SONNENBERG, D. BUCKHARDT, AND A. PERRICHOUD. Evidence for an augmented glucagon dependence of hepatic glucose production in cirrhosis of the liver. *J. Clin. Endocrinol. Metab.* 54: 961–968, 1981.
171. KELLOGG, E. W., AND I. FRIDOVICH. Superoxide, hydrogen peroxide and singlet oxygen in lipid peroxidation by a xanthine oxidase system. *J. Biol. Chem.* 250: 8812–8816, 1975.
172. KELLOGG, E. W., AND I. FRIDOVICH. Liposome oxidation and erythrocyte lysis by enzymatically-generated superoxide and hydrogen peroxide. *J. Biol. Chem.* 252: 6721–6727, 1977.
173. KELTY, R. H., A. H. BAGGENSTOSS, AND H. R. BUTT. The relation of the regenerated nodule to the vascular bed in cirrhosis. *Gastroenterology* 15: 285–295, 1950.
174. KEY, J. A. Blood vessels of a gastric ulcer. *Br. Med. J.* 2: 1464–1471, 1950.
175. KITANO, S. K., K. INOKUCHI, K. SUGIMACHI, AND N. KOYANAGI. Hemodynamic and morphological changes in the stomach of portal hypertensive rats. *Eur. Surg. Res.* 13: 227–235, 1981.
176. KITANO, S. N., K. KOYANASI, K. SUGIMACHI, M. KOBAYASHI, AND K. INOKUCHI. Mucosal blood flow and modified vascular responses to norepinephrine in the stomach of rats with liver cirrhosis. *Eur. Surg. Res.* 14: 221–230, 1982.
177. KIVILAAKSO, E., D. FROMM, AND W. SILEN. Relationship between ulceration and intramural pH of gastric mucosa during hemorrhagic shock. *Surgery St. Louis* 84: 70–79, 1978.
178. KLASS, A. A. The treatment of superior mesenteric artery occlusion: a reappraisal. *Can. Med. Assoc. J.* 93: 309–312, 1965.
179. KOCK, N. G., S. TIBLIN, AND W. G. SCHENK. Modification by glucagon of the splanchnic vascular responses to activation of the sympathetic adrenal system. *J. Surg. Res.* 11: 12–17, 1971.
180. KRENITSKY, T. A., J. V. TUTTLE, E. L. CATTAU, AND P. WANG. A comparison of the distribution and electron acceptor specialties of xanthine oxidase and aldehyde oxidase. *Comp. Biochem. Physiol. B Comp. Biochem.* 49: 687–703, 1974.
181. KUIDA, H., R. P. GILBERT, L. B. HINSHAW, J. G. BRUNSON, AND M. B. VISSCHER. Species differences in effect of gram-negative endotoxin on circulation. *Am. J. Physiol.* 200: 1197–1202, 1961.
182. KULLMANN, R., AND H. G. JUNK. Differential sympathetic response during coronary occlusion. *Res. Exp. Med.* 160: 317–320, 1973.
183. KWAAN, H. C., A. COCCO, A. I. MENDELOFF, AND T. ASTRUP. Fibrinolytic activity in the normal and inflamed rectal mucosa. *Scand. J. Gastroenterol.* 4: 441–445, 1969.
184. LAINE, G. A., AND H. J. GRANGER. Permeability of intestinal capillaries in chronic arterial hypertension (Abstract). *Microvasc. Res.* 21: 248, 1981.
185. LANCIAULT, G., W. F. FANG, E. D. JACOBSON, AND J. C. BOWEN. Evaluation of potential agents for treatment of nonocclusive mesenteric ischemia in dogs. *Circ. Shock* 3: 239–246, 1976.
186. LANCIAULT, G., AND E. D. JACOBSON. The gastrointestinal circulation. *Gastroenterology* 71: 851–873, 1976.
187. LANZAFAME, R. J., J. O. NAIM, Z. M. TOMKIEWICZ, AND J. R. HINSHAW. The effect of heparin on intestinal survival in experimental small intestinal ischemia. *Curr. Surg.* 40: 438–440, 1983.
188. LEUNG, F. W., M. ITOH, K. HIRABAYASHI, AND P. H. GUTH. Role of blood flow in gastric and duodenal mucosal injury in the rat. *Gastroenterology* 88: 281–289, 1985.
189. LEUNG, F. W., A. ROBERT, AND P. H. GUTH. Gastric mucosal blood flow in rats after 16,16-dimethyl prostaglandin $E_2$ given at a cytoprotective dose. *Gastroenterology* 88: 1948–1953, 1985.
190. LEVINE, B. A., H. V. GASKILL III, AND K. R. SIRINEK. Gastric mucosal blood flow. *J. Trauma* 23: 278–284, 1983.
191. LEVINE, B. A., W. H. SCHWEISINGER, AND K. R. SIRINEK. Cimetidine prevents reduction in gastric mucosal blood flow

during shock. *Surgery St. Louis* 84: 113–119, 1978.
192. LEY, K., AND K. E. ARFORS. Changes in micromolecular permeability by intravascular generation of oxygen-derived free radicals. *Microvasc. Res.* 24: 25–33, 1982.
193. LIARD, J. F. Regional blood flows in salt loading hypertension in the dog. *Am. J. Physiol.* 240 (*Heart Circ. Physiol.* 9): H361–H367, 1981.
194. LIGUMSKY, M., F. KARMELI, P. SHARON, U. ZOI, F. COHEN, AND D. RACHMILEWITZ. Enhanced thromboxane $A_2$ and prostacyclin production by cultured rectal mucosa in ulcerative colitis and its inhibition by steroids and sulfasalazine. *Gastroenterology* 81: 444–449, 1981.
195. LILLEHEI, C. W., AND O. H. WANGENSTEEN. Effect of celiac ganglionectomy upon experimental peptic ulcer formation. *Proc. Soc. Exp. Biol. Med.* 68: 369–372, 1948.
196. LILLEHEI, R. C., J. K. LONGERBEAM, J. H. BLOCH, AND W. G. MANAX. The modern treatment of shock based on physiological principles. *Clin. Pharmacol. Ther.* 5: 63–101, 1964.
197. LILLEHEI, R. C., J. K. LONGERBEAM, J. H. BLOCH, AND W. G. MANAX. The nature of experimental irreversible shock with its clinical implications. In: *Shock*, edited by S. G. Hershey. Boston, MA: Little, Brown, 1964, p. 139–205.
198. LILLIHEI, R. C., J. K. LONGERBEAM, J. H. BLOCK, AND W. G. MANAX. The nature of irreversible shock: experimental and clinical observations. *Ann. Surg.* 160: 682–710, 1964.
198a. LINTERMANS, J. P., A. J. APPEL, R. S. BLOOM, G. L. MULLINS, AND W. G. GUNTHEROTH. Mesenteric blood flow and vascular volume in hemorrhagic shock. *Am. J. Physiol.* 212: 482–487, 1967.
199. LUCAS, P. D., AND J. M. FOY. Effects of experimental diabetes and genetic obesity on regional blood flow in the rat. *Diabetes* 26: 786–792, 1977.
200. LUNDGREN, O. Studies in blood flow distribution and countercurrent exchange in the small intestine. *Acta Physiol. Scand. Suppl.* 303: 1–42, 1967.
201. LUNDGREN, O., AND J. SVANVIK. Mucosal hemodynamics in the small intestine of the cat during reduced perfusion pressure. *Acta Physiol. Scand.* 88: 551–562, 1973.
202. LYNCH, T. A., W. L. HIGHLY, AND A. G. WORTON. Gastric ulcers induced by phenylephrine in certain pharmaceutical compositions. *J. Pharm. Sci.* 53: 1077–1081, 1964.
203. MACKENZIE, G. J., S. H. TAYLOR, D. C. FLENLEY, A. H. MCDONALD, H. P. STAUNTON, AND K. W. DONALD. Circulatory and respiratory studies in myocardial infarction and cardiogenic shock. *Lancet* 2: 825–832, 1964.
204. MACLEAN, L. D., W. G. MULLIGAN, A. P. N. MACLEAN, AND J. N. DUFF. Patterns of septic shock in man—a detailed study of 56 patients. *Ann. Surg.* 166: 543–562, 1967.
205. MACPHERSON, B. R., AND C. J. PFEIFFER. Experimental colitis. *Digestion* 14: 425–452, 1976.
206. MADDEN, J. L., J. M. LORE, F. P. GEROLD, AND J. M. RAVID. Pathogenesis of ascites and the consideration of its treatment. *Surg. Gynecol. Obstet.* 99: 385–391, 1954.
206a. MALLIANI, A., P. J. SCHWARTZ, AND A. ZANCHETTI. A sympathetic reflex elicited by experimental coronary occlusion. *Am. J. Physiol.* 217: 703–709, 1969.
207. MANKU, M. S., D. F. HORROBIN, S. C. CUNNANE, A. I. ALLY, M. KARAMAZYN, R. A. KARAMALI, R. O. MORGAN, K. D. NOCHOLSON, AND W. E. BARNETTE. Prostaglandins $E_1$, $E_2$ and $I_2$: evidence for three distinct actions in vascular smooth muscle. *Biochem. Biophys. Res. Commun.* 83: 295–299, 1978.
208. MARCHESINI, G., G. BIANCHI, M. ZOLI, C. DONDI, G. FORLANI, A. MELLI, V. BUS, P. VANNINI, AND E. PISI. Plasma amino acid response to protein ingestion in patients with liver cirrhosis. *Gastroenterology* 85: 283–290, 1983.
209. MARCO, J., J. DIEGO, M. L. VILLANEUVA, J. DIAZ-FIERROS, I. VALVERDE, AND J. M. SEGOVIA. Elevated plasma glucagon levels in cirrhosis of the liver. *N. Engl. J. Med.* 289: 1107–1111, 1973.
210. MARKLUND, S. Distribution of CuZn superoxide dismutase and Mn superoxide dismutase in human tissue and extracellular fluids. *Acta Physiol. Scand.* 492: 19–24, 1980.
211. MARSTON, A., M. T. PHEILS, M. L. THOMAS, AND B. C. MOISON. Ischaemic colitis. *Gut* 7: 1–15, 1966.
212. MCCAY, P. B. Vitamin E: interactions with free radicals and ascorbate. *Annu. Rev. Nutr.* 5: 323–340, 1985.
213. MCCORD, J. M. Free radicals and inflammation: protection of synovial fluid by superoxide dismutase. *Science Wash. DC* 185: 529–531, 1974.
214. MCCORD, J. M., K. WONG, S. H. STOKES, W. F. PETRONE, AND D. ENGLISH. Superoxide and inflammation: a mechanism for the anti-inflammatory activity of superoxide dismutase. *Acta Physiol. Scand. Suppl.* 492: 25–30, 1980.
215. MCGREEVEY, J. M., AND F. G. MOODY. Protection of gastric mucosa against aspirin-induced erosions by enhanced blood flow. *Surg. Forum* 28: 357–360, 1977.
216. MCGREGOR, D. D., AND F. H. SMIRK. Vascular responses in mesenteric arteries from genetic and renal hypertensive rats. *Am. J. Physiol.* 214: 1429–1433, 1968.
217. MCINDOE, A. H. Vascular lesions of portal cirrhosis. *Arch. Pathol.* 5: 23–42, 1928.
218. MCNEILL, J. R., R. D. STARK, AND C. V. GREENWAY. Intestinal vasoconstriction after hemorrhage: roles of vasopressin and angiotensin. *Am. J. Physiol.* 219: 1342–1347, 1970.
219. MEAD, J. F. Free radical mechanisms of lipid damage and consequences for cellular membranes. In: *Free Radicals in Biology*, edited by W. A. Pryor. New York: Academic, 1976, vol. 1, p. 51–68.
220. MENGUY, R., AND Y. F. MASTERS. Gastric mucosal energy metabolism and "stress ulceration." *Ann. Surg.* 180: 538–548, 1974.
221. MERSEREAU, W. A., AND E. J. HINCHEY. Effect of gastric acidity on gastric ulceration induced by hemorrhage in the rat, utilizing a gastric chamber technique. *Gastroenterology* 64: 1130–1135, 1973.
222. MESSEILI, F. H., J. GENEST, W. NORVACZYNDKI, O. KIRCHEL, M. HONDA, Y. LATOUR, AND G. DUMONT. Splanchnic blood flow in essential hypertension and in hypertensive patients with renal artery stenosis. *Circulation* 51: 1114–1119, 1975.
223. MÓZSIK, G., T. JÁVOR, G. TÓTH, T. ZSOLDOS, AND A. TIGYI. Interrelationships between the gastric cytoprotective effects of vitamin A and B-carotene and the gastric mucosal superoxide dismutase activity in rats. *Acta Physiol. Hung.* 64: 315–318, 1984.
224. MÓZSIK, G., T. JÁVOR, T. ZSOLDOS, AND A. TIGYI. The interrelationships between the development of ethanol-, HCl-, NaOH- and NaCl-induced gastric mucosal damage and the gastric mucosal superoxide dismutase activity in the rats. *Acta Physiol. Hung.* 64: 309–314, 1984.
225. NEDZEL, A. J. Experimental production of gastric ulcers in dogs by inducing vascular spasm with pitressin. *Am. J. Dig. Dis.* 10: 283–291, 1943.
226. NG, K. K. F., S. DUFFEY, W. J. LOUIS, AND A. E. DOYLE. Interaction of angiotensin II with catecholamines in the circulation of the dog and cat. *Clin. Sci. Mol. Med.* 51: 4515–4545, 1976.
227. NISHIYAMA, K., A. NISHIYAMA, AND E. D. FROHLICH. Regional blood flow in normotensive and spontaneously hypertensive rats. *Am. J. Physiol.* 230: 691–698, 1976.
228. NORLÉN, K., L. RENTZHOG, AND S. WIKSTRÖM. Hemodynamic effects of phenoxybenzamine and volume replacement in segmental ischemia of the rat small intestine. *Acta Chir. Scand.* 144: 299–305, 1978.
229. NORLÉN, K., L. RENTZHOG, AND S. WIKSTRÖM. The effect of dopamine in segmental ischemia of the small intestine in the rat. *Acta Chir. Scand.* 144: 313–320, 1978.
230. NOVELLI, G. P., C. CORTESINE, AND E. PAGNI. The role of splanchnic adrenergic vasoconstriction in the development of irreversibility of hemorrhagic shock. *Adv. Exp. Biol. Med.* 9: 103–116, 1969.
230a. NYHOF, R. A., G. A. LAINE, G. A. MEININGER, AND H. J. GRANGER. Splanchnic circulation in hypertension. *Federation Proc.* 42: 1690–1693, 1983.
231. OBERG, B. Aspects on the reflex control of capillary filtration

transfer between blood and interstitial fluid. *Med. Exp.* 9: 49–61, 1963.
232. O'BRIEN, P., AND W. SILEN. Effects of bile salts and aspirin on the gastric mucosal blood flow. *Gastroenterology* 64: 246–251, 1973.
233. OHMAN, U. The effects of luminal distension and obstruction on the intestinal circulation. In: *Physiology of the Intestinal Circulation,* edited by A. P. Shepherd and D. N. Granger. New York: Raven, 1984, p. 321–334.
234. PAGE, D. L., J. B. CAUFIELD, J. A. KASTOR, R. W. DESANCTIS, AND C. A. SNODERS. Myocardial changes associated with cardiogenic shock. *N. Engl. J. Med.* 285: 133–137, 1971.
235. PAMNANI, M. B., G. SIMON, AND H. W. OVERBECK. Increased mesenteric blood flow and decreased mesenteric venous compliance in dogs with chronic perinephritic hypertension. *Proc. Soc. Exp. Biol. Med.* 161: 397–401, 1979.
236. PARKS, D. A., G. B. BULKLEY, D. N. GRANGER, B. R. HAMILTON, AND J. M. MCCORD. Ischemic injury in the cat small intestine: role of superoxide radicals. *Gastroenterology* 82: 9–14, 1982.
237. PARKS, D. A., AND D. N. GRANGER. Ischemia-induced vascular changes: role of xanthine oxidase and hydroxyl radicals. *Am. J. Physiol.* 245 (*Gastrointest. Liver Physiol.* 8): G285–G289, 1983.
238. PARKS, D. A., AND D. N. GRANGER. Effects of catalase on ischemia-induced vascular permeability changes in the small intestine. *Gastroenterology* 84: 1207–1212, 1984.
239. PARKS, D. A., AND D. N. GRANGER. Contributions of ischemia and reperfusion to mucosal lesion formation. *Am. J. Physiol.* 250 (*Gastrointest. Liver Physiol.* 13): G749–G753, 1986.
240. PARKS, D. A., AND E. D. JACOBSON. Intestinal ischemia. In: *Pathophysiology of the Splanchnic Circulation,* edited by D. N. Granger, P. R. Kvietys, and J. A. Barrowman. Boca Raton, FL: CRC, 1987, vol. 1, p. 125–140.
241. PARKS, D. A., A. K. SHAH, AND D. N. GRANGER. Oxygen radicals: effects on intestinal vascular permeability. *Am. J. Physiol.* 247 (*Gastrointest. Liver Physiol.* 10): G167–G172, 1984.
242. PARRATT, J. R. Neurohumoral agents and their release in shock. In: *Handbook of Shock and Trauma. Basic Science,* edited by B. M. Altura, A. M. Lefer, and W. Schumer. New York: Raven, 1983, vol. 1, p. 311–336.
243. PARVING, H. H., AND F. GYNTELBERG. Transcapillary escape rate of albumin and plasma volume in essential hypertension. *Circ. Res.* 32: 643–651, 1973.
244. PATART, O., M. DESNOS, G. LEROY, Y. LAURU, M. MOGENET, M. GARBAY, A. BARRILON, AND A. GERBAUX. Nécrose hémorragique du tube digestif au cours d'une intoxication digitaleque massive. *Nouv. Presse Med.* 10: 1489–1491, 1981.
245. PATTERSON, R. Laboratory models of reagenic allergy. *Prog. Allergy* 13: 332–407, 1969.
246. PAVEK, K. Anaphylactic shock in the monkey: its hemodynamics and mediators. *Acta Anaesthesiol. Scand.* 21: 293–307, 1977.
247. PAYNE, J. G., AND J. C. BOWEN. Hypoxia of canine gastric mucosa caused by *Escherichia coli* sepsis and prevented with methylprednisolone therapy. *Gastroenterology* 80: 84–93, 1981.
248. PEARCE, R. M., AND A. B. EISENBREY. The physiology of anaphylactic "shock" in the dog. *J. Infect. Dis.* 7: 565–576, 1910.
249. PICAZO, J. (editor). *Glucagon in Gastroenterology and Hepatology: Pharmacological, Clinical and Therapeutic Implications.* Lancaster, UK: MTP, 1982.
250. PRICE, A. B. Overlap in the spectrum of non-specific inflammatory bowel disease—colitis indeterminate. *J. Clin. Pathol.* 31: 567–577, 1978.
251. PRICE, W. E., G. V. ROHRER, AND E. D. JACOBSON. Mesenteric vascular diseases. *Gastroenterology* 57: 599–604, 1969.
252. PROCTOR, P. H. Free radicals and disease in man. *Physiol. Chem. Phys. Med. NMR* 16: 175–195, 1984.
253. RACHMILEWITZ, D., M. LIGUMSKY, A. HAIMOVITZ, AND A. J. TREVES. Prostanoid synthesis by cultured peripheral blood mononuclear cells in inflammatory disease of the bowel. *Gastroenterology* 82: 673–679, 1982.
254. RAVID, M., D. VAN-DYK, J. BERNHEIM, AND I. KEDAR. The protective effect of dimethyl sulfoxide in experimental ischemia of the intestine. *Ann. NY Acad. Sci.* 411: 100–104, 1983.
255. REES, M., J. G. PAYNE, AND J. C. BOWEN. Naloxone reverses tissue effects of live *Escherichia coli* sepsis. *Surgery* 91: 81–86, 1982.
256. REEVES, T. B. A study of the arteries supplying the stomach and duodenum and their relation to ulcers. *Surg. Gynecol. Obstet.* 30: 374–382, 1920.
257. RICCI, J. L., H. A. SLOVITER, AND M. M. ZIEGLER. Intestinal ischemia: reduction and mortality utilizing intraluminal perfluorochemical. *Am. J. Surg.* 149: 84–92, 1985.
258. RICHARDSON, J. D., M. H. MAX, L. M. FLINT, W. SCHWEISINGER, M. HOWARD, AND J. B. AUST. Bleeding vascular malformations of the intestine. *Surgery St. Louis* 3: 430–436, 1978.
259. RITCHIE, W. P., JR. Acute gastric mucosal damage induced by bile salts, acid and ischemia. *Gastroenterology* 68: 699–707, 1975.
260. RITCHIE, W. P., JR., AND K. J. CHERRY. Influence of hydrogen ion concentration on bile acid-induced acute gastric mucosal ulcerogenesis. *Ann. Surg.* 189: 637–645, 1979.
261. RITCHIE, W. P., JR., AND R. P. FISHER. Studies on the pathogenesis of "stress ulcers"; electrical potential differences and ionic fluxes across canine gastric mucosa during hemorrhagic shock. *J. Surg. Res.* 3: 173–176, 1972.
262. RITCHIE, W. P., JR., AND E. W. SHEARBURN III. Influence of isoproterenol and cholestyramine on acute gastric mucosal ulcerogenesis. *Gastroenterology* 73: 62–65, 1977.
263. ROBINSON, J. W. L., AND U. MIROVITCH. The roles of intraluminal oxygen and glucose in the protection of the rat intestinal mucosa from the effects of ischemia. *Biomedicine Paris* 27: 60–67, 1977.
264. ROKITANSKY, C. *Lehrbuch der pathologischen Anatomie.* Vienna: Braumüller, 1855, vol. I.
265. ROTHE, C. F., F. C. SCHWENDENMANN, AND E. E. SELKURT. Neurogenic control of skeletal muscular vascular resistance in hemorrhagic shock. *Am. J. Physiol.* 204: 925–932, 1963.
266. RUFFIN, J. M., AND I. W. BROWN, JR. The significance of hemorrhagic or pigment spots as observed by gastroscopy. *Am. J. Dig. Dis.* 10: 60–70, 1943.
267. RUTHERFORD, R. B., J. V. BALES, R. S. TROW, AND G. M. GRAVES. Comparison of hemodynamic and regional blood flow changes at equivalent states of endotoxin and hemorrhagic shock. *J. Trauma* 16: 886–897, 1976.
268. SAEGESSER, F., H. LOOSLI, J. W. L. ROBINSON, AND U. ROENSPIES. Ischemic diseases of the large intestine. *Int. Surg.* 66: 103–117, 1981.
269. SAID, S. I. Vasoactive peptides: state of the art review. *Hypertension* 5, Suppl. 1: 17–26, 1983.
270. SCHINDLER, R., AND R. I. BOXMEIER. Mucosal changes accompanying gastric ulcer: a gastroscopic study. *Ann. Int. Med.* 13: 693–699, 1939.
271. SCHOENBERG, M. H., E. MUHL, D. SELLIN, M. YOUNES, F. W. SCHILDBERG, AND U. HAGLUND. Postivopotensive generation of superoxide free radicals—possible role in the pathogenesis of the intestinal mucosal damage. *Acta Chir. Scand.* 150: 301–309, 1984.
272. SCHUTZ, C. B. The etiology of gastric and duodenal ulcers. *J. Am. Med. Assoc.* 96: 2182–2185, 1931.
273. SCHWAIGER, M., J. D. FONDACARO, AND E. D. JACOBSON. Effects of glucagon, histamine, and perhexiline on the ischemic canine mesenteric circulation. *Gastroenterology* 77: 730–735, 1979.
274. SEAMAN, K. L., AND C. V. GREENWAY. Loss of hepatic venous responsiveness after endotoxin in anesthetized cats. *Am. J. Physiol.* 246 (*Heart Circ. Physiol.* 15): H658–H663, 1984.
275. SEYDE, W. C., L. MCGOWAN, N. LUND, B. DULING, AND D. E. LONGNECKER. Effects of anesthetics on regional hemodynamics in normovolemic and hemorrhaged rats. *Am. J. Physiol.* 249 (*Heart Circ. Physiol.* 18): H164–H173, 1985.

276. SHANBOUR, L. L., AND E. D. JACOBSON. Digitalis and the mesenteric circulation. *Am. J. Dig. Dis.* 17: 826–828, 1972.
277. SHANBOUR, L. L., E. D. JACOBSON, G. F. BROBMANN, AND L. B. HINSHAW. Effects of ouabain on splanchnic hemodynamics in the rhesus monkey. *Am. Heart J.* 81: 511–515, 1971.
278. SHEPHERD, A. P., AND D. N. GRANGER. *Physiology of the Intestinal Circulation.* New York: Raven, 1984.
279. SHEPHERD, A. P., C. C. MAO, AND E. D. JACOBSON. The role of cyclic AMP in mesenteric vasodilation. *Microvasc. Res.* 6: 332–344, 1973.
280. SHERIVIN, R., P. JOSHI, R. HENDLER, P. FELIG, AND H. O. CONN. Hyperglucagonemia in Laennec's cirrhosis. The role of portal systemic shunting. *N. Engl. J. Med.* 290: 239–242, 1974.
281. SHORE, L. Interrelations between vasopressin and the renin-angiotensin system. *Federation Proc.* 38: 2267–2271, 1979.
282. SHUTE, K. Effect of intraluminal oxygen on experimental ischemia of the intestine. *Gut* 17: 100–107, 1976.
283. SIEGEL, J. H., F. B. CERRA, B. COLEMAN, I. GIOVANNINI, M. SHETYE, J. R. BORDER, AND R. H. MCMENAMY. Physiological and metabolic correlations in human sepsis. *Surgery St. Louis* 86: 163–193, 1979.
284. SIKULER, E., D. KRAVETZ, AND R. J. GROSZMANN. Evolution of portal hypertension and mechanisms involved in its maintenance in a rat model. *Am. J. Physiol.* 248 (*Gastrointest. Liver Physiol.* 11): G618–G625, 1985.
285. SIMON, G., M. B. PAMNANI, J. F. DUNKEL, AND H. W. OVERBECK. Mesenteric hemodynamics in early experimental renal hypertension in dogs. *Circ. Res.* 36: 791–798, 1975.
286. SIMONS, M. A., F. G. MOODY, AND M. G. TORMAS. Effects of carbenoxolone on gastric mucosal permeability and blood flows in the dog. *Gastroenterology* 71: 603–609, 1976.
287. SKILLMAN, J. J., S. A. GOULD, R. S. K. CHUNG, AND W. SILEN. The gastric mucosal barrier: clinical and experimental studies in critically ill and normal man and in the rabbit. *Ann. Surg.* 172: 564–574, 1930.
288. SMITH, P. R., D. J. DAWSON, AND C. H. J. SWAN. Prostaglandin synthetase activity in acute ulcerative colitis: effects of treatment with sulphasalazine, codeine phosphate and prednisalone. *Gut* 20: 802–805, 1979.
289. SNEDEGARD, G., R. BJORN, AND K. E. ARFORS. Anaphylaxis in the monkey: hemodynamics and blood flow distribution. *Acta Physiol. Scand.* 106: 191–198, 1979.
290. SNEDEGARD, G., B. REVENAS, AND T. SALDEEN. Anaphylaxis in the monkey: hematological and histological findings. *Int. Arch. Allergy Appl. Immunol.* 25: 11–18, 1979.
291. STARK, R. D., J. R. MCNEILL, AND C. V. GREENWAY. Sympathetic and hypophyseal roles in the splenic response to hemorrhage. *Am. J. Physiol.* 220: 837–840, 1971.
292. SVANES, K., K. A. LEIKNES, J. VARHAUG, AND O. SCREIDE. Aspirin damage to ischemic gastric mucosa in shocked cats. *Scand. J. Gastroenterol.* 14: 633–644, 1979.
293. SVANES, K., J. E. VARHANG, P. HOLM, A. BAKKE, AND I. ROMSLO. Effects of hemorrhagic shock in gastric blood flow and acid secretion in cats. *Acta Chir. Scand.* 147: 81–88 1981.
294. SWAN, K. G., R. W. BARTON, AND D. G. REYNOLDS. Mesenteric hemodynamics during endotoxemia in the baboon. *Gastroenterology* 61: 872–876, 1971.
295. SWAN, K. G., AND D. G. REYNOLDS. Splanchnic blood flow in experimental shock. In: *The Fundamental Mechanisms of Shock,* edited by L. B. Hinshaw and B. G. Cox. New York: Plenum, 1972, p. 87–103.
296. SWAN, K. G., H. H. TROUT III, AND D. G. REYNOLDS. Endotoxemia and large intestinal blood flow from subhuman primates. *Circ. Shock* 4: 369–377, 1979.
297. TEMMAR, M. M., M. E. SAFAR, J. A. LEVINSON, J. M. TOTOMOUKONO, AND A. C. SIMON. Regional blood flow in borderline and sustained essential hypertension. *Clin. Sci.* 60: 653–658, 1981.
298. TEPPERMAN, B. L., AND E. D. JACOBSON. Circulatory factor in gastric ulcers. In: *Peptic Ulcers,* edited by F. P. Brooks. New York: Churchill Livingstone, 1985, p. 261–278.
300. TOBIA, A. J., J. Y. LEE, AND G. M. WALSH. Regional blood flow and vascular resistance in the spontaneously hypertensive rat. *Cardiovasc. Res.* 8: 758–762, 1974.
301. TOBIA, A. J., G. M. WALSH, A. S. TADEPALLI, AND J. Y. LEE. Unaltered distribution of cardiac output in the conscious young spontaneously hypertensive rat: evidence for uniform elevation of regional vascular resistances. *Blood Vessels* 11: 287–294, 1974.
302. TREAT, E., H. B. ULANO, AND E. D. JACOBSON. Effects of intra-arterial ouabain on mesenteric and carotid hemodynamics. *J. Pharmacol. Exp. Ther.* 179: 144–148, 1971.
303. TYLER, G., R. A. CLARK, AND E. D. JACOBSON. Nonocclusive intestinal ischemia treated with intraarterial infusion of prostaglandin E1. *Cardiovasc. Interventional Radiol.* 5: 16–19, 1982.
304. ULANO, H. B., E. TREAT, L. L. SHANBOUR, AND E. D. JACOBSON. Selective dilation of the constricted superior mesenteric artery. *Gastroenterology* 62: 39–47, 1972.
305. ULRYCH, M. Plasma volume decrease and elevated Evans blue disappearance rate in essential hypertension. *Clin. Sci. Mol. Med.* 45: 173–181, 1973.
306. VIRCHOW, R. Historisches, Kritisches and Positives zue Lehre der Unterleibsaffektionen. *Virchows Arch. Pathol. Anat. Physiol. Klin. Med.* 5: 632–650, 1853.
307. VOROBIOFF, J., J. E. BREDFELDT, AND R. J. GROSZMANN. Hyperdynamic circulation in portal-hypertensive rat model: a primary factor for maintenance of chronic portal hypertension. *Am. J. Physiol.* 244 (*Gastrointest. Liver Physiol.* 7): G52–G57, 1983.
308. WALLENTIN, I. Studies on intestinal circulation. *Acta Physiol. Scand. Suppl.* 279: 1–38, 1966.
309. WANG, S. C., AND R. R. OVERMAN. A neurogenic factor in experimental traumatic shock. A summary of recent studies including observations on procainized and spinal dogs. *Ann. Surg.* 129: 207–222, 1949.
310. WATTS, D. T. Adrenergic mechanisms in hypovolemic shock. In: *Shock and Hypotension,* edited by L. C. Mills and J. H. Moyer. New York: Grune & Stratton, 1965, p. 385–391.
311. WEIDNER, M. G., M. ALBRECHT, AND G. H. A. CLOWES. Relationship of myocardial function to survival after oligemic hypotension. *Surgery St. Louis* 55: 73–84, 1964.
312. WEIL, M. H., L. D. MACLEAN, M. B. VISSCHER, AND W. W. SPINK. Studies on the circulatory changes in the dog produced by endotoxin from gram negative micro-organisms. *J. Clin. Invest.* 35: 1191–1198, 1956.
313. WEIL, M. H., AND H. N. NISHIJIMA. Cardiac output in bacterial shock. *Am. J. Med.* 64: 920–922, 1978.
314. WEIL, M. H., AND W. W. SPINK. A comparison of shock due to endotoxin with anaphylactic shock. *J. Lab. Clin. Med.* 50: 501–515, 1957.
314a. WHIPPLE, A. O. The problem of portal hypertension in relation to the hepatospleenopothies. *Ann. Surg.* 122: 449–475, 1945.
315. WHITE, F. N., G. ROSS, L. BARAJAS, AND E. D. JACOBSON. Hemodynamics of endotoxin shock in the rat and the effects of phenoxybenzamine. *Proc. Soc. Exp. Biol. Med.* 122: 1025–1029, 1966.
316. WHITTLE, B. J. R. Mechanisms underlying gastric mucosal damage induced by indomethacin and bile salts and the actions of prostaglandins. *Br. J. Pharmacol.* 60: 455–461, 1977.
317. WIGGERS, C. J. The functional consequences of coronary occlusion. *Ann. Int. Med.* 23: 158–169, 1945.
318. WILKINS, R. W., J. W. CULBERTSON, AND A. A. RYMUT. The hepatic blood flow in resting hypertensive patients before and after splanchnicectomy. *J. Clin. Invest.* 31: 529–531, 1952.
319. WINSLOW, E. J., H. S. LOEB, S. H. RAHIMTOOLA, S. KAMATH, AND R. M. GUNNAR. Hemodynamic studies and results of therapy in 50 patients with bacteremic shock. *Am. J. Med.* 54: 421–432, 1973.
320. WITTE, C. L., Y. C. CHUNG, M. N. WITTE, O. F. STERLE, AND W. R. COLE. Observations on the origin of ascites from experimental extrahepatic portal congestion. *Ann. Surg.* 170: 1002–1015, 1969.
321. WITTE, C. L., AND M. H. WITTE. Splanchnic circulatory and tissue fluid dynamics in portal hypertension. *Federation Proc.*

42: 1685–1689, 1983.
322. WITTE, C. L., M. H. WITTE, G. BAIN, W. P. MOBLEY, AND D. MORTON. Experimental study of hyperdynamic vs. stagnant mesenteric blood flow in portal hypertension. *Ann. Surg.* 179: 304–310, 1974.
323. WITTE, C. L., M. H. WITTE, AND A. E. DUMONT. The portal triad in hepatic cirrhosis. *Surg. Gynecol. Obstet.* 146: 965–974, 1978.
324. WITTE, C. L., M. H. WITTE, AND A. E. DUMONT. Lymph imbalance in the genesis and perpetuation of the ascites syndrome in hepatic cirrhosis. *Gastroenterology* 78: 1059–1068, 1980.
325. WITTE, M. H., C. L. WITTE, AND A. E. DUMONT. Physiologic factors involved in the causation of cirrhotic ascites. *Gastroenterology* 61: 742–750, 1971.
326. WOLF, E. A., AND D. S. SUMNER. Redistribution of intestinal blood flow during hypotension. *Surg. Forum* 24: 20–22, 1973.
327. WOOLF, A. C. Techniques of post mortem angiography of the stomach. *Br. J. Radiol.* 23: 8–12, 1950.
328. WYLER, F., R. F. FORSYTH, A. S. NIES, J. M. NEUTZE, AND K. L. MELMON. Endotoxin-induced regional circulatory changes in the unanesthetized monkey. *Circ. Res.* 24: 777–786, 1969.
329. YOUNES, M., M. H. SCHOENBERG, H. JUNG, B. B. FREDHOLM, U. HAGLUND, AND F. W. SCHILDBERG. Oxidative tissue damage following regional intestinal ischemia and reperfusion in the cat. *Res. Exp. Med.* 184: 259–264, 1984.
330. YU, Y. M., L. C. C. YU, AND C. C. CHOU. Distribution of blood flow in the intestine with hypertonic glucose in the lumen. *Surgery St. Louis* 78: 520–525, 1975.
331. ZETTERSTRÖM, B. E. M. Effect of denervation on blood flow in the dog spleen during haemorrhagic shock. *Acta Chir. Scand.* 139: 111–116, 1973.

# CHAPTER 48

# Gastrointestinal lymphatics

J. A. BARROWMAN — *Department of Medicine, Memorial University of Newfoundland, St. John's, Newfoundland, Canada*

P. TSO — *Departments of Physiology, Biophysics, and Medicine, University of Tennessee Center for the Health Sciences, Memphis, Tennessee*

## CHAPTER CONTENTS

Historical Aspects
Anatomical Considerations
  Interstitium
  Structure of lymphatics
    Initial lymphatics
    Collecting lymphatics
    Central lymphatic trunks
  Lymphaticovenous anastomoses
  Lymphatics of gastrointestinal organs
    Salivary glands
    Esophagus
    Stomach
    Small intestine
    Pancreas
    Colon
    Liver and gallbladder
General Physiological Considerations
  Formation of lymph
  Filling of initial lymphatics
  Role of lymph in tissue homeostasis
  Composition of lymph
  Modification of lymph by lymphatic vessels and nodes
  Propulsion of lymph in collecting vessels
Investigative Techniques
  Cannulation of lymph vessels
  Lymph fistula studies in the human
  In vitro studies of gastrointestinal lymphatics
  Micropuncture of intestinal mucosal lymphatics
Lymph from Gastrointestinal Organs
  Salivary glands
  Esophagus and stomach
  Small intestine
    Flow of small intestinal lymph
    Intestinal fluid absorption
    Intestinal secretion and lymph flow
    Transport of absorbed water-soluble substances by intestinal lymphatics
    Intestinal lipid absorption
    Gastrointestinal hormones in lymph
    Lymphatic transport of drugs and other xenobiotic substances
    Lymphatic transport of proteins of intestinal origin
  Colon
  Pancreas
  Liver
    Liver microcirculation
    Liver lymph flow
    Proteins of liver lymph
    Lipids of liver lymph
    Pathophysiology of liver lymph
      Hepatic congestion
      Cirrhosis
      Ascites in cirrhosis
      Cholestasis
  Pathophysiology of Gastrointestinal Lymphatics
    Primary intestinal lymphangiectasia
    Secondary intestinal lymphangiectasia
    Intestinal lymphangiectasia secondary to heart disease
    Experimental interruption of intestinal lymphatics
    Inflammatory bowel disease
    Acute pancreatitis
    Miscellaneous conditions involving gastrointestinal lymphatics

---

ALTHOUGH THE ALIMENTARY TRACT lymph vessels, specifically those of the small intestine, were those components of the lymphatic system first recognized by early investigators, the participation of the gastrointestinal lymphatic system as an integral part of the physiology of the digestive system has received relatively scant attention. Like lymphatics of other regions of the body, the gastrointestinal lymphatics contribute to the maintenance of homeostasis of the interstitial fluid composition and pressure and the return of extravasated plasma protein to the blood circulation. In addition, gastrointestinal lymphatics participate in a specific fashion in alimentary tract function. For example, in the process of lipid absorption, the essential role of lymphatics is illustrated by the impairment of lipid assimilation in intestinal lymphangiectasia. This chapter, which is concerned with lymph and lymphatics and not with the lymphoid tissues of the gut, describes the anatomical features of the lymphatics of the alimentary system and its general physiological functions together with the specific participation of the lymphatics in the function of the organs comprising the digestive tract. Finally, in a short pathophysiology section, the way in which deranged lymphatic function contributes to or results from various digestive diseases is discussed.

## HISTORICAL ASPECTS

Although credit is generally given to the great Renaissance schools of medicine in Italy for the discovery of lymphatic vessels, the writings of physicians in the fourth and third centuries B.C. suggest that these vessels had been identified and speculations made as to their function at that time. Both Aristotle and Hippocrates had described vessels in the mesentery that may well have been lymphatics, but the descriptions given by Erasistratus and Herophilus of the Alexandrian school of medicine leave little doubt that these scholars had identified these vessels. An example can be found in Galen's quotation from Erasistratus: "for on dividing the epigastrium and along with it the peritoneum, we may see arteries, on the mesentery of sucking kids full of milk." It has been alleged by Celsus that these observations were made in vivisection experiments that included human subjects. Herophilus, according to Galen, described mesenteric lymph nodes to which a proportion of the lymphatic vessels drained. It was generally believed that mesenteric lymphatic vessels ultimately drained to the liver. For nearly 2,000 years nothing further was added to the scientific knowledge of the lymphatic system. The Renaissance, which embraced both arts and sciences, saw a surge of activity in the field that established the basis for our modern concepts of the function of the lymphatic system.

The first significant event in the rediscovery of the lymphatic system was the description by Eustachio, anatomist in Rome during the mid-sixteenth century, of the thoracic duct of the horse. He recognized that this vessel drained into the left subclavian vein but was not clear as to its origin. In 1622 Gaspar Aselli of Pavia investigated the mesenteric lymphatic vessels of the dog. He was able to distinguish these vessels quite clearly from nerves in the mesentery, and he showed that they were more prominent in fed than in fasted animals, correctly inferring that intestinal lymphatics were concerned with the transport of absorbed nutrients. Aselli studied the same lymphatic vessels in a number of other species but not in the human. His thesis *De Lactibus sive lacteis venis* was published posthumously by two of his friends in 1627 and contains a number of beautiful colored woodcuts, among the earliest colored illustrations in medical literature. His figures show these lymphatic vessels draining to a large lymph node in the mesentery, and from there he believed that the absorbed nutrients were taken, in accordance with Galenic theory, to the liver for the concoction of blood. It appears that a year after publication of Asellius' thesis, Brechet in 1628 first saw mesenteric lymphatic vessels in the human. These vessels were described by Vesling of Padua in 1634, and his illustrations of human mesenteric lymphatics were the first of their kind.

Jean Pecquet of Dieppe in 1649 provided the link between Eustachio's thoracic duct and Asellius' mesenteric lymphatics by describing the receptaculum chyli or cisterna chyli. An appreciation of the lymphatic system as a functioning unit with flow from tissues to the main central lymph trunks, the cisterna chyli and thoracic duct, and thence to the bloodstream came from the prolific work of the Swede, Olaf Rudbeck of Uppsala, who did a series of ~400 experiments in several animals (cats, dogs, calves, sheep, goats, and wolves). He was able to describe lymphatic vessels arising from the large intestine and rectum that drained to the cisterna chyli. Rudbeck also discovered lymphatic vessels arising from the esophagus and in the limbs. Unlike the turbid lymph of small intestinal origin, lymph from other organs is clear and would be harder to recognize. Perhaps Rudbeck's most important contribution was the recognition that the lymphatic system functions as a unit, draining lymph from various tissues to the major trunks, and, importantly, he demonstrated that lymph does not flow toward the liver, a notion that had been an article of faith since the time of the Alexandrian school of medicine. A celebrated dispute arose between Rudbeck and the Dane, Thomas Bartholin, who, working independently, had come to conclusions similar to those of Rudbeck. There are some suggestions that George Joliffe, working in Cambridge between 1642 and 1658, may have made several of the discoveries attributed to Rudbeck and Bartholin before either of these workers. Unfortunately his publications have been lost and one has to rely on citations of his contemporaries. Some of his work was reported by the anatomist Glisson in 1654.

Frederick Ruysch published in 1665 his beautifully illustrated monograph *Dilucidatio vavularum in vasis lymphaticis et lacteis*, which contained the results of a detailed study of the valves of lymphatic vessels that had been examined mainly by dissection techniques but probably also by intravascular injections. Certainly he had been studying blood vessels by the injection of a solidifying wax and controlled his injections with the microscope.

By the end of the seventeenth century the anatomy of the lymphatic system was fairly clear, though studies in the eighteenth century by such distinguished investigators as Paolo Mascagni using injection techniques and detailed in his atlas of 1787, *Vasorum lymphaticorum corporis humani*, extended the understanding of the topography of the system. At the beginning of the eighteenth century, too, the notion of fluid flow from peripheral to central lymph vessels was established, and the stage was set for clarification of the physiological role of lymph formation and flow.

The achievements of the eighteenth century belong largely to the British schools of medicine, in particular the Hunterian schools of anatomy in London. It was William Hunter who proposed that the lymphatics form a common system concerned with absorption of fluid from various tissues. In one of his introductory anatomy lectures, Hunter wrote in 1774

> I think I have proved, that the lymphatic vessels are the absorbing vessels, all over the body; that they are the same as the lacteals; and that these altogether, with the thoracic duct constitute one great system, dispersed through the whole body for absorption; and this system only does absorb and not the veins; that it serves to take up, and convey, what there is to be made or mixed with the blood, from the skin, from the internal cavities or surfaces whatever.

William Hewson, a distinguished pupil of William Hunter, made a study of the comparative anatomy of lymphatics in birds, fish, and reptiles in addition to mammals and also gave an early description of lymphocytes in lymph. These observations, together with injection studies using colored materials, were reported in his *Experimental Inquiries* in 1774. Hewson's work was extended in the latter half of the eighteenth century by another pupil of William Hunter, William Cruickshank. Hunter and his pupils believed that the initial lymphatic capillary vessels were closed, and in this contention they differed from many of their contemporaries who believed that these vessels were in some way continuous with small blood vessels or that they formed open-ended tubes draining serous and other cavities. It was a century later that studies by such investigators as Ranvier in 1897, using injection techniques, confirmed the hypothesis that lymphatic vessels form a closed system.

The formulation of the principles governing transcapillary fluid movement and the formation of tissue fluid and lymph linked with the name of Ernest Starling is the culmination of early investigations of lymphatic physiology and is a suitable point to conclude this brief historical introduction. This proposal, advanced at the end of the nineteenth century, provides the functional link between the blood circulatory system and lymph. It incorporated some aspects of the "filtration theory" of Carl Ludwig (295), who regarded interstitial fluid and lymph as an ultrafiltrate of blood generated by the hydrostatic pressure in the microcirculation and reflecting regional blood flow. This theory was challenged by Heidenhain (204), who proposed as an alternative the notion that capillary endothelium actively secretes fluid under the influence of various lymphagogues. Starling's theory (420, 421) recognized the importance of the colloid osmotic pressure generated by intravascular plasma protein to which the capillary wall is relatively impermeable. This concept of a balance between hydrostatic and oncotic forces in determining transcapillary fluid transfer has been repeatedly validated by experiment. For a detailed account of the history of the discovery of the lymphatic system and recognition of its functions, see the reviews by Mayerson (308) and Lord (294).

## ANATOMICAL CONSIDERATIONS

### Interstitium

Lymph forms as interstitial or tissue fluid and its solutes enter initial lymph vessels. This interstitial fluid percolates through a complex noncellular domain composed of polymeric molecules that support the cells. Examination of the physical characteristics of this matrix shows that it is not simply a static supporting structure but has dynamic responses to physiological changes in the tissues. Histological and biochemical studies indicate that the composition of the interstitium differs substantially in different organs.

The main components of the interstitial structure are bundles of collagen fibers and glycosaminoglycan chains, mechanically entangled and cross-linked, producing a gellike structure (100, 184). Collagen fibers are rather stiff, having tensile strengths ~1/6 those of mild steel (92). In addition to glycosaminoglycans, some elastin fibers and single collagen fibers are found between the collagen bundles. Hyaluronic acid, the main interstitial glycosaminoglycan, is a polymer of $N$-acetylglucosamine and glucuronic acid; its molecular weight can range from a few thousand to several million. Some cross-linking occurs beween hyaluronic acid and collagen and other proteins in the interstitium, creating a complex interstitial mesh. An important property of this glycosaminoglycan gel is that, although it can resist compression, it tends to fall apart when stretched, the result of rupture of weak cross-linking forces and disentanglement of the chains. Because hyaluronic acid is anionic, areas of negative charge exist within the gel (184).

Glycosaminoglycans immobilize interstitial fluid, with the result that the hydraulic conductivity of the interstitium as a whole is normally very low. Dilution of the hyaluronic acid concentration of the interstitium by matrix hydration greatly increases the hydraulic conductivity. For example, doubling of the interstitial volume is estimated to increase the hydraulic conductance more than a thousandfold (100, 184).

A recent study with a sensitive radioassay for hyaluronate has shown that the concentration of hyaluronate in thoracic duct lymph of rats and fetal sheep and lumbar and popliteal lymph in adult sheep is ~10 times higher than that in plasma, suggesting that some hyaluronate may normally break loose from the interstitium and reach the circulation via lymph (264). It is probably removed from the blood by the liver. It has been calculated that as much as 5–10 mg of hyaluronate may pass through the human thoracic duct daily.

Within the normally hydrated gel, clusters of fluid vacuoles with diameters of 60–100 nm are recognized (151). These channels represent the free component of interstitial fluid, whereas the remainder is in the immobilized form. This arrangement of interstitial fluid (largely immobilized in a gel structure) can be viewed as advantageous to tissues in optimizing the diffusion of nutrients and waste to and from the cells. Compacted cells with no supporting matrix of this type would impede the access of nutrients to cells distant from the exchange blood vessels, whereas cells bathed in excessive amounts of free fluid would have their nutrient supply limited by the slow diffusion of these molecules through a bulky aqueous phase, as happens in edematous tissues (184).

The term *prelymphatics* has been coined to describe nonendothelialized fluid-filled channels seen in the interstitia of certain tissues. These channels are thought to end at interendothelial gaps of lymph vessels (84, 95). The nature and importance of these channels are presently unclear. Another important property of the matrix of the interstitium is its ability to exclude macromolecular solutes from a portion of the space available to water. Plasma proteins cannot fit into certain parts of the meshwork with high matrix density. For example, albumin is excluded from 35%–40% of the space available to water in the normally hydrated small intestinal interstitium (172). The degree of exclusion of albumin is consistent with a matrix perforated by pores of 20-nm radius and indicates that the rate of diffusion of albumin in the intestinal interstitium is reduced by more than one-third of its velocity in water because of the frictional interaction between the albumin molecule and the matrix. Stimulation of net transmucosal water absorption increases interstitial volume and reduces the degree of albumin exclusion by the intestinal interstitium—results consistent with the notion that the degree of exclusion of a molecule is inversely proportional to matrix hydration. This reduction in albumin exclusion during absorption is the result of an expanded matrix whose pores appear to exceed 100 nm in radius.

Although some measurements of physical parameters of the interstitium of gastrointestinal tissues have been made, little is known about the structure of individual interstitia. The histological appearance of the submucosa of the alimentary tract suggests a loose structure, and this compartment may have a relatively high compliance. One interstitial space that has received much attention is the perisinusoidal space of Disse in the liver. This space lies between the sinusoidal endothelium and the hepatocytes; it is ~500 nm deep. It has a loose appearance, containing a few collagen fibers and occasional lipoprotein particles. From the highly porous appearance of the discontinuous endothelium of the sinusoidal wall, it is inferred that the protein concentration of fluid in this space is comparable to that of plasma.

An assumption frequently made in studies of transcapillary fluid and solute exchange is that the composition of interstitial fluid and lymph is identical. As described above, there appear to be domains of restricted access to proteins and channels of free fluid. Moreover, evidence has recently been presented of yet another form of nonhomogeneity in interstitial fluid composition. With microspectrophotometry, Friedman and Witte (146) have found that the protein content of interstitial fluid in the perimicrovascular area in a rat ileal mesentery preparation is ~50% of plasma protein concentration in the regions of the arterioles and ~60% in the venular area. From the perimicrovascular sites the protein concentrations decline exponentially to a minimum of ~30% at average distances of 72 $\mu$m and 144 $\mu$m from the arteriolar and venular sites, respectively. These observations emphasize the importance of the dimensions and geometry of the interstitial space and the anatomical relationships between capillaries and lymphatics in determining lymph flow and composition.

## Structure of Lymphatics

INITIAL LYMPHATICS. Initial lymphatics are fine vessels ranging in length from 100 to 500 nm and have only a single endothelial cell layer. For reviews of their structure, see refs. 16, 17, 25, 79–87, 95, 241, 307, 354, 369. These vessels have an irregular shape; when fully distended their diameters range from 15 to 75 $\mu$m. The endothelium of initial lymph vessels is somewhat thicker than capillary endothelium and, unlike certain capillaries, lymphatics do not have fenestrated endothelium. In contrast to the complete basement membrane of blood capillary endothelium, the basement membrane of lymphatic endothelial walls is characteristically fragmented or incomplete. In some areas, no basement membrane is discernible. Anchoring filaments, bundles of connective tissue fibrils ~10 nm thick, are attached to the abluminal aspect of the endothelial cell membrane and pass into and around collagen bundles of the interstitium and possibly attach to other cells (269, 270). Their role has been the subject of much speculation: one likely possibility is that they serve to prevent collapse of the lymphatic vessel when excess tissue fluid accumulates and its hydrostatic pressure rises (95, 96, 241); they may also be involved in the opening of intercellular gaps facilitating the uptake of fluid, solutes, and particles into the vessel (95). In contrast with blood capillaries, initial lymphatics have no associated pericytes.

There has been recent interest in the distribution of charged sites on lymphatic endothelial membranes. A high density of anionic sites has been identified in relation to intercellular junctions in diaphragmatic lymphatics (268). In renal lymphatics, anionic sites predominate on the luminal aspect of the endothelium, with few charged sites present on the abluminal membrane (239).

Various types of junction between lymphatic endothelial cells are recognized (86). These include tight junctions, in which the outer laminae of the plasma membranes of two adjacent cells fuse over a short area, and close junctions, where the gap between the cells is ~6 nm. In other areas, the membranes of adjacent cells run closely parallel over a considerable distance separated by a gap of ~20 nm. Open junctions, usually with gaps of ~0.1 μm or occasionally greater, are also quite frequent. Many electron micrographs show initial lymphatics as collapsed vessels with convoluted, interdigitated intercellular regions, whereas in other areas the cells may simply seem to overlap over a short distance. It is these latter regions that can probably form open junctions. Open junctions are much less frequently observed in collecting lymph vessels. Three-dimensional reconstructions from electron micrographs show a special type of open junction formed by processes of lymphatic endothelium that enclose channels from the interstitium to the lymphatic lumen running along the long axis of the vessel. This type of junction has been observed in the submucosal lymphatics of the small intestine (16, 17). The importance of open junctions is dramatically demonstrated by the observation of particulate lipid passing through these channels in the initial lymphatic vessels of the small intestinal mucosa during fat absorption (Fig. 1).

An alternative route for transport of quanta of fluid and solutes from the interstitium to the lymphatic lumen is via transendothelial vesicular transport. Smooth vesicles ~70 nm in diameter are a feature of the endothelial cells and are estimated to account for ~35% of the nonnuclear cytoplasmic volume (80). Some are seen fusing with either the luminal or abluminal cell membrane. Calculations suggest that the

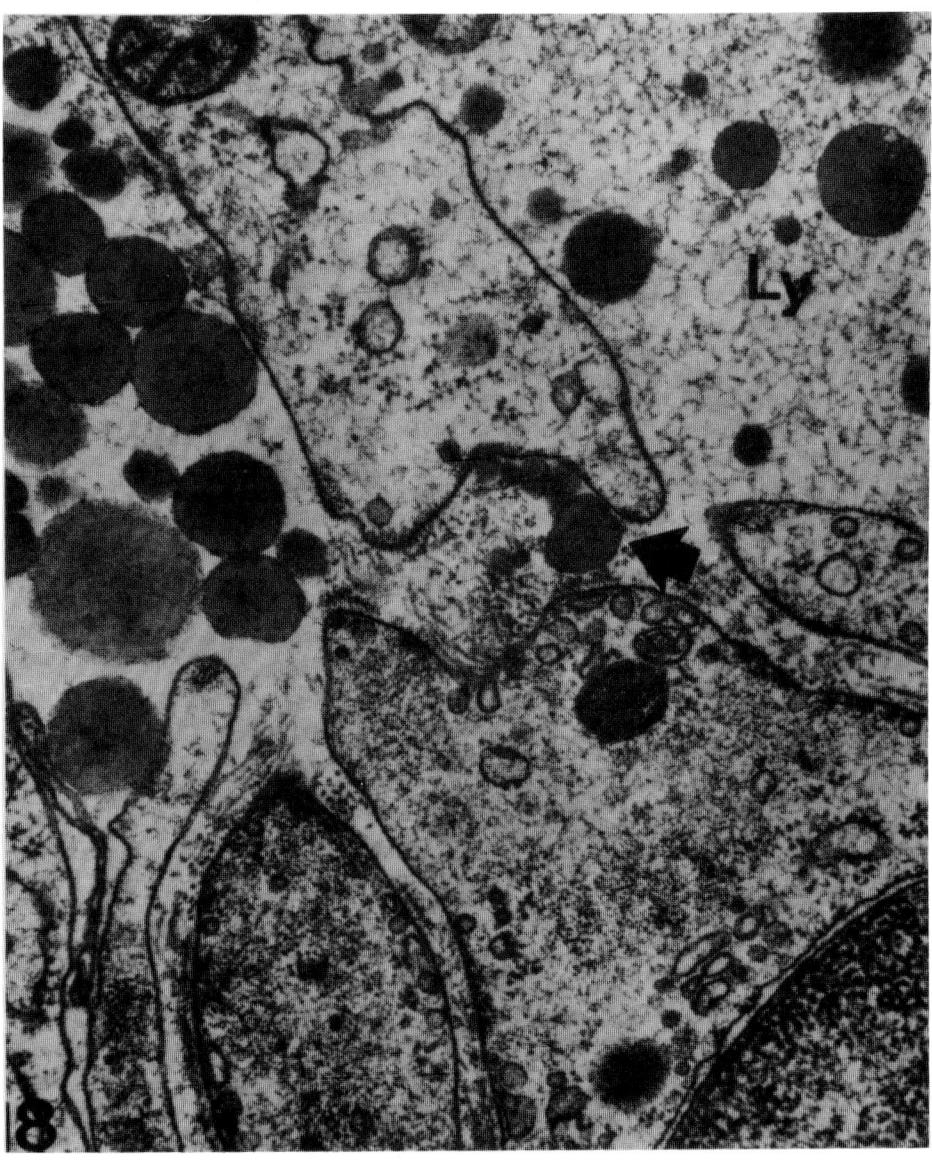

FIG. 1. Chylomicrons in rat small intestine entering lymphatic vessels (Ly) by moving between gaps (*arrow*) that develop between cytoplasmic extensions of endothelial lining of vessel. × 30,600. [From Sabesin and Frase (388).]

contribution of vesicular transport to total lymphatic uptake of fluid and solutes is rather small. Lymphatic endothelium also takes up foreign particles in larger phagocytic vesicles, and these are retained in the cell. During chylomicron uptake by lymphatics, endothelial vesicles account for a small proportion of the total transport. Chylomicrons are taken up by vesicles similar in size to phagocytic vesicles, but in this case the particles are transported across the cell (79, 113, 114, 347).

COLLECTING LYMPHATICS. Fine initial lymph vessels progressively merge as they pass centrally, forming collecting vessels whose function is the transport of lymph to the large central vessels, the cisterna chyli, and the thoracic duct. New elements appear in the vessel wall, including an internal elastic lamina, which is often incomplete (76). The endothelial basement membrane becomes more complete, and smooth muscle and connective tissue also appear. The amounts of smooth muscle in collecting lymphatic vessels vary among different species. In rats, mice, and guinea pigs, in which spontaneous contractility of these vessels is readily observed, there is abundant smooth muscle in the medium-sized (100- to 200-$\mu$m diam) and smaller (50-$\mu$m diam) vessels. In other species such as cats, the smooth muscle elements are less conspicuous (76). In bovine mesenteric lymphatics, the smooth muscle is arranged in three layers, an inner longitudinal, middle circumferential, and an external longitudinal layer (339).

Valves are a prominent feature of all but the finest of the mammalian lymphatic vessels, though they are not found in fish and amphibians. They are generally considered bicuspid [Fig. 2; (158, 241)] but have also been described as thin funnels or truncated cones (265, 499). These valves are anchored to the vessel wall with mesenteric-like folds or buttresses, and the smooth muscle elements of the vessel wall are characteristically thin at the site of the valve attachment (5). The valves divide lymphatic vessels into segments, and the term *lymphangion* has been applied to a segment bounded by two adjacent valves. These lymphangions have been regarded as individual pumping units (322, 323).

The innervation of lymphatic vessels has been described since the late eighteenth century. For example, Cruickshank in 1790 (103) showed that the thoracic duct receives branches from the vagus and intercostal nerves. In more modern times, Vajda (461) described an outer adventitial plexus of myelinated fibers that he proposed as having a sensory function and an inner plexus of smaller unmyelinated fibers concentrated near the origin of the valves. Good documentation of these structures, however, is lacking. Histochemical techniques have demonstrated cholinergic and adrenergic fibers in guinea pig mesenteric lymphatics (6). It has been proposed that there are sensory elements in lymphatic walls concerned with the reflex contract-

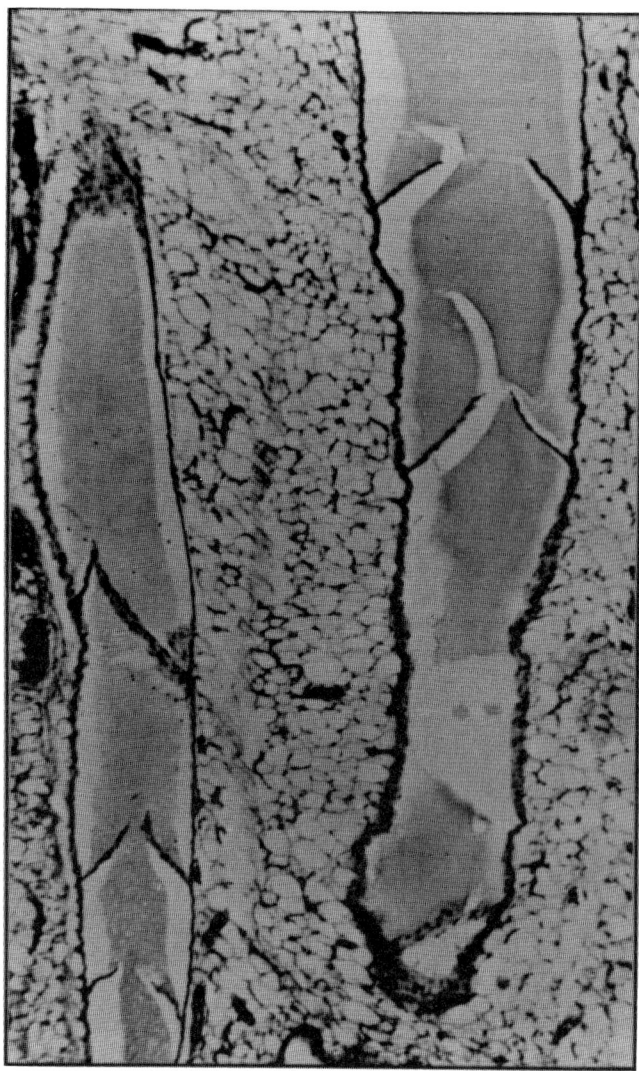

FIG. 2. Lymphatic valves in slightly dilated lymphatic vessels in rabbit mesentery. Low-power magnification. [From Kalima (241).]

ile response of the vessels to luminal distension (see ref. 461), though spontaneous contractility of lymphatics is not abolished by the nerve-blocking agent tetrodotoxin (316). Vasoactive intestinal peptide–immunoreactive nerves, which may have an inhibitory function with respect to contractility, have been demonstrated in bovine mesenteric lymphatics by histochemical techniques (343).

CENTRAL LYMPHATIC TRUNKS. In addition to smooth muscle, a connective tissue adventitial layer is found in these major vessels. The internal elastic lamina seen in collecting vessels disappears in the thoracic duct. Vasa vasorum are found in the adventitial layer of major lymphatics (340).

*Lymphaticovenous Anastomoses*

In addition to the jugulosubclavian tap, a number of lymphaticovenous anastomoses, mainly involving abdominal vessels, have been described in several species. Early studies demonstrated such communications in South American monkeys (407) and in wild rats (233). Gelatin injections in the monkeys showed lymphatic communications with the inferior vena cava and the renal vein. These monkeys, like the sloth, a species with extensive intra-abdominal lymphaticovenous communications, do not possess a cisterna chyli or thoracic duct (18). In rats, Job (233) demonstrated lymphaticovenous communications with the inferior vena cava at the level of the renal veins, most readily observed in pregnant animals, but in laboratory rats these channels are demonstrated only after ligation of the cisterna chyli. It has been postulated, however, that such communications could account for the observation that lymph flow in the main intestinal lymphatic vessel cannulated close to the cecum is almost as great as that in the thoracic duct, whereas occlusion of the ileocolic lymph trunk diminishes thoracic duct flow only slightly (348).

In sheep, lymphaticovenous anastomoses are nonexistent or uncommon, because $^{131}$I-labeled albumin is almost quantitatively recovered in the thoracic duct after infusion into a mesenteric vessel (203). If the thoracic duct is ligated, the appearance of radiolabeled albumin in the blood after intralymphatic infusion is very slow, but after 5 days, rapid transport of the label to blood indicates the development of lymphaticovenous communications. Similar observations have been made in cats and dogs (43, 78, 271). Lymphaticovenous communications in the abdomen have also been described in the human (442–444). The region of the renal veins is the most common site of abdominal lymphaticovenous communications in mammals. It is likely that potential anastomotic channels are normally present and that these open in response to increased intralymphatic pressure when major lymph trunks are obstructed. This should also be borne in mind in evaluating experimental evidence for lymphaticovenous anastomoses, because injection techniques are prone to create artifacts.

*Lymphatics of Gastrointestinal Organs*

SALIVARY GLANDS. A branching system of intraglandular lymphatics whose smallest branches begin at the level of the striated ducts was described by Klein (252). The vessels follow both the ducts and the blood vascular system within the gland. The initial lymph vessels seem to drain the interstitial spaces around the secretory end-pieces and intercalated ducts but do not penetrate between the secretory end-pieces. Other authors report similar findings (217, 430, 472). Papp and Fodor (350), using experimental lymphatic congestion, found initial lymph vessels in dog salivary glands lying very close to the smallest ducts and the secretory end-pieces.

A detailed study of the human parotid lymphatic system describes a branched system with initial lymphatics located in the connective tissue stroma surrounding a primary lobule, that is, a group of secretory end-pieces drained by a second-order striated duct (430). In the rabbit, Wenzel (472) has described networks of lymphatic vessels surrounding the salivary ducts and the blood vessels. Anastomotic vessels running laterally link these two systems. Like most other investigators, he found initial lymphatics in this species only at the level of the primary lobule and not in relation to the individual secretory end-pieces. Lymphatic vessels leave the salivary glands in relation to either the blood vessels or salivary duct. These vessels are commonly multiple (253).

ESOPHAGUS. Although lymphatics draining the esophagus were recognized in the mid-seventeenth century by Rudbeck, present-day literature on the subject is sparse. Most interest focuses on the lymph nodes involved in the dissemination of carcinoma of the esophagus. These include various mediastinal groups of nodes such as the chains of lymph glands related to the trachea. The thoracic duct serves as a major drainage route of esophageal lymph (435).

STOMACH. The anatomical arrangement of gastric lymphatic vessels within the stomach wall has been studied by various injection techniques (21, 22, 117, 379, 386). Technical difficulties in these methods have led to confusion in interpretation of the findings. In various species a rich network of lymphatic microvessels has been described in the interglandular space of the mucosa and in the muscularis externa by such methods, but some authors have failed to find these networks. For example, a study by Renyi-Vamos and Szinay (379), in which serial sections of resected human stomach were examined, failed to find a microlymphatic network in the muscularis externa. With in vivo microscopy after microinjection of a fluorescein-albumin conjugate, Nagata and Guth (331) recently demonstrated a lymphatic network at the base of the mucosa and superficial submucosa of the rat stomach. These networks were drained by larger lymph vessels running through the deep submucosa and muscularis externa to extragastric lymphatic vessels on the greater and lesser curvatures. These extragastric vessels with diameters of 50–340 $\mu$m contained valves and showed spontaneous contractility. As Renyi-Vamos and Szinay had found in the human stomach, no lymphatic network was discernible in the muscularis externa. In the human gastric mucosa, lymphatic vessels seem to be rather sparse and largely confined to the deeper parts of the mucosa (290). The arrangement of the lymphatic vessels draining the stomach and the associated lymph nodes has recently been described in detail in the human and other species (130).

SMALL INTESTINE. The best-characterized lymphatics of the gastrointestinal system are the vessels of the small intestinal mucosa. A central lacteal, the initial lymphatic of the mucosa runs axially along the intestinal villus to drain into a plexus of submucosal lymphatics of relatively large diameter. The lacteal, like other initial lymphatics, has only a single layer of endothelium, but associated smooth muscle cells that lie in the same axis confer contractile properties on the villus and the central lymph vessel, facilitating lymphatic filling and lymph propulsion (23, 113, 354). Anchoring filaments are reported to be relatively infrequent in the initial lymphatics of the intestinal villi (114), though they are found in submucosal lymphatics. There are conflicting reports on the frequency of open interendothelial junctions in the lymphatics of the intestinal villi. Generally in active tissues, where there is much motion or variation in tissue fluid pressure (e.g., in the intestine), interendothelial gaps in lymph vessels are common. However, Dobbins and Rollins (114) found that only 2% of the junctions they examined in intestinal villi were open. Others have described more frequent open junctions in this area (79, 95, 96, 347, 354). In a more recent study, the lymphatics of the submucosa and serosal-muscular layer of the small intestine have been examined. A complex extracellular route into the lymphatics, consisting of channels enclosed by processes of the lymphatic endothelium running in the long axis of the lymph vessel, has been described by Azzali (16, 17). A loose thick layer of connective tissue invests these lymph vessels.

PANCREAS. There is some uncertainty as to whether initial lymph vessels in this tissue arise in relation to individual acini, though Foldi et al. (140) have described such vessels lying close to the basement membrane of acinar cells. Injection studies, on the other hand, have failed to define these vessels and suggest that lymphatics reach only interlobular areas (159, 185). Lymphatic vessels do not penetrate the islets of Langerhans.

COLON. Colonic lymph vessels are generally rather inconspicuous (462). A network of horizontally arranged vessels located in the deeper one-third of the mucosa, draining to larger vessels that constitute a submucosal network of valved vessels, has been described (243, 258). This network links with vessels that traverse the muscle layer. A morphological study (212), including mucosal dye injections, intra-arterial infusion of silver nitrate–india ink mixtures, and electron microscopy, demonstrated a double layer of lymphatic channels in the colonic mucosa of dogs. The superficial layer lies just below the mucosal surface and the deeper layer just above the muscularis mucosae. The deeper layer corresponds to the network described by others. A few lymph vessels were also identified running parallel with the colonic glands. Electron-microscopic features of colonic lymph vessels (deficient basement membrane, marked overlapping of endothelial cells, and loose intercellular junctions) are similar to those of other initial lymph vessels. In a light- and electron-microscopic study of the human colon, on the other hand, a lymphatic network has been demonstrated just superficial to, within, and deep to the muscularis mucosae, but no lymphatics could be seen between the glands in the mucosa (135).

LIVER AND GALLBLADDER. There appear to be two major drainage routes for liver lymph. In dogs, vessels at the porta hepatis that drain to the cisterna chyli account for ~80% of hepatic lymph flow, whereas lymph vessels accompanying the hepatic veins collect the remaining 20% (383). A major set of portal vessels drains the right lobe in dogs, whereas a small accessory system drains the left lobe. In rats, it has been noted in some animals that anastomotic connections exist between the major hilar hepatic lymph trunk and the main intestinal lymph trunk (280). This poses a problem for investigators attempting to obtain pure lymph samples from either organ.

Within the liver, no initial lymph vessels can be found within the lobule. Initial vessels appear to arise in the portal tracts and, less conspicuously, in the region of the hepatic venules (99). These lymph vessels are thought to drain the space of Disse, a major interstitial space of the liver, as well as the interstitial spaces immediately surrounding these lymph vessels. A lymphatic network is also found close to the liver capsule. It consists of a complex three-layer arrangement. In dogs, this system does not appear to communicate with the deeper vessels that drain the hepatic parenchyma (432).

In the gallbladder, three interconnected lymphatic plexuses are described (97, 115, 478): a mucosal or subepithelial plexus lying rather deep in the mucosa, a perimuscular plexus, and a subserosal plexus. The distribution of lymphatics in the mucosa suggests that they may not play an important role in the transport of fluid absorbed by the gallbladder (compare colonic mucosa). The vessels of the subserosa drain into vessels running close to the cystic duct. In cats, the high flow and high-protein concentration of gallbladder lymph suggest the possibility of anastomotic connections between liver and gallbladder lymphatic vessels (311, 428, 478), and this has been confirmed with india ink injection studies (311). There is also evidence, from india ink injection studies, for communications between pancreatic and biliary tract lymphatics in dogs (470).

GENERAL PHYSIOLOGICAL CONSIDERATIONS

Although Starling had acknowledged that capillaries are not impermeable to proteins, it was Cecil Drinker in the 1930s who emphasized the magnitude of the transcapillary movement of protein. The principal function of the lymphatic system is to return to the blood vascular compartment the protein and fluid that have leaked from the circulation (119, 121). The return of protein is more important; if protein from interstitial fluid were selectively returned by the lymphatic vessels, the fluid remaining in the interstitium would readily be reabsorbed into the capillaries as a result of the transcapillary oncotic pressure gradient. It has been estimated that in 24 h, 50% or more of the total circulating plasma protein escapes from the blood vascular compartment and is returned by the lymphatics (see reviews by Mayerson, refs. 306, 307). At any time there is a greater quantity of albumin in the interstitial fluid than in the intravascular compartment.

*Formation of Lymph*

In organs that are not concerned with transepithelial movement of fluid, the flow of lymph is dependent on the rate of formation of interstitial fluid from the blood vessels of the microcirculation. This applies to tissues such as skeletal muscle and in the gastrointestinal tract to the submucosa and muscularis of the gut. On the other hand, where there is transepithelial movement of fluid, either as absorption or secretion or both, another factor comes into play in the generation of the interstitial fluid. Thus in the mucosa of the gastrointestinal tract the interstitium serves as a mixing pool for capillary filtrate together with fluid absorbed from the gut lumen, whereas in secretory states fluid is drawn from the interstitial compartment to provide for secretion. The latter consideration also applies to digestive glands such as the salivary glands and pancreas that are engaged in the transepithelial movement of large volumes of secretion.

Net fluid filtration or absorption across the exchange vessels of the microcirculation is determined by the physical forces operating across the capillary wall (355) and expressed in the Starling force balance (421)

$$J_{v,c} = K_{f,c} [(P_c - P_t) - \sigma_d (\pi_p - \pi_t)] \quad (1)$$

where $J_{v,c}$ is the net rate of capillary filtration (positive value) or absorption (negative value), $K_{f,c}$ is the capillary filtration coefficient, $P_c$ is the capillary hydrostatic pressure, $P_t$ is the interstitial fluid pressure, $\sigma_d$ is the osmotic reflection coefficient, $\pi_p$ is the plasma oncotic pressure, and $\pi_t$ is the interstitial oncotic pressure. In most tissues at rest, $(P_c - P_t)$ exceeds $(\pi_p - \pi_t)$, thus $J_{v,c}$ is a positive value, that is, the capillaries are in a filtering state and this is reflected as the resting lymph flow ($J_L$) that is equal to $J_{v,c}$ and that maintains a constant degree of hydration of the tissue. Table 1 gives estimates for the resting lymph flow, that is, the net transcapillary fluid filtration rate in various gastrointestinal tissues and in skeletal muscle. It can be seen that alimentary tract organs, and particularly the salivary glands, have very high resting lymph flows compared with skeletal muscle, and this presumably reflects the high density of the gastrointestinal capillaries, which are of the fenestrated type.

TABLE 1. *Resting Lymph Flows in Organs of the Alimentary Tract and Skeletal Muscle*

| Organ | Lymph Flow, ml/min·100 g |
|---|---|
| Stomach | 0.06 |
| Small intestine | 0.045 |
| Colon | 0.015 |
| Pancreas | 0.009 |
| Liver | 0.05 |
| Salivary glands | 0.42 |
| Skeletal muscle | 0.005 |

[Data from Granger and Barrowman (165).]

The Starling force equation allows prediction of changes in the transcapillary fluid filtration and lymph flow in response to disturbances of these physical parameters. For example, with an acute elevation of venous pressure (e.g., acute portal hypertension), enhanced intestinal lymph flow occurs as a result of a net increase in the transcapillary hydrostatic pressure gradient (330, 491). Increases of as much as 30-fold over basal lymph flow have been observed with acute elevations of venous pressure of 30 mmHg in the small intestine (174). A similar event occurs in the colon (381). Reduction of the hydrostatic pressure that would occur in arterial hypotension from hemorrhage leads to a reduction in lymph flow (173). Plasma dilution (hypoproteinemia) enhances lymph flow by reduction of transcapillary oncotic pressure gradient (174, 175).

*Filling of Initial Lymphatics*

Lymph forms as interstitial fluid enters the initial lymphatics. Its composition at this point may not correspond to that of lymph in central channels, because modification of its composition may occur en route in lymph nodes. Ultrastructural studies suggest that most fluid, solutes, and particles enter the lymphatics through open interendothelial cell junctions, though a minor amount passes by vesicular transport through endothelial cells.

What forces determine the uptake of fluid from the interstitium to the initial lymph vessels? This is an area of contention: three mechanisms have been proposed—*1*) a hydrostatic pressure gradient, *2*) an oncotic pressure mechanism, and *3*) vesicular transport through the endothelium. The latter is unlikely to be of great quantitative importance. Accurate measurements of the hydrostatic and oncotic pressures in the interstitium and initial lymph vessels are needed to establish the relative importance of each of these mechanisms. The hydrostatic pressure theory is the most generally accepted (for reviews see refs. 2, 196). However, a problem is posed by the observation that in most tissues the hydrostatic pressure of tissue fluid is a negative value or close to zero (2), whereas direct micropuncture of initial lymphatic vessels usually yields slightly positive values (499).

A modification of the hydrostatic pressure theory suggests that filling is achieved by intermittent increases in tissue fluid pressure due to contraction of local smooth or skeletal muscle (e.g., villus contraction in small intestinal mucosa) or local vasomotion (226, 500). This, together with an intermittent suction effect from the lymphatic side as a result of contractile activity of the collecting lymphatics coupled with a flap-valve effect at the interendothelial cell gaps, could create transient gradients of pressure favoring the filling of initial vessels. For such a suction effect, competence of lymphatic valves is required, and studies suggest that these valves can withstand pressures in excess of 50 mmHg (339). In support of the hydrostatic pressure theory is the observation that small intestinal lymph flow is related to steady-state interstitial fluid pressure (Fig. 3). It can be seen that there is an abrupt change in the relationship between interstitial volume and interstitial fluid pressure at about +3 mmHg, which presumably reflects a sudden change in the compliance of the interstitial matrix. These data suggest that as tissue fluid accumulates and its hydrostatic pressure increases, lymph flow is enhanced, driven by the increment in pressure. However, this theory leaves the low resting lymph flow unexplained, and perhaps under these circumstances the suction mechanism is more important. A degree of continuous motility in the resting intestine may also play a part. For further review of the hydrostatic pressure theory, see the publication by Adair and Guyton (2).

The oncotic pressure theory (82) is based on the notion that the protein concentration in initial lymphatics is substantially greater than that of interstitial fluid, creating an osmotic pull that exceeds the observed contrary hydrostatic pressure gradient. During tissue compression, total tissue pressure rises and is transmitted to the lymph vessel. Ultrafiltration of fluid to the tissues across closed interendothelial junctions concentrates macromolecules in the lymph. At the same time some lymph is driven centrally. During a relaxation phase the concentrated protein in the lymphatics exerts an osmotic pull, despite the fact that intercellular junctions have opened. There is little evidence to support this oncotic pressure hypothesis. The demonstration that samples of lymph and interstitial fluid obtained by micropuncture have similar protein concentrations argues against this mechanism of lymphatic filling (387).

*Role of Lymph in Tissue Homeostasis*

The highly permeable nature of the capillary wall with respect to fluid and crystalloids exposes the tissues to the possibility of excessive fluid accumulation. Thus a transient increase in capillary pressure or a fall in plasma oncotic pressure predisposes to an increase in capillary filtration. These disturbances are offset by alterations in Starling forces acting across the capillary wall and by an increase in lymph flow, the result of which is the establishment of a new steady state in terms of interstitial fluid formation and dispersal with a slightly more hydrated interstitium. When a rise in capillary pressure occurs as a result of a rise in venous pressure or there is a fall of the intravascular oncotic pressure (plasma dilution), increased capillary filtration results. Fluid accumulates in the interstitium and raises interstitial fluid pressure. This enhances lymphatic filling and lymph flow and, by opposing capillary hydrostatic pressure, resists further filtration. At the same time the excess tissue fluid dilutes interstitial fluid protein, provided the osmotic reflection coefficient of the microcirculation is greater than zero; this increases the transcapillary oncotic pressure gradient. Enhanced lymph flow and these alterations in Starling forces all oppose further capillary filtration and are collectively termed the *edema safety factor* (439).

The contribution of each of these factors in opposing further edema of the tissues can be estimated in a given organ. Table 2 presents data showing that the relative contribution of each factor varies in different tissues. In the three tissues compared in this table, it can be seen that no contribution is made by a change

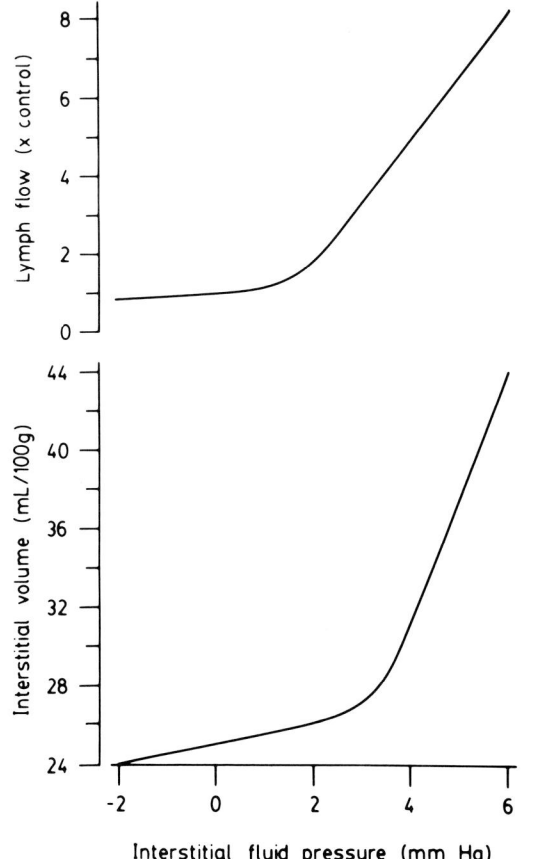

FIG. 3. Relations between lymph flow, interstitial fluid volume, and interstitial fluid pressure in small intestine of cat. [From Granger and Barrowman (165).]

TABLE 2. *Estimated Contributions of Extravascular Factors in Opposing Increased Microvascular Hydrostatic Pressure*

|  | Liver | Small Intestine | Colon |
|---|---|---|---|
| Increment in microvascular hydrostatic pressure, mmHg | 15.0 | 13.2 | 12.0 |
| Increased protein osmotic pressure differences, mmHg | 0 | 4.9 | 6.2 |
| Increased perimicrovascular fluid pressure, mmHg | 9.6 | 6.3 | 5.3 |
| Increased lymph flow, mmHg | 5.4 | 2.0 | 0.5 |

[Data from Laine et al. (261), Mortillaro and Taylor (330), and Richardson et al. (381).]

in transmicrovascular oncotic pressure in the liver, because the sinusoidal membrane is essentially freely permeable to all species of plasma protein. In the liver, the apparently low compliance of the tissue causes a marked increase in interstitial fluid pressure in response to venous pressure elevation and sinusoidal filtration (261). This serves to oppose further filtration and increases the rate of lymph flow. In the small intestine and colon, lymph flows play more minor roles; in particular, colonic lymph flow contributes little to the edema safety factor. When the disturbing force is very great the opposition to the edema safety factor is ultimately overwhelmed at a net change in transcapillary forces termed the *total safety factor*; in the small intestine this value is between 12 and 15 mmHg (123, 330). In the liver the total safety factor is much lower (~1–2 mmHg) (261). At this value gross liver edema leads to transcapsular fluid filtration and ascites. The corresponding effect that occurs at ~12 mmHg in the small intestinal mucosa is filtration secretion, where interstitial fluid escapes into the lumen of the intestine. When interstitial fluid pressure of the small intestinal mucosa rises 4–5 mmHg, large channels open at the villus tips, allowing free passage of fluid and macromolecules into the intestinal lumen (109, 167, 197). These effects in the intestine and liver can either be regarded as additional edema safety factors or the result of failure of the more conventional safety factors.

## Composition of Lymph

Plasma proteins cross the capillary walls to diffuse through the interstitium and return to the circulation via the lymph. The studies of Grotte et al. (193, 194) and Mayerson et al. (309) provide evidence that the lymph-to-plasma protein concentration ratio ($C_L/C_P$) for macromolecules is inversely proportional to the size of the individual molecule. This has allowed analysis of the permeability characteristics of the capillary wall to macromolecules with the assumption that there is no filtration of these macromolecules at the lymphatic endothelial wall. More recently, however, it has been demonstrated that the shape and electrical charge of the molecule also influence the transcapillary passage of macromolecules. A full account of this is discussed in the chapter by Taylor and Granger (440) in the 1984 edition of the *Handbook* section on the cardiovascular system.

In terms of lymph composition, the $C_L/C_P$ of proteins correlates fairly closely with the molecular size of each protein species. This is illustrated in Table 3, which presents data showing the molecular size and $C_L/C_P$ for a series of plasma protein fractions in cat intestinal lymph. For total protein, $C_L/C_P$ in gastrointestinal lymph in most species is between 0.50 and 0.65, though estimates in the rat are lower, 0.36–0.44 (440). The $C_L/C_P$ of protein-bound substances also depends on the lymph-to-plasma (L/P) ratio of the binding protein. For substances of <10,000 mol wt that are not bound to protein, the concentrations in lymph and plasma are similar (474).

### Modification of Lymph by Lymphatic Vessels and Nodes

Discrepancies between lymph flows in peripheral and central lymph trunks suggest the possibility of fluid transfer from lymph during its passage centrally (348). Lymph vessels are relatively impermeable to plasma proteins, as judged by high recovery of radio-labeled albumin in the thoracic duct after infusion into a peripheral lymph vessel (357). This argues against a significant loss of lymph volume by bulk transfer through lymphaticovenous anastomoses. Attempts to define the permeability of lymphatics to macromolecules suggest that molecules >20,000 mol wt are completely retained within the lymphatics (74).

However, there is a considerable amount of evidence that the lymph nodes act as fluid exchangers, and it is possible that a similar exchange goes on with blood in the vasa vasorum of the larger lymph vessels. The extent of exchange may be a function of the rate of flow of lymph and the anatomical nature of the lymph:blood barrier in nodes and vessels.

As long ago as 1934, Drinker et al. (120), using a popliteal node preparation, demonstrated the loss of small solutes from lymph during passage across the

TABLE 3. *Molecular Size and $C_L/C_P$ of Nine Plasma Protein Fractions in Cat Intestinal Lymph and Plasma*

| Fractions | Stokes-Einstein Radius, Å | $C_L/C_P$* |
|---|---|---|
| I | 37.5 | 0.50 |
| II | 38 | 0.45 |
| III | 39 | 0.43 |
| IV | 42 | 0.35 |
| V | 45 | 0.26 |
| VI | 76 | 0.24 |
| VII | 96 | 0.25 |
| VIII | 107 | 0.23 |
| IX | 120 | 0.21 |

* Lymph-to-plasma protein concentration ratio. [Data from Granger and Taylor (181a).]

node. Many investigators have shown a rise in lymph protein concentration in postnodal versus prenodal lymph. More recently Adair et al. (3) and Adair and Guyton (1) have obtained evidence supporting the notion that Starling forces operate to balance hydrostatic and oncotic pressures across the lymph:blood barrier in nodes. When artificial lymph of high protein concentration is infused into a prenodal lymphatic, the protein concentration of the postnodal lymph is found to be lower, whereas a dilute prenodal lymph is concentrated with respect to protein by the node. The equilibrium protein concentration is thought to represent the concentration that generates an oncotic pressure sufficient to balance the hydrostatic pressure in the fluid exchanger, that is, the lymph node. In addition to these alterations, immunoglobulins and lymphocytes enter the lymph in the nodes.

*Propulsion of Lymph in Collecting Vessels*

Although the forces responsible for uptake of fluid into initial lymphatic vessels are not clearly understood, various mechanisms are recognized that drive lymph centrally along the collecting vessels. Extrinsic factors include external compression as a result of mechanical activity of smooth and skeletal muscle. Mechanical forces are also set up by vasomotor activity in tissues, creating alterations in pressure in these tissues. This activity, vasomotion, causes substantial periodic volume displacements in the tissues. Studies of a skin preparation in rats show that the average period of arteriolar vasomotor cycles is ~20 s (226). As mentioned, this phenomenon may have a major role in filling the initial lymphatics but may also, by compression of small lymph vessels, force lymph along these channels. With all forms of external compression, the central propulsion of lymph is strongly dependent on the competence of the valves.

Contractile activity of lymphatic vessels has been recognized since the late eighteenth century (103). Lymph *hearts* are found in lower orders such as reptiles and amphibians. Observations in vivo and in vitro have documented a rhythmic contractility of lymphatic vessels in many mammalian species, including the human (250, 285, 339). The contractions observed in vivo have a peristaltic appearance. The extent of lymphatic contraction is considerable, because the lumen of the vessel can be almost completely obliterated during a contraction.

From in vitro observations such as those of McHale and Roddie (316) in isolated bovine lymphatics, an intrinsic mechanism is responsible, at least in part, for lymphatic contractility. The contractile activity of a segment of a lymph vessel has many of the features of the cardiac cycle. That is, a systole, consisting of an isometric contraction, is followed by an ejection phase that is succeeded by a diastole, consisting of isometric relaxation and filling. Because tetrodotoxin does not interfere with the contractile activity of the vessel, the mechanism of cell contraction probably does not depend on nervous activity (316). However, external controls also operate because spontaneous lymphatic vasomotion in the rat mesentery is abolished by spinal anesthesia (20, 318). In studies with sheep there have been regular rhythmic contractions of various unobstructed lymph vessels, with frequencies of $\leq 30$/min, creating pressures as high as 25 mmHg (198). Obstructed lymph vessels can generate pressures as great as 60 mmHg. A strong correlation between lymph flow and contractility has suggested a myogenic response to lymphatic distension. Good evidence for a myogenic pump mechanism in mesenteric lymphatics has been obtained with micro-occlusion techniques [Table 4; (201)]. In the bat's wing preparation, a correlation between interstitial fluid volume and lymphatic pumping has been demonstrated; it has been proposed that pumping by initial lymphatic vessels is sensitive to this parameter rather than interstitial fluid pressure (213).

Values for the resting membrane potential of the smooth muscle of bovine mesenteric lymphatics range between $-33$ and $-57$ mV (15, 338). A single action potential lasting ~3 s appears to precede a contraction of ~750 ms (15).

Lymphatic smooth muscle is responsive to a number of pharmacological agents (341). Adrenergic and cholinergic nerve fibers are found in the walls of lymphatic vessels (6, 315). There is very little evidence, however, that cholinergic activity plays any role in the regulation of lymphatic contractility. On the other hand, $\alpha$-adrenergic receptor activity seems to be important (15, 317, 318). Norepinephrine increases the frequency of lymphatic contractions in isolated bovine lymphatic vessels (8, 303). The stimulatory effects of norepinephrine are suppressed by $\alpha$-receptor blockade (303, 342). Isoprenaline, a $\beta$-agonist, has a relaxant effect, reducing the frequency of spontaneous contractions (303, 342). Isoprenaline causes hyperpolarization of lymphatic smooth muscle membranes that, in part at least, involves an increase in outward $K^+$ current (9). Electrical field stimulation studies, together with selective blocking agents, suggest that norepinephrine is probably a physiological regulator of lymphatic contractile function (342). Vasoactive intestinal polypeptide has been proposed as an inhibitory neurotransmitter to lymphatic smooth muscle, because it abol-

TABLE 4. *Downstream Micro-Occlusion in Collecting Lymphatics*

|  | Before Occlusion | During Total Occlusion |
|---|---|---|
| Contraction frequency, min$^{-1}$ | 7 ± 2 | 12 ± 2 |
| Maximum lymph pressure, cmH$_2$O | 16 ± 4.7 | 35 ± 5 |
| Minimum lymph pressure, cmH$_2$O | 4.1 ± 1.1 | 15 ± 6.4 |
| Maximum vessel diameter, μm | 89 ± 42 | 146 ± 83 |
| Minimum vessel diameter, μm | 53 ± 24 | 110 ± 28 |

Values represent mean ± S.D. in mesentery of rat and guinea pig. [Data from Zweifach and Schmid-Schonbein (500).]

ishes contractions induced by bradykinin in isolated lymphatic smooth muscle preparations (343). Of the autacoids, bradykinin is a very powerful tonic vasoconstrictor, whereas histamine can enhance contractility, but at nonphysiological concentrations (236).

There is evidence that lymphatic vessels can synthesize certain prostaglandins that have vasomotor effects on lymphatic vessels at very low concentrations. Some [e.g., prostaglandin $F_{2\alpha}$ ($PGF_{2\alpha}$)] are powerful stimulants of contractility, whereas others (prostaglandin E) are strong inhibitors. The overall effects of these chemical mediators of inflammatory processes on lymphatic vascular activity and lymph flow is presently unclear (237).

## INVESTIGATIVE TECHNIQUES

Morphological studies have employed light and electron microscopy. In conjunction with physiological investigations, these techniques have afforded information on the function of initial lymphatics. A good example of this is the uptake of particulate material (e.g., chylomicrons) by these vessels (79, 388). Radiological visualization of the lymphatic system involves subcutaneous injection of dyes followed by cannulation of the colored lymphatic vessels and infusion of contrast medium. Satisfactory methods for lymphangiography of gastrointestinal lymphatics, however, are not presently available.

### Cannulation of Lymph Vessels

Much of our knowledge of lymphatic physiology is derived from studies where major lymph trunks have been cannulated in various species. Most laboratory animals have been studied; in Australia the sheep has been extensively used. Both acute and chronic lymphatic fistulas can be created. In addition to measurement of flows and composition of lymph, cannulation allows pressure and contractility studies. In studies of the permeability of blood capillaries, lymph has been widely used as a reflection of interstitial fluid composition.

In early investigations glass cannulas were used in anesthetised animals, but the development of soft polyethylene and polyvinyl chloride tubing has greatly facilitated these investigations and allowed studies on conscious animals. The lymphatics of the rat have been used more than any other species since Bollman and colleagues (57) described the creation of chronic cisterna chyli, intestinal lymph trunk, and hepatic lymphatic fistulas. The use of restraining cages for the animals has been necessary (56), though some investigators have used harnesses and other devices, obviating the need for restraint (438). The majority of investigations of gastrointestinal lymphatic function have focused on the transport of absorbed lipids by intestinal vessels.

The techniques for the intestinal lymph vessels and cisterna chyli in the rat are relatively easy, but hepatic lymphatic fistulas are difficult because the vessel has a diameter of only 0.75 mm. It has been found helpful to put a temporary ligature around the common bile duct to facilitate the identification of the hepatic lymph vessels. The use of cyanoacrylate glues has greatly increased the success in setting up these difficult preparations. A method for obtaining prenodal and postnodal hepatic lymph in the anesthetized rat has recently been described (284).

Surgical procedures for the long-term studies of thoracic duct fistulas in rats have been described (153). Two techniques, thoracic duct shunt and thoracic duct side (T tube) fistula, allow repetitive sampling while preserving physiological conditions. The average lymph flows were 0.044 ml/min (shunts) and 0.042 ml/min (side fistulas), respectively. The animals remain in good general health with minimal loss of lymph and lymphocytes. The thoracic duct shunt is a difficult technique, but the T-tube fistula is no more difficult than the technique described by Bollman et al. (57).

Despite the usefulness of the lymph-fistula rat model, there are problems associated with this preparation. First, there are considerable anatomical variations in the lymphatic system between individual animals; accessory ducts or communicating vessels with other lymph ducts make it difficult to assess the completeness of lymph collection from a region. In ~60% of laboratory rats, a communicating vessel that connects the hepatic lymph trunk with the major mesenteric lymph vessel has been demonstrated. Second, one must often accept a compromise between completeness and the purity of the lymph being collected from a region. For instance, the cannulation of the mesenteric lymph duct collects fairly pure lymph from the gastrointestinal tract, with only infrequent contamination from the hepatic lymph duct, which can be obviated. The drawback, however, is that it does not drain all the lymph from the gastrointestinal tract even when the accessory duct is tied. On the other hand, the thoracic lymph duct drains almost all gastrointestinal lymph but also collects lymph from other organs. O'Morchoe and O'Morchoe (346) have shown in dogs that as much as 50% of the thoracic duct lymph flow may be of renal origin. Third, the lymph-fistula rats as described by Bollman et al. (57) require restraint, the stress of which undoubtedly affects the animal. A different type of problem associated with lymph fistulas is a technical one: clots form in the cannula. The coating of the plastic cannula with tridodecylmethyl ammonium chloride (TDMAC)-heparin complex seems to obviate the problem. It is a common observation that if clot formation can be avoided in the first postoperative day by maintaining high lymph flows, the chances of clots forming on subsequent days are relatively small. Lymphatic drainage results in considerable loss of electrolyte, protein, glucose, and other nutrients. The electrolyte loss in thoracic duct–fistula rats, ~5 meq of sodium per day (29), can be compensated either by intravenous infusion or oral feeding of an electrolyte solution. The protein loss in lymph-fistula rats is considerable, the albumin loss being more profound than that of globulins. Tilney and Murray (446) observed a modest fall in plasma protein concentration despite accurate replacement of lymph protein and fluid. Other solutes, like glucose, will also be lost in considerable quantities, because the concentration of glucose in lymph is comparable to that in plasma (29).

## Lymph Fistula Studies in the Human

Early investigations involved subjects with lymph fistulas or chylothorax. More recently there has been interest in the use of thoracic duct fistulas in patients for the removal of lymphocytes and for the treatment of acute pancreatitis. There are numerous descriptions of the preparation of chronic lymph fistulas in humans (see refs. 39, 293, 473–475). Fish et al. (139) have kept thoracic duct fistulas open in patients for periods of ≤150 days. Recently Green et al. (186) have studied the apolipoprotein composition of the chylomicrons they have collected from patients with chyluria.

## In Vitro Studies of Gastrointestinal Lymphatics

Lee and colleagues (272, 279, 280, 288) have described in vitro systems in which blood and the lymph vessels of rat small intestine segments were cannulated. These models have been used extensively for studying water absorption of the small intestine.

Many investigations of lymphatic contractility and the pharmacology and electrophysiology of lymphatic smooth muscle have employed in vitro preparations of bovine mesenteric lymphatics. For example, McHale and Roddie (316) have described a method for perfusion of a 28-mm length of one of these vessels for contractility studies.

## Micropuncture of Intestinal Mucosal Lymphatics

Lee (275, 278) has described the technique of micropuncture of the central lacteal of intestinal villi in vitro and in vivo and has used this successfully to obtain small samples of lymph for chemical analysis and to measure pressures in these initial lymphatics.

## LYMPH FROM GASTROINTESTINAL ORGANS

Table 1 presents the best available estimates of lymph flow from gastrointestinal organs in the resting state, that is, from the stomach and intestine in the nonsecreting, nonabsorbing state and at standardized venous pressures.

## Salivary Glands

Relatively little information is available regarding salivary lymph flow and composition, but the basal rate of lymph formation appears to be extremely high compared with other organs of the digestive system (253). The salivary glands are remarkable in that they can secrete enormous amounts of fluid relative to their weight, implying a large transcapillary fluid movement derived from greatly enhanced blood flow during secretory activity. Fifteenfold increases in salivary gland blood flow are reported during maximal secretion (141). There is little information about lymph flow from the salivary glands under such circumstances. In cat submandibular gland lymph, the L/P for albumin has been reported to be 0.25 and for immunoglobulin G (IgG) to be 0.19 (253).

## Esophagus and Stomach

The inaccessibility of the lymphatic vessels of the esophagus has prevented studies of its lymph. For similar reasons, only a few investigations have been carried out on gastric lymph. From the resting stomach of rabbits, gastric lymph flow has been estimated to be 0.06 ml·min$^{-1}$·100 g$^{-1}$ (40). In a single dog, Aune (14) has reported changes in lymph flow and composition in response to such agents as acetylcholine, scopolamine, histamine, and secretin. When gastric secretion is stimulated with acetylcholine or histamine, gastric lymph flow falls; this probably reflects a dehydration of the interstitium as fluid is withdrawn to supply the secretory process. A similar effect is observed in the small intestine in response to active secretagogues such as vasoactive intestinal polypeptide. With micropuncture techniques Bruggeman (67) collected dog gastric lymph, finding an L/P for total plasma protein of 0.51. The L/P data for various protein species in this study are presented in Table 5, indicating the sieving properties of the gastric microcirculation. Dithiothreitol, a sulfhydryl reducing agent that breaks the gastric mucosal barrier, had no significant effect on the composition of gastric lymph, though Wood and Davenport (489) found that it caused a reduction in the osmotic reflection coefficients for albumin and fibrinogen, indicating an in-

TABLE 5. *Lymph-to-Plasma Protein Ratios of Dog Gastric Lymph*

|  | $C_L/C_P$ |
|---|---|
| Total protein | 0.51 |
| Albumin | 0.68 |
| Globulins | 0.42 |
| $\alpha_1$-Globulins | 0.49 |
| $\alpha_2$-Globulins | 0.62 |
| $\beta$-Globulin | 0.35 |
| $\gamma$-Globulin | 0.46 |
| Fibrinogen | 0.39 |

[Data from Bruggeman (67).]

crease in capillary permeability to these macromolecules. In contrast to the data of Bruggeman, an L/P for total protein in canine gastric lymph of 0.80 has been obtained in the resting stomach (249). This fell to 0.69 when the pylorus was ligated and the stomach distended with air, possibly reflecting a diversion of blood from the relatively permeable microcirculation of the mucosa/submucosa to the less permeable capillaries of the muscularis.

In cats, Perry et al. (361) reported an L/P for total protein of 0.50. Flow rate of lymph in a major trunk on the lesser curve was 5 $\mu$l/min. Raising gastric venous pressure led to a fall in L/P for various plasma proteins, allowing an assessment of pore sizes of gastric capillaries.

*Small Intestine*

With respect to lymphatic physiology of the various gastrointestinal organs, the largest amount of information is available about the small intestine. This is due to the relative ease of access to its major lymph trunks and the interest in the transport function of lymph during fat absorption. Like other regions of the gut, the small intestine is made up of three layers: muscularis, submucosa, and mucosa. In many studies of lymph flow from this organ, it is assumed that the major contribution arises from the mucosa, an assumption that seems reasonable in view of the greater density of capillaries and high blood flow in this region; the mucosal capillaries are of the fenestrated type. Further support for this notion comes from the recent demonstration that in the rat small intestine the protein concentration in the villus lymphatic is the same as that in collecting lymph vessels (495), suggesting that no significant alteration in composition occurs as contributions from submucosa and muscularis are added to the initial mucosal lymph. Because lymph from these regions might be expected to have a lower protein concentration, it appears that their contributions are relatively small.

FLOW OF SMALL INTESTINAL LYMPH. The flow rate of intestinal lymph is highly variable. An estimate of the basal flow rate in the nonabsorbing, nonsecreting intestine is given in Table 1. Various physiological and pathophysiological states and pharmacological agents alter the flow. These are listed in Table 6. These various factors are discussed in the next sections.

INTESTINAL FLUID ABSORPTION. The large volumes of fluid and solutes that are periodically absorbed from the small intestine would quickly accumulate as gross mucosal edema in the absence of efficient routes of disposal (viz., the blood capillaries and lymphatics). It can be seen from Table 1 that the flow of lymph from the small intestine at rest (i.e., where minimal transepithelial movement of fluid is occurring) is relatively high and is thought to reflect net transcapillary filtration. This resting filtration state of the intestinal capillaries is capable of reversal to an absorbing state during fluid uptake from the intestinal lumen (178). A recent study in rats, however, has raised the question of whether lymph flow in the main intestinal trunk represents net transcapillary filtration in the intestine. All the lymph flowing in this vessel could be accounted for by lymph derived from the tissues of the mesenteric pedicle, and it was concluded from this

TABLE 6. *Physiological and Pathological Conditions and Pharmacological Agents Known to Alter Intestinal Lymph Flow*

| Conditions and Drugs That Increase Lymph Flow | Ref. | Conditions and Drugs That Decrease Lymph Flow | Ref. |
| --- | --- | --- | --- |
| Portal hypertension, acute and chronic | 127, 330, 491 | Vasoactive intestinal polypeptide | 168 |
| Plasma dilution | 174, 175, 282 | Theophylline | 168 |
| Fluid absorption | 25, 164 | Vasopressin | 370 |
| Enhanced motility | 274, 277, 283, 285 | Acetylcholine | 283 |
| Epinephrine | 283 | Eserine | 283 |
| Isoproterenol | 179 | Serotonin | 283 |
| Cholecystokinin | 177, 456 | Hemorrhage | 173 |
| Prostaglandin $E_1$ | 180 | Hypertonic glucose | 291 |
| Furosemide | 436 | Decreased motility | 285 |
| Mannitol | 436 | Sympathetic nerve stimulation | 166 |
| Fat absorption | 64, 410, 457, 485 | | |
| Inflammation | 165 | Morphine | 36, 274 |
| Luminal distension | 169 | Na pentobarbital | 222, 283, 368 |
| Tissue compression | 169 | Cholera toxin | 168, 174, 289 |
| Bradykinin | 179 | Carcinoid serum | 168 |
| Histamine | 329 | Net fluid secretion | 174 |
| Secretin | 177, 267 | | |
| Glucagon | 170 | | |
| Ricinoleic acid | 168 | | |
| Ethacrynic acid | 436 | | |
| Ethanol | 24 | | |

study that in the nonabsorbing intestine lymph flow is zero (286). This interesting observation requires further investigation.

The focal point for an understanding of the factors governing the disposal of absorbed fluid in the intestine is the mucosal interstitium. During absorption, interstitial volume increases in proportion to net fluid absorption rate (Fig. 4). This is associated with a rise in hydraulic conductivity of the interstitial matrix (100, 184). This latter change allows small alterations in interstitial fluid pressure to move fluid through the interstitium to blood and lymph vessels. Interstitial volume expansion also reduces the exclusion of macromolecules (172) and enhances diffusive movement of these molecules. The increase in interstitial fluid volume is accompanied by a rise in the hydrostatic pressure of tissue fluid. This can be demonstrated indirectly as a rise in villus lymphatic pressure by micropuncture measurements (279). Because initial lymphatics are highly permeable, lymphatic pressures probably reflect interstitial pressures. A rise in interstitial fluid pressure during fluid absorption can also be shown indirectly by calculations from the Starling force equation applied to the absorbing versus the nonabsorbing state (178). The rise in interstitial fluid pressure provides the main filling force for lymphatics that do not collapse in the face of this pressure increase. By altering the transcapillary hydrostatic pressure gradient, the rise in interstitial fluid pressure also contributes to the forces that convert capillaries that at rest were filtering to the absorbing state.

The dilution of the interstitial fluid protein by incoming fluid is further amplified by a reduction of exclusion of plasma protein in the interstitium. These factors alter markedly the transcapillary oncotic pressure gradient to favor strongly absorption by the capillaries. Reduction of the protein concentration of interstitial fluid probably plays no part in lymphatic filling.

The relationship between the rate of fluid absorption and changes in hydrostatic and oncotic pressure of interstitial fluid is not a simple one. It appears that a sudden change in the compliance of the interstitium occurs as interstitial volume increases [Figs. 3 and 4; (165, 330)]. At low interstitial volumes (low absorption rates) compliance is low ($\sim 0.4$ ml·mmHg$^{-1}$·100 g$^{-1}$). The corresponding interstitial fluid pressures are $-2$ to $+3$ mmHg. Thus as absorption rate increases within this range of low interstitial volumes, hydrostatic pressures rise rapidly. This favors lymphatic filling rather than capillary absorption because of greater hydraulic conductance of the lymphatic vessel wall. Above 3 mmHg interstitial pressure, the compliance of the interstitium undergoes an abrupt increase, probably the result of a physical alteration in the interstitial structure.

The changes in the oncotic pressure of tissue fluid (estimated from the oncotic pressure of lymph) during increasing rates of fluid absorption are not linear either. A sharp fall in tissue fluid oncotic pressure occurs at absorption rates $>0.30$ ml·min$^{-1}$·100 g$^{-1}$ (Fig. 5). The explanation for this sudden change may also reside in a sudden alteration in interstitial compliance over a narrow range of net fluid absorption.

In summary, at low rates of absorption of fluid from the intestinal lumen, the low compliance of the interstitium results in a substantial increase in hydrostatic pressure favoring lymphatic filling, whereas at high absorption rates (high compliance state) the dominant force is the reduction in tissue fluid oncotic pressure. This force, acting exclusively on the capillaries, favors absorption of fluid by the bloodstream.

It it well known that during fluid absorption from the intestine the flow of intestinal lymph increases. Attempts to assign fixed proportions of fluid transported by lymphatic versus blood vascular routes have led to widely disparate estimates varying between 1% and 85% (29, 37, 68, 94, 164, 273, 276, 280, 288, 332, 335, 409). The foregoing consideration lead one to expect that the proportion would vary with fluid absorption rate and that the blood vascular route would predominate, especially at high absorption rates. At fluid absorption rates of 0.2 ml·min$^{-1}$·100 g$^{-1}$, blood and lymphatic transport account for similar proportions; above this, the blood vascular route predominates (Fig. 6).

It is possible that there exists in the mucosa a small compartment of the interstitium that is functionally

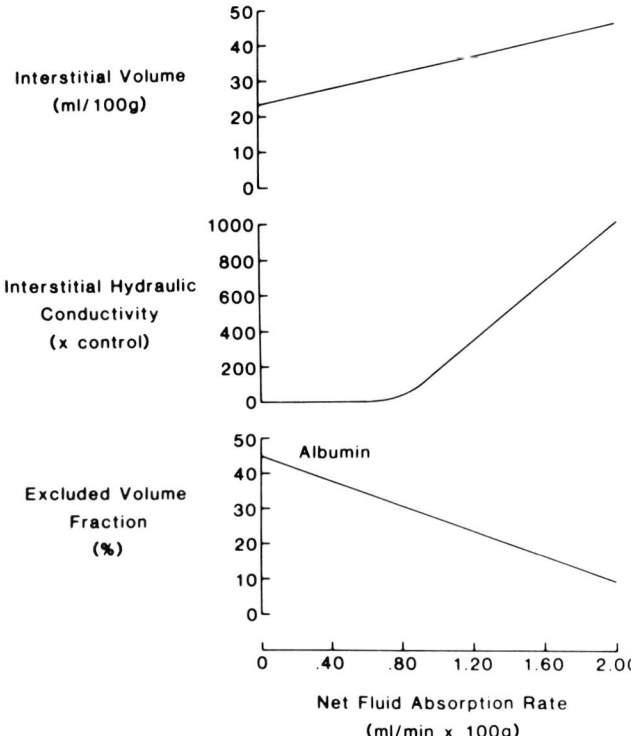

FIG. 4. Effects of net fluid absorption rate on intestinal interstitial volume, interstitial hydraulic conductivity, and excluded volume fraction of albumin. [From Granger et al. (182).]

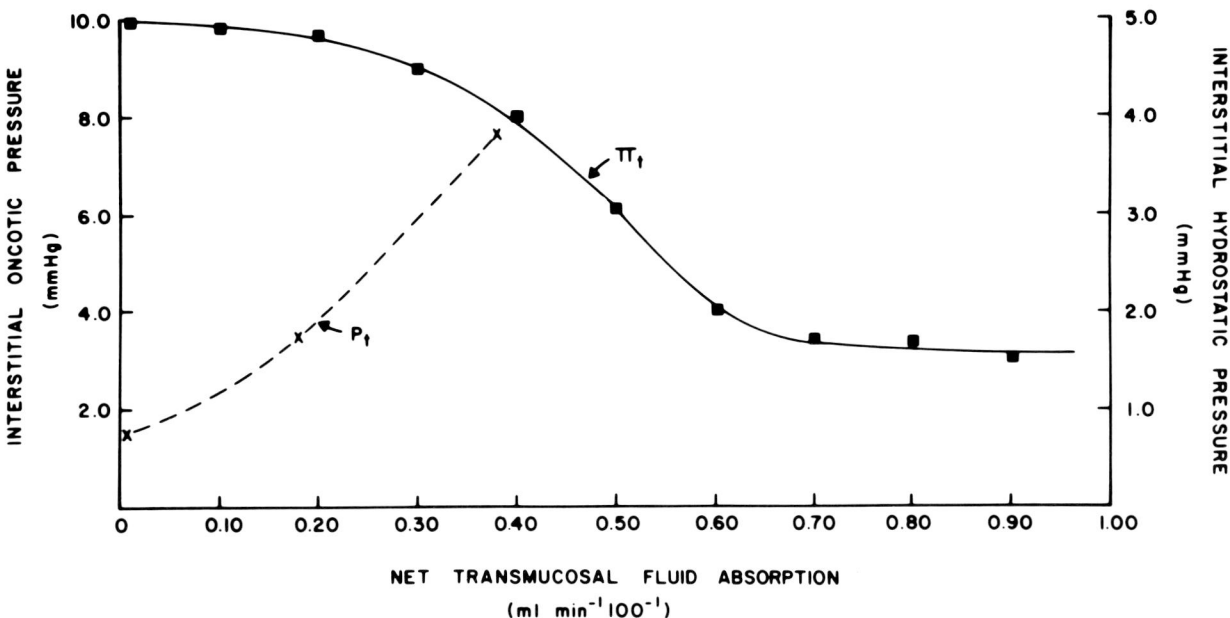

FIG. 5. Influence of net fluid absorption rate on intestinal interstitial oncotic ($\pi_t$) and hydrostatic ($P_t$) pressures. Micropuncture data (X) obtained in rats. [From Granger et al. (182).]

separated from the large interstitial space of the villus (491). This is a juxtacapillary space with a depth of 2 $\mu$m lying between the basement membrane of the epithelium and the fenestrated face of the subepithelial capillaries (Fig. 7). This interstitial space is much smaller than the 50-$\mu$m-deep general mucosal interstitial compartment (from the base of the enterocyte to the central lymphatic vessel) and is the first space exposed to incoming fluid. If such a functionally distinct compartment exists, this would enhance the importance of the blood capillaries in fluid transport, because a large rise in interstitial fluid pressure would be anticipated in this very small compartment during fluid absorption. This hypothesis, however, has not been tested.

INTESTINAL SECRETION AND LYMPH FLOW. In addition to its normally predominant absorptive function, the intestine is also engaged in fluid secretion. Four mechanisms are recognized as enhancing intes-

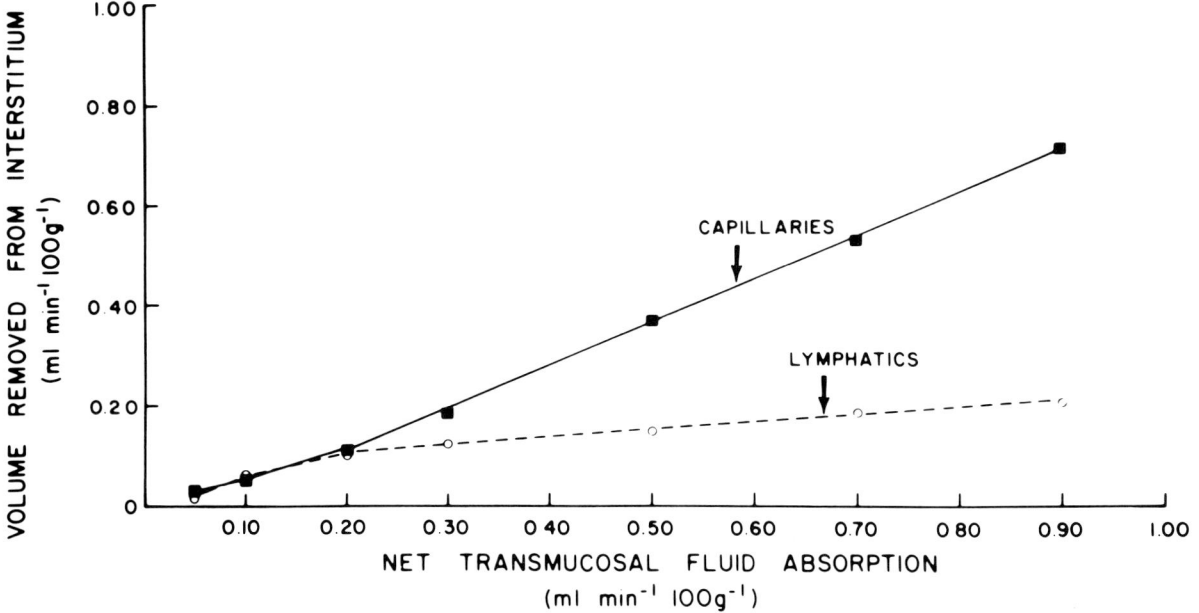

FIG. 6. Steady-state relations between rate of removal of absorbed fluid by intestinal capillaries and lymphatics and net fluid absorption rate. [From Granger et al. (182).]

tinal secretion: increased luminal osmolality, active electrolyte secretion, decreased electrolyte absorption, and increased hydrostatic pressure in the mucosal interstitium. Clinical examples of each of these four are, respectively, lactase deficiency, cholera, celiac disease, and plasma volume expansion. When fluid is actively secreted, for example by a cAMP-mediated process in the mucosa in cholera, the secretion consists of water and electrolytes and contains no protein (165, 168, 174). On the other hand, with filtration secretion created by a rise in hydrostatic pressure of interstitial fluid, the secretion entering the intestinal lumen by paracellular pathways contains protein in the same concentration as in the interstitium (165, 168, 174). One can predict that lymph flow from the intestine will be affected by both active secretion and filtration secretion. In active secretion the mucosal epithelium will draw on the interstitium for fluid, reducing tissue fluid hydrostatic pressure and reducing lymphatic filling and lymph flow; with filtration secretion the opposite will occur.

These predictions are borne out by experimental observation. Thus active secretagogues, such as cholera toxin, theophylline, vasoactive intestinal polypeptide, and human carcinoid serum, all reduce intestinal lymph flow while provoking a protein-free water and electrolyte secretion by the intestinal mucosa (168).

Direct measurements show that villus lacteal pressure and presumably villus interstitial pressure are reduced by cholera toxin (281, 289).

Filtration secretion may result from acute portal hypertension or plasma dilution through an increase in interstitial fluid formation. When these produce an imbalance of ~12 mmHg or more in transcapillary Starling forces, filtration secretion occurs (123, 330). When interstitial fluid pressure rises 4–5 mmHg, channels open in the mucosal membrane at the villus tips that allow passage of fluid and solutes as large as albumin (109, 167, 197). With plasma volume expansion intercellular spaces expand, and with the filtration secretion produced by vasoactive agents, such as $PGE_1$ and glucagon, erosions of villus tips can be demonstrated; these channels allow free escape of interstitial fluid into the intestinal lumen (170, 180). The capillary force perturbations that initiate these changes initially cause enhanced lymph flow, but when these low-resistance channels open in the mucosal membrane, lymph flow falls as excess interstitial fluid follows the pathway of lower resistance (174, 180). Recent microscopic studies of rat jejunal mucosa (287) have demonstrated leakage of lymph under certain circumstances from the central villus lymph vessels through channels in the villus tip. The significance of this observation, however, remains obscure.

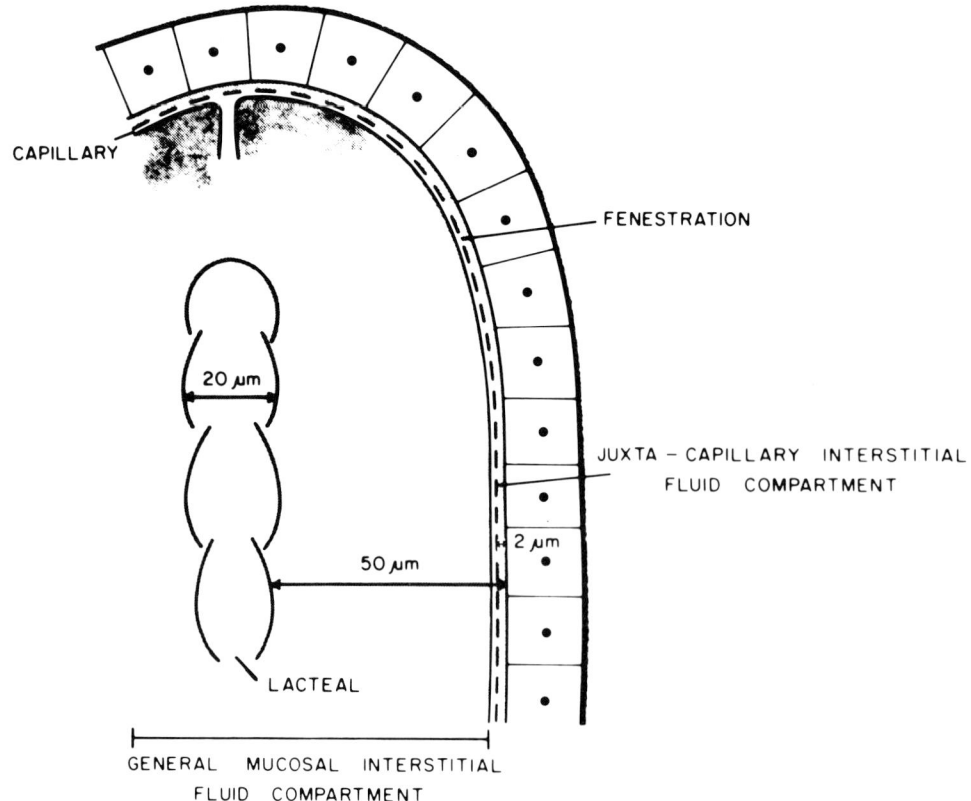

FIG. 7. Anatomical scheme of blood and lymph microcirculation in an intestinal villus. [From Granger (164).]

TRANSPORT OF ABSORBED WATER-SOLUBLE SUBSTANCES BY INTESTINAL LYMPHATICS. Although there is evidence for lymphatic transport of absorbed macromolecules and particulate material, including lipoprotein particles, there is no evidence that lymph plays any role in transport of small water-soluble molecules such as glucose (206, 221, 263, 399) or amino acids (363) or in the transport of minerals such as iron (133, 364, 378) and copper (422).

INTESTINAL LIPID ABSORPTION. Lipid assimilation is that aspect of gastrointestinal function in which lymphatics play their most specific role. Dietary lipid, which is chiefly triglyceride, undergoes a partial hydrolysis to monoglycerides and fatty acids in the intestinal lumen under the action of pancreatic lipase, and these split products are absorbed by a passive process by the enterocyte (see refs. 26, 62, 63, 358, 441, 450). A binding protein in the microvillous membrane is probably involved in promoting the uptake of fatty acids (426). The mucosal uptake of fatty acids and monoglycerides is facilitated by their association with bile salts in polymolecular aggregates (micelles and liposomes) that act to overcome the resistance of the unstirred water layer on the enterocyte surface to the diffusion of these poorly water-soluble substances to the microvillus membrane (411).

Other lipid species, phospholipids and cholesterol of biliary and dietary origin, are also solutes in bile salt–lipid micelles, as are trace nutrient lipids such as the fat-soluble vitamins and lipophilic xenobiotics. The translocation of fatty acids in the enterocyte is thought to be facilitated by a specific intracellular fatty acid–binding protein (337). Resynthesis of triglyceride occurs in the smooth endoplasmic reticulum (211) chiefly by the monoglyceride pathway, that is, reacylation of 2-monoglyceride with two fatty acyl–coenzyme A molecules (235). Where monoglyceride is in short supply, triglyceride is synthesized by the alternative $\alpha$-glycerophosphate pathway that utilizes glycerol-3-phosphate to which two fatty acyl–coenzyme A molecules are added to yield phosphatidic acid that is subsequently converted to triglyceride with a third fatty acyl–coenzyme A molecule. The resynthesized triglyceride droplets in the smooth endoplasmic reticulum acquire a surface coat of phospholipid and lipoprotein, the latter synthesized in the rough endoplasmic reticulum (187); the coated triglyceride droplets are subsequently transferred to the cisternae of the Golgi apparatus where glycosylation of the protein component occurs (248, 394). There is some preliminary evidence that the nonionic surfactant Pluronic L-81 may interfere with this transfer step (451, 453). In the Golgi apparatus the final assembly of chylomicrons occurs (372, 374). These spherical particles, 75–600 nm in diameter, contain a liquid triglyceride core comprising 86%–92% of the mass of the particle. Other major components located principally on the surface of the particle include cholesterol ester (1%–2%), free cholesterol (~1%), protein (~1%), and phospholipid (6%–8%). Trace amounts of nonpolar lipids such as fat-soluble vitamins and foreign lipophilic compounds are found as solutes in the core triglyceride. The protein covers ~10%–20% of the surface, whereas the phospholipid covers 80% or more. Triglyceride lipids reflect dietary lipid composition, and chylomicron size is related to the flux of lipid across the enterocyte and is maximal at high rates of absorption. The fatty acid composition of chylomicron cholesterol ester and phospholipid, however, bears little relationship to dietary fatty acid species, and the phospholipid of chylomicrons appears to be largely derived from biliary sources.

The synthesis of apolipoproteins in the enterocyte is of great importance in the process of lipid absorption. In the autosomal recessive disorder abetalipoproteinemia, the inability of the enterocyte to synthesize the apolipoprotein results in a block of lipid transport in the cell, with accumulation of lipid droplets in membrane-bound compartments within the cell (163, 254, 391). No chylomicrons appear in the lamina propria or the villus lymphatics. An animal model of this disease has been created with the protein synthesis inhibitor puromycin in rats (389). It appears that the enzymes of triglyceride synthesis are less susceptible to protein synthesis inhibition, and the histological appearances of triglyceride accumulation in the enterocyte are similar to those in abetalipoproteinemia. The puromycin model of abetalipoproteinemia, however, has been criticized chiefly because of the nonspecific effects of protein synthesis inhibition and other actions of puromycin, such as impairment of gastric emptying (145, 371, 375). Studies with another inhibitor of protein synthesis, acetoxycycloheximide, demonstrate the importance of concurrent mucosal protein synthesis in the process of lipid absorption and transcellular transport (155, 156), but a good animal model of abetalipoproteinemia is not presently available.

From the Golgi complex, chylomicrons move in membrane-bound vesicles to the basolateral cell membrane. Inhibition of microtubule function with colchicine interferes with this step (157). The particles, singly or in groups, leave the cell by exocytosis into the lateral intercellular spaces, a process that depends on calcium ions. During fat absorption, large numbers of chylomicrons can be seen accumulating in the intercellular space above the enterocyte basement membrane (388). This entire process of lipid absorption from gut lumen to intercellular space takes ~10–12 min (232, 454). There are several excellent reviews that describe the above process of lipid uptake and cellular processing in detail (see, e.g., ref. 441).

*Chylomicrons from enterocyte to lacteal.* Chylomicrons must first pass across the basement membrane of the enterocyte before penetrating the lamina propria of the intestinal mucosa. Electron-microscopic studies suggest that the chylomicrons pass across transient gaps opening in the membrane, but appearances of accumulation of chylomicrons behind the membrane indicate that the basement membrane offers considerable resistance to chylomicron flow (Fig. 8). The particles are too large to enter capillaries and must travel ~50 μm through the interstitium of the villus. One might anticipate that the interstitium will offer considerable resistance to the passage of these relatively large particles. The interstitium behaves as a mesh with pores of ~25-nm radius in the nonhydrated state, increasing to ~100 nm in the hydrated state. Most chylomicrons are clearly larger (≦600 nm) than these pores, and it is necessary to postulate the existence of a few fluid-filled channels of larger dimensions for the bulk transfer of these particles. It is probable that mucosal interstitial hydration is considerably increased during fat absorption, and this would facilitate the movement of chylomicrons to the lacteal. Recently Tso et al. (454) have shown in rats that the chylomicron appearance time—the time between placement of radioactive fatty acid in the intestinal lumen and the appearance of radioactive lipid in the central lacteal—is related to the rate of lymph flow, reaching a minimum of 13.6 min at high lymph flows. This minimum time, which probably represents the time required for intracellular processing of the fatty acid, agrees well with other estimates for this process (232). These data suggest that the rate of chylomicron transfer to the lymph is dependent on the state of hydration of the mucosal interstitium. Subsequent studies demonstrate that the reduced chylomicron appearance time produced by hydration (expansion) of the mucosal interstitium results from diminished resistance of the interstitial matrix to chylomicron movement rather than decreased transit time due to an enhanced convective flux of chylomicrons (452).

Chylomicrons enter the lacteal mainly by intercellular pathways, though vesicular transport through endothelial cells has also been shown (79). The main force for chylomicron uptake is probably a hydrostatic pressure gradient driving interstitial fluid into the lymphatic vessel held open by anchoring filaments.

*Partition of absorbed lipid between portal venous blood and intestinal lymph.* Since studies in the 1950s, it has been thought that absorbed long-chain fatty acids, that is, 12–carbon atom chain length and longer,

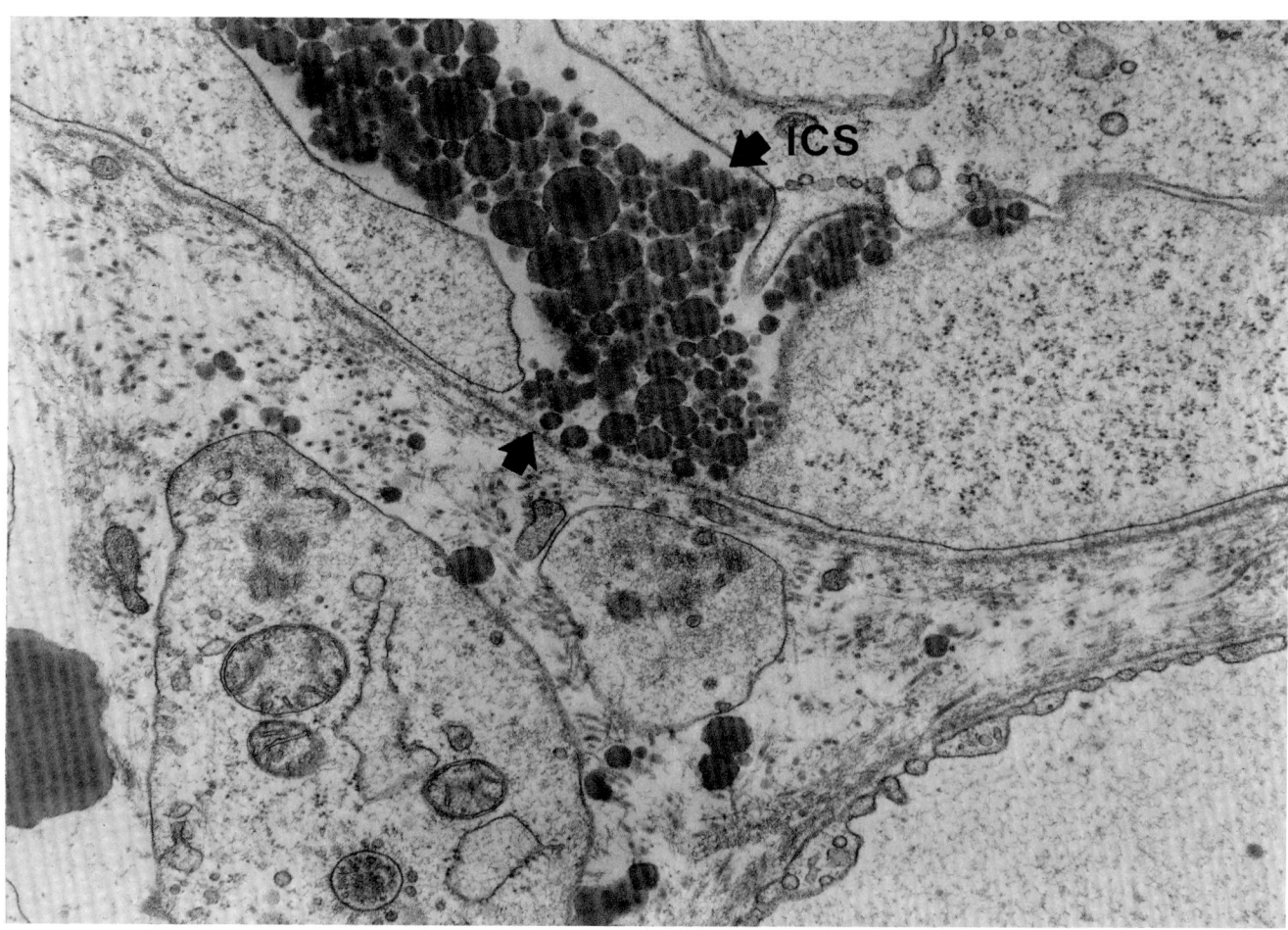

FIG. 8. Chylomicrons accumulating in distended intercellular space (ICS) between two enterocytes. Intact basement membrane (*arrow*) forms barrier separating absorptive epithelial cells and intercellular space from lamina propria. × 27,600. [From Sabesin and Frase (388).]

are resynthesized in the enterocyte and transported as chylomicron triglyceride, whereas shorter-chain fatty acids leave the enterocyte in the unesterified form and enter portal venous blood bound to proteins (38, 44, 49, 50, 61, 88, 377). A proportion of absorbed medium-chain fatty acids, however, appears in lymph (45). For example, ≦16% of absorbed decanoic acid appears in rat thoracic duct lymph esterified as triglyceride and phospholipid and 15%–55% of absorbed dodecanoic acid is recovered in rat intestinal lymph. There is some evidence that the concomitant feeding of long-chain triglyceride with medium-chain triglyceride increases the proportion of medium-chain fatty acids that are recovered in lymph (19). Early studies showed that only minor proportions of fatty acids of >14–carbon atom chain length were transported in portal venous blood.

The partition principle is still essentially correct, but recent studies suggest that the partition is governed by several complex factors. In a study with rats, McDonald et al. (313) showed that substantial amounts of long-chain fatty acids are transported from the rat intestine by portal venous blood. At low rates of delivery of fatty acid to the intestine, as much as 58% of linoleic acid and 69% of linolenic acid bypass the lymphatic route; only 28% of stearic acid, however, is carried by portal venous blood. At higher rates of fat absorption, proportionally more of a fatty acid species is carried by lymph. Thus both the rate of absorption and the degree of saturation of the fatty acid play a part in the partition.

In situations where mucosal handling of fatty acids is abnormal, the proportion of long-chain fatty acids transported by the portal venous route is increased. Thus in puromycin-treated rats with impairment of mucosal synthesis of lipoproteins, absorbed oleic acid is diverted to the portal vein (246). Where bile salt concentrations in the intestinal lumen are subnormal, long-chain fatty acids are similarly diverted to the portal vein (60, 148, 390). In rats with bile fistulas, oleic acid absorption is depressed and the major portion is transported by the portal vein. This effect, which can be reversed by supplying taurocholate, is probably due to defective mucosal esterification of the fatty acid due to bile salt deficiency. Feeding 2-ethyl-$n$-hexanoic acid to rats may also interfere with the mucosal esterification of absorbed long-chain fatty acids channeling a greater proportion of the fatty acids into the portal vein in the unesterified form (225). Morgan and Borgström (326) have shown that during the assimilation of labeled triglyceride in rats with a bile fistula the proportion of fatty acid to monoglyceride absorbed was increased compared with rats with an intact biliary system. The explanation for this is unknown. Sterols such as cholesterol are primarily transported in lymph after their absorption (89, 448), though a study in rats has demonstrated that minor amounts are carried in portal venous blood (320). As with fatty acids, it seems likely that, in the absence of bile, reesterification of cholesterol in the enterocyte is defective and some free cholesterol may enter portal venous blood in protein-bound form.

Fat-soluble vitamins are transported in intestinal lymph largely as solutes in the triglyceride core of chylomicrons (26, 142). After feeding carotene or retinol, the principal form of vitamin A found in intestinal lymph is retinyl palmitate (48, 161, 219, 266). Absorbed vitamins D are present in lymph mainly in the unesterified form, partly incorporated into chylomicrons and partly bound to protein (122, 144, 392, 393). Tocopherols, similarly, occur in the unesterified form in lymph (46, 234, 359). Of the vitamins K, phylloquinone (vitamin $K_1$) is chiefly transported in lymph (47, 229), whereas menadione (vitamin $K_3$) is transported by both portal venous blood and lymph (321).

Although lymph is the major route for fat-soluble vitamin transport, substantial amounts of the vitamins and their more polar derivatives pass into portal venous blood. This applies to retinol (102, 137, 214) and to some extent to tocopherol, whereas a large proportion of 25-hydroxycholecalciferol and 1,25-dihydroxycholecalciferol are transported by the blood (215, 297, 312, 413–415).

Certain circumstances seem to favor portal venous transport of fat-soluble vitamins. As with long-chain fatty acids and sterols, bile salt deficiency enhances portal venous transport of vitamin A (148). It has been suggested that feeding cholecalciferol with medium-chain triglyceride diverts the vitamin to the portal venous blood (365), and Hollander (214) has observed that the concurrent absorption of polyunsaturated long-chain fatty acids appears to divert some absorbed retinol from the lymphatic to the portal venous route.

*Lymph lipid during fasting.* The major lipoprotein particles transported in intestinal lymph after a mixed lipid meal are chylomicrons. However, when fatty acids are fed in the form of phospholipid, the major particles in lymph are very-low-density lipoproteins (VLDL) that have a diameter of 20–80 nm (34). During fasting, intestinal lymph continues to transport lipid at a low rate, mainly in the form of VLDL. It is estimated that the intestine contributes ~30% of circulating VLDL. This lipid has been considered to be derived chiefly from biliary lipids. This conclusion has been based on the effects of biliary diversion and cholestyramine administration on intestinal lipid synthesis and lymphatic transport (336). More recently it has been suggested that pancreaticobiliary secretions contain factors that stimulate intestinal triglyceride synthesis. Substrates derived from plasma may be a major source of triglyceride of VLDL secreted by the intestine in the fasting state (255). There is some similarity between the apoprotein composition of VLDL and chylomicrons, though there are certain quantitative differences in the proportions of the proteins. For example, human intestinal VLDL contains apoA-IV, apoA-II, apoB, apoE, and the C peptides.

The apoB and apoA-IV content is greater and the apoC content less than in chylomicrons (187).

The general similarity of the composition of the two classes of particle has, in the past, been considered to indicate that VLDL and chylomicrons represent a single family of particles with varying proportions of lipid. That is, in the fasting state with low rates of lipid transport VLDL predominate, whereas chylomicrons are predominant at high rates of lipid transport. This is probably not correct. There certainly seems to be a proportion of intestinal VLDL that is distinct from chylomicron particles, because there is only limited mixing of chylomicrons and VLDL-sized particles in secretory vesicles from rat enterocytes (296). Furthermore, feeding fatty acids in the form of phospholipid selectively stimulates VLDL formation (34). A recent study by Tso et al. (453), using the nonionic surfactant Pluronic L-81 that selectively inhibits chylomicron formation in the enterocyte, provides further evidence that there may be separate pathways of chylomicron and VLDL assembly and transport in the enterocyte.

*Intestinal lymph flow and fat absorption.* An interesting aspect of intestinal lymph flow is the increase that occurs during fat absorption. An increased protein flux in lymph is also observed, indicating enhanced transcapillary movement of plasma proteins (64, 410, 457, 485). These phenomena are observed with both long- and medium-chain triglyceride feeding (457); thus they are independent of the route of transport of the absorbed lipid. Intraluminal digestion of long-chain triglyceride is necessary, because pancreatic exclusion abolishes the effects of feeding the lipid (458). Neither the changes in the intestinal microcirculation responsible for the increased fluid and protein flux nor the mechanisms bringing them about have been fully established. There is a well-recognized increase in splanchnic blood flow in the postprandial period (91), and there is evidence that capillary recruitment occurs. Although the increased fluid transport in lymph might be due to capillary recruitment, the enhanced plasma protein flux suggests that, in addition, there is an increase in intestinal capillary permeability. Studies of the microcirculation of the cat ileum have shown that intraluminal lipids increase capillary permeability, as judged by a fall in the osmotic reflection coefficient. Pore-size analyses suggest that the permeability change is largely due to an increase in the size of large pores, the radius increasing from ~20 to 30 nm (177). An increase in interstitial hydration that leads to enhanced interstitial fluid formation and lymph flow could be regarded as advantageous in facilitating the movement of bulky lipoprotein particles, the chylomicrons, through the lamina propria of the mucosa toward the lacteal. Furthermore, the increased movement of plasma proteins from blood to interstitium to lymph could make substantial amounts of albumin available for the transport of unesterified fatty acids.

The mechanisms of these effects are incompletely understood. Gastrointestinal hormones such as cholecystokinin and secretin, which are liberated postprandially, have vasodilator actions on the splanchnic circulation (91) but no demonstrable effect on intestinal capillary permeability of the type observed in the cat ileal microcirculation with fat feeding (177). Prostaglandins do not seem to be involved and, though some experimental studies suggest a role for histamine, the evidence is conflicting (177, 487). The hormone neurotensin, which is released by intraluminal fat, is a splanchnic vasodilator at the concentrations reached postprandially and causes an increase in intestinal capillary permeability similar to that observed after fat feeding (202). Neurotensin may, therefore, be at least partly responsible for the lymph changes. Probably the lymph changes after fat feeding are the result of a combination of vasodilation and increased capillary permeability due to various gastrointestinal hormones released postprandially (91) and possible also due to net fluid absorption from the intestinal lumen resulting from the processes of fat digestion and absorption.

Intestinal lymph flow is enhanced by ethanol feeding in rats, and this is associated with increased transport of dietary lipids (24). Chronic ethanol feeding, however, appears to inhibit these acute effects. The mechanisms involved are unknown.

*Bile acid transport in intestinal lymph.* The enterohepatic circulation of bile acids is a remarkably efficient process that relies on active bile salt absorption in the distal ileum and passive absorption, particularly of the less polar dihydroxy bile acids, in the proximal small intestine. Efficient hepatic extraction of portal blood results in only small concentrations of bile acids in systemic blood compared with portal venous blood. Studies in rats suggest that the lymphatic pathway is not important for bile acid transport, because only 0.4% of a radioactive oral dose of taurocholate could be recovered from intestinal lymph (416). A recent study of the magnitude of bile acid flux via lymphatics has documented a significant postprandial increase in lymphatic flux of bile salts in the rat. In terms of systemic blood bile salt concentrations, however, the lymphatic contribution is negligible, because the hourly lymphatic flux is only 7 nmol, whereas the contribution resulting from incomplete hepatic extraction of bile salts from portal venous blood is roughly 7 $\mu$mol/h (32). In both systemic and portal venous blood, the concentration of cholate is greater than chenodeoxycholate, but in lymph from cisterna chyli, chenodeoxycholate predominates. This indicates that filtration from plasma or a substantial contribution from liver lymph is unlikely to account for lymphatic bile salt flux in the cisterna. It is not clear why chenodeoxycholic acid predominates in lymph; this bile acid is substantially absorbed in the upper small intestine, thus it is possible that lymph from this region may make a quantitatively more important contribution to cisternal lymph than lymph from the distal ileum. In the human, a similar preponderance of dihydroxy bile acids has been demonstrated in lymph (134). Calculations of bile acid flux via thoracic duct lymph show that only ~0.2% of absorbed bile acids follow the lymphatic route, results that are comparable to those in the rat. Bile acids are transported in both blood and lymph chiefly bound to albumin.

GASTROINTESTINAL HORMONES IN LYMPH. Before the advent of radioimmunoassays for gastrointestinal peptides in biological specimens, a few studies with various bioassays had indicated the presence of gut hormones in lymph (see ref. 25). The significance of this rests on the possibility that by bypassing the liver, lymph would deliver these hormones to the peripheral circulation without the opportunity for hepatic extraction. In the postprandial period, a marked rise in the concentration of a gastric secretagogue(s) in lymph has been demonstrated (247). However, subsequent studies have suggested that no significant amounts of gastrin are transported in postprandial lymph (93, 314). In human thoracic duct lymph, cholecystokinin-like activity was found to increase after duodenal infusion of sorbitol (429).

A recent study by Chen et al. (90) has documented the presence of various gastrointestinal peptides measured by radioimmunoassay in canine thoracic duct lymph and a rise in their concentrations in the postprandial period (Table 7). However, simultaneous measurement of portal venous plasma samples showed higher concentrations. Taking the high flow rate of portal venous blood versus intestinal lymph into account, it would require a high degree of hepatic inactivation for the lymphatic route to assume any significance in the postprandial rise in peripheral venous blood of these peptides.

LYMPHATIC TRANSPORT OF DRUGS AND OTHER XENOBIOTIC SUBSTANCES. In general terms, the degree of lipophilicity of foreign substances appears to determine the route of transport of these compounds from the small intestine, the more lipid-soluble compounds favoring the lymphatic route. When considering the role of small intestinal lymphatics in the absorption of drugs and other xenobiotics, however, it is important to recognize that the metabolic activity of the enterocyte, which has the capacity to carry out various phase I and phase II reactions, may modify the absorbed substance and be responsible for rerouting to the portal venous blood (in the form of more polar metabolites) highly lipophilic compounds that might be expected to be carried primarily by lymph. For example, after benzo(a)pyrene is instilled into a small intestinal loop, a large proportion of the compound is found as polar metabolites in venous blood draining the loop (53). Clearly the importance of lymphatic transport of foreign compounds rests on the fact that the liver is bypassed, allowing extensive systemic distribution of the compound. However, if a compound is partitioned between portal venous blood and lymph, the proportion transported by the lymphatics may be comparatively small considering the disparity of mesenteric blood and lymph flow (roughly, a 500-fold difference).

There are comparatively few studies of drug transport by intestinal lymph. Among those shown to be at least partly transported by lymph are p-aminosalicylic acid and tetracycline (108). The highly lipophilic antimycotic agent naftifine is transported to a substantial extent by intestinal lymph as a chylomicron solute. Its metabolites are largely transported in portal venous blood. Diversion of intestinal lymph greatly reduces systemic blood concentrations of naftifine (191). A number of lipid-soluble drugs, however, appear to be transported almost exclusively by portal venous blood. These include ethynyl-estradiol-3-cyclopentyl ether (152), digitoxin (33, 345), and proscillaridin A (11).

Various steroid hormones less hydrophobic than ethynyl estradiol-3-cyclopentyl ether are also carried mainly by the portal venous route. These include 17-methyl estradiol (54), 17-$\alpha$-methyl testosterone (224), cortisone acetate (55), and hydrocortisone and testosterone (205). In humans, testosterone undecanoate is partly metabolized in the intestinal epithelium during absorption, and the parent compound and a major metabolite, 5 $\alpha$-dihydrotestosterone undecanoate, are partly transported in the lymph (218).

Intestinal lymphatic transport of lipophilic toxic xenobiotics is of considerable current interest. Among those that are at least partly transported in intestinal lymph are benzo(a)pyrene (71, 376), 7, 12–dimethyl benzanthracene (195, 228, 259), 3-methylcholanthrene, and aminostilbene derivatives (244), polychlorinated biphenyls (72, 498), pentachlorophenol (477), and dichlorodiphenyltrichloroethane (DDT) (367). Sieber et al. (406) have studied the lymphatic transport of various xenobiotics, including benzene, benzoic acid, aniline, p-aminobenzoic acid, salicylic acid, phenanthrene, estradiol, testosterone, digoxin, hexanoic acid, hexylamine, hexanol, antipyrine, izoniazid, and caffeine. All these compounds appear to be chiefly transported by the portal venous route, whereas octadecanol and p,p$^1$-DDT (1,1$^1$-(2,2,2-trichloroethylidene)bis[4-chlorobenzene]) are selectively taken up by intestinal lymph.

TABLE 7. *Concentrations of Various Gastrointestinal Peptides in Canine Thoracic Duct Lymph*

| Peptides | Fasting | Postprandial |
|---|---|---|
| Gastrin, pg/ml | 21.4 | 49.0 |
| Neurotensin, pg/ml | 11.1 | 33.0 |
| Vasoactive intestinal polypeptide, pg/ml | 14.0 | 31.0 |
| Substance P, pg/ml | 8.0 | 12.0 |
| Bombesin, pg/ml | 15.0 | 46.0 |

[Data from Chen et al. (90).]

Compounds such as DDT, 7,12-dimethyl benzanthracene, benzo(a)pyrene, and polychlorinated biphenyls are transported as solutes in chylomicrons. However, a recent study (71) has shown that absorbed benzo(a)pyrene in lymph is associated to a greater extent with low-density lipoproteins (LDL) than with either VLDL or high-density lipoproteins (HDL). The different handling of nutrient lipids and lipophilic xenobiotics is illustrated by the fact that when benzo(a)pyrene is fed in a nutrient lipid solution, chylomicrons of lymph during the first 2 h after intraduodenal infusion are highly contaminated with benzo(a)pyrene, but in the subsequent hours the concentration of benzo(a)pyrene in the chylomicrons falls progressively, suggesting the possibility that metabolism of the xenobiotic by the enterocyte is increasing, rerouting the compound, as metabolites, to portal venous blood (260).

The nature of the concurrently administered nutrient lipid appears to determine the extent of lymphatic transport of a lipophilic xenobiotic. Thus a much greater lymphatic transport of absorbed DDT occurs when it is fed as a solute in a long-chain triglyceride vehicle than in a medium-chain triglyceride oil (349).

Deak and Csáky (106) have reported an interesting study of the factors determining the partition of absorbed compounds between blood and lymph pathways, concluding that lipid solubility per se is not the major determinant but rather the molecular size of a compound or the size of the particle (e.g., lipoprotein) with which it is associated. Using fluorescein isothiocyanate-labeled dextrans of varying molecular size, Yoshikawa et al. (493) have concluded that a threshold exists between 17,500 mol wt and 39,000 mol wt for fluorescein-labeled dextrans, above which transfer to lymph rather than blood is favored. These same authors have reported that the intestinal absorption and lymphatic transport of human fibroblast interferon is promoted by feeding the drug in mixed lipid-synthetic surfactant micelles (494).

It has long been claimed that small amounts of particulate matter can be absorbed by the intestine and transported in both portal venous blood and lymph (465). A recent study in rats has demonstrated the presence of certain types of ingested asbestos fiber, chrysotile and crocidolite, in thoracic duct lymph (398). The physical properties of these stiff sharp fibers presumably enable them to penetrate tissues relatively easily.

LYMPHATIC TRANSPORT OF PROTEINS OF INTESTINAL ORIGIN. The major source of protein of intestinal lymph, as with lymph from all regions of the body, is the plasma. A small proportion of lymph protein, however, is derived from intestinal sources (Table 8).

The protein components of lipoprotein molecules of intestinal lymph are derived either from the enterocyte, synthesized during lipid absorption and during fasting, or are preformed proteins already present in blood and lymph (41). In the latter category are apoproteins E and C (apoE, apoC). Chylomicrons, the major lipoprotein particles of intestinal lymph in the postprandial period, have as their major apoproteins in humans and rats apoB, 24,000 mol wt (~10%); apoA-IV, 46,000 mol wt (~10%); apoE, 35,000 mol wt (~5%); apoA-I, 28,000 mol wt (15%–35%); and the lower mol wt apoC group (45%–50%) (186, 187). Recently another species, apoA-V, 59,000 mol wt, has been described in rats (136). In humans and rats, the intestine synthesizes apoB, apoA-I, apoA-IV, and, in small amounts, apoC-II. In the human, the intestine also synthesizes apoA-II. The intestine is a major synthetic source of apoA-IV (187). For example, in the rat the intestine accounts for >60% of the total body synthesis of apoA-IV (187).

Small amounts of enzymes of intestinal origin appear in intestinal lymph. The best studied of these is alkaline phosphatase. This enzyme, derived from the microvillous membrane of the enterocyte, appears in lymph during lipid absorption (52). From studies with protein synthesis inhibitors, it seems that new synthesis of alkaline phosphatase occurs during the process of fat absorption (154). This seems to be related to the process of intercellular transport of lipid and/or the synthesis of lipoproteins. Another enzyme of intestinal origin appearing in intestinal lymph during fat absorption is diamine oxidase (486). Its functions in this process are unknown.

A major component of the body's lymphoid system is located in the gastrointestinal tract (GALT, the gastrointestinal-associated lymphoid tissue). This is generally divided into three components: Peyer's patches, intraepithelial lymphocytes, and the plasma cells and lymphocytes of the lamina propria of the mucosa. These plasma cells chiefly express immunoglobulins of the IgA class. It has been shown that in canine mesenteric lymph, 60%–90% of the IgA is derived from mucosal plasma cells (459). Similarly, it has been shown in a number of species that the IgA concentrations in mesenteric lymph are several times greater than those of plasma; for example, IgA concentrations in rat mesenteric lymph are greater than 13 times those of plasma (460). It thus appears that mesenteric lymphatics are a route of primary transport of newly synthesized IgA to the blood, and it has

TABLE 8. *Proteins and Polypeptides of Intestinal Lymph*

| Protein/Polypeptide | Source |
| --- | --- |
| Plasma proteins | Blood-capillary filtration |
| Lipoproteins | Enterocytes, blood |
| Enzymes of mucosal epithelium | Enterocytes |
| Gut regulatory peptides | Mucosal endocrine cells, enteric neurons |
| Immunoglobulins | Mucosal plasma cells |
| Ingested proteins | Intestinal lumen |

been calculated that 90%–97% of the IgA of mesenteric lymph is synthesized by intestinal plasma cells.

Ingested proteins are extensively hydrolyzed in the intestinal lumen, and the adult mammalian intestine is largely impermeable to protein-sized molecules. However, small amounts of protein do cross the epithelial surface and are carried in intestinal lymph (25, 467). Interest in this phenomenon chiefly centers on the antigenic properties of these large molecules. Certain conditions favor the transport of macromolecules (including antigens and toxins) across the epithelial barrier; these conditions include impaired intraluminal digestion, disruption of the mucosal barrier, and reduced local synthesis of IgA that would normally complex with antigenic molecules. The access of intact antigenic molecules even in small amounts to the systemic circulation presumably accounts for certain food allergies. Early observations indicated that egg white proteins (7) and the toxins of *Clostridium botulinum* (304) can gain access to the circulation by way of intestinal absorption and lymphatic transport. More recent studies have demonstrated this route of transport of a small percentage of a dose of horseradish peroxidase (40,000 mol wt) (468), elastase (24,000 mol wt) (245) and serum albumin (68,000 mol wt) (469). The relative proportions of an absorbed macromolecule removed by lymphatics and capillaries depend mainly on the size of the molecule (25).

The gut in the newborn of certain species is able to absorb macromolecules. This is important in the passive transfer of immunity via ingested immunoglobulins of colostrum. This mechanism has been extensively studied in cows, horses, pigs, and sheep. Lymph is the major transport route of these immunoglobulins (98, 403, 412). Not only natural substances such as colostrum globulins but also foreign macromolecules such as polyvinylpyrrolidone (160,000 mol wt) are absorbed by the newborn calf intestine and transported in intestinal lymph (200).

## COLON

There are comparatively few studies of colonic lymph. Under control (empty lumen) conditions, canine colonic lymph flow is $\sim 15$ $\mu$l·min$^{-1}$·100 g$^{-1}$ and has a protein concentration of 3.5 g/100 ml and an L/P of 0.52 (258, 381). As mentioned in *Lymphatics of Gastrointestinal Organs*, COLON, p. 1740, colonic lymphatics are relatively inconspicuous on histological examination. In a study of the permeability characteristics of the colonic microcirculation, it has been shown that, as in the small intestine, elevation of venous pressure increases colonic lymph flow and protein flux and the transcapillary oncotic pressure gradient, whereas the $C_L/C_P$ falls (381). Compared with the small intestinal lymph, however, colonic lymph flow plays a relatively unimportant part in preventing interstitial edema of the large intestine consequent on venous pressure elevation, that is, contributing only $\sim 4\%$ of the total edema safety factor in response to an estimated increment of 12 mmHg in microvascular hydrostatic pressure (381).

Colonic lymph, similarly, appears to take little part in the disturbances of hydration of the mucosal interstitium during net transmural fluid movement. In an isolated autoperfused canine colon preparation, stimulation of active fluid absorption and secretion produced no change in colonic lymph flow, lymph protein flux, or lymph oncotic pressure (258). Thus volume and hydrostatic pressure changes of the colonic mucosal interstitium do not appear to alter colonic lymph flow, in contrast with the situation in the small intestine where net fluid absorption enhances lymph flow (178), and active fluid secretion (in response, for example, to cholera toxin) diminishes lymph flow (174). Because colonic lymph plays no part in the transport of absorbed fluid, the considerable amounts of fluid absorbed by the normal colon must all enter the capillaries. The relative paucity of colonic mucosal lymphatics may account for this.

## PANCREAS

Little information is available on this subject. In 1971, Papp and his colleagues (352, 353) succeeded in collecting canine pancreaticoduodenal lymph, demonstrating that its pH is higher than that of arterial blood and measuring lipase output in response to pancreatic secretagogues.

The flow of lymph from the resting dog pancreas is low, being estimated at 0.009 ml·min$^{-1}$·100 g$^{-1}$ tissue (257). This is in striking contrast to the high lymph flows obtained from salivary glands. This low pancreatic lymph flow does not represent the total resting transcapillary filtration rate, because the basal secretion rate of the pancreas, 0.005 ml·min$^{-1}$·100·g$^{-1}$, should be added to give a net transcapillary filtration rate of $\sim 0.014$ ml·min$^{-1}$·100 g$^{-1}$ (176). Capillary hydrostatic pressure in the pancreas is very low, $\sim 3$ mmHg, probably the result of an extensive portal circulation in the gland (257, 292). The observed rate of capillary filtration in the pancreas is low compared with its capillary filtration coefficient, which indicates a low net filtration pressure across the capillaries. The calculated tissue fluid pressure ($P_t$) is remarkably low (ca. $-6.6$ mmHg), suggesting a dry interstitium. In light of this very low $P_t$, it is difficult to understand why lymph flows from the resting pancreas at all.

Pancreatic secretion can be driven by secretin to a level $\sim 30$ times the basal net transcapillary filtration rate (257). To provide this fluid, it has been proposed that an increase in capillary surface area or changes in the interstitial forces, such as a rise in tissue fluid oncotic pressure, are responsible. To elucidate the mechanisms, one would need to obtain flow rates and lymph samples during active pancreatic secretion. Hitherto these data have not been obtained.

From many older studies with indirect methods, it has been suggested that under certain circumstances pancreatic enzymes enter lymph and thence reach the systemic blood. These investigations generally relied on measurements of increases in pancreatic enzymes in thoracic duct lymph in response to pancreatic secretagogues, in some cases in combination with agents such as morphine that increase the resistance to pancreatic juice flow to the duodenum (30, 125, 129, 353, 464). The quantitative importance of this route for transport of pancreatic enzymes to the blood is dubious.

## LIVER

### Liver Microcirculation

The major microvascular bed in the liver is the sinusoidal system, in which hepatic arterial and portal venous blood mix in a proportion of ~30:70. The microscopic appearance of the sinusoid suggests that it is a highly porous structure allowing free access of most plasma solutes to the hepatocyte surface (for reviews see refs. 209, 238, 479, 480). No basement membrane is recognized in relation to human or rat sinusoidal endothelium. Wisse (479) has described the vessel as lined by fenestrated endothelium with no diaphragm closing the fenestrae. The diameter of the apertures of the sinusoids is reported to range between 0.1 and 0.5 $\mu$m, though some very large fenestral openings (0.5–2.0 $\mu$m) are also seen. Beneath the endothelium lies the space of Disse, a major interstitial space of the liver that has a depth of ~0.5 $\mu$m. The space dilates greatly when hepatic venous pressure is increased (58). There is free communication between the space of Disse and the interstitial spaces around the central veins and in the portal tracts. The contents of the space include a few bundles of collagen fibers, small fat-storing cells, and some VLDL particles. The microvilli of the hepatocytes, which form a boundary of this space, are occasionally seen in electron micrographs passing across the space and penetrating the apertures of the sinusoidal endothelium.

The free access of plasma to the perisinusoidal space of Disse through the fenestrae of the sinusoidal endothelium has led to the concept of a paravascular space, which in dogs has been estimated to be ~6% of the liver weight (162). In the portal tracts a few branches from the interlobular arteries give rise to a dense capillary network, the peribiliary capillary plexus, which surrounds the bile ductule and which drains by short venous vessels to the sinusoids. These capillaries are of the continuous type (447).

Liver lymph is generally considered to arise from the sinusoidal filtrate in the space of Disse (25, 65, 66), though morphological evidence to support this is not available. Modification of the sinusoidal filtrate would result from its mixing with the filtrate from the peribiliary capillary plexus in the portal tract. From morphological considerations, it is likely that the protein concentration of the filtrate from the peribiliary capillaries is lower than that of the sinusoidal filtrate. The relative magnitude of the contributions of the two types of filtrate to hepatic lymph, however, is unknown, though many investigators assume that the peribiliary capillary filtrate contributes <10% of the total liver lymph flow.

### Liver Lymph Flow

Hepatic lymph makes a major contribution to thoracic duct flow. In the dog this contribution has been estimated to be as large as 25%–50% (73, 334) and in the cat ~30% (327). Accurate estimates of total hepatic lymph flow, however, are difficult to obtain. The extreme sensitivity of hepatic lymph flow to venous pressure elevation such as may occur during any form of manipulation of the liver and the difficulty in ensuring complete liver lymph collection as a result of the anatomical disposition of the vessels are major obstacles to measuring total liver lymph flow. Bollman and his colleagues (57), who pioneered chronic lymph fistula preparations in the rat, found flows of ~5 ml/24 h, similar to values obtained by others (147, 300, 455). Rabbit hepatic lymph flows range between 0.8 and 12 ml/h in anesthetized animals (107), and in calves Shannon and Lascelles (402) have reported flow rates of 0.64 ml·kg$^{-1}$ body wt·h$^{-1}$. For various species, a figure of 0.4–0.6 ml·kg$^{-1}$ liver·min$^{-1}$ has been reported (66); because liver blood flow is ~1 liter·kg$^{-1}$ liver·min$^{-1}$, the ratio of liver lymph to blood flow is 1:2,000. This can be compared with a ratio of 1:1,000 for small intestine (183).

### Proteins of Liver Lymph

Of all the regional lymphs, that from the liver has the highest protein concentration. Table 9 presents data for the $C_L/C_P$ of hepatic lymph for various species, whereas Tables 10 and 11 present the $C_L/C_P$ for various plasma protein species in the rabbit and the dog. From these data one can conclude that there is some permselectivity of the blood/lymph barrier in the liver, though the anatomical basis for this selectivity is not clear. In most tissues other than the liver

TABLE 9. *Lymph-to-Plasma Total Protein Concentration Ratios for Hepatic Lymph in Various Species*

| Species | $C_L/C_P$ | Ref. |
| --- | --- | --- |
| Dog | 0.95 | 261 |
| Cat | 0.80 | 171 |
| Rat | 0.68 | 147 |
| Rabbit | 0.86 | 101 |
| Calf | 0.81 | 402 |
| Sheep | 0.76 | 328 |

TABLE 10. *Lymph-to-Plasma Concentration Ratios for Hepatic Lymph of Various Proteins in the Rabbit*

| Protein | $C_L/C_P$ |
|---|---|
| Albumin | 0.95 |
| $\alpha$-Globulin | 0.75 |
| $\beta$-Globulin | 0.71 |
| $\gamma$-Globulin | 0.74 |

[Data from Woolley and Courtice (490).]

TABLE 11. *Lymph-to-Plasma Concentration Ratios for Hepatic Lymph of Various Plasma Protein Species in the Dog*

| Protein | Approximate Mol Wt | $C_L/C_P$ |
|---|---|---|
| Orosomucoid | 44,000 | 0.874 |
| Albumin | 69,000 | 0.833 |
| Transferrin | 90,000 | 0.773 |
| $I_gG_{2ab}$ | 160,000 | 0.650 |
| $\alpha_2$-Macroglobulin | 820,000 | 0.506 |
| IgM | 1,000,000 | 0.471 |

[Data from Dive et al. (110).]

$C_L/C_P$ for plasma proteins falls progressively as capillary filtration rate increases; this is termed the *washdown* effect (440). At very high lymph flows, $C_L/C_P$ reaches a minimum independent of capillary filtration rate. This phenomenon has been used to define the permeability characteristics of the capillaries to plasma proteins. In the normal liver the converse occurs, and $C_L/C_P$ rises toward unity at high lymph flows, suggesting a loss of permselectivity of the blood/lymph barrier (171). This phenomenon is discussed later in this section.

Although filtration from the plasma is the major source of liver lymph protein, a number of early studies raised the question of whether lymph provides a major route of delivery of newly synthesized protein, notably albumin, from the hepatocyte to the circulation. More recent investigations with radiolabeled albumin, $\gamma$-globulin, and fibrinogen have indicated that hepatic lymph proteins are largely derived from plasma (10, 417, 490). One can regard the space of Disse as a mixing pool for filtered plasma protein and newly synthesized protein secreted by the hepatocyte. If proteins are freely exchangeable across the sinusoidal wall, the transport of newly synthesized molecules of albumin by blood and lymph will be broadly determined by the relative flow rates in these two systems.

*Formation of Liver Lymph*

Although it is presently not possible to make a separate study of transcapillary fluid and solute filtration from the sinusoidal and peribiliary microcirculation, morphological considerations lead one to expect considerable differences in the balance of Starling forces operating in these two cases. In view of the high degree of porosity of the sinusoidal wall, one would anticipate that no effective transsinusoidal oncotic pressure gradient exists (i.e., $\sigma_d$ would be close to zero); thus small increments in hydrostatic pressure would lead to brisk filtration. This is borne out by a 10- to 20-fold increase in protein-rich lymph flow in the thoracic duct observed nearly a century ago by Starling in response to constriction of the suprahepatic inferior vena cava (420). In animals subjected to hepatic venous obstruction, a marked dilatation of the space of Disse (58) accompanies engorgement of the central veins and sinusoids. The continuous endothelium of the peribiliary capillary plexus, which probably has sieving properties similar to those of the capillaries of skeletal muscle, would be expected to filter a relatively protein-poor fluid.

From measurements of portal and hepatic venous pressures and hepatic interstitial fluid pressure in the dog liver, Laine et al. (261) have concluded that sinusoidal hydrostatic pressure normally lies between 5.8 and 7.0 mmHg and that 90% of an increment of hepatic venous pressure is transmitted back to the sinusoids. Using capsules, these same authors have estimated that 70% of a rise in sinusoidal pressure is transmitted to the interstitial fluid pressure, suggesting a low interstitial compliance in the liver. This in turn drives liver lymph flow up, thus the main edema safety factors in the liver in response to a small increment in venous pressure are a rise in tissue hydrostatic pressure and a brisk lymph flow (see Table 2).

In most tissues, experimental reduction of plasma oncotic pressure produces a greater increment in lymph flow than does elevation of venous pressure. In the liver, however, the converse is true (171), an indication of the extremely low reflection coefficient of the sinusoidal endothelium.

As can be seen from Table 9, the ratio $C_L/C_P$ for plasma proteins in liver lymph is high, but Tables 10 and 11 also present data that demonstrate that there is some selectivity of the blood/lymph barrier in the liver toward these macromolecules. From studies in which the hepatic artery was ligated, Szabo and Magyar (431) proposed that there is a degree of restriction to macromolecules at the sinusoidal membrane. Nevertheless on ultrastructural evidence, the sinusoidal wall is unlikely to act as the sieve except for very large molecules of molecular weight >1,000,000 and particles such as lipoproteins (209). With an intravenous infusion of polymethacrylate particles as large as 70 nm in diameter (of the same order of size as VLDL), Grotte et al. (193, 194) have shown that some of these particles can pass from plasma to hepatic lymph. A possible explanation for the selectivity of the hepatic blood/lymph barrier is that it is mainly due to the sieve properties of the peribiliary capillaries. Their permeability characteristics are likely to resemble those of other continuous capillary beds, though this has never been examined. Figure 9 illustrates the relation between molecular size of various proteins and the ratios of their $C_L/C_P$ to that of albumin. It can be seen that although permselectivity is present under normal conditions, this disappears at elevated venous pressures, the converse of what happens in other tissues such as the small intestine. A possible explanation for this observation is that in the liver the sieve is located not in the sinusoidal wall but in the interstitium. It is known that the hepatic interstitium can exclude a proportion of albumin and other macromolecules (28) and thus may function as a sieve. When the interstitium is greatly hydrated, its mesh would open and its sieving properties would be abolished. As already discussed, sinusoidal filtration is very sensitive to venous pressure elevation, whereas peribiliary capillaries could be expected to be less affected by such a change. Thus the loss of permselectivity at high venous pressures may represent a disproportionate contribution by sinusoidal filtrate to liver lymph.

Another possible filter is the wall of the initial lymphatics. Unless liver lymphatics are different from those of other tissues, however, this is unlikely. Data of Rutili and Arfors (387), who demonstrated that the protein concentration of interstitial fluid and lymph in initial vessels in subcutaneous tissue were similar, argue against a significant filtration effect at the lymphatic wall, although this question can only be settled by a study of the permeability characteristics of the initial lymphatic vessels of the liver.

The idea of the hepatic interstitial matrix as the permselective barrier between blood and lymph is attractive, but to establish this as the mechanism will require methods for studying independently the permeability characteristics of the sinusoids and the peribiliary capillaries.

*Lipids of Liver Lymph*

The liver, like the intestine, is an important source of plasma lipoproteins. The liver is the major contributor to plasma VLDL, whereas the intestine and liver share in contribution to plasma HDL. From studies with cultured hepatocytes, it has been proposed that the liver may also secrete LDL (35). Lipoprotein particles synthesized in the hepatocyte are released by exocytosis into the space of Disse (238), from which they may have restricted access to the blood or may travel in hepatic lymph. Thus sampling hepatic lymph affords an opportunity to study nascent lipoproteins derived from the hepatocyte. Until recently little was known about lipid and lipoproteins of hepatic lymph. Friedman and colleagues (147) reported that rat lymph had cholesterol concentrations approximately two-thirds those of plasma. The fatty acid output from rat liver via lymph has been estimated at 2-3 $\mu$eq/h, whereas the sinusoidal blood transports 100-150 $\mu$eq/h (31). Studies in rabbits, sheep, and calves have

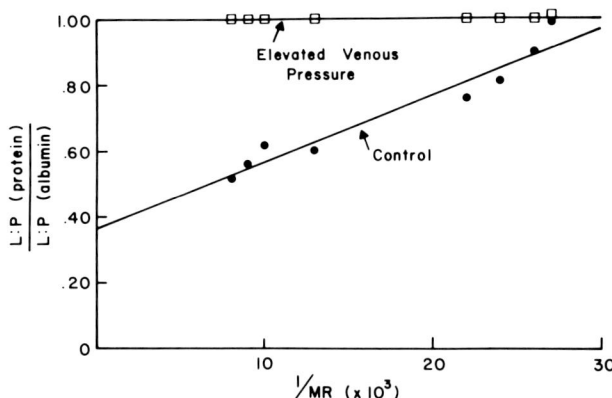

FIG. 9. Relation between lymph-to-plasma protein concentration ratio (L/P) normalized to albumin ratio and reciprocal of molecular radius (MR) in cat liver. [Data from Granger et al. (171).]

shown that the triglyceride, phospholipid, and cholesterol concentrations in hepatic lymph are ~70% those of plasma (4, 101).

A recent study in rats with chronic hepatic lymph fistulas has shown that the L/P for triglyceride, phospholipid, and cholesterol are ~59%, 57%, and 79%, respectively (455). The output of triglyceride in liver lymph is estimated, in this preparation, to be <1% of the total liver triglyceride output. Agarose gel electrophoresis of liver lymph shows two principal lipoproteins, $\alpha$-migrating HDL and hepatic VLDL that migrates between the plasma and pre-$\beta$-lipoproteins. Although hepatic lymph and plasma VLDL are of similar size (~60 nm diam), there are significant differences in their chemical composition. Hepatic lymph VLDL has significantly less apoC than plasma VLDL, and the apoB of hepatic VLDL exists mainly as the small apoB$_{240K}$ (~240,000 mol wt), whereas the apoB of plasma VLDL is composed equally of apoB$_{240K}$ and apoB$_{330K}$ (~330,000 mol wt). Interestingly, hepatic lymph VLDL has a higher apoB$_{240K}$-to-apoB$_{330K}$ ratio than VLDL obtained from isolated perfused rat liver (301). It is possible that a small fraction of the apoB$_{240K}$-rich VLDL particles tends to be retained by the endothelial lining of the liver sinusoids and contributes disproportionately to hepatic lymph. This observation tends to favor the hypothesis that newly secreted hepatic VLDL particles contain either apoB$_{240K}$ or apoB$_{330K}$.

*Pathophysiology of Liver Lymph*

HEPATIC CONGESTION. The effects on liver lymph flow of acute hepatic congestion resulting from hepatic venous obstruction have already been described. The liver in a plethysmograph responds in 5-15 min to venous obstruction by swelling (188, 189). Vascular distension is followed by increased filtration, hepatic edema (i.e., distension of the space of Disse), and transcapsular fluid filtration. This filtrate has a protein concentration of ~80% of that of plasma. In the clinical situation, acute hepatic venous obstruction leads to swelling of the liver and rapid accumulation of excess fluid in the peritoneal cavity as ascites with a high protein content. Although high liver lymph flow accompanies this, the transcapsular filtration represents the failure of liver lymph flow to compensate for the high filtration rate across the sinusoidal wall. On the other hand, chronic hepatic venous obstruction leads to fibrotic changes in the liver, developing first in the centrizonal regions. This eventually links with the fibrous tissue of neighboring centrizonal areas, producing changes described as cardiac cirrhosis. At a later stage, fibrosis extends to involve the portal zones. Other changes are also observed: collagen is deposited in the space of Disse and a basement membrane develops in relation to the sinusoidal endothelium (385, 396). This "capillarization" of the sinusoids results in these vessels taking on the appearances of continuous capillaries. The histologic changes in the liver in chronic congestion lead to obstruction to blood flow and reduced sinusoidal permeability with portal hypertension. This in turn leads to increased fluid filtration in the splanchnic bed, with increased intestinal lymph flow and a contribution to the ascitic fluid from the intestinal microcirculation (481). This contribution contains lower concentrations of protein than that of the transcapsular filtrate from the liver in acute hepatic venous congestion, though the protein concentration of the transcapsular filtrate in chronic congestion could be expected to be reduced as a result of capillarization of the sinusoids (385). The hemodynamic changes in chronic hepatic congestion thus bear some resemblance to those in cirrhosis.

CIRRHOSIS. Greatly elevated hepatic and intestinal lymph flows are a well-recognized feature of hepatic cirrhosis and other forms of portal hypertension (127). These effects are attributable to hydrostatic pressure disturbances in the hepatic and splanchnic microcirculations resulting from obstruction to blood flow at the sinusoidal and postsinusoidal level, together with increased arterial inflow into the splanchnic vascular bed. At the same time capillarization of the sinusoids alters the permeability characteristics of these vessels (27, 207, 209, 396). These changes further contribute to the development of hypertension in the splanchnic vascular bed. In a study of rats with carbon tetrachloride–induced cirrhosis, intestinal and liver lymph flows were increased 3- and 30-fold, respectively, over control values (27). Analysis of $C_L/C_P$ suggested that capillary permeability in the small intestine during sustained portal hypertension is similar to that in normal animals but that the ordinarily highly permeable blood/lymph barrier of the liver becomes restrictive in cirrhosis.

ASCITES IN CIRRHOSIS. Two filtrates, from the hepatic and from the splanchnic microcirculations, contribute variable proportions of fluid and protein in cirrhotic ascites. The protein concentration of the fluid, usually between 5 and 20 g/liter, is chiefly determined by the proportions of these two contributions (481). Various factors alter these proportions. These include the stage in evolution of the disease process and surgical procedures designed to decompress the hypertensive splanchnic vascular bed. The primary disturbance is the result of hypertension of these two microcirculations. Hypoalbuminemia, which is common in cirrhosis, contributes relatively little, because the washdown of protein concentration in the transcapillary filtrate from the splanchnic microcirculation at high filtration rates widens the transcapillary oncotic pressure gradient, thus opposing further filtration (483). Zimmon et al. (496), however, have provided evidence for the delivery of a proportion of newly synthesized albumin to the ascitic fluid from the liver in cirrhosis that would favor further fluid accumulation in the peritoneal cavity. This movement of albumin from the hepatocytes to the peritoneal cavity probably by the transcapsular route might be the result of a reduced sinusoidal permeability from capillarization.

The peritoneal cavity is primarily drained by diaphragmatic lymphatics that contribute to flow in the right lymph duct. Ordinarily the flow in the right lymph duct is one-twentieth that of the thoracic duct (432). The rate of fluid absorption from the peritoneal cavity has been shown to be a function of the pressure of the ascitic fluid, though at high pressures compression of the hepatic veins and intra-abdominal lymphatics complicates this relationship (497).

In cirrhotic ascites, therefore, intestinal and hepatic lymph flows are greatly elevated but are insufficient to prevent accumulation of intraperitoneal fluid, and even increased flow through the diaphragmatic lymphatics and right lymph duct is unable to clear the collected fluid.

In addition to altered Starling forces in the pathogenesis of ascites, it is recognized that there is abnormal renal salt and water retention under endocrine control, though its relation to the hemodynamic disturbances is unclear. Several theories attempt to unify these various factors, but analysis of these is beyond the scope of this chapter. One theory, however, that of lymph imbalance, put forward by Witte et al. (482), concentrates on the discrepancy between the rate of fluid input into the peritoneal cavity and its rate of return to blood via lymphatics; thus in early cirrhosis as portal venous pressure rises, intestinal lymphatics and the thoracic duct remove progressively more interstitial fluid from the gut while the diaphragmatic lymphatics take up any surplus fluid from the peritoneal cavity. Due to the relatively low transport capacity of the right lymph duct, clearance of the peritoneal cavity fails and a discrepancy between fluid leaving the circulation and returning to it arises. Certain lymphatic factors may contribute to the problem, including incompetence of the valves of distended mesenteric lymphatics, scarring with obliteration of diaphragmatic lymphatics, and flow resistance between the thoracic duct and the venous system at the jugulosubclavian tap. According to this theory, depletion of intravascular volume would lead to activation of the renin-angiotensin system, resulting in salt and water retention. In support of this theory (see ref. 482) are the observations that surgical procedures that reduce portal venous pressure (portacaval shunts) or improve lymph drainage (by insertion of a wide-bore peritoneal-venous shunt) restore salt and water homeostatic mechanisms to normal, suppressing the renin-angiotensin system. Refashioning the thoracic duct–venous junction has a similar effect. Support for the theory has also been obtained from estimates of lymphatic conductance (flow rate per unit pressure difference) in cirrhotic patients with and without ascites (208).

CHOLESTASIS. Biliary obstruction leads to enhanced liver lymph flow (107, 147). Experimental data suggest that in humans and in dogs hepatic lymph may be a significant route of transport of bile pigments to the blood during the early phases of acute biliary obstruction (51, 77, 124, 126, 160, 199, 299, 310, 382, 401, 476, 484). In chronic biliary obstruction, however, the bile pigment of lymph is probably derived from the plasma by transcapillary filtration. Similarly in early acute biliary obstruction, bile salt transport via lymph rises to 70 times the values observed in the normal situation (433, 434). It is possible that in early biliary obstruction, bile constituents leak into the interstitial space of the portal tracts and gain ready access to initial liver lymphatics.

## PATHOPHYSIOLOGY OF GASTROINTESTINAL LYMPHATICS

In some measure, lymphatics are involved in any pathological process. An important example is their role in the dissemination of epithelial malignant tumors arising in the gut and its associated structures. This section chiefly considers the role of disordered lymphatic function in the pathogenesis of selected gastrointestinal diseases.

### Primary Intestinal Lymphangiectasia

This condition, a form of protein-losing enteropathy, was first described by Waldmann et al. in 1961 (466). Although not well characterized, the condition is believed to result from congenital structural abnormalities in the lymphatics of the intestinal wall or its mesentery, resulting in impaired drainage of the initial mucosal lymphatic vessels. The disorder has also been observed in dogs (75, 138, 356). It is frequently associated with congenital lymphatic abnormalities in other regions such as the limbs, thus asymmetric peripheral lymphedema may also be present. Chylous effusions in the pleural or peritoneal cavity are occasionally associated with intestinal lymphangiectasia. The condition has been considered to be rare, but more recently it has been suggested that if the diagnosis is suspected and investigations are pursued, it may prove to be not uncommon (384, 463). If only a small segment of the intestine is affected, there may be no clinical disturbance that would warrant investigation. Although the condition generally affects the small intestine, it may also involve the large intestine and in some instances occur only in the colon (190, 227, 395). Little is known about the pathogenesis of the primary form of lymphangiectasia, though some studies in humans and dogs suggest that developmental abnormalities of lymphatic vessels may be heritable; it is proposed that an autosomal dominant gene with complete penetrance and variable expressivity is responsible (132, 356, 488).

The affected segments of the intestine often have a brownish pigmentation due to deposition of lipofuscin in the muscle. The central lymphatics of the intestinal villi are dilated (143) and filled with protein and lipid-rich lymph, and the villi are clubbed as a result of mucosal edema; submucosal lymphatics are dilated. Occasionally the mucosa ulcerates. Mucosal biopsy shows lipid particles in the mucosal interstitium, in the dilated lymph vessels, and in macrophages in the lamina propria. Foamy PAS (periodic acid–Schiff)-positive and lipofuscin-laden macrophages and occasional multinucleated giant cells are found in the lamina propria adjacent to lymphatics. Electron-microscopic changes in the endothelium of the mucosal lymphatics in intestinal lymphangiectasia (i.e., increase in basement membrane material and the presence of prominent intracellular fibrils, with increased amounts of collagen associated with the vessels) have been considered to reflect sustained high pressure within the lymphatics (111).

Intestinal lymphangiectasia should be distinguished from lymphangiectatic cysts of the small intestine. These latter are generally confined to the submucosa and have been said to occur in 20% of necropsies. No PAS-positive macrophages are found in the lamina propria in this condition (405).

The clinical features and biochemical disturbances of intestinal lymphangiectasia can be explained by impaired lymphatic transport function together with efflux or transudation of mucosal interstitial fluid and lymph across the intestinal epithelial membrane. Both by intubation (424) and direct endoscopy (12), chylous fluid has been found in the small intestinal lumen and radiographic contrast medium has been shown leaking into the gut at lymphangiography (59). A recent report describes the intestinal leak of contrast medium during abdominal lymphoscintigraphy with $^{99m}$Tc antimony colloid in a patient with intestinal lymphangiectasia (418).

The condition, although mostly affecting children and young adults, has been described in older patients.

Gastrointestinal symptoms are generally mild, though abdominal pain, nausea, vomiting, and diarrhea with steatorrhea can occur. Severe protein depletion can lead to hypoproteinemic edema; in children, nutritional problems can cause impaired growth. The enteric loss of protein leads to a reduced concentration of all species of plasma protein, notably albumin, as a result of its relatively long half-life (231). Serum calcium is low and concentrations of immunoglobulins in plasma are reduced, which, together with a loss of lymphocytes, leads to demonstrable defects of immunological function (427). The degree of steatorrhea is variable, whereas tests of carbohydrate absorption are generally normal.

Diagnosis is made by demonstration of protein-losing enteropathy and by mucosal biopsy showing the pathological features just described. Various isotope techniques with radiolabeled proteins or dextrans have been employed to demonstrate abnormal intestinal protein loss, the most popular at present being the $^{51}$Cr excretion test. Fecal clearance of endogenous $\alpha_1$-antitrypsin, however, offers considerable promise as a simpler means of demonstrating protein-losing enteropathy (360).

Other than in a few cases where a short affected segment of the small intestine can be resected or a lymphovenous anastomosis can be created where there is a localized anomaly (324), the treatment consists of reduction of the dietary load of long-chain triglyceride (231). This is effective not only in reducing the lipid required to be transported by the lymphatics but also reduces intestinal lymph formation, because fat feeding is a powerful intestinal lymphagogue. A clear increase in the half-life of endogenous albumin results from a low-fat diet (Fig. 10). Substitution of medium-chain triglyceride in the diet improves nutrition (216, 445), though from animal studies it might be anticipated to have less effect than overall reduction of dietary fat on enteric protein loss, because medium-chain triglycerides, like long-chain triglycerides, enhance intestinal lymph flow and lymphatic protein flux (457). In some patients, dietary or parenteral supplementation of trace nutrients (e.g., fat-soluble vitamins) may be necessary.

*Secondary Intestinal Lymphangiectasia*

Any pathological process that results in obstruction of major lymph trunks draining the intestine leads to secondary intestinal lymphangiectasia (143). In this category are inflammatory processes such as tuberculosis or Crohn's disease involving the intestine or mesentery and inflammation of the retroperitoneal tissues. The latter group includes chronic pancreatitis and retroperitoneal fibrosis. Neoplasia, notably lymphoma, is also an important cause of intestinal lymphatic obstruction. Intestinal lymphangiectasia has also been said to occur in Behçet's disease (13); the pathogenesis of lymphangiectasia in this condition is

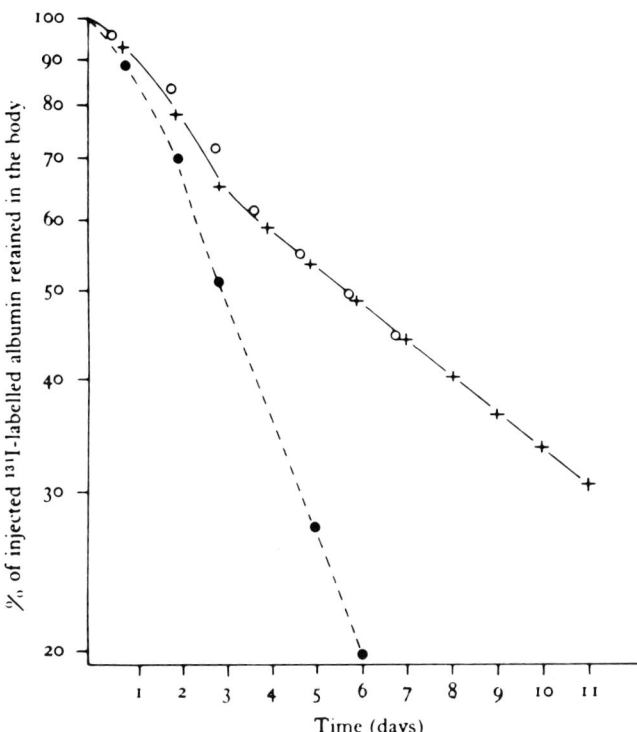

FIG. 10. Turnover of $^{131}$I-labeled albumin in patient with intestinal lymphangiectasia. *Closed circles* represent decay while patient was on 70 g/day fat diet. *Open circles* and *crosses* represent albumin decay on low-fat diet (5 g/day). [From Jeffries et al. (231).]

unclear. Although filariasis commonly affects the lymphatics draining the lower limbs and scrotum, obstruction of intestinal lymphatics by microfilariae has been documented as a cause of secondary intestinal lymphangiectasia (319). In hypobeta-lipoproteinemia, fat-containing macrophages occupying mesenteric lymph nodes have been considered to be a cause of lymphatic obstruction and lymphangiectasia (112). A moderate degree of secondary intestinal lymphangiectasia is observed in Whipple's disease (449); this may also be the result of infiltration of lymph nodes with PAS-positive macrophages similar to those found in the intestinal mucosa in this disease.

In cirrhotic patients with evidence of enteric loss of plasma proteins, intestinal lymphangiectasia has been observed in small intestinal biopsies (70), and in rats with carbon tetrachloride–induced cirrhosis a similar change has been documented (325). Partial obstruction of the portal vein leads to a striking dilatation of lymphatics of the intestinal mucosa (492). Treatment of the various underlying diseases in secondary intestinal lymphangiectasia may relieve the obstruction.

*Intestinal Lymphangiectasia Secondary to Heart Disease*

Various cardiac lesions have been shown to be associated with intestinal lymphangiectasia and gastrointestinal protein loss. These include constrictive pericarditis, cardiomyopathies, and some congenital heart diseases (105, 116, 230, 240). Two explanations for this effect have been put forward. Systemic venous hypertension, by impeding thoracic duct lymph flow, would lead to back pressure in the lymphatic system with incompetence of valves and consequent dilatation of initial lymph vessels in the intestinal mucosa together with mucosal edema. The alternative explanation proposes that portal venous hypertension, resulting from hepatic congestion, leads to enhanced capillary filtration in the splanchnic bed and overload of lymphatics. In various forms of portal hypertension, intestinal lymph flow is greatly increased, with intestinal mucosal edema and lymphangiectasia frequent, though not invariable, findings. The numbers of lymphatic vessels in the mesentery are also increased. Interestingly, thickening of the muscle of the mesenteric and intestinal lymph vessels has been observed in patients with cirrhosis and heart failure, suggesting a response to sustained raised intralymphatic pressure (380). It is probable that both of these mechanisms operate in heart disease. Experimental constrictive pericarditis has been shown to cause a rise in pressure in the thoracic duct and dilatation of the vessel (42). In some cases, involvement of the thoracic duct in the fibrosing process may cause direct obstruction to lymph flow (400, 437). Ligation of the thoracic duct in dogs leads to increased enteric loss of labeled macromolecules from the circulation (302).

*Experimental Interruption of Intestinal Lymphatics*

In a study of lymphatic drainage of the dog colon, Sterns and Vaughan (423) resected the lymphatics responsible for the drainage of the rectosigmoid region. This produced local intestinal edema that resolved partially or completely over three weeks when collateral lymphatic circulation had become established, as demonstrated by the opacification of nonregional lymph nodes after injection of radiographic contrast medium into the bowel segment.

It has proved difficult to create experimental models of intestinal lymphangiectasia, because obstruction of lymph vessels leads to the opening of lymphatic collaterals and lymphaticovenous anastomoses (241, 242). The latter channels open in response to raised intralymphatic pressure. Since lymphangiectasia has been described on several occasions in dogs, attempts have been made to create the condition in this species by ligation of major lymph trunks and injection of sclerosants, a technique first described by Drinker in the 1930s (119). Bank et al. (23) were unable to reproduce the histological appearance of lymphangiectasia with this combination, but Danese et al. (104, 150) were successful when complete interruption of the small intestinal lymphatic drainage was achieved with ligation and extensive intralymphatic injection of sclerosants. Short-term obstruction of ileal lymphatics in rats produces edema and hyperemia of the mucosa with dilatation of the central villus lymph vessel. Chronic lymphatic obstruction leads to marked inflammation with prominent accumulation of chronic inflammatory cells, appearances somewhat reminiscent of Crohn's disease. It is of interest that enhanced enteric losses of circulating macromolecules have been observed in animals with lymphatic interruption but without histological evidence of intestinal lymphangiectasia (302). It seems that lymphedema and transudation of a protein-rich fluid into the gut lumen is a common response to partial lymphatic obstruction and that the histological appearance of intestinal lymphangiectasia represents a complete obstruction with no effective compensatory mechanisms decompressing the lymphatic vessels.

*Inflammatory Bowel Disease*

Edema is a prominent histopathological feature of all forms of inflammatory bowel disease (220, 251). The pathogenesis of this edema is complex. There is evidence that capillary permeability is enhanced as a result of local liberation of chemical mediators of inflammation such as histamine, serotonin, bradykinin, and other such substances (251). Bacterial endotoxins may also produce enhanced vascular permeability to protein (251), as may oxygen free radicals derived from leukocyte activity (192). Increases in capillary hydrostatic pressure also contribute to intestinal edema in inflammatory bowel disease. Vascular congestion, particularly in the mucosa-submucosa layers, is marked in active disease (220), and blood flow to the colon in patients with inflammatory bowel disease has been shown by isotope washout methods to be increased two to six times. Hulten et al. (220) have established that in active colitis colonic blood flow may reach 1,500 ml/min (i.e., ~30% of the cardiac output), though during the late fibrosing stages of the idiopathic inflammatory bowel diseases colonic blood flow may actually fall below normal values. The enhanced lymph flow in experimental colonic inflammation in dogs (333) is probably the result of a combination of increased capillary hydrostatic pressure and increased capillary permeability. Sheppard and Sterns (404) have demonstrated increased lymphatic clearance of albumin from the dog colon in experimental colitis.

The extent to which abnormalities of lymphatic drainage play a part in edema of the intestine in inflammatory bowel disease is not clear. In Crohn's disease, lymphatic dilatation in all layers of the bowel wall, notably the submucosa, is a feature of the condition. It has frequently been suggested that an element of lymphatic obstruction from inflammatory changes in adjacent tissues and lymph nodes may be involved. Endothelial swelling in small blood vessels and lymphatics is often present. In addition, a defect in function of intestinal lymphatic vessels may occur in Crohn's disease. In ultrastructural studies, changes have been described in the initial lymphatics that may indicate decreased permeability of these vessels (256). These include a lack of open intercellular junctions noted in normal lymphatics, the development of a more complete thick basement membrane, and the accumulation of protein-rich fluid in the interstitium, suggesting a permeability barrier at the lymphatic wall. Whether these changes are primary or are secondary to lymphatic hypertension or are produced by the inflammatory process (e.g., in response to some chemical mediator) is not known, nor is it clear where such changes would fit into the overall pathological process.

*Acute Pancreatitis*

In both acute interstitial (edematous) pancreatitis and necrotizing (hemorrhagic) pancreatitis, there is gross edema of the gland (262, 397). Distended lymphatics are prominent as in any acutely inflamed tissue (223) and suggest enhanced transcapillary fluid filtration, the result of hyperemia and increased microvascular permeability (118). In sheep, experimental acute pancreatitis is accompanied by a rise in thoracic duct lymph flow with a fall in the protein concentration of the lymph (298). The explanation of this effect is not known. It seems unlikely that lymphatic obstruction plays a primary role in the pathogenesis of acute pancreatitis, but some evidence suggests that lymphatic obstruction may aggravate the autodigestive process by allowing the accumulation of toxic products in the tissue (351).

In the early stages of acute pancreatitis, considerable amounts of pancreatic enzymes and tissue digestion products are drained from the gland by both venous blood and lymph (305). The pattern of disseminated fat necrosis has been observed to follow the route of lymph drainage (362). The enzymes form macromolecular complexes with their digestion products [e.g., trypsin-antitrypsin (344)], and these large molecular aggregates tend to drain into lymphatics rather than capillaries. Papp et al. (352) have shown that, in experimental acute pancreatitis in dogs, the levels of lipase in pancreaticoduodenal lymph exceed those of portal venous blood. The early rise in serum amylase and lipase in acute pancreatitis is not prevented by thoracic duct drainage, but after 1 h, when serum levels of the enzymes have stabilized, lymph diversion markedly reduces these concentrations, suggesting that there is an important contribution via lymph to circulating enzymes at this stage of the condition (408).

Drainage of these various substances from the pancreas seems to be beneficial in that obstruction of lymph flow in experimental acute pancreatitis in dogs and rabbits increases the inflammatory process (128, 351). Early in the course of experimental pancreatitis in dogs, lymph flow is markedly enhanced, but subsequently this falls as lymphatic vessels are obstructed by coagulated proteins or red cell aggregates that presumably aggravate the tissue damage (408). It has been suggested that thoracic duct drainage in patients with acute pancreatitis might be beneficial in preventing reabsorbed vasoactive substances from reaching the circulation (69). In a study of patients with acute alcoholic pancreatitis, however, this has not been found to be true (425).

*Miscellaneous Conditions Involving Gastrointestinal Lymphatics*

Chylous mesenteric cysts are relatively uncommon entities thought to represent congenital or acquired obstructive lesions of lymphatics of the area. It is possible that developmental anomalies related to lymphaticovenous communications in the mesentery are responsible (131).

Similarly developmental and acquired lymphatic obstruction of abdominal lymphatics can result in chylous ascites (143, 250). This condition has to be distinguished from pseudochylous ascites in which phospholipid-protein material derived from degenerating cells in inflammatory and neoplastic intra-abdominal disease creates a turbid fluid. In chylous ascites, the fluid contains chylomicrons and high triglyceride concentrations. Malignant obstruction of major lymph trunks is a frequent cause (143). Other causes include inflammatory processes, trauma, intestinal lymphangiectasia, and cirrhosis. In the last case, it is believed that chylous ascites results from rupture of distended subserosal lymphatics, a consequence of portal hypertension. Chylous ascites can be chronic, in which case the cause is generally neoplastic, or acute, when a demonstrable cause can be found in no more than 50% of cases. Causes include obstruction of abdominal lymph trunks, rupture of chylous cysts, and trauma, often surgical. In some patients the condition does not recur after drainage. Peritoneovenous shunts have occasionally been successful, and it has been reported that a dietary regime that replaces long-chain triglycerides with medium-chain triglycerides will alleviate the condition by reducing the load on intestinal lymph (471).

A hereditary disorder in mice in which chylous ascites develops in 11%–17% of newborn heterozygous ragged (Ra+) mice has been described (210). These animals show no ascites at birth, but they accumulate chylous fluid in the peritoneal cavity after suckling. The wall of the intestine is pale and thickened, and the submucosa is distended with fat droplets. Mesenteric lymphatic vessels are dilated and tortuous, but a site of leakage of lymph into the abdominal cavity is not readily apparent. No lymphatic abnormalities are found in other areas in these animals.

Chyluria results from situations in which a major lymph trunk communicates with the urinary tract. It is frequently observed in infection with microfilariae. Patients with chyluria have afforded investigators the opportunity to study human intestinal lymph indirectly, in particular its apolipoprotein spectrum (187).

Preparation of this chapter was supported in part by National Institutes of Health grants HL-30553 and AM-32288.

## REFERENCES

1. ADAIR, T. H., AND A. C. GUYTON. Modification of lymph by lymph nodes. II. Effect of increased lymph node venous blood pressure. *Am. J. Physiol.* 245 (*Heart Circ. Physiol.* 14): H616–H622, 1983.
2. ADAIR, T. H., AND A. C. GUYTON. Lymph formation and its modification in the lymphatic system. In: *Experimental Biology of the Lymphatic Circulation*, edited by M. G. Johnston. Amsterdam: Elsevier, 1985.
3. ADAIR, T. H., D. S. MOFFAT, A. W. PAULSEN, AND A. C. GUYTON. Quantitation of changes in lymph protein concentration during lymph node transit. *Am. J. Physiol.* 243 (*Heart Circ. Physiol.* 12): H351–H359, 1982.
4. ADAMS, E. P. Transport and Metabolism of Long Chain Fatty Acids in the Sheep. Canberra: Australian National Univ., 1964. PhD thesis.
5. ALBERTINE, K. H., L. M. FOX, AND C. C. C. O'MORCHOE. The morphology of canine lymphatic valves. *Anat. Rec.* 202: 453–461, 1982.
6. ALESSANDRINI, C., R. GERLI, G. SACCHI, L. IBBA, AND A. M. FRUSCHELLI. Cholinergic and adrenergic innervation of mesenteric lymph vessels in guinea pig. *Lymphology* 14: 1–6, 1981.
7. ALEXANDER, H. L., K. SHIRLEY, AND D. ALLEN. The route of ingested egg white to the systemic circulation. *J. Clin. Invest.* 15: 163–167, 1936.
8. ALLEN, J. M., N. G. MCHALE, AND B. M. ROONEY. Effect of norepinephrine on contractility of isolated mesenteric lymphatics. *Am. J. Physiol.* 244 (*Heart Circ. Physiol.* 13): H479–H486, 1983.
9. ALLEN, J. M., H. L. A. IGGULDEN, AND N. G. MCHALE. α-Adrenergic inhibition of bovine mesenteric lymphatics. *J. Physiol. Lond.* 374: 401–411, 1986.
10. ALPER, C. A., J. H. PETERS, A. G. BIRTCH, AND F. H. GARDNER. Haptoglobin synthesis. I. In vivo studies of the production of haptoglobin, fibrinogen and γ-globulin by the canine liver. *J. Clin. Invest.* 44: 574–581, 1965.
11. ANDERSSON, K. E., B. BERGDAHL, H. DENCKER, AND G. WETTRELL. Activities of proscillaridin A in thoracic duct lymph after single doses in man. *Acta Pharmacol. Toxicol.* 40: 280–284, 1977.
12. ASAKURA, H., S. MIURA, T. MORISHITA, S. AISO, T. TANAKA, T. KITAHORA, M. TSUCHIYA, Y. ENOMOTO, AND Y. WATANABE. Endoscopic and histopathological study on primary and secondary intestinal lymphangiectasia. *Dig. Dis. Sci.* 26: 312–320, 1981.
13. ASAKURA, H., A. MORITA, T. MORISHITA, M. TSUCHIYA, Y. WATANABE, AND Y. ENOMOTO. Histopathological and electron microscopic studies of lymphangiectasia of the small intestine in Behçet's disease. *Gut* 14: 196–203, 1973.
14. AUNE, S. The lymphatics of the stomach. In: *The Physiology of Gastric Secretion*, edited by L. S. Semb and J. Myren. Baltimore, MD: Williams & Wilkins, 1968, p. 15–17.
15. AZUMA, T., T. OHHASHI, AND M. SAKAGUCHI. Electrical activity of lymphatic smooth muscles. *Proc. Soc. Exp. Biol. Med.* 155: 270–273, 1977.
16. AZZALI, G. Ultrastructure of small intestine submucosal and serosal-muscular lymphatic vessels. *Lymphology* 15: 106–111, 1982.
17. AZZALI, G. The ultrastructural basis of lipid transport in the absorbing lymphatic vessel. *J. Submicrosc. Cytol.* 14: 45–54, 1982.
18. AZZALI, G., AND L. J. A. DIDIO. The lymphatic system of *Bradypus tridactylus*. *Anat. Rec.* 153: 149–160, 1965.
19. BACH, A., AND P. METAIS. Graisses à chaînes courtes et moyennes: aspects physiologiques, biochimiques, nutritionels et thérapeutiques. *Ann. Nutr. Aliment.* 24: 75–144, 1970.
20. BAEZ, S. Pressure and flow relations in the lymphatic system. In: *Experimental Biology of the Lymphatic Circulation*, edited by M. G. Johnston. Amsterdam: Elsevier, 1985. (Cited by Zweifach, B. W. and Schmid-Schonbein.)
21. BALASHOV, V. N. Intraorganic lymphatic system of stomach in some species of amphibia and reptiles (Engl. abstract). *Arkh. Anat. Gistol. Embriol.* 52: 57–64, 1967.
22. BALASHOV, V. N. Senile changes in intraorgan lymphatic bed of the human stomach (Engl. abstract). *Arkh. Anat. Gistol. Embriol.* 55: 11–16, 1968.
23. BANK, S., G. FISHER, I. N. MARKS, AND A. GROLL. The lymphatics of the intestinal mucosa. A clinical and experimental study. *Am. J. Dig. Dis.* 12: 619–632, 1967.
24. BARAONA, E., AND C. S. LIEBER. Intestinal lymph formation and fat absorption: stimulation by acute ethanol administration and inhibition by chronic ethanol feeding. *Gastroenterology* 68: 495–502, 1975.
25. BARROWMAN, J. A. *Physiology of the Gastrointestinal Lymphatic System*. Cambridge, UK: Cambridge Univ. Press, 1978. (Monogr. of Physiol. Soc. No. 33.)
26. BARROWMAN, J. A. Intestinal Absorption of the Fat-Soluble Vitamins: Physiology and Pharmacology. In: *Handbook of Experimental Pharmacology*, edited by T. Z. Csaky. Berlin: Springer-Verlag. 1984, vol. 70, pt. 1, chapt. 17.
26a. BARROWMAN, J. A., AND D. N. GRANGER. Hepatic lymph. In: *Hepatic Circulation in Health and Diseases*, edited by W. W. Lautt. New York: Raven, 1981, p. 137–152.
27. BARROWMAN, J. A., AND D. N. GRANGER. Effects of experimental cirrhosis on splanchnic microvascular fluid and solute exchange in the rat. *Gastroenterology* 87: 165–172, 1984.
28. BARROWMAN, J. A., M. A. PERRY, P. R. KVIETYS, AND D. N. GRANGER. Exclusion phenomenon in the liver interstitium. *Am. J. Physiol.* 243 (*Gastrointest. Liver Physiol.* 6): G410–G414, 1982.
29. BARROWMAN, J. A., AND K. B. ROBERTS. The role of the lymphatic system in the absorption of water from the intestine of the rat. *Q. J. Exp. Physiol.* 52: 19–30, 1967.
30. BARTOS, V., V. BRZEK, J. GROH, AND O. KELLER. Alterations in human thoracic duct lymph in relation to the function of the pancreas. *Am. J. Med. Sci.* 252: 31–38, 1966.
31. BAXTER, J. H. Routes of glyceride delivery from liver to plasma in the rat. *Am. J. Physiol.* 218: 790–796, 1970.
32. BECKETT, G. J., AND I. W. PERCY-ROBB. Bile salt transport in intestinal lymph of the rat. *Eur. J. Clin. Invest.* 12: 23–27, 1982.
33. BEERMAN, B., AND K. HELLSTRÖM. The efficacy of lymph drainage in the elimination of orally administered digitoxin and digoxin. *Pharmacology Basel* 6: 17–21, 1971.
34. BEIL, F. W., AND S. M. GRUNDY. Studies on plasma lipoproteins during absorption of exogenous lecithin in man. *J. Lipid Res.* 21: 525–536, 1980.
35. BELL-QUINT, J., AND T. FORTE. Time-related changes in the synthesis and secretion of very low density, low density and high density lipoproteins by cultured rat hepatocytes. *Biochim. Biophys. Acta* 663: 83–98, 1981.
36. BENNETT, S., P. SHEPHERD, AND W. J. SIMMONDS. The effect of alterations in intestinal motility induced by morphine and atropine on fat absorption in the rat. *Aust. J. Exp. Biol. Med. Sci.* 40: 225–231, 1962.
37. BENSON, J. A., JR., P. R. LEE, J. F. SCHOLER, K. S. KIM, AND J. L. BOLLMAN. Water absorption from the intestine via portal and lymphatic pathways. *Am. J. Physiol.* 184: 441–444, 1956.
38. BERGSTROM, S., R. BLOMSTRAND, AND B. BORGSTROM. Route of absorption and distribution of oleic acid and triolein in the rat. *Biochem. J.* 58: 600–604, 1954.
39. BIERMAN, H. R., R. L. BYRON, K. H. KELLY, R. S. GILFILLAN, L. P. WHITE, N. E. FREEMAN, AND N. L. PETRAKIS. The characteristics of thoracic duct lymph in man. *J. Clin. Invest.* 32: 637–649, 1953.
40. BILL, A. Regional lymph flow in unanaesthetized rabbits. *Uppsala J. Med. Sci.* 84: 129–136, 1979.
41. BISGAIER, C. L., AND R. M. GLICKMAN. Intestinal synthesis, secretion and transport of lipoproteins. *Annu. Rev. Physiol.* 45: 625–636, 1983.
42. BLALOCK, A., AND C. S. BURWELL. Thoracic duct lymph

pressure in concretio cordis: experimental study. *J. Lab. Clin. Med.* 21: 296–297, 1935.
43. BLALOCK, A., C. S. ROBINSON, R. S. CUNNINGHAM, AND M. E. GRAY. Experimental studies on lymphatic blockage. *Arch. Surg.* 34: 1049–1071, 1937.
44. BLOMSTRAND, R. The intestinal absorption of linoleic-1-$^{14}$C acid. *Acta Physiol. Scand.* 32: 99–105, 1954.
45. BLOMSTRAND, R. Transport form of decanoic acid-1-$^{14}$C in the lymph during intestinal absorption in the rat. *Acta Physiol. Scand.* 34: 67–70, 1955.
46. BLOMSTRAND, R., AND L. FORSGREN. Labelled tocopherols in man. Intestinal absorption and thoracic-duct lymph transport of DL-alpha-tocopheryl-3,4-$^{14}$C$_2$ acetate, DL-alpha-tocopheramine-3,4-$^{14}$C$_2$, DL-alpha-tocopherol-(5-methyl-$^3$H) and N-(methyl-$^3$H)-DL-gamma tocopheramine. *Int. Z. Vitaminforsch.* 38: 328–344, 1968.
47. BLOMSTRAND, R., AND L. FORSGREN. Vitamin K$_1$-$^3$H in man. Its intestinal absorption and transport in the thoracic duct lymph. *Int. Z. Vitaminforsch.* 38: 45–64, 1968.
48. BLOMSTRAND, R., AND B. WERNER. Studies on the intestinal absorption of radioactive $\beta$-carotene and vitamin A in man. *Scand. J. Clin. Lab. Invest.* 19: 339–345, 1967.
49. BLOOM, B., I. L. CHAIKOFF, AND W. O. REINHARDT. Intestinal lymph as pathway for transport of absorbed fatty acids of different chain lengths. *Am. J. Physiol.* 166: 451–455, 1951.
50. BLOOM, B., I. L. CHAIKOFF, W. O. REINHARDT, C. ENTENMAN, AND W. G. DAUBEN. The quantitative significance of the lymphatic pathway in transport of absorbed fatty acids. *J. Biol. Chem.* 184: 1–8, 1950.
51. BLOOM, W. The role of lymphatics in the absorption of bile pigment from the liver in early obstructive jaundice. *Bull. Johns Hopkins Hosp.* 34: 316–320, 1923.
52. BLUESTEIN, M., J. MALAGELADA, W. LINSCHEER, AND W. H. FISHMAN. Enzymology of alkaline phosphatase of rat intestine following fatty acid infusion. *J. Histochem. Cytochem.* 18: 679, 1970.
53. BOCK, K. W., U. C. VON CLAUSBRUCH, AND D. WINNE. Absorption and metabolism of naphthalene and benzo($a$)pyrene in the rat jejunum in situ. *Med. Biol.* 57: 262–264, 1979.
54. BOCKLAGE, B. C., H. J. NICHOLAS, E. A. DOISY, W. H. ELLIOTT, S. A. THAYER, AND E. A. DOISY. Synthesis and biological studies of 17-methyl-$^{14}$C-estradiol. *J. Biol. Chem.* 202: 27–37, 1953.
55. BOCKLAGE, B. C., E. A. DOISY, JR., W. H. ELLIOTT, AND E. A. DOISY. Absorption and metabolism of cortisone -4-$^{14}$C acetate. *J. Biol. Chem.* 212: 935–939, 1955.
56. BOLLMAN, J. L. A cage which limits the activity of rats. *J. Lab. Clin. Med.* 33: 1348, 1948.
57. BOLLMAN, J. L., J. C. CAIN, AND J. H. GRINDLAY. Techniques for collection of lymph from liver, small intestine or thoracic duct of the rat. *J. Lab. Clin. Med.* 33: 1349–1352, 1948.
58. BOLTON, C., AND W. G. BARNARD. The pathological occurrences in liver in experimental venous stagnation. *J. Pathol. Bacteriol.* 34: 701–709, 1931.
59. BOOKSTEIN, J. J., A. B. FRENCH, AND H. M. POLLARD. Protein-losing gastroenteropathy: concepts derived from lymphangiography. *Am. J. Dig. Dis.* 10: 573–581, 1965.
60. BORGSTROM, B. On the mechanism of intestinal fat absorption. V. The effect of bile diversion on fat absorption in the rat. *Acta Physiol. Scand.* 28: 279–286, 1953.
61. BORGSTROM, B. Transport form of $^{14}$C-decanoic acid in portal and inferior vena cava blood during absorption in the rat. *Acta Physiol. Scand.* 34: 71–74, 1955.
62. BORGSTROM, B. Fat digestion and absorption. In: *Biomembranes. Intestinal Absorption*, edited by D. H. Smyth. New York: Plenum, 1974, vol. 4, pt. B, p. 555–620.
63. BORGSTROM, B. Phospholipid absorption. In: *Lipid absorption: Biochemical and Clinical Aspects*, edited by K. Rommel, H. Goebell, and R. Böhmer. Lancaster, UK: MTP, 1976, p. 65–72.
64. BORGSTROM, B., AND C. B. LAURELL. Studies on lymph and lymph-proteins during absorption of fat and saline by rats. *Acta Physiol. Scand.* 29: 264–280, 1953.
65. BRADLEY, S. E. Hepatic lymph formation—basic mechanism and dysfunctions. In: *Problems in Liver Diseases*, edited by C. S. Davidson. New York: Stratton (Intercont. Med. Book Co.), 1981, p. 53–65.
66. BRAUER, R. W. Liver circulation and function. *Physiol. Rev.* 43: 115–213, 1963.
67. BRUGGEMAN, T. M. Plasma proteins in canine gastric lymph. *Gastroenterology* 68: 1204–1210, 1975.
68. BRUNSSON, I., S. EKLUND, M. JODAL, O. LUNDGREN, AND H. SJÖVALL. The effect of vasodilation and sympathetic nerve activation on net water absorption in the cat's small intestine. *Acta Physiol. Scand.* 106: 61–68, 1979.
69. BRZEK, V., AND V. BARTOS. Therapeutic effect of prolonged thoracic duct lymph fistula in patients with acute pancreatitis. *Digestion* 2: 43–50, 1969.
70. BUHAC, J., AND J. JARMOLYCH. Histology of the intestinal peritoneum in patients with cirrhosis of the liver and ascites. *Dig. Dis. Sci.* 23: 417–422, 1978.
71. BUSBEE, D. L., C. O. JOE, P. W. RANKIN, R. L. ZIPRIN, AND R. R. WILSON. Benzo($a$)pyrene uptake by lymph: a possible transport mode for immunosuppressive chemicals. *J. Toxicol. Environ. Health* 13: 43–51, 1984.
72. BUSBEE, D. L., J. H. YOO, J. O. NORMAN, AND C. O. JOE. Polychlorinated biphenyl uptake and transport by lymph and plasma components. *Proc. Soc. Exp. Biol. Med.* 179: 116–122, 1985.
73. CAIN, J. C., J. H. GRINDLAY, J. L. BOLLMAN, E. V. FLOCK, AND F. C. MANN. Lymph from liver and thoracic duct: an experimental study. *Surg. Gynecol. Obstet.* 85: 559–562, 1947.
74. CALNAN, J. S., O. R. RIVERO, S. FILLMORE, AND L. MERCURIUS-TAYLOR. Permeability of normal lymphatics. *Br. J. Surg.* 54: 278–285, 1967.
75. CAMPBELL, R. S., D. BROBST, AND G. BISGARD. Intestinal lymphangiectasia in a dog. *J. Am. Vet. Med. Assoc.* 153: 1051–1054, 1968.
76. CARLETON, H. M., AND H. W. FLOREY. The mammalian lacteal: its histological structure in relation to its physiological properties. *Proc. R. Soc. Lond. B Biol. Sci.* 102: 110–118, 1927.
77. CARLSTEN, A., Y. EDLUND, AND O. THULESIUS. Bilirubin, alkaline phosphatase and transaminases in blood and lymph during biliary obstruction in the cat. *Acta Physiol. Scand.* 53: 58–67, 1961.
78. CARLSTEN, A., AND T. OLIN. The route of the intestinal lymph to the bloodstream. *Acta Physiol. Scand.* 25: 259–266, 1952.
79. CASLEY-SMITH, J. R. The identification of chylomicra and lipoproteins in tissue sections and their passage into jejunal lacteals. *J. Cell Biol.* 15: 259–277, 1962.
80. CASLEY-SMITH, J. R. The dimensions and numbers of small vesicles and the significance of these for endothelial permeability. *J. Microsc.* 90: 251–268, 1969.
81. CASLEY-SMITH, J. R. The transportation of large molecules, by small vesicles, through the endothelium. In: *Progress in Lymphology II*, edited by M. Viamonte et. al. Stuttgart, FRG: Thieme, 1970, p. 255–260.
82. CASLEY-SMITH, J. R. The role of the endothelial intercellular junctions in the functioning of the initial lymphatics. *Angiologica* 9: 106–131, 1972.
83. CASLEY-SMITH, J. R. In: *The Inflammatory Process*, edited by B. W. Zweifach, L. Grant, and R. T. McCluskey. New York: Academic, 1973, vol. 2, p. 161–204.
84. CASLEY-SMITH, J. R. The functioning and interrelationships of blood capillaries and lymphatics. *Experientia Basel* 32: 1–12, 1976.
85. CASLEY-SMITH, J. R. Are the initial lymphatics normally pulled open by the anchoring filaments? *Lymphology* 13: 120–129, 1980.
86. CASLEY-SMITH, J. R. The structure and functioning of the blood vessels, interstitial tissues, and lymphatics. In: *Lymphangiology*, edited by M. Foldi and J. R. Casley-Smith. Stuttgart, FRG: Schattauer, 1983, p. 27–164.

87. CASLEY-SMITH, J. R., AND B. J. GANNON. Intestinal microcirculation: spatial organization and fine structure. In: *Physiology of the Intestinal Circulation*, edited by A. P. Shepherd and D. N. Granger. New York: Raven, 1984.
88. CHAIKOFF, I. L., B. BLOOM, B. P. STEVENS, W. O. REINHARDT, W. G. DAUBEN, AND J. F. EASTHAM. Pentadecanoic acid-5-$^{14}$C: its absorption and lymphatic transport. *J. Biol. Chem.* 190: 431–435, 1951.
89. CHAIKOFF, I. L., B. BLOOM, B. P. STEVENS, W. O. REINHARDT, W. G. DAUBEN, AND J. F. EASTHAM. $^{14}$C-cholesterol. I. Lymphatic transport of absorbed cholesterol -4-$^{14}$C. *J. Biol. Chem.* 194: 407–412, 1952.
90. CHEN, Y. K., H. M. RICHTER, K. A. KELLY, J. M. JAY, AND V. L. W. GO. Postprandial gastrin, neurotensin, vasoactive intestinal peptide, substance P and bombesin output in canine thoracic duct lymph. *Gastroenterology* 86: 1046, 1984.
91. CHOU, C. C., AND P. R. KVIETYS. Physiological and pharmacological alterations in gastro-intestinal blood flow. In: *The Measurement of Splanchnic Blood Flow*, edited by D. N. Granger and G. B. Bulkley. Baltimore, MD: Williams & Wilkins, 1981, p. 475–509.
92. CHVAPIL, M. *Physiology of Connective Tissue*. London: Butterworths, 1967, p. 14.
93. CLENDINNEN, B. G., D. D. REEDER, AND J. C. THOMPSON. The role of thoracic duct lymph in gastrin transport and gastric secretion. *Gut* 14: 30–34, 1973.
94. CODE, C. F., AND D. W. PICKARD. The importance of the lymphatic system in the absorption of water from the intestine *J. Physiol. Lond.* 231: 40P–41P, 1973.
95. COLLAN, Y., AND T. V. KALIMA. The lymphatic pump of the intestinal villus of the rat. *Scand. J. Gastroenterol.* 5: 187–196, 1970.
96. COLLAN, Y., AND T. V. KALIMA. Topographic relations of lymphatic endothelial cells in the initial lymphatic of the intestinal villus. *Lymphology* 7: 175–184, 1974.
97. COLLAN, Y., J. NICKELS, AND T. V. KALIMA. Lymphatics of the gallbladder mucosa in pigs, an electron microscope study. In: *Lymphology*, edited by P. Malek, V. Bartos, H. Weissleder, and M. H. Witte. Stuttgart, FRG: Thieme, 1979, p. 30–33. (Proc. 6th Int. Congr.)
98. COMLINE, R. S., H. E. ROBERTS, AND D. A. TITCHEN. Route of absorption of colostrum globulin in the newborn animal. *Nature Lond.* 167: 561–562, 1951.
99. COMPARINI, L. Lymph vessels of the liver in man. *Angiologica* 6: 262–274, 1969.
100. COMPER, W. D., AND T. C. LAURENT. Physiologic function of connective tissue polysaccharides. *Physiol. Rev.* 58: 255–315, 1978.
101. COURTICE, F. C. The flow and composition of hepatic lymph in the normal and hypercholesterolaemic rabbit. *Aust. J. Exp. Biol. Med. Sci.* 38: 403–412, 1960.
102. CRAIN, F. D., F. J. LOTSPEICH, AND R. F. KRAUSE. Biosynthesis of retinoic acid by intestinal enzymes of the rat. *J. Lipid Res.* 8: 249–254, 1967.
103. CRUICKSHANK, W. *The Anatomy of the Absorbing Vessels of the Human Body*. London: G. Nicol, 1790.
104. DANESE, C. A., M. GEORGALAS-PENESIS, A. E. KARK, AND D. A. DREILING. Studies of the effects of blockage of intestinal lymphatics. I. Experimental procedure and structure alterations. *Am. J. Gastroenterol.* 57: 541–546, 1972.
105. DAVIDSON, J. D., T. A. WALDMANN, D. S. GOODMAN, AND R. S. GORDON. Protein-losing gastro-enteropathy in congestive heart failure. *Lancet* 1: 899–902, 1961.
106. DEAK, S. T., AND T. Z. CSÁKY. Factors regulating the exchange of nutrients and drugs between lymph and blood in the small intestine. *Microcirc. Endothelium Lymphatics* 1: 569–588, 1984.
107. DEL RIO LOZANO, I., AND W. H. H. ANDREWS. Some relationships between the lymphatic system, the biliary system and the blood vascular system in the liver of the rabbit. *Q. J. Exp. Physiol.* 51: 324–335, 1966.
108. DE MARCO, T. J., AND R. R. LEVINE. Role of the lymphatics in the intestinal absorption and distribution of drugs. *J. Pharmacol. Exp. Ther.* 169: 142–151, 1969.
109. DIBONA, D. R., L. C. CHEN, AND G. W. G. SHARP. A study of intercellular spaces in the rabbit jejunum during acute volume expansion and after treatment with cholera toxin. *J. Clin. Invest.* 53: 1300–1307, 1974.
110. DIVE, C. C., A. C. NADALINI, AND J. F. HEREMANS. Origin and composition of hepatic lymph proteins in the dog. *Lymphology* 4: 133–139, 1971.
111. DOBBINS, W. O. The intestinal mucosal lymphatic in man. A light and electron microscopic study. Electron microscopic study of the intestinal mucosa in intestinal lymphangiectasia. *Gastroenterology* 51: 994–1017, 1966.
112. DOBBINS, W. O. Hypo-$\beta$-lipoproteinemia and intestinal lymphangiectasia. A new syndrome of malabsorption and protein-losing enteropathy. *Arch. Intern. Med.* 122: 31–38, 1968.
113. DOBBINS, W. O. Intestinal mucosal lacteal in transport of macromolecules and chylomicrons. *Am. J. Clin. Nutr.* 24: 77–90, 1971.
114. DOBBINS, W. O., AND E. L. ROLLINS. Intestinal mucosal lymphatic permeability: an electron microscopic study of endothelial vesicles and cell junctions. *J. Ultrastruct. Res.* 33: 29–59, 1970.
115. DOGIEL, A. Über die Beziehungen zwischen Blut- und Lymphgefässen. *Arch. Mikrosk. Anat. Entw. Mech. Org.* 22: 608–615, 1883.
116. DOLLE, W., G. A. MARTINI, AND F. PETERSEN. Idiopathic familial cardiomegaly with intermittent loss of protein into the gastro-intestinal tract. *Dtsch. Med. Wochenshr.* 87: 1333–1338, 1962.
117. DONINI, I. Sur la fine distribution des vaisseaux lymphatiques dans l'estomac humain (Engl. abstract). *Acta Anat.* 23: 289–311, 1955.
118. DREILING, D. A. The lymphatics, pancreatic ascites and pancreatic inflammatory disease. A new therapy for pancreatitis. *Am. J. Gastroenterol.* 53: 119–131, 1970.
119. DRINKER, C. K., AND M. E. FIELD. *Lymphatics, Lymph and Tissue Fluid*. Baltimore, MD: Williams & Wilkins, 1933.
120. DRINKER, C. K., M. E. FIELD, AND H. K. WARD. The filtering capacity of lymph nodes. *J. Exp. Med.* 59: 393–405, 1934.
121. DRINKER, C. K., AND J. M. YOFFEY. *Lymphatics, Lymph, and Lymphoid Tissue*. Cambridge, MA: Harvard Univ. Press, 1941.
122. DUELAND, S., J. I. PEDERSEN, P. HELGERUD, AND C. A. DREVON. Transport of Vitamin $D_3$ from rat intestine. *J. Biol. Chem.* 257: 146–150, 1982.
123. DUFFY, P. A., D. N. GRANGER, AND A. E. TAYLOR. Intestinal secretion induced by volume expansion in the dog. *Gastroenterology* 75: 413–418, 1978.
124. DUMONT, A. E. Icteric thoracic duct lymph. Significance in patients with manifestations of obstructive jaundice. *Ann. Surg.* 178: 53–58, 1973.
125. DUMONT, A. E., H. DOUBILET, AND J. H. MULHOLLAND. Lymphatic pathway of pancreatic secretion in man. *Ann. Surg.* 152: 403–409, 1960.
126. DUMONT, A. E., H. DOUBILET, C. L. WITTE, AND J. H. MULHOLLAND. Disorders of the biliary-pancreatic system: observations on lymph drainage in jaundiced patients. *Ann. Surg.* 153: 774–780, 1961.
127. DUMONT, A. E., AND J. H. MULHOLLAND. Flow rate and composition of thoracic duct lymph in patients with cirrhosis. *N. Engl. J. Med.* 263: 471–474, 1960.
128. DUPONT, J. M., AND J. LITVINE. Le facteur lymphatique dans les pancréatites experimentales. *Acta Chir. Belg.* 63: 687–697, 1964.
129. DUPREZ, A., S. GODART, R. PLATTEBORSE, J. LITVINE, AND J. M. DUPONT. La voie de dérivation interstitielle et lymphatique de la secretion exocrine du pancréas. *Bull. Acad. R. Med. Belg.* 3: 691–706, 1963.
130. DUROVICOVA, J., AND V. MUNKA. Lymph drainage from stomach. In: *Lymphology*, edited by P. Malek, V. Bartos, H. Weissleder, and M. H. Witte. Stuttgart, FRG: Thieme, 1979, p. 33–35. (Proc. 6th Int. Congr. Lymphology.)

131. ELLIOTT, G. B., M. R. KLIMAN, AND K. A. ELLIOTT. Persistence of lymphaticovenous shunts at the level of the microcirculation. Their relationship to "lymphangioma" of mesentery. *Am. Surg.* 172: 131–136, 1970.
132. ESTERLY, J. R. Congenital hereditary lymphedema. *J. Med. Genet.* 2: 93–96, 1965.
133. EVERETT, N. B., W. E. GARRETT, AND B. S. SIMMONS. Lymphatics in iron absorption and transport. *Am. J. Physiol.* 178: 45–48, 1954.
134. EWERTH, S., I. BJORKHEM, K. EINARSON, AND L. OST. Lymphatic transport of bile acids in man. *J. Lipid Res.* 23: 1183–1186, 1982.
135. FENOGLIO, C. M., G. I. KAYE, AND N. LANE. Distribution of human colonic lymphatics in normal, hyperplastic and adenomatous tissue. *Gastroenterology* 64: 51–66, 1973.
136. FIDGE, N. H., AND P. J. MCCULLAGH. Studies on apoproteins of rat lymph chylomicrons: characterization and metabolism of a new chylomicron-associated apoprotein. *J. Lipid Res.* 22: 138–146, 1981.
137. FIDGE, N. H., T. SHIRATORI, J. GANGULY, AND D. S. GOODMAN. Pathways of absorption of retinal and retinoic acid in the rat. *J. Lipid Res.* 9: 103–109, 1968
138. FINCO, D. R., J. R. DUNCAN, W. D. SCHALL, B. E. HOOPER, F. W. CHANDLER, AND K. A. KEATING. Chronic enteric disease and hyproproteinaemia in nine dogs. *J. Am. Vet. Med. Assoc.* 163: 262–271, 1973.
139. FISH, J. C., H. E. SARLES, A. T. MATTINGLY, M. V. ROSS, AND A. R. REMMERO. Preparation of chronic thoracic duct lymph fistulas in man and laboratory animals. *J. Surg. Res.* 9: 101–106, 1969.
140. FOLDI, M., J. KEPES, AND G. SZABO. Data quoted in: *Lymphatics and Lymph Circulation* (2nd ed.), by I. Rusznyak, M. Foldi, and G. Szabo, Oxford, UK: Pergamon, 1967.
141. FOLKOW, B., AND E. NEIL. *Circulation.* London: Oxford Univ. Press, 1971.
142. FORSGREN, L. Studies on the intestinal absorption of labelled fat-soluble vitamins (A, D, E, and K) via the thoracic duct lymph in the absence of bile in man. *Acta Chir. Scand. Suppl.* 399, 1969.
143. FRANK, B. W., AND F. KERN. Intestinal and liver lymph and lymphatics. *Gastroenterology* 50: 677–683, 1968.
144. FRASER, R., AND E. KODICEK. Investigations on vitamin D esters synthesized in rats. *Biochem. J.* 106: 485–496, 1968.
145. FRIEDMAN, H. I., AND R. R. CARDELL. Effects of puromycin on the structure of rat intestinal epithelial cells during fat absorption. *J. Cell Biol.* 52: 15–40, 1972.
146. FRIEDMAN, J. J., AND S. WITTE. Protein concentration gradients in the interstitial space. *Microvasc. Res.* 29: 220, 1985.
147. FRIEDMAN, M., S. O. BYERS, AND C. OMOTO. Some characteristics of hepatic lymph in the intact rat. *Am. J. Physiol.* 184: 11–17, 1956.
148. GAGNON, M., AND A. M. DAWSON. The effect of bile on vitamin A absorption in the rat. *Proc. Soc. Exp. Biol. Med.* 127: 99–102, 1968.
149. GALLAGHER, N., J. WEBB, AND A. M. DAWSON. The absorption of $^{14}C$ oleic acid and $^{14}C$ triolein in bile fistula rats. *Clin. Sci.* 29: 73–82, 1965.
150. GEORGALAS-PENESIS, M., C. A. DANESE, C. WASTELL, A. E. KARK, AND D. A. DREILLING. Studies of the effects of blockade of intestinal lymphatics. II. Metabolic considerations. *Am. J. Gastroenterol.* 58: 15–21, 1972.
151. GERSH, I., AND H. R. CATCHPOLE. The nature of ground substance of connective tissue. *Perspect. Biol. Med.* 3: 282, 1960.
152. GIANNINA, T., B. G. STEINETZ, AND A. MELI. Pathway of absorption of orally administered ethynyl estradiol-3-cyclopentyl ether in the rat as influenced by vehicle of administration. *Proc. Soc. Exp. Biol. Med.* 121: 1175–1179, 1966.
153. GIRARDET, R. E. Surgical techniques for long-term studies of thoracic duct circulation in the rat. *J. Appl. Physiol.* 39: 682–688, 1975.
154. GLICKMAN, R. M., D. H. ALPERS, G. D. DRUMMEY, AND K. J. ISSELBACHER. Increased lymph alkaline phosphatase after fat feeding: effects of medium chain triglycerides and inhibition of protein synthesis. *Biochim. Biophys. Acta* 201: 226–235, 1970.
155. GLICKMAN, R. M., AND K. KIRSCH. Lymph chylomicron formation during the inhibition of protein synthesis. Studies of chylomicron apoproteins. *J. Clin. Invest.* 52: 2910–2920, 1973.
156. GLICKMAN, R. M., K. KIRSCH, AND K. J. ISSELBACHER. Fat absorption during inhibition of protein synthesis: studies of lymph chylomicrons. *J. Clin. Invest.* 51: 356–363, 1972.
157. GLICKMAN, R. M., J. L. PEROTTO, AND K. KIRSCH. Intestinal lipoprotein formation: effect of colchicine. *Gastroenterology* 70: 347–352, 1976.
158. GNEPP, D. R., AND F. H. Y. GREEN. Scanning electron microscopic study of canine lymphatic vessels and their valves. *Lymphology* 13: 91–99, 1980.
159. GODART, S. Lymphatic circulation of the pancreas. *Bibl. Anat.* 7: 410–413, 1965.
160. GONZALEZ-ODDONE, M. V. Bilirubin, bromsulfalein, bile acids, alkaline phosphatase and cholesterol of thoracic duct lymph in experimental regurgitation jaundice. *Proc. Soc. Exp. Biol. Med.* 63: 144–147, 1946.
161. GOODMAN, D. S., R. BLOMSTRAND, B. WERNER, H. S. HUANG, AND T. SHIRATORI. The intestinal absorption and metabolism of vitamin A and $\beta$-carotene in man. *J. Clin. Invest.* 45: 1615–1623, 1966.
162. GORESKY, C. A. The interstitial space in the liver: its partitioning effect. In: *Capillary Permeability*, edited by C. Crone and N. A. Lassen. Copenhagen: Munksgaard, 1970, p. 415–430. (Alfred Benzon Symp. II. Roy. Danish Acad. Sci. & Letters, 1969.)
163. GOTTO, A. M., R. I. LEVY, K. JOHN, AND D. S. FREDRICKSON. On the protein defect in a-$\beta$-lipoproteinemia. *N. Engl. J. Med.* 284: 813–818, 1971.
164. GRANGER, D. N. Intestinal microcirculation and transmucosal fluid transport. *Am. J. Physiol.* 240 (*Gastrointest. Liver Physiol.* 3): G343–G349, 1981.
165. GRANGER, D. N., AND J. A. BARROWMAN. Microcirculation of the alimentary tract. I. Physiology of transcapillary fluid and solute exchange. II. Pathophysiology of edema. *Gastroenterology* 84: 846–868; 1035–1059, 1983.
166. GRANGER, D. N., J. A. BARROWMAN, S. L. HARPER, P. R. KVIETYS, AND R. J. KORTHUIS. Sympathetic stimulation and intestinal capillary fluid exchange. *Am. J. Physiol.* 247 (*Gastrointest. Liver Physiol.* 10): G279–G283, 1984.
167. GRANGER, D. N., B. H. COOK, AND A. E. TAYLOR. Structural locus of transmucosal albumin efflux in canine ileum: a fluorescence study. *Gastroenterology* 71: 1023–1027, 1976.
168. GRANGER, D. N., R. CROSS, AND J. A. BARROWMAN. Effects of various secretagogues and human carcinoid serum on lymph flow in the cat ileum. *Gastroenterology* 83: 896–901, 1982.
169. GRANGER, D. N., P. R. KVIETYS, N. A. MORTILLARO, AND A. E. TAYLOR. Effect of luminal distension on intestinal transcapillary fluid exchange. *Am. J. Physiol.* 239 (*Gastrointest. Liver Physiol.* 2): G516–G523, 1980.
170. GRANGER, D. N., P. R. KVIETYS, W. H. WILBORN, N. A. MORTILLARO, AND A. E. TAYLOR. Mechanisms of glucagon-induced intestinal secretion. *Am. J. Physiol.* 239 (*Gastrointest. Liver Physiol.* 2): G30–G38, 1980.
171. GRANGER, D. N., T. MILLER, R. ALLEN, R. E. PARKER, J. C. PARKER, AND A. E. TAYLOR. Permselectivity of the liver blood-lymph barrier to endogenous macromolecules. *Gastroenterology* 77: 103–109, 1979.
172. GRANGER, D. N., N. A. MORTILLARO, P. R. KVIETYS, G. RUTILI, J. C. PARKER, AND A. E. TAYLOR. Role of the interstitial matrix during intestinal volume absorption. *Am. J. Physiol.* 238 (*Gastrointest. Liver Physiol.* 1): G183–G189, 1980.
173. GRANGER, D. N., N. A. MORTILLARO, M. A. PERRY, AND P. R. KVIETYS. Autoregulation of intestinal capillary filtration. *Am. J. Physiol.* 243 (*Gastrointest. Liver Physiol.* 6): G475–G483, 1982.
174. GRANGER, D. N., N. A. MORTILLARO, AND A. E. TAYLOR.

Interactions of intestinal lymph flow and secretion. *Am. J. Physiol.* 232 (*Endocrinol. Metab. Gastrointest. Physiol.* 1): E13–E18, 1977.

175. GRANGER, D. N., R. E. PARKER, E. W. QUILLEN, R. A. BRACE, AND A. E. TAYLOR. Lymph flow transients. In: *Lymphology*, edited by P. Malek, V. Bartos, H. Weissleder, and M. H. Witte. Stuttgart, FRG: Thieme, 1979, p. 61–64. (Proc. 6th Int. Congr.)

176. GRANGER, D. N., M. A. PERRY, AND P. R. KVIETYS. The microcirculation and fluid transport in digestive organs. *Federation Proc.* 42: 1667–1672, 1983.

177. GRANGER, D. N., M. A. PERRY, P. R. KVIETYS, AND A. E. TAYLOR. Permeability of intestinal capillaries: effects of fat absorption and gastrointestinal hormones. *Am. J. Physiol.* 242 (*Gastrointest. Liver Physiol.* 5): G194–G201, 1982.

178. GRANGER, D. N., M. A. PERRY, P. R. KVIETYS, AND A. E. TAYLOR. Capillary and interstitial forces during absorption in the cat small intestine. *Gastroenterology* 86: 267–273, 1984.

179. GRANGER, D. N., P. D. I. RICHARDSON, AND A. E. TAYLOR. Effects of isoprenaline and bradykinin on capillary filtration in the cat ileum. *Br. J. Pharmacol.* 67: 361–366, 1979.

180. GRANGER, D. N., J. S. SHACKLEFORD, AND A. E. TAYLOR. Prostaglandin $E_1$-induced filtration secretion in the feline ileum. *Am. J. Physiol.* 236 (*Endocrinol. Metab. Gastrointest. Physiol.* 5): E788–E798, 1979.

181. GRANGER, D. N., AND A. E. TAYLOR. Permselectivity of intestinal capillaries. *Physiologist* 23: 47–52, 1980.

181a. GRANGER, D. N., AND A. E. TAYLOR. Permeability of intestinal capillaries to endogenous macromolecules. *Am. J. Physiol.* 238 (*Heart Circ. Physiol.* 7): H457–464, 1980.

182. GRANGER, D. N., M. ULRICH, D. A. PARKS, AND S. L. HARPER. Transcapillary exchange during intestinal fluid absorption. In: *Physiology of the Intestinal Circulation*, edited by A. P. Shepherd and D. N. Granger. New York: Raven, 1984, p. 211–221.

183. GRANGER, D. N., J. D. VALLEAU, R. E. PARKER, R. S. LANE, AND A. E. TAYLOR. Effects of adenosine on intestinal hemodynamics, oxygen delivery and capillary fluid exchange. *Am. J. Physiol.* 235 (*Heart Circ. Physiol.* 4): H707–H719, 1978.

184. GRANGER, H. J. Physico chemical properties of the extracellular matrix. In: *Tissue Fluid Pressure and Composition*, edited by A. R. Hargens. Baltimore, MD: Williams & Wilkins, 1981.

185. GRAU, H., AND E. TAHER. Histologische Untersuchungen uber das innere Lymphgefäss System von Pancreas und Milz. *Berl. Muench. Tieraerztl. Wochenschr.* 78: 147–151, 1965.

186. GREEN, P. H. R., R. M. GLICKMAN, C. D. SAUDEK, C. B. BLUM, AND A. R. TALL. Human intestinal lipoproteins: studies in chyluric subjects. *J. Clin Invest.* 64: 233–242, 1979.

187. GREEN, P. H. R., J. W. LEFKOWITCH, R. M. GLICKMAN, J. W. RILEY, E. QUINET, AND C. B. BLUM. Apolipoprotein localization and quantitation in the human intestine. *Gastroenterology* 83: 1223–1230, 1982.

188. GREENWAY, C. V. Hepatic fluid change. In: *Hepatic Circulation in Health and Disease*, edited by W. W. Lautt. New York: Raven, 1981, p. 153–167.

189. GREENWAY, C. V., AND R. D. STARK. Hepatic vascular bed. *Physiol. Rev.* 51: 23–65, 1971.

190. GRIFFEN, W. O., R. P. BELIN, R. W. FURMAN, A. LIEBER, J. W. SCHAEFER, AND L. D. DUBILIER. Colonic lymphangiectasia: a report of two cases. *Dis. Colon Rectum* 15: 49–54, 1972.

191. GRIMUS, R. C., AND I. SCHUSTER. The role of the lymphatic transport in the enteral absorption of naftifine by the rat. *Xenobiotica* 14: 287–294, 1984.

192. GRØGAARD, B., D. PARKS, D. N. GRANGER, J. M. MCCORD, AND J. O. FORSBERG. Effects of ischemia and oxygen radicals on mucosal albumin clearance in intestine. *Am. J. Physiol.* 242 (*Gastrointest. Liver Physiol.* 5): G448–G454, 1982.

193. GROTTE, G. Passage of dextran molecules across the blood-lymph barrier. *Acta Chir. Scand. Suppl.* 211: 1–84, 1956.

194. GROTTE, G., L. JUHLIN, AND N. SANDBERG. Passage of solid spherical particles across the blood-lymph barrier. *Acta Physiol. Scand.* 50: 287–293, 1960.

195. GRUBBS, C. J., AND R. C. MOON. Transport of orally administered 9,10-dimethyl-1,2,-benzanthracene in the Sprague-Dawley rat. *Cancer Res.* 33: 1785–1789, 1973.

196. GUYTON, A. C., A. E. TAYLOR, AND R. A. BRACE. A synthesis of intestinal fluid regulation and lymph formation. *Federation Proc.* 35: 1881–1885, 1976.

197. HAKIM, A. A., AND LIFSON, N. Effects of pressure on water and solute transport by dog intestinal mucosa in vitro. *Am. J. Physiol.* 216: 276–284, 1969.

198. HALL, J. G., B. MORRIS, AND G. WOOLLEY. Intrinsic rhythmic propulsion of lymph in the unanaesthetized sheep. *J. Physiol. Lond.* 180: 336–349, 1965.

199. HANZON, V. Liver cell secretion under normal and pathologic conditions studied by fluorescence microscopy on living rats. *Acta Physiol. Scand. Suppl.* 28: 101, 1952.

200. HARDY, R. N. The influence of specific chemical factors in the solvent on the absorption of macromolecular substances from the small intestine of the newborn calf. *J. Physiol. Lond.* 204: 607–632, 1969.

201. HARGENS, A. R., AND B. W. ZWEIFACH. Transport between blood and peripheral lymph in intestine. *Microvasc. Res.* 11: 89–101, 1976.

202. HARPER, S. L., J. A. BARROWMAN, P. R. KVIETYS, AND D. N. GRANGER. Effect of neurotensin on intestinal capillary permeability and blood flow. *Am. J. Physiol.* 247 (*Gastrointest. Liver Physiol.* 10): G161–G166, 1984.

203. HEATH, T. Pathways of intestinal lymph drainage in normal sheep and in sheep following thoracic duct occlusion. *Am. J. Anat.* 115: 569–580, 1964.

204. HEIDENHAIN, R. Versuche und Fragen zur Lehre von der Lymphbildung. *Pfluegers Arch. Gesamte Physiol. Menschen Tiere* 49: 209–301, 1891.

205. HELLMAN, L., H. L. BRADLOW, E. L. FRAZELL, AND T. F. GALLAGHER. Tracer studies of the absorption and fate of steroid hormones in man. *J. Clin. Invest.* 35: 1033–1044, 1956.

206. HENDRIX, B. M., AND J. E. SWEET. A study of amino nitrogen and glucose in lymph and blood before and after the injection of nutrient solutions in the intestine. *J. Biol. Chem.* 32: 299–307, 1917.

207. HENRIKSEN, J. H. Permselectivity of the liver blood-lymph (ascitic fluid) barrier to macromolecules in decompensated cirrhosis: relation to calculated pore-size. *Clin. Physiol. Oxford* 3: 163–171, 1983.

208. HENRIKSEN, J. H. Estimation of lymphatic conductance. A model based on protein-kinetic studies and haemodynamic measurements in patients with cirrhosis of the liver and in pigs. *Scand. J. Clin. Lab. Invest.* 45: 123–130, 1985.

209. HENRIKSEN, J. H., T. HORN, AND P. CHRISTOFFERSEN. The blood-lymph barrier in the liver. A review based on morphological and functional concepts of normal and cirrhotic liver. *Liver* 4: 221–232, 1984.

210. HERBERTSON, B. M., AND M. E. WALLACE. Chylous ascites in newborn mice. *J. Med. Genet.* 1: 10–23, 1964.

211. HIGGINS, J. A., AND R. J. BARRNETT. Fine structural localization of acyltransferases. The monoglyceride and $\alpha$-glycerophosphate pathways in intestinal absorptive cells. *J. Cell Biol.* 50: 102–120, 1971.

212. HIRASHIMA, T., D. KUWAHARA, AND M. NISHI. Morphology of lymphatics in the canine large intestine. *Lymphology* 17: 69–72, 1984.

213. HOGAN, R. D., AND J. L. UNTHANK. The initial lymphatics as sensors of interstitial fluid volume. *Microvasc. Res.* 31: 317–324, 1986.

214. HOLLANDER, D. Retinol lymphatic and portal transport: influence of pH, bile and fatty acids. *Am. J. Physiol.* 239 (*Gastrointest. Liver Physiol.* 2): G210–G214, 1980.

215. HOLLANDER, D., E. RIM, AND D. MORGAN. Intestinal absorption of 25-hydroxyvitamin $D_3$ in unanaesthetised rat. *Am. J. Physiol.* 236 (*Endocrinol. Metab. Gastrointest. Physiol.* 5): E441–E445, 1979.

216. HOLT, P. R. Dietary treatment of protein loss in intestinal lymphangiectasia. *Pediatrics* 34: 629–635, 1964.

217. HOLTZLOHNER, E., AND C. NIESSING. Die Drusentatigkeit bei Nervenreizung 5. Lebenbeobachtungen an Zellen, Lymphspal-

ten und Kapillaren der Unterkieferdruse. *Z. Biol.* 97: 563–572, 1936.
218. HORST, H.-J., W. J. HOLTJE, M. DENNIS, A. COERT, J. GEELEN, AND K. D. VOIGT. Lymphatic absorption and metabolism of orally administered testosterone undecanoate in man. *Klin. Wochenschr.* 54: 875–879, 1976.
219. HUANG, H. S., AND D. S. GOODMAN. Vitamin A and carotenoids. I. Intestinal absorption and metabolism of $^{14}$C-labeled vitamin A alcohol and $\beta$-carotene in the rat. *J. Biol. Chem.* 240: 2839–2844, 1965.
220. HULTEN, L., J. LINDHAGEN, O. LUNDGREN, S. FASTH, AND C. AHREN. Regional intestinal blood flow in ulcerative colitis and Crohn's disease. *Gastroenterology* 72: 388–396, 1977.
221. HUNGERFORD, G. F. Effect of adrenalectomy and hydrocortisone on lymph glucose in rats. *Proc. Soc. Exp. Biol. Med.* 100: 754–756, 1959.
222. HUNGERFORD, G. F., AND W. O. REINHARDT. Comparison of effects of sodium pentobarbital or ether-induced anesthesia on rate of flow and cell content of rat thoracic duct lymph. *Am. J. Physiol* 160: 9–14, 1950.
223. HUTH, F. Special pathology of the lymphovascular system. In: *Lymphangiology*, edited by M. Foldi and J. R. Casley-Smith. Stuttgart, FRG: Schattauer, 1983, p. 243–250.
224. HYDE, P. M., E. A. DOISY, W. H. ELLIOTT, AND E. A. DOISY. Absorption of enterally administered 17-$\alpha$-methyl-$^{14}$C-testosterone and its metabolites. *J. Biol. Chem.* 209: 257–263, 1954.
225. HYUN, S. A., G. V. VAHOUNY, AND C. R. TREADWELL. Portal absorption of fatty acids in lymph and portal vein–cannulated rats. *Biochim. Biophys. Acta* 137: 296–305, 1967.
226. INTAGLIETTA, M., AND J. F. GROSS. Vasomotion, tissue fluid flow and the formation of lymph. *Int. J. Microcirc. Clin. Exp.* 1: 55–65, 1982.
227. IVEY, K., L. DENBESTEN, T. H. KENT, AND J. A. CLIFTON. Lymphangiectasia of the colon with protein loss and malabsorption. *Gastroenterology* 57: 709–714, 1969.
228. JANSS, D. H., AND R. C. MOON. Absorption of intragastrically administered 7,12-dimethylbenzanthracene (Abstract). *Federation Proc.* 29: 817, 1970.
229. JAQUES, L. B., G. J. MILLER, AND J. W. T. SPINKS. The metabolism of the K vitamins. *Schweiz. Med. Wochenschr.* 84: 792–796, 1954.
230. JEEJEEBHOY, K. N. Cause of hypoalbuminaemia in patients with gastrointestinal and cardiac disease. *Lancet* 1: 343–348, 1962.
231. JEFFRIES, G. H., A. CHAPMAN, AND M. H. SLEISENGER. Low fat diet in intestinal lymphangiectasia. *N. Engl. J. Med.* 270: 761–766, 1964.
232. JERSILD, R. A. A time sequence study of fat absorption in the rat jejunum. *Am. J. Anat.* 118: 135–162, 1966.
233. JOB, T. T. Lymphatico-venous communications in the common rat and their significance. *Am. J. Anat.* 24: 467–491, 1918.
234. JOHNSON, P., AND W. F. R. POVER. Intestinal absorption of alpha tocopherol. *Life Sci.* 1: 115–117, 1962.
235. JOHNSTON, J. M. Triglyceride biosynthesis in the intestinal mucosa. In: *Lipid Absorption: Biochemical and Clinical Aspects*, edited by K. Rommel, H. Goebell, and R. Böhmer. Lancaster, UK: MTP, 1976, p. 85–94.
236. JOHNSTON, M. G. Involvement of lymphatic collecting ducts in the physiology and pathophysiology of lymph flow. In: *Experimental Biology of the Lymphatic Circulation*, edited by M. G. Johnston. Amsterdam: Elsevier, 1985.
237. JOHNSTON, M. G., A. KANALEC, AND J. L. GORDON. Effects of arachidonic acid and its cyclo-oxygenase and lipoxygenase products on lymphatic vessel contractility in vitro. *Prostaglandins* 25: 85–98, 1983.
238. JONES, A. L., AND D. L. SCHMUCKER. Current concepts of liver structure as related to function. *Gastroenterology* 73: 833–851, 1977.
239. JONES, W. R., C. C. C. O'MORCHOE, H. M. JAROSZ, AND P. J. O'MORCHOE. Distribution of charged sites on lymphatic endothelium. *Lymphology* 19: 5–14, 1986.
240. KAIHARA, S., H. NISHIMURA, T. AOYAGI, H. KAMEDA, AND H. UEDA. Protein-losing gastroenteropathy as a cause of hypoproteinaemia in constrictive pericarditis. *Jpn Heart J.* 4: 386–394, 1963.
241. KALIMA, T. V. The structure and function of intestinal lymphatics and the influence of impaired lymph flow on the ileum of rats. *Scand. J. Gastroenterol. Suppl.* 6: 10, 1971.
242. KALIMA, T. V., AND Y. COLLAN. Intestinal villus in experimental lymphatic obstruction. Correlation of light and electron microscopic findings with clinical diseases. *Scand. J. Gastroenterol.* 5: 497–510, 1970.
243. KAMEI, Y. The distribution and relative location of the lymphatic and blood vessels in the mucosa of the rabbit colon. *Nagoya Med. J.* 15: 223–238, 1969.
244. KAMP, J. D., AND H.-G. NEUMANN. Absorption of carcinogens into the thoracic duct lymph of the rat: aminostilbene derivatives and 3-methylcholanthrene. *Xenobiotica* 5: 717–727, 1975.
245. KATAYAMA, K., AND FUJITA, T. Studies on biotransformation of elastase. II. Intestinal absorption of $^{131}$I-labelled elastase in vivo. *Biochim. Biophys. Acta* 288: 181–189, 1972.
246. KAYDEN, H. J., AND M. MEDICK. The absorption and metabolism of short and long chain fatty acids in puromycin-treated rats. *Biochim. Biophys. Acta* 176: 37–43, 1969.
247. KELLY, K. A., R. W. IKARD, L. M. NYHUS, AND H. N. HARKINS. Gastric secretagogues in postprandial thoracic duct lymph. *Am. J. Physiol.* 205: 85–88, 1963.
248. KESSLER, J. I., P. NARCESSIAN, AND D. MAUDLIN. Biosynthesis of lipoproteins by intestinal epithelium. Site of synthesis and sequence of association of lipid, sugar and protein moieties. *Gastroenterology* 68: 1058, 1975.
249. KEYL, M. J., A. C. K. CHANG, AND R. T. DOWELL. Constituents of lymph from the non-secreting stomach of the dog. *Lymphology* 14: 118–121, 1981.
250. KINMONTH, J. B. *The Lymphatics. Diseases, Lymphography and Surgery.* Baltimore, MD: Williams & Wilkins, 1972.
251. KIRSNER, J. B., AND R. G. SHORTER. *Inflammatory Bowel Disease.* Philadelphia, PA: Lea & Febiger, 1975.
252. KLEIN, E. On the lymphatic system and the minute structure of the salivary glands and pancreas. *Q. J. Microsc. Sci.* 22: 154–175, 1882.
253. KOO, A., L. H. SMAJE, AND P. D. SPENCER. Low permeability to macromolecules of the fenestrated capillaries in the submandibular gland. *Bibl. Anat.* 20: 301–304, 1981.
254. KOSTNER, G. M. Apo $\beta$-deficiency (a-$\beta$-lipoproteinaemia): a model for studying the lipoprotein metabolism. In: *Lipid Absorption: Biochemical and Clinical Aspects*, edited K. Rommel, H. Goebell, and R. Böhmer. Lancaster, UK: MTP, 1976.
255. KOTLER, D. P., Y. F. SHIAU, AND G. M. LEVINE. Effects of luminal contents on jejunal fatty acid esterification in the rat. *Am. J. Physiol.* 238 (*Gastrointest. Liver Physiol.* 1): G414–G418, 1980.
256. KOVI, J., H. D. DUONG, AND C. T. HOANG. Ultrastructure of intestinal lymphatics in Crohn's disease. *Am. J. Clin. Pathol.* 76: 385–394, 1981.
257. KVIETYS, P. R., J. M. MCLENDON, G. B. BULKLEY, M. A. PERRY, AND D. N. GRANGER. The pancreatic circulation: intrinsic regulation. *Am. J. Physiol.* 242 (*Gastrointest. Liver Physiol.* 5): G596–G602, 1982.
258. KVIETYS, P. R., W. H. WILBORN, AND D. N. GRANGER. Effects of net transmucosal volume flux on lymph flow in the canine colon. Structural-functional relationship. *Gastroenterology* 81: 1080–1090, 1981.
259. LAHER, J. M., G. A. CHERNENKO, AND J. A. BARROWMAN. Studies of the absorption and enterohepatic circulation of 7,12-dimethylbenzanthracene in the rat. *Can. J. Physiol. Pharmacol.* 61: 1368–1373, 1983.
260. LAHER, J. M., M. W. RIGLER, R. D. VETTER, J. A. BARROWMAN, AND J. S. PATTON. Similar bioavailability and lymphatic transport of benzo(a)pyrene when administered to rats in different amounts of dietary fat. *J. Lipid Res.* 25: 1337–1342, 1984.
261. LAINE, G., J. T. HALL, S. H. LAINE, AND H. J. GRANGER. Transsinusoidal fluid dynamics in canine liver during venous

hypertension. *Circ. Res.* 45: 317–323, 1979.
262. LAMPEL, M., AND H. F. KERN. Acute interstitial pancreatitis in the rat induced by excessive doses of a pancreatic secretagogue. *Virchows Arch. Pathol. Anat. Physiol.* 373: 97–117, 1977.
263. LARGIS, E. E., AND F. A. JACOBS. Effects of phlorizin on glucose transport into blood and lymph. *Biochim. Biophys. Acta* 225: 301–307, 1971.
264. LAURENT, U. B. C., AND T. C. LAURENT. On the origin of hyaluronate in blood. *Biochem. Internat.* 2: 195–199, 1981.
265. LAUWERYNS, J. M., A. BARET, AND L. BOUSSAUW. The pulmonary lymphatics: macroscopic and microscopic studies. *Am. Rev. Resp. Dis.* 101: 448–450, 1970.
266. LAWRENCE, C. W., F. D. CRAIN, F. J. LOTSPEICH, AND R. F. KRAUSE. Absorption, transport and storage of retinyl -15- $^{14}$C palmitate-9,10-$^{3}$H in the rat. *J. Lipid Res.* 7: 226–229, 1966.
267. LAWRENCE, J. A., D. BRYANT, K. B. ROBERTS, AND J. A. BARROWMAN. Effect of secretin on intestinal lymph flow and composition in the rat. *Q. J. Exp. Physiol.* 66: 297–305, 1981.
268. LEAK, L. V. Distribution of cell surface charges on mesothelium and lymphatic endothelium. *Microvasc. Res.* 31: 13–30, 1986.
269. LEAK, L. V., AND J. F. BURKE. Fine structure of the lymphatic capillary and the adjoining connective tissue area. *Am. J. Anat.* 118: 785–809, 1966.
270. LEAK, L. V., AND J. F. BURKE. Ultrastructural studies on the lymphatic anchoring filaments. *J. Cell Biol.* 36: 129–149, 1968.
271. LEE, F. C. The establishment of collateral circulation following ligation of the thoracic duct. *Bull. Johns Hopkins Hosp.* 33: 21–31, 1922.
272. LEE, J. S. Flows and pressures in lymphatic and blood vessels of intestine in water absorption. *Am. J. Physiol.* 200: 979–983, 1961.
273. LEE, J. S. Role of the mesenteric lymphatic system in water absorption from rat intestine in vitro. *Am. J. Physiol.* 204: 92–96, 1963.
274. LEE, J. S. Motility lymphatic contractility and distension pressure in intestinal absorption. *Am. J. Physiol.* 208: 621–627, 1965.
275. LEE, J. S. A micropuncture study of water transport by dog jejunal villi in vitro. *Am. J. Physiol.* 217: 1528–1533, 1969.
276. LEE, J. S. Role of lymphatic system in water and solute transport from rat intestine in vitro. *Q. J. Exp. Physiol.* 54: 311–321, 1969.
277. LEE, J. S. Contraction of villi and fluid transport in dog jejunal mucosa in vitro. *Am. J. Physiol.* 221: 488–495, 1971.
278. LEE, J. S. Glucose concentration and hydrostatic pressure in dog jejunal villus lymph. *Am. J. Physiol.* 226: 675–681, 1974.
279. LEE, J. S. Lymph capillary pressure of rat intestinal villi during fluid absorption. *Am. J. Physiol.* 237 (*Endocrinol. Metab. Gastrointest. Physiol.* 6): E301–E307, 1979.
280. LEE, J. S. Lymph flow during fluid absorption from rat jejunum. *Am. J. Physiol.* 240 (*Gastrointest. Liver Physiol.* 3): G312–G316, 1981.
281. LEE, J. S. Lymph pressure in intestinal villi and lymph flow during fluid secretion. In: *Tissue Fluid Pressure and Composition*, edited by A. R. Hargens. Baltimore, MD: Williams & Wilkins, 1981.
282. LEE, J. S. Intestinal transudation, secretion and lymph flow during volume expansion in the rat. *Am. J. Physiol.* 244 (*Gastrointest. Liver Physiol.* 7): G668–G674, 1983.
283. LEE, J. S. Relationship between intestinal motility, tone, water absorption and lymph flow in the rat. *J. Physiol. Lond.* 345: 489–499, 1983.
284. LEE, J. S. Hepatic lymph flow and protein concentration during intravenous saline infusion and intestinal fluid absorption. *Microvasc. Res.* 27: 370–378, 1984.
285. LEE, J. S. Lymphatic contractility. In: *Physiology of the Intestinal Circulation*, edited by A. P. Shepherd and D. N. Granger. New York: Raven, 1984, p. 201–210.
286. LEE, J. S. Lymph flow, lymph protein concentration, and protein output from rat small intestine. *Am. J. Physiol.* 248 (*Gastrointest. Liver Physiol.* 10): G670–G675, 1985.
287. LEE, J. S. Tissue fluid pressure, lymph pressure and fluid transport in rat intestinal villi. *Microvasc. Res.* 31: 170–183, 1986.
288. LEE, J. S., AND K. M. DUNCAN. Lymphatic and venous transport of water from rat jejunum: a vascular perfusion study. *Gastroenterology* 54: 559–567, 1968.
289. LEE, J. S., AND J. W. SILVERBERG. Effect of cholera toxin on fluid absorption and villus pressure in dog jejunal mucosa. *Gastroenterology* 62: 993–1000, 1972.
290. LEHNERT, T., R. A. ERLANDSON, AND J. J. DECOSSE. Lymph and blood capillaries of the human gastric mucosa. A morphologic basis for metastasis in early gastric carcinoma. *Gastroenterology* 89: 939–950, 1985.
291. LEVINE, S. E., D. N. GRANGER, R. A. BRACE, AND A. E. TAYLOR. Effect of hyperosmolality on vascular resistance and lymph flow in the cat ileum. *Am. J. Physiol.* 234 (*Heart Circ. Physiol.* 3): H14–H20, 1978.
292. LIFSON, N. Use of microspheres to measure intraorgan distribution of blood flow in the splanchnic circulation. In: *Measurement of Blood Flow: Application to the Splanchnic Circulation*, edited by D. N. Granger and G. B. Bulkley. Baltimore, MD: Williams & Wilkins, 1981, p. 177–194.
293. LINDER, E., AND R. BLOMSTRAND. Technic for collection of thoracic duct lymph of man. *Proc. Soc. Exp. Biol. Med.* 97: 653–657, 1958.
294. LORD, R. S. A. The white veins: conceptual difficulties in the history of the lymphatics. *Med. Hist.* 12: 174–184, 1968.
295. LUDWIG, C. *Lehrbuch der Physiologie des Menschen.* Leipzig: Winter, 1858.
296. MAHLEY, R. W., B. D. BENNETT, D. J. MORRE, M. E. GRAY, W. THISTLETHWAITE, AND V. S. LEQUIRE. Lipoproteins associated with the Golgi apparatus isolated from epithelial cells of rat small intestine. *Lab. Invest.* 25: 435–444, 1971.
297. MAISLOS, M., J. SILVER, AND M. FAINARU. Intestinal absorption of vitamin D sterols: differential absorption into lymph and portal blood in the rat. *Gastroenterology* 80: 1528–1534, 1981.
298. MALIK, A. B., R. J. MULLINS, P. S. BARIE, D. R. BELL, AND B. C. LEE. Thoracic duct lymph flow after pancreatitis: role in circulatory collapse. *Adv. Shock Res.* 8: 81–91, 1982.
299. MALLET-GUY, P., J. MICHOULIER, AND S. BAEV. In: *The Biliary System*, edited by W. Taylor. Philadelphia, PA: Davis, 1965.
300. MANN, J. D., AND G. M. HIGGINS. Lymphocytes in thoracic duct, intestinal and hepatic lymph. *Blood* 5: 177–190, 1950.
301. MARSH, J. B., AND C. E. SPARKS. Hepatic secretion of lipoproteins in the rat and the effect of experimental nephrosis. *J. Clin. Invest.* 64: 1229–1237, 1979.
302. MARSHALL, W. H., T. NEYAZAKI, AND H. L. ABRAMS. Abnormal protein loss after thoracic duct ligation in dogs. *N. Engl. J. Med.* 273: 1092–1094, 1965.
303. MAWHINNEY, H. J. D., AND I. C. RODDIE. Spontaneous activity in isolated bovine mesenteric lymphatics. *J. Physiol. Lond.* 229: 339–348, 1973.
304. MAY, A. J., AND B. C. WHALER. The absorption of *Clostridium botulinum* type A toxin from the alimentary canal. *Br. J. Exp. Pathol.* 39: 307–316, 1958.
305. MAYER, A. D., M. AIREY, J. HODGSON, AND M. J. MCMAHON. Enzyme transfer from pancreas to plasma during acute pancreatitis. The contribution of ascitic fluid and lymphatic drainage of the pancreas. *Gut* 26: 876–881, 1985.
306. MAYERSON, H. S. The lymphatic system. *Sci. Am.* 208: 80–90, 1963.
307. MAYERSON, H. S. The physiologic importance of lymph. In: *Handbook of Physiology. Circulation*, edited by W. F. Hamilton. Washington, DC: Am. Physiol. Soc., 1963, sect. 2, vol. II, chapt. 30, p. 1035–1073.
308. MAYERSON, H. S. Three centuries of lymphatic history—an outline. *Lymphology* 2: 143–150, 1969.
309. MAYERSON, H. S., C. G. WOLFRAM, H. H. SHIRLEY, JR., AND K. WASSERMAN. Regional differences in capillary permeability. *Am. J. Physiol.* 198: 155–160, 1960.

310. Mayo, C., and C. H. Greene. Studies in the metabolism of the bile. IV. The role of the lymphatics in the early stages of the development of obstructive jaundice. *Am. J. Physiol.* 89: 280–288, 1929.
311. McCarrell, J. D., S. Thayer, and C. K. Drinker. The lymph drainage of the gall bladder together with observations on the composition of liver lymph. *Am. J. Physiol.* 133: 79–81, 1941.
312. McDonald, G. B., K. W. Lau, A. L. Schy, J. E. Wergedal, and D. J. Baylink. Intestinal metabolism and portal venous transport of 1,25(OH)$_2$D$_3$, 25(OH)D$_3$ and vitamin D$_3$ in rat. *Am. J. Physiol.* 248 (*Gastrointest. Liver Physiol.* 11): G633–G638, 1985.
313. McDonald, G. B., D. R. Saunders, M. Weidman, and L. Fisher. Portal venous transport of long chain fatty acids absorbed from rat intestine. *Am. J. Physiol.* 239 (*Gastrointest. Liver Physiol.* 2): G141–G150, 1980.
314. McGuigan, J. E., B. M. Jaffe, and W. T. Newton. Immunochemical measurements of endogenous gastrin release. *Gastroenterology* 59: 499–504, 1970.
315. McHale, N. G. Innervation of the lymphatic circulation. In: *Experimental Biology of the Lymphatic Circulation*, edited by M. G. Johnston. Amsterdam: Elsevier, 1985.
316. McHale, N. G., and I. C. Roddie. The effect of transmural pressure on pumping activity in isolated bovine lymphatic vessels. *J. Physiol. Lond.* 261: 255–269, 1976.
317. McHale, N. G., and I. C. Roddie. The effect of catecholamines on pumping activity in isolated bovine mesenteric lymphatics. *J. Physiol. Lond.* 338: 527–536, 1983.
318. McHale, N. G., I. G. Roddie, and K. D. Thornbury. Nervous modulation of spontaneous contractions in bovine mesenteric lymphatics. *J. Physiol. Lond.* 309: 461–472, 1980.
319. McMahon, M. T., and G. R. Neale. Protein losing enteropathy possibly due to filariasis. *Proc. R. Soc. Med.* 62: 1043–1044, 1969.
320. McMahon, M. T., G. Neale, and G. R. Thompson. Lymphatic and portal venous transport of alpha-tocopherol and cholesterol. *Eur. J. Clin. Invest.* 1: 288–294, 1971.
321. Mezick, J. A., R. K. Tompkins, and D. G. Cornwell. Absorption and intestinal lymphatic transport of $^{14}$C-menadione. *Life Sci.* 7: 153–158, 1968.
322. Mislin, H. Experimental detection of automatism of lymph vessels. *Experientia Basel* 17: 29–30, 1961.
323. Mislin, H. Active contractility of the lymphangion and coordination of lymphangion chains. *Experientia Basel* 32: 820–822, 1976.
324. Mistilis, S. P., and A. P. Skyring. Intestinal lymphangiectasia. Therapeutic effect of lymph venous anastomosis. *Am. J. Med.* 40: 634–641, 1966.
325. Miura, S., H. Asakura, Y. Munakata, K. Kobayashi, M. Yashioka, T. Morishita, and M. Tsuchiya. Lymphatic role in the pathogenesis of fat malabsorption in liver cirrhosis in rats. *Dig. Dis. Sci.* 27: 1030–1036, 1982.
326. Morgan, R. G. H., and B. Borgström. The mechanism of fat absorption in the bile fistula rat. *Q. J. Exp. Physiol.* 54: 228–243, 1969.
327. Morris, B. The hepatic and intestinal contributions to the thoracic duct lymph. *Q. J. Exp. Physiol.* 41: 318–325, 1956.
328. Morris, B. Cited in: *Lymphatics, Lymph and the Lymphomyeloid Complex*, edited by M. Yoffey, and F. C. Courtice. London: Academic, 1970, p. 234.
329. Mortillaro, N. A., D. N. Granger, P. R. Kvietys, G. Rutili, and A. E. Taylor. Effects of histamine and histamine antagonists on intestinal capillary permeability. *Am. J. Physiol.* 240 (*Gastrointest. Liver Physiol.* 3): G381–G386, 1981.
330. Mortillaro, N. A., and A. E. Taylor. Interaction of capillary and tissue forces in the cat intestine. *Circ. Res.* 39: 348–358, 1976.
331. Nagata, H., and P. H. Guth. In vivo observation of the lymphatic system in the rat stomach. *Gastroenterology* 86: 1443–1450, 1984.
332. Nelson, R. A., and C. F. Code. Absorbed water and intestinal lymph flow (Abstract). *Federation Proc.* 28: 462, 1969.
333. Nesis, L., and E. E. Sterns. Lymph flow from the colon under varying conditions. *Ann. Surg.* 177: 422–427, 1973.
334. Nix, J. T., F. C. Mann, J. L. Bollman, J. H. Grindlay, and E. V. Flock. Alterations of protein constituents of lymph by specific injury to the liver. *Am. J. Physiol.* 164: 119–122, 1951.
335. Novan, A. Water absorption from the intestine via portal and lymphatic pathways in rats. *Proc. Soc. Exp. Biol. Med.* 117: 317–320, 1964.
336. Ockner, R. K., F. B. Hughes, and K. J. Isselbacher. Very low density lipoproteins in intestinal lymph: origin composition and role in lipid transport in the fasting state. *J. Clin. Invest.* 48: 2079–2088, 1969.
337. Ockner, R. K., and J. A. Manning. Fatty acid–binding protein in small intestine. Identification, isolation and evidence for its role in cellular fatty acid transport. *J. Clin. Invest.* 54: 326–338, 1974.
338. Ohhashi, T., T. Azuma, and M. Sakaguchi. Transmembrane potentials in ovine lymphatic smooth muscle. *Proc. Soc. Exp. Biol. Med.* 159: 350–352, 1978.
339. Ohhashi, T., T. Azuma, and M. Sakaguchi. Active and passive mechanical characteristics of bovine mesenteric lymphatics. *Am. J. Physiol.* 239 (*Heart Circ. Physiol.* 2): H88–H95, 1980.
340. Ohhashi, T., S. Fukushima, and T. Azuma. Vasa vasorum within the media of bovine mesenteric lymphatics. *Proc. Soc. Exp. Biol. Med.* 154: 582–586, 1977.
341. Ohhashi, T., Y. Kawai, and T. Azuma. The responses of lymphatic smooth muscles to vasoactive substances. *Pfluegers Arch.* 375: 183–188, 1978.
342. Ohhashi, T., N. G. McHale, I. C. Roddie, and K. D. Thornbury. Electrical field stimulation as a method of stimulating nerve or smooth muscle in isolated bovine mesenteric lymphatics. *Pfluegers Arch.* 388: 221–226, 1980.
343. Ohhashi, T., J. A. Olschowka, and D. M. Jacobowitz. Vasoactive intestinal peptide inhibitory innervation in bovine mesenteric lymphatics. *Circ. Res.* 53: 535–538, 1983.
344. Ohlsson, K. Experimental pancreatitis in the dog. Appearance of complexes between proteases and trypsin inhibitors in ascitic fluid, lymph and plasma. *Scand. J. Gastroenterol.* 6: 645–652, 1971.
345. Oliver, G. C., J. Cooksey, C. Witte, and M. Witte. Absorption and transport of digitoxin in the dog. *Circ. Res.* 29: 419–423, 1971.
346. O'Morchoe, C. C. C., and P. J. O'Morchoe. Renal contribution to thoracic duct lymph in dogs. *J. Physiol. Lond.* 194: 305–315, 1968.
347. Palay, S. L., and L. J. Karlin. An electron microscopic study of the intestinal villus. *J. Biophys. Biochem. Cytol.* 5: 363–384, 1959.
348. Paldino, R. L., and C. Hyman. Relationship between lymphatic and blood flow in various structures in the abdominal cavity. *Proc. Soc. Exp. Biol. Med.* 117: 904–910, 1964.
349. Palin, K. J., C. G. Wilson, S. S. Davis, and A. J. Phillips. The effect of oils on the lymphatic absorption of DDT. *J. Pharm. Pharmacol.* 34: 707–710, 1982.
350. Papp, M., and I. Fodor. Lymphatic system of the salivary glands. In: *Lymphatics and Lymph Circulation* (2nd ed.), edited by I. Rusznyak, M. Foldi, and G. Szabo. Oxford, UK: Pergamon, 1967.
351. Papp, M., E. Nemeth, I. Feuer, and I. Fodor. Effect of an impairment of lymph flow on experimental acute pancreatitis. *Acta Med. Acad. Sci. Hung.* 11: 203–208, 1958.
352. Papp, M., E. P. Nemeth, and E. J. Horvath. Pancreaticoduodenal lymph flow and lipase activity in acute experimental pancreatitis. *Lymphology* 4: 48–53, 1971.
353. Papp, M., S. Ormai, E. J. Horvath, and I. Fodor. The effect of secretin and pancreozymin on pancreatico-duodenal lymph flow and lipase activity in normal dogs and on thoracic duct lymph flow and lipase activity in rats with chronic pancreatitis. *Lymphology* 4: 67–73, 1971.
354. Papp, M., P. Rohlich, I. Rusznyak, and I. Toro. An

electron microscopic study of the central lacteal in the intestinal villus of the cat. *Z. Zellforsch. Mikrosk. Anat.* 57: 475–486, 1962.
355. PAPPENHEIMER, J. R., AND A. SOTO-RIVERA. Effective osmotic pressure of the plasma proteins and other quantities associated with the capillary circulation in the hindlimbs of cats and dogs. *Am. J. Physiol.* 152: 471–491, 1948.
356. PATTERSON, D. F., W. MEDWAY, H. LUNGINBUHL, AND S. CHACKO. Congenital hereditary lymphedema in the dog. 1. Clinical and genetic studies. *J. Med. Genet.* 4: 145–152, 1967.
357. PATTERSON, R. M., C. L. BALLARD, K. WASSERMAN, AND H. S. MAYERSON. Lymphatic permeability to albumin. *Am. J. Physiol.* 194: 120–124, 1958.
358. PATTON, J. S. Gastrointestinal lipid digestion. In: *Physiology of the Gastrointestinal Tract*, edited by L. R. Johnson. New York: Raven, 1981, p. 1123–1146.
359. PEAKE, I. R., H. G. WINDMUELLER, AND J. G. BIERI. A comparison of the intestinal absorption, lymph and plasma transport, and tissue uptake of $\alpha$- and $\gamma$-tocopherols in the rat. *Biochim. Biophys. Acta* 260: 679–688, 1972.
360. PERRAULT, J., AND H. MARKOWITZ. Protein-losing gastroenteropathy and the intestinal clearance of serum $\alpha_1$-antitrypsin. *Mayo Clin. Proc.* 59: 278–279, 1984.
361. PERRY, M. A., W. J. CROOK, AND D. N. GRANGER. Permeability of gastric capillaries to small and large molecules. *Am. J. Physiol.* 241 (*Gastrointest. Liver Physiol* 4): G478–G486, 1981.
362. PERRY, T. T. Role of lymphatic vessels in transmission of lipase in disseminated pancreatic fat necrosis. *Arch. Pathol.* 43: 456–465, 1947.
363. PETERS, T. J., AND M. T. MACMAHON. The absorption of glycine and glycine-oligopeptides by the rat. *Clin. Sci.* 39: 811–821, 1970.
364. PETERSON, R. E., AND J. D. MANN. Transport of radioactive iron in intestinal lymph. *Am. J. Physiol.* 169: 763–766, 1952.
365. PIHL, O., F. L. IBER, AND W. G. LINSCHEER. The enhancement of vitamin $D_3$ absorption in man by medium and long chain fatty acids. *Clin. Res.* 18: 462, 1970.
366. PLAUTH, W. H., T. A. WALDMANN, R. D. WOCHNER, N. S. BRAUNWALD, AND E. BRAUNWALD. Protein-losing enteropathy secondary to constrictive pericarditis in childhood. *Pediatrics* 34: 636–648, 1964.
367. POCOCK, D. M. E., AND A. VOST. DDT absorption and chylomicron transport in the rat. *Lipids* 9: 374–381, 1974.
368. POLDERMAN, H., J. D. MCCARRELL, AND H. K. BEECHER. Effect of anaesthesia on lymph flow (local procaine, ether and pentobarbital sodium). *J. Pharmacol. Exp. Ther.* 78: 400–406, 1943.
369. PULLINGER, B. D., AND H. W. FLOREY. Some observations on the structure and function of lymphatics: their behaviour in local oedema. *Br. J. Exp. Pathol.* 16: 49–61, 1935.
370. QUILLEN, E. W., D. N. GRANGER, AND A. E. TAYLOR. The effects of arginine-vasopressin on capillary filtration in the cat ileum. *Gastroenterology* 72: 474–478, 1977.
371. REDGRAVE, T. G. Inhibition of protein synthesis and absorption of lipid into thoracic duct lymph of rats. *Proc. Soc. Exp. Biol. Med.* 130: 776–780, 1969.
372. REDGRAVE, T. G. Association of Golgi membranes with lipid droplets (prechylomicrons) from within epithelial cells during absorption of fat. *Aust. J. Exp. Biol. Med. Sci.* 49: 209–224, 1971.
373. REDGRAVE, T. G. The role of chylomicron formation of phospholipase activity of intestinal Golgi membranes. *Aust. J. Exp. Biol. Med. Sci.* 51: 427–434, 1973.
374. REDGRAVE, T. G. Formation and metabolism of chylomicrons. In: *Gastrointestinal Physiology IV*, edited by J. A. Young. Baltimore, MD: University Park, 1983, vol. 28, p. 103–130. (Int. Rev. Physiol. Ser.)
375. REDGRAVE, T. G., AND D. B. ZILVERSMIT. Does puromycin block release of chylomicrons from the intestine? *Am. J. Physiol.* 217: 336–340, 1969.
376. REES, E. D., P. MANDELSTAM, J. Q. LOWRY, AND H. LIPSCOMB. A study of the mechanism of intestinal absorption of benzo($a$)pyrene. *Biochim. Biophys. Acta* 225: 96–107, 1971.
377. REISER, R., AND M. J. BRYSON. Route of absorption of free fatty acids and triglycerides from the intestine. *J. Biol. Chem.* 189: 87–91, 1951.
378. REIZENSTEIN, P. G., E. P. CRONKITE, L. M. MEYER, AND E. A. USENIK. Lymphatics in intestinal absorption of vitamin $B_{12}$ and iron. *Proc. Soc. Exp. Biol. Med.* 105: 233–236, 1960.
379. RENYI-VAMOS, F., AND G. SZINAY. Das lymphgefäss system des Magens und sein Verhalten bei Ulcus ventriculi. *Acta Morphol. Acad. Sci. Hung.* 4: 353–365, 1954.
380. REZA RAFII, M. Mesenteriale Lymphgefäss veranderungen bei Leberzirrhose und Rechtscherz Insuffienz. Morphologische Beitrage. *Fortschr. Med.* 90: 1295–1298, 1972.
381. RICHARDSON, P. D. I., D. N. GRANGER, D. MAILMAN, AND P. R. KVIETYS. Permeability characteristics of colonic capillaries. *Am. J. Physiol.* 239 (*Gastrointest. Liver Physiol.* 2): G300–G305, 1980.
382. RITCHIE, H. D., J. H. GRINDLAY, AND J. L. BOLLMAN. Surgical jaundice: experimental evidence against the regurgitation theory. *Surg. Forum* 7: 415–418, 1956.
383. RITCHIE, H. D., J. H. GRINDLAY, AND J. L. BOLLMAN. Flow of lymph from the canine liver. *Am. J. Physiol.* 196: 105–109, 1959.
384. ROBERTS, S. H., AND A. P. DOUGLAS. Intestinal lymphangiectasia: the variability of presentation. A study of five cases. *Q J. Med.* 45: 39–48, 1976.
385. ROBERTS, S. H., D. L. KEPKAY, AND J. A. BARROWMAN. Proteins of ascitic fluid in constrictive pericarditis. *Am. J. Dig. Dis.* 23: 844–848, 1978.
386. RUSZNYAK, I., M. FOLDI, AND G. SZABO. *Lymphatics and Lymph Circulation* (2nd ed.). New York: Pergamon, 1967.
387. RUTILI, G., AND K. E. ARFORS. Protein concentration in interstitial and lymphatic fluids from the subcutaneous tissue. *Acta Physiol. Scand.* 99: 1–8, 1977.
388. SABESIN, S. M., AND S. FRASE. Electron microscopic studies of the assembly, intracellular transport and secretion of chylomicrons by rat intestine. *J. Lipid Res.* 18: 496–511, 1977.
389. SABESIN, S. M., AND K. J. ISSELBACHER. Protein synthesis inhibition: mechanism for the production of impaired fat absorption. *Science Wash. DC* 147: 1149–1151, 1965.
390. SAUNDERS, D. R., AND A. M. DAWSON. The absorption of oleic acid in the bile fistula rat. *Gut* 4: 254–260, 1963.
391. SCANU, A. M., L. P. AGGERBECK, A. W. KRUSKI, C. T. LIM, AND H. J. KAYDEN. A study of the abnormal lipoproteins in abetalipoproteinaemia. *J. Clin. Invest.* 53: 440–453, 1974.
392. SCHACHTER, D., J. D. FINKELSTEIN, AND S. KOWARSKI. Pathways of transport and metabolism of $^{14}$C-vitamin $D_2$ in the rat. *J. Clin. Invest.* 42: 974–975, 1963.
393. SCHACHTER, D., J. D. FINKELSTEIN, AND S. KOWARSKI. Metabolism of vitamin D. I. Preparation of radioactive vitamin D and it intestinal absorption in the rat. *J. Clin. Invest.* 43: 787–796, 1964.
394. SCHACHTER, H. The subcellular sites of glycosylation. *Biochem. Soc. Symp.* 40: 57–71, 1974.
395. SCHAEFER, J. W., GRIFFEN, W. O., AND L. D. DUBILIER. Colonic lymphangiectasis associated with a potassium depletion syndrome. *Gastroenterology* 55: 515–521, 1968.
396. SCHAFFNER, F., AND H. POPPER. Capillarization of hepatic sinusoids in man. *Gastroenterology* 44: 239–242, 1963.
397. SCHMIDT, H., AND W. CREUTZFELDT. Etiology and pathogenesis of pancreatitis. In: *Gastroenterology*, edited by H. L. Bockus. Philadelphia, PA: Saunders, 1976, p. 1005–1019.
398. SEBASTIEN, P., R. MASSE, AND J. BIGNON. Recovery of ingested asbestos fibers from the gastrointestinal lymph in rats. *Environ. Res.* 22: 201–216, 1980.
399. SEIFERT, J., H. PROLS, K. MESSMER, R. BUCKLEIN, G. LOB, H. MEHNERT, AND W. BRENDEL. Concentration and transport of different sugars in the lymph of the thoracic duct and in blood of the portal vein in dogs after enteral and parenteral administration. *Digestion* 12: 221–231, 1975.
400. SERVELLE, M., Y. BOUVRAIN, R. TRICOT, J. SOULIE, H. TUR-

PYN, F. FRENTZ, C. CORNU, AND C. NADIM. Lymphatic circulation in constrictive pericarditis. *J. Cardiovasc. Surg.* 7: 182–200, 1966.
401. SHAFIROFF, B. G. P., H. DOUBILET, AND W. RUGGIERO. Bilirubin resorption in obstructive jaundice. *Proc. Soc. Exp. Biol. Med.* 42: 203–205, 1939.
402. SHANNON, A. D., AND A. K. LASCELLES. The intestinal and hepatic contributions to the flow and composition of thoracic duct lymph in young milk-fed calves. *Q. J. Exp. Physiol.* 53: 194–205, 1968.
403. SHANNON, A. D., AND A. K. LASCELLES. Lymph flow and protein composition of thoracic duct lymph in the newborn calf. *Q. J. Exp. Physiol.* 53: 415–421, 1968.
404. SHEPPARD, M. S., AND E. E. STERNS. The role of vascular and lymph capillaries in the clearance of interstitially injected albumin in acute and chronic inflammation of the colon. *Surg. Gynecol. Obstet.* 139: 707–711, 1974.
405. SHILKIN, K. B., B. J. ZERMAN, AND J. B. BLACKWELL. Lymphangiectatic cysts of the small bowel. *J. Pathol. Bacteriol.* 96: 353–358, 1968.
406. SIEBER, S. M., V. H. COHN, AND W. T. WYNN. The entry of foreign compounds into the thoracic duct lymph of the rat. *Xenobiotica* 4: 265–284, 1974.
407. SILVESTER, C. F. On the presence of permanent communications between the lymphatic and the venous system at the level of the renal veins in adult South American monkeys. *Am. J. Anat.* 12: 447–460, 1911.
408. SIM, D. N., A. DUPREZ, AND M. C. ANDERSON. Modifications apportées au débit et a la composition de la lymphe du canal thoracique par la pancréatite experimentale chez le chien. *Acta Gastro-Enterol. Belg.* 29: 235–247, 1966.
409. SIMMONDS, W. J. The effect of fluid, electrolyte and food intake on thoracic duct lymph flow in unanaesthetized rat. *Aust. J. Exp. Biol. Med. Sci.* 33: 285–300, 1954.
410. SIMMONDS, W. J. Some observations on the increase in thoracic duct lymph flow during intestinal absorption of fat in unanaesthetized rats. *Aust. J. Exp. Biol. Med. Sci.* 33: 305–313, 1955.
411. SIMMONDS, W. J. Uptake of fatty acid and monoglyceride. In: *Lipid Absorption: Biochemical and Clinical Aspects*, edited by K. Rommel, H. Goebell, and R. Böhmer. Lancaster, UK: MTP, 1976, p. 51–64.
412. SIMPSON-MORGAN, M. W., AND T. C. SMEATON. The transfer of antibodies by neonates and adults. *Adv. Vet. Sci. Comp. Med.* 16: 355–386, 1972.
413. SITRIN, M. D., K. L. POLLACK, AND M. J. G. BOLT. Intestinal absorption of 1,25-dihydroxy-vitamin $D_3$ in the rat. *Am. J. Physiol.* 248 (*Gastrointest. Liver Physiol.* 10): G718–G725, 1985.
414. SITRIN, M. D., K. L. POLLACK, M. J. G. BOLT, AND I. H. ROSENBERG. Comparison of vitamin D and 25-hydroxyvitamin D absorption in the rat. *Am. J. Physiol.* 242 (*Gastrointest. Liver Physiol.* 5): G326–G332, 1982.
415. SITRIN, M. D., K. L. POLLACK, AND I. H. ROSENBERG. Intestinal absorption of 1-25-$(OH)_2$ vitamin $D_3$ (1,25-$D_3$) in the rat. *Gastroenterology* 80: 1288, 1981.
416. SJOVALL, J., AND I. AKESSON. Intestinal absorption of taurocholic acid in the rat. *Acta Physiol. Scand.* 34: 273–278, 1955.
417. SMALLWOOD, R. A., E. A. JONES, A. CRAIGIE, S. RAIA, AND V. M. ROSENOER. The delivery of newly synthesized albumin and fibrinogen to the plasma in dogs. *Clin. Sci.* 35: 35–43, 1968.
418. SOUCY, J. P., M. C. EYBALIN, R. TAILLEFER, A. LEVASSEUR, AND G. JOBIN. Lymphoscintigraphic demonstration of intestinal lymphangiectasia. *Clin. Nucl. Med.* 8: 535–537, 1983.
419. STALDER, H., AND G. JOLIAT. Blood in the lymph (hemochylia) and intestinal lymphangiectasia associated with Lutembacher's syndrome. *Am. J. Med.* 55: 99–104, 1973.
420. STARLING, E. H. The Arris and Gale lectures on the physiologic factors in the causation of dropsy. *Lancet* 1: 1267–1270, 1896.
421. STARLING, E. H. On the absorption of fluids from the connective tissue spaces. *J. Physiol. Lond.* 19: 312–326, 1896.
422. STERNLIEB, I., C. J. A. VAN DEN HAMER, AND S. ALPERT. Role of intestinal lymphatics in copper absorption. *Nature Lond.* 216: 824, 1967.
423. STERNS, E. E., AND G. E. R. VAUGHAN. The lymphatics of the dog colon. *Cancer* 26: 218–231, 1970.
424. STOELINGA, G. B. A., P. J. J. VAN MUNSTER, AND J. P. SLOOFF. Chylons effusions into the intestine in a patient with protein-losing gastroenteropathy. *Pediatrics* 31: 1011–1018, 1963.
425. STONE, H., T. C. FABIAN, AND E. S. MORRIS. Failure of thoracic duct drainage to ameliorate life-threatening physiologic derangements of acute alcoholic pancreatitis. *South. Med. J.* 76: 613–614, 1983.
426. STREMMEL, W., G. LOTZ, G. STROHMEYER, AND P. D. BERK. Identification, isolation, and partial characterization of a fatty acid binding protein from rat jejunal microvillus membranes. *J. Clin. Invest.* 75: 1068–1076, 1985.
427. STROBER, W., R. D. WOCHNER, P. P. CARBONE, AND T. A. WALDMANN. Intestinal lymphangiectasia: a protein-losing enteropathy with hypogammaglobulinaemia, lymphocytopenia, and impaired homograft rejection. *J. Clin. Invest.* 46: 1643–1656, 1967.
428. SUDLER, M. T. The architecture of the gall bladder. *Bull. Johns Hopkins Hosp.* 12: 126–128, 1901.
429. SVATOS, A., V. BARTOS, AND V. BRZEK. The concentration of cholecystokinin in human lymph and serum. *Arch. Int. Pharmacodyn.* 149: 515–520, 1964.
430. SVIRIDOVA, I. K. Intraorganic lymphatic bed of the human parotid salivary gland (translation) *Arkh. Anat. Gistol. Embriol.* 59: 10–18, 1970.
431. SZABO, G., AND Z. MAGYAR. Effect of obstruction of the hepatic artery on the composition of hepatic lymph. *Acta Med. Acad. Sci. Hung.* 25: 153–156, 1968.
432. SZABO, G., Z. MAGYAR, AND F. JAKAB. The lymphatic drainage of the liver capsula and hepatic parenchyma. *Res. Exp. Med.* 166: 193–200, 1975.
433. SZABO, G., Z. MAGYAR, AND F. JAKAB. Bile constituents in blood and lymph during biliary obstruction. I. The dynamics of absorption and transport of bile acids and bilirubin. *Lymphology* 8: 29–36, 1975.
434. SZABO, G., Z. MAGYAR, AND A. SZENTIRMAI, F. JAKAB, AND K. MIHALY. Bile constituents in blood and lymph during biliary obstruction. II. The absorption and transport of bile acids and bilirubin. *Lymphology* 8: 36–42, 1975.
435. SZABO, L. E., S. KARACSONYI, AND Z. PATAKY. Uber den funktionellen Lymphkreislauf des Osophagus. *Acta Chir. Hung.* 4: 85–91, 1962.
436. SZWED, J. J., D. R. MAXWELL, R. ELLIOTT, AND L. R. REDLICH. Diuretics and small intestinal lymph flow in the dog. *J. Pharmacol. Exp. Therap.* 200: 88–94, 1977.
437. TAKASHIMA, T., AND N. TAKEKOSHI. Lymphographic evaluation of abnormal lymph flow in protein-losing gastroenteropathy secondary to chronic constrictive pericarditis. *Radiology* 90: 292–295, 1968.
438. TASKER, R. R. The collection of intestinal lymph from normally active rats. *J. Physiol. Lond.* 115: 292–295, 1951.
439. TAYLOR, A. E. Capillary fluid filtration. Starling forces and lymph flow. *Circ. Res.* 49: 557–575, 1981.
440. TAYLOR, A. E., AND D. N. GRANGER. Exchange of macromolecules across the microcirculation. In: *Handbook of Physiology. The Cardiovascular System*, edited by E. M. Renkin and C. C. Michel. Bethesda, MD: Am. Physiol. Soc., 1984, sect. 2, vol. IV, pt. 1, chapt. 11, p. 467–520.
441. THOMSON, A. B. R., AND J. M. DIETSCHY. Intestinal lipid absorption: major extracellular and intracellular events. In: *Physiology of the Gastrointestinal Tract*, edited by L. R. Johnson. New York: Raven, 1981, p. 1147–1220.
442. THREEFOOT, S. A. Gross and microscopic anatomy of the lymphatic vessels and lymphatico-venous communications. *Cancer Chemother. Rep.* 52: 1–20, 1968.
443. THREEFOOT, S. A., W. T. KENT, AND B. F. HATCHETT. Lym-

phatico-venous and lymphatico-lymphatic communications demonstrated by plastic corrosion models of rats and by postmortem lymphangiography in man. *J. Lab. Clin. Med.* 61: 9-22, 1963.
444. THREEFOOT, S. A., AND M. F. KOSSOVER. Lymphaticovenous communications in man. *Arch. Int. Med.* 117: 213-223, 1966.
445. TIFT, W. L., AND J. K. LLOYD. Intestinal lymphangiectasia. Long term results with MCT diet. *Arch. Dis. Child.* 50: 269-276, 1975.
446. TILNEY, N. L., AND J. E. MURRAY. Chronic thoracic duct fistula: operative technique and physiologic effects in man. *Ann. Surg.* 167: 1-8, 1968.
447. TOMPKINS, C. L., AND H. J. GRANGER. Ultrastructure of the peribiliary capillary. *Microvasc. Res.* 21: 261, 1981.
448. TREADWELL, C. R., AND G. V. VAHOUNY. Cholesterol absorption. In: *Handbook of Physiology. Alimentary Canal. Intestinal Absorption*, edited by C. F. Code. Washington, DC: Am. Physiol. Soc., 1968, sect. 6, vol. III, chapt. 72, p. 1407-1438.
449. TRIER, J. S. Whipple's disease. In: *Gastrointestinal Disease*, edited by M. H. Sleisenger and J. S. Fordtran. Philadelphia, PA: Saunders, 1983.
450. TSO, P. Gastrointestinal digestion and absorption of lipid. *Adv. Lipid Res.* 21: 143-186, 1985.
451. TSO, P., J. A. BALINT, M. B. BISHOP, AND J. B. RODGERS. Acute inhibition of intestinal lipid transport by Pluronic L-81 in the rat. *Am. J. Physiol.* 241 (*Gastrointest. Liver Physiol.* 4): G487-G497, 1981.
452. TSO, P., J. A. BARROWMAN, AND D. N. GRANGER. Importance of interstitial matrix hydration in intestinal chylomicron transport. *Am. J. Physiol.* 250 (*Gastrointest. Liver Physiol.* 12): G497-G500, 1986.
453. TSO, P., D. S. DRAKE, D. D. BLACK, AND S. M. SABESIN. Evidence for separate pathways of chylomicron and very low density lipoprotein assembly and transport by rat small intestine. *Am. J. Physiol.* 247 (*Gastrointest. Liver Physiol.* 10): G599-G610, 1984.
454. TSO, P., V. PITTS, AND D. N. GRANGER. Role of lymph flow in intestinal chylomicron transport. *Am. J. Physiol.* 249 (*Gastrointest. Liver Physiol.* 11): G21-G28, 1985.
455. TSO, P., J. B. RAGLAND, AND S. M. SABESIN. Isolation and characterization of lipoprotein of density <1.006 g/ml from rat hepatic lymph. *J. Lipid Res.* 24: 810-820, 1983.
456. TURNER, S. G., AND J. A. BARROWMAN. The effects of cholecystokinin on intestinal lymph flow in the rat. *Can. J. Physiol. Pharmacol.* 59: 1393-1396, 1977.
457. TURNER, S. G., AND J. A. BARROWMAN. Intestinal lymph flow and lymphatic transport of protein during fat absorption. *Q. J. Exp. Physiol.* 62: 175-180, 1977.
458. TURNER, S. G., AND J. A. BARROWMAN. Enhanced intestinal lymph formation during fat absorption: the importance of triglyceride hydrolysis. *Q. J. Exp. Physiol.* 63: 255-264, 1978.
459. VAERMAN, J.-P., AND J. F. HEREMANS. Origin and molecular size of immunoglobulin-A in the mesenteric lymph of the dog. *Immunology* 18: 27-38, 1970.
460. VAERMAN, J.-P., C. ANDRE, H. BAZIN, AND J. F. HEREMANS. Mesenteric lymph as a major source of serum IgA in guinea pigs and rats. *Eur. J. Immunol.* 3: 580-584, 1973.
461. VAJDA, J. Innervation of lymph vessels. *Acta Morph. Acad. Sci. Hung.* 14: 197-208, 1966.
462. VAJDA, J., AND C. LERANTH. The lymphatic system of the large intestine. *Acta Morphol. Acad. Sci. Hung.* 15: 257-263, 1967.
463. VARDY, P., E. LEBENTHAL, AND H. SCHWACHMAN. Intestinal lymphangiectasia. A reappraisal. *Pediatrics* 55: 842-851, 1975.
464. VEGA, R. E., H. E. APPERT, AND J. M. HOWARD. The effects of secretin in stimulating the output of amylase and lipase in the thoracic duct of the dog. *Ann. Surg.* 166: 995-1001, 1967.
465. VOLKHEIMER, G., F. H. SCHULZ, A. LINDENAU, AND U. BEITZ. Persorption of metallic iron particles. *Gut* 10: 32-33, 1969.
466. WALDMANN, T. A., J. L. STEINFELD, T. F. DUTCHER, J. D. DAVIDSON, AND R. S. GORDON. The role of the gastrointestinal system in 'idiopathic' hypoproteinemia. *Gastroenterology* 41: 197-207, 1961.
467. WALKER, W. A. Intestinal transport of macromolecules. In: *Physiology of the Gastrointestinal Tract*, edited by L. R. Johnson. New York: Raven, 1981, p. 1271-1289.
468. WARSHAW, A. L., W. A. WALKER, R. CORNELL, AND K. J. ISSELBACHER. Small intestinal permeability to macromolecules. Transmission of horseradish peroxidase into mesenteric lymph and portal blood. *Lab. Invest.* 25: 675-684, 1971.
469. WARSHAW, A. L., W. A. WALKER, AND K. J. ISSELBACHER. Protein uptake by the intestine: evidence for absorption of intact macromolecules. *Gastroenterology* 66: 987-992, 1974.
470. WEINER, S., L. GRAMATICA, L. D. VOEGLE, R. L. HAUMAN, AND M. C. ANDERSON. Role of the lymphatic system in the pathogenesis of inflammatory disease in the biliary tract and pancreas. *Am J. Surg.* 119: 55-61, 1970.
471. WEINSTEIN, L. D., G. T. SCANLON, AND J. HERSH. Chylous ascites: management with medium-chain triglycerides and exacerbation by lymphangiography. *Am. J. Dig. Dis.* 14: 500-509, 1969.
472. WENZEL, J. Untersuchungen über das innere Lymphgefässsystem der Speicehldrusen beim Kaninchen. *Z. Mikrosk. Anat. Forsch.* 76: 226-243, 1967.
473. WERNER, B. Thoracic duct cannulation in man. I. Surgical technique and a clinical study on 79 patients. *Acta Chir. Scand. Suppl.* 353: 1-32, 1965.
474. WERNER, B. The biochemical composition of the human thoracic duct lymph. *Acta Chir. Scand.* 132: 63-76, 1966.
475. WERNER, B. Thoracic duct cannulation in man. II. A followup study on 22 patients. *Acta Chir. Scand.* 132: 93-105, 1966.
476. WHIPPLE, G. H., AND J. H. KING. The pathogenesis of icterus. *J. Exp. Med.* 13: 115-135, 1911.
477. WILSON, R. D., R. L. ZIPRIN, D. E. CLARK, AND M. H. ELLISALDE. Absorption of pentachlorophenol by the ovine lymphatic system: a technical note. *Vet. Hum. Toxicol.* 24: 12-15, 1982.
478. WINKENWERDER, W. L. A study of the lymphatics of the gallbladder of the cat. *Bull. Johns Hopkins Hosp.* 41: 226-238, 1927.
479. WISSE, E. An electron microscopic study of the fenestrated endothelial lining of rat liver sinusoids. *J. Ultrastruct. Res.* 31: 125-150, 1970.
480. WISSE, E., R. B. DE ZANGER, K. CHARELS, P. VAN DER SMISSEN, AND R. S. MCCUSKEY. The liver sieve: considerations concerning the structure and function of endothelial fenestrae, the sinusoidal wall and the space of Disse. *Hepatology Baltimore* 5: 683-692, 1985.
481. WITTE, C. L., M. H. WITTE, W. R. COLE, Y. C. CHUNG, V. R. BLEISCH, AND A. E. DUMONT. Dual origin of ascites in hepatic cirrhosis. *Surg. Gynecol. Obstet.* 129: 1027-1033, 1969.
482. WITTE, C. L., M. H. WITTE, AND A. E. DUMONT. Lymph imbalance in the genesis and perpetuation of the ascites syndrome in hepatic cirrhosis. *Gastroenterology* 78: 1059-1068, 1980.
483. WITTE, C. L., M. H. WITTE, K. KINTNER, W. R. COLE, AND A. E. DUMONT. Colloid osmotic pressure in hepatic cirrhosis and experimental ascites. *Surg. Gynecol. Obstet.* 133: 65-71, 1971.
484. WITTE, M. H., A. E. DUMONT, N. LEVINE, AND W. R. COLE. Patterns of distribution of sulfobromophtalein in lymph and blood during obstruction to bile flow. *Am. J. Surg.* 115: 69-74, 1968.
485. WOLLIN, A., AND L. B. JAQUES. Plasma protein escape from the intestinal circulation to the lymphatics during fat absorption. *Proc. Soc. Exp. Biol. Med.* 142: 1114-1117, 1973.
486. WOLLIN, A., AND L. B. JAQUES. Increased diamine oxidase activity in the intestinal lymph of rats on fat ingestion. *Can. J. Physiol. Pharmacol.* 52: 760-762, 1974.
487. WOLLIN, A., AND L. B. JAQUES. Blocking of olive oil induced plasma protein escape from the intestinal circulation by histamine antagonists and by a diamine oxidase releasing agent. *Agents Actions* 6: 589-592, 1976.
488. WOOD, J. E., J. R. ESTERLING, AND V. A. MCKUSICK. Genetic,

clinical and physiologic observations in Milroy's disease. *Circulation* 22: 834–842, 1960.
489. WOOD, J. G., AND H. W. DAVENPORT. Measurement of canine gastric vascular permeability to plasma proteins in the normal and protein-losing states. *Gastroenterology* 82: 725–733, 1982.
490. WOOLLEY, G., AND F. C. COURTICE. The origin of albumin in hepatic lymph. *Aust. J. Exp. Biol. Med. Sci.* 40: 121–128, 1962.
491. YABLONSKI, M. E., AND N. LIFSON. Mechanism of production of intestinal secretion by elevated venous pressure. *J. Clin. Invest.* 57: 904–915, 1976.
492. YOFFEY, J. M., AND F. C. COURTICE. *Lymphatics, Lymph and the Lymphomyeloid Complex.* New York: Academic, 1970.
493. YOSHIKAWA, H., K. TAKADA, AND S. MURANISHI. Molecular weight dependence of permselectivity to rat small intestinal blood-lymph barrier for exogenous macromolecules absorbed from lumen. *J. Pharmacobio-Dyn.* 7: 1–6, 1984.
494. YOSHIKAWA, H., K. TAKADA, S. MURANISHI, Y. SATOH, AND N. NARUSE. A method to potentiate enteral absorption of interferon and selective delivery into lymphatics. *J. Pharmacobio-Dyn.* 7: 59–62, 1984.
495. ZAWIEJA, D., AND B. J. BARBER. A comparison of protein concentration in villi and collecting lymphatics of rats. *Microvasc. Res.* 29: 262, 1985.
496. ZIMMON, D. S., M. ORATZ, R. KESSLER, S. S. SCHREIBER, AND M. A. ROTHSCHILD. Albumin to ascites: demonstration of a direct pathway bypassing the systemic circulation. *J. Clin. Invest.* 48: 2074–2078, 1969.
497. ZINK, J., AND C. V. GREENWAY. Control of ascites absorption in anaesthetized cats: effects of intraperitoneal pressure, protein, and furosemide diuresis. *Gastroenterology* 73: 1119–1124, 1977.
498. ZIPRIN, R. L., M. H. ELISSALDE, D. E. CLARK, AND R. D. WILSON. Absorption of polychlorinated biphenyl by the ovine lymphatic system. *Vet. Hum. Toxicol.* 22: 305–308, 1980.
499. ZWEIFACH, B. W., AND J. W. PRATHER. Micromanipulation of pressure in terminal lymphatics in the mesentery. *Am. J. Physiol.* 228: 1326–1335, 1975.
500. ZWEIFACH, B. W., AND G. W. SCHMID-SCHONBEIN. Pressure and flow relations in the lymphatic system. In: *Experimental Biology of the Lymphatic Circulation*, edited by M. G. Johnston. Amsterdam: Elsevier, 1985.

INDEX

# Index

Abdominal prevertebral ganglia, neuroanatomy of, 520–521
Abomasum
    anatomy, 1250–1258
    embryonic development of, 1226
    functions of, 1225–1226
Absorption
    intestinal mucosal blood flow, 1430
    ruminant animals, 1229–1230
Acetylcholine (Ach)
    biliary tract pharmacology, 1105–1106
    in calcium channels, 180–181
    colonic motility, 954
    in colonic muscle
        electropharmacology, 257–259
        myenteric plexus regulation, 261
    dorsal motor nucleus and, 648–649
    electropharmacology of, 204
    enteric nervous system
        adrenergic control, 411–412
        autoreceptor modulation, 411
        bradykinin, 414
        cholinergic control, 414–419
        fast EPSPs and, 492–493
        GABA, 413–414
        histamine, 414
        neurotransmission, 409–414
        purinergic compounds, 412
        release factors, 410
        serotonin and, 413
        slow EPSPs, 393, 499
        slow IPSPs, 505
        synaptosomes, 422–423
        transmitter role of, 395
    exocrine gland circulation and, 1576–1577
    gastric muscle arrhythmia and, 197–198
    gastrointestinal blood flow, 1668–1669
    gastrointestinal electrophysiology, 182–183
        excitatory junction potentials, 450–451
    gastrointestinal motility
        intermediolateral cell column ($S_{2-3}$), 653–654
        in nTS, 658
        nucleus ambiguus, 652
        sympathetic preganglionic neurons, 656
    hepatic circulation, 1543
    internal anal sphincter
        regulation, 1011–1012
        sacral autonomic nerves, 1038–1039
    intestinal blood flow and motility, 1486–1490
        intramural tension, 1496
    intestinal smooth muscle
        receptor activation, 223–226
        receptor-evoked responses, 237–238
    lower esophageal sphincter
        disorders, 16
        relaxation, 995
    mesenteric artery
        excitatory junction potentials (EJP), 1615
        responses to, 1612–1614
    mesenteric vein, 1623
    in motor neurons, 388
    muscarinic receptors
        modulation of, 731
        release in enteric nervous system, 728
    nonocclusive intestinal ischemia, 1717
    nonvesicular enteric neurotransmission, 405
    portal vein, 1627
    in potassium channels, 180
    presynaptic inhibition, 394
    release of substance P, 772
    release by tachykinins, 770–771
    ruminant animals, 1271
    slow-wave research, 189
    VIP transmission
        in prevertebral ganglia, 566
[$^3$H]Acetylcholine, enteric synaptosomes, 422–423
Acetylcholinesterase (AChe)
    in dorsal motor nucleus of the vagus, 648
    enteric nervous system, 420
Acetylsalicylic acid (ASA), MAPC and, 1157–1158
Achalasia, 16–17
Acid secretion (gastric)
    aminopyrine clearance, 1355–1356
    blood flow stimulation, 1391–1392
        prostaglandins and, 1389–1390
    gastric emptying and, 923–924
    muscarinic receptors and, 729
Acinus vessel, microcirculation, 1521–1522
Actin filaments
    intestinal muscle
        dense body and band penetration, 114, 119, 122, 124
        embryonic development of, 131–132
        structure and function, 121–124
    skeletal muscle contraction, 276
$\alpha$-Actinin, localization at intestinal dense bands, 114–115
Action currents. *See* Action potentials; Slow waves
Action potentials
    colonic muscle
        characteristics of, 255–256
        propagation of, 267–268
    enteric nervous system, 488–489
        extracellular recording of, 466–468
    gastrointestinal muscle electrophysiology, 195–196
    historical research, 29–32
    from inferior mesenteric ganglia, 536–537
    intestinal smooth muscle, 229–230
        phasic contraction and, 226
        tetrodotoxin and, 228
    ionic mechanism of slow waves, 195
    mesenteric artery, 1611, 1617–1618
    mesenteric vein, 1622, 1624
    prevertebral ganglia, antidromic response and, 550–551
    rhythmicity in gastrointestinal cells, 166
    slow-wave activity, variations in, 193
    in small intestine, 46–48
    spontaneous in portal vein, 1625–1626
    terminology background on, 825–827
    voltage-clamp studies, 170–171
    of isolated cells, 167–169
Activation
    gastrointestinal smooth muscle, 274–275, 284–286
        electrical stimulation methods, 284–285
        patterns of, 284
        uniformity of, 284
    in intestinal smooth muscle, 221–223
        calcium currents, 222
        depolarization, 221–222

Activation (*continued*)
    outward current, 222–223
Active secretion, net fluid secretion and, 1455–1456
Active transport, sodium-potassium pump, 149–151
    ionic dependence of, 149
    number of pump sites, 150–151
    stoichiometry and electrogenicity, 149–150
Adenine nucleotides
    enteric nervous system, 422
    purinergic receptors and, 742
Adenosine
    enteric nervous system
        cholinergic nerves, 412
        neurotransmitter mechanism, 501
    exocrine gland circulation, 1575–1576
    hepatic arterial buffer response, 1525–1527
    intestinal mucosa blood flow, 1407
        small solute permeability, 1457
    postprandial intestinal hyperemia and, 1425
        neurohormonal control, 1698
Adenosine diphosphate (ADP)
    mesenteric artery, neuromuscular transmission, 1621
    ribosylation with cholera toxin, 1155
    small intestine
        early research, 64
Adenosine monophosphate (AMP)
    mesenteric artery neuromuscular transmission, 1621
    small intestine, 64
Adenosine triphosphate (ATP)
    colonic motility, 956
    enteric nervous system, 305, 423
    gastrointestinal neuromuscular transmission, 444–445
    inhibitory motor transmission, 389–390
    internal anal sphincter motor activity, 1035
    mesenteric artery
        neuroeffector transmission pharmacology, 1619–1620
        neuromuscular transmission, 1621
    purinergic receptors and, 742–743
    small intestine, 64
Adenosine 5′-triphosphate
    gastrointestinal neuromusclar transmission, 448–449
        excitatory junction potentials, 452–453
Adenylate cyclase, receptor-ligand binding and, 717–718
    *See also* Second messenger mechanisms
Adhesion to cells, enteric neuron development and, 334–336
Adjuvants, intestinal mucosal blood flow, 1438–1439
Adrenergic agonists
    in colonic muscle, 258–259
    electropharmacology of, 203–204
    internal anal sphincter, 1036–1037
$\alpha$-Adrenergic agonists, in ruminant animals, 1271
Adrenergic antagonists, lower esophageal sphincter activity, 890–891
$\alpha$-Adrenergic antagonists, internal anal sphincter regulation, 1011
Adrenergic drugs
    biliary tract pharmacology, 1106–1108
    colonic motility, 955
    mesenteric artery, neuromuscular transmission, 1620
Adrenergic innveration
    enteric nervous system, 420–422
        cholinergic system, 411–412
    gastric blood flow control, 1383
    gastrointestinal blood flow
        norepinephrine, 1669–1678
    intestinal smooth muscle activity, 233–234
    lower esophageal sphincter, 16–17
    mesenteric circulation and, 1607
    neuromuscular transmission, 443
        muscarinic receptors and, 729
        muscle coat adrenergic neurons, 441–443
        neuromodulation, 444–445
        nonsphincteric muscles, 444
        sphincteric muscles, 443–444
        sympathetic cotransmission, 444–445
    in small intestine, 62–63
Adrenergic receptors
    agonists, 1036–1037
    exocrine gland circulation, 1588–1589
    gastrointestinal motility, 733–739
        $\alpha$-adrenoreceptor mechanisms, 737–738
        $\beta$-adrenoreceptor–mediated mechanisms, 738–739
        classification of, 735–737
        innervation functions, 733–735
        postreceptor mechanisms, 737–738
        sympathetic pathways, 733
    vomiting reflex, 1192
$\alpha$-Adrenergic receptors
    classification of, 735–736
    colonic motility, 955
    functions of, 736–737
    gallbladder pharmacology, 1107
    hepatic blood flow and, 1524
    mesenteric artery, 1612
    smooth muscle inhibition, 737–738
    submucosal arterioles
        cotransmission, 1658–1660
        tension development, 1652–1653
$\alpha_2$-Adrenergic receptors, 738
$\beta$-Adrenergic receptors
    classification, 736–737
    effect on voltage recordings, 168
    extrinsic hepatic arterial flow regulation, 1528–1529
    functions of, 737
    gallbladder pharmacology, 1107
    gastrointestinal blood flow
        neurohormonal control, 1674–1678
    internal anal sphincter regulation, 1011
    intestinal smooth muscle, inhibitory effect, 239–240
    lower esophageal sphincter, 995–996
    mechanisms of, 738–739
    mesenteric artery, 1612
$\beta_2$-Adrenergic receptors, colonic motility, 955
Afferent (sensory) innervation
    colon, rectum and internal anal sphincter
        sacral fibers, 1027–1028
    esophageal and sphincter innervation, 867
    gastrointestinal motility, 593
        area postrema, 646
        dorsal root ganglia, 646
        nucleus tractus solitarius (nTS), 646
        pelvic fibers, 632, 634
        pudendal fibers, 634–636
        sympathetic fibers, 632–635
        vagal fibers, 629–632
    nonvagal, 609
    pelvic floor muscles, 1030
        dysfunction, 1047
    receptive relaxation and, 672
    rectum and anal canal
        dysfunction, 1047
        lumbar sympathetic afferents, 1045–1046
        sacral somatic afferents, 1045
        sacral visceral afferents, 1044–1046
    vomiting reflex, 1188–1190
Afterload, force-velocity curve in smooth muscle shortening, 308
Afterspike hyperpolarization
    prevertebral ganglia, 546–547
    of sympathetic neurons, 548–549
Aganglionosis. *See* Hirschsprung's disease
Age, mucosal blood flow and, 1393
Agonists
    adrenergic receptors, 734–736
    biliary tract pharmacology, 1104–1104
    drug-receptor response quantitation

antagonists and, 722
  as multiple transmitters, 722
  for κ-receptors, 781–782
  for μ-receptors, 780
  muscarinic receptors, 727–728
    binding of, 729–731
    modulation of, 731
  for opiate receptors, potency ranking for, 780–781
  purinergic receptors and, 743–744
  receptor mechanics and
    mathematics of, 716–717
  serotonin receptors, 739–740
  smooth muscle contractions, 726
β-Agonists
  colonic motility, 955
  intestinal villi motility, 979
AH/type neuron, 392
  enteric nervous system, presynaptic inhibition, 510
  serotonin immunoreactivity, 393
AH/type 2 neurons
  enteric nervous system, 485
    action potentials, 488–489
    fast EPSPs in, 492
    forskolin application, 500–501
    myenteric inhibitory neurotransmitters, 505–507
    schematic diagram, 502
    slow EPSP gating mechanism, 503
    tachykinin action and, 770–771
Alcohol metabolism, hepatic arterial buffer response, 1527
Alimentary tracts, interstitial cells of Cajal in, 381
Alipoproteins, lymph flow and composition, 1751
Alternate transmitter hypothesis
  neuroeffector transmission pharmacology, 1619–1620
Alternating current (AC), gastrointestinal smooth muscle activation, 285
American trypanosomiasis. See Chaga's disease
Amino acids
  in area postrema, 701
  in dorsal motor nucleus of the vagus, 650–651
  intestinal blood flow and motility, 1489–1490
  receptors, 603–604
  sequences,
    in motilin, 792
    peptides and, 759–760
    tachykinins, 766
γ-Aminobutyric acid. See GABA
Aminopeptidase, enteric nervous system, 420
4-Aminopyridine, in prevertebral ganglions, 545
Aminopyrine clearance, 1351
  acid secretion, 1355
  gastric blood flow measurements, 1393–1394
  initial studies, 1354–1356
  mucosal blood flow, 1377
  in nonsecreting stomach, 1356–1358
  pH partition hypothesis and, 1360–1361
  theoretical background, 1352–1354
  total blood flow and, 1356
[$^{14}$C]Aminopyrine clearance
  human gastric hemodynamics, 1359–1360, 1396
  resting and stimulated parietal cells, 1361
p-Aminosalicylic acid, lymph transport, 1755
Amphibian stomach, electrical activity, 200
Ampulla of Vater
  embryonic development, 1057
  gross anatomy, 1056
  structure, 1057–1058
Amygdala
  gastrointestinal motility
    neural input and output, 662–663
    stimulation and lesion of, 663–664
  neuronal inputs and outputs, 659
Anal canal

anatomy, 940
  See also External and Internal anal sphincters
Analog storage oscilloscopes, 282
Analog tape recorder, 282
Analog-to-digital converters, 283
Anal progression, regulation by intestinal muscle, 217
Anal sphincter
  anatomy and innervation, 1008–1012
  colonic motility
    external anal sphincter (EAS), 959–960
    internal anal sphincter (IAS), 957–959
  early research
    animal studies, 77–78
    human studies, 78–79
  integrated behavior with rectum, 79–80
  myoelectric activity, 844–845
  vasoactive intestinal polypeptide (VIP) action on, 780
  See also Internal and External anal sphincters
Anaphylactic shock,
  hepatic circulation, 1551
  intestinal circulation and, 1719
ANAPP$_3$ (arylazidoaminopropionyl-ATP)
  mesenteric artery, neuroeffector transmission pharmacology, 1619–1620
  purinergic receptors and, 743–744
  submucosal arteriole cotransmission, 1658–1659
Anastomoses
  intestinal motility and blood flow, 1478
  lymphaticovenous, 1738–1739
Anemia hypoxemia, neonatal intestinal circulation, 1601
Anesthesia, intestinal mucosal blood flow, 1438–1439
Aneurysms, intestinal blood flow and, 1724
Angiotensin
  colonic motility, 956
  in enteric neurons, 395
  gastrointestinal blood flow, neurohormonal control of, 1682–1683
  hepatic circulation, 1530, 1545
Angiotensin II
  cardiogenic shock, 1719
  emesis and, 701–702
  hypovolemic shock, 1718
  intestinal mucosal blood flow, 1437–1438
Anorectal inhibitory reflex, 1009–1010
Anorectum
  defecation and, 1044–1046
  motor dysfunction, 1047
Anoxia, intestinal blood flow and motility, 1512
Antagonist potency (pA$_2$), 767–768
Antagonists
  adrenergic receptors, 735–736
  α-adrenergic receptors, 1655–1656
  agonists and drug-receptor response quantitation, 721
  biliary tract pharmacology, 1104–1105
    CCK compounds, 1114–1115
  bombesin, 799
  cholecystokinin, gut and brain receptors, 760
  cholinergic muscarinic, 1106
  drug-receptor response quantitation, 722
  gastrin-releasing peptide, 799
  motilin, 793
  muscarinic receptors, 727–728
    binding of, 729–731
  neuromedin K, 767
  neurotensin, 797
  for opiate receptors, 783–784
  purine, submucosal arterioles, 1659–1660
  purinergic receptors and, 743–744
  receptor mechanics and, 717
  β-receptor, intestinal villi motility, 979
  serotonin receptors, 739–740
  substance K, 767

Antagonists (*continued*)
  substance P, 767–768
    action in stomach, 773–774
  tachykinins, 767–768
  for vasoactive intestinal polypeptide, 777
Anterograde tracing, parasympathetic neural pathways, 628
Antibiotics, colonic motility, 957
Anticholinergics
  colonic motility, 955–956
  junctional zone peristalsis, 884
  ruminant animals, gastroduodenal junction, 1272
Anticholinesterases in motor neurons, 388
Anticoagulants, nonocclusive intestinal ischemia, 1716
Antidiarrheal agents, opiate receptors and, 791–792
Antidiuretic hormone (ADH)
  gastrointestinal blood flow, 1683
  hemorrhagic hypotension, 1696
Antidromic response, prevertebral ganglia, 550–551
Antiemetics, 707–708
Antiperistalsis
  colonic motility, 943–944
  ileocolic junction, 68–70
  in ruminant animals, 1240
Antipyrylazo III, $Ca^{2+}$ measurement with, 147
Antral slow waves, 193
Antral transport function, gastric emptying, 921
Antropyloric grinder, gastric emptying, 917–918
Antropyloric motor response, 927–928
Antropyloroduodenal flow resistance, gastric emptying, 919–921
Antrum
  distension, gastric relaxation and, 927
  during gastric emptying, 920–921
  microvascular structure, 1307
  motility, retching and vomitus expulsion, 1182–1185
  surgical perturbation, small intestine regulation, 1206
  vomiting, myoelectric events, 1186–1187
Apamin
  inhibitory motor transmission, 389–390
  intestinal smooth muscle inhibitory effect, 239
Appendix, anatomy of, 940
Aqueorin technique
  $Ca^{2+}$ measurement with, 147
  gastrointestinal smooth muscle contraction, 288–290
Arachidonic acid
  enteric neurotransmission, 409
  gastric blood flow control, 1389
    pathways of, 1390–1391
  in machrophages, 365–366
Area postrema
  afferent vagal nerve fibers and, 629–632
  emesis and
    anterograde labeling, 700
    efferent projections and, 700–701
    physiology of, 702–705
    structure of, 698–701
    transmitter localization and binding sites, 701
  gastrointestinal motility, 646
  single neuron responses, 703–704
Arginine vasopressin, in prevertebral ganglia, 574
Arsenazo III, $Ca^{2+}$ measurement with, 147
Arterial chemoreceptors, gastrointestinal blood flow, 1694–1695
Arterial flow regulation, hepatic
  autoregulation, 1527
  buffer response, 1525–1527
  extrinsic, 1528–1531
  intrinsic, 1524–1528
  metabolic control, 1525
Arterial hypoxia, intestinal mucosal blood flow alterations, 1414–1416
Arterial pressure
  intestinal mucosa blood flow, 1408
    autoregulation, 1408–1411
    reduction, capillary-interstitial interaction, 1446–1448
Arterial resistance, hepatic circulation, 1541–1543
Arteriolar feedback, intestinal mucosal blood flow, 1424
Arterioles
  intramural organization and structure, 1637
  submucosal
    contraction initiation, 1650–1653
    innervation of, 1637–1641
    integration in, 1653–1654
    neuromuscular transmission, 1644–1645
    passive electrical properties, 1640–1644
    sympathetic nerve stimulation, 1645–1646
Arteriovenous anastomoses
  small intestine, 1309–1310
  submucosal microvessel circulation, 1373–1374
Arteriovenous malformations, intestinal blood flow and, 1723–1724
Arteriovenous oxygen content difference
  intestinal blood flow and motility
    compartmental blood flow, 1506–1507
Arylazidoaminopropionyl ATP (ANAPP$_3$), 448–449
*Ascaris suum*, 1148–1149
Ascending colon, anatomy, 940
ATPase
  skeletal muscle contraction, 276
  sodium pump activity and, 150
Atropine
  colonic motility, 954
    and blood flow, 1498–1500
      myenteric potential oscillations, 255
      vasodilatation, 1668
  electropharmacology of, 204
  esophageal peristalsis, 881
  gastric muscle arrhythmia and, 197
  gastrin receptors, 761
  lower esophageal sphincter innervation, 990
  noncholinergic excitatory motor transmission, 388–389
  receptor locus and functional coupling, 719
Attachment plaque. *See* Intermediate junction
Audio tape recorder, 282
Auerbach's plexus
  esophageal motility, 866
  interstitial cells of Cajal (ICC) and, 352–366
    functions of, 359–364
    future research developments, 364–366
    longitudinal muscle nerves and, 376–378
    nerve bundle contacts, 355–358
    origin and nature of, 359
    other interstitial cells and, 357–359
    relationship to smooth muscle, 357
    staining methods for, 352–354
    ultrastructural features, 354–355
  nervous control of LES, 14
  vasculature of, 1304
Augmented stretch resistance, relaxation mechanics, 316
Autacoids
  biliary tract pharmacology, 1108–1111
  collecting lymphatics, 1745
  postprandial intestinal hyperemia and, 1427–1429
Autonomic drugs, colonic motility, 954
Autonomic innervation
  colon, rectum, and internal anal sphincter
    lumbar sympathetic innervation, 1026
    sacral afferent fibers, 1027–1028
    sacral parasympathetic innervation, 1026–1027
  enteric system, 58–60
  exocrine gland circulation, 1572–1574
  gallbladder function, 1073
  gastric blood flow control
    parasympathetic nervous system, 1383–1385
    parasympathetic-sympathetic interaction, 1385
    sympathetic nervous system, 1382–1383

gastrointestinal innervation, 594–595
mesenteric circulation and, 1606
neuromuscular junction, 436, 439–440
sacral
    colon and rectal motor activity, 1039
    internal anal sphincter motor activity, 1038–1039
sphincter of Oddi function, 1088
sympathetic preganglionic neurons and, 533–534
Autonomic neuropathy, gastrointestinal dysfunction, 928
Autoreceptors
    enteric nervous system, 421
        modulation, 411
    mesenteric artery, neuromuscular transmission, 1620–1621
Autoregulation
    capillary pressure
        capillary-interstitial interaction, 1446–1448
        sympathetic stimulation, 1448–1449
    hepatic arterial buffer response, 1527–1528
    intestinal mucosa blood flow, 1408–1411
    mucosal blood flow and, 1392
    pressure-flow, exocrine gland circulation, 1570–1571
Autoregulatory escape
    extrinsic hepatic arterial flow regulation, 1528–1529
    intestinal blood flow, neurohormonal control of, 1672–1673
Avian gastrointestinal motor function
    ceca motility, 1295–1296
    esophagus and crop motility, 1286–1287
    gross anatomy, 1283–1286
        cecum, rectum and cloaca, 1285–1286
        esophagus and crop, 1283
        glandular stomach, 1283–1284
        liver and pancreas, 1286
        mouth and pharynx, 1283
        muscular stomach, 1284–1285
        small intestine, 1285
    ileum motility, 1295
    motility studies, 1286
    passage rate of ingesta, 1298
    prehension and swallowing, 1286
    rectal motility, 1296–1298
    stomach and duodenum
        fowl motility patterns, 1287–1289
        fowl motility regulation, 1289–1292
        raptor motility patterns, 1292–1295
        raptor motility regulation, 1292–1295
Axoaxonic synapse, enteric neurotransmission, 406
Axodendritic synaptic contacts, 526
Axons
    in dorsal motor nucleus, 647
    intramuaral arterioles, 1639–1640
    of pelvic neurons, 653
    in principal ganglia cells, 524, 526
    submucosal arterioles, sympathetic nerve stimulation, 1653–1654
    terminals in prevertebral ganglia, 527
    varicosities, ICC DMP and, 372

Backdiffusion of hydrogen ions, ulcerogenesis and, 1722
"Backward theory" of portal hypertension, 1720
Bacterial overgrowth syndrome
    future research trends, 1170–1171
    metabolic by-products, 1170
    small intestine motility alterations, 1167–1171
Balloon kymography
    colonic motility, 943
    internal anal sphincter, 957
Band-pass filtering, myoelectric activity analysis, 825
Barium
    esophageal motility, 869
    in intestinal smooth muscle
        action potential discharge and, 222
        potassium channel activity, 220
    swallowing research, 2–3
Barium ions ($Ba^{2+}$)
    lower esophageal sphincter, basal tone, 993
    potassium channel properties, 174
    in prevertebral ganglions, resting membrane potential modulation, 545
Baroreceptors, gastrointestinal blood flow, 1690–1692
Basal lamina
    intestinal capillaries, 1326–1327
    in intestinal muscle, 118–120
        embryonic development of, 131
        terminal apparatus, 120–121
Basal sphincter pressure
    lower esophageal sphincter
        genesis of, 888–890
        measurement techniques, 887
        mechanical factors, 888
        muscle tone, 888–890
    upper esophageal sphincter, 871
Basal tone
    lower esophageal sphincter, 990–994
        nontetanic tone, 992
        tetanic tone (tonus tetanus), 992
Basement membranes, exocrine gland circulation, 1580
Basic electrical rhythm. *See* Slow waves
BAY K 8644
    calcium channel properties, 177–178
    in intestinal smooth muscle
        action potentials and, 222
        calcium channels and, 220
Beaumont, William, 187
Bed nucleus of stria terminalis (BNST)
    gastrointestinal motility
        neural input and output, 662–663
        stimulation and lesion of, 663–664
    neuronal inputs and outputs, 659–660
Benzo(*a*)pyrene, lymph transport, 1755
Bethanechol
    biliary tract pharmacology, 1105–1106
    ruminant animals, gastroduodenal junction, 1272
B-fibers, in sympathetic preganglionic nerves, 532
Bicarbonate, LES control, 14
Biebl loops, small intestine, 49–51
Bile acids
    colonic motility, 957
    diarrhea and, 1168
    hepatic bile flow, 1070
Bile flow
    biliary duct system, 1055
    hepatic circulation and, 1521
    intestinal lymph flows, 1754–1755
    postprandial intestinal hyperemia, 1419
        neurohormonal control, 1698
    prevertebral ganglion and, 536
Bile salts, MAPC activity, 1162–1163
Bile-stained vomitus, 1185–1186
Biliary tract
    gastric emptying and, 914–916
    pharmacology
        adrenergic drugs, 1106–1108
        anatomy, 1103–1104
        autacoids, 1108–1111
        cholinergic drugs, 1105–1106
        neuropeptides, 1111–1124
Biliary tract motility
    abnormal function, 1090–1095
        gallbladder disorders, 1090–1091
        pancreatic sphincter of Oddi dysfunction, 1095
        sphincter of Oddi, 1091–1095
    common duct function, 1074–1077
    cystic duct function, 1074
    electromyography, 1064–1065

Biliary tract motility (continued)
  flow measurements, 1062
  gallbladder function, 1070–1074
  gross anatomy, 1056–1061
    component structures, 1057–1058
    embryonic development, 1056–1057
    extrinsic nerves, 1057
  hepatic bile secretion, 1067–1070
  historical research, 1055–1056
  imaging studies of, 1061–1062
  manometry, 1062–1064
  microscopic anatomy, 1058–1060
    innervation, 1059–1060
    muscle and mucosa, 1058–1059
  pharmacology, 1066–1067
  scintigraphy, 1065–1066
  sonography, 1066
  species variations, 1060–1061
  sphincter of Oddi, 1077–1088
    animal function studies, 1080–1088
    human functions, 1077–1080
    Poiseuille's law, 1077
Billroth surgical procedures
  B-I (type I), 1199
    Maki procedure, 1205
    stomach motility, 1203–1207
  B-II (type II), 1199
    conversion to B-I, 1207
    Polya-Reichel procedure, 1205
    postoperative effects, 1200
    stomach motility, 1203–1207
Biogenic amines
  gastric blood flow control, 1385–1387
  ruminant animals, pharmacology, 1270
Biomarkers, reticuloruminant contractions, 1232–1233
Bipolar recording methods, myoelectric activity, 824
Blood flow
  compartmental
    intestinal blood flow and motility, 1505–1507
    intestinal motility and, 1483, 1486
  exocrine gland circulation
    extrinsic regulation, 1588–1589
    intrinsic regulation of, 1569–1572
  extramural and intramural circuits, 1605–1606
  gastric, 1382–1391
    acid secretion and, 1391–1392
    age and, 1393
    autoregulation, 1392
    biogenic amines, 1385–1387
    disruption of, 1393–1397
    eating and, 1392–1393
    gross flow measurement, 1376
    hormonal control, 1387–1388
    leukotrienes, 1390–1391
    measurement techniques, 1376–1382
    motility and, 1393
    mucosal barrier disruption, 1393–1394
    mucosal blood flow measurements, 1376–1381
    neural control, 1382–1385
    prostaglandins, 1389–1390
    pulse pressure, 1393
    stomach wall modification, 1375–1376
  gastrointestinal
    acetylcholine, 1668–1669
    anastomotic connections, 1478
    angiotensin, 1682–1683
    antidiuretic hormone, 1683
    arterial chemoreceptors, 1694–1695
    arteriovenous malformations, 1723–1724
    cardiac mechanoreceptors, 1692–1694
    cholecystokinin, 1687
    colon, 1497–1500
    diabetes mellitus, 1723
    dumping syndrome and secretory disorders, 1724
    enkephalins, 1678
    epinephrine, 1683–1684
    gastrin and pentagastrin, 1684–1685
    glucagon and enteroglucagon, 1685–1686
    hemodynamic changes, 1478
    hemorrhagic hypotension, 1695–1697
    high-pressure baroreceptors, 1690–1692
    history, 1475–1476
    hormone candidates for, 1682–1687
    hypertension, 1723
    hypoxia and, 1509–1513
    inflammatory bowel disease, 1721
    integrated hormone/neurotransmitter responses, 1690–1700
    intestinal luminal distension, 1502–1509
    ischemic injury, 1713–1718
    microvascular anatomy, 1476–1478
    miscellaneous disorders, 1724
    motilin, 1686
    neuropeptide Y, 1678–1679
    neurotensin, 1689
    norepinephrine, 1669–1678
    peptide histidine isoleucine (PHI), 1679
    peptide YY, 1686–1687
    pharmacology and innervation, 1486–1497
    portal hypertension, 1720–1721
    postprandial hyperemia, 1697–1700
    schematic of factors, 1483–1484
    secretin, 1686
    serotonin, 1687–1689
    shock, 1718–1720
    somatostatin, 1689–1690
    small intestine, 1478–1486
    stomach, 1500–1502
    substance P, 1680
    ulcers, 1721–1723
    vasoactive intestinal polypeptide, 1680–1682
  hepatic
    anatomy and microcirculation, 1520–1522
    liver mass and, 1524
    pressure-volume relationship, 1537–1539
    uptake measurement, 1535–1537
    vascular resistance and, 1522–1531
  intestinal mucosa
    anesthesia and adjuvants, 1438–1439
    angiotensin II and vasopressin, 1437–1438
    arterial blood gas and hematocrit alterations, 1414–1416
    arterial pressure alterations, 1408–1411
    capillary filtration coefficient, 1442–1443
    capillary hydrostatic pressure, 1443–1444
    capillary-interstitial interaction, 1445–1456
    countercurrent exchange, 1430–1433
    future research, 1462
    interstitial hydrostatic pressure, 1444
    intestinal transport, 1429–1430
    intrinsic regulation and oxygenation, 1406–1429
    laparotomy and visceral manipulation, 1439
    lymph flow, 1441–1442
    macromolecule exchange, 1457–1459
    osmotic reflection coefficient, 1444
    permeability factors, 1459–1462
    postprandial intestinal hyperemia, 1416–1429
    reactive hyperemia, 1413–1414
    respiration and blood gases, 1439
    small solutes, 1456–1457
    temperature and, 1439–1440
    transcapillary fluid and solute exchange, 1441–1456
    transcapillary oncotic pressure gradient, 1444–1445
    vascular capacitance, 1433–1434
    vasoactive agents and oxygen uptake, 1434–1437, 1440
    venous pressure elevation, 1411–1413

limbic and skeletal, 1417
measurement comparison of techniques, 1365–1366
neonatal intestinal
  hemodynamics and oxygenation, 1597–1598
  intrinsic regulation, 1599–1602
  neural regulation, 1598–1599
pancreatic vasoactive agents, 1586–1587
portal, 1519–1520
salivary glands, vasoactive agents and, 1584–1585
small intestine
  gut wall distribution and, 1483–1485
  intramural tension, 1494–1496
Blood gases
  hepatic circulation, pH and, 1530–1531
  intestinal mucosal blood flow
    arterial, 1414–1416
    respiration and, 1439
Blood vessels
  cable constants, 1610
  electrophysiology of, 1608–1609
Blood volume
  hepatic, 1537–1551
  intestinal, 1540–1541
  pulmonary, 1539–1540
Bolton-Hunter labeling, tachykinin receptors, 766
Boltzmann equations, calcium channel properties, 177–178
Bolus deviation, surgical perturbation and, 1202–1203
Bombesin
  biliary tract pharmacology, 1118–1119
  colon innervation, 942
  enteric nervous system
    cholinergic system, 419
    slow EPSPs, 498
  gastrin-releasing endocrine cells, 392
  lower esophageal sphincter regulation, 998
  pharmacology, 799–800
  in prevertebral ganglia, 570–571
  pyloric sphincter regulation, 1002
Bradycardia, nucleus ambiguus activation and, 643–644
Bradykinin
  collecting lymphatics, 1745
  colonic motility, 956
  enteric cholinergic system, 414
  intestinal blood flow and motility, 1486–1488, 1491–1492
    smooth muscle receptor-evoked response, 239
  postprandial intestinal hyperemia and, 1428
Brain centers
  gastrointestinal motility, 929–930
  *See also* Central nervous system
Brain-gut neural circuitry and gastrointestinal motility, 665–672
Brain stem
  emesis and, 704
  gastrointestinal motility
    dorsal motor nucleus and, 637, 642–643
    nucleus ambiguus and, 644–645
  mastication and swallowing, 686
Brain tumors, emesis and, 707
8-brcAMP
  channel activation with, 181
  enteric nervous system, intraneuronal elevation, 501
Brunner's glands
  avian structure, 1285
  microvasculature, 1315–1316, 1318
    drainage routes, 1315, 1318
  vasculature of, 1304, 1306
Brush-border injury, 1168
Brush-border membranes, sodium-hydrogen exchange, 157–158
Bursa of Fabricius, 1286
Burst-type neurons
  early research, 67
  enteric nervous system, 471–475
    burst generation, 471–472

    functional significance, 475
    pharmacology, 475
    spike waveforms, 473
    statistical parameters, 471
    temperature change, 472–473
    unit interactions, 473–475
  mechanosensitive unit conversion to, 480–481

Cable constants
  mammalian blood vessels, 1610
  portal vein, 1626
Cable model of electrical control activity, 854–857
  gastric muscle electrophysiology, 212–213
Cable properties
  multidimensional analysis of, 206–207
  one-dimensional analysis of, 206
Cadmium ions ($Cd^{2+}$), in intestinal smooth muscle, 223
Caerulein
  biliary tract pharmacology, 1116–1117
  enteric nervous system, slow EPSPs, 498–499
  internal anal sphincter regulation, 1012
  links with gastrin and CCK, 759–760
  in ruminant animals
    pancreaticobiliary secretions, 1263–1264
    pharmacology, 1271
Caffeine, intestinal smooth muscle receptor-evoked response, 239
Calcitonin, esophageal peristalsis, 884
Calcitonin gene-related peptide (CGRP)
  enteric nervous system, 395
    slow EPSPs, 499–500
  esophageal and sphincter innervation, 867
  peristalsis, 884
  in prevertebral ganglia, 568, 571–572
    immunoreactivity, 559–560
  in sensory neurons, 395
Calcium ions ($Ca^{2+}$)
  action potentials, 166–167
  biliary tract pharmacology, CCK and, 1115
  channels, 176–179
    cholinergic regulation of, 180–181
    in intestinal smooth muscle, 220–222
    potassium channel properties, 171–173
    voltage dependence of, 203
  in colonic muscle, excitation-contraction coupling, 257
  enteric nervous system
    calmodulin and, 408
    norepinephrine release factors, 420–421
  extracellular, in tissue, 144
  fundus electrical events, 199
  gastrin-CCK receptors, postreceptor mechanisms, 764–765
  gastrointestinal blood flow
    norepinephrine, 1669–1670
  gastrointestinal smooth muscle contraction, 286–289
    cell membrane entry, 287–288
    free cytoplasmic, 288
    protein regulation by, 289–295
  influence on relaxation mechanisms, 313
  intestinal blood flow and motility, 1492–1493
  intestinal smooth muscle
    action potentials and, 229–230
    currents, action potentials and, 222
    intracellular concentration increases in, 236–237
    measurement of, 143
    muscarinic receptor activation, 223–226
    potassium channel and, 219–220
    sodium-calcium exchange and, 152, 154–156
  intracellular, 407
    electroprobe microanalysis of, 146
  ionic mechanism of slow waves, 194–195
  ionophore A23187, 180
  lower esophageal sphincter

Calcium ions ($Ca^{2+}$) (*continued*)
    basal tone, 992–993
        muscle tone, 888–889
    mesenteric artery, excitatory junction potentials, 1615–1616
    optical measurement of, 147
    parasite-induced alterations, small intestine, 1143–1144
    passive ion movements, 148–149
    in plasmalemma and endoplasmic reticulum, 151–154
    pyloric sphincter regulation, 1001–1002
    receptor
        ligand binding and, 717–718
        postreceptor mechanisms, 723
    role in dispersion techniques, 164
    role in presynaptic autoinhibition, 406
    skeletal muscle contraction, 276
    submucosal arterioles, 1644–1645
        potential-dependent calcium entry, 1650–1651
    voltage-clamp studies, 169
    voltage recordings of isolated cells, 167–169
$Ca^{2+}$-binding protein, contractile protein regulation, 291–293
Calcium-channel blockers, 289
Calcium chloride, intestinal blood flow
    and motility, 1492–1493
Calmodulin (CaM)
    binding with calcium pump, 152
    enteric neurotransmission, 408
Calomel electrodes, slow-wave research, 188
cAMP
    $\alpha$-adrenoreceptors and, 737
    channel activation with, 181
    diarrhea and, 1153–1154
    enteric nervous system, intraneuronal elevation, 501
    gastrin-CCK receptors, 765
    influence on relaxation mechanisms, 313
    intracellular control systems, 407
    muscarinic postreceptor events, 732
    receptors and, 723
*Campylobacter jejuni*, 1166–1167
Cannon, Walter B., historical research by, 2–3
Cannon's point, ileocolic junction, 69–70
Capacitance
    hemorrhagic hypotension, 1697
    hepatic circulation
        blood volume, 1539
        vessel constriction, 1543–1546
    intestinal mucosal blood flow, 1433–1434
    transducers, 280–282
Capillaries
    basal lamina, 1326–1327
    colonic, 1329
    continuous and fenestrated walls, 1320–1321, 1324
    exocrine gland circulation ultrastructure, 1578, 1580
    intestinal mucosa, 1406–1408
        cross section, 1319, 1323
        density, 1437
    junctions in, 1324–1327
    muscularis externa, 1372–1373
    net fluid absorption, 1452–1453
    structure and permeability, 1328
Capillary filtration coefficient ($K_{fc}$)
    gastrointestinal blood flow, antidiuretic hormone and, 1683
    hemorrhagic hypotension, 1696–1697
    intestinal blood flow, 1408
        luminal distension, 1507–1509
        nervous vasoconstriction, 1676
        neurohormonal control of, 1672
        transcapillary fluid and solute exchange, 1442–1444
        venous pressure ($P_v$), 1411–1413
    net fluid absorption, 1453
Capillary hydrostatic pressure ($P_t$)
    lymph flow and composition, 1748
    net fluid absorption, 1450–1452

    pancreatic lymph and, 1757–1758
Capillary pressure ($P_c$)
    autoregulation, 1446–1448
    exocrine gland circulation, 1582
    intestinal mucosal blood flow, 1445–1446
Capsaicin
    neurotransmission in prevertebral ganglia, 558–559
    in sensory neurons, 395
        tachykinin action, 771–772
Carbachol
    electropharmacology of, 204
        in colonic muscle, 257–258
    internal anal sphincter regulation, 1011–1012
Carbohydrates, postprandial intestinal hyperemia, 1419–1420
Cardiac glycosides, cardiogenic shock, 1719
Cardiac mechanoreceptors, gastrointestinal blood flow, 1692–1694
Cardiac orifice, lower esophageal sphincter, 885–886
Cardiac output, splanchnic nerve stimulation, 1549
Cardiac preload, drug response and, 1548–1550
Cardiac receptors, vomiting reflex, 1190
Cardiogenic shock, intestinal circulation and, 1718–1719
Cardiopulmonary bypass surgery, mucosal blood flow and, 1393
Cardiospasm of lower esophageal sphincter, 16
Cardiovascular system, compared with gastrointestinal system, 821–823
Carotid artery
    neonatal intestinal circulation, 1598–1599
    salivary gland circulation, 1566
Carotid sinus pressure, gastrointestinal blood flow, 1691–1692
Castor oil, MAPC activity, 1162
Catalase, nonocclusive intestinal ischemia, 1715
Catecholamines
    colonic motility, 954
    in dorsal motor nucleus of the vagus, 648–650
    early research, 63
    enteric nervous system
        cholinergic system, 412
        slow IPSPs, 507–508
    gastric blood flow control, 1385–1386
    gastrointestinal motility
        in nTS, 657–658
        sympathetic preganglionic neurons, 656
    hepatic circulation, 1543–1546
    small intestine, early research, 64
Cathartic colon, gastrointestinal neuromuscular transmission, 456
Cationized ferritin, exocrine gland circulation, 1580–1581
Cations, measurement techniques, 141
Caudad mass movement, myoelectric activity, 850–852
Caveolae
    arteriole structure, 1637
    impact on cell membrane, 108–109
    intestinal muscle cells, 109, 112–113, 115
        embryonic development of, 131
        extracellular space markers, 113
        intramembrane particles, 113–114
        sarcoplasmic reticulum and, 112
        space density, 113
CCK. *See* Cholecystokinin and derivatives
Cecum
    anatomy, 940
    avian structure, 1285–1286
        motility in, 1295–1296
    parasite-induced alterations, 1146–1147
    ruminant animals
        motility patterns, 1267–1268
        structure, 1266–1267
Celiac artery
    gastric circulation, 1372
    pancreatic circulation and, 1566
    stomach vasculature, 1302–1303
Celiac ganglion
    cholinergic inputs and, 551

neuroanatomy of, 520–521
slow EPSP in, 554–555
substance P in, 557
Cell coupling
mesenteric artery, 1608–1610
mesenteric vein, 1623
portal vein, 1626
Cell cultures
enteric nervous system, 338–344
human neurons, 344
rat neurons, 338–344
Cell junctions
in intestinal muscle, 115–121
basal lamina and cell-to-stroma junctions, 118–120
embryonic development of, 133
gap junctions, 115–118
intermediate junctions, 118
Cells
intestinal
embryonic development of, 131–133
structural changes during contraction, 126–127
size and shape, smooth muscle shortening, 306
Cell-to-cell coupling
electrical event propagation, 205
ICC DMP and, 372–373
slow-wave generation, 192
slow wave and spike potentials, small intestine, 54–55
Cell-to-stroma junction, in intestinal muscle, 118–120
Cell-to-tendon junction, in intestinal muscle, 119–121
Cellular force production, contractile protein regulation, 294–295
Cellular ion content, measurement of, 142–143
Cell viability, role in electrophysiological studies, 164
Central autonomic neurons, 654
Central nervous system (CNS)
defecation and colonic motility, 961–963
deglutition and, 685–697
diagram of nuclei in, 624
emesis and, 697–708
gastric blood flow control, 1382
gastrointestinal afferent innervation, 594–595
gastrointestinal motility
brain-gut neural circuitry, 665–672
center stimulation, 637–646
*See also* specific neural centers, 637–646
key concepts in, 672–673
neural inputs and outputs, 658–663
neuroanatomical description, 647–658
nuclei stimulation and lesion, 663–665
research background, 621–623
retrograde neuronal tracing techniques, 623–637
gastrointestinal tract, 593–94
hepatic circulation control by, 1520
ruminant forestomach motility, 1248
vomiting reflex, 1190
Centrioles, in intestinal muscle, 115
Cerebral cortex and gastrointestinal motility
neural input and output, 662–663
nucleus tractus solitarius pathway, 668
Onuf's nucleus pathway, 669
stimulation and lesion of, 663
Cesium ions ($Cs^{2+}$), 222
in intestinal smooth muscle
action potentials and, 222
C-fibers, in sympathetic preganglionic nerves, 532
cGMP
$\alpha$-adrenoreceptors and, 737
biliary tract pharmacology, 1115
diarrhea and, 1154
gastrin-CCK receptors, 765
intracellular control systems, 407
muscarinic postreceptor events, 732
receptors and postreceptor mechanisms, 723

*Chabertia ovina*, parasite-induced alterations
small intestine, 1137
stomach, 1134
Chaga's disease
esophageal alterations, 1133–1134
megaesophagus and megacolon, 1147
parasite-induced alterations, 1135–1136
Chemical control, defined, 818–819
Chemical neurotransmission, enteric nervous system, 491–511
fast EPSPs, 491–493
fast IPSPs, 503–504
presynaptic inhibition, 508–511
slow EPSPs, 493–503
slow IPSPs, 504–508
Chemoceptive trigger zone, emesis and, 698
Chemoreceptors
arterial, gastrointestinal blood flow, 1694–1695
gastrointestinal afferent innervation, 595–596
vomiting reflex, 1189
Chemotherapy-induced emesis, 706–707
Chloride-bicarbonate exchange, in smooth muscle, 156–157
Chloride ($Cl^-$) channels, 179–180
electron-probe microanalysis of, 145
gastrointestinal neuromuscular transmission
excitatory junction potentials, 449–451
permeability, 438, 440–442
in intestinal smooth muscle, 223
passive ion movements, 148–149
submucosal arterioles, excitatory junction potentials, 1646–1648
VIP transmission, 566
$\beta$-Chlornaltrexamine (b-CNA), 783–784
Cholangiography, biliary tract function, 1061–1062
Cholecystography, biliary tract function, 1061
Cholecystokinin (CCK)
in area postrema, 701
biliary tract pharmacology, 1111–1115
pancreatic polypeptide and, 1122–1123
secretin and, 1117
VIP and, 1117
colonic motility, 953, 956
innervation, 942
cystic duct function, 1074
in dorsal motor nucleus of the vagus, 650
enteric nervous system
cholinergic system, 417–418
slow EPSPs, 498–499
slow IPSPs, 506
exocrine gland circulation
functional hyperemia, 1575, 1577
metabolic regulation of, 1569
gallbladder function, 1066, 1070–1072
gastric blood flow and secretion, 1500–1501
gastric emptying, 41–42
antropyloroduodenal flow resistance, 920–921
proximal stomach tonic contractions, 919
gastrointestinal blood flow, 1687
gastrointestinal motility, 928
intermediolateral cell column ($S_{2-3}$), 654
intestinal blood flow and motility, 1492
colon, 1497–1500
lower esophageal sphincter, 891–892
regulation, 997–998
parasite-induced imbalance of, 1147
postprandial intestinal hyperemia and, 1425–1426
serotonin and, 1428
in prevertebral ganglion, 566–570
slow EPSP, 555
pyloric sphincter regulation, 1002–1003
receptors
gastrin-linked, 759–761
locus of action, 762–764

Cholecystokinin (*continued*)
  in ruminant animals
    gastric emptying, 1257–1258
    gastroduodenal junction, 1276
    sphincter of Oddi, 1066–1067, 1103–1104
    species differences, 1060
$^{125}$I-Cholecystokinin, 763
Cholecystokinin-2, biliary tract pharmacology, 1113–1114
Cholecystokinin-3, biliary tract pharmacology, 1113–1114
Cholecystokinin-4
  gastrointestinal blood flow, 1687
  in prevertebral ganglion, 567
Cholecystokinin-7
  analogue potencies, 761
  biliary tract pharmacology, 1112–1114
  receptor interaction, 761
Cholecystokinin COOH-terminal octapeptide (CCK-8)
  avian motility regulation, 1290–1291
  biliary tract pharmacology, 1111–1115
    gastrin and, 1115–1116
    prostaglandin interaction, 1109
    sphincter of Oddi dysfunction, 1092–1093
  in enteric nervous system, 395
    cholinergic system, 416–417
  exocrine gland circulation
    functional hyperemia and, 1577–1579
  gallbladder function, 1070
  gastrointestinal blood flow
    neurohormonal control, 1682, 1687
  gastrointestinal correlates of vomiting, 1191
  intestinal blood flow and motility
    intramural tension and, 1495–1496
  postprandial intestinal hyperemia and, 1426
  in prevertebral ganglion, 567
  receptors, 761–764
  in ruminant animals, 1238
    pancreaticobiliary secretions, 1263–1264
    pharmacology, 1271
Cholecystokinin-12, in prevertebral ganglion, 567
Cholecystokinin-27–33, 568
Cholecystokinin-30–33, 568
Cholecystokinin-33
  biliary tract pharmacology, 1111–1115
  CCK receptor action, 763
Cholecystomy, gallbladder function and, 1091
Choledochoduodenal junction
  myoelectric activity and, 847–848
  opiate receptors, 790
Choleragen, intestinal motility, 1156
Choleragenoid, intestinal motility, 1156
Cholestasis, liver lymph and, 1762
[$^3$H]Choline, enteric cholinergic system, 410
Choline acetyltransferase (ChAt)
  colonic motility, 953
  in dorsal motor nucleus of the vagus, 648
  gastrointestinal blood flow, 1668–1669
  gastrointestinal motility, 652
  in motor neurons, 388
  of rat enteric neurons, 339, 341–342
Cholinergic agonists
  in colonic muscle
    electropharmacology, 257–258
  effect on calcium channels, 180–181
  effect on potassium channels, 180
  effect on voltage recordings, 168
  electropharmacology of, 204
  internal anal sphincter, 1038–1039
  intestinal smooth muscle activity, 233–234
  mesenteric artery, 1613–1614, 1620
  potassium channel studies, 174–176
Cholinergic antagonists
  lower esophageal sphincter activity, 890–891

Cholinergic drugs
  gallbladder and sphincter of Oddi activity, 1105–1106
  intestinal blood flow and motility, 1488–1490
Cholinergic innervation
  colonic motility, 954
  in dorsal motor nucleus of the vagus, 648
  esophageal peristalsis, 880–882
  gastrointestinal motility, 652
  internal anal sphincter, motor activity, 1035
  lower esophageal sphincter, 990
  motor neurons, 388
  postprandial hyperemia and, 1422
  prevertebral ganglia, 551–554
  ruminant animals, 1276–1276
  sacral autonomic nerves, 1039
  in small intestine, 62–63
Cholinergic receptors
  lower esophageal sphincter contractions, 995–996
  vomiting reflex, 1192
Chorda lingual nerve, salivary gland circulation and, 1573–1574, 1576
Chrommaffin cells, structure and function, 527–529
Chronic constipation, gastrointestinal neuromuscular transmission, 456
Chylomicrons
  initial lymphatics, 1737–1738
  lymph flow and composition, 1751–1752
Chylous ascites, 1765
Chylous mesenteric cysts, 1765
Chyluria, 1765
Chyme
  intestinal villi motility, 980–981
  luminal stimulus, intestinal mucosal blood flow and, 1418–1419
  postprandial hyperemia and, vasoactive action by, 1421
Chymotrypsin, substance P hydrolysis, 393
Cinematography, early colon research, 72–73
Cineradiography
  common duct function, 1079
  sphincter of Oddi function, 1078–1079, 1083–1084
Circular muscle
  colonic motility, 947–948
    action potentials and, 256
    electrical coupling with longitudinal layers, 266–267
    innervation of, 260
    resting potential and, 252–253
    slow-wave propagation and, 262–265
  deep muscle plexus in, 367
  development of, 129–130
  dominant in cecum, 103–104, 110
  electrical control activity in anal sphincter, 844
  interstitial cells of Cajal and, 373–374
    colonic, 378–379
  intestinal
    cell size and shape, 108–109, 112
    cholinergic innervation, 234–235
    passive electrical properties, 228–229
    slow-wave origin and propagation, 231–233
    ultrastructure of, 104, 107
  in muscle coat, 103–104
  opiate receptors, 785–786
    in small intestine, 787–788
  slow-wave generation, 192
    ICC AP role in, 361–364
  small intestine microvascular anatomy, 1476–1478
  substance P action on, 769
  tension receptors and, 608–609
  thickness ratio to longitudinal muscle, 103
Circulatory shock, ulcerogenesis and, 1722
Cirrhosis
  ascites in, 1761–1762
  liver lymph and, 1761
Cloaca, avian structure, 1285–1286

Clonidine, interaction with substance P, 772
*Clostridium botulinum*, 1757
*Clostridium difficile*, 1165
*Clostridium perfringens*
    parasite-induced motility, 1149
    repetitive bursts of action potentials, 1164
Co-EDTA, extracellular space measurement, 142
Collagen
    fibril distribution in extracellular space, 106, 109
    intestinal muscle
        embryonic development of, 131
        helical pattern in submucosa, 128–129
        hypertrophy, 135
        structural changes during contraction, 127
        in submucosa, 128–130
    link with muscle cells, 106
Collagenase, role in dispersion techniques, 164
Collecting lymphatics
    downstream microocclusion, 1744
    structure, 1738
    valves, 1738–1739
Collecting venules, small intestine anatomy, 1477
Colocolonic inhibitory reflex, 540–541
Colon
    anatomy, 940–942
        human gross structure, 940
        muscular walls, 941
        nerves of, 941–942
    blood flow, vascular response pattern, 1676–1677
    bombesin action and, 800
    connections with inferior mesenteric ganglion, 539–540
    early research
        aganglionosis:megacolon, 83–84
        animal studies, 72
        cinematography, 72–73
        electrical studies, 84
        electromyography, 79
        image intensification, 73–74
        neurological deficits, 79–81
        psychosomatic factors, 84–86
        roentgen observations, 71–72
        spinal and higher control, 81–82
        surgical intervention, 84
        tandem balloon method, 71
    embryonic development of, 940
    gastrin-releasing peptide, 800
    giant migrating contractions in, 851–852
    haustration, 72
    historical research, 68–86
        aganglionosis megacolon, 83–84
        defecation and continence, 77–83
        ileocolonic junction and antiperistalsis, 68–70
        movement analysis, 70–74
        nervous control of movements, 74–77
        psychosomatic factors, 84–86
    innervation
        early research, 74–77
        parasympathetic innervation, 1026–1027
        sacral afferent fibers, 1027–1028
        schematic representation, 78–79
        sympathetic neural pathways, 629–630
    interstitial cells of Cajal and, 375–381
        association with longitudinal muscle, 376–378
    ischemia
        inflammatory bowel disease, 1721
        nonocclusive intestinal ischemia, 1715
    lumbar sympathetic innervation, 1026
        electrical stimulation, 1036–1037
        interruption, 1037–1038
    lymphatics, 1757
        structure, 1740
    microvasculature, 1315–1316, 1320–1321
    motilin in, 794
    motor activity. *See* Colonic motility
    myoelectric activity
        peptides in, 1030–1031
        spatial and temporal patterns, 834–838
    opiate receptors, 790–791
    parasite-induced alterations, 1146–1147
    parasympathetic neural pathways, 627
    postoperative inertia, 1201
    postprandial hyperemia and, 1420
    proctocolectomy, 1216–1218
    retrograde tracing of dorsal motor nucleus, 641
    surgical perturbations of, 1216–1218
    tachykinin actions in, 776
    tonic inhibitory drive to, 533
    vascular supply and drainage, 1303, 1329
    vasoactive intestinal polypeptide action on, 779–780
    vomiting and, 1185–1186
Colonic motility
    anal sphincters, 957–960
        external, 959–960
        internal sphincter, 957–959
    blood flow and, 1497–1500
        acetylcholine, 1668
        lumen pressure and, 1505
    cephalic phase in eating response, 960
    colonic phase in eating response, 961
    defecation and, 961–963
    eating and, 1046
    drugs and, 955–957
        adrenergic drugs, 955
        antibiotics, 957
        anticholinergic agents, 955–956
        ATP, 956
        bile acids, 957
        GABA, 956
        laxatives, 956–957
        morphine, 956
        polypeptides, 956
        prostaglandins, 956
    dysfunction, 963–966, 1047
        aganglionosis, 963–965
        diarrhea and constipation, 965
        diverticulosis, 963
        irritable colon syndrome, 965–966
        rectal incontinence, 966
        sacral autonomic nerves, 1039
    eating and defecation, 1046
    electrical activity model, 268–269
    electrical event propagation, 262–268
        electrical coupling, 262
        fast transients and action potentials, 267–268
        longitudinal and circular muscle layers, 266–267
        myenteric potential oscillations, 265–266
        slow-wave propagation, 262–265
    endogenous substance electropharmacology, 257–262
        adrenergic agonists, 258–259
        cholinergic agonists, 257–259
        paracrine substances, 259
        peptides, 259
    evolution of, 939–940
    excitable events in, 253–256
        action potentials, 255–256
        myenteric potential oscillations, 254–255
        slow electrical oscillations, 253
        slow waves, 253–254
    excitation-contraction coupling, 256–257
        pacemaker cells in, 268
        research background on, 251
        resting membrane potential, 251–253
            electrogenic pump and, 252–253
            values for, 251–252

Colonic motility (*continued*)
    spontaneous neural activity, 259–262
    transmural and extrinsic nerve stimulation, 259–262
  gastric emptying, 960–961
  gastric phase in eating response, 960
  gross contraction and flow patterns, 943–946
  hormonal control, 966–967
  human studies, 949–951
  intestinal phase in eating response, 960–961
  mass movement, 945
  motor functions of, 818
  myogenic factors, in contractions, 946–952, 966–967
  neurogenic factors, 952–955, 966–967
    autonomic drug response, 954
    extrinsic nervous control, 954–955
    intrinsic nerve stimulation, 954
    morphological studies, 952–953
    peristaltic reflex, 953
    tonic neurogenic inhibition, 953–954
  peripheral reflexes and, 536–542
  prolonged residence and mixing, 944–945
  rhythmic contractions, 945–946
  ruminant animals, 1266–1270
    cecal motility patterns, 1267–1268
    functional organization, 1266–1267
    neural influences, 1269
    pelleted feces formation, 1268–1269
  slow waves, contractions and flows, 951–952
  stress and, 963
  study methods, 942–943
  sympathetic nervous system, 661–662, 670–671
  tonic contractions, 536, 946
Colonic-rectal distension, 1041–1043
Colonmetrogram, 946
Common bile duct
  diameter measurements with sonography, 1066
  electromyography, 1064
  embryonic development, 1056–1057
  function studies, 1074–1077
    dilatation, 1075–1076
  gross anatomy, 1056
  hepatic bile flow, 1068–1070
  innervation, 1059
  manometry and, 1062–1063
  muscle and mucosal structure, 1058
  opening pressure, 1080
  peristalsis, 1084–1086
  species anatomical differences, 1060–1061
  structure, 1057
  T-tube manometry, 1063
Compartmental blood flow, intestinal blood flow and motility, 1483, 1486, 1505–1507
Competition binding studies, muscarinic receptor modulation and, 729–731
Compliance
  hepatic blood volume, 1537–1538
  viscoelastic systems, 321
Computer systems, gastrointestinal muscle mechanics, 283
Conductance change, in smooth muscle neurotransmission, 438, 440–442
Conduction
  defined, 205–206
  velocities
    determination of slow-wave origin, 207–208
    enteric nervous system, 483
    gastric muscle electrophysiology, 207
    prevertebral ganglion, 532
Congenital malformation, intestinal muscle, 133
Constant-field equation, slow-wave genesis and conduction, 53–54
Constant-flow preparation, intestinal blood flow and motility, 1478
  hypoxia and, 1510–1511

  luminal distension, 1505
  tonic contractions, 1482–1483
Constipation
  colonic motility and, 965
  opiate receptors and, 791–792
Continence
  defecation and, 962–963
  early research, 77–83
  external anal sphincter and, 959–960
  rectal, 962–963
  sphincteric, 962–963
Continuous electrical response activity, 836
Contractile electrical complex, 836–838
Contraction
  colonic motility
    interaction with slow waves, 951–952
    rhythmicity of, 945–946
    tonic contractions, 946
  gastrointestinal smooth muscle
    controlling conditions of, 273–275
    elastic components, 275
    isometric conditions, 274
    isotonic conditions, 274–275
    mechanical models of, 275
    regulation of, 286–295
  of intestinal muscle
    collagen fiber arrangement during, 128–129
    in vitro studies of, 226–227
    structural changes during, 125–127
  on and off, esophageal peristalsis, 880–882
  periodic, 25
  reflex, lower esophageal sphincter, 895–896
  rhythmicity, nerves and, 65
  segmental, slow-wave mechanism and, 231
  skeletal muscle mechanisms, 276
  small intestine, research on, 49–51
  smooth muscle mechanics, 125–127
    stiffness in contracting muscle, 299–306
Contraction phase, colonic motility and blood flow, 1497–1500
Cooling, gastrointestinal smooth muscle activation, 285
Core-conductor model of excitability, 209–213
Cotransmission
  gastrointestinal neuromuscular transmission, 444–445
  research background on, 435–436
  submucosal arterioles, 1658–1660
Coulter counter technique, 724
Countercurrent mechanism
  hydrogen clearance, 1363–1364
  intestinal mucosal blood flow, 1430–1433
    anatomical basis, 1430
    countercurrent multiplier, 1433
    evidence for, 1432–1433
    theory, 1430–1432
  nonocclusive intestinal ischemia, 1713–1715
Creep, in viscoelastic systems, 319–320
Cricopharyngeus muscle
  esophageal motility, 870
Crohn's disease
  colonic ischemia, 1721
  gastrointestinal neuromuscular transmission, 457
  lymphatic drainage, 1764–1765
Crop, avian motility, 1283, 1286–1287
Crossbridge hypothesis
  contractile protein regulation, 293–294
  contracting muscle stiffness, 299–300
  influence on relaxation, 314–315
  length-tension curve, 298–299
Culture techniques, background on, 331–332
Current clamp techniques, 545–548
Cyclic adenosine monophosphate. *See* cAMP
Cyclooxygenase
  gastric blood flow control, 1389

MAPC and, 1157–1159
Cystic duct
  function studies, 1074
  innervation, 1059
  muscle and mucosal structure, 1058
  structure, 1057
Cytoplasmic $Ca^{2+}$, potassium channel properties, 173–174
Cytoplasmic release mechanism, nonvesicular enteric neurotransmission, 405

D 600, calcium channel properties and, 179
Deep muscular plexus, interstitial cells of Cajal and, 366–373
Defecation
  anorectal and pelvic floor musculature, 1044–1046
    sacral parasympathetic efferent fibers, 1046
    visceral and somatic afferent fibers, 1044–1046
  colonic motility, 961–963
    eating and, 1046
    continence and, 962–963
    early research and, 77–83
    ruminant animals, pellet formation, 1267–1269
    sacral parasympathetic efferent fibers, 1046
Deglutition. *See* Swallowing
Degradation
  bombesin, 799
  gastrin-releasing peptide, 799
  of neurotensin, 797
Dendrites
  in dorsal motor nucleus, 647
  in principal ganglia cells, 524, 526
Dendrons, of pelvic neurons, 653
Denervation effects, enteric nervous system, 511
Dense bands, in intestinal muscle
  cell size and shape, 109, 111, 113–115, 119, 122
  embryonic development of, 131, 133
Dense bodies
  contractile protein regulation, 294
  intestinal muscle
    embryonic development of, 131, 133
    structure and distribution, 124–125
Dense patches. *See* Dense bands
Depolarization
  cholinergic innervation, 235
  gastrointestinal electrophysiology
    diastolic, 192
    ionic channel studies, 181–183
    smooth muscle activation, 286
  intestinal smooth muscle, 236
  potassium channel properties, 174–176
  resting membrane potentials and, 190
  voltage recordings of isolated cells, 167–168
  *See also* Slow depolarization
Dermorphans as opiate source, 780
Descending colon, anatomy, 940
Desmosomes, intestinal villi motility, 975
Detergent treatment
  contractile protein regulation, 292
  gastrointestinal smooth muscle activation, 286
Diabetes mellitus
  gallbladder function and, 1090–1091
  gastrointestinal neuromuscular transmission, 454, 456
  intestinal blood flow and, 1723
Diacylglycerol (DAG)
  enteric neurotransmission, 409
  intestinal smooth muscle, 237
  receptor-evoked responses, 237
Diarrhea
  colonic motility and, 965
  fast gastric emptying and, 1200
  historical research, 1153–1154
    animal studies, 1153–1155
  mechanisms of, 1168–1170
  parasite-induced motility, 1149–1150
  surgical perturbations
    with drainage operation, 1213
    truncal vagotomy, 1209
Dibenamine, lower esophageal sphincter, 17
Dibutyryl cAMP, channel activation with, 181
DIDS, chloride-bicarbonate exchange, 156–157
Diet, intestinal villi structure and, 977
Differential excitability, enteric nervous system, 483–484
Differentiated properties
  enteric neurons
    long afterhyperpolarization, 336–337
    slow synaptic potentials, 336
    tissue culture, 335–336
  of interstitial cells of Cajal, 371, 382
  rat enteric neurons, 399–341
Diffusion potential, resting membrane potential and, 189–190
Digestion, gastric mixing, 21–23
Digitalis, cardiogenic shock, 1719
Digital storage oscilloscopes, 282
Digital-to-analog converters, 283
Dihydroxyphenylalanine (Dopa), in rat enteric neurons, 341
Dipeptidyl peptidase IV, enteric nervous system, 420
4-Diphenylacetoxy-N-methylpiperidine methiodide (4-DAMP), 727
Direct current (DC), smooth muscle activation, 285
Discrete electrical response activity (DERA), 835–836
Disease states, gastrointestinal neuromuscular transmission, 453–457
Dispersion techniques
  cell evaluation, 164–166
  enzymatic techniques, 163–164
Dissections, enteric nervous system, 469–470
Distal stomach, motor activity, 911–912
Distributing arteriole
  small intestine anatomy, 1476–1477
  *See also* Submucosal arteriole
Dithiothreitol, lymph flow and composition, 1746–1747
Diverticular disease
  gastrointestinal neuromuscular transmission, 456
  of colon, 963
DMO, sodium-hydrogen exchange and, 157
DMPP (1,1-Dimethyl-4-phenylpiperazinium)
  enteric cholinergic system
    acetylcholine release, 416
    somatostatin, 417
  gastrointestinal neuromuscular transmission
    excitatory junction potentials, 450–451
    internal anal sphincter, motor activity, 1035
    secretomotor transmission, 392
Dogiel classification of enteric nervous system
  ganglion, 478–479
  intracellular recordings, 482–483
Dopamine
  in area postrema, 701
  in dorsal motor nucleus of the vagus, 648–649
  influence on rumination, 1239
  lower esophageal sphincter activity, 891
  nonocclusive intestinal ischemia, 1717
  in SIF cells, 529
Dopaminergic receptors, vomiting reflex, 1191
Doppler beat frequency, 1346
Doppler effect, laser Doppler volcimetry, 1344
Doppler frequency shift, 1345
Doppler frequency spectra, 1346
Dorsal motor nucleus of the vagus
  amygdala connections to, 663
  columnar organization of, 626–627
  gastrointestinal motility
    neuronal inputs and outputs, 658–660
    parasympathetic centers, 637–643
    pathway to esophageal sphincters, 671–672

Dorsal motor nucleus of the vagus (*continued*)
    pathway to periventricular hypothalamus, 668–669
    neuroanatomy of, 647–651
    parasympathetic neural pathway
        in colon, 627–628
        in esophagus, 625
        in stomach, 625–626
    receptive relaxation and, 672
Dorsal reticular formation, deglutition and, 688
Dorsal root ganglia, gastrointestinal motility, 646
Dose-response curves, smooth muscle contractions, 725–726
DPDTSP (substance P antagonist), 451
"Driver-follower" discharge, burst-pattern generation, 474–475
Drop recording, intestinal blood flow and motility, 1479
Duct of Santorini, embryonic development, 1057
Dumping syndrome, 1200
    intestinal blood flow and, 1724
    postsurgical, 1200
    vagotomy
        with drainage operation, 1213
        surgical perturbations, 1209
Duodenal brake mechanism, 1252–1255
Duodenal bulb, in ruminant animals, 1262–1263
Duodenogastric reflux, during interdigestive period, 913–914
Duodenum
    avian motility patterns, 1287–1289
    microvasculature, 1315–1316, 1318
    motility inhibition, 536
    transection, 1213
    vascular supply and drainage, 1303
Dynorphin
    biliary tract pharmacology, 1120–1121
    in enteric neurons, 395
        cholinergic system, 418–419
    in prevertebral ganglia, 569–570
    receptor locus and functional coupling, 719

Eating
    colonic motility and defecation and, 1046
    hepatic circulation, 1531
    ileocecal sphincter characteristics, 1004–1006
    intestinal villi motility, 980–981
    mucosal blood flow and, 1392–1393
    ruminant animals, 1275–1276
    sphincter of Oddi function, 1086–1088
Edema formation
    inflammatory bowel disease, 1764–1765
    intestinal mucosal blood flow
        capillary-interstitial interaction, 1445–1446
Edema safety factor, lymph and tissue homeostasis, 1742–1743
Effective dose ($ED_{50}$), electropharmacology of pentagastrin, 204
Effectors
    enteric nervous system activation, 501–502
    neuromuscular transmission and, 436
Efferent innervation
    esophageal motility, 866–867
    forestomach motility, 1247–1248
    pelvic floor muscle, 1028–1030
    vomiting reflex, 1190–1191
EGTA
    potassium channel properties, 171
    separation of extracellular $Ca^{2+}$, 144
*Eimeria magna*, parasite-induced alterations
    cecum, colon and rectum, 1147
    small intestine, 1139, 1145
    in stomach, 1134
*Eimeria nieschulzi*, parasite-induced alterations
        small intestine, 1139
        in stomach, 1134
Elastic fibers
    in intestinal muscle, 106–107, 111
        basal lamina and, 119

    in taeniae, 106–108, 110–111
Elastic modulus, viscoelastic systems, 321
Elastic tissue
    common duct function, 1075
    gastrointestinal smooth muscle, 275
Electric action potentials, avian motility, 1288
Electrical arrhythmias, gastric muscle electrophysiology, 196–198
Electrical control activity (ECA)
    anal sphincters, 844–845
    analysis of, 825
    caudad mass movement, 850–852
    choledochoduodenal junction, 847–848
    colon control, 76
    colon and rectum, 834–835
    defined, 818–819
    disruption during vomiting, 1186–1187
    esophagus, 838–842
    gallbladder, 849–850
    gastroduodenal junction, 845–846
    ileocolonic junction, 848–849
    lower esophageal sphincter, 843–844
    nausea and, 1193–1194
    phasic contractions
        spatial control, 821–823
    relaxation-oscillator vs. cable model, 852–857
        passive conduction, 852
        regenerative propagation, 852–853
        relaxation-oscillator propagation, 853–857
    reticuloruminant contractions, 1234–1235
    small intestine, 830–834
        frequency plateau and variable frequency regions, 831, 833
        mean frequency criterion, 831–832
    smooth contractions
        temporal control, 818–820
    in stomach, 827–830
    terminology background, 827
    transthoracic vagotomy and, 1208–1209
    vomiting, 850
    *See also* Slow waves
Electrical coupling
    in colonic muscle, 262
        circular and longitudinal layers, 266–267
    in intestinal smooth muscle, 227–229
    submucosal arterioles, 1643–1644, 1647
Electrical response activity (ERA)
    anal sphincters, 844–845
    analysis of, 825
    choledochoduodenal junction, 847–848
    colon and rectum
        continuous electrical response activity, 836
        discrete electrical response activity, 835–836
    esophagus, 838–842
    gallbladder, 849–850
    ileocolonic junction, 849
    lower esophageal sphincter, 843–844
    phasic contractions, spatial control, 821–823
    smooth contractions, temporal control, 818–820
    terminology background, 827
    vomiting, 850, 1187
Electrical stimulation
    CNS influence on gastrointestinal motility, 623
    colonic motility and blood flow, 1498–1500
    enteric cholinergic system, 410
    gastrointestinal blood flow, 1670–1671
    gastrointestinal motility
        dorsal motor nucleus, 637–641
        in nucleus ambiguus, 643–644
        smooth muscle activation, 284–286
    sacral autonomic nerves, colon and rectal activity, 1039
    shortening force-velocity curve, 311
    in stomach, ECA frequencies, 829–830
    swallowing reflex, 868

"Electric insulator," gastroduodenal junction, 56
Electrodes, in myoelectric activity recordings, 823–825
Electrogenic pump, 149–150
  resting membrane potentials and, 190
  in colonic muscle, 252–253
Electromotive force, small intestine gradient, 58
Electromyography
  biliary tract function, 1064–1065
  colon control, 79
  pelvic floor skeletal muscle, 1033–1034
  reticuloruminant contractions, 1232–1233
  sphincter of Oddi function, 1078–1079
  upper esophageal sphincter, 871–872
Electron microscopy, $Ca^{2+}$ distribution
  measurement with, 145
Electrophysiology of rat enteric neurons, 339
Eledoisin
  intestinal blood flow and motility, 1491
  prevertebral ganglia neurotransmission, 559
Embryonic development, intestinal musculature, 129–133
Emesis. *See* Vomiting
Endopeptidase, enteric nervous system, 419
Endoplasmic reticulum, calcium pumps in, 151–154
Endorphin in prevertebral ganglia, 560–564
Endoscopic retrograde cholangiopancreatography (ERCP),
    sphincter of Oddi function, 1063–1064, 1079–1080
Endoscopic sphincterotomy, 1095
Endotoxin
  hepatic circulation, 1551
  mucosal injury, 1394
  septic shock and, 1719
End-plate potential (EPP), mesenteric artery, 1615
Enkephalin
  in area postrema, 701
  colonic motility and blood flow, 1499–1500
  in dorsal motor nucleus of the vagus, 649
  enteric nervous system, 395
    cholinergic system, 418–419
    intracellular recordings, 485
  gastrointestinal blood flow, 1678
  gastrointestinal innervation, 1030–1031
  gastrointestinal motility
    in nTS, 657–658
    sympathetic preganglionic neurons, 656–657
  noncholinergic excitatory motor transmission, 389
  in prevertebral ganglia, 560–564
  δ-receptors and, 781
*Entamoeba histolytica*, substances derived from, 1147
Enteric nervous system
  associative neurons, 387
  autonomic connections, early research, 58–64
  cell cultures
    human neurons, 344
    modulation of synaptic interactions, 344
    rat neurons, 338–344
    retention of differentiated properties, 339–341
    synaptic interactions, 341
  coexistence of putative transmitters, 396
  culture studies
    advantages of, 344–345
    limitations of, 344
    techniques, 331–332
  electrical and synaptic behavior
    AH/type 2 neurons, 485
    burst-type units, 471–475
    cell body electrical behavior, 486–491
    chemical neurotransmission, 491–511
    conduction velocity, 483
    denervation effects, 511
    differential excitability, 483–484
    dissections, 469–470
    electrophysiological classification, 485–486
    extracellular recordings, 466–468, 470–481
    fast EPSPs, 491–493
    fast IPSPs, 503–504
    histoanatomical factors, 482–483
    intracellular recordings, 468–469, 481–485
    mechanosensitive neurons, 476–480
    morphine and enkephalin, 485
    presynaptic inhibition, 508–511
    refractory period, 483
    research background, 465–466
    single-spike units, 480–481
    slow EPSPs, 493–503
    slow IPSPs, 504–508
    S/type 1 neurons, 485–486
    tetrodotoxin and, 485
    type 3 neurons, 486
    type 4 neurons, 486
    unit classification of, 470
  electrical parameters, 486
  embryonic development, 332–333
  future research on, 396–397
  gastrointestinal correlates of vomiting, 1191
  glia, properties of, 338
  MAPC, 1159–1161
  motor neurons, 387
  muscarinic receptors in, 728
  neuroneuronal synapse transmission, 392–396
    fast excitatory synaptic potentials, 392
    inhibitory synaptic potentials, 394
    neurochemical transmission, 395–396
    neuromuscular junction actions, 394–395
    presynaptic inhibition at, 394
    sensory neurons, 395
    slow excitatory synaptic potentials, 392–394
  organotypic culture, 332–333
  postprandial hyperemia, 1699
  secretomotor, 391–392
  sensory neurons, 387
  serotonin receptors and, 741–742
  tissue culture, 333–338
    absent or rare differentiated properties, 336–337
    cell culture, 338–344
    enteric glia properties, 338
    fast response to substance P, 337–338
    GABA neurons, 337
    muscarinic receptor distribution, 338
    preferred growth substrates, 335–336
    retention of differentiated properties, 335–336
  transmitter research, 387–388
  historical background on, 387–388
  vasculature of, 1304
  vasodilator, 391
  *See also* Associative neurons; Motor neurons; Sensory neurons
Enteric plexus in small intestine
  Schofield's diagram, 62
  structure of, 61–62
Enterocyte membrane, diarrhea mechanisms, 1171–1172
"Enterogasterone," 36, 41–42
Enterogastric inhibitory reflex, 36
  prevertebral ganglion and, 535–536
  ruminant animals, 1254–1255
Enterogastric reflux, postoperative, 1200
Enteroglucagon, gastrointestinal blood flow, 1685–1686
"Enterograph," 35
Enterotoxins
  bacterial-induced motility, 1153–1171
  parasite-induced motility, 1149–1150
Enzymes, parasite-induced substances, 1147
Epilepsy, emesis and, 707
Epinephrine
  in area postrema, 701
  in colonic muscle, electropharmacology, 258–259

Epinephrine (*continued*)
  in dorsal motor nucleus of the vagus, 648–649
  enteric cholinergic system, 412
  gastric blood flow control, 1386
  gastrointestinal blood flow, 1683–1684
  influence on rumination, 1239
  intestinal blood flow and motility, 1488
    villous motility, 979
  slow-wave research, 189
  sphincter of Oddi pharmacology, 1107–1108
Epithelial receptors, ruminant forestomach motility, 1249–1250
EPSPs. *See* Excitatory postsynaptic potentials
Equilibrium model of hepatic circulation, 1520
    substrate uptake, 1532–1534
    venous model, 1532–1534
Equilibrium potentials, in prevertebral ganglion cells, 542–543
Eructation, 1239–1242
Escape phenomenon, gastrointestinal blood flow, 1683
*Escherichia coli*
  enterotoxin, MAPC stimulation, 1161
  parasite-induced motility, 1149
  repetitive bursts of action potentials
    heat-stable toxins, 1165–1166
    invasive strains, 1163–1164
  septic shock and, 1719
Esophageal achalasia and atresia, 1724
Esophageal body structure
  central peristaltic control, 875–877
  junctional zone peristalsis, 884
  longitudinal muscle layer, 884–885
  muscular anatomy, 873–874
  muscularis mucosa and, 884–885
  peripheral peristaltic control, 877
    contraction-inhibition correlates, 882–884
    electrical stimulation studies, 879–880
    latency and latency gradient, 882–883
    localized distension, 877–878
    neurotransmitters, 883–884
    on and off contractions, 880–882
    smooth muscle, 877–884
    vagal efferent stimulation, 878–879
  pressure profile, 874–875
Esophageal groove
  Flourens' illustration, 1228–1229
  functions of, 1228
  ruminant stomach, 1226
Esophageal inhibition, 875
Esophageal motility, 817
  anatomy and, 866
  deglutition reflex, 867–869
  nausea and vomiting, 1179–1182
  peristalsis, 10–12
    abnormal, 12
  research methods, 869–870
  *See also* Lower and Upper esophageal sphincters
Esophageal propulsive force, 875
Esophagus
  anatomy of, 865–866
  avian motility and structure, 1283, 1286–1287
  bombesin action and, 799
  "curling of," 12
  distension and gastric relaxation, 927
  gastrin-releasing peptide action in, 799
  human studies, 5–8
  innervation of, 866–867
    afferent innervation, 867
    dorsal motor nucleus of the vagus, 671–672
    efferent innervation, 866
    interstitial cells of Cajal, 867
    intrinsic innervation, 866–867
    nucleus ambiguus pathways, 671–672
    parasympathetic neural pathways in, 623–625
    peripheral innervation of, 695
    retrofacial nucleus pathways, 671–672
    sympathetic neural pathways, 628–629
    *See also* Lower and Upper esophageal sphincters
  interstitial cells of Cajal and, 374–378, 382, 867
  lymph flow and composition, 1746–1747
  lymph structure, 1739
  motilin in, 793
  muscles and nerves of, 8–9
  myoelectric activity, 838–842
    smooth muscle, 838–842
    striated muscle, 838
  opiate receptors and, 786
  parasite-induced alterations, 1133–1134
  sphincters. *See* Lower and Upper esophageal sphincters
  surgical perturbations of, 1202–1203
  tachykinin action on, 772–773
  vascular supply and drainage, 1302
  vasoactive intestinal polypeptide action in, 778–779
Estrogen, biliary tract pharmacology, 1123–1124
Evoked field potential, deglutition and, 688, 690
Exchange vessels, hemorrhagic hypotension, 1697
Excitability model, gastric muscle electrophysiology, 209–218
Excitation-contraction coupling
  in colonic muscle, 256–257
  gastric muscle electrophysiology, 200–203
    mechanical threshold, 200–201
    myogenic propagation regulation, 208–209
    slow waves and, 191
    voltage-tension relationship, 202–203
  smooth muscle contractions, 725
  sodium-calcium exchange and, 155
Excitatory junctional currents (EJCs), submucosal arterioles, 1646–1648
Excitatory junction potentials (EJP)
  in colonic muscle, parasympathetic stimulation, 260
  deglutition and, 695
  fundus electrical events, 198–199
  gastrointestinal neuromuscular transmission
    adrenergic neuromodulation, 444
    ionic basis for, 449–451
  intestinal smooth muscle, nerve-evoked responses, 233–235
  mesenteric artery, 1614–1615
    neuroeffector transmission pharmacology, 1618–1619
  mesenteric circulation, functional differences
    in artery and vein, 1627–1628
  mesenteric vein, 1623
    neuroeffector transmission pharmacology, 1625
  neuromuscular transmission and, 436
    in gastrointestinal tract, 437
  portal vein, 1626–1627
  submucosal arterioles, 1645–1646
    cotransmission, 1658–1660
    norepinephrine, 1656–1658
    pharmacology of, 1654–1660
    quantal content, 1647–1650
    time course, 1646–1648
    transmitter identification, 1656–1660
Excitatory postsynaptic potentials (EPSP)
  deglutition and, 694
  enteric nervous system, 341–342
    intracellular recordings, 483
  fast. *See* Fast excitatory postsynaptic potentials
  gastrointestinal motility, 656
  receptor locus and functional coupling, 720
  serotonin receptors, in enteric nervous system, 741
  slow. *See* Slow excitatory postsynaptic potentials
  small intestine, early research, 68
Excitatory receptors
  burst-pattern generation, 471
  $Ca^{2+}$ intracellular concentration, 236–237
  intestinal smooth muscle

mechanisms of, 236–238
Excitatory synaptic potentials (ESP)
  fast, 392
  slow, 392–394
  See also Excitatory postsynaptic potentials (EPSP)
Exercise
  hepatic circulation, 1551
  limbic and skeletal blood flow and, 1417
Exocrine glands. See Pancreas; Salivary glands
Exocytosis, gastrointestinal blood flow, 1669–1670
Exorphins, as opiate source, 780
Exponential elastic bodies, 320–321
External anal sphincter (EAS)
  colonic motility, 959–960
  electrical activity in, 1033–1034
  electromyographic recordings, 1040, 1042
  pudendal motor pathways, 1040, 1042
  somatic innervation, supraspinal pathways, 1040–1042
  structure, 988–989
Extracellular material, intestinal muscle, 105–108
Extracellular recording techniques
  electrical control activity (ECA), 820
  enteric nervous system, 466–468, 470–481
    burst-type units, 471–475
    mechanosensitive neurons, 476–480
    Pt-Ir electrodes, 466–467
    single-spike unitds, 480–481
    unit classification, 470
Extracellular space
  hepatic circulation, 1553
  intestinal muscle, caveolae and, 113
  measurement of, 141, 142
    ionic content in tissue, 141–142
  slow-wave genesis and conduction, 53–54
Extracontractions, in ruminant animals, 1240
Extramural circulation. See Mesenteric circulation
Extrinsic innervation
  avian muscular stomach, 1285
  biliary tract, 1057
  colonic motility, 259–262, 954–955
  forestomach motility, 1247–1248
  gastrointestinal motility, 927–928
  lower esophageal sphincter, 990
  small intestine, 61

Falck-Hill technique, intramural arteriole innervation, 1637–1638
Faraday constant, potassium channel properties, 172
Fast excitatory postsynaptic potentials (fast EPSPs)
  enteric nervous system, 491–493
    ionic mechanisms, 492
    neurotransmitters, 492–493
    presynaptic inhibition, 509–510
    rundown of, 493
  prevertebral ganglia, 537–540, 544, 551–554
Fast Fourier transform (FFT)
  contractile electrical complex (CEC), 837
  myoelectric activity analysis, 825
Fasting
  lymph lipids during, 1753–1754
  See also Eating
Fast inhibitory postsynaptic potentials (fast IPSPs)
  enteric neurons, 503–504
Fast transients, in colonic muscle, 267–268
Fat absorption, in lymph flows, 1754
Fat hydroxylation, diarrhea and, 1168
Fat-soluble vitamins, lymph flow and composition, 1753
Feedback mechanism
  enteric nervous system, 421
  gastrointestinal motility, 929–930
  presynaptic autoinhibition, 406
Fenestrae (intestinal), 1319, 1321–1322
  permeability, 1328

Fermentation, ruminant stomach, 1228–1229
Fiber bundles in small intestine, 55
Fiber dissection, gastrointestinal afferent innervation, 598
Fibroblasts
  ICC DMP and, 371
  in intestinal muscles, 127–129
Fick principle
  aminopyrine clearance, 1354–1356
  hepatic circulation, 1533–1534
  pH trapping, 1354
Filaments
  intestinal muscle, 121–125
    actin filaments, 121–125
    dense bodies, 124–125
    intermediate filaments, 124
    myosin filaments, 124
Filtration secretion, net fluid secretion and, 1453–1454
Fixation techniques, gastric microvasculature, 1381
Flexor reflexes, 1044
Floating ultramicroelectrode, 52
Flow-limited solutes, intestinal mucosal blood flow, 1429–1430
Flow measurement, biliary tract function, 1062
Fluid exchange
  hepatic circulation, 1552
  hepatic nerve stimulation and, 1554–1555
  in liver, drug effects on, 1554
  reabsorption of in liver, 1553–1554
Fluorescence histochemistry technique, 1638–1639
Fluorescence microscopy
  gastric blood flow control
    histamine and, 1387
    microvasculature, 1381
Follower-type cells, early research, 67
Food propulsion, ruminant digestion, 1230–1231
Force change/length change ratio
  contracting muscle stiffness, 300–305
  exponential elastic bodies, 320–321
Force plateau, tetanus level, 303–305
Force transducers in gastrointestinal muscle studies
  frequency response, 278–279
  long-term stability, 279–280
  noise, 280
  transducer mass and stiffness, 279
Force transients in smooth muscle, 305–306
Force-velocity curve
  isotonic contraction and, 274
  smooth muscle shortening, 306–309
  length and, 309
Forestomach
  motility, 1230–1250
  nervous control of, 1256–1250
    extrinsic contractions, 1247–1248
    gastric centers, 1248
    intrinsic contractions, 1246–1247
    visceral sensory mechanisms, 1248–1250
Forskolin, in enteric nervous system, 500–501
"Forward theory" of portal hypertension, 1720–1721
Fowl
  anterior mesenteric artery
    cell coupling in, 1610
    neuromuscular relationships in, 1620–1622
  motility regulation, 1289–1292
  stomach and duodenum, 1287–1289
Free diffusion models, passive ion movements, 147–149
Frequency compensation, gastric muscle electrophysiology, 208–209
Frequency/current (f/I) curve
  afterspike hyperpolarization, 547, 549
  prevertebral ganglia, 546–547
Frequency plateaus, relaxation-oscillator models, 211–212
Frothy bloat, reticulorumen contractions, 1241–1242
β-Funaltrexamine (b-FNA), 783–784

Functional bowel syndrome, slow-wave activity, 951
Fundamental contractile response, gastrointestinal smooth muscle, 274–275
Fundus, electrical events of, 198–199
Fura 2, Ca$^{2+}$ measurement with, 147

GABA ($\gamma$-aminobutyric acid)
  colonic motility, 953, 956
  enteric nervous system, 337, 395
    cholinergic system, 413–414
    slow IPSPs, 506–507
  gastrointestinal motility
    blockaded in nucleus ambiguus, 644
    hypothalamic pathway of, 668–669
    nucleus ambiguus, 652
  in prevertebral ganglion cells, 543
[$^3$H]GABA, enteric cholinergic system, 413
GABA-T enzyme, gastrointestinal motility, 652
Galanin
  in dorsal motor nucleus of the vagus, 650
  enteric nervous system, 395
    slow IPSPs, 507
  pharmacology of, 800
Gallbladder
  abnormal function, 1090–1091
  bile flow, 1070–1074
  bombesin action and, 800
  electromyography, 1064
  embryonic development, 1056–1057
  gastrin-releasing peptide, 800
  gross anatomy, 1056
  hyperkinesia, 1090
  hypokinesia, 1090–1091
  innervation, 1059
    extrinsic, 1057
  lymphatic structure, 1740
  manometry of, 1062–1064
  motilin and, 1067
  muscle and mucosal structure, 1058
  myoelectric activity, 849–850
  obstruction disorders, 1071–1072
  opiate receptors, 790
  overview of functions, 1088–1089
  pharmacology, 1066, 1104–1105
    adrenergic drugs, 1106–1108
    caerulein, 1116–1117
    cholecystokinin, 1111–1113
    cholinergic drugs, 1105–1106
    gastrin, 1115–1116
    histamine, 1110–1111
    motilin, 1121–1122
    opiates, 1119–1121
    pancreatic polypeptide, 1122–1123
    prostaglandins, 1109
    serotonin, 1110
    sex hormones, 1123–1124
    somatostatin and bombesin, 1118–1119
    substance P, 1123–1124
    VIP, GIP, glucagon, and secretin, 1117–1118
  in ruminant animals, pancreaticobiliary secretions, 1263
  sonography, 1066
  structure, 1057
  vasoactive intestinal polypeptide (VIP) action on, 779
  vomiting and, 1185–1186
Gamma-photon camera, biliary tract function, 1065–1066
Gap junctions
  in colonic muscle, 262, 947
  discovery of, 54–55
  interstitial cells of Cajal
    ICC AP, 360
    ICC CM cells, 360
    ICC DMP, 360, 368–369
  intestinal muscle, 115–118, 133
    distribution irregularities, 116
    electrical pathways, 228–229
    hypertrophy, 135
    mechanical strength, 116–117
  intestinal villi motility, 975
  mesenteric artery cell coupling, 1608–1610
  neuromuscular transmission and, 436
  schematic diagram, 54–55
  slow-wave generation, 192
  ultrastructure, 116, 118
Gastric acid secretion. *See* Acid secretion
Gastric barostat, proximal stomach tonic contractions, 919
Gastric centers, forestomach motility, 1248
Gastric circulation
  acid secretion and, 1391–1392
  age and blood flow changes, 1393
  anatomy, 1372–1376
    blood flow modification, 1375–1376
    lymphatic system, 1376
    microvessels, 1372–1375
    supplying vessels, 1372
  autoregulation, 1392
  blood flow control, 1382–1391
  blood flow measurements, 1376–1382
    gross flow, 1376
    mucosal blood flow, 1376–1381
  disruption of
    acid backdiffusion, 1393–1394
    human hemodynamic measurements, 1396–1397
    hypothermia and, 1395–1396
    ischemic injury, 1395
    mucosal injury, 1394–1395
    nicotine and smoking, 1396
    portal hypertension, 1396
  eating and, 1392–1393
  gastric motility and, 1393
  historical research, 1371–1372
  microvasculature, 1381–1382
  pulse pressure, 1393
  *See also* Gastrointestinal blood flow
Gastric emptying
  colonic motility and, 960–961
  declining phase and transition to interdigestive activity, 916
  delayed, postoperative, 1200
  duodenogastric reflux during, 913–914
  early postcibal period, 914–915
  fat in diet, 34
  gravity and body position, 921–922
  historical research, 18–42, 36–40
    anxiety, rage, or distress, 22, 24
    gastric mixing and digestion, 21–23
    human studies, 37–39
    humoral control, 41–42
    mechanisms of control, 40–42
    nervous control, 40–41
    patterns, 36–37
    peristalsis, 19–20
    pyloric sphincter, 35–36
    receptive relaxation, 20–21
    solids, 39–40
  intestinal motility, 924–925
  of liquids, 37–39
  measurement techniques, 38–39
  mechanics of, 40–42, 917–921
    antral transport function, 921
    antropyloric grinder, 917–918
    antropyloroduodenal flow resistance, 919–921
    proximal stomach tonic contractions, 918–919
  parietal force measurements, 910–912
  patterns of, 36–40
  plateau phase, 915–916

profile, 916–917
pyloric sphincter, 32–36
    as gate, 32–34
rapid
    postoperative, 1200
    vagotomies and, 1213
regulation of, 922–924
    acid, 923
    energy density of meal, 922–924
    interaction with gastric secretion, 924
    nutrient digestion products, 922–923
    osmolality, 923
    solid particle characteristics, 923–924
    volume of meal, 923
ruminant animals, 1255–1258
    adult ruminants, 1256–1258
    milk-fed animals, 1255–1256
sensory innervation, 593
small bowel transit measurement, 925–926
solids, 39–40
surgical perturbation, 1203–1207
swallowing, 914
Gastric mixing and digestion, 21–23
Gastric muscle electrophysiology
    conduction velocity measurements, 207–208
    electrical event propagation, 205–209
    endogenous electropharmacology, 203–205
    excitability and propagation models, 209–213
    excitable events in, 191–200
    excitation-contraction coupling, 200–203
    fundus electrical events, 198–199
    future research, 213
    historical background, 187–189
    myogenic propagation regulation, 208–209
    postoperative, 1200
    resting membrane potential, 189–190
Gastric pacemaker, 30–32
    antral contractions, 928
    gastrointestinal motility, 927
Gastric resection
    mortality and ulcer recurrence, 1201
    stomach motility, 1203–1207
Gastric secretion. *See* Acid secretion
Gastric syncytium, electrical event propagation, 205–206
Gastrin
    biliary tract pharmacology, 1115–1116
    in dorsal motor nucleus of the vagus, 649
    electropharmacology of, 204
    gastrointestinal blood flow, 1387
        neurohormonal control, 1684–1685
    gastrointestinal motility, 928
        receptors, 761–762
    intestinal blood flow and motility
        intramural tension and, 1495–1496
    lower esophageal sphincter control, 14
    postprandial intestinal hyperemia and, 1425–1426
    proximal stomach tonic contractions, 919
    receptors, CCK-linked, 759–761
    in ruminant animals, gastric emptying, 1258
Gastrin heptadecapeptide, colonic motility, 956
Gastrinlike peptides, ruminant control with, 1238
Gastrin-releasing peptide
    endocrine cells, 392
    enteric nervous system, 395
        cholinergic system, 419
        neurotransmission, 392
        slow EPSPs, 498
    pharmacology, 799–800
Gastritis, iced saline gastric lavage for, 1395
Gastrocolic reflex, 960–961
Gastroduodenal inhibitory reflex, peripheral
    pathways for, 540–541
Gastroduodenal junction. *See* Pyloric sphincter
Gastroenteroanastomosis, 1199
Gastroenterostomy
    history of, 1199
    mortality and ulcer recurrence, 1200
Gastroesophageal junction motility, retching and vomitus expulsion, 1171–1172
Gastroesophageal reflux, lower esophageal sphincter function, 17–18
Gastroesophageal ring, 885
Gastrogastric reflex, in ruminant animals, 1256–1258
Gastrointestinal afferent innervation
    adaptation rate, 614
    electrophysiology of, 596–597
    functional significance, 614–616
        stimuli transduction, 611–613
    in-series tension receptors, 605–609
        longitudinal vs. circular muscle location, 608–609
        nonvagal afferent pathways, 609
        regional differences, 606–608
        response characteristics, 605–606
        resting discharge, 605–606
    methodology of research, 596–598
    sensory code, 596
    single-unit recordings, 596–597
    spontaneous activity in, 613–614
Gastrointestinal-associated lymphoid tissue (GALT), 1756–1757
Gastrointestinal blood flow
    aminopyrine clearance, 1351–1352
        comparison with other techniques, 1358–1360
        initial studies, 1354–1355
        invalid assumptions, 1360–1361
        use in nonsecreting stomach, 1356–1358
    anastomotic connections, 1478
    aneurysms, 1724
    arteriovenous malformations, 1723–1724
    cholecystokinin, 1687
    colon, 1497–1500
    comparison of measuring techniques, 1364–1365
    diabetes mellitus, 1723
    dumping syndrome, 1724
    esophageal achalasia and atresia, 1724
    established neurotransmitters, 1667–1678
        acetylcholine, 1668–1669
        enkephalins, 1678
        neuropeptide Y, 1678–1679
        norepinephrine, 1669–1678
        peptide histidine isoleucine, 1679
        substance P, 1680
        vasoactive intestinal polypeptide, 1680–1682
    hemodynamic measurements, 1478
    history, 1475–1476
    hormones, 1682–1686
        angiotensin, 1682–1683
        antidiuretic hormone, 1683
        epinephrine, 1683–1684
        gastrin and pentagastrin, 1684–1685
        glucagon and enteroglucagon, 1685–1686
        motilin, 1686
        peptide YY, 1686–1687
        secretin, 1686
    hydrogen clearance
        history of, 1361–1362
        limits of, 1363–1364
        locally generated hydrogen, 1364
        principles of, 1362–1363
    hypertension, 1723
    hypoxia and, 1509–1513
    inflammatory bowel disease, 1721
    integrated responses, 1690–1700
        arterial chemoreceptors, 1694–1695
        cardiac mechanoreceptors, 1692–1694

Gastrointestinal blood flow (*continued*)
    hemorrhagic hypotension, 1695–1697
    high-pressure baroreceptors, 1690–1692
    postprandial hyperemia, 1697–1700
  intestinal luminal distension, 1502–1509
  ischemic injury, 1713–1718
    management of, 1715–1717
    nonocclusive intestinal ischemia, 173–1715
    occlusive disease, 1717–1718
  laser-Doppler volcimetry, 1343–1351
    evaluations, 1347–1351
    history, 1343–1344
    linearity, 1347–1349
    motion noise, 1351
    quantitative use, 1350–1351
    spatial selectivity and volume of measurement, 1348–1350
    theory, 1344–1347
  microsphere measurement techniques, 1335–1343
    gastric circulation, 1342–1343
    intramural flow in intestine, 1336–1342
  microvascular anatomy, 1476–1478
  neurotensin, 1689
  pH trapping techniques, 1351–1354
  pharmacology and innervation, small intestine, 1486–1497
  portal hypertension, 1720–1721
  reflux esophagitis, 1724
  secretory disorders, 1724
  serotonin, 1687–1689
  shock, 1718–1720
  small intestine, 1478–1485
  somatostatin, 1689–1690
  stomach, 1500–1502
  ulcers, 1721–1723
  vasculitis, 1724
Gastrointestinal correlates of nausea, 1194
Gastrointestinal correlates of vomiting, 1182–1185
Gastrointestinal fill, ruminant animals, 1275–1276
Gastrointestinal inhibitory polypeptide (GIP)
  biliary tract pharmacology, 1117–1118
  blood flow
    intramural tension and, 1495–1496
    neurohormonal control, 1686
  postprandial intestinal hyperemia and, 1426
  pyloric sphincter regulation, 1003
Gastrointestinal lymphatics. *See* Lymphatics, gastrointestinal
Gastrointestinal motility
  adrenergic receptors and, 733–739
  anesthesia and, 1202
  avian motor function
    esophagus and crop, 1286–1287
    gross anatomy, 1283–1286
    ileum, cecum, and rectum, 1295–1298
    passage rate, 1298
    prehension and swallowing, 1286
    regulation, 1289–1290
    research methods, 1286
    stomach and duodenum, 1287–1295
  blood flow. *See* Gastrointestinal blood flow
  bombesin action and, 799–800
  central nervous system control
    brain-gut neural circuitry, 665–672
    key concepts, 672–674
    neuroanatomy. *See also* specific centers and nuclei, 647–658
    neuronal inputs and outputs, 658–663
    nuclei stimulation and lesion, 663–665
    research background, 621–623
    retrograde neuronal tracing techniques, 623–637
    *See also* specific pathways and centers, 623–628
  cerebral control, 929–930
  drug pharmacology and, 715–746
  gastric emptying, opiates and sex hormones, 926
  gastrin-releasing peptide, 799–800
  historical research, 18–42
    emotional enhancement, 24
    pacemaker and action potentials, 29–32
    periodic activity, 24–29
    pyloric sphincter, 32–36
    small intestine, 42–68
  hormonal control, 928–929
  interdigestive period, 912–914
    motor patterns of stomach, 912–913
  intrinsic and extrinsic nervous systems, 927–928
  in vitro studies, 277–278
  in vivo observation, 277
  mucosal blood flow and, 1393
  neurotensin and pharmacology, 797–799
  opiate receptors, 788–790
    immune system and, 791
  parasite infections
    cecum, colon, and rectum, 1146–1147
    esophagus, 1133–1134
    gastrointestinal hormone imbalances, 1147
    inflammation, 1148–1149
    parasite-derived substances, 1147
    small intestine, 1134–1146
    stomach, 1134
  pharmacology
    isolated smooth muscle preparations, 723–726
    muscarinic receptors, 726–733
    postreceptor mechanism agents, 722–723
    receptor function and classification, 715–722
  postresection effects, 1199–1200
    paresis, 1201–1202
  purinergic receptors, 742–746
  ruminant animals, 1225
    cecal motility patterns, 1267–1268
    colonic motility, 1266–1270
    duodenal brake mechanism, 1252–1255
    duodenal bulb function, 1262–1263
    eructation, 1239–1242
    forestomach motility, 1230–1250
    forestomach nervous control, 1245–1250
    forestomach pharmacology, 1270–1272
    gastric emptying, 1255–1258
    gastroduodenal junction pharmacology, 1272–1275
    hormonal influences, 1239
    mammalian herbivore stomach, 1226–1230
    nervous control of rumination, 1237–1239
    pancreaticobiliary secretions, 1263–1264
    pelleted feces formation, 1268–1269
    pharmacology, 1269–1276
    regurgitation mechanism, 1236–1237
    reticular groove mechanisms, 1243–1245
    reticulorumen contractions, 1231–1236
    small intestine motility, 1258–1266
    stomach motility, 1250–1258
  serotonin receptors, 739–742
  smooth muscle control of, 926–927
  somatostatin and, 794–795
  vasoactive intestinal polypeptide, 777–780
  vomiting and, 1179–1193
    adrenergic receptor, 1192
    antrum and small intestine, 1182–1185
    central integration, 1190
    cholinergic receptors, 1192
    colon and gallbladder, 1185–1186
    digestive tract motor activity, 1192
    dopaminergic receptors, 1191
    efferent innervation, 1190–1191
    esophagus, 1179–1181
    independence from retching and vomitus expulsion, 1187–1188
    motor events, 1179–1186
    myoelectric events, 1186–1187

NANC receptors, 1192–1193
    nausea, 1193–1194
    neural control, 1188–1191
    neuropharmacology, 1191–1193
    opiate receptors, 1191–1192
    peptidergic receptors, 1193
    prodromal signs of, 1194–1195
    proximal stomach, 1181–1183
    retrograde giant contraction function, 1188
    sensory receptors and afferent pathways, 1188–1190
    serotonergic receptors, 1192
Gastrointestinal muscle
    compared with cardiovascular system, 821–823
    composition and structure, 163
    dispersion testing, cell viability, 164
    electrophysiology of
        agonists' effects on channels, 180–181
        dispersion techniques, 163–166
        ionic channels and, 181–183
        rhythmicity in cellular preparations, 166–167
        voltage-clamp studies of isolated cells, 169–180
        voltage recordings from isolated cells, 167–169
    mechanical properties
        direct study of gut movement and motility, 277–278
        force transducers for, 278–280
        instrumentation for study, 278–283
        isolated muscle preparations, 278
        isometric behavior, 276–277, 283–306
        isotonic behavior, 277, 306–312
        length (position) transducers, 280–282
        recording devices for, 282–283
        relaxation of, 312–317
    nausea mechanisms and, 1193–1194
    neurotransmission
        adrenergic transmission, 441–445
        in disease states, 453–457
        excitatory junction potentials in, 437
        excitatory nerve transmission, 449–453
        future research, 457
        historical background, 435–436
        inhibitory junction potentials, 436, 438
        inhibitory nerve transmission, 445–449
    sensory innervation, 593–616
    smooth muscle
        contraction conditions, 273–275
        historical background, 273
Gastrointestinal vasculature. *See* Vasculature of alimentary tract
Gaussian distribution, microsphere blood flow measurements, 1340–1341
Geometric compensation, gastric muscle electrophysiology, 208–209
Giant migrating contraction, 850–852
Glandular stomach, avian structure, 1283–1284
Glia fibrillary acidic protein (GFAP), 338
Glial cells
    enteric neuron development and, 334–336
    ICC AP cells and, 359
    interstitial cells of Cajal as, 382
Glucagon
    biliary tract pharmacology, 1117–1118
    gastrointestinal blood flow, 1388
        neurohormonal control, 1685–1686
    hepatic circulation, 1530
    intestinal blood flow and motility, 1492
    nonocclusive intestinal ischemia, 1717
Glucocorticosteroids, nonocclusive intestinal ischemia, 1716
Glucoreceptors, gastrointestinal afferent innervation, 601–603
Glucose transport
    intestinal mucosal blood flow
        glucose-mediated absorptive hyperemia, 1423–1424
        intestinal villi motility, 985

Glutamate, gastrointestinal motility, 638, 642
Glutathione peroxidase (GPO), nonocclusive intestinal ischemia, 1715
Glycerol, contractile protein regulation, 292
Glycosaminoglycans, intestinal lymphatics, 1735–1736
Goldman-Hodgkin-Katz equation
    enteric nervous system potentials, 487
    submucosal arteriole resting potential, 1643–1644
Golgi apparatus
    in ICC AP, 354–355, 357
    in intestinal muscle, 115
    lymph flow and composition, 1751
    neuropeptide Y in, 576
Golgi staining methods
    for ICC AP, 353
    for ICC DMP, 370
Goresky model of hepatic circulation, 1520
    substrate uptake, 1532
Gravimetric techniques, intestinal mucosal blood flow, 1442–1443
GTP-binding protein, intestinal smooth muscle, 237
Guanine nucleotides, agonist binding sites and, 730–731
5'-Guanylylimidodiphosphate [Gpp-(NH)p]
    agonist binding sites and, 730–731

$H_2$-receptor antagonists
    gastric blood flow control, 1386–1387
*Haemonchus contortus*, parasite-induced alterations
    small intestine, 1137–1138
    in stomach, 1134
Hairpin vessel arrangement, intestinal mucosal blood flow
    countercurrent exchange, 1430–1433
    nonocclusive intestinal ischemia, 1714
Halothane anesthesia, intestinal mucosal blood flow, 1438–1439
Hartmann's pouch, structure, 1057
Haustral shuttling, 74
Haustrations
    in cecum, 103–104, 106, 110
    embryonic development, 940
Hawks, gastric motility, 1295
Heartburn and lower esophageal sphincter function, 17–18
Heart disease, intestinal lymphangiectasia, 1763–1764
Heat clearance technique, mucosal blood flow measurement, 1380–1381
Heavy meromyosin (HMM), contractile protein regulation, 290–291
Heidenhain pouches, pH trapping, 1354
Hematocrit, intestinal mucosal blood flow alterations, 1414–1416
Hemigastrectomy, proximal stomach function, 1206
Hemodynamics
    exocrine gland circulation and, 1568–1569
    hepatic circulation and, 1520
    techniques for human studies, 1396–1397
Hemorrhage
    hepatic blood flow, 1531
        venous bed response, 1550–1551
    mucosal injury, 1394
    neurohormonal control of, 1695–1697
    *See also* Hypovolemic shock; Cardiogenic shock
Henderson-Hasselbalch equation, 1353–1354
Hepatic arterial buffer response, 1525–1527
Hepatic artery anatomy and microcirculation, 1520–1521
Hepatic bile flow, 1067–1070
Hepatic blood flow
    anatomical structure, 1519–1520
    blood volume, 1537–1551
        active capacitance vessel constriction, 1543–1546
        cardiac preload control and drug response, 1548–1550
        distribution and mobilization by sympathetic nerves, 1539–1540
        passive changes in, 1541–1543
        reflex control of venous bed, 1546–1548
        species differences in, 1539–1541

Hepatic blood flow (continued)
    terminology and normal values, 1537–1539
    venous bed responses, 1550–1551
  congestion, liver lymph and, 1760–1761
  fluid exchange, 1551–1555
    drugs and, 1554
    filtered fluid reabsorption, 1553–1554
    filtration and interstitial fluid sites, 1552–1553
    nerve stimulation and, 1554–1555
  microcirculation, 1520–1522
    blood supply origin and distribution, 1520–1521
  nervous control of, 1528–1529
  pooling, 1543
  substrate uptake and, 1531–1537
    blood flow measurement, 1535–1537
    equilibrium model, 1532–1533
    Goresky model, 1532
    model comparisons, 1534–1535
    parallel tube model, 1534
  vascular resistance and, 1522–1531
    extrinsic arterial flow regulation, 1528–1531
    intrinsic arterial flow regulation, 1524–1528
    sinusoidal pressure, 1522–1524
  venous response, 1520
Hepatic blood volume
  blood flow and, 1537–1551
  external pressure, 1541–1542
  flow and arterial resistance, 1541
  flow redistribution, 1542
  regional distribution and mobilization, 1539–1540
  values for splanchnic parameters, 1539
  venous resistance, 1542–1543
Hertwig's rule of nuclear-to-plasma ratio constancy
  principal ganglia cells, 524
Hexahydrosiladifenidol, muscarinic receptors, 728
High-density lipoprotein (HDL), in liver lymph, 1760
Hill equation, force-velocity curve, 308–309
Hirschprung's disease, 83–84
  colonic motility, 963–965
  gastrointestinal neuromuscular transmission, 453–455
  internal anal sphincter function and, 1009–1010
Histamine (5-HT)
  biliary tract pharmacology, 1110–1111
  enteric nervous system, 395
    cholinergic system, 414
    slow EPSPs, 496–498
    slow IPSPs, 505–506
  exocrine gland circulation and, 1576
  gastric blood flow control, 1386–1387
  hepatic circulation, 1542
  intestinal smooth muscle, receptor-evoked response, 239
  mechanosensitive neurons, 477–478
  postprandial intestinal hyperemia and, 1428
  ruminant animals, 1264–1266
    gastroduodenal junction, 1274–1276
Homeostasis, lymph and, 1742–1743
Hooke's law, viscoelastic systems, 317
Hormones
  defecation and, 1046
  gastric blood flow control, 1387–1388
  gastrointestinal blood flow
    families of, 1678–1679
    neurohormonal control of, 1682–1686
  hepatic circulation, 1530
  impact on gastrointestinal motility, 13–14
  influence on rumination, 1239
  intestinal blood flow and motility, 1486–1488
  lower esophageal sphincter regulation, 996–998
    table of, 892
  in lymph, 175
  pancreatic blood flow and, 1574–1575
  parasite-induced imbalances, 1147
  postprandial intestinal hyperemia and, 1425–1427
  proximal stomach tonic contractions, 919
  in ruminant animals, 1257–1258
  sphincter of Oddi function, 1080
  *See also* Sex hormones; specific hormone substances
Horseradish peroxidase (HRP) technique
  CNS influence on gastrointestinal motility, 623
  emesis, 700–701
  mechanosensitive neuron research, 478
5-HTP, ruminant animals, 1274–1275
Humoral factors
  hepatic circulation, 1529–1530
  internal anal sphincter regulation, 1012
  intestinal villi motility, 976, 978–979, 981
  lower esophageal sphincter regulation, 996–998
  pyloric sphincter regulation, 1002–1003
  ruminant animals, 1275–1276
Hunger contractions, historical research, 26–29
Hyaluronate, intestinal lymphatics, 1735–1736
Hydraulic conductivity (capillary) ($L_p$), 1443
Hydrogen clearance
  aminopyrine clearance and, 1359–1360
  history, 1361–1362
  human gastric hemodynamics, 1397
  hydrogen polarography principle, 1362
  Kety-Schmidt method, 1362–1363
  local generation of, 1365
  microsphere measurement and, 1363–1364
  mucosal blood flow measurement, 1378–1379
  tissue saturation and uptake, 1364
Hydrogen ions ($H^+$), gastrin receptors and, 762
11-Hydroperoxyeicosatetraenoic acid (11-HPETE), 1159
6-Hydroxydopamine, inhibitory synaptic potentials, 394
12-Hydroxyeicosatetraenoic acid (12-HETE), 1159
*Hymenolepis nana*
  parasite-induced alterations
    motility, 1149
    small intestine, 1136
Hypercapnia partial pressure of $CO_2$ ($P_{CO_2}$)
  intestinal blood flow and motility, 1494
    arterial hypoxia, 1415–1416
Hyperemia
  active, intestinal motility and blood flow, 1483–1486
  deflation, intestinal blood flow and motility, 1503–1504
  functional, exocrine gland circulation, 1572–1574
  glucose-mediated absorptive, 1423–1424
  jejunal, 1420
  postocclusive, 1527–1528
  postprandial intestinal
    intestinal mucosal blood flow, 1416–1429
    neonatal circulation, 1600
    neurohormonal control, 1697–1700
  poststimulation, 1588
  reactive
    exocrine gland circulation, 1571
    intestinal mucosal blood flow, 1413–1414
Hyperkinesia, gallbladder function and, 1090
Hyperosmolality
  exocrine gland circulation
    functional hyperemia, 1576
    metabolic regulation of, 1569
  postprandial hyperemia, 1698–1699
  tissue
    intestinal mucosal blood flow and, 1418
    postprandial hyperemia and, 1422
Hyperplasia
  exocrine gland circulatory adjustments and, 1577–1578
  intestinal muscle, 133–134
Hyperpolarization
  intestinal smooth muscle, 236
  *See also* Slow hyperpolarization
Hyperpolarizing afterpotentials, 488–489

Hyperpolarizing potentials
  slow EPSPs, 494–495
  slow IPSPs, 504
Hypertension
  arterial, 1409–1410
    hepatic circulation, 1551
    portal, 1396, 1720–1721
    small intestine changes during, 1723
    venous intestinal blood flow, 1413
Hypertonicity, intestinal blood flow and motility, 1492–1494
Hypertrophy, intestinal musculature, 133–135
Hypoalbuminemia, liver lymph and, 1761–1762
Hypoemia, reactive hyperemia and, 1414
Hypogastric nerves, colon, rectum, and internal anal sphincter, 1036
Hypoglossal nucleus, deglutition and, 692
Hypokinesia, gallbladder function and, 1090–1091
Hypopharynx, upper esophageal sphincter and, 870
Hypotension
  hemorrhagic, 1695–1697
  neonatal intestinal circulation, 1601–1602
Hypothalamus
  colonic motility and, 661, 955
  gastrointestinal motility, 664–665
    paraventricular nucleus, 664–665
  neuronal inputs and outputs, 658–665
  paraventricular area, 668–669
Hypothermia, gastric circulation, 1395
Hypotonic stomach, stomach resection, 1204
Hypovolemic shock, gastrointestinal circulation, 1718–1720
Hypoxemia
  intestinal blood flow and motility, 1494
  neonatal intestinal circulation, 1600–1601
Hypoxia
  intestinal blood flow and motility, 1509–1513
  nonocclusive intestinal ischemia, 1713–1714
  vasodilation and exocrine gland circulation, 1571
Hysteresis
  gallbladder function, 1062
  viscoelastic systems, 321

IJP. See Inhibitory junction potential
Ileocecal sphincter (ICS)
  anatomy and innervation, 1003–1004
  excitatory process, 1005–1006
  functional characteristics, 988, 1004–1006
  opiate receptors, 790
  regulation of, 1006–1008
Ileocolic junction
  antiperistalsis, 68–70
  competence, 69–70
  innervation and behavior, 70
  myoelectric activity, 848–849
Ileocolic sphincter, surgical perturbation of, 1214–1216
Ileum
  avian motility in, 1295
  intestinal blood flow and motility, 1494–1496
  postprandial intestinal hyperemia, 1419
  vascular supply and drainage, 1303
Ileus, postoperative effects, 1201–1202
Image intensification, early colon research, 73–74
Image-splitting micrometry, gastrointestinal pharmacology, 724
Imaging studies, biliary tract function, 1061–1062
Iminodiacetic acid (IDA) and biliary tract function, 1065–1066
Immune system, opiate receptors and, 791
Immunoglobulin A
  bacterial overgrowth syndrome, 1167–1168
  lymphatic transport and, 1756–1757
Immunoneutralization experiments, inhibitory motor transmission, 390–391
Indicator-dilution (fractional extraction)
  mucosal blood flow, 1377–1378
Indomethacin
  gastric muscle arrhythmia and, 197–198
  MAPC and, 1157–1158
  prostaglandin inhibition, 205
Inferior esophageal sphincter, 885
Inferior mesenteric ganglion
  arginine vasopressin in, 574
  cholecystokinin in, 569
  cholinergic inputs and, 551
  colon innervation, 539, 942
  neuroanatomy of, 520–521
  slow EPSP in, 554–556
Inferior thyroid artery, 1302
Inflammation, gastrointestinal, parasite-induced, 1148–1149
Inflammatory bowel disease
  colonic ischemia, 1721
  lymphatic drainage and, 1764–1765
Infundibulum (gallbladder), 1057
Inhibitor 3-isobutyl-1-methylxanthine (IBMX)
  enteric nervous system, 422
  intraneuronal elevation, 501
Inhibitory junction potential (IJP), 883–884
  colonic muscle innervation, 260
  deglutition and, 695
  in esophagus, VIP action and, 778
  fundus electrical events, 198–199
  gastrointestinal neuromuscular transmission, 445–449
    adenosine 5′-triphosphate, 448–449
    adrenergic neuromodulation, 444
    gut wall inhibitory neurons, 446–447
    ionic basis for, 446
    neurotensin, 448
    nonadrenergic, noncholinergic, 437, 441
    putative neurotransmitters, 446–449
    vasoactive intestinal polypeptide (VIP) and, 446–448
  inhibitory motor transmission, 389–390
  intestinal smooth muscle nerve-evoked responses, 233–235
  neuromuscular transmission, 436, 438
  tachykinins and, 770
Inhibitory motor transmission, 389–391
Inhibitory postsynaptic potentials (IPSPs)
  deglutition and, 694
  gastrointestinal motility, 656
  nonnoradrenergic, 394
  in prevertebral ganglia, 529, 555
  See Slow and Fast inhibitory postsynaptic potentials
Inhibitory substances, intestinal smooth muscle, 239–240
Inhibitory synaptic actions
  burst-pattern generation, 471
  in enteric neurons, 343–344
Initial lymphatics
  filling of, 1741–1742
  liver lymph, 1760
  structure, 1736–1738
Initial segment, enteric nervous system, 481–482
Injection techniques for gastric blood flow
  control studies, 1385–1386
  microvasculature, 1381
Inositol phosphates
  intestinal smooth muscle, 237
  receptors and, 723
Inositol phospholipids, enteric neurotransmission, 408–409
Inositol trisphosphate, 287
In-series tension receptors, 605–609
  longitudinal vs. circular muscle location, 608–609
  nonvagal afferent pathways, 609
  regional differences, 606–608
  response characteristics, 605–606
  resting discharge, 605–606
Inspiratory resistance breathing (IRB), 1693–1694
Insufflation in ruminant animals, 1240–1241

Insulin hypoglycemia, influence on rumination, 1239
Intercalated cells of Ferter. *See* Interstitial cells of Cajal
Intercalation hypothesis, 372
Intercellular junctions
  exocrine gland circulation, 1580
  permeability of, 1325–1326
  transcapillary exchange, 1324–1326
Interdigestive myoelectric complex, 45–46, 912
  declining phase, 916
Intermediate filaments, intestinal muscle, 124
Intermediate junctions
  contractile protein regulation, 294–295
  in intestinal muscle, 118
    hypertrophy, 135
Intermediolateral cell column
  levels $S_{2-3}$, 645
    neuroanatomy, 653–654
  thoracolumbar
    gastrointestinal motility, 646
    neuroanatomy, 654–657
Intermediolateral nucleus pars funiculus (IMLf)
  gastrointestinal motility, 654
  opioid peptides, 562
  prevertebral ganglion pathways, 530–531
Intermediolateral nucleus pars principalis (IMLp)
  gastrointestinal motility, 654
  neurotensin in, 572
  opioid peptides in, 562
  prevertebral ganglion pathways, 530–531
Intermediolateralis (IML), 530–531
Internal anal sphincter (IAS)
  colonic motility, 957–959
  electrical activity of, 1032–1033
  functional characteristics, 1008–1010
  innervation studies, 958–959
  lumbar sympathetic innervation, 1026
    electrical stimulation, 1036–1037
    interruption, 1037–1038
  motor activity, 1031–1033
    adrenergic receptor agonists, 1036–1037
  regulation of, 1010–1012
  sacral innervation
    afferent fibers, 1027–1028
    cholinergic agonists, 1038–1039
    electrical stimulation, 1038
    parasympathetic innervation, 1026–1027
  structure, 988–989
  *See also* External anal sphincter
Interstitial cells of Cajal (ICC)
  Auerbach's plexus association (ICC AP), 352–366
    cytodifferentiation in, 359
    in esophagus and stomach, 374–378
    functions of, 359–364
    future research on, 364–366
    nerve bundle contacts, 355–358
    origin and nature of, 359
    pharmacological properties of, 364–366
    relationship with other ICC, 357–359
    staining methods methylene blue, 352–354
    ultrastructure, 354–356
  characteristics of, 350–351
  coated muscle association (ICC CM), 103, 105, 373–374
    relationship to ICC AP, 359
  colonic muscle, 375–381
    functions of, 379–381
    longitudinal muscle coat and Auerbach's plexus, 376–378
    myenteric potential oscillations, 255
    with submuscular plexus, 378–379
  deep muscular plexus association (ICC DMP), 366–373
    functions of, 371–373
    general organization, 366–370
    origin and nature of, 371
    relationship to ICC AP, 358–359
    staining methods for, 369–370
    ultrastructure, 370–371
  in esophagus and stomach, 374–378
    functions of, 375
    general organization, 374–375
    innervation, 867
    ultrastructural investigations, 382
  glial characteristics of, 382
  historical background, 349
  improved staining methods for, 382
  neuromuscular transmission and, 436, 440
  nonadrenergic, noncholinergic nerve response, 382
  recent research trends on, 382–383
  rhythmicity in gastrointestinal cells, 166
  slow-wave generation, 382
  in small intestine, 127–129, 351–374
  subcerous compartment association (ICC SS), 366
  summary of research on, 381
  terminology and location, 351–353
Interstitial hydrostatic pressure ($P_t$)
  exocrine gland circulation, 1582–1583
  hepatic circulation, 1552–1553
  intestinal mucosa blood flow
    transcapillary fluid and solute exchange, 1444
    venous pressure ($P_v$), 1411–1413
Interstitium
  intestinal lymphatics, 1735–1736
  net fluid absorption, 1449–1450, 1453–1454
Intestinal fluid absorption, lymph flow and composition, 1747–1749
Intestinal gradient, small intestine, 56–58
Intestinal inhibitory reflex, intestinal blood flow and motility, 1491
Intestinal luminal distension
  capillary filtration coefficient, 1507–1509
  compartmental blood flow, 1505–1507
  lymph flow, 1508–1509
  oxygen consumption, 1505–1507
  total blood flow, 1503–1505
Intestinal mucosa
  microcirculation
    anesthesia and adjuvants, 1438–1439
    angiotensin II and vasopressin, 1437–1438
    arterial blood gases and hematocrit, 1414–1416
    arterial pressure alterations, 1408–1411
    background, 1405
    capillary filtration coefficient, 1442–1443
    capillary hydrostatic pressure, 1443–1444
    capillary-interstitial interaction, 1445–1456
    countercurrent exchange, 1430–1433
    future research, 1462–1463
    interstitial hydrostatic pressure, 1444
    intestinal transport and, 1429–1430
    intrinsic blood flow regulation and oxygenation, 1406–1429
    laparotomy and visceral manipulation, 1439
    lymph flow, 1441–1442
    macromolecule exchange, 1457–1459, 1462
    osmotic reflection coefficient, 1444
    permeability factors, 1459–1462
    postprandial hyperemia, 1416–1429
    reactive hyperemia, 1413–1414
    respiration and blood gases, 1439
    small solutes, 1456–1457
    Starling exchange hypothesis, 1441
    temperature and, 1439–1440
    transcapillary fluid and solute exchange, 1441–1456
    transcapillary oncotic pressure gradient, 1444–1445
    vascular capacitance, 1433–1434
    vasoactive agents and oxygen uptake, 1434–1437, 1440
    venous pressure elevation, 1411–1413

Intestinal muscle
  arrangement of, 103–105
  cell junctions, 115–121
    basal lamina and cell-to-stroma junctions, 118–120
    gap junctions, 115–118
    intermediate junctions, 118
    terminal apparatus and cell-to-tendon junctions, 119–121
  development of, 129–133
  electrophysiology, 217–241
    single smooth muscle properties, 217–219
    in vitro electrical and mechanical activity, 226–240
  extracellular materials, 105–108
  filaments, 121–125
    actin filaments, 121–124
    dense bodies, 124–125
    intermediate filaments, 124
    myosin filaments, 124
  hypertrophy, 133–135
    growth potential, 133
  nerve bundles in, 127–128
  nonmuscle cells in, 127–128
  organization of, 217–218
  smooth muscle cells, 108–115
    caveolae, 109, 112–113, 115
    cell size and shape, 108–109
    dense bands, 109, 111, 113–115, 119, 122
    mitochondria and organelles, 115
    permeability and receptor activation, 224
    sarcoplasmic reticulum, 111, 115, 119, 122
    single smooth muscle properties, 219–226
  structural changes during contraction, 125–127
  submucosa, 128–130
Intestinal refluxes, avian motility, 1288–1290
Intestinal transport function, gastric emptying, 921
Intestinal villi
  blood flow
    microcirculation, 1319, 1322
    neurohormonal control of, 1673–1674
  lymph flow, 1319, 1322
  microvasculature, 1309–1311
    anatomy, 1477
    capillary plexus, 1312, 1316
    countercurrent arrangements, 1312–1314
    fluid absorption by, 1312
    fountain pattern, 1317
    lymphatic drainage, 1314–1315
    models of, 1312, 1314
    species differences, 1312–1313, 1314–1315
  motility
    anatomy and contractile patterns, 975–976
    contraction frequency distribution, 977
    historical research, 975–976
    intrinsic nerves, 979–980
    nervous control, 976–980
    neuroeffector and humor factors, 976, 978–979
    nutrient absorption, 984–985
    parasympathetic control, 976–977
    pendular movements, 976
    physiological implications, 981–985
    pistonlike contractions, 976–977
    postprandial regulation, 980–981
    regulation of, 976–981
    sympathetic nervous control, 977, 979
    villous blood flow and, 983–984
  *See also* Blood flow, intestinal mucosa
Intestinointestinal reflex
  prevertebral ganglion and, 534–536
  small intestine, functions of, 61
Intra-arterial vasodilator therapy, nonocclusive intestinal ischemia, 1716
Intracellular acetylcholinesterase (iAChe), 339, 341
Intracellular control systems
  enteric neurotransmission and, 407–409
    calmodulin, 408
    inositol phospholipids, 408–409
    protein phosphorylation, 407
  slow-wave genesis and conduction, 53–54
  sodium-hydrogen exchange, pH function and, 158
Intracellular ion concentration, calculation for, 142–143
Intracellular pathways for neurotensin action, 799
Intracellular recordings
  colonic muscle, slow-wave activity, 255
  electrical control activity (ECA), 820
  enteric nervous system, 468–469, 481–485
    bridge circuits, 468–469
    conduction velocity, 483
    differential excitability, 483–484
    histoanatomical factors, 482–483
    morphine and enkephalin, 485
    refractory period, 483
    tetrodotoxin and, 485
  esophageal contraction and inhibition, 882–883
  gastrointestinal neuromuscular transmission, 437, 441–442
  somatostatin and gastrointestinal motility, 795
Intraganglionic laminar endings, 608–609
  esophageal and sphincter innervation, 867
Intrahepatic pressure, 1544
Intraluminal pressure
  avian gastrointestinal motility, 1286
  common duct function, 1075
  peripheral reflex activity and, 537–539
  rectum and internal anal sphincter, 1032
Intramembrane particles
  in gap junctions, 116–117
  intestinal muscle hypertrophy, 135
Intramural blood flow
  excitatory junction potentials, 1646–1650
    pharmacology, 1654–1660
  innervation, 1637–1641
  intestinal mucosal blood flow, 1437
  neuromuscular transmission, 1635, 1637
  organization and structure, 1636–1637
  submucosal arterioles
    contraction initiation in, 1650–1653
    integration in, 1653–1654
    neuromuscular transmission, 1644–1645
    passive electrical properties of, 1640–1644
    sympathetic nerve stimulation, 1645–1646
Intramural nerves
  electrical stimulation, 879–880
  esophageal and sphincter innervation, 867
  tension
    luminal distension, 1505
    pharmacology, 1494–1496
Intraspinal pathways
  gastrointestinal motility, 661
  for prevertebral ganglia, 531–532
Intrasyncytial recordings, voltage recordings of isolated cells, 168
Intravital microscopy
  biliary tract function, 1062
  sphincter of Oddi function, 1088
Intrinsic clearance, hepatic circulation, 1532–1534
Intrinsic innervation
  colonic motility, 954
  esophageal and sphincter innervation, 866–867
  forestomach motility, 1246–1247
  gastrointestinal motility, 927–928
  internal anal sphincter motor activity, 1035
  intestinal villi motility, 979–980
  postprandial hyperemia and, 1421–1422
Intrinsic vasoregulation, 1570–1572
In vitro arterial strips, gastric microvasculature, 1381–1382
In vitro electrical/mechanical activity
  in intestinal smooth muscle, 226–240

In vitro electrical/mechanical activity (*continued*)
    acetylcholine and muscarinic receptor stimulants, 237–238
    action potentials, 229–230
    active and passive properties, 227–233
    background on, 226–227
    electrical coupling between cells, 227–229
    excitatory and inhibitory junction potentials, 233–235
    excitatory receptor mechanisms, 236–238
    receptor-evoked responseses, 236–236
    slow waves, 230–233
    substance P and, 238–239
In vivo animal studies of slow-wave activity, 188–189
In vivo studies
    gastric blood flow control
        microvasculature, 1381
        vagus nerve stimulation, 1384
    intestinal smooth muscle electrical properties, 227
Inward current, in intestinal smooth muscle, 221–222
Iodoantipyrine clearance, mucosal blood flow measurement, 1380
Ion channels
    in colonic slow waves, 254
    enteric nervous system
        circuit model for, 495–496
        fast EPSPs and, 492
        slow EPSPs, 495–496
    gastrointestinal muscle cells, 141–158
        active transport, 149–152
        chemical analysis, 141–143
        electron microscopy and X-ray microanalysis, 145–146
        electrophysiology, 181–183
        exchange mechanisms, 152, 154–158
        ion-sensitive microelectrodes, 146
        optical properties, 147
        neuromuscular transmission, 446, 449–451
        passive movements, 147–149
        permeability, 438, 440–442
        tissue tracer content, 143–145
    muscarinic postreceptor events, 731–732
    in prevertebral ganglion cells, 542–543
    receptors
        ligand binding and, 717
        postreceptor mechanisms, 722–723
    single intestinal smooth muscle cell and, 219–226
    in slow waves, 194–195
    sodium pumping, 149
    *See also* specific channels, e.g., Potassium channel
Ionizing radiation, emesis and, 705–706
Ion-replacement studies
    action potentials in gastric muscle, 196
Ion-sensitive microelectrodes, 146
Irregular spiking activity (ISA)
    ruminant animals, 1253–1254
        mixing vs. propelling activity, 1261–1262
        nervous control, 1264
        periodic activity, 1258–1261
Irritable bowel syndrome (IBS)
    gastrin-CCK receptors and, 765
    gastrointestinal neuromuscular transmission, 456–457
    muscarinic pharmacology, 732–733
Irritable colon syndrome, 85–86, 965–966
Ischemia
    colonic, 1721
    gastrointestinal blood flow
        management of, 1715–1717
        nonocclusive intestinal, 1713–1715
        occlusive disease, 1717–1718
    intestinal blood flow and motility, 1511–1512
    ulcers and, 1721–1722
Ischemia-perfusion injury, 1395
Isolated cells
    electrical load in, 181–182
    voltage-clamp studies, 169–180
    calcium channel properties, 176–179
    chloride channel properties, 179–180
    microelectrode studies, 169–170
    potassium channel properties, 171–176
    whole-cell current and patch-clamp technique, 170–171
    voltage recordings on, 168–169
Isometric conditions
    gastrointestinal muscle mechanics, 274, 283–306
        $Ca^{2+}$ and 289–295
        contractile activity regulation, 286–295
        intrinsic regulatory mechanisms, 286–289
        length-tension relationship, 276–277, 295–299
        smooth muscle activation, 284–286
        stiffness of contracting muscle, 299–306
    relaxation mechanics, 315–316
    smooth muscle, 724
Isometric quick-stretch technique, 300
Isoprenaline, enteric nervous system, 422
Isoproterenol
    channel activation with, 181
    hepatic circulation, 1542–1543, 1549
    inhibitory motor transmission, 390
    nonocclusive intestinal ischemia, 1717
    ulcer prevention and, 1722
Isotonic conditions
    gastrointestinal muscle contraction, 274–275
        force-velocity curve, 277
        length and force-velocity curve, 309
        regulation of shortening velocity, 309–311
        smooth muscle shortening, 306–312
    relaxation properties, 313–314, 316–317
    smooth muscle shortening, 306–312
Isotonic quick-release technique, 300–301

Jejunal interposition, 1207
Jejunum
    intestinal blood flow and motility, 1480–1481
    postprandial hyperemia and, 1420
    vascular structure
        supply and drainage, 1303
        volume and dimensions, 1322
Junctional adrenergic hypothesis, 1620

$K^+$. *See* Potassium channels
Kallidin, intestinal blood flow and motility, 1491
Kallikrein
    exocrine gland circulation and, 1570
    functional hyperemia and, 1576
Kety-Schmidt method of hydrogen clearance, 1362–1363
Kinin, exocrine gland circulation, 1570
    functional hyperemia and, 1576
Kock's reservoir, construction of, 1216–1218
Koilin, avian muscular stomach, 1284–1285
$^{85}Kr$-clearance technique
    gastric blood flow control, 1384
    human gastric hemodynamics, 1396

Labeled–amino acid mapping, 700–701
Lability and smooth muscle contractions, 726
Lactate dehydrogenase studies, intestinal mucosal blood flow, 1459
Lanthanum ions ($La^{3+}$)
    binding with calcium pump, 152
    tissue tracing with, 143–144
Laparotomy
    gastrointestinal motility and, 1202
    intestinal mucosal blood flow, 1439
Laplace's law
    exocrine gland circulation, 1570
    pacemaker potentials and action potentials, 29–32
Large-amplitude fast EPSPs, 492
Large intestine. *See* Colon

Laser-Doppler velocimetry (LDV)
  computer-based, 1346–1348
  flowmeter comparisons, 1347–1351
  gastrointestinal tract variations, 1347–1351
    linearity, 1347–1350
    motion noise, 1351
    quantitative use of, 1350–1351
  history, 1343–1344
  lack of reproducibility, 1350
  mucosal blood flow measurement, 1380
  reactive hyperemia and motility artifacts, 1351–1352
  schematic of, 1346–1347
  theory, 1344–1347
Latch bridges, shortening force-velocity curve, 311
Latch phenomenon, lower esophageal sphincter, 888–889
Latency
  esophageal peristalsis, 882–883
    on and off contractions, 880–882
  lower esophageal sphincter, 995
  relaxation-oscillator models, 212
Law of conservation of mass, 1354
Laxatives and colonic motility, 956–957
Length constant, mammalian blood vessels, 1610
Lengthening of gastrointestinal cells, 165
Length (position) transducers
  gastrointestinal muscle mechanics, 279–282
    isotonic lever systems, 280
    position detectors, 279, 281–282
Length-tension relationship
  contracting muscle stiffness, 301, 303
  ileocecal sphincter regulation, 1006–1008
  parasite-induced alterations, 1140, 1143–1146
    small intestine, 1140, 1143–1146
  smooth muscle contraction and, 295–298
    active curve, 296, 298–299
LES. See Lower esophageal sphincter
Leu-enkephalin
  colonic motility, 953
  emesis and, 701–702
  esophageal peristalsis, 884
  gastrointestinal motility
    intermediolateral cell column ($S_{2-3}$), 653–654
    nucleus ambiguus, 652
  in prevertebral ganglion, 562–563
Leukotrienes
  biliary tract pharmacology, 1109–1110
  gastric blood flow control, 1390–1391
Lieberkuhn's crypts, avian structure, 1285
Ligand binding studies
  receptors, 717–718
    mathematical analysis of, 721–722
  opiate receptors, 785
  serotonin receptors, 739–740
  smooth muscle contractions, 725–726
Light meromyosin, protein regulation, 290–291
Lipids
  liver lymph, 1760
  lymph flow and composition, 1751–1755
  postprandial intestinal hyperemia, 1420
Lipoxygenase, gastric blood flow control, 1390–1391
Lissauer's tract, afferent nerve fiber distribution, 632
Lithium
  electrical activity of muscularis mucosa, 200
  intestinal smooth muscle, 194–195, 230–231
Liver
  avian structure, 1286
  gastrointestinal afferent innervation, 596
  lymphatic structure, 1740
  lymph in, 1758–1762
    cholestasis, 1762
    cirrhosis, 1761–1762
    formation of, 1759–1760

hepatic congestion, 1760–1761
microcirculation, 1758
proteins of, 1758–1759
Long afterhyperpolarizations (LAH), 336–337
Longitudinal muscle
  in cecum, 103–104, 110
  in colonic muscle, 941
    electrical coupling with circular layers, 266–267
    fast transient and action potential propagation, 267–268
    innervation of, 260
  electrical control activity in, 844
  esophagus
    myoelectric activity, 841–842
    peristalsis, 884–885
  interstitial cells of Cajal, 376–378
  in intestinal smooth muscle
    passive electrical properties, 228–229
    slow-wave origin and propagation, 231–233
  lower esophageal sphincter, 886
  in muscle coat, 103–104
  opiate receptor activation, 785–786
  slow-wave generation, 192
  small intestine
    microvascular anatomy, 1476–1478
    opiate receptors, 788
  substance P action on, 769
  tension receptors and, 608–609
  thickness ratio to circular muscle, 103
Long-train vagal efferent nerve stimulation, 878–879
Low-density lipoproteins (LDL)
  liver lymph, 1760
  lymph flow and, 1756
Lower esophageal sphincter (LES)
  basal sphincter pressure genesis, 888–890
  basal tone, 991–994
  efferent motor innervation, 866
  functional state, 988
  gastrointestinal motility, 641
  high-pressure zone, 991
  historical research, 12–18
    disorders of, 16–17
    heartburn and gastroesophageal reflux, 17–18
    humoral influences, 13–14
    nervous control of, 14–16
  inhibitory pathway neurotransmitters, 894–895
    synaptic transmitters, 894–895
  innervation, 989–990
  interstitial cells of Cajal research and, 374–375
  muscarinic receptors in, 727
  muscle tone genesis, 890–892
    anatomy, 885–886
    cholinergic and adrenergic antagonists, 890–891
    circulating excitatory hormone activity, 891–892
    early postcibal period, 914
    excitatory biological agents, 891
    tonic excitatory nerve activity, 890–891
  myoelectric activity, 842–844
  neurotransmitters
    effect on tone, 994–996
    vasoactive intestinal polypeptide (VIP), 883–884
  opiate receptors and, 786
  parasite-induced alterations, 1133–1134
  pressure profile, 886–888
  reflex contractions, 895–896
  reflex relaxation, 893–894
    cellular basis, 893
    esophageal distension, 894
    swallow-induced, 893–894
  regulation, humoral and hormonal factors, 996–998
  resting pressure modulation, 892–893
    table of hormone and neuropeptide effects, 892
  surgical perturbation, 1202–1203

Lower esophageal sphincter (LES) (*continued*)
   tachykinin action in, 772–773
Lower motor neuron dysfunction, 1047
Lumbar sympathetic innervation
   colon, rectum, and IAS activity, 1036–1038
     electrical stimulation, 1036–1037
     interruption of pathways, 1037–1038
   defecation and, 1045–1046
   internal anal sphincter schematic of, 1037
Luminal distension, intestinal motility and blood flow, 1483, 1485
Luminal stimuli, intestinal hyperemia and, 1418–1420
Lymph, composition of, 1743
Lymphangiectasia
   lipid assimilation impairment, 1733–1734
   primary intestinal, 1762–1763
   secondary intestinal, 1763
   secondary to heart disease, 1763–1764
Lymphangion, 1738–1739
Lymphatic endothelial membranes, 1736–1737
Lymphaticovenous anstomoses, 1738–1739
Lymphatic protein flux, 1329
Lymphatics
   gastrointestinal, 1376
     acute pancreatitis, 1765
     cannulation technique, 1745–1746
     central trunks, 1738
     chylous ascites, 1765
     chyluria, 1765
     collecting lymphatics, 1738–1739
     colon, 1740, 1757
     esophagus, 1739, 1746–1747
     experimental interruption, 1764
     fistula studies, 1746
     gallbladder, 1740
     heart disease–related lymphangiectasia, 1763–1764
     historical background, 1733–1735
     inflammatory bowel disease, 1764–1765
     initial lymphatics, 1736–1738, 1741–1742
     interstitium, 1735–1736
     in vitro studies, 1746
     liver, 1740, 1758–1762
     lymphaticovenous anastomoses, 1738–1739
     lymph formation, 1741, 1743
     micropuncture studies, 1746
     pancreas, 1740, 1757–1758
     primary intestinal lymphangiectasia, 1762–1763
     propulsion in collecting vessels, 1744–1745
     salivary glands, 1739, 1746
     secondary intestinal lymphangiectasia, 1763
     small intestine, 1739–1740, 1746–1757
     stomach, 1739, 1746–1747
     tissue homeostasis, 1742–1743
     vessel and node modification, 1743–1744
   *See also* Collecting lymphatics; Initial lymphatics
Lymph flow
   exocrine gland circulation and, 1567–1568
   hepatic circulation, 1553
   intestinal blood flow and motility, 982–984
     edema safety factors, 1445–1446
     luminal distension, 1508–1509
     lymph-to-plama solute concentration ratio (L/P), 1457–1458
     transcapillary fluid and solute exchange, 1441–1442
   net fluid absorption, 1451–1455
   portal hypertension, 1721
   resting rates, 1741
Lymph hearts, 1744
Lymph-to-plasma protein concentration ratio (L/P)
   colonic lymph, 1757
   exocrine gland circulation, 1583
   intestinal mucosal blood flow
     capillary reflection coefficients, 1458–1459
     lymph flow, 1457–1458
     protein flux, 1460
   liver lymph, 1758–1760
   lymph flow and composition, 1743, 1746–1747
     protein fractions, 1743

Macromolecules
   exocrine gland circulation, 1588
   intestinal mucosal blood flow, 1457–1458
     exchange pathways, 1462
Macrophage-like cell (MLC)
   ICC AP and, 357–359, 365
   ICC DMP and, 371
Macula communicans. *See* Gap junction
Magnesium ions ($Mg^{2+}$)
   agonist binding sites and, 730–731
   ATPase activity, 150–151
   burst-pattern generation, 471
   measurement of in smooth muscle, 143
Main arteriole, small intestine anatomy, 1476–1477
Malabsorption, small intestine resection, 1214–1216
Maldigestion, small intestine resection, 1214–1216
Mammalian blood vessels, electrophysiology of, 1608–1609
Mammalian herbivore stomach, 1226–1230
   anatomy, 1226–1227
   gastric form and relative volumes, 1227–1228
   species differences, 1227
Manganese ions ($Mn^{2+}$)
   in intestinal smooth muscle
     action potentials and, 229–230
     outward current, 223
Mann-Bollman fistula, 66–67
Manometry
   biliary tract function, 1062–1064
   colonic motility, 943
   parasite-induced alterations
     cecum, colon and rectum, 1146–1147
     small intestine, 1135–1136
   sphincter of Oddi function, 1078–1079
Mass movement, colonic motility and, 945
Mast cells, tachykinin action and, 772
Maximum force potential (MFP), relaxation mechanics, 315–316
Maxwell configuration
   gastrointestinal smooth muscle, 275
   viscoelastic systems, 318, 320
McN-A 343 muscarinic agonist, 727
Meal-to-pellet interval (MPI), raptor gastric motility, 1292–1295
Mean motility index (MMI), 1496
Mechanical threshold
   in colonic muscle, 257
   gastric muscle excitation-contraction coupling, 200–202
   voltage-tension relationship and, 202–203
Mechanoreceptors
   adaptation rate, 614
   cardiac, 1692–1694
   deglutition and, 688
   early research, 67–68
   functional significance, 615
   gastrointestinal afferent innervation, 595–596
   ICC DMP and, 372
   lower esophageal sphincter, 990
   rectal mucosa, 962
   ruminant forestomach motility, 1249–1250
   vomiting reflex, 1188–1190
Mechanosensitive neurons
   enteric nervous system, 476–480
     conversion to burst patterns, 480–481
     fast-adapting units, 479
     neuroanatomy, 478–479
     pharmacology, 477–478
     receptive fields, 478
     slowly adapting units, 476–477
     spike waveforms, 476–477, 480

tonic-type units, 479–480
Meckel's diverticulum, avian structure, 1285
Medulla
    neuronal inputs and outputs, 659
    pathways, deglutition and, 688–689, 696–697
Medullary reticular nuclei, 664
Megacolon
    aganglionosis, 83–84
    in Chagas' disease, 1147
    congenital. See Hirschsprung's disease
Meissner's plexus
    esophageal motility, 866
    vasculature of, 1304
Membrane-associated dense bodies. See Dense bands
Membrane hyperpolarization, esophageal peristalsis, 883–884
Membrane potential
    enteric nervous system, 486–487
    internal anal sphincter (IAS), 1008–1010
    lower espohageal sphincter
        basal tone, 993
        neurotransmitters, 995–996
    mesenteric artery, 1608
    in prevertebral ganglion, 562–563
    pyloric sphincter regulation, 1001–1002
    regenerative propagation, 852–853
    resting, mesenteric vein, 1622
    role in electrophysiological studies, 164–165
    smooth muscle contraction and, 819–820
    submucosal arterioles
        calcium entry, 1650–1651
        sympathetic nerve activity and, 1654
    voltage recordings of isolated cells, 167
Membrane rectification, 1611
Membrane time constant, mammalian blood vessels, 1610
Mesenchymal cells, as origin of intestinal muscle cells, 130–131
Mesenteric artery
    action potentials, 1611
    active membrane properties, 1611
    autonomic neurotransmitters, 1612–1614
        acetylcholine, 1613–1614
        norepinephrine, 1612–1613
    cell coupling, 1608–1610
    colon vasculature, 1303
    fowl anterior
        cell coupling, 1610
        neuromuscular relationships in, 1620–1622
    intramural blood vessels and, 1637
    jejunum and ileum vasculature, 1303
    membrane rectification, 1611
    nerve stimulation responses, 1614–1618
        $Ca^{2+}$ dependence, 1615–1616
        excitatory junction potentials, 1614–1615
        facilitation and summation, 1616
        neurally evoked action potentials, 1617–1618
        slow depolarization, 1618
        slow hyperpolarization, 1618
        spontaneous excitatory junction potentials (SEJPs), 1616–1617
    neuroeffector transmission pharmacology, 1618–1620
        excitatory juntion potentials, 1618–1619
        slow depolarization, 1619–1620
        slow hyperpolarization, 1620
    nonmammalian species, 1621–1622
    prejunctional effects on neuromuscular transmission, 1620–1621
    resting membrane potential, 1608
Mesenteric circulation
    colonic musculature, 941
    density and, 1607
    innervation of, 1606–1608
    junctional cleft width, 1607
    neuromuscular differences between artery and vein, 1627–1628
Mesenteric receptors, 609–611
    adaptation rate, 614
    functional significance, 615–616
    response characteristics, 611
    spontaneous activity, 610–611
Mesenteric vein
    action potentials, 1622
    function, 1605–1606
    neuroeffector transmission pharmacology, 1625
    passive membrane properties, 1622–1623
        action potentials, 1624
        autonomic transmitter substances, 1623
        excitatory junction potentials, 1623
        nerve stimulation and, 1623–1625
        slow depolarization, 1624–1625
    resting membrane potential, 1622
Metabolic condition of cells
    muscarinic postreceptor events, 731–732
    role in electrophysiological studies, 165
Metabolic regulation, exocrine gland circulation, 1569
Metabolism hypothesis
    intestinal mucosa blood flow, 1406–1407
        autoregulation, 1409
        reactive hyperemia, 1414
    neonatal intestinal circulation, 1599–1602
    postprandial hyperemia and, 1422–1425
Metabolites, 1673–1674
Met-enkephalin
    biliary tract pharmacology, 1119
    colonic motility, 956
    esophageal peristalsis, 884
    gastric blood flow control, 1388
    intestinal blood flow and motility, 1496
    receptor locus and functional coupling, 719
$\alpha,\beta$-Methylene-ATP, submucosal arterioles, 1659
Methylene blue stain
    interstitial cells of Cajal (ICC), 350–354
        advantages of, 382
        slow-wave observations with, 361–362
Michaelis-Menten equation, hepatic circulation models, 1532–1534
Microelectrode research
    gastrointestinal afferent innervation, 598
    ion sensitivity, 146
    peristaltic reflex, 66–68
    in smooth muscle research, 219
    voltage-clamp studies, 169–170
Microsphere measurement technique
    aminopyrine clearance and, 1358
    gastric circulation, 1342–1343
        vagus nerve stimulation, 1384
    gastrointestinal blood flow, 1335–1343
        intramural distribution, 1338–1339
        Lifson equation, 1337
        measurement principles, 1335–1336
        microsphere migration, 1339–1340
        microsphere shunting, 1340–1342
        microsphere size, 1336–1339
        reference organ approach, 1336
        sieving effect, 1340–1341
    mucosal blood flow measurement, 1377–1378
Microvascular anatomy
    gastrointestinal motility and, 1476–1478
    permeability characteristics, 1316, 1318–1329
    exocrine gland circulation, 1583, 1585, 1588
Microvascular vasospasm, nonocclusive intestinal ischemia, 1716
Micturition, external anal sphincter motor activity, 1041–1042
Migrating action-potential complex (MAPC)
    bacterial motility alterations, 1154–1163
        bile salts, 1162–1163
        castor oil and ricinoleic acid, 1162
        choleragen and choleragenoid, 1156
        cholera toxin, 1155–1156
        control mechanisms, 1162–1163

Migrating action-potential complex (MAPC) (*continued*)
  enteric nervous system and, 1159–1161
  *Escherichia coli* enterotoxin, 1161
  future research, 1163
  historical research, 1156–1157
  in vitro studies, 1161
  prostaglandins, 1157–1159
  *Salmonella*, 1161–1162
  vasoactive intestinal peptide (VIP), 1162
  bacterial overgrowth syndrome, 1168–1170
  parasite-induced motility, 1149
  small intestine, 1138–1145
Migrating myoelectrical complexes (MMC)
  bacterial overgrowth syndrome, 1167–1171
  biliary tract function, 1088–1089
  diarrhea and, 1154
  gallbladder function, 1072–1073
  hepatic bile flow, 1068–1070
  6-hydroxydopamine and, 1160–1161
  ileocecal sphincter characteristics, 1004–1005
  intestinal blood flow and motility, 1481–1482
  lower esophageal sphincter
    basal pressure fluctuations, 887
    contractions, 896, 991
    peptide regulation, 997–998
  MAPC and, 1161–1163
  parasite-induced alterations, 1137–1145
  postoperative paresis, 1201–1202
  pyloric sphincter electrical activity, 1000–1001
  ruminant animals
    duodenal brake mechanism, 1252–1255
    gastric emptying, 1255–1258
    5-hydroxytryptamine, 1264–1266
    mixing vs. propelling activity, 1261–1262
    nervous control, 1264
    pancreaticobiliary secretions, 1263–1264
    small intestinal motility, 1261–1262
  small intestine research, 46–49, 1137–1145, 1216
  surgical perturbations
    small intestine, 1213–1216
    truncal vagotomy, 1209–1211
Miniature excitatory junction potential, 1617
Mitochondria in intestinal muscle, 115
  embryonic development of, 131
  hypertrophy, 135
Mitosis, intestinal muscle hypertrophy, 134–135
Mixed-cation-selective channels, 220
Mixed synaptic potentials, in enteric neurons, 342–343
Mixing contractions, reticuloruminant contractions, 1232, 1235
MMF/APC ratio (microsphere-measured mucosal blood flow/aminopyrine clearance ratio), 1359
*Moniliformis dubius*, inflammation from, 1148–1149
Monopolar recording methods, myoelectric activity, 824
Morphine
  biliary tract pharmacology, 1119–1120
  colonic motility, 956
  enteric nervous system, 485
  gastric blood flow control, 1388
Morphological properties, enteric neurons, 339
Motilin
  biliary tract function, 1067, 1121–1122
  colonic motility, 956
  gallbladder function, 1072
  gastrointestinal blood flow, 1686
    norleucine interaction, 1388
  gastrointestinal motility, 928
  lower esophageal sphincter, 998
  pharmacology of, 792–794
    amino acid sequences, 792
    antagonists and, 793
    receptors, 792–793
    sites and mechanisms of action, 793–794
  proximal stomach tonic contractions, 919
  pyloric sphincter regulation, 1003
  small intestine, 47–49
Motility index
  intestinal blood flow and motility, 1489–1490
  mean motility index, 1496
Motility-regulating neurons, 532–533
Motion sickness, 705–706
Motor function, in gastrointestinal tract, 817–818
Motor neurons
  excitatory, 387
  inhibitory neurons, 387
  to muscle, 388–392
    cholinergic motor neurons, 388
    enteric inhibitory transmission, 389–391
    enteric secretomotor, 391–392
    enteric vasodilator neurons, 391
    gastrin-releasing endocrine cell transmission, 392
    noncholinergic excitatory motor transmission, 388–389
  secretomotor neurons, 387
  vasodilatory neurons, 387
Mouth, avian structure, 1283
Mucin layer, bacterial overgrowth syndrome, 1167
Mucosa
  blood flow
    acid secretion, 1391–1392
    autoregulation, 1392
    constant flow and variable pressure, 1381
    eating and, 1392–1393
    heat clearance, 1380–1381
    indicator-dilution techniques, 1377–1378
    inert-gas clearance technique, 1378–1379
    injury and, 1394–1395
    iodantipyrine clearance, 1380
    laser-Doppler velocimetry, 1348–1350, 1380
    $pK_a$ clearance techniques, 1376–1377
    prostaglandins and, 1389–1390
    reflectance spectrophotometry, 1379–1380
    venous pressure and, 1413
  disintegration in occlusive disease, 1717–1718
  energy metabolism and, 1394–1395
  injury, 1168
  microvessel circulation in, 1374–1375
    colon and, 1315–1316, 1320
    duodenum, 1315, 1318
    esophageal, 1306–1307
    small intestine, 1308–1315
    stomach, 1307–1308
  plexus, biliary tract, 1059
  receptors
    adaptation rate, 614
    amino acid receptors, 603–604
    chemosensitivity, 600–604
    functional significance, 614–615
    gastrointestinal afferent innervation, 595–596, 598–604
    glucoceptors, 601–603
    mechanosensitivity, 598–600
    multimodal receptors, 600–601
    quality-specific chemoreceptors, 601–604
    receptive fields, 600
    spontaneous activity, 598
    thermoreceptors, 604
Mucosal (Shatzki) ring, 885
Multidimensional models, gastric electrophysiology, 212–213
Multihaustral propulsion, 74–75
Muscarinic agonists
  enteric nervous system, 338, 421–422
    cholinergic system, 411
    presynaptic inhibition, 509–510
  in intestinal smooth muscle, 223–226
    receptor-evoked responses, 237–238
    locus of action, 728–729

modulation of, 729–731
  agonist exposure, 731
  by ions and guanine nucleotides, 730–731
 in motor neurons, 388
 noncholinergic excitatory motor transmission, 388–389
 postreceptor events, 731–732
 subtypes, 726–728
 therapeutic application of, 732–733
$M_2$ muscarinic receptors, 881–882
Muscle-bath studies, biliary tract function, 1066
Muscle coat
 anatomy of, 103
 circular, cytoarchitecture, 368
 circular/longitudinal thickness ratio, 103
 ICC AP location in, 351–353
 intestinal electrical activity in, 226–227
 microvessel circulation, 1372–1373
 spiral structure postulated, 103
 structure and function, 103–104
 thickness variations in, 103
Muscle microvessels, 1304
Muscle-myenteric plexus (MPLM), 409–411
Muscle receptors
 functional significance, 615
 gastrointestinal afferent innervation, 595–596
  in-series tension receptors, 604–609
Muscularis externa. *See* Muscle coat
Muscularis mucosa
 blood flow measurement, 1348–1350
 cell size and shape, 108
 electrical activity of, 199–200
 esophageal peristalsis, 884–885
 intestinal blood flow, venous pressure and, 1413
 microsphere measurement, 1343
 structure and function, 104, 108
 substance P action on, 772–773
 vasculature of, 1304–1305
 vasoactive intestinal polypeptide (VIP) action on, 779
Muscularis propria, esophageal motor function, 866
Muscular plexus, biliary tract, 1059
Myenteric neurons
 $\alpha_2$-adrenoceptors and, 738
 ICC AP in, 364–365
 inhibitory synaptic potentials, 394
 intestinal smooth muscle activity, 234
 muscarinic receptors in, 728
  ACh release, 728
 synaptic vesicles and, 336–337
 transmitter-related properties, 339–341
Myenteric plexus
 anorectal and pelvic floor muscle, 1047
 in colon, 941, 953
  nerve bundles in, 941–942
 culture studies of, 331–332
 diarrhea mechanisms, 1172
 enteric nervous system
  inhibitory neurotransmitters, 505–507
  slow IPSPs, 504
 opiate receptors in, 780–781
 pacemaker potentials and action potentials, 29–32
 parasympathetic innervation, 1026–1027
 tissue culture of, 333–335
Myenteric potential oscillations
 colonic muscle, 254–255
  circular/longitudinal layer electrical coupling, 266–267
  motoneurons and, 261
  propagation of, 265–266
Mylohyoid muscle, primary peristalsis, 868
Myoelectric activity
 analytical methods, 825
 esophageal motility, 869–870
 intestinal blood flow and motility, 1481

 neural control and, 844–845
 parasite-induced alterations, 1137–1145
 recording methods for, 823–825
 relaxation-oscillator vs. cable models, 852–857
  passive conduction, 852
  regenerative propagation, 852–853
  relaxation-oscillator propagation, 853–857
 research background, 817–818
  terminology, 825–827
 spatial and temporal patterns, 827–850
  colon and rectum, 834–838
  esophagus, 838–842
  gallbladder, 849–850
  organ junctions, 845–859
  small intestine, 830–834
  sphincters, 842–845
  stomach, 827–830
 special situation contractions, 850–852
  caudad mass movement, 850–852
  vomiting, 850
Myogenic hypothesis
 exocrine gland circulation, 1569–1570
 intestinal mucosa blood flow, 1406–1408, 1484–1486
  reactive hyperemia, 1414
 neonatal intestinal circulation, 1599–1602
Myosin
 contractile protein regulation, 290–291
 intestinal muscle
  heavy chain development, 131, 133
  ratio with actin filaments, 122–124
  structure and function, 124
 phosphorylation, basal sphincter muscle tone, 888
 skeletal muscle contraction, 276
Myosin light-chain kinase (MLCK)
 contractile protein regulation, 291–293
 relaxation mechanisms, 312–313
 shortening force-velocity curve, 311

NA/- cells
 somatostatin and neuropeptide Y, 574, 577
 VIP transmission and, 565
$Na^+$. *See* Sodium ($Na^+$) channels
Naloxone
 biliary tract pharmacology, 1121
 noncholinergic excitatory motor transmission, 389
NA/NPY cells
 neuropeptide Y in, 574, 576–577
 VIP transmission and, 565
NA/SOM
 somatostatin in, 574, 577
 VIP transmission and, 565
Natural-flow preparation, 1478
Nausea
 defined, 1193–1194
 reversed peristalsis, 45
Neonatal intestine
 fasting state, hemodynamics and oxygenation, 1597–1598
 intrinsic regulation of circulation, 1599–1602
  hypotension response, 1601–1602
  hypoxemia response, 1600–1601
  response to feeding, 1600
 neural regulation of circulation, 1598–1599
 reflex control of circulation, 1598–1599
Nernst equation, 1643–1644
Nerve fibers
 ICC AP and, 355–357
 in intestinal muscles, 127–129
Nerve growth factor, background on, 331–332
Nerve net analogy, enteric nervous system, 58–60
Nerves
 muscarinic receptors in, 728–729
 role in intestinal smooth muscle activity, 233–234

Nerves (*continued*)
  tachykinin action, 770
    sensory nerves, 771–772
Net fluid absorption
  capillary-interstitial interaction, 1449–1453
    capillary filtration coefficient, 1453
    capillary pressure ($P_c$), 1452–1453
    interstitial hydrostatic pressure, 1450–1451
    interstitium and, 1449–1450
    lymphatics and, 1451–1453
    oncotic forces, 1450, 1452–1453
    osmotic reflection coefficient, 1453
    solute mobility, 1450
    Starling forces, 1453–1454
  lymph flow and composition, 1747–1749
  postprandial hyperemia, neurohormonal control, 1699
Net fluid secretion
  capillary-interstitial interaction, 1453–1456
    active secretion, 1455–1456
    filtration secretion, 1453–1455
Net inward current, 182
Neural control
  defined, 818–819
  myoelectric activity and, 844–845
Neurally evoked action potentials, 1617–1618
Neural reflex, colonic motility and blood flow, 1499–1500
Neuroantagonists, cholera-induced secretion and motility, 1159
Neuroeffectors, intestinal villi motility, 976, 978–979
Neurogenic dysfunction, anorectal and pelvic floor muscles, 1047
Neurokinin A, neurotransmission in prevertebral ganglia, 559
Neuromedin K
  discovery of, 765–766
  potency sequences for, 766–767
Neuromedin N, neurotensin and, 797
Neuromodulation
  adrenergic, in gastrointestinal tract, 444–445
  research background on, 435–436
Neuromuscular junction in enteric neurons, 394–395
Neuromuscular transmission
  electrophysiology of, 436–441
    autonomic neuromuscular junction, 436, 439–440
    effector structure, 436
    recording techniques, 436–438, 441–442
  gastrointestinal tract
    adrenergic, 441–445
    disease states, 453–457
    excitatory nerve transmission, 449–453
    future research, 457
    inhibitory nerve transmission, 445–449
  ion permeability and conductance changes, 438, 440–442
Neuroneuronal synapses
  enteric neurons, 392–396
  presynaptic inhibition, 394
Neuropathology of Hirschsprung's disease, 964–965
Neuropeptide-degrading enzymes
  enteric cholinergic system, 419–420
    acetylcholinesterase, 410
    aminopeptidase, 420
    dipeptidyl peptidase IV, 420
    endopeptidase, 419
    peptidyl dipeptidase A, 419–420
Neuropeptide K
  capsaicin and, 771–772
  discovery of, 765–766
  prevertebral ganglia neurotransmission, 559
Neuropeptides
  biliary tract pharmacology, 1111–1124
    bombesin and somatostatin, 1118–1119
    caerulein, 1116–1117
    cholecystokinin-gastrin family, 1111–1115
    gastrin, 1115–1116
    motilin, 1121–1122
    opiates, 1119–1121
    pancreatic polypeptide, 1122–1123
    secretin, VIP, glucagon, and GIP, 1117–1118
    sex hormones, 1123–1124
    substance P, 1123–1124
  enteric cholinergic system, 414–419
  lower esophageal sphincter pressure
    acetylcholine release, 414–419
    table of, 892
Neuropeptide synaptic vesicles, 423
Neuropeptide Y
  in dorsal motor nucleus of the vagus, 650
  in enteric neurons, 396
  gastrointestinal blood flow
    coexistence with norepinephrine, 1679
    neurohormonal control, 1678-16779
  gastrointestinal neuromuscular transmission, 444–445
  in prevertebral ganglia, 574–577
  in submucosal arterioles, 1639–1640
Neurotensin
  colonic motility, 956
  dorsal motor nucleus and, 626–627, 650
  enteric nervous system, 396
    slow EPSPs, 400
    slow IPSPs, 5–6
  gastrointestinal blood flow, 1388, 1689
  gastrointestinal motility, 929
    sympathetic preganglionic neurons, 656–657
  gastrointestinal neuromusclar transmission
    excitatory junction potentials, 453
    putative inhibitory neurotransmission, 448
  inhibitory motor transmission, 390–391
  interaction with substance P, 772
  intestinal smooth muscle, 239
  pharmacology of, 795–799
    antagonists, 797
    degradation, 797
    gastrointestinal motility, 797–799
    intracellular pathways, 799
    receptors, 795–797
  postprandial intestinal hyperemia and, 1426
  in prevertebral ganglia, 571–573
  receptor locus and functional coupling, 719
Neurotransmission
  autonomic, mesenteric artery, 1612–1614
  colonic motility, 953
  in dorsal motor nucleus of vagus, 648–651
  in enteric neurons
    acetylcholine release, 410–414, 422
    acetylcholinesterase, 420
    adrenergic system, 420–422
    aminopeptidase, 420
    calmodulation activity, 408
    cholecystokinin, 417–418
    cholinergic system, 409–414
    coexistence of, 344
    depeptidyl peptidase IV, 420
    dynorphins and enkephalins, 418–419
    endopeptidase, 419
    enteric synaptosomes, 422–423
    historical background, 403–404
    inositol phospholipids, 408–409
    intracellular control activation, 407–409
    mechanism of release, 404–405
    modulation of transmitter release, 405–409
    neuroactive peptides, 414–419
    neuropeptide-degrading enzymesm, 419–420
    nonsynaptic transmitter release, 405
    nonvesicular hypothesis, 405
    norepinephrine release, 420–421
    peptidyl dipeptidase A, 419–420
    presynaptic modulation, 405–407

protein phosphorylation, 407–408
research on, 387–388
somatostatin, 417
substance P, 416–417
transsynaptic modulation, 407
vasoactive intestinal peptide, 414–416
vesicular release mechanism, 404–405
vs. neuromodulator, 404
esophageal peristalsis, 883–884
gastrointestinal blood flow, 1667–1683
gastrointestinal motility, distribution in nuclei, 651
Hirschsprung's disease, 964–965
lower esophageal sphincter, 994–996
inhibitory pathways, 894–895
in nucleus ambiguus, 652
in prevertebral ganglia, 556–577
responses to in enteric neurons, 341
small intestine, early research, 64
Neutral red clearance, human gastric hemodynamics, 1396
Nexuses. *See* Gap junctions
Nicotine
biliary tract pharmacology, 1105–1106
gastric circulation and, 1396
internal anal sphincter regulation, 1011–1012
Nicotinic fast EPSPs, 392
enteric nervous system, 341–342, 492–493
Nifedipine
hepatic circulation, 1549
submucosal arterioles, 1658–1659
IXth (ninth) nerve
deglutition and, 687–688
motor neurons of, 692
*Nippostrongylus brasiliensis*
inflammation from, 1148–1149
parasite-induced alterations, small intestine, 1137, 1143–1144
Nissl granules, in principal ganglia cells, 524
Nociceptors
functional significance, 615–616
gastrointestinal afferent innervation, 595–596
Nonadrenergic inhibitory nerves, 954
Nonadrenergic, noncholinergic nervous system (NANC)
biliary tract pharmacology, 1105–1106
drug-receptor response quantitation, 721
esophageal and gastric ICC, 375
gallbladder innervation, 1059
internal anal sphincter regulation, 1012
motor activity, 1035
interstitial cells of Cajal, 382
ICC DMP and, 373
lower esophageal sphincter, 990
prostaglandin and, 997
relaxation, 995
mesenteric artery, 1621
muscarinic receptors and, 729
postprandial hyperemia and, 1422
purinergic receptors and, 742–743
ruminant animals, 1254–1255
sacral autonomic nerves
colon and rectum motor activity, 1039
slow EPSP, in prevertebral ganglion, 555
sphincter of Oddi innervation, 1059–1060
vomiting reflex, 1192–1193
Noncholinergic excitatory motor transmission, 388–389
Noncholinergic nerves, esophageal peristalsis, 880–882
Nonmuscle cells
intestinal muscle hypertrophy, 135
in intestinal muscles, 127–129
Nonocclusive intestinal ischemia, gastrointestinal blood flow, 1713–1715
Nonsynaptic transmitter release, 405
Nonvesicular hypothesis, 405
Noradrenergic synaptosomes, 423

Norepinephrine (NE)
action potentials, 1611
adrenergic neuromuscular transmission
neuromodulation with, 444
nonsphincteric muscles, 444
$\alpha$-adrenoreceptors and, 734
in area postrema, 701
chloride channel properties, 180
in colonic muscle, electropharmacology, 258–259
in dorsal motor nucleus of the vagus, 648–649
enteric nervous system, 396
cholinergic system, 412
presynaptic inhibition, 509
release factors, 420–421
slow IPSPs, 506
gastrointestinal blood flow
adrenergic vascular innervation, 1669–1670
coexistence with neuropeptide Y, 1679
intestines, 1671–1673
stomach, 1677–1678
in vitro studies, 1670–1671, 1674–1678
in vivo studies, 1671–1674
hepatic circulation, 1542–1543
autoregulatory escape, 1529
hepatic nerve stimulation, 1520
inhibitory synaptic potentials, 394
intermediolateral cell column ($S_{2-3}$), 654
internal anal sphincter regulation, 1012
intestinal villi motility, 979
lower esophageal sphincter, 995
mechanosensitive neurons, 477–478
mesenteric artery
neuroeffector transmission pharmacology, 1618–1619
responses to, 1612–1613
mesenteric circulation
blood vessel density, 1607
functional differences in artery and vein, 1627–1628
functional implications, 1608
mesenteric vein, 1623
portal vein, 1626–1627
sphincter of Oddi pharmacology, 1107–1108
submucosal arterioles
excitatory junction potentials, 1656–1658
receptor-activated tension, 1652–1653
Norleucine motilin, gastric blood flow control, 1388
Nucleus ambiguus
amygdala connections to, 663
deglutition and, 692
gastrointestinal motility
neuronal inputs and outputs, 660
pathway to esophageal sphincters, 671–672
retrograde tracing studies, 643–645
motor nerves in, 692
neuroanatomy of, 651–652
parasympatheic neural pathway
in esophagus, 625
in stomach, 625–627
Nucleus intercalatus pars paraependymalis (ICP$_e$), 530–531
opioid peptides, 562
Nucleus intercalatus spinalis (IC)
gastrointestinal motility, 654
opioid peptides, 562
pathways to prevertebral ganglion, 530–531
Nucleus retroambiguus
gastrointestinal motility
electrical stimulation studies, 645
neuronal inputs and outputs, 660
neuroanatomy of, 652–653
parasympatheic neural pathway, 625
Nucleus tegmentalis laterodorsalis, 660
Nucleus tractus solitarius (nTS)
afferent pathways, 594–595

Nucleus tractus solitarius (nTS) (*continued*)
    dorsal motor nucleus connections, 647–648
    vagal nerve fibers and, 629–632
  amygdala connections to, 663
  deglutition and, 687–688
  gastrointestinal motility, 668
    afferent pathways in, 646
    dorsal motor nucleus and, 637–641
    neural input and output, 662–663
    neuroanatomy, 657–658
    nucleus ambiguus and, 660
    stimulation and lesions of, 664
  receptive relaxation and, 672
Null potential, submucosal arterioles, 1646
Nutrients
  absorption by intestinal villi, 984–985
  products of, 922–923

Obelin, $Ca^{2+}$ measurement with, 147
Obex, gastrointestinal motility, 637
Occlusive intestinal ischemia, 1717–1718
Occupation theory of receptor action, 715–716
Off-response, lower esophageal sphincter, 994–995
Omasum
  absorption function, 1229–1230
  body motility index, 1243
  cyclical activity, 1242–1243
Oncotic pressure
  lymph flow and composition, 1748
  net fluid absorption, 1450–1453
On-response, lower esophageal sphincter, 994
Onuf's nucleus
  colon innervation, 942
  gastrointestinal motility
    cerebral cortex pathway, 669
    electrical stimulation studies, 645
  neuroanatomy of, 653–654
  parasympathetic neural pathways, 628
  pelvic floor muscles, 1028–1030
  pudendal nerve efferent fibers and, 669–670
Open junctions, initial lymphatics, 1737–1738
Opiates
  biliary tract pharmacology, 1119–1121
  intestinal motility and, 926
  intestinal mucosal blood flow, 1438–1439
  pharmacology of, 780–792
    degradation of, 782
    drug design and, 791–792
    functions in ileum, 785–786
    gastrointestinal motility and, 786–791
    immune system and, 791
    locus of receptors, 782
    mechanism of action, 784–785
    natural opiates, 780
    postreceptor coupling, 785
    potential endogenous ligands, 785
    receptor types, 780–782
Opioid peptides
  degradation of, 782
  enteric nervous system, slow IPSPs, 505
  cholinergic system, 418–419
  lower esophageal sphincter, 998
  noncholinergic excitatory motor transmission, 389
  pharmacology, 780
  in prevertebral ganglia, 561
Opioid receptors
  ruminant animals, pharmacology, 1270–1272
  vomiting reflex, 1191–1192
Orad propagation, 196–197
  gastric slow waves, 191–192
  voltage-tension relationship, 202
Organ baths, 283, 285–286

Organelles
  in intestinal muscle, 115
    hypertrophy, 135
Organ junctions
  myoelectric activity and, 845–849
    choledochoduodenal junction, 847–848
    gastroduodenal junction (pylorus), 845–846
    ileocolonic junction, 848–849
Organotypic culture, enteric nervous system, 332–333
Oscilloscopes, gastrointestinal muscle mechanics, 282
Osmolality
  gastric emptying and, 923
  intestinal villi motility, 981
Osmotic reflection coefficient
  exocrine gland circulation, 1583
  intestinal mucosal blood flow
    plasma proteins, 1459–1460
    transcapillary fluid and solute exchange, 1444
  net fluid absorption, 1453
Otolith integrity, emesis and, 705–706
Ouabain
  contribution to resting potential
    in colonic muscle, 252–253
  slow-wave generation, 192
  sodium pump activity and, 150
Outward current, action potentials and, 222–223
Overstretch, length-tension curve, 297–298
Owls, gastric motility, 1292–1295
Oxidative metabolism
  intestinal mucosal blood flow, 1435–1437
  ruminant animals, 1266
Oxygenation
  exocrine gland circulation, 1568–159
    intrinsic regulation of, 1569–1572
  intestinal mucosa blood flow, 1406–1408
Oxygen delivery-to-demand ratio, 1410
Oxygen extraction, 1410
Oxygen free radicals, 1395
  nonocclusive intestinal ischemia, 1713–1715
Oxygen uptake
  hepatic arterial buffer response, 1527
  intestinal mucosal blood flow
    arterial pressure reduction, 1410–1411
    steady-state relation, 1411
    vasoactive agents and, 1434–1435
  postprandial intestinal hyperemia and, 1422–1423
Oxytocin, 656–657

Pacemaker activity
  gastric slow waves, 191–192
  gastrointestinal electrophysiology, 182
  structure of, 349–350
Pacemaker cells
  in colonic muscle, 268
  interstitial cells of Cajal
    colonic, 380–381
    ICC AP as, 360, 362–363
  in prevertebral ganglia, 548
Pacesetter potentials
  in gastric slow waves, 191, 827
  historical research, 29–32
  postoperative paresis, 1201–1202
  pyloric sphincter, 999–1000
  surgical perturbations
    resection, 1204–1207
    truncal vagotomy, 1207–1208
  *See also* Slow waves
Pacinian corpuscles, gastrointestinal afferent pathways, 609–611
Pancreas
  avian structure, 1286
  lymphatics, 1757–1758
    structure, 1740

periodic activity, 24–25
Pancreatic circulation
  basal hemodynamics and oxygenation, 1568–1569
  blood vessels
    extraglandular, 1565–1566
    intraglandular, 1566–1567
  extrinsic blood flow regulation, 1588–1589
  functional hyperemia, 1572–1577
    extrinsic factors, 1576–1577
    intrinsic metabolic factors, 1574–1576
    mediators of, 1574–1577
  hyperplasia circulatory adjustments, 1577–1578
    transcapillary fluid and solute exchange, 1578–1588
  hypoxic vasodilation, 1571
    venous pressure elevation, 1571–1572
  intrinsic regulation, 1569–1572
    kallikrein-kinin regulation, 1570
    metabolic regulation, 1569
    myogenic regulation, 1569–1570
    reactive hyperemia, 1571
    vasoregulation, 1570–1572
  lymph vessels, 1567–1568
  nerves, 1568
  sympathetic nerve stimulation, 1588–1589
  vasoactive agents, 1586–1587
Pancreatic duct
  muscle and mucosal structure, 1058
  species anatomical differences, 1060–1061
  structure, 1057
Pancreaticobiliary secretions, 1263–1264
Pancreatic polypeptide
  avian motility regulation, 1290–1291
  biliary tract pharmacology, 1122–1123
  gastrointestinal blood flow, 1686
  in ruminant animals, 1258
Pancreatitis
  lymphatic drainage, 1765
  sphincter of Oddi function, 1091
Papaverine, nonocclusive intestinal ischemia, 1716
Parabrachial nucleus, 664
Paracrine substances, 259
Parallel elastic property, 275
Parallel tube model of hepatic circulation, 1520
  substrate uptake, 1534
*Parascaris equorum*, inflammation from, 1148–1149
Parasite infections
  esophageal alterations, 1133–1134
  motility changes
    gastrointestinal hormone imbalances, 1147
    inflammation, 1148–1149
    parasite-derived substances, 1147
  small intestine, 1134–1146
  stomach alterations, 1134
Parasympathetic innervation
  colon and rectum, 1026–1027
  exocrine gland circulation, 1573–1574, 1576–1577
  gastric blood flow control, 1383–1385
  gastrointestinal motility, 623–628
    in colon, 627–628
    dorsal motor nucleus of the vagus, 637–643
    in esophagus, 623–625
    intermediolateral cell column–$S_{2-3}$, 645
    nucleus ambiguus, 643–645
    retrofacial nucleus and nucleus retroambiguus, 645
    in small intestine, 627
    in stomach, 625–627
  ileocecal sphincter regulation, 1007
  internal anal sphincter regulation, 1011, 1026–1027
  intestinal villi motility, 976–977
  muscarinic receptors in, 728–729
  sacral efferent fibers, 1046
Paravascular nerve stimulation, 1606, 1614–1618

Paraventricular nucleus
  dorsal motor nucleus and, 626–627
  neuronal inputs and outputs, 658–659
Partial pressure of oxygen ($P_{O_2}$)
  exocrine gland circulation, 1569–1570
    functional hyperemia, 1575
  intestinal mucosa blood flow, 1406
    arterial hypoxia, 1415
    metabolic hypothesis, 1407
    myogenic hypothesis, 1408
    neurohormonal control of, 1673–1674
    oxygen uptake and, 1435
  nonocclusive intestinal ischemia, 1714
  postprandial intestinal hyperemia and, 1424–1425
    neurohormonal control, 1698
  ulcerogenesis and, 1722
Partition principle, lymph flow and composition, 1753
Passive conduction, electrical control activity (ECA), 852
Passive electrical properties, in intestinal smooth muscle, 220–221
Passive ion movements, 147–149
Passive membrane properties, mesenteric vein, 1622–1623
Patch-clamp technique
  single-cell research with, 240
  voltage-clamp studies, 170–171
pCA concept, contractile protein regulation, 292
$pD_2$ logarithm, drug-receptor response quantitation, 721
Pelleted feces formation in ruminant animals, 1267–1269
Peltier effect, gastrointestinal muscle mechanics, 283
Pelvic floor
  motor dysfunction, 1047
  skeletal muscle motor activity, 1033–1035
    flexor reflexes, 1044
    force measurements, 1034–1035
    histochemiocal studies, 1034
    phasic isotonic contractions, 1034
    somatic nerves, 1040–1044
    somatic reflexes, 1040
    supraspinal pathways, 1040–1042
    viscerosomatic reflexes, 1041–1044
  somatic innervation to skeletal muscle, 1028–1030
Pelvic-hypogastric ganglion
  cholinergic inputs and, 552–553
  neuroanatomy of, 520–521
  slow EPSPs in, 555
Pelvic nerves
  afferent fibers, gastrointestinal motility, 632
  colonic motility and blood flow, 942, 1498–1500
  gastrointestinal afferent innervation, 595
  internal anal sphincter regulation, 1010–1011
Pendular movements of small intestine, 42–48
Pentagastrin
  in colonic muscle, 259
  gastric blood flow and secretion, 1500–1501
  gastric muscle arrhythmia and, 197–198
  gastrin receptors and, 761–762
  gastrointestinal blood flow, neurohormonal control, 1684–1685
  gastrointestinal motility, 928
  in ruminant animals
    pancreaticobiliary secretions, 1263–1264
    pharmacology, 1271
Peptide histidine isoleucine
  in enteric neurons, 396
  gastrointestinal blood flow, 1679
  pharmacology, 776–777
Peptide histidine methionine (PHM), 776–777
Peptidergic receptors, vomiting reflex, 1193
Peptides
  in area postrema, 701
  colonic motility, 953
  in colonic muscle, 1030–1031
  effect on voltage recordings, 168
  electropharmacology of, 204–205, 259

Peptides (*continued*)
  gastrointestinal motility, 653–654
  ileocecal sphincter regulation, 1008
  internal anal sphincter regulation, 1012
  lower esophageal sphincter regulation, 997–998
  in lymph, 175
  muscarinic receptors and, 729
  pharmacology, 792–800
    neurotensin family, 795–799
  postprandial intestinal hyperemia and, 1425–1427
  *See also* specific peptides
Peptide YY
  colonic motility, 956
  gastrointestinal blood flow, 1686–1687
  in prevertebral ganglion, 575
Peptidyl dipeptidase A, enteric nervous system, 419–420
Perfusion pressure reduction, 1602
Perhexiline, nonocclusive intestinal ischemia, 1717
Periarterial ganglia, neuroanatomy of, 521–522
Pericytic venule, 1326
Periductular capillary plexus, 1567
Periodic activity
  gastrointestinal motility, 24–29
  historical research, 24–29
    contractions, 25
      hunger contractions, 26–29
      periodic sounds, 26
    small intestine, 45
Periodic sounds, 26
Peripheral afferent nerves, 661
Peripheral reflexes
  colon control, 76–77
  prevertebral ganglion and, 534–542
    substance P and, 560
Peristalsis
  central esophageal control, 875–877
  colonic motility, 944
  deglutition and, 695
  distension-induced, 876
  emptying phase, 66
  esophageal, 10–12
    abnormal, 12
      longitudinal muscle layer, 884–885
      muscularis mucosa, 884–885
      surgical perturbation, 1202–1203
  functions of nerves in, 65–66
  gastric emptying, 19–20
  historical background on, 187–188
  ICC DMP and, 372
  intestinal smooth muscle and, 219
  junctional zone, 884
  peripheral esophageal control
    smooth muscle, 877–884
    striated muscle, 877
  preparatory phase, 66
  primary, 8
    deglutition reflex, 868
    striated esophageal muscle, 876
    surgical perturbation, 1203
    swallow-induced response, 874–875
  secondary, 8
    distension-induced responses, 875
    surgical perturbation, 1203
  slow potential change research on, 240–241
  slow-wave mechanism and, 231
  small intestine, 43–44
  sphincter of Oddi function, 1081–1083
  tertiary, 9
  *See also* Retrograde giant contraction
Peristaltic propulsive force, esophageal motility, 870
Peristaltic reflex
  colonic motility, 953

  early research on, 66–68
  small intestine, 64–68
Peritoneal dialysis, 1319
Perivascular nerve stimulation
  mesenteric artery, 1614–1618
  mesenteric circulation and, 1606
Permeability
  intestinal mucosal blood flow
    factors influencing, 1459–1462
    small solute permeability, 1456–1457
  ionic channels, 238
Permeability–surface area product (PS product)
  exocrine gland circulation, 1577, 1585, 1588
  intestinal blood flow and motility, 1489
pH
  changes in ruminant animals, 1253–1254
  heartburn and gastroesophageal reflux, 17–18
  hepatic circulation, blood gases and, 1530–1531
  intestinal villi motility, 981
  luminal, intestinal mucosal blood flow and, 1418
  partition hypothesis
    aminopyrine clearance, 1360–1361
    comparison with other methods, 1358–1360
    in nonsecreting stomach, 1356–1357
    two-compartment model, 1353–1354, 1360–1361
  trapping techniques, 1351–1354
    theoretical background, 1352–1354
Phagocytotic activity, in intestinal muscle, 115
Pharmacological stimulation, 285, 287
Pharyngoesophageal sphincter
  in achalasia, 16
  disorders of, 9–10
  historical research, 9–10
Pharynx, avian structure, 1283
Phasic contractions
  in colonic muscle, 256–257
  control of, 818–823
    spatial control, 821–823
    temporal control, 818–821
  gastrointestinal smooth muscle activation, 284
  ileocolonic junction, 849
  in intestinal smooth muscle, 226–227
    tetrodotoxin and, 228
  pelvic floor skeletal muscle, 1040
  research background, 817–818
  ruminant animals, 1267–1269
  sphincter of Oddi, 1078–1080, 1089
    abnormal propagation, 1093–1094
Phasic-firing neurons, prevertebral ganglia, 546–548
Phenoxybenzamine
  nonocclusive intestinal ischemia, 1716
  submucosal arterioles and, 1655–1656
Phentolamine, chloride channel properties, 180
L-Phenylalanine
  gastrointestinal blood flow, 1687
  postprandial hyperemia, 1699
Phorbol esters, 237
Phosphatidic acid, enteric neurotransmission, 409
Phosphatidylinositol
  enteric neurotransmission, 408–409
  tachykinins and, 769
Phospholipid turnover, 237
Photodetectors, Doppler frequency shifts, 1346
Photoelectric force transducer, 279–280, 281–282
Photon-tissue interactions, laser-Doppler velocimetry, 1345–1346
Physostigmine
  colonic motility, 1497–1500
  gastric blood flow and secretion, 1500–1501
  intestinal blood flow and motility, 1486–1488, 1490
Pirenzepine, muscarinic receptors, 727–728
$pK_a$ clearance technique, 1376–1377

Plasmalemmal vesicles
　calcium pumps in, 151–154
　exocrine gland circulation, 1580
Plateau potential
　in colonic muscle, 258
　gastric muscle excitation-contraction coupling, 201–202
Plexuses
　avian muscular stomach, 1285
　intramural vasculature, 1304
*Plexus muscularis profundus*
　*See* Deep muscular plexus
$P_{Na}/P_K$ ratio, neuromodulation of, 543–544
Poiseuille's law, 1077
Polypeptides
　colonic motility, 956
　lymphatic transport of, 1756–1757
Pons, role in deglutition, 689–690
Pontine reticular formation, 665
Portal blood flow
　liver mass and, 1519–1520
　lymph flow and composition, 1752–1753
Portal hypertension, 1720–1721
　gastric circulation and, 1396
Portal vein
　cell coupling, 1626
　function, 1605–1606
　nerve stimulation response, 1626
　neurotransmitter response, 1626–1627
　spontaneous action potentials, 1625–1626
Positive-pressure ventilation (PPV), 1693–1694
Postganglionic sympathetic neurons
　adrenergic receptors and, 733
　gastrin receptors and, 761
Postprandial hyperemia
　intestinal mucosal blood flow
　　anticipatory/ingestion phase, 1417
　　autacoids, 1427–1429
　　digestion/absorption phase, 1417
　　hormones and peptides, 1425–1427
　　intrinsic nerves, 1421–1422
　　localization of, 1417–1418
　　luminal stimuli and, 1418–1420
　　mechanisms of, 1420–1429
　　metabolic factors, 1422–1425
　　vasoactive action by chyme, 1421
　neurohormonal control, 1697–1700
Poststimulus depolarization, 235
Postsynaptic membrane, in prevertebral ganglions, 544
Postsynaptic potentials (PSP)
　in enteric neurons, 342–343
　*See also* Excitatory and Inhibitory postsynaptic potentials
Potassium ($K^+$) channels
　$Ca^{2+}$-dependence and 488–489
　cholinergic regulation of, 180
　contribution to resting potential, 252–253
　electron-probe microanalysis of, 145–146
　enteric nervous system
　　equilibrium potential, 487–488
　　slow IPSPs, 504–505
　esophageal peristalsis, 882–883
　exocrine gland circulation, 1575–1576
　gastrin-CCK receptor modulation, 764
　gastrointestinal smooth muscle activation, 286
　intestinal blood flow and motility, 1492–1493
　in intestinal smooth muscle, 218–219
　　action potentials and, 229–230
　　active properties of, 221–222
　　outward current, 222–223
　ionic mechanism of slow waves, 195
　lower esophageal sphincter
　　basal tone, 992–993
　membrane and equilibrium potential changes, 150
　mesenteric artery
　　acetylcholine stimulation, 1613–1614
　　action potentials, 1611
　　norepinephrine stimulation of, 1612–1613
　permeability, 438, 440–442
　$\mu$-receptor and, 784
　single intestinal smooth muscle cell and, 218–220
　slow-potential-sensitive, 220
　submucosal arterioles, 1642–1643
　substance P action and, 771
　VIP transmission in prevertebral ganglia, 565–566
　voltage-clamp studies
　　single-channel studies, 171–174
　　whole-cell studies, 174–176
Potassium-42 technique, mucosal blood flow measurement, 1377
Precapillary sphincter
　hemorrhagic hypotension, 1696–1697
　intestinal mucosa, 1406–1408
　small intestine anatomy, 1477
Precapillary-to-postcapillary resistance ratio ($R_a/R_v$)
　capillary-interstitial interaction, 1447–1448
　intestinal mucosa blood flow, 1409
Preganglionic sympathetic neurons, 662
Pregnancy
　biliary tract pharmacology, 1123–1124
　gallbladder function and, 1090–1091
Prehension, avian gastrointestinal motility, 1286
Prelymphatics, 1736
Preproenkephalin A, 561
Preproenkephalin B, 561
Prepro-opiomelanocortin, 561
$\alpha$-Preprotachykinin, 766
$\beta$-Preprotachykinin, 766
Pressure electrodes, esophageal contraction and inhibition, 882–883
Pressure profiles
　esophageal body, 874–875
　lower esophageal sphincter, 886–888
　　basal pressure fluctuations, 886–887
　upper esophageal sphincter, 871
Pressure transducers, 1381
Pressure-volume relationships, 1433–1434
Presynaptic feedback mechanisms, 421
Presynaptic inhibition
　enteric nervous system, 508–510
　neuroneuronal synapses, 394
Presynaptic modulation
　enteric neurotransmission, 405–407
　　autoinhibition, 406
　　nonsynaptic inhibition, 406–407
Prevertebral ganglia
　electrophysiology, 542–549
　　afterspike hyperpolarizations, sympathetic neurons, 548–549
　　modification of firing patterns, 548
　　neuromodulation of resting membrane potential, 543–545
　　resting membrane potential, 542–543
　　sympathetic neuronal firing patterns, 545–548
　gastrointestinal correlates of vomiting, 1191
　innervation of, 530–542
　　spinal preganglionic neurons, 530–534
　　visceral afferent fibers, 534–542
　neuroanatomy of, 519–530
　　abdominal, 519
　　celiac ganglion, 520–521
　　chromaffin cell structure and function, 527–529
　　chromaffin SIF cells, 522–523
　　components, 522–530
　　inferior mesenteric ganglion, 520–521
　　pelvic-hypogastric plexus, 520–521
　　principal ganglion cells, 522–527
　　satellite cells, 522, 524, 529–530
　　superior mesenteric ganglion, 520–521

Prevertebral ganglia (*continued*)
  neurotransmitters in, 556–577
    bombesin, 570–571
    calcitonin gene-related peptide, 571–572
    cholecystokinin, 566–570
    dynorphin, 569–570
    enkephalins and endorphin, 560–564
    neurotensin, 571–573
    serotonin, 572–573
    somatostatin and neuropeptide Y, 574–577
    substance P, 556–560
    vasoactive intestinal polypeptide, 564–566
    vasopressin, 573–574
  research background on, 519–520
  synaptic transmission, 549–556
    fast transmission, 551–554
    slow transmission, 554–556
Primary cycle movement, 1232, 1234
Principal ganglion cells
  structure and function, 523–527
  substance P lacking in, 558
Proctocolectomy, 1216–1218
Prodromal signs of vomiting, 1194–1195
Progesterone, biliary tract pharmacology, 1123–1124
Prokinetic drugs, muscarinic pharmacology, 632–633
Propagation
  defined, 205–206
  gastric muscle electrophysiology models, 209–218
Propulsive behavior, parasite-induced alterations, 1140–1146
Prostacyclin (PCI), opiate receptors and, 782
Prostacyclin$_2$ (PGI$_2$), 1429
Prostaglandins
  biliary tract pharmacology, 1108–1110
  colonic motility, 956
    electropharmacology, 259
  deglutition and, 695
  electropharmacology of, 205
  esophageal peristalsis, 884
  exocrine gland circulation
    extrinsic regulation of, 1588–1589
    functional hyperemia and, 1576
  gastric blood flow control, 1389–1390
  ileocecal sphincter regulation, 1008
  intestinal smooth muscle, 239
  lower esophageal sphincter regulation, 891, 996–997
  macrophage-like cell as source of, 365–366
  MAPC and, 1157–1159
  mesenteric artery, neuromuscular transmission, 1620–1621
  postprandial intestinal hyperemia and, 1428–1429
  pyloric sphincter regulation, 1003
  receptor locus and functional coupling, 719–720
  tachygastria, 1211
  ulcer prevention and, 1722
Prostaglandins D$_2$
  intestinal blood flow and motility, 1489
  intramural tension, 1496
Prostaglandins E, biliary tract pharmacology, 1108–1109
Prostaglandins E$_1$ (PGE$_1$)
  lower esophageal sphincter regulation, 996–997
  nonocclusive intestinal ischemia, 1716–1717
  pyloric sphincter regulation, 1003
Prostaglandins E$_2$
  gastric muscle arrhythmia and, 197–198
  gastrointestinal motility, 928
  hepatic circulation, 1530
  intestinal blood flow and motility, 1492
  ruminant animals
    pharmacology, 1271
Prostaglandins E$_{2\alpha}$, pyloric sphincter regulation, 1003
Prostaglandins F, 1108–1109
Prostaglandin F$_{2\alpha}$
  ileocecal sphincter regulation, 1008

  lower esophageal sphincter activity, 891, 996–997
  MAPC and, 1157–1158
  RBAP activity, 1166
Protein
  contractile, 289–295
  intestinal mucosal blood flow and, 1417
    fluxes, 1460–1461
  lymphatic transport of, 1756–1757
  phosphorylation, 407–408
  postprandial intestinal hyperemia, 1419–1420
Protein kinase, 1157–1159
  MAPC/prostaglandins interaction, 1157–1159
Protein kinase C
  enteric neurotransmission, 409
  intestinal smooth muscle, 237
Protein-losing enteropathy, 1762–1763
Proximal colon, nervous control of, 75–76
Proximal stomach
  motility, 910
    retching and vomitus expulsion, 1181–1183
    vagal innervation, 927
    surgical perturbations, 1205–1206
    tonic contractions during gastric emptying, 919
Pseudorumination, 1238
Psychosomatic factors, colon research, 84–86
P-type axons, 373
Puborectalis, electrical activity in, 1033–1034
Pudendal nerve
  afferent fibers
    gastrointestinal motility, 634–636
    spinal reflex and, 669–670
  efferent fibers, Onuf's nucleus, 669–670
  motor neurons, 1028–1030
Pull-through manometry
  lower esophageal sphincter measurements, 887–888
  sphincter of Oddi function, 1078–1079, 1081
Pulmonary blood volume, 1539–1540
Pulse pressure, mucosal blood flow and, 1393
Purine
  enteric cholinergic system, 412
    nucleotides and nucleosides, slow IPSPs, 507
Purinergic compounds
  enteric cholinergic system, 412
  mesenteric artery, 412
  neuromuscular transmission, 1621
Purinergic receptors
  gastrointestinal motility
    classification, 744–745
    functions, 742
    nonadrenergic gut inhibition, 742–743
    P$_1$ receptors, 744–745
    P$_2$ receptors, 745
    postsynaptic activity, 744–746
    presynaptic activity, 744
Purines
  exocrine gland circulation, 1569
  gastrointestinal neuromuscular transmission, 453
P$_1$ purinoceptor, 744–745
P$_2$ purinoceptor, 745
Putative inhibitory neurotransmitters, 468
  in enteric neurons, 396
  gastrointestinal neuromusclar transmission, 446–449
Pyloric reconstruction, 1207
Pyloric sphincter
  acid and fat control, 36
  anatomy and innervation, 998–999
  functional characteristics, 999–1000
  gastric emptying and, 34–36
  gate keeper analogy, 32–36
  high-pressure zone, 999
  historical research, 32–36, 187–188
    acid and fat control, 36

Cannon's admirable mechanism, 32–34
  gastric emptying, 35–36
myoelectric activity and, 845–846
regulation, 1001–1003
  frequency of stimulation, 1002
  humoral regulation, 1002–1003
  neural control, 1002
  relaxation during electrical field stimulation, 1002–1003
ruminant animals, 1720, 1272–1275
slow-wave conduction, 55–56
stomach-duodenal electrical activity and, 1000–1001
  ringlike contractions and waves, 1000–1001
structure and function, 998–1003
surgical perturbation, 1206
Pyloroplasty, surgical perturbations from, 1209
Pylorus
  during gastric emptying, 919–921
  myoelectric activity and, 845–846
  opiate receptors and, 787
  ruminant animal motor patterns of activity, 1251–1252
  surgical perturbation, 1206
  tachykinin action in, 775

Quantal transmitter release, 1669–1670
Quick-release method, isotonic, 308
Quick stretch phenomenon, 285
Quin 2, $Ca^{2+}$ measurement with, 147

Radiation-induced emesis, 705–706
Radiography, colonic motility, 942–943
Radioisotope techniques, 869
Radiolabeled inert gas washout, 1379
Radioligand binding studies, 737
Raphe nuclei, 660
Raptor motility patterns, 1292–1295
Rat enteric neuron cell cultures, 338–344
Receptive relaxation
  gastric emptying, 20–21
  pathways for, 672
  surgical perturbations and, 1208–1209
Receptor-evoked response
  intestinal smooth muscle, 235–236
    acetylcholine and muscarinic receptor, 237–238
    excitatory receptor mechanisms, 236–238
    inhibitory substances, 239–240
    substance P, 238–239
Receptor-operated channels, 224
Receptor plates, in principal ganglia cells, 526
Receptors
  abdominal, vomiting reflex, 1189–1190
  activation
    in intestinal smooth muscle, 223–226
    submucosal arterioles, 1651–1653
  adrenergic, vomiting reflex and, 1192
  biliary tract pharmacology, 1120
  bombesin, 799
  cholinergic, vomiting reflex and, 1192
  classification of, 715–722
    gastrin-CCK receptors, 759–761
    heterogeneity, 760–761
    preferring receptors, 660
  deglutition and, 688
  δ-receptors, 781
  dopaminergic, vomiting reflex and, 1191
  drug-receptor response quantitation, 720–722
    multiple transmitters, 722
    in vitro studies, 721
    in vivo studies, 720–721
  functional studies, 715–720
  γ-receptors
    norepinephrine, 1656–1658
    submucosal arterioles, 1655–1656
  gastrin-CCK, 759–761
    applied pharmacology of, 765
    modulation of, 764
    postreceptor mechanisms, 764–765
  gastrin-releasing peptide, 799
  gastrointestinal afferent innervation, 595–596
    muscle receptors, 604–609
  hepatic venous bed, 1545–1546
  histamine, 1386
  κ-receptors, 781–782
    cellular properties, 784–785
    ligands for, 785
  ligand binding studies, 717–718
  locus of
    CCK receptors, 762–764
    gastrin, 761–762
    in vivo and ex vivo studies, 718–720
  modulation of activity, 614
  motilin, 792–793
  μ-receptors, 781
    cellular properties, 784
    ligands for, 785
  muscarinic, 726–733
  neurotensin, 795–797
  nonadrenergic, noncholinergic receptors, 1192–1193
  opiates, 780–782
    postreceptor coupling, 785
    vomiting reflex and, 1191–1192
  peptidergic receptors, 1193
  postreceptor mechanisms, 722–723
  quantitation of drug-receptor response, 720–722
    multiple transmitters, 722
    in vitro studies, 721–722
    in vivo studies, 720–721
  ruminant forestomach motility, 1248–1250
  sensory, vomiting reflex, 1188–1190
  serosal and mesenteric, 609–611
  serotonergic, 1192
  somatostatin, 794
  to tachykinins, 766–768
  for vasoactive intestinal polypeptide, 777
  *See also* specific receptors, e.g., Serotonin receptors
Rectal continence, 962–963
Rectal incontinence, 966
Rectal mucosa, mechanoreceptors in, 962
Rectification, membrane, 1611
Rectoanal reflexes, 1035
Rectum
  anatomy, 940
  avian motility in, 1285–1286, 1296–1298
  electrical activity of, 1032–1033
  integrated behavior with sphincter, 79–80
  lumbar sympathetic innervation, 1026
    electrical stimulation, 1036–1037
    interruption, 1037–1038
  motor activity, 1031–1033
    sacral autonomic nerves, 1039
  musculature, defecation and, 1044–1046
  myoelectric activity, 834–838
  parasite-induced alterations, 1146–1147
  sacral afferent fibers, 1027–1028
  sacral parasympathetic innervation, 1026–1027
  vascular system of, 1304
Re-elongation of gastrointestinal cells, 165
Reference organ size, 1336
Reflectance-spectrophotometry technique
  human gastric hemodynamics, 1396–1397
  mucosal blood flow, 1379–1380
Reflex contractions, lower esophageal sphincter, 895–896
Reflex increases, upper esophageal sphincter pressure, 873
Reflex relaxation
  lower esophageal sphincter, 893–894

Reflex relaxation (*continued*)
  cellular basis of, 893
    swallow-induced, 893–894
  upper esophageal sphincter, 873
Reflex responses, hepatic venous bed, 1546–1548
Reflex visceroinhibition, 534
Reflux esophagitis, 1724
Refractory period, 483
Regenerative propagation, 852–853
Regular spiking activity (RSA)
  ruminant animals, 1253–1254
    mixing vs. propelling activity, 1261–1262
    nervous control, 1264
    periodic activity, 1258–1261
Regurgitation
  defined, 1193
  in ruminant animals, 1236–1237
  *See also* Vomiting
Relaxation
  biomechanical mechanisms of, 312–313
  crossbridge states during, 314–315
  gastrointestinal muscle mechanics
    biochemical mechanisms, 312–313
    crossbridge states, 314–315
    isometric relaxation, 315–316
    isotonic relaxation, 316–317
    smooth muscle, 312–317
  isotonic properties, 316–317
Relaxation-oscillator model of propagation, 209–213
  electrical control activity (ECA), 853–857
  limitations of, 210–211
Remak's nerve, 1286
Renal blood flow, digestion and, 1417
Repetitive bursts of action potentials (RBAP)
  bacterial motility alterations, 1163–1167
    *Campylobacter jejuni*, 1166–1167
    *Clostridium difficile*, 1165
    *Clostridium perfringens* A enterotoxin, 1164
    *Escherichia coli* heat-stable toxins, 1165–1166
    invasive *Escherichia coli*, 1163–1164
    *Shigella dysenteriae* 1, 60R enterotoxin, 1164
  bacterial overgrowth syndrome, 1168–1170
Repolarization
  action potentials in gastric muscle, 196
  gastrointestinal electrophysiology, 181–183
  potassium channel properties, 174–176
Resistance vessels, 1695–1696
Respiration, intestinal mucosal blood flow and, 1439
Resting discharge, in-series tension receptors, 605–606
Resting membrane potential
  anatomical variations in slow-wave, 192–193
  colonic muscle, 251–253
    electrogenic pump and, 252–253
    reported values for, 251–252
  diffusion potential and, 189–190
  enteric nervous system, 487
  gastric muscle electrophysiology, 189–190
  mesenteric artery, 1608
  mesenteric vein, 1622
  prevertebral ganglion cells, 542–544
  role in electrophysiological studies, 164–165
  submucosal arterioles, 1640–1643
  voltage-tension relationship and, 203
Resting pressure, lower esophageal sphincter, 892–893
Resting tone, upper esophageal sphincter, 872–873
Retching, esophageal motility, 1179–1182
Retention time, ruminant digestion, 1230–1231
Reticular groove mechanisms, 1243–1245
  reticulorumen contraction inhibition, 1244–1245
Reticulo-omasal orifice, 1230–1231
Reticulorumen
  absorption function, 1229–1230
  cyclical contractions of, 1231–1236
    electrical activity, 1234–1235
    electromyographic recordings, 1240–1241
    measurement of, 1231–1233
    mechanical activity, 1233–1234
    pharmacology, 1269–1270
    primary cycle movements, 1231
    ruminating behavior and, 1236
    sleep patterns and, 1236
  dorsal sac, 1235–1236
  motility, 1230–1231
  posterior dorsal sac, 1235–1236
Reticulum, ruminant, embryonic development of, 1226
Retrofacial nucleus
  gastrointestinal motility
    electrical stimulation studies, 645
    neuronal inputs and outputs, 660
    pathway to esophageal sphincters, 671–672
  neuroanatomy of, 651, 652–653
  parasympathetic neural pathway
    in esophagus, 623–625
    in stomach, 625–627
Retrograde giant contraction (RGC)
  apomorphine dose and, 1184
  characteristics under different conditions, 1185
  electrical control activity and, 1186–1187
  emesis and, 1182–1184
  enteric nervous system, 1191
  functions of, 1188
  nausea and, 1193–1194
  small intestine, 44–45
Retrograde motility, ruminant animals, 1251–1252
Retrograde peristaltic contraction, 1184
Retrograde tracing techniques, 628
Reversed peristalsis. *See* Retrograde giant contraction
Rhythmicity
  colonic motility, 947
  in colonic slow waves, 254
  in gastrointestinal cells, 166–167
  intestinal blood flow and motility, 1478–1482
    luminal distension, 1505
  in principal ganglia cells, 524
  slow-wave generation, 192
Ricinoleic acid
  fat hydroxylation, 1168
  MAPC activity, 1162
Roentgenological observations, 2–3
Rostral pons, gastrointestinal motility, 664–665
Roux gastrojejunostomy, 1207
Rubidium-86 technique, 1377
Rumblings and periodic contractions, 25
Rumen, embryonic development, 1226
Ruminal acidosis, 1235
Ruminant animals
  embryonic development of stomach, 1226
  gastrointestinal motility
    absorption adaptation, 1229–1230
    anatomy, 1226–1227
    colonic motility, 1266–1270
    early research, 1225–1226
    eructation, 1239–1242
    fermentation adaptation, 1228–1229
    forestomach motility, 1230–1250
    forestomach nervous control, 1245–1250
    hormonal influences, 1239
    liquid digesta diversion, 1227–1229
    mammalian herbivore stomach, 1226–1230
    morphological adaptation to bulky food, 1226–1228
    nervous control of rumination, 1237–1239
    omasum cyclical activity, 1242–1243
    pharmacology, 1269–1276
    recticulorumen contractions, 1231–1236

regurgitation mechanism, 1236–1237
retention time and food propulsion, 1230–1231
reticular groove mechanisms, 1243–1245
rumination events, 1236–1239
small intestinal motility, 1258–1266
solid digesta breakdown, 1227
stomach motility, 1250–1258
grazing vs. browsing species, 1230
neonatal intestine, 1597–1598
"Ruminating center," 1238

Sacral innervation
autonomic nerves
cholinergic agonists, 1038–1039
colon and rectum motor activity, 80–81, 1039
electrical stimulation, 1038
somatic afferents, defecation and, 1045
spinal cord
gastrointestinal motility, 660
parasympathetic neural pathways, 627–628
visceral afferents, defecation and, 1044–1046
Salivary glands
avian structure, 1283
circulation
anatomical considerations, 1565–1566
blood flow regulation, 1588–1589
sympathetic nerve stimulation, 1588–1589
functional hyperemia, 1572–1574
extrinsic factors, 1576–1577
intrinsic factors, 1574–1576
hemodynamics and oxygenation, 1568–1569
hyperplasia circulatory adjustments, 1577–1578
intraglandular portal schematic, 1566–1567
intrinsic regulation of blood flow and oxygenation, 1569–1572
hypoxic vasodilation, 1571
kallikrein-kinin regulation, 1570
metabolic regulation, 1569
myogenic regulation, 1569–1570
pressure-flow autoregulation, 1570–1571
reactive hyperemia, 1571
venous pressure elevation, 1571–1572
nerves, 1568
pharmacology, 1589
transcapillary fluid and solute exchange, 1578–1588
capillary and interstitial interaction, 1583
capillary pressure, 1582
interstitial fluid pressure, 1583–1583
microvascular permeability, 1583–1588
net capillary filtration rate, 1580–1583
oncotic pressure gradient, 1583
osmotic reflection coefficient, 1583
ultrastructural basis of, 1578, 1580
lymphatics
flow and composition, 1746
structure, 1739
vessel structure, 1567–1568
vasoactive agents and, 1584–1585
*Salmonella enteritidis*, 1719
*Salmonella typhimurium*, 1161–1162
Sarcoplasmic reticulum
association with caveolae, 112
gastrointestinal smooth muscle contraction, 287–288
in intestinal muscle
calcium ion accumulation, 115
cell size and shape, 111, 115, 119, 122
embryonic development of, 131
$Na^+$ activity in, 145
Satellite cells, structure and function, 529–530
Schwann cells, in intestinal muscles, 127–129
Scintigraphy, biliary tract function, 1065–1066
Scleroderma, esophageal peristalsis, 12
Secondary cycle movement, in ruminant animals, 1240

Second-messenger mechanisms,
diarrhea mechanisms, 1171–1172
gastrin-CCK receptor, 764–765
receptors
ligand binding and, 717
postreceptor mechanisms, 722–723
Second-order neurons, 595
Secretagogues
lymph flow and composition, 1750
net fluid secretion and, 1453–1454
Secretin
biliary tract pharmacology, 1117–1118
exocrine gland circulation, 1575, 1577–1578
gallbladder function, 1070
gastric blood flow control, 1388
gastric emptying, 41–42
gastrointestinal blood flow, 1686
intestinal blood flow and motility, 1495–1496
lower esophageal control, 14
parasite-induced imbalance of, 1147
postprandial intestinal hyperemia and, 1425–1426
pyloric sphincter regulation, 1002–1003
Secretomotor neurons, enteric, 391–392
Secretory disorders, intestinal blood flow and, 1724
Secretory inhibition, mucosal blood flow and, 1392
Segmentation
early terminology, 64–68
of small intestine, 42–43
Sensory nerves
enteric nervous system, 395
gastrointestinal afferent innervation, 596
motility pathways, 629–636
pelvic afferent nerve fibers, 632, 634
pudendal afferent nerve fibers, 634–636
sympathetic afferent nerve fibers, 632–635
vagal afferent nerve fibers, 629–632
in vagal or spinal sensory ganglia, 395
visceral nerves and, 594–595
Sensory receptors, vomiting reflex, 1188–1190
Septa
of intestinal circular muscle, 105–106
connections with submucosa, 128
Septic shock, intestinal circulation, 1719
Series elastic component
active state in smooth muscle, 303
contracting muscle stiffness, 301
gastrointestinal smooth muscle, 275
Serosal receptors, 609–611
adaptation rate, 614
functional significance, 615–616
gastrointestinal afferent innervation, 595–596
response characteristics, 611
ruminant forestomach motility, 1249–1250
spontaneous activity, 610–611
Serotonergic receptors, vomiting reflex, 1192
Serotonergic synaptosomes, 423
Serotonin
in area postrema, 701
biliary tract pharmacology, 1110
colonic motility, 953
blood flow, 1498–1500
in dorsal motor nucleus of the vagus, 650
enteric cholinergic system, 413
in enteric neurons, 396
transmitter role, 396
gastrointestinal blood flow
neurohormonal control, 1698–1690
vasoactive intestinal polypeptide (VIP) and, 1681–1682
gastrointestinal motility
in nTS, 658
sympathetic preganglionic neurons, 656
interaction with substance P, 772

Serotonin (*continued*)
  intestinal blood flow and motility, 1486–1488, 1492
  postprandial intestinal hyperemia and, 1428
  presynaptic inhibition, 394
  in prevertebral ganglia, 572–573
  receptors
    action on enteric nerves, 741
    action on smooth muscle, 741
    D receptors, 739–740
    gastrointestinal motility, 739–742
    M receptors, 739–740
    nerve locus and function, 739
    receptor classification, 739–740
    therapeutic considerations, 742
  slow excitatory synaptic potentials
    enteric neurons, 393
    in prevertebral ganglion, 555
  small intestine, 63–64
[$^3$H]Serotonin, 413
  enteric cholinergic system, 413
Sex hormones, intestinal motility and, 926
*Shigella dysenteriae*
  parasite-induced motility, 1149
  repetitive bursts of action potentials (RBAP), 1164
Shock
  hepatic blood flow, 1531, 1551
  *See also* Cardiogenic shock; Circulatory shock; Hypovolemic shock; Septic shock
Short bowel syndrome, small intestine resection, 1214–1216
Shortening velocity, regulation of, 309–311
SIF. *See* Small intensely fluorescing cells
Sigmoid colon
  anatomy, 940
  early research, 73–74
    continence, 83
    defecation control, 81–82
Signal transduction, slow EPSPs, 499–501
Single-cell research
  force transients, 305–306
  gastrointestinal muscle studies, 278
  smooth muscle pharmacology, 723–726
Single-channel studies
  in intestinal smooth muscle, 223
  potassium channels, 171–174
    electrical activity models, 183
Single smooth muscle cell
  intestinal muscle
    acetylcholine and muscarinic receptors, 237–238
    action potential, 229–230
    active properties, 221–223
    background information, 217–219
    electrical coupling, 227–229
    excitatory/inhibitory junction potentials, 233–235
    excitatory receptor mechanisms, 236–238
    inhibitory substances, 239–240
    in vitro studies
      electrical/mechanical activity, 226–240
      passive and active properties, 227–233
    ionic channel complement, 219–220
    passive electrical properties, 220–221
    potassium-selective channels, 217–218
    properties of, 219–226
    receptor activation response, 223–226, 235–240
    slow-wave activity, 230–233
    substance P action, 239–240
Single-spike units, enteric nervous system, 480–481
Single-unit recordings, gastrointestinal afferent innervation, 596–597
Sinusoidal-perfusion model of hepatic circulation, 1522–1524, 1534
SITS tracer, enteric nervous system, 482
Skeletal muscle, contraction mechanism, 276
Sliding-filament/crossbridge hypothesis

contractile protein regulation, 293–294
length-tension curve, 298–299
Slow depolarization
  mesenteric artery, 1618–1620
  mesenteric vein, 1624–1625
Slow electrical oscillations, in colonic muscle, 253
Slow excitatory postsynaptic potentials (slow EPSPs)
  in colonic muscle, 254–255
  enteric nervous system, 336, 493–503
    acetylcholine, 499
    bombesin, gastrin-releasing peptide and VIP, 498
    calcitonin gene-related peptide, 499
    cAMP intraneuronal elevation, 501
    cholecystokinin and caerulein, 498–499
    circuit specificity, 502–503
    effector activation, 501–502
    excitability augmentation, 494
    forskolin, 500–501
    gating mechanism, 503
    histamine neurotransmitter, 496, 498
    hyperpolarizing afterpotentials, 494–495
    ionic mechanisms, 495–496
    membrane depolarization, 494
    neurotensin, 499
    neurotransmitters, 496–499, 501
    presynaptic inhibition, 510
    signal transduction, 499–501
    somatostatin, 499
    spike trains and, 494
    substance P neurotransmitter, 496–498
  noncholinergic, 556–557
  opiate receptors and, 782
  in prevertebral ganglia, 554–556
  substance P and, 558
  tachykinin action and, 770–771
Slow hyperpolarization, mesenteric artery, 1618, 1620
Slow inhibitory postsynaptic potetntials (slow IPSPs)
  colonic muscle, 254–255
  enteric nervous system, 336, 504–508
    catecholamines, 507–508
    cholecystokinin, 506
    GABA, 506–507
    galanin, 507
    histamine, 505–506
    myenteric inhibitory neurotransmitters, 505–507
    myenteric plexus, 504
    neurotensin, 506
    norepinephrine, 506
    opioid peptides, 505
    presynaptic inhibition, 510
    purine nucleotides and nucleosides, 507
    somatostatin, 506
    submucosal inhibitory neurotransmitters, 507–508
    submucosal plexus, 504–505
  tachykinin action and, 770–771
Slow noncholinergic synaptic potentials (SNSP), 342–343
Slow-transit constipation, 456
Slow waves
  amphibian stomach electrical activity, 200
  amplitude and contractile force, 201–202
  anatomical variations in, 192–193
  avian motility, 1288–1290
    cecum, colon, and rectum, 1295–1298
  basic electrical rhythm (BER), 827
  colonic motility
    characteristics of, 253–254
    circular muscle, 948–949
    contraction and flow interactions, 951–952
    frequency gradients, 254
    human studies, 949–952
    innervation patterns and, 260–261
    propagation of, 262–265

relationship with myenteric potential oscillation, 266
smooth muscle, 947
conduction-velocity measurements of, 207–208
electrical signs of gradient, 57–58
fiber bundles, 55
in gastric muscles, 191–195
    anatomical variations in, 192–194
    cellular mechanism, 192
    frequency regulation, 192
    ionic mechanism of, 194–195
    origin of, 191–192
    plateau phase, 191
    upstroke depolarization, 191
gastroduodenal junction conduction, 55–56
genesis and conduction, 53–54
historical background on, 187–189
internal anal sphincter, 1008–1010
interstitial cells of Cajal, 380–382
    ICCAP role in, 360–364
intestinal blood flow and motility, 1511–1512
intestinal smooth muscle
    activity during contraction, 227
    gradient, 233
    mechanism of, 230–231
    muscarinic receptor response and, 238
    origin and propagation, 231–233
    relationship of spikes to, 227
    synchronous discharge of, 231–232
ionic mechanism of, 194–195
pyloric sphincter function, 1001
rectum and internal anal sphincter, 1032–1033
rhythmicity in gastrointestinal cells, 166
small intestine
    electrophysiology, 51–56
    research on, 49–51
    transection, 1213
sphincter of Oddi function, 1082–1083
stomach research, 29–30
surgical perturbations, 1205–1207
    terminology background on, 826–827
upstroke and plateau components, 188
*See also* Contractile electrical complex
Small axon bundles, mesenteric circulation and, 1606–1607
Small bowel, transit measurements in, 925–926
Small intensely fluorescing (SIF) cells
    content of, 529
    innervation of, 528–529
    neuropeptide Y in, 576
    opioid peptides in, 561–562
    paracrine role of, 522–523
    physiological role of, 529
    type I cells, 528
    type II cells, 528
        role in slow IPSP, 529
    *See also* Chromaffin cells
Small intestine
    avian structure, 1285
    blood flow
        glucagon and, 1685–1686
        neonatal hemodynamics and oxygenation, 1597–1598
            intrinsic regulation of, 1599–1602
            neural regulation of, 1598–1599
            neurohormonal control of, 1671–1673
    bombesin action and, 800
    gastrin-releasing peptide, 800
    historical research, 42–68
        Boldyreff's research, 45–49
        cholinergic and adrenergic nerves, 62–63
        enteric nervous system, 58–64
        interdigestive myoelectric complex, 45–46
        intestinal gradient, 56–58
        migrating complex control, 46–49
        peristalsis, 43–44, 64–68
        reversed peristalsis, 44–45
        segmentation, 42–43
        slow waves, spikes, and contractions, 49–56
    interstitial cells of Cajal (ICC) in, 351–374
    lymphatic structure, 1739–1740
    lymph flow and composition, 1747–1757
        bile acid transport, 1754–1755
        chylomicrons from enterocyte to lacteal, 1751–1752
        drug transport and, 1755–1756
        fasting levels, 1753–1754
        fat absorption, 1754
        hormones and, 1755
        intestinal fluid absorption, 1747–1749
        intestinal lipid composition, 1751–1755
        intestinal secretion, 1749–1750
        portal venous blood, 1852⅛855
        proteins, 1756–1757
        water-soluble transport, 1751
    microvascular anatomy, 1476–1477
    microvasculature. *See* Intestinal villi
    motilin in, 793–794
    motility. *See* Small intestine motility
    myoelectric activity, spatial and temporal patterns, 830–834
    neurotensin action, 798–799
    opiate receptors and
        local effects, circular muscle, 787–788
        local effects, longitudinal muscle, 788
        nonlocal administration, 788
    parasite-induced alterations, 1134–1146
        length-tension relationships, 1140, 1143–1146
        manometric measurements, 1135–1136
        myoelelectric measurements, 1137–1145
        transit measurements, 1136–1139
        in vitro measurements, 1140–1146
    parasympathetic neural pathways, 627
    somatostatin and, 794–795
    surgical perturbations of
        resection, 1214–1216
        transection of, 1213–1214
        vagotomy, 1216
    sympathetic neural pathways, 629
    tachykinin actions in, 775–776
    vasculature
        capillary wall ultrastructure, 1319, 1321–1327
        charge barrier to transcapillary exchange, 1327
        fenestrae, 1319, 1321–1322
        junctions, 1324–1327
        permeability characteristics, 1319, 1322
        structure-capillary permeability correlation, 1328
        vesicles, 1321–1324
    vasoactive intestinal polypeptide (VIP) action in, 778–779
    *See also* Intestinal mucosa
Small intestine motility
    bacterial enterotoxins
        bacterial overgrowth syndrome, 1167–1171
        historical research, 1153–1154
        migrating action-potential complex (MAPC), 1154–1163
        repetitive bursts of action potentials (RBAP), 1163–1167
    luminal flow and absorption, 924–925
    postoperative inertia, 1201
    retching and vomitus expulsion, 1182–1185
    in ruminant animals, 1258–1266
        duodenal bulb motor function, 1262–1263
        5-hydroxytryptamine, 1264–1266
        mixing vs. propelling activity, 1261–1262
        nervous control, 1264
        pancreaticobiliary secretions, 1263–1264
        periodic activity, 1258–1261
Small solutes
    permeability
        exocrine gland circulation, 1583, 1585, 1588

Small solutes (*continued*)
    intestinal mucosal blood flow, 1456–1457
Smoking
    gastric circulation and, 1396
    *See also* Nicotine
Smooth muscle
    $\alpha$-adrenoceptor inhibition of, 737–738
    anorectal and pelvic floor muscles, 1025–1026
        dysfunction, 1047
    arteriolar, autoregulation in, 1529
    biochemistry of, 219
    $Ca^{2+}$ accumulation in, 143, 151–152, 178–179
    CCK receptors and, 763–764
    central esophageal peristalsis, 876–877
    $Cl^-$ equilibrium potential, 143
    collagen content of, 106
    colonic motility, 946–947
    contractile protein regulation, 293–294
    contracting muscle stiffness, 303–305
        length-tension curve, 295–298
    esophageal
        myoelectric activity, 838–842
        "on and off" contractions, 841
    gallbladder function, 1071
    gastrin receptors and, 761–762
    gastrointestinal motility
        contraction conditions, 273–275
        force transducers, 278–280
        gut movement and motility, 277–278, 926–927
        instrumentation for, 278–283
        isolated muscle preparations, 278
        isometric behavior, 276–277, 283–306
        isotonic behavior, 277, 306–312
        length (position) transducers, 280–282
        models of, 275
        recording devices, 282–283
        relaxation of, 312–317
    ICC AP and, 357, 359
        excitatory influence of, 362–363
    ICC DMP and, 370–371
    ileocecal sphincter regulation, 1006–1008
    internal anal sphincter, 1010–1012
    intestinal, 108–115
        blood flow and motility during ischemia, 1512
        caveolae, 109, 112–113, 115
        cell size and shape, 108–109
        dense bands, 109, 111, 113–115, 119, 122
        embryonic development of, 132–133
        gap junction scarcity in, 116–117
        mitochondria and organelles, 115
        sarcoplasmic reticulum, 111, 115, 119, 122
        structure and function, 105, 125–127
    intramural arterioles, 1637
    ion permeability and conductance changes, 438, 440–442
    isotonic shortening, 306–312
        force-velocity curve, 306–309
        length and force-velocity curve, 309
        limits to, 306
        regulation of shortening velocity, 309–312
        velocity transients, 309
    lymphatic, 1744
    muscarinic receptors in, 728–729
    neurotensin inactivation by, 797
    parasite-induced alterations
        inflammation, 1149
        small intestine, 1140–1145
    peripheral esophageal control
        contraction-inhibition correlates, 882–883
        intramural nerve stimulation, 879–880
        latency and latency gradient, 882–883
        localized distension, 877–878
        neurotransmitters, 883–884
        on and off contractions, 880–882
        peristalsis, 877–884
        vagal efferent stimulation, 878–879
    pyloric sphincter regulation, 1001–1002
    relaxation of, 312–317
        biomechanical mechanisms, 312–313
        isotonic properties, 316–317
        mechanical properties, 313–316
    ruminant stomach, 1227
    serotonin receptors and, 741
    single-cell preparation
        gastrointestinal pharmacology, 723–726
        properties of, 217–219
    slow-wave generation, 192
    sodium-hydrogen exchange, 158
    submucosal arterioles, 1643–1644, 1647
    tachykinin action on, 768–770
    voltage recordings of isolated cells, 167–168
S neurons and serotonin immunoreactivity, 393
Sodium channel ($Na^+$)
    calcium channel properties and, 179
    frequency distribution of, 145–146
    gastrin-CCK receptor modulation, 764
    intestinal smooth muscle, 220
        current studies, 223
        slow-wave mechanism and, 230–231
    ionic mechanism of slow waves, 194–195
    measurement of, 146
    muscarinic receptors, agonist binding sites and, 730–731
    passive ion movements, 148–149
    permeability, 438, 440–442
    submucosal arterioles, 1641–1643
        potential-dependent calcium entry, 1651
    transmembrane movement of, 143–144
    VIP transmission, prevertebral ganglia, 566
Sodium-calcium exchange, 152, 154–156
Sodium-hydrogen exchange, 157–158
Sodium-potassium pump ($Na^+$-$K^+$-ATPase)
    colonic muscle resting potential, 252–253
    enteric cholinergic system, 410–411
    exchange mechanisms and, 152, 154–158
        calcium extrusion, 152, 154–156
        chloride-bicarbonate exchange, 156–157
        sodium-calcium exchange, 152, 154–156
        sodium-hydrogen exchange, 157–158
        sodium-sodium exchange, 152
    intestinal mucosal blood flow, 1431–1432
    intestinal smooth muscle, 230, 233
    ionic dependence of, 149
    number of pump sites, 150–151
    receptors and postreceptor mechanisms, 723
    resting membrane potentials and, 190
    slow-wave generation, 192
    stoichiometry and electrogenicity, 149–150
Sodium-sodium exchange, 152
Solute exchange
    intestinal mucosal blood flow, 1441–1456
    net fluid absorption, 1450
Somatic reflexes, pelvic floor skeletal muscle, 1040
Somatostatin
    biliary tract pharmacology, 1118–1119
    colonic motility, 953
    in dorsal motor nucleus of the vagus, 649
    enteric nervous system, 396
        cholinergic system, 417
        slow EPSPs, 499
        slow IPSPs, 506
    gastric blood flow control, 1388
    gastrointestinal blood flow, 1689–1690
    gastrointestinal motility
        intermediolateral cell column ($S_{2-3}$), 654
        sympathetic preganglionic neurons, 656–657

pharmacology of, 794–795
in prevertebral ganglia, 574–577
in ruminant animals, 1258
gastroduodenal junction, 1274
Somatostatin-like peptide, gastrointestinal innervation, 1031
Sonography, biliary tract function, 1066
Space constant, mammalian blood vessels, 1610
Space of Mall, hepatic vascular junctions, 1526
Space sickness, 705–706
SPANTIDE antagonist, 767
substance P and, 770
Special situation contractions
research background, 817–818
*See also* Antiperistalsis; Retrograde giant contraction
Sphincter ampullae structure, 1057–1058
Sphincter choledochus structure, 1057–1058
Sphincter of Lutkens,
function studies, 1074
muscle and mucosal structure, 1058
Sphincter of Oddi
abnormal function, 1091–1095
biliary dysfunction, 1092–1095
abnormal phasic contractions, 1093–1094
early research, 1055–1056
paradoxical contraction to CCK-8, 1092–1093
sphincter spasm, 1092
tachyoddia, 1094–1095
cholinergic drugs, 1105–1106
drop counter measurements, 1083–1084
dysfunction and treatment, 1095
dyskinesia, 1092
electromyography, 1064–1065
function studies, 1077–1088
animal studies, 1080–1088
human studies, 1077–1080
manometry, 1063
Poiseuille's law, 1077
hepatic bile flow, 1068–1070
high-pressure zone, 1081–1082
innervation, 1059–1060
motilin and, 1067
muscle and mucosal structure, 1058–1059
pancreatic dysfunction, 1095
peristalsis, 1083–1086
pharmacology, 1066–1067, 1104–1105
adrenergic drugs, 1107–1108
caerulein, 1116–1117
cystokinin, 1113–1115
gastrin, 1116
histamine, 1108, 1111
motilin, 1122
opiates, 1119–1121
pancreatic polypeptide, 1123
pregnancy and sex hormones, 1124
prostaglandins, 1109–1110
serotonin, 1110
somatostatin and bombesin, 1119
substance P, 1124
VIP, GIP, glucagon, and secretin, 1118
phasic pressure waves, 1078
resistance of, flow measurements, 1062
sonography and, 1066
species differences, 1060–1061, 1103
stenosis, 1091–1092
structure, 1057
Sphincteric function
adrenergic neuromuscular transmission in, 443–444
continence, 962–963
future research trends, 1012–1013
myoelectric activity, 842–845
structure and, 987–988
synchronous nature of, 987

*See also* specific sphincter muscles
Sphincteroplasty, 1095
Sphincterotomy, 1095
gallbladder function and, 1091
Sphincter pancreaticus
muscle and mucosal structure, 1059
structure, 1057–1058
Spike activity, terminology background on, 826–827
Spike-burst activity
in colon and rectum, 837, 949
gallbladder function, 1071
ruminant animals, 1268
sphincter of Oddi function, 1086–1088
Spike potentials
gastrointestinal muscle electrophysiology, 195–196
genesis and conduction, 53–54
ileocecal sphincter regulation, 1006–1008
lower esophageal sphincter, 992–994
postoperative paresis, 1202
pyloric sphincter, 999
coupling with stomach, 1000
ruminant animals, 1269
small intestine
electrophysiology, 51–56
research on, 49–51
surgical perturbation, stomach resection, 1204–1205
Spike waveforms
burst-pattern generation, 473
mechanosensitive neurons, 476–477
tonic-type mechanosensitive neurons, 480
Spinal cord
anorectal and pelvic floor muscles, 1047
defecation and, 1046
gastrointestinal motility
inputs to, 664
sympathetic centers and, 670–671
sympathetic centers, gastrointestinal motility and, 646
Spinal preganglianic neurons, 530–534
Spinal reflex, pudendal nerve afferent fibers and, 669–670
Spiral colon, ruminant animals, 1266–1269
Splanchnic circulation
blood vessels, 1606
components of, 1605–1606
gastric blood flow control, 1383, 1396
hemodynamics in, 1416–1417
hepatic circulation, 1542
hypertension and, 1723
hypovolemic shock, 1718
neonatal intestinal circulation
direct stimulation, 1598
transection, 1598
pooling with septic shock, 1719
portal hypertension, 1720
*See also* Intramural blood vessels
Splanchnic nerves
afferent units, 609–610
blood vessel control, 1606
gastrointestinal afferent innervation, 595
small intestine, 61
vomiting reflex, 1189
Spontaneous action potentials
in colonic muscle, 259–262
portal vein, 1625–1626
rhythmicity in gastrointestinal cells, 166
Spontaneous excitatory junction potentials (SEJPs)
mesenteric artery, 1616–1617
submucosal arterioles
cotransmission, 1659
quantal content, 1647–1650
Spontaneous oscillatory potentials, enteric nervous system, 490–491
Spontaneous spike discharge, enteric nervous system, 484–485

Spontaneous transient outward currents (STOC)
  calcium channel properties, 178
  in intestinal smooth muscle, 225–226
  potassium channel properties, whole-cell studies, 174–176
  rhythmicity in gastrointestinal cells, 166
Sprue, gallbladder function and, 1091
Starling force equation
  liver lymph and cirrhosis ascites, 1761–1762
  lymph flow, 1741
Starling hypothesis
  intestinal mucosal blood flow
    capillary membrane parameters, 1445
    transcapillary fluid and solute exchange, 1441
  net fluid secretion and, 1455–1456
  transcapillary fluid exchange, exocrine gland circulation, 1580
Station pull-through technique
  lower esophageal sphincter
    basal pressure measurements, 887–888
Steady-state activation, calcium channel properties, 177–178
Stenosis hypothesis, parasite-induced inflammation, 1148–1149
Steroid hormones, lymph transport, 1755
Stiffness
  relaxation mechanics and, 316
  smooth muscle contraction, 299–306
    force transients, 305–306
    measurement of, 300–301
    stretch mechanics, 301–305
  viscoelastic systems, 321
Stoichiometry of sodium pumping, 149–150
Stomach
  arterial supply of, 1372
  avian motility
    muscle structure, 1284–1285
    patterns, 1287–1289
  blood flow
    adrenergic receptors, 1677–1678
    ischemia and, 1512–1513
    modification, 1375–1376
  bombesin action and, 799–800
  capillary system in, 1303, 1305
  functional division of, 909–912
  gastric blood flow and secretion, 1500–1502
  gastrin-releasing peptide action in, 799–800
  glandular (avian), 1283–1284
  interstitial cells of Cajal and, 374–378
  lymphatic structure, 1739
  lymph flow and composition, 1746–1747
  mammalian herbivore, 1226–1230
  microvascular anatomy, 1306–1309, 1477–1478
  motilin in, 793
  myoelectric activity, 827–830
  neurotensin action, 798
  Openchowski's scheme of nervous control, 14–15
  opiate receptors and, 786–787
  parasite-induced alterations, 1134
  parasympathetic neural pathways in, 625–627
  proximal. See Proximal stomach
  somatostatin and, 794–795
  surgical perturbations of, 1203–1213
    bypass operation, 1204
    drainage/vagotomy operations, 1212–1213
    resection, 1203–1207
    selective vagotomy, 1211–1212
    truncal vagotomy, 1207–1211
    vagotomy, 1207–1213
  sympathetic neural pathways, 629
  tachykinin action in, 773–774
  vascular supply and drainage, 1302–1303
    permeability, 1328–1329
    structure, 1328
  vasoactive intestinal polypeptide (VIP) action on, 779
  vasodilatation in, 1668
Stomach motility, 817–818
  ruminant animals, 1250–1258
Storage oscilloscopes, gastrointestinal muscle mechanics, 282
Strain, viscoelastic systems, 321
Strain-gauge transducers
  avian gastrointestinal motility, 1286
  colonic motility studies, 955
  pelvic floor skeletal muscle activity, 1034–1035
Stress
  colonic motility and, 963, 966–967
  gastrointestinal motility and, 22, 24
Stressed volume, hepatic circulation and, 1537–1539
Stress relaxation, viscoelastic systems, 318–321
Stretch
  contracting muscle stiffness, 301–304
  ICC DMP and, 372
Striated muscle
  central esophageal peristalsis, 876
  esophageal myoelectric activity, 838
  pelvic floor innervation, 1028–1030
  peripheral esophageal peristalsis, 877
  upper esophageal sphincter, 870
Strip-chart recorders, gastrointestinal muscle mechanics, 282
Strontium ions ($Sr^{2+}$)
  in intestinal smooth muscle, 222
  lower esophageal sphincter, 993
S/type 1 neurons
  enteric nervous system, 485–486
    action potentials, 489–490
    fast EPSPs in, 491
    myenteric inhibitory neurotransmitters, 505–507
Subcellular membranes in smooth muscle, 155–156
Subcerous compartment of interstitial cells of Cajal (ICC-SC), 366
Submucosa
  blood flow control, 1383
  circular colon muscle and slow-wave propagation, 263–265
  intestinal blood flow, venous pressure and, 1413
  in intestinal muscles, 128–130
  microsphere measurement
    migration, 1337–1339
    size and distribution, 1343
  microvessel circulation, 1373–1374
  vasculature of, 1304–1306
    interamural arterial and venous plexuses, 1305–1306
Submucosal arterioles
  blood flow control, 1383
  contraction initiation, 1650–1653
    potential-dependent calcium entry, 1650–1651
    receptor-activated tension development, 1651–1653
  excitatory junction potentials (EJP)
    cotransmission, 1658–1660
    norepinephrine, 1656–1658
    pharmacology of, 1654–1660
    quantal content, 1647–1650
    time course, 1646–1647
  innervation of, 1639–1641
  integration in, 1653–1654
  membrane potentials and diameter changes, 1652–1653
  neuromuscular transmission, 1644–1645
  passive electrical properties of, 1640–1644
    electrical coupling, 1643–1644
    resting potential, 1640–1643
  sympathetic nerve stimulation, 1645–1646
Submucosal plexus
  $\alpha_2$-adrenoceptors and, 738
  culture studies of, 331–332
  enteric nervous system
    inhibitory neurotransmitters, 507–508
    slow IPSPs, 394, 504–505
  interstitial cells of Cajal and, 378–379
  slow excitatory synaptic potentials, 393–394

Substance K
  actions of in small intestine, 775–776
  capsaicin and, 771–772
  degradation of, 768–769
  discovery of, 765–766
  enteric cholinergic system, 416–417
  numbered peptide sequences, 769
  potency sequences for, 766–767
Substance P
  in area postrema, 701
  biliary tract pharmacology, 1124
  Bolton-Hunter labeling, 766
  capsaicin and, 771–772
  in colonic muscle
    blood flow, 1499–1500
    electropharmacology, 259, 776
    motility, 953, 956
  degradation of, 768–769
  in dorsal motor nucleus of the vagus, 649–650
  effect on calcium channels, 181
  effect on potassium channels, 181
  enteric nervous system
    acetylcholine release, 416–417
    extracellular recording of, 468
    fast responses to, 337–338
    slow EPSPs, 496–498
    transmitter role of, 396
  in esophagus, 772–773
    peristalsis, 884
  exocrine gland circulation and functional hyperemia, 1577
  gastrointestinal blood flow, 1680
    depolarization, 182–183
  gastrointestinal motility, 928
    excitatory junction potentials, 450–452
    intermediolateral cell column ($S_{2-3}$), 654
    in nTS, 657–658
    sympathetic preganglionic neurons, 656–657
  internal anal sphincter regulation, 1012
  intestinal motility, 981
    receptor-evoked response, 239–240
  lower esophageal sphincter regulation, 998
  in mast cells, 772
  in nerves, 770–771
  nociceptive function of, 559–560
  noncholinergic excitatory motor transmission, 388–389
  numbered peptide sequences, 769
  opiate receptors and, 782
  pharmacology, 765–766
  postprandial intestinal hyperemia and, 1426–1427
  potassium conductance and, 771
  potency sequences for, 766–767
  prevertebral ganglia, neurotransmission, 556–561
  in pylorus, 775
  ruminant animals, 1271
    gastroduodenal junction, 1272
  secretomotor transmission, 391–392
  in sensory neurons, 395
  slow excitatory postsynaptic potentials
    enteric neurons, 393
    in prevertebral ganglion, 555
  in small intestine, 775–776
  smooth muscle, 768–770
  in stomach, 774–776
Substance P-like peptide, 1031
Substrates
  hepatic blood flow, 1531–1537
    equilibrium model, 1532–1534
    Goresky model, 1532
    parallel tube model, 1534
Sucrose gap technique, colonic muscle action potentials, 256
Superior laryngeal nerve (SLN)
  deglutition and, 687–688
  afferent fiber projection, 688–691
  group I and II neurons in, 692, 694
Superior mesenteric artery (SMA)
  intestinal blood flow and motility
    occlusion and hypoxia, 1511–1512
  pancreatic circulation and, 1566
  postprandial hyperemia and, 1417
Superior mesenteric ganglion
  cholinergic inputs and, 551
  neuroanatomy of, 520–521
Superior mesenteric vein, intestinal blood flow and motility, 1511–1512
Superoxide dismutase, nonocclusive intestinal ischemia, 1715
Supraspinal pathways
  anorectal and pelvic floor muscles
    dysfunction, 1047
  gastrointestinal motility, 661–662
  pelvic floor skeletal muscle, 1040–1042
Suprathreshold synaptic potential, 526
Surface area-to-volume ratio
  intestinal smooth muscle cells, 108
  ion permeability and, 141
  submucosal arterioles, 1641–1642
Surgical perturbations
  gastrointestinal motility
    colon, 1216–1218
    esophagus, 1202–1203
    historical research, 1199–1202
    small intestine, 1213–1216
    stomach, 1203–1213
  historical research on, 1199–1201
  nonocclusive intestinal ischemia, 1715–1717
Swallow-induced relaxation response
  esophageal body, 874–875
  lower esophageal sphincter, 893–894
Swallowing
  avian gastrointestinal motility, 1286
  buccal phase of, 685–686
  central pattern generator, 3–5, 695–697
  cortical stimulation of, 690–691
  defined, 685
  esophageal phase of, 686
  gastrointestinal response to, 914
  historical research, 2–18
    Cannon's roentgenological observations, 2–3
    esophageal peristalsis, 5–8, 10–12
    functional innervation, 8–9
    lower esophageal sphincter, 9–10, 12–18
    swallowing reflex, 3–5
  motor mechanisms of, 691–695
  neural organization scheme, 4
  pharyngeal phase of, 686
  phases of, 685–686
  pressures and bolus movement, 6–7
  reflex, 3–5, 867–869
  research background, 683–686
  sensory components, 686–688
    central nervous system, 688–691
  upper esophageal sphincter
    central organization of, 869
    initiation of, 868–869
    pressure profile, 871
Sympathetic innervation
  adrenergic receptors and, 733
  afferent fibers, 632–635
  capillary-interstitial interaction, 1448–1449
  colon, rectum, and internal anal sphincter, 1026
  exocrine gland circulation, 1568, 1588–1589
  functional hyperemia, 1573–1574
  gastric blood flow control, 1382–1383
    histamine and, 1387
  gastrointestinal blood flow, 1675–1676

Sympathetic innervation (continued)
  norepinephrine, 1669
  gastrointestinal motility
    in colon, 629–630
    in esophagus, 628
    in small intestine, 629
    in stomach, 629
  hepatic circulation, 1543–1546
  hypovolemic shock, 1718
  ileocecal sphincter regulation, 1007
  internal anal sphincter, 1010–1011, 1026
  intestinal blood flow and motility, 1490–1491
    smooth muscle activity, 234
    villous motility, 977, 979
  intramural arterioles, 1639–1640
    varicosities, 1639–1641
  lower esophageal sphincter, 16–17, 990
  muscarinic receptors in, 728–729
  in prevertebral ganglions, 545–548
  pyloric sphincter regulation, 1002
  submucosal arterioles, 1645–1646
Synaptic interactions
  in enteric neurons, 341–344
    fast nicotinic synaptic potentials, 341–342
    inhibitory actions, 343–344
    mixed potentials, 343
    modulation of, 344, 404
    slow noncholinergic synaptic potentials, 342–343
  lower esophageal sphincter inhibitory pathways, 894–895
  neuroneuronal syapses, 392–396
  prevertebral ganglia, 549–551
Synaptosomes
  enteric nervous system, 422–423
    noradrenergic, 423
    serotonergic, 423
Synctia, core-conductor models of, 212
Syncytial sink, 181–182

Tachycardia, and omasal contractions, 1242–1243
Tachygastria, 196–197
  surgical perturbations and, 1208
Tachykinins
  actions of, 768–776
  in colon, 776
  degradation, 768
  in esophagus, 772–773
  gastrointestinal motility, 772–776
  guinea pig ileum and taenia coli studies, 768–772
  pharmacology, 765–776
  prevertebral ganglia neurotransmission, 559–560
  in pylorus, 775
  receptors to, 766–768
  in small intestine, 775–776
  smooth muscle, 768–770
  in stomach, 773–774
Tachyoddia, 1094–1095
Taenia coli
  colonic musculature, 941
  contraction, length-tension curve, 297–298
  elastic fibers in, 106–108, 110–111
  functions of, 104
  intestinal structure, 125–127
    cell size and shape, 108
  longitudinal muscle in, 103–104, 106, 110
  slow-wave genesis and conduction, 53
  smooth muscle in
    calcium channels and, 220
    sodium-calcium exchange and, 154–156
*Taenia taeniaeformis*, 1147
Tape recorders, 282–283
Taste buds, avian structure, 1283
TEA. *See* Tetraethylammonium ions

Temperature
  burst-pattern generation, 472–473
  intestinal mucosal blood flow, 1439–1440
Tension receptors
  ruminant forestomach motility, 1249–1250
  spontaneous activity in, 613
Terminal apparatus, intestinal muscle cells, 119–121
Terminal ground plexus, mesenteric circulation and, 1606
Tetracarboxylic dyes, $Ca^{2+}$ measurement with, 147
Tetraethylammonium (TEA) ions
  intestinal smooth muscle action potentials, 222, 229–230
  ionic mechanism of slow waves, 195
  lower espohageal sphincter, 992
  potassium channel properties, 170
    single intestinal smooth muscle cell, 220
    whole-cell studies, 176
  in prevertebral ganglions, 544–545
  pyloric sphincter regulation, 1001–1002
  slow-wave frequency regulation, 192
  submucosal arterioles, calcium entry, 1650–1651
  voltage recordings of isolated cells, 167
Tetrodotoxin (TTX)
  biliary tract pharmacology, 1104–1105
  CCK receptors, 762
  colonic muscle, 255
    electropharmacology, 258–259
  enteric nervous system
    cholinergic system, 410
    intracellular recordings, 485
    vasodilator neurons, 391
  gastrin receptors, 761
  gastrointestinal blood flow, 1681–1682
  gastrointestinal neuromuscular transmission, 446, 448
  in intestinal smooth muscle, 228
  lower espohageal sphincter, 993–994
  mesenteric artery, 1615–1616
  receptor locus and functional coupling, 719
  sphincter of Oddi function, 1081–1082
  submucosal arterioles, calcium entry, 1650–1651
  voltage recordings of isolated cells, 167–169
Thermopile technique, intestinal blood flow and motility, 1479
Thermoreceptors, gastrointestinal afferent innervation, 595–596, 604
Thick muscle pairs, avian muscular stomach, 1284–1285
Thiry-Vella loop
  colonic motility, 961
  periodic activity, 24–25
Thoracic duct shunt, cannulation of lymph vessels, 1745–1746
Thoracic duct side (T tube), cannulation of lymph vessels, 1745–1746
Thoracolumbar nerves,
  intermediolateral cell column ($S_{2-3}$), 654–657
  pathways to prevertebral ganglion, 530–531
Thorax receptors, vomiting reflex, 1190
Thyrotropin-releasing hormone (TRH)
  in dorsal motor nucleus of the vagus, 650
  muscarinic receptor modulation and, 731
Tissue culture
  background on, 331–332
  enteric nervous system, 333–338
    absent or rare differentiated properties, 336–337
    enteric glial properties, 338
    fast responses to substance P, 337–338
    GABA neurons, 337
    muscarinic receptor distribution, 338
    preferred growth substrates, 335–336
    retention of differentiated properties, 335–336
  ICC AP studies and, 363–364
Tissue tracer, ionic content in, 143–145
Tissue variables, receptor mechanics and, 716–717
Tissue volume, intestinal blood flow, 1676–1677
Tomita chamber apparatus, 206

Tomita's hypothesis, interstitial cells of Cajal, 380
Tongue, buccal phase of deglutition, 685
Tonic contractions
   colonic motility, 946
      neurogenic inhibition, 953–954
      gastrointestinal smooth muscle activation, 284
      intestinal blood flow and motility, 1482–1483
         ions and hypertonicity, 1492–1494
      lower esophageal sphincter, 991
         excitatory nerve activity, 890
      mechanosensitive units, 479–480
      pelvic floor skeletal muscle, 1040
      prevertebral ganglia, 546–547
         modification of, 548
      proximal stomach during gastric emptying, 919
      research background, 817–818
      sphincter of Oddi rhythmicity, 1089
Total-body hypothermia, gastric circulation and, 1395
Total peripheral resistance (TPR), septic shock and, 1719
Total safety factor, lymph and tissue homeostasis, 1743
Total tissue content estimating techniques, 141–142
Touch receptors, deglutition and, 688
Tracer-flux analysis, ionic permeabilities, 109
Transcapillary fluid exchange ($K_f$)
   charge barrier to, 1327
   exocrine gland circulation
      capillary exchange ultrastructure, 1578, 1580
      capillary filtration coefficient, 1581–1582
      net capillary filtration rate, 1580–1582
      Starling hypothesis, 1580
   intestinal mucosal blood flow
      capillary filtration coefficient, 1442–1443
      capillary hydrostatic pressure, 1443–1444
      capillary-interstitial interaction, 1445–1456
      interstitial hydrostatic pressure, 1444
      lymph flow, 1441–1442
      oncotic pressure gradient, 1444–1445
      osmotic reflection coefficient, 1444
      Starling hypothesis, 1441
   intestinal vesicles, 1321–1322
   lymphatics, 1735
Transcapillary oncotic pressure gradient
   exocrine gland circulation, 1583
   intestinal mucosal blood flow, 1444–1445
Transient ruminal stasis, 1235
Transit measurements, parasite-induced alterations in small intestine, 1136–1139
Transmembrane potential
   resting membrane potential, 189
   role in electrophysiological studies, 165
Transmission, defined, 205–206
Transmural nerve stimulation in colonic muscle, 259–262
Transsynaptic modulation, 407
Transverse colon anatomy, 940
*Trichinella spiralis*
   hormonal imbalances, 1147
   inflammation from, 1148–1149
   parasite-induced alterations
      motility, 1149
      small intestine, 1136–1142
*Trichostrongylus axei*
   alterations in small intestine, 1137
   alterations stomach, 1134
Tris [tris(hydroxymethyl)aminomethane], intestinal smooth muscle, 230–231
*Trypanosoma cruzi*
   parasite-induced alterations
      cecum, colon, and rectum, 1146–1147
      small intestine, 1135–1136
   substances derived from, 1147
Trypsin, role in dispersion techniques, 163–164
T-tube manometry, common duct pressure, 1063

TTX. *See* Tetrodotoxin
Two-component analogue model, gastrointestinal smooth muscle mechanics, 275
Type 3 neurons in enteric nervous system, 486
   forskolin application, 500–501
Type 4 neurons in enteric nervous system, 486
   forskolin application, 500–501
Tyramine, sphincter of Oddi pharmacology, 1107–1108
Tyrosine hydroxylase (TH), in rat enteric neurons, 341

Ulcerative colitis
   colonic ischemia, 1721
   gastrointestinal neuromuscular transmission, 456
Ulcers
   Billroth surgical procedures for, 1199–1201
   ischemia and, 1721–1722
   recurrence rate
      reconstructive surgery and, 1207
      vagotomies and, 1211–1213
   stomach microvasculature and, 1307–1308
Unstressed volume
   hepatic circulation, 1544–1545
   values for splanchnic parameters, 1538–1539
Upper esophageal sphincter (UES)
   anatomy, 870–871
   control of, 872–873
   efferent motor innervation, 866
   function and structure, 989
   myoelectric activity, 842
   pressure profile, 871–872
Uptake measurement technique, hepatic blood flow, 1535–1537

Vagotomy
   drainage operations and, 1212–1213
   emesis and, 1182–1183
   esophageal peristalsis, 1203
   gallbladder function and, 1090–1091
   gastric blood flow control and, 1384–1385
   gastrointestinal motility, 638–641
   highly selective, 1213
   mortality and ulcer recurrence, 1200–1201
   proximal stomach, 1211–1212
   in ruminant animals, 1264
   selective, 1211–1212
   small intestine, 1216
   truncal
      restoration phases, 1209–1210
      surgical perturbations from, 1207–1212
   ulcer therapy with, 1200–1201
Vagovagal reflex system, forestomach motility, 1245–1246
Vagus nerve
   afferent fibers, 629–632
   avian muscular stomach, 1285
   biliary tract pharmacology, 1106
   efferents, 878–879
   esophageal and sphincter innervation, 866
   gastric blood flow control, 1383–1385
   gastrointestinal afferent innervation, 594
   intestinal blood flow and motility, 1490–1491
   lower esophageal sphincter, 990
   motor neurons of, 692
   neuronal inputs and outputs, 660
   pancreatic blood flow and, 1574–1575
   pyloric sphincter regulation, 1002
   reticulorumen contractions, 1241–1242
   vomiting reflex, 1189
Valves of Heister
   function studies, 1074
   structure, 1057
Valvula ileocecocolica (valvula Bauchini), 1003
Van der Pol solutions, relaxation-oscillator models, 210–212
Varicosities, in intestinal muscles, 127–129

Vascular resistance
   hemorrhagic hypotension, 1695–1696
   hepatic blood flow and, 1522–1531
   sympathetic nerve stimulation and, 1635
"Vascular steal" mechanism, 1425
"Vascular waterfall" phenomenon, 1412–1413
Vasculature of alimentary tract
   functions of, 1301–1302
   future research trends, 1329–1330
   intestinal muscles, 127–129
   microvascular ultrastructure, 1316, 1318–1329
      colon, 1329
      small intestine, 1319, 1322–1328
         *See also* Intestinal villi
      stomach, 1328–1329
   organization, 1302–1316
      enteric neural plexus vasculature, 1304
      intramural distributive vessels, 1304
      mucosal microvessels, 1306–1316
      muscle microvessels, 1304
      submucosal microvessels, 1304, 1306
      vascular supply and drainage, 1302–1303
Vasculitis, intestinal blood flow and, 1724
Vasoactive agents
   intestinal mucosal blood flow, 1434–1437, 1486–1488
   pancreatic circulation, 1586–1587
   salivary gland blood flow, 1584–1585
Vasoactive intestinal polypeptide (VIP)
   antagonists, 777
   biliary tract pharmacology, 1117–1118
   colon innervation, 942, 1030
   colonic motility and blood flow, 953, 1499–1500
   enteric nervous system
      acetylcholine release, 414–416
      slow EPSPs, 498
      transmitter role of, 396
   esophageal peristalsis, 883–884
   exocrine gland circulation and
      functional hyperemia and, 1576–1577
   gallbladder
      function, 1070
      innervation, 1059
   gastric blood flow control, 1387, 1500–1501
   gastrointestinal blood flow
      neurohormonal control, 1680–1682
      serotonin interaction with, 1681–1682
   gastrointestinal motility
      intermediolateral cell column ($S_{2-3}$), 654
   gastrointestinal neuromusclar transmission
      putative inhibitory neurotransmission, 446–448
   genome coding for, 776
   ICC DMP and, 373
   immunoreactivity and, 1030
   inhibitory motor transmission, 389–390
   internal anal sphincter
      motor activity, 1035
      regulation, 1012
   lower esophageal sphincter
      inhibitory action, 895
      regulation, 998
   MAPC activity, 1162
   motility control, 777–780
      colon, 779–780
      in esophagus, 778–779
      gallbladder, 779
      internal anal sphincter, 780
      small intestine, 778–779
      in stomach, 779
   muscarinic receptor modulation and, 731
   pharmacology of, 776–777
   in prevertebral ganglion, 564–566, 568
      slow EPSP in, 555
   postprandial intestinal hyperemia and, 1427
   receptors, 777
   in ruminant animals, 1258, 1271
   secretomotor transmission, 391
Vasoconstriction
   intestinal blood flow and motility, 1492
      oxidative metabolism, 1436–1437
   steady state of, 1675
   submucosal arterioles, 1653–1654
Vasodilatation
   acetylcholine-induced gastrointestinal blood flow, 1668
   enteric, 391
   intestinal blood flow and motility, 1492
   intestinal mucosal blood flow
      capillary density and, 1437
      intramural distribution, 1437
      oxidative metabolism, 1435–1437
Vasopressin
   cardiogenic shock, 1719
   gastric blood flow control, 1387–1388
   hemorrhagic hypotension, 1696
   hypovolemic shock, 1718
   intestinal mucosal blood flow, 1437–1438
   in prevertebral ganglia, 572–573
Velocity transients, 309
Venous constriction
   cardiac output and, 1549
   hepatic circulation, 1544
   intestinal mucosal blood flow, 1434
      rhythmic contractions, 1480–1482
Venous pressure ($P_v$)
   elevation
      capillary-interstitial interaction, 1446
      exocrine gland circulation, 1571–1572
      hepatic, profiles of, 1523
      intestinal mucosa blood flow, 1408
         response to elevation, 1411–1413
   portal, capillary pressure in exocrine glands, 1582
Venous resistance, hepatic circulation, 1542–1543
Venous system, cardiovascular reflexes, 1548
Ventromedial hypothalamus, 1382
Venules, structure in small intestine, 1637–1638
Very-low-density lipoproteins
   liver lymph, 1760
   in lymph flows, 1753–1754
Vesicles
   channels, 1322, 1324
   small intestinal microvasculature, 1321–1322
Vesicoanal reflexes, internal anal sphincter
   motor activity, 1035
Vesicular release mechanism in enteric neurons, 404–405
*Vibrio cholerae*
   diarrhea and, 1154
   enterotoxin motility alterations, 1155–1156
   parasite-induced motility, 1149
Villikinin, 981
Villous motility. *See* Intestinal villi, motility
Villous pump mechanism, 981–983
Viniculin, localization at intestinal dense bands, 114–115
Visceral afferent fibers, 534–542
Visceral muscle
   cell size and shape, 108–109
   collagen concentration in, 106
   intestinal mucosal blood flow, 1439
Visceral nerves, 594–595
Visceroinhibitory nerves, 530–534
Viscerosomatic reflexes
   colonic-rectal distension, 1041
   electrophysiological studies, 1042–1043
   micturition, 1041–1042
   operant conditioning, 1042, 1044

Viscoelastic systems
  behavior of, 318–321
  components, 317–318
Voight configuration
  gastrointestinal smooth muscle mechanics, 275
  viscoelastic systems, 318, 320
Voltage-clamp studies
  action potentials in gastric muscle, 196
  isolated gastrointestinal cells
    calcium channel properties, 176–179
    chloride channels, 179–180
    microelectrode studies, 169–170
    potassium channel properties, 171–176
    whole-cell and patch-clamp technique, 170–171
  slow-wave generation, 192
Voltage-dependent intestinal smooth muscle, 230
Voltage recordings
  agonist effects on, 168
  isolated gastrointestinal cells, 167–169
Voltage-tension relationships, 202–203
Vomiting (emesis), 697–708
  area postrema
    physiology of, 701
    structure, 698–701
    transmitter localization and binding sites, 701
  brain tumors, 707
  chemotherapy-induced, 706–707
  defined, 697
  epilepsy, 707
  esophageal motility, 1179–1182
  gastrointestinal correlates of, 1182–1185
    independence from retching and vomitus expulsion, 1187–1188
  gastrointestinal motility
    antrum and small intestine, 1183–1185
    central integration, 1190
    colon and gallbladder, 1185–1186
    efferent innervation, 1190–1191
    esophagus and sphincters, 1179–1182
    nausea mechanisms, 1193–1194
    neural control, 1188–1191
    neuropharmacology, 1191–1193
    prodromal signs of, 1194–1195
    proximal stomach, 1181–1183
    retrograde giant contraction, 1188
    sensory receptors and afferent pathways, 1188–1190
  motion and space sickness, 705–706
  myoelectric activity, 850, 1186–1187
  neural circuitry for, 698
  pharmacology of, 707–708
  radiation-induced, 705–706
  species differences in, 697
  vomiting center or central pattern generator, 703–705

Washdown effect, liver lymph, 1759
Waterfall phenomenon, hepatic blood flow and, 1523–1524
Water transport, intestinal villi motility, 985
Weight loss and surgical perturbation, 1214–1216
Well-stirred model of hepatic circulation, 1532–1534
Wheat germ agglutinin–conjugate horseradish peroxidase, 659
Wheatstone bridge, in force transducer, 279–280
Whole-cell current, voltage-clamp studies, 170–171
Window current, calcium channel properties, 177–178

Xanthine oxidase
  colon countercurrent exchange mechanism, 1715
  ischemic gastric injury, 1395
X-ray microanalysis, $Ca^{2+}$ distribution, 145

Young's modulus, viscoelastic systems, 321

ZIO (zinc iodide/osmic acid) staining
  Interstitial cells of Cajal, 350
    for ICC AP, 353
    ICC CM research, 373–374
    for ICC DMP, 370
    ICC SS and, 366
Zollinger-Ellison syndrome, 765